VASCULAR PATHOLOGY

VASCULAR PATHOLOGY

VASCULAR PATHOLOGY

EDITED BY

W.E. Stehbens

MB, BS, MD (Syd.), DPhil (Oxon.), FRCPA, FRCPath

Emeritus Professor and Foundation Chairman of Department of Pathology, Wellington School of Medicine, University of Otago, and concurrently Foundation Director of the Malaghan Institute of Medical Research, Wellington, New Zealand. Formerly Professor of Pathology, Albany Medical College of Union University, Albany, New York, and previously Professor of Pathology, Washington University of St. Louis, Missouri, USA

and

J.T. Lie

MB, BS, MD (Melb.), MS (Minn.), FACC, FACA, FACR, FCCP, FSVMB

Professor and Director, Division of Anatomic Pathology, University of California Davis School of Medicine and University of California Davis Medical Center, Sacramento, California. Formerly, Professor of Pathology, Mayo Medical School and Mayo Graduate School of Medicine, Rochester, Minnesota, USA

CHAPMAN & HALL MEDICAL
London · Glasgow · Weinheim · New York · Tokyo · Melbourne · Madras

Published by Chapman & Hall, 2–6 Boundary Row, London SE1 8HN, UK

Chapman & Hall, 2–6 Boundary Row, London SE1 8HN, UK

Blackie Academic & Professional, Wester Cleddens Road, Bishopbriggs, Glasgow G64 2NZ, UK

Chapman & Hall GmbH, Pappelallee 3, 69469 Weinheim, Germany

Chapman & Hall USA, One Penn Plaza, 41st Floor, New York NY 10119, USA

Chapman & Hall Japan, ITP-Japan, Kyowa Building, 3F, 2-2-1 Hirakawa-cho, Chiyoda-ku, Tokyo 102, Japan

Chapman & Hall Australia, Thomas Nelson Australia, 102 Dodds Street, South Melbourne, Victoria 3205, Australia

Chapman & Hall India, R. Seshadri, 32 Second Main Road, CIT East, Madras 600 035, India

First edition 1995

© 1995 Chapman & Hall

Typeset in 10/12 Sabon by Best-set Typesetter Ltd., Hong Kong
Printed in Great Britain at the Alden Press, Oxford

ISBN 0 412 48640 7

Apart from any fair dealing for the purposes of research or private study, or criticism or review, as permitted under the UK Copyright Designs and Patents Act, 1988, this publication may not be reproduced, stored, or transmitted, in any form or by any means, without the prior permission in writing of the publishers, or in the case of reprographic reproduction only in accordance with the terms of the licences issued by the Copyright Licensing Agency in the UK, or in accordance with the terms of licences issued by the appropriate Reproduction Rights Organization outside the UK. Enquiries concerning reproduction outside the terms stated here should be sent to the publishers at the London address printed on this page.

The publisher makes no representation, express or implied, with regard to the accuracy of the information contained in this book and cannot accept any legal responsibility or liability for any errors or omissions that may be made.

A catalogue record for this book is available from the British Library

Library of Congress Catalog Card Number: 94-69665

∞ Printed on acid-free text paper, manufactured in accordance with ANSI/NISO Z39.48-1992 (Permanence of Paper).

CONTENTS

List of Contributors	xi
Preface	xiii
Acknowledgements	xiv

1 General features, structure, topography and adaptation of the circulatory systems — 1
W.E. Stehbens

1.1	Basic topography of the vascular system	1
1.2	Arteries	2
1.3	Special structural features of arteries	7
1.4	Veins	9
1.5	The terminal vascular bed	9
1.6	The pulmonary circulation	9
1.7	The cerebral circulation	10
1.8	Anatomical variations of peripheral vascular patterns	11
1.9	Naturally occurring collateral circulation	12
1.10	Angiogenesis	13
1.11	Postnatal angiogenesis	15
1.12	Circulatory changes during maturation	15
1.13	Arteriomegaly	16
1.14	Misuse of terminology	16
	References	18

2 Congenital anomalies of blood vessels and their complications — 21
J.E. Edwards and J.L. Titus

2.1	Communication between aorta and pulmonary arterial system	21
2.2	Systemic arteries	27
2.3	Pulmonary arteries	47
2.4	Systemic veins	50
2.5	Pulmonary veins	53
	References	59

3 Thrombosis and vascular trauma — 63
W.E. Stehbens

3.1	Haemostasis and thrombosis	64
3.2	Thrombogenesis	65
3.3	Virchow's triad	67
3.4	Arterial thrombosis	70
3.5	Venous thrombi	72
3.6	Atypical thrombosis	73
3.7	Sequelae of thrombosis	73
3.8	Trauma	80
3.9	Vibrating tool disease	81
3.10	Iatrogenic trauma	82
3.11	Trauma, repair and intimal proliferation	82
3.12	Thrombogenic hypothesis of atherogenesis	83
	References	85

4	**Connective tissue components of the blood vessel wall in health and disease**	**89**
	S.P. Robins and C. Farquharson	
	4.1 Vessel wall constituents	89
	4.2 Degradation and turnover	108
	4.3 Biomechanical properties	110
	4.4 Abnormalities of connective tissue in disease	111
	4.5 Concluding remarks	121
	References	121
5	**Pathology of blood vessels in metabolic disorders**	**129**
	R. Subramanian, R. Virmani and V.J. Ferrans	
	5.1 Diseases of carbohydrate metabolism	129
	5.2 Diseases of lipid metabolism	137
	5.3 Diseases of amino acid and protein metabolism	147
	5.4 Diseases of mineral and vitamin metabolism	163
	References	166
6	**Atherosclerosis and degenerative diseases of blood vessels**	**175**
	W.E. Stehbens	
	6.1 Nomenclature of degenerative vascular diseases	175
	6.2 Atherosclerosis	175
	6.3 Aetiology of atherosclerosis	225
	6.4 Medial degeneration of the aorta (medionecrosis)	252
	6.5 Diseases of small blood vessels	253
	6.6 Miscellaneous degenerative changes	257
	6.7 Phlebosclerosis	258
	6.8 Lymphangiosclerosis	260
	6.9 Vascular calcification	260
	6.10 Miscellaneous diseases	262
	References	262
7	**Biochemistry and cell biology of atherogenesis**	**271**
	H.F. Hoff	
	7.1 LDL localization in arteries	271
	7.2 Lipoprotein quantification in arteries	276
	7.3 Physicochemical characterization of lipoprotein in arteries	286
	7.4 Functional characteristics of lipoproteins in human arteries	293
	7.5 Physical and functional properties of other lipoproteins	301
	7.6 Large lipid-rich particles isolated from atherosclerotic lesions – structure and function	304
	7.7 Conclusions	308
	References	308
8	**Histochemistry and immunochemistry of vascular disease**	**313**
	D.V. Parums	
	8.1 Histochemistry of vascular disease	313
	8.2 Immunocytochemistry of vascular disease	315
	References	326
9	**Inflammation and atherosclerosis**	**329**
	D.V. Parums	
	9.1 Inflammation and atherogenesis	329
	9.2 Macrophages, oxidized lipids and atherosclerosis	333
	9.3 Chronic inflammation and advanced atherosclerosis	336
	9.4 Chronic periaortitis as a local complication of advanced atherosclerosis	346
	References	349

10 Aneurysms
W.E. Stehbens
    10.1   Definitions   353
    10.2   Aneurysms of the aorta   355
    10.3   Pulmonary artery aneurysms   368
    10.4   Extracranial carotid and vertebral arterial aneurysms   369
    10.5   Aneurysms of the subclavian artery   370
    10.6   Aneurysms of the iliac and femoral arteries   370
    10.7   Popliteal aneurysms   370
    10.8   Aneurysms of the splanchnic arteries   371
    10.9   Complications of aneurysms   374
    10.10   Aneurysms of the cerebral circulation   377
    10.11   Traumatic aneurysms of peripheral arteries   400
    10.12   Mycotic (septic embolic) aneurysms   401
    10.13   Neoplastic (oncotic) aneurysms   403
    10.14   Dissecting aneurysms of peripheral arteries   404
    10.15   Aneurysms of the microcirculation   407
    10.16   Venous aneurysms   407
    10.17   Thoracic duct aneurysms   408
    10.18   False aneurysms   408
    10.19   Iatrogenic aneurysms   408
    10.20   Miscellaneous and unusual aneurysms   409
    References   409

11 Atheroembolism: clinical and experimental aspects
B.A. Warren
    11.1   Clinical aspects   415
    11.2   Experimental aspects   425
    References   433

12 Cerebrovascular disease
W.E. Stehbens
    12.1   Cerebrovascular mortality and epidemiology   437
    12.2   Carotidynia   439
    12.3   Tortuosity, coiling, kinking and anatomical displacement   439
    12.4   Vascular compression   440
    12.5   Cerebral atherosclerosis   441
    12.6   Murmurs   441
    12.7   Cerebrovascular insufficiency   442
    12.8   Cerebral infarction or encephalomalacia   444
    12.9   Other ischaemic lesions   454
    12.10   Ischaemic lesions of the spinal cord   458
    12.11   Intracranial and intraspinal haemorrhage   460
    12.12   Spinal extradural haematoma   462
    12.13   Subdural haematoma   462
    12.14   Spinal subdural haematoma   467
    12.15   Subarachnoid haemorrhage   467
    12.16   Spinal subarachnoid haemorrhage   469
    12.17   Intracerebral haemorrhage   469
    12.18   Intraventricular haemorrhage   482
    12.19   Intraspinal haemorrhage   482
    12.20   Miscellaneous conditions   482
    References   485

13 Diseases of the veins and lymphatic vessels, including angiodysplasias — 489
H.J. Leu and J.T. Lie

- 13.1 Venous malformations — 489
- 13.2 Degenerative venous diseases — 493
- 13.3 Circulatory venous disturbances — 499
- 13.4 Inflammatory venous diseases — 504
- 13.5 Malformations of the lymphatic vessels — 506
- 13.6 Degenerative disorders of lymphatic vessels — 509
- 13.7 Circulatory disorders of lymphatic vessels — 510
- 13.8 Inflammatory disease of lymphatic vessels — 511
- 13.9 Neoplasias of lymphatic vessels — 511
- References — 514

14 Abnormal arteriovenous communications and fistulae — 517
W.E. Stehbens

- 14.1 Haemodynamics of arteriovenous fistulae — 519
- 14.2 Traumatic arteriovenous fistulae and communications — 522
- 14.3 Left-to-right arterial shunts (systemic artery–pulmonary artery shunt) — 524
- 14.4 Congenital arteriovenous communications of the extremities — 525
- 14.5 Vascular anomalies of the central nervous system — 528
- 14.6 Arteriovenous communications and fistulae of the brain — 530
- 14.7 Aetiology of arteriovenous communications — 539
- 14.8 Carotid cavernous fistula — 540
- 14.9 Associated intracranial and extracranial arteriovenous communications — 541
- 14.10 Extracranial arteriovenous communications and fistulae — 542
- 14.11 Carotid–jugular fistulae — 542
- 14.12 Vertebral arteriovenous fistulae — 542
- 14.13 Arteriovenous communications of the spinal cord — 542
- 14.14 Extradural, vertebral and calvarial lesions — 544
- 14.15 Ataxia telangiectasia (Louis–Bar syndrome) — 544
- 14.16 Pulmonary arteriovenous communications — 544
- 14.17 Coronary arteriovenous communications — 545
- 14.18 Splanchnic arteriovenous communications — 545
- 14.19 Therapeutic arteriovenous shunts — 546
- 14.20 Arteriovenous communications and tumours — 546
- 14.21 Venous varicosities — 547
- 14.22 Venous aneurysms and angiomas — 548
- 14.23 Significance of arteriovenous shunts — 549
- References — 550

15 Systemic hypertension and related vascular diseases — 553
Section A: *T.F. Lüscher, G. Noll and R.R. Wenzel*

- 15.1 Pathophysiology of hypertension — 553
- 15.2 Vascular causes of secondary hypertension — 559
- 15.3 Clinical manifestations and complications of hypertension — 564
- References — 567

Section B: *J. Churg and M.H. Goldstein*

- 15.4 Reactive changes in blood vessels — 571
- 15.5 Complications of hypertension — 576
- 15.6 Complications of therapy of hypertension — 580
- 15.7 Portal hypertension — 582
- References — 583

16	**Pulmonary hypertension and related vascular diseases** *W.D. Edwards*	**585**
	16.1 General features	585
	16.2 Normal pulmonary vasculature	585
	16.3 Acute and subacute pulmonary hypertension	588
	16.4 Chronic pulmonary hypertension	590
	16.5 Chronic precapillary pulmonary hypertension	596
	16.6 Chronic postcapillary pulmonary hypertension	605
	16.7 Primary pulmonary hypertension	607
	16.8 Open lung biopsy	615
	16.9 Related vascular disorders	617
	References	618
17	**Systemic, pulmonary and cerebral vasculitis** *J.T. Lie*	**623**
	17.1 Definition	623
	17.2 Etiology and pathogenesis	623
	17.3 Clinicopathological classification	623
	17.4 Giant cell arteritides	625
	17.5 Polyarteritis group of systemic vasculitis	630
	17.6 Pulmonary angiitis and granulomatosis	637
	17.7 Cerebral vasculitis	645
	References	653
18	**Buerger's disease (thromboangiitis obliterans)** *S. Shionoya, H.J. Leu and J.T. Lie*	**657**
	18.1 Historical perspective	657
	18.2 Etiology and pathogenesis	658
	18.3 Epidemiology	659
	18.4 Clinical and angiographic characteristics	660
	18.5 Pathology	661
	18.6 Buerger's disease of blood vessels in unusual locations	675
	18.7 Conclusion	677
	References	678
19	**Non-atherosclerotic and non-vasculitic diseases of coronary arteries** *R. Virmani, A. Farb and A.P. Burke*	**679**
	19.1 Pathophysiology of coronary circulation	680
	19.2 Disease categories and their consequences	682
	19.3 Summary	693
	References	695
20	**Diagnostic angiography, imaging and interventional radiology** *A.W. Stanson*	**699**
	20.1 Imaging modalities	699
	20.2 Morphology	699
	20.3 Arterial diseases	700
	20.4 Arterial intervention	720
	20.5 Venous diseases	723
	20.6 Venous intervention	726
	References	728

21 Neoplasms of large blood vessels and tumor angiogenesis — 729
A.P. Burke and R. Virmani
   21.1 Tumors of large arteries — 729
   21.2 Neoplasms of veins — 734
   21.3 Tumor angiogenesis — 736
   References — 737

22 Tumors and tumefactions of peripheral blood vessels — 739
E.A. Montgomery and J.F. Fetsch
   22.1 Reactive lesions of peripheral vessels — 739
   22.2 Benign vascular tumors — 749
   22.3 Lesions of indeterminate biologic potential — 760
   22.4 Malignant vascular tumors — 764
   References — 776

Index — 787

CONTRIBUTORS

Dr Allen Burke
Department of Cardiovascular Pathology
Department of Defense
Armed Forces Institute of Pathology
Washington, DC 20306-6000
USA

Dr Jacob Churg
Department of Pathology
Barnert Memorial Hospital
680 Broadway
Patterson, NJ 07514
USA

Dr Jesse E. Edwards
St Paul Heart and Lung Center
255 North Smith Avenue, Suite 200
St Paul, MN 55102
USA

Dr William D. Edwards
Mayo Clinic, Hilton-1142
200 First Street, S.W.
Rochester, MN 55905
USA

Dr Andrew Farb
Department of Cardiovascular Pathology
Department of Defense
Armed Forces Institute of Pathology
Washington, DC 20306-6000
USA

Dr Colin Farquharson
Institute of Animal Physiology and Genetics Research
Edinburgh Research Station
Roslin, Midlothian EH25 9PS
Scotland
UK

Dr Victor J. Ferrans
National Institutes of Health
Building 10, Room 7N-236
Bethesda, MD 20892
USA

Dr John F. Fetsch
Staff Pathologist
Department of the Army
Armed Forces Institute of Pathology
16 Alaska Avenue
Washington, DC 20306-6000
USA

Dr Marvin H. Goldstein
Mount Sinai School of Medicine
1225 Park Avenue
New York, NY 10128
USA

Dr Henry F. Hoff
Department of Cell Biology
Research Institute – NC10
The Cleveland Clinic Foundation
9500 Euclid Avenue
Cleveland, OH 44195
USA

Professor Hans Jörg Leu
CH-6986
Novaggio
Switzerland

Professor J.T. Lie
Department of Pathology
UC Davis Medical Center
2315 Stockton Boulevard
Sacramento, CA 95817
USA

Professor Thomas F. Lüscher
Professor of Medicine
Medizinische Universitatsklinik Kardiologische
   Abteilung
Inselspital
CH-3010 Bern
Switzerland

Dr Elizabeth A. Montgomery
Department of Pathology
Georgetown University
Room 105, Basic Science Building
3900 Reservoir Road, N.W.
Washington, DC 20007-2197
USA

Dr Georg Noll
Medizinische Universitatsklinik Kardiologische
 Abteilung
Inselspital
CH-3010 Bern
Switzerland

Dr Dinah V. Parums
Department of Histopathology
Royal Postgraduate Medical School
Hammersmith Hospital
DuCane Road
London W12 ONN
UK

Dr Simon P. Robins
Rowett Research Institute
Bucksburn
Aberdeen, Scotland AB2 0SB
UK

Professor Shigehiko Shionoya
Japan International Co-Operation Agency (JICA)
JICA Project Team Leader
Sanjay Gandhi Post Graduate Institute of Med. Sci.
Adm. Block, Raebareli Road
Lucknow 226001, India;
Emeritus Professor of Surgery
 Nagoya University School of Medicine
Nagoya, Japan

Dr A.W. Stanson
Department of Diagnostic Radiology
Mayo Clinic
200 First Street, S.W.
Rochester, MN 55905
USA

Professor W.E. Stehbens
Department of Pathology
Malaghan Institute of Medical Research
Wellington School of Medicine
P.O. Box 7343
Wellington South
New Zealand

Dr Ramiah Subramanian
Medical Officer
Food and Drug Administration (HFZ-450)
Division of Cardiovascular, Respiratory and
 Neurological Devices
1390 Piccard Drive
Rockville, MD 20850
USA

Dr Jack L. Titus
St Paul Heart & Lung Center
225 North Smith Avenue, Suite 200
St Paul, MN 55102
USA

Dr Renu Virmani
Chair, Department of Cardiovascular Pathology
Department of Defense
Armed Forces Institute of Pathology
Washington, DC 20306-6000
USA

Professor B.A. Warren
Department of Anatomic Pathology
Prince Henry Hospital
Little Bay NSW 2036
Australia

Dr René R. Wenzel
Medizinische Universitatsklinik Kardiologische
 Abteilung
Inselspital
CH-3010 Bern
Switzerland

PREFACE

This book was conceived and developed because of our conviction that in a human suffering from any malady, effective clinical management must be based ultimately on sound knowledge of the pathology of the disease. Vascular diseases are the major cause of mortality and morbidity in the technologically and economically developed countries, with hypertension, coronary artery disease, cerebrovascular disease, aortorenal and peripheral vascular diseases and venous thromboembolism accounting for more deaths annually than all other causes combined.

It has been more than 365 years since the recognition of the existence and function of venous valves that led to the discovery, in 1628, of unidirectional flow of blood in the circulation by William Harvey. Great strides have been made in our knowledge of molecular medicine, vascular biology, surgical sciences and hemodynamics and this is reflected by the proliferation in the past two to three decades of texts on vascular medicine, vascular surgery and circulatory biomechanics. What has not been available until now is an English language textbook solely and entirely devoted to the pathology of vascular disease. We hope this book will fill the void and should become the standard reference for the health care professional; it will be most valuable to the pathologist, vascular physician and vascular surgeon, neurologist and neurosurgeon, rheumatologist, vascular radiologist, epidemiologist and researcher in vascular medicine and biological sciences.

This multiauthored book is designed to provide a comprehensive, well illustrated and extensively referenced text on vascular pathology important to the practice of medicine in every subspecialty area. To accomplish this goal, we have been fortunate to solicit contributions from an international group of authors from six countries; some are young and others not so young, but all are recognized and well respected authorities in their respective fields. The diversity of experience and depth of knowledge of our contributors are amply exemplified by the different writing styles and presentations of individual chapters. The length of each chapter is, of course, dictated by the content of the designated topic. We consider such diversity the strength of our book rather than a distraction and any attempt by the editors to enforce uniformity and unanimity would be contrived and unimaginative. The views expressed in the different chapters are at times at variance as is inevitable in a multiauthored book but this will focus attention on the controversial subjects, facilitate the evolution of further knowledge and stimulate interest in vascular pathology which is so important in every branch of modern day medicine.

Early chapters cover the topography and adaptation of the circulatory system; congenital anomalies; thrombosis and trauma; vascular connective tissue proteins; and metabolic disorders. This is followed by chapters dealing first with atherosclerosis and degenerative diseases of blood vessels, including morphology, biochemistry, cell biology, histochemistry, immunochemistry and inflammatory and immunologic response of atherosclerosis; and secondly, chapters on arterial aneurysms; atheroembolism; cerebrovascular disease; diseases of the veins and lymphatics including angiodysplasia and arteriovenous communications. The final group of chapters includes systemic and pulmonary hypertension, vasculitides, non-atherosclerotic and non-vasculitic coronary artery disease, diagnostic angiography, imaging and interventional radiology, neoplasms of the great vessels and tumour angiogenesis, and finally tumour and tumefactions of peripheral blood vessels. Because each individual chapter stands alone and is completely self-contained, some overlap of topics is inevitable; however, this has been kept to a minimum and, together, they comprise a contemporary treatise on the pathology of vascular diseases.

William E. Stehbens

ACKNOWLEDGEMENTS

Our sincere appreciation is due to all the contributors to this book for making their time and expertise available to produce this volume. We thank the publishing companies and the many authors who have so willingly given permission for reproduction of their illustrations and data used in the compilation of the text. We are grateful to Dr Peter Altman of Chapman & Hall, for his assistance and advice during the preparation of the book, and also to the subeditorial and production team at Chapman & Hall, and Jennifer Bew and Michèle Clarke for their expert and patient editorial work in the final production of the book.

W.E.S. is grateful to Mrs J. Todd and Miss G. Dennis for their assistance with the typing and extends special thanks to Mrs Jean Stehbens for her encouragement, interest and assistance in so many ways that were indispensable in the preparation of the book.

J.T.L. is grateful for the secretarial help of Lisa Schwab and Susan Miller of Rochester, Minnesota and Suzanne Miranda and Janelle Hernandez of Sacramento, California. This book is dedicated to Margaret, Penelope, Simon and Andrew Lie for their love and support and the untold hours I have taken from them.

1 GENERAL FEATURES, STRUCTURE, TOPOGRAPHY AND ADAPTATION OF THE CIRCULATORY SYSTEM

William E. Stehbens

In the evolution of complex metazoa, an animal beyond a certain limiting size requires a circulatory system to assist in the maintenance of homeostatic conditions for constituent cells and tissues. This is done by:

1. providing an adequate, rapid supply of well oxygenated blood to the tissues to cater for metabolic and hormonal needs according to functional requirements under physiological and pathological conditions with variation from organ to organ, site to site and moment to moment;
2. removing metabolic end products [1];
3. assisting in thermal regulation.

The circulation of blood within the vascular system is maintained principally by the heart and assisted by gravity, contractions of voluntary muscles and the windkessel action of proximal elastic arteries. Characteristically in circulatory systems the most active parts preferentially receive most blood [2]. John Hunter [3] enunciated the cardinal principle of the circulatory system: 'to maintain a circulation sufficient for the part and no more'. The complex mechanisms by which this is achieved are not understood.

Since William Harvey's logical exposition of the circulatory system and Malpighi's demonstration of the capillary link between arteries and veins, a considerable body of knowledge appertaining to physiological control of the circulation has been amassed. The structure of blood vessels varies according to tissue function and requirements but control of the structural differentiation of vessels is not well understood. The effect of circulating blood on angiogenesis, on the topographical and architectural design of the vascular system and on vascular pathology was relatively neglected until recent years. The vascular system is continuously subjected to hydrodynamic forces and is not immune to their effects. It is considerably more complex than simple mechanical circulation units because of the need for biological response to altered physiological conditions and its inherent ability to repair and compensate for changing physiological requirements and pathological states whether short or long term or primarily of the vessels themselves or of the related tissues. Blood vessels permit and facilitate the transmural passage of gases, nutrients, metabolites and hormones for normal physiology and growth, and transport cells and humoral agents essential for defence, detoxification and tissue repair. The adaptability of the circulatory system is remarkable in that both its organization and development have proven constantly adequate to permit evolution, whilst simultaneously retaining the ability to repair, proliferate and differentiate, such functions being mandatory for the survival of the individual and the various animal species.

1.1 Basic topography of the vascular system

The circulatory system consists of the heart and the systemic and pulmonary circulations. Descriptions of their detailed anatomical course and relationships, available in current textbooks, will not be dealt with here but some of their general anatomical features of relevance to the pathology of the circulatory system will be discussed.

The systemic circulation is designed to supply well oxygenated blood to the entire body at high pressure, with veins returning blood from individual microcirculatory beds to the right atrium. The pulmonary circulation delivers systemic venous blood to the lungs for gaseous exchange and oxygenation in the pulmonary microcirculation. Its veins return oxygenated blood to the left atrium for subsequent delivery to the systemic circulation. The portal venous systems in the alimentary system, the kidneys and adenohypophysis are specialized circulations adapted for specific functional requirements.

The fetal circulation is specifically modified for intrauterine life. The circulation of the placenta and umbilical vessels serves adequately the temporary needs of the fetus and together with changes initiated immediately after birth, is of immense interest to the haemodynamicist constituting a profitable avenue of future research.

1.2 Arteries

Arteries, being supply vessels, divide progressively into smaller channels. The total cross-sectional area increases progressively as they branch, minimizing the steady drop of pressure as the blood flows peripherally. The topography of arterial branching varies with site and organ supplied [1].

While John Hunter [3] asserted that arteries generally take a direct course from their origin to their destination, there are innumerable exceptions to this dictum, such as the carotid siphon and the tortuous course of the vertebral artery. Hunter attributed such exceptions to the need for reducing blood momentum and presumably pulse pressure in intracerebral arteries. The consensus view is that such configurations are designed to dampen the pulse pressure without significantly reducing mean pressure and flow rate. However, the effect could be fortuitous with the pattern dependent on fetal development after the principal channels have been determined. Large arteries generally pursue a relatively direct course within loose fascial planes to allow for pulsation and tortuosity and on the flexural surfaces of joints to obviate undue stretching.

Arteries have thicker walls than veins and the low-pressure pulmonary arteries are slightly thinner than vessels of corresponding diameter from the systemic circulation. In any vascular bed the calibre and pressure seem to determine wall thickness. However, cerebrospinal arteries, despite the high pressure and high velocity, are considerably thinner than extracranial arteries, the reason being obscure. Within the cerebrospinal circulation size again correlates with wall thickness.

Thoma's first histomechanical law indicates a relationship between arterial size and the rate of blood flow per unit of cross-sectional area which is generally proportional to the size of the capillary bed supplied [4]. In humans progressive arteriectasis with age due to mural degeneration must be taken into account for there is disproportionate, uneven enlargement of the arterial lumen [1]. Calibre ultimately depends on the volume of blood flow carried by the artery: the smaller the artery, the greater the economy of mural constituents, although this is counterbalanced by the greater resistance to flow and loss of energy consequent upon increased arboriz-

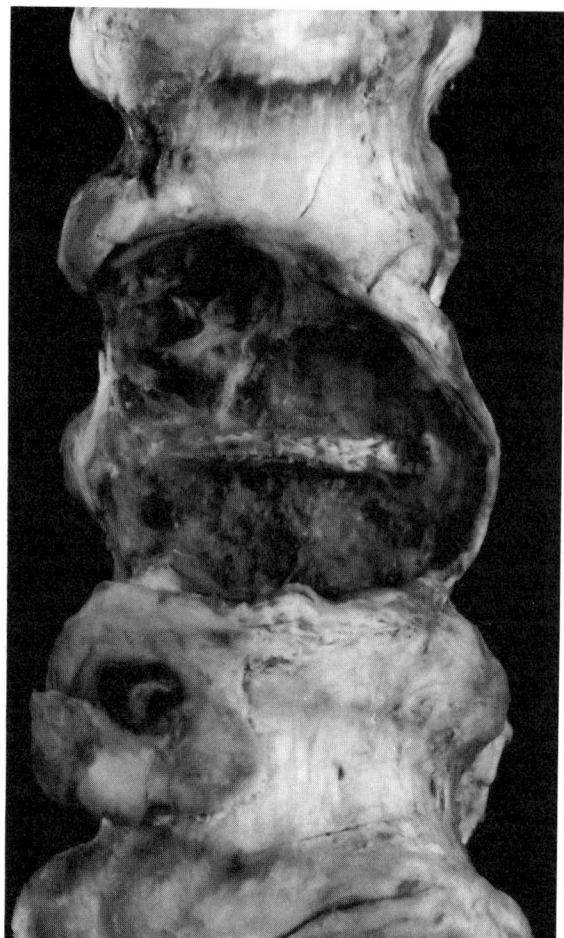

Figure 1.1 Vertebral bodies displaying erosion due to an abdominal aortic aneurysm. Note the greater erosion of the cancellous bone than of the intervertebral disc.

ation and greater frictional surface area. Disturbed or turbulent flow is less likely in vessels of small calibre and generally the optimal design prevails.

Compression of other anatomical structures by blood vessels is in all probability due to atherosclerosis, ectasia or tortuosity with secondary displacement of the vessel such as in the S-shaped course of the atherosclerotic basilar and vertebral arteries compressing cranial nerves, or the intense grooving of the subcostal surface of the ribs by tortuous intercostal arteries in coarctation of the aorta. Alternatively, it can be due to altered anatomical relationships as with aneurysmal dilatation. The most well known examples are:

1. the compression–erosion of the vertebral bodies and to a lesser extent the intervertebral discs by an aortic aneurysm (Figure 1.1);
2. compression of the recurrent laryngeal nerve by an aneurysm of the aortic arch;
3. cranial nerve palsies associated with cerebral aneurysms especially of the internal carotid artery.

With age in some individuals there may be a downward movement of the kidney such that an accessory renal artery may compress the uretopelvic junction resulting in hydronephrosis and hypertension.

The topography of the arterial tree strongly influences the nature of blood flow in the circulation. Each bifurcation or branching, by splitting and deflecting the stream, can be regarded as an obstacle to the free flow of blood. Most bifurcations are asymmetrical or unequal and unions of branches forming a common stem (e.g. vertebrobasilar junctions) are also unequal and though such configurations predominate in the venous system, these anastomoses have not been studied in depth.

The method of arterial arborization varies with the organ or part supplied. Mathematical analyses of the arborization patterns have been heavily dependent on the accuracy and detail of the available data. The actual configuration of each branching site is important haemodynamically particularly in respect of the angle of bifurcation, the size of the branches, the changes in cross-sectional area at the fork and proximity of other branches and even the fusiform dilatation known as the carotid sinus.

1.2.1 ANGLE OF BIFURCATION

Most investigators have focused on angles of bifurcation which generally conform to the principle of minimal work. The angle formed by the stem to the plane of the two branches, though ignored, was recently found to be virtually 0°, thus being in the same plane as would be expected [5]. Some slight curvature could modify the intimal thickening about the forks and pathological conditions could produce curvature secondarily.

Hunter [3] considered the angle of branching was determined by the functional needs of the part and that the angle varied to provide a velocity of flow sufficient for each vascular bed. He found the angle of branching tended to be wider or more obtuse and sometimes was actually recurrent near the heart, becoming increasingly acute distally. In 1879 Roux [6] estimated that the angle formed by a branch with the axis of the parent stem varied with the relative calibre of the branch. In general, the larger the branch the smaller was the angle and vice versa. In the analogous bronchial arborization the angles of branching are a function of the cross-sectional area of the branches with the tendency being towards maintenance of efficient dichotomy with minimal wind resistance. The angles are proportionately larger in smaller peripheral bronchi [7].

General rules governing arterial bifurcations have been formulated:

1. If an artery bifurcates into two equal branches, such branches form equal angles with the axis of the parent stem.
2. In an unequal branching the major branch forms a smaller angle with the axis of the parent stem than the lesser branch, the angle increasing as the calibre of the branch decreases.
3. Small branches that scarcely affect the calibre of the parent stem arise at a relatively wide angle (70° to 90°) [8].

Clark [9] essentially confirmed these observations in the tadpole tail, also observing that when one branch enlarged due to augmented flow, there was a concomitant change in the angle formed by the branches, the parent stem conforming with the hypothesis of Roux [6]. It is known that the proportional size of vessels can change from postnatal life to maturity in association with disparate growth of tissues. These anatomical alterations and the changed physical stresses to which the branches are subjected seem to allow modification of the fork in conformity with the above findings [10].

In later life haemodynamic forces still appear to play an important role in determining branch size and the configuration of arterial forks with the bifurcation angle approximating the optimal angle for efficiency. Murray [11] confirmed the laws of Roux. In a mathematical analysis he considered arterial forks and the confluence of veins conformed to the principle of minimal work. Calculations put the minimal theoretical angle of an arterial bifurcation at about 75°. Angles varied within wide limits with most not conforming to this ideal. According to Murray the bifurcation of the pulmonary trunk was too wide and that of the aortic bifurcation too narrow (60° to 75°). Murray also indicated that the workload required to overcome the inertia of the blood is significant when the velocity is high and therefore the larger the animal the larger the aorta has to be in comparison with the rest of the vascular system and with the normal blood flow.

It has been estimated mathematically that the optimum angle at the junction of the two vertebral arteries to form the basilar is theoretically 70°54′ [12]. The average angle of union is approximately 64°30′ (range 34° to 118°), but Stopford [13] found the two vertebral arteries were equal in only 8% of the specimens. Therefore, the angle is also variable and is thus likely to alter flow conditions substantially [14]. In general flow disturbances are more frequent when the angle of bifurcation or union is large.

In a study of arterial forks from humans, rabbits and pigs [5,15], the bifurcation angles and branch diameters and angles which the axes of the branches made with that of the parent stem, compared favourably with the predicted optimal values. There was some biological scatter as anticipated but the relatively good agreement led the authors to conclude that the architecture of the fork was governed by certain physiological principles designed to maintain minimum drag and energy loss. However, Hutchins *et al.* [16] found no relationship between the branch angle and vessel calibre in human coronary arteries, an unexplained exception.

Measurements of such angles are taken at autopsy mostly from middle-aged and elderly subjects whose vessels, affected by varying degrees of atherosclerosis, are not necessarily representative of the angles at birth or early maturity. Atherosclerotic changes could account for the wide variation so often observed.

1.2.2 CROSS-SECTIONAL AREA AT THE FORK

At the approach to a bifurcation, one would expect the lumen to be partitioned by mural indentations in order to divide the blood stream proportionately according to the volume capacity of the branches without significant variation in cross-sectional area. Thoma [17] claimed that enlargement of the lumen occurred at all forks especially in the microcirculation. Wiggers [18] referred to an Indian club enlargement allegedly designed to avert turbulence, whilst Willis [19] thought the arterial lumen enlarged concentrically immediately before the lumen divided. However, by measuring the cross-sectional area of step-serial sections through a series of arterial forks distended with a gelatin–barium sulphate mixture under physiological pressures, considerable distortion of the circular lumen was demonstrated before, during and immediately after the actual bifurcation [20]. As the blood proceeds peripherally, the contour of the lumen changes from a circular to an oval profile with slight focal thickening of the three layers of the wall on the flattened surfaces where stress concentration is a recognized phenomenon. The flattening becomes an indentation with more pronounced mural thickening and the lumen assumes a dumb-bell shape immediately proximal to the apex or actual division of the lumen (Figure 1.2). The cross-sectional area at this site can undergo considerable, variable expansion to as much as 219% of the proximal cross-sectional area. This ampulla-like expansion in an equal bifurcation is symmetrical but not concentric as Willis [19] alleged. The greatest enlargement occurs within 1 to 2 mm proximal to the apex or crotch whilst the facial and dorsal surfaces approximate only slightly as facial and dorsal extensions of the flow divider encroach on the lumen [20]. This configuration constitutes an elliptical diffuser and is probably asymmetrical more often than not. The medial walls of the daughter branches immediately beyond the apex are initially flattened with the branches providing D-shaped profiles but rapidly assume a circular contour (Figure 1.2). The lateral (transverse) measurement or width of the fork within the final 3 to 4 mm proximal to the apex can increase by as much as 50 to 80%.

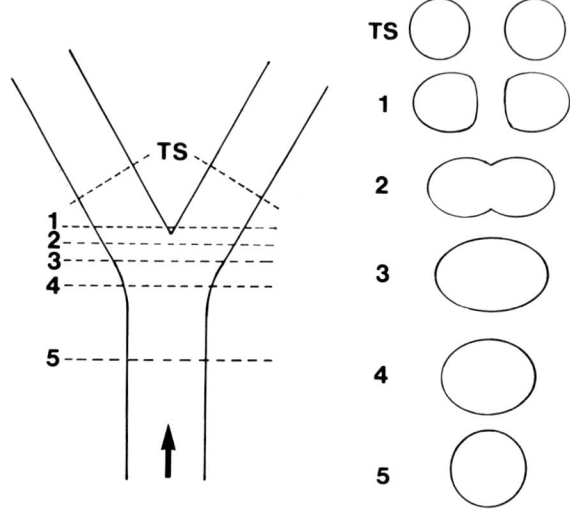

Figure 1.2 Changes in the cross-sectional area at different levels (1–5) through an arterial fork. TS transverse sectional profiles of the daughter branches beyond the bifurcation whereas the numerals represent the cross-sectional profiles relative to the axis of the parent stem. (Redrawn from Stehbens [107].)

Lateral or side branches are associated with slight mural thickening proximal to the ostium concomitantly with the lumen becoming egg-shaped in cross-section. The cross-sectional area expands laterally to a greater or lesser extent depending on the size of the branch and its angle of bifurcation, whilst facial and dorsal extremities of the flow divider project into and gradually partition the lumen. The cross-section of the vessel presents an eccentric aneurysm-like bulge or diverticulum which increases the cross-sectional area by 20% in small branches and by more than 100% in large wide angled branches. Sections immediately distal to the apex again show flattening and on occasion slight invagination with some intimal thickening before the lumen resumes a circular profile. In longitudinal sections the flow divider or apex overrides the proximal stem to ensure diversion of blood into the branch. The allegation that pulmonary arteries are elliptical in cross-section rather than circular [21] can be attributed to the configuration in rapidly dichotomizing branches. It is inconceivable, however, that any physiological advantage would be derived from arteries of such shape or that the internal pressure would not tend to produce a circular outline in cross-section.

Zamir and Brown [10] analyzed angiograms of 137 arterial bifurcations from multiple sources and reported that the position of the apex of the flow dividers was consistent with an optimum model of a bifurcation in which the apex lies on a streamline which distributes the flow from the parent artery in proportion to the diameter of the two branches. This is at one with the observation that the apex overrides the flux of blood in the parent vessel [1,20], an architectural feature sometimes ignored in theoretical modelling of arterial forks.

1.2.3 AREA RATIO (BRANCHING COEFFICIENT)

The area ratio or branching coefficient is the ratio of the sum of the cross-sectional areas of the two daughter branches to that of the parent stem. In arborization of the arterial tree, even though the size of the main trunk progressively tapers, the total cross-sectional area progressively increases as blood flows peripherally. This increase is said to offset the loss of pressure due to increased friction consequent upon the progressive increase in intimal surface. The ratio is therefore usually greater than one, the optimal value is 1.26 and the radius of each branch in an equal bifurcation to that of the parent stem is 0.794 [22,23]. Hamilton [24] found that in practice the value of the area ratio approximated 1.33. The proportion of the pulse wave reflected from arterial forks has been related to the area ratio [25] and Gosling et al. [26] predicted the minimum reflection at a bifurcation would occur at an area ratio of 1.15 and at a trifurcation of 1.25. Newman et al. [27] reported that the proportion of the wave reflected and the size of the standing wave increased progressively with divergence from the optimal values and accentuation of the oscillatory pressure stresses on the vessel wall.

Estimates of the area ratio for the human aortic bifurcation have varied from 0.734 to unity for adults [17,28,29], but Gosling et al. [26] reported an area ratio of 1.11 at birth with a progressive decrease with age. According to Dinnar [30] it is about 1.15 in infancy, 0.8 to 0.9 at the fourth decade and less in the fifth which indicates narrowing rather than expansion and also increased peripheral rigidity and increased wave reflection with increased systolic pressure. Lallemand et al. [31] alleged that low values reported for the aortic bifurcation indicated a propensity for atherosclerosis but it is more likely to be the effect rather than the cause.

A reduction in the area ratio of human aortae has also been calculated in subjects with angiographic evidence of atherosclerosis. This is consistent with the area ratio of 1.18 found in 19 young persons [32] and a similar observation has been made for the coronary artery area ratios [16]. Another study [33] found coronary artery area ratios to be 1.179 with higher values for the higher order coronary branchings and asymmetrical branchings. The aorto-iliac area ratios were only 0.848 suggesting moderately severe atherosclerosis. From angiograms and resin casts, Caro et al. [34] calculated a value of less than or only slightly greater than one for large proximal arteries. Variation in such measurements obviously depends on the technique and accuracy of mensuration. Since intimal thickening in the distal aorta at birth can be almost half the thickness of the media, its width, if not offset by some aortic dilatation, will affect the area ratio. Thus, the value of the area ratio in man is also dependent on the severity of atherosclerosis and the balance between intimal thickening and ectasia. The whole range of progressive change from the fetus to atherosclerotic adult needs to be investigated taking into consideration the severity of atherosclerotic involvement.

The area ratio ranged from 1.16 to 1.35 (mean 1.23) for the aortic bifurcation in the dog and in the cockerel it was 1.05 to 1.28 (mean 1.16) [26]. In cockerels with dietary-induced fat-containing lesions, the area ratio of the aorta was only 0.86, the reduction being attributed to increased distensibility in the experimental animals [27]. Since the dietary-induced lesions do not exhibit the medial thinning of atherosclerosis, the reduction in area ratio may really be caused by intimal encroachment on the lumen in the absence of the usual medial yield or tendency to ectasia.

Thoma [17] emphasized the need to avoid measurements too close to the fork and area ratios can vary within wide limits depending on the site of measurement [20]. Angiographic measurements will often be unreliable. Determination of cross-sectional areas from fixed distended vessels is probably more accurate although some error from shrinkage in the preparation of sections can be expected. The cross-sectional area will vary with the pulse cycle and any acquired weakness of the wall tends to yield most at the peak of systolic pulse pressure and under high pressure fixation of vessels *in vitro*.

The complicating factor in the measurement of area ratios in man or in lower animals with moderate to severe atherosclerosis is that the respective severity of intimal thickening and ectasia will affect measurements. Allegations that a low value suggests a propensity for atherosclerosis become meaningless. The area ratio will unquestionably affect flow at the fork or junction and this in turn affects intimal thickening and overt atherosclerosis. Walburn et al. [35] found that the critical Reynolds numbers in symmetrically branched tubes decreased from 2100 at a ratio of 0.8 to 1200 for a ratio of 1.4. Lighthill [36] estimated 1.2 was the critical value above which flow separation was likely to occur but more attention should be given to variations in the cross-sectional area in the plane perpendicular to the blood flow because divergence of the wall from the main flux will lead to flow instability and the consequences thereof. Investigation should determine to what extent the tendency to ectasia and increase in the cross-sectional area at the fork are acquired and also the variation in the functional area ratio during the pulse cycle and with variations in vasomotor tone.

The observation that changes in the cross-sectional area at forks and area ratios greater than 1.0 give arterial bifurcations the structure of eccentric symmetrical or asymmetrical diffusers, led to the hypothesis that under certain conditions physiological murmurs may be generated at such forks [1].

1.2.4 MURMURS

Murmurs or bruits in the circulatory system are frequent and constitute a valuable clinical sign often associated with well-known pathological lesions. Frequent causes are pulmonary or aortic valvular stenoses, coarctation of the aorta, patent ductus arteriosus, arteriovenous shunts, compression of the subclavian artery by a cervical rib and, particularly, acquired stenoses due to atherosclerosis. Murmurs may thus herald serious pathological lesions.

The exact mechanism of murmur production in the circulatory system has not been resolved. Laminar flow is silent and sound generation is rarely detectable on the exterior of a tube in which there is turbulent flow. Rushmer and Morgan [37] consider that the most common type of murmur develops in the vicinity of turbulent jets produced by high velocity flow through narrow orifices. The sound is thought to be generated by fluctuations in pressure associated with eddy currents striking the vessel downstream from the orifice or stenosis without dominant frequencies. The vibration of the wall may be transmitted through the tissues to the skin surface and for sound to be heard in this way the wall must vibrate [38]. In the above clinical examples flow is through a narrow orifice or jet into a wider channel or chamber. The murmurs are often associated with a palpable thrill and the energy involved must be considerable. Those murmurs in humans that signify a pathological stenosis and jet flow are usually harsh and blowing in quality and have the characteristics of grossly turbulent flow.

Murmurs are generated over the pregnant uterus, the mammary gland during lactation and the thyroid gland in thyrotoxicosis. A murmur over the skull in Paget's disease of bone has been attributed to a significant arteriovenous shunt associated with augmented flow in the calvarium. These murmurs, considered to be physiological bruits, are regarded as hyperkinetic in type. Some are associated with reduced viscosity as in anaemia – the so-called haemic murmurs which disappear on correction of the anaemia. Orbital bruits are frequent in subjects on maintenance haemodialysis and are attributed to anaemia and general vascular dilatation [39]. These are soft murmurs or hums and are generally considered to be of no clinical significance. Their detection and differentiation depend on the auditory acuity of the individual observer. There can be difficulty in determining the site of origin and a need exists for objective analysis of the physical characteristics of such murmurs and correlation with their source and mechanism.

Murmurs over the head have been detected in auscultation in chronic hydrocephalus, acute inflammation of the brain and cerebral abscess. In acute leptomeningitis the increased blood flow and vasodilatation are demonstrable angiographically and the murmur may disappear following therapy. Murmurs have been detected during an attack of migraine but no underlying cause can be found in many instances, especially in children. Bruits can be evoked at times by contralateral carotid compression which would increase arterial flow on the side of the skull being auscultated. Wadia and Monckton [40] suggested that certain variations or even asymmetry of the circle of Willis might be responsible but the size of the vessels concerned does not support such a concept. These authors found spontaneous bruits in up to 80% of 4–5-year-old children, diminishing to 10% in 10-year-old children with a slower flow up to 15 years (4%). The bruits were mainly unilateral. Yet more than 30% of 10-year-old children have either a spontaneous bruit or one that can be evoked by carotid compression. This incidence falls to about 22% at 15 years of age.

Bruits in the neck are frequent having been found in 87% of adults over 60 years of age [4]. Cervical bruits were found in 40% of 70 healthy medical students with a mean age of 23 years [42].

There is no agreement regarding the nature of soft physiological murmurs emanating from the vascular system though they are usually regarded as benign and of no pathological significance. Physiological murmurs are not understood but their occurrence in hyperkinetic states with vasodilatation and reduced viscosity indicate dependence on the Reynolds number. It is likely these factors only accentuate naturally occurring flow disturbances of insufficient energy to produce audible sound [1]. Flow disturbances associated with stenoses, jets and arteriovenous fistulae appear in conjunction with severe degenerative changes which have been attributed to the effect of vibrations on the vessel wall and the induction of mechanical fatigue. If this is true, then lesser vibrations associated with physiological murmurs may contribute to the overall changes in the vessel wall.

Flow at arterial forks simulates jet flow into a symmetrical or asymmetrical lateral diffuser because of the antrum-like dilatation of the stem immediately before the division of the lumen into the two daughter branches [1]. The increase in cross-sectional area varies with the branch and the angle of bifurcation, being greatest at wide angles and particularly at the common carotid bifurcation due to the presence of the carotid sinus which is, in effect, a fusiform dilatation. Flow under such circumstances is likened to an organ pipe in which sound is produced by a jet edge effect with alternating vortex shedding on either side of the reed. The apex of the fork (Figure 1.3) would constitute the wedge in the

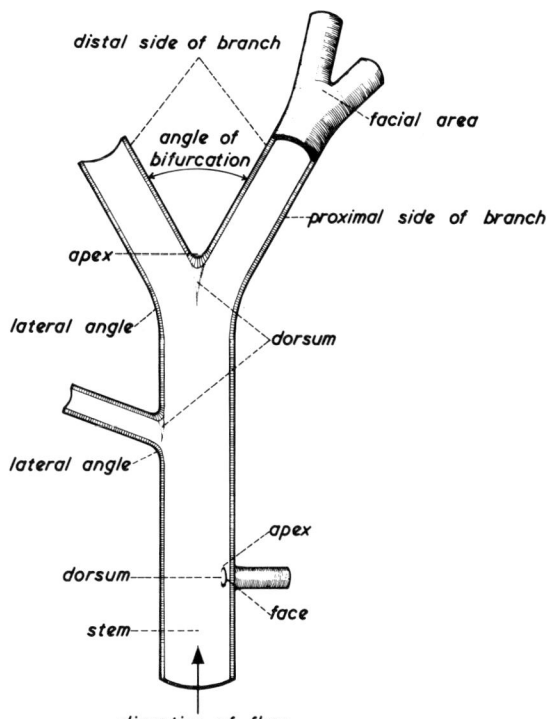

Figure 1.3 Anatomical nomenclature of sites about forks of vessels. Apex is the crotch of the fork or carina and the apical angle is the angle of bifurcation. The lateral angles are those subtended by the daughter branches and the parent stem. The face is the uppermost surface of the stem near the fork between the entrances of the two branches and is the uppermost extremity of the crescentic flow divider. The dorsum is the corresponding region on the reverse side of the fork. (Reproduced with permission from Stehbens [108].)

flux of blood. This would not require high velocity flow but the sound intensity would depend on blood velocity and viscosity and the architecture of the fork. This could account for physiological murmurs. Venous hums may emanate from junctions of tributaries where vortex shedding is particularly likely to occur [14]. Eccentrically placed wedges in the flow generate asymmetrical vortices which conceivably could account for the asymmetrical intimal proliferation over the crescentic flow divider of small side branches of the aorta and iliofemoral arteries. This seems to be the most plausible explanation for the soft, musical, physiological murmur. To suggest that such murmurs have no effect on the blood vessel wall is conjecture. The possibility of a chronic subtle influence being exerted cannot be excluded.

Aneurysms in general have no audible bruit but several authors using appropriate amplification have detected low amplitude, low frequency murmurs, often musical and associated with berry aneurysms [43,44]. It has been suggested that the two sides of the entrance to the aneurysm would constitute two wedges and induce vortex shedding on either side of each wedge [1,46].

Such a phenomenon could account for the intimal thickening on either side of the aneurysmal sac and at times the augmented thickening at the entrance.

1.3 Special structural features of arteries

Any investigator commencing a study of a vascular bed should initially study the normal anatomy, anatomical variations and structure of the vessels concerned. If not readily available such data should be obtained before investigations proceed. Different species at times have anatomical and structural peculiarities.

1.3.1 THE INTIMA

The structure of arteries varies according to the circulatory bed and in this respect it is important to adhere to standardized and well accepted nomenclature and definitions. For example the intima of arteries has been defined at least since 1858 in the first edition of Gray's *Anatomy* [46] and subsequently in textbooks of histology as the inner layer of the arterial wall, consisting of the endothelium, the internal elastic lamina and the intervening tissue. There is already confusion in the literature [47] but unless all adhere to a universal established definition, scientific communication becomes impossible internationally, temporally and between disciplines. It is inappropriate for a committee to redefine the intima or any other structure without adequate reason.

1.3.2 MEDIAL ELASTIC LAMELLAR UNITS

In the aorta and elastic arteries, the media consists of multiple fenestrated sheets of lamellae of elastic tissue, somewhat thinner than the internal elastic lamina if still present. In the intervening space are smooth muscle cells circularly arranged, possibly with a slight helical orientation. In between these muscle cells are obliquely arranged collagen and interconnecting bands or fibrils of elastic tissue between the elastic laminae forming as it were small compartments in which the smooth muscle cells (enveloped in their basement membranes) lie in a proteoglycan matrix. This arrangement of multiple lamellar units [48,49] distributes the stresses as well as maintaining cohesion and viscoelastic properties of the wall. Wolinsky and Glagov [48] reported that the number of lamellar units in the thoracic aortas of several mammals was nearly proportional to the aortic radius regardless of species or variation in wall thickness. They estimated that the average tension per lamellar unit, relatively constant irrespective of the species, ranged by a factor of about 3.

Peripherally the lamellar structure of the aorta is lost and except in cerebral arteries there is considerably more elastic tissue in the adventitia and not just a single external elastic lamina at the junction of the media and adventitia. There is usually a transitional stage between the elastic and muscular architectures although it can be relatively abrupt on occasions.

An elastic sponge-like skeleton in the media of cerebral arteries, not previously recognized by light microscopy, is in a way similar to but much less pronounced than that in the aortic media though without distinct elastic laminae [50]. On the inner surface of the internal elastic lamina are fold-like protrusions of elastic tissue. The medial elastic tissue in extracranial muscular arteries is much more pronounced.

Different species have structural peculiarities [51] often associated with size and behavioural characteristics of the individual species.

1.3.3 MEDIAL DEFECTS OF FORBUS OR MEDIAL RAPHES

In 1930 Forbus [52] drew attention to wedge-shaped adventitial invaginations into the media as far as the internal elastic lamina at the apex or crotch of cerebral arterial forks of a stillborn infant. He inappropriately labelled them 'medial defects', alleging that they were *loci minoris resistentiae*, where berry aneurysms are prone to occur. Such a label implied congenital or maldevelopmental weakness but no such mechanical or structural weakness has ever been demonstrated. Finding in a fetus such a discontinuity of the medial musculature where cerebral aneurysms occur, he assumed a cause and effect relationship. His observation and alleged causality were used to substantiate the congenital hypothesis of cerebral berry aneurysms.

The adventitial wedges consist of adventitial tissue (Figure 1.4) and often require serial histological sections to verify their presence. They tend to be smaller in neonates and at times only partially interrupt the media. They are particularly prone to occur in acute angles not only at the apex or crotch, but at the lateral angles and at junctions. They appear to be of universal occurrence in the cerebral circulation and in extracranial splanchnic arteries of man and the other mammals (Figure 1.5) so far examined [53,54]. In the cerebral circulation they are found at major arterial forks where berry aneurysms occur and at forks in more peripheral smaller arteries where aneurysms are extremely rare [54]. In internal carotid and middle cerebral artery bifurcations they increase in frequency with age and thus are not all congenital, i.e. present at birth [54]. Since some are acquired postnatally, it can be concluded that they may be acquired, that they appear to be universal in man and other mammals examined, and that their histological distribution is quite different from that of the berry type aneurysm of which they have been alleged to be the cause or major contributing factor.

It is important to be aware of the existence of these

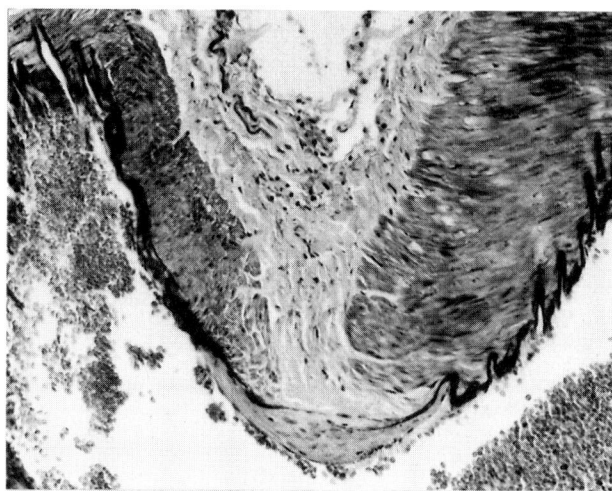

Figure 1.4 Medial raphe at apex of a cerebral arterial fork. Note the apical thickening, loss of elastica and the adventitial reinforcement. (Reproduced with permission from Stehbens [109].)

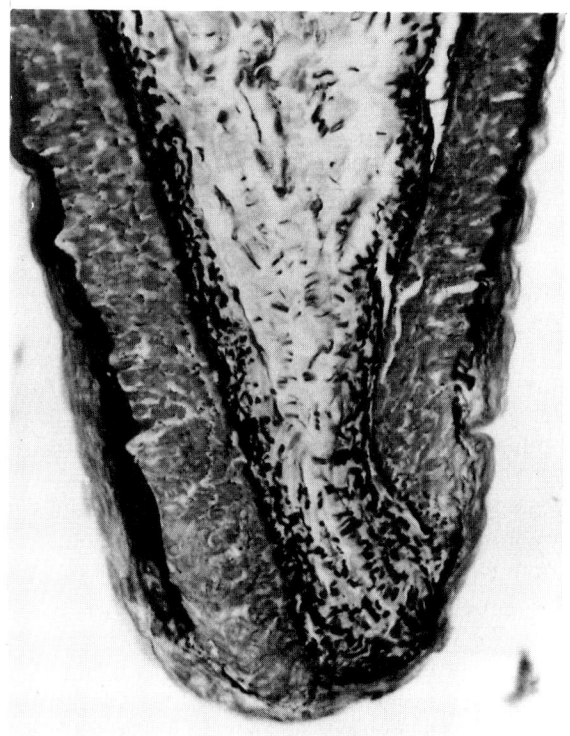

Figure 1.5 Medial raphe at apex of the renal arterial fork of a rabbit. Note the intimal thickening and deficient internal elastic lamina. (Reproduced with permission from Stehbens [108].)

medial raphes for at times they have been mistaken for scars. The raphes have been considered as reinforcements such as at the bow of a boat [55,57] and they also act in the capacity of a raphe where during vasoconstriction, especially at acute angles, the medial muscle of the adjoining arterial walls of the daughter branches would be pulling in almost opposite directions. Biologically, whenever muscles pull in opposing directions, they have attachment to a bone, tendon or fibrous raphe. The so-called 'medial defects' of Forbus [52] should therefore be regarded as medial raphes and not as sites of *loci minoris resistentiae* [58]. The term 'medial defect' should be abandoned and regarded as an historical allusion and unwarranted speculation.

1.4 Veins

All veins are thin-walled vessels, with those of the cerebrospinal circulation thinner than other tissues. Even so, the walls of veins vary according to their site, those of the lower limb being relatively thicker than other veins such as in the splanchnic circulation. Their thin walls and low pressure make them particularly vulnerable to external pressure occlusion by tumours, strangulated hernias, or at times by pathological arteries and as the result of the torsion of a loop of bowel or vascular pedicle. These conditions, by preventing drainage, may lead to haemorrhagic infarction in the absence of adequate collateral flow.

Veins are designed to return blood to the heart under low pressure but being more numerous than arteries and with many interconnecting vessels, they provide an extensive, variable interconnecting drainage. Because of this variability, in general only major veins have specific anatomical names. Many are cylindrical while others, except when grossly distended, are somewhat flattened or elliptical and some intracranial sinuses may by triangular in section. General anatomical patterns are maintained but the topography in monozygous twins is not identical [54]; Edwards [59] noted the extreme individual variability of tributaries of the inferior vena cava.

Anastomoses are much more frequent between veins than between the corresponding arteries and the union of their tributaries and the venous valves with their sinuses produce the principal configurations that affect flow in the venous circulation. The veins constitute a physiological reservoir of considerable size, their cross-sectional area progressively diminishing as the heart is approached. The extent to which venous topography is determined by haemodynamic forces, vagaries of flow and physiological requirements during development is unknown and difficult to investigate.

Venous pressures are generally much lower than arterial pressures but it is frequently not appreciated that the pressure about the ankle in the standing position may be 100 mmHg and is considerably higher during the Valsalva manoeuvre (up to 200 mmHg).

The low flow rate and blood pressure seem to be responsible for the less severe degenerative changes in the venous circulation but thin walls, the vulnerability of superficial veins to injury and the plentiful collateral circulation are responsible for the particular features of venous involvement in many human diseases and also for their participation in the spread of the disease.

1.5 The terminal vascular bed

As peripheral arteries continue to arborize they become progressively smaller, eventually terminating in arterioles, the small supply channels with a muscular media, thin adventitia and no elastic tissue. Arterioles then supply the microvascular or capillary bed, in turn drained by a series of vessels progressively uniting to form small veins. Controversy surrounds the topography of the microvascular bed, the interconnecting vessels and the size and nomenclature of the respective components. Disagreement may be attributed in part to the natural variability in pattern, vascularity and functional requirements. It is difficult to conceive of a regular topographical pattern for the microcirculatory bed for in general the smaller the vessel the greater is the anatomical variability. The arterioles, the terminal ramifications of the arterial circulation, are of particular interest in this survey. Flow in the microcirculation *in vivo* is fascinating and some of its aspects are applicable to the macrocirculation [60].

There is considerable variation in capillary density in different tissues even within the one organ. This vascularity seems to be directly related to functional or metabolic need. A variable proportion of the capillary bed may be actively perfused during a period of rest or diminished function. Evidence indicates that in the absence of pathological changes the circulatory system is always adequate for functional requirements.

Arteriovenous anastomoses of variable size, known to exist in the microcirculation, are believed to function as a means of shunting blood directly from arterioles to venules. The lumen of those in the heart has been found to vary from 70 to 170 µm, in the lung from 10 to 750 µm, in the stomach about 165 µm and in the spleen 300 µm. Particularly numerous in the skin, these arteriovenous anastomoses function in thermal regulation in the skin, rabbit ear and superficial parts, by diverting blood from the capillary bed [61]. They may also function as a type of pressure safety valve controlling pressure in the microcirculation. By varying blood flow to the microcirculation they affect blood flow through the larger feeding arteries and may have a cumulative effect of significance.

1.6 The pulmonary circulation

The pulmonary circulation differs from the systemic circulation in that during fetal life it is partially bypassed by means of the foramen ovale and ductus arteriosus, a situation reversed at birth or shortly thereafter. Other important differences are the lower blood pressure within the pulmonary arterial tree and the double arterial blood supply, of particular importance in occlusive pulmonary vascular disease.

The pulmonary trunk and major arteries are relatively constant but the topography of the peripheral distributing arteries displays much variability consistent with their size [62] and as in the systemic circulation, their topography seems to be determined by haemodynamics and the vagaries of blood flow. The circumference of the pulmonary artery in the child is 1 to 2 cm greater than that of the aorta [63], but is 1 to 5 cm less in the adult, the difference being most notable after the age of 40 years, no doubt due to progressive aortic ectasia.

The medial thickness of the pulmonary artery is equal to that of the aorta in the fetus, since the blood pressures are comparable and the disposition of the medial elastic laminae is also similar [64] apart from minor differences [62]. The ratio of the thickness of the pulmonary artery to that of the aorta falls from 1.0 at birth to 0.4–0.8 within 6 to 24 months after birth. However the pulmonary blood pressures fall postnatally and the aortic configuration of the pulmonary artery changes to a more loose, open appearance with interrupted laminae and short segments and clubbed terminations [62] by the age of 2 years. The adult pattern is said to consist of multiple, thin, fragmented and non-parallel laminae with zones of lamellar compression, but the possibility of progressive degenerative changes contributing to these observations must not be dismissed. Both the pulmonary artery and the aorta increase substantially in size during physical maturation and the number of elastic laminae also increases.

After birth the pulmonary muscular arteries increase in diameter with growth and maturation. The media is thinner than in the systemic circulation. Pulmonary arterioles consist of little more than endothelium and a thin elastic lamina with no significant media or adventitia. They are consequently difficult to distinguish from venules. These architectural changes in the elastic and muscular arteries of the pulmonary tree can be regarded as physiological adaptation to a lower pressure and lower peripheral resistance. One must be sceptical about the loss of continuity of elastic laminae for such 'fragmentation' also occurs in the aorta especially in middle age. It should not be considered as a type of disuse atrophy. Elastic laminae in occluded non-functional arteries can persist indefinitely. They do not disappear as one might expect [54] and it is doubtful whether there is such an entity as disuse atrophy of elastin.

Individuals born at high altitudes have pulmonary hypertension from birth. It has been attributed to relative hypoxia at low barometric altitudes. As a consequence the normal postnatal transition of the pulmonary elastic arteries does not occur and elastic arteries retain their aortic configuration. Such a phenomenon may be accepted as adaptation but other sequelae, pathological in nature including intimal thickening and overt atherosclerosis are pathological rather than adaptive changes.

1.7 The cerebral circulation

The brain is supplied by four arteries, each of which has a sigmoid tortuosity prior to entering the skull where they converge on the interpeduncular fossa as if it were a hilum. They anastomose with each other and give rise to long tenuous branches which spread out and ramify over the surface of the brain, giving off small branches to supply the parenchyma. Thus the main branches are long and reduce only slowly in calibre; only very small branches ever enter brain substance.

Drainage of blood is via superficial leptomeningeal veins emptying into the dural venous sinuses. The deeper portions of the cerebrum drain via the deep transcerebral veins into the subependymal collecting veins, the largest vessels within the brain parenchyma and then into the great cerebral vein of Galen which also drains into the dural sinus circulation. The terminal leptomeningeal arteries have anastomoses with the small branches in neighbouring arterial supply areas and likewise the small venous tributaries have anastomoses, as is consistent with their small calibre.

The spinal cord in man derives its blood supply from a number of sources and in like fashion the arteries and veins anastomose freely over the surface of the cord, but again in the absence of some vascular abnormality only very small vessels are found within the cord substance.

Cerebrospinal blood vessels are unique in that their walls are much thinner than extracranial arteries of comparable size. This is demonstrable macroscopically as blood clots and air bubbles, and overt atherosclerosis can be seen through the transparent walls of cerebral arteries. Microscopically the arteries are muscular in type (Figure 1.6). At birth the intima consists of an endothelial layer and a prominent internal elastic lamina with no demonstrable intervening tissue histologically except at branching sites where, like all the distributing arteries, there is intimal proliferation (pads or cushions) [65]. The media is thinner than that of extracranial arteries and contains a fine elastic sponge-like skeleton [51]. The width of the adventitia is considerably less than in extracranial arteries and contains relatively little elastica, the fibrils being very sparse without definite external elastic laminae. There are no vasa vasorum until atherosclerosis is prominent. The collagen is less dense and there is no perivascular supporting tissue, making cerebral vessels comparatively easy to dissect and frozen sections free from contaminating adipose fat. The reason for this unique structure is unknown. There are also differences in the sympathetic nervous control and the blood velocity angiographically is faster in

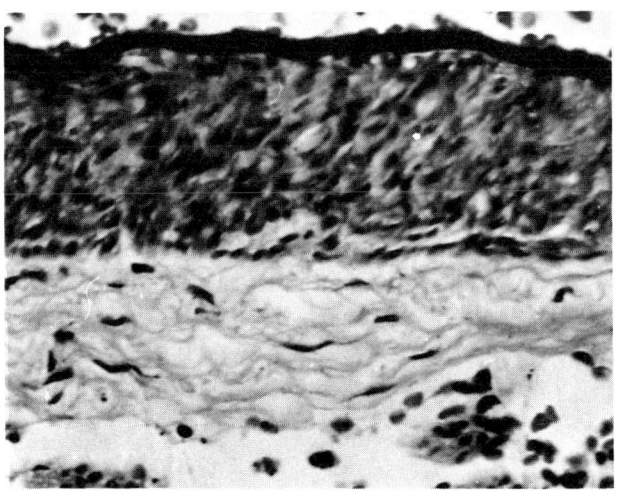

Figure 1.6 Histological section of a neonatal cerebral artery with a prominent internal elastic lamina (black) above and virtually no elastic tissue in the media and thin adventitia. (Verhoeff's elastic stain and eosin.)

cerebral arteries than in the external carotid circulation.

These architectural peculiarities of the cerebral arteries are important and help explain some pathological lesions prone to affect the central nervous system. They indicate the need for investigators to ensure they are conversant with peculiarities of the particular vessel or vascular bed under study.

1.8 Anatomical variations of peripheral vascular patterns

Anatomical variation in the circulatory system is of interest to the anatomist because of possible embryological and physiological significance. Of practical importance to the surgeon, to pathologists and to physiologists, variations may have haemodynamic consequences. In any vascular bed the topographical distribution of large vessels is likely to be individualistic although overall the relative constancy of the vessel distribution is quite remarkable. Anatomy texts do not reveal the true frequency of variations. Only detailed study of individual vascular beds provides a realistic appraisal of the variability. Abbie [66] considered topographical variation of the arterial circulation to be consistent with the principle of economy of distribution and convenience of source. This dictum is valid in the developing embryo when the arterial pattern is being determined by the competition of the many channels for supremacy from the primordial vascular plexus [67]. However some variations are secondary events, occurring later than the mural differentiation of major channels. Postnatal alterations in the arterial tree can occur due to disparate growth of an organ or part thereof and to changes in functional demands of individual tissues.

The innumerable variations of the adult circulatory system and the occurrence of arterial and venous anastomoses are generally attributed to events at their origin from the primitive capillary network. Some variations are more frequent than others. Many are modifications of the common or 'normal' developmental pathway, and may represent vascular patterns existing in lower animals. Other variations have no counterpart in ontogeny or in other lower animals and owe their existence to utility and mechanical advantage. Experimentally any slight interference with the primitive capillary plexus results in anatomical variations with compensatory enlargement of alternate pathways [68]. This adaptability is probably one of the most remarkable and characteristic features of embryogenesis [69]. Some variations, especially of large vessels, are disadvantageous. The reason they have arisen is obscure and assumptions are unwise until more is known of embryonic and fetal angiogenesis and possible factors leading to such unfortunate variations. Aberrant development of an organ or part, even if only in shape, results in some modification of vascular supply and drainage. Adaptation of blood supply seems to be the secondary event [11].

Evans [67] in explaining vascular variations declared that it cannot be doubted that hydrodynamic factors determine which vessels of the primitive plexus become supply and drainage channels, permitting the possibility of variation in the position of the trunk and the area served by it. Whilst duplicated arteries are frequent in embryology, duplications and plexiform vessels in adults are not necessarily survivals of embryonic conditions for many are secondary formations and minor differences in the angles of origin can greatly favour or hinder their acquisition of a dominant role in the contest of trunks serving the same field.

Anatomical variations of distributing arteries are often regarded as developmental anomalies, particularly in the cerebral circulation where the main basal arteries exhibit considerable variation in size and symmetry. Variations of the superficial cortical arteries, more common than those of the major arteries at the base of the brain, have received little attention. The arterial topography of the circle of Willis is highly individualistic [54,70] as are the coronary [71] and subclavian arterial trees [72] and also, it seems, the mesenteric circulation and other vascular beds.

Available evidence indicates that anatomical variations of veins of almost any site, if studied in detail, display individualistic topography [59,73,74]. Speculations concerning the significance of these cerebral vascular variations can be applied equally to the systemic circulation. Chance, chemical, physical and haemodynamic factors, as well as vagaries of flow and minor differences in the angles of bifurcations in the primordial microcirculation, could determine dominance or otherwise in major channel development. Study of vascular beds in identical twins is a means of determining the extent to which genetic factors operate during angiogenesis. Such twins do not have identical circles of Willis, nor are their retinal circulations or superficial veins of the forearm identical and, like fingerprints, the topography is individualistic and determined during angiogenesis although the vascular pattern can vary postnatally during maturation [54]. Lower animals also exhibit individuality of the circulatory tree. Suggestions that a set pattern is determined by anatomical, text-book type diagrams or that such variations are associated with hypothetical mural weaknesses or defects leading to the formation of arterial aneurysms or arteriovenous fistulae are scientifically unacceptable [54]. It is difficult to exclude all anatomical variations of the arterial tree from the category of congenital or developmental abnormalities, particularly in regard to some variations of the aorta or possibly of the coronary arteries (such as the origin of a coronary artery from the pulmonary artery). Such variations could be primarily genetic or alternatively secondary to another anomalous condition whether primary, secondary or even acquired or environmental *in utero*. There is no more reason for believing that arterial variation has such significance than that it pertains to topographical variations of veins or even smaller vessels. Unsubstantiated assumptions cannot be accepted despite difficulties in disproving them.

Anatomical variations influence the severity of atherosclerosis and its complications [1]. Since atherosclerosis is more pronounced in large vessels in any circulatory bed, a variation in which one vessel is compensatorily enlarged enhances the progression of the disease in that vessel. For instance, theoretically, if one internal carotid artery supplies blood to both anterior cerebral arteries as well as the homolateral middle and posterior cerebral arteries, one would expect enhanced atherosclerosis in that internal carotid because of the greater mural tension due to its larger calibre. Likewise atherosclerosis would be less severe in the contralateral internal carotid and in the proximal segment of the contralateral anterior cerebral arteries. The predisposition to atherosclerosis is inherent in the calibre of the artery and the associated haemodynamic stress. Moreover small components of the circle of Willis would limit the availability of collateral flow in cases of sudden occlusion of an artery thus affecting the size and distribution of a cerebral infarct. This in turn would increase the likelihood of such variation being noticed in clinicopathological studies. Other examples point to the need for confirmatory studies as illustrated by the heightened risk of coronary occlusion and myocardial infarction [71] in subjects with right or left coronary artery dominance. In recent years it has become apparent that imbalance at a cerebral arterial fork and participation in collateral flow is associated with degenerative changes in the arterial wall and aneurysm formation [75]. Such changes are regarded as atherosclerotic. It can be deduced that development of such changes may be enhanced by pathological lesions either in the neck or in the more peripheral circulation that are associated with either increased or decreased flow [76,77].

1.8.1 HYPOPLASIA AND APLASIA

'Hypoplasia' (for example, of an internal carotid artery) is a term applied to unusually small arteries. It may be either unilateral or bilateral. There is no evidence of impaired cerebral development and other arteries are compensatorily larger and provide collateral blood flow to the area of distribution of the internal carotid artery. This collateral flow may come either from other arteries supplying the brain or from some unusual source such as branches of the internal maxillary artery. Such 'hypoplasia' may be the result of some disease process or an unknown circumstance even *in utero*. There is no evidence at present that arteries fail to develop and enlarge as required given the time to do so. This is a characteristic of blood vessels that persists throughout life and it is wise to be sceptical about the use of 'aplasia' and 'hypoplasia' in reference to arteries. Such alleged states are more likely to be secondary to some other event or disease process. Variation in the size of arteries usually depends on the area of blood supply rather than on any deficiency of the artery wall itself.

1.9 Naturally occurring collateral circulation

Collateral circulation is the naturally occurring vascular pathway secondary or subsidiary to the principal route generally taken by the blood. In cases of vascular obstruction, circuitous alternative pathways may develop in addition to naturally occurring collaterals (see section 3.7.1). Alternate more circuitous pathways are dependent on pre-existing vascular anastomoses, some of which are large and capable of providing or dispensing blood instantaneously if necessary. Other alternate pathways depend on anastomoses of small calibre with terminal ramifications of neighbouring vessels in 'watershed regions'. On occasions these are more vulnerable and therefore sites of serious vascular complications, whether arterial or venous. Interarterial anastomoses between terminal branches of adjoining arteries suggest some overlap in territories of adjacent arterial supply with the border zone or watershed area supplied on one occasion by one artery and on another occasion by the other artery, depending on the haemodynamics prevailing at the time.

When the paths of two arteries eventually converge as

the result of the changing position of developing tissues supplied (anterior cerebral arteries), development of anastomoses is probably inevitable, as in the case of the anterior communicating artery. In other instances, muscular contractions may narrow smaller arteries or inhibit run off via the microcirculation, thereby leading to diversion of blood into alternate pathways which enhances the development of anastomoses. It is likely that haemodynamic factors during embryogenesis and postnatal development are responsible for the development and enlargement of many potential collaterals.

There has been much speculation on the significance of the anastomotic polygon or circle of Willis. Once it was considered to be a mechanism of ensuring blood flow to the brain, then as a mechanism for mixing the blood and even as a distributor station. In reality it is probably an anastomotic circle that developed as the result of proximity of the chief arteries of supply, changing haemodynamics during ontogeny and functioning as an important potential collateral pathway in cerebrovascular pathology. Patency of the collateral arterial circulation is probably maintained by periodic demands for collateral flow. It is likely that haemodynamic factors are also responsible for the development and maintenance of venous anastomoses and hence venous collateral pathways [13].

Perhaps the most extreme example of arterial collateral circulation is seen in coarctation of the aorta, in which the tortuosity of the collaterals is dramatic. Having so much redundant vessel wall rather than the arteries pursuing a more direct course must be regarded as unphysiological.

Veins display more numerous anastomoses than arteries and consequently collateral circulation is in most situations readily available. However, with large vessels such as an occlusion of a large vein like the inferior vena cava, the large tortuous and indeed varicose collateral veins over the abdomen are equally dramatic. In portal venous obstruction, the collateral circulation develops where there are anastomoses between the systemic and portal circulations (cardio-oesophageal junction, diaphragm, anal canal, retroperitoneum, umbilicus), and these venous collaterals become extremely dilated and varicose with a propensity for rupture (oesophageal varices, haemorrhoids). A similar phenomenon is common in the lower limb (varicose veins).

One of the most fascinating naturally occurring collateral circulations is the controversial system of vertebral veins, which Batson [78] divided into three intercommunicating divisions: first, the internal vertebral epidural venous network; the second or intermediate network consisting of veins within the bones of the vertebral column itself, and the third or outer division, the external vertebral venous plexus. These plexuses have communications with each other and also with testicular, prostatic, iliac and sacral veins and the inferior vena cava. There are also communications with the retroperitoneum, the renal vasculature, and the mammary, pulmonary, intercostal, clavicular and humeral veins, and the superior vena cava and intracranial sinuses. By simulating coughing or the Valsalva manoeuvre it is possible to show transfer of radio-opaque dye from the pelvic vessels to the vertebral system of veins, with dye entering the thoracic spine and intercostal veins. With injections into small mammary veins in a female cadaver, dye entered the head of the humerus, the clavicle, cervical vertebrae, skull, intracranial venous sinuses, the azygos vein and superior vena cava. Subsequent studies and reviews suggest that these vertebral plexuses of veins are a potential source of haematogenous spread of tumour cells or even infections under certain physiological conditions allowing retrograde flow [78–80].

1.10 Angiogenesis

All blood vessels develop initially from primitive undifferentiated mesenchyme, primarily mesodermal in origin although possibly ectodermal to some extent about the neural tube [81]. In embryos of higher animals, these vascular anlagen appear first about the body stalk and the wall of the yolk sac but intraembryonic vessels soon develop from the mesenchyme. According to Sabin [82,83] angioblasts divide and proliferate to form dense syncytial masses linked by delicate cytoplasmic processes to adjoining cell masses. Vacuolization was said to commence within these syncytial masses. By confluence and extension of vacuoles a lumen develops lined by peripheral angioblasts which become the endothelium. Some angioblasts separate off, multiply and differentiate into circulating blood cells within the lumen. These endothelial tubes contain a plasma-like fluid which Sabin thought was formed by angioblast disintegration. Ultrastructural studies have since revealed that angioblastic masses are not syncytial and it is unlikely that the lumen results from central liquefaction [84]. The proteinaceous fluid in the intercellular sinusoidal spaces may be secreted or accumulate by osmosis [85]. A vascular plexus soon develops, spreads and interconnects with other plexuses.

The primordial blood capillary plexus is the source from which all arteries, veins and capillaries are derived, constituent parts displaying considerable irregularity in size and form. Large arteries and vessels are usually laid down as a capillary plexus initially rather than as a single trunk-like form even when the vessel is apparently genetically predetermined [67]. Once an intensive primordial capillary plexus develops, further growth probably ensues by sprouting of capillary buds, as seen in the rabbit ear chamber. There is extensive development of primordial blood vessels before the heart induces circulation of the blood [82,83].

Differentiation of mesenchymal cells into angioblasts in early angiogenesis is presumably genetically determined. The early embryonic vascular pattern with its paired symmetrical vessels, intersegmental vessels and aortic arches is apparently also genetically determined. Tissue factors responsible for stimulating capillary invasion of tissues and the mechanism by which blood vessels serve such needs are uncertain. Local tissue factors can influence capillary proliferation throughout life. Some embryonic tissues are angiotactic probably due to similar angioblastic substances present in tumours of adults but it is unlikely that a single substance governs such growth. The underlying control mechanisms and cytokines are probably a complex, finely tuned system of inter-related pharmacokinetic agents.

The growth or development of the capillary network in any area seems to be secondary to the development of embryonic organs and tissues, functional needs determining vascular growth. The orderly growth of such organs is probably genetically determined with vascular supply a secondary event. Drainage and supply channels then develop from the most convenient source at the time of embryonic development, a sequence consistent with Shellshear's concept of functional constancy of arterial supply [86]. Subsequent shift in the position of an organ sometimes accounts for the distal origin of its supply in the adult anatomy (e.g. the aortic origin of the testicular arteries just distal to the origin of the renal arteries). By enlargement of some channels and coincidental dwindling of others, supply and drainage channels arise within each vascular bed. Some major arterial and venous channels can develop and exist for a time in the absence of a beating heart [9,87].

Involution of vessels is probably associated with a redistribution of endothelial cells among the walls of other vessels rather than by means of cell degeneration or atrophy [88]. Alternatively the vessels may not disappear but instead lose the prominent position they held in embryonic life and remain as part of the capillary bed having served temporary needs, paralleled by the elaboration of others. The vascular apparatus reacts continuously and adequately in a sensitive manner according to tissue requirements and is uninfluenced by the nature of its subsequent morphology [69]. The final topography of the vascular system owes much to the haemodynamic forces to which the primordial circulation is subjected. As such, it is automatic and inevitable though some variations may be fortuitous and secondary to changing environmental conditions. There is no certainty as to the stage when hereditary factors predominate or when haemodynamic factors take over.

Whilst haemodynamic factors probably determine which vessels of the capillary plexus become supply or drainage channels, the specific haemodynamic parameters responsible are uncertain. Augmented flow is associated with increased diameter. Venous drainage may have much in common with river morphology for the lower flow rates and pressure permit a more plexiform topography amongst the collecting veins. Thoma [89] formulated rules which he considered responsible for the growth of blood vessels including the metabolic rate. Thoma's histomechanical laws state:

1. The increase in size of the lumen of a vessel (or the increase or decrease in the surface of the vessel wall) depends on the rate of blood flow. (In practice, the surface ceases to grow when the blood current acquires a definitive rate; the vessel increases in size when this rate is exceeded, becomes smaller when the blood flow is slowed, and disappears when it is finally arrested.)
2. The growth in thickness of the vessel wall is dependent upon its tension. Further, the tension of the wall is dependent upon the diameter of the lumen of the vessel and the blood pressure.
3. Increase of blood pressure in the capillary areas leads to the formation of new capillaries.

Thoma believed the first law to be the most important and indicated that an interrelationship exists between the blood velocity and size of the vessel under physiological and pathological conditions. It presumes a specific velocity for each vessel whether artery or vein. However consistent this theory may be with current knowledge, the mechanism by which a vessel increases in girth with augmented flow is unknown. Clark [9] believed increase in size of the vessel was dependent more on volume flow and this seems plausible. The second law also appears to be in general accord with our knowledge of the vascular system. The third law being conjecture is as yet unproven. Clark [9] doubted its validity believing that capillary sprouts grew just as often from the venous end of the capillary bed as from the arterial end. It is more likely that capillary sprouting is dependent on biochemical factors including metabolites and tissue breakdown products rather than biophysical parameters. There is a need to test these histomechanical laws experimentally.

The effect of haemodynamics on the differentiation of vessels from small to large channels provides the possibility of considerable variation in topography and the exact position of a specific trunk, its branches and their area of supply. Functional adaptation is characteristic of the developing human vascular system, permitting modification of old paths and the development of new alternate pathways. Once a relatively definitive pattern is established in relation to the visceral anlagen, the enlarging vessels lose their transitory nature and progressively undergo differentiation of their walls in response to the augmented haemodynamic stresses associated with blood flow. However, even then their relative sizes may vary due to changing demands and the variable growth of parts of the body or organs.

According to Evans [67] delay in the acquisition of the arterial coats is to prevent limitation of the primitive endothelial channels in giving off new channels. However, the possibility is that the haemodynamic stresses on the vessels requiring reinforcement and mural differentiation may coincide fortuitously with the establishment of the definitive adult localization of skeletal and visceral anlagen which thereafter increase in size and functional activity without significant rearrangement of anatomical relationships.

Histological differentiation of blood vessel walls is said to commence initially about the aorta and extend peripherally in the fourth month when the embryo is 40 mm in length [89]. However, some periaortic mesenchymal condensation has been observed at 11 mm and some muscle and elastica at 35 mm [53] when definitive arterial topography may not be finalized. Differentiation of the wall develops from within outwards with the appearance of a fine internal elastic lamina and elongation and multiplication of medial muscle cells. Elastic fibrils appear in the media and an external elastic lamina forms to differentiate media from adventitia, the latter being the last to differentiate with large collagenous bundles becoming prominent in the seventh and eighth month. Vasa vasorum arise from the proximal ends of the aortic branches and supply the mesenchyme and eventually the outer media and adventitia of vessels requiring additional blood supply.

Very little is known of the mechanisms underlying the differentiation of the perivascular mesenchyme into the definitive connective tissues though haemodynamic stresses play a significant role. Differentiation of smooth muscle and elastica appears to be influenced by pulsatile blood pressure. An implanted tube subjected to pulsatile internal pressure becomes ensheathed by muscle-like cells but no elastic tissue forms [90]. In an acardiac parasitic twin the aortic wall resembled a peripheral muscular artery [89]. In another acardiac twin, presumably also parasitic, there were no elastic lamellae in the aortic media [91]. Other aspects of the architecture of the arterial tree are beyond our present knowledge, notably the relatively abrupt transition from the elastic-type aorta to the muscular type of its small branches and particularly the unique structure of cerebrospinal arteries.

There has been little interest in the differentiation of walls of veins apart from the valves [92] which are indispensable for venous return. In general the development of the vascular system is adequate for each stage of embryogenesis and currently it would appear that major defects are of non-vascular tissues to which the vasculature adapts to compensate rather than the reverse. Alleged persistence of undifferentiated portions of the primordial vasculature leading to the formation of cerebral (berry) aneurysms or of 'arteriovenous malformations', are unsubstantiated assumptions that have no place in modern scientific medicine [1,54].

1.11 Postnatal angiogenesis

Postnatal angiogenesis is essentially similar to that in the embryo after the establishment of a capillary plexus and in the absence of perivascular mesenchyme. The growth rate of the capillary network varies from 0.1 to 0.6 mm/day and with the temperature and environment to which the animals are exposed [93]. The differentiation of capillary channels into arterioles and venules occurs rapidly, but muscle cell origin is unknown. Speculation is that either they may extend peripherally from more proximal pre-existing vasculature or that they arise *in situ* from proliferation of some multi-potential or parent stem cell. Capillary proliferation is a characteristic of the vascular system throughout life during repair and organization together with regression and atrophy of some channels during resolution. This stage of devascularization is exemplified by progressive change from pink to white in scar tissue over three months. The development of a capillary network and its extension is seen most conveniently in the healing phase of a rabbit ear chamber. In practice arterial channels larger than arteries, such as those in a recanalized thrombus, do not differentiate but acquire the architecture normally observed during development and maturation in the young. They display degenerative changes with much intimal proliferation and poor elastic tissue production, doubtless due to their participation in collateral flow which is associated with accentuated vascular degeneration. Such changes may well affect superficial vessels in those parts of adult mammals exposed to different types of trauma, injury or pathological occlusion throughout life.

1.12 Circulatory changes during maturation

Changes in the circulation and blood occur at birth when placental circulation gives way to one of independent existence. When umbilical arteries and the ductus arteriosus close, the ascending aorta and arch enlarge and the respective sizes of the iliac arteries are modified in accordance with altered functional requirements. Even so they may still display distinct evidence of the role they played *in utero* [94]. These topographical alterations are regarded as adaptation on the part of the infant to the change in its environment, there being no evidence of any immediate secondary pathological consequence on the part of the vascular system. As the infant grows to maturity, arteries increase in length, calibre and wall thickness without significant change in mural architecture except for an increase in the number of lamellar units in the aorta. The relative calibre of many arteries changes in accordance with the functional requirements since there are disproportionate growth rates of some organs or parts thereof during physical maturation.

In the cerebral circulation, there is alteration in the comparative size and configuration of the circle of Willis postnatally because of the disproportionate enlargement of the cerebellum. Voluntary muscle exhibits an unduly large increase in proportion to body weight and therefore the topography of the vascular tree in respect to size and position of the branches also alters during maturation. This is well seen in the subclavian artery [72]. However, it does not follow that all concomitant changes in blood vessels during maturation are *a priori* manifestations of adaptation.

1.13 Arteriomegaly

Pronounced ectasia, noted in the cerebral arteries of patients with acromegaly and possibly analogous to splanchnomegaly, has been regarded as systemic since it also occurs in coronary arteries [95]. This 'arteriomegaly', as it has been called, can be associated with tortuosity and even kinking. Naturally it has been linked with pituitary growth hormone but not all acromegalics are affected. Hypertension is often present but this too can occur without arteriectasis [95]. Cerebral aneurysms have also been found in acromegalics [95]. The significance of the ectasia or 'arteriomegaly' is uncertain but many of the features suggest degenerative changes that could still be secondary to and aggravated by the accompanying hypertension. There is need for more data on the extent of vessel involvement in acromegaly, the effect of pituitary growth hormone on angiogenesis and blood vessels, their size compared to physiological requirements and the pathological changes.

1.14 Misuse of terminology

Loose usage or misuse of words should be avoided in science as it not only misrepresents but misleads and can impede scientific progress. The alleged medial defect of Forbus [52] is a case in point and this allegation of weakness of the medial raphe hindered progress and influenced thinking adversely for decades.

Arterialization is a macroscopic term suggesting that the vein is arterialized when its basic architecture is unaltered although its wall is thickened macroscopically. Likewise, venization of an artery is mural thinning macroscopically without architectural change to that of a vein. It is likely too that the use of these terms delayed thorough investigation of the vascular changes associated with arteriovenous shunts.

For some years adaptation and remodelling have been used in reference to changes in arteries and some clarification of the correct usage of these terms is in order. This is not merely a matter of semantics but of scientific exactitude which is essential to avoid misrepresentation that can mislead and beguile trusting and less discerning readers.

1.14.1 PHYSIOLOGICAL ADAPTATION AND REMODELLING

The term adaptation is used in many senses in medicine and biology. It is the process of adjustment of an individual or organism to altered environmental conditions. It is used in regard to sensory adaptation, social and behavioural adaptation and the augmented pigmentation and epidermal thickening in response to light. It may also occur by natural selection resulting in improved survival and reproductive success as the result of an evolutionary genetic change. By a process of behavioural or physiological changes the individual may enhance survival within the environment. It can involve an acquired biochemical adaptation to a specific dietary constituent or even some noxious agent. However, adaptation implies a beneficial physiological response to a new or altered environment or even functional activity.

A physiological response or reflex, such as vasodilatation due to increased demand for blood by the tissues, should not be designated as an adaptive response, even though adaptation is often used in reference to reflex optical changes to light and dark. Adaptation also is a physiological response and implies a change or alteration of the organ, tissue, or perhaps a functional biochemical response to a more prolonged alteration in the environment or new conditions to which the body is exposed. It is implicit that alterations that occur are advantageous, allowing the individual to cope better with environmental changes that would otherwise be detrimental. They do not include pathological changes or complications involving loss of integrity of the tissue or organ which may occur if insufficient time is allowed for the individual to respond appropriately, i.e. to adapt.

Some arteries increase in size and proportionately more than other vessels during growth and maturation and even beyond because of unequal growth rates of some organs or parts thereof. However, they enlarge by an increase in the lumen and wall thickness with proliferation of cellular elements and production of more elastin, collagen and interstitial matrix but without significant change in mural architecture, yet in most of the intima the endothelium is applied to the internal elastic lamina without discernible intervening tissue histologically. The vessels grow and no doubt the capillary bed enlarges as required by the growing and maturing animal but this is a slow insidious change allowing tissues time for the necessary alterations and strengthening of the wall. In this sense the vessels adapt to the growing functional demand of the tissues they serve.

The term 'adaptation' must not be used inappropriately without adequate justification. Every tissue response is not a manifestation of physiological adaptation, nor is the term appropriate for an inflammatory response to bacterial invasion or to repair damage in response to trauma, injury or some loss of tissue integrity even though these constitute biological reactions essential for survival of the species. Use of the term adaptation for a biological reaction to any disease process is incorrect usage and the dividing line between physiological adaptation and pathology depends on the criteria of beneficial versus detrimental or retrogressive change.

Recently it was alleged [96–98] that the radius of the artery proximal to an arteriovenous fistula, after a temporary increase in wall shear stress due to augmented flow, enlarges as an adaptive response until the wall shear stress is restored to the normal level of about 15 dynes/cm^2. Yet within two to five days after creation of the fistula, tears appear in the internal elastic lamina, sometimes with endothelial disruption and thrombosis, and become so extensive and numerous as to render the elastic remnants of relatively little functional value [99,100]. Underlying elastic laminae in the media may also tear, fragment and disappear as medial thinning and atrophy progress. It is easy to accept vasodilatation as a physiological response and natural growth of the blood vessel with new tissue formation to strengthen the wall in the longer term whilst maintaining normal architecture as adaptation, but this is not what happens. When the altered conditions are associated with progressive degenerative changes in the elastic tissue and muscle and loss of integrity of the vessel with tortuosity, aneurysm formation and atherosclerosis [77], adaptation is an inappropriate designation.

Moreover, the calculated mean shear stress may remain relatively constant for a while but it does not follow that the destructive changes to the mural architecture are physiological responses and it is unlikely that the mean shear stress, even if valid, is as important as the pulsatile changes in shear stress. It is unlikely also that the mean shear stress governs vascular calibre, intimal proliferation and other compensatory morphological alterations in the arterial wall. Furthermore, no consideration has been given to the simultaneous changes in the anastomosed vein [96;97] in which these concepts of adaptation would not be tenable. Initially there may be hypertrophy of the medial musculature, which can be regarded as physiological adaptation, but the loss of elastic tissue and development of a thick intima, irregular dilatation and atherosclerosis are pathological responses.

In a recent Special Report of the American Heart Association [47] intimal thickening in the neonate was labelled as adaptive and allegedly due to physiological change in pulse rate, blood pressure, arterial geometry, flow rate and resistance to flow in distal vascular segments. Since this intimal proliferation is universal and occurs in other animals, it might be considered to support the allegation. However, intimal thickening develops from 26 weeks *in utero* at specific sites about the arterial forks of cerebral arteries suggestive of haemodynamic localization [65], so it is unlikely that such proliferation can be regarded as a manifestation of adaptation, since even at birth there is evidence of mural thinning, loss or gaps in the internal elastic lamina which was intact at an earlier age, and evidence of vesiculogranular degeneration of smooth muscle cells with progressive accumulation of matrix vesicles [101]. Such degenerative changes are inconsistent with a physiological adaptive response and the fibromusculoelastic intimal thickening is widely acknowledged as an early stage of atherosclerosis with which it merges without any sharp line of demarcation and with the same topographical distribution.

Meyer *et al.* [94] also attributed many of the intimal changes prior to birth and in postnatal life to haemodynamic stress but nevertheless regarded them as physiological responses. However, when the internal elastic lamina forms *in utero* only to be torn, fragmented or disappear (such being acknowledged characteristics of degenerative changes [102]), the media to become thinned [103] and the muscle cells to undergo vesiculogranular disintegration, these changes must be regarded as degenerative and it is difficult to accept the reparative intimal thickening and elastic tissue proliferation that follow as manifestations of physiological adaptation. Blood vessels enlarge if the functional need increases and this is well seen during growth and maturation, but to assume that stresses exceeding some marginal level or continued usage have no effect on the blood vessel wall is probably having excessive faith in the absolute perfection of Nature's handiwork.

Remodelling also implies an adaptive response and is observed during physical maturation or some reproductive function, such as relative enlargement or diminution of calibre of an artery due to altered functional demand or the modifications of the female body and genital tract due to the reproductive cycle. However, remodelling is also used in reference to substantial changes in the blood vessel wall that are essentially pathological or manifestations of atherosclerosis.

There is retention of a relatively circular lumen in the presence of intimal thickening and atherosclerosis whether these are eccentrically or unevenly circumferentially located when the vessel is fixed under pressure. An eccentric thickening is associated with medial thinning and the wall may bulge somewhat externally rather than encroach on the circular lumen. This medial thinning has in the past been regarded as a type of pressure atrophy. Thoma [17] considered intimal proliferation to be compensatory in nature on account of angiomalacia or medial weakness with dilatation of the lumen. This in turn slowed the blood and allowed intimal thickening to return the lumen to a relatively constant diameter and profile. In recent years this phenomenon has been attributed to the recognized need of the blood vessel to maintain a constant theoretical optimal shear stress as calculated post mortem, whereby slowing of the flow associated with dilatation would result in adaptive intimal proliferation [96] or remodelling. These interpretations remain conjectural, not explaining all the available data and overlooking the fact that shear stress is pulsatile, variable in location and direction, can vary during the pulse cycle and can even be reversed. In longitudinal section of pressure-fixed vessels or in angiograms, there is often some distortion of the lumen, and 'nipping' or stenosis at the orifices of aortic branches is common [104]. This is not adaptation and progressive diminution in the area ratio of the aortic bifurcation is not consistent with this concept.

It is recognized that bone adapts to the applied stresses with some bone remodelling following healing with angulation at a fracture site and stress concentration. Similar remodelling may occur to some extent in the case of intimal tears with organization of thrombus and intimal proliferation filling in regions about the base of an intimal flap whilst leaving a residual irregularity of the intimal surface. Though knowledge of various vasoactive substances or mediators produced by endothelium and smooth muscle cells [105] has increased, how these interact and the complex pharmacological control mechanisms are obscure, but the mural cells must respond to altered local conditions and stresses which undoubtedly play a major role in determining the consistent and specific localization of intimal thickenings. Retrogressive changes appear to be superimposed when the stresses become excessive, they are applied too rapidly, there is a combination of the two, or there is a cumulative effect of chronic low-grade repetitive stresses on the connective tissues. If the tissue wall is not architecturally designed to withstand the stresses under artificial (experimental or therapeutic) conditions, then this would augment or accelerate the retrograde changes. There appear to be limits to adaptation, for prolonged exposure may eventually result in disadvantageous responses or pathological change.

In studies of stress deprivation of bones and ligaments [106], there is a substantial reduction in failure load and modulus of elasticity. The effect of exercise experimentally has resulted in improved structural properties of bone due to cortical hypertrophy rather than qualitative improvement but such responses do not necessarily indicate the long-term functional state or mechanical durability due to repetitive loading. Whether the changes are applicable to blood vessels is uncertain but they would appear to support the contention that the vessel wall responds within reasonable limits to physiological stress.

The term adaptation is often used in an evolutionary sense to indicate that the mural architecture is so very well designed in order to meet the functional and mechanical requirements of the tissue most efficiently rather than as a physiological response to an altered physiological or even a pathological state, but the term essentially means a physiological response of benefit to the individual and not a compensatory repair process in response to a destructive force or mechanical failure of the vessel wall.

References

1. Stehbens, W.E. (1979) *Hemodynamics and the Blood Vessel Wall*, C.C. Thomas, Springfield.
2. Bayliss, L.E. (1960) *Principles of General Physiology*, vol. 2, Longmans, London, p. 578.
3. Palmer, J.F. (1835) *The Works of John Hunter, F.R.S.*, vol. 3, Longman, Rees, Orme, Brown, Green and Longman, London.
4. Woollard, H.H. and Harpman, J.A. (1937) The relation between size of the artery and the capillary bed in the embryo. *J. Anat.*, 72, 18–22.
5. Zamir, M., Wrigley, S.M. and Langille, B.L. (1983) Arterial bifurcations in the cardiovascular system of a rat. *J. Gen. Physiol.*, 81, 325–35.
6. Roux, W. (1879) Ueber die Bedeutung der Ablenkung des Arterienstammes bei der Astabgabe. *Zeitschr. Naturwiss.*, 13, 321–37.
7. Horsfield, K. and Cumming, G. (1967) Angles of branching and diameters of branches in the human bronchial tree. *Bull. Math. Biophys.*, 29, 245–59.
8. Thompson, D.W. (1942) *On Growth and Form*, Cambridge University Press, Cambridge, pp. 948–57.
9. Clark, E.R. (1918) Studies on the growth of blood vessels in the tail of the frog larvae, by observation and experiment on the living animal. *Am. J. Anat.*, 23, 37–88.
10. Zamir, M. and Brown, N. (1983) Internal geometry of arterial bifurcations. *J. Biomechanics*, 16, 857–63.
11. Murray, C.D. (1925–1926) The physiological principle of minimum work applied to the angle of branching at arteries. *J. Gen. Physiol.*, 9, 835–41.
12. Turner, R.S. (1957) A comparison of theoretical with observed angles between the vertebral arteries at their junction to form the basilar. *Anat. Rec.*, 129, 243–53.
13. Stopford, J.S.B. (1915) The arteries of the pons and medulla oblongata. *J. Anat. Physiol.*, 50, 131–64.
14. Stehbens, W.E. and Stehbens, G.R. (1985) Flow in glass models simulating vascular junctions under steady flow conditions. *Quart. J. Exp. Physiol.*, 70, 515–26.
15. Zamir, M. and Brown, N. (1982) Arterial branching in various parts of the cardiovascular system. *Am. J. Anat.*, 163, 295–307.
16. Hutchins, G.M., Miner, M.M. and Boitnott, J.K. (1976) Vessel caliber and branch-angle of human coronary artery branch-points. *Circ. Res.*, 38, 572–6.
17. Thoma, R. (1896) *Text-Book of General Pathology* (transl. by A. Bruce), vol. 1, Adam and Charles Black, London.
18. Wiggers, C.J. (1949) *Physiology in Health and Disease*, 5th edn, Lea and Febiger, Philadelphia.
19. Willis, G.C. (1954) Localizing factors in atherosclerosis. *Canad. Med. Ass. J.*, 70, 1–8.
20. Stehbens, W.E. (1974) Changes in the cross-sectional area of the arterial fork. *Angiology*, 25, 561–75.
21. Attinger, E.O. (1963) Pressure transmission in pulmonary arteries related to frequency and geometry. *Circ. Res.*, 12, 623–41.
22. Rashevsky, N. (1955) Organic form as determined by function. *Ann. N.Y. Acad. Sci.*, 63, 442–53.
23. Rashevsky, N. (1960) *Mathematical Biophysics. Physico-mathematical Foundations of Biology*, vol. 2, 3rd edn, Dover Publications, New York, pp. 292–305.
24. Hamilton, W.F. (1949) Regulation of arterial pressure, in *A Textbook of Physiology*, (ed. J.F. Fulton), Saunders, Philadelphia, pp. 750–5.

25. Womersley, J.R. (1958) Oscillatory flow in arteries. II. The reflection of the pulse wave at junctions and rigid inserts in the arterial system. *Phys. Med. Biol.*, **2**, 313–23.
26. Gosling, R.G., Newman, D.L., Bowden, N.L.R. and Twinn, K.W. (1971) The area ratio of normal aortic junctions. Aortic configuration and pulse wave reflection. *Br. J. Radiol.*, **44**, 850–3.
27. Newman, D.L., Gosling, R.G. and Bowden, N.L.R. (1971) Changes in aortic distensibility and area ratio with the development of atherosclerosis. *Atherosclerosis*, **14**, 231–40.
28. Beales, J.S.M. and Steiner, R.E. (1972) Radiological assessment of arterial branching coefficients. *Cardiovasc. Res.*, **6**, 181–6.
29. Arnot, R.S. and Louw, J.H. (1973) The anatomy of the posterior wall of the abdominal aorta. Its significance with regard to hypoplasia of the distal aorta. *S. Afr. Med. J.*, **47**, 899–902.
30. Dinnar V. (1981) *Cardiovascular Fluid Dynamics*, CRC Press Inc., Boca Raton, Florida, pp. 98–9.
31. Lallemand, R.C., Brown, K.G.E. and Boulter, P.S. (1972) Vessel dimensions in premature atheromatous disease of aortic bifurcation. *Br. Med. J.*, **2**, 255–7.
32. Hardy-Stashin, J., Meyer, W.W. and Kaufman, S.L. (1980) Branching coefficient (area ratio) of the human aortic bifurcation determined in distended specimens. *Atherosclerosis*, **37**, 388–402.
33. Papageorgiou, G.L., Jones, B.N., Redding, V.J. and Hudson, N. (1990) The area ratio of normal arterial junctions and its implications in pulse wave reflections. *Cardiovasc. Res.*, **24**, 478–84.
34. Caro, C.G., Fitzgerald, J.M. and Schroter, R.C. (1971) Atheroma and arterial wall shear. Observation, correlation and proposal of a shear dependent mass transfer mechanism for atherogenesis. *Proc. Roy. Soc. London (Biol)*, **117**, 109–59.
35. Walburn, F.J., Blick, E.F. and Stein, P.D. (1979) Effect of the branch-to-trunk area ratio on the transition to turbulent flow: implications in the cardiovascular system. *Biorheology*, **16**, 411–17.
36. Lighthill, M.J. (1972) Physiological fluid dynamics: a survey. *J. Fluid Mech.*, **52**, 475–97.
37. Rushmer, R.F. and Morgan, C. (1968) Meaning of murmurs. *Am. J. Cardiol.*, **21**, 722–30.
38. McDonald, D.A. (1957) Murmurs in relation to turbulence and eddy formation in the circulation. *Circulation*, **16**, 278.
39. Lancer, S.R., Gutierrez, L.F. and Pillay, V.K.G. (1975) Orbital bruits in patients on maintenance haemodialysis. *Br. Med. J.*, **2**, 481.
40. Wadia, N.H. and Monckton, G. (1957) Intracranial bruits in health and disease. *Brain*, **80**, 492–509.
41. Hammond, J.H. and Eisinger, R.P. (1962) Carotid bruits in 1000 normal subjects. *Arch. Int. Med.*, **109**, 563–5.
42. Rennie, L., Ejrup, B. and McDowell, F. (1964) Arterial bruits in cerebrovascular disease. *Neurology*, **14**, 751–6.
43. Ferguson, G.G. (1972) Physical factors in the initiation, growth, and rupture of human intracranial saccular aneurysms. *J. Neurosurg.*, **37**, 666–77.
44. Olinger, C.P. and Wasserman, J.F. (1977) Electronic stethoscope for detection of cerebral aneurysm, vasospasm and arterial disease. *Surg. Neurol.*, **8**, 298–313.
45. Stehbens, W.E. (1975) Flow in glass models of arterial bifurcations and berry aneurysms at low Reynolds numbers. *Quart. J. Exp. Physiol.*, **60**, 181–92.
46. Gray, H. (1858) *Anatomy. Descriptive and Surgical*, 1st edn, (facsimile), J.W. Parke & Son, Leicester, p. 308.
47. Stary, H.C., Blankenhorn, D.H., Chandler, A.B. *et al.* (1992) A definition of the intima of human arteries and of its atherosclerosis-prone regions. *Arteriosclerosis Thrombosis*, **12**, 120–34.
48. Wolinsky, H. and Glagov, S. (1967) A lamellar unit of aortic medial structure and function in mammals. *Circ. Res.*, **20**, 99–111.
49. Clark, J.M. and Glagov, S. (1985) Transmural organization of the arterial media. The lamellar unit revisited. *Arteriosclerosis*, **5**, 19–34.
50. Yamazoe, N., Hashimoto, N., Kikuchi, H. *et al.* (1990) Study of the elastic skeleton of intracranial arteries in animal and human vessels by scanning electron microscopy. *Stroke*, **21**, 765–70.
51. Berry, C.L., Germain, J. and Lovell, P. (1974) Comparison of aortic lamellar unit structure in birds and mammals. *Atherosclerosis*, **19**, 47–59.
52. Forbus, W.D. (1930) On the origin of miliary aneurysms of the superficial cerebral arteries. *Bull. Johns Hopkins Hosp.*, **47**, 239–84.
53. Stehbens, W.E. (1959) Medial defects of the cerebral arteries of man. *J. Pathol. Bacteriol.*, **78**, 179–85.
54. Stehbens, W.E. (1972) *Pathology of Cerebral Blood Vessels*, C.V. Mosby, St Louis.
55. Bremer, J.L. (1943) Congenital aneurysms of the cerebral arteries. *Arch. Pathol.*, **35**, 819–31.
56. Du Boulay, G.H. (1965) Some observations on the natural history of intracranial aneurysms. *Br. J. Radiol.*, **38**, 721–57.
57. Du Boulay, G.H. (1967) The natural history of intracranial aneurysms. *Am. Heart J.*, **73**, 723–9.
58. Stehbens, W.E. (1981) Aetiology of cerebral aneurysms. *Lancet*, **2**, 524–5.
59. Edwards, E.A. (1951) Clinical anatomy of lesser variations of the inferior vena cava: and a proposal for classifying the anomalies of this vessel. *Angiology*, **2**, 85–99.
60. Stehbens, W.E. (1967) Observations on the microcirculation in the rabbit ear chamber. *Quart. J. Exp. Physiol.*, **52**, 150–6.
61. Mescon, H., Hurley, H.J. and Moretti, G. (1956) The anatomy and histochemistry of the arteriovenous anastomosis in human digital skin. *J. Invest. Dermatol.*, **27**, 133–45.
62. Harris, P. and Heath, D. (1962) *The Human Pulmonary Circulation*, Livingstone, Edinburgh.
63. Brenner, O. (1935) Pathology of the vessels of the pulmonary circulation. *Arch. Int. Med.*, **56**, 211–37.
64. Heath, D., Wood, E.H., Du Shane, J.W. and Edwards, J.E. (1959) The structure of the pulmonary trunk at different ages and in cases of pulmonary hypertension and pulmonary stenosis. *J. Pathol. Bacteriol.*, **77**, 443–56.
65. Stehbens, W.E. (1960) Focal intimal proliferation in the cerebral arteries. *Am. J. Pathol.*, **36**, 289–301.
66. Abbie, A.A. (1934) The morphology of the forebrain arteries, with especial reference to the evolution of the basal ganglia. *J. Anat.*, **68**, 433–70.
67. Evans, H.M. (1912) The development of the vascular system, in *Manual of Human Embryology*, vol. 2, (eds F. Keibel and F.P. Mall), Lippincott, Philadelphia, pp. 570–709.
68. Levenson, G.E. and Nelsen, O.E. (1967) Experimentally induced variations in vitelline artery development and circulatory pattern in the early chick embryo. *J. Morphol.*, **123**, 313–27.
69. Streeter, G.L. (1918) The developmental alterations in the vascular system of the brain of the human embryo. *Contrib. Embryol. Carneg. Inst.*, **24**, 5–38.
70. Stehbens, W.E. (1963) Aneurysms and anatomical variation of cerebral arteries. *Arch. Pathol.*, **75**, 45–64.
71. Schlesinger, M.J. (1940) Relation of anatomic pattern to pathologic conditions of the coronary arteries. *Arch. Pathol.*, **30**, 403–15.
72. Bean, R.B. (1905) A composite study of the subclavian artery in man. *Am. J. Anat.*, **4**, 303–8.
73. Milloy, F.J., Anson, B.J. and Cauldwell, E.W. (1962) Variations in the inferior vena caval veins and in the renal and lumbar communications. *Surg. Gynec. Obst.*, **115**, 131–42.
74. Davis, R.A., Milloy, F.J. and Anson, B.J. (1958) Lumbar, renal, and associated parietal and visceral veins based upon a study of 100 specimens. *Surg. Gynec. Obstet.*, **107**, 1–22.
75. Hazama, F. and Hashimoto, N. (1987) An animal model of cerebral aneurysms. *Neuropath. Appl. Neurobiol.*, **13**, 77–90.
76. Stehbens, W.E. (1990) The lipid hypothesis and the role of hemodynamics in atherogenesis. *Progr. Cardiovasc. Dis.*, **33**, 119–36.
77. Stehbens, W.E. (1992) Experimental induction of atherosclerosis associated with femoral arteriovenous fistulae in rabbits on a stock diet. *Atherosclerosis*, **95**, 127–35.
78. Batson, O.V. (1957) The vertebral vein system. *Am. J. Roentgenol.*, **78**, 195–212.
79. Batson, O.V. (1942) The role of the vertebral veins in metastatic processes. *Ann. Int. Med.*, **16**, 38–45.
80. Herlihy, W.F. (1947) Revision of the venous system; the role of the vertebral veins. *Med. J. Aust.*, **1**, 661–72.
81. Harvey, S.C. and Burr, H.S. (1926) The development of the meninges. *Arch. Neurol. Psychiat.*, **15**, 545–67.
82. Sabin, F.R. (1917) Origin and development of the primitive vessels of the chick and the pig. *Contrib. Embryol. Carneg. Inst.*, **6**, 61–124.
83. Sabin, F.R. (1917) Preliminary note on the differentiation of angioblasts and the method by which they produce blood vessels, blood-plasma and red blood-cells as seen in the living chick. *Anat. Rec.*, **13**, 199–204.
84. Gonzales-Cruzzi, F. (1971) Vasculogenesis in the chick embryo. An ultrastructural study. *Am. J. Anat.*, **130**, 441–60.
85. Haynes, R.H. and Rodbard, S. (1962) Arterial and arteriolar systems: biophysical principles and physiology, in *Blood Vessels and Lymphatics*, (ed. D.J. Abramson), Academic Press, New York, pp. 26–61.
86. Shellshear, J.L. (1930) The arterial supply of the cerebral cortex in the chimpanzee (*Anthropopithecus troglodytes*). *J. Anat.*, **65**, 45–87.
87. Knower, H.M. (1907) Effects of early removal of the heart and arrest of the circulation on the development of frog embryos. *Anat. Rec.*, **1**, 161–5.
88. Congdon, E.D. (1922) Transformation of the aortic arch system during the development of the human embryo. *Contrib. Embryol. Carneg. Inst.*, **14**, 47–110.
89. Arey, L.B. (1963) The development of peripheral blood vessels, in *The Peripheral Blood Vessels*, (eds J.L. Orbison and D.E. Smith), Williams and Wilkins, Baltimore, pp. 1–16.
90. Glagov, S., Rowley, D.A. and Wolinsky, H. (1968) Connective tissue layers resembling arterial media formed around implanted pulsating tubes. *Am. J. Pathol.*, **52**, 25a (abstract).
91. Bloch, E.H. and McCuskey, R.S. (1973) The cardiovascular system, in *Histology*, 3rd edn, (eds R.O. Greep and L. Weiss), McGraw-Hill, New York, pp. 315–37.
92. Kampmeier, O.F. and Birch, C.LaF. (1926–1927) The origin and devel-

opment of the venous valves, with particular reference to the saphenous district. *Am. J. Anat.*, **38**, 451–99.
93. Florey, H.W. (1958) *General Pathology*, 2nd edn, Lloyd-Luke, London, pp. 378–409.
94. Meyer, W.W., Walsh, S.Z. and Lind, J. (1980) Functional morphology of human arteries during fetal and postnatal development, in *Structure and Function of the Circulation*, vol. 1, (eds C.J. Schwartz, N.T. Werthessen and S. Wolf), Plenum Press, New York, pp. 95–379.
95. Weir, B. (1992) Pituitary tumors and aneuryms: case report and review of the literature. *Neurosurgery*, **30**, 585–91.
96. Zarins, C.K., Zatina, M.A., Giddens, D.P. *et al.* (1987) Shear stress regulation of artery lumen diameter in experimental atherogenesis. *J. Vasc. Surg.*, **5**, 413–20.
97. Glagov, S., Vito, R., Giddens, D.P. and Zarins, C.K. (1992) Microarchitecture and composition of artery walls: relationship to location, diameter and the distribution of mechanical stress. *J. Hypertension*, **10**, S101–4.
98. Kamiya, A. and Togawa, T. (1980) Adaptive regulation of wall shear stress to flow change in the canine carotid artery. *Am. J. Physiol.*, **239**, H14–21.
99. Greenhill, N.S. and Stehbens, W.E. (1983) Scanning electron-microscopic study of experimentally-induced intimal tears in rabbit arteries. *Atherosclerosis*, **49**, 119–26.
100. Greenhill, N.S. and Stehbens, W.E. (1987) Scanning electron microscopic study of the afferent arteries of experimental femoral arteriovenous fistulae in rabbits. *Pathology*, **19**, 22–7.
101. Stehbens, W.E. (1975) Cerebral atherosclerosis. Intimal proliferation and atherosclerosis in the cerebral arteries. *Arch. Pathol.*, **99**, 582–91.
102. Harvey, W.H. (1906) Studies upon the influence of tension in the degeneration of elastic fibres of buried aortae. *J. Exp. Med.*, **8**, 388–9.
103. Levene, C.I. (1956) The pathogenesis of atheroma of the coronary arteries. *J. Pathol. Bacteriol.*, **72**, 83–86.
104. Cluroe, A.D., Fitzjohn, T.P. and Stehbens, W.E. (1992) Combined pathological and radiological study of the effect of atherosclerosis on the ostia of segmental branches of the abdominal aorta. *Pathology*, **24**, 140–5.
105. Gibbons, G.H. and Dzan, V.J. (1990) Endothelial function in vascular remodelling, in *The Endothelium: An Introduction to Current Research*, (ed. J.B. Warren), Wiley-Liss, New York, pp. 81–93.
106. Akeson, W.H., Garfin, S., Amiel, D. and Woo, S.L.-Y. (1989) Para-articular connective tissue in osteoarthritis. *Seminars Arthr. Rheum.*, **18**, 41–50.
107. Stehbens, W.E. (1981) Arterial structure at branches and bifurcations with reference to physiological and pathological processes, including aneurysm formation, in *Structure and Function of the Circulation*, (eds C.J. Schwartz, N.T. Werthessen and S. Wolf), Plenum Publ. Co., New York, pp. 667–93.
108. Stehbens, W.E. (1963) The renal artery in normal and cholesterol-free rabbits. *Am. J. Pathol.*, **43**, 969–85.
109. Stehbens, W.E. (1983) Etiology and pathogenesis of intracranial berry aneurysms, in *Intracranial Aneurysms: A Text and Atlas*, (ed. J.L. Fox), Springer-Verlag, New York, pp. 358–95.

2 CONGENITAL ANOMALIES OF BLOOD VESSELS AND THEIR COMPLICATIONS

Jesse E. Edwards
and Jack L. Titus

In a consideration of anomalies of blood vessels, it is appropriate to divide both the arteries and veins into systemic and pulmonary types. Congenital anomalies of the arteries will be presented in three major sections. The first concerns the subject of connections between the aorta and the pulmonary arterial system, while the two following sections will consider separately intrinsic anomalies of the systemic arteries and of the pulmonary arteries. The final two sections discuss the systemic and pulmonary veins.

2.1 Communication between aorta and pulmonary arterial system

Communication between the aorta and pulmonary arterial system may take one of several forms, including patent ductus arteriosus, aortopulmonary window (aortopulmonary septal defect), persistent truncus arteriosus and origin of pulmonary arterial supply from aorta.

2.1.1 PATENT DUCTUS ARTERIOSUS

The ductus arteriosus extends between the origin of the left pulmonary artery, proximally, to the underside of the aorta at the junction of the aortic arch and descending aorta, distally.

It is probable that this structure normally closes shortly after birth through vasospasm. In this state, the vessel, upon dissection, is patent. It is commonly accepted that anatomic patency of the ductus, after one month after birth, is an abnormality [1].

Functionally, patent ductus is somewhat comparable to ventricular septal defect in that there are the obstructive and non-obstructive types. The obstructive or classical patent ductus is associated with a differential pressure between the aorta and pulmonary arterial system and is comparable to a small ventricular septal defect. The non-obstructive patent ductus arteriosus often is called the wide type of ductus arteriosus and is comparable to the large, non-obstructive ventricular septal defect.

In classical patent ductus arteriosus and in the wide patent ductus, the shunt initially is left-to-right and continuous. In classical ductus arteriosus, a differential in pressure is maintained between the aorta and pulmonary arterial system (Figure 2.1(a)). In this condition, as with small ventricular septal defect, the stream of flow through the ductus arteriosus has a jet-like quality. At sites of impact of the jet, infected pulmonary endarteritis with the chance of aneurysm formation may occur.

In wide patent ductus arteriosus (Figure 2.1(b)), pulmonary hypertension is associated with changes in the pulmonary arterial bed, as in large ventricular septal defect. Left ventricular failure may occur in infancy or childhood. If survival occurs, the ultimate appearance of significantly obstructive pulmonary vascular disease may be associated with a right-to-left shunt through the ductus arteriosus [2,3] (Figure 2.1(c)). Since the flow of desaturated blood tends to flow into the descending aorta ('reversing ductus'), the oxygen saturation of blood in the lower part of the body is lower than that in the upper [4]. Significant changes of this type may be apparent as differential cyanosis in which the toes are blue, while the fingers are not.

Aneurysms of a pulmonary artery may complicate patent ductus arteriosus. Among these are the mycotic type from infection and the dissecting type from the pulmonary hypertension [5].

2.1.2 AORTOPULMONARY SEPTAL DEFECT

Aortopulmonary septal defect, or AP window, is characterized as a wide opening between the ascending aorta and pulmonary trunk. The two semilunar valves

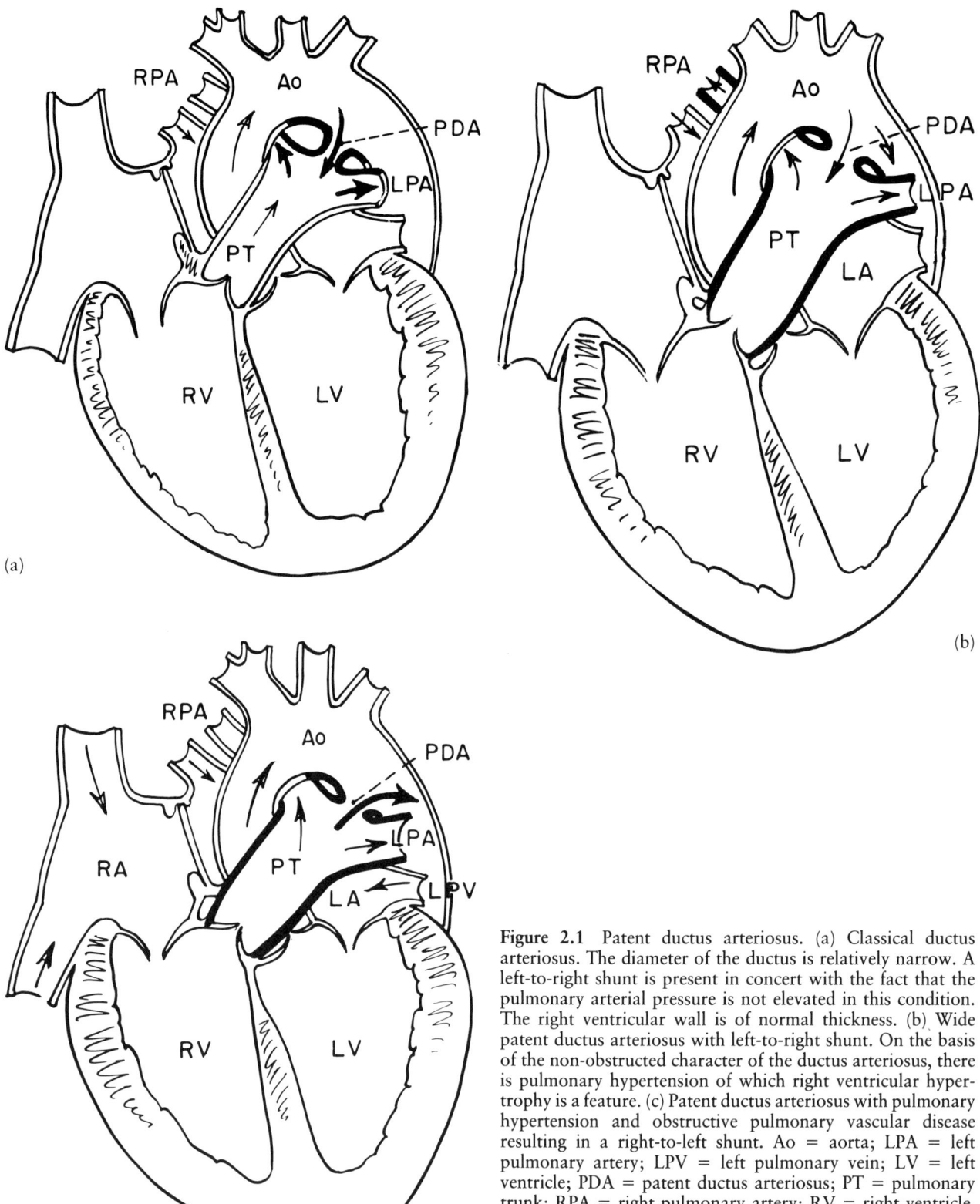

Figure 2.1 Patent ductus arteriosus. (a) Classical ductus arteriosus. The diameter of the ductus is relatively narrow. A left-to-right shunt is present in concert with the fact that the pulmonary arterial pressure is not elevated in this condition. The right ventricular wall is of normal thickness. (b) Wide patent ductus arteriosus with left-to-right shunt. On the basis of the non-obstructed character of the ductus arteriosus, there is pulmonary hypertension of which right ventricular hypertrophy is a feature. (c) Patent ductus arteriosus with pulmonary hypertension and obstructive pulmonary vascular disease resulting in a right-to-left shunt. Ao = aorta; LPA = left pulmonary artery; LPV = left pulmonary vein; LV = left ventricle; PDA = patent ductus arteriosus; PT = pulmonary trunk; RPA = right pulmonary artery; RV = right ventricle. (Reproduced with permission from Edwards and Edwards [133].)

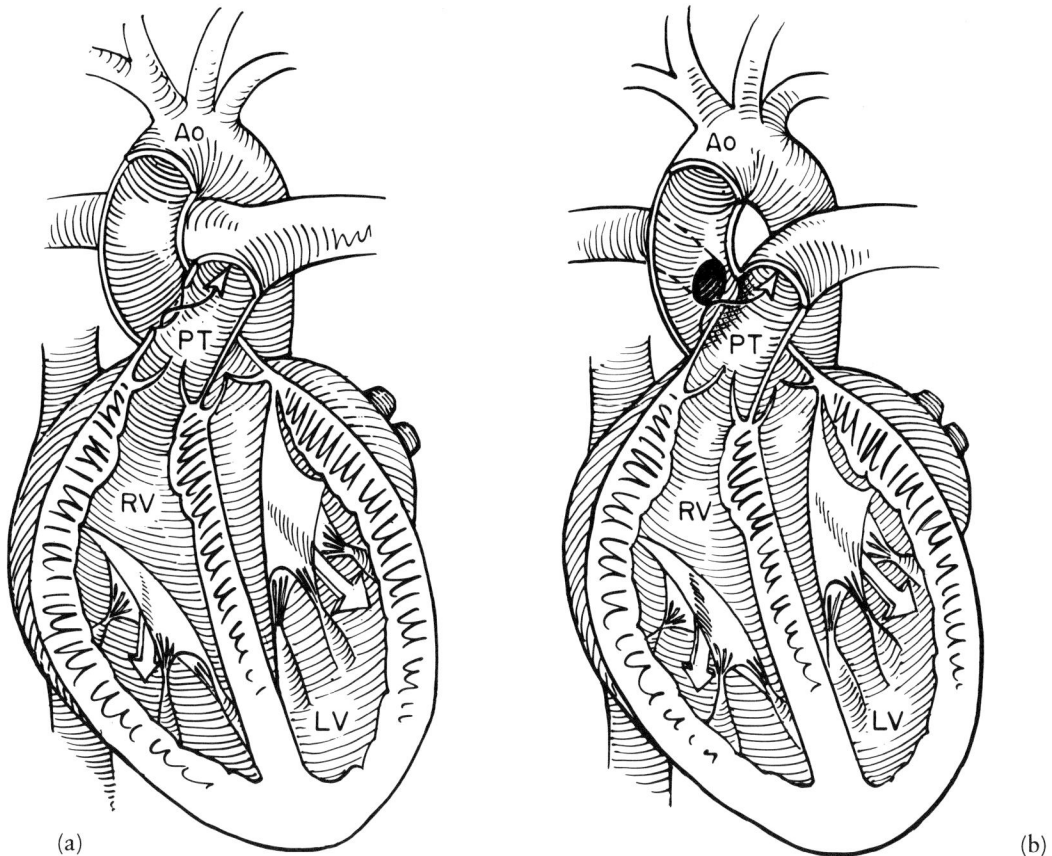

Figure 2.2 Aortopulmonary defect. (a) Proximal type of defect in which the defect lies between the left side of the ascending aorta and the right side of the pulmonary trunk. (b) Distal defect. The defect lies between the left posterolateral wall of the ascending aorta and the junction of the right pulmonary artery from the pulmonary trunk. Ao = aorta; LV = left ventricle; PT = pulmonary trunk; RV = right ventricle.

are present, and the relationship between the great arteries is normal (Figure 2.2). Usually, the defect is of sufficient width to constitute an unobstructed opening between the great arteries leading to hemodynamics and secondary changes comparable to those of wide patent ductus arteriosus [6]. Mori and associates [7] proposed an anatomic classification of aortopulmonary septal defect as follows:

- *Type I ('proximal defect')*: In this condition, the defect lies between the left side of the ascending aorta and the right side of the pulmonary trunk (Figure 2.2(a)).
- *Type II ('distal defect')*: The defect lies between the left posterolateral wall of the ascending aorta and the junction of the right pulmonary artery with the pulmonary trunk (Figure 2.2(b)).
- *Type III ('total defect')*: The defect involves the entire length of the pulmonary trunk from immediately above the semilunar valve to the level of its bifurcation near the proximal portion of the right pulmonary artery.

Aortopulmonary window commonly occurs without associated anomalies (75% as observed by Neufeld and associates [6]). Among the uncommonly present anomalies associated with aortopulmonary window is patent ductus arteriosus. Less commonly, anomalous coronary arterial origin, tetralogy of Fallot [8] and ventricular septal defect [9] are associated. In contrast to the findings of Neufeld and co-workers [6], Kutscher and van Mierop [10] showed that approximately one half of the cases of aortopulmonary window were associated with another cardiovascular anomaly, such as interrupted aortic arch, Type I, or preductal coarctation.

2.1.3 PERSISTENT TRUNCUS ARTERIOSUS

Persistent truncus arteriosus is characterized by one arterial vessel arising from the ventricular base. The vessel is equipped with a semilunar valve and gives rise to the coronary arteries. Above this, the pulmonary arterial supply arises from the single artery beyond which the vessel continues as the ascending aorta. A

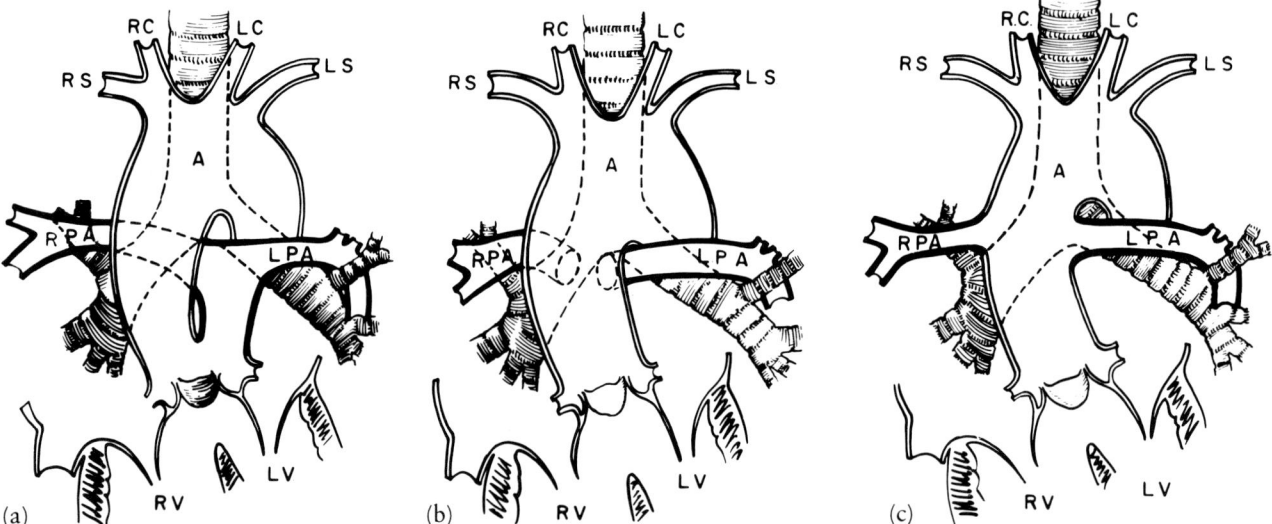

Figure 2.3 Persistent truncus arteriosus of various types. (a) Type I. (b) Type II. (c) Type III. A = aorta; LC = left carotid artery; LS = left subclavian artery; LPA = left pulmonary artery; LV = left ventricle; RC = right carotid artery; RS = right subclavian artery; RPA = right pulmonary artery; RV = right ventricle. (Reproduced with permission from Edwards and McGoon [134].)

ventricular septal defect is present at the base of the heart. In 1949, Collett and Edwards [11] proposed an anatomic classification of persistent truncus arteriosus into four types. These are defined as follows:

- *Type I*: The truncus is partially subdivided by an incomplete septum, yielding a pulmonary trunk, usually of restricted length, and ascending aorta. The pulmonary trunk then divides into left and right pulmonary arteries (Figure 2.3(a)).
- *Type II*: Persistent truncus arteriosus type II is the most common type. It is characterized by independent origins of the right and left pulmonary arteries from the posterior wall of the truncus arteriosus (Figure 2.3(b)).
- *Type III*: This is the least common of the first three types of truncus arteriosus. It is characterized by origin of each pulmonary artery from the homolateral side of the truncus (Figure 2.3(c)).
- *Type IV*: In the review of Collett and Edwards [11], reported cases were identified in which a single artery arose from the base of the heart. No pulmonary arteries arose from this vessel which then continued as the aorta. The pulmonary arterial supply came from branches (bronchial arteries) arising from the descending aorta.

Subsequently, Sotomora and Edwards in 1978 [12] found that in cases essentially of the Type IV truncus, the pulmonary arteries usually are identifiable at the pulmonary hili. For this reason and other considerations, Type IV truncus generally is not recognized today.

Usually, regardless of type, the truncus arteriosus arises above a ventricular septal defect, straddling the ventricular septum. Origin of the truncus from the right ventricle, either predominantly or entirely, occurs in up to 80% of the cases [13–15]. The latter situation is, however, rare.

The semilunar valve of the truncus arteriosus may have one, two, three or four cusps. In the study of Butto and associates [15], the per cent of cusps in the truncus valve among 53 specimens was one cusp in 4%, two cusps in 32%, three cusps in 49% and four cusps in 15%. It is to be emphasized that a tricuspid semilunar truncal valve is the most common type, occurring in about half of the cases studied. The basic structural form or secondary changes in the truncal valve may be responsible either for stenosis or for insufficiency, the latter process being more common than the former [16,17].

Variations in coronary arterial origin are commonly observed in persistent truncus arteriosus. Anderson, McGoon and Lie [18] studied the coronary arterial patterns in 34 specimens of truncus arteriosus. When three truncal sinuses were present, these authors considered the sinuses to be anterior left, anterior right and posterior. In almost half of the cases, the left coronary artery arose from the posterior sinus and the right artery from the right anterior right sinus. In 13% of cases, the right artery arose from the posterior sinus and the left artery from the anterior left sinus. Other variations of sporadic frequency were noted. It was emphasized by these authors that commonly the right coronary artery gives off prominent branches to the anterior aspect of the ventricles.

Shrivastava and Edwards [19] noted that when two coronary arterial origins were present, the left artery arose somewhat more posteriorly than in the normal heart. A single coronary artery was seen in four of 30 cases (13%). Among the variations observed were high origin of one or both coronary arterial ostia. Angular origin of a coronary artery was observed in one of the series of Butto and colleagues [15]. Origin of the posterior descending artery from the left coronary arterial system ('left dominance') was found in about 32% of cases of Shrivastava and Edwards [19].

Associated anomalies of the major arteries of the thorax are common in persistent truncus arteriosus. Among these are right aortic arch, interruption of the aortic arch, and absence of one major pulmonary artery. Butto *et al.* [15] found in 47 cases, in which the state of the aortic arch was known, that it was left-sided in 28 (59%), right-sided in 14 (30%) and interrupted in five cases (11%). Respective percentages in the series of Van Praagh and Van Praagh [20] were 58, 21 and 19%. Bharati and associates [21] observed 34 cases (19%) of right aortic arch among 180 specimens with persistent truncus arteriosus. The usual type of right aortic arch is that without a retroesophageal segment, as is the usual right aortic arch associated with the tetralogy of Fallot. The branching of the right aortic arch usually is that of the mirror image type. Butto *et al.* [15] observed that two of 14 cases with right aortic arch had an aberrant aortic origin of the left subclavian artery.

Absence of the ductus arteriosus is commonly observed (up to 50%) among cases of persistent truncus with an intact aortic arch [20].

Absence of a pulmonary artery, usually on the side of the aortic arch, was observed during cardiac catheterization in 17 of 126 patients reported by Mair and associates [22]. In seven, the right pulmonary artery was absent, and in 10 the left was absent. They pointed out that obstructive pulmonary vascular disease is apt to occur in the lung with the intact pulmonary artery and at an earlier age than in the lungs of patients with truncus arteriosus and both pulmonary arteries present. Bharati and associates [21] observed 10 cases with absence of a pulmonary artery in the usual sense. In this circumstance, the arterial supply to the homolateral lung was either through 'distal ductal origin' of the pulmonary artery or through bronchial arteries.

A large variety of associated anomalies other than the ones presented herein have been observed in truncus arteriosus. The report of Bharati *et al.* [21] has a comprehensive presentation of associations as observed in 180 autopsied cases.

In cases of persistent truncus arteriosus not treated surgically, survival beyond infancy is uncommon. Exceptional cases have been reported, among which is that of Silverman and Scheinesson of a man of 43 years [23]. In the files of the Registry of Cardiovascular Disease of United Hospital, St Paul, are four cases of truncus each of which had lived longer than usual, including one patient aged 53 years. In each case, pulmonary vascular disease was advanced, with plexiform lesions present.

2.1.4 ORIGIN OF PULMONARY ARTERIAL SUPPLY FROM AORTA

Situations in which one or both pulmonary arteries do not originate from the pulmonary trunk are considered in those with patent pulmonary trunk and those with atretic or non-identifiable (absent) pulmonary trunk.

(a) With patent pulmonary trunk

The pulmonary trunk may be patent when one or both pulmonary arteries do not originate from it, but arise from the aorta.

One pulmonary artery anomalous origin

With unilateral anomalous pulmonary arterial origin from the aorta and the pulmonary trunk patent, the latter vessel does not bifurcate. It leads to one lung, the opposite lung being supplied by the 'absent' pulmonary artery. The artery to the lung that does not arise from the pulmonary artery (i.e. the absent pulmonary artery) may originate from one of three sources. These are: the ascending aorta [24] (Figure 2.4(a)); the distal segment of the ductus arteriosus (*distal ductal origin*) (Figure 2.4(b)), or the descending aorta.

In distal ductal origin [12], the anomalous pulmonary artery arises from the aorta or a subclavian artery. The primary stem of the vessel is considered to be derived from the aortic end of the sixth aortic arch of that side. For a particular pulmonary artery so arising, the site of its stem depends upon the pulmonary artery involved and the side of the aortic arch. Thus, a pulmonary artery arising on the homolateral side as the aortic arch arises from the arch. The pulmonary artery contralateral to the aortic arch arises from the base of the homolateral subclavian artery (Figure 2.5). When there is distal ductal origin of a pulmonary artery, its proximal segment is composed of ductal tissue and is usually more narrow than the more distal segments of the artery.

Pool and associates [24] made an extensive study of the subject of unilateral origin of a pulmonary artery from the aorta. They found that the unilateral pulmonary arterial absence was about equally divided between the two sides, and in nearly half of the cases no other cardiovascular anomaly was associated. When tetralogy of Fallot was associated with absence of a pulmonary artery, it was always the left artery that was absent.

When the arterial supply to the involved lung originates from the descending aorta, it is usual that multiple

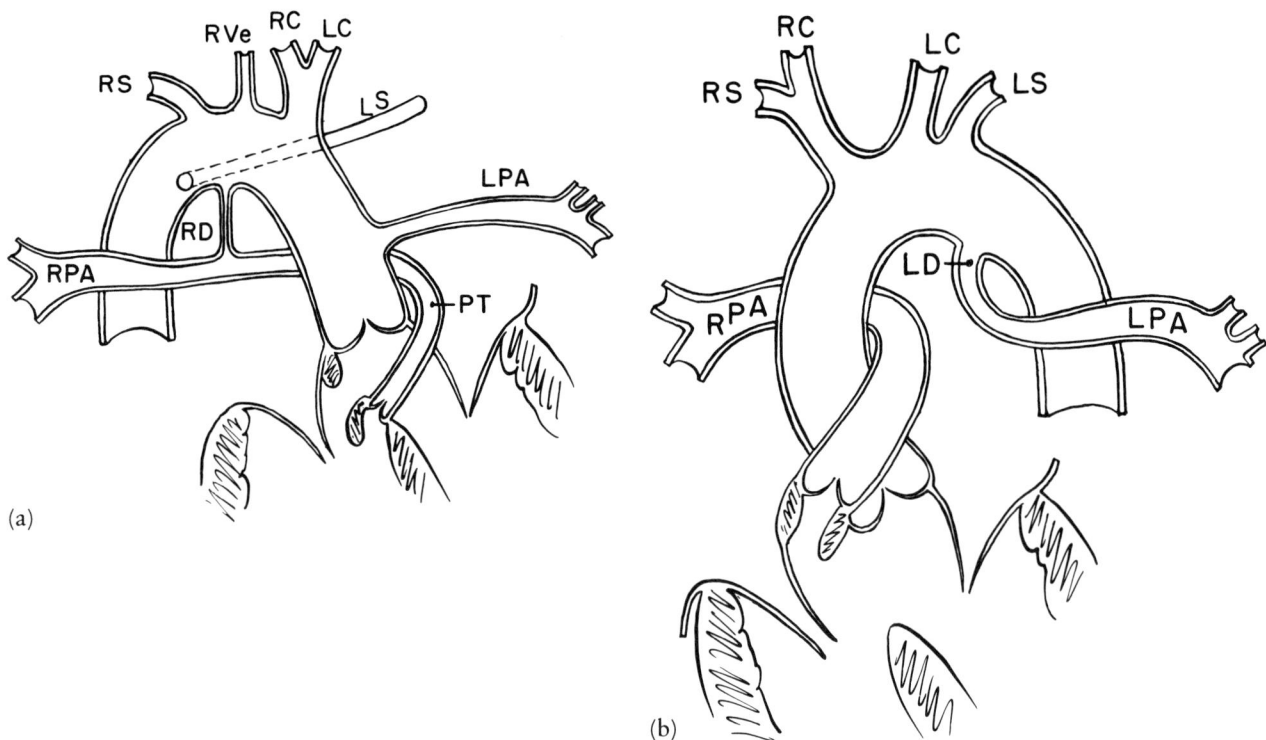

Figure 2.4 (a) Origin of left pulmonary artery from ascending aorta. A right aortic arch is present. A right ductus arteriosus extends between the right aortic arch and the right pulmonary artery. The left subclavian artery arises anomalously from the aorta. (b) Left pulmonary artery has distal ductal origin from left-sided aortic arch. The right pulmonary artery is in continuity with the pulmonary trunk. LD = left ductus; RD = right ductus; LPA = left pulmonary artery; RPA = right pulmonary artery; RS = right subclavian artery; RC = right common carotid artery; LC = left common carotid artery; LS = left subclavian artery; RC = right ductus arteriosus; RVe = right vertebral artery. (Reproduced with permission from Sotomora and Edwards [12].)

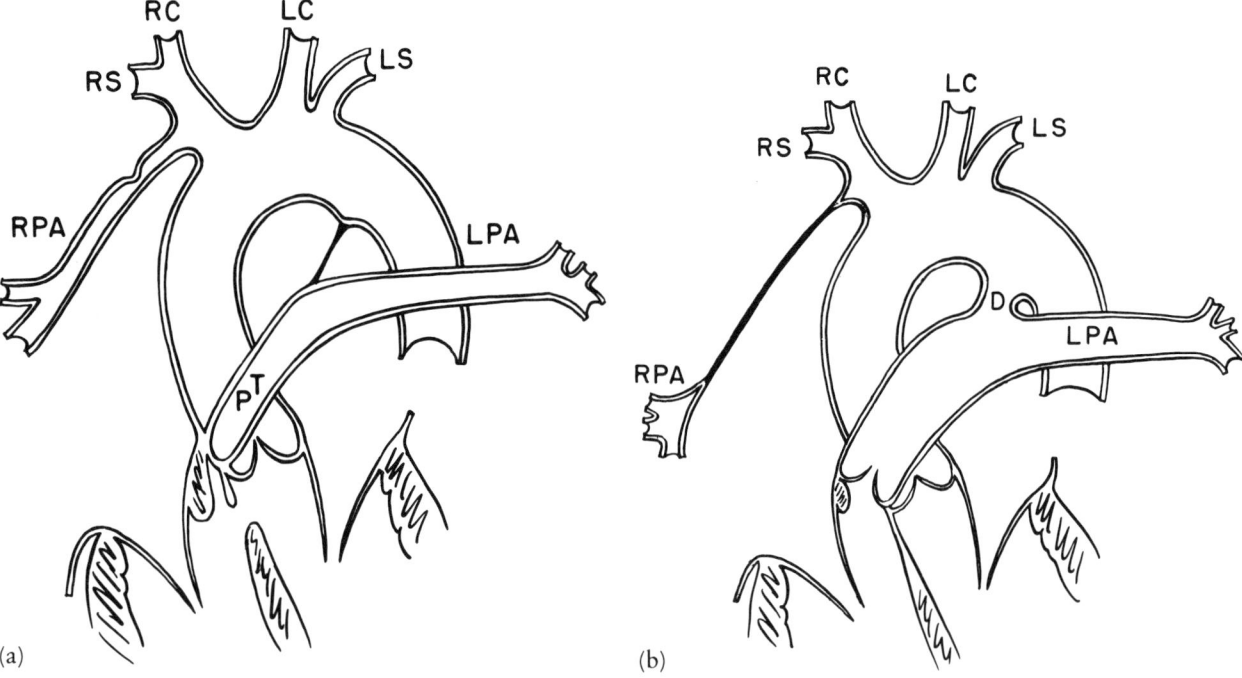

Figure 2.5 Distal ductal origin of the right pulmonary artery. (a) Left aortic arch. The right pulmonary artery arises from the right ductus arteriosus which, in turn, takes origin from the base of the right subclavian artery. The vessel shows a focus of narrowing but is basically patent. (b) Distal ductal origin of the right pulmonary artery associated with left aortic arch. The vessel arises from the subclavian artery. The ductal segment and the proximal part of the right pulmonary artery are atretic. At the pulmonary hilus the right pulmonary artery is patent. D = ductus arteriosus; LC = left carotid artery; LPA = left pulmonary artery; LS = left subclavian artery; PT = pulmonary trunk; RC = right carotid artery; PRA = right pulmonary artery; RS = right subclavian artery. (Reproduced with permission from Sotomora and Edwards [12].)

branches arise. When the anomalous supply is from either the ascending aorta or of the distal ductal type, only one vessel passes to the lung of that side. Origin of the right pulmonary artery from the ascending aorta is much more common than origin of the left artery from that segment of aorta. The vessel characteristically is about the same width as a normal pulmonary artery [25]. Richardson and associates [26] referred to this condition as a variation of the aortopulmonary defect or window.

In absence of a pulmonary artery, the entire cardiac output passes through the normally arising artery into the homolateral lung [24]. In infants, pulmonary hypertension of the side with the normal artery is usually present. In the opposite lung, the arterial pressure depends upon whether or not there is an effective narrowing in the channel between the aorta and the pulmonary vascular bed of the side with the anomalous arterial supply.

Both pulmonary arteries anomalous origin

In the condition in which pulmonary arteries cannot be identified proximal to the hili of the lungs, bronchial arteries from the aorta are present. These bronchial arteries usually connect to an identifiable pulmonary artery at the lung hilus [12]. This condition in the past was termed persistent truncus arteriosus type IV, but more appropriately is considered atresia of pulmonary arteries with bronchial arterial supply to the lungs.

Bilateral distal ductal origin of pulmonary arteries is a rare situation in which the pulmonary trunk is present and simply appears to continue as a ductus arteriosus. Neither pulmonary artery arises from the pulmonary trunk. In the case described by Bricker and associates [27], the right pulmonary artery arose from the aorta just proximal to the origin of the innominate artery, while the left pulmonary artery arose from the aorta distal to the ductal insertion into the aorta. In 1980, Beitzke and Shinebourne [28] described the angiograms in a newborn in whom the pulmonary trunk arose from the right ventricle. This vessel, without branching, connected with the descending aorta through a patent ductus arteriosus. The right and left pulmonary arteries arose from the ascending aorta through a common stem.

(b) **With atretic or absent pulmonary trunk**

When the pulmonary trunk is absent or atretic, and there are two pulmonary arteries, it is important to determine whether the two pulmonary arteries arise from near a common stem, a state called *confluent origin*, or each of the pulmonary arteries arise some distance from the other, so-called *non-confluence*. A common example of confluent origin of the pulmonary arteries is atresia of the proximal pulmonary trunk, with each pulmonary artery arising in continuity with the opposite artery. The blood supply to the pulmonary arterial confluence is through a patent ductus arteriosus. When non-confluence of the origin of the pulmonary arteries exists, it is common that bilateral distal ductal origin of the pulmonary arteries is present, or that on one side there may be distal ductal origin, while on the other the pulmonary arterial supply is derived from bronchial arteries.

2.2 Systemic arteries

Discussion of anomalies of the systemic arterial system is divided into those of the aorta and the coronary arteries.

2.2.1 AORTA

Anomalies of the aorta are classified as those causing obstruction, those with communication with other vessels or cardiac chambers, and those that are characterized by abnormal course and/or branching.

(a) **Aortic obstruction**

Obstructive anomalies may occur in any segment of the aorta.

Ascending aorta

Supravalvular aortic stenosis is obstruction of the ascending aorta. Three types are identified: the hour-glass form, the hypoplastic form, and the membranous form [29] (Figure 2.6).

The **hour-glass type** has the following features. As the name implies, the exterior of the ascending aorta exhibits an hour-glass deformity. Histologically, the media is thick and exhibits irregularity, with a tendency toward a mosaic pattern. The intima at the site of greatest narrowing is thickened. The site of greatest narrowing of the aortic lumen includes the level of the upper aspects of the aortic cusps. Uncommonly, the upper edge of an aortic cusp is adherent to the aortic intima at the site of the lesion. This has been demonstrated to involve the right aortic cusp, thereby excluding the right coronary artery from direct communication with the aortic lumen. In a case observed by the authors, this condition was associated with origin of the left circumflex coronary artery from the right coronary artery (Figure 2.7).

The **hypoplastic type** of supravalvular aortic stenosis is characterized by abnormal thickness of the entire ascending aorta, the thickness making a corresponding narrowing of the entire length of the involved aortic segment. The pulmonary trunk may share in the process.

The **membranous type** is characterized by the presence

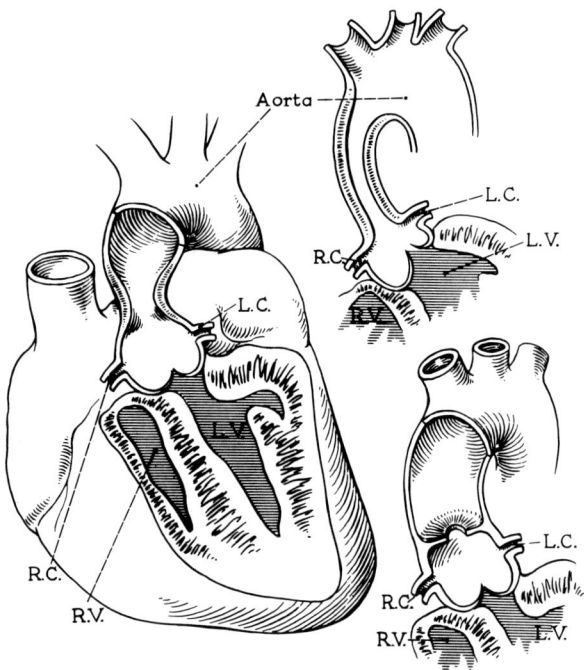

Figure 2.6 Three types of supravalvular aortic stenosis. (a) The hour-glass type is the most common variety. (b) The hypoplastic type. (c) The membranous type. LC = left coronary artery; LV = left ventricle; RC = right coronary artery; RV = right ventricle. (Reproduced with permission from Edwards [135].)

of fibrous strands attached to the aortic intima and crossing the lumen of the aorta.

Any case with significant obstruction of the aorta results in major concentric hypertrophy of the left ventricle. Stenosis of the branches of the aortic arch is common, as is peripheral pulmonary arterial obstruction. Supravalvular aortic stenosis has been associated with the Williams syndrome that includes infantile hypercalcemia and peculiar (elfin) facies. Jones and Smith [30] pointed out that this syndrome is commonly associated with growth deficiency, mild microcephaly with mental deficiency and altered patterns of facial development. Supravalvular aortic stenosis is not universally associated with any of the patterns of Williams syndrome [30].

Blieden and co-workers [31] described a developmental complex that, in its full expression, includes supravalvular aortic and pulmonary stenosis, stenosis of branches of the aorta and pulmonary artery, dysplasia of valves and stenosis of the coronary arterial ostia. Valvular dysplasia, when present, tends to cause stenosis of the semilunar and regurgitation of the atrioventricular valves. Some of the elements of the complex may not be present.

Secondary effects of supravalvular aortic stenosis include premature coronary atherosclerosis and, uncommonly, infected endarteritis, and aortic dissection.

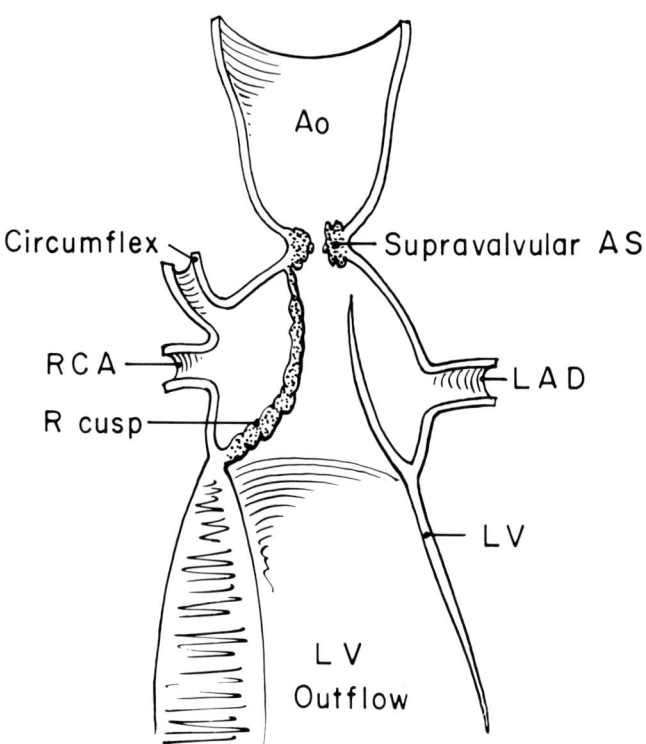

Figure 2.7 Hour-glass type of supravalvular aortic stenosis with adhesion of the right aortic cusp to the aortic lesion. In this instance, the right coronary artery arises from the right aortic sinus, while the circumflex coronary artery arises from the right artery. Each of the vessels involved are exteriorized from the aortic lumen by the adhesion of the right aortic cusp to the aortic lesion. Ao = aorta; AS = aortic stenosis; LAD = left anterior descending coronary artery; LV = left ventricle; R = right; RCA = right coronary artery.

Associated valvular disease occurs, especially with the hypoplastic type [31].

Hypoplasia of the ascending aorta is a pronounced, uniform narrowing of the ascending aorta in which the structure of the wall of the vessel is normal histologically. This state is classical for congenital aortic stenosis or atresia, most pronounced in the latter. It should not be considered an aortic anomaly, but rather a secondary consequence of the aortic valvular anomaly.

Aortic arch

In the fetus, the isthmus is the narrow segment lying between the origin of the left subclavian artery and the entrance of the ductus. This narrow segment reflects the passage of the major quantity of blood from the arch into the vessels supplying the brain, proximally, and flow of blood into the descending aorta through the ductus arteriosus, distally. Normally, the narrow state of the isthmus gradually gives way to a near-normal caliber postnatally.

The condition **tubular hypoplasia** is usually present

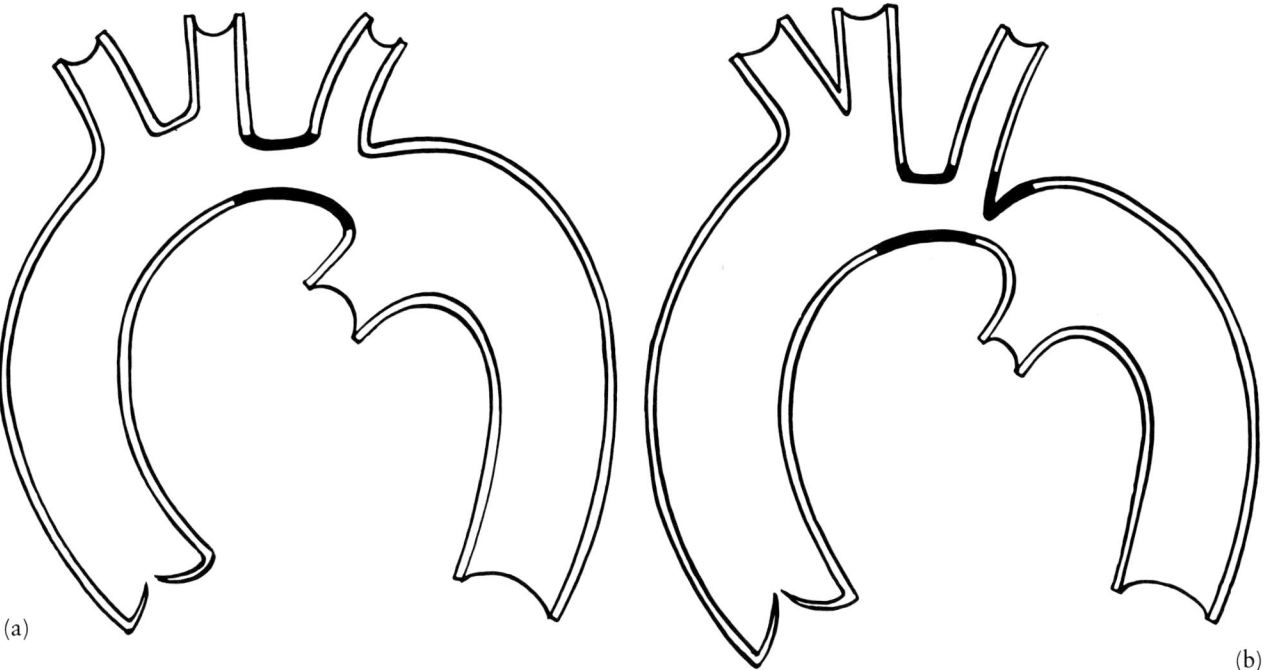

Figure 2.8 Tubular hypoplasia of the aortic arch. (a) In this case, the lesion lies in the segment between the left common carotid and left subclavian arteries. (b) The condition of tubular hypoplasia of the aortic arch is associated with classical coarctation of the aorta in this instance.

either in the segment of the aortic arch between the innominate artery and the left common carotid, or between the left common carotid and the left subclavian arteries. The condition is associated with normal histologic pattern. The state of narrowing varies from being significant (sometimes called long segment coarctation) to unobstructive. The condition may be isolated (Figure 2.8(a)) or be associated with the classical morphologic features of coarctation of the aorta (Figure 2.8(b)).

Coarctation of the aortic arch refers to the uncommon condition in which classical features of aortic coarctation are present due to narrowing of the arch between the origins of the left common carotid and left subclavian arteries. In this condition, the left subclavian artery exhibits anatomic 'subclavian lag', joining the aorta distal rather than proximal to the ductal connection with the aorta [32].

Junction of arch and descending aorta (classical coarctation)

The anatomic features of classical coarctation include location of major congenital obstruction of the aorta at the junction of the arch and descending aorta (Figure 2.9). The lesion is characterized by a ridge caused primarily by abnormal medial tissue. The ridge involves the anterior, superior and posterior aspects of the aorta at the general zone of the junction of the ductus arteriosus, or ligamentum arteriosum, with the aorta. Corresponding to the site of the true ridge of coarctation, there is a depression in the external adventitial aspect of the aorta, most evident on the superior aspect (greater curve) of the descending aorta. This deformity is exaggerated by the intrinsic narrow state of the aorta at the obstruction, post-stenotic dilatation distal, and dilatation of the aorta proximal to the obstruction. The aortic lumen lies eccentrically near the lower wall of the aorta. The caliber of the aortic lumen at the site of coarctation varies but is narrower than the aortic lumen elsewhere [33].

Among the anomalies associated with typical coarctation, the most consistent is congenital bicuspid aortic valve. In the report of Becker and associates [34] the frequency was 46%, but it has been observed in more than two-thirds of some studies. The congenital bicuspid aortic valve varies in structure [34], so that examples of congenital bicuspid valve may be misinterpreted as an acquired bicuspid aortic valve.

Variations of branching of the aortic arch and the relationship to the coarctation occur. Aberrant right subclavian artery in association with a left aortic arch, which occurs in about 0.5% of the population, probably has a similar frequency in cases with aortic coarctation. In the authors' experience, when this arterial variation occurs with aortic coarctation, the right subclavian artery arises proximal to the coarctation in about one half of the cases and distal to the aortic obstruction in the other half (Figure 2.10).

In established coarctation, rich collateral circulation develops and may carry normal volumes of blood of

30 CONGENITAL ANOMALIES OF BLOOD VESSELS

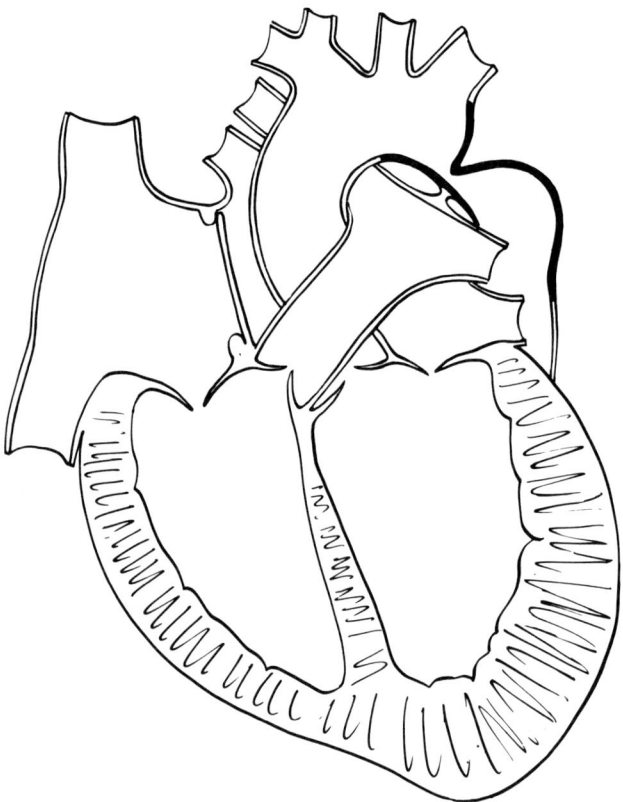

Figure 2.9 Classical coarctation of the aorta. The lesion lies distal to the left subclavian artery and is represented by an infolding of the superior wall of the aorta which causes the aortic lumen to be eccentric and narrowed. Dilatation of the left subclavian artery and post-stenotic dilatation of the aorta may yield a so-called figure-of-three pattern in roentgenograms. (Reproduced with permission from Edwards and Edwards [133].)

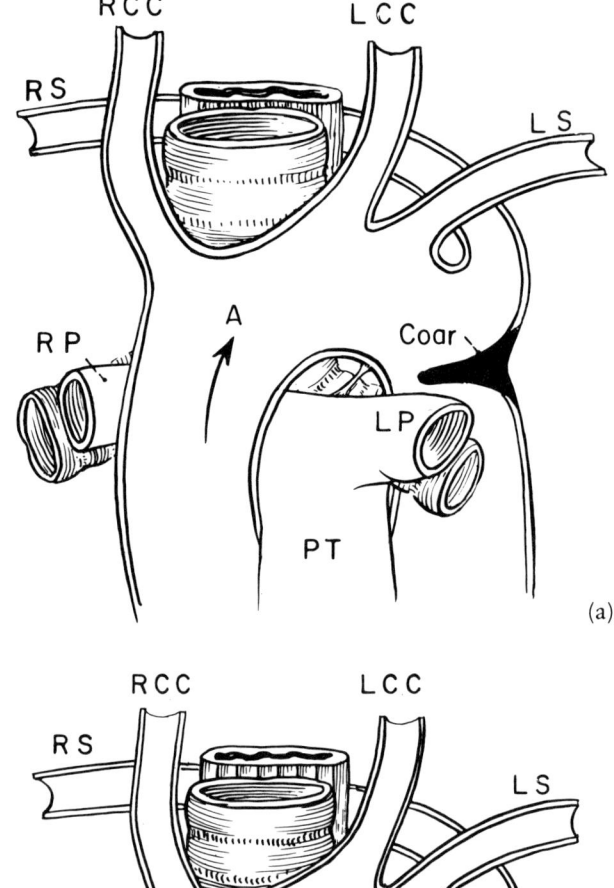

Figure 2.10 Aberrant right subclavian artery associated with coarctation of the aorta. (a) The aberrant right subclavian artery arises from the proximal compartment of the aorta. (b) The right subclavian artery arises from the distal compartment of the aorta. A = aorta; Coar = coarctation; LCC = left common carotid artery; LP = left pulmonary artery; LS = left subclavian artery; PT = pulmonary trunk; RCC = right common carotid artery; RP = right pulmonary artery; RS = right subclavian artery.

that part of the body supplied by the arterial system below the level of the coarctation. The primary sources of collateral flow around the obstruction in the aorta are the subclavian arteries. Essentially, there are two systems, the anterior, supplying the lower extremities, and the posterior, supplying the abdominal viscerae [36] (Figure 2.11).

The specific consequences and complications of aortic coarctation, in general, are related in part to the age of the patient when they occur. They also tend to be related to the position of the coarctation with respect to the ductus arteriosus. Preductal coarctation tends to be complicated by left ventricular failure in early infancy. When the coarctation lies distal to the ductus arteriosus, symptoms usually are not present in the neonatal period. Exclusive of hypertension, symptoms may be absent for many years until some specific complication results. The associated hypertension is systolic in the proximal compartment and diastolic in both proximal and distal compartments.

Aneurysms of the arterial system may complicate coarctation. These include the aorta [37] (Figures 2.12–2.15), the circle of Willis, the anterior spinal artery, and, rarely, the arch branches.

In coarctation, two sites of intravascular infection may occur (Figures 2.14, 2.15). More common is that

SYSTEMIC ARTERIES 31

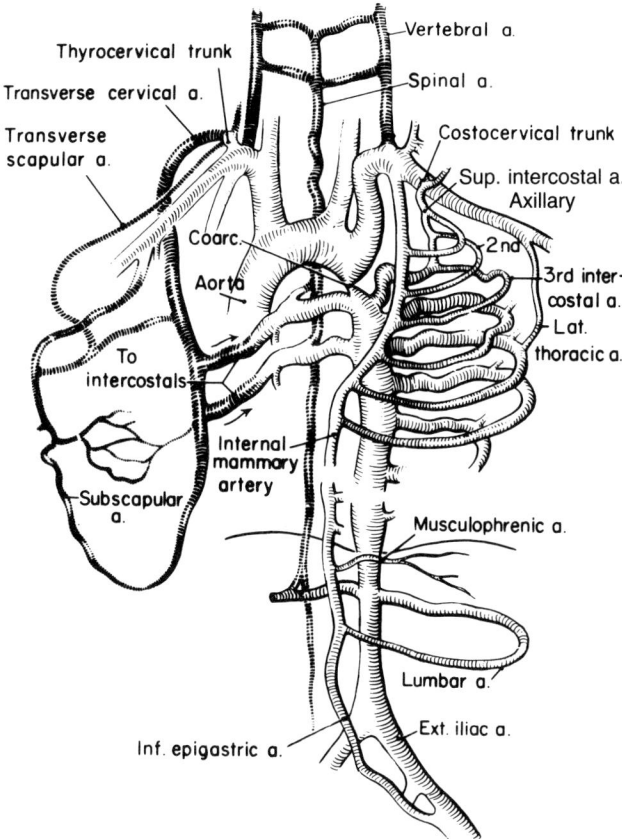

Figure 2.11 Collateral circulation in coarctation of the aorta. The anterior system is shown in the right side of the illustration, and the posterior system is shown in the left side of the illustration. Each system takes origin with the subclavian arteries. The anterior system is composed of the internal mammary artery and the superior and inferior epigastric arteries which ultimately terminate in the external iliac artery. The posterior system of collaterals is also derived from the subclavian arteries and makes use of the parascapular vessels. The latter have communications with the intercostal arteries from the descending aorta. a = artery; Coarc. = coarctation; Ext. = exterior; Inf. = inferior; Lat. = lateral; Sup. = supreme. (Reproduced with permission from Edwards and Edwards [133].)

of the frequently associated congenital bicuspid aortic valve. Occasionally, infection may occur at the site of jet impact in the aorta distal to the coarctation. Aortic valvular insufficiency may complicate the congenital bicuspid valve, either infected or non-infected. Mitral insufficiency is an uncommon association.

Thoracic and abdominal aortic coarctation

Obstruction of either the lower thoracic or the abdominal aorta may occur as congenital anomalies, but many cases are acquired in nature. In 1973, two cases of abdominal coarctation were reported and the literature reviewed 110 other cases that were considered to be of congenital nature, excluding cases thought to be

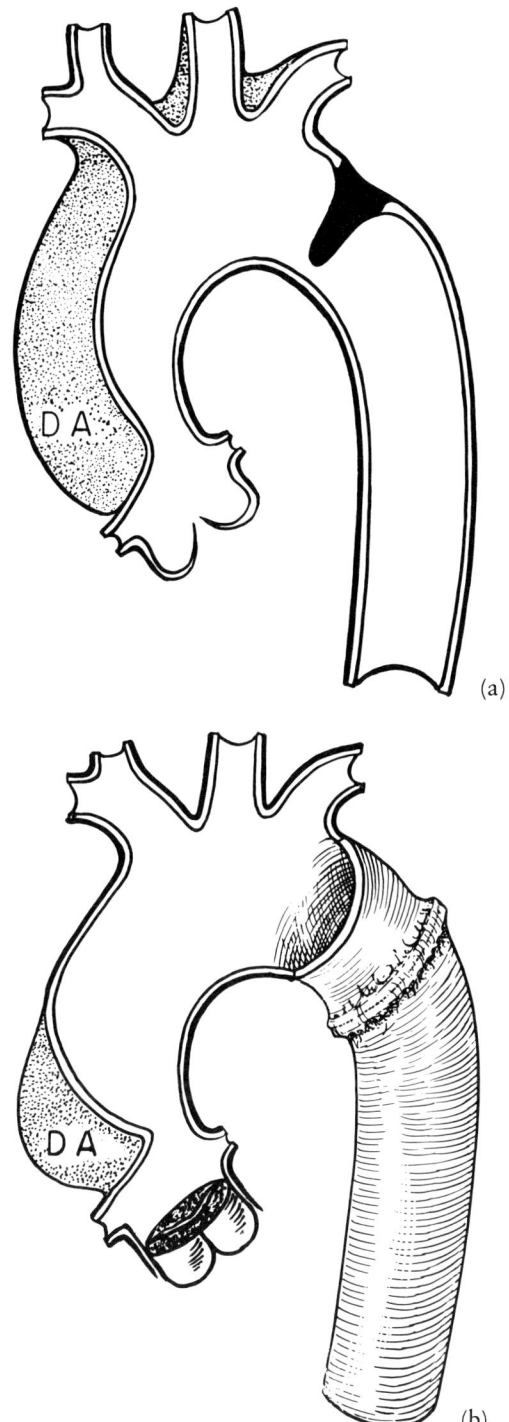

Figure 2.12 Coarctation of the aorta and aortic dissection in the ascending portion. (a) Coarctation with acute dissection involving the ascending aorta and aortic arch. (b) Dissection of the aorta in an example of coarctation previously treated surgically. DA = dissecting aneurysm. (Reproduced with permission from Edwards [37].)

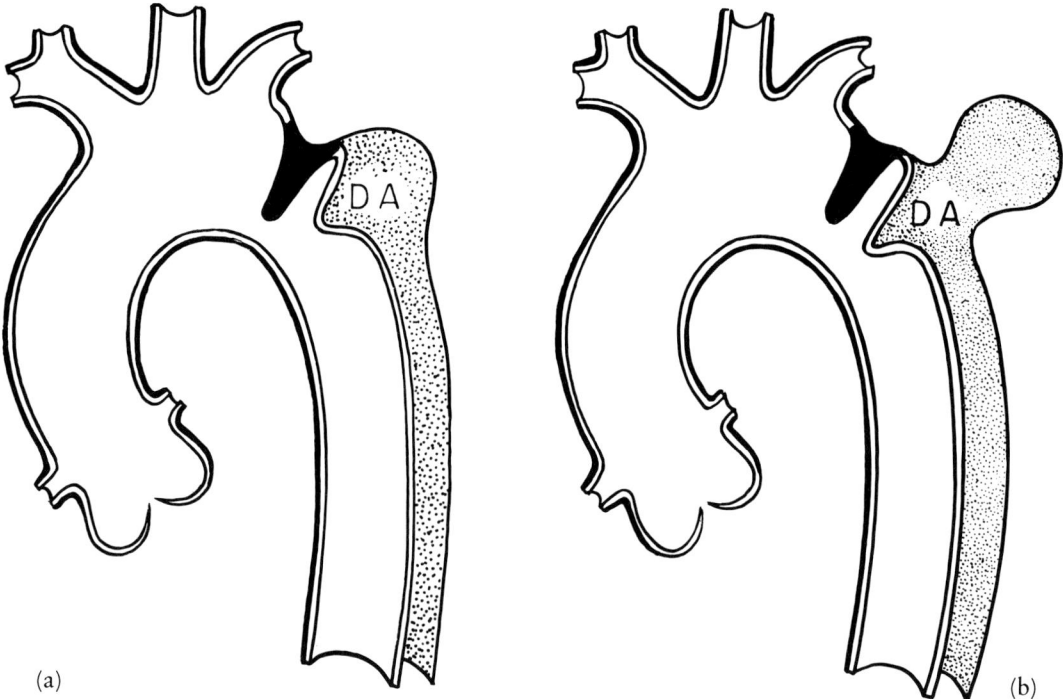

Figure 2.13 Coarctation of the aorta with aortic dissection beginning distal to the coarctation. (a) The dissection begins distal to the coarctation and is restricted to the lower compartment of the aorta. (b) The dissection begins distal to the coarctation and is associated with saccular aneurysm at the site of the initial tear. DA = dissecting aneurysm. (Reproduced with permission from Edwards [37].)

acquired [38]. These authors found that congenital coarctation of the abdominal aorta favored the female (62%). The most common type (35%) was in relation to the renal arteries and involved a short segment of aorta; a diffuse form (21%) involved the aorta both proximally and distally to the renal arterial origins.

Interruption of aortic arch

The ultimate in aortic obstruction is interruption of the aortic arch. Classically, there is no continuity between the ascending aorta and the descending aorta. Rarely is there an atretic segment between the two compartments. In the classical state, the aortic arch ends either after giving off the three branches of the arch or, most frequently, distal to the origin of the left common carotid artery. The descending aorta is supplied by a patent ductus arteriosus. The ductus is usually single and most often left-sided. Uncommonly, the ductus is right-sided, and, rarely, bilateral ducti arteriosi are present.

A classification of interruption of the aortic arch with left ductus arteriosus into three types depends upon the level of interruption of the arch [39]. In each, the descending aorta is fed by a left-sided ductus arteriosus. Type A is characterized by interruption of the arch distal to the left subclavian artery (Figure 2.16(a)). In Type B, the interruption of the arch lies between the left common carotid and left subclavian arteries. In this type, the left subclavian artery arises from the descending aorta (Figure 2.16(b)). In Type C, the left common and subclavian arteries arise from the descending aorta.

Variations of the above-listed patterns occur, the most common being that in which the right subclavian artery is aberrant. This may occur either in Type A or B (Figure 2.16(c),(d)). In Type B with aberrant right subclavian artery, both subclavian arteries arise from the descending aorta (Figure 2.16(d)). Isolation of the left subclavian artery may be observed but is uncommon (Figure 2.17).

Although there are rare cases of interruption of the aortic arch without intracardiac anomalies, classically intracardiac anomalies are associated [40], especially communication between the ventricles or single ventricle. The most common associated anomaly is **ventricular septal defect**. In at least half of the cases of interruption of the aortic arch the ventricular septal defect is so situated as to be in a subpulmonary position, allowing for biventricular origin of the pulmonary trunk. Associated with this defect is a spur of muscle that is interposed between the aortic origin and the ventricular septal defect. This muscle bundle is so positioned as to cause subaortic stenosis distal to the ventricular septal defect [41]. A congenitally bicuspid aortic valve is common, occurring in about 50% of the cases with interruption of the aortic arch.

SYSTEMIC ARTERIES 33

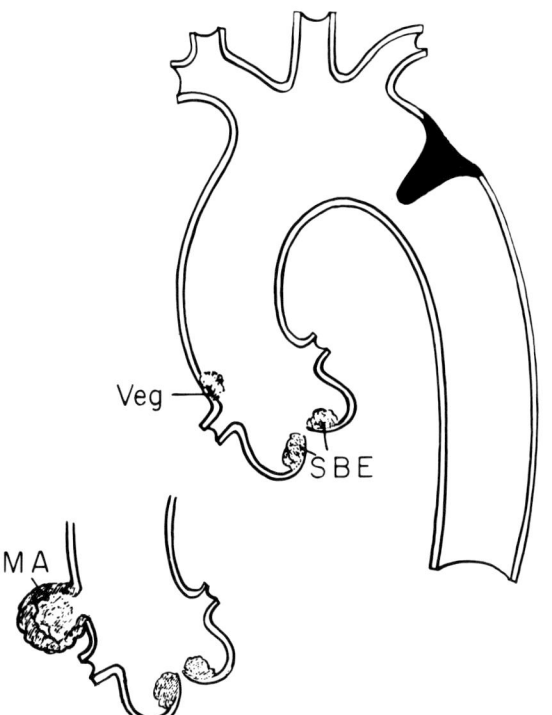

Figure 2.14 Coarctation of the aorta with bacterial endocarditis of the bicuspid aortic valve. The main body of the illustration shows the site of primary vegetative process on the aortic valve. A secondary vegetation appears on the wall of the aorta. In the insert, the process shown in the main body of the illustration has extended to form a mycotic aneurysm of the ascending aorta. The latter may rupture into surrounding structures such as the right atrium or right ventricle. MA = mycotic aneurysm; SBE = primary vegetative process; Veg = vegetation. (Reproduced with permission from Edwards [37].)

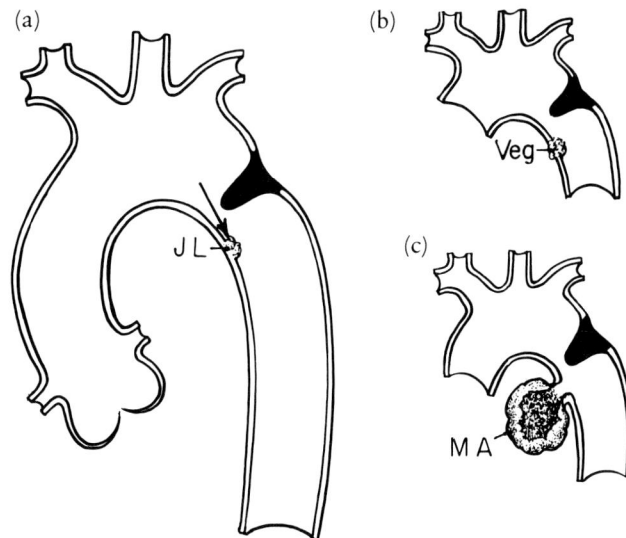

Figure 2.15 Infection of the aorta at the site of a jet lesion distal to the coarctation. (a) Distal to the coarctation, on the wall opposite the deformity, is the site of a jet lesion. (b) The site of the jet lesion is infected with a vegetation evident. (c) The vegetative infective process has led to mycotic aneurysm of the aorta distal to the coarctation. JL = jet lesion; MA = mycotic aneurysm; Veg. = vegetation.

It is uncommon that interruption of the aortic arch is associated with a right ductus arteriosus rather than a left. The patterns are mirror images of the various forms with left ductus arteriosus including the presence of a right descending aorta in association with right ductus arteriosus. In cases of right ductus arteriosus there is a tendency for right-sided bronchial obstruction to be caused by the right ductus arteriosus [42] (Figure 2.18).

Interruption of aortic arch with bilateral ducti arteriosi was described by Blatchford and associates [43]. The condition created a vascular ring causing compression of the trachea and esophagus.

(b) Communications of aorta with adjacent structures other than the pulmonary arterial system

Aortic sinus aneurysm

Congenital aneurysm of an aortic sinus is usually observed in the adult. While it is impossible to tell when the aneurysmal state started, it is probable that the congenital form implies an inborn localized tendency for aneurysm like that in congenital aneurysm of the circle of Willis. The classical, essential pathologic process is a separation of the aortic media from the aortic annulus. This results in a displacement upward of the aortic media, leaving myocardial tissue to support the involved sinus [44]. Aneurysm results. Uncommonly, the fundamental pathologic process is a 'slippage' of the media of the wall of the sinus rather than an abrupt discontinuity between the aortic media and annulus.

Usually, the congenital aortic sinus aneurysm is a solitary lesion of an aortic sinus. The two most common sites for sinus aneurysms are the posterior and the right aortic sinuses [45] (Figure 2.19(a),(b)). Involvement of the left aortic sinus is rare [46]. The gross morphologic appearance is a thin-walled, fibrous sac bulging into the related cardiac chamber. Classically, aneurysm of the posterior aortic sinus presents into the right atrium (Figure 2.19(a)), while that of the right aortic sinus presents into the right ventricle [47] (Figure 2.19(b)). Aneurysm of the right aortic sinus may have associated ventricular septal defect, with the defect lying subjacent to the aortic valve.

The major complication of aortic sinus aneurysm is rupture with development of a left-to-right shunt. Infection may complicate and cause rupture of a congenital aortic sinus aneurysm. Such a mycotic aneurysm may rupture into a cardiac chamber. In a given case it may be difficult to distinguish whether rupture preceded or followed infection of the aneurysm.

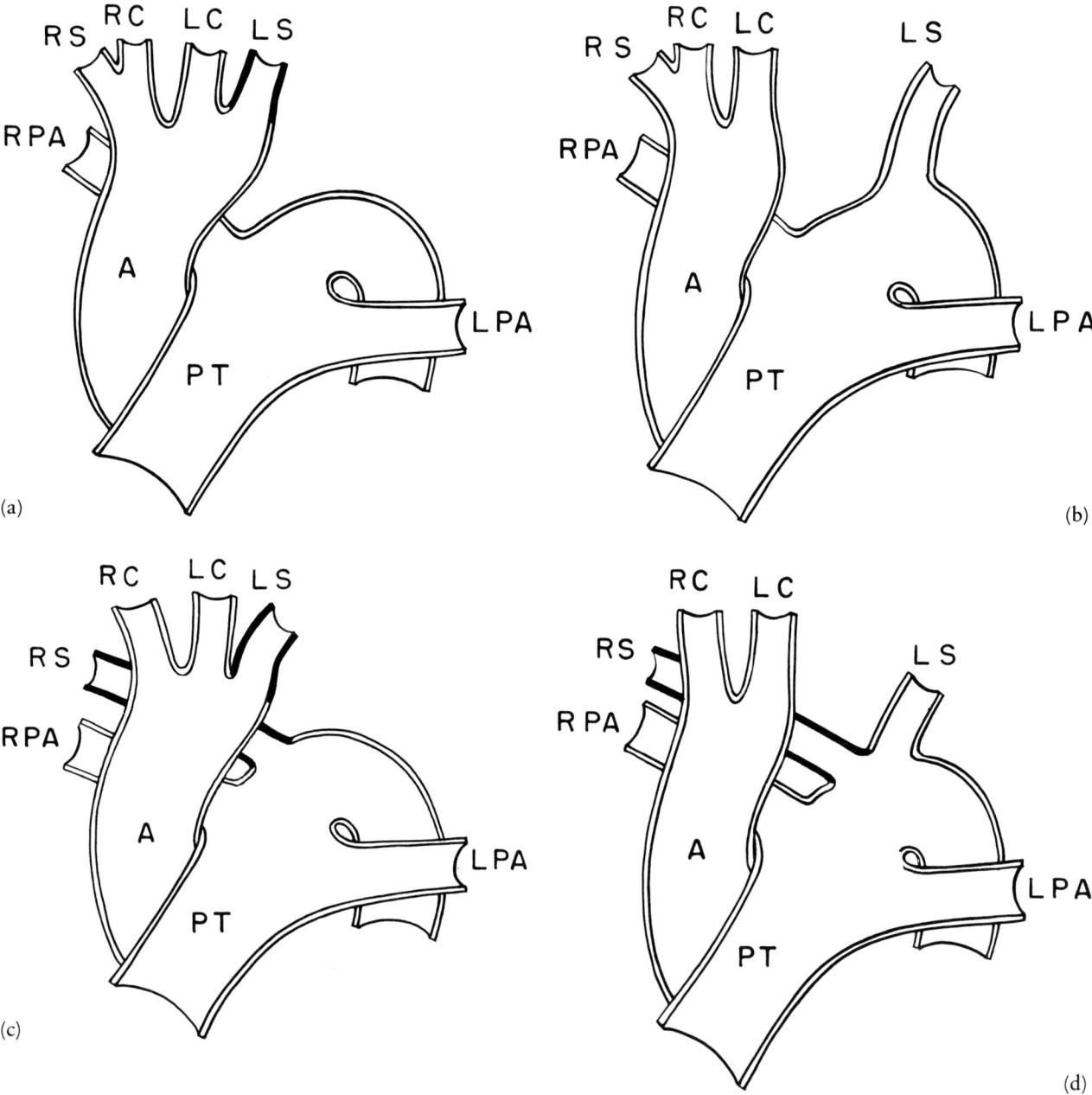

Figure 2.16 Interruption of aortic arch. (a) Type A. The interruption is distal to the left subclavian artery. The descending aorta continues from the ductus arteriosus arising from the pulmonary trunk. (b) Type B. The interruption is between the left common carotid and left subclavian arteries so that the left subclavian artery arises from the distal aorta which is supplied by the ductus arteriosus. (c) Interruption of aortic arch, type A, with aberrant origin right subclavian artery. (d) Interruption of the aortic arch, type B, with aberrant origin of the right subclavian artery. A = aorta; LC = left carotid artery; LPA = left pulmonary artery; LS = left subclavian artery; PT = pulmonary trunk; RC = right carotid artery; RPA = right pulmonary artery; RS = right subclavian artery. (Reproduced with permission from Moller and Edwards [40].)

Aorto-left ventricular tunnel

This was named by Levy and associates in 1963 [47] and is characterized by a channel starting in the ascending aorta, just above the levels of the coronary arterial origins and terminating in the left ventricle near the aortic valve. Tuna and Edwards [49] indicated that the tunnel was responsible for inadequate support of the aortic origin in a manner similar to that in ventricular septal defect (Figure 2.20). This finding supports the surgical proposal that the treatment should consist not only of closing the channel but also of supporting the aortic origin to avoid valvular insufficiency.

SYSTEMIC ARTERIES 35

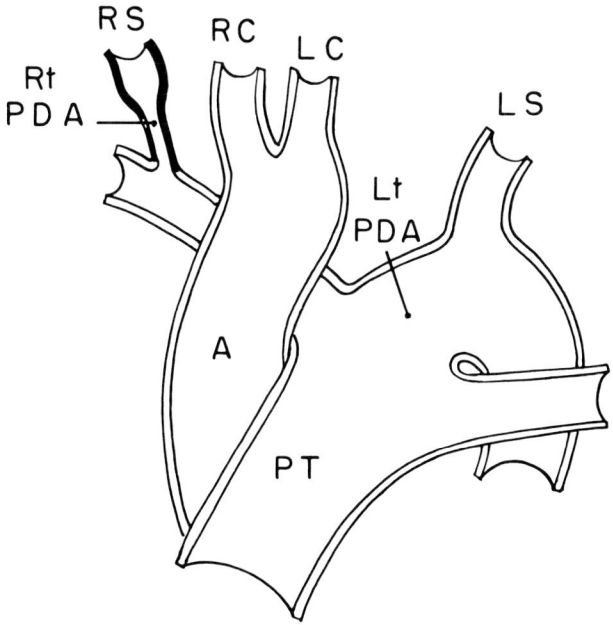

Figure 2.17 Interruption of aortic arch, type B, associated with isolation of the right subclavian artery. In this situation, the right subclavian artery is connected to the right pulmonary artery through a right ductus arteriosus. A = aorta; LC = left carotid artery; LS = left subclavian artery; Lt PDA = left patent ductus arteriosus; PT = pulmonary trunk; RC = right carotid artery; RS = right subclavian artery; Rt PDA = right patent ductus arteriosus.

(c) Abnormal course and/or branching of aortic arch

Abnormalities of the embryologic development and maturation of the primitive aortic arch system can yield many anatomic patterns. Some of these may cause symptoms of tracheal and/or esophageal obstruction. Both known and as yet unidentified anatomic patterns of normal and abnormal course and branching of the aortic arch result from normal or abnormal development.

Hypothetical double aortic arch of Edwards

This will classify the developmental relationships between the described types of aortic arches and their branches [50]. In this construct, each arch has independent origins of the homolateral common carotid and subclavian arteries (Figure 2.21). A ductus arteriosus is present on each side [50], running between the aortic arch and the pulmonary artery of that side. This structure represents a pattern from which, by deviation of the descending aorta to the right or left, and disappearance of one ductus, four families of aortic arch result. Each of the hypothetical subdivisions (families) are characterized by double aortic arch with (Figure 2.22):

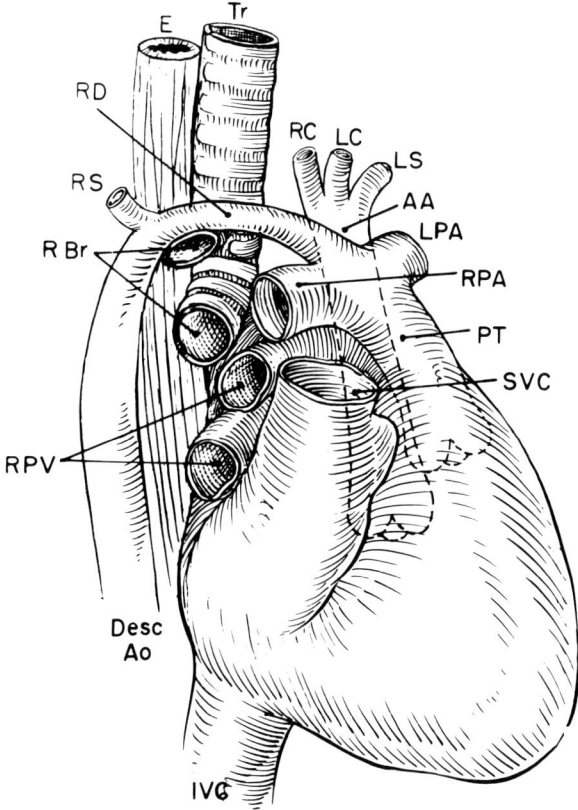

Figure 2.18 Interruption of the aortic arch with right ductus arteriosus. Compression of right upper bronchus by the right ductus arteriosus. AA = ascending aorta; Desc. Ao = descending aorta; E = esophagus; IVC = inferior vena cava; LPA = left pulmonary artery; LS = left subclavian artery; PT = pulmonary trunk; R Br = right bronchi; RC and LC = right and left common carotid arteries; RPA = right pulmonary artery; RPV = right pulmonary veins; RS = right subclavian artery; SVC = superior vena cava; Tr = trachea. (Reproduced with permission from Pierpont [42].)

- left ductus present and left descending aorta
- right ductus present and right descending aorta
- left ductus present and right descending aorta
- right ductus present and left descending aorta

From any of these, by interruption of one or another site or sites, different known anomalies and postulated forms may be derived. In the following discussion, the different anatomic patterns that may be derived from these hypothetical patterns representing the four families of hypothetical aortic arches are presented; they constitute anomalies of the aortic arch.

With intact arch or arches

When one or both aortic arches are intact, the possible anatomic patterns are double aortic arch, patent left arch and patent right aortic arch.

The usual **double aortic arch** had the structure of the hypothetical form shown in Figure 2.22(a) and may be

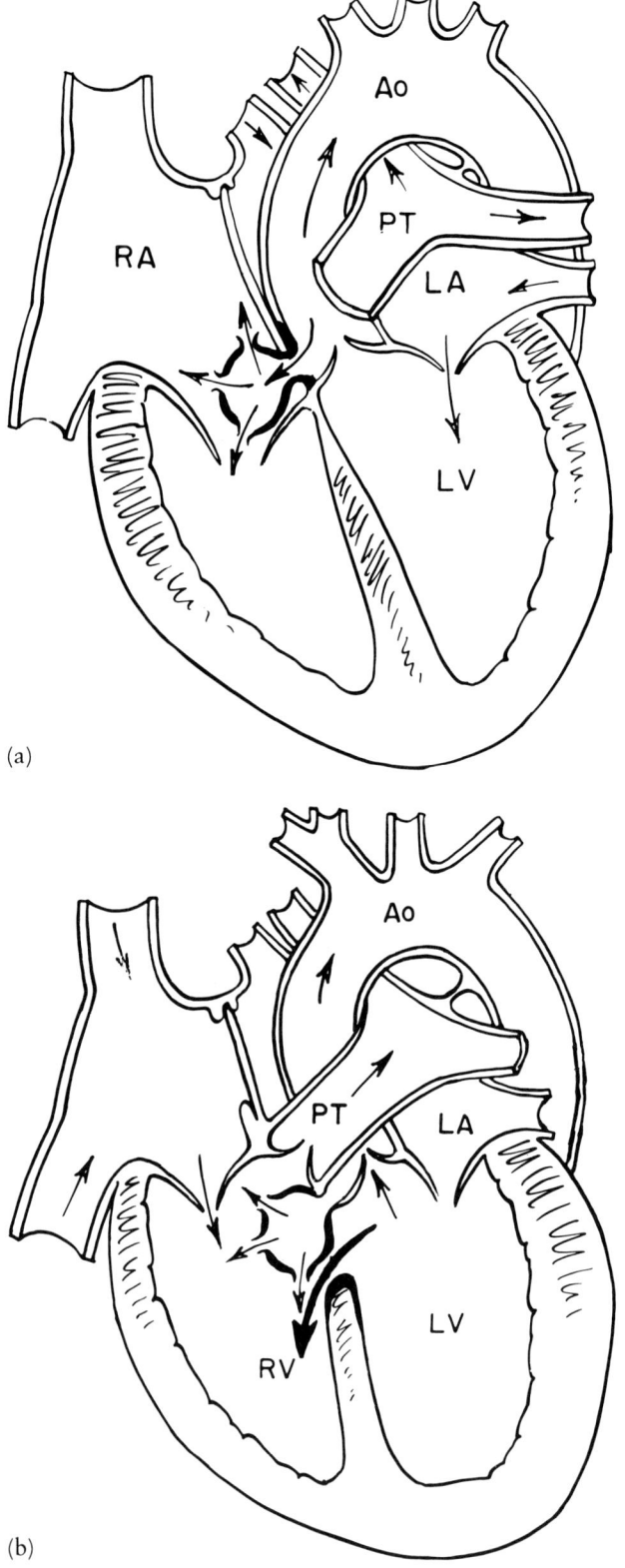
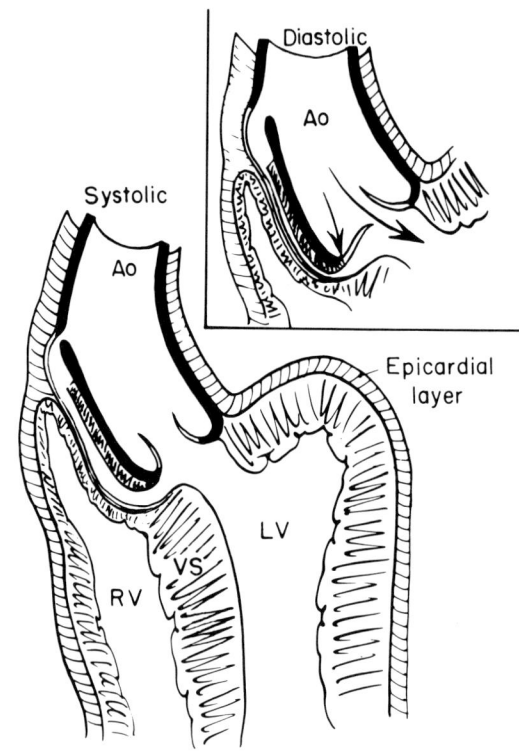

Figure 2.20 Aortic-left ventricular tunnel. In the main body of the illustration, the anomaly in the systolic phase is shown. This reveals the channel between the left ventricle and the ascending aorta. The insert shows that during diastole the unsupported aortic root moves out of optimal position so that there is improper apposition of the aortic cusps, allowing for aortic regurgitation. Ao = aorta; LV = left ventricle; RV = right ventricle; VS = ventricular septum. (Reproduced with permission from Tuna and Edwards [49].)

Figure 2.19 Congenital aneurysm of aortic sinus. (a) The aneurysm arises from the posterior aortic sinus and presents into the right atrium. An aortic-right atrial shunt results when rupture of the aneurysm occurs. (b) Congenital aneurysm of the right aortic sinus leads from the aorta into the outflow tract of the right ventricle. As illustrated, a ventricular septal defect subjacent to the aortic origin commonly is associated with this type of aortic sinus aneurysm. Ao = aorta; LA = left atrium; LV = left ventricle; PT = pulmonary trunk; RA = right atrium; RV = right ventricle. (Reproduced with permission from Edwards and Edwards [133].)

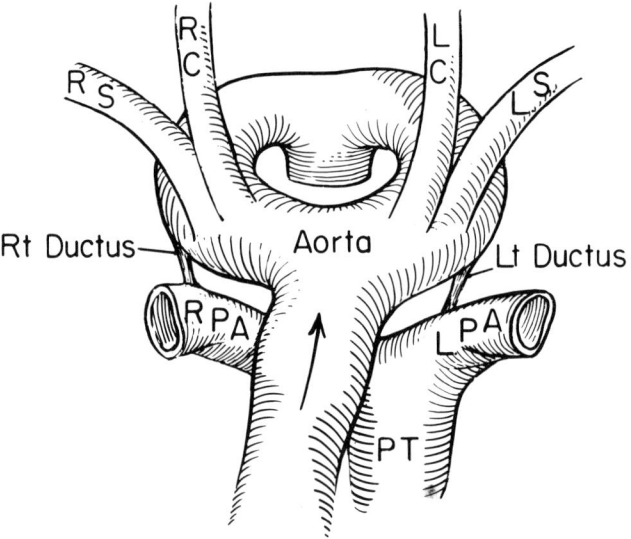

Figure 2.21 Hypothetical double aortic arch as described by Edwards [50]. There are two aortic arches. Each gives rise to independent origins of the carotid and subclavian branches. A ductus arteriosus extends between each aortic arch and the homolateral pulmonary artery. LC = left carotid artery; LS = left subclavian artery; Lt = left; LPA = left pulmonary artery; PT = pulmonary trunk; RC = right carotid artery; RS = right subclavian artery; Rt = right; RPA = right pulmonary artery.

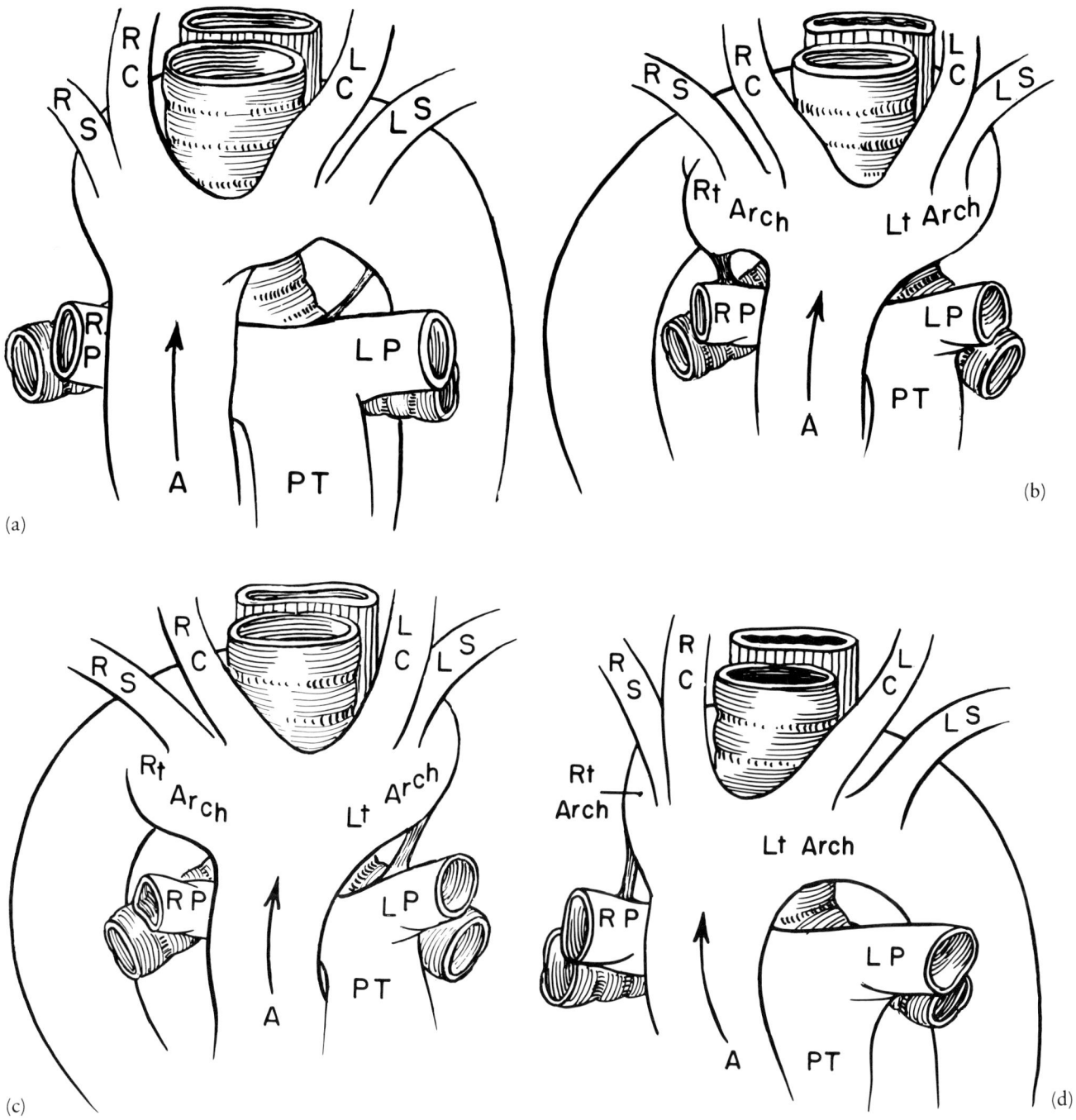

Figure 2.22 Variations in the hypothetical double aortic arch illustrated in Figure 2.21 by virtue of loss of one ductus arteriosus, and shifting of the descending aorta to one side or the other. (a) Double aortic arch with left ductus arteriosus and left descending aorta. (b) Mirror image of (a) characterized by right ductus arteriosus and right descending aorta. (c) Left ductus arteriosus and right descending aorta. (d) Right ductus and left descending aorta. A = aorta; LC = left carotid artery; LP = left pulmonary artery; LS = left subclavian artery; Lt = left; PT = pulmonary trunk; RC = right carotid artery; RP = right pulmonary artery, RS = right subclavian artery; Rt = right.

responsible for tracheal and esophageal obstruction. In this condition, the ascending aorta bifurcates into two arches, the left passing over the left main bronchus, while the right passes over the right bronchus. The right arch then passes behind the esophagus to join the left-sided descending aorta. A left ductus arteriosus or ligamentum arteriosum is present. This runs from the left pulmonary artery to the distal part of the left arch. The arch branching is as follows: from each arch, the homolateral common carotid and subclavian arteries arise independently from before (anterior) and backward (posterior), respectively. There is no

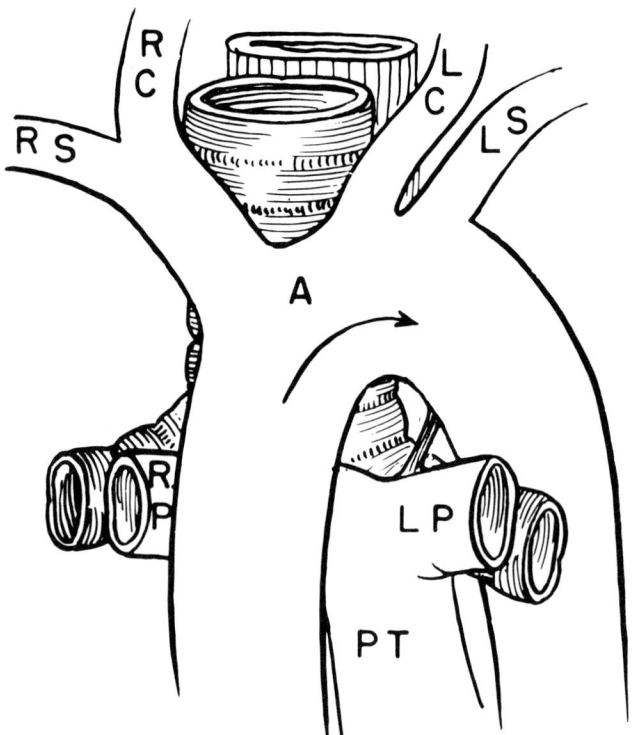

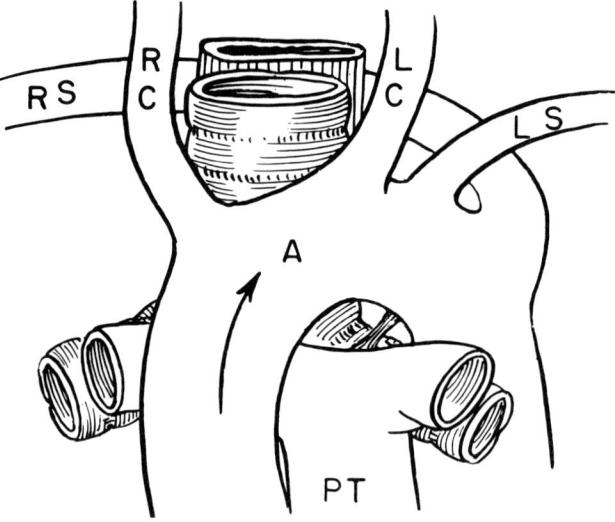

Figure 2.24 Interruption of right arch of Figure 2.22(a) at a level between the right common carotid and right subclavian arteries results in aberrant right subclavian artery arising from the left aortic arch as illustrated. Abbreviations as in Figure 2.22.

Figure 2.23 Interruption of a hypothetical double aortic arch of Figure 2.22(a) at a level distal to the origin of the right subclavian artery yields the pattern of the normal aorta with left aortic arch and left ductus arteriosus. Abbreviations as in Figure 2.22.

innominate artery. In classical double aortic arch, each arch is patent, with the right arch being wider than the left arch.

Most patients born with double aortic arch manifest tracheal and/or esophageal obstruction. The major basis for this is the relatively narrow ring of the aortic arches that encircles the trachea and esophagus. Additionally, the ductus arteriosus may pull and hold the pulmonary arterial bifurcation against the anterior aspect of the trachea.

In instances of **left-sided aortic arch**, the descending aorta is usually left-sided. The anatomic patterns are derived from the double aortic arch with left-sided ductus arteriosus and left descending aorta. In this section, intact left aortic arch will be considered when associated with left-sided descending aorta. When left aortic arch has a left descending aorta, a normal aortic arch exists. Its development may be viewed to result from interruption of the hypothetical right aortic arch (Figure 2.22) distal to the origin of the right subclavian artery (Figure 2.23). This results in creation of an innominate artery as a branch of the normal aortic arch. While this pattern is not associated with any specific condition, it has been claimed that in some cases the innominate artery may cause symptoms of compression of the anterior wall of the trachea.

Variations in origin of systemic branches from the left aortic arch are fairly common. In all except one the branches arise from the vertex of the arch. The most common of these is aortic origin of the left vertebral artery just proximal to origin of the left subclavian artery rather than origin from the subclavian artery. The other common variation is that in which only two arteries arise from the vertex of the aortic arch. From anterior to posterior, these are a common stem for the origin of the innominate and left common carotid arteries followed by origin of the left subclavian artery.

Aberrant right subclavian artery results from division of the hypothetical right arch (Figure 2.22(a)) between the right common carotid and subclavian arteries. Aberrant origin of the right subclavian artery from the left aortic arch occurs in about 0.5% of subjects with left aortic arch. The vessel arises distal to the origin of the left subclavian artery from the posterior aspect of the aorta. From its origin, characteristically, the aberrant right subclavian artery courses from its aortic origin upward and towards the right, passing behind the esophagus (Figure 2.24). The position of the aberrant right subclavian artery with respect to the esophagus may be responsible for peculiar complications. For example, an aneurysm of the artery may rupture into the esophagus. A sharp foreign body in the esophagus may penetrate both the esophagus and aberrant artery so as to lead to major arterial hemorrhage into the esophagus [51]. In a case observed by one of us, aortic dissection occurred in a case with aberrant right subclavian artery. The intramural hematoma of the aortic media extended into the media of the aberrant right subclavian artery.

SYSTEMIC ARTERIES 39

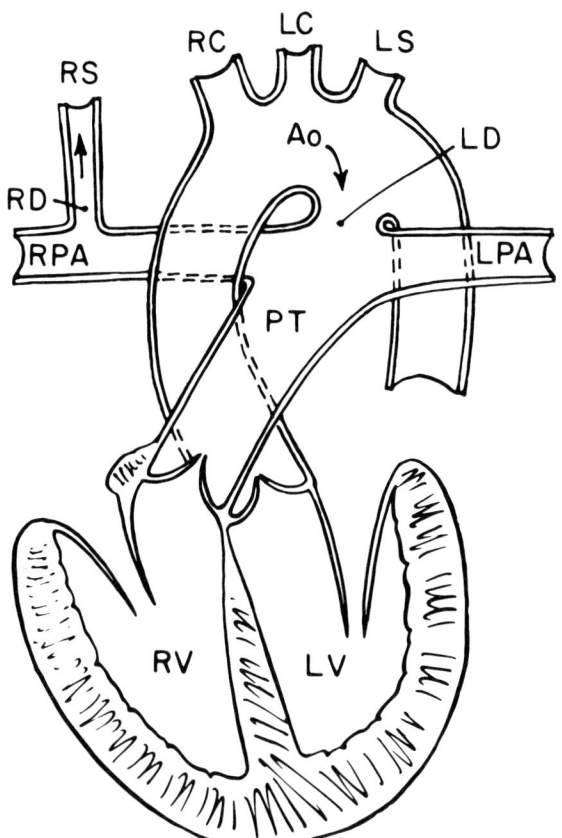

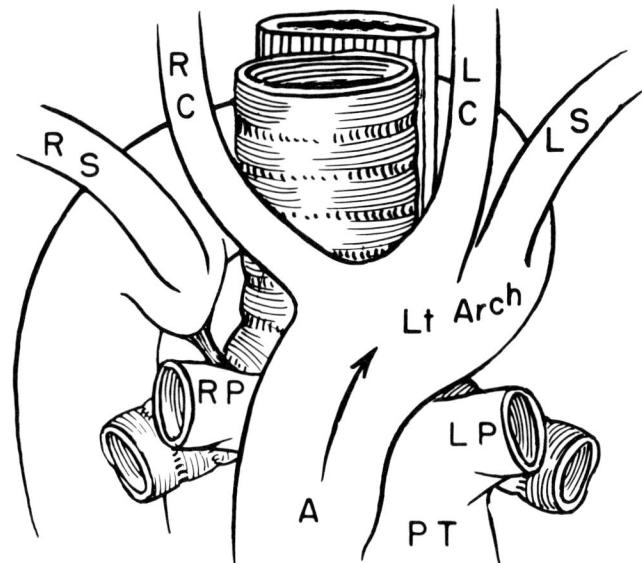

Figure 2.26 Left aortic arch with retroesophageal segment and right descending aorta. This pattern is a cause of constriction of the trachea and esophagus. It may be viewed as resulting from the hypothetical double aortic arch shown in Figure 2.22(b) by interruption of the right arch between the origins of the right common carotid and right subclavian arteries. Abbreviations as in Figure 2.22.

Figure 2.25 Isolation of right subclavian artery. Referring to Figure 2.22(a) an interruption of the right arch between the right common carotid and right subclavian origins and also distal to the union of the right ductus with the right arch results in the right subclavian artery being isolated and joined through the right ductus arteriosus with the right pulmonary artery. Ao = aorta; LC = left carotid artery; LD = left ductus; LPA = left pulmonary artery; LS = left subclavian artery; LV = left ventricle; PT = pulmonary trunk; RC = right carotid artery; RD = right ductus; LPA = right pulmonary artery; RS = right subclavian artery; RV = right ventricle.

The resulting mass compressed the right sympathetic chain causing Horner's syndrome.

Isolation of right subclavian artery may be considered to result from changes in the primitive type of hypothetical double aortic arch (Figure 2.21) in which there is a ductus arteriosus on each side. Deviation of the descending aorta to the left and division of the right arch at two sites, namely between the common carotid and subclavian arteries and distal to the right ductus arteriosus causes loss of the connection of the right subclavian artery to the aorta. The resulting pattern is that of a left arch from which, from before, backwards, arise the right common carotid, left common carotid and left subclavian arteries. The right subclavian artery is 'isolated', arising from the right pulmonary artery through the intervening right ductus arteriosus (Figure 2.25). Isolation of a subclavian artery is un-

common. The isolated subclavian artery arises contralateral to the intact aortic arch. While this condition may be associated with the tetralogy of Fallot, it may appear as an isolated anomaly [52]. Supply of blood to the territory of the isolated subclavian artery comes primarily through collateral branches of the contralateral subclavian artery via vertebral and parascapular arterial branches and ramifications of other branches of the subclavian arteries.

The left aortic arch may have a right descending aorta. Appropriate division in the pattern shown in Figure 2.22(b) of the right aortic arch between its carotid and subclavian branches results in a left aortic arch which passes behind the esophagus to join the right-sided descending aorta. The right subclavian artery arises as the fourth branch of the aorta from a diverticulum that receives the right ductus arteriosus. There is no innominate artery, the left common carotid and subclavain arteries arising from the intact left aortic arch. In the case described by one of us in 1948 [53], symptomatic esophageal compression was present (Figure 2.26).

Right aortic arch may be associated either with a right or left descending aorta. The various known or hypothetical anatomic patterns are mirror images of instances with left aortic arch. The patterns with the characteristic of right arch with right descending aorta are more common than right aortic arch with left descending aorta. The pattern of right aortic arch with

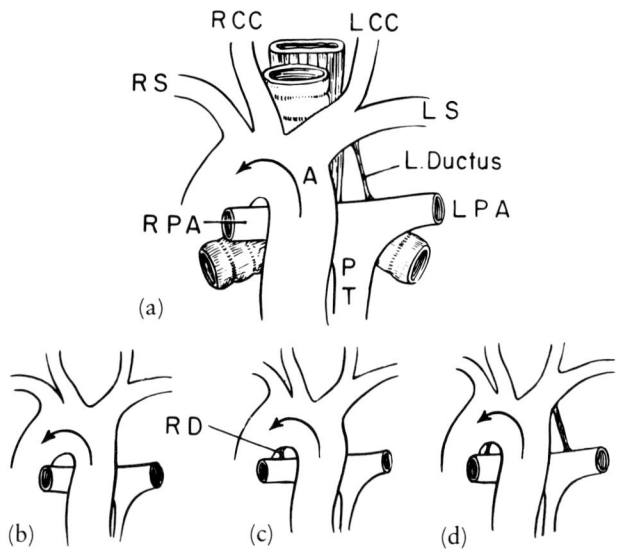

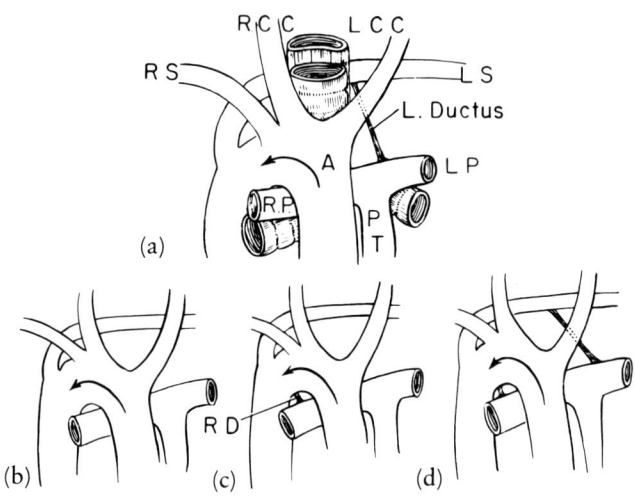

Figure 2.27 Right aortic arch without retroesophageal segment and with right-sided descending aorta. This is associated with mirror image branching. This condition is commonly associated with tetralogy of Fallot. Variations with regard to the ductus arteriosus may occur. (a) Left ductus present; (b) no ductus present; (c) right ductus present; (d) bilateral ducti arteriosi. A = aorta; L. Ductus = left ductus; LCC = left common carotid artery; LPA = left pulmonary artery; LS = left subclavian artery; PT = pulmonary trunk; RCC = right common carotid artery; RD = right ductus; RPA = right pulmonary artery; RS = right subclavian artery.

Figure 2.28 Right aortic arch without retroesophageal segment and with right descending aorta associated with aberrant left subclavian artery. In each instance, the artery passes behind the esophagus. As with Figure 2.27, variations may occur with regard to the presence or absence of the ductus arteriosus, as shown in the lower panel of diagrams. Abbreviations as in Figure 2.27.

right descending aorta has the important feature that there is no retroesophageal segment of aorta [54]. These anomalies are derivatives of the primitive hypothetical aortic arch as shown in Figure 2.22(b). Usually, they are associated with congenital heart disease, of which the most common type is the tetralogy of Fallot. Variations occur with respect to the ductus. In some cases, there is retention of the hypothetical double aorta with bilateral ductus arteriosus. In others, neither ductus is retained, while in some cases only one ductus is retained.

If the left of the hypothetical double aortic arch is divided beyond the origin of the left subclavian artery, the resulting pattern is that of so-called **mirror image branching of right aortic arch without retroesophageal segment** (Figure 2.27). The branches of the right aortic arch from before, backwards, are the left innominate artery, the right common carotid artery and the right subclavian artery. The descending aorta gradually deviates to the left, so that the aortic hiatus in the diaphragm is in normal position. A ligamentum arteriosum or ductus arteriosus may run from the origin of the left subclavian artery, above, to the left pulmonary artery, below. The pattern just described is the most common type of right aortic arch in the tetralogy of Fallot.

Right aortic arch with right descending aorta and aberrant left subclavian artery (Figure 2.28) depends upon division of the left arch of the primitive hypothetical double aortic arch between the left common carotid and subclavian arteries. The left subclavian artery is retroesophageal. Whether or not features of esophageal obstruction are present depends primarily on whether or not a left ductus arteriosus is present. Without this structure being present, the situation is comparable to that of the usual aberrant right subclavian artery. If a left ductus is present, the aberrant left subclavian artery is held against the esophagus, and symptoms of esophageal obstruction may result. A right-sided ductus may be present or absent.

Right aortic arch with isolation of the left subclavian artery (Figure 2.29) is the mirror image of the isolated right subclavian artery described previously. This pattern is derived from altering the primitive hypothetical double aortic arch by division of the left arch anterior to the origin of the left subclavian artery and distal to the union of the left ductus with the left aortic arch. This pattern is the least common type of right aortic arch seen in the tetralogy of Fallot. A right ductus may be present or absent.

Right aortic arch with left descending aorta may be understood more clearly by reference to the hypothetical double aortic arch with left ductus and left descending aorta (Figure 2.22(a)). The pattern of right aortic arch with left descending aorta results from division of the hypothetical left arch between the left common carotid and subclavian arteries (Figure 2.30). The resulting condition which may be called **right aortic arch with retroesophageal segment** is the most common type of right aortic arch in instances of right aortic arch without

SYSTEMIC ARTERIES 41

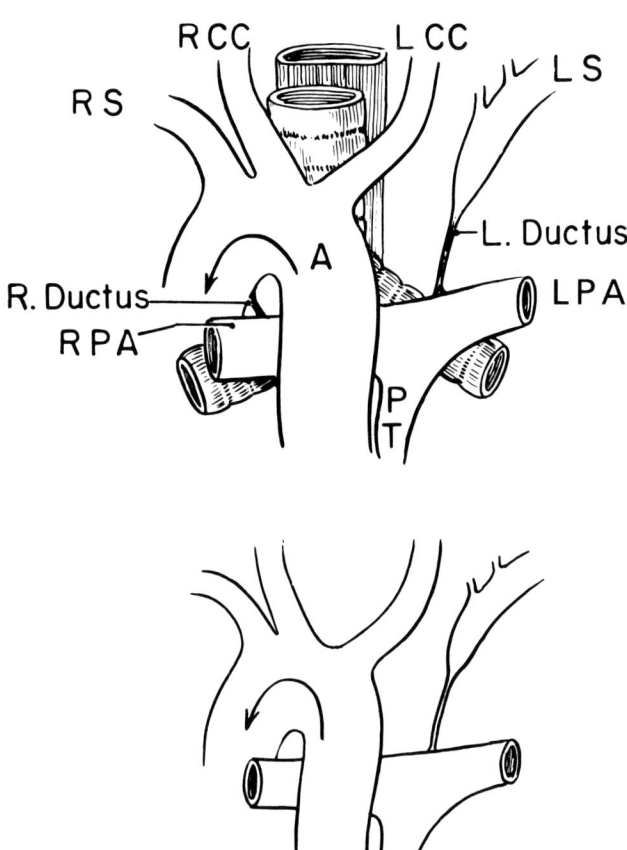

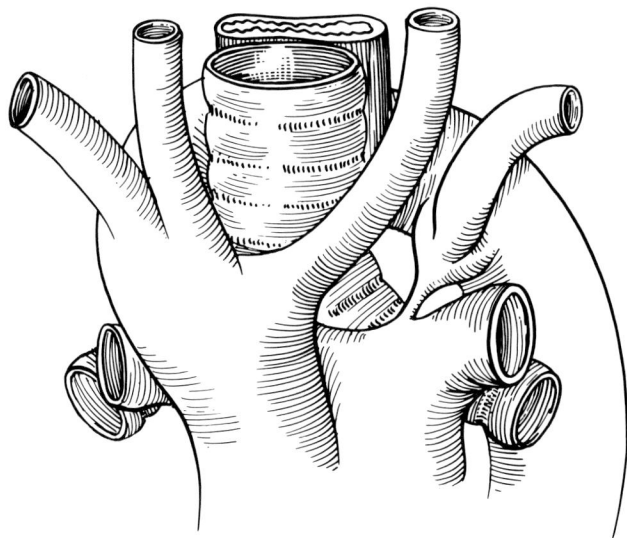

Figure 2.30 Right aortic arch with retroesophageal segment and left-sided descending aorta. The left subclavian artery arises as the fourth branch of the aortic arch. The condition is the result of altering the hypothetical double aortic arch shown in Figure 2.22(a) by division of the left arch between the origins of the carotid and subclavian arteries.

Figure 2.29 Isolation of left subclavian artery associated with right aortic arch. The anomaly results from division of the hypothetical double aortic arch shown in Figure 2.22(b) by division of the left arch both proximal to the origin of the left subclavian artery and distal to the ductus arteriosus. (a) The right ductus is also present. (b) The right ductus is absent. Abbreviations as in Figure 2.27.

congenital heart disease. This pattern often causes compression of the esophagus by the retroesophageal segment of the right aortic arch. The anterior aspect of the trachea may be compressed by the bifurcation of pulmonary trunk as it is held against the trachea by the left ductus arteriosus, the latter running between the left pulmonary artery, inferiorly, and the site (often a diverticulum) of origin of the left subclavian artery, above. Symptoms of esophageal and/or tracheal obstruction may be present or absent. If symptomatic, symptoms tend to develop during infancy. When symptoms occur, the accepted surgical treatment is division of the ductus arteriosus or ligamentum arteriosum.

A word of caution needs to be considered in discussing this anomaly. It is to be recognized that angiography for right aortic arch with left descending aorta (discussed above) will yield essentially the same picture as double aortic arch with atresia of the left arch between the origins of the left common carotid and left

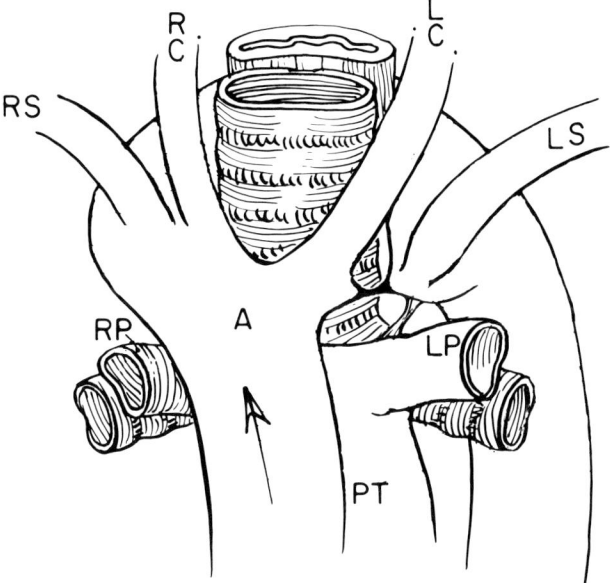

Figure 2.31 Double aortic arch with atresia of the left arch between the left common carotid and left subclavian arteries. This is an important pattern, since it may give rise to the identical angiographic features seen in the anomaly illustrated in Figure 2.30. A = aorta; LC = left carotid artery; LP = left pulmonary artery; LS = left subclavian artery; PT = pulmonary trunk; RC = right carotid artery; RP = right pulmonary artery; RS = right subclavian artery.

subclavian arteries (Figure 2.31). Since such a finding may be considered to indicate a right aortic arch, during surgical exploration it is vital that search for an atretic segment be made. If present, this must be divided.

42 CONGENITAL ANOMALIES OF BLOOD VESSELS

Otherwise, misjudged double aortic arch would be left untreated.

(b) Exceptional patterns

In unusual cases instead of a single ductus arteriosus, two such vessels, so-called double ductus, are present. Another rare state is 'subclavian artery lag' in which the left subclavian artery arises from the descending aorta distal to the level of origin of the ductus arteriosus.

Double ducti arteriosi

Reference to the hypothetical double aortic arch shows a ductus arteriosus on each side (Figure 2.21). Usually, one disappears, but rarely both are present. With double ductus, the ductus related to the intact arch joins the homolateral arch just distal to the site of origin of the subclavian artery. When the ductus is on the side with a divided arch, there is usually an innominate artery on that side. The ductus of that side runs from the base of the subclavian artery, above, to the homolateral pulmonary artery, below. An example of this type has been reported [55]. In an unreported case observed by the late Dr Michael Korns, the primary cardiac anomaly was aortic atresia with intact ventricular septum. A left aortic arch and patent left ductus were present. To the right of the hypoplastic ascending aorta was a narrow vessel that ran between the base of the right subclavian, above, and the right pulmonary artery, below. This vessel was interpreted as a right ductus, the case representing an example of double ductus. In isolation of a subclavian artery, the isolated subclavian artery arises from the homolateral ductus arteriosus on the opposite side of the aortic arch. Among cases with distal ductal origin of a pulmonary artery, there is usually a classical ductus on the side opposite the vessel with distal ductal origin.

Subclavian lag

In early stages of development, the subclavian arteries arise from the homolateral dorsal aorta caudal to the site of insertion of the homolateral sixth aortic arch which becomes, in part, the ductus arteriosus. By the time of birth, the relative positions of these vessels change, so that on the left side the subclavian artery comes to originate proximal to the ductal insertion. If a primitive state persists, in which the left subclavian artery arises distal to the ductal insertion, the state may be called subclavian lag. This uncommon state is seen when coarctation of the aorta lies between the left common carotid and subclavian arteries (Figure 2.32). It has also been observed in some cases of distal ductal origin of a pulmonary artery.

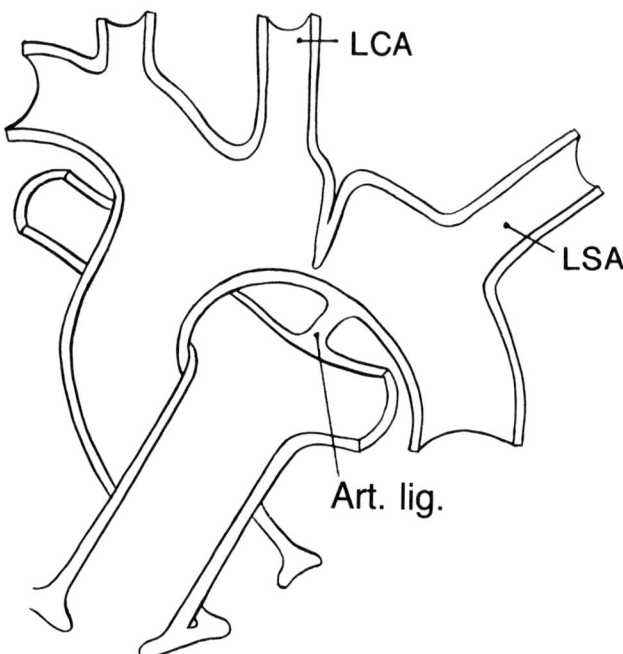

Figure 2.32 Coarctation of the aorta between the origins of the left common carotid and left subclavian arteries. The process is associated with so-called subclavian lag in which the ligamentum arteriosum (or ductus arteriosus) is proximal to the left subclavian artery. Art. lig. = ligamentum arteriosum; LCA = left carotid artery; LSA = left subclavian artery.

Cervical arch

When there is a right aortic arch, either alone or as part of a double aortic arch, the right arch may lie unusually high in the thorax, creating the so-called cervical aortic arch. In this state, its pulsation may be evident at the supraclavicular area. No special functional abnormalities of right aortic arches that present in this fashion occur.

2.2.2 CORONARY ARTERIES

Anomalies of the coronary vessels encompass a large variety of conditions. They will be discussed in two groups, namely coronary arteries originating from the aorta, and all or part of the coronary arterial system originating from a pulmonary artery.

(a) Arteries originating from aorta

Ectopic origin of coronary artery

Ectopic origin of a coronary artery from the aorta is a term appropriately applied to two states: *high origin* and *origin from a 'wrong aortic sinus'*. In high origin, the vessel arises above the appropriate aortic sinus. From its high origin (Figure 2.33), the vessel has a sharp angle with the aortic wall as it descends toward the level

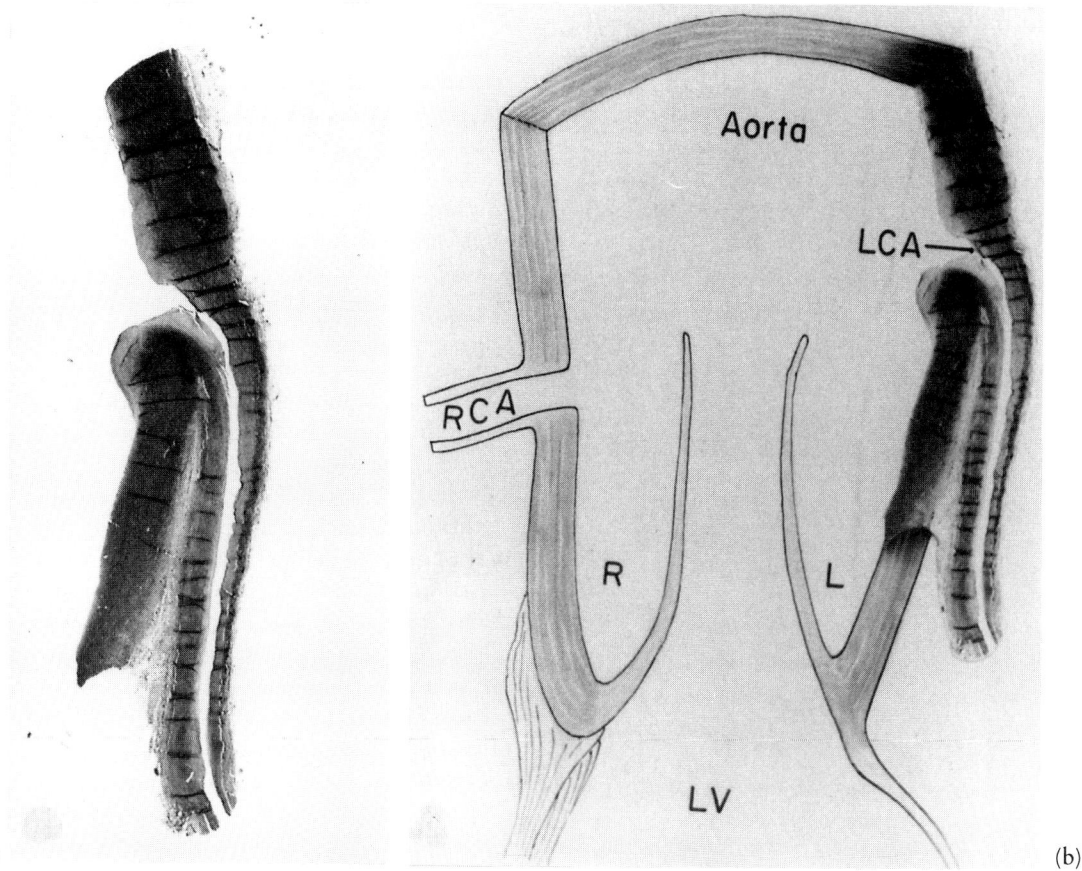

(a)   (b)

Figure 2.33 High origin of the left coronary artery. The origin of the left coronary artery in a high position yields an acute angle between the aorta and the arterial wall as shown in (a). In (b), the photomicrograph illustrated in (a) is used to create a collage showing not only the high origin but also the relative angular origin of the high, ectopic origin left coronary artery. L = left aortic sinus; LCA = left coronary artery; LV = left ventricle; R = right aortic sinus; RCA = right coronary artery. (Reproduced with permission from Tuna [136].)

of normal origin. The sharp angle of origin creates a flap composed of adjacent parts of aorta and coronary artery. It has been postulated that this flap may cause stenosis of the arterial ostium during diastole. Signs of ischemic disease may be apparent in that region of the left ventricle supplied by the abnormally arising coronary artery [56,57] (Figure 2.33). Several possibilities exist for a coronary arterial segment arising from the 'wrong' sinus (Figure 2.34). The most common pattern is that the left circumflex artery arises from the right aortic sinus, or occasionally from the right coronary artery. The anterior descending coronary artery arises from the left aortic sinus. From its ectopic origin, the left circumflex proceeds along the posterior and left lateral aspects of the ascending aorta to reach the left atrioventricular sulcus. Isolated cases of sudden death have been observed among subjects with this condition.

Less common than the condition just described is that in which the right coronary artery arises from the left aortic sinus and that in which the left coronary artery arises from the right aortic sinus (Figure 2.34). In each of these conditions, the ectopically arising artery often passes between the ascending aorta and pulmonary trunk as it courses from its origin to either the right atrioventricular sulcus (for the right artery), or the anterior interventricular sulcus (for the left coronary artery). At the ectopic origin, the coronary artery makes an acute angle with the aorta, yielding a flap composed of the aorta and the artery. Sudden death, usually during exercise, has been observed among individuals with ectopic origin of the right or the left coronary artery. It is claimed that sudden death is more likely when the ectopically arising artery is the left.

Single coronary artery

When the entire coronary arterial system connects with the aorta and there is only one coronary arterial ostium in the aorta, the condition is single coronary artery. Numerous patterns of distribution and branching from a single coronary artery occur. One of these is presence

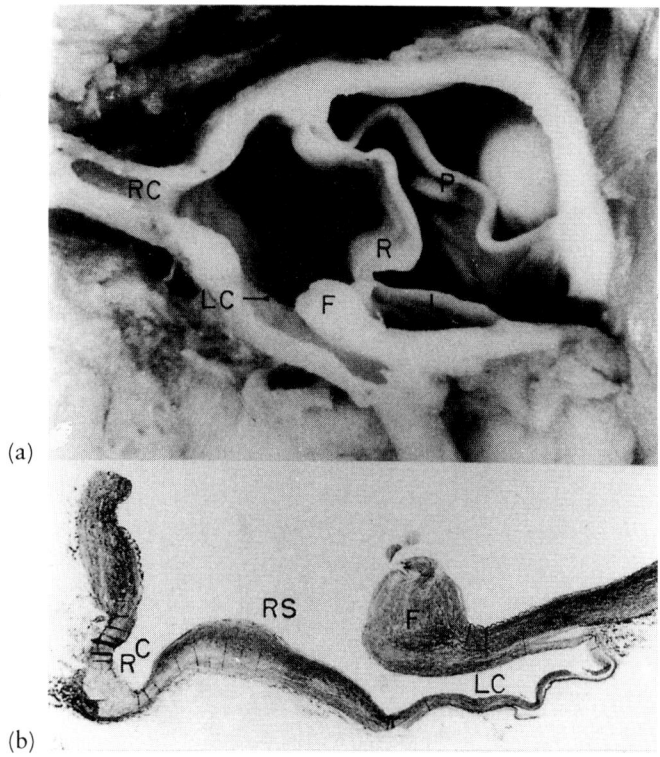

Figure 2.34 Origin of a coronary artery from the 'wrong' sinus. (a) The aortic valve and coronary arteries are viewed from above. The right coronary artery arises from the right aortic sinus, as does the left coronary artery. The left coronary artery arising anomalously makes an acute angle with the aorta, with a flap of tissue protruding into the ostium of the left coronary artery. (b) Photomicrograph of right aortic sinus. The flap formed by the anomalously arising left coronary artery is considered to be a basis for diastolic obstruction of the anomalously arising left coronary artery. RS = right aortic sinus; F = flap; LC = left coronary artery; RC = right coronary artery; L, P and R = left, posterior and right aortic cusps, respectively. (Reproduced with permission from Mahowald et al. [137].)

of the usual arteries, with the ostium of one being atretic and not identifiable [58]. Through collaterals, the artery that does not communicate with the aorta receives its blood supply from the artery that does arise from the aorta. A common pattern is that one of the vessels has a normal origin and the 'absent' vessel arises from it. From this origin, for example, an 'absent' left coronary artery may course in the epicardium across the right ventricular infundibulum to reach an appropriate location.

Stenosis of origin

In some cases of so-called single coronary artery, the 'absent' vessel may be, in part, identified as an atretic strand without an associated sign of an ostium in the aorta. In a case described by Price and associates [59], an infant presented with clinical features like those in origin of the left coronary artery from the pulmonary trunk with the exception that studies did not demonstrate communication of left coronary artery and pulmonary trunk. The basis for arterial stenosis was a proliferative process of the artery, including its ostium. In the ascending aorta there may be histologic features displaying a mosaic pattern suggesting a *forme fruste* of supravalvular aortic stenosis.

Communication of a coronary artery with a vessel or cardiac chamber

The condition in which two usual coronary arteries arise from the aorta but one communicates with a vessel (either the coronary sinus or the pulmonary trunk) or a cardiac chamber [60] (Figure 2.35) generally has clinical significance. In the classical situation, the parent vessel of the communication is as wide as the branch leading to the communication. Beyond the communicating branch the artery is of normal diameter or more narrow. In the dilated segment it is not uncommon that one or more saccular aneurysms may develop. These are often of the pseudoaneurysm type, with gaps in the media and foci of calcium being common.

Since the communications are essentially of the arteriovenous type, the conditions exist for the development of collateral flow into the low pressure areas distal to the communication. Contribution of flow into the site of shunt come from branches of the coronary system not involved in the primary communication, as well as from mediastinal vessels that communicate with coronary arteries in the visceral pericardium over the ascending aorta.

Communications of coronary arterial source with the left ventricle tend to be multiple, while those to the other chambers or pulmonary trunk tend to be single. In instances of coronary arterial communications with the pulmonary trunk it is common that collaterals from both coronary systems contribute to the shunt. This results in an arcade of vessels over the base of the heart and pulmonary trunk (Figure 2.36).

It is recognized that in pulmonary atresia with intact ventricular septum and competent tricuspid valve, there may be numerous communications between the right ventricle and the coronary arterial system. Similarly, multiple communications may exist between the left ventricle and coronary arterial system in instances of aortic atresia, intact ventricular septum and competent mitral valve.

(b) Coronary arteries originating from the pulmonary trunk

One or both coronary arteries may arise from the pulmonary arterial system. The most common conditions are anomalous origin from the pulmonary trunk.

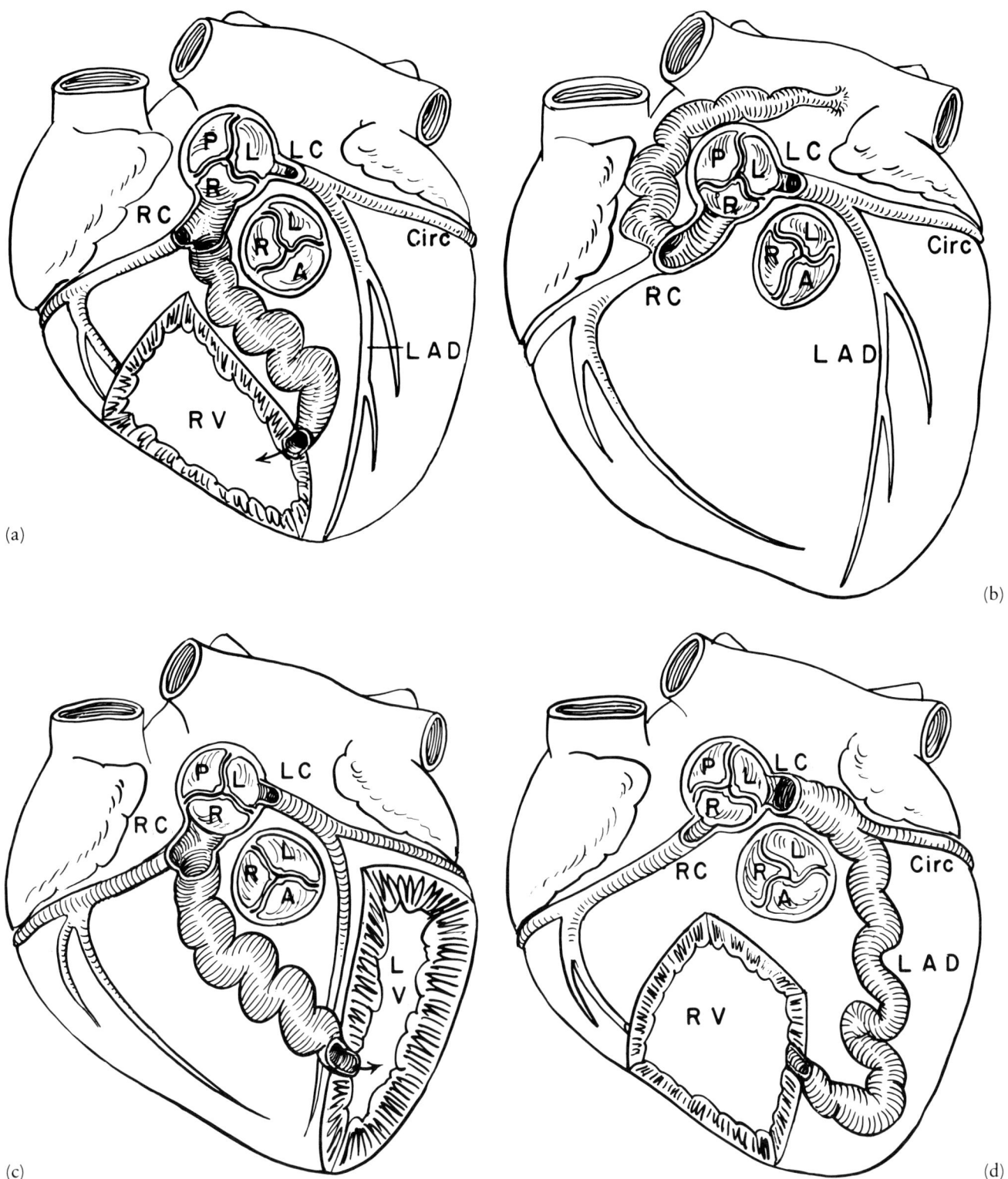

Figure 2.35 Examples of anomalous communication of a coronary artery with a cardiac chamber. (a) Right coronary artery communicating with right ventricle; (b) right coronary artery communicating with left atrium; (c) right coronary artery communicating with left ventricle; (d) anterior descending coronary artery communicating with right ventricle. Circ = circumflex coronary artery; LAD = left anterior descending coronary artery; LC = left coronary artery; RC = right coronary artery; RV = right ventricle; P, A, R, and L = posterior, anterior, right and left cusp, respectively. (Reproduced with permission from Vlodaver et al. [138].)

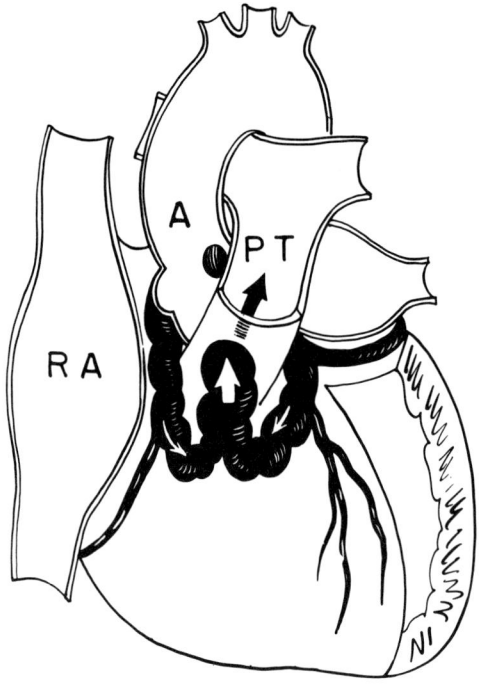

Figure 2.36 Anomalous origin of a coronary artery from the pulmonary trunk communicating with branches of normally arising right and left coronary arteries. A = aorta; PT = pulmonary trunk; RA = right atrium.

Uncommonly, the anomalous origin of a coronary artery may be from the right pulmonary artery rather than from the pulmonary trunk. Another uncommon form is origin of the anterior descending coronary artery from the pulmonary trunk, while the left circumflex artery arises from the aorta.

Left coronary artery

Origin of the left coronary artery from the pulmonary trunk is the most common anatomic pattern when part of the coronary system arises from the pulmonary arterial system (Figure 2.37). The consequence of the anomaly is based upon ischemic disease in the distribution of the left coronary artery. During fetal life, when there are equal pressures in the aorta and pulmonary trunk, the direction and volume of coronary flow is normal. After birth, with the normal fall in pulmonary arterial pressure, reduced flow occurs into the myocardium normally supplied by the anomalous artery; commonly, little or no flow occurs from the pulmonary trunk into the left coronary artery (Figure 2.37(a)). A collateral system is developed in which multiple pre-existent connections between ramifications of the left and right coronary arterial systems become enlarged. Flow occurs from the right coronary system into the bed of the left coronary system, so that blood from the aortic-arising right coronary artery is carried into the ramifications of the left system. From the left coronary system, some of the blood is shunted into the pulmonary trunk (Figure 2.37(b)). As a consequence of this 'short circuiting' of blood that is characteristic of arteriovenous fistula, the left ventricular myocardium is ischemic.

The functional consequences of origin of a coronary artery from the pulmonary arterial system include myocardial infarction, mitral regurgitation and varying degrees of left ventricular failure. While some newborns die from this condition, commonly patients may not manifest any clinically recognized abnormality until about three months of age. Pain while feeding, failure to thrive and cardiac enlargement are among the manifestations that first lead to suspicion of a cardiac problem. Certain functional abnormalities may characterize age groups as reported by Wesselhoeft and associates [61]. During infancy, symptomatic patients exhibit anginal symptoms or signs of congestive heart failure. In children and older infants, mitral insufficiency is a common form of presentation. Older children and adults may have a continuous murmur on the basis of left-to-right shunts through collaterals between the right and left coronary arterial systems. Sudden death may occur in some adults.

Right coronary artery

Anomalous origin of the right coronary artery from the pulmonary trunk is both less common and less troublesome than anomalous origin of the left coronary artery. Commonly, the condition is observed in adults either at autopsy or at angiography. While it is commonly taught that origin of the right coronary artery from the pulmonary trunk is a benign condition, it is interesting that of the reported cases it is not uncommon that the subjects are relatively young men who died suddenly and unexpectedly [62].

Both coronary arteries

Origin of both coronary arteries from the pulmonary trunk is a rare condition. Without certain associated anomalies, death classically occurs in the neonatal period [63]. Feldt and associates [64] reported the case of a 7-year-old girl in whom the entire coronary arterial system, through a single coronary artery, arose from the pulmonary trunk. This feature was not identified until an associated ventricular septal defect (preoperative pulmonary arterial pressure 100/42) was closed. After this procedure, appropriate circulation could not be maintained and death occurred.

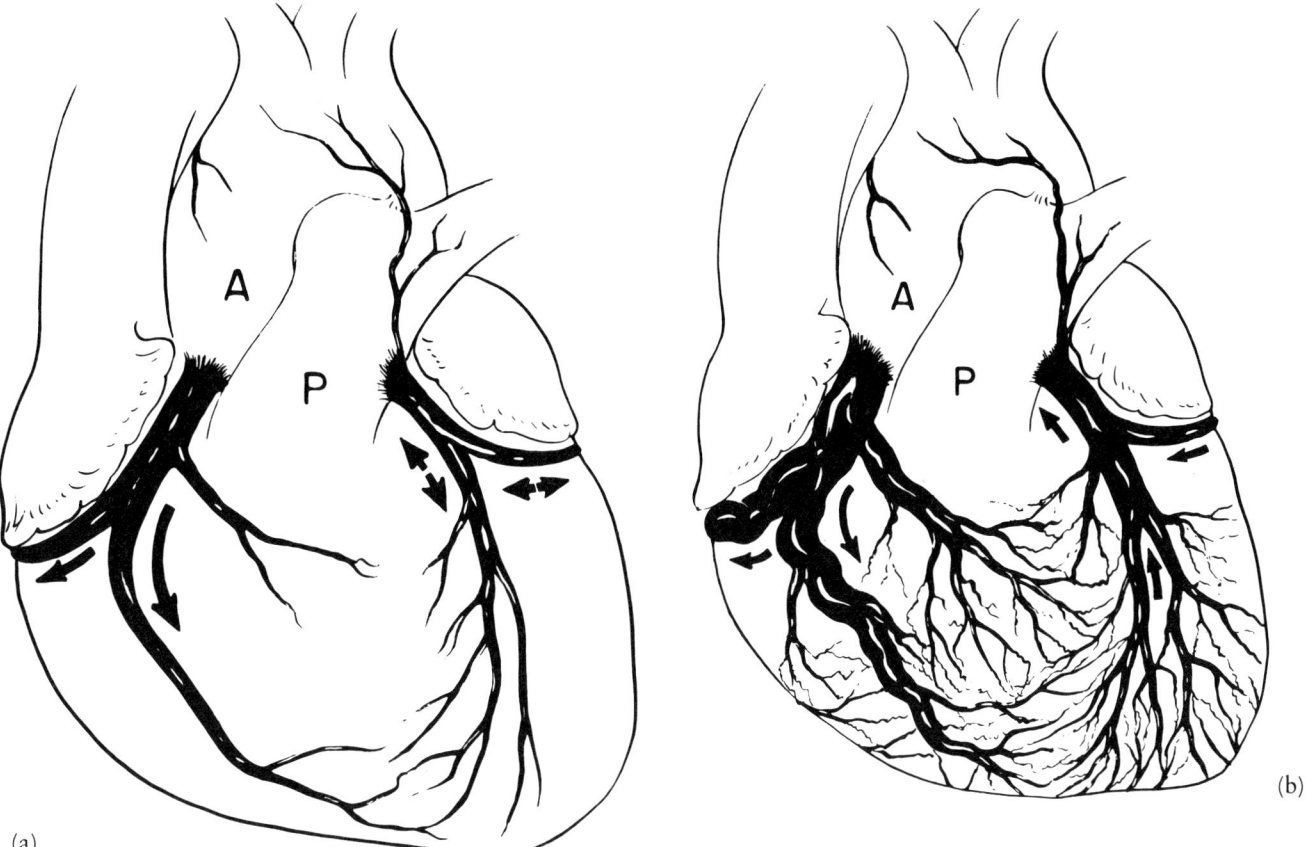

Figure 2.37 Origin of left coronary artery from the pulmonary trunk. Arrows in relation to the left coronary arterial branches indicate the direction of flow under certain circumstances. (a) Mainly in the young, there may be flow from the pulmonary trunk into the left coronary arterial system. (b) In the established situation of major collateral flow between the two coronary arteries, the flow is from the right coronary artery, through collateral branches into the left system, with ultimate delivery of aortic blood into the pulmonary trunk. A = aorta; P = pulmonary trunk.

2.3 Pulmonary arteries

2.3.1 PULMONARY TRUNK

Among the anomalies of the pulmonary trunk are idiopathic dilatation, obstruction of the lumen, communication with the aorta and origin of coronary arteries from this segment of the pulmonary arterial system. The latter two subjects have been presented in earlier sections.

(a) Idiopathic dilatation

The pulmonary trunk may be dilated as a consequence either of elevated hemodynamic pressure or flow, or response to pulmonary stenosis (post-stenotic dilatation). Idiopathic dilatation of the pulmonary trunk, as the name implies, is not associated with the usual causes just named. The condition may be a *forme fruste* of the Marfan syndrome [65], with histologically demonstrable cystic medial necrosis [66]. Pulmonary valvular insufficiency, usually well tolerated [67], has been observed in 29 and 25% of cases reported by Brayshaw and Perloff [68] and by Ishikawa and Seki [69], respectively. This condition may represent a complication of the dilated state of the pulmonary trunk. Pulmonary valvular insufficiency, if present, is well tolerated by the patient.

(b) Luminal obstruction

Obstruction of the lumen of the pulmonary trunk may be either stenosis or atresia. Atresia and certain forms of stenosis of the pulmonary trunk characteristically are associated with an intracardiac anomalous state, usually ventricular septal defect and other features of the tetralogy of Fallot. In such an association, stenosis of the pulmonary trunk takes the form of a more or less uniform narrow caliber to the vessel where the wall is normal. When atresia involves the entire length of the vessel, the atretic vessel may be represented by an identifiable cord-like structure, or no such structure may be found (Figure 2.38). The left and right pulmonary arteries are identifiable as confluent vessels. If the

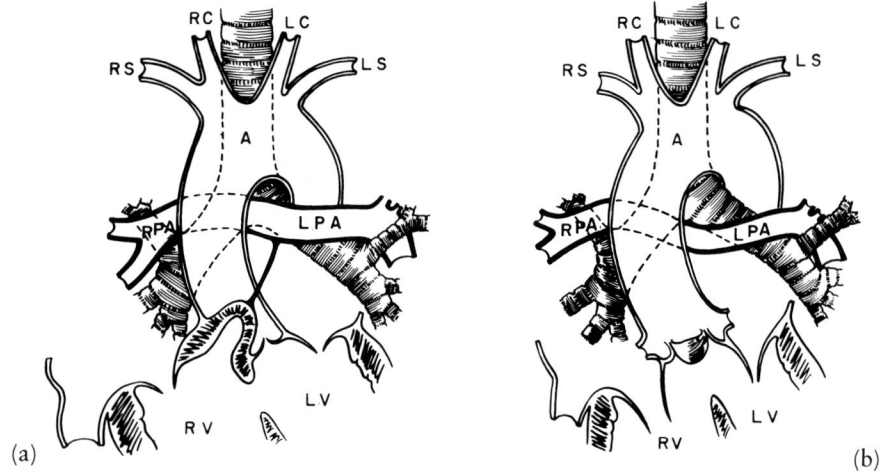

Figure 2.38 Ventricular septal defect associated with atresia of the pulmonary trunk. (a) The pulmonary trunk is identified as an atretic cord. (b) The pulmonary trunk is not identifiable. A = aorta; LC = left carotid artery; LPA = left pulmonary artery; LS = left subclavian artery; LV = left ventricle; RC = right carotid artery; RPA = right pulmonary artery; RS = right subclavin artery; RV = right ventricle. (Reproduced with permission from Edwards and McGoon [139].)

pulmonary trunk cannot be identified and the left and right pulmonary arteries are shown to exhibit 'distal ductal origin' (see previous discussion), the single arterial vessel at the base of the heart is considered to be a **solitary aortic trunk** [70].

In the absence of intracardiac malformations, stenosis of the pulmonary trunk usually is part of the syndrome of supravalvular aortic stenosis. The changes are uniform thickening of the media of the pulmonary trunk with corresponding encroachment upon the lumen. The process in the pulmonary trunk commonly is associated with the hypoplastic type of supravalvular aortic stenosis [71]. Stenosis of peripheral pulmonary arteries may be associated.

2.3.2 PULMONARY ARTERIAL BRANCHES

The pulmonary arterial branches are subject to anomalous origin, stenosis or atresia.

(a) Anomalous origin

The subject of anomalous origin of pulmonary arterial branches from the aorta has been covered in an earlier section of this chapter. In this section, those anomalies of pulmonary arteries in which the pulmonary arteries arise from the pulmonary trunk will be covered.

In **crossed pulmonary arteries**, the pulmonary arteries arise either from the pulmonary trunk or from a persistent truncus arteriosus in such a way that the ostia of the two branches are malplaced (Figure 2.39). The right pulmonary artery arises to the left of and at a lower level than the origin of the left pulmonary artery. Having such origins, the pulmonary arteries cross one another as they proceed to their respective lungs

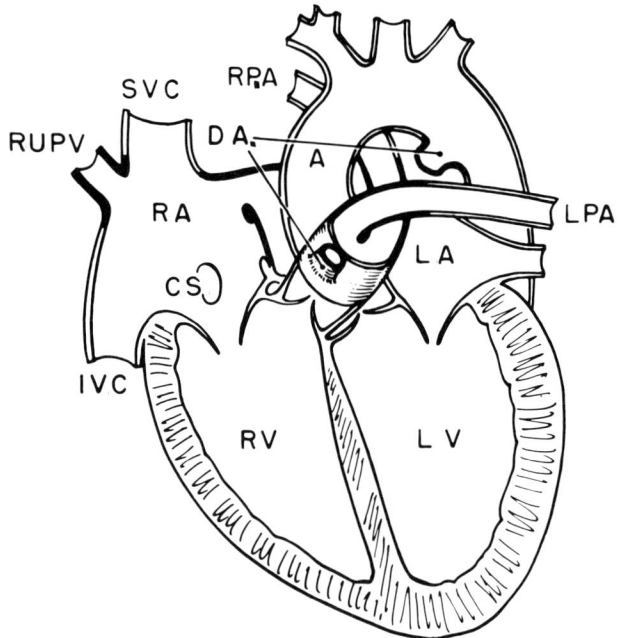

Figure 2.39 Crossed pulmonary arteries from a case in which an atrial septal defect was associated with anomalous connection of right upper pulmonary vein to the right atrium. LPA and RPA = left and right pulmonary arteries, respectively; A = aorta; CS = coronary sinus; DA = ductus arteriosus; IVC = inferior vena cava; LA = left atrium; LPA = left pulmonary artery; LV = left ventricle; RA = right atrium; RPA = right pulmonary artery; RUPV = right upper pulmonary vein; RV = right ventricle; SVC = superior vena cava. (Reproduced with permission from Edwards [140].)

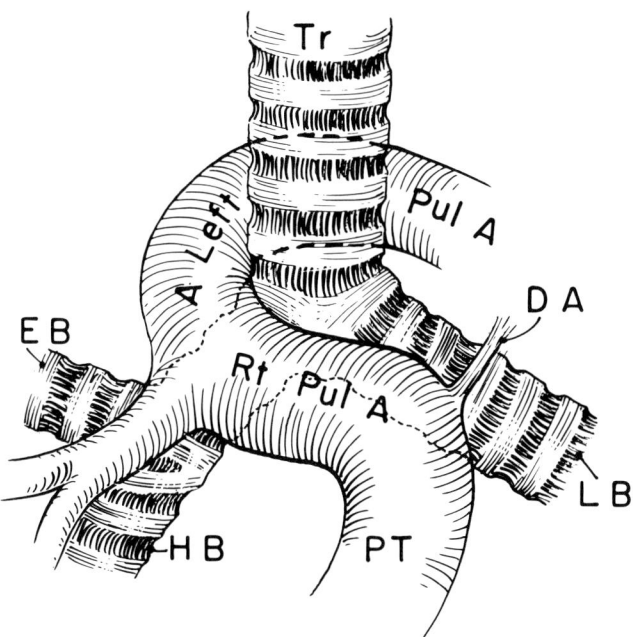

Figure 2.40 Pulmonary vascular sling associated with normal branching of the trachea. The left pulmonary artery arises from the right pulmonary artery and passes in the angle between the trachea and the right main bronchus to cross toward the left lung. PT = pulmonary trunk; EB and HB = eparterial and hyparterial bronchi of right lung, respectively; LB = left main bronchus; Rt = right; Pul A = pulmonary artery; Tr = trachea; DA, ductus arteriosus. (Reproduced with permission from Jue et al. [74].)

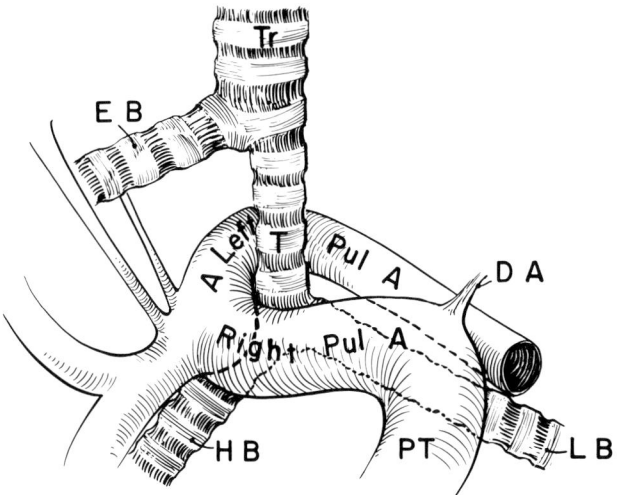

Figure 2.41 Pulmonary arterial sling associated with bronchus suis. The eparterial bronchus (bronchus suis) arises independently from the trachea. Under this circumstance, the angle over which the anomalous left pulmonary artery passes is formed by the lower segment of the trachea and the origin of the hyparterial (intermediate) bronchus. DA = ductus arteriosus; EB = eparterial bronchus; T and Tr = trachea; HB = hyparterial bronchus; LB = left bronchus; Pul A = pulmonary artery; PT, pulmonary trunk. (Reproduced with permission from Jue et al. [74].)

[72,73]. The ductus arteriosus occupies a normal position, originating from the proximal segment of the left pulmonary artery. When the condition of crossed pulmonary arteries is associated with persistent truncus arteriosus, reported cases usually have associated interruption of the aortic arch [72]. No functional abnormality is attributed to crossed pulmonary arteries.

Pulmonary vascular sling is characterized by origin of the left pulmonary artery from the right pulmonary artery [74,75]. After its origin, the left pulmonary artery proceeds posteriorly over the angle formed by the origin of the right main bronchus and trachea. The left pulmonary artery then turns towards the left lung, passing between the trachea, in front, and the esophagus, behind, to the hilus of the left lung (Figure 2.40). Indentation of the anterior aspect of the esophagus is a characteristic roentgenographic feature of this condition. If the right bronchial tree has the anomaly of **bronchus suis** in which the right upper bronchus arises from the trachea before the trachea bifurcates into the left main stem and the right intermediate bronchi, the anomalous left pulmonary artery passes over the intermediate bronchus (Figure 2.41). Congenital heart disease may be associated with pulmonary vascular sling, the most common type being the tetralogy of Fallot [76].

(b) Obstruction

Obstruction of pulmonary arterial branches may take the form of stenosis or atresia.

Stenosis

Stenosis involving pulmonary arterial branches is characterized by focal obstruction or obstructions that may involve the origins of the main pulmonary arterial branches and/or one or more foci in secondary and tertiary branches. Localized pulmonary stenosis is uncommon. D'Cruz and associates [77] found only 84 cases among approximately 2000 patients in whom diagnostic cardiac catheterization, angiocardiography, or both, had been done. Delaney and Nadas [78] during a 7-year experience at the Children's Medical Center, Boston, found only 17 cases among subjects between the ages of 9 months and 13 years. From limited published data on the condition, the process appears to be caused by focal intimal proliferation that encroaches upon the lumen. MacMahon and associates [79] additionally observed medial thickening of involved peripheral segments.

Using angiographic data, D'Cruz and associates [77] divided the lesions into four types: localized stenosis with poststenotic dilatation, segmental stenosis, diffuse hypoplasia and multiple peripheral stenoses. These authors observed that among their 84 cases the stenosis was unilateral in 32 (38%) and bilateral in 52 (62%). Association with maternal rubella has been recognized [80]. Association with cardiovascular anomalies is more common (about two-thirds of cases) than with normally developed hearts. Commonly associated anomalies include ventricular septal defect and pulmonary valvular stenosis [77,78]. Less common conditions are supravalvular aortic stenosis, aortic coarctation, and the tetralogy of Fallot [81]. When not associated with intracardiac anomalies, pulmonary arterial stenosis, if severe, may be confused with primary pulmonary hypertension [82].

Atresia

Atresia of a pulmonary arterial branch may be focal or diffuse. Diffuse atresia of a pulmonary artery often, but not universally, is associated with atresia of the pulmonary trunk and with the intracardiac features of the tetralogy of Fallot. In pulmonary arteries that show 'distal ductal origin of a pulmonary artery', atresia may be present either in focal or diffuse nature. Regardless of the site of origin of a diffusely atretic pulmonary artery, whether from the pulmonary trunk or by distal ductus origin, there is usually patency of the vessel at the pulmonary hilus [12].

2.4 Systemic veins

The clinical implications of anomalies of the systemic veins related to the heart vary. Some may have little or no functional effect. Others are associated with marked systemic arterial desaturation [83].

2.4.1 SUPERIOR VENA CAVAL SYSTEM

The most common anomaly involving the superior vena caval system is that in which there are two (right and left) superior venae cavae. Among such cases there are two basic patterns, one in which the left superior vena cava joins the coronary sinus, the condition commonly called persistent left superior vena cava, and the other in which each superior vena cava joins the homologous atrium, the condition commonly called bilateral superior venae cavae or junction of left superior vena cava with left atrium.

(a) Persistent left superior vena cava

In this condition [84], the left internal jugular vein, after joining the left subclavian vein, descends as a left superior vena cava. It descends anteriorly to the left pulmonary hilus above which the hemiazygos vein joins

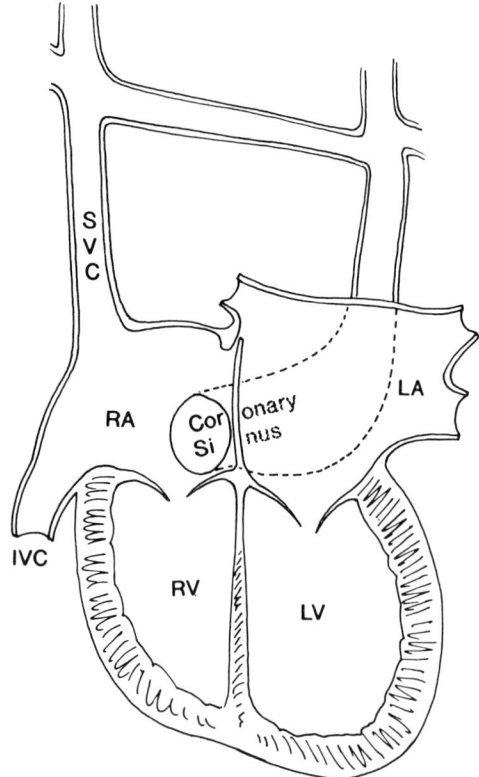

Figure 2.42 Classic example of persistent left superior vena cava. The left cava joins the coronary sinus from which blood is delivered to the right atrium. IVC = inferior vena cava; LA = left atrium; LV = left ventricle; RA = right atrium; SVC = superior vena cava.

it. As this vein lies near the heart, it descends from near the base of the left atrial appendage along the posterior aspect of the left atrial wall to reach the left atrioventricular sulcus. Here, it blends with the lateral extremity of the coronary sinus. The latter is unusually wide (Figure 2.42). In normal hearts not having a persistent patent left superior vena cava, the atretic remnant of the lower left superior vena cava lies along the posterior aspect of the left atrium as a cord called the obliterated vein of Marshall. In some normal hearts, there may be persistence only of the terminal part of the left superior vena cava, represented as a patent vein running from the lower aspect of the obliterated vein of Marshall to the lateral aspect of the coronary sinus. Such a vein is termed the oblique vein of Marshall.

It is estimated that among subjects without congenital heart disease the incidence of classical persistent left superior vena cava is about 0.3% [85]. Among individuals with congenital heart disease, the incidence is probably higher, being estimated to occur in the range of 2.8–4.3% [86].

The situation with regard to a 'bridging vein' between the two superior venae cavae varies. In about 40% of cases with persistent left superior vena cava, a bridging vein is absent, while in the remainder it is present.

An uncommon variation in the anatomic pattern of persistent left superior vena cava is that in which the lower segment of the right superior vena cava is either absent, or less commonly represented by an atretic strand. In this pattern, the blood from the right innominate vein is carried into the persistent left superior vena cava through a 'bridging innominate vein' [87]. We have, rarely, observed this variation in normally formed hearts.

(b) Left superior vena cava to left atrium

When the left superior vena cava joins the left atrium, it does so near the base of the left atrial appendage. This state is most common in the asplenic and polysplenic syndromes. In the asplenic syndrome, the atrial septum is represented by a strand which, for practical purposes, equals the presence of no atrial septum. Raghib and associates [88] described a syndrome in which the left superior vena cava joined the left atrium of a four chambered heart. Associated with this venous anomaly was absence of the coronary sinus and an atrial septal defect at the usual location of the ostium of the coronary sinus. In this congenital syndrome, persistent common atrioventricular canal may be present. In that case, the atrial septal defects of the two conditions join and form one large defect in the lowermost part of the atrial septum.

2.4.2 INFERIOR VENA CAVA

Anomalies of the inferior vena cava are uncommon. The subject has been reviewed and a classification offered by Edwards [89]. The more common anomalies are a bilateral state and left-sided inferior vena cava.

(a) Continuity with azygos or hemiazygos vein ('interruption of inferior vena cava')

In this condition, superior to the union of the renal veins, the inferior vena cava deviates posteriorly to the right to join the azygos vein (Figure 2.43), accounting for the term 'azygos continuity of the inferior vena cava'. The azygos vein joins the superior vena cava in the usual position. The hepatic veins unite to form a common hepatic vein which joins the right atrium at the usual location of the inferior vena caval ostium. Classically, azygos continuity of the inferior vena cava is associated with polysplenia and its related cardiovascular anomalies [90]. In the authors' experience, the one exception was observed in a dog in which one spleen was present, and there was inferior vena caval continuity with the azygos vein. The portal vein was absent, and the venous drainage of the abdominal viscerae was into the inferior vena caval system [91].

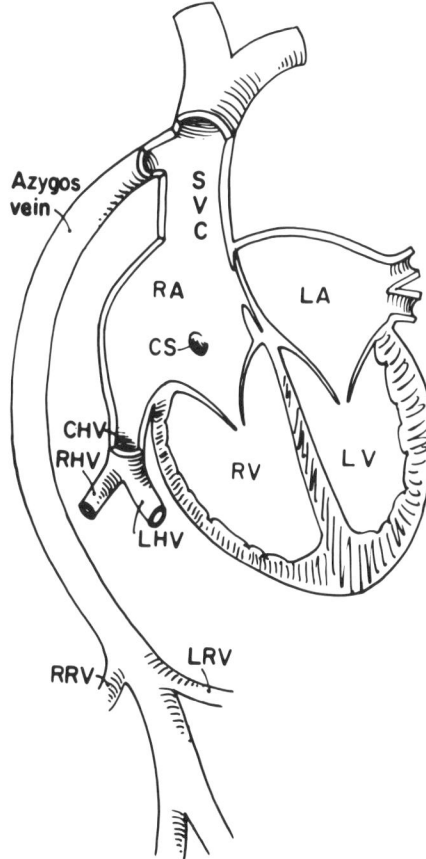

Figure 2.43 Continuity of inferior vena cava with azygos vein, so-called interruption of the inferior vena cava. Hepatic veins join to form a common vein which, in turn, leads to the right atrium. CHV = common hepatic vein; CS = coronary sinus; LA = left atrium; LHV = left hepatic vein; LRV = left renal vein; LV = left ventricle; RA = right atrium; RHV = right hepatic vein; RV = right ventricle; RRV = right renal vein; SVC = superior vena cava.

A comparable state also occurs when the inferior vena cava is left-sided. In this circumstance, the inferior vena cava joins the hemiazygos vein. The latter joins a left superior vena cava which, in turn, terminates in the coronary sinus (Figure 2.44).

(b) Termination in left atrium

In 1961, Meadows and associates [92] found by angiographic study in a cyanotic man that the drainage of all of the inferior vena caval blood was into the left atrium. The authors considered their case the second reported one of inferior vena caval connection with the left atrium in the absence of intracardiac anomalies. The earlier case was that of Gardner and Cole [93]. Iatrogenically, the inferior vena cava may be carried into the left atrium during closure of an atrial septal defect at the fossa ovalis. Cyanosis not present preoperatively becomes manifest postoperatively [94].

52 CONGENITAL ANOMALIES OF BLOOD VESSELS

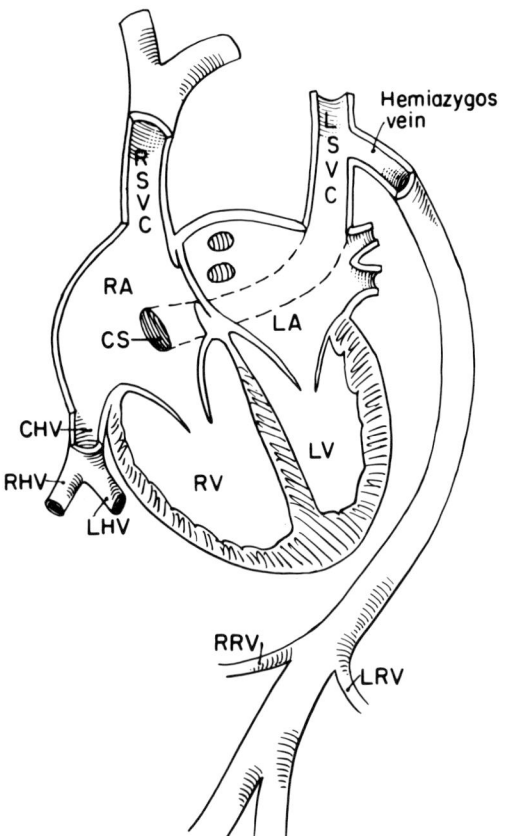

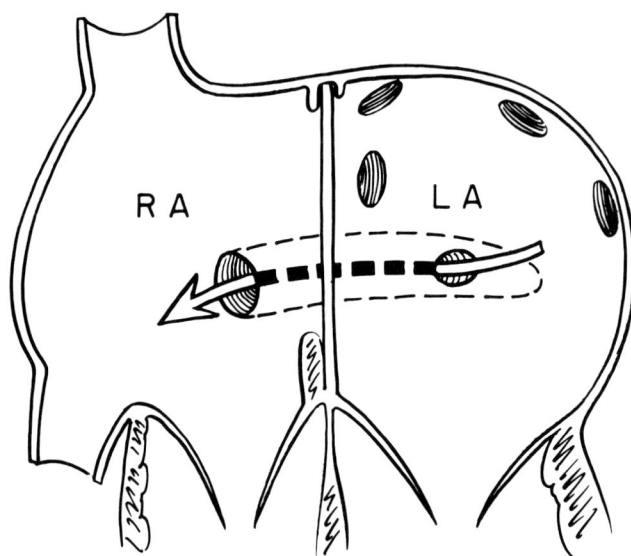

Figure 2.44 Left-sided inferior vena cava showing continuity with the hemiazygos vein. The latter, in turn, joins the left superior vena cava which terminates in the coronary sinus. Abbreviations as in Figure 2.43. LSVC and RSVC = left and right superior venae cavae, respectively.

Figure 2.45 Communication of coronary sinus with the left atrium. The anterior wall of the coronary sinus and the corresponding part of the posterior wall of the left atrium are absent, allowing the left atrial cavity to communicate with the coronary sinus. The illustration shows one such communication. In some cases, several openings of the type shown here are present. LA = left atrium; RA = right atrium.

2.4.3 BOTH VENAE CAVAE TERMINATING IN LEFT ATRIUM

Rarely, both venae cavae join the left atrium [95,96]. Cyanosis is common. In the case of Gueron and associates [97] involving an extremely cyanotic 15-year-old boy, the condition was associated with an atrial septal defect and a hypoplastic right atrium. Correction resulted from removal of the atrial septum and replacement with an atrial septum of pericardial tissue. The case of Miller and associates [98] was similar, with the exceptions that the coronary sinus drained into the left atrium and the left, rather than the right, superior vena cava drained into the left atrium. Repair was similar in both cases.

2.4.4 CORONARY SINUS

Anomalies of the coronary sinus are uncommon. Some of the conditions may be considered as anatomic variants rather than anomalies.

(a) Termination of left superior vena cava

In section 2.4.1(a), it was pointed out that a persistent left superior vena cava usually terminates in the left extremity of the coronary sinus (Figure 2.42). In this state, the coronary sinus is unusually wide [99]. Accentuation of the width of the coronary sinus also occurs in those cases of the polysplenic cardiac syndrome in which there is inferior vena caval continuity with the hemiazygos vein and the presence of a left superior vena cava [90].

(b) Communication with a coronary artery

Among the anomalies of the coronary arteries is coronary arterial–coronary sinus communication (fistula). In this state, the coronary sinus is wide on the basis of abnormal delivery of arterial blood into it. Major complications are congestive cardiac failure and myocardial infarction in the territory of the involved artery [100].

(c) Communication with left atrium

The main portion of the coronary sinus is in the upper part of the atrioventricular sulcus in relation to the left atrium. An unusual anomaly is that in which one or more openings are present between the coronary sinus and left atrium [101] (Figure 2.45). Without associated anomalies, the functional results of such communication seems to be trivial. In instances of atresia of an atrioventricular valve and an inadequate opening in the atrial septum, the communication may serve as a vital channel for delivery of blood from one atrium to the other.

(d) Atresia of right atrial ostium

Uncommonly, the right atrial ostium of the coronary sinus is atretic. Usually, this results from union of the edges of the Thebesian valve with the lining of the orifice. Two possible categories of channels exist for delivery of blood from the coronary sinus to the atria. Less commonly, there is an associated persistent left superior vena cava [102]. Through this, the coronary sinus blood is carried retrograde in the left superior vena cava, across the bridging innominate vein into the right superior vena cava and finally to the right atrium. More commonly, a left superior vena cava is absent. Blood from the coronary sinus appears to be delivered through connections of Thebesian veins with each atrium. Rarely, an associated communication between the coronary sinus and the left atrium (see above) allows emptying of the coronary sinus.

(e) Absence

When a left superior vena cava joins the left atrium directly, there is no coronary sinus. In those cases with a recognizable atrial septum there is an atrial septal defect at the usual location of the right atrial ostium of the coronary sinus. Most instances of absence of the coronary sinus occur in two conditions. One of these is the syndrome described by Raghib and associates [88] of union of the left superior vena cava with the left atrium, absence of the coronary sinus and atrial septal defect. The other is that seen in the splenic cardiac anomalies, particularly asplenia [103]. When there are bilateral superior venae cavae, junction of a left superior with the left atrium is less common in polysplenia than in asplenia [104].

2.5 Pulmonary veins

Anomalies of the pulmonary venous system include anomalous connections, stenosis and pulmonary veno-occlusive disease.

2.5.1 ANOMALOUS CONNECTIONS

Anomalous connections of pulmonary veins embrace a wide variety of conditions, including anomalous connection between one (partial) or all (total) of the pulmonary veins and systemic veins or the right atrium, and anomalous connection between pulmonary veins either of the same or contralateral lung.

(a) Partial anomalous connection

In the classical situation of partial anomalous pulmonary venous connection, one or more pulmonary veins terminate anomalously, while the other pulmonary veins join the left atrium normally. The condition may be simply an isolated condition of non-specific form or where partial anomalous connection of the pulmonary venous system forms part of a syndrome.

Non-specific forms

Uncommonly, a pulmonary vein, usually the left upper vein, connects anomalously, usually to the left innominate vein. Less commonly, the right upper vein joins the superior vena cava. No specific intracardiac anomaly is associated, although an atrial septal defect at the fossa ovalis may be present. Classically, there is minor disturbance in circulatory efficiency.

Anomalous right pulmonary veins and sinus venosus atrial septal defect

Most commonly in this syndrome, veins from the right upper lobe fail to join the left atrium and instead join either the superior vena cava or the right atrium near the superior vena caval–right atrial junction (Figure 2.46). An atrial septal defect superior to the fossa ovalis and straddled by the superior vena cava is part of this developmental complex. The functional effects are like those of atrial septal defect [105]. Repair may lead to injury of the sinoatrial node.

Scimitar syndrome

Here, a crescent-shaped vein of the right lung descends to join the inferior vena cava (Figure 2.47). The curvature recognized in thoracic roentgenograms accounts for the name applied to the condition [106]. The presence of a vein of the right lung leading to the inferior vena cava usually is part of a syndrome that includes hypoplasia of the right lung and pulmonary arteries, maldevelopment of the bronchial system and part of the arterial supply of the right lung derived from systemic arteries [107,108]. The mediastinal structures may be shifted to the right depending upon the degree of hypoplasia of the right lung. The atrial septum may be intact [109] and show a valve-competent foramen ovale or, uncommonly, an atrial septal defect [109].

The hypoplastic right lung may exhibit one, two or three lobes. In some instances, the broncho-arterial relationships in the right lung are essentially mirror images of those in the left lung. This formation was observed in two of four cases of the scimitar syndrome studied by Gikonyo and associates [110]. Abnormalities in bronchial branching are common. Diverticula of

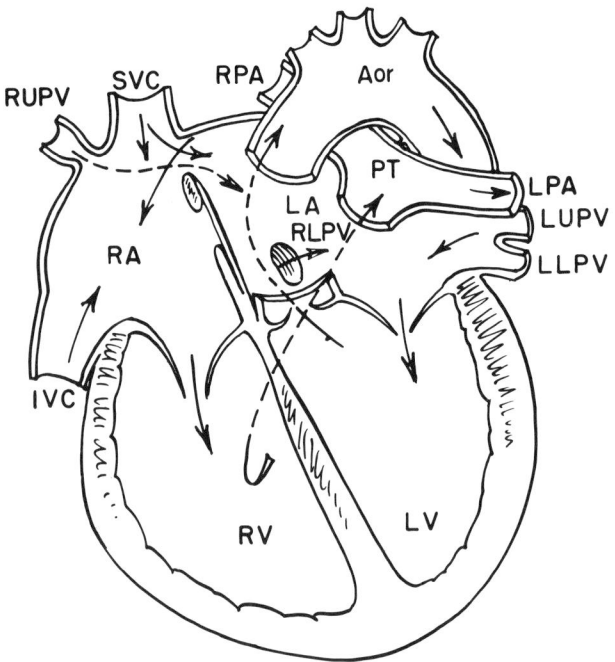

Figure 2.46 Communication of right upper pulmonary vein with right atrium in sinus venosus atrial septal defect. Aor = aorta; IVC = inferior vena cava; LA = left atrium; LPA = left pulmonary artery; LLPV = left lower pulmonary vein; LUPV = left upper pulmonary vein; LV = left ventricle; PT = pulmonary trunk; RA = right atrium; RPA = right pulmonary artery; RUPV = right upper pulmonary vein; RV = right ventricle; SVC = superior vena cava. (Reproduced with permission from Edwards [140].)

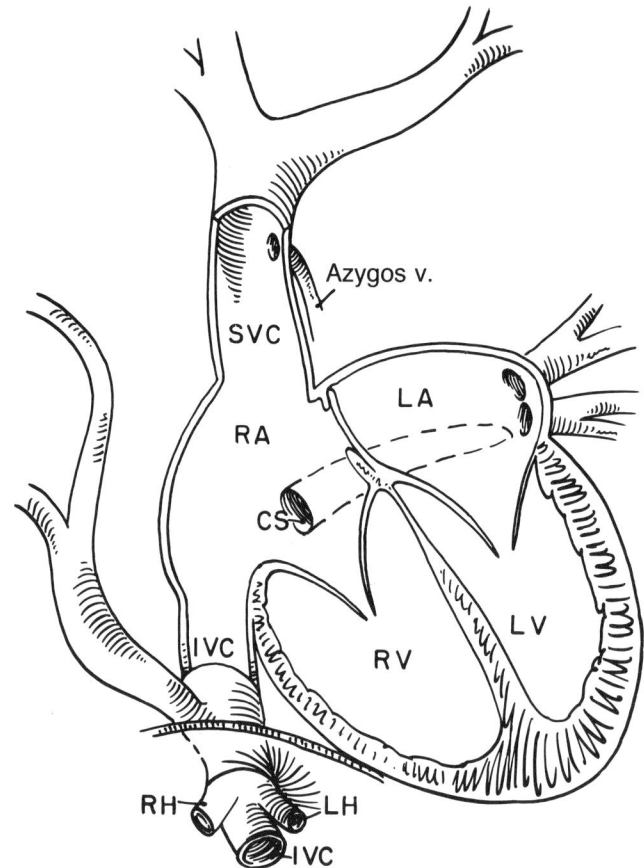

Figure 2.47 Scimitar syndrome: termination of the right lower pulmonary vein in the inferior vena cava. Azygos v. = azygos vein; CS = coronary sinus; IVC = inferior vena cava; LA = left atrium; LH and RH = left and right hepatic veins, respectively; LV = left ventricle; RA = right atrium; RV = right ventricle; SVC = superior vena cava; v = vein. (Reproduced with permission from Edwards [140].)

bronchi according to Halasz and associates [107] are acquired changes secondary to infection. It appears that all units of the lung are supplied by bronchi and are aerated, thereby excluding from consideration the subject of pulmonary sequestration. It is common, however, as with sequestration of the lung, that the right lung receives, but not necessarily exclusively, arterial supply from the aorta by multiple branches arising either from the lower thoracic or, more commonly, from the abdominal aorta. The upper part of the right lung usually is supplied by a hypoplastic pulmonary artery. In the segments supplied by systemic arteries the arterial branches in the lung follow the course of the pulmonary arteries.

The abnormal vein of the scimitar syndrome descends in the major fissure and receives tributaries from one, two or three lobes. Usually it pierces the diaphragm to join the nearby inferior vena cava, but in some instances, connection to the inferior vena cava occurs above the diaphragm. In rare cases, there have been two anomalous veins side by side. In the review of Kiely and co-workers [108], in each of eleven patients the scimitar vein was believed to drain all the lobes on the right, but in eight others all or part of the right upper lobe drained into the left atrium. The right lower lobe always had abnormal drainage. In a case of Frye and associates [109], the scimitar vein joined the common hepatic vein in an instance in which the inferior vena cava showed 'azygos continuity'. In two cases observed at operation by Mohiuddin and associates [111], the scimitar vein had a branch connecting to the left atrium, either directly or through a post-atrial chamber. Scimitar syndrome has apparently been observed on the left side [112]. Diaphragmatic anomalies have been described in about 20% of cases.

Congenital heart disease has been associated with the scimitar syndrome in about 25% of the reviewed cases [108,110] of all ages. Among neonates, the frequency of associated congenital heart disease is higher, being 56% in the study of Gikonyo and coworkers [110]. These authors pointed out that the presence of congenital heart disease may be a major factor in bringing patients to medical attention earlier than those patients without associated congenital heart disease. This concept was supported by the study of Jue and associates [113], in which of 22 patients in the pediatric age with the scimitar syndrome, 36% had congenital heart disease.

Frye and associates [109] emphasized that variations occur from conditions just discussed. These include a normal right lung and absence of the commonly present aberrant arteries to the right lung from the aorta. In some cases, a prominent curved vein in the right pulmonary field of chest roentgenograms is not necessarily a pulmonary vein joining the inferior vena cava. Among such cases are anomalous connection between the veins of one lobe to another [114]. In the case of Dische and associates [115], in a subject with a horseshoe lung, the right pulmonary veins joined the right atrium.

Right pulmonary veins in polysplenic cardiac syndrome

In polysplenia, it is common, though not universal, that anomalous pulmonary venous connection to the right atrium may occur. This may involve all of the pulmonary veins or only the right pulmonary veins.

(b) **Total anomalous connection**

Total anomalous pulmonary venous connection refers to the state in which the entire pulmonary venous compartment is connected to the systemic venous system, either at a systemic vein or to the right atrium. Although the types usually are classified on an anatomic basis, the functional consequences also are dependent on the presence or absence of obstruction to pulmonary venous flow. Accordingly, obstructions will be considered in the different anatomic types. Classification of total anomalous pulmonary venous obstruction uses the anatomic site of termination of pulmonary venous blood. Three types, considered the usual, are supracardiac, cardiac and infracardiac. A fourth type includes variations from those three common types.

Supracardiac

In the supracardiac types of total pulmonary venous connection, the usual pulmonary veins leave the lungs. In the mediastinum, these join a common pulmonary venous recess or chamber-like structure. From the upper aspect of the common pulmonary venous recess, a vein (emanating vein) ascends to terminate in a systemic vein of the upper portion of the thorax. In order of decreasing frequency these terminations are the left innominate vein (Figure 2.48), the superior vena cava and the azygos vein [116].

In anomalous connection to the left innominate veins, the emanating vein ascending from the common pulmonary venous recess has been called the vertical vein as it ascends to terminate in the left lateral aspect of the left innominate (sometimes called bridging) vein.

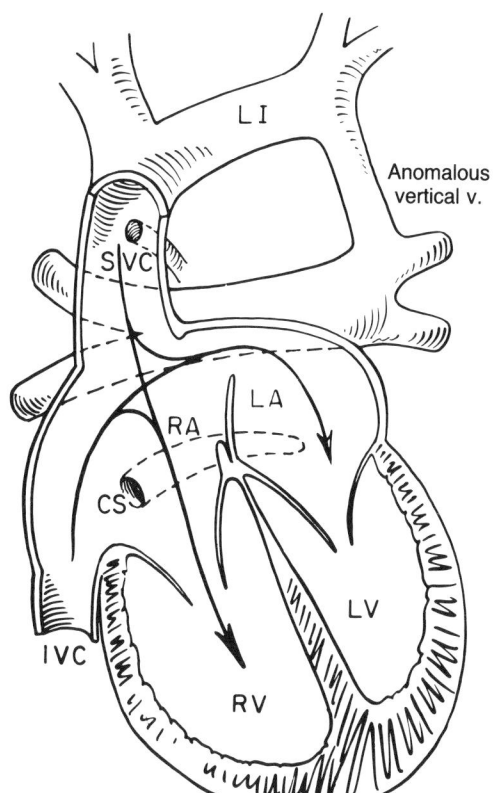

Figure 2.48 Total anomalous pulmonary venous connection to the left innominate vein. Abbreviations as in Figure 2.47; LI = left innominate vein. (Reproduced with permission from Edwards [140].)

Classically, the ascending vein runs anterior to the left pulmonary hilus. As a consequence of the delivery of all of the pulmonary venous blood into the left innominate vein, the latter is uncommonly wide. It may be evident as a radiologic supracardiac shadow which, together with that of the heart, forms the so-called 'figure of eight' or 'snowman shadow'. The ascending vertical vein has been called a left superior vena cava, but for several reasons we prefer to refer to this as an ascending vertical vein.

In those cases of total anomalous pulmonary venous connection to the left innominate vein when the ascending vertical vein is not narrow and runs anterior to the pulmonary hilus, there usually is no sign of pulmonary venous obstruction. If the ascending vein runs between the left pulmonary artery, anteriorly, and left bronchus, posteriorly, signs of pulmonary venous obstruction are common. These result primarily from compression of the ascending vein by a 'hemodynamic vise' [117]. The ascending vein, regardless of its course, may show focal zones of intimal tissue proliferation that cause stenosis [118,119].

Total anomalous pulmonary venous connection to the superior vena cava usually involves the right superior vena cava; rarely the connection is to a true persistent

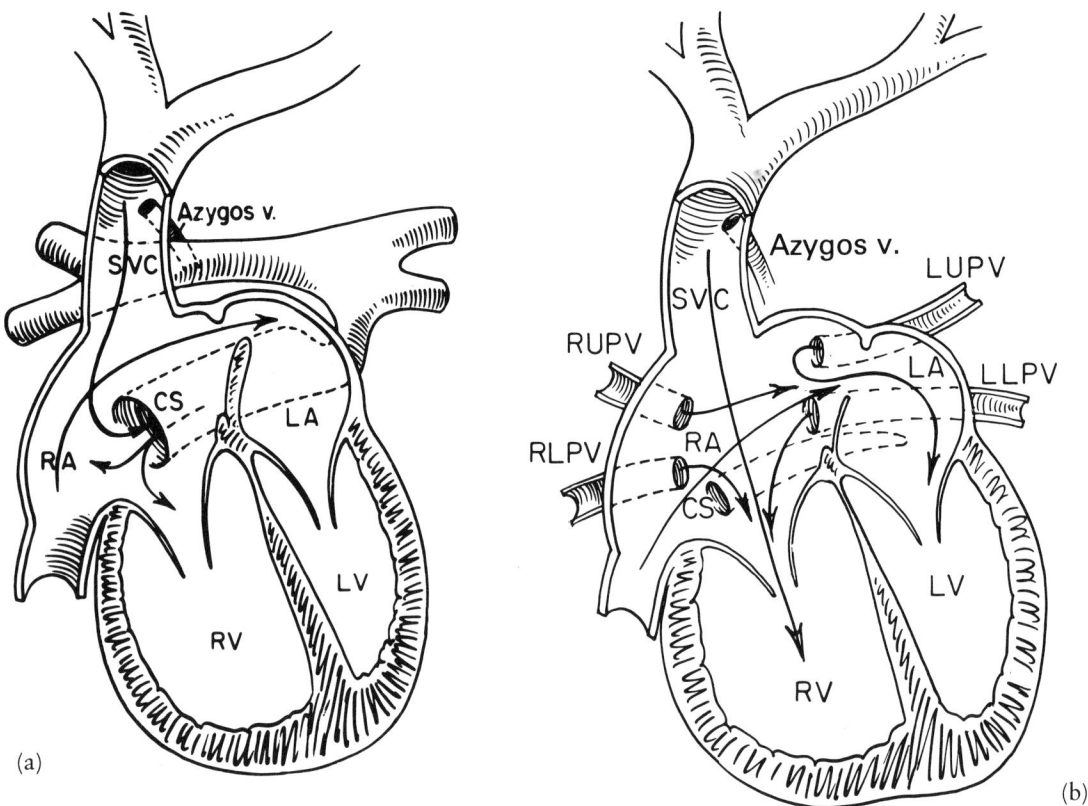

Figure 2.49 (a) Total anomalous pulmonary venous connection to the coronary sinus. (b) Total anomalous pulmonary venous connection to the right atrium (RA) from a case of polysplenia. Abbreviations as in Figure 2.47; LLPV and LUPV = left lower and left upper pulmonary veins, respectively; RLPV and RUPV = right lower and right upper pulmonary veins, respectively. (Reproduced with permission from Edwards [140].)

left superior vena cava that terminates in the coronary sinus. Total anomalous pulmonary venous connection to the superior vena cava usually is not attended by features of pulmonary venous obstruction. When present, it results either from intrinsic stenosis of the emanating vein, or from an associated hemodynamic vise because the anomalous vein passes between the right pulmonary artery and right bronchus.

Total anomalous pulmonary venous connection to the azygos vein is rare.

Cardiac

Total anomalous pulmonary venous connection of the cardiac types are two in number. In one, the pulmonary venous blood is carried into the coronary sinus (Figure 2.49(a)). In the other, the individual pulmonary veins connect anomalously to the right atrium (Figure 2.49(b)). In total anomalous pulmonary venous connection to the coronary sinus, the basic anatomic arrangement is like that in the other types of connection to a systemic vein. The pulmonary venous confluence is drained by a channel that opens into the coronary sinus. The coronary sinus is huge, resembling a separate cardiac chamber.

Usually, the right atrial ostium of the coronary sinus is wide, so that pulmonary venous obstruction is not a feature of this anomaly. The second form of the cardiac type of total anomalous pulmonary venous connection is that in which the pulmonary veins individually join the right atrium without forming an extra cardiac confluence. The condition might be viewed as the veins making normal connections with the atrial portion of the heart except that the atrial septum is misplaced to the left. Pulmonary venous obstruction does not occur. This type of total anomalous pulmonary venous connection appears to be restricted to the polysplenic cardiac syndrome.

Infracardiac

The infradiaphragmatic types of total anomalous pulmonary venous connection share certain features. A confluence of pulmonary veins as seen in the supracardiac types is present. Usually, one vein (the emanating vein) leaves the confluence, descends beside the esophagus, and enters the abdominal cavity, alongside the esophagus through the esophageal hiatus of the diaphragm. In the abdominal cavity, variations occur as

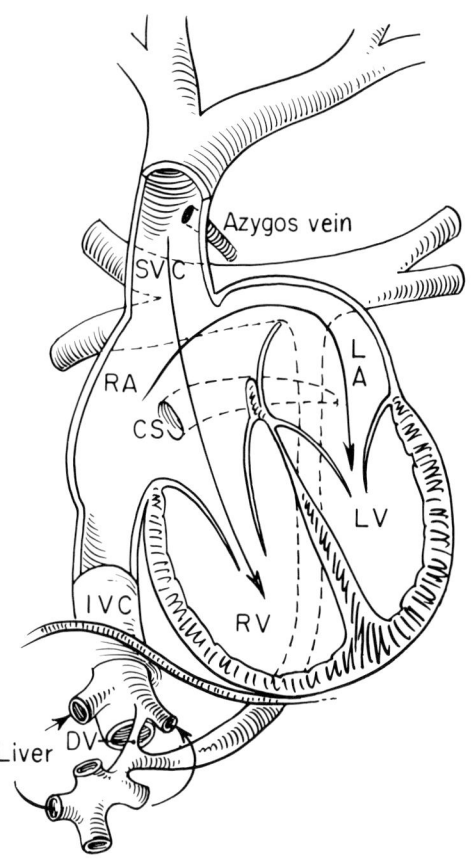

Figure 2.50 Total anomalous pulmonary venous connection to the ductus venosus. Abbreviations as in Figure 2.47; DV = ductus venosus. (Reproduced with permission from Edwards [140].)

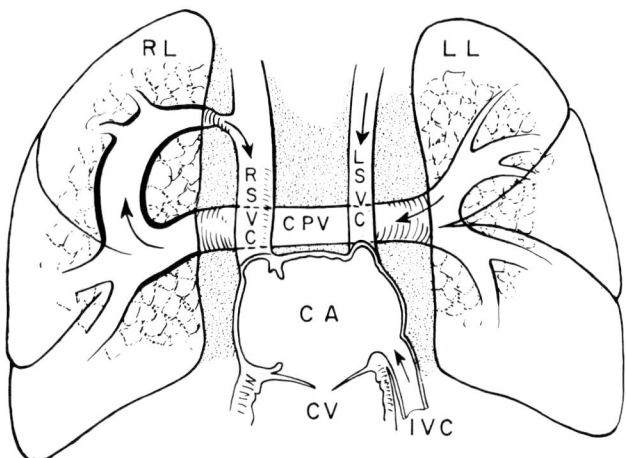

Figure 2.51 Anomalous connection of pulmonary veins from both lungs to right superior vena cava, from a case of asplenia with a common atrium. A vein crosses the mediastinum to connect the veins of both lungs. CA = common atrium; CPV = common pulmonary vein; IVC = inferior vena cava; LL = left lung; LSVC = left superior vena cava; RL = right lung; RSVC = right superior vena cava. (Reproduced with permission from Everhart et al. [114].)

to site of termination of the descending vein. Common sites of termination are the ductus venosus and the portal vein (Figure 2.50). Less commonly, the left gastric or the superior mesenteric vein may be the site of termination. Uncommonly, the descending vein may branch and have more than one site of delivery of pulmonary venous blood. A rare exception to the solitary descending trunk, as observed by Kanjuh and associates [121], is characterized by two pulmonary venous confluences, one for each lung. From each confluence, a separate vein descends through the diaphragm, one to terminate in the portal vein and the other in the ductus venosus. Infradiaphragmatic total anomalous pulmonary venous connection usually is associated with severe, major pulmonary venous obstruction.

Variations from the usual types

These are characterized by one of three basic features [121]: multiple levels of termination with one or more trunk per level; one level of termination by two trunks; solitary trunk with subdivisions and multiple terminations.

From our laboratory was reported a condition which we termed atresia of the common pulmonary vein [122]. The individual pulmonary veins joined to form a confluence as in classical total anomalous pulmonary venous connection. The variation from the classical condition is that no gross vein emanates from the confluence. It is probable that the pulmonary venous drainage is from many hilar veins that join multiple veins in the esophageal wall. Major pulmonary venous hypertension is characteristic.

It is uncommon that there are gross connections within a given lung between veins of one lobe and another. Usually, such connections are within the substance of the lung and are not apparent from extraparenchymal dissections. Such connections result from obstruction in major venous channels. The obstruction may be in a lobar vein or within the heart, as was demonstrated by Shone and Edwards in instances of mitral atresia [123]. In some such instances there may be anomalous termination of a pulmonary vein in a systemic vein.

Pulmonary veins may connect to the contralateral lung, when there is no outlet for blood from one lung. There may be both intrapulmonary connections between veins of one lung and also a vein from one lung may cross the mediastinum to enter the opposite lung and terminate in a vein in the second lung (Figure 2.51). In observed cases, intrapulmonary venous connections of the second lung have been present, and ultimately anomalous connection with a systemic vein, thereby completing a complex route for the flow of blood from each lung [124].

A connection may exist between the left atrium and a

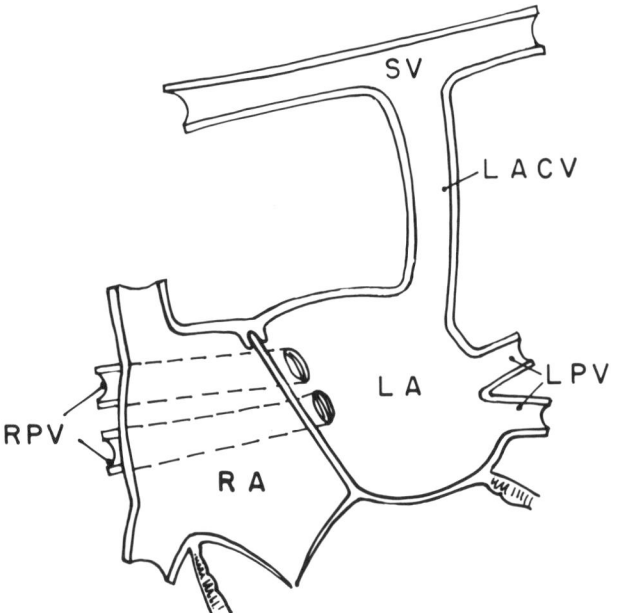

Figure 2.52 Mitral atresia with levoatriocardinal vein. The latter leads from the left atrium to a systemic vein derived from the cardinal venous system. LA = left atrium; LACV = levoatriocardinal vein; LPV = left pulmonary vein; RA = right atrium; RPV = right pulmonary vein; SV = systemic vein. (Reproduced with permission from Edwards [140].)

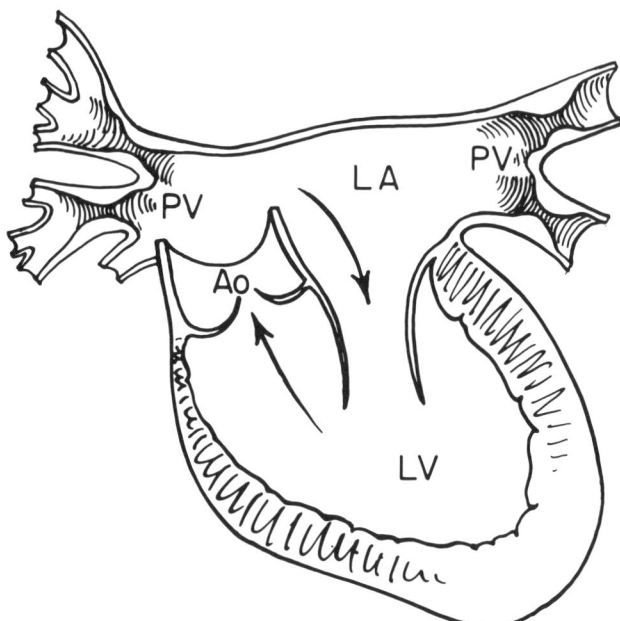

Figure 2.53 Stenosis of individual pulmonary veins. Shown in the illustration is stenosis of each pulmonary vein as it joins the left atrium. In the syndrome of stenosis of individual pulmonary veins, one or any combination of pulmonary venous obstruction may be present. Ao = aorta; LA = left atrium; LV = left ventricle; PV = pulmonary vein.

systemic vein. The connecting vein is termed a **levoatriocardinal vein**. The basis is the following. In mitral and/or aortic atresia, pulmonary venous flow is obstructed because of the primary anomaly. Additional obstruction occurs when the foramen ovale channel is either narrow or prematurely closed. The obstructive phenomenon developing fairly early may result in venous collaterals. Some of these may extend from the definitive pulmonary veins to systemic veins [123]. A variation of this state is developmental incorporation into the left atrium of the collaterals with normal development of the left atrium. The anatomic feature is a vein from left atrium to a systemic vein, which is a derivative of the cardinal venous system. This arrangement was the basis for naming the vein a levoatriocardinal vein in 1950 [125] (Figure 2.52), although similar cases reported earlier were cited. A different basis for the development of a classical levoatriocardinal vein was described by Eliot and associates [126]. They noted that with obstruction of the right atrial ostium of the coronary sinus, a vein extended from the coronary sinus to the left atrium.

2.5.2 STENOSIS OR ATRESIA OF INDIVIDUAL PULMONARY VEINS

Stenotic lesions at the junctions of pulmonary veins with the left atrium may involve one or more of any of the pulmonary veins (Figure 2.53), as stenosis of individual pulmonary veins [127]. The lesion, as far as we are aware, was first described in 1951 by Reye in an 8-year-old girl [128]. The lesion, characteristically, is limited in extent to the site of junction of the involved pulmonary vein with the left atrium [127–129]. It is characterized by intimal proliferation. In some instances, individual pulmonary veins also may be hypoplastic. The secondary effect of this condition depends upon the degree of obstruction and the number of veins involved. When the condition causes hemodynamic disturbance, the latter is associated with the morphologic changes of pulmonary venous hypertension. These are right ventricular hypertrophy, medial hypertrophy of muscular pulmonary arteries, pulmonary congestion and dilatation of pulmonary and pleural lymphatics. Shrivastava and associates [130] reported a case with atresia of the pulmonary veins in one lung and pulmonary veno-occlusive disease in the other lung.

2.5.3 PULMONARY VENO-OCCLUSIVE DISEASE

Pulmonary veno-occlusive disease is characterized by obstruction of pulmonary venules and small veins in the lungs. The lesions may be represented either by nonspecific fibrous intimal proliferative process or by the presence of intraluminal channels resembling organized thrombi [131]. The fact that most of the patients are infants or children favors a congenital basis. Nevertheless, exceptional cases in adults occur.

The condition is associated with pulmonary hypertension. Since usually there are no associated congenital anomalies and also since the pulmonary arterial wedge pressure is not elevated [132], pulmonary veno-occlusive disease has been included as one of the three forms of clinical primary pulmonary hypertension.

An important and major difference between pulmonary veno-occlusive disease and the other forms of clinical primary pulmonary hypertension are the findings of pulmonary venous hypertension in pulmonary veno-occlusive disease. These include pulmonary capillary engorgement and tortuosity, dilatation of pleural and pulmonary lymphatics, pulmonary hemosiderosis and medial hypertrophy of vessels in the precapillary segments. In the other forms of primary pulmonary hypertension, these features of pulmonary venous hypertension are not present.

References

1. Moss, A.J. Emmanouilides, G. and Duffie Jr, E.R. (1963) Closure of the ductus arteriosus in the newborn infant. *Pediatrics*, **32**, 25–30.
2. Heath, D., Helmholz Jr, F.H., Burchell, H.B. *et al.* (1958) Graded pulmonary vascular changes and hemodynamic findings in cases of atrial and ventricular septal defect and patent ductus arteriosus. *Circulation*, **18**, 1155–66.
3. Heath, D., Swan, H.J.C., Du Shane, J.W. and Edwards, J.E. (1958) Relation of medial thickness of small muscular pulmonary arteries to immediate postnatal survival in patients with ventricular septal defect or patent ductus arteriosus. *Thorax*, **13**, 267–71.
4. Chesler, E., Moller, J.H. and Edwards, J.E. (1968) Anatomic basis for delivery of right ventricular blood into localized segments of the systemic arterial system. Relation to differential cyanosis. *Am. J. Cardiol.*, **21**, 72–80.
5. D'Aunoy, R. and Von Haam, E. (1934) Aneurysm of the pulmonary artery with patent ductus arteriosus (Botallo's duct); report of two cases and review of the literature. *J. Path. Bact.*, **38**, 39–60.
6. Neufeld, H.N., Lester, R.G., Adams Jr, P. *et al.* (1962) Aorticopulmonary septal defect. *Am. J. Cardiol.*, **9**, 12–25.
7. Mori, K., Ando, M., Takao, A. *et al.* (1978) Distal type of aortopulmonary window. Report of 4 cases. *Br. Heart J.*, **40**, 681–9.
8. Perez-Martinez, V.M., Burgueros, M.A., Quero, M. *et al.* (1976) Aorticopulmonary window associated with tetralogy of Fallot. Report of one case and review of the literature. *Angiology*, **27**, 526–34.
9. Tandon, R., da Silva, C.L., Moller, J.H. and Edwards, J.E. (1974) Aorticopulmonary septal defect coexisting with ventricular septal defect. *Circulation*, **50**, 188–91.
10. Kutscher, L.M. and Van Mierop, L.H.S. (1987) Anatomy and pathogenesis of aorticopulmonary septal defect. *Am. J. Cardiol.*, **59**, 443–7.
11. Collett, R.W. and Edwards, J.E. (1949) Persistent truncus arteriosus: a classification according to anatomic types. *Surg. Clin. N. Amer.*, **29**, 1245–70.
12. Sotomora, R.F. and Edwards, J.E. (1978) Anatomic identification of so-called absent pulmonary artery. *Circulation*, **57**, 624–33.
13. Crupi, G., Maccartney, F.J. and Anderson, R.H. (1977) Persistent truncus arteriosus: a study of 66 autopsy cases with special reference to definition and morphogenesis. *Am. J. Cardiol.*, **40**, 569–78.
14. Thiene, G., Bortolotti, U., Gallucci, V. *et al.* (1976) Anatomical study of truncus arteriosus communis with embryological and surgical considerations. *Br. Heart J.*, **38**, 1109–23.
15. Butto, F., Lucas Jr, R.V. and Edwards, J.E. (1986) Persistent truncus arteriosus: pathologic anatomy in 54 cases. *Pediat. Cardiol.*, **7**, 95–101.
16. Gelband, H., Van Meter, S. and Gersony, W.M. (1972) Truncal valve abnormalities in infants with persistent truncus arteriosus: a clinicopathologic study. *Circulation*, **45**, 397–403.
17. Gerlis, L.M. Wilson, N., Dickinson, D.F. and Scott, O. (1984) Valvar stenosis in truncus arteriosus. *Br. Heart J.*, **54**, 440–5.
18. Anderson, K.R., McGoon, D.C. and Lie, J.T. (1978) Surgical significance of the coronary arterial anatomy in truncus arteriosus communis. *Am. J. Cardiol.*, **41**, 76–81.
19. Shrivastava, S. and Edwards, J.E. (1977) Coronary arterial origin in persistent truncus arteriosus. *Circulation*, **55**, 551–4.
20. Van Praagh, R. and Van Praagh, S. (1965) The anatomy of common aorticopulmonary trunk (truncus arteriosus communis) and its embryological implications: a study of 57 necropsy cases. *Am. J. Cardiol.*, **16**, 406–25.
21. Bharati, S., McAllister Jr, H.A., Rosenquist, G.C. *et al.* (1974) The surgical anatomy of truncus arteriosus communis. *J. Thor. Cardiovasc. Surg.*, **67**, 501–10.
22. Mair, D.D., Ritter, D.G., Danielson, G.K. *et al.* (1977) Truncus arteriosus with unilateral absence of a pulmonary artery. Criteria for operability and surgical results. *Circulation*, **55**, 641–7.
23. Silverman, J.J. and Scheinesson, G.P. (1966) Persistent truncus arteriosus in a 43-year-old man. *Am. J. Cardiol.*, **17**, 94–96.
24. Pool, P.E., Vogel, J.H.K. and Blount Jr, S.G. (1962) Congenital unilateral absence of a pulmonary artery. The importance of flow in pulmonary hypertension. *Am. J. Cardiol.*, **10**, 706–32.
25. Duncan, W.J., Freedom, R.M., Olley, P.M. and Rowe, R.D. (1981) Two-dimensional echocardiographic identification of hemitruncus: anomalous origin of one pulmonary artery from ascending aorta with the other pulmonary artery arising normally from the right ventricle. *Am. Heart J.*, **102**, 892–6.
26. Richardson, J.V., Doty, D.B., Rossi, N.P. and Ehrenhaft, J.L. (1979) The spectrum of anomalies of aortopulmonary septation. *J. Thor. Cardiovasc. Surg.*, **78**, 21–27.
27. Bricker, D.L., King, S.M. and Edwards, J.E. (1975) Anomalous aortic origin of the right and left pulmonary arteries in a normally septated truncus arteriosus. *Chest*, **68**, 591–4.
28. Beitzke, A. and Shinebourne, E.A. (1980) Single origin of right and left pulmonary arteries from ascending aorta, with main pulmonary artery from right ventricle. *Br. Heart J.*, **43**, 363–5.
29. Peterson, T.A., Todd, D.B. and Edwards, J.E. (1965) Supravalvular aortic stenosis. *J. Thor. Cardiovasc. Surg.*, **50**, 734–41.
30. Jones, K.L. and Smith, D.W. (1975) The Williams elfin facies syndrome. A new perspective. *J. Pediat.*, **86**, 718–23.
31. Blieden, L.C., Lucas Jr, R.V., Carter, J.B. *et al.* (1974) A developmental complex including supravalvular stenosis of the aorta and pulmonary trunk. *Circulation*, **49**, 585–90.
31. Clagett, O.T., Kirklin, J.W. and Edwards, J.E. (1954) Anatomic variations and pathologic changes in 124 cases of coarctation of the aorta. *Surg. Gynec. Obstet.*, **98**, 193–214.
33. Edwards, J.E., Christensen, N.A., Clagett, O.T. and McDonald, J.R. (1948) Pathologic considerations in coarctation of the aorta. *Proc. Mayo Clin.*, **23**, 324–32.
34. Becker, A.E., Becker, M.J. and Edwards, J.E. (1970) Anomalies associated with coarctation of aorta. Particular reference to infancy. *Circulation*, **41**, 1067–75.
35. Waller, B.F., Carter, J.B., Williams Jr, H.J. *et al.* (1973) Bicuspid aortic valve. Comparison of congenital and acquired types. *Circulation*, **48**, 1140–50.
36. Edwards, J.E., Clagett, O.T., Drake, R.L. and Christensen, N.A. (1948) The collateral circulation in coarctation of the aorta. *Proc. Mayo Clin.*, **23**, 333–9.
37. Edwards, J.E. (1973) Aneurysms of the thoracic aorta complicating coarctation. *Circulation*, **48**, 195–201.
38. Ben-Shoshan, M., Rossi, N.P. and Korns, M.E. (1973) Coarctation of the abdominal aorta. *Arch. Pathol. Lab. Med.*, **95**, 221–5.
39. Celoria, G.C. and Patton, R.B. (1959) Congenital absence of the aortic arch. *Am. Heart J.*, **58**, 407–13.
40. Moller, J.H. and Edwards, J.E. (1965) Interruption of aortic arch. Anatomic patterns and associated cardiac malformations. *Amer. J. Roentgenol.*, **95**, 557–72.
41. Becu, L.M., Tauxe, W.N., DuShane, J.W. and Edwards, J.E. (1955) A complex of congenital cardiac anomalies: ventricular septal defect, biventricular origin of the pulmonary trunk and subaortic stenosis. *Am. Heart J.*, **50**, 901–11.
42. Pierpont, M.E.M., Zollikofer, C.L., Moller, J.H. and Edwards, J.E. (1982) Interruption of the aortic arch with right descending aorta. A rare condition and a cause of bronchial compression. *Pediat. Cardiol.*, **2**, 153–9.
43. Blatchford III, J.W., Franciosi, R.A., Singh, A. and Edwards, J.E. (1987) Vascular ring in interruption of the aortic arch with bilateral patent ductus arteriosus. *J. Thor. Cardiovasc. Surg.*, **94**, 596–9.
44. Edwards, J.E., Burchell, H.B. and Christensen, N.A. (1956) Specimen exhibiting the essential lesion in aneurysm of the aortic sinus. *Proc. Mayo Clin.*, **31**, 407–12.
45. Sakakibara, S. and Konno, S. (1962) Congenital aneurysm of the sinus of Valsalva. Anatomy and classification. *Am. Heart J.*, **63**, 405–24.
46. Eliot, R.S., Wolbrink, A. and Edwards, J.E. (1963) Congenital aneurysm of the left aortic sinus. A rare lesion and a rare cause of coronary insufficiency. *Circulation*, **28**, 951–6.
47. Edwards, J.E. and Burchell, H.B. (1957) Pathologic anatomy of deficiencies between the aortic root and the heart, including aortic sinus aneurysms. *Thorax*, **12**, 125–39.
48. Levy, M.J., Lillehei, C.W., Anderson, R.C. *et al.* (1963) Aortico-left ventricular tunnel. *Circulation*, **27**, 841–53.
49. Tuna, I.C. and Edwards, J.E. (1988) Aortico-left ventricular tunnel and aortic insufficiency. *Ann. Thorac. Surg.*, **45**, 5–6.

50. Edwards, J.E. (1953) Malformations of the aortic arch system manifested as 'vascular rings'. *Lab. Invest.*, **2**, 56–75.
51. Edwards, B.S., Edwards, W.D., Connolly, D.C. and Edwards, J.E. (1984) Arterial-esophageal fistulae developing in patients with anomalies of the aortic arch system. *Chest*, **86**, 732–35.
52. Nath, P.H., Castaneda-Zuniga, W., Zollikofer, C. *et al.* (1981) Isolation of a subclavian artery. *Am. J. Roentgenol.*, **137**, 683–8.
53. Edwards, J.E. (1948) Retro-esophageal segment of the left aortic arch, right ligamentum arteriosum and right descending aorta causing a congenital vascular ring about the trachea and esophagus. *Proc. Mayo Clin. Cardiol.*, **23**, 108–16.
54. Knight, L. and Edwards, J.E. (1974) Right aortic arch. Types and associated cardiac anomalies. *Circulation*, **50**, 1047–51.
55. Kelsey, J.R., Gilmore, C.E. and Edwards, J.E. (1953) Bilateral ductus arteriosus representing persistence of each sixth aortic arch. Report of a case. *Arch. Pathol. Lab. Med.*, **55**, 154–61.
56. Radley-Smith, R., Yacoub, M., Durrer, D. *et al.* (1980) Anomalous origin of left coronary artery from anterior aortic sinus: Potential cause of characterisation and surgical treatment (Abstr.). *Br. Heart J.*, **43**, 120–1.
57. Virmani, R., Chun, P.K., Goldstein, R.E. *et al.* (1984) Acute takeoffs of the coronary arteries along the aortic wall and congenital coronary ostial valve-like ridges: association with sudden death. *J. Am. Coll. Cardiol.*, **3**, 766–71.
58. Blake, H.U., Manion, W.C., Mattingly, T.W. and Baroldi, G. (1964) Coronary artery anomalies. *Circulation*, **30**, 927–40.
59. Price, A.C., Lee, D.A., Kagan, K.E. and Baker, W.P. (1973) Aortic dysplasia in infancy simulating anomalous origin of the left coronary artery. *Circulation*, **48**, 434–7.
60. Upshaw Jr, C.B. (1962) Congenital coronary arteriovenous fistula. Report of a case with an analysis of seventy-three reported cases. *Am. Heart J.*, **63**, 399–404.
61. Wesselhoeft, H., Fawcett, J.S. and Johnson, A.L. (1968) Anomalous origin of the left coronary artery from the pulmonary trunk. Its clinical spectrum, pathology, and patho-physiology, based on a review of 140 cases with seven further cases. *Circulation*, **38**, 403–25.
62. Nelson-Piercy, C., Rickards, A.F. and Yacoub, M.H. (1990) Aberrant origin of the right coronary artery as a potential cause of sudden death: successful anatomical correction. *Br. Heart J.*, **64**, 208–10.
63. Roberts, W.C. (1962) Anomalous origin of both coronary arteries from the pulmonary artery. *Am. J. Cardiol.*, **10**, 595–600.
64. Feldt, R.H., Ongley, P.A. and Titus, J.L. (1965) Total coronary arterial circulation from pulmonary artery with survival to age seven: report of case. *Mayo Clin. Proc.*, **40**, 539–43.
65. Golden, R.L. and Lakin, H. (1959) The *forme fruste* in Marfan's syndrome. *New Engl. J. Med.*, **260**, 797–801.
66. Tung, H.L. and Liebow, A.A. (1952) Marfan's syndrome. Observations at necropsy: with special reference to medionecrosis of the great vessels. *Lab. Invest.*, **1**, 382–406.
67. Ramsey, H.W., de la Torre, A., Linhart, J.W. *et al.* (1967) Idiopathic dilatation of the pulmonary artery. *Am. J. Cardiol.*, **20**, 324–30.
68. Brayshaw, J.R. and Perloff, J.K. (1962) Congenital pulmonary insufficiency complicating idiopathic dilatation of the pulmonary artery. *Am. J. Cardiol.*, **10**, 282–6.
69. Ishikawa, T. and Seki, I. (1965) Idiopathic dilatation of the pulmonary artery; report of a case and review of the literature. *Jpn. Heart J.*, **6**, 273–83.
70. Manhoff Jr, L.J. and Howe, J.S. (1949) Absence of the pulmonary artery: A new classification for pulmonary arteries of anomalous origin. Report of a case of absence of the pulmonary artery with hypertrophied bronchial arteries. *Arch. Pathol. Lab. Med.*, **48**, 155–70.
71. Blieden, L.C., Lucas Jr, R.V., Carter, J.B. (1974) A developmental complex including supravalvular stenosis of the aorta and pulmonary trunk. *Circulation*, **49**, 585–90.
72. Jue, K.L., Lockman, L.A. and Edwards, J.E. (1966) Anomalous origins of pulmonary arteries from pulmonary trunk ('crossed pulmonary arteries'). Observation in a case with 18 trisomy syndrome. *Am. Heart J.*, **71**, 807–12.
73. Becker, A.E., Becker, M.J. and Edwards, J.E. (1970) Malposition of pulmonary arteries (crossed pulmonary arteries) in persistent truncus arteriosus. *Am. J. Roentgenol.*, **110**, 509–14.
74. Jue, K.L., Raghib, G., Amplatz, K. *et al.* (1965) Anomalous origin of the left pulmonary artery from the right pulmonary artery; report of 2 cases and review of the literature. *Am. J. Roentgenol.*, **95**, 598–610.
75. Clarkson, P.M., Ritter, D.G., Rahimtoola, S.H. *et al.* (1967) Aberrant left pulmonary artery. *Am. J. Dis. Child.*, **113**, 373–7.
76. Gikonyo, B.M., Jue, K.L. and Edwards, J.E. (1989) Pulmonary vascular sling: Report of seven cases and review of the literature. *Pediat. Cardiol.*, **10**, 81–9.
77. D'Cruz, I.A., Agustsson, M.H., Bicoff, J.P. *et al.* (1964) Stenotic lesions of the pulmonary arteries. Clinical and hemodynamic findings in 84 cases. *Am. J. Cardiol.*, **13**, 441–50.
78. Delaney, T.B. and Nadas, A.S. (1964) Peripheral pulmonic stenosis. *Am. J. Cardiol.*, **13**, 451–61.
79. MacMahon, H.E., Lee, H.Y. and Stone, P.A. (1967) Congenital segmental coarctation of pulmonary arteries (an anatomic study). *Am. J. Pathol.*, **50**, 15–25.
80. Esterly, J.R. and Oppenheimer, E.H. (1967) Vascular lesions in infants with congenital rubella. *Circulation*, **34**, 242–8.
81. Beuren, A.J., Schulze, C., Eberle, P. *et al.* (1964) The syndrome of supravalvular aortic stenosis, peripheral pulmonary stenosis, mental retardation and similar facial appearance. *Am. J. Cardiol.*, **13**, 471–83.
82. Snitcowsky, R., Toledo, A.N., Zaniolo, W. *et al.* (1964) Severe pulmonary artery hypertension due to an anomaly of the pulmonary arteries. *Am. J. Cardiol.*, **13**, 542–6.
83. Mazzucco, A., Bortolotti, U., Stellin, G. and Gallucci, V. (1990) Anomalies of the systemic venous return: a review. *J. Card. Surg.*, **5**, 122–33.
84. Winter, F.S. (1954) Persistent left superior vena cava. Survey of world literature and report of thirty additional cases. *Angiology*, **5**, 90–132.
85. Geissler, W. and Albert, M. (1956) Persistierende linke obere Hohlvene und Mitralstenose. *Zschr. Ges. Inn. Med.*, **11**, 865–74.
86. Loogen, F. and Rippert, R. (1958) Anomalien der grossen Korper und lungenvenen. *Z. Kreislaufforsch.*, **47**, 677–90.
87. Karnegis, J.N., Wang, Y., Winchell, P. and Edwards, J.E. (1964) Persistent left superior vena cava, fibrous remnant of the right superior vena cava and ventricular septal defect. *Am. J. Cardiol.*, **14**, 573–7.
88. Raghib, G., Ruttenberg, H.D., Anderson, R.C. *et al.* (1965) Termination of left superior vena cava in left atrium, atrial septal defect, and absence of coronary sinus. A developmental complex. *Circulation*, **31**, 906–18.
89. Edwards, E.A. (1951) Clinical anatomy of lesser variations of the inferior vena cava; and a proposal for classifying the anomalies of this vessel. *Angiology*, **2**, 85–99.
90. Ongley, P.A., Titus, J.L., Khoury, G.H. *et al.* (1965) Anomalous connection of pulmonary veins to right atrium associated with anomalous inferior vena cava, situs inversus and multiple spleens: a developmental complex. *Mayo Clin. Proc.*, **40**, 609–24.
91. Hickman, J., Edwards, J.E. and Mann, F.C. (1949) Venous anomalies in a dog. I. Absence of the portal vein. II. Continuity of the lower inferior vena cava with the azygos vein. *Anat. Rec.*, **104**, 137–46.
92. Meadows, W.R., Bergstrand, I. and Sharp, J.T. (1961) Isolated anomalous connection of a great vein to the left atrium. The syndrome of cyanosis and clubbing, 'normal' heart, and left ventricular hypertrophy on electrocardiogram. *Circulation*, **24**, 669–76.
93. Gardner, D.L. and Cole, L. (1955) Long survival with inferior vena cava draining into left atrium. *Br. Heart J.*, **17**, 93–7.
94. Mustard, W.T., Firor, W.B. and Kidd, L. (1964) Diversion of the venae cavae into the left atrium during closure of atrial septal defects. *J. Thor. Cardiovasc. Surg.*, **47**, 317–24.
95. Gautam, H.P. (1968) Left atrial inferior vena cava with atrial septal defect. *J. Thor. Cardiovasc. Surg.*, **55**, 827–9.
96. Black, H., Smith, G.T. and Goodale, W.T. (1964) Anomalous inferior vena cava draining into the left atrium associated with intact interatrial septum and multiple pulmonary arteriovenous fistulae. *Circulation*, **29**, 258–67.
97. Gueron, M., Hirsh, M. and Borman, J. (1969) Total anomalous systemic venous drainage into the left atrium. *J. Thor. Cardiovasc. Surg.*, **58**, 570–4.
98. Miller, G.A.H., Ongley, P.A., Rastelli, G.C. and Kirklin, J.W. (1965) Surgical correction of total anomalous systemic venous connection: report of case. *Mayo Clin. Proc.*, **40**, 532–8.
99. Mantini, E., Grondin, C.M., Lillehei, C.W. and Edwards, J.E. (1966) Congenital anomalies involving the coronary sinus. *Circulation*, **33**, 317–27.
100. Liberthson, R.R., Sagar, K., Berkoben, J.P. *et al.* (1979) Congenital coronary arteriovenous fistula. Report of 13 patients, review of the literature and delineation of management. *Circulation*, **59**, 849–54.
101. Rose, A.G., Beckman, C.B. and Edwards, J.E. (1974) Communication between coronary sinus and left atrium. *Br. Heart J.*, **36**, 182–5.
102. Harris, W.G. (1960) A case of bilateral superior vena cava with a closed coronary sinus. *Thorax*, **15**, 172–3.
103. Ruttenberg, H.D., Neufeld, H.N., Lucas Jr, R.V. *et al.* (1964) Syndrome of congenital cardiac disease with asplenia. Distinction from other forms of congenital cyanotic cardiac disease. *Am. J. Cardiol.*, **13**, 387–406.
104. Peoples, W.M., Moller, J.H. and Edwards, J.E. (1983) Polysplenia: a review of 146 cases. *Pediat. Cardiol.*, **4**, 129–37.
105. Davia, J.E., Cheitlin, M.D. and Bedynek, J.L. (1973) Sinus venosus atrial septal defect: analysis of fifty cases. *Am. Heart J.*, **85**, 177–85.
106. Neill, C.A., Ferencz, C., Sabiston, D.C. and Sheldon, H. (1960) The familial occurrence of hypoplastic right lung with systemic arterial supply and venous drainage 'scimitar syndrome'. *Bull. Johns Hopkins Hosp.*, **107**, 1–21.
107. Halasz, N.A., Halloran, K.H. and Liebow, A.A. (1956) Bronchial and arterial anomalies with drainage of the right lung into the inferior vena cava. *Circulation*, **14**, 826–46.
108. Kiely, B., Filler, J., Stone, S. and Doyle, E.F. (1967) Syndrome of anomalous venous drainage of the right lung to the inferior vena cava. A review of 67 reported cases and three new cases in children. *Am. J.*

Cardiol., **20**, 102–16.
109. Frye, R.L., Krebs, M., Rahimtoola, S.H. *et al.* (1968) Partial anomalous pulmonary venous connection without atrial septal defect. *Am. J. Cardiol.*, **22**, 242–50.
110. Gikonyo, D.K., Tandon, R., Lucas Jr, R.V. and Edwards, J.E. (1986) Scimitar syndrome in neonates: report of four cases and review of the literature. *Pediat. Cardiol.*, **6**, 193–7.
111. Mohiuddin, S.M., Levin, H.S., Runco, V. and Booth, R.W. (1966) Anomalous pulmonary venous drainage. A common trunk emptying into the left atrium and inferior vena cava. *Circulation*, **24**, 46–51.
112. Kenanoglu, A. and Tuncbilek, E. (1978) Accessory diaphragm in the left side. *Pediat. Cardiol.*, **7**, 172–4.
113. Jue, K.L., Amplatz, K., Adams Jr, P. and Anderson, R.C. (1966) Anomalies of great vessels associated with lung hypoplasia. *Am. J. Dis. Child.*, **111**, 35–44.
114. Everhart, F.J., Korns, M.E., Amplatz, K. and Edwards, J.E. (1967) Intrapulmonary segment in anomalous pulmonary venous connection. Resemblance to scimitar syndrome. *Circulation*, **35**, 1163–9.
115. Dische, M.R., Teixeira, M.L., Winchester, P.H. and Engle, M.A. (1974) Horseshoe lung associated with a variant of the 'scimitar' syndrome. *Br. Heart J.*, **36**, 617–20.
116. Paster, S.B., Swensson, R.E. and Yabek, S.M. (1977) Total anomalous pulmonary venous connection. Report of ten cases and review of the literature. *Pediat. Radiol.*, **6**, 132–40.
117. Elliott, L.P. and Edwards, J.E. (1962) The problem of pulmonary venous obstruction in total anomalous pulmonary venous connection to the left innominate vein. *Circulation*, **25**, 913–15.
118. Carey, L.S. and Edwards, J.E. (1963) Severe pulmonary venous obstruction in total anomalous pulmonary venous connection to the left innominate vein. Report of case. *Am. J. Roentgenol.*, **90**, 593–8.
119. Chia, B.-L., Tan, N.-C. and Tan, L.K.A. (1974) Total anomalous pulmonary venous drainage. Case presenting with prominent right supraclavicular thrill and loud continuous murmur. *Am. J. Cardiol.*, **34**, 850–3.
120. Bonham Carter, R.E., Capriles, M. and Noe, Y. (1969) Total anomalous pulmonary venous drainage. A clinical and anatomical study of 75 children. *Br. Heart J.*, **31**, 45–51.
121. Kanjuh, V.I., Katkov, H., Singh, A. *et al.* (1989) Atypical total anomalous pulmonary venous connection; two channels leading to infracardiac terminations. *Pediat. Cardiol.*, **10**, 115–20.
122. Lucas, R.V., Woolfrey, B.F., Anderson, R.C. *et al.* (1962) Atresia of the common pulmonary vein. *Pediatrics*, **29**, 729–39.
123. Shone, J.D. and Edwards, J.E. (1964) Mitral atresia associated with pulmonary venous anomalies. *Br. Heart J.*, **26**, 241–9.
124. Sutherland, R.D., Korns, M.E., Pyle, R.R. and Edwards, J.E. (1970) Intrapulmonary vein contributing a segment of venous supply of contralateral lung. *Chest*, **57**, 182–4.
125. Edwards, J.E. and DuShane, J.W. (1950) Thoracic venous anomalies. I. Vascular connection of the left atrium and the left innominate vein (levoatriocardinal vein) associated with mitral atresia and premature closure of the foramen ovale. II. Pulmonary veins draining wholly into the ductus venosus. *Arch. Pathol. Lab. Med.*, **49**, 517–37.
126. Eliot, R.S., Wang, Y., Elliott, L.P. *et al.* (1963) Partial anomalous pulmonary venous connection, ventricular septal defect, and anomalous communication of left atrium with coronary sinus. *Am. Heart J.*, **66**, 542–51.
127. Edwards, J.E. (1960) Congenital stenosis of pulmonary veins. Pathologic and developmental considerations. *Lab. Invest.*, **9**, 46–66.
128. Reye, R.D.K. (1951) Congenital stenosis of the pulmonary veins in their extrapulmonary course. *Med. J. Aust.*, **1**, 801–2.
129. Sade, R.M., Freed, M.D., Matthews, E.C. and Castaneda, A.R. (1979) Stenosis of individual pulmonary veins. Review of the literature and report of a surgical case. *J. Thor. Cardiovasc. Surg.*, **67**, 953–62.
130. Shrivastava, S., Moller, J.H. and Edwards, J.E. (1986) Congenital unilateral pulmonary venous atresia with pulmonary veno-occlusive disease in contralateral lung: an unusual association. *Pediat. Cardiol.*, **7**, 213–19.
131. Wagenvoort, C.A. (1976) Pulmonary veno-occlusive disease: entity or syndrome? *Chest*, **69**, 82–6.
132. Carrington, C.B. and Liebow, A.A. (1970) Pulmonary veno-occlusive disease. *Hum. Pathol.*, **1**, 322–4.
133. Edwards, B.S. and Edwards, J.E. (1987) Classification, in *Adult Congenital Heart Disease*, (ed. W.C. Roberts), F.A. Davis, Philadelphia.
134. Edwards, J.E. and McGoon, D.C. (1973) Absence of anatomic origin from heart of pulmonary arterial supply. *Circulation*, **47**, 393–8.
135. Edwards, J.E. (1965) Pathology of left ventricular outflow tract obstruction. *Circulation*, **31**, 586–99.
136. Tuna, I.C., Bessinger, F.B., Ophoven, J.P. and Edwards, J.E. (1989) Acute angular origin of left coronary artery from aorta: an unusual cause of left ventricular failure in infancy. *Pediat. Cardiol.*, **10**, 39–43.
137. Mahowald, J.M., Blieden, L.C., Coe, J.I. and Edwards, J.E. (1986) Ectopic origin of a coronary artery from the aorta. Sudden death in 3 of 23 patients. *Chest*, **89**, 668–72.
138. Vlodaver, Z. *et al.* (1975) *Coronary Arterial Variations in the Normal Heart and in Congenital Heart Disease*, Academic Press, New York, p. 171.
139. Edwards, J.E. and McGoon, D.C. (1973) Absence of anatomic origin from heart of pulmonary arterial supply. *Circulation*, **47**, 393–8.
140. Edwards, J.E. (1979) Congenital pulmonary vascular disorders, in *Pulmonary Vascular Disorders*, (ed. K.M. Moser), Marcel Dekker, New York, pp. 527–71.

3 THROMBOSIS AND VASCULAR TRAUMA

William E. Stehbens

Thrombosis is the *in vivo* formation of an intravascular solid or semisolid mass (thrombus) comprised of blood constituents and is distinguishable macroscopically and histologically from clots formed by coagulation [1]. A mass formed from the constituents of the blood *in vitro* or within the cardiovascular system after death is a clot. The process of coagulation is essentially the formation of fibrin and is an integral aspect of thrombogenesis. Thrombus and clot are often used synonymously but the difference is more than semantic. Thrombosis is an essential biological and physiological reaction to prevent haemorrhage and as such plays a life-saving role in injury and repair. It is an integral stage of haemostasis which has been essential for the evolution of the cardiovascular system and indeed of man. On the other hand this function of thrombosis on a foreign surface initiates malign consequences under certain pathological conditions and deaths associated with thromboembolic phenomena have increased substantially in aging populations of the world. When a pathological event, it is secondary to another pathological change or lesion whether a mural defect, trauma, inflammation or an intravascular foreign surface.

In routine autopsies at a general hospital up to 60% of cadavers have thrombi in the veins of the pelvis and lower limbs [2] and a similar percentage has emboli in the pulmonary arteries. Thrombi also occur in otherwise healthy middle-aged and young persons postoperatively or in the puerperium but in general thromboembolic phenomena are less prevalent in the young. Given the nature of thrombosis and the prevalence and morbidity of atherosclerosis, many middle-aged and elderly persons must harbour symptomless mural thrombi on areas of ulcerated atherosclerosis. However, occlusive arterial thrombosis is a major complication playing a leading role in the cause of death and disability from that disease. Nationally and geographically thromboembolic phenomena have a distribution similar to that for coronary heart disease and severe atherosclerosis.

Under physiological conditions endothelium is antithrombogenic to maintain fluidity of the blood. Blood within a segment of blood vessels isolated by two ligatures coagulates slowly and may remain fluid for days if the vessel is left *in situ* and *in vivo* [3] or if the blood is held in a glass vessel smeared with vaseline. However, ligation of the vessel causes trauma, even if minimal, and deposition of some thrombus would be expected, much depending on the care taken in dissection and ligation of the vessel. Rapid coagulation occurs in the vessel if it is traumatized. Under physiological conditions fluidity of the circulating blood is maintained without coagulation, platelet activation or haemorrhage by means of a well controlled and balanced interaction between endothelium, platelets, the coagulation system and antithrombogenic and thrombolytic mechanisms.

Care should be taken in differentiating between thrombi and clots and yet this elementary, essential difference is ill understood by many graduates. Platelet thrombi tend to be gelatinous, granular and not readily removed. Ante-mortem thrombi are therefore usually attached to the wall. The established thrombus is dry and tends to have a dull surface as has the underlying vessel wall. In the gross state, the thrombus is said to have a pale or white head and is usually mottled, whilst the tail, formed rapidly and by propagation, is mostly red with usually some laminated white streaks of fibrin. In general the veins are distended by the thrombus which forms a cast of the vessel in its physiologically distended state and consequently does not collapse or retract but pouts or protrudes from the cut surface. Infected thrombi are softer, more friable and may be frankly purulent, whilst the vessel wall and surrounding tissues show signs consistent with infection.

Post-mortem clots are usually loose casts of non-distended veins, moist, shiny, rubbery, readily removed and uniformly red (resembling redcurrant jelly). They consist simply of coagulated blood but if sedimentation occurs prior to clotting, the clot will be dark red in the

Vascular Pathology. Edited by W.E. Stehbens and J.T. Lie. Published in 1995 by Chapman & Hall, London. ISBN 0 412 48640 7

dependent part and yellow in the uppermost portion due to coagulated plasma (chicken fat clot). The line of demarcation is usually sharp.

3.1 Haemostasis and thrombosis

Severe injury to a blood vessel, such as partial or complete severance, results in bleeding into the tissues. This is at least partially diminished within seconds by vasoconstriction. Extravasated blood infiltrates the interstices of the surrounding tissues and coagulates, tending to restrict further infiltration and increasing the interstitial pressure within the perivascular tissue. In this way it can impede blood flow unless there is an open avenue of escape to the exterior or into a body cavity or possibly into a neighbouring vessel of lower pressure.

With such injuries or less severe trauma without much blood loss, platelets adhere to the damaged and exposed tissues of the wall producing the primary platelet thrombus. If the hole in the wall is small, it may be sealed by a platelet plug but if large and in the absence of intervention, fatal haemorrhage can ensue. The initiating lesion may be a spontaneous non-traumatic tear or ulceration, associated with weakening of the connective tissues, but the thrombotic process is the same.

The initial event in thrombosis is the deposition of a layer of platelets on the damaged blood vessel wall (Figure 3.1) or a foreign surface within the vascular system. This is the primary platelet thrombus [4], which appears pale, granular and semitransparent or gelatinous. In arteries with a high velocity it may have a smooth surface but in a vein the surface may be rough and granular. The factors determining whether this primary platelet thrombus progresses to the fully developed occlusive thrombus have not all been ascertained but the major events and known chemical mediators of the intrinsic and extrinsic systems of platelet aggregation and thrombosis are reviewed elsewhere [5,6].

The basic structure of such a thrombus was well described by Hadfield [4]. In essence coralline thrombus grows out from the platelet thrombus and consists of a series of roughly parallel laminae orientated across the stream and bent somewhat in the direction of flow (Figures 3.2 and 3.3). These laminae (lines or striae of Zahn) consist of platelet aggregates with an occasional leucocyte. Leucocytes and a fibrin mesh then form a cover over the surface of the platelet laminae whilst the intervening stagnant blood coagulates (Figure 3.4). The laminae continue to grow out into the lumen anastomosing with neighbouring striae providing cohesion and strength to the thrombus to resist disintegration and fragmentation by the flowing blood. Retraction and condensation of the thrombus releases serum containing thrombin and other clotting factors so helping to perpetuate growth of the thrombus. The surface of the

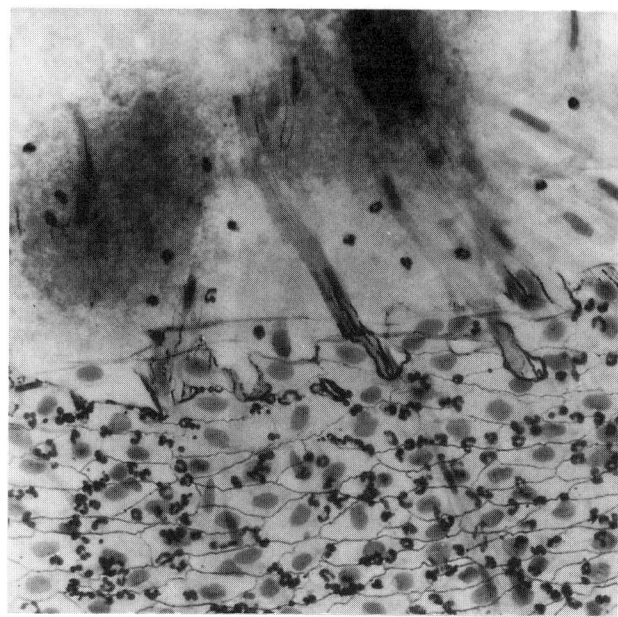

Figure 3.1 *En face* preparation of venous endothelium from a rabbit. Leucocytes are adhering to endothelial cells outlined by silver lines due to experimental phlebitis but platelet masses are adhering in the upper portion of the wall denuded of endothelium. (Haematoxylin and silver nitrate.) (Reproduced with permission from Stehbens [10].)

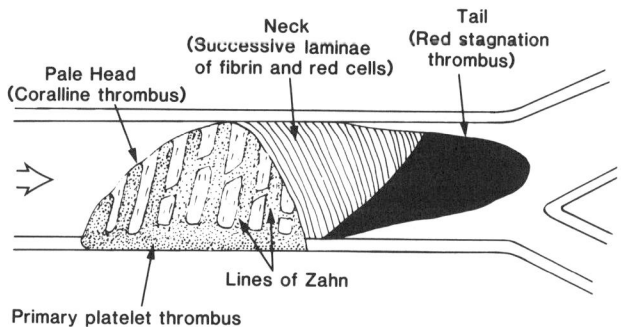

Figure 3.2 Diagram of the formation of a thrombus in an arterial segment. The open arrow indicates direction of flow. (Redrawn from Hadfield [4].)

thrombus at this stage has a series of flow-induced transversely orientated closely set ridges [4] in much the same manner as windswept sand or a river bed with alternating parallel ridges and hollows. The first ridge leads to the formation of the second and so on [7]. This corrugated appearance is observed at times on the surface of some flat mural thrombi on the aortic surface or within an aneurysmal sac although these are not necessarily lines of Zahn. As the coralline thrombus grows into the lumen producing some degree of obstruction, successive laminae of fibrin and red cells form a deep red laminated occluding clot on the downstream side of the coralline thrombus (Figure 3.2). Following

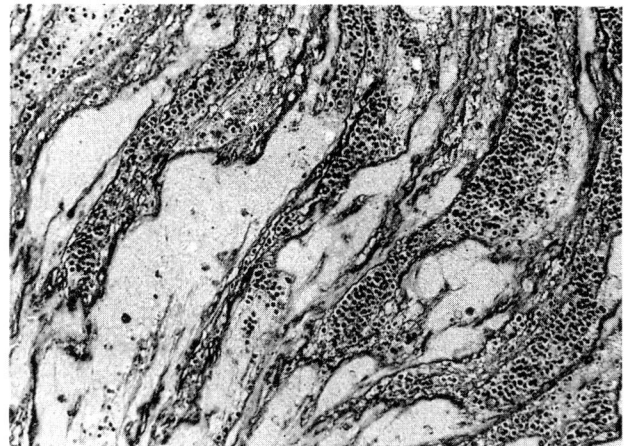

Figure 3.3 Low magnification of the lines of Zahn (pale zones) extending upwards with a layer of dark staining fibrin at their borders and intervening coagulated blood containing a concentration of leucocytes. (Phosphotungstic acid haematoxylin.)

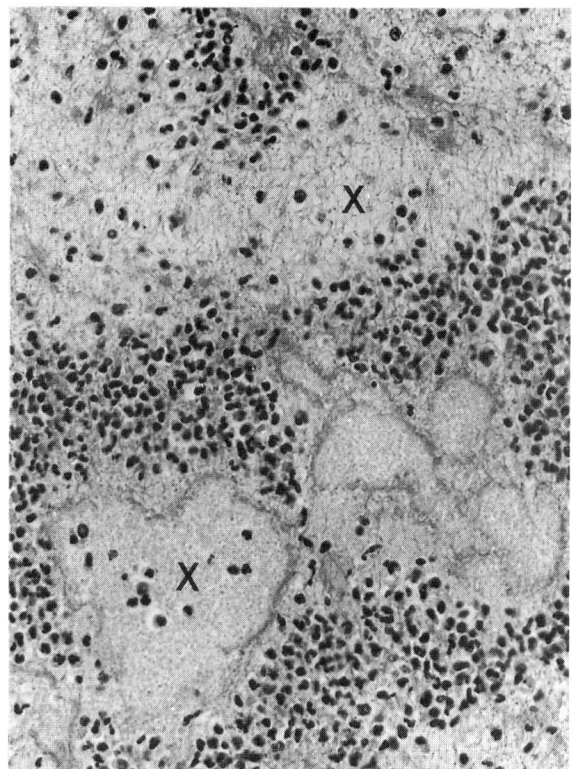

Figure 3.4 High magnification demonstrating granular appearance of lines of Zahn (X) containing a few leucocytes and enveloped in a layer of fibrin with coagulated blood and leucocytes in the intervening areas. (Haematoxylin and eosin.)

occlusion of the lumen, red stagnation thrombus propagates as far as the next large branch or tributary. The red tail, which is elastic, rapidly forms then shrinks (syneresis), permitting it to float relatively freely though anchored to the occlusive thrombus.

The time sequence of events is difficult to determine and would appear to vary from person to person. The thrombus may remain mural for some time, possibly regressing with thrombolytic activity and a fast blood flow, only to progress once more with adverse changes in flow and in the blood. If the thrombus is present for some time, organization commences and will be found in the oldest area of the thrombus.

The tail may grow to a considerable length in veins, possibly potentiated by immobility of the limb. Due to movement in the column of blood, currents are likely and the propagated thrombus in the stagnant column of blood between the head and the next branch or tributary is not uniformly red as laminae of fibrin deposits lie parallel or in eccentric whorls.

In veins when the tail of propagated thrombus lies in front of the flow from a large tributary, the rounded end rapidly becomes coated with platelets. This platelet mass then initiates deposition of more coralline thrombus until the tributary is virtually obstructed and propagation continues to the next tributary and so on. The anoxia of an occluded vessel results in damage or death of endothelial cells.

Retrograde thrombus with the characteristics of red stagnation thrombus may also form on the distal side of an occlusive venous thrombus. Extensive stagnation thrombi can form in this way in the lower limbs. Macroscopic examination of the red stagnation thrombus forming a cast of the distended vessel reveals pale mottling or rib-like markings enabling it to be distinguished from post-mortem clots.

Continual movement, even that from the neighbouring pulsing artery, together with some drag effect at the free end results in fragmentation and embolism. Since the propagated thrombus proximal to the pale head often extends up the femoral to the iliac veins, this red tail is possibly more likely to break off, e.g. when a subject sits up in bed and flexes the thigh. Transverse cuts in the calf muscles may reveal residual thrombi pouting loosely from distended veins left behind after embolism of thrombus from the more proximal reaches of the venous tree.

Such factors as (1) dilution of mediators, (2) hepatic clearance of activated clotting factors, (3) appearance or increase in specific inhibitors, (4) consumption of coagulation factors and (5) fibrinolytic activity may all participate in inhibiting undue growth of the haemostatic plug or of the thrombus but currently control of this protective mechanism is beyond present knowledge.

3.2 Thrombogenesis

From early experimental evidence it became evident that platelets play a dominant role in early thrombogenesis. In non-inflamed and growing vessels in transparent

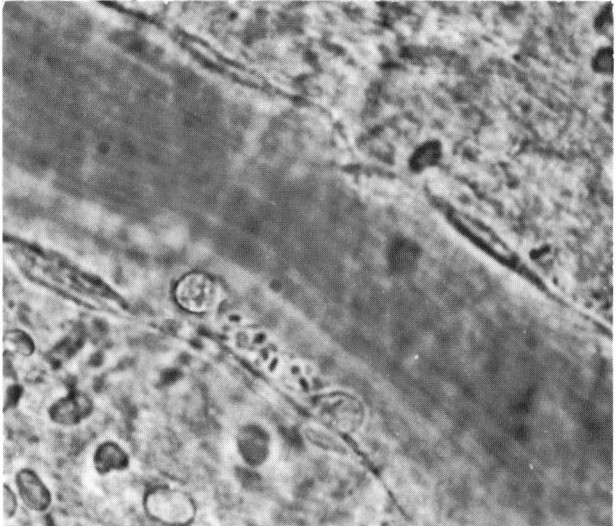

Figure 3.5 Two leucocytes and a cluster of adherent platelets forming a small leucocyte–platelet microthrombus in a venule within a rabbit ear chamber. (Flow is from top left to bottom right.)

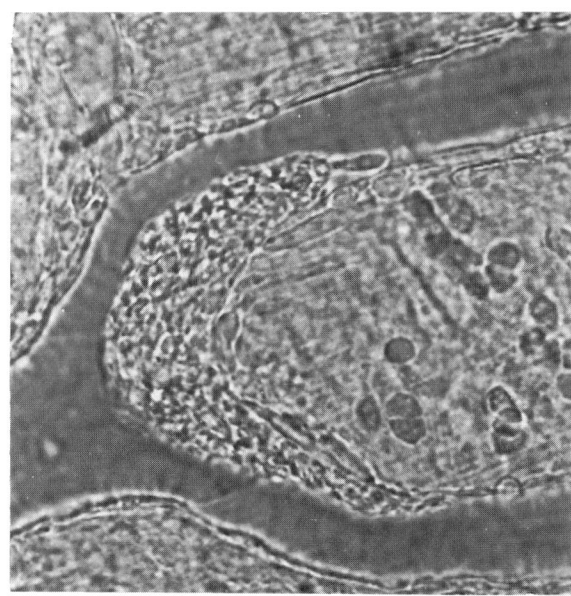

Figure 3.6 Large embolic thrombus (caught at a fork) consisting mostly of platelets. Individual platelets are distinguishable and give the thrombus a granular appearance. Flow is from left to right. (Reproduced with permission from Stehbens [57].)

chambers inserted in rabbit ears, platelets are small biconvex refractile discs. When flow is stationary, they exhibit Brownian movement in plasma with no tendency to aggregate or adhere to endothelium or other cellular constituents of the blood [8]. Even though seen at times in the marginal plasma zone of flowing blood, they exhibit no propensity to adhere to endothelium and at branching sites they are seen to strike the wall without adhering [9]. They rarely adhere to endothelium and then only at a very localized point of attachment. The platelet may be washed away only to be replaced by another platelet or a small chain of platelets, but this phenomenon does not appear to be progressive. They will, however, from time to time adhere to leucocytes rolling along or adherent to the wall (Figure 3.5). Platelet sticking to leucocytes is accentuated by mild trauma and small leucocyte–platelet thromboemboli develop often in a transient manner [8]. With time these circulatory disturbances are resolved as normal flow is restored. Since minimal trauma is required such leucocyte–platelet aggregations must be reversible. There is no evidence that a microthrombus once initiated institutes an irreversible train of events causing further endothelial damage, increased permeability, occlusive thrombosis or proliferation of subendothelial tissues. Indeed this phenomenon of leucocyte–platelet thrombosis is so readily induced that if microthrombi were progressive, life would be impossible because, during a lifetime, soft tissues and superficial vessels are constantly subjected to many and more severe injuries both accidental and iatrogenic.

Leucocyte–platelet thromboembolism is accentuated by the intravenous administration of particulate matter, lipopolysaccharides, methocel, bacteria, fat emulsions and some pharmacological agents, causing a greatly enhanced tendency for platelets to form large aggregates and to adhere to leucocytes [9]. The platelets still do not adhere to endothelium and within a few hours there is again restitution of flow. Some thrombi form long tenuous tails predominantly of aggregated platelets but still with no tendency for these sticky platelets to adhere to endothelium. Intermittent embolic shedding during enlargement or resolution of a thrombus is characteristic and influenced by flow conditions. Some leucocyte–platelet microthrombi become caught temporarily at forks (Figure 3.6) but these too wash away without evidence of altered behaviour of the underlying endothelium.

In *en face* preparations of rabbit veins [10], platelet sticking occurs where endothelium is desquamated or severely damaged (Figure 3.1). In severely inflamed veins, platelets stick at interendothelial cell gaps where endothelial cells have separated. Moreover in cell cultures of endothelium, even when injured and incubated with platelet-rich plasma, platelets exhibit little tendency to adhere to endothelial cells and there is no distortion of platelet shape or platelet release [11,12]. In ultrastructural studies of trauma-induced microthrombosis, platelets covered stomata or areas of endothelial denudation [13,14]. There was at times apposition of platelets and microthrombi with endothelium but this does not of necessity indicate adhesion.

Ultrastructurally platelets exhibit no deformation in

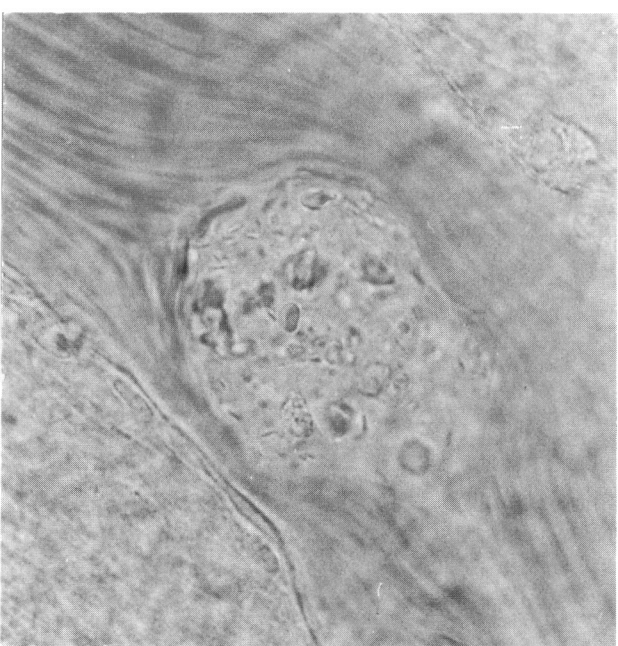

Figure 3.7 Large microthrombus in a large venule in a rabbit ear chamber. A few individual platelets and blood cells are distinguishable but the hyaline and semitransparent appearance of the thrombus is due to the close packing and application of platelets one to another giving the appearance of viscous metamorphosis. (Reproduced with permission from Silver and Stehbens [8].)

shape and the contact between platelets is limited but subsequently platelets gradually apply themselves to one another and to leucocytes with consequent alteration in shape. Dendritic forms, degranulation and rearrangement of the granulomere location are not observed in these early stages. There is amorphous material surrounding platelets in this aggregated state but whether it is microprecipitation of fibrin, other flocculated plasma proteins or glycoproteins contributing to the stickiness of platelets is unknown. Platelets and leucocytes with the occasional entrapped red cell become closely packed with platelet pseudopodia-like prolongations interdigitating with neighbouring platelets [14]. This stage probably corresponds to the hyaline microthrombi (viscous metamorphosis) *in vivo* (Figure 3.7), which proceeds to degranulation with release of several pharmacological mediators 5-hydroxytryptamine, platelet factor IV, adenosine diphosphate (ADP) which is a powerful platelet aggregating agent and thromboxane A2, a vasoconstrictor which promotes further platelet aggregation and platelet release. Histologically considerable fibrin deposition occurs around the platelet masses contributing to the stability of the haemostatic plug.

In recent years a large number of highly specialized proteins of the endothelial and smooth muscle cells, platelets, the blood plasma, vascular matrix and cell surface receptors have been shown to promote pharmacological activities of importance in haemostasis and in the intrinsic and extrinsic coagulation pathways [5,6,15,16]. Some of these proteins exert multiple interactions but just how their potential activities fit into the field of coagulation and thrombosis is not understood at present. Likewise variations within individuals and sometimes biochemical disorders involving defective activities of these mediators and some as yet to be discovered will affect the final outcome to a variable degree. In most instances the complex interplay of these substances must be under a remarkable and complex regulatory system that checks and balances individual contributions from the initial stickiness of platelets to the formation of the haemostatic plug and occlusive thrombus. In addition, the endothelium secretes fibrinolysin and the circulating blood contains thrombolysins and various antagonists or inhibitors, whilst the blood flow dilutes and washes away mediators. Further knowledge of this seemingly finely balanced and controlled pharmacodynamic biological event will continue to be elucidated for years to come. Obviously quantitative variation of these mediators can upset the equilibrium, thereby enhancing progression of the thrombus [17].

3.3 Virchow's triad

For more than one hundred years, three factors (Virchow's triad) have been considered to play vital roles in thrombogenesis: changes in the vessel wall, flow and composition of the blood and in more recent times much emphasis has been placed on flow disturbances.

3.3.1 THE VESSEL WALL

The endothelium maintains a non-thrombogenic surface on its luminal aspect by producing a variety of pharmacological agents to maintain its surface free of thrombus [18,19] but little is known of the interrelationships, conditions or half-life of these activities. All the experimental evidence suggests that mural thrombosis is promoted only where endothelium is denuded [10] and that platelets adhere to underlying tissues particularly collagen fibrils [20,21] but also basement membranes, elastin and elastic tissue microfibrils (mediated by von Willebrand factor (vWF)) [22–24]. In perfusion chambers platelet adhesion to subendothelial tissue has been found to be enhanced by the presence of other blood cells [25].

Nothing is known of the ultimate fate of the many small platelet and platelet–leucocyte microemboli that must form every day. Some platelets break off and appear to remain unchanged but whether there is a platelet disaggregating factor or whether this occurs by mechanical buffeting in the circulation is not known.

However, the experimentally induced platelet aggregate can develop into hyaline thrombus [9]. Whether hyaline thrombi are associated with endothelial damage is uncertain. Such thrombi and emboli, seemingly in an irreversible state, may be progressively cleared by a combination of thrombolysis and phagocytosis of platelet and cellular remnants.

In the aorta, mural thrombi are remarkably common in middle-aged and elderly humans and are attributable to intimal tears, cracks and ulcerations. Most individuals of this age group must be leading everyday lives despite such lesions and the emboli they shed. Similarly, in coronary and cerebral arteries, mural and occlusive thrombi arise secondarily to intimal tears, ulcerations or superficial intimal erosions [26–31]. The few exceptions may be variously accounted for by artefact, the difficulty in cutting serial sections of thrombi *in situ* in the presence of grossly atherosclerotic calcified arteries, the difficulty in demonstrating superficial intimal or endothelial damage and the possibility that emboli may be mistaken for thrombosis *in situ*. Scanning electron microscopy of endarterectomy specimens has revealed the presence of superficial ulcerations and microthrombi beyond the capabilities of naked eye inspection [32]. Not only could such lesions provide emboli for transient ischaemic attacks but such small lesions could occur in other atherosclerotic lesions. Thrombosis in aneurysms has also been attributed to tears of the aneurysm wall [33].

In lower animals, spontaneous thrombotic lesions from any cause are rare but can be due to arteritis, trauma or parasites. Nevertheless, thrombotic lesions superimposed on severe atherosclerosis can occur [34] and the infrequency of thrombi in young humans is attributable to the lesser severity of atherosclerosis.

Thrombosis in veins is extremely common in humans particularly in the elderly. It can be readily understood why thrombosis complicates any inflammatory or traumatic lesion or neoplastic involvement of veins. The high incidence of venous thrombosis in humans in the older age groups seems to be due to phlebosclerosis which develops *pari passu* with atherosclerosis of arteries in increasingly aging populations of affluent countries [35]. In view of the frequency of thrombosis in varicose veins with or without arteriovenous shunts, these lesions must also contribute to the incidence. Flow disturbances and stresses to which venous valves are subjected must in the long term exert some effect and contribute to the thrombi forming within the venous valve sinuses. Thrombotic occlusions associated with periodic trauma and pregnancies would contribute to varicose collaterals and subsequently thrombosis. The natural history of thrombosis in the veins of the lower limb has never been studied in detail to determine the endothelial and intimal integrity, which cannot be assessed adequately by conventional histology. Even so the ease with which endothelial injury occurs, for example even by compression of a vein, suggests that minor subclinical injuries to veins must be frequent and undetected.

3.3.2 FLOW

Stasis of blood flow has long been considered a factor in thrombosis because of its frequency in veins and aneurysms in which relative stasis has been considered important. Reduced venous flow rates and a propensity for thrombosis occur in patients immobilized postoperatively, in the puerperium and in those with congestive cardiac failure, debilitating and often terminal conditions including cancer (especially of the pancreas). Reduction in postoperative thrombosis has followed early ambulation. The greater frequency of venous thrombosis in the soleus muscle than in the gastrocnemius has been attributed to slower flow rates in the soleus [2]. Prolonged immobility in the elderly predisposes to venous thromboses in the legs as when watching television, during prolonged air flights, etc. and particularly in paralysed legs of stroke victims [36].

There is said to be a relationship with myocardial infarction. In one study of subjects with confirmed myocardial infarction, the incidence of deep vein thromboses was 38% in those not treated with anticoagulants and 5.5% in those treated, but the incidence was 60% in severely ill patients irrespective of therapy [37]. Such thrombosis, when seen in young severely ill and often malnourished children is called marantic thrombosis and can occur in a dural sinus.

The likely contribution of phlebosclerosis in stroke victims and the elderly is substantiated by the rarity of venous thrombosis in children postoperatively and in young paraplegics after recovery from the initial trauma. The lines of Zahn develop only in flowing blood. It was once believed that cellular constituents of the blood remained in the central axial stream and that flow reduction or eddy currents enabled platelets to enter the marginal plasma zone to adhere to damaged endothelium. In larger vessels with faster flow rates and a wider marginal plasma zone, flow disturbances are thought to facilitate platelet contact with the wall and subsequent thrombosis. The importance of platelet contact with the wall has been overemphasized and the non-thrombogenic surface of endothelium has been overlooked. Angiographically flow retardation in the deep veins of the legs occurs without thrombosis ensuing [38,39] and experimentally blood remains fluid *in vivo* for a long time in vessels isolated from the general circulation when the intima is intact [1].

Platelet sticking and thrombosis follow endothelial denudation in a rabbit iliac artery within two minutes. Basal platelets are partially degranulated but within 40 minutes only a thin monolayer of platelets remains. This appears to be non-thrombogenic and apparently limits thromboembolism [40]. Severe injuries can be associated with larger thrombi which may become occlusive. Rheological parameters affect both development and fragmentation of the thrombus *in vitro* [40]. High blood flow rates minimize thrombus formation perhaps due to shear stress with only a thin layer of platelets and leucocytes associated with experimental arterial intimal tears [41,42]. Shear stresses may prevent sedimentation and adherence of platelets and microthrombi to the vessel wall, thereby enhancing dispersal of emboli. When shear forces are less than the cohesive forces holding the cellular constituents to one another and to the vessel wall, the thrombus is likely to grow. Flow is of importance in supplying thrombogenic factors and in their removal from the platelets and thrombus but little is known of such influences. Studies of shear stress *in vitro* do not take into account the alternating nature of such stresses nor the vagaries of flow which include at times flow reversal.

Platelets are of particular importance at high, i.e. arterial blood flow, velocities and function independently of coagulation [43]. Thrombus growth and stability are normal and even increased in patients with fibrinogen deficiency, suggesting that fibrin is not crucial for early platelet thrombus stability and platelet to platelet cohesion may be potentiated by von Willebrand factor [44]. Fibrin on the other hand appears to require stagnant blood [43] but must contribute to the overall cohesion of the thrombus.

Disturbed flow has been invoked as a potent factor in producing thrombi no doubt due to their frequency in aneurysms, varicose veins, venous valve sinuses, and in arteriovenous communications. Consequently vortices or eddy currents have been considered the flow pattern most conducive to thrombogenesis. The deposition of platelets has been likened to sediment deposition in meandering streams and many authors [45–47], who have studied platelet behaviour and deposition in extracorporeal flow chambers, have extrapolated to thrombosis *in vivo* and the localization and development of atherosclerosis [47–50]. The thrombogenic surface of the flow chamber is ignored and the topography of the deposition is dissimilar to that of early proliferative lesions [26]. Thrombosis whether in arteries or veins is not merely a matter of silting of platelets as has been suggested [51] and implied. Observations on vascular forks and unions in the microcirculation did not reveal any predilection to platelet sticking and platelets exhibited no morphological change or tendency to adhere to the endothelium or to one another when swirling in vortices [26]. No leucocytes, red cells, carbon particles or droplets of lipid emulsions stuck or sedimented in eddy currents or areas of separation. Microthrombosis exhibited no predilection for forks or junctions in the microcirculation [9].

Therefore, the inescapable conclusion is that sedimentation in meandering streams and deposition of platelets in extracorporeal flow models are not applicable to the mammalian circulatory system because of the special antithrombogenic properties of vascular endothelium. All available experimental evidence indicates that platelet sticking to intact endothelium is not the primary event.

The effect of flow on the vessel wall where flow disturbances occur has been overlooked. There is need to explain the spontaneous disruption of the vessel wall under physiological flow conditions and the reason why pressures required to tear or burst their walls by far exceed those encountered even under extreme conditions of stress. The most plausible explanation for the occurrence of thrombus in pathological lesions, where vortex shedding or turbulence occurs, is loss of tensile strength due to essential engineering failure of the connective tissues caused by enhanced vibratory or alternating stresses as arises in the post-stenotic dilatation [26,52] and the stress fractures of bones and tendons.

3.3.3 CHANGES IN COMPOSITION OF THE BLOOD

The frequency of postoperative and puerperal venous thrombosis in non-ambulant patients led to the concept of blood hypercoagulability but this is a vague term. Nevertheless, a number of conditions is associated with an enhanced tendency to thrombosis. Wright [53] demonstrated an increase in the platelet count and adhesiveness to one another and to foreign surfaces *in vitro* which coincided with the maximal incidence of postoperative thrombosis, a shortened prothrombin time, increased prothrombin and lengthened circulation time. Since that time there has been a marked increase in our knowledge of the mediators of thrombosis and coagulation. Stasis and changes in the vessel wall probably occur concomitantly and factors increasing blood coagulability have not significantly influenced experimental thrombogenesis [20]. Polycythaemia rubra vera, macroglobulinaemia, haemoglobinopathies, inherited deficiency of antithrombin III, haemoconcentration, thrombocytosis, increased blood viscosity and high levels of coagulation factors (particularly factors, V, VII, VIII and X) are frequently associated with clinical thrombosis [54]. There is also some evidence that race is important but racial differences coexist usually with many other concomitant changes. Disseminated cancer especially of the pancreas is alleged to predispose to a thrombotic diathesis and smoking too has been incriminated. Again this is controversial and age and nutrition have to be considered as such subjects are usually old, poorly nourished and bedridden. There is in addition increased aggregability of platelets with age [55]. The concept of hypercoagulability is attractive but as yet there is little evidence that haematological tests can detect those who are at greatest risk.

In women taking oral contraceptive medication there is a propensity to aseptic thromboembolic phenomena. The risk is believed to be associated with a high oestrogen content and either arterial or venous thromboses occur. The thromboses not infrequently affect the central nervous system with thrombosis of leptomeningeal arteries or veins, thrombotic occlusion of a dural sinus [56] and also veins in the lower limb and less frequently of the viscera. The pathogenesis of these events is still unknown.

As indicated above, leucocyte–platelet thromboembolism can be induced in the microcirculation by the intravenous injection of a variety of substances as also occurs in anaphylaxis [57]. Associated with these changes there is often a variable degree of red cell aggregation. When this is severe, red cells adhere forming large red cell masses, a condition known as sludging of the erythrocytes, in which there may be acanthocytosis or the red cells may be of normal shape. This red cell aggregation can cause severe stasis or even widespread obstruction in the microcirculation that cannot be recognized as such by light microscopy but gives the impression merely of congestion. It is associated with hyperviscosity and increased sedimentation rate. By definition these red cell masses can be regarded as thrombi and occur in anaphylaxis, malaria and after a fatty meal. There are grades of the condition, which if present must accentuate the ischaemia induced by conventional thrombosis and embolism by virtue of the slow flow and mircrocirculatory obstruction.

There has been much interest regarding dietary fat augmenting the tendency to thrombosis. This has involved *in vitro* studies and as yet there is no positive scientific evidence that the ingestion of fat increases the tendency to conventional thrombosis apart from a temporary effect on erythrocytes. This thesis is said to be supported by epidemiological evidence although a recent review of this topic [58], like that of Renaud [59] some years ealier, concluded that there is insufficient information available on the various dietary fatty acids and their effects on lipid biosynthesis and metabolism to reach a definite conclusion. More recent interest has centred on the role of dietary (*n*-3) polyunsaturated fatty acids in lowering total blood cholesterol and low density lipoprotein (LDL) cholesterol, but in reducing the propensity for thrombosis [58] the evidence is not strong [60]. Alimentary hyperlipaemia is said to inhibit fibrinolysis [61]. The importance of transient and reversible postprandial haematological changes in the long term is uncertain and counter effects and biological adaptation to prevent vascular damage from occurring after every meal seem highly probable. Many dietary constituents including fish oils may have varied effects (mostly *in vitro*) on the many biochemical mechanisms in thrombogenesis or coagulation but it does not follow that their continued or increased ingestion will bring about perpetual enhancement of the corresponding effect *in vivo*. Even if it were so, the effect is a secondary one on thrombosis rather than on the initiating factor which is a disrupted vessel wall due to atherosclerotic fragility or some other vascular disease.

Lipoprotein(a) (Lp(a)) refers to a family of lipoprotein particles closely related to or variants of LDL, the protein moiety of apolipoprotein-B100, being linked by disulphide bonds to one or two molecules of apolipoprotein(a) which is similar to the fibrinolytic zymogen plasminogen. The molecular similarity has led to the suspicion that elevated blood levels of Lp(a) may suppress normal fibrinolytic activity by competing with plasminogen for cell-surface binding and thus enhance thrombosis. At present it is unknown whether Lp(a) has any effect on the fibrinolytic system *in vivo* and as yet the physiological role of these lipoprotein particles is uncertain. It is therefore speculative to invoke a thrombus enhancing effect for Lp(a). Likewise it has been suggested that elevated blood levels of plasminogen activator inhibitor-1 (PAI-1) promote thrombotic disease [62] but again this would be a secondary effect and not the initial mural lesion leading to thrombosis as far as is known.

When a segment of jugular vein is dissected free and its tributaries ligated followed by an infusion of aged homologous or heterologous mammalian serum into a distant vein and a minute later a segment of jugular vein isolated between clamps, a red thrombus develops to form a cast in the occluded segment and in the area distally where stasis is incomplete [63]. Subsequent studies have demonstrated that the serum contained activated clotting factors that promote coagulation and in the experimental model stasis allows clotting to occur without dilution and inactivation of the clotting factors that normally occur with blood flow. Though trauma was not specifically excluded, this has been considered a model of the red stagnation thrombus that occurs distal to a venous thrombus.

3.4 Arterial thrombosis

Arterial thrombi are usually pale with a slightly translucent appearance or are mixed in type. Thrombosis in the aorta can at times be very extensive and as is consistent with the distribution of atherosclerosis, most thrombi occur in the infrarenal segment of the aorta (Figure 3.8). Multiple mural thrombi are frequent and the ulcers often have undermined edges, probably accounting for recurrent embolic phenomena. A characteristic feature of the development of a thrombus is the continual shedding of emboli followed by its growth in a cyclical manner. Some large mural thrombi cover areas

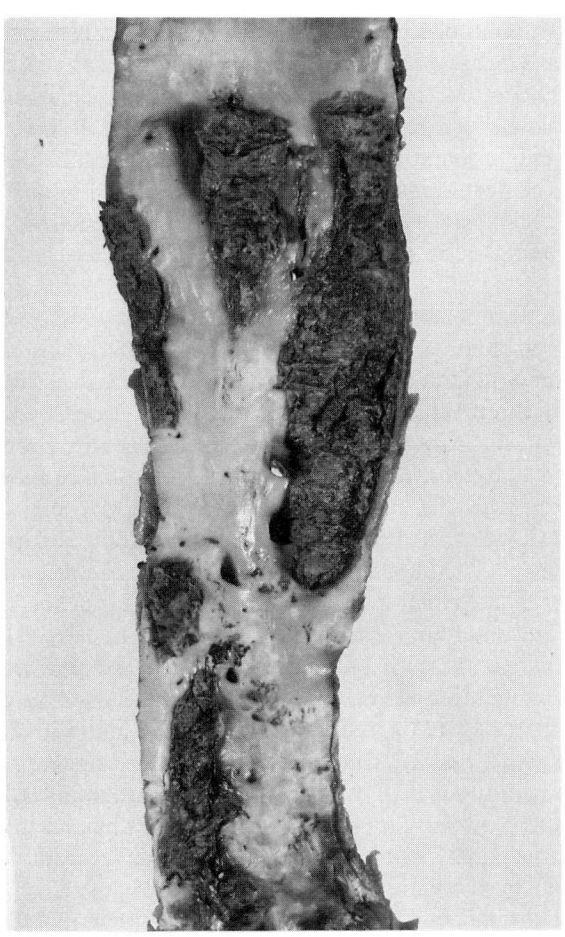

Figure 3.8 Abdominal aorta exhibiting extensive multiple mural thrombi.

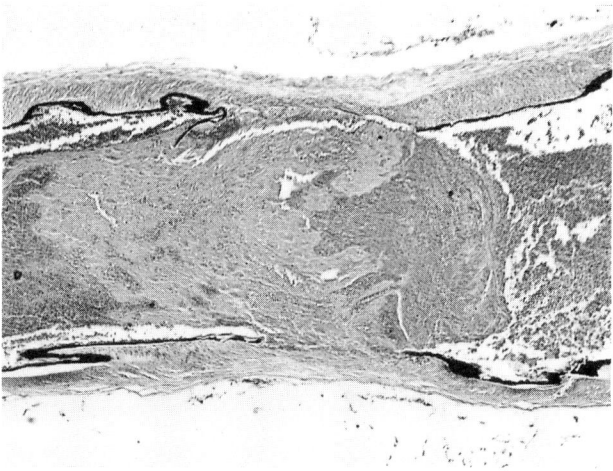

Figure 3.9 Thrombotic occlusion of a cerebral artery at the site of a spontaneous circumferential tear of the internal elastic lamina which has retracted with only minimal dissection between the lamina and the media. (Verhoeff's elastic stain and eosin.)

of 5 cm or more and have a relatively smooth surface sometimes with a laminated pattern. If there is an early fusiform aneurysm, its surface too may be covered with thrombus which is often red with a rough or ragged surface. Thrombotic occlusion of the abdominal aorta is rare and is usually in a severely atherosclerotic distal aorta.

The lower limbs are affected more often than is clinically recognized, thrombotic occlusion being twice as common as coronary thrombosis and it is only the large collateral circulation that accommodates this frequency of thrombosis and the showers of emboli that must originate in the aorta.

Coronary artery thrombi usually involve only a limited length of the artery with little propagation, probably because of the plentiful branchings. In thick-walled arteries the thrombus cannot be localized without sectioning or opening the artery and in the presence of severe atherosclerosis, often with calcification, artefactual damage occurs readily. For this reason thrombi are probably often overlooked. Mural thrombi could give rise to multiple emboli with transient ischaemic attacks providing a varied clinical picture and being responsible for the controversy regarding the incidence of thrombosis and the sequence of events in myocardial infarction [64]. The thrombus is almost invariably sited over an atherosclerotic plaque in which there is a tear or an ulceration. Blood may have extended into the atheromatous debris perhaps excavating the wall and causing some atheroembolism.

Arterial thrombi do not often propagate unless the artery has a long unbranched segment distal to the thrombotic occlusion, e.g. a red thrombus may be found distal to the carotid sinus in the internal carotid artery occlusion and also in the vertebral artery [65]. It can occur in the coronary arteries but propagation is usually of limited extent.

Thrombi in cerebral arteries are not nearly as frequent as in the coronary circulation and embolic lesions probably predominate with thrombosis *in situ* frequently being extracranial rather than intracranial. Atherosclerosis is usually the underlying mural factor responsible. Dissecting aneurysm of a cerebral artery is usually associated with a tear of the internal elastic lamina and a variable degree of subintimal dissection (between the internal elastic lamina and media). Thrombotic occlusion may complicate these lesions even when the dissection is of limited extent (Figure 3.9).

Thrombi in the common carotid arteries and the carotid sinus may be of considerable size and non-occlusive. It is likely that these thrombi may remain mural for many months since the carotid ulcers can be responsible for transient embolic attacks for a long time prior to occlusion or possibly healing. The incidence of healing in arterial thrombi is uncertain.

Thrombi associated with inflammation or frank infection are usually quite friable and the wall is not typical of atherosclerosis. There is usually other evidence of the inflammatory or infective disorder.

Thrombosis within the heart, either within the chambers or on the valves is of frequent occurrence and a major source of arterial emboli but is not dealt with in this text. The characteristic laminated thrombus within arterial aneurysms is a special instance in which organization is usually limited and the thrombus develops over an expanding wall (Chapter 10).

3.5 Venous thrombi

At autopsy venous thrombi are commonly seen in vessels of the lower limb and pelvis. The thrombi generally form in large or medium-sized veins of the lower limb of venous sinuses and at sites where eddying is likely such as in the soleal veins, particularly the large sinuses and where there is a change of direction on compression [66]. It has been alleged that the underlying endothelium is normal but this seems most doubtful and Short [35] found that the early sites of thrombi in the lower limb were on areas of intimal thickening similar to that of arteries, in the venous sinuses and at the crescentic edge at the junction with tributaries. These occurred in the posterior tibial veins rather than in veins within the soleus muscle. The possible relationship to haemodynamics is apparent. Thrombi have also been found in venous sinuses in the iliofemoral veins. When small, they consist predominantly of platelets but when larger they are pale or mixed thrombi, sometimes several sinuses being affected. They progressively enlarge until the vein is occluded. This is then followed by red stagnation thrombus distally, but it can also propagate proximally. Much will depend on the venous anatomy. The red tail (stagnation thrombus) formed in this way is also likely to be loosely attached to the vein wall, to become disconnected and embolize.

There has been controversy as to whether thrombus in the deep veins of the leg commences proximally with retrograde propagation or distally in the calf or even the foot with anterograde propagation. There is little doubt that thrombi may commence in venous sinuses in the thigh or calf as demonstrated by autopsy studies [67–70], thus accounting for variation in the clinical recognition of deep vein thrombosis and the lack of gross oedema in some subjects. In an autopsy investigation [71] 73% of the venous thrombi arose in large veins of the thigh and pelvis and not all in the small veins of the calf and foot as was once believed.

Sevitt [51] found a predilection for six sites in the lower limbs:

1. iliac veins, generally the external iliac just above the inguinal ligament;
2. the common femoral vein including the mouth of the medial and lateral circumflex veins;
3. the termination of the deep femoral vein usually at a valve cusp at the ostium;
4. the popliteal vein near the adductor ring;
5. the posterior tibial vein;
6. the intramuscular veins of the calf, especially the veins in the soleus muscle.

The thrombi occur independently of one another and can be bilateral. Up to four small thrombi were observed in an individual. Organization was common deep in the sinus along the wall adjacent to the line of attachment of the cusp. Fat globules were observed with thrombi in two specimens and were attributed to fat embolism in the past. The red stasis thrombus is more prominent distally but with the head of the thrombus firmly attached, it cannot embolize. The propagation thrombus on the proximal side is that which is more likely to embolize because it tends to float free.

Kakkar et al. [72], in a clinical study, found postoperative deep vein thrombosis commenced in the calf and propagated proximally. Within 72 hours at least one third had lysed spontaneously. It is possible that pale thrombus may be deposited on the proximal end of propagated thrombus and that when this has occluded the proximal branch, further proximal spread may occur in like manner.

Thrombi in the pelvis, either in the periprostatic plexus or in veins of the internal female genitalia are frequent and usually subclinical. The legacy of pelvic thrombi is revealed by the incidence of phleboliths radiologically.

Thrombosed veins are often incorrectly referred to as thrombophlebitis and this may be true in subjects with recurrent or prolonged intravenous therapy where there may be iatrogenic damage or mild infection of the venous wall. More often it is merely thrombosis and a mild inflammatory response is the early phase of resolution and organization.

In any severely ill patient, possibly because of the senescence, phlebosclerosis and immobility, venous thrombosis must be considered as a potential complication. Clinical conditions with a particular propensity for deep vein thrombosis of the lower limbs include old age, the puerperium, post-surgical status, congestive cardiac failure, prolonged immobilization, severe infections and marasmus, endocrine contraception, myocardial infarction, carcinomatosis and peripheral vein disease. Since some thrombi in venous sinuses are found incidentally at autopsy and often partially or wholly organized, it is possible that predisposing conditions may contribute to their enlargement and propagation as terminal events following immobilization.

3.6 Atypical thrombosis

Platelets will adhere to foreign material inserted, injected or escaping into the circulation. This has become a common feature in these days of cardiovascular prostheses and intravenous drug abusage associated with impurities and lack of hygiene. It is also a feature of homologous tissue embolism, atheroembolism and neoplastic invasion of blood vessels. Microthrombi may also occur in the microcirculation as small peripheral vessels in various inflammatory disorders, immunological reactions, overwhelming septicaemia and disseminated intravascular coagulation. The similarity of some of these disorders to the response to intravenous infusion of particulate matter or high molecular weight polysaccharides, referred to as the macromolecular haematologic syndrome of Hueper, is quite remarkable [26,73,74].

3.7 Sequelae of thrombosis

A mural thrombus in an artery or vein will be subjected to thrombolytic activity. Plasma normally contains the pro-enzyme plasminogen, and a low concentration of plasminogen activator which is synthesized by the vascular endothelium and can convert plasminogen to the potent fibrinolytic enzyme plasmin [75]. This is normally a slow process because the plasminogen activator has a low affinity for free plasminogen and the plasmin so produced is inactivated rapidly mostly by α_2-antitrypsin. When fibrin is formed intravascularly in a thrombus, plasminogen and its activator bind rapidly to it and the plasminogen is rapidly converted to plasmin in concentration to digest the fibrin into soluble fibrin degradation products. In the bound form the plasmin is protected from degradation by α_2-antiplasmin [75]. Activated Hageman factor and kallikrein can both convert plasminogen to plasmin. The ultimate balanced control of these factors in the fibrinolytic system is not well understood, nor the mechanism by which platelet aggregation is reversed at least before irreversible viscous metamorphosis occurs.

Just how much thrombus is lysed in this manner is uncertain but if the fate of experimental pulmonary emboli is an indicator, most will disappear though this takes time. The quantity not lysed will be incorporated in the intima and endothelialization and organization will proceed. There is no evidence that mural thrombi in veins produce eccentric plaques although such has been assumed to be the case in arteries. Eccentric plaques in arteries form by peripheral extension of the lateral intimal thickenings at arterial bifurcations but it cannot be denied that a mural thrombus may contribute to a plaque, the extent being unknown. If the mural thrombus remains small, healing may occur but further tearing and thrombosis can arise at a later date. The kinetics of such tears and variability of the clinical picture was well depicted by Davies and Thomas [31].

Whether a thrombus becomes occlusive depends on several factors. In general the larger the vessel diameter, the less is the likelihood of progression to occlusion regardless of whether the vessel is an artery or vein and thus occlusive thrombi are rare in the aorta and venae cavae. More severe pathology will also favour occlusion as probably will the quantity of surface area involved. The mobility, physical characteristics and surface irregularities of the vessel may also be of importance. A high flow rate is probably the most effective deterrent to thrombus growth and occlusion. In the case of an artery, impaired run-off which could be due to widespread embolism may predispose to occlusion by reducing the blood flow and velocity.

Thrombi about heart valve prostheses can form rapidly in the agonal phase in the presence of congestive cardiac failure. It is therefore possible that pre-existing arterial and venous thrombi elsewhere may enlarge more readily in an agonal state and become occlusive as well as being a source of emboli.

Complete arterial thrombotic occlusion can have serious consequences which depend on the duration of the occlusion, size of the artery, its anatomy, the vulnerability of the tissue supplied, pathological state of the collateral circulation, cardiac haemodynamics and even anaemia. Infarction of vital tissues is the dreaded sequel. If the patient survives, a series of possible consequences follows. Factors to be considered in arterial occlusion or stenosis include:

- Site of occlusion and size of vessel
- Nature and extent of the occlusion
- Rapidity of onset of occlusion
- Transient or permanent
- Collateral circulation
- Pathology of collateral vessels
- Haemodynamics – local and general
- Haematological status
- Oxygen carrying capacity of the blood
- Age of the subject
- Coexistent diseases
- Fibrinolysis
- Organization of thrombus
- Recanalization
- Susceptibility of tissue supplied
- Ischaemia or infarction

Contraction of the thrombus possibly aided by fibrinolytic activity may result in reopening the lumen to restore flow (Figure 3.10) even though it may remain minor. Occlusion may redevelop followed by propagation of the red thrombus proximally and distally but this is usually limited in arteries being dependent on the

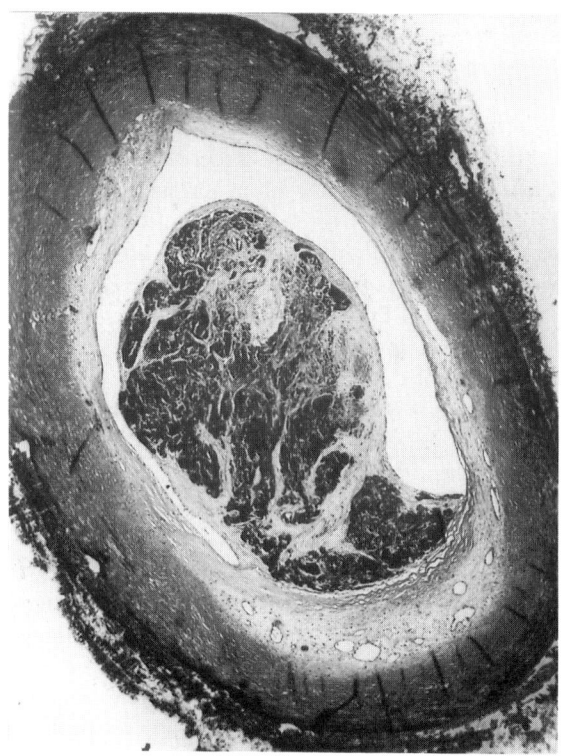

Figure 3.10 Organizing mural thrombus partially occludes lumen of a coronary artery. This could also have resulted from contraction of the thrombus and thrombolytic activity partially restoring patency of the lumen. Note vascularization of the thickened intima. (Haematoxylin and eosin.) (Reproduced with permission from Vlodaver and Edwards [137].)

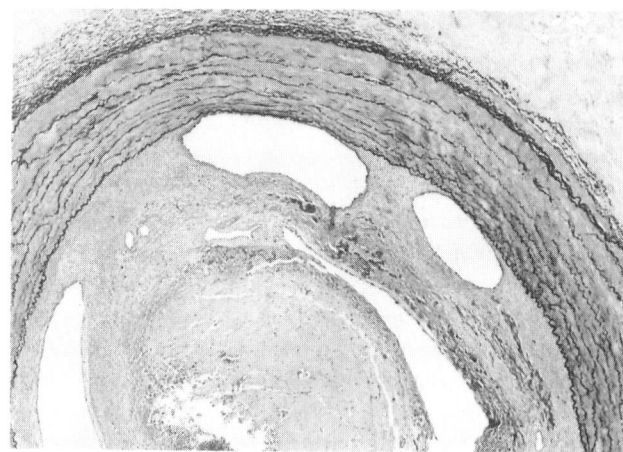

Figure 3.11 Organized thrombus in an experimental artery displaying larger channels than usual. Vessels of this size provide better flow than usual but this does not preclude serious ischaemia distally. (Verhoeff's elastic stain and eosin.)

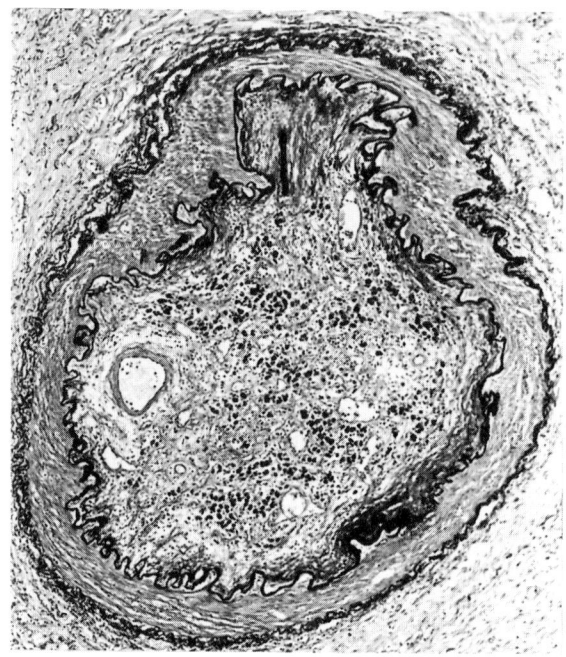

Figure 3.12 Organized thrombus in an experimental artery. The partially collapsed lumen is filled with fibrous tissue, blood vessels and siderophages. Note the thickened wall of the large vessel in the organized thrombus. (Verhoeff's elastic stain and eosin.)

anatomy of the arterial tree, the pathological state of the vessels and the degree of stagnation. However, it can propagate beyond the nearest branches and even occlude several branches [76].

In an experimental study [79] it was found that if a thrombus remains occlusive for more than the first few days, it will probably remain occluded and proceed to organization. Once organization has occurred the residual artery or vein is thin, contracted and white, firm and cord-like. The new vessels within the occluded lumen and wall are usually small and provide little collateral flow. Occasionally the lumen may be subdivided into channels of reasonable size (Figure 3.11) but not often. Many vessels in the lumen are thin walled and sinusoidal and one or two arterial channels have thickened walls but a poor arterial architecture, little elastic tissue and a small lumen (Figure 3.12). Atheromatous debris is usually not present, and appears to be cleared rather rapidly whereas it incites relatively little response in atherosclerosis unless the lipid herniates into the adventitia. The prevalence of siderophages reflects the inclusion of red cells in the thrombus that occluded the lumen and there are usually some round cells present in the loose connective tissue.

In distal arteries occluded by emboli, as in the cerebral leptomeningeal vessels, ghosts of the arteries persist, and the media and lumen are replaced by loose hyaline fibrous tissue possibly with a small vessel and a few siderophages (Figure 3.13). The elastic tissue of the occluded vessel remains. Larger arteries, when occluded, continue to exist as a thin firm white cord and histological examination reveals its nature. An elastic stain aids in the recognition.

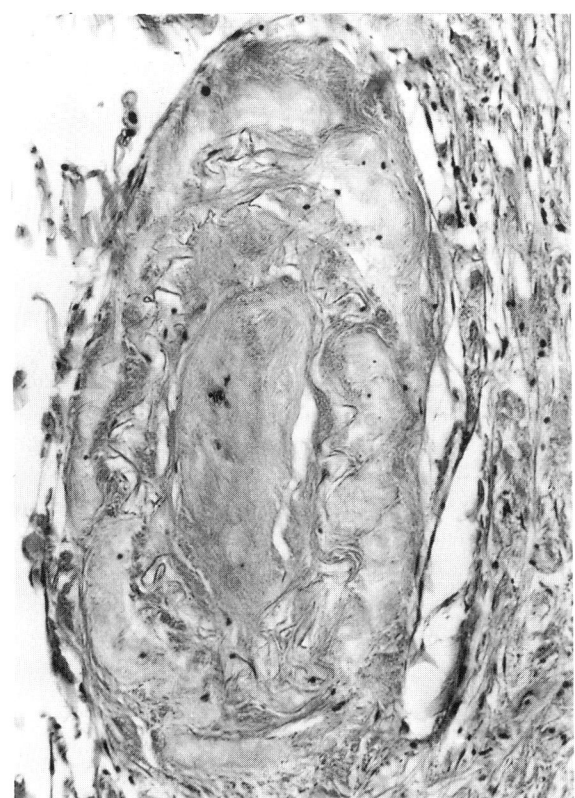

Figure 3.13 Old occluded arteries replaced by a cellular hyaline connective tissue without surviving muscle fibres. The original elastic tissue persists. (Haematoxylin and eosin.)

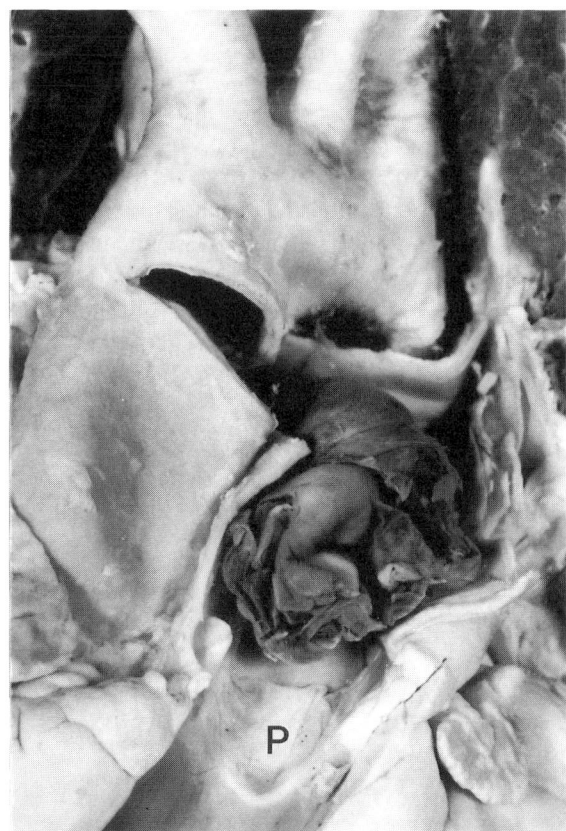

Figure 3.14 Massive pulmonary embolism occluding the bifurcation of the pulmonary trunk. A pulmonary valve cusp is at P.

Veins are more likely to become occluded by thrombus rather than remaining mural. Distal to the thrombus, congestion and oedema are likely although often absent in deep vein thrombosis in the legs. There may be progression to severe congestion and ultimately multiple haemorrhages become confluent if the collateral circulation is inadequate such as with haemorrhagic infarction of the brain or kidney. This is essentially similar to torsion of a pedicle or a polypoid tumour or when a loop of bowel becomes constricted so that there is venous obstruction but arterial flow continues.

Deep vein thrombosis in the lower limbs is often silent. Some subjects have oedematous swelling with pain and tenderness but the swelling may not occur until the leg is in the dependent position. Even if one leg is swollen the thrombosis is usually bilateral. Most fatal pulmonary emboli come from iliac or femoral veins. When the leg is intensely swollen and violaceous often with ecchymoses, there is usually massive occlusion of the iliofemoral veins, the risk of pulmonary embolism is high, the cause of the thrombosis is nearly always clear and amputation for gangrene may be necessary.

White leg (or phlegmasia alba dolens) is a swollen oedematous leg associated with iliofemoral vein thrombosis, occurring most often on the left side and in the third trimester of pregnancy, in the puerperium or after extensive pelvic surgery. It has been postulated that the secondary inflammatory response associated with organization may occlude lymphatic channels thus accentuating the oedema.

Most pulmonary emboli being relatively small are clinically silent but the major catastrophe with deep vein thrombosis in the pelvis and lower extremities is of course massive pulmonary embolism (Figure 3.14) which is more often misdiagnosed than diagnosed correctly. On occasions the main trunk at the bifurcation may be virtually occluded such as by a saddle embolus. More than half the pulmonary arterial flow must be occluded for the clinical syndrome of massive pulmonary embolism to appear. Such an event is rare in the young, but has been reported in infants with congenital heart disease, recent surgery, indwelling catheters, sepsis and prolonged immobility [78]. Neither the sensitivity (20.3%) nor the predictive value (46.7%) of a death certificate diagnosis of pulmonary embolism is high [79].

It is important to appreciate that experimental pulmonary emboli can be lysed rapidly but not necessarily completely. It is also of importance to accept that experimental emboli are often clots rather than pale thrombi or mixed thrombi. In humans emboli can be progressively lysed, the size being an important factor. Monitoring of emboli has revealed minimal effect within seven days and substantial improvement by 10 to 21 days. Some subjects between 14 and 34 days were normal angiographically and haemodynamically [80]. Medium-sized naturally occurring emboli in the lung have been found to be organized within four months and the emboli are reduced in size and transformed into thin strings or bands of connective tissue which remain for a long time. Emboli elsewhere seem to behave in a similar manner often in association with ischaemic changes and without the hypertensive effects of pulmonary emboli.

The direct effect of repetitive emboli on a specific organ or tissue must be considered, for a percentage of these emboli may produce microscopic zones of ischaemia, some possibly permanent. Multiple small fibrotic scars may occur in the heart or the brain and, in an experimental model, hypertension due to renal ischaemia was reported [81]. Similarly repetitive pulmonary embolism results in pulmonary hypertension but the mechanisms are different.

3.7.1 COLLATERAL CIRCULATION

Collateral vessels may be classified as those that naturally exist (see Section 1.9) and those which develop secondarily when there is an impediment or obstruction to flow through the usual more direct channels. There is often considerable enlargement of pre-existing collateral channels with provision of additional significant flow through unusual or even newly formed pathways.

The capacity of the circulatory system to circumvent sites of pathological obstruction by means of development of a collateral circulation is evident in many disease states. The general topography of collateral circulations is often remarkably similar from animal to animal even though the efficacy will vary. Most emphasis has been on arterial collaterals. Venous anastomoses are in general more numerous than those of the arterial tree and the consequences of venous obstruction are usually not as serious as those following occlusion of a major artery. Capillary beds are continuous with neighbouring capillary plexuses but such anastomoses are of relatively little practical value in acute vascular occlusion, although in chronic vascular insufficiency they have the potential to contribute significantly to an alternative collateral pathway.

In many viscera, the existing collateral vessels are generally too small to supply sufficient blood to maintain functional viability of an organ in the event of a sudden occlusion of a major artery. Interarterial anastomoses or arterial arcades in some vascular beds (such as in the mesentery) are so numerous and variable that no attempt has been made to name or classify them. Such anastomotic pathways may at times be a distinct disadvantage for occlusion or stenosis of one vessel may so alter normal blood pressure gradients as to result in the diversion of blood from one tissue (such as the brain) to another perhaps less crucial tissue. This phenomenon is referred to as a 'vascular steal', such as the subclavian steal [33]. Variations of the steal phenomenon involving the central nervous system are reviewed in section 12.7.2. Other vascular beds can be similarly affected if normal pressure gradients are significantly altered. Arteriovenous fistulae can and do steal blood from other tissues, initiating a reversal of the direction of blood flow in arteries which ultimately come to feed the arteriovenous shunt.

When blood flow to a part is compromised by any sudden occlusion of the arterial supply, the function and survival of the tissue become dependent on flow through the pre-existing collateral circulation. The effectiveness of this collateral circulation depends on:

1. the size of the anastomoses;
2. the occlusion pattern as regards the nature and site of obstruction and the involvement of the collaterals;
3. the functional needs of the tissue;
4. general factors affecting the blood flow and blood content [82] as they relate to velocity;
5. neural and metabolic factors which may but do not necessarily influence the collateral circulation.

Blood flow through the collateral circulation rarely equals that through the major arteries supplying the area [83]. When it is adequate the tissue survives in part or in whole and if it is inadequate the tissue dies or the function of the tissue (e.g. myocardium) is seriously compromised. Infarcts do not usually involve the entire territory normally supplied by the occluded vessel, and the amount of infarcted tissue varies with the individual and is dependent on the anatomy of the vascular supply and its collaterals. If the tissue survives, the collateral circulation will enlarge. If the occlusion is gradual, collateral circulation will develop but only after the stenosis reduces the lumen of the vessel by some 80–90%, at which stage there is an effect on the pressure gradient and blood flow [84]. Further reduction of the lumen results in a steep fall in blood flow and an increase in the pressure gradient which is considered the primary stimulus to development of collaterals.

The arterial collateral circulation consists essentially of:

1. an artery or arteries originating on the proximal side of the arterial obstruction with the direction of flow lying towards the anastomoses (the afferent pathway) [85];
2. those arteries with reversed flow carrying blood from the anastomoses to the main arteries beyond the obstruction (the efferent vessels);

3. the mid-zone region or watershed area where the essential small anastomoses exist [83,85].

The mid-zone region is normally supplied by both vessels where the anastomoses between them customarily occur. The reconstituted pathway may be extremely circuitous and before the blood ultimately reaches its destination, intermediate anastomoses may have been incorporated.

The change from a single large vessel to multiple channels of smaller calibre is always associated with diminution in blood flow proportional to the radius of the collateral vessels. In practice, flow through collaterals is rarely equal to that through the normal arteries of supply unless there are interarterial or intervenous anastomoses. The nature of the anastomoses is of considerable importance. The additional resistance to flow is not significantly affected by the simple union of two major vessels as in the circle of Willis. It can be significantly increased when the anastomoses are established by a retiform plexus of very small vessels as occurs in moyamoya disease.

Following an occlusion of an artery there are at least two phases in the establishment of the collateral circulation. Initially in the acute phase, there is a critical period in which flow to the distal tissues depends on the pre-existing state of the collaterals. In the chronic stage there is a considerable enlargement of collateral vessels, some of which may be newly acquired or at least not previously demonstrable. On occlusion of a major artery, a fall in blood pressure distal to the obstruction and in the distal part of the collateral pathways creates a pressure gradient which can be accentuated by an increase in pressure proximally. Consistent with hydrodynamic laws, blood flows from a high to a low pressure area and so it traverses the stem or afferent vessels, the fine anastomotic vessels of the mid-zone, and the re-entrant or efferent vessels, until eventually it reaches the main artery beyond the occlusion. There is thus a reversal of blood flow through some of the anastomotic network of small vessels in the intermediate region or mid-zone, in the larger re-entrant vessels and possibly also in part of the parent trunk itself immediately distal to the occlusion. The mid-zone region of the collateral pathway provides the greatest resistance to flow on account of the greatly increased surface area of contact. If the mid-zone anastomoses are large thereby offering minimal resistance, the flow may be sufficient to prevent infarction. In this regard blood viscosity is probably of negligible importance because of its limited variability.

Following acute occlusion of the femoral artery in dogs, a fall in blood pressure to a non-pulsatile level between 35 and 60 mmHg has been recorded. A feeble pulse is restored within four to six seconds, followed by progressive increase in systolic, diastolic and pulse pressures, until within one minute of occlusion the systolic pressure equals approximately the diastolic pressure prior to occlusion. Thereafter, there is a slower progressive increase until a plateau or maximum level is reached (up to eight minutes) at which time the systolic pressure is slightly higher than the pre-occlusion diastolic level and the pulse pressure is close to half its original value. Such levels have been maintained for as long as four months [86]. The re-establishment of pulsations in the arteries distal to the occlusion was demonstrated angiographically to coincide with the opening up or dilatation of anastomoses in the pre-existing collateral pathway. Tissue oxygen in the calf muscle dropped to a mean of about 90% of the control level (range of 84–95%) within a few minutes, and then slowly rose to normal values within eight minutes. However, viability of the lower limb may be maintained by a blood pressure of only 22 mmHg and low flow rates, whereas the metabolic needs of such tissues as the brain and heart could not be met with such paltry flow conditions [87]. Increased workload serves to aggravate the inadequacy although increased pressure increases collateral flow.

Following ligation of a major artery to a limb, the limb temperature, presumably because of the reduced blood flow, falls to that of the room. After eight to 15 hours, the temperature returns within the next hour to that of the opposite limb. Experimental evidence indicates that the collateral vessels are initially constricted during the period of reduced flow and that ganglionectomy to interrupt the efferent vasomotor nerves relieves the vasoconstriction and collateral vessels then dilate [88]. Thus in a biological system, apart from the hydrodynamic laws, other factors such as nervous control of vasomotor activity, the metabolic activity of the tissue and the muscular activity and elasticity of the walls of collateral vessels all modify vessel calibre and volume flow and thereby play a role in establishing the collateral circulation which may vary from time to time until a definite equilibrium is achieved [89]. Even when an equilibrium is reached, the volume flow rate is always less than that originally prevailing because of the reduced blood pressure distally and the increased peripheral resistance in the collateral pathways. The presence of severe atherosclerosis of accessory sources of blood supply further jeopardizes distal limbs.

During the second phase the vessels in the collateral pathways increase in calibre and mural hypertrophy develops [89]. Different rates of growth (calibre and length) are known to occur, the small vessels of the mid-zone increasing proportionately more than those of the stem and re-entrant vessels [85]. The growth of collateral circulation is more prominent in the young than in adults. There has been much debate as to whether the development of the collateral circulation is merely the enlargement of pre-existing channels or the further proliferation of vessels, for quite large channels develop in rather unusual locations. Experimental evidence indicates that the development encompasses both methods.

Mitotic activity in endothelial, medial and adventitial cells occurs in collateral vessels following experimental coronary occlusion. The enhanced mitotic activity is maximal at three weeks but persists for eight weeks postoperatively. This proliferative activity is always most pronounced in the small vessels of the mid-zone [90]. The newly developed collateral vessels are rarely of comparable size to the stem or to re-entrant vessels in man or in experimental animals.

The anastomotic channels in the human heart are generally less than 350 µm in diameter but as the result of the augmented flow in coronary artery disease, may enlarge to a diameter of 1 to 2 mm and characteristically become elongated, tortuous and even spiral [91]. Tortuosity is generally observed first in the intermediate zone and then progressively extends distally until the entire length of the efferent trunk is affected [89].

Although the mechanisms underlying the development of a collateral circulation are uncertain, four theories have been proposed.

1. *Tissue metabolites.* Tissue metabolites accumulate in an area suddenly deprived of its blood supply. Recovery of blood pressure and flow distally occurs too early for a significant increase in tissue metabolites to become apparent. Since the major factors establishing collateral flow are likely to be the same for arteries and veins, the theory would not satisfactorily explain development of venous collaterals.
2. *Increased tissue demand.* This is known to induce increased flow locally but the same criticisms apply to this hypothesis as to the preceding one.
3. *Neurogenic reflex vasodilation.* Sympathectomy improves the collateral circulation [86,88] possibly by increasing circulation to the ischaemic zone in general, by reducing the overall peripheral resistance distally.
4. *Pressure differential.* The pressure differential, established by occlusion of an artery resulting in a drop in blood pressure distally [86] and a variable increase proximally, will induce blood to flow along all available channels towards such an area. In an arteriovenous fistula the blood flows along direct and collateral arterial channels towards the fistula beyond which is the low pressure venous system. In the venous system, there is stagnation distally and resistance to flow along conventional venous pathways. With an increase in venous pressure distally, blood flows along collateral vessels in which the pressure is reduced and resistance to flow is less. Holman [92] considered this theory was the most likely to account for the establishment of a collateral circulation. He invoked the law of hydraulics, that flowing blood, like water, inevitably follows the path of least resistance. This concept is supported by the consequences of anomalous origin of the left coronary artery from the pulmonary artery. Under such circumstances, collaterals develop and blood flows from the right coronary artery with its high pressure into the low pressure left coronary artery and thence into the pulmonary artery.

Physical or haemodynamic factors appear to be the primary stimulus to the development of the collateral vessels but the precise reason for the dilatation of the anastomotic channels in the collateral pathway following an occlusive lesion of a major artery is not yet known. The chronic and progressive enlargement of collateral vessels associated with an arteriovenous fistula is apparently a response of the vessel walls to augmented haemodynamic stress associated with the greatly increased flow (hyperkinetic state) and to changes in blood pressure and profound degenerative changes in blood vessels participating in the shunt [93–95].

According to Thoma's histomechanical law [96] the increase in calibre of collateral vessels would ensue because of the increased blood velocity but this in itself is an inadequate explanation for it ignores both the underlying mechanism and the means by which an equilibrium is reached. In association with an increase in radius, blood velocity and pulse pressure in the collaterals, there will be an increased Reynolds number. It is suggested that the dilatation is due to yield of the vessel wall consequent upon fatigue associated with the flow disturbances and augmented pulse pressure. Certainly such a concept would satisfactorily explain the dilatation, elongation and tortuosity that characteristically occur in collateral vessels and also the severe degenerative changes, aneurysm formation and at times haemorrhage from rupture of collaterals [33,93–95]. Retarded development of collateral vessels would presumably result when the pressure differential was reduced following enlargement of the collaterals and further flow would be prevented by the greater peripheral resistance due to the larger surface area. The increase in diameter and pressure in the collaterals will lead to an increase in mural tension and proliferation of mural connective tissues but the control mechanism is quite unknown.

Collateral vessels have been found to regress within the first postoperative month after the performance of a coronary by-pass operation in dogs with a chronically occluded coronary artery [97]. However, no mention was made of structural changes in the walls or whether the tortuosity had disappeared. Redevelopment of collateral vessels follows occlusion of the bypass graft [98]. There is a tendency to maintain the velocity in an artery at near to normal levels, for a reduction in flow to a part is accompanied by a simultaneous reduction in the calibre of the artery as has been observed following amputation of a limb. Active constriction together with intimal thickening is said to occur [98]. A detailed analysis of these structural changes is required.

When a vein is occluded, the pressure distally is increased and low pressure is found proximal to the occlusion. The venous valves prevent backflow but the anastomoses are generally so liberal in the venous circulation that collaterals are usually present. Irregular dilatation and tortuosity ensue as the flow through the collaterals is increased until an equilibrium is obtained. Varicosities may become pronounced and there is a tendency to rupture often with severe haemorrhage. Collateral circulation may arise from one venous circulatory bed to other venous or portal circulations (or vice versa) and it is the watershed area that exhibits the varicosities.

Newly formed collateral vessels developed in the inflammatory reaction at the site of arterial ligation in the rabbit ear [99] but collateral vessels elsewhere appeared to have been enlarged pre-existing vessels. Later Lambert et al. [100] demonstrated angiographically the restoration of the continuity of divided arteries and veins in rabbit ears that had been nearly transected. The sequence of events following transection of the vessels is:

1. connections formed by side branches on either side of the incision;
2. invasion of the divided ends of the vessels by vascular granulation tissue that filled the wound;
3. continuity between the divided ends of the vessel attained through the capillary network in this granulation tissue in the wound and involving the ends of the vessels (as early as six days);
4. gradual enlargement of the most direct pathway with dwindling or disappearance of more remote connections.

Arteries are always connected to arteries and veins to veins even when lying in close proximity. There was proliferation of both muscle and elastic tissue in the newly formed arterial anastomoses and the pressure gradient across the line of division seemed to be a determining factor in the rate at which the reconnections developed although restoration of the continuity of the lumen and the development of the direct end-to-end channels regularly occurred earlier in veins than in arteries. It is not yet clear why arteriovenous anastomoses do not develop more frequently under such circumstances. When alternative collaterals are available, the shorter pathway is ultimately favoured whilst alternative pathways diminish in size, suggesting that the choice of vessel is determined by haemodynamic factors.

Whether or not distinctly new vessels develop other than at the site of thrombotic occlusion is uncertain, since even small vessels in the microcirculation may conceivably enlarge. New vessels certainly form in a thrombotic occlusion as part of the process of organization and it has been acknowledged that these can participate in a collateral circulation from the proximal to the distal end usually only to a limited extent.

Collateral vessels developing from the microcirculation enlarge as in angiogenesis, according to the physiological demand with the progressive and eventual dominance of vessels providing the most convenient path. Concomitantly the perivascular connective tissues would be endeavouring to produce a suitable mural architecture in the face of hydrodynamic stresses in excess of the physiological capabilities of vessels of that calibre. This is the possible explanation as to why the mural connective tissues of such vessels never seem to differentiate to produce a vessel of normal architecture.

There is evidence that the enlarged collateral vessels, subjected to augmented flow and pressure changes, characteristically become tortuous if not spiral. There has been much investigation into the topography, angiography, size, flow capacity and development of collateral vessels but little interest has been manifested in the structural changes in collateral vessels. Borgers et al. [101] reported the occurrence of necrotic lesions in the medial smooth muscle cells of developing collateral arteries together with intimal tears, intramural haemorrhage and leucocyte infiltration.

Venous varicosities participating in a collateral circulation exhibit phlebosclerosis and manifest a tendency to rupture and haemorrhage. This propensity for rupture of the vein itself and also of the underlying mucosa or even skin suggests an insidious, progressive loss of tensile strength seemingly attributable to the cumulative local stresses to which the vein and surrounding perivenous tissues are subjected. More than mere hydrostatic venous pressure would be required to rupture normal veins, perivenous tissue and the skin in particular. Vessels supplying arteriovenous fistulae exhibit gross degenerative changes commencing within a few days of the creation of the fistula [93–96]. In the small arteries and also in veins close to an experimental arteriovenous fistula and participating in the collateral flow, severe elastic tissue degeneration can be observed as well as considerable intimal thickening, the changes being consistent with atherosclerosis and phlebosclerosis respectively. The stresses applied to many collateral vessels would be less severe than in experimental fistulae and there is need for thorough investigation of the progressive changes that occur.

Arteries participating in the collateral circulation in subjects with aortic coarctation also exhibit gross tortuosity and degenerative changes and not infrequently develop saccular aneurysms. Such aneurysms have been observed on the intercostal arteries [33,102] and the anterior spinal artery [33].

Many cases have also been described often in young adults and children with multiple intracranial arterial occlusions with an extremely prominent compensatory collateral circulation at the base of the brain, in the basal ganglia and upper brain stem [103]. These cases have been referred to in Japan as examples of moyamoya disease (or rete mirabile). The vascular network consisting of a profuse collateral circulation secondary to occlusion of major cerebral arteries [33] is particularly prone to subarachnoid haemorrhage and aneurysm of these vessels. It would appear that haemorrhage from these small collateral vessels occurs only after the collateral circulation has been established for many years.

3.7.2 PHLEBOLITHS

Phleboliths are harmless calcified thrombi, mostly seen in the pelvic veins near the lower end of the ureters and in the periprostatic venous plexus. Phleboliths are prevalent in economically developed countries but rare in Africans and traditional Polynesians. In this respect they are comparable with the comparative prevalence of thromboembolic disorders. They have been observed in varicocoeles, splenic veins and in haemangiomas. Usually only 4 mm in diameter, they can measure up to 20 mm. Usually an average of about four but up to 20 can be found per person and then mostly in the middle-aged or elderly. The absence of bicuspid valves, and only remnants of ostial valves in the veins of adults suggest that the high pressures during coughing and straining (up to 140 mmHg) may contribute to the irregular dilatations and narrowings so prevalent in the pelvic venous circulation [104]. It is possible that remnants of torn valves could act as a nidus for thrombus which subsequently separates from the wall and is retained like a ball in a ball valve. The cell debris in the thrombus has a non-specific affinity for calcification and lipid, with the former predominating.

Ball thrombi have been reported in the carotid sinus and may be either free or attached to the wall by a pedicle [105]. Such thrombi would be prone to calcification and are known as arterioliths.

3.8 Trauma

Trauma is always associated with damaged blood vessels causing anything from bruising to fatal exsanguinating haemorrhage. The injuries may be of many sorts and injuries involving cerebral blood vessels are dealt with in Chapter 12.

Non-penetrating injuries of the aorta result from severe blows, crushing injuries or falls with sudden deceleration in the vertical or horizontal direction. Complete severance of the aorta may occur in falls from heights or a partial tear of the inner aspect can result in an aneurysm or dissection which is not extensive. The two most common sites for such tears are immediately beyond the origin of the left subclavian artery and just above the aortic valve. It is curious that these are the two common sites for the initiating tears of dissecting aneurysms. The injury may also occur proximal to the brachiocephalic artery. The false aneurysms and the dissections may require therapy and fatal haemorrhage may occur after a lag period. Lacerations of the midthoracic descending aorta are extremely rare. Such tears have been attributed to hyperextension of the spine though it is difficult to accept this as feasible. They are more likely to be associated with sudden deceleration in a vertical direction with the thoracic viscera being thrust upwards and the aorta being subjected to excessive elongation. Such injuries to the thoracic aorta, a consequence of motor vehicle accidents, are increasing in frequency. Most tears are linear involving partial or complete transection [106]. Tears are most often transverse since the aorta has less tensile strength to longitudinal stress than to transverse or lateral stress [107]. Depending on the nature of the injury, the aortic injuries may be multiple contusions or intimomedial lacerations with flaps and secondary thromboembolic phenomena as well as leakage. Hyperextension of the spine has been considered a cause of multiple transverse tears of the ventral surface of the abdominal aorta. The swallowing of sharp objects such as fish bones is a known hazard since they can penetrate the wall of the oesophagus and the adjacent aorta leading to aortitis and haemorrhage.

It is not usually appreciated that an atherosclerotic abdominal aorta in particular can be damaged by severe blunt injuries to the abdomen. Even deep palpation compressing the aorta against the vertebral bodies can cause brittle intimal lesions to crack leading to severe atheroembolism and thrombosis. However, most injuries to the abdominal aorta are due to penetrating wounds from knives or missiles and usually require urgent treatment to prevent fatal haemorrhage.

Injuries are likely to be multiple and the chest injuries may affect the heart, valves or coronary arteries. Blunt or penetrating injuries of smaller arteries may cause fatal haemorrhage from one or several arterial lesions but also from large veins which can entail equally serious consequences. Complete transection of an artery may cause less bleeding than a partial lateral tear because, with the former, vasoconstriction reduces blood loss, thus facilitating the formation of a haemostatic plug whilst lateral tears may bleed more since vasoconstriction is less effective. Traumatic aneurysm or arteriovenous shunts arise almost anywhere and the latter may contribute to cardiac failure. Sometimes the injury may lead to thrombotic occlusion and the consequences therefrom.

Blunt injuries to the chest can cause avulsion or laceration of the branches of the aortic arch and lesser injuries can result in post-traumatic aneurysms, usually not dissecting in type.

An unusual complication of road accidents and falls is renal artery thrombosis which may be bilateral and result in renal infarction. The renal arterial injuries close to their origin from the aorta have been attributed to the mobility of the kidneys: sudden deceleration results in a severe pull on the renal arteries with overstretching [108].

Blunt or penetrating injuries to the superior mesenteric artery are unusual but occur in civilian life. When the injury is to the trunk, surgical repair is imperative but injuries sustained more peripherally are of less consequence and can be repaired by ligatures because of the plentiful arterial anastomotic arcades that exist. Even these injuries can result in arteriovenous shunts with secondary portal hypertension.

It has been recognized that certain movements of the head including head traction can lead to impaired vertebral artery flow. Injuries to the neck and at times merely forcible manipulation of the head and neck can cause crushing injuries to the vertebral artery. It is thought that the vertebral artery in the region of the atlas and the atlanto-occipital membrane can be compressed by rotation of the head to the opposite side [33,65]. This may be accentuated by degenerative changes in the artery and also spinal osteoarthritis but can occur even in birth injuries. The thrombus may propagate upwards into the basilar artery with fatal results. The consequences are dependent on the collateral circulation, the respective sizes of the vertebral arteries and the extent of propagation of the thrombus.

Blunt trauma to the neck with or without spinal fracture can severely damage the carotid arteries. Some injuries of the internal carotid artery near the base of the skull may be due to excessive stretching and result in an intimomedial tear with limited dissection deep to the media and thus would be classified pathologically as a dissecting aneurysm. The superadded thrombus or emboli produces ischaemic lesions in the brain [109]. It is unlikely that hyperextension of the neck would cause such an injury. Whilst an occlusion may be asymptomatic, most subjects develop neurological deficit and many die (20 to 40%) [110]. Some lesions are of an embolic nature but there can be extensive thrombotic occlusion with propagation into the intracranial segment.

With trauma, damage to major blood vessels is always a serious consideration and unfortunately injuries are frequently multiple with tears to smaller vessels often missed. Bruising and swelling can easily mask more serious injuries. In those of the chest, the heart may be involved together with major vessels, and haemorrhage can also stem from ruptured abdominal viscera. Fractured bones, dislocations and nerve injuries must be sought. Transection of large vessels with massive bleeding is more easily recognized than lesser injuries such as contusions, lacerations and dissections which can lead to serious secondary complications. Secondary thrombosis with ischaemia distally in a limb can be readily overlooked and if uncorrected within 12 hours, can result in amputation or protracted infection and incapacitation. Post-traumatic thrombotic occlusion may take time to develop.

Traumatic aneurysms may not become manifest for months or years [111] and the pernicious arteriovenous aneurysm may become apparent insidiously only as the shunt enlarges, while the traumatic episode has been forgotten with the passage of time. Consequently serious vascular trauma must be considered at the time of injury and also during the recovery period. Superadded infection particularly in the presence of foreign bodies is a serious complication.

Chronic repetitive vascular injuries such as may result from the prolonged use of crutches can result in thrombosis with embolism and aneurysm of the axillary and brachial artery with ischaemia of the hand. These are often related to the presence of cervical ribs, anomalous fibrous bands or scalene muscle hypertrophy, but have also been attributed to compression of the axillary artery by the head of the humerus as well as compression of the thoracic outlet while pitching the ball [112]. The use of the dominant hand as a mallet may result in thrombosis of the ulnar artery as it passes over the hamate and sometimes the superficial volar arch and digital arteries are also occluded. Thrombosis of digital arteries also complicates baseball and handball games, the catching hand being affected. Axillary artery tears and secondary thrombosis are sustained by baseball pitchers due to the repetitive forces to which arm and shoulder are subjected for years.

3.9 Vibrating tool disease

Vibration white finger or Raynaud's phenomenon of occupational origin had been recognized since the 1950s and associated with vibrating tools. In subsequent years it was recognized that with longer exposure and more severe vibration as with impact percussion tools, the vascular changes were much more severe [113,114]. High speed vibrating tools such as chain saws, pneumatic drills and even light tools (pneumatic screw-drivers and nut-runners) used in engine assembling factories may be implicated [115]. The harmful effects depend not only on mechanical factors (frequency, energy) but on personal sensitivity and susceptibility. Bones exhibit vacuoles, cysts and exostoses especially of the carpal and metacarpal bones [115]. The disease is not limited to periodic ischaemic attacks of the fingers and has led to the title vibration-induced white finger; vibrating tool disease is a more apt title. Quite apart from the vibration-induced deafness, there is numbness, tingling and even pain in the hands, sensitivity to cold, loss of sensation, white fingers and trophic changes of the finger tips [116]. There is loss of manual dexterity and manipulative skills. The effect is cumulative eventually leading to stenotic intimal thickening of digital arteries, possibly with thrombosis and even gangrene of the tips of the fingers, osteoarthritis and peripheral neuropathy. The evidence is that the disease is irreversible and the vibration effect cumulative. Withdrawal from exposure has little effect and the disease may well deteriorate further [119]. The only objective test seems to be cold provocation. There may also be general psychosomatic symptoms which are difficult to evaluate [114] and if the legs are exposed to vibration, they too can be affected.

3.10 Iatrogenic trauma

Iatrogenic injuries can be relatively trivial or more severe as with angioplasty but it is often not fully appreciated that the passage of a cannula along an artery or vein will cause intimal injury of varying degree, sometimes perforation of the wall with severe haemorrhage and thrombotic episodes. Evans and Kerr [118] reported thrombotic arterial occlusion in 17% of cannulated patients and if the cannula was in position for more than six hours, this increased to 43%. By the end of the observation period, flow had returned in 19% of the occluded arteries. These thrombotic episodes are more common with right-sided cannulation than on the left. Thrombosis secondary to temporary venous catheters and secondary emboli is probably more frequent than is supposed but fortunately most are cleared by thrombolysis, although atheroembolism is a particular risk in elderly atherosclerotic subjects [119]. Inadvertent loss of cannulae within the vascular system occurs from time to time and can lead to secondary injuries to blood vessels and to heart valves which are then susceptible to bacterial endocarditis.

Infection by skin commensals is a serious risk with chronic central venous cannulation, occurring usually later in 7-16% of subjects and especially with hyperalimentation [120].

Surgical clamps in human surgery may cause serious injuries to blood vessels especially if atherosclerotic and with a high closing pressure [121].

The practice of angioplasty is becoming more widespread and the balloon catheter, by disrupting the stenotic wall like a bougie, must inevitably cause embolism of atheromatous debris, calcific particles or merely thrombi.

Thrombosis at the site of the angioplasty may result in early occlusion. The possibility of aneurysm formation is very real and the incidence may increase with time. Mural dissection is not unexpected. Fatal rupture appears to be infrequent although a periarterial haematoma due to perforation is more frequent. Embolism may impair the run-off and contribute to exacerbation of the ischaemia. Over a variable period of time restenosis may ensue due to repair tissue, organization of a mural thrombus and re-establishment of the atherosclerosis. Other complications peculiar to the form of angioplasty such as thermal injury and perforation by a wire probe will no doubt be increased with technological innovations.

X-irradiation causes increased permeability of arterioles, venules and capillaries and fibrinoid necrosis of small arteries resembling an arteritis possibly associated with thrombotic occlusion, fibrinous exudate or even haemorrhage. More protracted injuries of larger vessels cause extensive mural fibrosis with intimal proliferation, disruption of mural architecture, considerable adventitial fibrotic thickening with hyalinization and complete occlusion. Amyloid deposition occurs in the larger vessels and about capillary walls of the microcirculation.

3.11 Trauma, repair and intimal proliferation

Following microvascular surgery where the injury is far from minimal, re-endothelialization is usually complete within two weeks and at clamp sites even earlier. Reidy and Schwartz [122] induced minimal defined injuries to rat aortic endothelium and a single monolayer of platelets covered the breach. Longitudinal injuries were covered by endothelial replication but transverse injuries were covered by endothelial spreading within eight hours without replication. What happens to platelets is uncertain. They could be shed only to be phagocytosed within the circulation or could be phagocytosed *in situ*. In spontaneous tears (transverse or longitudinal) of the arterial internal elastic lamina often with endothelial disruption, there is intense endothelial replication within the confines of the tear with gradual resumption of the normal endothelial pattern over subsequent weeks [93,123].

Experimental injuries to venous endothelium cause deposition of platelets and a few leucocytes but thicker deposits of thrombus are present even though they may heal rapidly by endothelial replication. Curiously, endothelial repair of experimental injuries to arteries and veins is associated with multinucleated giant cells as they occur at arterial forks, experimental arteriovenous fistulae and in atherosclerosis, but this does not arise where spontaneous tears of the internal elastic lamina occur in afferent arteries feeding arteriovenous fistulae [123].

Considerable interest has been demonstrated in repair of the arterial wall following injuries of all types in the mistaken belief that mechanical endothelial injury initiates atherosclerosis. The minimal injuries to arteries causing endothelial denudation reported by Reidy and Schwartz [122] did not result in intimal proliferation. Arteriotomy in the rabbit common carotid artery results in intimal thickening along the suture line but not along clamp sites [124] suggesting that the severity of the injury is important but the severity is obviously difficult to quantify and to standardize experimentally.

Following endothelial denudation by a gentle stream of air passed through the carotid artery of rats sufficient to dry the surface [125], platelets adhered to the surface and oedema developed in the injured wall until endothelialization was complete within seven to ten days. After 14 days pronounced intimal proliferation appeared in the central region of the denuded zone and consisted of musculo-elastic tissue. Regression and condensation of the intimal thickening occurred within three months postoperatively. The authors attributed the proliferation to undefined factors from the lumen but recent data would suggest that many mitogenic factors including platelet-derived growth factor (PDGF) could be responsible. The experiment demonstrated that trauma-induced intimal thickening was an example of excessive proliferation or hyperplasia in the repair process only to be followed by some regression. This is a typical biological reaction as occurs with most tissues. The thickening is also much greater than a corresponding injury to a vein. The precise reason is unknown and the intima behaves differently from that occurring spontaneously about arterial forks.

The intimal thickenings at sites of arterial injury of diverse nature have been shown to be sites of predilection for dietary-induced lipid deposition and whereas the intimal thickening of forks is always susceptible to such lipid deposition, the former, after healing is complete, no longer exhibits any such predilection. Moreover, the intimal proliferation at forks and curvatures can be induced by haemodynamic stress experimentally [52].

It is apparent that endothelial loss alone does not necessarily cause intimal thickening as has been seen in association with elastic tears in the afferent arteries of experimental arteriovenous fistulae or about curvatures, although it may occur after a very long lag period and under continued stress. In a dissecting aneurysm the internal elastic lamina was stripped from half to at least three quarters of the circumference over a length of the middle cerebral artery, yet years later no significant intimal thickening was present despite increase in the size of the patient and the artery [126].

These observations suggest that the underlying stimulus to intimal proliferation is uncertain and that the intimal proliferation due to trauma differs from that spontaneously occurring at arterial forks which is intimately associated with atherosclerosis. There is no evidence that thrombosis plays any role in the pathogenesis of the intimal proliferation at forks. More severe experimental injuries or those in humans progressively acquire an endothelial covering and intimal proliferation of some degree invariably follows severe injuries such as surgical procedures. Even a prosthetic surface, or the lining of a false passage of an aortic dissecting aneurysm will in time develop a neointima. Likewise a false aneurysm lined by thrombus will also develop an neointima. Such vessels in humans are exposed to the stimuli that produce atherosclerosis and early changes may appear but there have been no ultrastructural studies of such changes. Severe experimental traumatic injuries may have thrombus but there is no evidence that they progress to atherosclerosis as it occurs in man.

3.12 Thrombogenic hypothesis of atherogenesis

The thrombogenic hypothesis as it is known currently postulates that thrombi forming within the vascular system become incorporated in the vessel wall and undergo fatty degeneration resulting in atherosclerosis.

Von Rokitansky [127] postulated that atherosclerosis was caused by encrustation of mural deposits from the blood, mostly fibrin, with atheromatous change and calcification considered secondary [128]. Inspissated mural thrombus can indeed merge with an ulcerated atherosclerotic aorta and without adequate histological techniques it is understandable that he could reach such a conclusion. More recently Leary [129] described acute fibrinoid necrosis of subendothelial tissue, which Clark et al. [130] interpreted as an organizing thrombus suggesting that repeated deposition of thrombus and organization could progress to atherosclerosis. This interpretation was not proof to others [131], but Duguid [132] was convinced that arterial thrombi formed fibrous intimal plaques indistinguishable from atherosclerosis and that red thrombus was especially prone to softening and fatty degeneration. Eccentric plaques and a suggestion of layering, particularly when the innermost region was infiltrated with fibrin, were used as evidence in support of the concept. Duguid's interpretation of morbid anatomy does not constitute scientific proof, there being no evidence that thrombus progresses to advanced atherosclerosis and its complications experimentally or in human pathology [133].

It is acknowledged that thrombosis is a complication of atherosclerosis and that organization of thrombus may contribute to the overall thickening of the intima and encroachment on the arterial lumen. From knowledge of emboli in human pathology this contribution may be nothing or very little since thrombolytic activity can clear most of the thrombus within days if not all in many instances. On the other hand, the role of thrombosis in the aetiology and pathogenesis of the early intimal proliferation which is a precursor or integral stage of atherosclerosis is without basic evidence and remains conjectural. Crucial to this question is whether or not platelets adhere to and form a thrombus on intact endothelium. All current evidence suggests this is not the case and that even if it were so, there is no evidence that thrombus plays a primary role in the initial intimal proliferation. All evidence indicates that thrombosis is a late secondary rather than the primary event.

The thrombogenic theory and its variants do not explain the initiation and pathogenesis of atherosclerosis, its topography or its complications. In summary the thrombogenic theory of the aetiology of atherosclerosis is not valid for the following reasons:

1. The endothelium is a non-thrombogenic surface and experimentally platelets *in vivo* under physiological conditions require some defect or discontinuity of the endothelium before adhering to the vessel wall.
2. The thrombogenic theory fails to explain the cause of the initial endothelial lesion resulting in mural thrombus, which is then secondary rather than primary.
3. Thrombus is a complication of end-stage atherosclerosis and its organization may contribute to the overall thickening of the intima and encroachment of the lumen but to an unknown degree.
4. There is no evidence that thrombosis occurs on normal arterial endothelium and most if not all non-embolic arterial occlusive thrombi are believed to be secondary to intimal disruption, the severity of which has been underestimated [31,134].
5. The cause of intimal tears and ulceration has received scant attention despite their being frequent and at times extensive in the aorta under physiological flow conditions. Attributed to an acquired fragility [26,34], they are analogous to stress (fatigue) fractures of bones and tendons of soldiers, joggers and sportsmen. The thrombus is a secondary phenomenon.
6. There is no evidence that thrombosis plays a role in the development of early intimal proliferation at forks, bends and junctions which are widely accepted as being a prelipid phase of atherosclerosis.
7. Intimal layering, though interpreted as episodic mural thrombosis with organization, is seen in fetuses and neonates and the eccentric thickening is but a peripheral extension of the intimal proliferation at the lateral angle of forks and is also seen in the cerebral arteries of sheep.
8. Aneurysms with laminated thrombus, cardiac valve vegetations and organizing occlusive arterial and venous thrombi do not undergo atheromatous degeneration. Venous thrombosis and pulmonary emboli have been found in 60% of autopsies, yet overt atheromatous degeneration does not parallel this incidence.
9. The presence of fibrin in the atherosclerotic wall does not indicate the entire plaque is derived from a mural thrombus.
10. The thrombogenic theory does not explain the topography of atherosclerosis, the variation in severity from vascular bed to vascular bed, nor the complications of atherosclerosis (tortuosity, ectasia, aneurysms, intimal tears and ulcerations).
11. Speculation that platelet aggregation, induced haemodynamically or otherwise, consistently injures the arterial wall at specific anatomical sites of both low and high shear stress about arterial forks and induces intimal proliferation by the release of a mitogenic factor or under the influence of other mediators, and that such lesions progress to advanced disease, is unproven, implausible and incompatible with life. Leucocyte–platelet microthrombi must form in many tissues (veins, venules and the microvasculature) daily in view of the ease with which they occur in the rabbit ear chamber indicating that they must resolve rapidly without ill-effects. If it were not so, atherosclerosis would be widespread in man and all other mammals at the site of every arterial and venous injury.
12. Embolism of experimental clots and fibrin emboli do not lead to atherosclerosis nor its complications.
13. Since thrombi are found in the veins of the lower limb in some 60% of patients at autopsy in a general hospital, atherosclerosis would be much more severe in those vessels if the thrombogenic theory were valid.
14. The thrombogenic theory fails to explain the occurrence of lipid in the vessel wall and the other ultrastructural changes characteristic of atherosclerosis.
15. Atheromatous embolism with superadded thrombosis does not progress to atherosclerosis but is readily distinguishable from atherosclerosis of the host artery.
16. Advanced atherosclerotic lesions are rare in the cardiac chambers and valve cusps despite the frequency of mural thrombi and intima-like thickening of the endocardium particularly in the left atrium.
17. Thrombi on cardiac valves heal by fibrotic thickening of the cusps with calcification and not by atheromatous degeneration.
18. Thromboemboli are uncommon pathologically in the first two decades and are usually secondary events of middle and old age.

To assume that thrombus contributes substantially to the atherosclerotic plaque is conjecture and there is no evidence that large thrombi (aneurysms, heart, veins) degenerate into caseous atheromatous material nor proof that a mural thrombus precedes lipid-containing atherosclerotic lesions [133]. Moreover, the thrombogenic hypothesis does not explain the pathogenesis of atherosclerosis including all the histological and ultrastructural changes, the complications including intimal tears, ulcerations and aneurysms with which mural or occlusive thrombosis occurs secondarily.

The fate of experimental thrombi has been reviewed elsewhere [133] and conclusions reached were that neither the thrombi nor thrombotic lesions of the vessel wall resulted in atherosclerosis, that in the process of organization the presence of minimal lipid was a temporary event and that an extensive lipid content was achieved by inducing hypercholesterolaemia. The lipid content of experimental thromboemboli did not have the characteristics of spontaneous atherosclerosis, and the lipid diminished with the duration of the experiment with the lesion progressively losing its lipophilia [135]. Lipid accumulation and calcification can be expected in a chronic necrotic thrombus because the cell debris has an affinity for lipid and mineralization but the conditions necessary for each are unknown. Hence an old ball thrombus in the pelvic veins becomes calcified but does not become atheromatous. Moreover, experimental thrombotic lesions of arteries are not progressive and do not comply with the specific criteria for experimental atherosclerosis [135].

References

1. Wessler, S. and Stehbens, W.E. (1971) Thrombosis, in *Thrombosis and Bleeding Disorders*, (eds N.U. Bang, F.K. Beller, E. Deutsch and E.F. Mammen), Thieme, Stuttgart, pp. 488–98.
2. Gibbs, N.M. (1957) Venous thrombosis of the lower limbs with particular reference to bed-rest. *Br. J. Surg.*, 45, 209–36.
3. Thoma, R. (1896) *Text-Book of General Pathology* (transl. by A. Bruce), vol. 1, Adam and Black, London, pp. 278–84.
4. Hadfield, G. (1950) Thrombosis. *Ann. Roy. Coll. Surg. Engl.*, 6, 219–34.
5. Harker, L.A. (1987) Role of platelets and thrombosis in mechanisms of acute occlusion and restenosis after angioplasty. *Am. J. Cardiol.*, 60, 20B–28B.
6. Bithell, T.C. (1993) The physiology of primary hemostasis, in *Wintrobe's Clinical Hematology*, 9th edn, vol. 1, (eds G.R. Lee, T.C. Bithell, J. Foerster et al.), Lea & Febiger, Philadelphia, pp. 540–65.
7. Aschoff, L. (1912) Thrombose und Sandbankbildung. *Beiträge Pathol. Anat.*, 52, 205–12.
8. Silver, M.D. and Stehbens, W.E. (1965) The behaviour of platelets *in vivo*. *Quart. J. Exp. Physiol.*, 50, 241–7.
9. Stehbens, W.E. (1972) Platelet behaviour in the microcirculation: interaction with other formed elements and endothelium. Trans. of II Congress International Society Thrombosis and Haemostasis, Suppl. 51, *Thrombosis: Risk Factors and Diagnostic Approaches*, Schattauer, New York, pp. 177–82.
10. Stehbens, W.E. (1965) Reaction of venous endothelium to injury. *Lab. Invest.*, 14, 449–59.
11. Mustard, J.F., Glynn, M.F., Hovig, T. et al. (1967) Platelets, blood coagulation and thrombosis, in *Physiology of Hemostasis and Thrombosis*, (eds S.A. Johnson and W.H. Seegers), C.C. Thomas, Springfield, pp. 288–326.
12. Wechezak, A.R., Holbrook, K.A., Way, S.A. et al. (1979) Platelet adherence in endothelial cell cultures. *Blood Vessels*, 16, 35–42.
13. French, J.E., Macfarlane, R.G. and Sanders, A.G. (1964) The structure of haemostatic plugs and experimental thrombi in small arteries. *Br. J. Exp. Pathol.*, 45, 467–74.
14. Stehbens, W.E. and Biscoe, T.J. (1967) The ultrastructure of early platelet aggregation *in vivo*. *Am. J. Pathol.*, 50, 219–43.
15. Preissner, K.T. and Jenne, D. (1991) Vitronectin: a new molecular connection in haemostasis. *Thromb. Haemostasis*, 66, 189–94.
16. Coller, B.S. (1991) Platelets in cardiovascular thrombosis and thrombolysis, in *The Heart and Cardiovascular System*, (eds H.A. Fozzard, E. Haber, R.B. Jennings et al.), Raven Press, New York, pp. 219–73.
17. Wiman, B. and Hamsten, A. (1990) The fibrinolytic enzyme system and its role in the etiology of thromboembolic disease. *Semin. Thromb. Hemostasis*, 16, 207–16.
18. Warren, B.A. (1963) Fibrinolytic properties of vascular endothelium. *Br. J. Exp. Pathol.*, 44, 365–72.
19. Gryglewski, R.J., Botting, R.M. and Vane, J.R. (1988) Mediators produced by the endothelial cell. *Hypertension*, 12, 530–48.
20. Spaet, T.H. and Erichson, R.B. (1966) The vascular wall in the pathogenesis of thrombosis. *Thromb. Diath. Haemorrh.* (suppl. 21), 67–86.
21. Stemerman, M.B. (1978) Atherosclerosis: the etiologic role of blood elements and cellular changes. *Cardiovasc. Med.*, 3, 17–36.
22. Sheppard, B.L. and French, J.E. (1971) Platelet adhesion in the rabbit abdominal aorta following the removal of the endothelium: a scanning and transmission electron microscopical study. *Proc. Roy. Soc. Lond. B*, 176, 427–32.
23. Ts'ao, C.H. and Glagov, S. (1970) Platelet adhesion to subendothelial components in experimental aortic injury. Role of fine fibrils and basement membrane. *Br. J. Exp. Pathol.*, 51, 423–7.
24. Niewiarowski, S. and Rao, A.K. (1983) Contribution of thrombogenic factors to the pathogenesis of atherosclerosis. *Progr. Cardiovasc. Dis.*, 26, 197–222.
25. Baumgartner, H.R. and Haudenschild, C. (1972) Adhesion of platelets to subendothelium. *Ann. N.Y. Acad. Sci.*, 201, 22–36.
26. Stehbens, W.E. (1979) *Hemodynamics and the Blood Vessel Wall*, C.C. Thomas, Springfield.
27. Drury, R.A.B. (1954) The role of intimal haemorrhage in coronary occlusion. *J. Pathol. Bacteriol.*, 67, 207–15.
28. Stehbens, W.E. (1963) Contentious features of coronary occlusion and atherosclerosis. *Bull. Postgrad. Com. Med. Univ. Sydney*, 19, 216–25.
29. Chapman, I. (1965) Morphogenesis of occluding coronary artery thrombosis. *Arch. Pathol.*, 80, 256–61.
30. Constantinides, P. (1966) Plaque fissures in human coronary thrombosis. *J. Atheroscl. Res.*, 6, 1–17.
31. Davies, M.J. and Thomas, A.C. (1985) Plaque fissuring – the cause of acute myocardial infarction, sudden ischaemic death, and crescendo angina. *Br. Heart J.*, 53, 363–73.
32. Hertzer, N.R., Beven, E.G. and Benjamin, S.P. (1977) Ultramicroscopic ulceration and thrombi of the carotid bifurcation. *Arch. Surg.*, 112, 1394–402.
33. Stehbens, W.E. (1972) *Pathology of the Cerebral Blood Vessels*, C.V. Mosby, St Louis.
34. Stehbens, W.E. (1986) Vascular complications in experimental atherosclerosis. *Progr. Cardiovasc. Dis.*, 29, 221–37.
35. Short, R.D.H. (1954) Orientation of structure of thrombi in the deep veins of the leg in man. *J. Pathol. Bacteriol.*, 68, 41–54.
36. Warlow, C., Ogston, D. and Douglas, A.S. (1976) Deep venous thrombosis of the legs after strokes. Part 1. Incidence and predisposing factors. *Br. Med. J.*, 1, 1178–83.
37. Nicolaides, A.N., Kakkar, V.V., Renney, J.T.G. et al. (1971) Myocardial infarction and deep-vein thrombosis. *Br. Med. J.*, 1, 432–4.
38. Stanton, J.R., Freis, E.D. and Wilkins, R.W. (1949) Acceleration of linear flow in deep veins of lower extremity of man by local compression. *J. Clin. Invest.*, 28, 553–8.
39. McLachlin, A.D., McLachlin, J.A., Jory, T.A. et al. (1960) Venous stasis in the lower extremities. *Ann. Surg.*, 152, 678–85.
40. Baumgartner, H.R. and Muggli, R. (1976) Adhesion and aggregation: morphological demonstration and quantitation *in vivo* and *in vitro*, in *Platelets in Biology and Pathology*, (ed. J.L. Gordon), North-Holland, Amsterdam, pp. 23–60.
41. Paik, W.C.W. and Lalich, J.J. (1968) The relation of aortic intimal tears to thrombosis in rats fed β-aminoproprionitrile. *Lab. Invest.*, 19, 174–80.
42. Greenhill, N.S. and Stehbens, W.E. (1983) Scanning electron-microscopic study of experimentally induced intimal tears in rabbit arteries. *Atherosclerosis*, 49, 119–26.
43. Baumgartner, H.R. (1973) The role of blood flow in platelet adhesion, fibrin deposition, and formation of mural thrombi. *Microvascular Res.*, 5, 167–79.
44. Baumgartner, H.R. and Sakariassen, K.S. (1985) Factors controlling thrombus formation on arterial lesions. *Ann. N.Y. Acad Sci.*, 454, 162–77.
45. Shionoya, T. (1927) Studies in experimental extracorporeal thrombosis. II. Thrombus formation in normal blood in the extracorporeal vascular loop. *J. Exp. Med.*, 46, 13–17.
46. Shionoya, T. (1927) Studies in experimental extracorporeal thrombosis. III. Effects of certain anticoagulants (heparin and hirudin) on extracorporeal thrombosis and on the mechanism of thrombus formation. *J. Exp. Med.*, 46, 19–26.
47. Murphy, E.A., Rowsell, H.C., Downie, H.G. et al. (1962) Encrustation

and atherosclerosis: the analogy between early *in vivo* lesions and deposits which occur in extracorporeal circulations. *Canad. Med. Assoc. J.*, 87, 259–74.
48. Downie, H.G., Murphy, E.A., Rowsell, H.C. *et al.* (1963) Extracorporeal circulation: a device for the quantitative study of thrombus formation in flowing blood. *Circulation Res.*, 12, 441–8.
49. Smith, R.L., Blick, E.F., Coalson, J. *et al.* (1972) Thrombus production by turbulence. *J. Appl. Physiol.*, 32, 261–4.
50. Stein, P.D. and Sabbah, H.N. (1974) Measured turbulence and its effect on thrombus formation. *Circulation Res.*, 35, 608–14.
51. Sevitt, S. (1960) Aetiology and pathogenesis of deep vein thrombosis. *Lancet*, 1, 384–5.
52. Stehbens, W.E. (1990) The lipid hypothesis and the role of hemodynamics in atherogenesis. *Progr. Cardiovasc. Dis.*, 33, 119–36.
53. Wright, G.P. (1950) *An Introduction to Pathology*, Longmans Green, London.
54. Kernoff, P.B.A. (1989) Thrombosis and antithrombotic therapy, in *Postgraduate Haematology*, 3rd edn, (eds A.V. Hoffbrand and S.M. Lewis), Heinemann Professional Publishing, Oxford, pp. 672–95.
55. Meade, T.W., Vickers, M.V., Thompson, S.G. *et al.* (1985) Epidemiological characteristics of platelet aggregability. *Br. Med. J.*, 290, 428–31.
56. Atkinson, E.A., Fairburn, B. and Heathfield, K.W.G. (1970) Intracranial venous thrombosis as complications of oral contraception. *Lancet*, 1, 914–18.
57. Stehbens, W.E. (1969) Effects of adrenalin and anaphylaxis on the aggregation of the cellular constituents of the blood *in vivo*. *Quart. J. Exp. Physiol.*, 54, 41–8.
58. Nordøy, A. and Goodnight, S.H. (1990) Dietary lipids and thrombosis. Relationship to atherosclerosis. *Arteriosclerosis*, 10, 149–63.
59. Renaud, S. (1969) Thrombotic, atherosclerotic and lipemic effects of dietary fats in rats. *Angiology*, 20, 657–69.
60. Stehbens, W.E. (1993) *The Lipid Hypothesis of Atherogenesis*, R.G. Landes Pub. Co., Austin.
61. Greig, H.B.W. (1956) Inhibition of fibrinolysis by alimentary lipaemia. *Lancet*, 2, 16–18.
62. Dawson, S. and Henney, A. (1992) The status of PAI-1 as a risk factor for arterial and thrombotic disease: a review. *Atherosclerosis*, 95, 105–17.
63. Wessler, S. (1963) Stasis, hypercoagulability, and thrombosis. *Fed. Proc.*, 22, 1366–70.
64. Stehbens, W.E. (1985) Relationship of coronary artery thrombosis to myocardial infarction. *Lancet*, 2, 639–42.
65. Carpenter, S. (1961) Injury of neck as cause of vertebral artery thrombosis. *J. Neurosurg.*, 18, 849–53.
66. Sevitt, S. (1974) The structure and growth of valve-pocket thrombi in femoral veins. *J. Clin. Pathol.*, 27, 517–28.
67. Barker, N.W., Nygaard, K.K., Walters, W. *et al.* (1941) A statistical study of postoperative venous thrombosis and pulmonary embolism. *Proc. Staff Meet. Mayo Clin.*, 16, 33–7.
68. Cotton, L.T. and Clark, C. (1965) Anatomical localization of venous thrombosis. *Ann. Roy. Coll. Surg. Engl.*, 36, 214–24.
69. Stein, P.D. and Evans, H. (1967) An autopsy study of leg vein thrombosis. *Circulation*, 35, 671–81.
70. Beckering, R.E. and Titus, J.L. (1969) Femoro-popliteal venous thrombosis and pulmonary embolism. *Am. J. Clin. Pathol.*, 52, 530–7.
71. McLachlin, J. and Paterson, J.C. (1951) Some basic observations on venous thrombosis and pulmonary embolism. *Surg. Gynec. Obstet.*, 93, 1–8.
72. Kakkar, V.V., Howe, C.T., Flanc, C. *et al.* (1969) Natural history of postoperative deep-vein thrombosis. *Lancet*, 2, 230–2.
73. Hueper, W.C. (1942) Macromolecular substances as pathogenic agents. *Arch. Pathol.*, 33, 267–90.
74. Hueper, W.C. (1945) The relation between etiology and morphology in degenerative and sclerosing vascular diseases. *Biol. Sympos.*, 11, 1–42.
75. Anderson, J.R. (1985) Disturbances of blood flow and body fluids, in *Muir's Textbook of Pathology*, 12th edn, (ed. J.R. Anderson), Edward Arnold, London, pp. 10.1–10.47.
76. Falk, E. (1991) Coronary thrombosis: pathogenesis and clinical manifestations. *Am. J. Cardiol.*, 68, 28B–35B.
77. Allison, P.R. and Dunnil, M.S. (1968) Recanalization of systemic thrombi. *J. Cardiovasc. Surg.*, 9, 383–91.
78. Byard, R.W. and Cutz, E. (1990) Sudden and unexpected death in infancy and childhood due to pulmonary thromboembolism. *Arch. Pathol. Lab. Med.*, 114, 142–4.
79. Dismuke, S.E. and Vander Zwaag, R. (1984) Accuracy and epidemiological implications of the death certificate diagnosis of pulmonary embolism. *J. Chr. Dis.*, 37, 67–73.
80. Dalen, J.E., Banas, J.S., Brooks, H.I. *et al.* (1969) Resolution rate of acute pulmonary embolism in man. *New Engl. J. Med.*, 280, 1194–9.
81. Moore, S. and Mersereau, W.A. (1965) Micro-embolic renal ischemia and hypertension. *Canad. Med. Ass. J.*, 92, 221–4.
82. Edwards, E.A. (1958) The anatomy of collateral circulation. *Surg. Gynec. Obstet.*, 107, 183–94.
83. Edwards, E.A. and Le May, M. (1955) Occlusion patterns and collaterals in arteriosclerosis of the lower aorta and iliac arteries. *Surgery*, 38, 950–63.
84. Brice, J.G., Dowsett, D.J. and Lowe, R.D. (1964) The effect of constriction on carotid blood-flow and pressure gradient. *Lancet*, 1, 84–5.
85. Longland, C.J. (1955) The collateral circulation of the limb. *Ann. Roy. Coll. Surg. Engl.*, 13, 161–76.
86. Winblad, J.N., Reemtsma, K., Vernhet, J.L. *et al.* (1959) Etiologic mechanisms in the development of collateral circulation. *Surgery*, 45, 105–17.
87. Strandness, D.E. (1969) *Collaeral Circulation in Clinical Surgery*, Saunders, Philadelphia, pp. 2–39.
88. Mulvihill, D.A. and Harvey, S.C. (1951) The mechanisms of the development of collateral circulation. *New Engl. J. Med.*, 204, 1032–4.
89. Cresti, M. and Steger, C. (1962) The correlation between the effects of morphology and function on the collateral circulation in the obliterative arteriopathy of the inferior limbs. *Angiology*, 13, 271–83.
90. Schaper, W., De Brabander, M. and Lewi, P. (1971) DNA synthesis and mitoses in coronary collateral vessels of the dog. *Circulation Res.*, 28, 671–9.
91. Levin, D.C., Kauff, M. and Baltaxe, H.A. (1973) Coronary collateral circulation. *Am. J. Roentgenol Rad. Ther. Nucl. Med.*, 119, 463–73.
92. Holman, E. (1968) *Abnormal Arteriovenous Communications*, C.C. Thomas, Springfield.
93. Stehbens, W.E. (1992) Experimental induction of atherosclerosis associated with femoral arteriovenous fistulae in rabbits on a stock diet. *Atherosclerosis*, 95, 127–35.
94. Greenhill, N.S. and Stehbens, W.E. (1983) Scanning electron-microscopic study of experimentally-induced intimal tears in rabbit arteries. *Atherosclerosis*, 49, 119–26.
95. Martin, B.J., Stehbens, W.E., Davis, P.F. *et al.* (1989) Scanning electron microscopic study of hemodynamically induced tears in the internal elastic lamina of rabbit arteries. *Pathology*, 21, 207–12.
96. Arey, L.B. (1963) The development of peripheral blood vessels, in *The Peripheral Blood Vessels*, (eds J.L. Orbison and D.E. Smith), Williams and Wilkins, Baltimore, pp. 1–16.
97. Cibulski, A.A., Lehan, E.H. and Timmis, H.H. (1973) Regression of intercoronary collateral vessels in mongrel dogs after coronary bypass grafting. *Am. J. Cardiol.*, 31, 480–3.
98. Callow, A.D., Aboulafia, E.D. and Ballas, P.E. (1961) The restrictive effect of bypass grafts upon the occluded major arterial channel and its collaterals. *Surgery*, 49, 26–34.
99. Bellman, S., Frank, H.A., Lambert, P.B. *et al.* (1959) Effects of selective occlusions of major trunks within an extensively anastomosing arterial system. *Angiology*, 10, 214–31.
100. Lambert, P.B., Frank, H.A., Bellman, S. *et al.* (1963) Observations on the recovery of divided arteries and veins. *Angiology*, 14, 121–33.
101. Borgers, M., Schaper, J. and Schaper, W. (1970) Acute vascular lesions in developing coronary collaterals. *Virch. Arch. Abt. A Pathol. Anat.*, 371, 1–11.
102. Sloan, R.D. and Cooley, R.N. (1953) Coarctation of the aorta. The roentgenologic aspects of one hundred and twenty-five surgically confirmed cases. *Radiology*, 61, 701–21.
103. Taveras, J.M. (1969) Multiple progressive intracranial arterial occlusions: a syndrome of children and young adults. *Am. J. Roentgenol.*, 106, 235–68.
104. Shemilt, P. (1972) The origin of phleboliths. *Br. J. Surg.*, 59, 695–700.
105. Ogata, J., Karasawa, J. and Nakagawara, J. (1987) Ball thrombi in carotid artery plaque. *Stroke*, 18, 959–60.
106. Iyengar, S.R.K., Charette, E.J.P., Lynn, R.B. *et al.* (1972) Traumatic rupture of the thoracic aorta. *Canad. J. Surg.*, 15, 350–9.
107. Heggtveit, H.A. (1992) Cardiovascular trauma, in *Cardiovascular Pathology*, 2nd edn, vol. 2, (ed. M.D. Silver), Churchill Livingstone, New York, 1335–66.
108. Steiness, F. and Thaysen, J.H. (1965) Bilateral traumatic renal-artery thrombosis. *Lancet* 1, 527–9.
109. Hughes, J.T. and Brownell, B. (1968) Traumatic thrombosis of the internal carotid arteries in the neck. *J. Neurol. Neurosurg. Psychiat.*, 31, 307–14.
110. Martin, R.F., Eldrup-Jorgensen, J., Clark, D.E. *et al.* (1991) Blunt trauma to the carotid arteries. *J. Vasc. Surg.*, 14, 789–95.
111. Townsend, J.N., Davies, M.K. and Jones, E.L. (1991) Fatal rupture of an unsuspected post-traumatic aneurysm of the thoracic aorta during pregnancy. *Br. Heart J.*, 66, 248–9.
112. Rohrer, M.J., Cardullo, P.A., Pappas, A.M. *et al.* (1990) Axillary artery compression and thrombosis in throwing athletes. *J. Vasc. Surg.*, 11, 761–9.
113. Taylor, W. and Palmear, P.L. (1975) *Vibration White Finger in Industry*. Academic Press, London, pp. 83–110.
114. Taylor, W. (1985) Vibration white finger: a newly prescribed disease. *Br. Med. J.*, 291, 921–2.
115. Van den Bossche, J. and Lahaye, D. (1984) X-ray anomalies occurring in workers exposed to vibration caused by light tools. *Br. J. Indust. Med.*, 41, 137–41.
116. Barker, N.W. and Hines, E.A. (1944) Arterial occlusion in the hands and

fingers associated with repeated occupational trauma. *Proc. Staff Meet. Mayo Clinic*, **19**, 345–9.
117. Futasuka, M., Veno, T. and Sakurai, T. (1985) Follow up study of vibration induced white finger in chain saw operators. *Br. J. Indust. Med.*, **42**, 267–71.
118. Evans, P.J.D. and Kear, J.M. (1975) Arterial occlusion after cannulation. *Br. Med. J.*, **2**, 197–9.
119. Ong, H.T., Elmsly, W.G., Friedlander, D.H. (1991) Cholesterol atheroembolism: an increasingly frequent complication of cardiac catheterization. *Med. J. Aust.*, **154**, 412–14.
120. Kaye, C.G. and Smith, D.R. (1988) Complications of central venous cannulation. *Br. Med. J.*, **297**, 572–3.
121. Slayback, J.B., Bowen, W.W. and Hinshaw, D.B. (1976) Intimal injury from arterial clamps. *Am. J. Surg.*, **132**, 183–8.
122. Reidy, M.A. and Schwartz, S.M. (1981) Endothelial regeneration. III Time course of intimal changes after small defined injury to rat aortic endothelium. *Lab. Invest.*, **44**, 301–8.
123. Jones, G.T., Martin, B.J., Stehbens, W.E. (1992) Tears in the afferent artery of experimental arteriovenous fistulae in rabbits. *Int. J. Exp. Pathol.*, **73**, 405–16.
124. Stehbens, W.E. (1973) Experimental arteriovenous fistulae in normal and cholesterol-fed rabbits. *Pathology*, **5**, 311–24.
125. Fishman, J.S., Ryan, G.B. and Karnovsky, M.J. (1975) Endothelial regeneration in the rat carotid artery and the significance of endothelial denudation in the pathogenesis of myointimal thickening. *Lab. Invest.*, **32**, 339–51.
126. Norman, R.M. and Urich, H. (1957) Dissecting aneurysm of the middle cerebral artery as a cause of acute infantile hemiplegia. *J. Pathol. Bacteriol.*, **73**, 580–2.
127. von Rokitansky, C. (1852) *Handbuch der Pathologischen Anatomie*, (trans. by G.E. Day), Sydenham, London.
128. Morgan, A.D. (1956) *The Pathogenesis of Coronary Occlusion*, Blackwell Scient. Pub., Oxford.
129. Leary, T. (1935) Coronary spasm as a possible factor in producing sudden death. *Am. Heart J.*, **10**, 338–44.
130. Clark, E., Graef, I. and Chasis, H. (1936) Thrombosis of the aorta and coronary arteries with special reference to the 'fibrinoid lesions'. *Arch. Pathol.*, **22**, 183–212.
131. Horn, H. and Finkelstein, L.F. (1940) Arteriosclerosis of the coronary arteries and the mechanism of their occlusion. *Am. Heart J.*, **19**, 655–82.
132. Duguid, J.B. (1955) Mural thrombosis in arteries. *Br. Med. Bull.*, **11**, 36–8.
133. Stehbens, W.E. (1992) The role of thrombosis and variants of the thrombogenic theory in the etiology and pathogenesis of atherosclerosis. *Progr. Cardiovasc. Dis.*, **34**, 325–46.
134. Davies, M.J. and Thomas, T. (1981) The pathological basis and microanatomy of occlusive thrombus formation in human coronary arteries. *Phil. Trans. Roy. Soc. Lond. B*, **294**, 225–9.
135. Friedman, M. and Byers, S.O. (1965) Immunity of the mature thromboatherosclerotic plaque to hypercholesterlaemia. *Br. J. Exp. Pathol.*, **46**, 539–44.
136. Stehbens, W.E. (1991) Koch's postulates and experimental atherosclerosis. *Med. Hypotheses*, **35**, 288–92.
137. Vlodaver, Z. and Edwards, J.E. (1971) Pathology of coronary atherosclerosis. *Progr. Cardiovasc. Dis.*, **14**, 256–74.

4 CONNECTIVE TISSUE COMPONENTS OF THE BLOOD VESSEL WALL IN HEALTH AND DISEASE

Simon P. Robins and Colin Farquharson

Connective tissue in blood vessel walls provides the structural framework necessary for the function of the vessel and also to accommodate the many different specialized cell types required to produce and replenish the fabric of the tissue. The connective tissue is by no means a passive structure, however, and there are active channels of communication through which the extracellular matrix influences cellular function. There are of course a multitude of functional requirements for blood vessels ranging from the high degree of physical stresses for arterial vessels close to the heart to the more subtle filtration functions necessary in the microvasculature. Consistent with this wide diversity of function, there is a wide range of connective tissue components in blood vessel walls, including collagens, elastin, proteoglycans, glycosaminoglycans and glycoproteins. The purpose of this review is to introduce the main biochemical features of these components and to examine briefly the mechanisms governing their synthesis, assembly and degradation. In addition, the characteristics of a series of disorders affecting the vasculature will be reviewed in relation to functional alterations, and recent progress in understanding the biochemical basis of these defects will be assessed.

4.1 Vessel wall constituents

Collagens represent the main protein constituents of blood vessels and much of this section will be devoted to the biosynthesis, structure and stabilization of the collagenous matrix. The biomechanical properties of the vessel wall, particularly of the major arteries, are crucially dependent on the elastic components, elastin and the associated glycoproteins, and a great deal of new information has been gained recently on the composition and structural assembly of these fibres.

4.1.1 COLLAGENS

(a) Classification of collagen types

Since the discovery in cartilage of a collagen (now designated type II), genetically distinct from that in skin, tendon and bone (type I collagen) in the late 1960s and the report of an additional fibrillar collagen (type III) in skin in 1973 [1], the number of different collagen types recognized has increased dramatically so that there are now at least 15 different types known. For some, however, the structures are known only as gene sequences and no associated protein has yet been isolated. The gene structure and characteristics of the different collagen types have been reviewed extensively in recent years [2,3], and will not be discussed in detail here. Although the different collagen types are designated by Roman numerals in the approximate order in which they were discovered, current knowledge suggests that classification according to their structure and likely function is more appropriate, as shown in Table 4.1. It is now recognized that the three major collagen types (I, II and III) represent about 70% of the total [4]. They are characterized by the presence of a long, continuous triple-helical structure with each chain comprising about 330 repeats of the amino acid sequence, $-Gly-X-Y-$, where X is often proline and Y is often hydroxyproline. These collagens, together with collagen types V and XI, comprise a class that may be referred to as fibrillar collagens. A second class of collagens appears to function primarily in modifying the properties of other collagen fibrils by associating with their surface. Because these collagens have shorter triple-helical segments interrupted by non-helical polypeptides, they have been referred to as FACIT collagens, or Fibril Associated Collagens with Interrupted Triple helix [5]. This group comprises

Table 4.1 Genetically distinct collagen types

Collagen type	Molecular structures	Representative tissue distribution
Fibril-forming		
I	(α1(I))$_2$α2(I)	Widespread; skin, bone, tendon, etc.
	[α1(I)]$_3$ (Type I trimer)	Minor component detected in skin, dentin
III	[α1(III)]$_3$	Blood vessels, skin, tendon, cornea, etc.
V	[α1(V)]$_3$; [α1(V)]$_2$α2(V) and α1(V)α2(V)α3(V)	Widespead; skin, tendon, cornea, ligament
II	[α1(II)]$_3$	Cartilage, vitreous humour, intervertebral disc
XI	α1(XI)α2(XI)α3(XI)	Cartilage
Fibril-associated collagens with interrupted triple-helices		
IX	α1(IX)α2(IX)α3(IX)	Cartilage, vitreous humour
XII	[α1(XII)]$_3$	Collagen I-containing tissues, cartilage
XIV	[α1(XIV)]$_3$	As for collagen XII
Sheet-forming collagens		
IV	[α1(IV)]$_2$α2(IV)	All basement membranes
	Molecules also containing α3(IV), α4(IV) and α5(IV)	Glomerular basement membrane
VIII	Probably [α1(VIII)]$_2$α2(VIII)	Descemet's membrane, blood capillaries
X	[α1(X)]$_3$	Growth plate cartilage
Specialized structures		
VI	α(VI)α2(IV)α3(IV)	Widespread; skin, vasculature, tendon ligament, cartilage
VII	[α1(VII)]$_3$	Dermal−epidermal junction

collagen types IX, XII and XIV (Table 4.1). A third group of collagens (types IV, VIII and X) may be classed as 'sheet-forming', although their precise function, particularly of the latter two types, is still unclear. Two other collagen types appear to have specialized structures that do not fit into the other groups; these are the beaded filament structure of collagen VI and the long, antiparallel dimers of collagen VII that form anchoring fibrils at the dermo-epidermal junction. New collagens continue to be discovered and collagen types XIII, XV and XVI, not included in Table 4.1, have so far been described primarily at the cDNA level [6,7,8] and there is little information about their supramolecular structure.

The major tissue distributions of the different collagen types are shown in Table 4.1. As the main collagens present in blood vessel walls are types I, III, IV, V, VI and VIII, discussion of the functions and structural assembly will be restricted mainly to these collagen types. Initially, however, it is pertinent to consider the biosynthesis and macromolecular assembly of the archetypal fibrillar collagen, type I, against which differences for other collagen types can be compared. The main functional role of collagen type I is to provide a structural framework through the formation of stable, interconnected fibrils. Rather than give a comprehensive account of collagen biochemistry, a few of the essential characteristics necessary for the molecule to accomplish this functional role will be highlighted.

(b) Structure, biosynthesis and assembly of fibrillar collagen

Collagen molecules within fibrils have three functional domains; namely, a central section in triple-helical conformation and two short non-helical segments at each end, referred to as telopeptides. The type I collagen molecule comprises two identical chains each having 1057 amino acid residues, denoted α1(I), and a third chain of 1039 residues derived from a different gene, α2(I). The helical section contains 1014 amino acids with Gly every third residue. This structure is dictated by the fact that, as the Gly residues radiate into the centre of the helix, any amino acid with a side chain grouping could not be accommodated sterically into the structure. Thus, as will be discussed in later sections, any genetic mutation leading to alteration of the Gly residue has a dramatic effect on the stability and structure of the collagen helix. Collagen type III differs from type I in that it is a homotrimer of three identical α-chains, with an uninterrupted triple helical section of 1023 residues in Gly−X−Y triplets. Another significant difference for collagen type III is the presence within the helix of cysteine residues which give rise to both intra- and intermolecular disulphide bonding.

Collagen is characterized by the large number of post-ribosomal modifications that occur; these are summarized in Table 4.2, together with the enzymes and some of the cofactors involved. A hydrophobic signal

Table 4.2 Stages of collagen biosynthesis

Biosynthetic step	Product – enzymes and cofactors involved
Intracellular	
Transcription of genomic DNA	Pre-messenger RNA
Processing of RNA (capping, polyadenylation and splicing)	Messenger RNA
Translation of mRNA	Pre-protoprocollagen (unhydroxylated)
Removal of 'signal' sequences	Protoprocollagen (unhydroxylated)
Hydroxylation of some proline and lysine residues	Accomplished by at least three separate enzymes requiring Fe^{2+}, α-ketoglutarate and ascorbate
Glycosylation of certain hydroxylysine residues	Accomplished by two glycosyl transferases requiring Mn^{2+}
Helix formation	Registration by association of C-propeptides involving a disulphide isomerase
Secretion of procollagen	An energy-consuming process involving microtubules
Extracellular	
Excision of the N- and C-terminal polypeptides	Removal *en bloc* of globular extension portions by at least two Ca^{2+}-dependent proteases giving soluble collagen monomers
Oxidative deamination of telopeptide lysine or hydroxylysine residues	Performed by lysyl oxidase, a Cu^{2+}-dependent enzyme requiring O_2 and an aromatic carbonyl
Formation of intermediate crosslinks	Spontaneous reactions giving Schiff bases and keto-amines
Maturation and aging	Alterations in crosslinking to give insoluble collagen fibres

peptide directs the nascent polypeptide chain into the secretory route from the cell by penetrating the membrane of the rough endoplasmic reticulum. Following the proteolytic removal of this peptide [9,10], the emerging chain is acted upon by a series of hydroxylases and glycosyl transferases. Hydroxylation of proline to 4-hydroxyproline is accomplished by a multisubunit enzyme, prolyl hydroxylase, for which the mechanisms have been studied in great detail [11]. The β-subunit of this enzyme has been shown to be the same polypeptide as the enzyme, protein disulphide isomerase [12], an enzyme that may be involved in expediting the correct registration and alignment of collagen chains for formation of the triple helix. The hydroxyproline residues are essential in stabilizing the helix through hydrogen bonding and when insufficient hydroxyproline is formed through inhibition of the enzyme with, for example, α,α'-dipyridyl, the helix is unstable at 37°C and under-hydroxylated, non-helical collagen builds up in the cell and is not secreted. The hydroxylase enzyme has been used in certain circumstances as a target for therapeutic agents to control fibrotic proliferation of collagen [13]. A separate enzyme, lysyl hydroxylase, acts through a similar mechanism to hydroxylate lysine residues at the 5 position [11]. The hydroxylysine residues produced are important in the crosslinking mechanisms of collagen (see below) and also as substrates for glycosylation enzymes. The formation of two types of O-linked hydroxylysine glycosides, galactosyl-hydroxylysine and glucosyl-galactosyl-hydroxylysine, is brought about by two transferase enzymes [14], but the function of these substituents remains obscure.

All enzyme modifications of the collagen within the cisternae of the rough endoplasmic reticulum cease after the triple helix has been formed. In some genetic disorders where mutations retard the formation of the helix, over-modification of the collagen chains can occur and these can be detected by their abnormal biochemical properties, such as their electrophoretic mobility [15]. Once formed, the triple-helical molecules have the ability to associate spontaneously to form fibrillar structures. Thus, a mechanism had to be found to explain these two potential problems in collagen biosynthesis; firstly, on how the three separate chains of collagen associate to register the start of the helix, and secondly, on how the collagen molecules are prevented from forming fibrils before being secreted from the cell. The answers came with the discovery that collagen is synthesized as a larger precursor molecule [16] with globular propeptide extensions at both the N- and C-terminal ends, so that the procollagen molecule initially produced is about 50% larger than fibrillar collagen. Sequence analyses, mostly by cDNA analysis, have shown that the N- and C-terminal propeptides of the human pro-α1(I) chain comprise 157 and 246 amino acids respectively, whereas the pro-α2(I) chain has a similar sized C-terminal propeptide but a much shorter N-terminal peptide of 57 residues. The large C-terminal domain of procollagen serves to register the three chains, initially through non-covalent interactions between the globular domains [17] and subsequently through disulphide bond formation [18]. Studies *in vitro* of the assembly of molecules containing only α(I) chains, collagen type I homotrimer, which can occur in small quantities in tissues [19], have shown that the more hydrophobic α2(I) chain is important in accelerating the entropy-driven self-assembly process [20]. Formation of the helix may also require an additional enzyme activity that induces changes in structure around prolyl residues, prolyl peptidyl *cis/trans* isomerase [21].

Some additional glycosylation reactions of procollagen, particularly the addition of asparagine-linked oligosaccharides in the C-terminal propeptide [22], occur before the procollagen is secreted via the Golgi apparatus. Although the procollagen extensions render the molecule soluble within the physiological environment, some association of the procollagen occurs in vacuoles that are secreted with the aid of cytoskeletal elements.

Not all of the newly synthesized collagen is secreted from the cell as some intracellular degradation is known to occur. Initial estimates from cell culture studies were that up to 40% was degraded within minutes of its synthesis [23]. Subsequent studies (reviewed in [24]) showed wide variations in different cell types and similarly large variations were observed *in vivo* in different tissues [25]. The concept has emerged of a basal level of intracellular degradation of about 10–15% with increased loss of newly synthesized material under certain circumstances. Whether the degradation is primarily lysosomal or occurs mainly in the rough endoplasmic reticulum and Golgi apparatus is uncertain [24]. The function of this process is also unclear but regulation of intracellular degradation could represent a mechanism for the rapid alterations in the rate of collagen deposition [26].

A critical step before fibril formation can occur is the removal of both terminal propeptides. This is accomplished extracellularly by two specific neutral proteases, procollagen N-proteinase and procollagen C-proteinase, both of which are Ca^{2+} dependent and require the presence of a triple-helical structure. The precise order of removal of the propeptides appears to be developmentally regulated and has an effect on the nature of the fibrils produced [27], but the implications of these experiments for the assembly *in vivo* are not completely understood. Although much useful information on the role of the propeptides in fibrillogenesis has been obtained using cell-free systems generating the required precursors [28], studies of fibril formation in tissues using the electron microscope have revealed the intricate involvement of the cell surface with fibrillogenesis [29]. Some additional protein components may also be required to enhance the removal of propeptides [30].

Newly formed collagen fibrils are soluble in salt solutions and dilute acid, and have no tensile strength. During maturation and aging, collagen fibres become increasingly insoluble, more refractory to the actions of enzymes and show progressive increases in tensile strength. These properties which are intrinsic to the function of the collagen are brought about mainly through the formation of intermolecular crosslinks, and this process will therefore be discussed in some detail.

(c) Crosslinking of collagen

Lysyl oxidase

The crosslinking process is initiated by the enzyme, lysyl oxidase, through the oxidation of specific lysine or hydroxylysine residues in the telopeptide regions. The enzyme is a copper-dependent amine oxidase requiring molecular oxygen and an aromatic carbonyl compound, the identity of which is still in doubt; both pyridoxal 5′-phosphate and PQQ have been suggested [31,32]. The same enzyme is responsible for amine oxidase activity on both collagen and elastin, although a number of isoforms have been isolated from tissues. The enzyme has little activity on soluble collagen and appears to require the presence of quarter-staggered fibrils [33]. These observations, combined with evidence that lysyl oxidase cannot penetrate within collagen fibrils but binds only to their surface, have led to the suggestion that there are distinct steric requirements for activity, perhaps involving sequences adjacent to the telopeptides in the fibril that are known to be conserved [34].

The complete derived amino acid sequence of human lysyl oxidase has been determined and the gene assigned to chromosome 5 [35,36]. As for the rodent lysyl oxidase nucleotide sequence, there was a very high degree of similarity with the sequence of the *ras* recision gene (rrg) which codes for a protein that counteracts the action of *ras* oncogene transformation [37]. These results suggest that lysyl oxidase and rrg are products of the same gene, although it is not yet known whether the anti-oncogenic properties of rrg are related to amine oxidase activity of the protein. It appears, however, that lysyl oxidase may also have a direct role in tumour suppression.

Reducible crosslink formation

The aldehydes produced through oxidative deamination undergo a series of reactions (summarized in Figure 4.1) to give both inter- and intramolecular crosslinks. All of these reactions are apparently spontaneous and occur as a result of the correct juxtaposition of the appropriate residues within the collagen fibril. As can be appreciated from Figure 4.1, the presence of either a lysyl or hydroxylysyl residue in the telopeptide has a profound effect on the nature of the crosslinks produced, and this single hydroxylation event represents a major factor in explaining the observed tissue specificity of crosslinking. Indeed, some early studies suggested that this hydroxylation reaction may be accomplished by a separate enzyme [38,39], reflecting the potential importance of the reaction by implying distinct control mechanisms. Recently, further evidence for a separate hydroxylation mechanism was obtained by peptide analysis of hypertrophic tendons where increased telopeptide hydroxylation was observed without any change in hydroxylation of lysines in the helix [40]. Of the two crosslinking

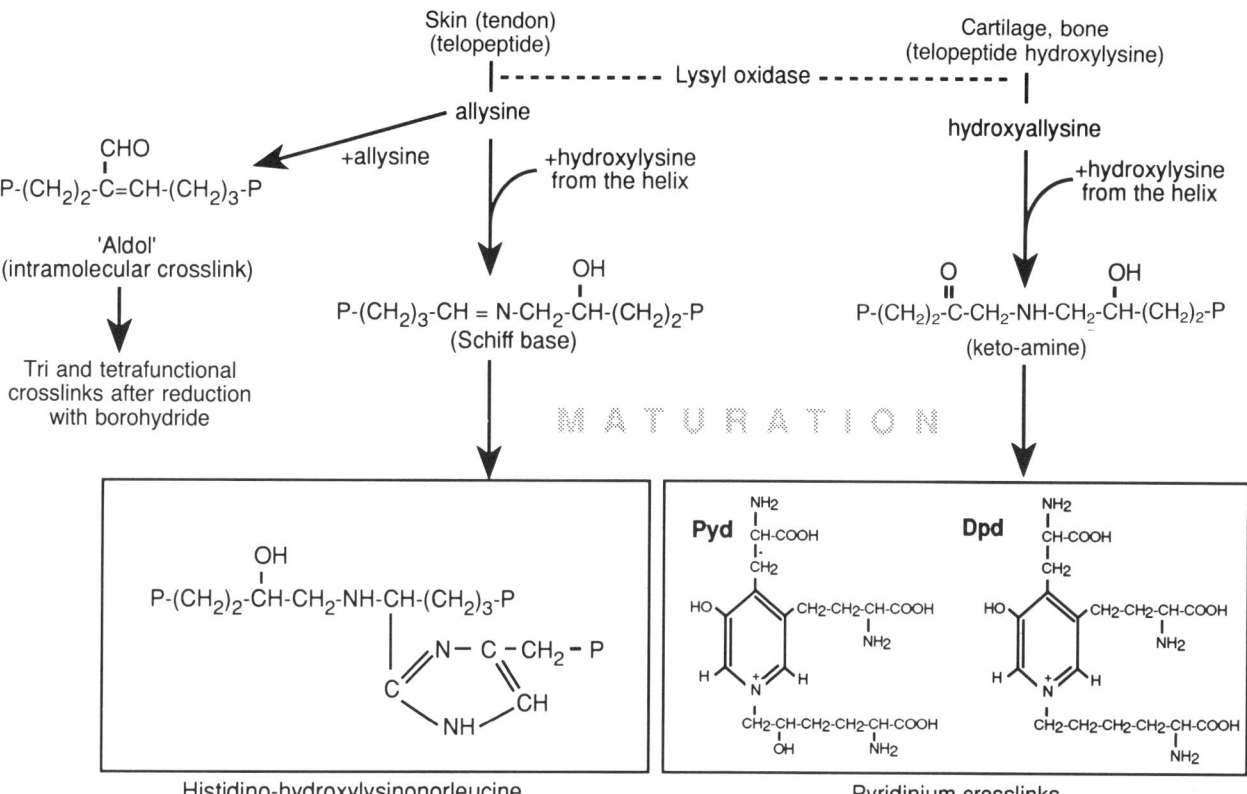

Figure 4.1 Tissue specificity in the formation of inter- and intramolecular crosslinks in fibrillar collagens.

pathways, that involving an oxidized lysyl residue (allysine) in the telopeptide is typified by skin collagen where reaction with hydroxylysine in the helix of an adjacent molecule gives rise to an aldimine (Schiff base). This —CH=N— bond achieves stabilization of the collagen fibril under physiological conditions but is very labile to the effects of heat and dilute acids, so that chemical modification by reduction with borohydride was necessary to facilitate its isolation as hydroxylysinonorleucine (HLNL). Where the telopeptide lysine residue is hydroxylated, as occurs in cartilage, bone and some tendons, reaction of hydroxylysine aldehyde (hydroxyallysine) with adjacent hydroxylysine or lysine residues gives rise initially to an aldimine but the presence of the hydroxyl group facilitates an Amadori rearrangement to give the oxo-imine compound, (hydroxy)lysino-5-oxonorleucine. The oxo-imines (also referred to as ketoamines) are more stable to heat and dilute acids than the aldimine bonds, thus explaining many of the differences in physicochemical properties of the tissue. Skin collagen from young animals is therefore completely soluble in dilute acetic acid whereas achilles tendon from the same animal is only partially soluble due to the presence of a higher proportion of stable oxoimine bonds.

The amount of the borohydride-reducible crosslinks in collagen increases during the rapid growth phase and thereafter declines with age [41]. These changes coincide with increases in the stability and tensile strength of the collagen, leading to the suggestion that the reducible components are intermediates that are transformed into more stable compounds. Several different types of modification of the reducible bonds have been suggested but it is now recognized that the major maturation product of the aldimine bond is histidino-hydroxylysinonorleucine (HHL), a trifunctional crosslink [42]. The formation of HHL involves the addition of a histidine residue across the double bond although the precise mechanism, which must include a reduction step, is still unclear. The predominant maturation product of the oxo-imine compounds are the 3-hydroxypyridinium crosslinks, pyridinoline (also referred to as hydroxylysyl-pyridinoline) and deoxy-pyridinoline (or lysyl-pyridinoline). Two mechanisms have been proposed for their formation [43,44] and, although these mechanisms are very similar chemically, they impose very different steric constraints on the arrangement of collagen fibrils. Thus, in proposing that pyridinoline is formed by reaction of two hydroxylysino-5-oxonorleucine crosslinks [43], only microfibrils in register could participate in this type of reaction. This mechanism would also result in an increase of one trifunctional crosslink for the loss of two bifunctional molecules, as measured experimentally using *in vitro* systems. The alternative mechanism [44] suggests that the bifunctional, oxo-imine crosslink could react with hydroxylysine aldehyde (as its enol tautomer) derived from the same molecule as the bifunctional aldehyde donor. This suggests that the pyridinium crosslinks may only act as a crosslink between two molecules.

Glycosylated forms of the reducible, bifunctional crosslinks have been indentified [45] showing that O-glycosylation of the participating hydroxylysine residue in the helix does not inhibit the formation of crosslinks. Consistent with this observation, a glycosylated form of pyridinoline was detected in alkali hydrolysates of cartilage [44] and 10–15% of the pyridinoline excreted in urine is glycosylated [46].

Other crosslinking components

In addition to the Schiff base compounds, lysine aldehyde reacts intramolecularly to form the aldol condensation product (Figure 4.1), that again was identified after reduction with borohydride. In borohydride-reduced tissues, the aldol has been shown to react with histidine and hydroxylysine residues to give a number of tri- and tetrafunctional compounds (reviewed in [47,48, 49]). The major component of this group is histidinohydroxymerodesmosine (HHMD). Some doubt exists, however, as to whether these compounds exist in non-reduced form as crosslinks in the tissue or whether they are artefacts of the chemical reduction procedure [50, 51]. The fact that different reducing agents give rise to different products [52] appears to strengthen this argument although this question remains unresolved. The concentrations of HHMD in reduced tissue also decline with age and it is clear that the aldol condensation product or the non-reduced form of multifunctional crosslinks undergoes modification to give components that have yet to be identified.

As the concentrations of crosslinks change with physiological age, comparison of different studies using different species is difficult. However, it is clear from a summary of the relatively few detailed studies available that cartilage collagen contains the highest concentrations of pyridinoline whereas, in bone collagen, the concentration of pyridinium crosslinks is only 10–30% of this value. This introduces an additional problem in that the concentrations of crosslinks are dependent not only on their rate of formation and maturation but also on the rate of turnover of the tissue. The relatively low concentrations of pyridinium crosslinks in bone may therefore result in part from the known high turnover rate of this tissue through the remodelling process. It is likely, however, that some maturation products of the oxo-imine bonds other than 3-hydroxy-pyridinium derivatives occur, and evidence for this has been obtained from several peptide studies where non-stoichiometric amounts of crosslink were obtained [53,54,55]. Following earlier work by Scott and colleagues [56], the possi-

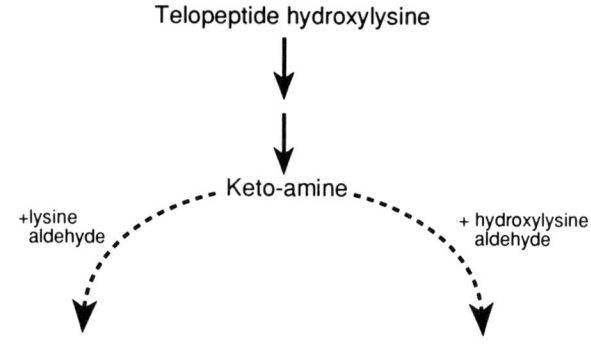

Figure 4.2 Possible alternative pathways of crosslinking in tissues containing telopeptide hydroxylysine to form pyridinium or pyrrolic compounds.

bility that pyrrolic crosslinks form an alternative maturation pathway has been proposed [57], as indicated in Figure 4.2. Peptides apparently containing pyrrolic crosslinks have been identified from both collagen types I and III [57,58,59] and the concentration in the bovine tendons showed a positive correlation with the biophysical properties [60]. The actual structure of the putative crosslink has not yet been elucidated and this topic still represents an area of active research. It is likely that a number of pyrrolic structures are produced through different mechanisms that may explain the apparent location of these compounds in skin collagen and elastin [59], neither of which has a significant proportion of hydroxylysine aldehyde-derived crosslinks.

Most studies of the collagen crosslinking in blood vessels have concentrated on the large arteries. Measurements of pyridinoline by ELISA in hydrolysates of samples taken at different sites of the thoracic aorta revealed a wide range of values that appeared to be related to the level of biophysical stresses experienced by the tissue. Thus, in a proximal site close to the aortic valve, the pyridinoline concentration was around 1.0–1.5 residues per molecule of collagen whereas, in the descending aorta, values of 0.3–0.5 residues per molecule were obtained [61]. Interestingly, there were no marked decreases in pyridinoline concentrations in the corresponding samples from age-matched patients with dissecting aneurysms [61]. Some deoxypyridinoline (not detected by the ELISA method) is present in aorta [62] and a reducible precursor of this crosslink, dehydrohydroxylysinonorleucine, detected in the ascending aorta has been shown to undergo age-related changes [63]. Measurement of the reducible compounds present in the matrix elaborated by human and porcine endothelial cells in culture revealed that the vascular endothelium contributes a proportion of the crosslinks, with the pyridinoline precursor, dihydroxylysinonorleucine being the most abundant [64].

Non-enzymatic glycosylation

The changes in lysine-derived crosslinks are referred to as maturational changes, the function of which is not fully understood but which may be associated with the requirements of growth remodelling and fibril organization within tissues. These essential changes are distinct from those associated with true aging or senescence that may be defined as deleterious to the proper functioning of the tissue. Non-enzymatic glycosylation appears to bring about the latter types of change and has led to the term Advanced Glycosylation End-products (or AGE products) which have been the subject of extensive research efforts over the past few years (reviewed in [65,66]). This topic is directly relevant to studies of aging and of the well recognized changes in connective tissues, particularly those of the vascular system, that occur in diabetes.

As a generally long-lived family of proteins, collagen is highly susceptible to the age-dependent reactions initiated by N-glycosylation of lysine and hydroxylysine residues. The primary products of the Maillard reaction in collagen were initially identified as borohydride-reduced adducts that were shown to increase with age [67]. More recently, much interest has focused on the possibility of further reaction of the fructosyl lysine produced to form chemical crosslinks. Evidence has accumulated that these reactions involve the formation of reactive dicarbonyl compounds from the Amadori products, in addition to other, non-crosslinking compounds such as carboxymethyl-lysine, which act as reporters of the degree of glycation reactions [68]. There is also evidence that metal-catalysed autoxidation reactions of glucose may provide an alternative mechanism for the oxidative modification of proteins [69].

Indirect evidence from experiments where collagenous tissues were incubated *in vitro* with high concentrations of glucose suggested that further stabilization was occurring in both fibrillar [70] and basement membrane collagens [71]. Elucidation of the crosslinking products has, however, proved extremely difficult as only small amounts of these compounds are produced and the use of model systems with high, non-physiological concentrations of glucose is susceptible to the production of artefacts. The work of Monnier and colleagues showed that the insolubilization reactions *in vitro* were much faster in the presence of pentose rather than glucose, and further analysis succeeded in isolating and identifying an adduct, apparently formed between lysine, ribose and arginine, which was given the trivial name, pentosidine [72]. Although this component has been detected in several connective tissues, including vascular tissues [73], the biosynthetic mechanism of formation has not been determined and the concentrations are generally at such low levels that the physiological relevance of the potential crosslinking has not been established. The carbohydrate precursors of pentosidine *in vivo* are unknown and mechanisms for reactions involving glucose, fructose and ascorbate have been proposed [74,75].

The detection of pyrrolic crosslinks in collagen has already been discussed in relation to the lysyl oxidase mediated crosslinks (section 4.1.1.c, p. 92). Other pyrrole derivatives have been characterized as products of nonenzymatic glycosylation and one has been designated, pyrraline [76,77]. This finding has naturally led to speculation that these compounds are related to the Ehrlich Chromogen crosslinks. The tissue specificity and localization of the Ehrlich Chromogen within the collagen fibril [57] suggest that there is no relationship between these pyrrolic compounds. Structural considerations support this view as reaction with the *p*-dimethylamino-benzaldehyde reagent requires a free 2 position on the ring which is not present in pyrraline. Definitive studies of the structure and biochemical derivation of these compounds in collagen is, however, necessary to resolve these questions.

(d) Functions of the different collagen types

Fibrillar collagens

As by far the major collagen in the body, the function of type I collagen is to provide structural support. It is now recognized, however, that collagen fibrils in tissues rarely consist of a single collagen type and the specialized functions in different tissues are accomplished by the modifying influences of other collagen types. In many soft tissues, for example, collagen III is known to form co-fibrils with collagen I as detected immunocytochemically [78] and the relative proportions of these two collagen types may control the fibril diameter. This effect may be partially derived from the slower metabolic processing rate of procollagen III as determined *in vivo* for skin [79], with the result that some N-propeptides become incorporated in the fibrils [80] and presumably sterically influence the attainable fibril diameter. More direct evidence for the formation of co-fibrils was provided by the isolation of crosslinked peptides from human leiomyoma containing both collagen I- and III-derived telopeptides linked with the helical regions of each collagen type [81].

Collagen types I and III probably constitute about 80–90% of the total collagens in blood vessels. The relative proportions and distribution of the two vary according to the species, the type of vessel and the location in the vessel. Generally, collagen I is present throughout arterial vessels but with larger amounts in the adventitia compared with the medial and intimal layers, as demonstrated for rat aorta by immunofluorescence staining (Figure 4.3). Collagen III shows a similar pattern except that relatively more intense staining is

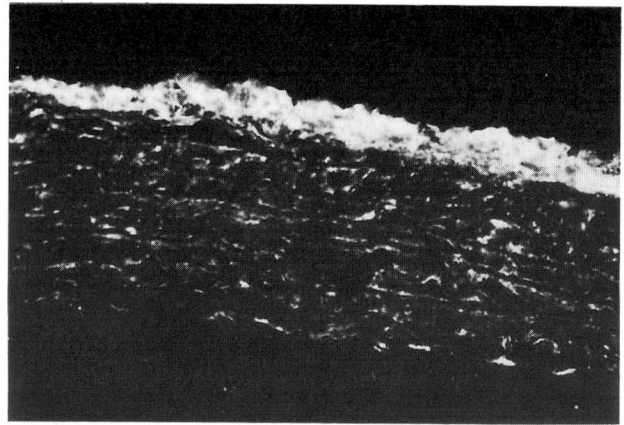

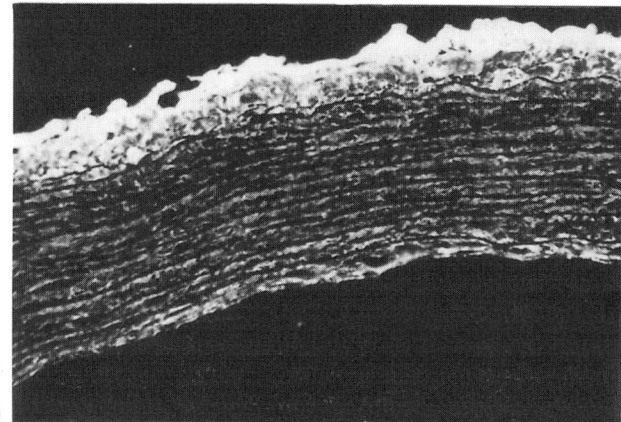

Figure 4.3 Immunostaining of rat aorta with type-specific anticollagen antibodies showing the localization of collagen type I(a) mainly in the adventitial layer (a), whereas collagen type III(b), also abundant in the adventitia, shows distinct staining in the medial and intimal layers (b).

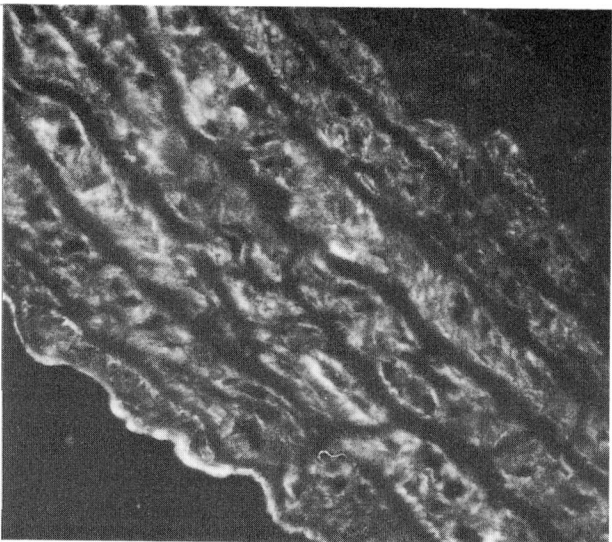

Figure 4.4 Immunostaining of rat aorta showing the distribution of collagen type V throughout the media between the elastic layers with strong staining of the intima (lower left) but virtually absent from the adventitia (upper right).

present in the media and intima (Figure 4.3). Studies of collagen distribution in human aorta have demonstrated an age dependency with very little interstitial collagen detected in the intima from young individuals [82] but a preponderance of collagen III staining in the intima of subjects aged 45–65 years [83]. Apparently conflicting results were obtained by analysis of marker peptides for collagen types I and III derived by digestion with cyanogen bromide [84], although the relatively large proportions of collagen I determined in the latter study may have resulted from intimal thickening in the subjects investigated.

Collagen types V and XI may also be considered as fibrillar collagens, as they have a long, uninterrupted triple-helical domain and extension peptides at both N- and C-terminal ends. Although quantitatively minor, collagen type V is present in virtually all non-cartilagenous tissues. Studies of its structure and assembly showed differences to collagen I in a much slower processing rate and the incomplete removal of the N-terminal propeptides [85]. Immunocytochemical studies have shown that collagen V can be stained only after disruption of the fibril structure [86], leading to speculation that this collagen may form thin fibrils that act as cores for the assembly of collagen type I. A corresponding function could be ascribed to collagen XI for the assembly of the major cartilage collagen, type II [87]. More recent evidence, however, reveals a much more complex situation with multiple forms of collagen V being described as having different chain compositions [85]. Thus, three main α-chains for collagen V are known, but these may occur as a homotrimer, $[α1(V)]3$, or as heterotrimeric molecules having a chain composition of either $[α1(V)]_2 α2(V)$ or $[α1(V)α2(V)α3(V)]$. Additional variants arising by alternative splicing of the mRNA may also occur. Further complications have arisen with the discoveries that collagen XI is not restricted to the cartilage system but is expressed in many other tissues [88], and that molecules containing both collagens V and XI chains may be formed [89].

In blood vessels, collagen V is associated primarily with the smooth muscle cell surface and with the subendothelial basement membrane [83,90,91]. Immunostaining of rat aorta with specific antibodies revealed strong staining of the smooth muscle between the elastic fibres with virtually no labelling in the adventitia (Figure 4.4).

FACIT collagens

This term, suggested by Olsen [92], refers to a group of fibril-associated collagens with interrupted triple helices that, as the name implies, do not form fibrils alone but interact with the major fibrillar collagens. This group comprises collagen types IX, XII and XIV, where collagen IX is essentially restricted to the cartilage system whereas the other two types appear to be homologous molecules interacting primarily with collagen I fibrils [93]. Most information on this group is derived from studies of collagen IX in cartilage which contains heterotrimeric molecules with the chain composition [α1(IX)α2(IX)α3(IX)]. This molecule has three collagenous domains with COL1 and COL2 interacting with the fibril and the third, COL3, protruding from the surface, as visualized by electron microscopy [87]. The non-collagenous domains are relatively short except for a 266 residue NC4 region at the N-terminus that is highly basic and may serve to mediate interactions of the collagen II fibrils with the glycosaminoglycans. Tissue variants of collagen IX occur both in the size of the NC4 region [94] and in the presence of a covalently attached glycosaminoglycan at the NC3 region of the α2(IX) chain [95]. Collagen IX is covalently attached to collagen II by the lysine-derived pyridinium crosslinks and studies of their location indicate an antiparallel arrangement of collagen IX with respect to the fibril, with crosslinking to both the N- and C-terminal telopeptides of collagen II [96].

Collagen type XII, initially discovered by sequencing cDNA from an embryonic chick library, exists as a homotrimer, [α1(XII)]₃, and has only two collagenous domains. The COL1 domain shows a high sequence similarity with COL1 of collagen IX, and this part of the molecule is believed to interact with the collagen I fibrils. There is a 190 kDa non-triple-helical domain (NC3) at the N-terminal end of each chain that adopts a cruciform appearance which has been detected by rotary shadowing. Collagen XII-like molecules have been localized by immunocytochemistry to the surface of banded fibrils [97] and this collagen type appears to provide interactions between the structural fibres and other matrix components. Collagen type XIV has been extracted from bovine skin and tendon and is also a homotrimer with similar characteristics to collagen XII [98].

Much more information on the tissue distribution and fibrillar interactions of these FACIT collagens is currently emerging, although their distribution in vascular tissues has not yet been studied in detail. It is already clear, however, that these collagens, and perhaps similar as yet unidentified molecules, will prove to have profound influences in mediating interactions of the major collagen fibrils with other components of the extracellular matrix.

Collagen type VI

This collagen was originally termed 'intimal collagen' following its isolation as short disulphide-bonded fragments from pepsin digests of vascular tissues [99]. The intractability of this collagen type in most physiological buffer solutions hampered extraction of the native molecule, but subsequent studies have shown that collagen VI is present in almost all soft tissues, often in relatively large amounts [100,101]. Although classified as a collagen, this component is essentially a glycoprotein with up to 25% by weight of carbohydrate and a collagenous triple helix that comprises less than one third of the molecule. Flanking the short triple helix are large globular extensions at both the N- and C-terminal ends. The molecule is usually a heterotrimer with three different chains, [α1(VI)α2(VI)α3(VI)], but there appears to be a variety of tissue isoforms resulting from alternative splicing of the mRNA and by proteolytic cleavage [102,103]. The assembly of collagen VI appears to be unique among the collagens as little proteolytic processing is required. The process, initiated intracellularly, involves lateral aggregation into dimers in a staggered antiparallel manner followed by association of the dimers in register to form tetramers. This secreted form associates extracellularly into the characteristic beaded filaments with a periodicity of 105 nm (Figure 4.5) visible in the electron microscope [104]. The molecule is stabilized by disulphide bonding and analysis of intact collagen VI from intervertebral discs using hyaluronidase treatment showed that no lysine-derived crosslinks were present [105].

Despite the wealth of structural information available for collagen VI, the function of the molecule is still uncertain. The ubiquitous nature of the collagen and its location particularly at pericellular sites [106] has led to the suggestion that collagen VI fibrils act as bridging networks between cells and the surrounding matrix. This hypothesis is strengthened by the fact that the collagen VI molecule has 11 arginine-glycine-aspartate (RGD) sequences that potentially interact with integrin receptors in the cell membrane [107]. Collagen type VI is also known to interact with other matrix macromolecules including hyaluronan [108] and the proteoglycan, decorin [109]. The presence of several isoforms of the molecule provides the scope for multiple functions in growth, development and remodelling of soft connective tissues.

Collagen type VIII

This collagen was originally detected in culture medium of aortic endothelial cells and termed 'endothelial cell' or EC collagen, for which a number of variants was proposed [110]. Subsequent studies, particularly of corneal endothelial cells [111], have revealed that collagen VIII is a member of the short-chain collagens that form sheet-like structures. Initially it was thought to be a homotrimeric molecule, but cloning and sequencing of the α1(VIII) collagen cDNA demonstrated a

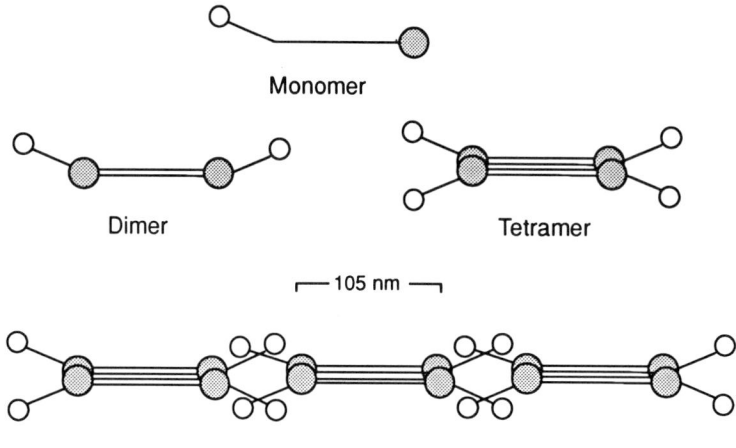

Figure 4.5 Schematic representation of the association of collagen VI molecules to form dimers and tetramers, and their subsequent aggregation to form beaded filaments.

helical domain having eight imperfections, together with a large C-terminal non-helical region and a shorter N-terminal extension peptide [112]. An α2(VIII) has now been described with similar structure [113] and the ratio of the two chains suggests that heterotrimers are produced of the form [α1(VIII)$_2$α2(VIII)], but direct confirmation of this arrangement has not yet been obtained.

There is a remarkable similarity between collagen VIII and collagen X, the latter being associated specifically with the hypertrophic chondrocytes in the growth plate [114]. This extends to over 50% similarity in nucleotide sequences and, interestingly, there are also similarities in sequence with the serum complement component, C1q [17]. Relatively little is known about the assembly and function of collagen VIII. This molecule appears to represent the major structural element of the hexagonal lattice observed in Descemet's membrane, the specialized basement membrane structure supporting corneal endothelial cells [115]. Similar hexagonal structures have been visualized *in vitro* for collagen X [116] in which molecules appear to aggregate through as yet unknown interaction between their C-terminal globular regions. Immunochemical studies have shown that collagen type VIII, as a component of most blood vessels, has a wide tissue distribution and is probably associated with the subendothelial basement membrane [117]. Recent studies have shown that rat mesangial cells also express collagen VIII which was localized to the media of large intrarenal arteries and to the capillary loops and mesangium of normal rat kidney [118]. These observations confirm the wider distribution of this collagen and suggest that the molecule functions to provide a three-dimensional organizational network for endothelial cells.

Collagen type IV

Following recognition of a distinct form of collagen extractable from basement membranes [119], there is now known to be a variety of molecular species [120] consistent with the wide distribution and functional requirements of these structures. Basement membranes are present at all epithelial and endothelial linings as well as surrounding specialized cell types such as muscle and nerve cells. This molecule occurs primarily as [α1(IV)$_2$α2(IV)] and has a major triple-helical domain about 350 nm in length with a large globular extension at the C-terminus (NC1 region) and a 30 nm helical N-terminal domain referred to as the 7S region. In the triple-helical domain, the —Gly—X—Y— sequence has short interruptions at over 20 points along the chain giving rise to very flexible monomers [121,122]. Newly synthesized collagen type IV monomers appear not to undergo proteolytic processing before assembly involving interactions at both the N- and C-terminal ends. Electron microscope studies using rotary shadowing have visualized spider-like structures formed by the antiparallel interactions of monomers through the 7S region. These structures then aggregate into a flexible, three-dimensional network formed by the head-to-head interactions of the NC1 regions. The structure is stabilized by disulphide bonds within both 7S and NC1 domains and by lysyl oxidase-mediated crosslinks that are present mainly as the reducible intermediate, hydroxylysino-5-oxo-norleucine [123]. No conversion of these compounds to form pyridinium crosslinks occurs in basement membrane collagen, presumably due to the lack of appropriate molecular packing, although it is conceivable that other as yet unidentified crosslink maturation products are formed.

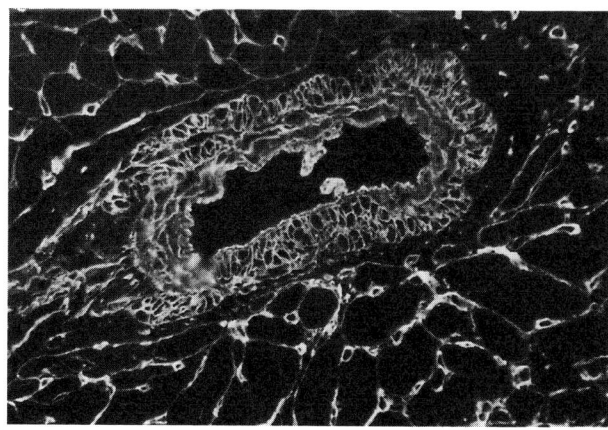

Figure 4.6 Immunostaining of rat coronary artery with antibodies specific for collagen type IV.

Collagen IV has been isolated from bovine and human aorta [124,125,126]. Immunolocalization confirms the presence of this collagen in the subendothelial basement membrane and those surrounding the smooth muscle cells (Figure 4.6). Consistent with this distribution, collagen IV synthesis *in vitro* has been demonstrated for both smooth muscle cells [127] and endothelial cells [128]. A number of isoforms of collagen IV have recently been described and there is now evidence for several other genetically distinct α-chains, designated α3(IV) to α5(IV), that appear to impart specialized functions since these are localized in specific basement membranes [129]. One of the main stimulators of this work has been characterization of various renal diseases involving basement membranes. Thus, the primary lesion in the autoimmune disease, Goodpasture syndrome, has been localized to the NC1 domain of the α3(IV) chain [130], and in Alport's syndrome, a familial nephritis, the main lesion was found to be due to a mutation in the α5(IV) chain [131]. Although there is a great deal of structural information on these isomorphic chains, little is known about their molecular composition *in vivo*.

Collagen type IV clearly functions as the main structural scaffold for basement membranes but the association with a large number of other macromolecules is essential to accomplish the diverse biological functions required of these structures. Thus, associations with laminin-entactin, heparan sulphate proteoglycans and many other minor components in a tissue-specific manner, combine to provide structures that act as cell-anchoring points, selective molecular sieving and direct the growth and development of tissues.

4.1.2 ELASTIN

Elastin is found in the extracellular matrix of the blood vessel wall in association with collagen and proteoglycans which are organized in a way that transfers stress throughout the vessel wall. Elastin is the most abundant protein of the major arteries that are subjected to large pulsatile pressure generated by cardiac contraction. In contrast, vessels that are subjected to less pressure are enriched with collagen and therefore stiffer and less pliable. Elastin is a crosslinked biopolymer with tensile properties similar to rubber and therefore its stretchability and subsequent recoil make it highly suitable for its role in providing elasticity to the blood vessel wall.

Elastin is the major protein of elastic system fibres which include elastic, elaunin and oxytalan fibres [132]. The elastic fibre consists of two distinct morphological components; large amounts of an elastin core, which is responsible for the elastic properties, surrounded by glycoprotein microfibrils, 10–12 nm in diameter. Elaunin fibres also contain both components but are composed predominantly of microfibrils with little amorphous elastin, whereas oxytalan fibres are exclusively bundles of microfibrils. The microfibrillar component comprises a number of high molecular weight glycoproteins. They are a 31 kDa microfibril-associated glycoprotein (MAGP), a 35 kDa protein with amine oxidase activity and fibrillin, a large 350 kDa glycoprotein (see section 4.1.3(c)). Collagen type VI was initially thought to be a microfibrillar protein but evidence now indicates that this collagen type is chemically and immunologically distinct from microfibril proteins [133]. During the formation of the chick aorta the smooth muscle cells of the arterial wall first synthesize bundles of oxytalan fibres and then deposit the amorphous elastin component between the microfibrils, which subsequently coalesce and form firstly the intermediate elaunin fibre and finally the mature elastic fibre. These histological observations have led to the conclusion that both oxytalan and elaunin fibres are precursors of the mature elastic fibre.

(a) Composition and biosynthesis

An understanding of elastin composition and of its synthesis and chemistry was initially thwarted by its extreme insolubility. Significant advances came about when a protein, now called tropoelastin, was isolated from copper-deficient animals and was found to have strong similarities to elastin. The amino acid profile of tropoelastin (M_r 72 000) is characterized by a high proportion (86%) of hydrophobic amino acids mainly glycine, alanine, proline, valine, leucine, iso-leucine and phenylalanine but no methionine, cysteine or histidine residues. In addition tropoelastin has, in contrast to elastin, a high content of lysine and no crosslinking amino acids desmosine and isodesmosine. Tryptic digests indicate the presence of large and small peptides with the latter rich in alanine and lysine residues, which form the crosslink regions. The amino acid sequence of the larger peptides demonstrates that, as for collagen, approximately every third residue is glycine. Although there is little homology of sequence a (Gly—Val—Pro)$_{13}$ repeat found in chick tropoelastin may indicate that elastin and collagen evolved from the same distant gene.

Tropoelastin is the primary translation product of elastin mRNA and is the soluble intermediate in the biosynthesis of the insoluble and highly crosslinked mature elastin. The mechanisms by which elastin synthesis is regulated are not well understood and although mechanical stimulation is involved cellular factors such as insulin-like growth factor-I, glucocorticoids, transforming growth factor-β, and 1,25-dihydroxyvitamin D$_3$ have also been implicated in its regulation at the pretranslational level. Although tropoelastin undergoes very little intracellular post-translational modification, hydroxylation of some proline residues does occur. The significance of this is unclear but it has been postulated that over-hydroxylation can impair the ability of tropoelastin to form fibres [134]. The secretion of tropoelastin from both smooth muscle and endothelial cells of the arterial wall follows the classical pathway for protein secretion via the Golgi apparatus and exocytotic processes. On secretion, tropoelastin is accreted to the elastic fibres and eventually crosslinked into the developing fibre. This process occurs without prior cleavage of the tropoelastin molecule although the presence of a larger pro-elastin polypeptide (90–140 kDa) was initially reported. Although it is realized that aggregation of secreted tropoelastin is necessary for subsequent crosslinking the process is poorly understood. It was proposed over 25 years ago that aggregation was a consequence of the interaction of tropoelastin molecules with the glycoprotein microfibrils which serve to align tropoelastin molecules in precise register for subsequent crosslinking. This theory of aggregation is supported by more recent studies but new evidence indicates that the tropoelastin monomer contains in its primary sequence sufficient information for self alignment. In addition, recent studies suggest that the regulation of elastogenesis is mediated at the cell surface by the elastin receptor [135]. The 67 kDa elastin receptor contains both a protein binding site that recognizes a hydrophobic sequence in elastin (VGVAPG) and a carbohydrate binding site. Binding of the highly glycosylated microfibrils to the receptor serves to lower the affinity of tropoelastin for its receptor and thereby directs the transfer of tropoelastin molecules to the microfibrils [136].

(b) Crosslinking of elastin

After secretion of the soluble tropoelastin monomers, the peptidyl lysine residues undergo oxidative deamination catalysed by the enzyme lysyl oxidase as previously described for collagen crosslinking (see section 4.1.1(c)). Unlike collagen, hydroxyallysine is not formed in elastin due to the lack of peptidyl hydroxylysine in tropoelastin and thus the crosslinks of elastin subsequently formed differ markedly from those found in collagen. The lysine residues susceptible to the actions of lysyl oxidase are present in pairs separated by two or three alanine residues. The two most abundant peptides, Lys-Ala-Ala-Lys and Lys-Ala-Ala-Ala-Lys are repeated 12 times in the polypeptide chain and form an α-helical conformation, with lysine residues extending from the same side of the helix. The tropoelastin molecules are appropriately juxtaposed bringing together the opposing lysine residues and, in the presence of lysyl oxidase, three of the lysine residues of the lysine–alanine clusters are converted to allysine (α-aminoadipic acid δ-semialdehyde). The fourth residue has an adjacent tyrosine or phenylalanine residue which inhibits its oxidation and therefore this lysine residue retains its amino group. Ultimately, through as yet unknown mechanisms, one of these unoxidized lysine residues reacts with three allysine residues to form, via a number of intermediate crosslinks, a pyridinium ring alkylated in four positions. The lysyl oxidase-mediated step appears to be the only enzymatic step involved in elastin crosslinking with the others probably occurring as spontaneous condensation reactions. Originally described over 30 years ago, this cyclic compound exists in elastin as two isomers which are referred to as desmosine and isodesmosine. These two structures (Figure 4.7) are now regarded as the mature tetrafunctional crosslinks of elastin [137]. Of the 38 lysine residues per tropoelastin molecule about 15 are present in desmosine and isodesmosine, 13 are present in the bi- and trifunctional intermediate crosslinks and six remain unoxidized in mature elastin [138]. The fate of the four remaining residues is unclear but they may be lost during analysis or present in as yet unidentified derivatives. The recent detection of a crosslink derived from 5 lysine residues [139] further indicates that the biochemistry of elastin crosslinks is not yet completely elucidated.

(c) Distribution and function of vascular elastin

In large arteries such as the aorta, elastin is the main structural protein, constituting approximately 60% of the dry weight. There are highly localized differences in the amount of elastin synthesized by the smooth muscle cells of the arterial tree which reflects the diverse properties of the vessel wall. In the intimal region of the vessel wall, elastin provides support for the endothelial cells in the form of the internal elastic membrane, whereas in the medial layer it forms concentric cylindrical sheets separated by layers of smooth muscle and collagen fibres (Figure 4.8; Plate 1). In addition to being

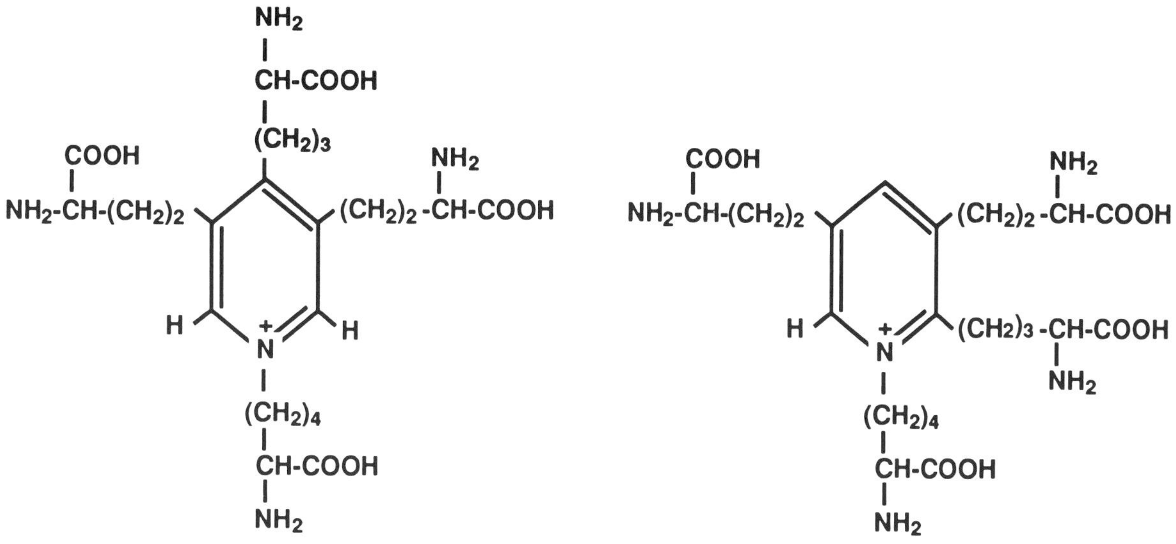

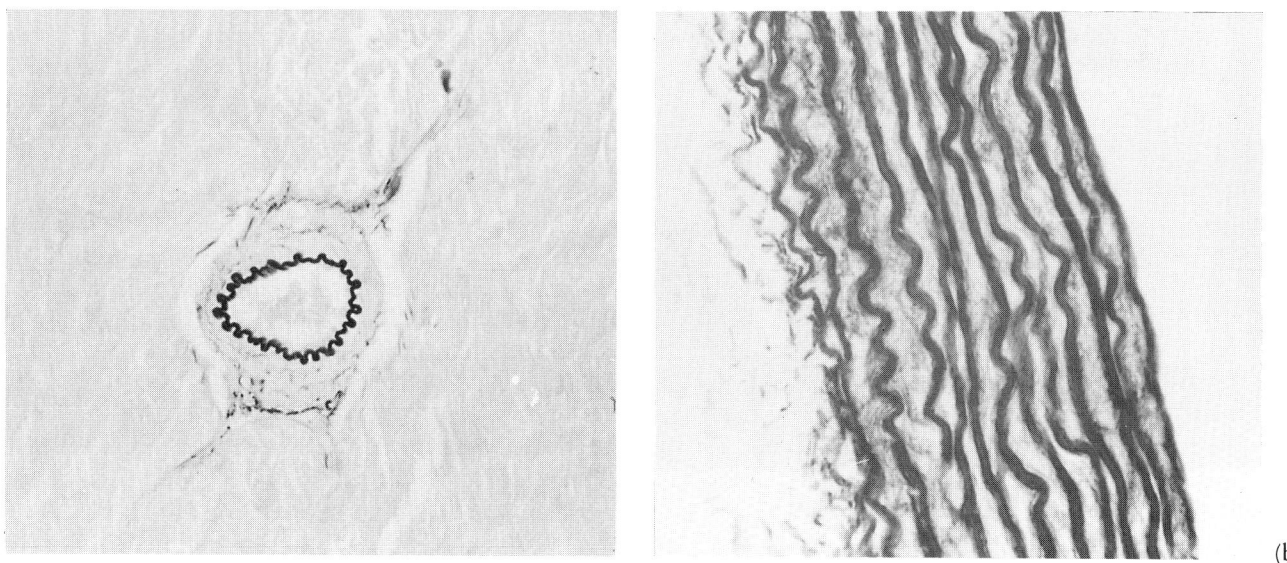

Figure 4.7 Structure of the desmosine crosslinks of elastin.

Figure 4.8 Localization of elastin with Weigert's stain showing (a) the inner elastic membrane of a coronary artery and (b) the elastic laminae of rat aorta. In (b) the adventitia is at the left.

present in the interlaminar space, collagen (type III) is distributed along and around the elastic fibres, whereas collagen type I appears to radiate from the surface of the elastic fibre [140,141]. The medial elastic sheets are interconnected by radially orientated interlaminar elastic fibres, which transfer stress throughout the vessel wall. Wolinsky and Glagov [142] referred to these 'sandwich' layers of elastin as medial lamellar units and regarded them as the fundamental unit of medial structure. These authors have reported in a series of papers a number of features characteristic of the medial units and these have been described in detail [143,144]. In sheep, there is a decrease in the number of medial lamellar units along the descending thoracic artery from the arch to the diaphragm, whereas in the abdominal aorta this decrease is not so marked. It has been hypothesized that the decrease in the thoracic lamellar units is due to 'peeling off' of elastin in the formation of the elastic intercostal and lumber arteries. Evidence suggests that a proportion of the elastic lamellae in the outer third of the aorta is continuous with the lamellar units of the intercostal arteries. The number of elastic lamellae in the intercostals is approximately equal to the number of 'missing' lamellae distal to the branch [145].

Marked differences exist in the elastin distribution at the proximal and distal lips of the aorta-branch junctions. This is clearly demonstrated at the junction between the elastic abdominal aorta and the large branching muscular arteries. In contrast to the abrupt junction at the proximal lip, where little elastin continues into the branch, the junction at the distal lip is characterized by more elastin overlapping into the muscular artery. This distribution in the distal lip demonstrates the need for a stiffer structure for a flow divider [145] and reflects the anisotropic properties of the arterial wall.

Recent findings [146] on the media of the rat aorta indicate that the innermost lamellae are thicker than those situated in the outer third and in addition the number of smooth muscle cell contacts is greater in the thicker lamellae. These data support the concept that there is a difference in the stress-resisting properties of the aortic wall between the outer and inner parts of the media with the innermost lamellae supporting the high tension. The authors suggest that due to the change in form, tearing may be expected at their junction and this may be critical in the location of aortic dissections.

Visualization of arterial elastin by scanning electron microscopy after removal of contaminating components by hot alkali treatment, indicates that the internal elastic membrane and the next few medial elastin layers are fenestrated sheets. The fenestrations in the media are larger than those of the internal elastic membrane with the size and density of those in the latter varying with location. In the lower abdominal canine aorta the size of the fenestrations is 2.23 ± 0.05 μm whereas in the upper thoracic aorta they measure 0.95 ± 0.03 μm [147]. The physiological importance of the elastic fenestrations is unclear but they may play a role in permeability and the development of atherosclerosis. Atherosclerotic plaques tend to develop at arterial bifurcations and it is at these locations that the fenestration size and density are increased [143,148]. Their role in permeability is difficult to assess as *in vivo* the fenestrations are filled with muscle and connective tissue components which all have different permeability coefficients [149]. Analysis of non-digested material would be required to address this question. The fenestrae of the internal elastic membrane allow endothelial–smooth muscle cell communication in the form of cytoplasmic projections. These myoendothelial contacts are potential sites for electrical and metabolic communication between the intima and the media, making the vessel wall a cohesive operational unit [150]. Break up of these contacts may be responsible for impairment of communication between the intima and media of the vessel wall in arteriosclerosis [151]. In contrast to the fenestrated sheets of the intimal side, the elastic layers of the adventitial side of the media are made up of thick elastic fibres forming a dense fibrous network.

Unlike collagen which is known to be distributed along lines of stress there is no direct evidence to suggest a relationship between stress and/or strain (stroke volume and pulse pressure) and elastin synthesis in the vessel wall. There are, however, a number of indirect observations to support such a relationship. Firstly, the internal elastic lamina is observed in large veins but not in smaller medium-sized vessels and, secondly, a fully developed internal elastic lamina and an abundance of medial elastin develops in veins upon transplantation to the coronary circulation. These two lines of evidence suggest that pulsatile flow and pressure may trigger the development of vascular elastic fibres.

The major biological property of elastin is its extreme extensibility. It can be extended to 200–300% of its original length and still recoil to its normal dimensions after removal of the deformation stress. It is this property of elastin that permits large arteries to distend in systole and recoil in diastole, properties which are necessary for constant blood flow to the microcirculation. These characteristics of elastin are largely due to the random coil conformation of its crosslinked polypeptide chains. This random coil arises from the unrestricted movement of the hydrophobic regions and results in a state of total disorder (maximum entropy). When subjected to stress or compression a degree of orientation of the polypeptide chains takes place and order is restored. This decrease in entropy results in the storage of free energy, which is necessary for elastic recoil. Therefore, when the external force is removed the elastic fibre follows thermodynamic principles and returns to a state of maximum disorder, i.e. the initial disordered random coil. A more detailed explanation of the mechanochemistry of elastin is given by Gosline and Rosenbloom [152].

4.1.3 GLYCOPROTEINS

There is an increasing number of structural glycoprotein macromolecules in the extracellular matrix that may be described as 'adhesive' because of their strong interactions with cell membranes and with other components of the matrix. These include fibronectin, vitronectin, laminin, entactin, tenascin and thrombospondin. Their distinction from the collagens is somewhat arbitrary as collagens are also glycoproteins to varying degrees and some, such as collagen type VI, have marked cell-binding capacity.

A full description of these glycoproteins is beyond the scope of this review but the purpose of this section is to provide an overview of their structure in relation to the known functions and interactions within the extracellular matrix. The grouping of these glycoproteins in this section does not suggest a common functionality; indeed, the examples discussed are located in such diverse structures as the extracellular matrix sur-

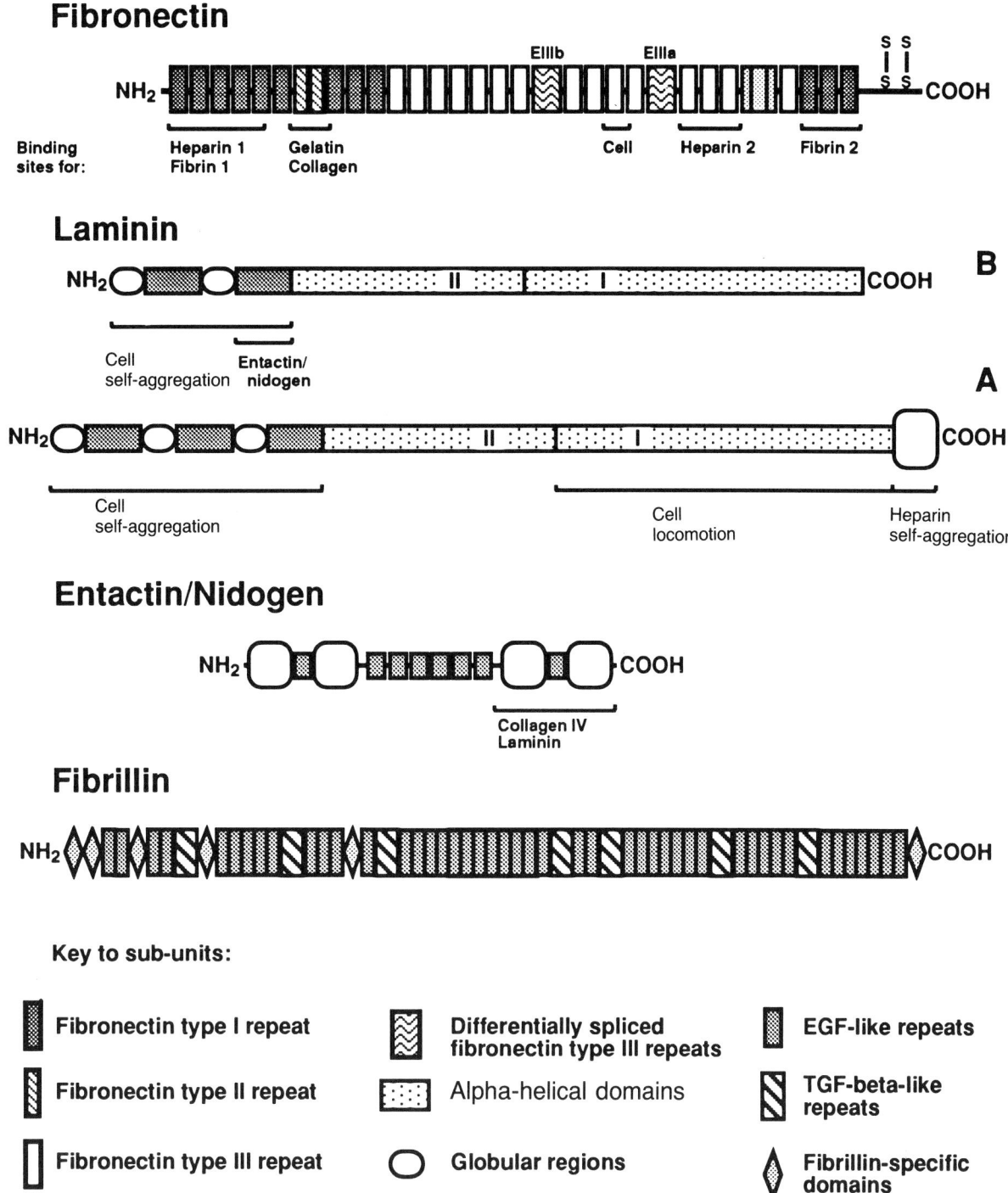

Figure 4.9 Sub-unit structure of glycoproteins.

rounding mesenchymal cells, in basement membranes and in elastic fibres. With the rapid increase in recent years in the amount of information on the primary structure of extracellular proteins, the concept has emerged of mosaic proteins containing well defined subunits that may appear in apparently unrelated proteins [153]. These structural elements or subunits are generally coded by discrete exons and the presence of particular motifs in the surrounding introns suggests that these extracellular proteins have evolved from a relatively small number of exons by exon shuffling, as originally proposed by Gilbert [154]. In computer jargon, this might be described as an 'evolutionary macro' that would allow the rapid evolution of a multitude of protein components with a wide variety of biochemical functions contributed by the unique assembly of different domains. The subunit structure of a number of structural glycoproteins is shown in Figure 4.9. Prominent among the different domain structures is the epidermal growth factor (EGF)-like repeats. Their presence serves to emphasize the dynamic nature of the interactions between cells and the extracellular matrix as it has been proposed that the EGF repeat sequences and other growth factor-related motifs in extracellular proteins may act as local signals for cellular growth and differentiation [155].

(a) Fibronectin

The subunit assembly of fibronectin results in two polypeptide chains about 2500 amino acid residues in length linked at the C-terminal end by disulphide bridges. There are multiple forms of the molecule arising from a single gene through variations in splicing of the mRNA. Thus, in the human plasma form of fibronectin secreted by hepatocytes, two subunits, termed EIIIa and EIIIb (see Figure 4.9), are absent, whereas these subunits are present in a cellular form synthesized by fibroblasts [156]. The fibronectin molecule has multiple biological activities that are located at different sites along the multidomain structure, thus potentially enabling simultaneous interactions between cells and several extracellular components. The cell-binding sites, located on most cell types, have been shown to be mainly of the Arg-Gly-Asp (RGD) type that interact with integrin receptors (reviewed in [157,158]). The binding site for denatured collagen type I (gelatin) that has been utilized for isolation of fibronectin also binds native collagen, but this interaction is much weaker and is not thought to be important *in vivo*. In addition, there are binding sites for glycosaminoglycans [159] and fibrin [160]. The tissue form of fibronectin therefore plays an important role in the cell migration and proliferation both in development and during tissue repair and remodelling.

As might be expected, fibronectin is widely distributed in vascular tissues and is synthesized by most mesenchymal cells. Immunocytochemical labelling of the aorta shows strong staining for fibronectin in the adventitial layer, distinct labelling throughout the medial layer associated with smooth muscle cells between the elastic laminae, and intense staining of the intima (Figure 4.10).

(b) Laminin

As a major component of basement membranes, laminin is a large glycoprotein for which the multidomain structure leads to multiple interactions with cells and other matrix constituents [161]. The molecule has three chains, an A chain of about 400 kDa and two B chains each of about 200 kDa, for which the full amino acid sequences are known [162]. This information together

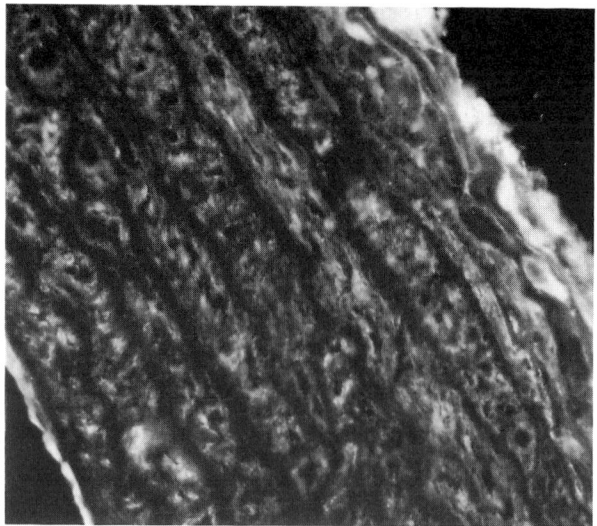

Figure 4.10 Localization of fibronectin in rat aorta by showing intense immunostaining in the intima (lower left), throughout the medial layer and in the adventitia (upper right).

with rotary shadowing studies has led to the proposal of a cruciform structure in which the short arms are contributed separately by the three chains and their C-terminal portions are combined in a disulphide-bonded, coiled-coil structure to form the long arm [163]. There are multiple cell-binding regions situated mainly in the globular domains of the short arms and a glycosaminoglycan binding region at the end of the long arm [164,165]. There is a number of isoforms of laminin many of which appear to be developmentally regulated [129] but their biological function is as yet unclear.

Laminin is associated with a 158 kDa component termed nidogen or entactin that has been shown to interact with laminin at a site on one of the B chains. This interaction occurs soon after translation of the two proteins and is thought to be necessary for the secretion of the laminin–entactin complex [166]. Entactin/nidogen is a protease sensitive, dumbbell-shaped molecule that also has cell attachment sites as well as binding sites for collagen type IV, which assist in the assembly of a three-dimensional complex in the basement membrane [120].

(c) Fibrillin

Fibrillin, a 350 kDa glycoprotein, is a major component of elastic microfibrils [167]. The extended subunit structure (Figure 4.9) gives rod-like molecules, about 150 nm in length and 2 nm wide as visualized in the electron microscope, that aggregate in a head-to-tail manner to form long flexible filaments [168]. The structure is characterized by the multiple repeats of EGF-like domains in which the three cystine bridges stabilize the β-turns within the molecule [169]. Recent evidence has shown that fibrillin may also interact with hyaluronan [168]. Cloning and sequencing have revealed a family of related fibrillin genes of which the major forms are located on chromosome 15, termed Fib-15, and on chromosome 5, termed Fib-5 [170,171]; these code for the glycoproteins, fibrillin-1 and fibrillin-2, respectively, although the latter has not been fully characterized. There is also evidence for a third component, fibrillin-3, for which the gene has been located on chromosome 17 [170,172]. There has recently been intense interest in fibrillin since the discovery in 1991 that the fibrillin on chromosome 15 was linked with Marfan syndrome (see section 4.4.1).

4.1.4 PROTEOGLYCANS

Proteoglycans (PGs) comprise a group of macromolecules which have a near ubiquitous distribution within tissues. Their location in both the plasma membrane and the extracellular matrix means that they, in conjunction with other matrix components, are strategically positioned to provide structural integrity to the tissues as well as mediating a plethora of cellular functions such as growth, differentiation, adhesion and migration. PGs are characterized by the covalent binding of multiple polysaccharide chains to the central polypeptide protein core along with N- and O-linked oligosaccharides. It is from these polysaccharide side chains, the glycosaminoglycans (GAGs), which vary in structure and composition, that the PGs have traditionally derived their name. More importantly the GAG side chains are regarded as the biologically important part of the PG and are responsible for the diverse number of functions attributed to these molecules. It is important to bear in mind that many of the proposed roles of PGs must be regarded as speculative and considering the diversity and abundance of these macromolecules many of their functions are yet to be elucidated.

(a) Proteoglycan synthesis and structure

The PG core proteins, of which several are known to exist, have received little attention, in comparison to their GAG side chains. This is a result of the difficulty in obtaining intact homogeneous core protein free of contaminating GAG side chains and also the poor immunogenicity of the PGs themselves. New methods for the deglycosylation of the core protein [173] and the advent of recombinant DNA technology [174] are now beginning to provide information on the amino acid sequence and peptide structure of the different protein cores that are known to exist. Such information has led to a new nomenclature for the PGs which is based on the make up of the protein core. Although PG core proteins can be grouped into distinct families based on their amino acid motif, this nomenclature, which is now becoming popular, has several limitations. The name conveys no information on the associated GAGs and it is possible that one name will describe several PGs that have a common protein core but different associated GAGs.

A great deal of information is known about the basic structure of the GAGs. Considering their size, their basic structure is relatively simple and easily understood. The GAG side chains comprise a linear sequence of characteristic disaccharide repeats strung together in a strictly alternating fashion. In most GAGs, the disaccharide repeat consists of an amino sugar, either D-glucosamine or D-galactosamine and a uronic acid, either D-glucuronic or L-iduronic acid. The only exception to this is keratan sulphate (KS), in which galactose replaces the urinortic acid residue. It would be an oversimplification, however, to conceive the GAGs as simple disaccharide repeats, as considerable complexity can be bestowed upon the component sugars. The structure of the GAG is rendered more complex by a series of sporadic enzymatic modifications of the monosaccharides. These modifications, accomplished by several epimerases and sulphotransferases, consist of N- and O-sulphation and the epimerization of glucuronic acid to iduronic acid yielding the final secretory product. The disaccharide units that make up the most common GAG structures, namely, chondroitin sulphate (CS), heparan sulphate (HS), dermatan sulphate (DS), KS, hyaluronic acid (HA) and heparin are listed in Table 4.3. HA differs from the other GAGs in the fact that it is neither covalently attached to a core protein nor subjected to further modifications by epimerases or sulphotransferases. It is likely that HA is formed by mechanisms different from the other protein-bound GAGs.

Following synthesis of the core protein in the endoplasmic reticulum, the synthesis of CSPG, DSPG, HSPG and heparin is initiated by the formation of a xylose–serine linkage. Xylose from UDP-xylose is transferred to serine hydroxyl residues situated in the protein core. Xylosyltransferase, the enzyme responsible for this reaction is located in the rough endoplasmic reticulum. The GAG-protein linkage (N-linked to asparagine) observed in KSPG is the kind used to attach complex polysaccharides of glycoproteins to protein but is not observed in any other PGs [175]. Chain synthesis of GAGs occurs in the Golgi apparatus where individual monosaccharides are transferred one by one from appropriate nucleotide sugar precursors, a process mediated by specific glycosyltransferases. The termination of chain elongation in CS is thought to be achieved by sulphation of terminal hexosamine residues, as CS chains ending in N-acetylgalactosamine 4-sulphate are unable to accept a glucuronic acid. GAG chain length varies significantly and the factors determining length are at present unclear [175,176].

Table 4.3 Composition of the major glycosaminoglycans

	Disaccharide repeat units		
	Amino sugar	Uronic acid	Sulphation
Hyaluronic acid	N-acetyl-D-glucosamine	D-glucuronic acid	None
Chondroitin 4-sulphate	N-acetyl-D-galactosamine	D-glucuronic acid	O-sulphate
Chondroitin 6-sulphate	N-acetyl-D-galactosamine	D-glucuronic acid	O-sulphate
Dermatan sulphate	N-acetyl-D-galactosamine	D-glucuronic acid or L-iduronic acid	O-sulphate
Heparin and heparan sulphate	N-acetyl-D-glucosamine or D-glucosamine	D-glucuronic acid or L-iduronic acid	O- and N-sulphate
Keratan sulphate	N-acetyl-D-glucosamine	D-galactose	O-sulphate

PGs that are secreted by cells can be divided into two classes based on their size and state of aggregation. The large aggregating PGs of cartilage are the most studied and they are considered the prototype of molecules of this type. An HA-binding region is located at the N-terminus and constitutes up to 33.0% of the core protein. This region binds specifically to HA which results in the formation of large macromolecular aggregates. The binding region also interacts with a link protein, which stabilizes and strengthens the HA and PG interaction [177]. This interaction leads to a change in the molecular shape of the link protein which can be detected immunologically. In the main, KS chains are concentrated adjacent to the HA binding region with CS chains attached to the remainder of the core protein. The vascular wall of the aorta also contains large aggregating CSPG (M_r: $1-2 \times 10^6$) with GAG chains of M_r approximately 43 000 containing a 6-sulphate to 4-sulphate ratio of approximately 2 [178]. These large aggregating PGs have a high water-binding capacity enabling tissues to resist enormous compressive forces. These properties undoubtedly play an important role in maintaining vessel shape and withstanding the pulsatile pressures of blood flow.

Non-aggregating PGs are generally smaller than their aggregating counterparts although within this former group there is a wide range of sizes and they are therefore often grouped into either small or large non-aggregating PGs. The amino acid composition of the core protein lacks both cystine and methionine residues which is consistent with their lack of aggregation since both amino acids are present in the HA binding region of aggregating PGs [179].

(b) **Proteoglycan families**

Aggrecan and versican

Both of these large aggregating PGs have been located in the aorta and found to be synthesized by vascular smooth muscle cells (VSMC) [180]. Aggrecan consists of both covalently bonded CS and KS. The abundant CS chains are attached in the middle two thirds of the molecule which is rich in serine–glycine repeats. The KS chains, of which there are approximately 100–150, are clustered into a region rich in serine, glycine and glutamic acid residues. Versican, unlike aggrecan, contains only CS side chains which are attached in a glutamic acid rich region in the middle of the protein core. Both versican and aggrecan have many similarities in the N- and C-terminal portions such as similar HA binding domains but their GAG regions are completely distinct from each other.

Biglycan, decorin and fibromodulin

These small non-aggregating interstitial PGs are characterized by a series of leucine rich repeats which may be characteristic of PGs that are involved in protein–protein interactions. Biglycan is located at the cell surface or the pericellular matrix of a number of specialized cell types including endothelial cells [181]. Also called proteoglycan-I it is made up of two CS or two DS GAGs attached to a 38 kDa core protein. The deduced core protein for the secreted form of vascular smooth muscle biglycan is composed of 10 leucine-rich repeating sequences similar to that present in biglycan of bone and cartilage [182]. Decorin (proteoglycan-II) is found associated with many cell types including endothelial and VSMC of the vessel wall. Decorin derived from VSMC is highly conserved at both the RNA and protein level between species [183]. It has associated with it a single CS or DS GAG chain attached to a protein core characterized by seven tandem leucine repeats. Situated within this repeat sequence is the consensus sequence NKISK which has been proposed to be the fibronectin-binding sequence of decorin [184]. Although its size varies due to differing chain length it is generally smaller than biglycan of the same tissue. It has been located by immunoelectron microscopy to the d and e bands of the D period of collagen [185]. The biological role of both decorin and biglycan is uncertain but they may modulate the biological effect of transforming growth factor-β [186]. Fibromodulin unlike biglycan and decorin contains asparagine-linked KS chains. Both decorin and fibromodulin bind to collagen, inhibiting collagen fibrillogenesis [187].

Syndecan, fibroglycan and glypican

These PGs are associated with the cell surface and syndecan and fibroglycan have cytoplasmic, transmembrane and extracellular domains. Syndecan is anchored to the cell via a membrane-spanning domain in the core protein [188] and the extracellular domain of this proteoglycan is substituted with both HS and CS GAGs. These GAGs function as a receptor for interstitial matrix components such as collagen (types I, III and V), thrombospondin and fibronectin whereas the cytoplasmic domain associates with the actin cytoskeleton. Without doubt this PG is intimately involved in both cell–cell and cell–matrix interactions. Although the extracellular domain of fibroglycan is distinct from that of syndecan it also interacts, via its HS chains, with both collagen type I and fibronectin. Glypican is anchored to the cell membrane by a covalent linkage to phosphotidylinositol [189]. This component is expressed by a number of cell types, including endothelial cells and through its HS chains it binds collagen type I, fibronectin and antithrombin III. It has been hypothesized that through these interactions, glypican may modulate the anticoagulant properties of the vascular wall. HS, found in all three membrane PGs inhibits arterial smooth muscle cell proliferation [190] and thus this GAG has attracted a great deal of interest in the possible treatment of atherosclerosis.

(c) **Function and distribution of proteoglycans in the vascular wall**

The blood vessel wall contains a mixture of PGs each located within discrete areas of the tissue reflecting the diverse and varied functions of these macromolecules within the vasculature. It has long been recognized that the PGs of the vascular wall are involved in a range of functions which include amongst others the control of viscoelasticity, permeability, thrombosis and lipid deposition. It is this latter property that has stimulated considerable interest as it has implications in the pathogenesis of atherosclerosis. Evidence has indicated that PGs may bind lipoproteins, thereby allowing them to be taken up by VSMC and macrophages.

More recent *in vitro* studies have indicated that vascular PGs are capable of influencing various properties of smooth muscle cells such as adhesion, morphology, proliferation, macromolecular arrangement and cytoskeletal α-actin organization [191]. Through their ability to interact and form complexes with other connective tissue proteins, PGs are considered essential for the deposition of the extracellular matrix of VSMC. In addition heparin and heparan sulphate proteoglycan are known to inhibit smooth muscle cell proliferation and this may be central to the low proliferation rate of these cells in the normal vessel wall.

CSPG, HSPG and DSPG are the predominant PGs within the vessel wall. Immunocytochemical studies indicate that CSPG is found enriched in the intimal layer with lesser amounts in the media. At these sites it is not closely associated with collagen, elastic fibres or the basal lamina material [192]. It is important to note that this PG is also found in the thickened intima of atherosclerotic blood vessels [192], which predisposes the vessel wall to further complications such as lipid accumulation and entrapment and formation of the fibrous plaque [193]. HSPG is present primarily within endothelial basement membranes and intercalated with the smooth muscle cell membrane [194,195], which reflects its role as a regulator in cell adhesion through interactions with other extracellular matrix components and the cytoskeleton [196]. DSPG is found in the interstitial space of the vessel wall and, in contrast to CSPG, is intimately associated with collagen fibrils [197]. Recent protein sequence analysis of the major DSPG of the aorta has indicated that this PG can be classified as a decorin molecule [198]. Further, and more detailed information on PG distribution has been obtained by the use of antibodies against enzymatically derived epitopes specific for PG types [199]. Such studies have indicated that in the thoracic aorta DSPG and C4S PG were distributed equally throughout the intercellular matrix of the media and adventitia, whereas the distribution of C6S PG displayed a concentration gradient (inner media > outer media > intima > adventitia). Although KS is not detected in the normal aorta by immunocytochemistry, blotted PG preparations suggest that masking by other matrix constituents or differences in the degree of sulphation (impairing antibody recognition) may occur in normal tissue [200].

Endothelial and VSMC in culture synthesize PGs similar to those found in the human aorta with endothelial cells synthesizing predominately HSPG, and VSMC producing mainly CS and DSPGs and little HSPG. Recent evidence by northern blotting analysis has indicated that these cells are capable of expressing transcripts homologous to biglycan, decorin, versican and aggrecan [180]. Differential expression of the small non-aggregating PGs, decorin and biglycan occurs in endothelial and VSMC. Bovine aortic smooth muscle cells express both decorin and biglycan transcripts whereas bovine aortic and human umbilical vein endothelial cells express transcripts for biglycan only [201]. The fact that VSMC but not endothelial cells express transcripts for collagen type I (a collagen known to react specifically with decorin) led these authors [201] to suggest that the differences in the expression of matrix proteins may be important in regulating the behaviour of endothelial and smooth muscle cells within the vascular wall.

It is interesting to note that although HSPG is secreted into the medium in small amounts, it is the predominant PG of the cell layer [202]. Arterial smooth muscle cells appear to be capable of synthesizing at least two forms of DSPG, one of which is enriched in glucuronic acid and another enriched in iduronic acid. It has been speculated that these two classes may differ in their ability to bind to collagen fibrils.

Although cell culture studies have advanced our understanding of the role of vessel wall PGs it is important to note that in culture a number of variables influences the amount and type of PG synthesized by endothelial and VSMC. PG synthesis differs depending on the physiological state of the cells (quiescent or dividing), the age of the donor animal and the type of substratum on which the cells are cultured. It is therefore important to bear these points in mind when comparing and interpreting results of cell culture investigations.

4.2 Degradation and turnover

For many years, collagen was considered as inert, a view that was established mainly from the very early studies using radiolabelling to assess collagen degradation rates (reviewed in [203]). With the multiplicity of collagen types currently recognized has come the realization that collagens, together with other matrix macromolecules, play a more important role in the regulation of cellular function. The composition of the extracellular matrix therefore has major effects on the growth, migration and differentiation of cells through cell membrane-mediated interactions. The manner in which the extracellular matrix is modified and remodelled is therefore an extremely important area of current research.

4.2.1 MECHANISMS OF DEGRADATION

The major pathway of connective tissue degradation is via a family of metal-dependent enzymes known as the matrix metalloproteinases (MMPs). Generally, these may be divided into three groups of closely related proteinases: the collagenases, the gelatinases and the stromelysins, depending on their substrate specificity. The main characteristics and substrate specificities of these enzymes are given in Table 4.4 but, as the matrix metalloproteinase nomenclature [204] is still hotly debated, the original assignments are given in addition to the MMP numbering. Most of the MMPs have been cloned and sequenced, and together they have the ability to degrade virtually all components of the extracellular matrix [205,206]. There are two members of the interstitial collagenase subclass (MMP-1 and MMP-8) that cleave all three chains of native fibrillar collagens at a site a quarter of the distance from the C-terminal end, as described originally by Gross [207]. The neutrophil-derived enzyme (MMP-8) cleaves collagen I at a faster rate than collagen III whereas the reverse is true for the interstitial collagenase, MMP-1. The stromelysins, as the name suggests, have a wide substrate specificity that includes fibronectin, proteoglycan core protein, laminin, elastin and some collagens. A third group of the MMP family, the gelatinases, again have a relatively wide substrate specificity but are characterized by their ability to cleave denatured collagens and intact collagen IV, although the latter activity may not be strong for the 72 kDa (MMP-2) and 92 kDa (MMP-9) enzymes [208]. A similar specificity has been proposed for MMP-7 or matrilysin that also is able to cleave elastin. A recent addition to the MMP family, isolated from mouse macrophages, has been designated murine macrophage elastase (MME) because of its marked elastolytic activity [209].

The MMPs have a similar modular structure centred around a catalytic domain containing the Zn^{2+} binding site, but with differences primarily in the N-terminal precursor region leading to the variations in substrate specificity. All enzymes, however, are synthesized as larger precursor molecules that require activation. Conversion from the latent to active form can be accomplished *in vitro* by organomercurial compounds, metal ions, oxidizing agents or thiol reagents, all of which appear to disrupt the disulphide-bonded structure in the propeptide and induce a conformational change that makes the active site sterically accessible. The process of activation *in vivo* is more complex and appears to involve a cascade of proteolytic events initiated by the activation of plasminogen. The plasmin produced cleaves the propeptide, particularly of prostromelysins and the stromelysins released can then activate the interstitial collagenase precursors; these processes are summarized in Figure 4.11. An added complication in the control of these processes, also depicted in Figure 4.11, is the presence of a series of inhibitors, both of the plasminogen activators and of the metalloproteinases. The MMPs can be inhibited by serum α2-macroglobulin and by specific tissue inhibitors of metalloproteinase (TIMP). The tissue inhibitors again probably represent a family of closely related proteins but two main forms of TIMP have been described. TIMP-1 (more generally known as TIMP) is a 30 kDa glycoprotein synthesized by most connective tissue cell types that binds irreversibly to the active form (but not the pro-enzymes) of the collagenase, stromelysin and gelatinase groups [210]. By contrast, TIMP-2 which exhibits about 40% identity in amino acid sequence to TIMP [211], is a non-glycosylated protein of about 21 kDa that appears to complex specifically with the low molecular mass gelatinase [212].

Table 4.4 Characteristics of matrix metalloproteinases

Enzyme	MMP no.	Synonym(s)	Approx. M_r	Extracellular matrix substrates
Interstitial collagenase	MMP-1	Fibroblast colagenase	55 kDa	Collagen types I, II, III, VII, VIII and X; limited cleavage of gelatins and proteoglycan core protein
Neutrophil collagenase	MMP-8	PMN collagenase	75 kDa	Essentially the same as interstitial enzyme (but see text)
Gelatinase A	MMP-2	Type IV collagenase	72 kDa	Gelatin; collagen types IV, V, VII, X and XI; elastin; fibronectin; PG core protein; telopeptides of fibrillar collagens
Gelatinase B	MMP-9	92 kDa gelatinase; 92 kDa type IV gelatinase	92 kDa	Gelatin; collagen types IV and V; elastin, PG core protein
Stromelysin 1 types	MMP-3	Proteoglycanase; Transin; Procollagenase activator	57 kDa	PG core protein; fibronectin; laminin; collagens III, IV, V, IX and X; propeptides of procollagens I, II and III; limited cleavage of elastin and gelatin
Stromelysin 2 types	MMP-10	Transin-2	55 kDa	Same as stromelysin 1
Matrilysin	MMP-7	PUMP-1	29 kDa	PG core protein; fibronectin; laminin; collagen IV; procollagen peptides; gelatin; elastin

MMP = matrix metalloproteinase; PG = proteoglycan; PMN = polymorphonuclear; PUMP = putative metalloproteinase.

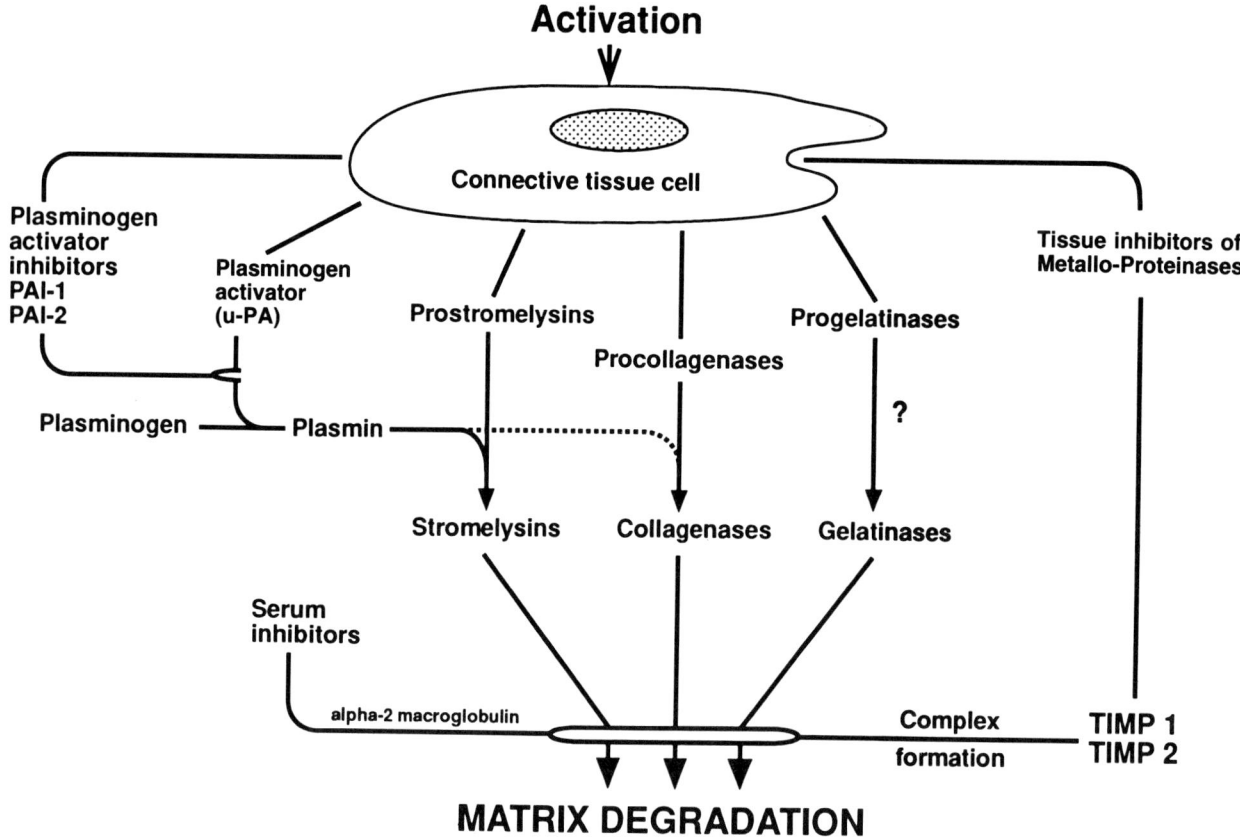

Figure 4.11 Scheme depicting the generation of active metalloproteinases for extracellular matrix degradation together with some of the inhibitory control pathways.

In addition to the plasmin-mediated pathway, degradation of essentially all components of connective tissue can be accomplished by release of the serine proteinases, elastase and cathepsin G, from polymorphonuclear leukocytes [213]. This mechanism is particularly relevant in inflammatory processes. Although the degradative mechanism discussed in this section occurs extracellularly, there is ultrastructural evidence for intracellular degradation following phagocytosis of connective tissue fragments, particularly in situations involving rapid turnover such as periodontal ligament [214] or wound healing [215]. Cell culture studies using specific inhibitors show that metalloproteinases are not involved in the phagocytic degradation [216] which is probably achieved through the action of lysosomal cathepsins.

4.2.2 REGULATION OF PROTEOLYSIS

From the foregoing discussion, it is evident that the regulation of connective tissue degradation is complex. Control can be exercised at many points, including regulation of MMP gene expression, and changes in the relative levels of activators and inhibitors of enzyme activity. These processes can be influenced by a large number of growth factors, oncogenes, prostaglandins and hormones. This topic has recently been reviewed comprehensively [206].

4.3 Biomechanical properties

From the previous sections, it is clear that the main contributors to the biomechanical properties of vascular tissues are the collagenous and elastin components. The glycoproteins, proteoglycans, and glycosaminoglycans are now known to have an important structural role in addition to their modifying influences on the organization of the major macromolecules. Experimental verification of the precise contributions of different components to the biomechanical properties of the tissue is, however, difficult and most studies in this area have naturally concentrated on well organized tissues, such as tendon, which comprises essentially a single collagen type making the results much easier to interpret [217].

In addition to analysis of tissue samples by generation of classical stress–strain curves, the technique of isometric tension has been widely used in which the tissue is heated at a constant rate whilst being held rigidly at a constant length, and the contractive forces generated by protein denaturation are measured. This procedure was particularly useful in early studies that demonstrated the dramatic effects in tendons of intermolecular collagen crosslinking [218], and analysis of the shapes of the isometric tension curves in different tissues indicated that these properties were derived mainly from the collagen type I and not from other collagen types or from the non-collagenous components [219]. The crucial effect of the lysyl oxidase-mediated crosslinks (see section 4.2.1(c)) in providing mechanical strength has recently been confirmed using an ingenious model system involving fibroblast culture within collagen gels to simulate the formation of a ligament [220]. Over a 12-week period, the breaking strength of these pseudoligaments increased over 30-fold but this increase was entirely sensitive to the lysyl oxidase inhibitor, β-amino-proprionitrile. This type of biosynthetic model appears to offer major opportunities in being able to document the contribution of various matrix components to mechanical properties as the accumulation of individual components can be directly measured and manipulated.

Several studies in recent years have attempted to relate localized changes in composition of arterial vessel walls with mechanical strength and the propensity for structural weakening in atherosclerotic lesions. The proportion of collagen type III relative to total fibrillar collagens was not related to fracture stress and was not different between the ulcerated and non-ulcerated plaques [221]. The total collagen content was greater in the plaque areas relative to the surrounding intima although, for the ulcerated lesions, there was a distinct decrease in collagen concentration at the centre of the plaque. From these results, it was concluded that the structural weakness arose primarily from defective organization of fibrillar collagen [221] but, as no biochemical measurements of crosslinking were made, this could also have been a contributory factor. The development of more sophisticated biomechanical testing systems applicable to small tissue samples will facilitate comparisons of lesions and the surrounding areas [222] that will allow more rigorous correlations with biochemical changes. Alterations brought about by non-enzymatic glycosylation have been shown to lead to increased stiffness in connective tissues [70] and may contribute to the increased risk of vascular disease in patients with diabetes. A study in which the biomechanical parameters, such as specimen thickness, were carefully controlled confirmed that aortic samples from patients with insulin-dependent diabetes exhibited decreased extensibility and increased stiffness compared with samples from age- and sex-matched controls [223]. There was, however, no direct link with the severity of atherosclerotic lesions in the thoracic aorta in this study.

The biochemical composition and structural organization of arterial walls are to a large extent dependent on the mechanical stresses imposed on them. Thus, alterations in the haemodynamic stresses can lead to compensatory changes at the cellular level in the intima [224]. In attempting to relate the biomechanical properties of vascular tissues to functional stresses, it will be necessary to combine the basic measurements of strength and stiffness with an understanding of the complex molecular signals involved in these processes. For example, studies *in vitro* have revealed that mechanical stresses have a profound influence in potentiating the mitogenic effects of angiotensins in rat smooth muscle cells [225]. Further experiments such as these will enable the effects of cellular interactions with the different extracellular matrix components to be established.

4.4 Abnormalities of connective tissue in disease

In this section, a number of diseases affecting connective tissue will be considered including some heritable disorders as well as nutritional and acquired diseases. The intention is not to attempt a comprehensive review of these disorders, but to provide an appreciation of current knowledge of their aetiology, with particular attention to the effects on the cardiovascular system.

4.4.1 MARFAN SYNDROME

Originally described in 1896 by the paediatrician, A.-B. Marfan, as 'a congenital malformation of the four limbs', this syndrome is now recognized as having a complex and variable phenotype. The pleiotropic nature of the disorder results in manifestations primarily in the cardiovascular, ocular and skeletal systems, but also in the pulmonary and central nervous systems, and in the skin and tissue fascia. The most common overt signs of the disease are a disproportionate skeleton with long legs and arms, frequently with arachnodactyly. The major cardiovascular features of the disorder are progressive aortic root dilatation, often leading to aneurysms and dissection, and mitral valve prolapse. Histologically, fragmentation and disruption of the elastic fibres is evident in the aortic wall; medial smooth muscle fibres are also fragmented with inclusions of collagen and other matrix constituents [226,227]. In many instances, these changes are very similar to those brought about by other factors deleteriously affecting cardiovascular function, such as haemodynamic stress, copper deficiency or lathyrism [228,229]. In the severe phenotype, mitral regurgitation can lead to congestive heart failure and pulmonary hypertension early in life [230]. Calcification of the mitral annulus often occurs in Marfan syndrome, distinguishing this condition from mitral valve prolapse in the general population [231].

(a) **Genetics and candidate genes**

Almost all available evidence suggests autosomal dominant inheritance of Marfan syndrome. For many years the wide-ranging connective tissue abnormalities defied all attempts to elucidate the primary cause of the disease, and there are many reports in the literature detailing specific abnormalities in the collagenous network, proteoglycans and glycosaminoglycans, and in the elastic fibres. The development of DNA probes for many of the candidate genes, together with polymorphic restriction sites within these probes, has facilitated linkage analysis in large families affected by Marfan syndrome. In this way, all of the major fibrillar collagens were excluded as being responsible for the primary abnormality [232–236], although there were clearly often secondary abnormalities in the properties and metabolism of collagen [237,238].

Because of the major ultrastructural alterations in the elastic fibres, particularly in the aortic media [239], attention has focused more recently on the proteins making up these fibres. Few common restriction-site polymorphisms were available for the elastin gene but this same approach for the microfibrillar component, fibrillin, culminated in the discovery by two independent groups that mutations of the fibrillin gene located on chromosome 15 represented the primary defect in Marfan syndrome [170,240]. Because of its chromosomal location, this gene is referred to as the fibrillin-15 or Fib-15 gene and its product of translation as fibrillin-1 (see section 4.1.3(c)). Part of the evidence leading to this discovery was from immunofluorescence studies using monoclonal antibodies against fibrillin, where sections of the dermis from affected individuals revealed much lower levels of the protein, and from culture of fibroblasts from the affected skin which produced abnormal elastic fibres [241]. To date, over 20 mutations in the fibrillin gene have been described and these generally are of two types [242]. Firstly, there are single point mutations that appear to affect particularly the EGF-like domains of fibrillin and often result in alterations of a cysteine residue to another amino acid. The EGF repeat units have six cysteine residues that participate in intramolecular disulphide bonding to maintain the β-pleated sheet conformation, so that removal of even a single cysteine has a large disruptive effect on the fibrillin molecule. The second type of mutation comprises exon deletion events and exon skipping due to splicing defects. As more fibrillin gene defects are described, the relationship between the location of the defect and the precise effects on the structure and assembly of elastic fibres can be deduced.

Cloning studies have revealed that, in addition to fibrillin-15 located on chromosome 15q-21, there is at least one other gene located on chromosome 5q23–31 [170,171]. The product of the fibrillin-5 gene has not, however, yet been fully identified. Linkage analysis using restriction fragment length polymorphisms in the fibrillin-5 gene has shown linkage with a Marfan-like disorder, contractural arachnodactyly, in three families [171]. Recently, an additional fibrillin-like protein has been described that contains multiple EGF repeats [243], but the structure has not yet been fully elucidated. As more of the family of these fibrillin genes are characterized and their relationship with other microfibrillar proteins is established, the chances of explaining the wide variety of tissue abnormalities in Marfan syndrome will be greatly enhanced.

There is evidence that, in a minority of patients with a Marfan or Marfan-like syndrome, there are no alterations in the known fibrillin genes and that some other component of, or associated with, the elastic fibre is involved. A group of 19 patients with the cardiovascular and skeletal abnormalities characteristic of Marfan syndrome, but with no ocular manifestations, has recently been described in which no linkage with the Fib-15 or Fib-5 genes was detected [244]; this group, therefore, appears to represent an overlapping but distinct disorder. As stated previously, studies of elastin abnormalities have been hampered by the lack of suitable markers but recent work, in which the assigment of the elastin gene to chromosome 7 was confirmed, also detected a repeat polymorphism in intron 17 of the gene that may be potentially useful in linkage studies of connective tissue diseases involving elastic tissues [245]. It has been suggested that the proteoglycan, decorin, may also be deficient in some patients with Marfan syndrome and that this may contribute to the complex phenotypic variations observed in this disease [246].

There are many other potential candidates for abnormalities in the elastic fibre, including lysyl oxidase [247] and a series of microfibril-associated glycoproteins [248–250]. Many of these components have been cloned and sequenced [251,252], thus facilitating evaluation of their structural role in elastic fibres. The fibulins represent another group of ubiquitous glycoproteins with a mosaic structure containing multiple EGF repeats, suggesting that the genes may also be potential candidates for connective tissue disorders. Strong staining with antibodies to fibulin-2 was observed in the subintimal layer of mouse aorta and in other blood vessels, whereas no significant staining for fibulin-1 was obtained [253]. None of these glycoproteins has, however, yet been linked to any disease and their function is unknown.

Table 4.5 Classification of the Ehlers–Danlos syndrome

Type	Major features	Inheritance	Primary defect
I	Joint laxity, hyperelastic skin	AD	Unknown
II	Less severe joint laxity, skin hyperelasticity	AD	Unknown
III	Joint laxity, some cardiac abnormalities	AD	Unknown
IV	Severe fragility of arteries and other internal organs	AD	Lack of normal collagen type III
V	Soft, doughy skin, severe cardiovascular defects	(XL)	Unknown
VI	Ocular defects, muscular hypotonia, arterial rupture is common	AR	Lack of lysyl hydroxylation in some patients
VII	Severe joint hypermobility	AD	Failure to remove N-terminal propeptides
VIII	Skin lesions, periodontal disease	AD	Unknown
IX	Skin laxity, cardiovascular defects	XL	Abnormal copper transport
X	Joint laxity	?	Possibly a defect in fibronectin

AD = autosomal dominant; AR = autosomal recessive; XL = X-linked.
EDS type IX, originally referred to as X-linked cutis laxa, is now classified as occipital horn syndrome (see text).

4.4.2 EHLERS–DANLOS SYNDROME

The Ehlers–Danlos syndrome (EDS) is a heterogeneous group of heritable disorders that affect the connective tissue in skin, blood vessels, joints and ligaments, and for which the clinical manifestations are well documented [254]. Generally, this disorder results in hypermobile joints, thin and fragile skin that is often hyperelastic, aortic fragility, and cardiovascular and intestinal abnormalities.

(a) Classification of the phenotype

The disorder has been classified according to clinical, genetic and biochemical criteria into about ten sub-types as shown in Table 4.5, although the heterogeneity of the disorder means that there is considerable overlap in the phenotype. The biochemical defects, where these have been elucidated, will be considered separately in the following section. The sub-types EDS I to III, which comprise about 90% of the total cases [255], differ mainly in their degree of involvement, EDS I being the most severe with marked joint laxity and hyperelastic skin, and often with aortic or bowel rupture. EDS II represents a mild form of the disorder that is often undiagnosed with limited joint laxity and few complications of the internal organs. In EDS III, there is moderately severe joint laxity with minimal skin involvement, but this type is more likely to have cardiac abnormalities such as mitral valve prolapse.

EDS IV is characterized by extreme fragility of the blood vessels and is referred to as the arterial type of EDS. Affected individuals may suffer severe, life-threatening complications that include spontaneous rupture of the arteries or other internal organs. In contrast to most other forms of the disease, there is little joint hypermobility and the skin is not hyperelastic but is thin and translucent.

The separate classification of EDS V is based primarily on its X-linked recessive mode of inheritance, distinct from most other EDS types with autosomal dominant inheritance. The occurrence of EDS V is rare but most affected individuals tend to have soft, doughy skin with only mild hyperelasticity. There are usually severe cardiovascular defects including floppy mitral and tricuspid valves.

EDS VI is characterized by the presence of severe ocular defects, often leading to retinal detachment, and by ligamentous laxity and severe muscular hypotonia that may be manifest as severe progressive kyphoscoliosis from birth. Arterial rupture is also common in this autosomal recessively inherited form of EDS. As discussed later, the biochemical findings have led to the classification of sub-types of EDS VI.

The major characteristic of EDS VII is the involvement of ligaments and joint capsule which results in excessive joint hypermobility, usually with congenital bilateral hip dislocation. Effects on the vascular system in this phenotype are usually less severe.

The EDS VIII phenotype affects mainly the skin with characteristic lesions on the shins, and there is an associated progression of dental disease. Again there are few effects on the cardiovascular system in this type.

EDS IX exhibits few of the 'classical' manifestations and this condition, now known to be a defect in copper transport [256], has been reclassified as occipital horn syndrome. This disease is characterized by loose rather than hyperelastic skin, and by cardiovascular defects that are similar to those observed in Menkes' disease (see section 4.4.5(e)).

(b) Biochemical defects

For many of the EDS types, the basic defect at the biochemical level has not been elucidated (Table 4.5). Generally, however, this disorder is believed to affect the structure and/or metabolism of collagenous macromolecules in the matrix. The wide variety of defects illustrates the complex post-ribosomal modifications to collagen with abnormalities at almost every stage of processing. Many of the EDS types are extremely rare and, as classification is often based on only one or two families, there are few cases where the link between the biochemical defect and severity of the phenotype can be unequivocally established.

In EDS IV, the primary defect is a lack of collagen type III and this accounts for the major effects of the disease being evident in the blood vessels, internal organs and skin which normally have relatively high amounts of this collagen. A variety of structural defects in collagen III have been characterized in EDS IV including point mutations replacing the triplet glycine residue and disrupting the helix [257-262], genomic deletions of one of the COL3A1 alleles [263,264] and point mutations within introns leading to abnormal splicing of the mRNA [265,266]. These defects often lead to slow helix formation, over-modification of the procollagen III and poor secretion of the molecule with accumulation intracellularly. The structural aberrations can also lead to an increased rate of intracellular degradation of the collagen [267]. The number of well characterized mutations in the COL3A1 gene is at present still too small to correlate the site of the mutation with the severity of the phenotype, as has been achieved for defects in the procollagen type I genes in osteogenesis imperfecta, where mutations nearer the C-terminal end tend to have a more severe effect.

The arterial vessels in EDS IV patients often have a small bore with a lower than normal collagen content [268] and, consequently, a relative increase in elastic fibres. There appear to be variable effects on the collagen fibril morphology, with decreased fibril diameters in adventitia and intima of some arteries but increased fibril size in the vena cava [268]. Much of the evidence for abnormal collagen III production has been obtained by culturing cells derived from affected individuals and there appears to be a good correlation with measurements *in vivo* of the amounts of the procollagen III N-terminal propeptide detected in serum [269].

Mutations in collagen type III may not always result in an EDS phenotype but these still have profound effects on blood vessels. Thus, two families with aortic aneurysms but without the clinical features of EDS, were shown to be carrying a single base mutation in the procollagen III gene [260]. Structural defects in procollagen III have also been found in patients with cerebral aneurysms [270], although other patients with this form of aneurysm appeared to show a more general defect in collagen secretion [271].

The biochemical basis of the defect in EDS V is unknown. Although a deficiency of lysyl oxidase has been reported [272], these results were prone to technical error [255] and subsequent analysis of four patients with EDS V showed that the amounts of the borohydride-reducible crosslinks in the skin were normal [273]. A defect in lysyl oxidase seems unlikely on biomechanical grounds as such a defect would be expected to affect elastin to a greater extent because of the larger number of oxidizable lysine residues present. Disruption of the elastin would presumably remove the ability for tissue recoil which is inconsistent with the observed properties in this condition.

Many patients with EDS VI have decreased lysyl hydroxylase activity as indicated by low tissue levels of hydroxylysine [274], and this appeared to be the main biochemical defect. The degree of hydroxylation varied between tissues and several possible explanations were put forward, including substrate specificity, the existence of tissue-specific enzymes and differences in cofactor concentrations. Further studies revealed patients with similar phenotypes but having normal tissue hydoxylysine concentrations, thus requiring reclassification of this EDS group such that those patients with low hydroxylysine were defined as sub-type EDS VIA and those with normal hydroxylation as type VIB [275]. The human gene for lysyl hydroxylase has recently been cloned and sequenced [276], and analysis of a family with EDS VIA revealed mutations in the lysyl hydroxylase gene [277,278]. Mutations in this gene were, however, not found in several other families with EDS VIA [277] and the contribution of differences in lysyl hydroxyase activity to this form of EDS remains in doubt. In this context, it should be remembered that, if there is a second form of lysyl hydroxylase acting on the telopeptide regions of collagen (see section 4.1.1(c)), then part of the heterogeneity of this disorder may arise through alterations in this enzyme.

The only other defined EDS group for which the prime biochemical defect has been elucidated is EDS VII, which is now known to involve a lack of removal of the type I procollagen N-propeptide. This arises mainly by mutations around the junctions of exon 6 in genes for both the proα1(I) and proα2(I) chains leading to deletion of this exon in the spliced mRNA [255]. As exon 6 codes for amino acid sequences at the junction of the N-propeptide and the telopeptide, this deletion removes the N-proteinase cleavage site and may also result in loss of the telopeptide lysine that participates in lysyl oxidase-mediated crosslinking. The collagen from these patients is therefore very soluble due to the lack of crosslinks [279] and the fibrils are irregular in shape as a result of the incorporation of the bulky N-propeptide [280]. A classification of sub-types has been made so that mutations affecting the proα1(I) and the proα2(I) chains are designated EDS VIIA and EDS VIIB, respectively. A further sub-type, EDS VIIC, has recently been described in which there is a deficiency of the N-proteinase enzyme itself rather than in the substrate [281,282]. This type closely resembles the animal disorder, dermatosparaxis, in which ribbon-like, poorly crosslinked fibrils are produced [283,284]. As for most other groups of EDS, type VII shows considerable heterogeneity and there are several cases of this phenotype in which the collagen processing appears to be normal.

4.4.3 CUTIS LAXA

Cutis laxa is primarily a skin disorder characterized by hyperelasticity and a lack of resilience, leading to the formation of pendulous folds of skin and an appearance of premature ageing in affected individuals. Histologically, there is fragmentation of elastic fibres in the dermis together with a decrease in their amounts [285]. The primary biochemical defect in this condition has not yet been established. Studies of cultured fibroblasts from affected individuals have shown there may be decreased elastin mRNA levels [286,287], but there was also evidence for alterations in translational or post-translational events [288]. There was also a report that fibroblasts from a patient with cutis laxa synthesized increased amounts of collagen type VI in culture [289], although subsequent studies showed that the defect was more likely to be over-production of a microfibrillar component, designated GP140 [133]. There is still no explanation as to why the effects on elastic fibres in cutis laxa are generally restricted to the skin and pulmonary system, but are not evident in the vasculature.

In addition to the heritable disease, there are acquired forms of cutis laxa where similar losses of elastic fibres in the dermis occur. One form, referred to as mid-dermal elastolysis, appears to be secondary to an inflammatory event as indicated by the presence of lymphocytes, macrophages and phagocytosed elastin fragments [290–292]. Changes similar to those in cutis laxa may also be observed in patients with Wilson's disease or cystinuria that are receiving long-term treatment with D-penicillamine. These effects are presumably mediated by deficiencies in elastin crosslinking, either through direct interaction of D-penicillamine with the precursor aldehydes or by chelation of the copper cofactor for lysyl oxidase. The D-penicillamine effects, particularly the dermal lesions, have also been likened to the changes that occur in pseudoxanthoma elasticum [293,294], although mineralization of the elastic fibres is not normally observed [295].

4.4.4 PSEUDOXANTHOMA ELASTICUM

Pseudoxanthoma elasticum (PXE) is an inherited disorder for which the main characteristic is progressive calcification of the elastic tissues in the skin, eyes and cardiovascular system. In contrast to cutis laxa, there is usually an increased production of elastic fibres in the skin, together with an increase in the deposition of glycosaminoglycans [296]. Despite extensive investigations using molecular biology and genetics, the primary biochemical defect is still uncertain. Immunohistological studies using both light and electron microscopy have shown abnormal elastic fibres in the lesions but also in areas without lesions, whereas collagen fibres were disrupted only in the lesional areas [297]. These observations suggest that the defect in PXE originates in the elastic fibres and that this gives rise to secondary changes in the collagen.

The significance of changes in glycosaminoglycan production in skin is also unclear. There have been a number of reports of altered patterns of these polyanions both in the tissue [298,299] and in fibroblast cultures from PXE skin [300], leading to the suggestion that aberrant synthesis or metabolism of these components is a causative factor of the disease. Such hypotheses, however, provide little explanation for the mineralization of elastic tissues. Addressing the latter point, abnormalities in vitamin D metabolites and in the vitamin-K linked gamma-carboxylation system have been invoked, but without any really substantial evidence. It is also possible that alterations in calcium affinities in elastic tissue may arise from specific mutations in one of the many glycoproteins, such as fibrillin, that contain EGF-like repeat units with calcium binding properties [301].

4.4.5 COPPER DEFICIENCY

Trace elements are now recognized as essential for a number of metabolic functions in the health and development of both man and animals. Of the many trace elements that exist, the biological role of copper has been one of the most thoroughly investigated and using animal models it is now well accepted this element is vital for the synthesis and structural maintenance of both collagen and elastin within the extracellular matrix of a variety of tissues including the blood vessel wall. The animal models have indicated that structurally weakened arteries are the major vascular defect in copper deficiency. This leads to aneurysm formation and subsequent rupture.

Although copper deficiency in humans is extremely rare, a number of cases occurring in infancy have been reported. Individuals found to be most at risk are those born preterm or those receiving prolonged total parenteral nutrition [302]. Apart from these few isolated cases the significance of copper deficiency in adults is unclear. The scarcity of specific pathological manifestations of copper deficiency in humans makes it difficult to assess the effect of copper deficiency on connective tissue proteins of the blood vessel wall. However, as the dietary intake of copper is thought to be less than the recommended 2–3 mg per day, a state of marginal copper deficiency may exist in a large proportion of the population. Such observations have led to the suggestions that inadequate copper nutrition may be a risk factor for arterial disease and ischemic heart disease [303].

(a) Sites of action in connective tissue metabolism

Copper owes its biological role to its incorporation into a number of metalloenzymes which are dependent on the element for normal activity. Of the 10 cuproenzymes that are known to exist we will limit our attention to lysyl oxidase (protein-lysine 6-oxidase; EC 1.4.3.13) which catalyses the oxidative deamination of peptidyl lysine and hydroxylysine residues in collagen and lysine residues in elastin. This is the first step in the covalent crosslinking of collagen and tropoelastin and results in the formation of insoluble collagen and elastin in the extracellular matrix. The enzyme was first isolated from chick bone but has now been purified from a number of tissues including the aorta [304]. Recently a number of laboratories has derived the amino acid sequence of both human [35,36] and rat [305,306] lysyl oxidase. Almost 90% of amino acids are identical between the two species and the carboxy terminus of the protein shows the greatest conservation. The carboxy region contains the copper-binding sites and is regarded as the catalytically active domain. Information has now been obtained on the structure, organization and regulation of the human lysyl oxidase gene [307]. Similar studies have assigned the human lysyl oxidase gene to chromosome 5 [35]. The current understanding of its properties and functions has recently been reviewed [308].

(b) Information from animal models

The large major blood vessels and in particular the aorta are very susceptible to the adverse effects of copper deficiency. The majority of the connective tissue abnormalities reported in the aorta has been related to disturbances in the arterial elastin, although alterations in other connective tissue components such as collagen and proteoglycans have also been implicated.

Abnormal morphology of arterial elastin has been observed in a number of copper-deficient species such as the rat, pig, chick, guineapig and rabbit. The elastic laminae of the copper-deficient vessels are irregular with considerable vacuolation, fraying and fragmentation (Figure 4.12). Ultrastructural irregularities in the structure of chick aortic elastin due to copper deficiency were first reported almost 30 years ago. Elastic fibre degeneration occurred in three steps. Initially, there was swelling of the elastic fibrils which was followed by dissolution of the associated matrix, giving a vacuolated appearance. The last retrograde step consisted of complete

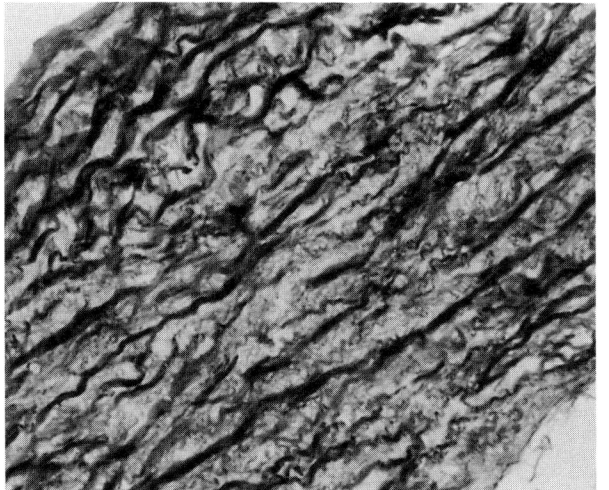

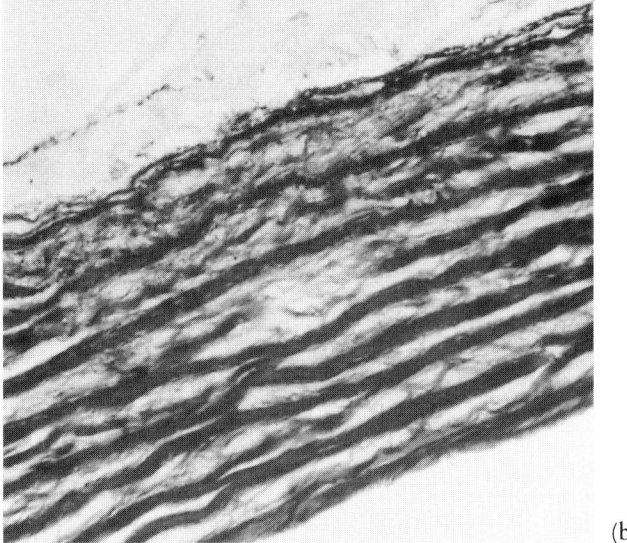

Figure 4.12 Disrupted elastic laminae in the aorta of copper-deficient rat (a) in comparison with the distribution for a copper-supplemented animal (b). The lumen of the vessel is bottom right (Weigert's stain).

dissolution of the matrix with the persistence of naked, swollen elastic fibrils [309]. These results were confirmed and extended by others [310]. Changes to the elastic lamina within the intima, media and adventitial regions of the rat aorta were found. The alterations include discontinuity of the internal elastic lamina which is comprised of clumps of elastin of irregular size and shape. Medial elastic lamina are narrower, more electron opaque, non-homogeneous in appearance and occasionally gapped. Discontinuities of the internal elastic lamina are the most commonly reported feature of elastic defects in copper deficiency. Carlton and Henderson [311] considered that the altered elastin was primary to the development of intramural haemorrhage, dissecting aneurysm and eventual rupture of the vessel. Rupture of the aorta, which was first reported in the copper-deficient chick [312] and subsequently in a number of other species such as the pig and guineapig, has never been reported in the copper-deficient rat. Of interest, the pig is the only species where both heart and aortic rupture have been reported in copper deficiency. These species differences are important when extrapolating animal data to humans.

In contrast to the elastic tissue abnormalities noted in the aorta of copper-deficient animals, similar lesions in the coronary arteries have generally not been observed [313], as shown in Figure 4.13. Where lesions have been observed, they have been restricted to the pig and the pathology was similar to that observed in the aorta. There was evidence of fragmentation of the internal elastic membrane, radially orientated fissures, infarction and rupture of the blood vessel [314]. These authors also emphasize the importance of the internal elastic lamina in maintaining the integrity of the vessel wall suggesting that the entire sequence of events noted in the coronary arteries may be a result of internal elastic membrane rupture. With the exception of the pig, it is somewhat difficult to explain why vascular elastin is unaltered while that of the endomysium which surrounds individual muscle fibres in the myocardium is severely disrupted in places by copper deficiency [313]. Apart from the coronary arteries and the aorta, little information exists on the effects of copper deficiency on other arteries. Degeneration of the internal elastic lamina has also been observed in the major arteries of the brain [315].

As previously mentioned the bulk of information on this topic is on the structural defects of elastic tissue. This may be because the elastic lamina is readily visualized histologically making any abnormality easily recognizable. There is, however, some limited evidence to suggest that both proteoglycans and collagen of the vessel wall are affected in copper deficiency. Both morphological and biochemical studies carried out over 30 years ago have indicated that copper deficiency results in an increase in total proteoglycans of the aorta wall. Recent studies have also indicated that the proteoglycans from copper-deficient rat aortas were of greater molecular size. Further, the concentration of isomeric chondroitin sulphates, particularly dermatan sulphate, was greater in deficient than control animals [316]. The increase in aortic proteoglycans may be due to the prolonged stretching of smooth muscle cells observed in copper-deficient rats, which can result in elevated levels of collagen and proteoglycan synthesis. Alternatively, as proteoglycans in the arterial wall are synthesized by smooth muscle cells and endothelial cells, the higher concentrations of proteoglycans may be a consequence of smooth muscle cell proliferation which is known to occur in copper deficiency.

These observations are similar to earlier findings in experimental atherosclerosis and to a response of cardiovascular connective tissue to injury. An apparent increase in collagen concentration and also in the repair of collagenous medial defects has been reported within the wall of affected blood vessels. This ability to repair vascular tears by scar tissue formation has been regarded to be essential for the extended survival of copper-deficient pigs. The newly formed collagen which may be due to cyclic stretching of smooth muscle cells and/or fibrous repair could explain the excessive salt-soluble collagen present in the aortas of copper-deficient chicks. An increase in collagen solubility due to a reduction in lysyl oxidase activity and a subsequent decrease in collagen crosslinking are also possible. There is, however, no strong morphological, mechanical or biochemical (see section 4.4.5(c)) evidence to suggest the formation of abnormal collagen in the aorta of copper-deficient animals.

An isolated report on the aorta of copper-deficient rats indicated that the basal lamina beneath the endothelial cells exhibited frequent disruptions in regions where collagen aggregation existed [310]. Although the results of Hunsaker have not been substantiated, early, apparently specific lesions have also been observed in the basement membranes of the heart, kidney and pancreas [313,317,318] of copper-deficient animals. Reasons for the extreme sensitivity of basement membranes to copper deficiency are unknown as is the pathological significance of this very early lesion.

A reduction in the tensile strength and rupture of the aorta of copper-deficient animals is mainly due to a decrease in elasticity of the vessel wall, which can be attributed to a decrease in the amount of elastin. The role of collagen in the altered mechanical properties of the copper-deficient aorta remains equivocal. Changes in the contractile properties of aortic smooth muscle cells from copper-deficient rats have also been reported

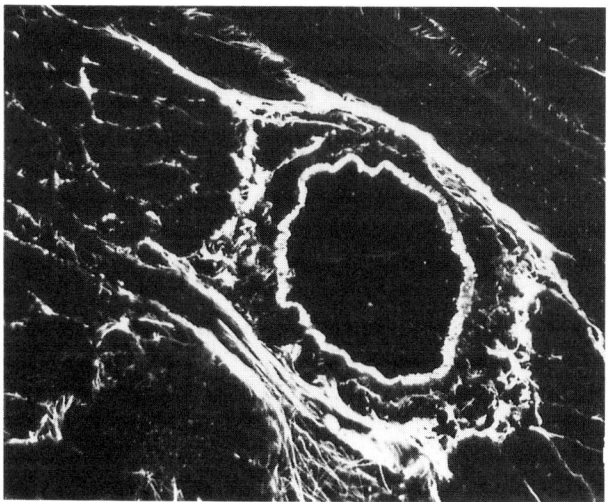

Figure 4.13 Immunostaining of elastin in the coronary artery of a copper-deficient rat showing a normal distribution in contrast to aortic tissue (Figure 4.12).

[319]. These changes, prolongation of contraction time and enhanced sensitivity to noradrenaline were regarded as compensatory mechanisms which served to protect the less elastic vascular walls of the copper-deficient animals.

(c) Effects on collagen and elastin crosslinking

As described in detail in sections 4.1.1(c) and 4.1.2(b), both elastin and collagen are crosslinked, providing these connective tissue proteins with the tensile strength necessary for the maintainance of proper function. The mature non-reducible crosslinks of elastin (desmosine and isodesmosine) and collagen (pyridinoline and deoxypyridinoline) are formed via a number of intermediate crosslinks by the initial actions of the copper-dependent enzyme, lysyl oxidase. As the structural defects noted in elastin and also possibly collagen of copper-deficient animals are considered to be due to a decrease in crosslinking, the paucity of studies detailing the effects of copper deficiency on collagen and elastin crosslinking within a number of tissues including the blood vessel wall is somewhat surprising. The elastin of the blood vessel wall is probably more prone to disruption by copper deficiency than collagen as, per unit mass, tropoelastin contains approximately 15 times more oxidisable lysine residues than type I collagen.

When animals are rendered copper deficient, covalent crosslinking of aortic elastin decreases, resulting in increased tissue concentrations of tropoelastin, and decreased quantities of mature elastin [320]. There is a reduction of 40% in the concentration of both isodesmosine and desmosine with a concomitant increase in the number of lysine residues [321]. Contrary to some observations elevated concentrations of aortic tropoelastin in copper deficiency did not influence the amounts of functional tropoelastin mRNA and therefore the potential for elastin synthesis was not impaired by copper deficiency [320]. These authors further suggest that the loss of aorta elastin from copper deficiency results from proteolysis of tropoelastin and partially crosslinked elastin.

Early studies reported increased solubility of aortic collagens in the copper-deficient pig [322] and chick [321] which is indicative of decreased crosslinking. We have, however, reported that the concentrations of both pyridinium crosslinks of the rat aorta are unaltered by copper deficiency [323]. These results taken together may partly explain why the aortas of the pig and chick but not the rat are susceptible to rupture in copper deficiency. Although lysyl oxidase activity is diminished by copper deficiency in the rat aorta, there is strong evidence to suggest that normal collagen crosslinking takes place even when lysyl oxidase activity is less than optimal. A reduction of at least 50% of normal activity was considered necessary to impair crosslink formation in order to produce clinically demonstrable disorders in the aneurysm-prone mottled mouse [324]. Thus, a decrease in lysyl oxidase activity cannot always be regarded as equivalent to a decrease in crosslink formation. Although copper-deficient rats do not have diminished levels of aortic collagen crosslinks they do display impaired collagen crosslinking in the heart (Table 4.6). This suggests that tissue-specific lysyl oxidase enzymes may exist, each with a different copper requirement for activity. Different forms of the enzyme have been detected in the human placenta, bovine lung and bovine aorta, with those in the latter tissue shown to be immunochemically distinct.

(d) Lathyrogens and connective tissue crosslinking

Of the two types of disorders that result from the consumption of lathyrogens one is confined largely to structural defects within both collagen and elastin. This type of lathyrism, osteolathyrism, is produced from substances in the sweet pea (*Lathyrus odoratus*) and singletary pea (*Lathyrus pusillus*). The active substance is β-aminopropionitrile (BAPN) and is essential for activity. Pinnell and Martin [325] were the first to

Table 4.6 Pyridinium crosslinks in the aorta and heart of normal and copper-deficient rats

			*Residues per collagen molecule**	
Tissue	Copper status	n	Pyridinoline	Deoxypyridinoline
Thoracic aorta	+	6	0.070 ± 0.013	0.008 ± 0.003
	−	6	0.068 ± 0.011^{NS}	0.010 ± 0.004^{NS}
Left ventricle	+	6	0.214 ± 0.025	0.014 ± 0.003
	−	6	$0.116 \pm 0.021^{***}$	$0.008 \pm 0.002^{***}$
Right ventricle	+	6	0.170 ± 0.020	0.015 ± 0.002
	−	6	$0.095 \pm 0.022^{***}$	$0.009 \pm 0.002^{***}$

* Expressed as mean ± SD. Significance of difference between normal and copper-deficient rats as determined by Student's *t*-test is given: NS = not significant; *** = $P < 0.001$.

indicate that the site of action of BAPN is the inhibition of lysyl oxidase activity. As BAPN intoxication leads to inhibition of crosslink formation, it is not suprising that the clinical and pathological manifestations are similar to those induced by copper deficiency. In the turkey aorta both copper deficiency and BAPN toxicity resulted in fragmentation of elastic lamellae and dissecting aneurysms. In addition, increased collagen solubility and decreased elastin content were a feature of both conditions. Disruption to the elastic laminae of the BAPN-treated mouse has also recently been observed, although the laminae of the media and not the adventitia are affected [326]. Not suprisingly, excess dietary copper does not counteract BAPN toxicity but after cessation of BAPN administration, lysyl oxidase activity, perhaps by resynthesis, returns to normal.

(e) Copper deficiency in human genetic diseases

The most extreme form of copper deficiency is observed in Menkes' disease, an X-linked condition that is probably homologous to the aneurysm-prone mottled mouse [324]. Inadequate crosslinking of collagen and elastin is thought to be responsible for the many features of the disease, which include elongation and dilation of arteries, leading to rupture and haemorrhage. Although the basic lesion in Menkes' disease remains to be defined it is thought to involve a generalized cellular abnormality in copper metabolism. Defects in both copper absorption and transport have been reported to result in abnormal copper distribution between organs and within cells. Danks [302] suggested that the connective tissue and other defects are simply due to inadequate supply of copper required for normal copper enzyme synthesis and activity.

Other genetic disorders such as occipital horn syndrome (previously referred to as Ehlers–Danlos syndrome type IX; section 4.4.2) and cutis laxa (section 4.4.3) exhibit low levels of lysyl oxidase activity which may in part be responsible for the connective tissue defects, possibly through impairment of collagen and elastin crosslinking, observed in these disorders.

4.4.6 ATHEROSCLEROSIS

Atherosclerosis is a disease of large- and medium-sized arteries that is characterized by a focal thickening of the intimal lining of the vessel wall, in association with the accumulation of fatty deposits. The lesions may be in the form of 'fatty streaks' where the presence of lipid-laden cells, foam cells, within the intima result in slightly raised yellowish patches on the aortic wall. This type of lesion is likely to be the precursor of the more definitive atherosclerotic lesion, the 'fibrofatty plaque', which comprises a fibrous cap containing dense connective tissue with a necrotic core of lipid deposits and cellular debris. The fibrous plaque causes narrowing of the artery and, with time, leads to increased necrosis and lipid accumulation, calcification and ulceration of the lesion culminating in thrombosis through the interaction of platelets with the exposed connective tissue components. The formation of atherosclerotic plaques therefore involves a large number of different cellular events including infiltration of macrophages and lymphocytes typical of an inflammatory event, proliferation of smooth muscle cells and calcification.

The pathogenesis of atherosclerosis is a subject of much debate but it is not intended here to review the various hypotheses in detail; a comprehensive discussion of this topic is given in other chapters of this volume. Although the widely advanced view is that the lesions generally are initiated by some form of injury to the endothelial lining of the vessel, it is likely that atherosclerosis is a multifactorial disease [327,328]. In many cases, the presence of the lesion causes structural weaknesses in the vessel wall leading to aneurysms. However, the commonly held view that atherosclerosis is the major cause of arterial aneurysms should probably be modified in view of the recent work on genetic predisposition to aneurysms in all types of artery that may arise from mutations in collagen type III [329], the primary defect in Ehlers–Danlos syndrome type IV (section 4.4.2).

The atherosclerotic lesion results in major changes in the extracellular matrix and alterations in the collagenous constituents, proteoglycans and the other matrix components will be considered separately.

(a) Collagen changes in atherosclerosis

Determination of the relative amounts of collagens I and III, the major fibrillar types, in the aorta has received considerable attention. This followed an early report by McCullagh and Balian [330] that collagen III constituted approximately 70% of the total collagen in the medial layer of normal arteries whereas collagen I predominated in the thickened intima of the lesion. On this basis, it was hypothesized that the aetiology of the lesion involved migration of smooth muscle cells into the lesion and 'transformation' into a more fibroblastic phenotype, synthesizing a greater proportion of collagen I [330]. The high proportion of collagen III detected by these workers was in fact a methodological artefact caused by the very low extraction of collagen from aorta using digestion with pepsin. Subsequent studies have confirmed that, even with multiple extractions with pepsin, only 25–50% of the collagen can be extracted and that collagen III is solubilized preferentially [126]. With the use of digestion with cyanogen bromide where a much higher proportion of the collagen is solubilized, analysis of marker peptides, separated by SDS-gel electrophoresis, has shown that the ratio of collagen I:III is generally between 2:1 and 3:1 in the media and that this proportion does not change significantly in the area of the plaque [84]. Thus, it is likely that smooth muscle cells migrating into the lesion cause thickening of the intima through a hyperplastic response rather than any transformation [331]. In a recent detailed study of collagen III:I ratios in different areas of the plaque in comparison with surrounding intima, there were no differences between the centre and periphery of the plaque, but considerable variations between individuals in the relative proportions of these collagens (20–40% type III) in the intima [221] that probably reflected differences in age, degree of intimal thickening and sampling site in the aorta. Comparison of paired samples from plaque and surrounding intima showed only marginal differences in the relative proportions of collagens I and III, with no differences between ulcerated and non-ulcerated plaques [221]. An immunohistochemical study of collagens in human atherosclerosis with type-specific antibodies also showed no changes in the relative proportions of collagens I and III in any stage of the disease from mild intimal thickening to the fibrous cap of the complicated lesion [82]. This study did, however, note marked increases in the preponderance of these collagens as the lesion became more severe, changes that were paralleled by increased intensities of staining for the collagen types IV, V and VI [82]. These observed changes in amounts of collagen types IV, V and VI are consistent with the results of biochemical analyses where the content of these collagens increased with progression of the fibrotic process [84,126,332]. In an experimentally induced atherosclerotic lesion in sheep, collagen VI exhibited a diffuse immunostaining throughout the vessel wall with more marked concentrations around the smooth muscle cells, and appeared to increase in amount with the severity of the lesion [333]. By contrast, the staining for collagen type IV was localized in the basement membranes in control tissue but declined as the lesion progressed [333]. These findings lend support to the view that collagen VI filaments act as a secondary network that provides cell–matrix interactions and aids the organization of the major fibrillar collagens [334].

(b) Proteoglycan changes in atherosclerosis

Although a quantitatively minor constituent of vascular tissues, proteoglycans have many important functions in the organization of other macromolecules in the matrix, platelet aggregation and regulation of fluid and electrolyte balance (section 4.3.4). In the context of the pathogenesis of atherosclerosis, alterations in the composition and structure of proteoglycans are believed to play a central role in the accumulation of plasma lipoproteins in the arterial wall [335,336]. Consistent with this hypothesis was the finding of selective interactions between low density lipoproteins (LDLs) and glycosaminoglycans (GAGs) of the arterial wall [337,338]. A large number of studies has confirmed that there is an increase in proteoglycan content in atherosclerosis, although some doubt exists as to the compositional changes [339]. A detailed study of proteoglycans extracted from normal and atherosclerotic human aorta showed that the atherosclerotic samples contained a higher proportion of dermatan sulphate relative to chondroitin and heparan sulphates, and density gradient centrifugation revealed that the these proteoglycans had a markedly reduced hydrodynamic size in comparison with samples extracted from control tissue [340]. In addition, GAGs extracted by papain digestion of the proteoglycans from atherosclerotic areas of the aorta exhibited a much stronger interaction with human LDL than the corresponding samples extracted from normal areas of the same artery [340]. These findings clearly indicate that the atherosclerotic process brings about either some structural modification of proteoglycans or a change in their biosynthesis.

Attempts to interpret the observed changes in proteoglycan biosynthesis in atherosclerosis are confounded by variations in the cellular origin of these macromolecules. Thus, proliferating smooth muscle cells are known to modulate proteoglycan synthesis, but in a manner that fluctuates depending on the age and physiological state of the cell [341,342]. In addition, endothelial cells in culture show a marked increase in sulphated proteoglycan synthesis in response to injury [341]. A study of arterial GAG synthesis by incorporation of radiolabelled glucosamine *in vitro* into the neointima of rabbit aorta following endothelial damage with a balloon catheter, showed increases in labelling of areas denuded of endothelium compared with the re-endothelialized areas or control tissue [343]. Similar experiments with samples from cholesterol-fed rabbits revealed an enhanced effect of hypercholesterolaemia on the retention of newly synthesized proteoglycans, particularly in the areas of aorta where re-formation of the endothelium had occurred [343]. These types of experiment therefore emphasize the importance of changes in proteoglycan synthesis in atherosclerosis. A large number of growth factors and hormones have been implicated in these processes, and a recent study of thickened intima of human coronary arteries has suggested that the changes in the proteoglycan layer correlate with the immunohistochemical localization of transforming growth factor-β [344].

(c) Changes in other matrix components in atherosclerosis

As a prominant feature of the disease is accumulation of collagenous and proteoglycan components, an important area of study has been the proteases responsible for the normal turnover and repair. As discussed previously (section 4.2.1), plasminogen activator inhibitor type 1

(PAI-1) plays a central role in the proteolytic cascade leading to degradation of the extracellular matrix components. In addition, PAI-1 inhibits fibrinolysis and modulates migration of smooth muscle cells [345,346]. A significant finding, therefore, was that endothelial injury caused an increased synthesis and accumulation of PAI-1 in rabbit aorta that was potentiated by cholesterol feeding [347]. This was accompanied by an increased synthesis and deposition in the fibrotic regions of the glycoprotein, vitronectin, which is known to stabilize PAI-1 [347]. These results suggest, therefore, that regulation of protease inhibitors may be an important contributory factor in the accumulation of matrix in the atherosclerotic lesion.

An increasing body of evidence suggests that accumulation of matrix in the neointima of atherosclerotic lesions is also a result of increased synthesis by smooth muscle cells mediated by macrophage-derived factors. Macrophages are known to produce a series of cytokines and growth factors, including transforming growth factor-β, tumour necrosis factor, interleukin-1 and γ-interferon [348], which increase production of collagen, fibronectin and other matrix components. A study of human pulmonary arteries using sequential immunohistochemistry and *in situ* hybridization demonstrated co-localization of macrophages with extracellular matrix gene expression in the thickened intima [349]. These results were obtained only for macrophages before their transformation into foam cells, a process that therefore appears to be associated with a change in secretory activity [349].

4.5 Concluding remarks

Major advances have been made in extracellular matrix biochemistry over the past few years. Part of this advance has emanated from the advent of molecular biology techniques that have provided some insights into the basic defects in diseases affecting the blood vessels. In addition, the extracellular matrix is now considered as an integrated unit where the different components exhibit multiple interactions with each other that in turn affect cellular activity. Many of the components of this system have been characterized in great detail and, in this review, we have necessarily been rather selective in dealing with the information available. A large number of questions remain, however, with regard to the functional interactions between matrix constituents and the regulation of their metabolism. This fascinating area of work therefore provides many more challenges for future research.

Acknowledgements

We acknowledge the support of the Scottish Office Agriculture and Fisheries Department.

References

1. Chung, E. and Miller, E.J. (1974) Collagen polymorphism. Characterization of molecules with the chain composition [α-1(III)]$_3$ in human tissues. *Science*, **183**, 1200–1.
2. Ramirez, F. and di Liberto, M. (1990) Complex and diversified regulatory programs control the expression of vertebrate collagen genes. *FASEB J.*, **4**, 1616–23.
3. Chu, M.-L. and Prockop, D.J. (1993) Collagen: gene structure, in *Connective Tissue and its Heritable Disorders*, (eds P. Royce and B. Steinmann), Wiley-Liss, New York, pp. 149–65.
4. Kuhn, K. (1987) The classical collagens: types I, II and III, in *Structure and Function of Collagen Types*, (eds R. Mayne and R.E. Burgeson), Academic Press, Orlando, pp. 1–42.
5. Ninomiya, Y., Castognola, P., Gerecke, D. *et al.* (1990) The molecular biology of collagens with short triple-helical domains, in *Extracellular Matrix Genes*, Academic Press, New York, pp. 79–125.
6. Pihlajaniemi, T. and Tamminen, M. (1990) The alpha 1 chain of type XIII collagen consists of three collagenous and four non-collagenous domains, and its primary transcript undergoes complex alternative splicing. *J. Biol. Chem.*, **265**, 16922–8.
7. Myers, J.C., Kivirikko, S., Gordon, M.K. *et al.* (1992) Identification of a previously unknown human collagen chain, alpha 1(XV), characterized by extensive interruptions in the triple-helical region. *Proc. Natl. Acad. Sci. USA*, **89**, 10144–8.
8. Pan, T.C., Zhang, R.Z., Mattei, M.G. *et al.* (1992) Cloning and chromosomal location of human alpha 1(XVI) collagen. *Proc. Natl. Acad. Sci. USA*, **89**, 6565–9.
9. Baker, R.K. and Lively, M.O. (1987) Purification and characterization of hen oviduct microsomal signal peptidase. *Biochemistry*, **26**, 8561–7.
10. Evans, E.A., Gilmore, R. and Blobel, G. (1986) Purification of microsomal signal peptidase as a complex. *Proc. Natl. Acad. Sci. USA*, **83**, 581–5.
11. Kivirikko, K., Myllyla, R. and Pihlajaniemi, T. (1989) Protein hydroxylation: prolyl 4-hydroxylase, an enzyme with four cosubstrates and a multifunctional subunit. *FASEB J.*, **3**, 1609–17.
12. Bassuk, J.A. and Berg, R.A. (1989) Protein disulphide isomerase, a multifunctional endoplasmic reticulum protein. *Matrix*, **9**, 244–58.
13. Hanauske-Abel, H.M. (1991) Prolyl 4-hydroxylase, a target enzyme for drug development. Design of suppressive agents and the in vivo effects of inhibitors and proinhibitors. *J. Hepatol.*, **13**, S8–S16.
14. Kivirikko, K.I. and Myllyla, R. (1979) Collagen glycosyl transferases. *Int. Rev. Connect. Tissue Res.*, **8**, 23–72.
15. Bonadio, J., Holbrook, K.A., Gelinas, R.E. *et al.* (1985) Altered triple helical structure of type I procollagen in lethal perinatal osteogenesis imperfecta. *J. Biol. Chem.*, **260**, 1734–42.
16. Martin, G.R., Byers, P.H. and Piez, K.A. (1975) Procollagen. *Adv. Enzymol.*, **42**, 167–91.
17. Brass, A., Kadler, K., Thomas, J. *et al.* (1992) The fibrillar collagens, collagen VIII, collagen X and the C1q complement proteins share a similar domain in their C-terminal non-collagenous regions. *FEBS Lett.*, **303**, 126–8.
18. Freedman, R.B. (1989) Protein disulphide isomerase: multiple roles in the modification of nascent secretory proteins. *Cell*, **57**, 1069–72.
19. Uitto, J. (1979) Collagen polymorphism. Isolation and partial characterization of alpha 1(I) trimer molecules in normal human skin. *Arch. Biochem. Biophys.*, **192**, 371–9.
20. McBride, D.J., Kadler, K., Hojima, Y. *et al.* (1992) Self-assembly into fibrils of a homotrimer of type I collagen. *Matrix*, **12**, 256–63.
21. Steinmann, B., Bruckner, P. and Superti-Furga, A. (1991) Cyclosporin A slows collagen triple-helix formation in vivo: indirect evidence for a physiological role of peptidyl-prolyl-cis-trans-isomerase. *J. Biol. Chem.*, **266**, 1299–303.
22. Clark, C.C. (1979) The distribution and initial characterization of oligosaccharide units on the COOH-terminal propeptide extensions of the pro-alpha 1 and pro-alpha 2 chains of type I procollagen. *J. Biol. Chem.*, **254**, 10798–802.
23. Bienkowski, R.S., Cowan, M.J., McDonald, J.A. *et al.* (1978) Degradation of newly synthesized collagen. *J. Biol. Chem.*, **253**, 4356–63.
24. Bienkowski, R.S. (1984) Intracellular degradation of newly synthesized collagen. *Collagen Rel. Res.*, **4**, 399–412.
25. McAnulty, R.J. and Laurent, G.J. (1987) Collagen synthesis and degradation in vivo. Evidence for rapid rates of collagen turnover with extensive degradation of newly synthesized collagen in tissues of the adult rat. *Collagen Rel. Res.*, **7**, 93–104.
26. Laurent, G.J. (1987) Dynamic state of collagen: pathways of collagen degradation in vivo and their possible role in regulation of collagen mass. *Am. J. Physiol.*, **252**, C1–C9.
27. Mellor, S.J., Atkins, G.L. and Hulmes, D.J.S. (1991) Developmental changes in the type I procollagen processing pathway in chick-embryo cornea. *Biochem. J.*, **276**, 777–84.
28. Kadler, K.E., Hojima, Y. and Prockop, D.J. (1987) Assembly of collagen fibrils de novo by cleavage of the type I pC-collagen with procollagen C-proteinase. Assay of critical concentration demonstrates that collagen self-

assembly is a classical example of an entropy-driven process. *J. Biol. Chem.*, **262**, 15696–701.
29. Birk, D.E. and Trelstad, R.L. (1985) Fibroblasts create compartments in the extracellular space where collagen polymerizes into fibrils and fibrils associate into bundles. *Ann. N.Y. Acad. Sci.*, **460**, 258–66.
30. Kessler, E. and Adar, R. (1989) Type I procollagen C-proteinase from mouse fibroblasts. Purification and demonstration of a 55-kDa enhancer glycoprotein. *Eur. J. Biochem.*, **186**, 115–21.
31. Levene, C., O'Shea, M. and Carrington, M. (1988) Protein lysine 6-oxidase (lysyl oxidase) cofactor: methoxatin (PQQ) or pyridoxal? *Int. J. Biochem.*, **20**, 1451–6.
32. Gallop, P., Paz, M., Fluckiger, R. et al. (1989) PQQ, the elusive coenzyme. *Trends Biochem. Sci.*, **14**, 343–6.
33. Cronlund, A.L., Smith, B.D. and Kagan, H.M. (1985) Binding of lysyl oxidase to fibrils of type I collagen. *Connect. Tissue Res.*, **14**, 109–19.
34. Fietzek, P.P., Allmann, H., Rauterberg, J. et al. (1977) Ordering of cyanogen bromide peptides of type III collagen based on their homology to type I collagen: preservation of sites for crosslink formation during evolution. *Proc. Natl. Acad. Sci. USA*, **74**, 84–6.
35. Hamalainen, E.R., Jones, T.A., Sheer, D. et al. (1991) Molecular cloning of human lysyl oxidase and assignment of the gene to chromosome-5q23.3–31.2. *Genomics*, **11**, 508–16.
36. Mariani, T.J., Trackman, P.C., Kagan, H.M. et al. (1992) The complete derived amino acid sequence of human lysyl oxidase and assignment of the gene to chromosome 5 (extensive sequence homology with the murine ras recision gene). *Matrix*, **12**, 242–8.
37. Kenyon, K., Contente, S., Trackman, P.C. et al. (1991) Lysyl oxidase and rrg messenger RNA. *Science*, **253**, 802.
38. Barnes, M.J., Constable, B.J. and Morton, L.F. (1974) Age-related variations in hydroxylation of lysine and proline in collagens. *Biochem. J.*, **139**, 461–8.
39. Royce, P.M. and Barnes, M.J. (1985) Failure of highly purified lysyl hydroxylase to hydroxylate lysyl residues in the non-helical regions of collagen. *Biochem. J.*, **230**, 475–80.
40. Gerriets, J.E., Curwin, S.L. and Last, J.A. (1993) Tendon hypertrophy is associated with increased hydroxylation of nonhelical lysine residues at two specific cross-linking sites in type-I collagen. *J. Biol. Chem.*, **268**, 25553–60.
41. Robins, S.P., Shimokomaki, M. and Bailey, A.J. (1973) The chemistry of the collagen crosslinks: age-related changes in the reducible components of intact bovine collagen fibres. *Biochem. J.*, **131**, 771–80.
42. Yamauchi, M., London, R.E., Guenat, C. et al. (1987) Structure and formation of a stable histidine-based trifunctional crosslink in skin collagen. *J. Biol. Chem.*, **262**, 11428–34.
43. Eyre, D.R. and Oguchi, H. (1980) Hydroxypyridinium crosslinks of skeletal collagens: their measurement, properties and a proposed pathway of formation. *Biochem. Biophys. Res. Commun.*, **92**, 403–10.
44. Robins, S.P. (1983) Crosslinking of collagen: isolation, structural characterization and glycosylation of pyridinoline. *Biochem. J.*, **215**, 167–73.
45. Robins, S.P. and Bailey, A.J. (1975) The mechanism of stabilization of the reducible intermediate crosslinks. *Biochem. J.*, **149**, 381–5.
46. Robins, S.P., Duncan, A. and Riggs, B.L. (1990) Direct measurement of free hydroxypyridinium crosslinks of collagen in urine as new markers of bone resorption in osteoporosis, in *Osteoporosis 1990*, Osteopress ApS, Copenhagen, pp. 465–8.
47. Eyre, D.R. (1987) Collagen cross-linking amino acids. *Methods Enzymol.*, **144**, 115–39.
48. Robins. S.P. (1988) Functional properties of collagen and elastin. *Bailliere's Clinical Rheumatology*, **2**, 1–36.
49. Last, J.A., Armstrong, L.G. and Reiser, K.M. (1990) Biosynthesis of collagen crosslinks. *Int. J. Biochem.*, **22**, 559–64.
50. Robins, S.P. and Bailey, A.J. (1973) The characterisation of Fraction C, a possible artifact produced during the reduction of collagen fibres with borohydride. *Biochem. J.*, **135**, 657–65.
51. Bernstein, P.H. and Mechanic, G.L. (1980) A natural histidine-based imminium cross-link in collagen and its location. *J. Biol. Chem.*, **255**, 10414–22.
52. Robins, S.P. and Bailey, A.J. (1977) Characterization of the products of reduction of skin, tendon and bone with sodium cyanoborohydride. *Biochem. J.*, **163**, 339–46.
53. Scott, P.G. (1980) A major intermolecular cross-linking site in bovine dentine collagen involving the alpha 2 chain and stabilising the 4D overlap. *Biochemistry*, **19**, 6118–24.
54. Robins, S.P. and Duncan, A. (1987) Pyridinium crosslinks of bone collagen and their location in peptides isolated from rat femur. *Biochim. Biophys. Acta*, **914**, 233–9.
55. Henkel, W., Glanville, R.W. and Greifendorf, D. (1987) Characterisation of a type-I collagen trimeric cross-linked peptide from calf aorta and its cross-linked structure. Detection of pyridinoline by time-of-flight secondary ion-mass spectrometry and evidence for a new cross-link. *Eur. J. Biochem.*, **165**, 427–36.
56. Scott, J.E., Hughes, E.W. and Shuttleworth, A. (1981) A collagen-associated Ehrlich chromogen: a pyrrolic cross-link? *Biosci. Rep.*, **1**, 611–18.
57. Kuypers, R., Tyler, M., Kurth, L.B. et al. (1992) Identification of the loci of the collagen-associated Ehrlich chromogen in type I collagen confirms its role as a trivalent cross-link. *Biochem. J.*, **283**, 129–36.
58. Scott, J.E., Qian, R., Henkel, W. et al. (1983) An Ehrlich chromogen in collagen cross-links. *Biochem. J.*, **209**, 263–4.
59. Kemp, P.D. and Scott, J.E. (1988) Ehrlich chromogens, probable crosslinks in elastin and collagen. *Biochem. J.*, **252**, 387–93.
60. Horgan, D.J., King, N.L., Kurth, L.B. et al. (1990) Collagen crosslinks and their relationship to the thermal properties of calf tendons. *Arch. Biochem. Biophys.*, **281**, 21–6.
61. Whittle, M.A., Robins, S.P., Hasleton, P.S. et al. (1987) Biochemical investigation of possible lesions in human aorta that predispose to dissecting aneurysms: pyridinoline crosslinks. *Cardiovasc. Res.*, **21**, 161–8.
62. Seibel, M.J., Robins, S.P. and Bilezikian, J.P. (1992) Urinary pyridinium crosslinks of collagen: specific markers of bone resorption in metabolic bone disease. *Trends Endocrinol. Metab.*, **3**, 263–70.
63. Halme, T., Peltonen, J., Sims, T.J. et al. (1986) Collagen in human aorta. Changes in the type III/I ratio and concentration of the reducible crosslink, dehydrohydroxylysinonorleucine in ascending aorta from healthy subjects of different age and patients with annulo-aortic ectasia. *Biochim. Biophys. Acta*, **881**, 222–8.
64. Levene, C., Heale, G. and Robins, S. (1989) Collagen cross-link synthesis in cultured vascular endothelium. *Br. J. Exp. Pathol.*, **70**, 621–6.
65. Baynes, J. (1991) Role of oxidative stress in development of complications in diabetes. *Diabetes*, **40**, 405–12.
66. Reiser, K.M. (1991) Nonenzymatic glycation of collagen in aging and diabetes. *Proc. Soc. Exp. Biol. Med.*, **196**, 17–29.
67. Robins, S.P. and Bailey, A.J. (1972) Age-related changes in collagen: the identification of reducible lysine-carbohydrate condensation products. *Biochem. Biophys. Res. Commun.*, **48**, 76–84.
68. Reiser, K., McCormick, R.J. and Rucker, R.B. (1992) Enzymatic and nonenzymatic cross-linking of collagen and elastin. *FASEB J.*, **6**, 2439–49.
69. Hunt, J.V., Smith, C.C.T. and Wolff, S.P. (1990) Autoxidative glycosylation and possible involvement of peroxides and free radicals in LDL modification by glucose. *Diabetes*, **39**, 1420–4.
70. Kent, M.J.C., Light, N.D. and Bailey, A.J. (1985) Evidence for glucose-mediated covalent cross-linking of collagen after glycosylation in vitro. *Biochem. J.*, **225**, 745–52.
71. Bailey, A., Wotton, S., Sims, T. et al. (1993) Biochemical changes in the collagen of human osteoporotic bone matrix. *Connect Tissue Res.*, **29**, 119–32.
72. Sell, D.R. and Monnier, V.M. (1989) Structure elucidation of a senescence cross-link from human extracellular matrix. *J. Biol. Chem.*, **264**, 21597–602.
73. Takahashi, M., Ohishi, T., Aoshima, H. et al. (1993) Pre-fractionation with cation exchanger for determination of intermolecular crosslinks, pyridinoline and pentosidine, in hydrolysates. *J. Liq. Chromatog.*, **16**, 1355–61.
74. Grandhee, S.K. and Monnier, V.M. (1991) Mechanism of formation of the Maillard protein cross-link pentosidine – glucose, fructose, and ascorbate as pentosidine precursors. *J. Biol. Chem.*, **266**, 11649–53.
75. Dyer, D.G., Blackledge, J.A., Thorpe, S.R. et al. (1991) Formation of pentosidine during nonenzymatic browning of proteins by glucose – identification of glucose and other carbohydrates as possible precursors of pentosidine in vivo. *J. Biol. Chem.*, **266**, 11654–60.
76. Njoroge, F.G., Fernandez, A.A. and Monnier, V.M. (1987) 3-D-Erythro-trihydroprolyl-1-neopentyl pyrrole-2-carboxaldehyde, a novel nonenzymatic browning product of glucose. *J. Carbohydrate Chem.*, **6**, 553–68.
77. Hayase, F., Nagaraj, R.H., Miyata, S. et al. (1989) Aging of proteins: Immunological detection of a glucose-derived pyrrole formed during Maillard reaction in vivo. *J. Biol. Chem.*, **264**, 3758–64.
78. Keene, D.R., Sakai, L.Y., Bachinger, H.P. et al. (1987) Type III collagen can be present on banded collagen fibrils regardless of fibril diameter. *J. Cell Biol.*, **105**, 2393–402.
79. Robins, S.P. (1979) Metabolism of rabbit skin collagen. *Biochem. J.*, **181**, 75–82.
80. Fleischmajer, R., Perlish, J.S., Burgeson, R.E. et al. (1990) Type I and type III interactions during fibrillogenesis. *Ann. N.Y. Acad. Sci.*, **580**, 161–75.
81. Henkel, W. and Glanville, R.W. (1982) Covalent crosslinking between molecules of type I and type III collagen. The involvement of the N-terminal, non-helical regions of the alpha 1(I) and alpha 1(III) chains in the formation of intermolecular crosslinks. *Eur. J. Biochem.*, **122**, 205–13.
82. Katsuda, S., Okada, Y., Minamoto, T. et al. (1992) Collagens in human atherosclerosis. Immunohistochemical analysis using collagen type-specific antibodies. *Arteriosclerosis Thromb.*, **12**, 494–502.
83. McCullagh, K.G., Duance, V.C. and Bishop, K.A. (1980) The distribution of collagen types I, III and V (AB) in normal and atherosclerotic human aorta. *J. Pathol.*, **130**, 45–55.
84. Morton, L.F. and Barnes, M.J. (1984) Collagen polymorphism in the normal and diseased blood vessel wall. Investigation of collagen types I, III and V. *Atherosclerosis*, **42**, 4–51.
85. Fessler, J.H. and Fessler, L.I. (1987) Type V collagen, in *Structure and Function of Collagen Types*, (eds R. Mayne and R.E. Burgeson), Academic Press, Orlando, pp. 81–103.

86. Birk, D.E., Fitch, J.M., Babiarz, J.P. et al. (1988) Collagen type I and V are present in the same fibril in avian corneal stroma. *J. Cell Biol.*, **106**, 999–1008.
87. Mendler, M., Eich-Bender, S.G., Vaugan, L. et al. (1989) Cartilage contains mixed fibrils of collagen types II, IX and XI. *J. Cell Biol.*, **108**, 191–7.
88. Bernard, M.P., Yoshioka, H., Rodriguez, E. et al. (1988) Cloning and sequencing of pro-alpha1 (XI) collagen cDNA demonstrates that type XI belongs to the fibrillar class of collagens and reveals that the expression is not restricted to cartilagenous tissue. *J. Biol Chem.*, **263**, 17159–66.
89. Niyibizi, C. and Eyre, D.J. (1989) Identification of the cartilage alpha 1(XI) chain in type V collagen from bovine bone. *FEBS Lett.*, **242**, 314–18.
90. Madri, J.A., Dreyer, B., Pitlick, F.A. et al. (1980) The collagenous components of the subendothelium: correlation of structure and function. *Lab. Invest.*, **43**, 303–15.
91. Gay, S., Martinez-Hernandez, A., Rhodes, R.K. et al. (1981) The collagenous exocytoskeleton of smooth muscle cells. *Collagen Rel. Res.*, **1**, 377–84.
92. Gordon, M.K. and Olsen, B.R. (1990) The contribution of collagenous proteins to tissue specific matrix assemblies. *Curr. Opin. Cell Biol.*, **2**, 833–8.
93. Van der Rest, M. and Garrone, R. (1991) Collagen family of proteins. *FASEB J.*, **5**, 2814–23.
94. Nishimura, I., Muragaki, Y., Hayashi, M. et al. (1990) Tissue-specific expression of type IX collagen. *Ann. NY Acad. Sci.*, **580**, 112–19.
95. Ayad, S., Marriott, A., Brierley, V.H. et al. (1991) Mammalian cartilage synthesizes both proteoglycan and non-proteoglycan forms of type IX collagen. *Biochem. J.*, **278**, 441–5.
96. Wu, J.J., Woods, P.E. and Eyre, D.R. (1992) Identification of cross-linking sites in bovine cartilage type IX collagen reveals an antiparallel type II–type IX molecular relationship and type IX to type IX bonding. *J. Biol. Chem.*, **267**, 23007–14.
97. Keene, D.R., Lunstrum, G.P., Morris, N.P. et al. (1991) Two type XII-like collagens localize to the surface of banded collagen fibrils. *J. Cell Biol.*, **113**, 971–8.
98. Dublet, B. and van der Rest, M. (1991) Type XIV collagen, a new homotrimeric molecule extracted from fetal bovine skin and tendon, with a triple helical disulfide-bonded domain homologous to type IX and type XII collagens. *J. Biol. Chem.*, **266**, 6853–9.
99. Timpl, R. and Engel, J. (1987) Type VI collagen, in *Structure and Function of Collagen Types*, (eds. R. Mayne and R.E. Burgeson), Academic Press, Orlando, pp. 105–53.
100. Trueb, B., Schreier, T., Bruckner, P. et al. (1987) Type VI collagen represents a major fraction of connective tissue collagens. *Eur. J. Biochem.*, **166**, 699–703.
101. Colombatti, A., Ainger, K. and Colizzi, F. (1989) Type VI collagen: high yields of a molecule with multiple forms of alpha 3 chain from avian and human tissues. *Matrix*, **9**, 177–85.
102. Saitta, B., Stokes, D.G., Vissing, H. et al. (1990) Alternative splicing of the human alpha 2(VI) collagen gene generates multiple mRNA transcripts which predict three protein variants with distinct carboxyl termini. *J. Biol. Chem.*, **265**, 6473–80.
103. Kielty, C., Boot-Handford, R., Ayad, S. et al. (1990) Molecular composition of type VI collagen. Evidence for chain heterogeneity in mammalian tissues and cultured cells. *Biochem. J.*, **272**, 787–95.
104. Bruns, R.R., Press, W., Engvall, E. et al. (1986) Type VI collagen in extracellular, 100-nm periodic filaments and fibrils: identification by immunoelectron microscopy. *J. Cell Biol.*, **103**, 393–404.
105. Wu, J.-J., Eyre, D.R. and Slayter, H.S. (1987) Type VI collagen of the intervetebral disc. Biochemical and electron-microscopic characterization of the native protein. *Biochem. J.*, **248**, 373–81.
106. Keene, D.R., Engvall, E. and Glanville, R.W. (1988) Ultrastructure of type VI collagen in human skin and cartilage suggests an anchoring function for this filamentous network. *J. Cell Biol.*, **107**, 1995–2006.
107. Aumailley, M., Mann, K., von der Mark, H. et al. (1989) Cell attachment properties of collagen type VI and Arg-Gly-Asp dependent binding to its alpha 2(VI) and alpha 3(VI) chains. *Exp. Cell Res.*, **181**, 463–74.
108. Kielty, C.M., Whittaker, SP., Grant, M.E. et al. (1992) Type VI collagen microfibrils: evidence for a structural association with hyaluronan. *J. Cell Biol.*, **118**, 979–90.
109. Bidnaset, D.J., Guidry, C., Rosenberg, L.C. et al. (1992) Binding of the proteoglycan decorin to collagen type VI. *J. Biol. Chem.*, **267**, 5250–6.
110. Sage, H., Pritzl, P. and Bornstein, P. (1980) A unique pepsin-sensitive collagen synthesized by aortic endothelial cells in culture. *Biochemistry*, **19**, 5747–55.
111. Benya, P.D. and Padilla, S.R. (1986) Isolation and characterization of type VIII collagen synthesized by cultured corneal endothelial cells. A conventional structure replaces the interrupted-helix model. *J. Biol. Chem.*, **261**, 4160–9.
112. Yamaguchi, N., Benya, P.D., van der Rest, M. et al. (1989) The cloning and sequencing of alpha 1(VIII) collagen cDNAs demonstrate that type VIII collagen is a short chain collagen and contains triple-helical and carboxyl-terminal non-triple-helical domains similar to those of type X collagen. *J. Biol. Chem.*, **264**, 16022–9.
113. Muragaki, Y., Jacenko, O., Apte, S. et al. (1991) The alpha 2(VIII) collagen gene – a novel member of the short-chain collagen family located on human chromosome 1. *J. Biol. Chem.*, **266**, 7721–7.
114. Kwan, A.P.L., Freemont, A.J. and Grant, M.E. (1986) Immunoperoxidase localization of type X collagen in chick tibiae. *Biosci. Rep.*, **6**, 155–62.
115. Sawada, H., Konomi, H. and Hirosawa, K. (1990) Characterization of the collagen in the hexagonal lattice of Descemet's membrane: its relation to type VIII collagen. *J. Cell Biol.*, **110**, 219–27.
116. Kwan, A.P.L., Cummings, C.E., Chapman, J.A. et al. (1991) Macromolecular organization of chicken type X collagen in vitro. *J. Cell Biol.*, **114**, 597–604.
117. Kittelberger, R., Davis, P.F., Flynn, D.W. et al. (1990) Distribution of type VIII collagen in tissues: an immunohistochemical study. *Connect. Tissue Res.*, **24**, 303–18.
118. Rosenblum, N.D., Briscoe, D.M., Karnovsky, M.J. et al. (1993) Alpha 1-VIII collagen is expressed in the rat glomerulaus and in resident glomerular cells. *Am. J. Physiol.*, **264**, F1003–10.
119. Kefalides, N.A. (1971) Isolation of a collagen from basement membranes containing three identical alpha-chains. *Biochem. Biophys. Res. Commun.*, **45**, 226–34.
120. Yurchenco, P.D. and Schittny, J.C. (1990) Molecular architecture of basement membranes. *FASEB J.*, **4**, 1577–88.
121. Brazel, D., Oberbaeumer, I.D.H., Babel, W. et al. (1987) Completion of the amino acid sequence of the alpha 1 chain of human basement membrane collagen (type IV) reveals 21 non-triplet interruptions located within the collagenous domain. *Eur. J. Biochem.*, **168**, 529–36.
122. Hostickka, S.L. and Tryggvason, K. (1988) The complete primary structure of the alpha 2 chain of human type IV collagen and comparison with the alpha 1(IV) chain *J. Biol. Chem.*, **263**, 19488–93.
123. Bailey, A.J., Sims, T. and Light, N. (1984) Cross-linking in type IV collagen. *Biochem. J.*, **218**, 713–23.
124. Mayne, R., Zettergren, J.G., Mayne, P.M. et al. (1980) Isolation and partial characterization of basement membrane-like collagens from bovine thoracic aorta. *Artery*, **4**, 262–80.
125. Leushner, J.R.A. and Haust, M.D. (1984) Characterization of basement membrane collagens of bovine aortae. *Atherosclerosis*, **50**, 11–27.
126. Murata, K., Motayama, T. and Kotake, C. (1986) Collagen types in various layers of the human aorta and their changes with the atherosclerotic process. *Atherosclerosis*, **251**, 251–62.
127. Sankey, E.A. and Barnes, M.J. (1984) Comparison of the collagenous products synthesized in culture by pig aortic endothelial and smooth muscle cells: variability in endothelial cell culture. *Biochem. J.*, **218**, 11–18.
128. Sage, H. and Bornstein, P. (1982) Endothelial cells from umbilical vein and a hemangioendothelioma secrete basement membrane largely to the exclusion of interstitial procollagens. *Arteriosclerosis*, **2**, 27–36.
129. Paulsson, M. (1992) Basement membrane proteins: structure, assembly and cellular interactions. *Crit. Rev. Biochem. Mol. Biol.*, **27**, 93–127.
130. Kalluri, R., Gunwar, S., Reeders, S.T. et al. (1991) Goodpasture syndrome. Localisation of the epitope for the autoantibodies to the carboxy-terminal region of the alpha 3(IV) chain of basement membrane. *J. Biol. Chem.*, **266**, 24018–24.
131. Barker, D.F., Hostikka, S.L., Zhou, J. et al. (1990) Identification of mutations in the COL4A5 collagen gene in Alport syndrome. *Science*, **248**, 1224–7.
132. Schwartz, E. and Fleischmajer, R. (1986) Association of elastin with oxytalan fibers of the dermis and with extracellular skin fibroblasts. *J. Histochem. Cytochem.*, **34**, 1063–8.
133. Ayad, S., Chambers, C.A., Berry, L. et al. (1986) Type VI collagen and glycoprotein MFPI are distinct components of the extracellular matrix. *Biochem. J.*, **236**, 299–302.
134. Barone, L.M., Faris, B., Chipman, S.D. et al. (1985) Alteration in the extracellular matrix of smooth muscle cells by ascorbate. *Biochim. Biophys. Acta*, **840**, 245–54.
135. Hinek, A., Wrenn, D.S., Mecham, R.P. et al. (1988) The elastin receptor: a galactoside-binding protein. *Science*, **239**, 1539–41.
136. Mecham, R.P. (1991) Elastin synthesis and fiber assembly. *Ann. N.Y. Acad. Sci.*, **624**, 137–46.
137. Rucker, R.B. and Murray, J. (1978) Cross-linking amino acids in collagen and elastin. *Amer. J. Clin. Nutr.*, **31**, 1221–36.
138. Rosenbloom, J. (1987) Elastin: an overview. *Meth. Enzymol.*, **144**, 172–96.
139. Starcher, B.C., Cook, G., Gallop, P.M., Henson, E. et al. (1987) Isolation and characterization of a pentameric amino acid from elastin. *Conn. Tissue Res.*, **16**, 15–25.
140. Farquharson, C. and Robins, S.P. (1989) Immunolocalistion of collagen types I and III in the arterial wall of the rat. *Histochem. J.*, **21**, 172–8.
141. Bartholemew, K. and Anderson, J.C. (1983) Investigation of relationships between collagens, elastin and proteoglycans in bovine thoracic aorta by immunofluorescence techniques. *Histochem. J.*, **15**, 1177–90.
142. Wolinsky, H. and Glagov, S. (1964) Structural basis for the static mechanical properties of the aortic media. *Circ. Res.*, **14**, 400–13.
143. Roach, M.R. (1983) The patterns of elastin in the aorta and large arteries

of mammals, in *Development of the vascular system*, Ciba Foundation symposium 100, London, pp 37–5.
144. Mecham, R.P., Stenmark, K.R. and Parks, W.C. (1991) Connective tissue production by vascular smooth muscle in development and disease. *Chest*, **99**, 43S–7S.
145. Roach, M.R. (1986) The structure and elastic properties of arterial junctions. *Conn. Tissue Res.*, **15**, 77–84.
146. Berry, C.L., Sosa-Melgarejo, J.A. and Greenwald, S.E. (1993) The relationship between wall tension, lamellar thickness, and intercellular junctions in the fetal and adult aorta: its relevance to the pathology of dissecting aneurysm. *J. Pathol.*, **169**, 15–20.
147. Song, S.H. and Roach, M.R. (1984) Comparison of fenestrations in internal elastic laminae of canine thoracic vessels. *Blood Vessels*, **21**, 90–97.
148. Roach, M.R. and Song, S.H. (1988) Arterial elastin as seen with scanning electron microscopy: a review. *Scanning Microsc.*, **2**, 994–1004.
149. Dunmore, P.J., Song, S.H. and Roach, M.R. (1990) A comparison of the size in the fenestrations in the internal elastic lamina as seen with the scanning electron microscope. *Can. J. Physiol. Pharmacol.*, **68**, 139–43.
150. Sosa-Melgarejo, J.A. and Berry, C.L. (1992) Myoendothelial contacts in the thoracic aorta of rat fetuses. *J. Pathol.*, **167**, 311–16.
151. Sosa-Melgarejo, J.A. and Berry, C.L. (1992) Myoendothelial contacts in arteriosclerosis. *J. Pathol.*, **167**, 235–9.
152. Gosline, J.M. and Rosenbloom, J. (1985) Elastin, in *Extracellular Matrix Biochemistry*, (eds. K.A. Piez and A.H. Reddi), Elsevier, Amsterdam, pp. 191–227.
153. Bork, P. (1991) Shuffled domains in extracellular proteins. *FEBS Lett.*, **286**, 47–54.
154. Gilbert, W. (1978) Why genes in pieces? *Nature*, **271**, 501.
155. Engel, J. (1989) EGF-like domains in extracellular matrix proteins: localized signals for growth and differentiation? *FEBS Lett.*, **251**, 1–7.
156. Gutman, A. and Kornblihtt, A.R. (1987) Identification of a third region of cell-specific alternative splicing in human fibronectin mRNA. *Proc. Natl Acad. Sci. USA*, **84**, 7179–82.
157. Yamada, K. (1989) Fibronectin domains and receptors, in *Fibronectin*, (ed. D.F. Mosher), Academic Press, San Diego, pp. 47–121.
158. Hynes, R.O. (1990) '*Fibronectin*', Springer, New York.
159. Yamada, K.M., Kennedy, D.W., Kimata, K. et al. (1980) Characterization of fibronectin interactions with glycosaminoglycans and identification of active proteolytic fragments. *J. Biol. Chem.*, **255**, 6055–63.
160. Richter, H. and Hoermann, H. (1983) A large cathepsin D-derived fragment from the central part of fibronectin subunit chains. *FEBS Lett.*, **155**, 317–20.
161. Engel, J. (1993) Structure and function of laminin, in *Molecular and Cellular Aspects of Basement Membranes*, (eds. D.H. Rohrbach and R. Timpl), Academic Press, San Diego, pp. 147–76.
162. Sasaki, M., Kleinman, H.K., Huber, H. et al. (1988) Laminin, a multidomain protein. The A chain has a unique globular domain and homology with basement membrane proteoglycan and the laminin B chains. *J. Biol. Chem.*, **263**, 16536–43.
163. Beck, K., Hunter, I. and Engel, J. (1990) Structure and function of laminin: anatomy of a multidomain glycoprotein. *FASEB J.*, **4**, 148–57.
164. Paulsson, M. (1992) The role of laminin in attachment, growth and differentiation of cultured cells: a brief review. *Cytotechnology*, **9**, 99–106.
165. Sung, U., Orear, J.J. and Yurchenco, P.D. (1993) Cell and heparin binding in the distal long arm of laminin. Identification of active and cryptic sites with recombinant and hybrid glycoprotein. *J. Cell Biol.*, **123**, 1255–68.
166. Wu, C., Friedmann, R. and Chung, A.E. (1988) Analysis of the assembly of laminin and the laminin-entactin complex with laminin chain specific monclonal and polyclonal antibodies. *Biochemistry*, **27**, 8780–6.
167. Sakai, L.Y., Keene, D.R. and Engvall, E. (1986) Fibrilin, a new 350-kD glycoprotein, is a component of extracellular microfibrils. *J. Cell Biol.*, **103**, 2499–509.
168. Kielty, C.M., Berry, L., Whittaker, S.P. et al. (1993) Microfibrillar assemblies of foetal bovine skin. Developmental expression and relative abundance of type VI collagen and fibrillin. *Matrix*, **13**, 103–12.
169. Dietz, H., Saraiva, J., Pyeritz, R. et al. (1992) Clustering of fibrillin (FBN1) missense mutations in Marfan syndrome patients at cysteine residues in EGF-like domains. *Hum. Mutat*, **1**, 366–74.
170. Lee, B., Godfrey, M., Vitale, E. et al. (1991) Linkage of Marfan syndrome and a phenotypically related disorder to two different fibrillin genes. *Nature*, **352**, 330–4.
171. Maslen, C.L., Corson, G.M., Maddox, B.K. et al. (1991) Partial sequence of a candidate gene for the Marfan syndrome. *Nature*, **352**, 334–7.
172. Christiano, A.M., Lebwohl, M.G., Boyd, C.D. et al. (1992) Workshop on pseudoxanthoma elasticum: molecular biology and pathology of the elastic fibers. Jefferson Medical College, Philadelphia, Pennsylvania, June 10, 1992. *J. Invest. Dermatol.*, **99**, 660–3.
173. Schwartz, N.B., Habib, G., Campbell, S. et al. (1985) Synthesis and structure of proteoglycan core protein. *Fed. Proc.*, **44**, 369–72.
174. Bourdon, M.A., Oldberg, A., Pierschbacher, M. et al. (1985) Molecular cloning and sequence analysis of chondroitin sulphate proteoglycan cDNA. *Proc. Natl Acad. Sci. USA*, **84**, 6770–4.
175. Roden, L., Koerner, T., Olson, C. et al. (1985) Mechanisms of chain initiation the biosynthesis of connective tissue polysaccharides. *Fed. Proc.*, **44**, 373–80.
176. Poole, A.R. (1986) Proteoglycans in health and disease: structures and functions. *Biochem. J.*, **236**, 1–14.
177. Neame, P.J., Christner, J.E. and Baker, J.R. (1987) Cartilage proteoglycan aggregates. The link protein and proteoglycan globular domains have similar structures. *J. Biol. Chem.*, **262**, 17768–78.
178. Chang, Y., Yanagishita, M., Hascall, V.C. et al. (1983) Proteoglycans synthesised by smooth muscle cells derived from monkey (*Macaca nemestrina*) aorta. *J. Biol. Chem.*, **258**, 5679–88.
179. Fellini, S.A., Kimura, J.H. and Hascall, V.C. (1981) Polydispersity of proteoglycans synthesised by chondrocytes from the Swarm rat chondrosarcoma. *J. Biol. Chem.*, **256**, 7883–9.
180. Asundi, V.K., Cowan K, Matzura, D. et al. (1990) Characterization of extracellular matrix proteoglycan transcripts expressed by vascular smooth muscle cells. *Eur. J. Cell Biol.*, **52**, 98–104.
181. Bianco, P., Fisher, L.W., Young, M.F. et al. (1990) Expression and localization of the two small proteoglycans, biglycan and decorin, in developing human skeletal and non-skeletal tissues. *J. Histochem. Cytochem.*, **38**, 1549–63.
182. Dreher, K.L., Asundi, V.K., Matzura, D. et al. (1990) Vascular smooth muscle biglycan represents a highly conserved proteoglycan within the arterial wall. *Eur. J. Cell Biol.*, **53**, 296–304.
183. Asundi, V.K. and Dreher, K.L. (1992) Molecular characterization of vascular smooth muscle decorin: deduced core regulation of gene expression. *Eur. J. Cell Biol.*, **59**, 314–21.
184. Schmidt, G., Hausser, H. and Kresse, H. (1991) Interaction of the small proteoglycan decorin with fibronectin. Involvement of the sequence NKISK of the core protein. *Biochem. J.*, **280**, 411–14.
185. Pringle, G.A. and Dodd, C.M. (1990) Immunodetection and microscopic localization of the core protein of decorin near the D-bands and E-bands of tendon collagen fibrils by use of monoclonal antibodies. *J. Histochem. Cytochem.*, **38**, 1405–11.
186. Yamaguchi, Y., Mann, D.M. and Ruoslahti, E. (1990) Negative regulation of transforming growth factor-beta by the proteoglycan decorin. *Nature*, **346**, 281–4.
187. Oldberg, A., Antonsson, P., Lindblom, K. et al. (1989) A collagen binding 59-kD protein (fibromodulin) is structurally related to the small interstitial proteoglycans, proteoglycan-S1 and proteoglycan-S2 (decorin). *EMBO J.*, **8**, 2601–4.
188. Kjellen, L., Petterson, I. and Hook, M. (1981) Cell-surface heparan sulphate: an intercalated membrane proteoglycan. *Proc. Natl Acad. Sci. USA*, **78**, 5371–5.
189. Carey, D.J. and Evans, D.M. (1989) Membrane anchoring of heparan sulphate proteoglycans by phosphotidylinositol and kinetics of synthesis of peripheral and detergent-solubilised proteoglycans in Schwann cells. *J. Cell Biol.*, **108**, 1891–9.
190. Ishihara, M., Fedarko, N.S. and Conrad, H.E. (1986) Transport of heparan sulphate into the nuclei of hepatocytes. *J. Biol. Chem.*, **261**, 13575–80.
191. Hamati, H.F., Britton, E.L. and Carey, D.J. (1989) Inhibition of proteoglycan synthesis alters extracellular matrix deposition, proliferation and cytoskeletal organization of rat aortic smooth muscle cells in culture. *J. Cell Biol.*, **108**, 2495–505.
192. Lark, M.W., Yeo, T.-K., Mar, H. et al. (1988) Arterial chondroitin sulphate proteoglycan: localisation with a monoclonal antibody. *J. Histochem. Cytochem.*, **36**, 1211–21.
193. Camejo, G. (1982) The interactions of lipids and lipoproteins with the intercellular matrix of arterial tissue: its possible role in atherogenesis. *Adv. Lipid Res.*, **19**, 1–53.
194. Clowes, A.W., Clowes, M.M., Gown, A.M. et al. (1984) Localisation of proteoheparin sulphate in rat aorta. *Histochemistry*, **80**, 379–84.
195. Kanwar, Y.S. and Farquhar, M.G. (1979) Presence of heparan sulphate in the glomerular basement membrane. *Proc. Natl Acad. Sci. USA*, **76**, 1303–7.
196. Woods, A., Couchman, J.R. and Hook, M. (1985) Heparan sulfate proteoglycans of rat embryo fibroblasts. A hydrophobic form may link cytoskeleton and matrix components. *J. Biol. Chem.*, **260**, 10872–9.
197. Volker, W., Schmidt, A. and Buddecke, E. (1986) Compartmentalization and characterization of different proteoglycans in bovine arterial wall. *J. Histochem. Cytochem.*, **34**, 1293–9.
198. Register, T.C., Wagner, W.D., Robbins, R.A. et al. (1993) Structural properties and partial protein sequence analysis of the major dematan sulphate proteoglycan of pigeon aorta. *Atheroclerosis*, **98**, 99–111.
199. Robbins, R.A., Wagner, W.D., Sawyer, L.M. et al. (1989) Immunolocalization of proteoglycan types in aortas of pigeons with spontaneous or diet-induced atherosclerosis. *Am. J. Pathol.*, **134**, 615–26.
200. Robbins, R.A., Wagner, W.D., Register, T.C. et al. (1992) Demonstration of a keratan sulphate-containing proteoglycan in atherosclerotic aorta. *Arterioscler. Thromb.*, **12**, 83–91.
201. Jarvelainen, H.T., Kinsella, M.G., Wight, T.N. et al. (1991) Differential expression of small chondroitin/dermatan sulfate proteoglycans, PG-I/

biglycan and PG-II/decorin, by vascular smooth muscle and endothelial cells in culture. *J. Biol. Chem.*, 266, 23274–81.
202. Ohishi, H., Hess, D., Kosakai, M. *et al.* (1988) Glycosaminoglycan content in neonatal rat aortic smooth muscle cell cultures. *Atherosclerosis*, 69, 61–8.
203. Robins, S.P. (1982) Turnover and corsslinking of collagen, in *Collagen in Health and Disease*, (eds J.B. Weiss and M.I.V. Jayson), Churchill Livingstone, Edinburgh, pp. 160–78.
204. Nagase, H., Barrett, A.J. and Woessner Jr, J.F. (1992) Nomenclature and glossary of the matrix metalloproteinases, in *Matrix Metalloproteinases and Inhibitors*, (eds H. Birkedal-Hansen, Z. Werb and H.G. Welgus), Gustav Fischer, Stuttgart, pp. 421–4.
205. Matrisian, L.M. (1992) The matrix-degrading metalloproteinases. *Bioessays*, 14, 455–62.
206. BirkedalHansen, H., Moore, W.G.I., Bodden, M.K. *et al.* (1993) Matrix metalloproteinases: a review. *Crit. Rev. Oral Biol. Med.*, 4, 197–250.
207. Gross, J. and Lapiere, C.M. (1962) Collagenolytic activity in amphibian tissues: a tissue culture assay. *Proc. Natl Acad. Sci. USA*, 54, 1197–204.
208. Mackay, A.R., Hartzler, J.L., Pelina, M.D. *et al.* (1990) Studies on the ability of 65-kDa and 92-kDa tumour cell gelatinases to degrade type IV collagen. *J. Biol. Chem.*, 265, 10628–34.
209. Shapiro, S.D., Griffin, G.L., Gilbert, D.J. *et al.* (1992) Molecular cloning, chromosomal localization and bacterial expression of a murine macrophage metalloproteinase. *J. Biol. Chem.*, 267, 4664–71.
210. Cawston, T.E. (1986) Protein inhibitors of metallo-proteinases in *Proteinases Inhibitors*, (eds A.J. Barrett and G. Salvesen), Elsevier, Amsterdam, pp. 589–610.
211. Stetler-Stevenson, W.G., Brown, P.D., Onisto, M. *et al.* (1990) Tissue inhibitor of metalloproteinases-2 (TIMP-2) mRNA expression in tumor cell lines and human tumor tissues. *J. Biol. Chem.*, 265, 13933–8.
212. Goldberg, G.I., Marmer, B.L., Grant, G.A. *et al.* (1989) Human 72-kilodalton type IV collagenase forms a complex with a tissue inhibitor of metalloprotinases designated TIMP-2. *Proc. Natl Acad. Sci. USA*, 86, 8207–11.
213. Weiss, S.J. (1989) Tissue destruction by neutrophils. *N. Engl. J. Med.*, 320, 365–76.
214. Melcher, A.H. and Chan, J. (1981) Phagocytosis and digestion of collagen by gingival fibroblasts in vivo: a study of serial sections. *J. Ultrastruct. Res.*, 77, 1–36.
215. McGaw, W.T. and Ten Cate, A.R. (1983) A role for collagen phagocytosis by fibroblasts in scar remodelling: an ultrastructural stereological study. *J. Invest. Dermatol.*, 81, 375–8.
216. Everts, V.R., Hembrey, R.M., Reynolds, J.J. *et al.* (1989) Metalloproteinases are not involved in the phagocytosis of collagen fibrils by fibroblasts. *Matrix*, 9, 266–76.
217. Vidiik, A. (1982) Mechanical properties of parallel-fibred collagenous tissues, in *Biology of Collagen*, (eds A. Vidiik and J. Vuust), Academic Press, London, pp. 237–55.
218. Allain, J.C., Le Lous, M., Bazin, S. *et al.* (1978) Isometric tension developed during heating of collagenous tissues. Relationships with collagen crosslinking. *Biochim. Biophys. Acta*, 533, 147–55.
219. Le Lous, M., Allain, J.-C., Cohen-Solal, L. *et al.* (1983) Hydrothermal isometric tension curves from different connective tissues: role of collagen genetic types and non-collagenous components. *Connect. Tissue Res.*, 11, 199–206.
220. Huang, D., Chang, T., Aggarwal, A. *et al.* (1993) Mechanisms and dynamics of mechanical strengthening in ligament-equivalent fibroblast-populated collagen matrices. *Ann. Biomed. Eng.*, 21, 289–305.
221. Burleigh, M., Briggs, A., Lendon, C. *et al.* (1992) Collagen types I and III, collagen content, GAGs and mechanical strength of human atherosclerotic plaque caps: span-wise variations. *Atherosclerosis*, 96, 71–81.
222. Lendon, C., Davies, M., Richardson, P. *et al.* (1993) Testing of small connective tissue specimens for the determination of the mechanical behaviour of atherosclerotic plaques. *J. Biomed Eng.*, 15, 27–33.
223. Oxlund, H., Rasmussen, L.M., Reassen, T.T. *et al.* (1993) Increased aortic stiffness in patients with type 1(insulin-dependent) diabetes mellitus. *Diabetologia*, 32, 748–52.
224. Glagov, S., Zarins, C., Masawa, N. *et al.* (1993) Mechanical functional role of non-atherosclerotic intimal thickening. *Front. Med. Biol. Eng.*, 5, 37–43.
225. Sudhir, K., Wilson, E., Chatterjee, K. *et al.* (1993) Mechanical strain and collagen potentiate mitogenic activity of angiotensin-II in rat vascular smooth muscle cells. *J. Clin. Invest.*, 92, 3003–7.
226. Takeichi, S. (1984) An autopsy case of Marfan syndrome with histochemical studies on the cardiovascular system. *Tokushima J. Exp. Med.*, 31, 33–9.
227. Stehbens, W.E., Delahunt, B. and Hilless, A.D. (1989) Early berry aneurysm formation in Marfan's syndrome. *Surg. Neurol.*, 31, 200–2.
228. Becker, A.E. and van Mantgem, J.-P. (1975) The coronary arteries in Marfan's syndrome: a morphological study. *Am. J. Cardiol.*, 36, 315–21.
229. Simpson, C.F., Boucek, R.J. and Noble, N.L. (1980) Similarity of aortic pathology in Marfan's syndrome, copper deficiency in chicks and beta-aminoproprionitrile toxicity in turkeys. *Exp. Mol. Pathol.*, 32, 81–90.
230. Marlow, N., Gregg, J.E.M. and Qureshi, S.A. (1987) Mitral valve disease in Marfan's syndrome. *Arch. Dis. Child.*, 62, 960–2.
231. Roberts, W.C. and Honig, H.S. (1982) The spectrum of cardiovascular disease in the Marfan syndrome: a clinico-morphological study of 18 necropsy patients and comparison to 151 previously reported necropsy patients. *Am. Heart J.*, 104, 115–35.
232. Tsipouras, P., Borresen, A.-L., Bamforth, S. *et al.* (1986) Marfan syndrome: exclusion of genetic linkage to the COL1A2 gene. *Clin. Genet.*, 30, 428–32.
233. Dalgleish, R., Hawkins, J.R. and Keston, M. (1987) Exclusion of the alpha 2(I) and alpha 1(III) collagen genes as the mutant loci in a Marfan syndrome family. *J. Med. Genet.*, 24, 148–51.
234. Ogilvie, D.J., Wordswoth, B.P., Priestley, L.M. *et al.* (1987) Segregation of all four major fibrillar genes in the Marfan syndrome. *Am. J. Human Genet.*, 41, 1071–82.
235. Francomano, C.A., Streeten, E.A., Meyers, D.A. *et al.* (1988) Marfan syndrome: exclusion of genetic linkage to three major collaen genes. *Am. J. Med. Genet.*, 29, 457–62.
236. Kainulainen, K., Savolainen, A., Palotie, A. *et al.* (1990) Marfan syndrome: exclusion of genetic linkage to five genes coding for connective tissue components in the long arm of chromosome 2. *Hum. Genet.*, 84, 233–6.
237. Priest, R.E., Moinuddin, J.F. and Priest, J.H. (1973) Collagen of Marfan syndrome is abnormally soluble. *Nature*, 245, 264–6.
238. Boucek, R.J., Noble, N.L., Gunja-Smith, Z. *et al.* (1981) The Marfan syndrome: a deficiency in chemically stable collagen crosslinks. *N. Engl J. Med.*, 305, 988–91.
291. Pereyja, A.J., Abraham, P.A., Carnes, W.H. *et al.* (1985) Marfan's syndrome: structural, biochemical and mechanical studies of the aortic media. *J. Lab. Clin. Med.*, 106, 376–83.
240. Dietz, H.C., Cutting, G.R., Pyeritz, R.E. *et al.* (1991) Marfan syndrome caused by recurrent de novo missense mutation in the fibrillin gene. *Nature*, 352, 337–9.
241. Hollister, D.W., Godfrey, M., Sakai, L.Y. *et al.* (1990) Immunohistologic abnormalities of the microfibrillar-fiber system in the Marfan syndrome. *N. Engl J. Med.*, 323, 152–9.
242. Sykes, B. (1993) Marfan gene dissected. *Nature Genet.*, 3, 99–100.
243. Rosenbloom, J., Abrams, W.R. and Mecham, R. (1993) Extracellular matrix 4: the elastic fiber. *FASEB J.*, 7, 1208–18.
244. Boileau, C., Jondeau, G., Babron, M. *et al.* (1993) Autosomal dominant Marfan-like connective-tissue disorder with aortic dilation and skeletal anomalies not linked to the fibrillin genes. *Am. J. Hum. Genet.*, 53, 46–54.
245. Foster, K., Ferrell, R., King, U.L. *et al.* (1993) Description of a dinucleotide repeat polymorphism in the human elastin gene and its use to confirm assignment of the gene to chromosome 7. *Ann. Hum. Genet.*, 57, 87–96.
246. Pulkkinen, L., Kainulainen, K., Krusius, T. *et al.* (1990) Deficient expression of the gene coding for decorin in a lethal form of Marfan syndrome. *J. Biol. Chem.*, 265, 17780–5.
247. Serafini-Fracassini, A., Ventrella, G., Field, M.J. *et al.* (1981) Characterization of a structural glycoprotein from bovine ligamentum nuchae exhibiting dual amine oxidase activity. *Biochemistry*, 20, 5424–31.
248. Gibson, M.A., Kumaratilake, J.S. and Cleary, E.G. (1989) The protein components of the 12-nanometer microfibrils of elastic and non-elastic tissues. *J. Biol. Chem.*, 264, 4590–8.
249. Kobayashi, R., Tashima, Y., Masuda, H. *et al.* (1989) Isolation and characterization of a new 36-kDa microfibril-associated glycoprotein from porcine aorta. *J. Biol. Chem.*, 264, 17437–44.
250. Bressan, G.M., Castellani, I., Colombatti, A. *et al.* (1983) Isolation and characterization of a 115,000 Da matrix-associated glycoprotein from chick aorta. *J. Biol. Chem*, 258, 13262–7.
251. Gibson, M.A., Sandberg, L.B. Grosso, L.E. *et al.* (1991) Complementary DNA cloning establishes microfibril-associated glycoprotein (MAGP) to be a discrete component of the elastin-associated microfibrils. *J. Biol. Chem.*, 266, 7596–601.
252. Horrigan, S.K., Rich, C.B., Streeten, B.W. *et al.* (1992) Characterization of an associated microfibril protein through recombinant DNA techniques. *J. Biol. Chem.*, 267, 10087–95.
253. Pan, T.C., Sasaki, T., Zhang, R.Z. *et al.* (1993) Structure and expression of fibulin-2, a novel extracellular matrix protein with multiple EGF-like repeats and consensus motifs for calcium binding. *J. Cell Biol.*, 123, 1269–77.
254. McKusick, V.A. (1972) The Ehlers–Danlos syndrome, in *Heritable Disorders of Connective Tissue*, 4th edn, C.V. Mosby, St Louis, pp. 292–371.
255. Steinmann, B., Royce, P.M. and Superti-Furga, A. (1993) The Ehlers–Danlos syndrome, in *Connective Tissue and its Heritable Disorders*, (eds P.M. Royce and B. Steinmann), Wiley-Liss, New York, pp. 351–407.
256. Beighton, P., De Paepe, A., Danks, D. *et al.* (1988) International nosology of heritable disorders of connective tissue, Berlin, 1986. *Am. J. Med. Genet.*, 29, 581–94.
257. Tromp, G., Kuivaniemi, H., Shikata, H. *et al.* (1989) A single base mutation that substitutes serine for glycine 790 of the alpha 1(III) chain of type III procollagen exposes an arginine and causes Ehlers–Danlos

syndrome IV. *J. Biol. Chem.*, **264**, 1349–52.
258. Tromp, G., Kuivaniemi, H., Stolle, C. *et al.* (1989) Single base mutation in the type III procollagen gene that converts the coden for glycine 883 to aspartate in a mild variant of Ehlers–Danlos syndrome IV. *J. Biol. Chem.*, **264**, 19313–7.
259. De Paepe, A., Nuytinck, L., Nicholls, A. *et al.* (1992) Study of a type III collagen protein defect in a patient with ecchymotic EDS: importance of the analysis of non-cutaneous connective tissues, in *Genetics of Hematological Disorders*, (eds C. Bartsocas and D. Loukopoulos), Hemisphere, Washington, pp. 267–74.
260. Kontuassari, S., Tromp, G., Kuivaniemi, H. *et al.* (1990) A mutation in the gene for type III procollagen (COL3A1) in a family with aortic aneurysms. *J. Clin. Invest.*, **86**, 1465–73.
261. Kontusaari, S., Tromp, G., Kuivaniemi, H. *et al.* (1992) Substitution of aspartate for glycine 1018 in the type III procollagen (COL3A1) gene causes type IV Ehlers–Danlos syndrome: the mutated allele is present in most blood leukocytes of the asymptomatic and mosaic mother. *Am. J. Hum. Genet.*, **51**, 497–507.
262. Johnson, P.H., Richards, A.J., Pope, F.M. *et al.* (1992) A COL3A1 glycine 1006 to glutamic acid substitution in a patient with Ehlers–Danlos syndrome type IV detected by denaturing gradient gel electrophoresis. *J. Inherit. Metab. Dis.*, **15**, 426–30.
263. Superti-Furga, A., Steinmann, B., Ramirez, F. *et al.* (1989) Molecular defects of type III procollagen in Ehlers-Danlos syndrome. *Hum. Gnenet.*, **82**, 104–8.
264. McGookey, D.J., Smith, A.C.M., Waldstein, G. *et al.* (1989) Mosaicism for a deletion in one of the type III collagen alleles indicates that the deletion occurred after identification of cells for recruitment to different cell lineages early in human development. *Am. J. Hum. Genet.*, **45**, A206.
265. Sillence, D.O., Chiodo, A.A., Campbell, P.E. *et al.* (1991) Ehlers–Danlos syndrome type IV: phenotypic consequences of a splicing mutation in one COL3A1 allele. *J. Med. Genet.*, **28**, 840–5.
266. Kuivaniemi, H., Kontusaari, S., Tromp, G. *et al.* (1990) Identical G(+1) to A mutation in three different introns of the type III procollagen gene (COL3A1) produce different patterns of RNA splicing in three variants of Ehlers–Danlos syndrome IV. An explanation for exon skipping with some mutations and not others. *J. Biol. Chem.*, **265**, 12067–74.
267. Thakker-Varia, S., Anderson, D., Kuivaniemi, H. *et al.* (1990) An exon deletion in type III procollagen mRNA is associated with intracellular degradation of the abnormal protein in a patient with Ehlers–Danlos syndrome type IV. *Matrix*, **10**, 249–50.
268. Crowther, M.A., Lach, B., Dunmore, P.J. *et al.* (1991) Vascular collagen fibril morphology in type IV Ehlers–Danlos syndrome. *Connect. Tissue Res.*, **25**, 209–17.
269. Steinmann, B., Superti-Furga, A., Joller-Jemelka, H. *et al.* (1989) Ehlers–Danlos syndrome type IV: a subset of patients distinguished by low serum levels of the amino-terminal propeptide of type III procollagen. *Am. J. Med. Genet.*, **34**, 68–71.
270. Majamaa, K., Savolainen, E.-R. and Myllyla, V.V. (1992) Synthesis of structurally unstable type III procollagen in patients with cerebral artery aneurysm. *Biochim. Biophys. Acta*, **1138**, 191–6.
271. Majamaa, K. and Myllyla, V.V. (1993) A disorder of collagen biosynthesis in patients with cerebral artery aneurysm. *Biochim. Biophys. Acta*, **1225**, 48–52.
272. Di Ferrante, N., Leachman, R.D., Angelini, P. *et al.* (1975) Lysyl oxidase deficiency in Ehlers–Danlos syndrome type V. *Connect. Tissue Res.*, **5**, 49–53.
273. Seigel, R.C., Black, C.M. and Bailey, A.J. (1979) Crosslinking of collagen in the X-linked Ehlers–Danlos type V. *Biochem. Biophys. Res. Commun.*, **88**, 281–7.
274. Pinnell, S.R., Krane, S.M., Kenzora, J.E. *et al.* (1972) A heritable disorder of connective tissue. Hydroxylysine-deficient collagen disease. *N. Engl J. Med.*, **286**, 1013–20.
275. McKusick, V.A. (1983) *Mendelian Inheritance in Man. Catalogs of Autosomal Dominant, Autosomal Recessive and X-linked Phenotypes*, 6th edn, Johns Hopkins University Press, Baltimore.
276. Hautala, T., Byers, M.G., Eddy, R.L. *et al.* (1992) Cloning of human lysyl hydroxylase: complete cDNA-derived amino acid sequence and assignment of the gene (PLOD) to chromosome 1p36.2–p36.2. *Genomics*, **13**, 62–69.
277. Hyland, J., Ala-Kokko, L., Royce, P. *et al.* (1992) A homozygous stop codon in the lysyl hydroxylase gene in two siblings with Ehlers–Danlos syndrome type IV. *Nature Genet.*, **2**, 228–31.
278. Hautala, T., Heikkinen, J., Kivirikko, K.I. *et al.* (1993) A large duplication in the gene for lysyl hydroxylase accounts for the type VI variant of Ehlers–Danlos syndrome in two siblings. *Genomics*, **15**, 399–404.
279. Eyre, D.R., Shapiro, F.D. and Aldridge, J.F. (1985) A heterozygous collagen defect in a variant of the Ehlers–Danlos syndrome type VII. Evidence for a deleted amino-telopeptide domain in the pro-alpha 2(I) chain. *J. Biol. Chem.*, **260**, 11322–9.
280. Cole, W.G., Evans, R. and Sillence, D.O. (1987) The clinical features of Ehlers–Danlos syndrome type VII due to a deletion of 24 amino acids from the pro alpha 1(I) chain of type I procollagen. *J. Med. Genet.*, **24**, 698–701.
281. Smith, L., Wertelecki, W., Milstone, L. *et al.* (1992) Human dermatosparaxis: a form of Ehlers–Danlos syndrome that results from failure to remove the amino-terminal propeptide of type I procollagen. *Am. J. Hum. Genet.*, **51**, 235–44.
282. Wertelecki, W., Smith, L. and Byers, P. (1992) Initial observations of human dermatosparaxis: Ehlers–Danlos syndrome type VIIC. *J. Pediatr.*, **121**, 558–64.
283. Lichtenstein, J.R., Martin, G.R., Kohn, L.D. *et al.* (1973) Defect in conversion of procollagen to collagen in a form of Ehlers–Danlos syndrome. *Science*, **182**, 298–330.
284. Bailey, A.J. and Lapiere, C.M. (1973) Effect of an additional peptide extension of the N-terminus of collagen from dermatosparatic calves on the cross-linking of the collagen fibres. *Eur. J. Biochem.*, **34**, 91–6.
285. Uitto, J. and Shamban, A. (1987) Heritable skin diseases with molecular defects in collagen or elastin. *Dermatol. Clin.*, **5**, 63–84.
286. Olsen, D., Fazio, M., Shamban, A. *et al.* (1988) Cutis laxa: reduced elastin gene expression in skin fibroblast cultures as determined by hybridizations with a homologous cDNA and an exon 1-specific oligonucleotide. *J. Biol. Chem.*, **263**, 6465–7.
287. Sephel, G., Byers, P., Holbrook, K. *et al.* (1989) Heterogeneity of elastin expression in cutis laxa fibroblast strains. *J. Invest. Dermatol.*, **93**, 147–53.
288. Fazio, M., Olsen, D. and Uitto, J. (1989) Skin aging: lessons from cutis laxa and elastoderma. *Cutis*, **43**, 437–44.
289. Crawford, S.W., Featherstone, J.A., Holbrook, K. *et al.* (1985) Characterization of a type VI collagen-related Mr-140 000 protein from cutis laxa fibroblasts in culture. *Biochem. J.*, **227**, 491–502.
290. Rae, V. and Falanga, V. (1989) Wrinkling due to mid-dermal elastolysis. Report of a case and review of the literature. *Arch. Dermatol.*, **125**, 950–1.
291. Brod, B., Rabkin, M., Rhodes, A. *et al.* (1992) Mid-dermal elastolysis with inflammation. *J. Am. Acad. Dermatol.*, **26**, 882–4.
292. Ortel, B., Rappersberger, K. and Konrad, K. (1992) Mid-dermal elastolysis in an elderly man with evidence of elastic fiber phagocytosis. *Arch. Dermatol.*, **128**, 88–90.
293. Bolognia, J. and Braverman, I. (1992) Pseudoxanthoma-elasticum-like skin changes induced by penicillamine. *Dermatology*, **184**, 12–18.
294. Narron, G., Zec, N., Neves, R. *et al.* (1992) Penicillamine-induced pseudoxanthoma elasticum-like skin change requiring rhytidectomy. *Ann. Plast. Surg.*, **29**, 367–70.
295. Burge, S. and Ryan, T. (1988) Penicillamine-induced pseudoxanthoma elasticum in a patient with rheumatiod arthritis. *Clin. Exp. Dermatol.*, **13**, 255–8.
296. Nelder, K.H. (1993) Pseudoxanthoma elasticum, in *Connective Tissue and its Heritable Disorders*, (eds P.M. Royce and B. Steinmann), Wiley-Liss, New York, pp. 425–36.
297. Lebwohl, M., Schwartz, E., Lemlich, G. *et al.* (1993) Abnormalities of connective tissue components in lesional and non-lesional tissue of patients with pseudoxanthoma elasticum. *Arch. Dermatol. Res.*, **285**, 121–6.
298. Longas, M.O., Wisch, P., Lebwohl, M.G. *et al.* (1986) Glycosaminoglycan of skin and urine in pseudoxanthoma elasticum: evidence for chondroitin-6-sulphate alterations. *Clin. Chim. Acta*, **155**, 227–36.
299. Walker, E., Frederickson, R. and Mayes, M. (1989) The mineralization of elastic fibers and alterations of extracellular matrix in pseudoxanthoma elasticum. Ultrastructure, immunocytochemistry, and X-ray analysis. *Arch. Dermatol.*, **125**, 70–6.
300. Tizzo-Costa, R., Baccarani-Contri, M., Cingi, M.R. *et al.* (1988) Pseudoxanthoma elasticum (PXE): ultrastructural and biochemical study on proteoglycan and proteoglycan-associated material produced by skin fibroblasts in vitro. *Coll. Relat. Res.*, **8**, 49–64.
301. Dietz, H.C., McIntosh, I., Sakai, L.Y. *et al.* (1993) Four novel FBN1 mutations: significance for mutant transcript level and EGF-like domain calcium binding in the pathogenesis of Marfan syndrome. *Genomics*, **17**, 468–75.
302. Danks, D.M. (1988) Copper deficiency in humans. *Ann. Rev. Nutr.*, **8**, 235–57.
303. Klevay, L.M. (1983) Copper and ischaemic heart disease. *Biol. Trace Elem. Res.*, **5**, 245–55.
304. Bronson, R., Calaman, S., Traish, A. *et al.* (1987) Stimulation of lysyl oxidase (EC 1.4.3.13) activity by testosterone and characterization of androgen receptors in cultured calf aorta smooth-muscle cells. *Biochem. J.*, **244**, 317–23.
305. Trackman, P.C., Pratt, A.M., Wolanski, A. *et al.* (1990) Cloning of rat aorta lysyl oxidase cDNA: complete codons and predicted amino acid sequence. *Biochemistry*, **29**, 4863–70.
306. Trackman, P.C., Pratt, A.M., Wolanski, A. *et al.* (1991) Cloning of rat aorta lysyl oxidase cDNA: complete codons and predicted amino acid sequence. *Biochemistry*, **30**, 8282.
307. Svinarich, D.M., Twomey, T.T., Macauley, S.P. *et al.* (1992) Characterization of the human lysyl oxidase gene locus. *J. Biol. Chem.*, **267**, 14382–7.
308. Kagan, H.M. and Trackman, P.C. (1991) Properties and function of lysyl oxidase. *Am. J. Respir. Cell. Mol. Biol.*, **5**, 206–10.
309. Simpson, C.F. and Harms, R.H. (1964) Pathology of the aorta of chicks fed a copper deficient diet. *Exp. Mol. Pathol.*, **3**, 390–400.

310. Hunsaker, H.A., Morita, M. and Allen, K.G.D. (1984) Marginal copper deficiency in rats. Aortal morphology of elastin and cholesterol values in first generation adult males. *Atherosclerosis*, **51**, 1–19.
311. Carlton, W.W. and Henderson, W. (1963) Cardiovascular lesions in experimental copper deficiency in chickens. *J. Nutr.*, **81**, 200–8.
312. O'Dell, B.L., Hardwick, B.C., Reynolds, G. *et al.* (1961) Connective tissue defects in the chick resulting from copper deficiency. *Proc. Soc. Exp. Biol. Med.*, **108**, 402–6.
313. Farquharson, C. and Robins, S.P. (1991) Immunolocalization of collagen types I, III and IV, elastin and fibronectin in copper-deficient rats. *J. Comp. Pathol.*, **104**, 245–55.
314. Coulson, W.F. and Carnes, W.H. (1963) Cardiovascular studies of copper deficient swine. V. The histogenesis of the coronary lesions. *Amer. J. Pathol.*, **43**, 945–54.
315. Stemmer, K.L., Petering, H.G., Murthy, L. *et al.* (1985) Copper deficiency effects on cardiovascular system and lipid metabolism in proteins and zinc. *Ann. Nutr. Metab.*, **29**, 332–47.
316. Radhakrishnamurthy, B., Ruiz, H., Dalferes, E.R. *et al.* (1989) Composition of proteoglycans in the aortas of copper-deficient rats. *Proc. Soc. Exp. Biol. Med.*, **190**, 98–104.
317. Fell, B.F., Farmer, L.J., Farquharson, C. *et al.* (1985) Observations on the pancreas of cattle deficient in copper. *J. Comp. Pathol.*, **95**, 573–90.
318. Fell, B.F., Farquharson, C. and Riddoch, G.I. (1987) Kidney lesions in copper deficient rats. *J. Comp. Pathol.*, **97**, 187–96.
319. Kitano, S. (1980) Membrane and contractile properties of rat vascular tissue in copper deficient conditions. *Circ. Res.*, **46**, 681–9.
320. Tinker, D., Geller, J., Romero, N. *et al.* (1986) Tropoelastin production and tropoelastin messenger RNA activity. Relationship to crosslinking in chick aorta. *Biochem. J.*, **236**, 17–23.
321. O'Dell, B.L., Bird, D.W., Ruggles, D.L. *et al.* (1966) Composition of aortic tissue from copper deficient chicks. *J. Nutr.*, **88**, 9–14.
322. Weissman, N., Shields, G.S. and Carnes, W.H. (1963) Cardiovascular studies on copper deficient swine. IV. Content and solubility of the aortic elastin, collagen and hexosamine. *J. Biol. Chem.*, **238**, 3115–18.
323. Farquharson, C., Duncan, A. and Robins, S.P. (1989) The effect of copper deficiency on the pyridinium crosslinks of mature collagen in the rat skeleton and cardiovascular sysytem. *Proc. Soc. Exp. Biol. Med.*, **192**, 166–71.
324. Rowe, D.W., McGoodwin, E.B., Martin, G.R. *et al.* (1977) Decreased lysyl oxidase activity in the aneurysm-prone, mottled mouse. *J. Biol. Chem.*, **252**, 939–42.
325. Pinnell, S.R. and Martin, G.R. (1968) The crosslinking of collagen and elastin: enzymatic conversion of lysine in peptide linkage to alpha-aminoadipic-delta-semialdehyde (allysine) by an extract from bone. *Proc. Natl Acad. Sci.*, **61**, 707–18.
326. Akita, M., Lee, S. and Kaneko, K. (1992) Electron microscopic observations of elastic fibres in the lung and aorta of tight-skin and beta-aminopropionitrile-fed mice. *Histol. Histopathol.*, **7**, 39–45.
327. Steinberg, D. (1987) Current theories of the pathogenesis of atherosclerosis, in *Hypercholesterolemia and Atherosclerosis. Pathogenesis and Prevention*, (eds D. Steinberg and J.M. Olefsky), Churchill Livingstone, New York, pp. 5–17.
328. Badimon, J., Fuster, V., Chesebro, J. *et al.* (1993) Coronary atherosclerosis. A multifactorial disease. *Circulation*, **87**(II), 3–16.
329. Kuivaniemi, H., Tromp, G. and Prockop, D.J. (1991) Mutations in collagen genes: causes of rare and some more common disease. *FASEB J.*, **3**, 2052–60.
330. McCullagh, K.G. and Balian, G. (1975) Collagen characterization and cell transformation in human atherosclerosis: *Nature*, **258**, 73–5.
331. Barnes, M.J. (1985) Collagen in atherosclerosis. *Collagen Rel. Res.*, **5**, 65–97.
332. Murata, K., Kotake, C. and Motoyama, T. (1987) Collagen species in human aorta with special reference to basement membrane associated collagens in the intima and media and their alterations with atherosclerosis. *Artery*, **14**, 229–37.
333. Kittelberger, R., Davis, P.F. and Stehbens, W.E. (1990) Type VI collagen in experimental atherosclerosis. *Experientia*, **46**, 264–7.
334. Mayne, R. (1986) Collagenous proteins of blood vessels. *Arteriosclerosis*, **6**, 585–93.
335. Wagner, W.D., Salisbury, B.G.J. and Rowe, H.A. (1986) A proposed structure of chondroitin 6-sulphate proteoglycans of human normal aorta and adjacent atherosclerotic plaque. *Arteriosclerosis*, **6**, 407–17.
336. Berenson, G.S., Radhakrishnamurthy, B., Srinivasan, S.R. *et al.* (1988) Arterial wall injury and proteoglycan changes in atherosclerosis. *Arch. Pathol. Lab. Med.*, **112**, 1002–10.
337. Camejo, G., Linden, T., Olsson, U. *et al.* (1989) Binding parameters and concentration modulate formation of complexes between LDL and arterial proteoglycans in serum. *Atherosclerosis*, **79**, 121–8.
338. Srinivasan, S.R., Radhakrishnamurthy, B., Vijayagopal, P. *et al.* (1991) Proteoglycans, lipoproteins, and atherosclerosis. *Adv. Exp. Med. Biol.*, **285**, 373–81.
339. Berenson, G.S., Radhakrishnamurthy, B., Srinivasan, S.R. *et al.* (1985) Proteoglycans and potential mechanisms related to atherosclerosis. *Ann. N.Y. Acad. Sci.*, **254**, 69–78.
340. Cherchi, G.M., Coinu, R., Demuro, P. *et al.* (1990) Structural and functional modifications of human aorta proteoglycans in atherosclerosis. *Matrix*, **10**, 362–72.
341. Wight, T.N. (1985) Proteoglycans in pathological conditions: atherosclerosis. *Fed. Proc.*, **44**, 381–5.
342. Merrilees, M.J., Campbell, J.H., Spanidies, E. *et al.* (1990) Glycosaminoglycan synthesis by smooth muscle cells of differing phenotype and their response to endothelial cell conditioned medium. *Atheroclerosis*, **81**, 245–53.
343. Alavi, M.Z., Wasty, F., Li, Z. *et al.* (1992) Enhanced incorporation of [14C]glucosamine into glycosaminoglycans of aortic neointima of balloon-injured and cholesterol-fed rabbits in vitro. *Atherosclerosis*, **95**, 59–67.
344. Merrilees, M.J. and Beaumont, B. (1993) Structural heterogeneity of the diffuse intimal thickening and correlation with distribution of TGF-beta 1. *J. Vasc. Res.*, **30**, 293–302.
345. Loskutoff, D.J., Sawdey, M. and Mimuro, J. (1989) Type 1 plasminogen activator inhibitor. *Prog. Hemostasis Thromb.*, **9**, 87–115.
346. Loskutoff, D.J. (1991) Regulation of PAI-1 gene expression. *Fibrinolysis*, **5**, 197–206.
347. Sawa, H., Sobel, B.E. and Fujii, S. (1993) Potentiation by hypercholesterolemia of the induction of aortic intramural synthesis of plasminogen activator inhibitor type 1 by endothelial injury. *Circ. Res.*, **73**, 671–80.
348. Nathan, C.F. (1987) Secretory products of macrophages. *J. Clin. Invest.*, **79**, 319–26.
349. Liptay, M.J., Parks, W.C., Mecham, R.P. *et al.* (1993) Neointimal macrophages colocalize with extracellular matrix gene expression in human atherosclerotic pulmonary arteries. *J. Clin. Invest.*, **91**, 588–94.

5 PATHOLOGY OF BLOOD VESSELS IN METABOLIC DISORDERS

Ramiah Subramanian, Renu Virmani and Victor J. Ferrans

Vascular abnormalities are important clinical and pathologic manifestations of many metabolic diseases. Vascular anatomic changes in metabolic diseases can consist of:

1. deposits of storage materials, which can involve either the vascular cells (endothelial cells, smooth muscle cells, other mesenchymal cells and neural elements) or the interstitium;
2. abnormalities in the composition of extracellular elements of vascular connective tissue, leading to either vascular thickening and luminal narrowing or to thinning, dilatation and formation of aneurysms;
3. proliferation of intimal smooth muscle cells;
4. alterations related to the induction or acceleration of atherosclerosis, which can involve the aorta and elastic or muscular arteries as well as the pulmonary circulation and the microcirculation in various organs.

In this chapter, vascular anatomic abnormalities related to metabolic diseases are reviewed according to their underlying biochemical defect. Disorders of carbohydrate metabolism are reviewed first, followed by diseases of lipid metabolism, amino acid and protein metabolism and mineral and trace element metabolism.

5.1 Diseases of carbohydrate metabolism

Vascular lesions in diseases of carbohydrate metabolism are reviewed under the following five categories: the glycogen storage diseases; the mucopolysaccharidoses; the mucolipidoses; the hyperoxalurias; and diabetes mellitus.

5.1.1 GLYCOGEN STORAGE DISEASES

None of the 12 types of glycogen storage disease is associated with clinically significant vascular disease. However, vascular anatomic lesions in type II glycogen storage disease (deficiency of acid maltase, a lysosomal enzyme) consist of deposits of morphologically and biochemically normal glycogen particles within lysosomes of endothelial and vascular smooth muscle cells (V.J. Ferrans, unpublished observations).

5.1.2 THE MUCOPOLYSACCHARIDOSES

The mucopolysaccharidoses (MPS) are characterized by deficiencies in lysosomal enzymes involved in degrading various acid mucopolysaccharides (AMP), compounds which presently are also referred to as proteoglycans. The consequences of such deficiencies are twofold: intracellular accumulations of AMP within lysosomes and complex abnormalities in the organization of connective tissue. Various combinations of these effects account for the different clinical manifestations of these disorders including storage phenomena in liver, central nervous system, cornea and other ocular tissues, musculoskeletal deformities and thickening of cardiac valves and blood vessels.

MPS II (Hunter syndrome) is transmitted as a sex-linked recessive disorder; the other types of MPS are transmitted as autosomal recessive disorders [1]. The term MPS V is no longer in use, as patients with this disorder have been reclassified as having MPS I-S. Genetic forms of MPS exist in animals: MPS I and VI in cats and MPS VII in dogs and mice.

(a) Mucopolysaccharidosis I

Three clinical subtypes of MPS I (α-L-iduronidase deficiency) occur: the Hurler syndrome (MPS I-H), the Scheie syndrome (MPS I-S) and the Hurler–Scheie syndrome (MPS I-HS).

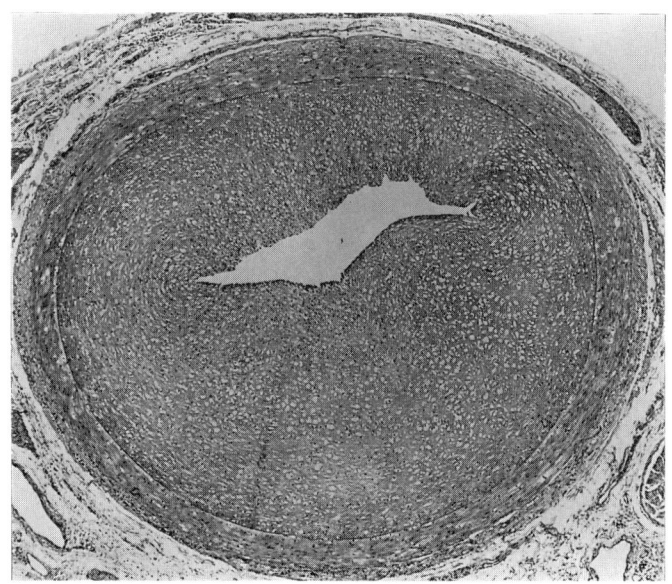

Figure 5.1 Left circumflex coronary artery of child with Hurler syndrome, showing marked luminal narrowing, caused by severe intimal thickening due to proliferation of vacuolated smooth muscle cells. The media is thin and is clearly demarcated from the intima by the internal elastic lamina. (Movat pentachrome stain.)

Patients with MPS I-H present with lumbar lordosis, stiffness of joints, hepatosplenomegaly short stature, clouding of the corneas, mental retardation, coarse facies, umbilical hernias, macroglossia and claw hand deformities.

Cardiovascular manifestations include myocardial involvement, endocardial fibroelastosis [2], pulmonary hypertension and valvular dysfunction, namely mitral and aortic valve regurgitation and asymmetric septal hypertrophy. Cardiovascular anatomic lesions in the Hurler syndrome involve the valves, endocardium, myocardium, coronary arteries and large systemic arteries [3-6] (Figures 5.1 and 5.2). The aortic and mitral valves are thickened and can undergo calcification, causing severe stenosis, in the Scheie syndrome. One patient with this syndrome who underwent mitral and aortic valve replacement had normal coronary arteries on cardiac catheterization [7].

In a study of 22 patients with MPS types I-IV [8], echocardiographic and ECG findings suggested an infiltrative cardiomyopathy owing to AMP deposition rather than to hypertrophy. Cardiac failure in MPS I-H and in other MPS types may be multifactorial and may reflect the coexistence of myocardial infiltration by AMP, valvular heart disease, endocardial thickening and myocardial ischemia secondary to coronary luminal narrowing.

The cardiac myocytes in MPS I-H contain AMP deposits in the form of clear, membrane-bound vacuoles, and stacks of parallel, dense lamellae presumed to represent glycolipids. The clear vacuoles are similar to those present in other types of MPS and represent sites from which AMP, which are extremely soluble, have dissolved during the fixation and processing of tissue for microscopic study. The biochemical defects leading to the storage of glycolipid material in the form of electron

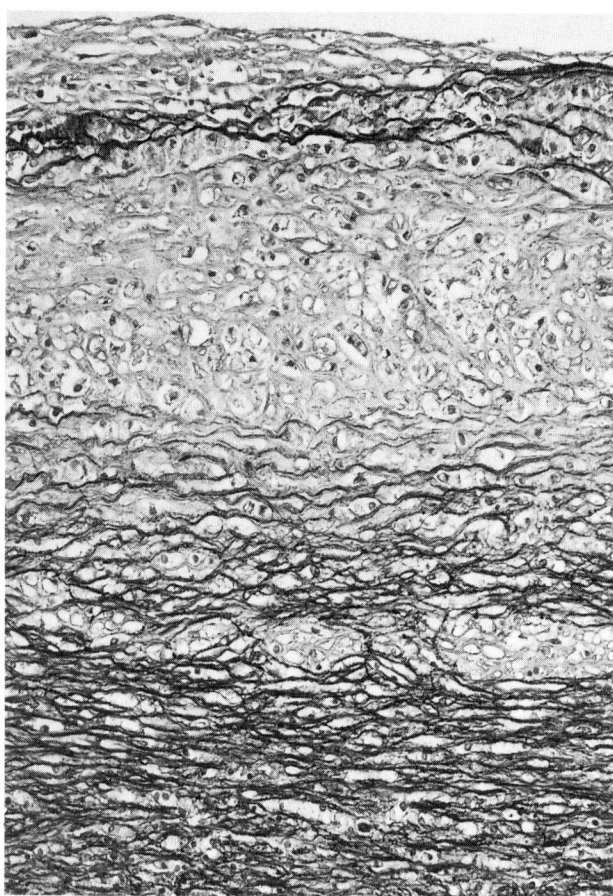

Figure 5.2 Aorta from patient with the Hurler syndrome. Numerous Hurler cells with large clear cytoplasm are present in the vascular wall. (Movat pentachrome stain.)

dense lamellae, which also have been observed in other MPS, have not been completely elucidated.

The myocardial interstitium and the cardiac valves contain large connective tissue cells (Hurler cells) that are filled with clear, membrane-bound vacuoles which are considered to represent sites of deposition of AMP. In addition to these cells small granular cells are also present and contain membrane-bound deposits of moderately dense amorphous material in which fragments of collagen fibrils are embedded [5].

The aorta and large systemic arteries have raised intimal plaques which are composed of Hurler cells, granular cells and abundant fibrous tissue. The Hurler syndrome is the cause of the most severe coronary arterial narrowing (Figure 5.1) in childhood [9]. However, myocardial infarction has not been noted in this syndrome. The large extramural coronary arteries are rigid and thickened, with severe, concentric luminal narrowing [10]. Coronary artery involvement was noted angiographically in five of seven children with the Hurler syndrome. There were either mild irregularities of the left main coronary artery or its first-order branches, or marked paucity of third-order branching of either the right or the left coronary artery [11]. In an autopsy study of six children with the Hurler syndrome, all major coronary arteries were found to have luminal narrowing of 76–100% in cross-sectional area [9]; 71% of the 5 mm-long segments studied had coronary narrowing exceeding 75%. The extent of the coronary narrowing is particularly noteworthy in view of the young age of the patients (mean, 9 years; range, 3–16 years) and the absence of clinical evidence of myocardial ischemia in all six patients.

The severe luminal narrowing of the large, extramural coronary arteries is caused primarily by thickening of the intima, which contains numerous smooth muscle cells, few Hurler cells and increased amounts of collagen [5,12] (Figure 5.1). Hurler cells are also found in the medial layers of these vessels and in some of the intramural coronary arteries. The intimal smooth muscle cells of large coronary arteries contain numerous clear vacuoles, a few lamellar bodies and only peripherally located contractile elements, and they have thickened basement membranes. The number of lamellar and electron-lucent cytoplasmic inclusions is larger in intimal than in medial smooth muscle cells. The clear cells and smooth muscle cells are surrounded by dense bundles of collagen of normal size and periodicity. The interstitial space also contains collagen, large deposits of basement membrane-like material, electron-dense granules and fine spicules of AMP [5,10].

The coronary artery lesions in adults with atherosclerosis differ from those in children with the Hurler syndrome. In the latter, these lesions tend to be concentric with central lumina. The lesions in the aorta (Figure 5.2) and peripheral arteries are less cellular and more fibrotic than those in the coronary vessels and resemble fibrous atherosclerotic plaques, but differ from the latter in that they contain a small number of Hurler cells which are similar to those typically found in various other tissues of patients with the Hurler syndrome [12]. Eight children with MPS I studied at one institution developed hypertension [13]. Five of these children also exhibited aortic coarctation. Important clinical and radiological findings were noted in these patients. The ascending aorta in one patient showed supravalvular stenosis and post-stenotic dilatation. Irregular wall lesions were present in the aortic arch in two patients. The descending thoracic aorta showed asymmetric wall lesions in three patients, with occlusion and irregularity of multiple intercostal arteries. All children had involvement of the abdominal aorta, consisting of multiple minor asymmetric wall lesions and/or abrupt concentric narrowing. Two patients had occlusion of lumbar arteries. In three patients, the major visceral arteries, including the celiac, superior and inferior mesenteric and renal arteries, had stenosis of their origins and/or irregular wall lesions in peripheral branches. Narrowing of the iliac arteries was seen in three patients. Autopsy in one patient showed diffuse narrowing of the coronary arteries. Yellowish streaks were noted on the intimal surface of the ascending aorta just above the aortic valve. On microscopic examination, AMP had expanded the intima of the coronary arteries; foamy macrophages and myointimal cells were present within the aortic intima.

A variant form of MPS I has been described in which α-L-iduronidase deficiency was noted in five patients who did not have the typical Hurler or Scheie phenotype [14]. No information was provided concerning vascular involvement in these patients.

Histochemical and electron microscopic studies of the brain and leptomeninges containing large blood vessels from seven patients with MPS I-H, I-S, II, and IIIA showed marked increases in mesenchymal elements and the generalized presence of characteristic lesions around cerebral veins and arteries [15]. The periadventitial spaces were greatly distended and filled with viscous fluid. Numerous mononuclear cells containing large cytoplasmic vacuoles which stained positively for AMP were also present.

Chan et al. [16] performed light and electron microscopic studies on the eyes of two patients with MPS I-H. They observed numerous fine fibrillogranular inclusions in a variety of cell types, including the endothelium and pericytes of different ocular tissues.

(b) Mucopolysaccharidosis II

MPS II (Hunter syndrome) is characterized by a deficiency of iduronate-2-sulfatase. Patients have stiff joints, short stature, coarse facial features and deafness.

Mental retardation is slow in onset and corneal clouding does not occur. The disease may range from clinically mild, with survival to adulthood, to severe, with death in the juvenile period. Cardiovascular lesions are less severe than those in MPS I-H. Increased diameter of the coronary arteries was noted on echocardiographic study in three patients with the Hunter syndrome as well as in one patient with the Scheie syndrome, one patient with the Sanfilippo syndrome and one with Maroteaux–Lamy syndrome [17]. In contrast one patient had thickening of the mitral, tricuspid and aortic valves but not of the coronary arteries and the aorta [18]. The aorta and the main coronary arteries also were normal at autopsy in a 19-year-old boy who had shown typical features of MPS II [18]. Coronary arterial lumina were widely patent in a 30-year-old male with MPS II and severe aortic stenosis and systemic lupus erythematosus [19]. Thickening of the cerebral arteries was noted at autopsy in a 19-year-old patient [20].

(c) Mucopolysaccharidosis III

Four types of MPS III (Sanfilippo syndrome) are recognized, which differ in enzymatic defect: deficiency of heparin sulfatase in type A, of N-acetyl-α-D-glucosaminidase in type B, of acetyl-COA:α-glucosaminide N-acetyltransferase in type C and of N-acetylglucosamine-6-sulfatase in type D. These subtypes are not clinically distinguishable. Manifestations of the disease are variable and include mental retardation, mild skeletal changes and usually no corneal clouding. Mitral valvular disease has been described in patients with type A [21,22]. Reports of type A did not describe coronary arterial pathology [21–23]. The aorta was normal in one patient [21] and showed minor changes in another [23]. One patient had subendothelial deposits of periodic acid-Schiff-positive material in small splenic arteries [21]. The significance of these deposits is unclear. Necropsy in a patient with biochemically proven type B showed slightly sclerotic aorta and coronary arteries [24]. Medial smooth muscle cells of systemic arteries were vacuolated and areas of intimal thickening in large and medium-sized arteries also contained vacuolated cells. Ultrastructural studies showed that some of the vacuoles in the clear cells were electron-lucent while others were filled with laminated osmiophilic material. Light and electron microscopic studies of the eyes of patients with MPS III type B revealed cytoplasmic, single membrane-bound vacuoles containing material in virtually every ocular tissue including endothelium [25].

(d) Mucopolysaccharidosis IV

Two subtypes of MPS IV (Morquio syndrome) are recognized which differ in the enzymatic defect: galactose-6-sulfatase in type A and β-D-galactosidase in type B. Manifestations of MPS IV include genu valgum, short trunk, prominent sternum and a short neck. Clouding of the corneas occurs late and progressive deafness is invariable. Aortic regurgitation has been noted clinically. Calcification of the pulmonary and aortic valve rings has been reported. Echocardiographic abnormalities found in MPS IV include thickening of the mitral and aortic valves, ventricular hypertrophy and asymmetric septal hypertrophy [26,27]. Thickening of the aorta, pulmonary trunk and coronary arteries has been noted [28,29]. The coronary arteries can be significantly narrowed due to prominent intimal sclerosis. Ultrastructural examination of the coronary arteries of a 15-year-old boy with Morquio syndrome revealed numerous intimal smooth muscle cells with vacuoles consistent with lysosomes. This was associated with marked deposition of collagen, elastin and basement membrane material [28].

(e) Mucopolysaccharidosis VI

MPS VI (Maroteaux–Lamy syndrome), caused by deficiency of N-acetylgalactosamine-4-sulfatase exists in at least three closely related forms. Growth retardation is prominent by 2 years of age. Coarsening of facial features is evident and corneal clouding is massive and striking. Aortic stenosis and regurgitation are the predominant lesions noted clinically. Although mitral and aortic valve involvement requiring double valvular replacement has been observed [30], we are not aware of detailed description of the pathology of the vascular system in MPS VI.

(f) Mucopolysaccharidosis VII

MPS VII (Sly syndrome) is caused by deficiency of β-glucuronidase. The clinical picture varies from a rapidly progressive infantile form, with severe mental retardation, skeletal deformities, stiff joints and cloudy corneas, to a milder juvenile form. One patient with MPS VII had systemic hypertension, aortic regurgitation and obstructive lesions in the aorta and major blood vessels. The abdominal aorta showed fibromuscular dysplasia associated with vacuolated cells and abundant extracellular deposits of AMP [31]. MPS VII also occurs in certain breeds of dogs and mice [32,33]. MPS VII in dogs is associated with thickening of the atrioventricular valves and deposits of AMP in valvular fibroblasts [34].

(g) Induced MPS

Heart valves in rats were shown to be involved in a mucopolysaccharidosis-like disorder induced by tilorone, a compound which stimulates interferon production and has antiviral and antitumor activities [35].

Vascular lesions have not been described in these animals. The storage of AMP has been attributed to impaired lysosomal degradation.

The antitrypanosomal drug suramin causes proteoglycan and sphingolipid accumulation in rats, simulating mucopolysaccharidosis. *In vitro*, suramin is a potent inhibitor of the lysosomal enzymes iduronate sulfatase, β-hexosaminidase A and GM_3-sialidase required for the degradation of GM_2 and GM_3 gangliosides, respectively [36].

5.1.3 THE MUCOLIPIDOSES

Patients with mucolipidoses exhibit clinical features of both lipidoses and mucopolysaccharidoses. All of the mucolipidoses are inherited as autosomal recessive traits. Four types of mucolipidoses are recognized, which differ clinically; however, the enzymatic defects in types II and III involve a similar deficiency. Urinary excretion of AMP is normal in patients with mucolipidoses.

(a) Mucolipidosis I

Mucolipidosis I (lipomucopolysaccharidosis or sialidosis) produces symptoms in the first year of life. The features are similar to those of the Hurler syndrome, with dysostosis multiplex, moderate mental retardation, visceromegaly, corneal clouding, retinal cherry-red spot, seizures, vacuolated lymphocytes and coarse inclusions in fibroblasts. These patients are deficient in glycoprotein sialidase activity [37]. One patient with mucolipidosis I had echocardiographic evidence of abnormality of the mitral valve [38]. We are not aware of detailed descriptions of cardiovascular pathology in mucolipidosis I.

(b) Mucolipidosis II

Mucolipidosis II (I-cell disease) is caused by deficiency of UDP-N-acetylglucosamine:N-acetylglucosamine-1-phosphate transferase and is characterized by coarse facial features, severe psychomotor retardation and striking dysostosis multiplex. Large pleomorphic inclusions are found in a variety of cell types. In the myocardium of one patient, cytoplasmic vacuoles with a lucent content were found in fibroblasts but not in myocytes [39]. However, morphological studies in a 2-year-old girl with I-cell disease showed changes in the myocardium and aorta. The cardiac myocytes contained vacuoles with either a clear content or lamellae and fingerprint-like structures. The atrioventricular valves were considerably thickened and contained foamy fibroblasts. The aorta showed thickening of the intima without atherosclerotic plaques. Nodular thickening of the mitral and aortic valves, as well as storage deposits in perivascular connective tissue cells, have also been described [40].

(c) Mucolipidosis III

Mucolipidosis III (pseudo-Hurler polydystrophy) is characterized by mild mental retardation, skleletal dysplasia, corneal clouding, coarse facies and joint contractures. Valvular heart disease has been noted in these patients, but no information is available regarding the pathology of blood vessels [41].

(d) Mucolipidosis IV

Mucolipidosis IV occurs most often in children of Ashkenazi Jewish descent. Corneal opacities and strabismus develop soon after birth. Hypotonia and psychomotor retardation become more evident after 6 months. Cytoplasmic inclusions composed of vesicles and concentric lamellae are present in a variety of cells including hepatocytes, neurons, conjunctival epithelial and goblet cells and fibroblasts [41].

Muscle and conjunctival biopsies from a 15-month-old boy with mucolipidosis IV revealed inclusions composed of membranous bodies with concentric lamellae in endothelial cells and skeletal muscle cells [42]. Numerous small, dense granules were observed in the smooth muscle cells of blood vessels in skin from 3 patients with mucolipidoses IV [43]. The lamellar inclusions in the smooth muscle cells also contained multitubular arrays. The lamellar structures showed a periodicity of 4.2 nm. This periodicity is similar to that of the lamellae found in Fabry's disease.

(e) Fucosidosis

At least three types of fucosidosis, all of which are autosomal recessive disorders, and are characterized by deficiency of alpha-L-fucosidase activity [44], are recognized. Some of the patients have features similar to those of Hurler syndrome, while others have angiokeratomas similar to those in Fabry's disease. We are not aware of cardiovascular involvement having been reported in fucosidosis; however, capillary endothelium of the skin has been noted to be involved (cytoplasmic vacuoles with a lucent or amorphous content) in patients with fucosidosis [45,46].

(f) Mannosidosis

Two forms of mannosidosis have been noted, both of which are autosomal recessive disorders [47]. They are α-mannosidosis, due to α-mannosidase deficiency and β-mannosidosis, due to β-mannosidase deficiency. One patient with α-mannosidosis had slight hepatosplenomegaly, muscular hypotonia, skeletal abnormalities, dilated cerebral ventricles and vacuolated lymphocytes

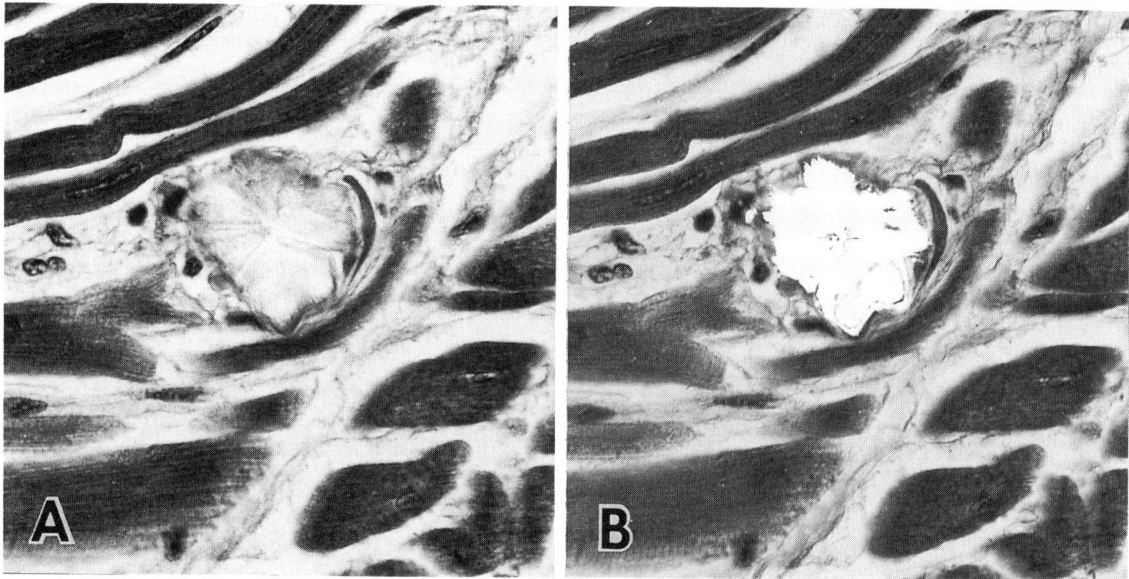

Figure 5.3 Bright field (A) and polarized light (B) micrographs of the same field in section of myocardium from patient with oxalosis. Highly birefringent crystals are present in the wall of an intramyocardial arteriole. (H & E stain.)

[48]. The clinical features of a 46-month-old boy with severe deficiency of β-mannosidase activity [49] resembled those of patients with Sanfilippo syndrome, fucosidosis, sialidosis and aspartylglucosaminuria. No detailed descriptions of cardiovascular pathology in patients with mannosidosis are available; however, capillary endothelial cells in skeletal muscle of two siblings with α-mannosidosis [50] contained cytoplasmic vacuoles with or without electron dense amorphous material.

5.1.4 THE HYPEROXALURIAS (OXALOSIS)

Deposits of oxalate crystals (oxalosis) are found in the myocardium and in the walls of blood vessels (Figure 5.3) in primary and secondary hyperoxaluria. Primary hyperoxaluria includes at least two rare disorders (type I and type II) of glyoxylate metabolism with autosomal recessive transmission [51]. The two types of oxalosis are clinically indistinguishable from one another and are characterized by high urinary oxalate excretion, bilateral oxalate urolithiasis and nephrolithiasis and extrarenal deposits of calcium oxalate. Death from renal failure occurs in childhood or early adult life.

Most patients with type I primary hyperoxaluria have a complete deficiency of alanine:glyoxylate aminotransferase (AGT), resulting in systemic accumulation of glyoxylate and excessive urinary excretion of oxalic, glycolic and glyoxylic acids. In normal human liver AGT is entirely peroxisomal. However, this enzyme is entirely mitochondrial in carnivores. Thus, type I hyperoxaluria is considered to be a peroxisomal disorder. Danpure *et al.* [52] have described two type I patients in whom the enzyme activity and immunoreactive protein were largely mitochondrial and not peroxisomal. In these patients, type I appears to be due, at least in part, to a unique 'traffic' defect, in which AGT is diverted to mitochondria rather than to peroxisomes. In type II primary hyperoxaluria, deficiency of D-glyceric dehydrogenase results in accumulation of hydroxypyruvate and excessive urinary excretion of oxalic and glyceric acids.

In both types of hyperoxaluria, all arteries are affected to some degree, muscular arteries more severely than elastic arteries. Smooth muscle cells of the arterial media are the most common sites of deposition of oxalate crystals in many organ systems. Calcium oxalate is identified as light yellow-brown, strongly birefringent crystals in routinely prepared sections stained with hematoxylin and eosin. These deposits are associated with degeneration and necrosis of the smooth muscle cells. Oxalate crystals in arterioles and capillaries often are larger than the vessel walls. They cause part of the wall to protrude into the lumen, which becomes narrowed or occluded. Raynaud's phenomenon, livido reticularis, acrocyanosis, spasm of large arteries, gangrene and intermittent claudication have been reported [53]. Embolization of material from massive intracardiac calcific deposits has been reported [54].

Secondary oxalosis resulting from chronic renal insufficiency has been reported to cause oxalate deposition, similar to that seen in primary oxalosis, in the heart and blood vessels [55–58]. Other causes of secondary oxalosis are:

1. ingestion of oxalic acid, oxalates or ethylene glycol;
2. intravenous feeding with xylitol and use or abuse

of the anesthetic methoxyflurane [59] (these two compounds are metabolized to oxalate);
3. enteric hyperoxaluria occurring in patients with extensive disease of the small bowel or resection of the small bowel [60];
4. pyridoxine deficiency [61].

Oxalate nephropathy has been noted in a Tibetan spaniel litter [62]. Since there was no exposure to agents capable of producing secondary hyperoxaluria and the histological findings were consistent, a primary hyperoxaluria was suspected in these animals. No information is available regarding the cardiovascular changes in these animals. Primary type II hyperoxaluria has also been described in cats [63].

5.1.5 DIABETES MELLITUS

The vascular manifestations of diabetes mellitus include accelerated atherosclerosis, with consequent regional ischemia and microangiopathy. Atherosclerosis tends to occur at an earlier age and with greater severity in diabetics than in non-diabetics [64]. The association between atherosclerosis and diabetes is firmly established. The hyperlipidemia that often accompanies diabetes mellitus is a major contributory factor. Coronary heart disease is the most important cause of death in patients with diabetes. Such patients also have a disproportionately high incidence of gangrene of the lower extremities, due to peripheral vascular disease [65]. A qualitative morphological difference between atherosclerotic lesions in non-diabetics and diabetics has not been shown convincingly. In addition to atherosclerosis, medial arterial calcification is also frequent in diabetic patients [66].

Diabetic microangiopathy includes arteriolosclerosis and capillary wall thickening. Arteriolosclerosis indicates a concentric hyaline thickening of arteriolar walls, identifiable predominantly in the kidneys, although other organs also may be affected. In the kidney, both the afferent and efferent arterioles may be involved, in contrast to afferent arterioles only in essential hypertension [67]. Other organs affected by arteriolosclerosis in diabetic patients include the pancreas, retina and the pericapsular zone of the adrenal glands [64]. In the pancreas, arteriolosclerosis has been thought to produce, by ischemia, patches of acinar degeneration (seen in the centers of the lobules).

Important aspects of the microangiopathy include various abnormalities of endothelial function. Among these are:

1. diminished endothelium-dependent relaxation and enhanced endothelium-dependent contraction [68];
2. thickening and alterations in the barrier function of the basement membranes of capillaries;
3. loss of pericytes;
4. formation of capillary microaneurysms;
5. various degrees of loss and proliferation of capillaries.

Thickening of the walls of capillaries in diabetics was first noted by Aagenaes and Moe [69] and is due to widening of the basement membrane by PAS-positive material. This abnormality is not specific for diabetes. The thickening of the capillary basement membranes in skeletal muscle has a positive correlation with the age of the patient and the duration of the hyperglycemia [70]. In needle biopsies of the quadriceps muscle, the average thickness of the capillary basement membranes, as measured in electron micrographs, was found to average 108 nm in non-diabetics, 240 nm in diabetics and 137 nm in prediabetics [71]. Feingold et al. [72] have noted that increase in the thickness of capillary basement membranes in muscle over a period of time may serve as a marker to detect individuals who are at increased risk of developing diabetes.

The most important sites of involvement by microangiopathy are the retina and the kidney (Figure 5.4), although these abnormalities also occur in the heart, nerve and other tissues. Changes in diabetic retinopathy include capillary microangiopathy with microinfarctions, exudates, edema and neovascularization. Diabetic retinopathy can be classified into non-proliferative ('background' retinopathy) and proliferative [73]. Dilatation of the veins is an early sign of background retinopathy. Microaneurysms are of capillary origin and may be saccular or fusiform. Intraretinal neovascularization and foci of bleeding are seen in proliferative retinopathy. A selective loss of pericytes in

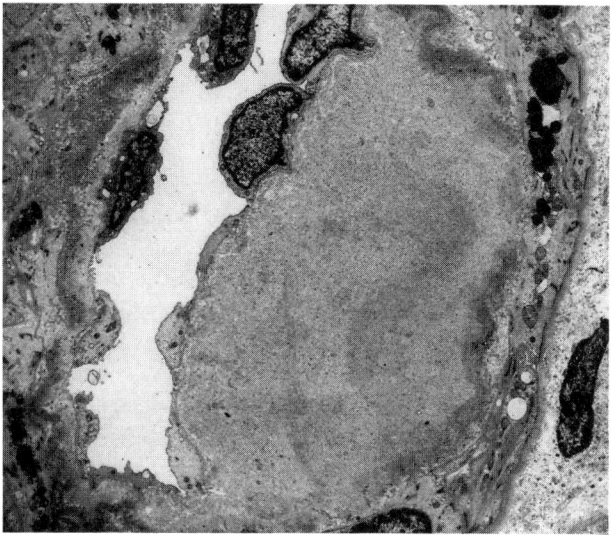

Figure 5.4 Electron micrograph of renal arteriole from patient with diabetes mellitus. The basement membrane is markedly thickened. (Uranyl acetate and lead citrate stain.)

retinal capillaries in diabetes is believed to weaken the capillary wall and predispose to the development of microaneurysms [73]. The terminal arterioles show hyaline thickening and luminal narrowing, changes which progress with increasing duration of the disease. Venous loops and varicosities are also present. Eventually there is loss of both endothelial cells and pericytes, with functionless, short capillaries in which only the basement membranes remain.

Several reports have also described thickening of capillary basement membranes in the myocardium in diabetic patients [74–77]. Ultrastructural observations on the basement membranes of small vessels from hearts of patients with diabetes revealed that the membranes of those with diabetes are nearly three times (mean 177 ± 15 nm) as thick as those in normal hearts (mean 62 ± 5 nm) [75]. Other changes, similar to those observed in the retina, also have been reported to occur in diabetic cardiac microangiopathy. Saccular and fusiform microaneurysms were present in three of six diabetic hearts, in contrast to none of eight control subjects [78]. Microaneurysms have not been described in other studies of diabetic hearts, although most of these studies have not utilized techniques for directly visualizing such lesions.

Cardiac dysfunction leading to heart failure has been found in certain patients with diabetes mellitus. This impaired function has been attributed to 'diabetic cardiomyopathy' and has been found to occur in the absence of hypertension or significant coronary atherosclerosis [79]. This cardiomyopathy has been variously thought to be due to microvascular changes, to metabolic abnormalities and to a combination of these two factors. However, a detailed investigation of the histological and histochemical characteristics of intramyocardial vessels in a group of patients with diabetes and in matched control subjects disclosed no lesions specific for this disease [80]. It should be pointed out, however, that the thickness of the capillary basement membrane in myocardium was not measured in the patients included in this study. Yarom et al. [81] have suggested that in diabetes there is an inadequate, ischemia-induced reactive angiogenesis (i.e. insufficient development of collateral vessels) in the myocardium. This may contribute towards increased myocardial vulnerability in further ischemic injury and perhaps to diabetic cardiomyopathy. Myocardial fibrosis may play a role in diastolic dysfunction in patients with 'hypertensive diabetic cardiomyopathy'. These patients manifest congestive heart failure in the absence of coronary artery disease [82]. Such interstitial fibrosis, has been thought to be responsible for impaired early diastolic dysfunction of the left ventricle in patients with diabetes mellitus alone [83].

Renal vascular changes in diabetes include atherosclerosis, arteriolosclerosis and glomerular changes. Renal artery atherosclerosis occurs at younger ages and with greater severity in diabetics than in non-diabetics. The arteriolosclerosis in diabetics is similar qualitatively to that in non-diabetics, but shows more distinctly segmental hyaline thickening of arteriolar walls, with progression to occlusion [64]. The arteriolar lesions are more frequent and severe in insulin-dependent diabetics. Glomerular involvement is a most important complication of diabetes mellitus and the reader is referred to an extensive review [84] for consideration of this topic.

Polyneuropathy also is a common complication of diabetes mellitus. Microangiopathy involving the blood supply to the peripheral nerves (vasa nervorum) is considered to play an important role in the pathogenesis of this polyneuropathy. Sural nerve biopsies from diabetics exhibited a small but statistically significant increase in the number of endothelial nuclei per capillary. This finding correlated with the severity of the neuropathy [85]. There was a statistically significant increase in the percentage of capillaries closed in diabetic patients with neuropathy as compared to those without neuropathy and control subjects.

The metabolic relationships between the hyperglycemia that characterizes diabetes mellitus and the microangiopathy that complicates this disorder are complex and poorly understood. Studies have been performed on the effect of high glucose levels on the metabolism of extracellular matrix proteins in cultures of endothelial cells and glomerular mesangial cells. These studies have shown that in both of these cell types the synthesis of basement membrane components, such as laminin, fibronectin and type IV collagen, increased in the presence of high concentrations of glucose [86]. *In vitro* studies have also determined that the production of basement membrane components by pericytes increases when glucose levels are elevated [87]. Sims [88] has reviewed evidence showing that following prolonged hyperglycemia there is thinning of the pericyte processes and isolation of pericytes within the basement membrane away from endothelial cells. In addition there is a decrease in the number of contacts between pericytes and endothelial cells, impairment of biochemical pathways in pericytes and a reduction in the number of pericytes, with an increase in the number of pericyte 'ghosts' within microvascular walls. Thus, these studies support the concept that hyperglycemia itself can result in abnormalities of connective tissue synthesis that can lead to microangiopathy. This concept is further substantiated by the facts that microangiopathy eventually develops in normal kidneys transplanted into diabetic patients, and that this complication also occurs in patients in whom diabetes mellitus results from the ingestion (accidental or suicidal) of a toxic agent. Feingold et al. [89] measured muscle capillary basement membrane thickness in controls, insulin-dependent diabetics and individuals with diabetes secondary to the ingestion of Vacor [N-3-pyridylmethyl-N'-p-nitrophenyl urea (PNU)], a rodenticide that induces destruction of the beta cells of the islets of Langerhans. The muscle capillary basement membrane width was increased to a similar extent in insulin-dependent diabetes and in Vacor diabetics.

Mordes and Rossini [90] have reviewed the features of diabetes mellitus in animals, including obese and non-obese animals with spontaneous disease and those with experimentally induced diabetes. The generalization can be made that such animals do not develop vascular changes and retinopathy similar to those observed in the human diseases. The reason for this appears to be the short duration of the diabetes in animal models of this disorder. Nevertheless, thickening of the basement membranes, frequently associated with nodules filled with fibrillar deposits, was noted in the retinal capillaries in spontaneously diabetic BB rats [91]. Thus, these animals may provide an useful model for the study of early vascular changes in diabetes.

The polyol pathway is considered to be of great importance in the pathogenesis of vascular complications of diabetes mellitus. In support of this concept is the finding that dogs with galactosemia (induced experimentally by the dietary intake of large amounts of galactose for a prolonged period of time) develop preproliferative and proliferative retinopathy as well as cataracts and renal vascular disease. The retinal changes are similar to those in human diabetic retinopathy and include degeneration of pericytes to form pericyte ghosts, uneven distribution of endothelial cells, thickening of the basement membranes of capillaries, microaneurysms, dot and blot hemorrhages, confluent hemorrhages, preretinal hemorrhages, broad areas of non-perfusion, occluded arterioles, large arteriovenous shunts, soft exudates (cytoid bodies), possible new vessel growth, intravitreous hemorrhages and partial posterior vitreous detachment [92]. Galactosemic dogs appear to represent the most important animal model of diabetic retinopathy [92,93].

5.2 Diseases of lipid metabolism

Diseases of lipid metabolism comprise a very large and heterogeneous group of disorders, which can be classified into diseases related to deficiencies in the activities of lysosomal enzymes of lipid metabolism; the hyperlipoproteinemias; the lipoprotein deficiencies and disorders of cholesterol, other sterols and phytanic acid metabolism.

5.2.1 DEFICIENCIES OF LYSOSOMAL ENZYMES OF LIPID METABOLISM

Vascular lesions related to lysosomal disorders of lipid metabolism have been observed in Fabry's disease, Gaucher's disease, Farber's disease and acid lipase deficiencies (Wolman's disease and cholesteryl ester storage disease) and lipofuscinosis.

(a) **Fabry's disease**

Fabry's disease (angiokeratoma corporis diffusum universale) is caused by deficiency of a lysosomal α-galactosidase A (ceramide trihexosidase) and has an X-linked recessive mode of inheritance. The genetic defect in Fabry's disease is complex and heterogeneous [94–96]. Among the diseases caused by deficiencies of lysosomal hydrolases active in lipid metabolism, Fabry's disease is the one in which cardiovascular involvement is most important, both clinically and pathologically. Fabry's disease is manifested by skin lesions (angiokeratomas), pain and paresthesias in the extremities and progressive renal and cardiac lesions. The latter include cardiac hypertrophy (often with asymmetric septal hypertrophy) and dilatation, congestive heart failure, anginal pain and systemic hypertension, all of which are related to the presence of deposits of ceramide trihexoside in lysosomes in endothelial cells, smooth muscle cells and pericytes throughout the vascular system, especially the coronary arteries, as well as in renal glomeruli and tubules, cardiac muscle cells, specialized tissues of the atrioventricular conduction system and valvular fibroblasts. In addition to these, areas of ectasia develop in small blood vessels in the skin and other organs, and microaneurysms are prominent in ocular vessels [97]. The aorta in one patient showed changes suggestive of cystic medial necrosis [98].

The deposits noted above are composed of irregularly shaped concentric or parallel lamellae (myelin figures) [99]. In ordinary histologic sections these deposits of ceramide trihexoside appear as vacuoles (Figure 5.5); in frozen sections (Figure 5.6), they are sudanophilic, PAS-positive and strongly birefringent. Large vessels show cellular proliferation and fibrosis in the intima, with concentric luminal narrowing. The thickened vessels tend to have a peculiar whitish color [100].

Lipid deposition in the vascular endothelium and media has been noted in conjunctival biopsies from patients with Fabry's disease [101]. Such deposits were also seen in the smooth muscle cells of the media and endothelial cells of the small and medium sized arteries of the choroid, retina, ciliary body and in endothelial cells and pericytes of retinal capillaries and choriocapillaries in a male patient with Fabry's disease [102] (Figure 5.6). Similar deposits were found in the vascular endothelium, smooth muscle and pericytes in the eye of a female carrier [103].

Smith et al. [104] described the histopathology and electron microscopy of the pulmonary vasculature in a 52-year-old man with Fabry's disease. Autopsy on this patient revealed accumulation of glycolipid in cardiac

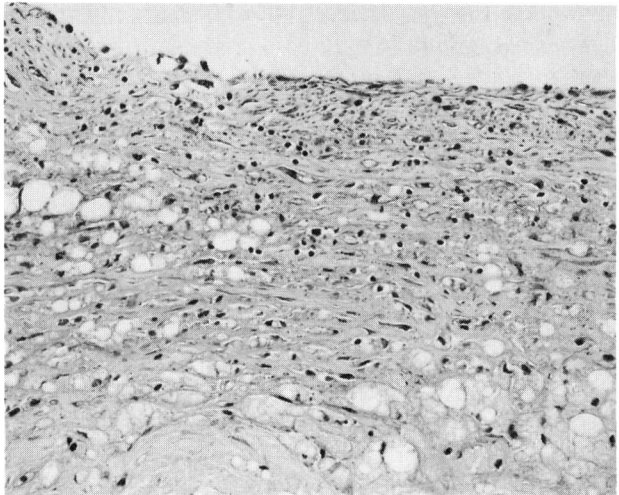

Figure 5.5 Portion of large epicardial coronary artery from patient with Fabry's disease, showing prominent vacuolization of intimal smooth muscle cells. (Movat pentachrome stain.)

and skeletal muscle, smooth muscle and endothelium of systemic blood vessels. The media of the muscular pulmonary arteries was hypertrophied and presented a striking bubbly appearance due to collections of small clear vesicles in the cytoplasm of the distended vascular smooth muscle cells. They stained positively with Luxol Fast blue and faintly with PAS in paraffin sections, and with Sudan black B in frozen sections. The same histological and staining reactions were seen in a thick zone of proliferation of intimal smooth muscle cells. Vesicles were also seen in pulmonary veins, venules and arterioles. Electron microscopy showed numerous electron-dense inclusions, composed of concentric lamellae, in pulmonary arteries, arterioles, veins and alveolar walls. Zebra bodies composed of parallel lamellae were also present. Zebra bodies and other lamellar inclusions were found in profusion in the smooth muscle cells of the media of muscular pulmonary arteries and veins and in the intimal cells, the endothelial cells of all pulmonary arteries and veins and within capillary endothelial cells. A biopsy specimen of an area of telangiectasia from a patient with Fabry's disease showed many cytoplasmic inclusions with lamellar internal structures in endothelial cells, pericytes and fibroblasts [105].

(b) Gaucher's disease

Gaucher's disease (glucosyl ceramide lipidosis), the most common of the metabolic diseases involving glycolipids, exists in three forms: infantile, juvenile and adult. These forms are transmitted in an autosomal recessive mode and are due to deficiency of glucocerebrosidase. This results in the accumulation of glucosyl ceramide in a variety of cell types, particularly in mononuclear phagocytes in liver and spleen. Neuronal storage occurs in the infantile form, in which early death results from rapid progression of the neurological manifestations. The adult form is compatible with long-term survival. The diagnosis is established on the basis of the finding of

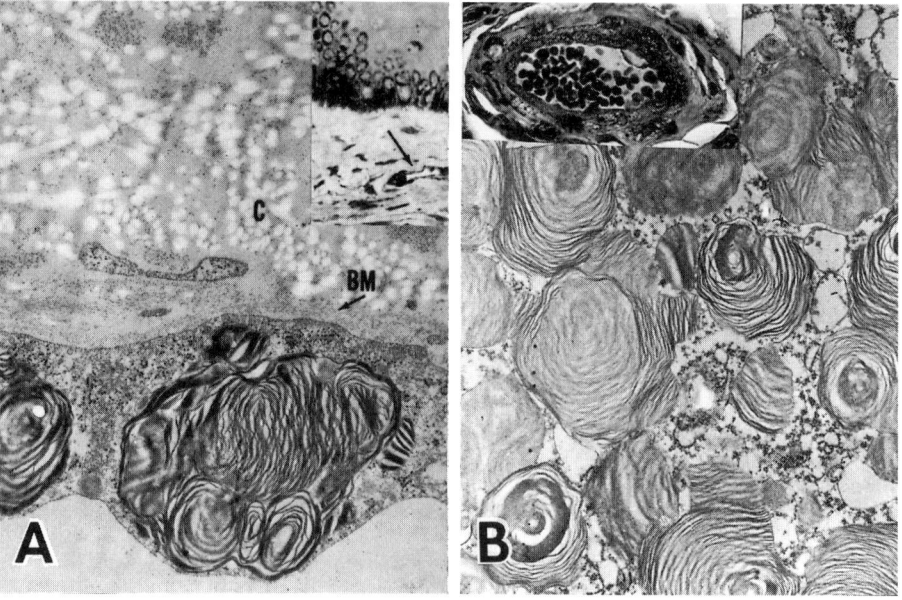

Figure 5.6 Light and electron micrographs of limbal (A) and choroidal (B) vessels in eye of patient with Fabry's disease. (A) Accumulation of lamellar material in endothelial cell (arrow in inset). BM = endothelial basement membrane; C = collagen. (Inset: p-phenylenediamine stain.) (B) Lipid deposits in vascular wall (inset). The electron micrograph shows numerous dense lamellae in medial smooth muscle cells. (×12 300.) (Inset: sudan black B stain, ×300.) (Courtesy of Dr L. Zimmerman, Armed Forces Institute of Pathology, Washington, DC.)

typical Gaucher cells in bone marrow aspirates or liver biopsy. The Gaucher cells are large and their cytoplasm shows a wrinkled appearance. Ultrastructural study of Gaucher cells demonstrates the presence of numerous elongated cytoplasmic inclusions that consist of membrane-bound accumulations of tubules that measure 20 nm in diameter.

Cardiac involvement by storage deposits does not occur in Gaucher's disease. However, patients with the adult form of Gaucher's disease have been reported to develop pulmonary hypertension and cor pulmonale as a consequence of occlusion of alveolar capillaries by Gaucher's cells derived from bone marrow [106]. We are not aware of comparable findings having been reported in other lysosomal disorders of lipid metabolism.

Significant vascular involvement has been reported in a few cases of biochemically confirmed Gaucher's disease. Uyama et al. [107] observed coronary and aortic atherosclerosis, severe perivascular fibrosis in leptomeningeal vessels, cardiac dilatation, hypertrophy and fibrosis and mitral and aortic valvular stenosis caused by fibrous thickening of the valves, in two adult patients with a variant form of Gaucher's disease in which the usual manifestations of this disorder were present only to a minimal degree (although typical Gaucher cells were found on light and electron microscopic study). Two other patients with Gaucher's disease were reported to have significant cardiovascular involvement. One of these, who had the neuronopathic form, had aortic and coronary intimal fibrosis [108]. The other had mitral and aortic valve disease [109]. It is to be noted that the lesions just described were not due to accumulations of Gaucher cells.

(c) Farber's disease

Farber's disease (disseminated lipogranulomatosis) is a lipidosis with autosomal recessive transmission. It exists in two forms, clinically severe and clinically mild, which differ in the severity and age of onset of symptoms. The enzymatic defect in the severe form involves a lack of acid ceramidase activity (a lysosomal enzyme that hydrolyzes ceramide to sphingosine and a free fatty acid) in viscera, leukocytes and cultured fibroblasts [110]. This defect results in high levels of ceramide and AMP in a variety of cell types and in the formation of granulomas with lipid-filled histiocytes. These granulomas give rise to the clinical symptoms of hoarseness, swollen joints, periarticular subcutaneous nodules and pulmonary infiltrates.

Involvement of the pericardium, cardiac valves, coronary arteries, aorta and pulmonary artery by yellow plaques has been noted [111–113]. Remarkable alterations in pulmonary, carotid and coronary arteries were seen in a 7-month-old with Farber's disease [114]. In addition to granulomatous changes, deposits considered to contain glycolipids were observed extracellularly in the intima, media and adventitia of these vessels. These deposits were associated with very severe thickening of the walls and luminal narrowing of the coronary arteries. Such deposits were also seen in perivascular areas in liver and skeletal muscle.

Ultrastructural studies of the granulomas [115] have described pleomorphic inclusions containing either parallel lamellae or curvilinear tubules (banana bodies) in a matrix. These tubules resemble those seen in Batten's disease [116]. Curvilinear bodies have been noted in the cytoplasm of fibroblasts and endothelial cells in skin biopsies [117] and zebra-like bodies have been noted in endothelial cells in the liver [118].

(d) Acid lipase deficiency

Wolman's disease and cholesteryl ester storage disease are two allelic diseases in which cholesteryl ester and triglycerides accumulate in lysosomes in a variety of tissues, due to deficient activity of an acid lipase which hydrolyses cholesteryl ester [119].

Wolman's disease is the more severe form. It is a recessive disorder and is associated with hypersplenism, calcification of the adrenals and death in infancy. Aortic intimal lipid deposition may be extensive [120]. Numerous histiocytes with foamy cytoplasm have been noted histologically in the aortic intima [121]. Cytoplasmic inclusions, which were round or spindle-shaped and surrounded by a double membrane, were present in the endothelial cells in a skin biopsy from a child with Wolman's disease [121].

Cholesteryl ester storage disease is the benign form of acid lipase deficiency and is compatible with adult life. Two patients with this disease had accelerated atherosclerosis at autopsy. One was 21-years-old and had aortic valvular stenosis, severe coronary arterial luminal narrowing and lesions in the circle of Willis, abdominal aorta and common iliac arteries [119] (Figures 5.7 and 5.8); the other died aged 9 and had a few elevated plaques in the ascending aorta [122]. An extremely benign variant of cholesteryl ester storage disease was diagnosed in two women aged 43 and 56 years [123]. The development of atherosclerosis in patients with cholesteryl ester storage disease has been attributed to the concomitant occurrence of type IIb hyperlipoproteinemia.

(e) Neuronal ceroid lipofuscinosis

The term neuronal ceroid lipofuscinosis refers to at least two disorders (also known as Batten's disease and Kuf's disease) which are characterized by the accumulation of a pigmented lipid material in most types of cells. Clinically, the patients have variable degrees of mental retardation, seizures, myoclonus, visual impairment and

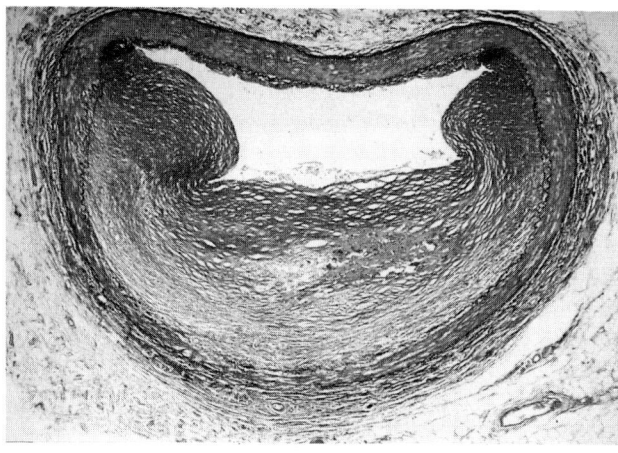

Figure 5.7 Cholesteryl ester storage disease. Section of coronary artery showing large atheromatous plaque. (Movat pentachrome stain.)

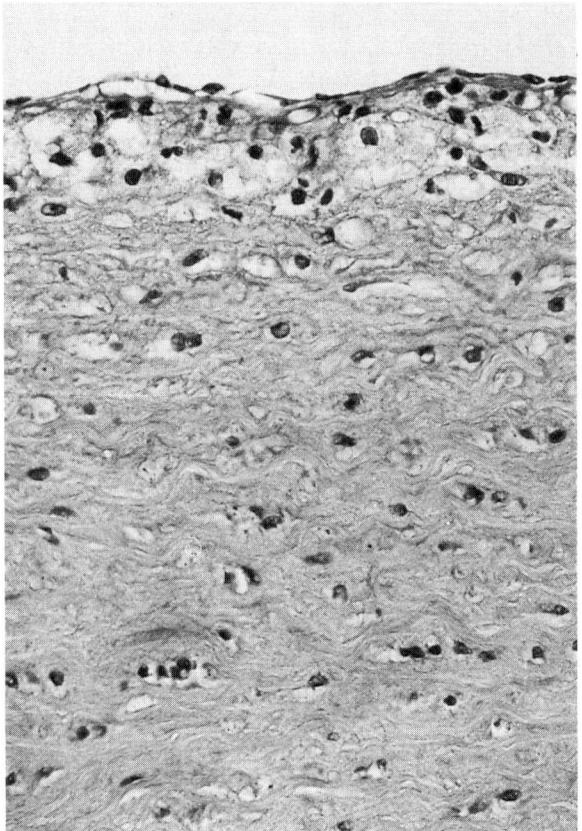

Figure 5.8 Aorta from patient with cholesteryl ester storage disease, showing accumulation of foam cells in the intima. (H & E.)

pigmentary degeneration of the retina. The stored material has histochemical features similar to those of lipofuscin (yellow-brown color, yellow-orange autofluorescence and positive reactions with lipid stains and the PAS technique). However, the ultrastructural appearance of this material differs from that of normal lipofuscin and consists of curvilinear bodies, rectilinear bodies and granular deposits [124]. The enzymatic defect has not been identified. However, lipofuscin is known to be a product of the lysosomal degradation of complex lipids, and for this reason the lipofuscinoses have been tentatively classified as lysosomal disorders. Vascular involvement in the lipofuscinoses appears to be limited to endothelial cells, which contain abnormal lysosomes with pigment deposits [46].

5.2.2 THE HYPERLIPOPROTEINEMIAS

The hyperlipoproteinemias have been classified into the following five types according to the nature of the lipoprotein particles which are present in increased concentrations in plasma: type I (chylomicrons); type II (low density lipoproteins or LDL); type III (intermediate density lipoproteins or IDL); type IV (very low density lipoproteins or VLDL) and type V (both VLDL and chylomicrons).

Hyperlipoproteinemias exist both as genetically transmitted (primary hyperlipoproteinemias) and as acquired disorders (secondary hyperlipoproteinemias) related to other systemic diseases. Disorders which are manifested by hyperlipoproteinemias and which result from single gene mutations include: familial lipoprotein lipase deficiency (type I hyperlipoproteinemia), familial hypercholesterolemia (type II hyperlipoproteinemia), dysbetalipoproteinemia (type III hyperlipoproteinemia), familial hypertriglyceridemia (type IV hyperlipoproteinemia), and multiple lipoprotein-type hyperlipidemia (familial combined hyperlipidemia or type V hyperlipoproteinemia).

Primary hyperlipoproteinemias of unknown etiology include polygenic hypercholesterolemia, sporadic hypertriglyceridemia and familial hyperalphalipoproteinemia. Secondary hyperlipoproteinemias may be associated with a variety of clinical disorders, the most frequent of which are diabetes mellitus, consumption of alcohol and ingestion of oral contraceptives [125].

As described below, the hyperlipoproteinemias, with the exceptions of familial lipoprotein lipase deficiency and familial hyperalphalipoproteinemias, represent risk factors for the development and progression of atherosclerotic lesions. However, no specific patterns of microscopic characteristics of these lesions have been recognized in any of the hyperlipoproteinemias, although in some instances (type II and type III), the topographic distribution of the atherosclerotic changes does show a relationship to the type of hyperlipoproteinemia.

(a) Familial lipoprotein lipase deficiency

Familial lipoprotein lipase deficiency is an autosomal recessive disorder that results from the absence or marked reduction in the activity of lipoprotein lipase. This enzyme is located in the plasma membrane of endothelial cells and hydrolyses chylomicrons. This defect in the metabolism of chylomicrons results in the massive accumulation of these particles in plasma, from which they are removed by cells of the mononuclear phagocyte system. The affected cells become greatly enlarged, have a foamy cytoplasm, with inclusions that contain chylomicrons in various stages of degradation and accumulate in liver, spleen and bone marrow.

Affected patients present in childhood with recurrent episodes of abdominal pain, eruptive xanthomas and small yellowish papules on pressure-sensitive areas. The abdominal pain is caused by pancreatitis due to hyperchylomicronemia, related to the ingestion of fat. Patients with familial lipoprotein lipase deficiency have no evidence of accelerated atherosclerosis and the only cardiac lesions described in these patients are yellow patches containing foam cells in the left atrial endocardium [126]. The accumulation of chylomicrons does not appear to be atherogenic.

(b) **Familial apoprotein CII deficiency**

Familial apoprotein CII deficiency is an autosomal recessive disorder due to the absence of apoprotein CII, an essential cofactor for lipoprotein lipase. This results in a syndrome similar to that of familial lipoprotein lipase deficiency.

(c) **Familial hypercholesterolemia**

Familial hypercholesterolemia is an autosomal dominant disorder resulting from a mutation in the gene for LDL receptors. These are located on the surfaces of certain cells types and control the intracellular entry of LDL. This constitutes an initial step in the regulation of LDL degradation and cholesterol synthesis [127]. The total plasma cholesterol is increased two- to threefold in heterozygotes and six- to eight-fold in homozygotes.

The homozygous and heterozygous forms differ in the severity and age of onset of clinical symptoms. These symptoms are related to acceleration of atherosclerosis and to deposition of cholesterol in vascular walls, cardiac valves and xanthomatous lesions. Extremely severe aortic and coronary atherosclerosis (Figure 5.9) develops in childhood in homozygous patients in association with tuberous and tendinous xanthomas and a high incidence of aortic valve disease. In homozygotes, coronary atherosclerosis frequently has its clinical onset before the age of 10; however, myocardial infarction has been reported as early as 18 months of age [125]. Myocardial infarction begins to occur in affected male heterozygotes in the third decade and peaks in the fourth and fifth decades, but in women this onset is delayed 10 years.

The atherosclerotic lesions are more severe in the

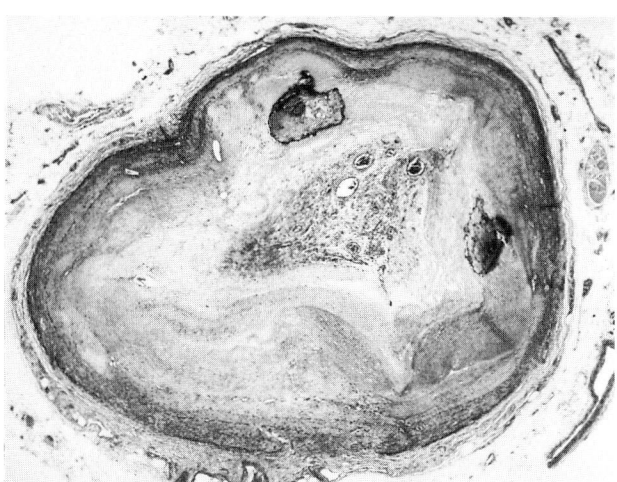

Figure 5.9 Coronary artery from patient with homozygous type II hyperlipoproteinemia, showing large, partially calcified plaque and luminal occlusion. (Movat pentachrome stain.)

ascending than in the abdominal aorta. This represents a reversal of the usual pattern of distribution of aortic atherosclerotic lesions. The involvement of the ascending aorta in homozygous patients can be so severe as to produce the clinical and angiographic picture of supravalvular aortic stenosis [128–130]. Atherosclerotic plaques have been reported to produce severe coronary ostial narrowing and myocardial infarction without significant coronary artery disease [125]. The aortic valve may be markedly stenosed by fibrous tissue, masses of foam cells and cholesterol clefts in the cusps [131,132]. Thickening of the mitral valve (causing both mitral stenosis and mitral regurgitation), pulmonary valve and endocardium by foam cells has also been reported [131,133]. Clinically significant accumulations of foam cells in cardiac valves are not a feature of the heterozygous form.

The coronary arteries show widespread proximal and distal disease, with frequent, clinically significant stenosis of the left main coronary artery [134]. Cerebral atherosclerosis in patients with familial hypercholesterolemia occurs later in life than does coronary artery disease and the reasons for this difference are not understood [135]. Atherosclerotic plaques also develop in the pulmonary trunk and its branches [131].

Absence of coronary ostial lesions together with only minimal irregularity of the left and right coronary arteries was noted on angiographic study in a 31-year-old woman with homozygous familial hypercholesterolemia. In contrast to this, this patient had severe atherosclerotic lesions involving the vertebral and internal carotid arteries, as well as moderate supravalvular aortic stenosis [136]. Certain differences in the morphology and distribution of lipid deposits in the cardiovascular system in familial hypercholesterolemia and atherosclerosis of other causes have been sum-

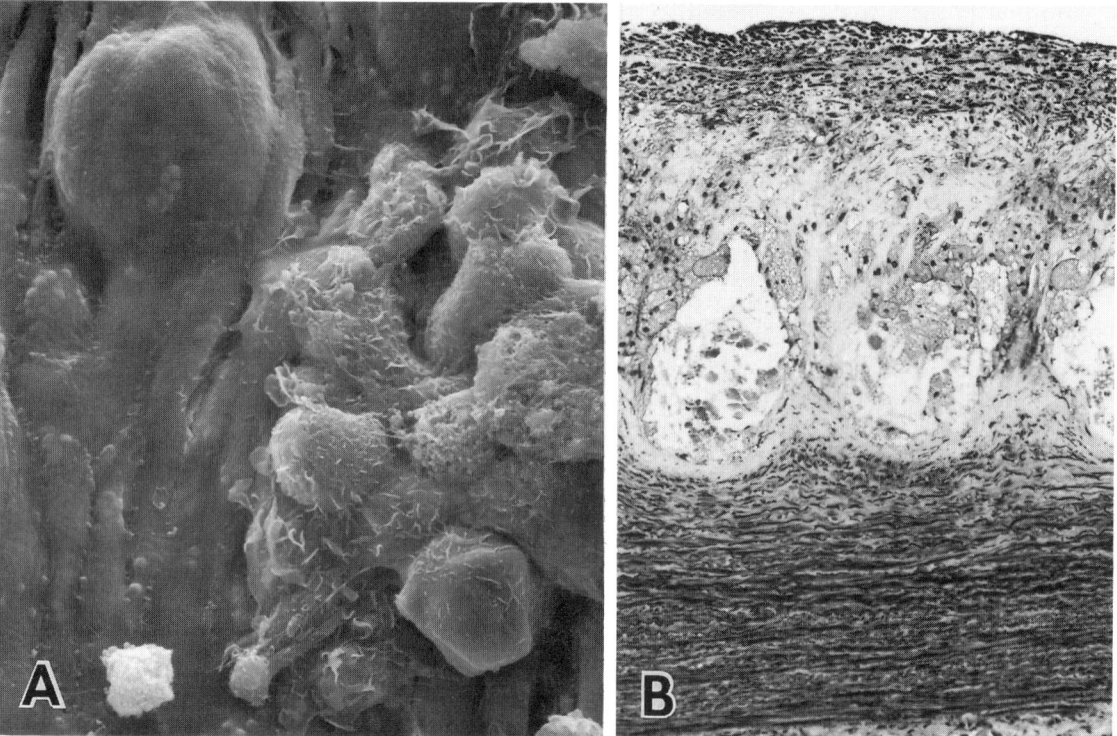

Figure 5.10 Scanning electron (A) and light (B) micrographs of aorta from Watanabe homozygous hyperlipidemic (WHHL) rabbit. (A) Subendothelial accumulation of foam cells has led to bulging, stretching and disruption of the endothelium. An aggregate of foam cells that are exposed to the surface is seen on the right. (B) Late lesion showing marked intimal thickening by atherosclerotic plaque containing foam cells, calcific and necrotic material with an overlying fibrous cap. (Movat pentachrome stain.)

marized by Stehbens [137]. However, the histologic appearance of the atherosclerotic plaques has been reported not to differ in patients with type II or type IV hyperlipoproteinemia or those with normal lipoprotein patterns [127,138,139]. These studies have been made using morphometric measurements in paraffin sections from which all lipids have been removed during tissue processing. Therefore, the amount of lipid present has been only inferred, and no large-scale, systematic study of the lipid materials present in such lesions has been reported. The planimetric studies of Roberts and associates have shown that fibrous tissue, rather than lipid or calcium deposits, is the major component of atherosclerotic plaques in the extramural coronary arteries, regardless of associated abnormalities in plasma lipoproteins [138]. This was also found to be true in a patient with homozygous familial hypercholesterolemia, in whom the coronary arterial lesions contained the highest percentage of fibrous tissue yet reported [140]. This finding was in sharp contrast with the expectation that such lesions might be predominantly composed of cholesterol deposits, as are the cutaneous xanthomas.

An animal model of familial hypercholesterolemia has been studied in a strain of rabbits, designated Watanabe heritable hyperlipidemic (WHHL) rabbits (Figures 5.10 and 5.11). The pattern of atherosclerosis in homozygous WHHL rabbits is similar to that in patients with familial hypercholesterolemia [141,142]. The earliest atherosclerotic lesions occur in the aortic arch at 2 months of age. Raised lesions are present in all portions of the aorta at 6 months. Advanced atherosclerotic plaques can be seen by 10 to 12 months. Coronary artery disease can be detected at 5 months and is most severe at the ostia, particularly of the left coronary artery. Virtually all rabbits have evidence of myocardial ischemia by 10 months.

(d) Familial dysbetalipoproteinemia

Familial dysbetalipoproteinemia (type III hyperlipoproteinemia) is characterized by increased plasma levels of IDL, triglycerides and cholesterol. The disorder is transmitted by a single gene mechanism, but its expression appears to require the presence of contributory environmental and/or genetic factors [125]. A mutation involving the gene that encodes the structure of apoprotein E, which is normally found in IDL and chylomicron remnants, has been identified in these patients. This apoprotein binds with very high affinity to both chylomicron remnant receptors and LDL recep-

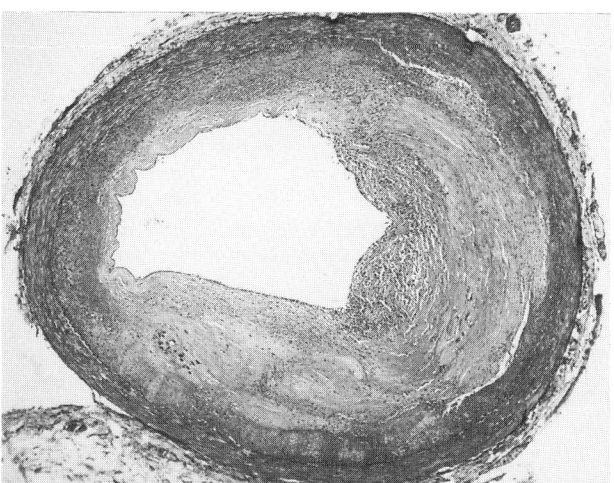

Figure 5.12 Coronary artery from patient with type III hyperlipoproteinemia. There is luminal narrowing associated with large fibrous plaque. (Movat pentachrome stain.)

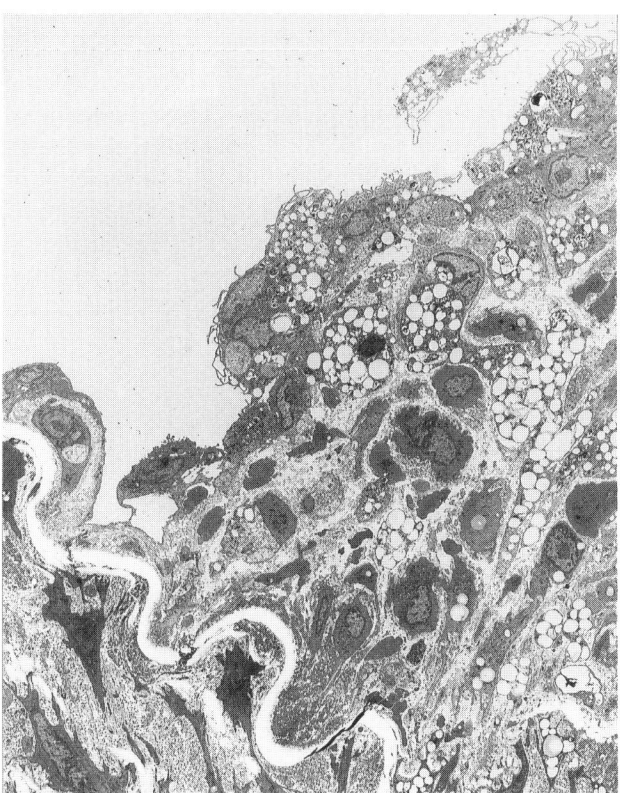

Figure 5.11 Electron micrograph of a late aortic lesion in WHHL rabbit, showing a plaque that consists of foam cells and smooth muscle cells with overlying disrupted endothelium.

tors. Apoprotein E thus mediates the rapid uptake of chylomicron remnants and IDL by the liver. The gene for apoprotein E is polymorphic. Type III hyperlipoproteinemia occurs only in individuals who are homozygous for the E^2 allele. The protein produced by the E^2 allele is defective in its ability to bind to the liver receptors that mediate the uptake of chylomicron remnants and IDL, as a result of which these particles accumulate in plasma [125]. Severe and fulminant atherosclerosis occurs involving the coronary arteries (Figure 5.12), the internal carotids and the abdominal aorta and its branches. In addition, peripheral vascular disease is severe. Two types of cutaneous xanthomas, palmar xanthomas and tuberous or tuberoeruptive xanthomas occur in these patients. The first necropsy observations in a patient with type III hyperlipoproteinemia described occlusion of the lumina of the major coronary arteries by deposits consisting primarily of foam cells [126,138]. However, subsequent reports [143–146] showed that the coronary arteries and saphenous vein bypass grafts had been occluded by atheromas that contained a scattering of foam cells and mononuclear cells. Of six patients with type III hyperlipoproteinemia who died from coronary artery disease, all had severe atherosclerosis of the aorta, major coronary arteries and common iliac arteries. Three of these patients had severe narrowing of the left main coronary artery. One patient had atypical coronary atherosclerotic plaques with increased numbers of foam cells. Immunoperoxidase staining of coronary atherosclerotic plaques from patients with type III hyperlipoproteinemia showed no difference in the location of apolipoproteins AI, AII, B, CI and CIII when compared to the plaques from patients with type II and type IV hyperlipoproteinemia or with normal lipoprotein values [147].

Apoprotein E-deficient mice have been created by homologous recombination in mouse embryonic stem cells [148]. On a low fat, low cholesterol diet these animals have markedly elevated plasma cholesterol levels compared with control animals and when challenged with a high fat diet, they develop a four-fold increase in plasma cholesterol level. This marked hypercholesterolemia is primarily due to elevated levels of VLDL and IDL. At 10 weeks of age, apo-E-deficient mice have already developed atherosclerotic lesions in the aorta and coronary and pulmonary arteries.

Apo-E-deficient mice generated by gene targeting were used [149] to test the hypothesis that lack of apoprotein B is expected to cause accumulation in plasma of cholesterol-rich remnants whose prolonged circulation should be atherogenic. The mutant mice had five times the normal plasma cholesterol and foam cell-rich deposits in the proximal aorta by age 3 months. These lesions progressed and caused severe occlusion of the coronary ostia by 8 months.

(e) **Familial hypertriglyceridemia**

Familial hypertriglyceridemia (type IV hyperlipoproteinemia) is an autosomal dominant disorder in which the plasma concentration of VLDL is elevated. Affected individuals manifest obesity, hyperglycemia and hyperinsulinemia. Hypertension and hyperuricemia are frequently seen. There is an increased incidence of atherosclerosis in patients with this disease [125].

(f) Multiple lipoprotein-type hyperlipidemia

Multiple lipoprotein-type hyperlipidemia (familial combined hyperlipidemia) is an autosomal dominant disorder. Three different lipoprotein patterns have been noted in affected individuals in a single family: hypercholesterolemia, with elevated levels of LDL (type 2), hypertriglyceridemia with elevated levels of VLDL (type 4), or both (type 5). These appear at puberty and continue throughout life. Patients with the disease develop, and have a strong family history of, premature atherosclerosis.

(g) Primary hyperlipoproteinemias of unknown etiology

Hyperlipoproteinemias of undetermined genetic transmittance include polygenic hypercholesterolemia, sporadic hypertriglyceridemia and familial hyperalphalipoproteinemia. Details of cardiovascular pathological changes in these diseases are not available at the present time.

Polygenic hypercholesterolemia

As the name implies, polygenic hypercholesterolemia results from a complex interaction of multiple genetic and environmental factors. In normal individuals there may be genetic polymorphisms in the proteins that govern the rates of intestinal absorption of cholesterol, the synthesis of bile acids and cholesterol and the synthesis or catabolism of LDL. Patients with polygenic hypercholesterolemia may have mild alterations in these proteins. Unfavorable combinations of these alterations and environmental challenges, such as diets high in cholesterol may result in polygenic hypercholesterolemia [125].

Sporadic hypertriglyceridemia

Endogenous hypertriglyceridemia with or without hyperchylomicronemia sometimes occurs sporadically in individuals without involvement of their relatives. Sporadic hypertriglyceridemia thus includes a heterogeneous group of affected individuals. Only on the basis of the family history can this condition be distinguished clinically from hypertriglyceridemia resulting from a single gene defect.

Familial hyperalphalipoproteinemia

Familial hyperalphalipoproteinemia is characterized by increased plasma levels of high density lipoproteins (HDL), also known as alphalipoproteins. In some families hyperalphalipoproteinemia is inherited as an autosomal dominant trait, but in others a polygenic mode of transmission is suspected. Hyperalphalipoproteinemia is associated with a slightly increased longevity and an apparent protection against myocardial infarction [125].

5.2.3 LIPOPROTEIN DEFICIENCIES

In contrast to the preceding disorders, which are due to increased levels of lipoproteins, the following group of disorders is associated with decreased levels of various lipoproteins in plasma. This group includes conditions characterized by hypoalphalipoproteinemia (deficiency of HDL); hypobetalipoproteinemia and abetalipoproteinemia.

(a) Hypoalphalipoproteinemias

Plasma HDL have alpha mobility on lipoprotein electrophoresis. Apolipoprotein AI and AII are the major constituents of HDL, while apolipoproteins B, Lp(a), CI, CII, CIII, D, E, F and G are minor constituents [150,151]. Epidemiologic studies have shown that plasma concentrations of HDL cholesterol are inversely associated with risk of premature atherosclerosis [152].

Several reports have characterized a group of inherited dyslipoproteinemias in which low levels of HDL and HDL cholesterol are present. The majority of these syndromes are associated with accelerated atherosclerosis [153–156]. These disorders are: familial apo-AI and CIII deficiency, Tangier disease, HDL deficiency with planar xanthomas, apo-AI$_{Milano}$, fish-eye disease, familial lecithin-cholesterol acyltransferase (LCAT) deficiency and familial hypoalphalipoproteinemia [150]. Coronary artery disease before 60 years of age has been observed in most HDL-deficient kindreds, but not in patients with apo-AI$_{Milano}$. Premature atherosclerosis also has been reported in probands for HDL deficiency with planar xanthomas and for familial hypoalphalipoproteinemia. The latter disorder has also been associated with strokes in children [150].

Several genetic disorders are associated with low levels of HDL and deficient LCAT activity in plasma. This enzyme plays a key role in the transfer of cholesterol from cells to plasma and its esterification and incorporation into HDL. This process is known as reverse cholesterol transport. Such disorders, the most important of which are familial LCAT deficiency and fish-eye disease, can be due to mutations in the LCAT gene or on the gene for its cofactor apo-AI [157]. In addition, LCAT activity has been found to be deficient although to a much lesser extent, in patients with Tangier disease and in many patients with clinical evidence of coronary artery disease, particularly in those with concomitant type 4 hyperlipoproteinemia. The contribution of this deficiency to the development of atherosclerosis remains a subject of great clinical importance [158]. Familial LCAT deficiency is an autosomal recessive disorder manifested by anemia with target cells, corneal opacity with arcus formation, proteinuria and progressive renal disease, and lipid deposits in bone marrow, renal glomeruli and other organs. The chemical composition of atheromatous lesions was found to be unusual in one patient with familial LCAT deficiency. The percentage of free cholesterol was high, while the percentage of esterified cholesterol was low, and the percentage composition of fatty acids esterified to cholesterol reflected the abnormal pattern found in plasma [159]. Deposition of lipid occurs in larger muscular arteries in association with hyalinization of the vessel wall and proliferation of intimal smooth muscle cells. In three patients with familial LCAT deficiency, electron microscopic examination revealed characteristic deposition of lipid material in the kidneys, especially in the glomeruli and vessel walls. In the glomeruli, osmophilic membrane fragments or lamellae forming vesicles or particles which contained an amorphous, mottled material were observed. The thickness of each dense lamella was about 35 Å and the interlamellar distance was about 30 Å. These structures were observed within the capillary lumina, in the capillary walls, beneath the endothelium and in the basement membranes, as well as in the mesangial regions and in Bowman's capsules. The membranes sometimes formed meshworks in the capillary lumina, capillary walls and mesangial regions. An amorphous material and cross-striated fibrils, about 200 Å in diameter and with a periodicity of about 60 Å, were seen in some capillary lumina and in mesangial regions. The endothelium often appeared to be detached or even completely lost in regions where the meshwork of membranes were lying close to the capillary walls. Foam cells with numerous neutral fat droplets were observed in the glomerular capillary lumina as well as in the interstitium. Arterioles showed deposits of membranous materials, and a marked thickening of the walls and hyalinization of the intima. Similar deposits were observed in larger muscular arteries. Hyalinization, foam cells and proliferation of smooth muscle cells were also noted in the arterial walls. Atherosclerotic plaques were not specifically examined. However, accumulations of lipid material, similar to those just described, were observed in all sections from renal and iliac arteries and aorta [160].

In spite of the early reports just cited, it is now believed that the risk for atherosclerosis in patients with familial LCAT deficiency and fish-eye disease is normal or only moderately increased. However, coronary artery disease was thought to be of increased severity in two patients with combined deficiency of apo-AI and apo-CIII [161].

Patients with fish-eye disease have marked corneal opacity (from which the name of the disease is derived) but do not have the renal disease typical of familial LCAT deficiency. In fish-eye disease the LCAT activity is absent in HDL- or apo-AI-containing proteoliposomes (α-LCAT activity) but is normal in VLDL and LDL (β-LCAT activity), resulting in near-normal *in vivo* ratios of nonesterified:esterified cholesterol [162]. In contrast, esterification of cholesterol in patients with familial LCAT deficiency is disturbed in all lipoprotein classes, and the ratio of non-esterified to esterified cholesterol is greatly increased.

Tangier disease

Tangier disease is transmitted in an autosomal codominant mode and is manifested by low plasma levels of HDL, LDL and total cholesterol. Patients with Tangier disease have accumulation of cholesteryl esters in various tissues, including tonsils (which are enlarged and orange-yellow in color), lymph nodes, thymus, bone marrow, intestinal mucosa, liver, spleen, skin and cornea. Plasma levels of HDL cholesterol and apo-AI are very low as a result of exceptionally rapid catabolism, rather than decreased synthesis of HDL [163–165].

Five of eight homozygotes older than 40 years had clinically significant atherosclerosis, with four having onset of symptoms before the age of 60 [150,166]. Obligate heterozygotes have HDL cholesterol levels 50% of normal [150,166,167].

Clinical evidence of cardiovascular disease was noted in seven of 14 heterozygotes older than 40 years, five of whom had onset of symptoms before the age of 60. However, no homozygous or heterozygous patient developed symptoms of cardiovascular disease before the age of 40 years. Thus, patients with Tangier disease are at some increased risk for premature vascular disease, but not to the extent expected from the extremely low plasma HDL cholesterol levels. This may be due to the fact that plasma LDL levels are significantly lower in patients with Tangier disease than in normal subjects. Therefore, these patients may be partially protected from the acceleration of atherosclerosis associated with low levels of HDL [150,166]. Despite the very low steady-state plasma levels of HDL, a high flux of HDL due to normal synthesis with markedly accelerated catabolism may permit some HDL-mediated removal of excess cholesterol from tissues (reverse cholesterol transport).

Cardiac morphologic findings in a patient with Tangier disease were reported by Mautner *et al.* [168]. The patient developed angina pectoris at the age of 59 years

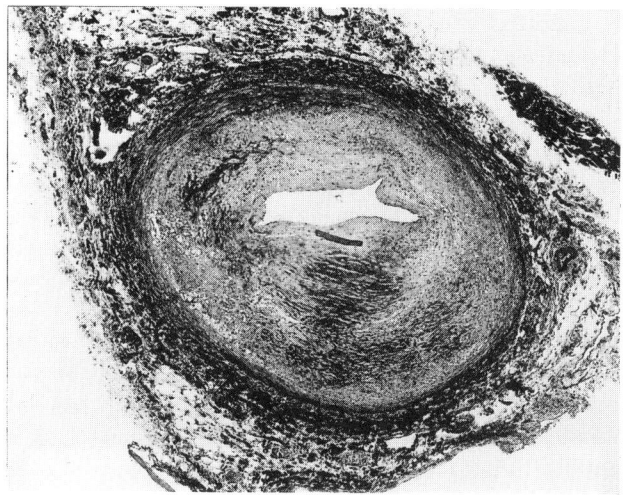

Figure 5.13 Narrowed left circumflex coronary artery of patient with Tangier disease. The plaque consists primarily of fibrous tissue. (Movat pentachrome stain.)

and angiography at that time disclosed severe coronary arterial narrowing. At 60 years the patient underwent saphenous vein coronary artery bypass grafting and died of pneumonia 12 years later. At autopsy, both the native coronary arteries and the saphenous vein grafts showed significant (>75%) cross-sectional luminal narrowing by atherosclerotic plaques (Figure 5.13). The plaques in the arteries were composed primarily of fibrous tissue. The distribution of oil red O-positive material in the coronary arteries and saphenous venous grafts was inhomogeneous and variable in location and amount, with this material present in the adventitia, media and plaques. Birefringent cholesteryl ester crystals were present in the smooth muscle cells in coronary arteries, the saphenous venous graft and ascending aorta. Aortic lesions and adjacent, normal-appearing areas of aorta from a 5-year-old boy with Tangier disease were studied ultrastructurally [169]. In lesions, lipid vacuoles and/or other cytoplasmic 'inclusions' (ultrastructurally considered to represent complex forms of lipids) were found on occasion in the endothelium but consistently involved the smooth muscle cells. Similar changes were present in the adjacent intima, but were less prominent and 'tapered off' distally. A moderate number of macrophages also contained cytoplasmic lipids but such cells entirely free of lipid inclusions were also observed. Many cisterns of rough endoplasmic reticulum in the smooth muscle cells of lesions were associated especially with cytoplasmic droplets and other forms of lipids.

A syndrome of HDL deficiency in chickens with a sex-linked mutation has been reported [170]. The mutants have a 70–90% reduction in plasma HDL cholesterol and apo-AI concentrations. Cholesterol feeding produced a significant increase in the area of the aorta with atherosclerosis lesions in both control and mutant chickens. The HDL deficiency in mutant chickens did not correlate with a higher lesion area or increased lesion thickness. Control and mutant chickens maintained on a low-fat, cholesterol-free diet for 3 years showed no significant difference in the area and thickness of the spontaneous aortic lesions at the end of the period. Thus in this model, spontaneous HDL deficiency was not associated with increased susceptibility to atherosclerosis [171].

(b) Familial disorders associated with low levels of low-density lipoprotein

Very low levels of LDL cholesterol have been found in patients with hypobetalipoproteinemia and abetalipoproteinemia. Recent studies have shown that hypobeta- and abetalipoproteinemia are a complex group of disorders related to abnormalities in B apoproteins. The larger form of apo-B, apo-B100, is produced by the liver and is a major component of serum VLDL and LDL. It contains a binding domain for LDL receptors. The smaller form, apo-B48, derived solely from the intestine, does not contain the LDL-receptor binding sequence. In both abetalipoproteinemia and homozygous hypobetalipoproteinemia, the plasma is nearly devoid of apolipoproteins B1 and B48.

Hypobetalipoproteinemia

Patients with hypobetalipoproteinemia usually do not manifest clinical symptoms. However, the condition has received attention because of its association with increased longevity and decreased coronary artery disease [172].

Abetalipoproteinemia

Abetalipoproteinemia (Bassen–Kornzweig syndrome) is characterized by acanthocytosis, absence of chylomicrons, malabsorption of fat, retinitis pigmentosa, external ophthalmoplegia and degenerative central nervous system disease which involves the cerebellum and resembles that seen in Friedreich's ataxia. The disease is recessively inherited and the metabolic defect is manifested by absence of all lipoproteins containing apo-B. Molecular genetic studies on two patients with abetalipoproteinemia have been described [173]. The defect in these two cases appears to be related to some aspect of lipoprotein assembly or secretion and does not involve the apolipoprotein B gene nor the synthesis or glycosylation of the apolipoprotein. Autopsy observations in one patient with Bassen–Kornzweig syndrome included fragmentation of the internal elastic lamina and marked intimal fibrous thickening, but without luminal narrowing, of coronary arteries [174]. There was considerable cardiomegaly and severe fibrosis of the myocardium and endocardium. In a patient with abetalipoproteinemia, microscopic examination showed that the retinal blood vessels were markedly sclerotic, with hyalinization of their walls and luminal narrowing [175].

5.2.4 DISEASES INVOLVING STORAGE OF CHOLESTEROL, OTHER STEROLS AND PHYTANIC ACID

(a) Cerebrotendinous xanthomatosis

Cerebrotendinous xanthomatosis is a rare lipid storage disease resulting from an autosomal recessive inherited defect of the hepatic mitochondrial steroid 26-hydroxylase. Clinically the disease is characterized by xanthomas in tendons, lung and brain, cataracts, subnormal intelligence, progressive cerebellar ataxia, spinal cord paresis and normal or low plasma cholesterol levels. The diagnosis is confirmed by the demonstration of abnormally elevated concentration of cholestanol or biliary alcohols in serum and urine, respectively [176]. Large amounts of cholestanol accumulate in various tissues. Premature atherosclerosis, including coronary artery disease, has been noted in a few patients with cerebrotendinous xanthomatosis. However, no detailed descriptions of the vascular pathology in this disorder are available [177–179].

(b) Refsum's disease

The term Refsum's disease refers to two syndromes related to deficient oxidation of phytanic acid, which accumulates in a number of tissues. The first of these syndromes, the adult form of Refsum's disease, is considered to involve a defect in the mitochondrial oxidation of phytanic acid by phytanic acid α-hydroxylase to pristanic acid. The second, designated as infantile Refsum's disease, is thought to be related to a defect further in the pathway of oxidation of phytanic acid. This defect has been reported to involve the oxidation of pristanic acid within peroxisomes [180]. The adult form of Refsum's disease is manifested by peripheral neuropathy, ataxia, retinitis pigmentosa and changes in skin and bones [181,182]. Aortic cystic medial necrosis has been reported in two patients with the adult form of Refsum's disease [183]. The relationship of these changes to the metabolic defect is unknown.

Patients with the infantile form of Refsum's disease have impaired vision and hearing from infancy and slowly progressive psychomotor deterioration [184]. Multiple defects of peroxisomal functions, involving very long chain fatty acid oxidation and bile acid metabolism, are present in these patients. Such defects are related to abnormal biogenesis of the peroxisomes (failure of the synthesized proteins to reach their destination in the peroxisomal matrix). Because of these multiple enzymatic defects, the infantile form of Refsum's disease is closely related to Zellweger's syndrome and adrenoleukodystrophy. No descriptions of cardiovascular pathology in infantile Refsum's disease are available.

5.3 Diseases of amino acid and protein metabolism

Vascular abnormalities associated with diseases of amino acid and protein metabolism are presented under the following categories: defects in the metabolism of individual amino acids, including ochronosis, homocystinuria and methylmalonic acidemia; diseases related to defective synthesis of components of connective tissue, i.e. elastic fibers (the Marfan syndrome, cutis laxa and pseudoxanthoma elasticum), the various types of collagens (osteogenesis imperfecta and the Ehlers–Danlos syndrome) and still unidentified components (Larsen's syndrome and the fragile X syndrome); diseases resulting from the extracellular accumulation of fibrillar proteins including amyloidosis and light-chain deposition disease; diseases caused by abnormalities in the synthesis of other specific proteins such as hemoglobin in the hemoglobinopathies and the heavy β-chain of cardiac myosin in hypertrophic cardiomyopathy, and finally diseases of uncertain etiology, including childhood progeria (Hutchinson–Gilford syndrome) and adult progeria (Werner's syndrome).

5.3.1 DISEASES OF AMINO ACID METABOLISM

Although disorders of amino acid metabolism are numerous, only two of these, ochronosis and homocystinuria, are know to lead to abnormalities of blood vessels. The relationship of homocystinuria to vascular complications is emphasized by their occurrence in patients with a defect in cyanocobalamin utilization that results in homocystinuria and methylmalonic acidemia.

(a) Ochronosis

Ochronosis, a manifestation of chronic alkaptonuria, results from the deposition of pigment produced by the oxidation and polymerization of homogentisic acid, an intermediate metabolite of tyrosine and phenylalanine [185,186]. It is manifested clinically by abnormalities of skin coloration, arthropathy and cardiovascular disease particularly aortic valvular stenosis (which can be the initial manifestation) [187]. The metabolic defect, a recessive trait, consists of deficient activity of homogentisic acid oxidase. Secondary or exogenous ochronosis can result from long-term use of hydroquinone-containing bleaching creams [188]. Ochronotic pigment appears bluish-black on gross examination and brownish in histologic sections. It is

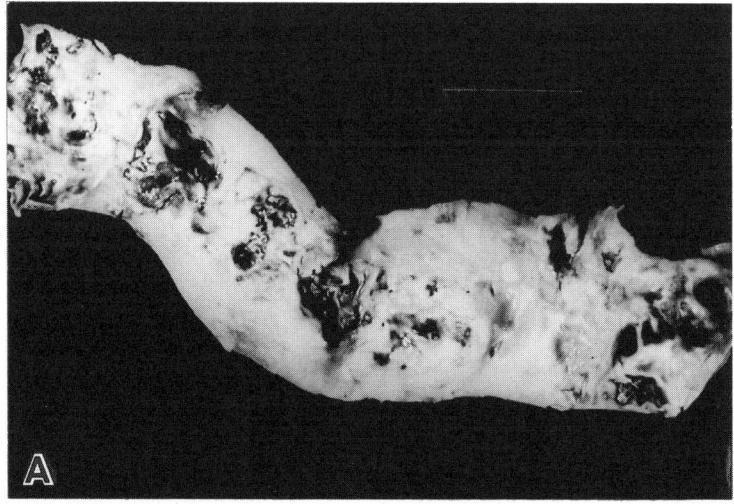

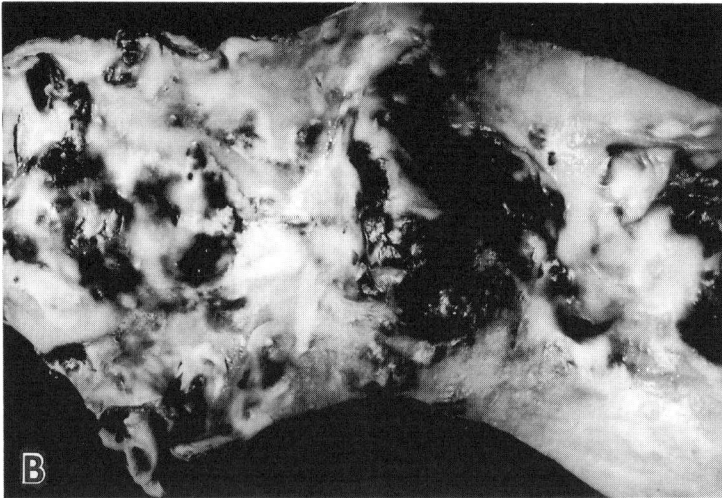

Figure 5.14 Ochronosis. Gross photos (A and B) of aorta showing dark deposits of ochronotic pigment (A). Higher magnification view (B) shows focal distribution of deposits.

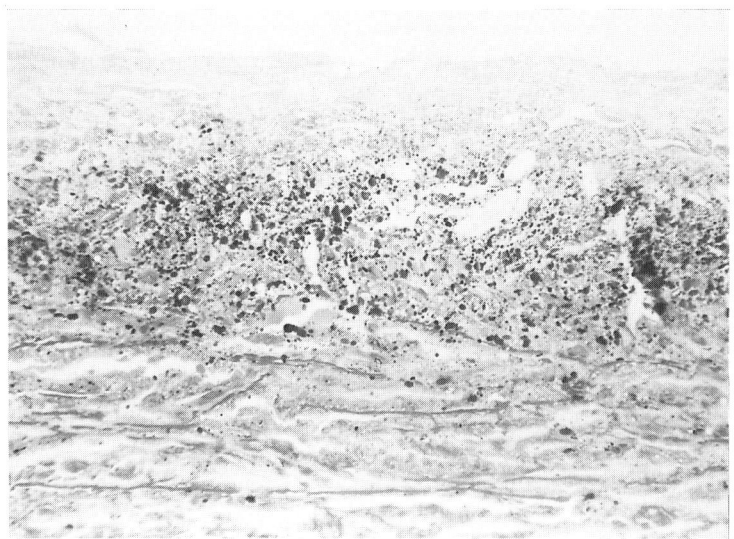

Figure 5.15 Aorta of patient with ochronosis, showing abundant intimal and medial deposits of ochronotic pigment. (1 μm-thick section of epoxy resin-embedded tissue, toluidine blue stain.)

deposited in cartilage, vertebral disks, and, to a lesser extent, in skin and sclerae. Heart valves and valvular annuli, especially the mitral and aortic valves, are sites of marked deposition of pigment. Also involved by pigment deposits are: the endocardium, particularly at the base and tips of the papillary muscles; areas of endocardial and pericardial thickening; the aorta [187] (Figures 5.14 and 5.15); the coronary arteries [189]

DISEASES OF AMINO ACID AND PROTEIN METABOLISM   149

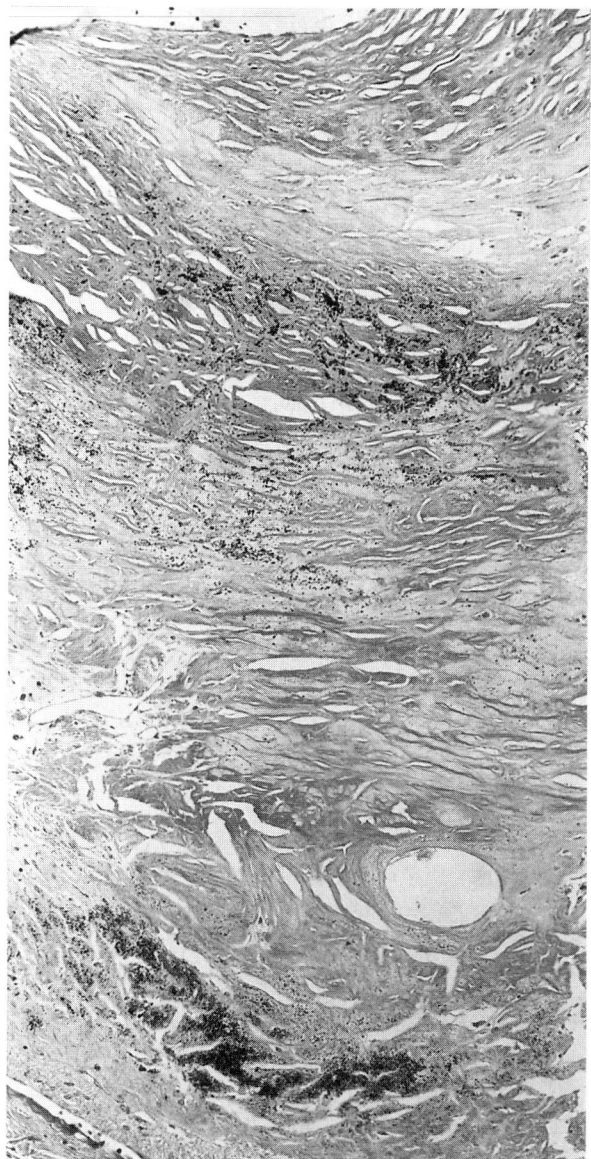

Figure 5.16 Coronary artery of patient with ochronosis, demonstrating ochronotic pigment in atheromatous plaque. (H & E stain.)

(Figure 5.16); other elastic and muscular arteries; veins and capillaries and myocardium, especially in areas of fibrosis [184,186,190,191] and in scars due to previous myocardial infarcts. Heavy pigmentation in cardiac valves and valvular annuli is frequently associated with calcific deposits [151,190,191]. Several patients with ochronosis have been reported to have aortic stenosis, with or without fusion of the commissures and with or without leaflet calcification [192–195]. It has been suggested that the presence of ochronotic pigment predisposes to valvular calcification [194]. Marked pigmentation also has been observed in calcified and non-calcified atheromatous plaques in aorta and other arteries, including coronary arteries [185,190,192,193].

Ochronotic pigment is deposited both intra- and extracellularly. Intracellular deposits occur in endothelial cells, fibroblasts, smooth muscle cells [194] and macrophages; they form small membrane-bound inclusions filled with electron-dense particles less than 100 nm in diameter [196]. Extracellular deposits form much larger, homogeneous granules in connective tissue [197]. These deposits, which are thought to resolve from breakdown of pigment-containing cells, affect all three layers of the arterial walls, especially the inner portion of the media.

(b) Homocystinuria

Homocystinuria, transmitted as an autosomal recessive trait, is caused by a defect in the activity of cystathionine synthetase, which converts homocysteine to cystathionine. This results in increased plasma levels of homocysteine (which can be reversibly converted to homocystine) and methionine, and in increased urinary excretion of homocystine. A clinically similar syndrome (Cbl-C)-type methylmalonic aciduria occurs in patients with a defect in the activation of vitamin B_{12}, which is necessary for the methylation of homocysteine. Homocystinuria is manifested by: mental retardation; seizures; skeletal deformities and ectopia lentis (similar to that seen in the Marfan syndrome) and occlusive vascular disease (the major cause of death). Lesions related to vascular disease include: cerebrovascular accidents; myocardial infarction; peripheral arterial occlusions; venous thromboses and pulmonary and systemic emboli [198]. Aortic thrombosis and aortic aneurysms also have been reported [199,200]. Veins, including cerebral cortical veins and sinuses, often are the sites of thromboses [201,202]. Histologically, the aorta shows intimal thickening and marked fragmentation of elastic fibers. Muscular arteries, including coronary arteries, demonstrate marked fibromuscular intimal thickening, fragmentation of the internal elastic lamina and medial fibrosis. These changes lead to severe luminal narrowing. Arterioles show prominent vacuolization of endothelial cells and proliferation of perivascular connective tissue [203–205].

The marked tendency of vessels in patients with homocystinuria to undergo thrombosis seems to be related to:

1. increase in platelet adhesiveness and consumption;
2. decrease in platelet survival time;
3. pronounced fragility of the endothelium, which tends to detach, thus predisposing to the formation of platelet thrombi on the denuded subendothelial connective tissue.

The vascular changes in homocystinuria are thought to result from increased plasma levels of homocysteine and can be reproduced in experimental animals by the administration of this compound [206].

(c) Vitamin B_{12} metabolic defect with methylmalonic acidemia and homocystinuria (Cbl-C type)

Cbl-C mutation is one of several metabolic defects which interfere with the intracellular availability of cobalamin (Vit B_{12}) moieties [207,208]. This specific mutation involves a deficiency of both methylfolate-H(4) methyltransferase and methylmalonyl CoA isomerase and therefore affects both cytosolic and intramitochondrial cobalamin utilization. It is characterized by methylmalonic aciduria, homocystinuria and hypomethioninemia. The clinical manifestations include lethargy, failure to thrive, feeding difficulties, megaloblastic anemia, mental retardation, seizures and retinal changes [209]. Brandstetter *et al.* [207] reported an infant with this disorder who presented with a bronchiolitis-like illness and developed cor pulmonale and right ventricular dilatation. Necropsy showed multiple pulmonary thromboemboli. These abnormalities were considered to be due to mechanisms similar to those in homocystinuria. Another patient with Cbl-C-type mutation had renal vascular lesions that were considered to be similar to those in thrombotic thrombocytopenic purpura.

5.3.2 DISEASES OF CONNECTIVE TISSUE

Included in this section are genetic disorders related to abnormal synthesis of extracellular connective tissue proteins, particularly those in collagenous and elastic fibers. The organization of the extracellular elements of connective tissue is a highly complex process that involves a multiplicity of steps, the most important of which are:

1. the intracellular synthesis of the individual connective tissue proteins;
2. the secretion of the proteins into the extracellular space;
3. biochemical modifications of the secreted proteins, including proteolytic cleavage of certain peptide segments, hydroxylation and glycosylation;
4. polymerization, crosslinking and assembly of the modified proteins into different types of fibrils;
5. assumption of the definitive arrangement of these fibrils and of their three-dimensional relationships with other types of connective tissue components.

In view of the number and complexity of these events, it is not surprising that a large variety of disorders result from biochemical defects in the synthesis and assembly of elastic fibers and collagen. This situation is further complicated by the findings that elastic fibers have two distinct components (elastin and microfibrils) and that at least 12 biochemically distinct types of collagen exist. Our knowledge of the biochemical and genetic abnormalities involved in these disorders is incomplete. Therefore, the present classification must be regarded as very tentative.

Connective tissue microfibrils can exist either independently or as a component of elastic fibers. Abnormalities involving these microfibrils occur in the Marfan syndrome and related disorders. Other abnormalities involving elastic fibers occur in cutis laxa and pseudoxanthoma elasticum, both of which are described in this section, as well as in Menkes' syndrome and in copper deficiency. The latter two disorders are related to abnormalities in copper metabolism (copper is a component of lysyl oxidase, the enzyme responsible for the crosslinking of both collagen and elastin) and are described in the section on vitamins and minerals.

Abnormalities in the synthesis of the collagens comprise a large heterogeneous group of disorders, many of which have been classified into two categories, namely, osteogenesis imperfecta and the Ehlers–Danlos syndrome. Several types of each of these disorders are recognized, and they vary according to the type of collagen defect and to the corresponding clinical manifestations. A biochemical defect still remains to be identified in other disorders involving connective tissue. Among these are the Larsen's syndrome and the fragile X syndrome.

A number of morphological abnormalities of collagen have been noted in the skin and other tissues of patients with various disorders of connective tissues. These include: unraveling (loosely arranged subunits of the fibrils), marked irregularities in diameter (fibrils that are normal in shape but have abnormally large or small diameters), and abnormal shapes, especially 'collagen hieroglyphs' or 'collagen flowers' (the term given to collagen fibrils that, when sectioned transversely, show an outline which resembles that of a flower with petals). None of these changes are specific for any given disorder of connective tissue. Collagen flowers have been noted in types I through III, V through VII and IX Ehlers–Danlos syndrome, pseudoxanthoma elasticum, type I osteogenesis imperfecta and cutis laxa. Mixtures of abnormally small and abnormally large collagen fibrils are present in these conditions and in Marfan syndrome [210].

(a) Marfan syndrome

The Marfan syndrome is characterized by musculoskeletal abnormalities, ectopia lentis and cardiovascular lesions, the most striking of which are dilatation of the aortic root and mitral and aortic regurgitation. Pulmonary emphysema often is also present. The inheritance is autosomal dominant and the phenotypic expression varies among different patients. Some patients (usually described clinically as having a forme fruste of the syndrome) present only part of the spectrum of clinical manifestations. The basic abnormality is a defect in the synthesis of connective tissue microfibrils. This defect involves mutations in the gene that encodes for fibrillin-1, a major glycoprotein component of microfibrils.

Two forms of fibrillin, fibrillin-1 and fibrillin-2, have been identified [211]. Mutations in the gene for fibrillin-1, which is located in chromosome 15, are responsible for the defect in two disorders: Marfan syndrome and hereditary ectopia lentis [212,213]. The mutations in the Marfan syndrome are heterogeneous and can result either in decreased production of normal fibrillin-1, due to a non-functioning allele or in production of an abnormal protein. The latter type of defect is associated with the more severe forms of the disease. Mutations in the gene for fibrillin-2, which is located in chromosome 5, cause congenital contractural arachnodactyly (Beals syndrome) which is characterized by flexion contractures of the joints rather than the loose jointedness of patients with the Marfan syndrome. Fibrillin has a molecular weight of 350 kD and has been immunolocalized to microfibrils. Ultrastructural studies have shown that elastic fibers contain two components: centrally located amorphous cores, formed by elastin and peripherally located microfibrils. Elastic tissue stains employed for the visualization of elastic fibers demonstrate the amorphous components. Developing elastic fibers have numerous microfibrils, but these are few in mature elastic fibers. It has been suggested that microfibrils play a crucial role in elastogenesis by forming a scaffold upon which the amorphous component of elastic fibers is deposited and organized. Microfibrils associated with elastin measure 100–130 Å in diameter and have a beaded appearance and hollow centers. The amorphous component remains unstained or is very lightly stained in electron microscopic preparations contrasted with uranyl acetate and lead citrate. This component, however, is darkly stained by the tannic acid method of Kajikawa [214].

Three patterns of cardiovascular involvement have been recognized in patients with the Marfan syndrome [215]:

1. saccular aneurysms of the ascending aorta;
2. dissection of the entire aorta;
3. mitral valvular prolapse, which may or may not be associated with aortic disease.

Saccular aneurysms involve the sinuses of Valsalva and the proximal tubular portion of the ascending aorta. They tend to rupture rather than to dissect [215]. Aneurysms in the Marfan syndrome also have been reported in the descending thoracic and abdominal aorta [216,217], pulmonary arteries [218], cerebral vessels [219], ductus arteriosus [220], internal carotid artery [221] and coronary arteries [222]. Microscopically (Figures 5.17–5.19), the walls of the aneurysms show severe fragmentation, atrophy and loss of elastic

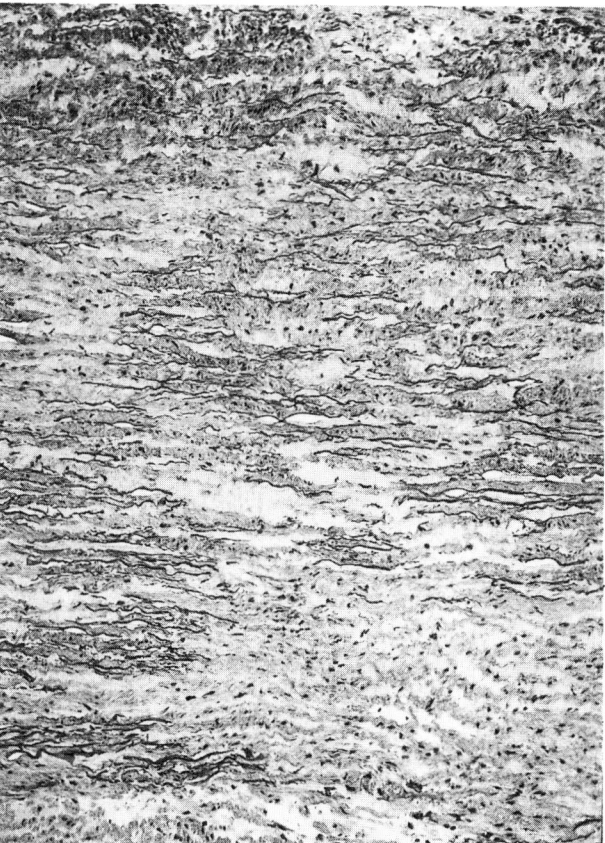

Figure 5.17 Section of aorta of patient with the Marfan syndrome. The elastic fibers in the media are severely disrupted and there is marked accumulation of proteoglycan material. (Movat pentachrome stain.)

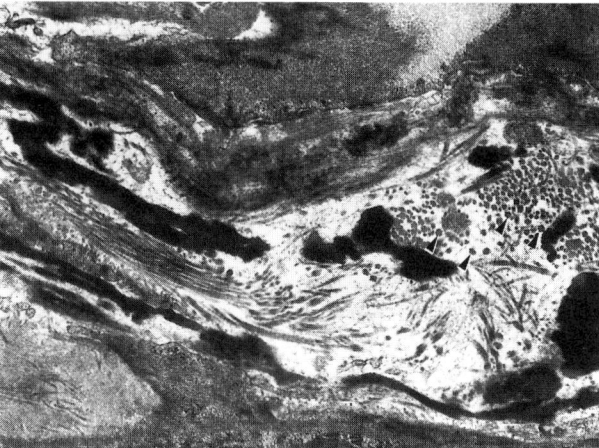

Figure 5.18 Electron micrograph of aorta of patient with the Marfan syndrome, showing various degrees of disruption of the amorphous components (which appear darkly stained) of the elastic fibers in the media. Irregularly shaped and stained amorphous components are associated with granular material. Note collagen 'flowers' (arrowheads). (Kajikawa stain.)

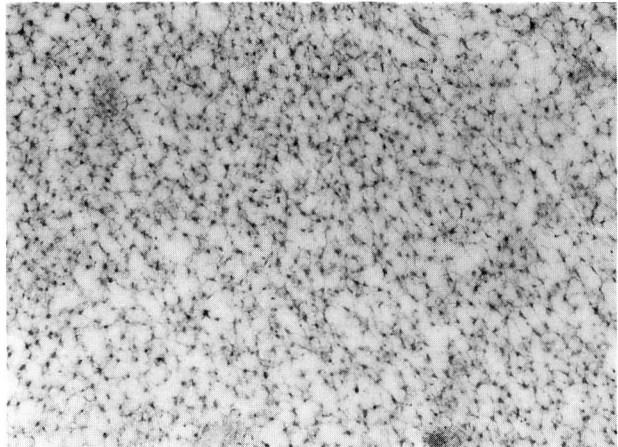

Figure 5.19 Electron micrograph showing marked accumulation of proteoglycan material in the aortic media of a patient with the Marfan syndrome. This material appears in the form of star-shaped granules, which often form a network. (Uranyl acetate and lead citrate stain.)

fibers and a pronounced increase in proteoglycans, which form large pools between the remaining elastic lamellae [223–225]. Increased vascularization of the media also has been described [222]. Although the accumulation of proteoglycans is well known to be a very striking microscopic manifestation of the Marfan syndrome, it is now regarded as a secondary phenomenon and its relationship to the basic metabolic defects is not understood. Alterations in the mechanical properties of the aorta, such as reduction in tensile strength, have been reported in patients with the Marfan syndrome [226,227] and reflect the structural and biochemical changes noted in this disorder. Diastolic and systolic cross-sectional areas of the ascending and descending thoracic aorta were determined by magnetic resonance imaging and two-dimensional echocardiography in children with Marfan syndrome and in age-matched controls [228]. The ascending aorta in 33% of patients with the Marfan syndrome had an abnormally low distensibility and a large diastolic luminal size [229].

Ultrastructural studies (Figure 5.19) of the aorta in patients with the Marfan syndrome have shown that the accumulations of proteoglycans form a meshwork of fine filaments and star-shaped granules that often are in close relationship to elastic and collagenous fibers [224,225]. Elastic fibers have a moth-eaten appearance. Their amorphous components show an increase in electron density and appear to degenerate into masses of dark granules. These changes are non-specific and have been observed in other conditions, including the senile elastoses. The microfibrils associated with elastin are decreased in number. Such a decrease is difficult to evaluate, as microfibrils normally are found in reduced numbers in mature elastic fibers (as opposed to their abundance in developing elastic fibers). In addition, it is very difficult to assess the occurrence of secondary degenerative changes in elastic fibers in aneurysmal walls. To a lesser extent, the microscopic changes just described may also be found in other arteries, including coronary arteries [225,230]; however, peripheral arterial disease is rarely of clinical significance in the Marfan syndrome [218].

According to Roberts [215], patients with the Marfan syndrome in whom aortic dissection occurs tend to have morphologically normal aortas, which only show changes comparable to those in age-matched control patients. Schlatmann and Becker [231,232] have shown that alterations of aging in normal aortas include the occurrence of changes of cystic medial necrosis or mucoid medial degeneration (defined as pooling of proteoglycans, fragmentation of elastic fiber, fibrosis and loss of nuclei). Thus, the differences between these changes in normal and abnormal aortas are quantitative rather than qualitative [231,232].

A particularly severe, rapidly progressive form of the Marfan syndrome has been reported in small children, in whom aortic dilatation and cardiac valvular lesions coexist with musculoskeletal deformities and with marked alterations in the structure of the aorta [233] similar to those observed in adults with the Marfan syndrome. One report [234] described a newborn who had features consistent with both Marfan syndrome and Beals syndrome, including severe arachnodactyly, hypermobility of the fingers, flexion contractures of elbow joints, hips, and knees, micrognathia, crumpled ears, rocker-bottom feet and loose, redundant skin. The aorta and the pulmonary trunk were dilated and all cardiac valves were regurgitant and myxomatous. The genetic implications of the apparent overlap of the features of these two syndromes remains to be assessed. Both fibrillin and decorin (a low molecular weight proteoglycan normally present in the extracellular matrix of connective tissue) are severely deficient in the skin of patients with neonatal Marfan syndrome [235,236]. Furthermore, the expression of these two components is very minimal in cultured skin fibroblasts from these patients [236]. These data have been interpreted as suggesting that at least some cases of neonatal Marfan syndrome are due to a severe defect in fibrillin and that the defect in decorin may be secondary but significantly contributory to this phenotypic manifestation.

A variety of congenital cardiovascular malformations has been observed in association with the Marfan syndrome; coarctation of the aorta and atrial septal defect are unusually frequent [218,237,238]. The relationship of these malformations to the metabolic defect in the Marfan syndrome is not known.

A congenital syndrome, similar in some respects (long thin extremities and laxity of joints and dilatation of the aorta and pulmonary artery) to the Marfan syndrome in humans has been described in calves [239]. Histopathologic studies of the aortic media of the affected calves demonstrated narrowed elastic lamellae separated by widened spaces. Electron microscopy showed elastic laminae that were irregular and thin. The amorphous components seemed less abundant so that microfibrils could be seen throughout the elastic fibers. Bovine Marfan syndrome, like the human disorder, is caused by a mutation in fibrillin, leading to defective synthesis of microfibrils [240].

(b) 9q34 duplication syndrome

Patients with the 9q34 duplication syndrome present with physical findings similar to those observed in Marfan syndrome and in congenital contractural arachnodactyly [241]. However, they have minimal or no cardiovascular complications and they can be clearly identified on the basis of cytogenetic studies, which show a chromosomal abnormality consisting of a duplication of 9q34.

(c) Cutis laxa

The term cutis laxa designates a heterogeneous group of disorders that affect elastic fibers and are characterized by loose, redundant, inelastic skin and a high incidence of emphysema, aortic dilatation and multiple hernias. Congenital and acquired types have been described. The congenital forms can be transmitted as autosomal dominant, autosomal recessive or X-linked disorders. The dominant form is not associated with cardiovascular lesions [242]. A deficiency of lysyl oxidase is involved in the pathogenesis of the X-linked type. This form of cutis laxa (previously known as type IX Ehlers–Danlos syndrome) is characterized by skin laxity and hyperelasticity, bladder diverticula, inguinal hernias and skeletal abnormalities including an occipital exostosis (occipital horn syndrome) [243]. This disease is related to deficient activity of lysyl oxidase. Copper concentrations are markedly elevated in cultured skin fibroblasts, but decreased in serum and hair. Serum ceruloplasmin levels are also low. This form of cutis laxa is allelic to Menkes' syndrome (section 5.4.2(b)) in which similar defects in copper transport have been recognized [244]. Interpretation of published reports on cardiovascular pathologic findings in cutis laxa is difficult because of the uncertainties related to the exact biochemical defects in the affected patients.

Emphysema and arterial disease are most prominent in the recessive form, in which the aortic root, the ascending aorta and the major branches of the aortic arch and the vertebral arteries are dilatated, elongated and tortuous [242,245–247]. Dilatation of the thoracic aorta also occurs in the acquired type [248,249]. Rupture of the thoracic aorta without aneurysm formation has been described in a patient with the acquired type [248]. Dilatation of the pulmonary artery, multiple stenosis in peripheral pulmonary arterial branches and tortuosity of the pulmonary veins have been reported in the congenital recessive form. [250]. Cor pulmonale in this syndrome can result from emphysema or from multiple pulmonary arterial stenosis [251].

Histologically, the affected vessels show a marked decrease in elastic fibers, which often appear fragmented and granular, and an increase in proteoglycans [252, 253]. On ultrastructural study, elastic fibers appear irregular in outline; abundant microfibrils and accumulations of electron dense granular material surround the amorphous component. The elastic fibers are not calcified [247,251,253,254]. Both the histologic and ultrastructural changes resemble those in the Marfan syndrome. In one patient with cutis laxa, study of the elastic fibers of the skin revealed normal microfibrils and abnormal, markedly decreased amorphous component [255]. Severe coronary arterial narrowing associated with an aortic aneurysm was reported in a small child diagnosed as having an acquired form of cutis laxa (Sweet's disease) [256]. The pathogenesis of this syndrome (postinflammatory elastolysis) remains unknown.

(d) Pseudoxanthoma elasticum

Pseudoxanthoma elasticum (PXE) is a systemic disorder manifested by cutaneous lesions, retinal angioid streaks, gastrointestinal hemorrhages, and fragmentation and calcification of elastic fibers. Studies of the transmission of the disorder have disclosed at least two forms of autosomal dominant and two forms of autosomal recessive inheritance. These forms differ in the incidence and severity of their cardiovascular manifestations [257]. The underlying biochemical defect is unknown. Cardiovascular manifestations result from enlargement and calcification of elastic fibers in endocardium and in the intima and media of muscular arteries [258]. These changes may be associated with premature atherosclerosis. The distinctive cardiac lesions are yellowish white endocardial plaques, which are composed of degenerated, calcified elastic fibers located in the deeper areas of the endocardium [259,260]. These lesions are more frequent and extensive in the atria than in the ventricles. The femoral, radial and ulnar arteries are among the most common sites of arterial calcification [258]. In spite of its abundant content of elastic fibers, the aorta is infrequently involved; however, almost complete occlusion of the ascending aorta by a calcific mass was reported in one patient [261]. Intimal calcification involves the internal elastic lamina and can progress to irregular discrete plaques, causing severe luminal narrowing of coronary arteries (Figure 5.20). Atherosclerotic plaques also can contribute to this luminal narrowing. Medial calcification is more uniformly dis-

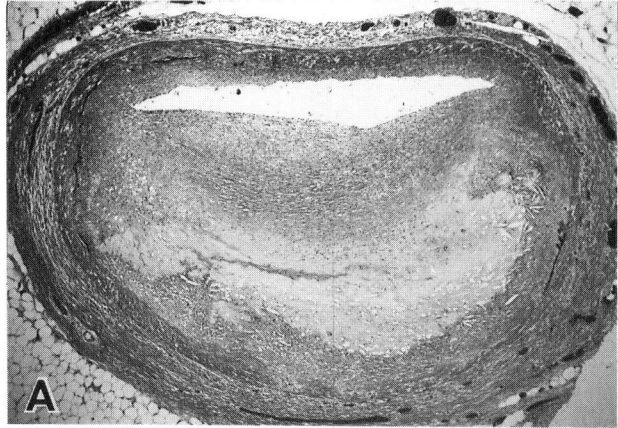
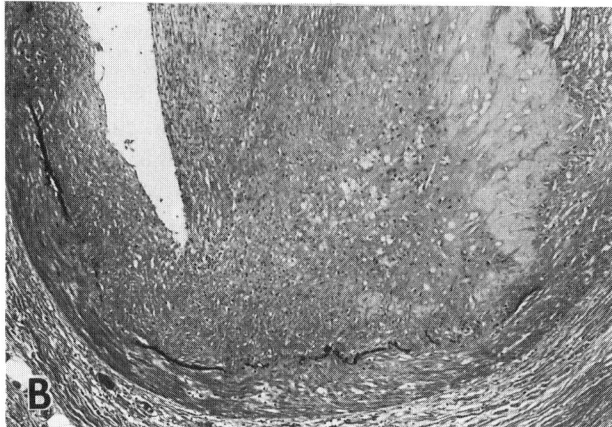

Figure 5.20 Sections of coronary artery of patient with pseudoxanthoma elasticum showing fibrous plaque associated with calcification of the elastic fibers (A). (B) High magnification view of calcified internal elastic lamina. (H & E stain.)

tributed, encompasses the entire circumference of the artery, and is not frequently associated with marked luminal narrowing [258]. There is extreme variation in the degree of coronary arterial disease. Sudden death in PXE has been associated with coronary arterial involvement [262] and with encasement of bundle branches by fibrous tissue [263]. Myocardial infarction is surprisingly infrequent [264].

On histological examination, the abnormal elastic fibers appear larger than normal, are disorganized and fragmented, and show strong basophilia in preparations stained with hematoxylin-eosin. The basophilia is due to the presence of calcific deposits, which involve the amorphous components of elastic fibers [265]. In the skin, the calcified elastic fibers showed electron-dense areas with granular structures. Mineralized elastic fibers contained very electron dense, needle-shaped apatite crystals. Degenerated elastic fibers are often surrounded by masses of fine filamentous material that might represent degraded absent elastin [226]. Lebwohl et al. [267] described the occurrence of premature atherosclerotic heart disease in four young patients with PXE. These authors pointed out that arterial grafts should not be used for coronary artery bypass surgery in patients with PXE because of possible calcification of the internal elastic laminae of the arteries.

(e) **Osteogenesis imperfecta**

Osteogenesis imperfecta is the name given to a group of generalized disorders of connective tissue that primarily affect bones, tendons, ligaments and dentin. It occurs in four forms [268,269], which differ in age of onset, phenotypic signs, mode of inheritance, severity of the bone fragility and resultant skeletal deformity [270–273]. Type II is the most severe form of the disease and is lethal in the perinatal period.

Osteogenesis imperfecta results from structural defects in collagen. In at least 90% of the cases this disorder is due to mutations of the genes encoding the α1(I) or α2(I) chain of type I collagen [274]. Most patients with osteogenesis imperfecta are heterozygous for mutations of the COL1A1 gene which encodes the α1(I) chain or the COL1A2 gene which encodes the α2(I) chain of type I collagen. Such patients have one normal allele and one mutant allele. The mild classic form of osteogenesis imperfecta, with grey-blue sclerae, mild bone fragility, premature deafness and normal dentition, is due to a functionless allele, usually of the COL1A1 gene [274]. The affected tissues contain about 50% of the normal amount of type I collagen. In contrast, tissues from patients with the moderate and severe forms of osteogenesis imperfecta usually contain a mixture of mutant and normal type I collagen [275,276]. Approximately 70 different structural mutations of the COL1A1 gene and 30 different structural mutations of the COL1A2 gene have been described. Correlations have been found between the type and site of the mutation and the severity of the phenotype [277].

Myxoid degeneration of the aortic valve and cystic medial necrosis of the aorta have been noted. Criscitiello et al. [278] described a decrease in the number of elastic lamellae in the aorta and pulmonary artery of a 50-year-old man with type I osteogenesis imperfecta. We are not aware of detailed descriptions of the cardiovascular pathology in patients with osteogenesis imperfecta type III or IV.

Overall, the most common valvular lesions in osteogenesis imperfecta are aortic regurgitation and combined aortic and mitral regurgitation, particularly in type 1 [279–285]. The aortic regurgitation results from dilation of the aortic root and deformity of the valvular cusps, which are abnormally translucent, weak and elongated. Aneurysms of the sinuses of Valsalva also occur. The aorta and valves show decreased amounts of fibrous connective tissue and elastic fibers, as well as areas of myxoid change [278,285–288].

Sigmund et al. [289] described a patient with osteogenesis imperfecta associated with isthmic coarctation of the aorta. Electron microscopic examination revealed damaged elastic fibers at the site of the coarctation. Skin and aorta from two patients with type II osteogenesis imperfecta were studied by light and electron microscopy and compared with similar samples from two normal human fetuses and one newborn child [290]. In the aortas of both patients collagen fibrils were significantly smaller than in controls; moreover, elastic lamellae were altered and consisted of roundish aggregates of elastin, massively permeated by proteoglycans.

Transgenic mouse models, expressing variously alterations in the COL1A1 gene have been developed [291–293]. Biochemical and pathological findings in these animals have provided direct evidence that the mutations result in osteogenesis imperfecta. One such mouse model [293] reproduces the typical features of mild osteogenesis imperfecta in humans. In two other models, the findings are similar to those in the mild (type I) osteogenesis imperfecta [291,292]. The cardiovascular lesions in these animals have not been described.

(f) Ehlers–Danlos syndrome

The Ehlers–Danlos syndrome is a heterogeneous group of 12 genetically distinct disorders of connective tissue synthesis, which differ in major clinical features, inheritance patterns and biochemical defects. The modes of inheritance are: autosomal dominant in types I–IV and VIII; X-linked recessive in types V; autosomal recessive in types VI, VII and X, and undetermined in types XI and XII. Types I, II and III are due to unknown biochemical defects; type IV, to deficient synthesis of type III collagen (several different defects have been found in different patients); type V, to a lysyl oxidase deficiency; type VI, to lysyl hydroxylase deficiency; type VII to a procollagen peptidase deficiency; type X, defective fibronectin and types VIII, XI and XII to unknown defects [294]. Type IX Ehlers–Danlos syndrome is now considered vacant and patients with this syndrome have been reclassified as having the X-linked recessive form of cutis laxa [269] (section 5.3.2(c)).

Biochemical study has shown that skin fibroblasts from a patient with type IV Ehlers–Danlos syndrome produced markedly diminished amounts of type III collagen [295]. Cells obtained from other, non-cutaneous tissues (including artery, vein and peritoneum) produced two forms of collagen α1(III) chains: a normal and a slow-migrating mutant form. The type III collagen molecules containing mutant chains which were over-modified had a lower thermal stability and were poorly secreted into the extracellular medium. Inability of cultured fibroblasts to produce type III collagen has also been noted in another patient with type IV Ehlers–Danlos syndrome [296].

Recent studies have disclosed defects in the synthesis and distribution of fibronectin in the extracellular matrix of skin and cultured fibroblasts as well as a decrease in the number of fibronectin receptors of the polymorphonuclear leukocytes in patients with types I, II and VI of Ehlers–Danlos syndrome. Tissue fibronectin has been found to be absent in the skin extracellular matrix in type X Ehlers–Danlos syndrome [297–299].

Cardiovascular lesions have been described in most of the types of Ehlers–Danlos syndrome [300]. Evaluation of cardiovascular findings in many of the reported patients is complicated because the clinical features of approximately half of the patients are difficult to classify as to exact type. There is a poor correlation between the severity of cardiac and extracardiac findings in patients with the Ehlers–Danlos syndrome [301]. Dissection of the aorta and tears in peripheral arteries have been reported in type I, the gravis form [302]. One patient with type II, the mitis form, had an atrial septal defect, congenital atrioventricular block, and an aneurysm of the ascending aorta [303]. Another patient had aneurysms of the brachial artery and abdominal aorta [304]. Major vascular complications are most common in patients with type IV, the ecchymotic, arterial, or Sack type [294,302–307] (Figure 5.21). These patients are predisposed to sudden death from rupture of the aorta or other major arteries or veins. They frequently have varicose veins, tortuous arteries, arterial aneurysms, and a prominent superficial venous pattern. Affected vessels are easily torn and may appear smaller than normal in size. Histologically, they show thinning of the wall, with a diffuse decrease in elastic tissue in the media, deposition of proteoglycans between the medial elastic lamellae, and a decrease in adventitial and medial collagen. They do not show changes of 'cystic medial necrosis'. Aortic rupture may be mediated by a tear in a previously undamaged, but thin and fragile portion of the vessel.

A rare finding associated with the Ehlers–Danlos syndrome is the occurrence of multiple congenital aneurysms of elastic and muscular arteries, including coronary arteries. Of four patients reported with these changes (which may represent a variant of type IV Ehlers–Danlos syndrome), three were 5–8 years old, and one was 42 years old. Only two of these patients demonstrated some of the other connective tissue abnormalities associated with the Ehlers–Danlos syndrome [308–310]. Histologic studies demonstrated a normal internal elastic lamina, distortion and clumping of medial elastic fibers, replacement of the outer third of the media by collagen and an increased amount of proteoglycans in the media. The media of the aorta and muscular arteries showed a decrease in the total amount of connective tissue, with separation and disruption of the collagen fibers. Medial smooth muscle cells in muscular arteries were decreased in numbers; in the aorta, they varied in size and arrangement. Recent

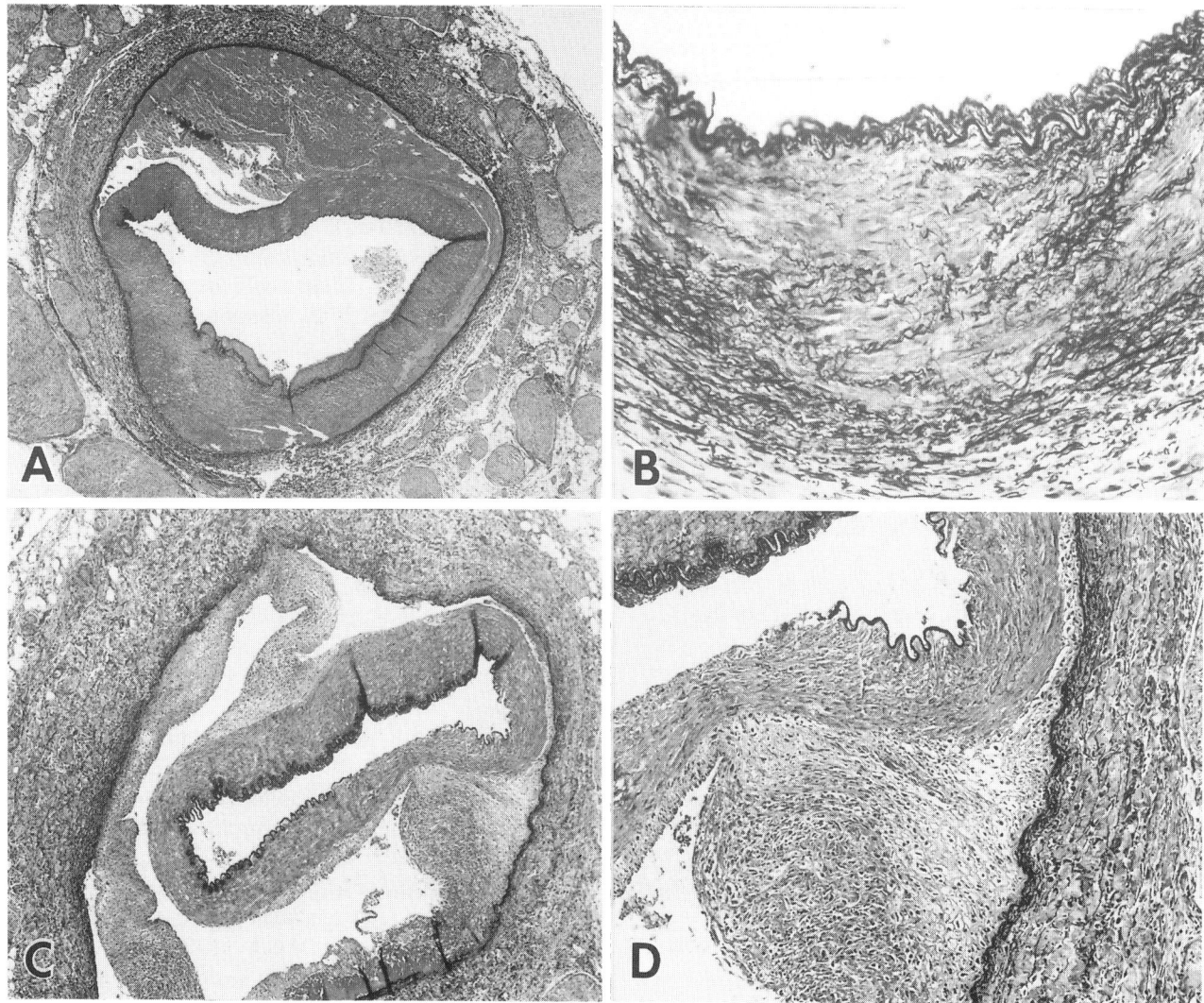

Figure 5.21 Four views of systemic arteries from 33-year-old man with probable type 4 Ehlers–Danlos syndrome. The patient died after developing multiple arterial dissections. (A) Celiac artery showing medial dissection. (B) Non-dissected area of axillary artery showing altered architecture of medial elastic fibers. (C) Axillary artery showing organizing dissection. (D) Higher magnification of organization of thrombus in area of dissection shown in (B). (Movat pentachrome stain.)

studies indicate that there may be further clinical and biochemical heterogeneity among patients with type IV [311]. Four subtypes (A, B, C and D) have been recognized [269].

Spontaneous carotid cavernous fistula and multiple arterial dissections were present in a 43-year-old patient with type IV Ehlers–Danlos syndrome [312]. In addition to the carotid cavernous fistula, the patient had independent dissections of the internal carotid artery at the site of the fistula and an intracavernous aneurysm of the contralateral internal carotid artery. There were dissections of major arteries, including the right renal, external iliac and femoral arteries and laceration of the right common iliac artery, but these arteries showed only mild histological abnormalities. Morphometric analysis of collagen from the aorta revealed an increase in large-sized fibers. This finding was considered to be consistent with deficiency of type III collagen. Rupture of the left renal artery and left common iliac artery was complicated by perforation of the sigmoid colon in one patient with type IV Ehers–Danlos syndrome [313]. Kitazono et al. [296] reported two patients with type IV Ehlers–Danlos syndrome who had myocardial infarctions which might have resulted from fragility of their coronary arteries. One of these patients also had spontaneous rupture of a brachial artery.

Microvascular involvement appears to be an additional manifestation of type IV Ehlers–Danlos syndrome [314]. Capillary microscopy of the nail folds, performed in two such patients, showed microangiopathy of the skin capillaries with microbleeding, microaneurysms and increased transcapillary diffusion.

Cardiovascular lesions reported in other types of Ehlers–Danlos syndrome include: mitral valvular prolapse in types V, VI, VIII, X and XI, aortic root dilatation in type X and sinus of Valsalva aneurysm in type XII [300].

(g) Larsen's syndrome

Larsen's syndrome is characterized by skeletal dysplasia with multiple joint dislocations and a characteristic facies. It is believed to be a generalized mesenchymal disorder affecting connective tissue and collagen formation [315]. The precise biochemical defect has not been delineated. Dominant and recessively inherited forms of the syndrome have been described [316]. Phenotypic differences between the dominant and the recessive type have not been delineated. A lethal type of Larsen-like syndrome has also been described [316]. Cardiac septal defects have been found to be associated with Larsen's syndrome [315]. Cardiovascular abnormalities in Larsen's syndrome include dilatation of the aorta, aortic regurgitation, tricuspid and mitral valve prolapse. A 3-year-old patient with the Larsen's syndrome had aortic valvular stenosis and regurgitation associated with severe dilatation of the ascending and descending thoracic aorta [317]. Another patient had aortic dilatation and an aneurysm of the ductus arteriosus [318]. Histologically, the wall of the aneurysm showed myxoid change and disruption of the elastic fibers. These changes were thought to resemble those reported in the Marfan syndrome. Dilatation of the aortic root and superior mesenteric artery and ectasia and marked tortuosity of the bifurcation of the common carotid artery, the intracranial portion of the internal carotid artery, and the proximal portion of the middle cerebral artery and anterior cerebral arteries were seen angiographically in one patient with Larsen's syndrome [319].

(h) Fragile X syndrome (Martin–Bell syndrome)

A high incidence of mitral valve prolapse and dilatation of the aortic root has been found in patients with the fragile X syndrome, a relatively common disorder characterized by mental retardation, long face, large and prominent ears, macro-orchidism, prognathism and a fragile site on the long arm of the X chromosome [320]. A metabolic defect in connective tissue is suspected but has not been identified [320,321]. The genetic abnormalities in the fragile X syndrome are characterized by heritable unstable DNA in a portion of the X chromosome, with methylation of the cytosine bases and inactivation of the FMR-1 gene. The mechanism by which this leads to the clinical expression of this syndrome is yet to be clarified [322]. Echocardiographic study of 23 patients with the fragile X syndrome showed aortic root dilatation in 12 patients and mitral valve prolapse in 5 [323]. Detailed cardiac evaluation was made in 40 asymptomatic patients with fragile X syndrome [324]. Of 34 male patients 19 had mitral valvular prolapse and seven of these also had mild dilatation of the aortic root. In contrast, aortic dilatation was absent and mitral valvular prolapse was present in only three of the seven female patients. An 18-year-old mentally impaired male with the fragile X syndrome died suddenly with viral pneumonia and myocarditis. At autopsy, generalized tubular hypoplasia of the aorta and a mild coarctation were discovered. The base of the mitral and tricuspid valves showed striking alterations in elastin distribution and structure by light microscopy. Local collagen alterations were also noted. Comparable changes were seen in the skin elastin as well as a severe depletion of proteoglycans [325].

5.3.3 DISEASES OF EXTRACELLULAR ACCUMULATION OF FIBRILLAR PROTEINS

(a) Amyloidosis

The term amyloidosis describes a large group of disorders which have as a common feature the formation of extracellular deposits of amloid fibrils. These fibrils (Figures 5.22, 5.23) are straight and non-branching, measure 7–10 nm in diameter, have an affinity for Congo red stain, show an X-ray diffraction pattern of β-pleated sheets, and are derived from soluble circulating proteins that are processed (partial proteolysis and polymerization) to convert them into insoluble deposits in organs that may be remote from the sites of synthesis of these proteins [326].

The amyloid fibrils are associated with the P component, which consists of doughnut-shaped, pentagonal structures that measure 9 nm in external diameter and contain globular subunits. This component is identical to a normal serum glycoprotein, has a molecular weight of 180–220 kDa and shows a striking structural homology with C-reactive protein, which is an acute-phase reactant [327]. Amyloid deposits often also contain sulfated proteoglycans [327]. The relationship of these two components of amyloid deposits to the formation of amyloid fibrils is unclear.

The diagnosis of amyloidosis must be confirmed by one or more of the following morphological criteria:

1. demonstration of green (dichroic) birefringence of the deposits after staining with Congo red;
2. electron microscopic identification of amyloid fibrils;
3. immunohistochemical staining using specific antisera for the identification of the type of amyloidogenic proteins [328].

The dichroism observed after Congo red staining is considered indicative of the highly ordered arrangement of the dye molecules, which become aligned along the

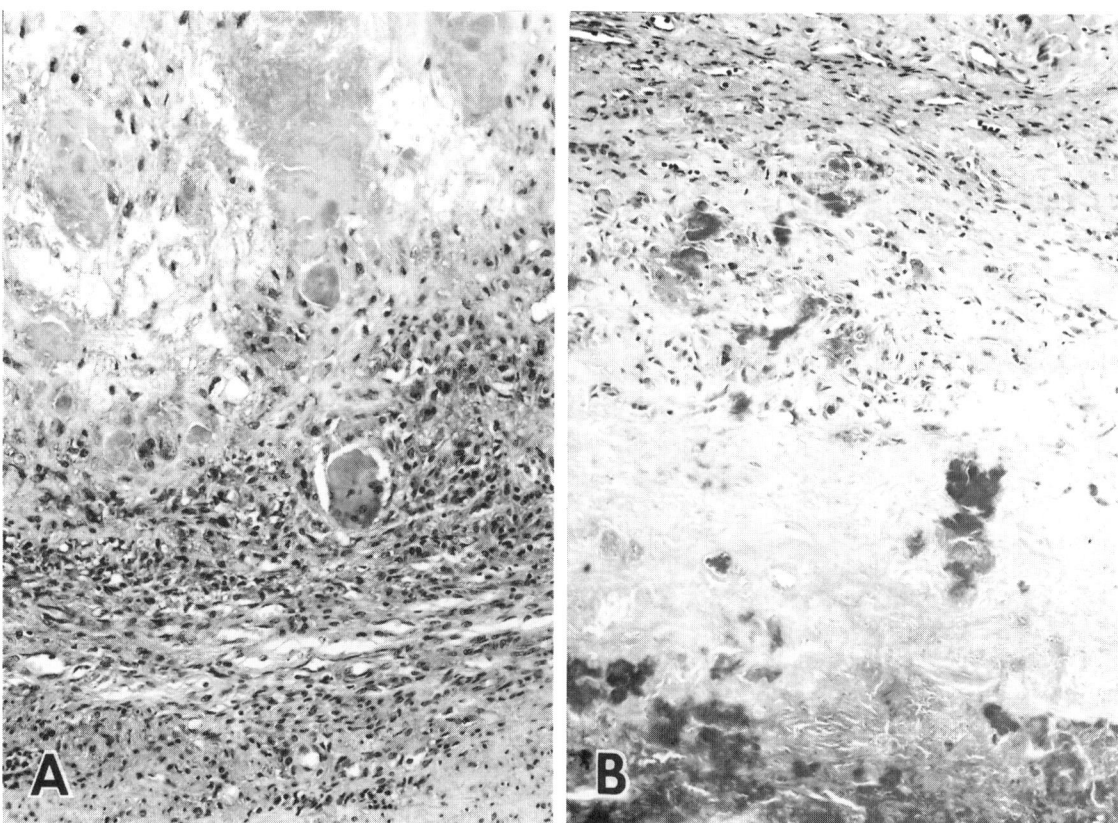

Figure 5.22 Aortic amyloidosis. Amyloid deposits are present in the intima and media. (A) H & E stain. (B) Congo red stain.

longitudinal axes of the amyloid fibrils. In some patients with 'amyloid' deposits derived from light chains (particularly κ chains) of immunoglobulins are not sufficiently organized to permit the binding of Congo red in an orderly fashion. Such deposits are regarded as resulting in 'light-chain deposition disease' and are considered separately in this review. The amyloidoses can be classified into systemic (involving several organ systems) and localized forms [327,329]. These two categories can be subdivided according to the nature of the precursor protein.

The systemic amyloidoses include:

1. AL amyloidosis (often referred to as primary amyloidosis), in which the amyloid deposits are derived from immunoglobulins and are associated with immunocyte dyscrasias;
2. AA amyloidosis or reactive systemic amyloidosis (secondary amyloidosis) associated with chronic inflammatory conditions, especially rheumatoid arthritis, in which the amyloid deposits are derived from a serum precursor known as serum amyloid-associated protein (SAA), which is synthesized in the liver and circulates in association with the HDL3 subclass of lipoproteins;
3. hemodialysis-associated amyloidosis, in which the deposits are derived from β2-macroglobulins;
4. the hereditary amyloidoses, including familial Mediterranean fever (related to AA protein in which the deposits also are derived from SAA) and the familial amyloid polyneuropathy (the amyloidoses in which the amyloid is derived from mutant forms of transthyretin); four types are recognized [330]: type 1 (Andrade or Portuguese type); type 2 (Rukovina type); type 3 (Van Allen type), and type 4 (Meretoja type).

The localized forms of amyloidosis include:

1. senile cardiac amyloidosis, which is related to transthyretin;
2. senile cerebral amyloidosis (Alzheimer's disease), related to β2-amyloid protein (also called A_4);
3. amyloidosis associated with abnormal secretion of a variety of polypeptide hormones and other proteins (such as calcitonin, atrial natriuretic factor and islet amyloid peptide).

AL amyloidosis, the most common form of amyloidosis, occurs in primary amyloidosis and multiple myeloma [331]. Both of the disorders are characterized by proliferation of plasma cells, which produce either whole immunoglobulin light chains or fragments thereof (mostly λ chains). These proteins are found in

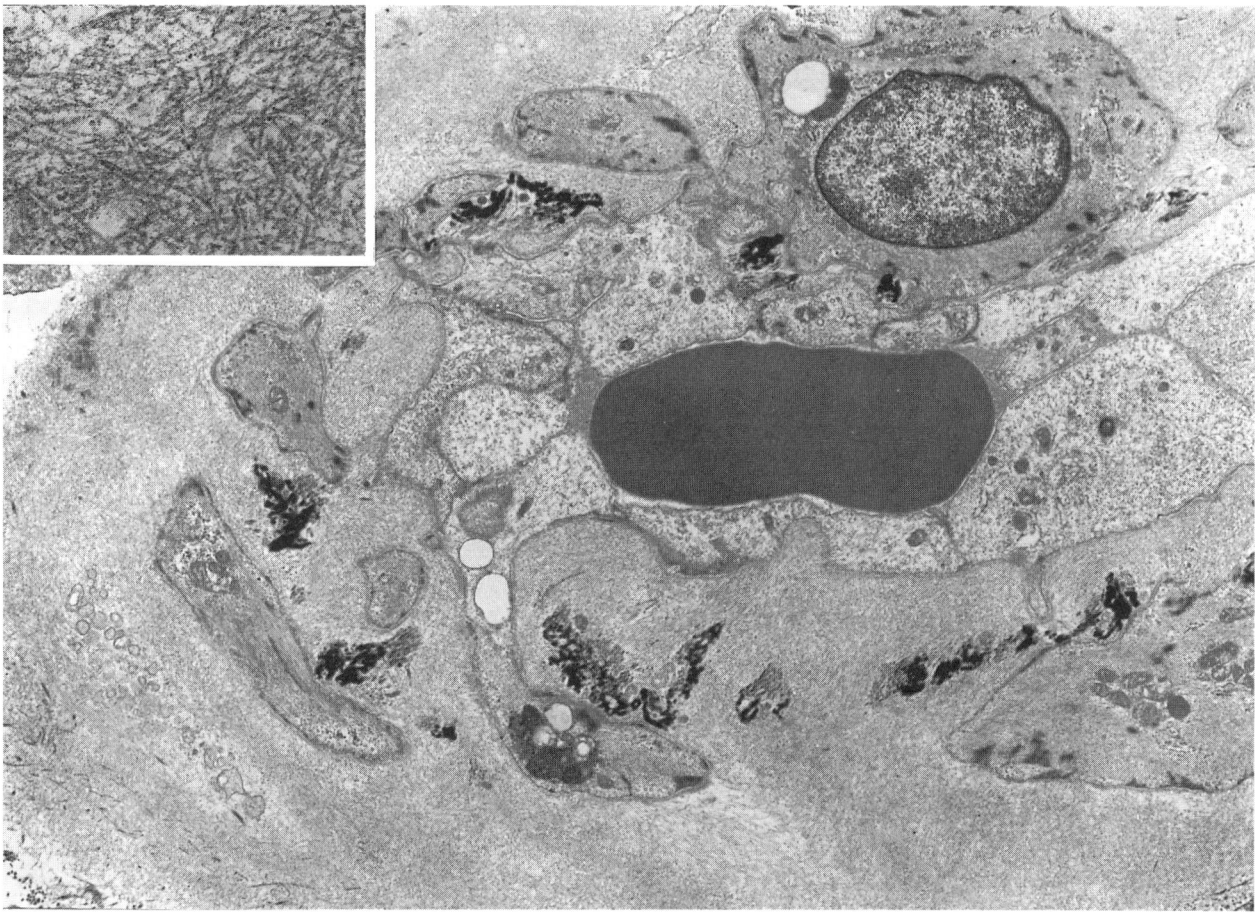

Figure 5.23 Electron micrograph of intramyocardial arteriole which is completely surrounded by deposits of amyloid fibrils. The elastic fibers appear darkly stained. (Kajikawa stain.) Inset shows high magnification view of the amyloid fibrils, which are straight and unbranched. (Uranyl acetate and lead citrate stain.)

the plasma or urine, or both, and are the source of the amyloid deposits. It can be difficult to distinguish between AL amyloidosis related to multiple myeloma and that caused by primary amyloidosis, since bone marrow plasmacytosis is found in both disorders. In myeloma, many of the clinical manifestations are related directly to the proliferation of the plasma cells, while in primary amyloidosis they are determined mainly by the organ dysfunction caused by the deposits of proteins synthesized by the plasma cells.

AA amyloidosis (reactive systemic or secondary amyloidosis) is most often associated with chronic inflammatory states, including familial Mediterranean fever, rheumatoid arthritis, tuberculosis and osteomyelitis. The mononuclear phagocyte system plays an important role in the pathogenesis of AA amyloid deposits by providing cytokine signals, mediated by interleukin-1 and interleukin-6, that regulate the expression of certain amyloid precursors and of proteolytic enzymes involved in the processing of amyloidogenic proteins. Deposits in AA amyloidosis lose their affinity for Congo red after treatment with $KMnO_4$, while those in other forms of amyloidosis retain their stainability.

The term ATTR amyloidosis refers to disorders associated with amyloid deposits that are derived from transthyretin, a plasma protein that migrates electrophoretically in the prealbumin fraction and functions as a carrier for circulating thyroxine and retinol. At least 20 different mutations (mostly single amino acid substitutions) are known to involve the structure of transthyretin [332]. Included among the syndromes resulting from these mutations are the various types of familial amyloid polyneuropathy and the senile forms of cardiovascular amyloidosis [332]. These were previously referred to as ASc amyloidosis.

Three forms of senile cardiovascular amyloidosis have been recognized on the basis of morphologic studies [328,333]:

1. senile aortic amyloidosis;
2. isolated atrial amyloidosis;
3. systemic senile amyloidosis with cardiovascular involvement.

Isolated atrial amyloidosis is related to deposits derived from atrial natriuretic factor, a polypeptide that is normally secreted by atrial myocytes and, to a much lesser extent, by ventricular myocytes [334]. The other two forms appear to correspond to TTR amyloidosis and have been previously recognized on the basis of immunohistochemical staining with antibodies directed against prealbumin [328]. In a series of 85 consecutive autopsies of patients ≥80 years of age, amyloid deposits were present in the aorta in all patients and occurred predominantly in the inner third of the media, appearing as either lumps or lines oriented parallel to the smooth muscle cells [333]. A very high frequency of aortic amyloidosis also has been reported in other studies of elderly patients [335,336,337]. Aortic amyloidosis in itself may not be functionally significant; however, cardiac amyloid deposits in the senile amyloidoses can result in significant cardiac dysfunction.

Regardless of the type of amyloidosis, cardiac amyloid deposits can occur in myocardial interstitium, conduction tissue, valves, endocardium, pericardium, and in small intramural coronary arteries, veins and capillaries. In the systemic amyloidoses, cardiac deposits are extremely common in primary or immunocyte-related amyloidosis but are less frequent in the secondary amyloidoses. Epicardial nerves are involved in patients with familial amyloidotic polyneuropathies [338,339]. Amyloid deposits often form rings around the cardiac muscle cells and capillaries. Deposits in coronary vessels involve all layers and can lead to luminal obliteration [338,340]. Amyloid fibrils can become aggregated just external to the capillary basement membranes or can completely replace them. In general, they tend to become less densely packed as the distance from the basement membrane increases. Amyloid fibrils must be distinguished from connective tissue microfibrils, which occur commonly in fibrotic hearts and vessels and are larger (13 nm in diameter) than amyloid fibrils.

In the familial neuropathic syndromes, amyloid deposits in blood vessels are prominent in the Portuguese type; myocardial interstitium is involved to a lesser extent. In familial Mediterranean fever, arterioles throughout the body are sites of amyloid deposition, but cardiac interstitial involvement is extremely rare. A syndrome of cerebral hemorrhage associated with amyloid deposits in cerebral arteries has been described in Iceland [338,341].

Various types of amyloidosis occur spontaneously in animals, including cats, dogs, horses, pigs and monkeys [342]. Hereditary amyloidosis, with severe renal involvement, occurs in Abyssinian cats. Systemic reactive amyloidosis develops in a variety of species in association with chronic infections, but is particularly prominent in horses used for the production of antisera, especially tetanus antitoxin. A syndrome of cyclic neutropenia in dogs is also associated with systemic amyloidosis. Deposits of amyloid material in neurons (neurofibrillary tangles), similar to those in humans with Alzheimer's disease, have been found in old dogs, bears and monkeys, and pancreatic insular amyloidosis has been identified in cats [342].

A transgenic mouse model of type 1 familial amyloidotic polyneuropathy has been developed by the introduction of the human mutant transthyretin gene [343]. In these transgenic mice, amyloid deposition in the gastrointestinal tract, cardiovascular system and kidneys was noted at 6 months after birth. At 24 months, the pattern of amyloid deposition was similar to that observed in patients with familial amyloidotic polyneuropathy. Amyloid deposits were shown to contain human mutant transthyretin and mouse serum amyloid P component. In the vascular system of these transgenic mice, initial amyloid deposits were observed just external to the basement membranes of capillaries and venules. Amyloid deposition in arterial walls occurred mostly in the advanced stage and was noted in the gastrointestinal tract, salivary glands, lung, liver, pancreas and skeletal muscles.

(b) Light-chain deposition disease

Under some circumstances, the amyloidogenic proteins (usually immunoglobulin light chains) in the blood do not polymerize into fibrils, but instead form amorphous deposits (Figure 5.24) that do not stain with Congo red or the other usual stains for amyloid. Excessive amounts of either kappa or lambda chains can be synthesized (sometimes together with fragments of heavy chains) in AL amyloidosis. Light-chain deposition occurs most frequently in association with multiple myeloma. It is characterized by rapidly progressive renal disease, cardiac involvement manifested by congestive heart failure and restrictive cardiomyopathy, hepatic disease and polyneuropathy [344–348]. The mechanism of tissue deposition in most cases of AL amyloidosis is related to post-secretory proteolysis of light chains that are secreted as normal-sized chains but are especially sensitive to proteolysis. Thus, the AL amyloid fibrils contain fragments of light chains that essentially correspond to the 'variable' regions of such chains [345]. This mechanism is different from that involved in light-chain deposition disease, in which it involves the synthesis of structurally abnormal immunoglobulin chains. The spectrum of alterations in these chains includes abnormal chain glycosylation, aberrations in chain length, and defects in the 'variable' region of the chain, which is considered critical for the formation of amyloid fibrils. These biochemical abnormalities favor deposition of amorphous rather than fibrillar material [344]. It has been suggested that the deposits in light-chain deposition disease contain variously altered 'constant' portions of the light chains [344]. An inter-

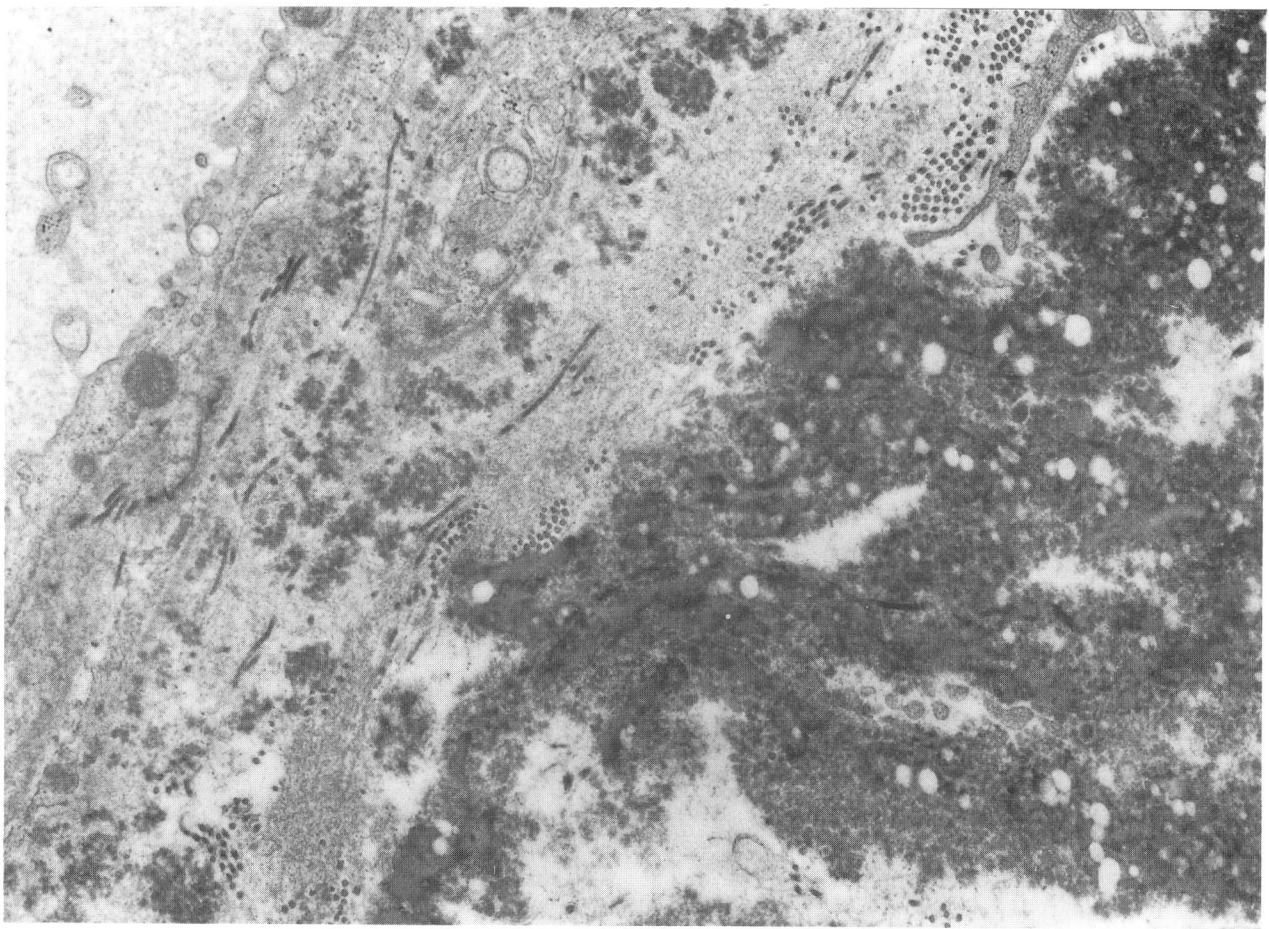

Figure 5.24 Electron micrograph of arteriole in endomyocardial biopsy specimen from patient with light chain deposition disease. Light chain deposits in the form of dark, amorphous material are present in the subendothelial space. (Uranyl acetate and lead citrate stain.)

mediate form, featuring both AL amyloidosis and light-chain deposition, has been reported in a patient in whom ultrastructural and immunohistochemical studies demonstrated amyloid deposits in the myocardium, tongue, walls of portal vein branches and synovium, as well as light-chain deposits in liver, spleen and bone marrow [349]. Light-chain deposits occurring in myocardium were identified ultrastructurally and immunohistochemically in a right ventricular endomyocardial biopsy specimen. These deposits were not evident on routine histopathologic examination; they were Congo red-negative and gave a positive reaction for kappa light chains and a negative reaction for lambda chains. They consisted of amorphous, electron-dense granules that formed discontinuous layers adjacent to the plasma membranes of cardiac myocytes, arteriolar endothelial and smooth-muscle cells, and neural elements [350].

5.3.4 DISEASES FROM ABNORMALITIES IN OTHER PROTEIN SYNTHESES

(a) Hemoglobinopathies

Cardiovascular pathologic changes in patients with hemoglobinopathies can be classified according to whether they are consequences of anemia or of sickling of erythrocytes. Patients with sickle cell disease (SS hemoglobin) often develop pulmonary vascular disease and pulmonary hypertension, which are related to multiple episodes of sickling and thrombosis in small pulmonary artery branches [351,352]. They also may have cerebrovascular disease, which results from sickling and thrombosis in small cerebral blood vessels and from narrowing and occlusion of large vessels. The latter changes are thought to be due to organization of thrombi and to fibromuscular proliferation (which occurs independently of thrombosis) [353,354]. Sites of cerebral vascular lesions in patients with sickle cell disease include ischemic and/or hemorrhagic infarction, intracerebral hemorrhage, cortical venous and/or sinus thrombosis and subarachnoid hemorrhage [355]. Sickling and thrombosis in sickle cell disease also develop in vessels in other organs, including the heart, spleen, kidney and retina. Conjunctival vessels may show striking degrees of tortuosity [356]. Coronary arteries with unusually large diameters have been observed in patients with sickle cell disease [357].

In comparison with patients with sickle cell disease, patients with sickle cell trait (SA hemoglobin) have much milder and infrequent episodes of visceral infarction and, as a rule, do not show chronic cardiovascular abnormalities [351]. However, sudden cardiac death and myocardial infarction due to coronary thrombosis have been reported in patients with sickle cell trait [358] and in non-anemic patients with sickling associated with less well defined abnormalities of hemoglobin types [358,359]. Patients with hemoglobin SC disease are more symptomatic than those with sickle cell trait, but have a lower incidence and severity of cardiovascular manifestations than do patients with sickle cell disease [351]; however, they frequently have pulmonary infarction [360] and much more severe retinal vascular occlusive disease than do patients with sickle cell disease [361].

Conjunctival vessels have been examined with a slit lamp and the abnormalities were graded in 77 patients with sickling disorders, including 48 with sickle cell anemia, 17 with sickle cell β-thalassemia and 12 with hemoglobin SC disease [362]. The abnormalities observed consisted of increased tortuosity and areas of segmental dilatation of the vessels. These abnormalities were more severe in patients with sickle cell disease homozygous for hemoglobin SS in whom they increased with age.

(b) Hypertrophic cardiomyopathy

The term hypertrophic cardiomyopathy refers to a group of conditions characterized by the development of cardiac hypertrophy without any known causative factors. Asymmetric hypertrophy of the ventricular septum (with or without obstruction to left or right ventricular outflow), is a common feature. Hypertrophic cardiomyopathy occurs as an isolated disorder (idiopathic hypertrophic cardiomyopathy) and in combination with a variety of systemic disorders. The biochemical abnormality in idiopathic hypertrophic cardiomyopathy is heterogeneous and involves various amino acid substitutions in the heavy chain of cardiac β-myosin. The genetic defect appears to vary among different affected families, and most frequently is localized to chromosome 14. In a high percentage of patients, the cardiac hypertrophy is associated with important anatomic abnormalities in the small

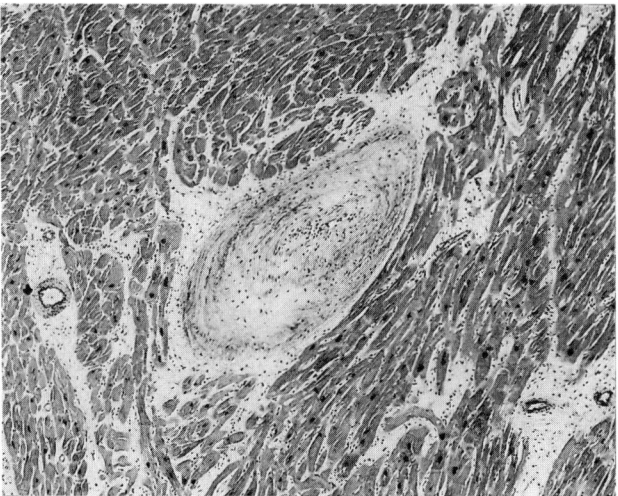

Figure 5.25 Small intramural coronary artery of patient with hypertrophic cardiomyopathy. Marked luminal narrowing is due to increased amounts of proteoglycan material and fibrous tissue with interspersed smooth muscle cells in the intima. (Movat pentachrome stain.)

intramural coronary arteries [363]. About 80% of patients with hypertrophic cardiomyopathy show narrowing of intramural coronary arteries (Figure 5.25). This tends to be maximal in the ventricular septum and is related to intimal and medial thickening by increased amounts of fibrous connective tissue, elastic tissue and smooth muscle cells, and adventitial fibrosis. These lesions can be of considerable clinical significance in the late stages of the disease, in which they can be the cause of cardiac dilatation, fibrosis and thinning of the left ventricular free wall. Their precise relationship to the cardiomyopathic process is unknown. They are not specific for hypertrophic cardiomyopathy [364].

5.3.5 DISEASES OF UNCERTAIN ETIOLOGY

(a) Childhood progeria

Patients with childhood progeria (Hutchinson–Gilford syndrome) develop hypertension, hypercholesterolemia, generalized arteriosclerosis and ischemic heart disease at a very early age; death follows cardiac complications during late childhood or adolescence. The mode of inheritance has not been clarified [365]. It is probable that most cases represent new, sporadic mutations. Recent studies suggest that the abnormal gene responsible for this disorder is located in chromosome 1 [366]. The biochemical defect in progeria is unknown. However, increased urinary excretion of hyaluronic acid has been a consistent finding in patients with this disorder. Some patients with progeria have multiple, small foci of myocardial necrosis and fibrosis, whereas others have large infarcts. Coronary atherosclerosis is usually severe, and the coronary ostia may be markedly narrowed. Calcification develops in aortic and mitral valvular leaflets, large extramural coronary arteries and cerebral arteries. Atheromatous changes are present in the aorta, pulmonary artery, and large and medium-sized systemic arteries [367–372]. Cerebrovascular disease also occurs in progeria syndrome [373,374]. Bilateral occlusions of the proximal internal carotid arteries and origins of the vertebral arteries were demonstrated by magnetic resonance angiography in a 4-year-old boy with progeria [375,376]. Wagle et al. [376] noted gyral edema and infarction in the distribution of the superior division of the right middle cerebral artery in a 6-year-old girl with progeria. The cause for the infarction was not apparent since magnetic resonance angiography demonstrated that the carotid bifurcations and the large intracranial arteries were normal.

(b) **Adult progeria**

Werner's syndrome, also known as adult progeria [377,378], has a number of clinical features, such as widespread atherosclerosis and calcification of the cardiac valves, which resemble those of childhood progeria. The abnormalities and growth delay in progeria are not apparent at birth, but progressively develop usually beginning in the first year of life. In Werner's syndrome however, the recognizable phenotype often is not apparent until the individuals are in their mid-teens to their twenties, and diagnosis is not usually made until they are in their thirties [378]. The mode of inheritance of Werner's syndrome appears to be autosomal recessive and increased consanguinity exists among the affected families. A 37-year-old female diagnosed as having Werner's syndrome developed insulin-dependent diabetes mellitus at age 30 and underwent bilateral femoral–popliteal bypass surgery at age 32 for circulatory insufficiency and below-knee amputation at age 37 for non-healing ankle ulcers. Another 37-year-old man with Werner's syndrome, who developed angina at age 32 and coronary arteriography at age 37, showed 50–90% obstruction of the coronary arteries [378].

5.4 Diseases of mineral and vitamin metabolism

Vascular abnormalities associated with metabolic disorders involving minerals and vitamins are presented in this section and comprise idiopathic infantile hypercalcemia (Williams–Beuren syndrome); disorders of copper metabolism, including Wilson's disease, Menkes' syndrome and dietary deficiency of copper; deficiency of Vitamin C and finally selenium–Vitamin E deficiency.

5.4.1 IDIOPATHIC INFANTILE HYPERCALCEMIA (WILLIAMS–BEUREN SYNDROME)

The Williams–Beuren syndrome is an autosomal dominant disorder which in its full clinical expression is manifested by mental and physical retardation, a typical elfin facies, dental malformations, hypercalcemia and supravalvular aortic stenosis [379,380,381,382]. The etiology of this syndrome remains undetermined as is the relationship between the hypercalcemia and the vascular alterations. Variability in the expression of the clinical manifestations has led to the description of separate aspects of the syndrome as two distinct entities: supravalvular aortic stenosis and infantile hypercalcemia [383]. Beuren [384] presented compelling evidence that supravalvular aortic stenosis and idiopathic infantile hypercalcemia are the same disorder. Other cardiovascular anomalies observed in this syndrome are: aortic regurgitation [385,386], pulmonary valvular stenosis [385–387], multiple stenoses of the peripheral branches of the pulmonary arteries [388], hypoplasia of the aorta [385], aortic coarctation [389,390], coarctation of systemic arteries other than the aorta [385,386], dilatation and tortuosity of the coronary arteries [385,386] and disarray of elastic lamellae and smooth muscle cells of the aortic media [382]. Luminal narrowing and medial calcification also occur in the coronary arteries (Figure 5.26). The total length of the ascending aorta is reduced, and the extent of this reduction is not related to the severity of the supravalvular aortic stenosis [380]. Atrial and ventricular septal defects [387], mitral regurgitation [382], calcification of the mitral annulus [388] and bicuspid aortic valve [385] also have been noted.

5.4.2 DISORDERS OF COPPER METABOLISM

Vascular abnormalities in disorders of copper metabolism have been described in Wilson's disease, Menkes' syndrome, and dietary deficiency of copper. This metal is an integral component of lysyl oxidase, the enzyme responsible for the formation of crosslinks of both elastin and collagen. This enzyme catalyzes the oxidative deamination of the ε-amino group in the lysyl and hydroxylysyl residues of collagen and lysyl residues of elastin. The resulting aldehydes undergo aldol condensation or Schiff base formation to yield covalent crosslinks of these proteins. Immunohistochemical studies have shown that lysyl oxidase in the vascular system is associated with collagen fibrils, elastic fibers, smooth muscle cells and fibroblasts [391]. For these reasons, deficient activity of lysyl oxidase is associated

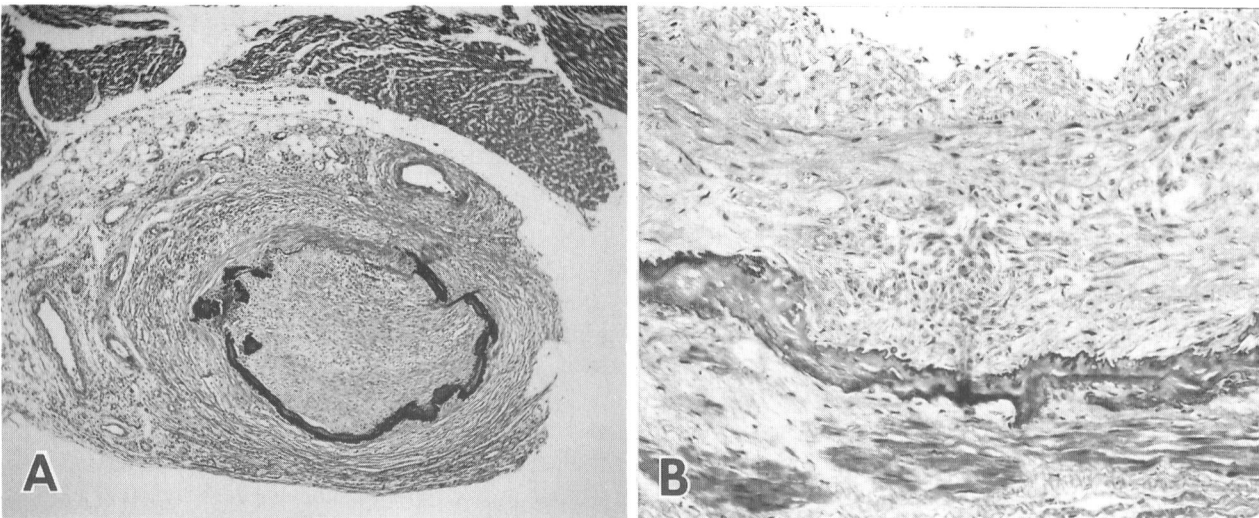

Figure 5.26 View of two coronary arteries from patients with idiopathic infantile hypercalcemia. (A) Epicardial coronary artery showing almost circumferential calcification in the media, with luminal obliteration by proliferation of intimal smooth muscle cells. (B) High power view of artery showing medial calcification with overlying smooth muscle cells surrounded by proteoglycan material. (Movat pentachrome stain.)

with structural abnormalities involving both elastin and collagen.

(a) Wilson's disease

Wilson's disease (hepatolenticular degeneration) is transmitted as an autosomal recessive trait and is characterized by cirrhosis of the liver, degenerative changes in the brain, especially in the basal ganglia, and Kayser–Fleischer rings in the cornea. Low serum copper concentrations, decreased serum ceruloplasmin levels and increased urinary copper excretion are observed, together with increased copper deposition in various tissues, mainly in the liver. The accumulation of copper in the liver is thought to result from abnormal copper export from the hepatocytes. A defect in copper export underlies both Wilson's disease (in which it involves mainly the hepatocytes) and Menkes' disease in which it affects other types of cells [392]. Although generalized vascular involvement has not been described in Wilson's disease, Factor et al. [393] noted intramyocardial small vessel sclerosis in nine patients with this condition.

(b) Menkes' syndrome

Menkes' syndrome is an X-linked disorder characterized by abnormal transport and cellular sequestration of copper. These changes result in defective crosslinking of collagen and elastin, due to impaired activity of lysyl oxidase [394]. Low levels of lysyl oxidase activity may be the result of disturbances in intracellular copper translocation and, consequently, of impaired incorporation of copper into lysyl oxidase. The basic defect in Menkes' syndrome involves a deficiency in the activity of a copper-transporting ATPase. The defect in lysyl oxidase activity is a secondary phenomenon [392]. The gene coding for this enzyme is located in the X-chromosome. The disorder is characterized principally by growth retardation, progressive cerebral degeneration, distinctive facial features, hypopigmentation of skin and hair, recurrent episodes of hypothermia and abnormal, kinky hair [395]. The cardiovascular lesions in this syndrome are characterized by widespread but patchy, degenerative changes in the arterial walls [396–399]. Grossly, the heart in Menkes' syndrome is normal. Superficial vessels often appear tortuous or dilated. Aneurysm formation often involves major arteries and veins and is associated with subintimal edema, marked collagenous thickening of the media and extensive loss of elastin and smooth muscle cells.

Arterial wall changes consist of fragmentation, splitting and reduplication of the internal elastic lamina, an abnormal increase in the amount of collagen throughout the vessel wall and a marked reduction in the number of smooth muscle cells. Involvement of coronary arteries is variable. The vascular lumina often are compromised and occasionally are obliterated [400,401]. Vascular changes constitute an important factor in the pathogenesis of central nervous system lesions in patients with Menkes' syndrome; however, cellular metabolic alterations more directly related to abnormalities of cellular copper metabolism also play important roles in this respect [402].

Ultrastructural study of the aorta in a patient with Menkes' syndrome showed that the elastic lamellae were poorly formed and were composed of clumps of elastin surrounded by large numbers of microfibrils. The aortic smooth muscle cells contained large aggregates of loosely arranged, flocculent, metachromatic material of unknown nature [403].

A murine homologue (mottled), of Menkes' disease has been described. Mottled cells in culture show cellular defects of copper export that are similar to those in Menkes' syndrome and result in a copper accumulation [392]. Alleles of the mottled locus show considerable phenotypic variability including the hair pigmentation defects of MO^{Pewter}, connective tissue defects of MO^{blotchy}, the neurologic defects MO^{brindled} and the prenatal lethality of MO^{tortoiseshell}. However, the pathology of the cardiovascular system in these models has not been reported in detail.

(c) Dietary deficiency of copper

Dietary deficiency of copper in various species of animals (rats, swine, miniature swine, steers, turkeys and chickens) induces myocardial hypertrophy, focal necrosis, aortic rupture and left ventricular aneurysms and rupture. These lesions are much more severe when the dietary deficiency is induced during the neonatal period. Such changes are associated with extensive alterations in the connective tissue network of the heart, and they resemble those induced by treatment with β-amino-propionitrile (BAPN), a lathyritic agent that inhibits lysyl oxidase [404].

5.4.3 VITAMIN C DEFICIENCY (SCURVY)

Ascorbic acid has many antioxidant functions and also plays a role in proline hydroxylation, an important step in collagen synthesis. Cardiovascular lesions reported in ascorbic acid deficiency consist of hemorrhagic phenomena, which have been shown in animals to result from disruption of capillary basement membranes, depletion of pericapillary collagen and separation of endothelial cell junctions [405]. In addition, right ventricular hypertrophy has been observed in several necropsy studies of children with scurvy [406].

5.4.4 DEFICIENCY OF SELENIUM AND VITAMIN E

Although numerous minerals and trace elements have been shown to be of importance in various aspects of cardiovascular disease, morphologically distinct cardiovascular lesions related to deficiency states involving these elements have been documented in man only in the case of selenium [407].

Deficiency of selenium and vitamin E results in a wide spectrum of clinical and pathologic changes, including necrosis of myocardium, skeletal muscle, liver, pancreas and central nervous system [408,409]. Selenium and vitamin E are components of the glutathione peroxidase

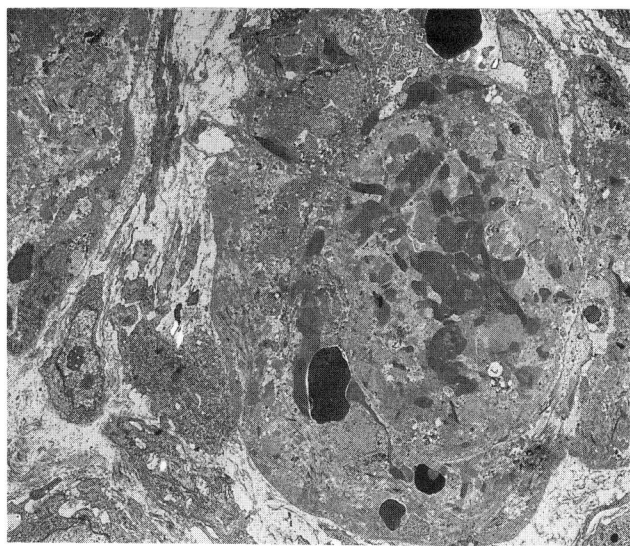

Figure 5.27 Fibrinoid necrosis is evident in myocardial arteriole of pig with deficiency of selenium and vitamin E (mulberry heart disease). (Electron micrograph, uranyl acetate and lead citrate stain.)

system, which plays an important role in preventing lipoperoxidative damage induced by oxygen-free radicals. The distribution and relative severity of the lesions due to deficiency of these two nutrients are related to the rate of their depletion, the concomitant presence of other pro-oxidant agents and the animal species.

In humans, selenium deficiency results in a peculiar type of dilated cardiomyopathy that occurs mostly in China (Keshan disease) in a zone in which the selenium content of the soil is very low [410]. In Western countries, this disorder occurs mainly in patients who have been maintained for long periods of time on total parenteral nutrition without supplements of selenium [411]. It is manifested by congestive heart failure or, less frequently, by sudden death or by embolic strokes related to cardiac mural thrombi. The microscopic appearance of the heart often is characteristic, showing large areas of myocardial necrosis with extensive myocytolysis. The resulting myocardial fibrosis can be very extensive [412–414].

While in humans this cardiomyopathy develops without associated vascular lesions, deficiency of selenium and vitamin E in pigs is manifested not only by necrosis of myocytes [408] but also by severe vascular alterations [409]. These consist of multiple areas of epicardial hemorrhages (for which reason this disorder is known as 'mulberry heart disease' in pigs), fibrinoid necrosis (Figure 5.27) of arterioles and fibrin microthrombi in capillaries. These vascular lesions also occur in kidney, intestine, liver, skeletal muscle, stomach and skin [415]. Such lesions tend to be more severe in pigs in which the disorder occurs spontaneously than in those in which it is induced experimentally. Ultrastructural study of the vascular lesions in the hearts of pigs with experimentally induced deficiency of selenium and vitamin E disclosed extensive granular deposits of serum proteins and masses of fibrin in arterioles in which fibrinoid was identified by light microscopy. Endothelial cells of these arterioles were loosely attached to each other. In arterioles with fibrin thrombi, the endothelium was disrupted. In mildly injured arterioles, increased endothelial permeability resulted in insudation of blood proteins into the vessel wall to produce accumulation of fibrinoid material. In severely injured vessels, endothelial integrity was destroyed, smooth muscle cells were necrotic and thrombosis had developed. Initiation of these arteriolar lesions was apparently the result of lipoperoxidative damage to endothelial cell membranes that lacked protection by selenium and vitamin E [409,416].

References

1. McKusick, V.A., Neufeld, E.F. and Kelly, T.E. (1978) The mucopolysaccharide storage diseases, in *The Metabolic Basis of Inherited Disease*, 4th edn, (eds B.J. Stanbury, B.J. Weingarten and D.S. Fredrickson), McGraw-Hill, New York, pp. 1282–1307.
2. Stephan, M.J., Stevens Jr, E.L., Wenstrup, R.J. *et al.* (1989) Mucopolysaccharidosis I presenting with endocardial fibroelastosis of infancy. *Am. J. Dis. Child.*, 143, 782–4.
3. Krovetz, L.J. and Schiebler, G.L. (1965) Cardiovascular manifestations of the Hurler syndrome. Hemodynamic and angiographic observations in 15 patients. *Circulation*, 31, 132–41.
4. Perkins, D.G., and Haust, M.D. (1982) Ultrastructure of the myocardium in the Hurler syndrome: possible relation to cardiac function. *Virchows Arch. Path. Anat.*, 394, 195–205.
5. Renteria, V.G., Ferrans, V.J. and Roberts, W.C. (1976) The heart in the Hurler syndrome: gross, histologic and ultrastructural observations in five necropsy cases. *Am. J. Cardiol.*, 38, 487–501.
6. Schieken, R.M., Kerber, R.E., Ionasescu, V.V. and Zellweger, H. (1975) Cardiac manifestations of the mucopolysaccharidoses. *Circulation*, 52, 700–5.
7. Butman, S.M., Karl, L. and Copeland, J.G. (1989) Combined aortic and mitral valve replacement in an adult with Scheie's disease. *Chest*, 96, 209–10.
8. Nelson, J., Shields, M.D. and Mulholland, H.C. (1990) Cardiovascular studies in the mucopolysaccharidoses. *J. Med. Genet.*, 27, 94–100.
9. Brosius, F.C. and Roberts, W.C. (1981) Coronary artery disease in the Hurler syndrome: qualitative and quantitative analysis of the extent of coronary narrowing at necropsy in six children. *Am. J. Cardiol.*, 47, 649–53.
10. Ferrans, V.J., and Boyce, S.W. (1983) Metabolic and familial and familial disease, in *Cardiovascular Pathology*, vol. 2, (ed. M.D. Silver), Churchill Livingstone, New York, pp. 945–1004.
11. Braunlin, E.A., Hunter, D.W., Krivit, W. *et al.* (1992) Evaluation of coronary artery disease in Hurler syndrome by angiography. *Am. J. Cardiol.*, 69, 1487–9.
12. Goldfischer, J.L., Coltoff-Schiller, B., Biempica, L. and Wolinsky, H. (1975) Lysosomes and the sclerotic arterial lesions in Hurler's disease. *Hum. Pathol.*, 6, 633–7.
13. Taylor, D.B., Blaser, S.I., Burrows, P.E. *et al.* (1991) Arteriopathy and coarctation of the abdominal aorta in children with mucopolysaccharidoses: imaging findings. *Am. J. Roentg.*, 157, 819–23.
14. Roubicek, M., Gehler, J. and Spranger, J. (1985) The clinical spectrum of α-L-iduronidase deficiency. *Am. J. Med. Genet.*, 20, 471–81.
15. Dekaban, A.S. and Constantopoulos, G. (1977) Mucopolysaccharidosis type I, II, IIIA and V. Pathological and biochemical abnormalities in the neural and mesenchymal elements of the brain. *Acta Neuropath.*, 39, 1–7.
16. Chan, C.C., Green, W.R., Manmenee, I.H. and Sack Jr, G.H. (1983) Ocular ultrastructural studies of two cases of Hurler syndrome (systemic mucopolysaccharidosis I-H). *Ophthalmic Paediatr. Genet.*, 2, 3–19.
17. Tada, A., Tanaka, A., Yasuda, M. *et al.* (1983) Cardiac manifestations of the mucopolysaccharidoses: periodical echocardiographic evaluation in six cases. *J. Cardiog.*, 13, 407–23.
18. Nagashima, K., Endo, H., Sakakibara, K. *et al.* (1976) Morphological and biochemical studies of a case of mucopolysaccharidosis II (Hunter Syndrome). *Acta Pathol. Jpn*, 26, 115–32.
19. Zimmerman, B., Lally, E.V., Sharma, S.C. *et al.* (1988) Severe aortic stenosis in systemic lupus erythematosus and mucopolysaccharidosis type II (Hunter's syndrome). *Clin. Cardiol.*, 11, 723–5.
20. Kurhara, M., Kumagai, K., Goto, K. *et al.* (1992) Severe type Hunter's syndrome. Polysomnographic and neuropathological study. *Neuropediatrics*, 23, 248–56.
21. Cain, H., Egner, E. and Kresse, H. (1977) Mucopolysaccharidosis III A (Sanfilippo disease type A). Histochemical, electron microscopical and biochemical findings. *Beitr. Pathol.*, 160, 58–72.
22. Herd, J.K., Subramanian, S. and Robinson, H. (1973) Type III mucopolysaccharidosis: report of a case with severe mitral valve involvement. *J. Pediatr.*, 82, 101–4.
23. Witting, C., Muller, K.M., Kresse, H. *et al.* (1975) Morphological and biochemical findings in a case of mucopolysaccharidosis type III A (Sanfilippo's disease type A). *Beitr. Pathol.*, 154, 324–38.
24. Shimamura, K., Hakozaki, H., Takahashi, K. *et al.* (1976) Sanfilippo B syndrome: a case report. *Acta Pathol. Jpn*, 26, 739–74.
25. Lavery, M.A., Green, W.R., Jabs, E.W. *et al.* (1983) Ocular histopathology and ultrastructure of Sanfilippo's syndrome, type III-B. *Arch. Ophthalmol.*, 101, 1263–74.
26. John, R.M., Hunter, D. and Swanton, R.H. (1990) Echocardiographic abnormalities in type IV mucopolysaccharidosis. *Arch. Dis. Child.*, 65, 746–9.
27. Gross, D.M., Williams, J.C., Caprioli, C. *et al.* (1988) Echocardiographic abnormalities in the mucopolysaccharide storage diseases. *Am. J. Cardiol.*, 61, 170–6.
28. Factor, S.M., Biempica, L. and Goldfischer, S. (1978) Coronary intimal sclerosis in Morquio's syndrome. *Virchows Arch. A (Path. Anat.)*, 379, 1–10.
29. Schenk, E.A. and Haggerty, J. (1964) Morquio's disease. A radiologic and morphologic study. *Pediatrics*, 34, 839–50.
30. Tan, C.T., Schaff, H.V., Miller Jr, F.A. *et al.* (1992) Valvular heart disease in four patients with Maroteaux–Lamy syndrome. *Circulation*, 85, 188–95.
31. Beaudet, A.L., DiFerante, N.M., Ferry, G.D. *et al.* (1975) Variation in the phenotypic expression of β-glucuronidase deficiency. *J. Pediatr.*, 86, 388–94.
32. Haskins, M.E., Otis, E.J., Hayden, J.E. *et al.* (1992) Hepatic storage of glycosaminoglycans in feline and canine models of mucopolysaccharidoses I, VI and VII. *Vet. Pathol.*, 29, 112–19.
33. Wolfe, J.H., Sands, M.S., Barker, J.E. *et al.* (1992) Reversal of pathology in murine mucopolysaccharidosis type VII by somatic cell gene transfer. *Nature*, 360, 749–53.
34. Haskins, M.E., Desnick, R.J., DiFerrante, N. *et al.* (1984) β-glucuronidase deficiency in a dog: a model of human mucopolysaccharidosis VII. *Pediatr Res.*, 18, 980–4.
35. Horstmann, G. and Lullman-Rauch, R. (1985) Mucopolysaccharidosis-like alterations in cardiac valves of rats treated with tilorone. *Virchows Arch. (Cell Path.)*, 48, 33–45.
36. Rees, S., Constantopoulos, G., Barranger, J.A. and Brady, R.O. (1982) Organomegaly and histopathology in an animal model of mucopolysaccharidosis induced by suramin. *Naunyn-Schmiederberg's Arch. Pharmac.*, 319, 262–70.
37. McKusick, V.A. (1990) Mucolipidosis 1, in *Mendelian Inheritance in Man. Catalogs of Autosomal Dominant, Autosomal Recessive and X-linked Phenotypes*, 9th edn, Johns Hopkins University Press, Baltimore, p. 1338.
38. Kelly, T.E., Bartoshesky, L., Harris, D.J. *et al.* (1981) Mucolipidosis I (acid neuraminidase deficiency). *Am. J. Dis. Child.*, 135, 703–8.
39. Kitagawa, H., Toki, J., Morimoto, T. *et al.* (1991) An autopsy case of I-cell disease. Ultrastructural and biochemical analyses. *Am. J. Clin. Pathol.*, 96, 262–6.
40. Okada, S., Owada, M., Sakiyama, T. *et al.* (1985) I-cell disease: clinical studies of 21 Japanese cases. *Clin. Genet.*, 28, 207–15.
41. Wenger, D. (1987) Defects in metabolism of lipids, in *Nelson Textbook of Pediatrics*. (eds R. Behrman and V. Vaughan), W.B. Saunders Co., Philadelphia, pp. 329–38.
42. Weitz, R., Kramer, I., Nissenkorn, I. *et al.* (1990) Muscle involvement in mucolipidosis IV. *Brain Dev.*, 12, 524–8.
43. Chitayat, D., Meunier, C.M., Hodgkinson, K.A. *et al.* (1991) Mucolipidosis type IV: clinical manifestations and natural history. *Am. J. Med. Genet.*, 41, 313–18.
44. McKusick, V.A. (1990) Fucosidosis, in *Mendelian Inheritance in Man. Catalogs of Autosomal Dominant, Autosomal Recessive and X-linked Phenotypes*, 9th edn, The Johns Hopkins University Press, Baltimore, pp. 1190–2.
45. Honjoh, M., Yamaguchi, S., Kohda, N. *et al.* (1985) Fucosidosis type 3 with angiokeratoma corporis diffusum. *J. Dermatol.*, 12, 174–82.
46. Carpenter, S. and Karpati, G. (1986) Lysosomal storage in human skeletal muscle. *Hum. Pathol.*, 17, 683–703.

47. McKusick, V.A. (1990) Mannosidosis, in *Mendelian Inheritance in Man. Catalogs of Autosomal Dominant, Autosomal Recessive and X-linked Phenotypes*, 9th edn, The John's Hopkins University Press, Baltimore, pp. 1305–6.
48. Ockerman, P.A. (1967) A generalized storage disorder resembling Hurler's syndrome. *Lancet*, 2, 239–41.
49. Wenger, D.A., Sujansky, E., Fennessey, P.V. and Thompson, J.N. (1986) Human beta-mannosidase deficiency. *N. Engl. J. Med.*, 315, 1201–5.
50. Kawai, H., Nishino, H., Nishida, Y. et al. (1985) Skeletal muscle pathology of mannosidosis in two siblings with spastic paraplegia. *Acta Neuropath.*, 68, 201–4.
51. McKusick, V.A. (1990) Oxalosis, in *Mendelian Inheritance In Man. Catalogs of Autosomal Dominant, Autosomal Recessive and X-linked Phenotypes*, 9th edn, Johns Hopkins University Press, Baltimore, pp. 1405–7.
52. Danpure, C.J., Cooper, P.J., Wise, P.J. and Jennings, P.R. (1989) An enzyme trafficking defect in two patients with primary hyperoxaluria type 1: peroxisomal alanine/glyoxylate aminotransferase rerouted to mitochondria. *J. Cell Biol.*, 108, 1345–52.
53. Dennis Jr, A.J. Hudson, J.B., Humphries, A.L. et al. (1980) Nitroglycerin as a remedy for peripheral vascular insufficiency associated with oxalosis. *Ann. Intern. Med.*, 92, 799–800.
54. Di Pasquale, G., Ribani, M., Andreoli, A. et al. (1989) Cardioembolic stroke in primary oxalosis with cardiac involvement. *Stroke*, 20, 1403–6.
55. Blackburn, W.E., McRoberts, J.W., Bhatena, D. et al. (1975) Severe vascular complications in oxalosis after bilateral nephrectomy. *Ann. Intern. Med.*, 82, 44–6.
56. Fayemi, A.O., Ali, M. and Braun, E.V. (1979) Oxalosis in hemodialysis patients: a pathologic study of 80 cases. *Arch. Pathol. Lab. Med.*, 103, 58–62.
57. Salyer, W.R. and Hutchins, G.M. (1974) Cardiac lesions in secondary oxalosis. *Arch. Intern. Med.*, 134, 250–2.
58. Hahlweg, G. and Orf, G. (1966) Sog. fibroplastische Myocarditis bei Oxalose. *Pathol. Microbiol. (Basel)*, 29, 1–7.
59. Novak, M.A., Roth, A.S. and Levine, M.R. (1988) Calcium oxalate retinopathy associated with methoxyflurane abuse. *Retina*, 8, 230–6.
60. Kiss, D., Meier, R., Gyr, K. and Wegmann, W. (1992) Secondary oxalosis following small bowel resection with kidney insufficiency and oxalate vasculopathy. *Schweiz. Med. Wochenschr.*, 122, 854–7.
61. Chaplin, A.J. (1977) Histopathological occurrence and characterization of calcium oxalate: a review. *J. Clin. Pathol.*, 30, 800–11.
62. Jansen, J.H. and Arnesen, K. (1990) Oxalate nephropathy in a Tibetan spaniel litter. A probable case of primary hyperoxaluria. *J. Comp. Pathol.*, 103, 79–84.
63. McKerrell, R.E., Blakemore, W.F., Heath, M.F. et al. (1989) Primary hyperoxaluria (L-glyceric aciduria) in the cat: a newly recognized inherited disease. *Vet. Rec.*, 125, 31–4.
64. Legg, M.A. and Harawi, S.J. (1985) The pathology of diabetes mellitus, in *Joslin's Diabetes Mellitus*, 12th edn, (eds A. Marble, L.P. Krall, R.F. Bradley et al.), Lea & Febiger, Philadelphia, pp. 298–331.
65. Warren, S., LeCompte, P.M. and Legg, M.A. (1966) *The Pathology of Diabetes Mellitus*, 4th edn, Lea & Febiger, Philadelphia; Arteriosclerosis in diabetes mellitus pp. 178–87; The heart pp. 188–98; Diabetic angiopathy pp. 310–23.
66. Everhart, J.E., Pettitt, D.J., Knowler, W.C. et al. (1988) Medial arterial calcification and its association with mortality and complications of diabetes. *Diabetologia*, 31, 16–23.
67. Bell, E.T. (1953) Renal vascular disease in diabetes mellitus. *Diabetes*, 2, 376–89.
68. Vallance, P., Calver, A. and Collier, J. (1992) The vascular endothelium in diabetes and hypertension. *J. Hypertens.*, 10 (suppl. 1), S25–S29.
69. Aagenaes, O. and Moe, H. (1961) Light and electron-microscopic study of skin capillaries of diabetics. *Diabetes*, 10, 253–9.
70. Kilo, C., Vogler, N. and Williamson, J.R. (1972) Muscle capillary basement membrane changes related to aging and to diabetes mellitus. *Diabetes*, 21, 881–905.
71. Siperstein, M.D., Unger, R.H. and Madison, L.L. (1967) Studies of muscle capillary basement membranes in normal subjects, diabetic and prediabetic patients. *J. Clin. Invest.*, 47, 1973–99.
72. Feingold, K.R., Browner, W.S. and Siperstein, M.D. (1989) Prospective studies of muscle capillary basement membrane width in prediabetics. *J. Clin. Endocrinol. Metab.*, 69, 784–9.
73. Green, W.R. (1985) Systemic diseases with retinal involvement: diabetic retinopathy, in *Ophthalmic Pathology*, vol. 2, 3rd edn, (ed. W.H. Spencer), W.B. Saunders Co., Philadelphia, pp. 1048–53.
74. Ledet, T. (1976) Diabetic cardiopathy. Quantitative histological studies of the heart from young juvenile diabetics. *Acta Pathol. Microbiol. Scand.*, 84, 421–8.
75. Silver, M.D., Huckell, V.F. and Lorber, M. (1977) Basement membranes of small cardiac vessels in patients with diabetes and myxoedema: preliminary observations. *Pathology*, 9, 213–20.
76. Crall Jr, F.V. and Roberts W.C. (1978) The extramural and intramural coronary arteries in juvenile diabetes mellitus: analysis of necropsy patients aged 19 to 38 years with onset of diabetes before age 15 years. *Am. J. Med.*, 64, 221–30.
77. Fischer, V.W., Barner, H.B. and Leskiw, M.L. (1979) Capillary basal laminar thickness in diabetic human myocardium. *Diabetes*, 28, 713–19.
78. Factor, S.M., Okun, E.M. and Minase, T. (1980) Capillary microaneurysms in the human diabetic heart. *N. Engl. J. Med.*, 302, 384–8.
79. Regan, T.J. and Weisse, A.B. (1978) The question of cardiomyopathy in diabetes mellitus. *Ann. Intern. Med.*, 89, 1000–2.
80. Sunni, S., Bishop, S.P., Kent, S.P. and Geer, J.C. (1986) Diabetic cardiomyopathy. A morphological study of intramyocardial arteries. *Arch. Pathol. Lab. Med.*, 110, 375–81.
81. Yarom, R., Zirkin, H., Stammler, G. and Rose, A.G. (1992) Human coronary microvessels in diabetes and ischaemia. Morphometric study of autopsy material. *J. Pathol.*, 166, 265–70.
82. Van Hoeven, K.H. and Factor, S.M. (1990) A comparison of the pathological spectrum of hypertensive, diabetic and hypertensive-diabetic heart disease. *Circulation*, 82, 848–55.
83. Minamoto, M., Shimizu, M., Suematsu, T. et al. (1990) Early diastolic dysfunction of the left ventricle and its relation to histopathological findings in patients with diabetes mellitus. *J. Cardiol.*, 20, 293–300.
84. Olson, J.L. (1992) Diabetes mellitus, in *Pathology of the Kidney*, vol. 3, 4th edn, (ed. R.H. Heptinstall), Little, Brown & Co., Boston, pp. 1715–1.
85. Dyck, P.J., Hansen, S., Karnes, J. et al. (1985) Capillary number and percentage closed in human diabetic sural nerve. *Proc. Natl Acad. Sci. USA*, 82, 2513–7.
86. Kreisberg, J.I. (1992) Hyperglycemia and microangiopathy. Direct regulation by glucose of microvascular cells. *Lab. Invest.*, 67, 416–26.
87. Ayo, S.H., Radnik, R.A., Garoni, J.A. et al. (1990) High glucose causes an increase in extracellular matrix proteins in cultured mesangial cells. *Am. J. Pathol.*, 136, 1339–48.
88. Sims, D.E. (1991) Recent advances in pericyte biology – implications for health and disease. *Can. J. Cardiol.*, 7, 431–43.
89. Feingold, K.R., Lee, T.H., Chung, M.Y. and Siperstein, M.D. (1986) Muscle capillary basement membrane width in patients with Vacor-induced diabetes mellitus. *J. Clin. Invest.*, 78, 102–7.
90. Mordes, J.P. and Rossini, A.A. (1985) Animal models of diabetes mellitus, in *Joslin's Diabetes Mellitus*, 12th edn, (eds A. Marble, L.P. Krall, R.P. Bradley et al.), Lea & Febiger, Philadelphia, pp. 110–37.
91. Vinores, S.A., Campochiaro, P.A., May, E.E. and Blaydes, S.H. (1988) Progressive ultrastructural damage and thickening of the basement membrane of the retinal pigment epithelium in spontaneously diabetic BB rats. *Exp. Eye Res.*, 46, 545–58.
92. Takahashi, Y., Wyman, M., Ferris III, F. and Kador, P.E. (1992) Diabetes-like preproliferative retinal changes in galactose-fed dogs. *Arch. Ophthalmol.*, 110, 1295–302.
93. Engerman, R.L. and Kern, T.S. (1993) Aldose reductase inhibition fails to prevent retinopathy in diabetic and galactosemic dogs. *Diabetes* 42: 820–5.
94. Bernstein, H.S., Bishop, D.F., Astrin, K.H. et al. (1989) Fabry disease: six gene rearrangements and an exonic point mutation in the alpha-galactosidase gene. *J. Clin. Invest.*, 83, 1390–9.
95. Kornreich, R., Bishop, D.F. and Desnick, R.J. (1990) Alpha-galactosidase A gene rearrangements causing Fabry disease. Identification of short direct repeats at breakpoints in an Alurich gene. *J. Biol. Clem.*, 265, 9319–26.
96. Laszlo, A., Torok, L., Havass, Z. and Bartos, Z. (1988–1989) Manifestations of angiokeratoma diffusum in a girl patient with heterozygous genotype for Fabry disease. *Acta Paediatr. Hung.*, 29, 331–6.
97. Le Bodic, M.F., Le Bodic, L., Buzelin, F. et al. (1978) Les lesions vaculaires de la maladie de Fabry. Etudes optique, histo-chimique et ultrastructurale. *Ann. Anat. Pathol. (Paris)*, 23, 23–39.
98. Becker, A.E., Schoorl, R., Balk, A.G. and van der Heide, R.M. (1975) Cardiac manifestations of Fabry's disease. Report of a case with mitral insufficiency and electrocardiographic evidence of myocardial infarction. *Am. J. Cardiol.*, 36, 829–35.
99. Ferrans, V.J., Hibbs, R.G. and Burda, C.D. (1969) The heart in Fabry's disease. A histochemical and electron microscopic study. *Am. J. Cardiol.*, 24, 95–110.
100. Scully, R.E., Mark, E.J. and McNeely, B.U. (1984) Case 2 – 1984. Case records of Massachusetts General Hospital. *N. Engl. J. Med.*, 310, 106–14.
101. Spaeth, A.L. and Frost, P. (1965) Fabry's disease: its ocular manifestations. *Arch. Ophthalmol.*, 74, 760–9.
102. Font, R.L. and Fine, B.S. (1972) Ocular pathology in Fabry's disease. Histochemical and electron microscopic observations. *Am. J. Ophthalmol.*, 73, 419–30.
103. Weingeist, T.A. and Blodi, F.C. (1971) Fabry's disease: ocular findings in a female carrier. *Arch. Ophthalmol.*, 85, 169–76.
104. Smith, P., Heath, D., Rodgers, B. and Helliwell, T. (1991) Pulmonary vasculature in Fabry's disease. *Histopathology*, 19, 567–9.
105. Inaoki, M., Otsuki, N., Ishise, S. et al. (1992) Two cases of Fabry's disease: a hemizygote with a point mutation in the alpha-galactosidase A gene and his relative. *J. Dermatol.*, 19, 481–6.

106. Roberts, W.C. and Fredrickson, D.S. (1967) Gaucher's disease of the lung causing severe pulmonary hypertension with associated acute recurrent pericarditis. *Circulation*, **35**, 783–9.
107. Uyama, E., Takahashi, K., Owada, M. *et al.* (1992) Hydrocephalus, corneal opacities, deafness, valvular heart disease, deformed toes and leptomeningeal fibrous thickening in adult siblings: a new syndrome associated with glucocerebrosidase deficiency and a mosaic population of storage cells. *Acta Neurol. Scand.*, **86**, 407–20.
108. Wilson, E.R., Barton, N.W. and Barranger, J.A. (1985) Vascular involvement in type 3 neuronopathic Gaucher's disease. *Arch. Pathol. Lab. Med.*, **109**, 82–4.
109. Tsutsumi, A. (1982) A case of Gaucher disease with corneal opacities. *Ganka Rhinshoiho*, **76**, 1730–3.
110. Zappatini-Tommasi, L., Dumontel, C., Guibaud, P. and Girod, C. (1992) Farber disease: an ultrastructural study. *Virchows Arch. A Pathol. Anat. Histopathol.*, **420**, 281–90.
111. Abul-Haj, S.K., Martz, D.G., Douglas, W.F. and Geperl, L.J. (1962) Farber's disease. Report of a case with observations on its histogenesis and notes on the nature of the stored material. *J. Pediatr.*, **61**, 221–32.
112. Battin, J., Vital, C. and Azanza, X. (1970) Une neurolipidose rare avec lesions nodulaires sous-cutanées et articulaires: la lipogranulomatose disseminée de Farber. *Ann. Dermatol. Syphiligr. (Paris)*, **97**, 241–8.
113. Farber, S., Cohen, J. and Uzman, L.L. (1957) Lipogranulomatosis: a new lipoglyco-protein 'storage' disease. *Mt Sinai J. Med.*, **24**, 816–37.
114. Molz, G. (1968) Farbersche Krankheit. Pathologisch-anatomische Befunde. *Virchows Arch. A Pathol. Anat.*, **344**, 86–99.
115. Dustin, P., Tondeur, M., Jonniaux, G. *et al.* (1973) La maladie de Farber. Etude anatomo-clinique et ultrastructurale. *Bull. Acad. R Med. Belg.*, **13**, 733–62.
116. Dal Canto, M.C., Rapin, I. and Suzuki, K. (1974) Neuronal storage disorder with chorea and curvilinear bodies. *Neurology (Minneapolis)*, **24**, 1026–32.
117. Schmoeckel, C. (1980) Subtle clues to diagnosis of skin diseases by electron microscopy. *Am. J. Dermatopath.*, **2**, 153–6.
118. Abenoza, P. and Sibley, R.K. (1987) Farber's disease: a fine structural study. *Ultrastruct. Pathol.*, **11**, 397–403.
119. Fredickson, D.S. and Ferrans, V.J. (1978) Acid cholesteryl ester hydrolase deficiency. (Wolman's disease and cholesteryl ester storage disease), in *The Metabolic Basis of Inherited Disease*, 4th edn, (eds J.B. Stanbury, J.B. Wyngaarden and D.S. Fredrickson), McGraw-Hill, New York, pp. 670–87.
120. Lowden, J.A., Barson, A.J. and Wentworth, P. (1970) Wolman's disease: a microscopic and biochemical study showing accumulation of ceroid and esterified cholesterol. *Can. Med. Assoc. J.*, **102**, 402–5.
121. Roytta, M., Fagerlund, A.S., Toikkanen, S. *et al.* (1992) Wolman disease: morphological, clinical and genetic studies on the first Scandinavian cases. *Clin. Genet.*, **42**, 1–7.
122. Beaudet, A.L., Ferry, G.D., Nichols Jr, B.L. and Rosenberg, H.S. (1977) Cholesterol ester storage disease: clinical, biochemical and pathological studies. *J. Pediatr.*, **90**, 910–14.
123. Elleder, M., Ledvinova, J., Cieslar, P. and Kuhn, R. (1990) Subclinical course of cholesterol ester storage disease (CESD) diagnosed in adulthood. *Virchows Arch. A Pathol. Anat. Histopathol.*, **416**, 357–65.
124. Dolman, C.L. and Chang, E. (1972) Visceral lesions in amaurotic familial idiocy with curvilinear bodies. *Arch. Path.*, **94**, 425–30.
125. Brown, M.S. and Goldstein, J.L. (1991) The hyperlipoproteinemias and other disorders of lipid metabolism, in *Harrison's Principles of Internal Medicine*, vol. 2, 12th edn, (eds J.D. Wilson, E. Braunwald, K.J. Isselbacher *et al.*), McGraw-Hill, New York, pp. 1814–25.
126. Roberts, W.C., Levy, R.I. and Fredrickson, D.S. (1970) Hyperlipoproteinemia. A review of the five types with first report of necropsy findings in type 3. *Arch. Pathol.*, **90**, 46–56.
127. Goldstein, J.L. and Brown, M.S. (1978) Familial hypercholesterolemia: pathogenesis of a receptor disease. *Johns Hopkins Med. J.*, **143**, 8–16.
128. Rothbard, S., Hagstrom, J.W. and Smith, J.P. (1967) Aortic stenosis and myocardial infarction in hypercholesterolemic xanthomatosis. *Am. Heart J.*, **73**, 687–92.
129. Stanley, P., Chartrand, C. and Davignon, A. (1965) Acquired aortic stenosis in a twelve-year-old girl with xanthomatosis. *N. Engl. J. Med.*, **273**, 1378–81.
130. Wennevold, A. and Jacobsen, JG. (1971) Acquired supravalvular aortic stenosis in familial hypercholesterolemia. A hemodynamic and angiographic study. *Am. J. Med.*, **50**, 823–7.
131. Barr, D.P., Rothbard, S. and Eder, H.A. (1954) Atherosclerosis and aortic stenosis in hypercholesterolemic xanthomatosis. *J. Am. Med. Assoc.*, **156**, 943–7.
132. McCleary, J.E., Brunsting, L.A. and Kennedy, R.L.J. (1959) Primary xanthoma tuberosum in children, with classification of xanthomas. *Pediatrics*, **23**, 67–75.
133. Maher, J.A., Epstein, F.H. and Hand, E.A. (1958) Xanthomatosis and coronary heart disease. Necropsy studies of two affected siblings. *Arch. Intern. Med.*, **102**, 437–42.
134. Bloch, A., Dinsmore, R.E. and Lees, R.S. (1976) Coronary arteriographic findings in type II and type IV hyperlipoproteinemia. *Lancet*, **1**, 928–30.
135. Postiglione, A., Nappi, A., Brunetti, A. *et al.* (1991) Relative protection from cerebral atherosclerosis of young patients with homozygous familial hypercholesterolemia. *Atherosclerosis*, **90**, 23–30.
136. Yamashita, S., Ueyama, Y., Funahashi, T. *et al.* (1986). A 31-year-old woman with homozygous familial hypercholesterolemia without significant lesions in the coronary arteries. *Atherosclerosis*, **62**, 117–22.
137. Stehbens, W.E. and Martin, M. (1991) The vascular pathology of familial hypercholesterolemia. *Pathology*, **23**, 54–61.
138. Roberts, W.C., Ferrans, V.J., Levy, R.I. and Fredrickson, D.S. (1973) Cardiovascular pathology in hyperlipoproteinemia. Anatomic observations in 42 necropsy patients with normal or abnormal serum lipoprotein patterns. *Am. J. Cardiol.*, **31**, 557–70.
139. Marais, A.D., Firth, J.C., Rose, A.G. and Berger, G.M. (1990) Fatal outcome of homozygous familial hypercholesterolemia in a black patient. A case report. *S. Afr. Med. J.*, **77**, 588–90.
140. Kragel, A.H. and Roberts, W.C. (1991) Composition of atherosclerotic plaques in the coronary arteries in homozygous familial hypercholesterolemia. *Am. Heart J.*, **121**, 210–11.
141. Atkinson, J.B., Swift, L.L. and Virmani, R. (1992) Watanabe heritable hyperlipidemic rabbits. Familial hypercholesterolemia. *Am. J. Pathol.*, **140**, 749–53.
142. Buja, L.M., Kita, T., Goldstein, J.L. *et al.* (1983) Cellular pathology of progressive atherosclerosis in the WHHL rabbit. An animal model of familial hypercholesterolemia. *Arteriosclerosis*, **3**, 87–101.
143. Amatruda, J.M., Margolis, S. and Hutchins, G.M. (1974) Type III hyperlipoproteinemia with mesangial foam cells in renal glomeruli. *Arch. Pathol.*, **98**, 51–4.
144. Cabin, H.S., Schwartz, D.E., Virmani, R. *et al.* (1981) Type III hyperlipoproteinemia. Quantification, distribution, and nature of atherosclerotic coronary arterial narrowing in five necropsy patients. *Am. Heart J.*, **102**, 830–5.
145. Gown, A.M., Hazzard, W.R. and Benditt, E.P. (1982) Type III hyperlipoproteinemia and atherosclerosis: a case report and reevaluation. *Human Pathol.*, **13**, 506–10.
146. Holimon, J.L. and Wasserman, A.J. (1971) Autopsy findings in type 3 hyperlipoproteinemia. *Arch. Pathol.*, **92**, 415–17.
147. Brewer Jr, H.B., Zech, L.A., Gregg, R.E. *et al.* (1983) Type III hyperlipoproteinemia: diagnosis, molecular defects, pathology and treatment. *Ann. Int. Med.*, **98**, 623–40.
148. Plump, A.S., Smith, J.D., Hayek, T. *et al.* (1993) Severe hypercholesterolemia and atherosclerosis in apolipoprotein E-deficient mice created by homologous recombination in ES cells. *Cell*, **71**, 343–53.
149. Zhang, S.H., Reddick, R.L., Piedrahita, J.A. and Maeda, N. (1992) Spontaneous hypercholesterolemia and arterial lesions in mice lacking apolipoprotein E. *Science*, **258**, 468–71.
150. Schaefer, E.J. (1984) Clinical, biochemical, and genetic features in familial disorders of high density lipoprotein deficiency. *Arteriosclerosis*, **4**, 303–22.
151. Brewer Jr, H.B., Gregg, R.E., Hoeg, J.M. and Fojo, S.S. (1988) Apolipoproteins and lipoproteins in human plasma: An overview. *Clin. Chem.*, **34**, 4–8.
152. Gordon, D.J. and Rifkind, B.M. (1989) High-density lipoprotein – the clinical implications of recent studies. *N. Engl. J. Med.*, **321**, 1311–16.
153. Ferrans, V.J. and Fredrickson, D.S. (1975) The pathology of Tangier disease. A light and electron microscopic study. *Am. J. Pathol.*, **78**, 101–58.
154. Haas, L.F. and Bergin, J.D. (1970) Alpha lipoprotein deficiency with neurological features. *Aust. Ann. Med.*, **19**, 76.
155. Hoffman, H.N. and Fredrickson, D.S. (1965) Tangier disease (familial HDL deficiency): clinical and genetic features in two adults. *Am. J. Med.*, **39**, 582–93.
156. Ordovas, J.M., Schaefer, E.J., Salem, D. *et al.* (1986) Apolipoprotein A-I gene polymorphism associated with premature coronary artery disease and familial hypoalphalipoproteinemia. *N. Engl. J. Med.*, **314**, 671–7.
157. Breslow, J.L. (1993) Genetics of lipoprotein disorders. *Circulation*, **87**, (Suppl. III), III-16–III-21.
158. Wallentin, L. and Moberg, B. (1982) Lecithin:cholesterol acyl transfer rate and high density lipoprotein level in coronary artery disease. *Atherosclerosis*, **41**, 155–65.
159. Stokke, K.T., Bjerve, K.S., Blomhoff, J.P. *et al.* (1974) Familial lecithin:cholesterol acyltransferase deficiency. Studies on lipid composition and morphology of tissues. *Scand. J. Clin. Lab. Invest.*, **137**, 93–100.
160. Hovig, T. and Gjone, E. (1974) Familial lecithin:cholesterol acyltransferase deficiency. Ultrastructural studies on lipid deposition and tissue reactions. *Scand. J. Clin. Lab. Invest.*, **137**, 135–46.
161. Norum, R.A., Lakier, J.B., Goldstein, S. *et al.* (1982) Familial deficiency of apolipoproteins A-I and C-III and precocious coronary artery disease. *N. Engl. J. Med.*, **306**, 1513–19.
162. Assman, G., von Eckardstein, A. and Funke, H. (1993) High density lipoproteins, reverse transport of cholesterol, and coronary artery disease. Insights from mutations. *Circulation*, 87 (suppl. III), III28–34.
163. Schaefer, E.J., Blum, C.B., Levy, R.I. *et al.* (1978) Metabolism of high-

density lipoprotein apolipoproteins in Tangier disease. *N. Engl. J. Med.*, **299**, 905–10.
164. Schaefer, E.J., Anderson, D.W., Zech, L.A. *et al.* (1981) Metabolism of high density lipoprotein subfractions and constituents in Tangier disease following the infusion of high density lipoproteins. *J. Lipid Res.*, **22**, 217–28.
165. Bojanovski, D., Gregg, R.E., Zech, L.A. *et al.* (1987) In vivo metabolism of proapolipoprotein A-I in Tangier disease. *J. Clin. Invest.*, **80**, 1742–17.
166. Schaefer, E.J., Zech, L.A., Schwartz, D.E. and Brewer Jr, H.B. (1980) Coronary heart disease prevalence and other clinical features in familial high density lipoprotein deficiency (Tangier disease). *Ann. Intern. Med.*, **93**, 261–6.
167. Assmann, G., Schmitz, G. and Brewer Jr, H.B. (1989) Familial high density lipoprotein deficiency: Tangier disease, in *The Metabolic Basis of Inherited Disease*, 6th (edn, eds C.R. Scriver, A.L. Beaudet, W.S. Sly and D Valle), McGraw-Hill, New York, pp. 1267–82.
168. Mautner, S.L., Sanchez, J.A., Rader, D.J. *et al.* (1992) The heart in Tangier disease. Severe coronary atherosclerosis with near absence of high-density lipoprotein cholesterol. *Am. J. Clin. Pathol.*, **98**, 191–8.
169. Haust, M.D. (1992) Aortic features in Tangier disease and pathogenetic considerations – Part I. Fatty dots and streaks. *Eur. J. Epidemiol.*, **8** (suppl. 1), 36–47.
170. Poernama, F., Schreyer, S.A., Bitgood, J.J. *et al.* (1990) Spontaneous high density lipoprotein deficiency syndrome associated with a Z-linked mutation in chickens. *J. Lipid Res.*, **31**, 955–63.
171. Poernama, F., Subramanian, R., Cook, M.E. and Attie, A.D. (1992) High density lipoprotein deficiency syndrome in chickens is not associated with an increased susceptibility to atherosclerosis. *Arterioscler. Thromb.*, **12**, 601–7.
172. Kwiterovich Jr, P.O. and Sniderman, A.D. (1983) Atherosclerosis and apoproteins B and A-I. *Prev. Med.*, **12**, 815–34.
173. Bouma, M.E., Beucler, I., Pessah, M. *et al.* (1990) Description of two different patients with abetalipoproteinemia: synthesis of a normal-sized apolipoprotein B-48 in intestinal organ culture. *J. Lipid Res.*, **31**, 1–15.
174. Dische, M.R. and Porro, R.S. (1970) The cardiac lesions in Bassen–Kornzweig syndrome. Report of a case, with autopsy findings. *Am. J. Med.*, **49**, 568–71.
175. Von Sallmann, L., Gelderman, A.H. and Laster, L. (1969) Ocular histopathologic changes in a case of α-beta-lipoproteinemia (Bassen–Kornzweig syndrome). *Doc. Ophthalmol.*, **26**, 451–60.
176. Baumgartner, R.W., Hauser, V., Grob, P. and Waespe, W. (1991) Cerebrotendinous xanthomatosis. *Schweiz. Med. Wschr.*, **121**, 858–64.
177. Salen, G. (1971) Cholesterol deposition in cerebrotendinous xanthomatosis. A possible mechanism. *Ann. Intern. Med.*, **75**, 843–51.
178. Schimschock, J.R., Alvord Jr, E.C. and Swanson, P.D. (1968) Cerebrotendinous xanthomatosis. Clinical and pathological studies. *Arch. Neurol.*, **18**, 688–98.
179. Kuriyama, M., Fujiyama, J., Yoshidome, H. *et al.* (1991) Cerebrotendinous xanthomatosis: clinical and biochemical evaluation of eight patients and review of the literature. *J. Neurol. Sci.*, **102**, 225–32.
180. Moser, H.W., Bergin, A. and Cornblath, D. (1991) Peroxisomal disorders. *Biochem. Cell Biol.*, **69**, 463–74.
181. Kahlke, W. (1967) Heredopathia atactica polyneuritiformis (Refsum's disease), in *Lipids and Lipidosis*, (ed. G. Schettler), Springer-Verlag, New York, pp. 352–81.
182. Refsum, S. (1975) Heredopathia atactica polyneuritiformis. Phytanic acid storage disease (Refsum's disease), in *Handbook of Clinical Neurology, Vol. 21, System Disorders and Atrophies Part I*, (eds P.J. Vinken and G.W. Bruyn), American Elsevier, New York, p. 181.
183. Allen, I.V., Swallow, M., Nevin, N.C. and McCormick, D. (1978) Clinico-pathological study of Refsum's disease with particular reference to fatal complications. *J. Neurol. Neurosurg. Psychiatry*, **41**, 323–32.
184. Torvik, A., Torp, S., Kase, B.F. *et al.* (1988) Infantile Refsum's disease: a generalized peroxisomal disorder. *J. Neurol. Sci.*, **85**, 39–53.
185. Galdston, M., Steele, J.M. and Dobrinerk, ●● (1952) Alkaptonuria and ochronosis. With a report of three patients and metabolic studies in two. *Am. J. Med.*, **13**, 432–52.
186. O'Brien, W.M., La Du, B.N. and Bunim, J.J. (1963) Biochemical, pathologic and clinical aspects of alcaptonuria, ochronosis and ochronotic arthropathy. *Am. J. Med.*, **34**, 813–38.
187. Kim, Y.I. and Daenen, W. (1992) Aortic valve replacement in cardiac ochronosis. *Eur. J. Cardiothorac. Surg.*, **6**, 625–6.
188. Menke, H.E., Dekker, S.K., Noordhoek, H.V. *et al.* (1992) Exogenous ochronosis, a little-known side effect of hydroquinone-containing ointments. *Ned. Tijdschr. Geneeskd.*, **136**, 187–90.
189. Kenny, D., Ptacin, M.J., Bamrah, V.S. and Almagro, U. (1990) Cardiovascular ochronosis: a case report and review of the medical literature. *Cardiology*, **77**, 477–83.
190. Cooper, J.A. and Moran, T.J. (1957) Studies on ochronosis. I. Report of case with death from ochronotic nephrosis. *Arch. Pathol.*, **64**, 46–53.
191. Levine, H.D., Parisi, A.F., Holdsworth, D.E. and Cohn, L.H. (1978) Aortic valve replacement for ochronosis of the aortic valve. *Chest*, **74**, 466–7.
192. Gould, L., Reddy, C.V., DePalma, D. *et al.* (1976) Cardiac manifestations of ochronosis. *J. Thorac. Cardiovasc. Surg.*, **72**, 788–91.
193. Lichtenstein, L. and Kaplan, L. (1954) Hereditary ochronosis. Pathologic changes observed in two necropsied cases. *Am. J. Pathol.*, **30**, 99–125
194. Gaines Jr, J.J. and Pai, G.M. (1987) Cardiovascular ochronosis. *Arch. Pathol. Lab. Med.*, **111**, 991–4.
195. Gaines, Jr, J.J. (1989) The pathology of alkaptonuric ochronosis. *Hum. Pathol.*, **20**, 40–6.
196. Pages, A. and Baldet, P. (1971) Ochronosis: aspects anatomo-cliniques et ultrastructuraux. *Ann. Anat. Pathol. (Paris)*, **16**, 27–45.
197. Attwood, H.D., Clifton, S. and Mitchell, R.E. (1971) A histological, histochemical and ultrastructural study of dermal ochronosis. *Pathology*, **3**, 115–21.
198. Grieco, A.J. (1977) Homocystinuria: pathogenetic mechanism. *Am. J. Med. Sci.*, **273**, 120–32.
199. Almgren, B., Eriksson, I., Hemmingsson, A. *et al.* (1978) Abdominal aortic aneurysm in homocystinuria. *Acta Chir. Scand.*, **144**, 545–8.
200. Carey, M.C., Donovan, D.E., Fitzgerald, O. and McAuley, F.D. (1968) Homocystinuria: A clinical and pathological study of nine subjects in six families. *Am. J. Med.*, **45**, 7–25.
201. Carson, N.A.J., Dent, C.E., Field, C.M.B. and Gaull, G.E. (1965) Homocystinuria. Clinical and pathological review of ten cases. *J. Pediatr.*, **66**, 565–83.
202. Gibson, J.B., Carson, N.A.J. and Neill, D.W. (1964) Pathological findings in homocystinuria. *J. Clin. Pathol.*, **17**, 427–37.
203. Hubert, J.P., Retif, J., Brihaye, J. and Flament-Durand, J. (1973) Etude anatomopathologique d'un cas d'homocystinurie. *Pathol. Eur.*, **8**, 113–26.
204. James, T.N., Carson, N.A. and Froggatt, P. (1974) De subitaneis mortibus. IV. Coronary vessels and conduction system in homocystinuria. *Circulation*, **49**, 367–74.
205. McCully, K.S. (1969) Vascular pathology of homocystinemia: implications for the pathogenesis of arteriosclerosis. *Am. J. Pathol.*, **56**, 111–28.
206. Harker, L.A., Slichter, S.J., Scott, C.R. and Ross, R. (1974) Homocystinemia: vascular injury and arterial thrombosis. *N. Engl. J. Med.*, **291**, 537–43.
207. Brandstetter, Y., Weinhouse, E., Splaingard, M.L. and Tang, T.T. (1990) Cor pulmonale as a complication of methylmalonic acidemia and homocystinuria (Cbl-C Type). *Am. J. Med. Genet.*, **36**, 167–71.
208. McKusick, V. (1990) *Mendelian Inheritance in Man. Catalogs of Autosomal Dominant, Autosomal Recessive and X-linked Phenotypes*, 9th edn, Johns Hopkins University Press, Baltimore, pp. 1526–7.
209. Cooper, B.A. and Rosenblatt, D.S. (1987) Inherited vitamin B_{12} defects. *Ann. Rev. Nutr.*, **7**, 308–12.
210. Holbrook, K.A. and Byers, P.H. (1982) Structural abnormalities in the dermal collagen and elastic matrix from the skin of patients with inherited connective tissue disorders. *J. Invest. Dermatol.*, **79**, 95–165.
211. Lee, B., Godfrey, M., Vitale, E. *et al.* (1991) Linkage of Marfan syndrome and a phenotypically related disorder to two different fibrillin genes. *Nature*, **352**, 330–4.
212. Dietz, H.C., Saraiva, J.M., Pyeritz, R.E. *et al.* (1992) Clustering of fibrillin (FBN 1) missense mutations in Marfan syndrome patients at cysteine residues in EGF-like domains. *Hum. Mutat.*, **1**, 366–74.
213. Ramirez, F., Lee, B. and Vitale, E. (1992) Clinical and genetic associations in Marfan syndrome and related disorders. *Mt Sinai J. Med.*, **59**, 350–6.
214. Kajikawa, K., Yamaguchi, T., Katsuda, S. and Miwa, A. (1975) An improved electron stain for elastic fibers using tannic acid. *J. Electr. Microsc.*, **24**, 287–9.
215. Roberts, W.C. (1979) Congenital cardiovascular abnormalities usually 'silent' until adulthood: morphologic features of the floppy mitral valve, valvular aortic stenosis, discrete subvalvular aortic stenosis, hypertrophic cardiomyopathy, sinus of Valsalva aneurysm and the Marfan syndrome, in *Congenital Heart Disease in Adults*, (ed. W.C. Roberts), F.A. Davis Co., Philadelphia, pp. 407–53.
216. Goertz, K., Diehl, A.M., Vaseenon, T. and Mattioli, L. (1978) A catastrophic complication. Acute dissection of an aortic aneurysm in a child with Marfan's syndrome. *J. Kansas Med. Soc.*, **79**, 115–17.
217. Houston, H.E. (1978) Abdominal aortic aneurysm in Marfan's syndrome. *J. Kentucky Med. Assoc.*, **76**, 492–3.
218. McKusick, V.A. (1955) The cardiovascular aspects of Marfan's syndrome: a heritable disorder of connective tissue. *Circulation*, **11**, 321–42.
219. Julien, J. and De Boucaud, D. (1971) Aneurysmes dans le system de la veine de Galien et syndrome de Marfan. *Bordeaux Med.*, **11**, 3245–52.
220. Crisfield, R.J. (1971) Spontaneous aneurysm of the ductus arteriosus in a patient with Marfan's syndrome. *J. Thorac. Cardiovasc. Surg.*, **62**, 243–7.
221. Latter, D.A., Ricci, M.A., Forbes, R.D. and Graham, A.M. (1989) Internal carotid artery aneurysm and Marfan syndrome. *Can. J. Surg.*, **32**, 463–6.
222. Fournier, C. (1977) Les lesions cardio-vasculaires du syndrome de Marfan. *Coeur Med. Interne*, **16**, 331–6.
223. Bolande, R.P. (1963) The nature of the connective tissue abiotrophy in the Marfan syndrome. *Lab. Invest.*, **12**, 1087–93.
224. Sabaik, M. and Eisenstein, R. (1977) Aortic lesions in Marfan syndrome. The ultrastructure of cystic medial degeneration. *Arch. Pathol. Lab. Med.*, **101**, 74–7.

225. Takebayashi, S., Kubota, I. and Takagi, T. (1973) Ultrastructural and histochemical studies of vascular lesions in Marfan's syndrome, with report of 4 autopsy cases. *Acta Pathol. Jpn*, **23**, 847–66.
226. Perejda, A.J., Abraham, P.A., Carnes, W.H. *et al.* (1985) Marfan's syndrome: structural, biochemical and mechanical studies of the aortic media. *J. Lab. Clin. Med.*, **106**, 376–83.
227. Abraham, P.A., Perejda, A.J., Carnes, W.H. and Uitto, J. (1982) Marfan syndrome. Demonstration of abnormal elastin in aorta. *J. Clin. Invest.*, **70**, 1245–52.
228. Savolainen, A., Keto, P., Hekali, P. *et al.* (1992) Aortic distensibility in children with the Marfan syndrome. *Am. J. Cardiol.*, **70**, 691–3.
229. Modesto, C., Cabrera, A., Pastor, E. *et al.* (1989) Patologia cardiovascular en el síndrome de Marfan. Estudio de 11 niños con ecocardiografía bidimensional. *Rev. Esp. Cardiol.*, **42**, 318–21.
230. Stelzig, H.H. and Kossling, F.K. (1967) Zur Pathologie der Aorta und der grossen arterien beim Marfan-Syndrome. *Frankf. Z. Pathol.*, **76**, 201–12.
231. Schlatmann, T.J. and Becker, A.E. (1977) Pathogenesis of dissecting aneurysm of aorta. Comparative histopathologic study of significance of medial changes. *Am. J. Cardiol.*, **39**, 21–6.
232. Schlatmann, T.J. and Becker, A.E. (1977) Histologic changes in the normal aging aorta: implications for dissecting aortic aneurysm. *Am. J. Cardiol.*, **39**, 13–20.
233. Mathieu, M., Labeille, B., Sevestre, H. *et al.* (1989) Marfan disease presenting in neonates with rapid cardiovascular failure. A propos of 2 cases. *Ann. Pediatr (Paris)*, **36**, 465–68.
234. Buntinx, I.M., Willems, P.T., Spitaels, S.E. *et al.* (1991) Neonatal Marfan syndrome with congenital arachnodactyly, flexion contractures, and severe cardiac valve insufficiency. *J. Med. Genet.*, **28**, 267–73.
235. Raghunath, M., Superti-Furga, A., Godfrey, M. and Steinmann, B. (1993) Decreased extracellular deposition of fibrillin and decorin in neonatal Marfan syndrome fibroblasts. *Hum. Genet.*, **90**, 511–5.
236. Superti-Furga, A., Raghunath, M. and Willems, P.J. (1992) Deficiencies of fibrillin and decorin in fibroblast cultures of a patient with neonatal Marfan syndrome. *J. Med. Genet.*, **29**, 875–8.
237. Eldridge, R. (1964) Coarctation in the Marfan syndrome. *Arch. Intern. Med.*, **113**, 342–9.
238. Marvel, R.J. and Genovese, P.D. (1951) Cardiovascular disease in Marfan's syndrome. *Am. Heart J.*, **42**, 814–25.
239. Besser, T.E., Potter, K.A., Bryan, G.M. and Knowlen, G.G. (1990) An animal model of the Marfan syndrome. *Am. J. Med. Genet.*, **37**, 159–65.
240. Potter, K.A., Hoffman, Y., Sakai, L.Y. *et al.* (1993). Abnormal fibrillin metabolism in bovine Marfan syndrome. *Am. J. Pathol.*, **142**, 803–10.
241. Allerdice, P.W., Eales, B., Onyett, H. *et al.* (1983) Duplication 9q34 syndrome. *Am. J. Hum. Genet.*, **35**, 1005–19.
242. Beighton, P. (1972) The dominant and recessive forms of cutis laxa. *J. Med. Genet.*, **9**, 216–21.
243. Kuivaniemi, H., Peltonen, L., Palotie, A. *et al.* (1982) Abnormal copper metabolism and deficient lysyl oxidase activity in heritable connective tissue disorder. *J. Clin. Invest.*, **69**, 730–3.
244. Levinson, B., Gitschier, Vulpe, C. *et al.* (1993) Are X-linked cutis laxa and Menkes disease allelic? *Nature Genet.*, **3**, 6.
245. Dingman, R.O., Grabb, W.C. and O'Neal, R.M. (1969) Cutis laxa congenita. Generalized elastolysis. *Plast. Reconstr. Surg.*, **44**, 431–5.
246. Hayden, J.G., Talner, N.S. and Klaus, S.N. (1968) Cutis laxa associated with pulmonary artery stenosis. *J. Pediatr.*, **72**, 506–9.
247. Wagstaff, L.A., Firth, J.C. and Levin, S.E. (1970) Vascular abnormalities in congenital generalized elastolysis (cutis laxa): report of a cases. *S. Afr. Med. J.*, **44**, 1125–7.
248. Harris, R.B., Heaphy, M.R. and Perry, H.O. (1978) Generalized elastolysis (cutis laxa). *Am. J. Med.*, **65**, 815–22.
249. Reed, W.B., Horowitz, R.B. and Beighton, P. (1971) Acquired cutis laxa. Primary generalized elastolysis. *Arch. Dermatol.*, **103**, 661–9.
250. Weir, E.K., Joffe, H.S., Blaufuss, A.H. and Beighton, P. (1977) Cardiovascular abnormalities in cutis laxa. *Eur. J. Cardiol.*, **5**, 255–61.
251. Goltz, R.W., Hult, A.M., Goldfarb, M. and Gorlin, R.J. (1965) Cutis laxa, a manifestation of generalized elastolysis. *Arch. Dermatol.*, **92**, 373–87.
252. Mehregan, A.H., Lee, S.C. and Nabai, H. (1978) Cutis laxa (generalized elastolysis). A report of four cases with autopsy findings. *J. Cutan. Pathol.*, **5**, 116–26.
253. Sayers, C.L., Goltz, R.W. and Mottiaz, J. (1975) Pulmonary elastic tissue in generalized elastolysis (cutis laxa) and Marfan's syndrome: a light and electron microscopic study. *J. Invest. Dermatol.*, **65**, 451–7.
254. Hashimoto, K. and Kanzaki, T. (1975) Cutis laxa. Ultrastructural and biochemical studies. *Arch. Dermatol.*, **111**, 861–73.
255. De Anda, G. and Vignale, R.A. (1984) Congenital cutis laxa. *Med. Cutan. Ibero Lat. Am.*, **12**, 1–5.
256. Muster, A.J., Bharati, S., Herman, J.J. *et al.* (1983) Fatal cardiovascular disease and cutis laxa following acute febrile neutrophilic dermatosis. *J. Pediatr.*, **102**, 243–8.
257. McKusick, V.A. (1990) Pseudoxanthoma elasticum, in *Mendelian Inheritance in Man. Catalogs of Autosomal Dominant, Autosomal Recessive and X-linked Phenotypes*, 9th edn, Johns Hopkins University Press, Baltimore, pp. 1443–4.
258. Goodman, R.M., Smith, E.W., Paton, D. *et al.* (1963) Pseudoxanthoma elasticum: a clinical and histopathological study. *Medicine*, **42**, 297–334.
259. Mendelsohn, G., Bulkley, B.H. and Hutchins, G.M. (1978) Cardiovascular manifestations of pseudoxanthoma elasticum. *Arch. Pathol. Lab. Med.*, **102**, 298–302.
260. Schachner, L. and Young, D. (1974) Pseudoxanthoma elasticum with severe cardiovascular disease in a child. *Am. J. Dis. Child.*, **127**, 571–5.
261. Milstoc, M. (1969) An unusual anatomo-pathologic aspect of a case with pseudoxanthoma elasticum. *Dis. Chest.*, **55**, 431–4.
262. Wilhelm, K. and Paver, K. (1972) Sudden death in pseudoxanthoma elasticum. *Med. J. Aust.*, **24**, 1363–5.
263. Huang, S., Kumar, G., Steele, H.D. and Parker, J.O. (1967) Cardiac involvement in pseudoxanthoma elasticum. Report of a case. *Am. Heart J.*, **74**, 680–6.
264. Cristol, R., Debray, J. and Aron, Mme (1972) Les manifestations cardiovasculaires du pseudo-xanthome elastique à propos d'un cas typique avec infarctus myocardique. *Ann. Med. Interne (Paris)*, **123**, 771–6.
265. Akhtar, M. and Brody, H. (1975) Elastic tissue in pseudoxanthoma elasticum. Ultrastructural study of endocardial lesions. *Arch. Pathol.*, **99**, 667–71.
266. Hausser, I. and Anton-Lamprecht, I. (1991) Early preclinical diagnosis of dominant pseudoxanthoma elasticum by specific ultrastructural changes of dermal elastic and collagen tissue in a family at risk. *Hum. Genet.*, **87**, 693–700.
267. Lebwohl, M., Halperin, J. and Phelps, R.G. (1993) Brief report: Occult pseudoxanthoma elasticum in patients with premature cardiovascular disease. *N. Engl. J. Med.*, **329**, 1237–9.
268. Sillence, D. (1981) Osteogenesis imperfecta: an expanding panorama of variants. *Clin. Orthop.*, **159**, 11–25.
269. Beighton, P., dePaepe, A., Danks, D. *et al.* (1988) International nosology of heritable disorders of connective tissue, Berlin, 1986. *Am. J. Med. Genet.*, **29**, 581–94.
270. Hortop, J., Tsipouras, P., Hanley, J.A. *et al.* (1986) Cardiovascular involvement in osteogenesis imperfecta. *Circulation*, **73**, 54–61.
271. Pope, F.M., Daw, C.M., Narcisi, P. and Richarde, A.R. (1989) Prenatal diagnosis and prevention of inherited abnormalities of collagen. *J. Inherit. Metab. Dis.*, **12**, 135–73.
272. Wheeler, V.R., Cooley, N.R. and Blackburn, W.R. (1988) Cardiovascular pathology in osteogenesis imperfecta type IIA with a review of the literature. *Pediatr. Pathol.*, **8**, 55–64.
273. White, N.J., Winearls, C.G. and Smith, R. (1983) Cardiovascular abnormalities in osteogenesis imperfecta. *Am. Heart. J.*, **106**, 1416–20.
274. Cole, W.G. (1993) Genetics of connective tissue disease. *Med. J. Aust.*, **158**, 678–80.
275. Lamande, S.R., Dahl, H.H., Cole, W.G. and Bateman, J.F. (1989) Characterization of point mutations in the collagen COL1A1 and COL1A2 genes causing lethal perinatal osteogenesis imperfecta. *J. Biol. Chem.*, **264**, 15809–12.
276. Bateman, J.F., Mascara, T., Chan, D. and Cole, W.G. (1984) Abnormal type I collagen metabolism by cultured fibroblasts in lethal perinatal osteogenesis imperfecta. *Biochem. J.*, **217**, 103–15.
277. Byers, P.H., Wallis, G. and Willing, M.C. (1991) Osteogenesis imperfecta: translation of mutation to phenotype. *J. Med. Genet.*, **28**, 433–42.
278. Criscitiello, M.G., Ronan, J.A., Besterman, E.M.M. and Schoenwetter, W. (1965) Cardiovascular abnormalities in osteogenesis imperfecta. *Circulation*, **31**, 255–62.
279. Cohen, I.M., Vieweg, W.V.R., Alpert, J.S. *et al.* (1977) Osteogenesis imperfecta tarda. Cardiovascular pathology. *West. J. Med.*, **126**, 228–31.
280. Heckman, B.A. and Steinberg, I. (1968) Congenital heart disease (mitral regurtitation) in osteogenesis imperfecta. *Am. J. Roentgen. Radium Ther. Nucl. Med.*, **103**, 601–7.
281. Melamed, R., Aygen, M.M. and Lowenstein, A. (1976) Osteogenesis imperfecta with mitral insufficiency due to ballooning of the mitral valve. A case report. *Isr. J. Med. Sci.*, **12**, 1325–8.
282. Pijoan de Beristain, C. (1973) Asociacion de insuficiencia aórtica con osteogenesis imperfecta, en dos sujetos de la misma familia. *Rev. Esp. Cardiol.*, **26**, 405–10.
283. Remigio, P.A. and Grinvalsky, H.T. (1970) Osteogenesis imperfecta congenita. Association with conspicuous extraskeletal connective tissue dysplasia. *Am. J. Dis. Child.*, **119**, 524–8.
284. Siggers, D.C. (1974) Osteogenesis imperfecta with aortic valve replacement. *Birth Defects*, **10**, 495–8.
285. Stein, D. and Kloster, F.E. (1977) Valvular heart disease in osteogenesis imperfecta. *Am. Heart J.*, **94**, 637–41.
286. Heppner, R.L., Babbit, H.I., Bianchine, J.W. and Warbasse, J.R. (1973) Aortic regurgitation and aneurysm of sinus of Valsalva associated with osteogenesis imperfecta. *Am. J. Cardiol.*, **31**, 654–7.
287. Weisinger, B., Glassman, E., Spencer, F.C. and Berger, A. (1975) Successful aortic valve replacement for aortic regurgitation associated with osteogenesis imperfecta. *Br. Heart J.*, **37**, 475–7.
288. Wood, S.J., Thomas, J. and Braimbridge, M.V. (1973) Mitral valve disease and open heart surgery in osteogenesis imperfecta tarda. *Br. Heart J.*, **35**, 103–6.

289. Sigmund, J., Sperl, W., Fink, F.M. and Stos, H. (1986) Aortenisthmusstenosen und Osteogenesis imperfecta. *Padiatr. Pathol.*, **21**, 343–9.
290. Pasquali-Ronchetti, I., Ouaglino, D., Baccarani-Contri, M. *et al.* (1986) Aortic elastin abnormalities in osteogenesis imperfecta type II. *Coll. Relat. Res.*, **6**, 407–11.
291. Stacey, A., Bateman, J., Choi, T. *et al.* (1988) Perinatal lethal osteogenesis imperferta in transgenic mice bearing an engineered mutant pro-alpha 1(I) collagen gene. *Nature*, **332**, 131–6.
292. Khillan, J.S., Olsen, A.S., Kontusaari, S., *et al.* (1991) Transgenic mice that express a mini-gene version of the human gene for type I procollagen (COL1A1) develop a phenotype resembling a lethal form of osteogenesis imperfecta. *J. Biol. Chem.*, **266**, 23373–9.
293. Bonadio, J., Saunders, T.L., Tsai, E. *et al.* (1990) Transgenic mouse model of the mild dominant form of osteogenesis imperfecta. *Proc. Natl. Acad. Sci. USA*, **87**, 7145–9.
294. Scully, R.E., Galdabini, J.J. and McNealy, B.U. (1979) Case 3–1979, presentation of a case (case records of the Masschusetts General Hospital). *N. Engl. J. Med.*, **300**, 129–35.
295. Nuytinck, L., Narcisi, P., Nicholls, A. *et al.* (1992) Detection and characterization of an overmodified type III collagen by analysis of non-cutaneous connective tissues in a patient with Ehlers–Danlos syndrome IV. *J. Med. Genet.*, **29**, 375–80.
296. Kitazono, T., Imaizumi, T., Imayama, S. *et al.* (1989) Two cases of myocardial infarction in type IV Ehlers–Danlos syndrome. *Chest*, **95**, 1274–7.
297. Shekhonin, B.V., Semiachkina, A.N., Makkaer, K.G.M. *et al.* (1988) Collagen type I, III, IV and V and fibronectin in skin biopsies of patients with Ehlers–Danlos syndrome and cutis laxa. *Arkh. Patol.*, **50**, 41–8.
298. Cutolo, M., Castellani, P., Borsi, L. and Zardi, L. (1986) Altered fibronectin distribution in cultured fibroblasts from patients with Ehlers–Danlos syndrome. *Clin. Exp. Rheumatol.*, **4**, 125–8.
299. Miura, S., Shirakami, A., Ohara, A. *et al.* (1990) Fibronectin receptor on polymorphonuclear leukocytes in families of Ehlers–Danlos syndrome and other hereditary connective tissue diseases. *J. Lab. Clin. Med.*, **116**, 363–8.
300. Wilson, J.H. and Moodie, D.S. (1986) Cardiac amyloidosis in a patient with Ehlers–Danlos syndrome type IV. *Cleveland Clin.*, **53**, 205–11.
301. Shohet, I., Rosenbaum, I., Frand, M. *et al.* (1987) Cardiovascular complications in the Ehlers–Danlos syndrome with minimal external findings. *Clin. Genet.* **31**, 148–52.
302. Beighton, P. (1968) Lethal complications of the Ehlers–Danlos syndrome. *Br. Med. J.*, **3**, 656–9.
303. Rotberg, T., Sanagustín, M.T., Salinas, L. and Macias, R. (1977) Síndrome de Ehlers–Danlos asociado a communicación interauricular, bloqueo A–V completo, aneurisma de aorta y crecimiento de ventrículo izquierdo (miocardiopatía). *Arch. Int. Cardiol. Mex.*, **47**, 562–71.
304. Burnett, H.F., Bledose, J.H., Char, F. and Williams, G.D. (1973) Abdominal aortic aneurysmectomy in a 17-year-old patient with Ehlers–Danlos syndrome: case report and review of the literature. *Surgery*, **74**, 617–20.
305. Barabas, A.P. (1972) Vascular complications in the Ehlers–Danlos syndrome, with special reference to the 'arterial type' or Sack's syndrome. *J. Cardiovasc. Surg.*, **13**, 160–7.
306. Schoolman, A. and Kepes, J.J. (1965) Bilateral spontaneous carotid-cavernous fistulae in Ehlers–Danlos syndrome. Case report. *J. Neurosurg.*, **26**, 82–6.
307. Umlas, J. (1972) Spontaneous rupture of the subclavian artery in Ehlers–Danlos syndrome. *Hum. Pathol.*, **3**, 121–6.
308. Imahori, S., Bannerman, R.M., Graf, C.J. and Brennan, J.C. (1969) Ehlers–Danlos syndrome with multiple arterial lesions. *Am. J. Med.*, **47**, 967–7.
309. Short, D.W. (1978) Multiple congenital aneurysms in childhood: report of a case. *Br. J. Surg.*, **65**, 509–12.
310. Williams, J.L. (1975) Multiple aneurysms in a child. *Proc. Roy. Soc. Med.*, **68**, 523–5.
311. Byers, P.H., Holbrook, K.A., McGillivray, B. *et al.* (1979). Clinical and ultrastructural heterogeneity of type IV Ehlers–Danlos syndrome. *Hum. Genet.*, **47**, 141–50.
312. Lach, B., Nair, S.G., Russell, N.A. and Benoit, B.G. (1987) Spontaneous carotid-cavernous fistula and multiple arterial dissections in type IV Ehlers–Danlos syndrome. *J. Neurosurg.*, **66**, 462–7.
313. Silva, R., Cogbill, T.H., Hansbrough, J.F. *et al.* (1986) Intestinal perforation and vascular rupture in Ehlers–Danlos syndrome. *Int. Surg.*, **71**, 48–50.
314. Superti-Furga, A., Saesseli, B., Steinmann, B. and Bollinger, A. (1992) Microangiopathy in Ehlers–Danlos syndrome type IV. *Int. J. Microcirc. Clin. Exp.*, **11**, 241–7.
315. Klenn, P.J. and Iozzo, R.V. (1991) Larsen's syndrome with novel congenital anomalies. *Hum. Pathol.*, **22**, 1055–7.
316. McKusick, V. (1990) Larsen syndrome, in *Mendelian Inheritance in Man. Catalogs of Autosomal Dominant, Autosomal Recessive and X-linked Phenotypes*, 9th edn, Johns Hopkins University Press, Baltimore, pp. 560, 1291, 1292.
317. Swensson, R.E., Linnebur, A.C. and Paster, S.B. (1975) Striking aortic root dilatation in a patient with Larsen syndrome, *J. Pediatr.*, **86**, 914–15.
318. Kiel, E.A., Frias, J.L. and Victorica, B.E. (1983) Cardiovascular manifestations in the Larsen syndrome. *Pediatrics*, **71**, 942–6.
319. Rasooly, R., Gomori, J.M. and BenEzra, D. (1988) Arterial tortuosity and dilatation in Larsen syndrome. *Neuroradiology*, **30**, 258–60.
320. Chudley, A.E. and Hagerman, R.J. (1987) Fragile X syndrome. *J. Pediatr.*, **110**, 821–31.
321. Opitz, J.M., Westphal, J.M. and Daniel, A. (1984) Discovery of a connective tissue dysplasia in the Martin–Bell syndrome. *Am. J. Med. Genet.*, **17**, 101–9.
322. Sutherland, G.R., Mulley, J.L. and Richards, R.I. (1993) Fragile X syndrome. The most common cause of familial intellectual handicap. *Med. J. Aust.*, **158**, 482–5.
323. Sreeram, N., Wren, C., Bhate, M. *et al.* (1989) Cardiac abnormalities in the fragile X syndrome. *Br. Heart J.*, **61**, 289–91.
324. Loehr, J.P., Synhorst, D.P., Wolfe, R.R. and Hagerman, R.J. (1986) Aortic root dilatation and mitral valve prolapse in the fragile X syndrome. *Am. J. Med. Genet.*, **23**, 189–94.
325. Waldstein, G. and Hagerman, R. (1988) Aortic hypoplasia and cardiac valvular abnormalities in a boy with fragile X syndrome. *Am. J. Med. Genet.*, **30**, 83–98.
326. Glenner, G.G., Ignaczak, T.F. and Page, D.L. (1978) The inherited systemic amyloidosis and localized amyloid deposits, in *The Metabolic Basis of Inherited Disease*, 4th edn, (eds J.B. Stanbury, J.B. Wyngaarden and D.S. Fredrickson), McGraw-Hill, New York, pp. 1308–39.
327. Kumar, V. (1989) Amyloidosis, in *Robbins Pathologic Basis of Disease*, 4th edn, (eds R.S. Cotran, V. Kumar and S.C. Robbins), WB Saunders Company, Philadelphia, pp. 210–20.
328. Olson, L.J., Gertz, M.A., Edwards, W.D. *et al.* (1987) Senile cardiac amyloidosis with myocardial dysfunction. Diagnosis by endomyocardial biopsy and immunohistochemistry. *N. Engl. J. Med.*, **317**, 738–42.
329. Sipe, J.D. (1992) Amyloidosis. *Ann. Rev. Biochem.*, **61**, 947–75.
330. Bosch, E. and Mitsumoto, H. (1991) Disorders of peripheral nerves, plexuses and nerve roots, in *Neurology in Clinical Practice*, vol. II, (eds W.H. Bradley, R.B. Daroff, G.M. Feniche and C.D. Marsden), Butterworth-Heinemann, Boston, pp. 1719–92.
331. Diebold, J. (1985) Letters to the case. *Pathol. Res. Pract.*, **180**, 200–1.
332. Koeppen, A.H., Wallace, M.R., Benson, M.D. and Altland, K. (1990) Familial amyloid polyneuropathy: alanine-for-threonine substitution in the transthyretin (prealbumin) molecule. *Muscle Nerve*, **13**, 1065–75.
333. Cornwell, G.G. III, Murdoch, W.L., Kyle, R.A. *et al.* (1983) Frequency and distribution of senile cardiovascular amyloid. A clinicopathologic correlation. *Am. J. Med.*, **75**, 618–23.
334. Johansson, B. and Westermark, P. (1990) The relation of atrial natriuretic factor to isolated atrial amyloid. *Exp. Mol. Pathol.*, **52**, 266–78.
335. Cornwell, G.G. III, Westermark, P., Murdoch, W. and Pitkanen, P. (1982) Senile aortic amyloid. A third distinctive type of age-related cardiovascular amyloid. *Am. J. Pathol.*, **108**, 135–9.
336. Schwartz, P.H., Wolfe, K.G., Bath, J.S. *et al.* (1977) Amyloidosis in human and animal pathology: a comparative study, in *Amyloidosis*, (eds O. Wegelius and A. Pasternack), Academic Press, London, pp. 71–102.
337. Iwata, T., Kamei, T., Uchino, F. *et al.* (1978) Pathological study on amyloidosis – relationship of amyloid deposits in the aorta to aging. *Acta Pathol. Jpn*, **28**, 193–203.
338. Buja, L.M., Khoi, N.B. and Roberts, W.C. (1970) Clinically significant cardiac amyloidosis. Clinicopathologic findings in 15 patients. *Am. J. Cardiol.*, **26**, 394–405.
339. James, T.N. (1966) Pathology of the cardiac conduction system in amyloidosis. *Ann. Intern. Med.*, **65**, 28–36.
340. Smith, R.R., Hutchins, G.M., Sack Jr, G.H. and Ridolfi, R.L. (1979) Ischemic heart disease secondary to amyloidosis of intramyocardial arteries. *Am. J. Cardiol.*, **44**, 413–17.
341. Mahloudji, M., Teasdall, R.D., Adamkiewicz, J.J. *et al.* (1969) The genetic amyloidosis with particular reference to hereditary neuropathic amyloidosis, Type II (Indiana or Rukavina type). *Medicine*, **48**, 1–37.
342. Cheville, N.F. (1988) *Introduction to Veterinary Pathology*, 1st edn, Iowa State University Press, Ames, Iowa, pp. 125–130.
343. Yi, S., Takahashi, K., Naito, M. *et al.* (1991) Systemic amyloidosis in transgenic mice carrying the human mutant transthyretin (Met 30) gene. *Am. J. Pathol.*, **138**, 403–12.
344. Ganeval, D., Mignon, F. and Homme, J.-L.P. (1981) Dépots de chaînes légères et d'immunoglobulines monoclonales: Aspects nephrologiques et hypothesies physiopathologiques. *Actualités nephrologiques de l'Hôpital Necker*. Flammarion Medicine-Sciences, Paris, p. 179.
345. Ganeval, D., Noel, L.H., Homme, J.L. *et al.* (1984) Light-chain-deposition disease: its relation with AL-type amyloidosis. *Kidney Int.*, **26**, 1–9.
346. Hoffman-Guilaine, C., Nochy, D., Tricottet, V. *et al.* (1984) La maladie des dépots de chaînes légères: une entité anatomopathologique. *Ann. Pathol.*, **4**, 105–13.
347. Laurent, M., Toulet, R. and Ramee, M.P. (1984) Maladie des chaînes légères avec myocardiopathie terminale. *Arch. Mal. Coeur.*, **78**, 943–6.
348. Randall, R.E., Williamson Jr, W.C. Mullinax, F. *et al.* (1976) Manifestations of systemic light chain deposition. *Am. J. Med.*, **60**, 293–9.

349. Kirkpatrick, C.J., Curry, A. and Galle, J. (1986) Systemic kappa light chain deposition and amyloidosis in multiple myeloma: novel morphological observations. *Histopathology*, **10**, 1065–76.
350. McAllister Jr, H.A. Seger, J., Bossart, M. and Ferrans, V.J. (1988) Restrictive cardiomyopathy with kappa light chain deposits in myocardium as a complication of multiple myeloma. *Arch. Pathol. Lab. Med.*, **112**, 1151–4.
351. Lindsay Jr, J. Meshel, J.C. and Patterson, R.H. (1974) The cardiovascular manifestations of sickle cell disease. *Arch. Intern. Med.*, **133**, 643–51.
352. Rubler, S. and Fleischer, R.A. (1967) Sickle cell states and cardiomyopathy. Sudden death due to pulmonary thrombosis and infarction. *Am. J. Cardiol.*, **19**, 867–73.
353. Merkel, K.H., Ginberg, P.L., Parker Jr, J.C. and Post, M.J. (1978) Cerebrovascular disease in sickle cell anemia: a clinical, pathological and radiological correlation. *Stroke*, **9**, 45–52.
354. Stockman, J.A., Nigro, M.A., Mishkin, M.M. and Oski, F.A. (1972) Occlusion of large cerebral vessels in sickle-cell anemia. *N. Engl. J. Med.*, **287**, 846–9.
355. Wood, D.H. (1978) Cerebrovascular complications of sickle cell anemia. *Stroke*, **9**, 73–5.
356. Harley, R.D. (1975) *Pediatric Ophthalmology*, WB Saunders Company, Philadelphia, p. 593.
357. Gerry Jr, J.L., Bulkley, B.H. and Hutchins, G.M. (1978) Clinicopathologic analysis of cardiac dysfunction in 52 patients with sickle cell anemia. *Am. J. Cardiol.*, **42**, 211–16.
358. Botreau-Roussel, P., Drobinski, G., Levy, R. et al. (1977) Infarctus du myocarde et drepanocytose heterozygote. A propos de 2 cas. *Arch. Mal. Coeur*, **70**, 141.
359. Fleischer, R.A. and Rubler, S. (1968) Primary cardiomyopathy in non-anemic patients. Association with sickle cell trait. *Am. J. Cardiol.*, **22**, 532–7.
360. Rowley, P.T. and Enlander, D. (1968) Hemoglobin S-C disease presenting as acute cor pulmonale. *Am. Rev. Respir. Dis.*, **98**, 494–500.
361. Chopdar, A. (1975) Multiple major retinal vascular occlusions in sickle cell haemoglobin C disease. *Br. J. Ophthalmol.*, **59**, 493–6.
362. Siqueira, W.C., Figueiredo, M.S., Cruz, A.A. et al. (1990) Conjunctival vessel abnormalities in sickle cell diseases: the influence of age and genotype. *Acta Ophthalmol.*, **68**, 515–18.
363. Maron, B.J. (1993) Hypertrophic cardiomyopathy. *Curr. Prob. Cardiol.*, **18**, 637–704.
364. Tanaka, M., Fujiwara, H., Onodera, T. et al. (1987) Quantitative analysis of narrowings of intramyocardial small arteries in normal hearts, hypertensive hearts, and hearts with hypertrophic cardiomyopathy. *Circulation*, **75**, 1130–9.
365. McKusick, V.A. (1990) Progeria, in *Mendelian Inheritance in Man. Catalogs of Autosomal Dominant, Autosomal Recessive and X-linked Phenotypes*, 9th edn, Johns Hopkins University Press, Baltimore, pp. 797–8.
366. Brown, W.T., Abdenur, J., Goonewardena, R. et al. (1990) Hutchinson–Gilford progeria syndrome: *Clin. Chromosom. Metab. Abnorm.*, **47**, A50 (abstr).
367. Atkins, L. (1954) Progeria. Report of a case with postmortem findings. *N. Engl. J. Med.*, **250**, 1065–9.
368. Gabr, M., Hashem, N., Hashem, M. et al. (1960) Progeria, a pathologic study, *J. Pediatr.* **57**, 70–7.
369. Makous, N., Friedman, S., Yakovac, W. and Mari, E.P. (1962) Cardiovascular manifestations in progeria. Report of clinical and pathologic findings in a patient with severe arteriosclerotic heart disease and aortic stenosis. *Am. Heart J.*, **64**, 334–6.
370. Manschot, W.A. (1950) A case of progeronanism (progeria of Gilford). *Acta Paediat. Scand.*, **39**, 158–164.
371. Rosenthal, I.M., Bronstein, I.P., Dallenbach, F.D. et al. (1956) Progeria. Report of a case with cephalometric roentgenograms and abnormally high concentrations of lipoproteins in the serum. *Pediatrics*, **18**, 565.
372. Talbot, N.B., Butler, A.M., Pratt, E.L. et al. (1945) Progeria. Clinical, metabolic and pathologic studies on a patient. *Am. J. Dis. Child.*, **69**, 267.
373. Naganuma, Y., Konishi, T., Hongou, K. et al. (1990) A case of progeria syndrome with cerebral infarction. *No To Hattatsu*, **22**, 71–6.
374. Baker, P.B., Baba, N. and Boesel, C.P. (1981) Cardiovascular abnormalities in progeria. Case report and review of the literature. *Arch. Pathol. Lab. Med.*, **105**, 384–6.
375. Smith, A.S., Wiznitzer, M., Karaman, B.A. et al. (1993) MRA detection of vascular occlusion in a child with progeria. *Am. J. Neuroradiol.*, **14**, 441–3.
376. Wagle, W.A., Haller, J.S. and Cousins, J.P. (1992) Cerebral infarction in progeria. *Pediatr. Neurol.* **8**, 476–7.
377. Epstein, C.J., Martin, G.M., Schultz, A.L. and Motulsky, A.G. (1966) Werner's syndrome: a review of its symptomatology, natural history, pathological features, genetics and relationship to natural aging process. *Medicine*, **45**, 177–221.
378. Brown, W.T., Kieras, F.J., Houck Jr, G.E. et al. (1985) A comparison of adult and childhood progerias: Werner syndrome and Hutchinson–Gilford progeria syndrome. *Adv. Exp. Med. Biol.*, **1990**, 229–44.
379. Grimm, T. and Wesselhoeft, H. (1980) Zur Genetik des Williams–Beuren-Syndroms und der isolierten Form der supravalvularen Aortenstenose (Untersuchungen von 128 Familien). *Z. Kardiol.*, **69**, 168–72.
380. Folger Jr, G.M. (1977) Further observations on the syndrome of idiopathic infantile hypercalcemia associated with supravalvular aortic stenosis. *Am. Heart J.*, **93**, 455–62.
381. Friedman, W.F. (1967) Vitamin D as a cause of the supravalvular aortic stenosis syndrome. *Am. Heart J.*, **73**, 718–20.
382. Hutchins, G.M., Mirvis, S.E., Mendelsohn, G. and Bulkley, B.H. (1978) Supravalvular aortic stenosis with parafollicular cell (C-cell) hyperplasia. *Am. J. Med.*, **64**, 967–73.
383. McKusick, V.A. (1990) Williams' syndrome, in *Mendelian Inheritance in Man. Catalogs of Autosomal Dominant, Autosomal Recessive and X-linked Phenotypes*, 9th edn, Johns Hopkins Press, Baltimore, pp. 483, 979–81.
384. Beuren, A.J. (1972) Supravalvular aortic stenosis: a complex syndrome with and without mental retardation. *Birth Defects Orig. Art. Ser. VIII* (5), 45–56.
385. Antia, A.U., Wiltse, H.E., Rowe, R.D. et al. (1967) Pathogenesis of the supravalvular aortic stenosis syndrome. *J. Pediatr.*, **71**, 431–41.
386. Garcia, R.E., Friedman, W.F., Kaback, M.M. and Rowe, R.D. (1964) Idiopathic hypercalcemia and supravalvular aortic stenosis. Documentation of a new syndrome. *N. Engl. J. Med.*, **271**, 117–20.
387. Jones, K.L. and Smith, D.W. (1975) The Williams elfin facies syndrome: a new perspective. *J. Pediatr.* **86**, 718–23.
388. Page Jr, H.L. Vogel, J.H. Pryor, R. and Blount Jr, S.G. (1969) Supravalvular aortic stenosis. Unusual observations in three patients. *Am. J. Cardiol.*, **23**, 270–7.
389. Kurlander, G.J., Petry, E.L., Taybi, H. et al. (1966) Supravalvual aortic stenosis. Roentgen analysis of twenty-seven cases. *Am. J. Roentgen. Radium Ther. Nucl. Med.*, **98**, 782–99.
390. Ottesen, O.E., Antia, A.N. and Rowe, R.D. (1966) Peripheral vascular anomalies associated with the supravalvular aortic stenosis syndrome. *Radiology*, **86**, 430–5.
391. Wakasaki, H. and Ooshima, A. (1990). Immunohistochemical localization of lysyl oxidase with monoclonal antibodies. *Lab. Invest.*, **63**, 377–84.
392. Vulpe, C. Levinson, B., Whitney, S. et al. (1993) Isolation of a candidate gene for Menkes disease and evidence that it encodes a copper-transporting ATPase. *Nat. Genet.*, **3**, 7–13.
393. Factor, S.M., Cho, S., Sternlieb, I. et al. (1982) The cardiomyopathy of Wilson's disease. Myocardial alterations in nine cases. *Virchows Arch. Pathol. Anat.*, **397**, 301–11.
394. Gacheru, S., McGee, C., Uriu-Hare, J.Y. et al. (1993) Expression and accumulation of lysyl oxidase, elastin and type I procollagen in human Menkes and mottled mouse fibroblasts. *Arch. Biochem. Biophys.*, **301**, 325–9.
395. Royce, P.M. and Steinmann, B. (1990) Markedly reduced activity of lysyl oxidase in skin and aorta from a patient with Menkes disease showing unusually severe connective tissue manifestations. *Pediatr. Res.*, **28**, 137–41.
396. Danks, D.M., Campbell, P.E., Stevens, B.J. et al. (1972) Menkes's kinky hair syndrome. An inherited defect in copper absorption with widespread effects. *Pediatrics*, **50**, 188–201.
397. Moon, H.R., Chi, J.G., Yeon, K.M. et al. (1987) Menks disease: an autopsy case with metal analysis of hair. *J. Korean Med. Sci.*, **2**, 75–83.
398. Olivares Lopez, J.L., Tosao Sanchez, A., Cerda, M.P. and Carpeto, F.J. (1989) Menkes syndrome: study of 2 new cases. *An. Esp. Pediatr.*, **31**, 380–4.
399. Uno, H., Arya, S., Laxova, R. and Gilbert, E.F. (1983) Menkes syndrome with vascular and adrenergic nerve abnormalities. *Arch. Pathol. Lab. Med.*, **107**, 286–9.
400. Martin, J.J., Flament-Durand, J., Farriaux, J.P. et al. (1978) Menkes kinky-hair disease. A report on its pathology. *Acta Neuropathol. (Berlin)*, **42**, 25–32.
401. Wheeler, E.M. and Roberts, P.F. (1976) Menkes's steely hair syndrome. *Arch. Dis. Child.*, **51**, 269–74.
402. Johnsen, D.E., Coleman, L. and Poe, L. (1991) MR. of progressive neurodegenerative change in treated Menkes' kinky hair disease. *Neuroradiology*, **32**, 181–2.
403. Oakes, B.W., Danks, D.M. and Campbell, P.E. (1976). Human copper deficiency: ultrastructural studies of the aorta and skin in a child with Menkes' syndrome. *Exp. Mol. Pathol.*, **25**, 82–98.
404. Borg, T.K., Klevay, L.M., Gay, R.E. et al. (1985) Alteration of the connective tissue network of striated muscle in copper deficient rats. *J. Mol. Cell Cardiol.*, **17**, 1173–83.
405. Gore, I., Wada, M. and Goodman, M.L. (1968) Capillary hemorrhage in ascorbic-acid-deficient guinea pigs. Ultrastructural basis. *Arch. Pathol.*, **85**, 493–502.
406. Follis Jr, R.H. (1942) Sudden death in infants with scurvy. *J. Pediatr.*, **20**, 347.
407. Follis Jr, R.H. (1956) The effects of nutritional deficiency on the heart: a review. *Am. J. Clin. Nutr.*, **4**, 107–16.
408. Van Vleet, J.F., Ferrans, V.J. and Ruth, G.R. (1977) Ultrastructural

alterations in nutritional cardiomyopathy of selenium-vitamin E deficient swine. I. Fiber lesions. *Lab. Invest.*, **37**, 188–200.
409. Van Vleet, J.F., Ferrans, V.J. and Ruth, G.R. (1977) Ultrastructural alterations in nutritional cardiomyopathy of selenium-vitamin E deficient swine. II. Vascular lesions. *Lab. Invest.*, **37**, 201–11.
410. Keshan Disease Research Group of the Chinese Academy of Medical Sciences, Beijing (1979) Epidemiologic studies on the etiologic relationship of selenium and Keshan disease. *Chinese Med. J.*, **92**, 477–82.
411. Baker, S.S., Lerman, R.H., Krey, S.H. *et al.* (1983) Selenium deficiency with total parenteral nutrition: reversal of biochemical and functional abnormalities by selenium supplementation: a case report. *Am. J. Clin. Nutr.*, **38**, 769–74.
412. Chen, X., Yang, G., Chen, J. *et al.* (1980). Studies on the relations of selenium and Keshan disease. *Biol. Trace Element Res.*, **2**, 91.
413. Ge, K., Xue, A., Bai, J. and Wang, S. (1983) Keshan disease – an endemic cardiomyopathy in China. *Virchows Arch. Pathol. Anat.*, **401**, 1–15.
414. Yu, W.H. (1982) A study of nutritional and bio-geochemical factors in the occurrence and development of Keshan disease. The 6th conference on prevention of rheumatic fever and rheumatic heart disease. *Jpn Circ. J.*, **46**, 1201–7.
415. Grant, C.A. (1961) Morphological and etiological studies of dietetic microangiopathy in pigs ('mulberry heart'). *Acta Vet. Scand.* (suppl. 3), 5–107.
416. Ferrans, V.J. and Van, Vleet, J.F. (1988) Cardiac lesions of selenium-vitamin E deficiency in animals, in *Myocarditis and Related Disorders*, (eds M. Sekiguchi, E.G.J. Olsen and J.F. Goodwin), Springer Verlag, Tokyo, pp. 294–7.

6 ATHEROSCLEROSIS AND DEGENERATIVE DISEASES OF BLOOD VESSELS

William E. Stehbens

6.1 Nomenclature of degenerative vascular diseases

The nomenclature of degenerative vascular diseases is confusing, there being no unanimity of opinion regarding classification or differentiation of one from another. Review of the pathology of these degenerative diseases during this century reveals:

1. lack of agreement on what constitutes the early stage of atherosclerosis;
2. difficulty in interpreting the intimal thickening seen in the fetus and neonate;
3. confusion over differentiation of sclerotic changes that increase in severity with age and the accumulation of caseous debris.

Many pathologists seem to have regarded the sclerotic changes in arteries as distinct from lipid-rich caseous lesions and this concept seems to be perpetuated even today because the presence of lipid is widely thought to be the hallmark or *sine qua non* of atherosclerosis. Investigators have attempted to elucidate aetiologies from end-stage disease particularly in respect of lipid deposition and calcification rather than taking the more logical approach of seeking, even macroscopically, the earliest demonstrable lesion. Difficulty was experienced in differentiating vascular disease from mere senescence with Osler [1] declaring that 'a man is only as old as his arteries'. Current views on the nomenclature of terms in common use are as follows.

Atheroma, derived from the Greek word *athere* for mush, draws attention to the pultaceous or caseous material of high lipid content in advanced intimal plaques. In recent years the disease has been referred to as **atherosclerosis** to emphasize the extensive sclerotic or fibrous tissue component of the lesion and, especially in American literature, atheroma is reserved for the advanced localized necrotic pultaceous lesion only. In British literature atheroma and atherosclerosis are still frequently used synonymously.

Arteriosclerosis literally means sclerosis or hardening of the arteries as if this were a manifestation of aging independent of atherosclerosis although, again, the two terms are often used synonymously. Arteriosclerosis, in a generic sense, includes atherosclerosis, Mönckeberg's sclerosis and sclerotic age-related changes of large and small peripheral distributing arteries. These small peripheral and parenchymal vessels are frequently neglected altogether in textbooks and their sclerotic changes have been referred to as diffuse hyperplastic sclerosis. Arteriosclerosis should be reserved for the sclerotic involvement of these small peripheral distributing arteries until their relationship to atherosclerosis has been clarified.

Arteriolosclerosis refers to the thickening, fibrosis and hyalinization of the walls of arterioles with narrowing of the lumen.

Phlebosclerosis literally means sclerosis or fibrosis of veins, thus distinguishing it from arterial degeneration. A convenient term, it should really encompass all venous changes from the earliest pathological thickening of the intima to overt atherosclerosis. It is not generally appreciated that these sclerotic changes may also manifest lipid accumulation and mineralization as in arteries. Phlebosclerosis is, in reality, venous atherosclerosis.

The continued lack of uniformity in terminology of degenerative vascular disease and the recent increase in knowledge of vascular pathology indicate the need for revision.

6.2 Atherosclerosis

Atherosclerosis is not a disease restricted to modern man. It was common in ancient Egyptian mummies [2] although there is no evidence that it was recognized as such even in later Greco-Roman times. The disease has been found in other preserved bodies in China but it was not described and recognized in the aorta and other arteries until the sixteenth century when exploratory autopsies were conducted in Europe. Many famous men of medicine have made observations on atherosclerosis and its complications but only during the present century has concentrated effort been focused on its aetiology and pathogenesis. Many theories of aetiology have been proffered since the turn of the century and currently knowledge is still very much in evolution. A satisfactory theory has to explain the cause, pathogenesis and complications and a unifying thread must interconnect the diverse observations already made.

Atherosclerosis, now the world's foremost medical problem and the inevitable fate of all human arteries, is of increasing concern because of the socioeconomic implications of the high morbidity and mortality of its complications in aging populations. Almost half of all deaths in technologically advanced countries are attributable to this chronic, slowly progressive, degenerative disease, recognized primarily in large arteries and associated with progressive intimal proliferation, the development of fibrofatty plaques, intimal tears and ulceration with secondary thromboembolism and aneurysmal dilatation with its sequelae.

Not always appreciated is that small arteries also exhibit medial thinning, musculoelastic intimal thickening with sclerosis, loss of elastica and hyalinization and also lipid accumulation, calcification and severe luminal stenosis. Moreover, atherosclerosis is not confined to arteries and veins but regularly involves the cardiac valves especially the anterior leaflet of the mitral valve, chordae tendineae [3] and occasionally the heart itself [4].

It is a universal disease in humans varying in severity from person to person and it is inappropriate to allege without substantial scientific evidence that some individuals have no atherosclerosis even in old age. Such allegations are probably based on superficial macroscopic inspection and on varying definitions. Atherosclerosis is not specific to humans nor even to mammals. It occurs in a wide variety of species, including herbivores. For a long time it has been known to occur in severe form in parrots, pigeons and more recently in chimpanzees and gorillas. Its severity in lower species is usually less than in humans. If it is acknowledged that the intimal fibromusculoelastic thickenings at arterial forks in humans are an early stage of atherosclerosis, then the disease is widespread in the animal kingdom, not only in mammals and birds but also in fish and reptiles. It is, therefore, illogical to speak of the incidence of atherosclerosis in humans and to compare atherosclerotic subjects with those allegedly unaffected.

Atherosclerosis may be divided into two stages for convenience. The first is the silent or quiescent phase of progressive development from the initial stage in infancy or *in utero* with slow inexorable progression until the second phase of complications is apparent, usually in the sixth decade or beyond (Figure 6.1). During this latter stage atherosclerosis becomes manifest clinically as coronary heart disease (CHD), cerebrovascular disease (CVD) or peripheral vascular disease (PVD). However, complications are not always clinically detectable.

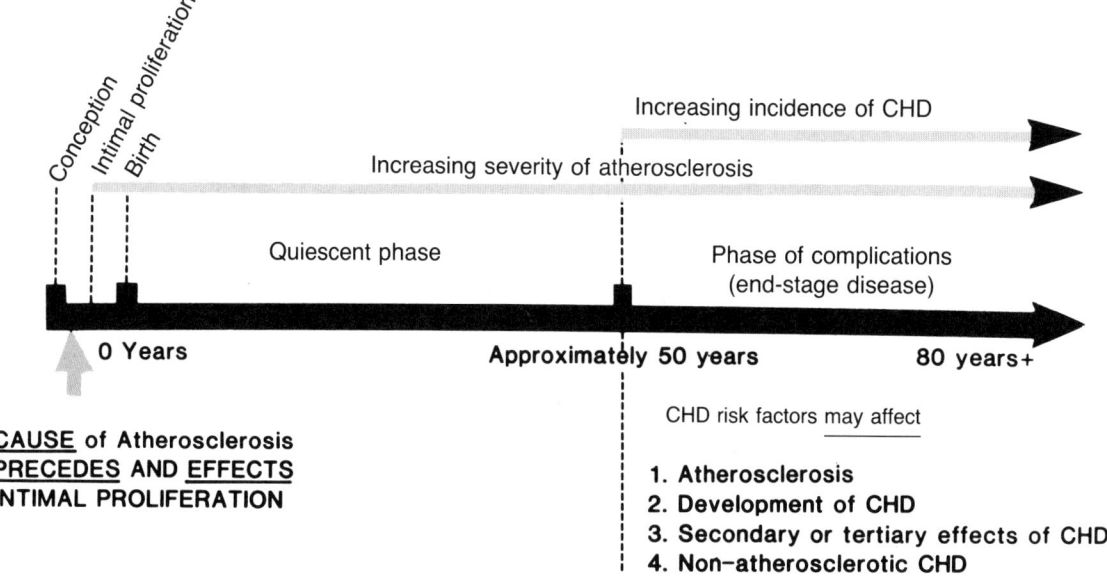

Figure 6.1 Diagram to illustrate the two phases of atherosclerosis in humans with reference to age, its inception with intimal proliferation, the quiescent phase, the development of complications about 50 years of age and their relationship to causation and risk factors for coronary heart disease (CHD). (Reproduced with permission from Stehbens [5].)

6.2.1 MORPHOLOGY OF THE AORTA AND ILIAC ARTERIES

Human atherosclerosis is known to be most severe in the aorta, particularly the abdominal segment and the orifices of the segmental branches being sites of predilection for severe involvement. In the neonate the ostia, like those in the rabbit aorta, are characterized by the sharp U-shaped distal lip of the flow divider which, when viewed *en face*, is elevated and overhangs the antrum-like ostium to ensure blood enters the branch. This configuration is associated with considerable lateral expansion in cross-sectional area of the lumen as blood approaches the flow divider [6]. Elsewhere the intimal surface is smooth, glistening and creamy in colour.

Even in infancy the ostia of the aortic segmental branches may, upon close inspection, exhibit slight deformation, i.e. relative encroachment on the ostium with rounding of the orifice, due particularly to thickening of the flow divider, elevation of the proximal or cardiac aspect of the ostium and slight irregularity of the aortic surface. There may be some slight transverse wrinkling of the aortic surface mostly on its posterior wall (Figure 6.2).

Progressively, small nodules or elevations often in a linear arrangement become more prominent on the posterior wall as yellow fatty dots and streaks (Figure 6.3). These lesions occur late in the first decade and also in the second and third decades. The age of onset varies. For the most part they are confined to the posterior surface of the descending aorta between the paired segmental branches or close to their lateral borders. The alignment of streaks or successive dots is in the long axis of the aorta. They spare the flow dividers and the aorta immediately distal and at times the lateral boundary of involvement diverges from a segmental ostium only to curve back towards the next ostium distally giving a slightly scalloped appearance to the pattern. Some dots may be found in the proximal aspect of the ostia of

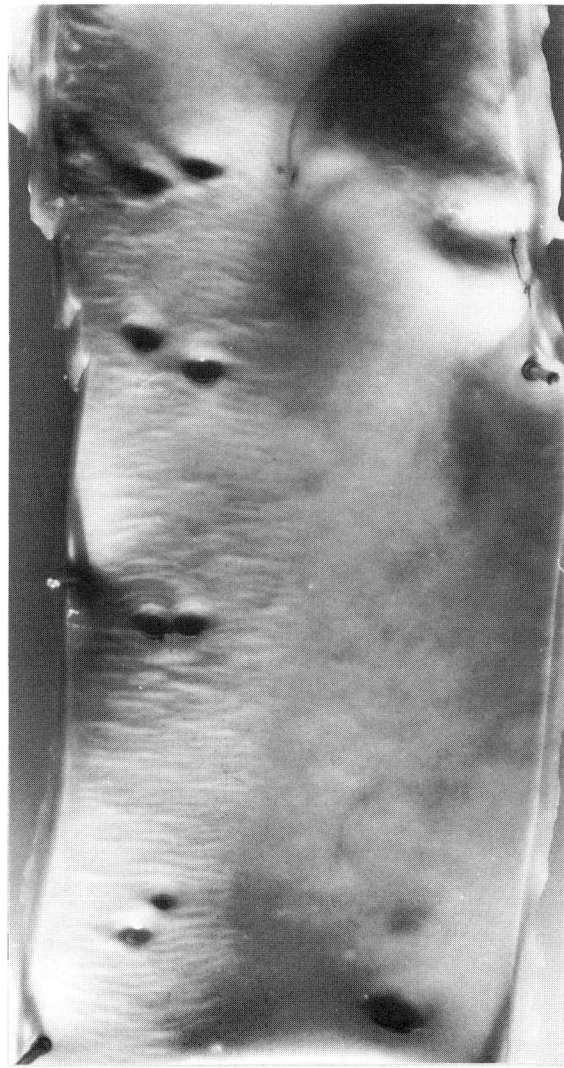

Figure 6.2 Segment of human aorta displaying transverse wrinkling of the intima along the posterior wall between the ostia of segmental branches. Flow is from above down.

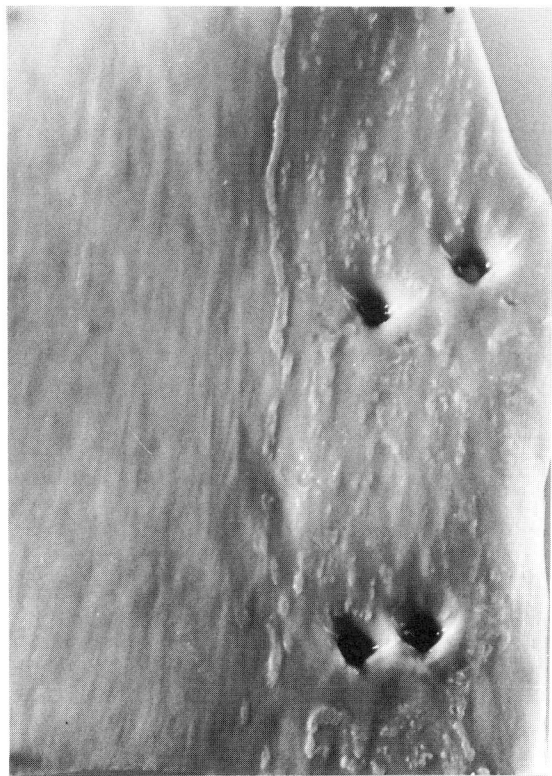

Figure 6.3 Segment of descending aorta displaying elevated fatty dots and streaks predominantly along the posterior wall from which the segmental branches arise. The crescentic edge of the flow divider and the aortic surface immediately below tend to be spared. Note the aortic surface elsewhere has a somewhat irregular surface. Flow is from above down.

segmental branches and in the larger branches arising from the arch and ventral and lateral aspects of the descending aorta. They also occur distally to the large abdominal branches. Fatty dots and streaks may or may not be slightly elevated above the general intimal surface and some elevations may not be yellow.

The surface becomes more irregular, the lumen insidiously expands and the recoil of the edges of a transversely transected aorta (*in situ*) diminishes. The fatty streaks enlarge and coalesce especially distally. These shade imperceptibly into the adjoining aortic surface and are usually not sessile or sharply demarcated like the xanthelasmatous appearance of the lesions of familial hypercholesterolaemia (FH). With progressive thickening of the intima in the distal aorta, the intimal surface posteriorly above the bifurcation becomes a whitish elevated plaque with disappearance of fatty streaks. The plaque shades imperceptibly into the adjoining aortic surface and extends into the external iliac arteries posteromedially. Similar elevated whitish plaques progressively involve the ostia of the aortic branches (Figure 6.4) and the two ostia of the paired segmental branches in the middle of the confluent plaque give the appearance of buttonholes. Fatty streaks are replaced by the progressive development of these plaques which may merge with those about neighbouring ostia.

It has been alleged without evidence that fatty streaks are reversible and disappear, no doubt because of the variation in age when seen at autopsy. There is controversy over the relationship of fatty streaks to atherosclerosis. Since fatty streaks precede fibrofatty plaques and they both affect the posterior wall, it is reasonable to accept that increased fibromuscular proliferation in the intima is responsible for the transformation and that the fatty streaks are an integral stage of atherosclerosis.

The ostia enlarge as the aorta grows, their relative size diminishing more in some aortas than in others but with increasing irregularity and deformity (Figure 6.5). The prominence of the flow divider is lost as is the antrum-like entrance to the branches. Emphasis has been given to stenosis of the ostia of the renal arteries but this also occurs at the entrance to the coronary and other aortic branches, the phenomenon being frequently recognized angiographically [7].

On the cut surface, yellow lipid is usually most prominent deep in the intima but gross lipid staining reveals the lipid to be much more extensive than *en face* staining suggests. Some fibrous plaques on sectioning reveal a variable amount of yellow caseous material without evidence of any fibrous stroma. Such lesions have been referred to as atheromata or atheromatous abscesses. The overlying intimal tissue varies in thickness.

Coarse transversely orientated wrinkling occurs particularly on the posterior or lateral surfaces of the aorta, more so in the abdominal than the thoracic segment but also on the posterior surface of the common iliac arteries. The extent of involvement varies and occurs independently of fatty streaks [7]. The wrinkling may be faint but on other occasions is quite distinct. Recognized in the last century, these wrinklings have been neglected in English literature. They are known variously as 'rhythmic structures' [8], aortic functional structures [9] and 'wave lines' [10] but these terms are inappropriate. They are best regarded as transverse wrinkling and there is little doubt they are fashioned by the flowing blood. They have been observed from the first to the eighth decade and their periodicity is relatively regular.

These wrinkles or corrugations are replaced by fibrous plaques which coalesce with those about the ostia sometimes forming an extensive fibrous plaque along the posterior aortic wall. Individual plaques may thus become less distinct although the aortic surface is irregular with elevations, depressions, wrinkling and creases. These changes progressively affect the entire circumference and also the aorta more proximally. Some regions may be yellowish due to the presence of lipid, other regions display greyish discoloration and are somewhat translucent following calcification and some may exhibit reddish, brown or black discolouration due to extravasation of blood into the intima around tears or ulceration (Figure 6.5). There is healing of many such tears which otherwise increase in size and extent often with undermined edges and a variable degree of thrombus over the denuded surface. Some tears may be

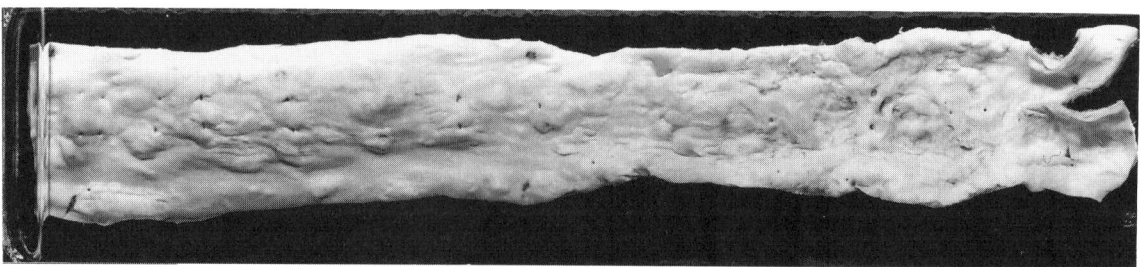

Figure 6.4 Descending aorta exhibiting irregular intimal surface with plaques involving the segmental paired ostia which are possibly narrower. Note the enlarged width of the distal aorta.

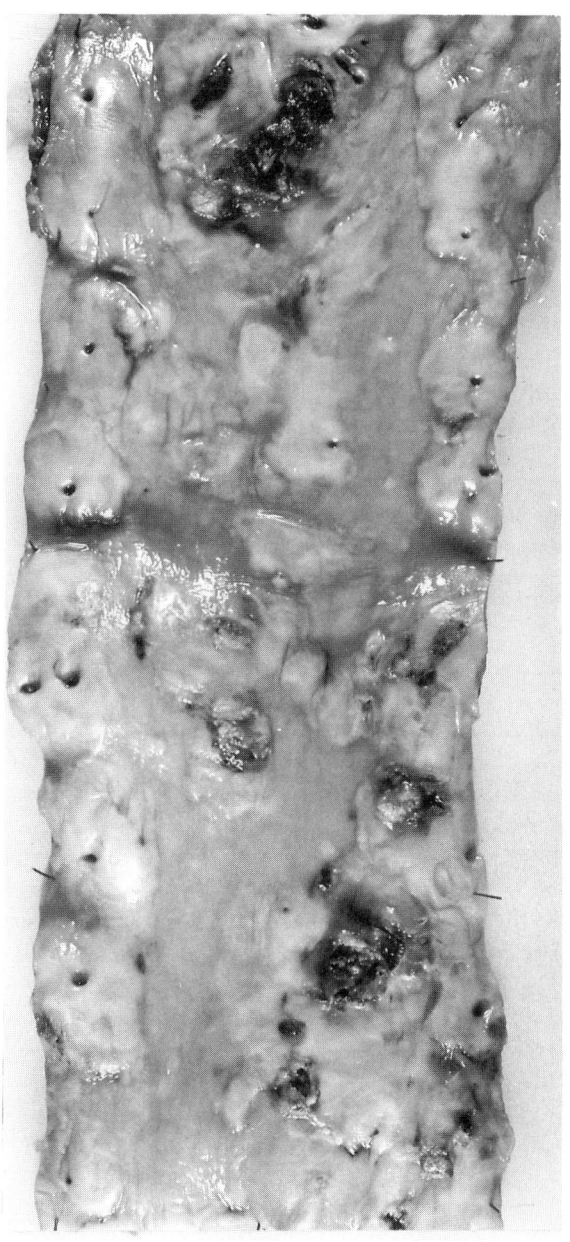

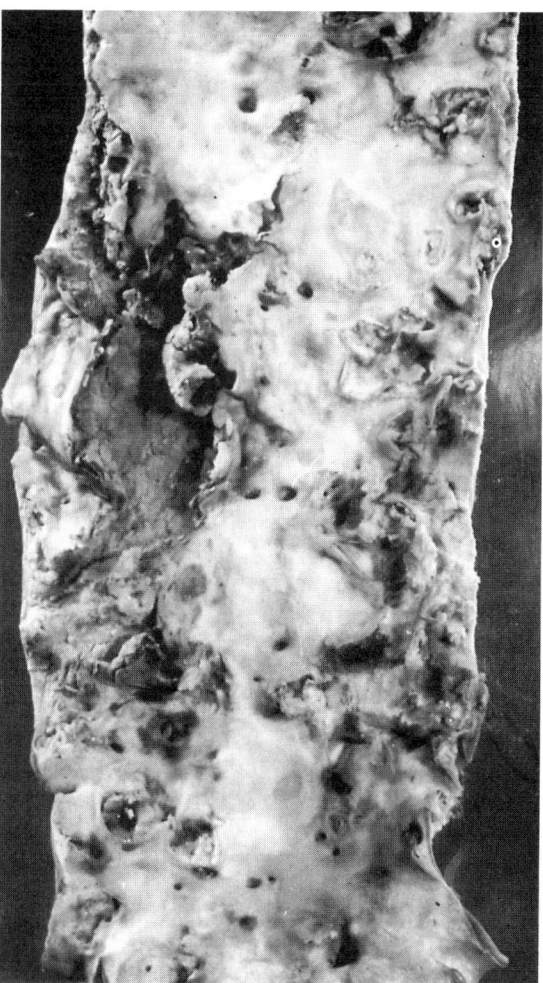

Figure 6.6 Advanced aortic atherosclerosis with gross ulceration, cracks and mural thrombosis on exposed intimal surface. Some ostia are lost in the ulceration. (Reproduced with permission from Stehbens [422].)

Figure 6.5 Segment of moderately severe atherosclerotic descending aorta opened posteriorly between the ostia of the segmental branches. Note their distorted orifices and the elevated plaques surrounding them. Ulceration and tears are present with superimposed thrombus and infiltration of neighbouring wall with blood.

large and irregular, some may simulate a crevice but the gross ulceration (Figure 6.6) with desquamation of large areas of intima must be associated with serious circulatory disturbances in the limbs. On opening some aortae and iliac arteries, the hard brittle inner part of the wall may separate from the outer portion, simulating partial endarterectomy and also demonstrating how easily such vessels could be injured by deep palpation.

Areas of ulceration may be coated with pale granular thrombus mixed with caseous cell debris. Larger thrombi have a variable amount of red thrombus admixed often with extravasation of blood into the adjoining wall. With excavation of the wall and especially with ectasia there may be large, flat, transversely ridged laminated thrombus. In advanced atherosclerosis with thrombus and ulceration, many ostia will be impossible to identify even if not completely obliterated [7]. Expansion of the remnants of the aortic wall in the base of an ulcer can result in a localized saccular aneurysm (Figure 10.8, p. 360).

With progressive development of these atherosclerotic changes, there may be some tortuosity and the circumference of the aorta enlarges. In some the functional lumen, seen angiographically, is grossly narrowed and irregular. When the aortae, opened longitudinally, are compared, the circumferential width does not always taper distally. Some specimens exhibit variable but localized widening above the bifurcation due to incipient aneurysmal dilatation (Figure 6.4). Some aortae display pronounced diffuse ectasia and tortuosity often in association with one or several small localized aneurysmal dilatations. Ectasia may involve the common iliac arteries which also exhibit severe atherosclerosis, often with widening of the angle of bifurcation and displacement of the iliac arteries but one or other iliac artery may be stenosed rather than ectatic.

The frequency of tears, ulceration and mural thrombosis in the abdominal aorta at autopsy indicates that many middle-aged and elderly individuals live with complicated but symptomless aortic lesions. It is fortunate that mural thrombi in the aorta rarely become occlusive and that emboli of thrombotic and atheromatous debris, which must frequently enter the iliofemoral arteries, usually cause so little disturbance clinically due to rapid clearance and a plentiful collateral circulation.

Traditionally the fatty dots and streaks were regarded as the earliest manifestation of atherosclerosis. Implicit in this concept was the acceptance that intimal thickening preceded the appearance of lipid. However, there is nothing sacrosanct about the concept of lipid being the initial indicator of disease and if lipid usually occurs in the deepest part of the intima, this histological intimal thickening must be considered a precursor or an earlier, integral stage of atherosclerosis [11].

An increasing number of investigators has regarded intimal proliferation or thickening at branching sites and its more diffuse distribution in the aorta as an early or pre-lipid stage of atherosclerosis. This concept has been reinforced by the 'intimal injury hypothesis' [12] whereby the initial demonstrable alteration is smooth-muscle proliferation in the intima and lipid accumulation is belatedly acknowledged as a secondary event. The logical approach must therefore be to examine the earliest intimal change. Unfortunately there is limited information available on aortic changes due to the size and the logistical difficulties in performing serial sections on large numbers of aortic specimens. Nevertheless, it is possible to draw together the following information.

The aortic intima has usually been represented as a significant portion (up to one fifth) of the total thickness of the wall. In the early fetus most of the aortic intima consists of an endothelial layer superimposed on a thick well formed internal elastic lamina (Figure 6.7) with presumably only elastic tissue microfibrils in the intervening space. There are intimal thickenings about orifices of branches and the internal elastic lamina is thin or absent beneath these (Figure 6.7). Such thickenings occur as early as 15 weeks. Elsewhere, even at 22 weeks, there are zones where the internal elastic lamina is thin or replaced by a network of thin elastic fibrils or reduplicated [13]. These intimal changes become diffuse but appear to extend particularly distal to the flow

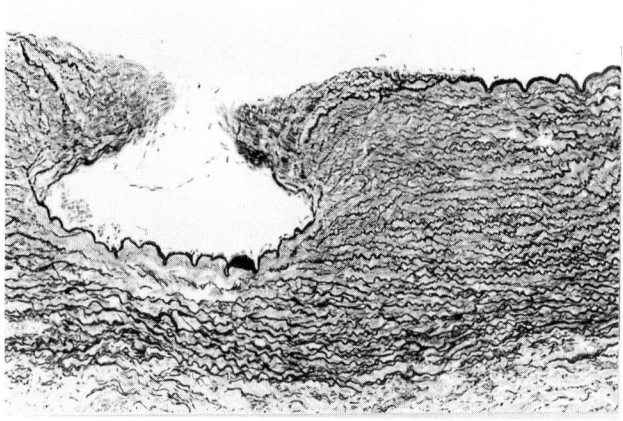

Figure 6.7 Early fetal aorta at orifice of segmental branch. Note the thick internal elastic lamina on the right and the intimal proliferation on either side of the branch on the left. Note the thinning and loss of the internal elastic lamina beneath the intimal proliferation. (Verhoeff's elastic stain and eosin.)

dividers. There has been no accurate localization of these intimal changes which appear to be similar to those studied in peripheral arteries. Overall, however, the thickening and cushions have a similar localization not only about the ostia but also along the lesser curvature of the aortic arch.

At the end of the fetal stage there is intimal musculoelastic proliferation in the ascending aorta with loss of the well formed internal elastic lamina. In the isthmus, little of the circumference has an internal elastic lamina and the prominent thickening about the lesser curvature of the arch is continuous with that extending distally from the insertion of the ductus arteriosus. In the descending aorta the internal elastic lamina is replaced by intimal proliferation which becomes progressively more pronounced distally with accentuation about the ostia. It may amount to one third of the total wall thickness with lipid in intimal smooth muscle cells [13]. Intimal proliferation extends into the ostia of the branches but rapidly tapers usually before the branch emerges from the adventitia. In the neonate the initial proliferation over the flow divider of the aortic bifurcation extends peripherally along the posteromedial wall of the common iliac arteries and transverse tears of the internal elastic lamina develop on the lateral aspect of the common iliac artery and the dorsomedial aspect of the internal iliac arteries.

In the infant, transverse folds or ridges are observed in large muscular arteries, possibly accentuated by retraction after their removal at autopsy. These are sites of transversely orientated elastic tears which increase in number and extent during the first two decades and form intricate patterns with smaller interconnecting tears. Even by the end of the first decade they are

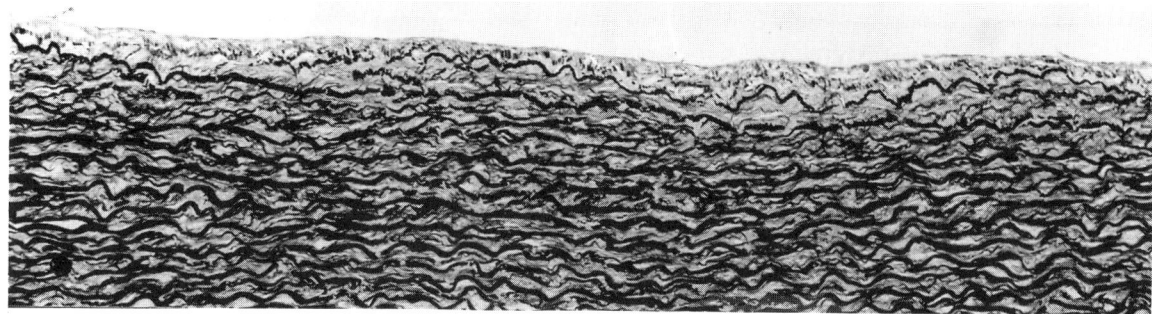

Figure 6.8 Early intimal thickening in infant with fibrillary elastic tissue in the intimal thickening. Note absence of a distinct internal elastic lamina. Medial elastic laminae are mostly continuous except the innermost laminae. (Verhoeff's elastic stain.)

extensive and exhibit calcification which commences at the edges of the tear and extends into the lamina but not into the floor of the gap in the elastica. These tears are similar to those that form *in utero* in the common and internal iliac arteries [14]. Smooth muscle cells and fibrillary elastic tissue appear in the gaps and progressively a layer of intimal thickening overgrows the elastic tears continuous with the intimal thickenings or cushions about the ostia and their peripheral extensions. It is uncertain whether these elastic tears develop in the aorta *in utero* since intimal changes have not been examined in detail from early fetal life. However, they have a similar disposition to the wrinkling seen macroscopically in the aorta (Figure 6.2).

It is likely that intimal proliferation over the flow divider extends distally ultimately to coalesce with that over the proximal aspect of the next segmental branch, thereby producing what appears to be diffuse thickening along the posterior aortic wall. This intimal proliferation, in the past regarded as an integral part of the vessel wall, is sometimes alleged to be a physiological adaptive response to alterations in flow, pressure and the haemodynamic stresses occurring naturally at such sites [15].

The aortic internal elastic lamina is thicker than the medial elastic laminae and diffuse intimal proliferation commences between it and the endothelium. Initially this tissue is loose with fibrillary elastic tissue and few cells. The internal elastic lamina becomes thinner, fragmented and disappears as the intima thickens (Figure 6.8). Initially the intima may simulate the lamellar units of the media making differentiation between intima and media difficult, though this can be facilitated by an elastic stain and by tracing the remnants of the internal elastic lamina. However, this appearance does not persist. Thickenings extend from the proximal aspect of branch sites in the aorta and iliac arteries into the ampulla-like dilatation as the wall diverges outwards into the branch. Over the flow divider they extend further downstream along the parent stem (from the crest of the flow divider) than in the entrance to the branch. Despite distinct intimal thickening about the aortic ostia, the thickening tapers rapidly in the branch.

Intimal proliferation progresses. The deep and more dense layer has been termed the musculoelastic layer and the superficial less compact almost oedematous subendothelial layer, the hyperplastic elastic layer, but these are variable and not always discernible. As the intima thickens, other indistinct elastic laminae may form with fuzzy fibrillary elastica often surrounding individual smooth muscle cells. The intimal thickening is invariably thickest near the orifices of branches. Away from the branches some regions appear thick and remain as compact fibromusculoelastic layers. The junction with the media is often indistinct. It is uncertain whether successive medial elastic laminae disappear as the intima thickens which is inevitable in later life.

In longitudinal sections through regions of macroscopic intimal wrinkling, the intima exhibits alternating hillocks and troughs (Figure 6.9) and the underlying internal elastic lamina is usually not identifiable. The denser musculoelastic mounds, often with prominent subendothelial elastic tissue, alternate with depressions beneath which the intima is loose and almost oedematous with a paucity of elastic tissue and muscle. These pale zones may be obliquely orientated with lipid and a few foam cells are occasionally present in the loose connective tissue deep to the floor of the troughs [9]. The underlying elastic tissue is often straight suggesting that these are not artifactual due to medial contraction or longitudinal shortening. Loose intimal proliferation develops as a separate layer superimposed on the floor of these troughs (Figure 6.9(b),(c)). With further extension it becomes continuous over both mounds and troughs which in this way become masked by further intimal proliferation and fibrosis.

The appearance is reminiscent of the much larger transverse wavy pattern on the sea floor and windswept sands. No doubt the hydrodynamic forces responsible are similar in both locations despite pathogenetic mechanisms in the arterial wall being quite different. Occurring at a young age they may precede fatty streaks. The internal elastic lamina underlying these

182 ATHEROSCLEROSIS AND DEGENERATIVE DISEASES

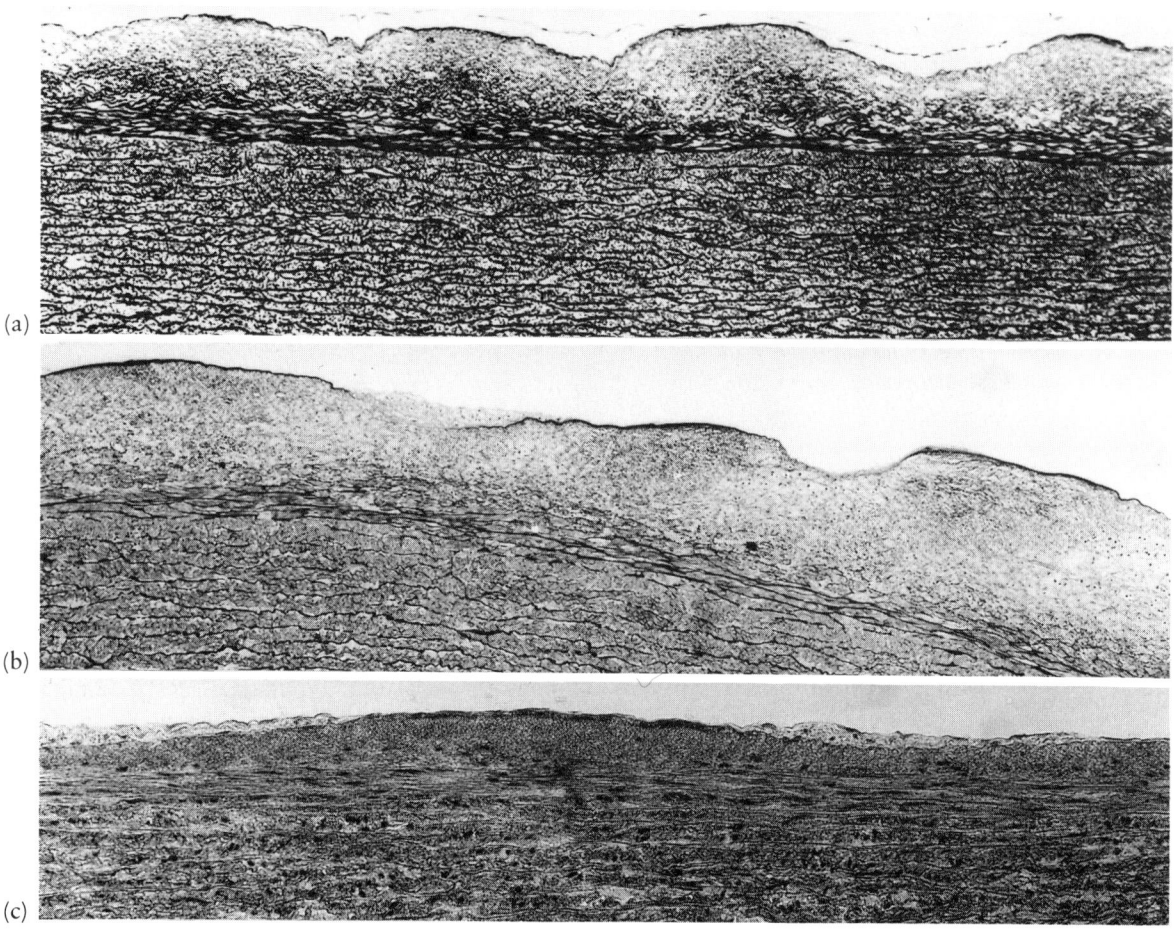

Figure 6.9 Longitudinal sections through segments of the aorta with intimal wrinkling. The ridges have denser musculoelastic tissue than beneath the valleys and subendothelial elastic tissue is more pronounced over the crests of the ridges in (a) and (b). In (b) loose intimal tissue has developed in one valley and in both valleys in (c). This loose intimal layer ultimately extends over the ridges as well. In (c) (frozen section) subendothelial dark staining material over the crest of the ridge is lipid. ((a), (b) Verhoeff's elastic tissue stain and eosin; (c) haematoxylin and fat stain.)

ridges is absent or so indistinct as to prevent correlation with the transverse tears in the internal elastic lamina seen in the iliac, internal carotid and muscular arteries. Hydrodynamic forces that produce the elastic tears may be those that induce the formation of the transverse wrinkling. The size of the mounds and their periodicity vary, being greater in older subjects than in infants. A similar phenomenon is commonly seen within the ostium of segmental branches of the aorta [7]. One mound is situated over the crescentic ridge or apex, with a concentration of elastic tissue often forming strange shapes with looser relatively acellular tissue to the sides. Another or several may occur on the adjacent surface of the daughter branch where the flux of blood entering the branch impinges. They have been likened to the ridges and depressions of a jet lesion [7]. The extension of the intimal proliferation distally from the flow divider along the parent stem often exhibits undulations in histological sections.

Darkly stained oval nuclei accumulate in the loose subendothelial intimal tissue of fatty dots or streaks and are probably monocytes (Figure 6.10). At this time lipid stains reveal positively stained droplets at the poles of the nuclei of some smooth muscle cells. There may be a hazy faint positive lipid staining reaction in the interstitial matrix and the intima, which may or may not be slightly thicker in that region and is continuous with similar thickening of the adjacent aortic surface. The dense foam cell infiltration seen in early lesions of the cholesterol-fed rabbit and FH do not occur (Figure 6.11). In more advanced lipid accumulations a few foam cells with oval darkly stained nuclei may be loosely scattered in the intima or in small aggregates either subendothelial in position or deeper in the intima. Interstitial lipid is more pronounced (Figure 6.12) and the affected area is wider and usually slightly thicker. Smooth muscle cells still contain large lipid droplets at the poles of the muscle nuclei and there may be both intracellular and extracellular lipid in the innermost aspect of the media. Metachromasia, usually more

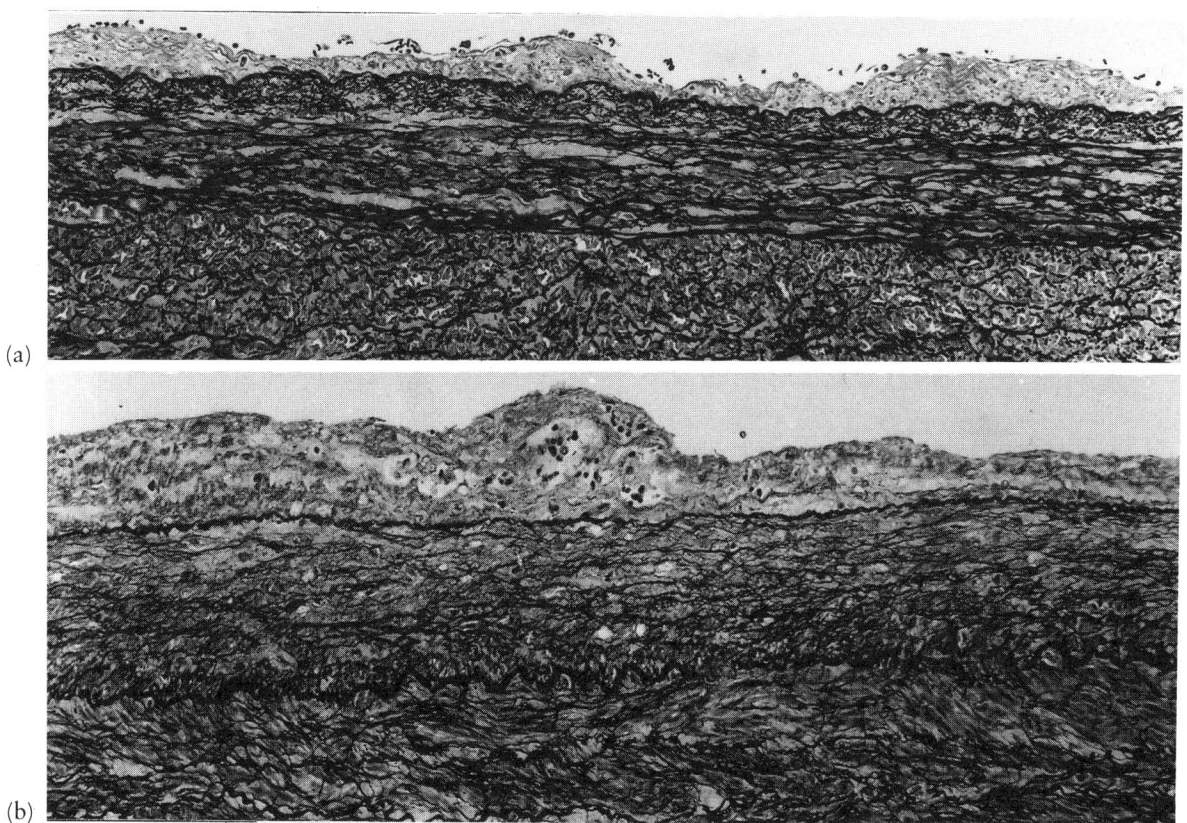

Figure 6.10 Longitudinal sections of descending aorta displaying a deeper musculoelastic layer of the intima. In (a) there are a few dark nuclei of monocytes and irregularity of the surface. In (b) there is also surface irregularity but more extensive infiltration of the superficial intimal layer with dark-staining nucleated cells (probably monocytes) with more in the central raised zone (fatty dot or streak). (Verhoeff's elastic stain.)

pronounced in the media than in the intimal thickening or fatty streaks, suggests dissociation between the appearance of lipid and proteoglycan accumulation. Immunohistochemical evidence of fibrin infiltration has been demonstrated [16].

Extracellular fat may be closely related to elastic laminae deep in the intima (Figure 6.13) but this is mostly a feature of older individuals rather than adolescents. However, the elastic tissue beneath such fatty deposits is usually thin and consists of discontinuous or frayed fibrillary laminae.

The musculoelastic tissue merges with the media. Even the innermost medial elastic laminae are fragmented and fibrillary. Stages of lipid accumulation from fatty streaks to overt atherosclerosis are readily observed as the intima thickens and fibromuscular proliferation with relatively little elastic tissue develops beneath the endothelium. Some aortic intima contains quite dense musculoelastic thickening in the absence of lipid.

Progressive intimal thickening is associated with increased fibrosis, loss of cellularity and elastic tissue and gross hyalinization of the intima. Diffuse extracellular lipid droplets, incorrectly regarded as an aging phenomenon [17], can be extensive in such zones and foam cells are frequently not numerous (Figure 6.14). As the zone of lipid accumulation increases, the centre often tends to break down and is lost in processing due to loss of cohesion of matrix connective tissue. Simultaneously a more cellular proliferation with little elastic tissue develops internal to the lipid but progressively this too becomes fibrotic and hyalinized (Figure 6.15). Some intimal lamination, often separated by a hazy poorly stained elastic lamina, may be apparent. Calcific granules, coalescing to form large calcified plaques, are often associated with zones of acellular hyaline tissue or with accumulations of necrotic debris and cholesterol clefts. Such zones are at times sharply demarcated as if within an intimal cavity containing no connective tissue matrix. Some cholesterol clefts about the margins may be surrounded wholly or partly by foreign body giant cells (Figure 6.16) together with a variable number of lipophages. Lymphocytes and plasma cells may be scattered in the intima in advanced disease. Lipid in smooth muscle cells is not a prominent feature in end-stage disease.

Haemosiderin-laden macrophages indicate previous haemorrhage and extensive laminated zones of fibrin may be present in the innermost intima. A subendothelial

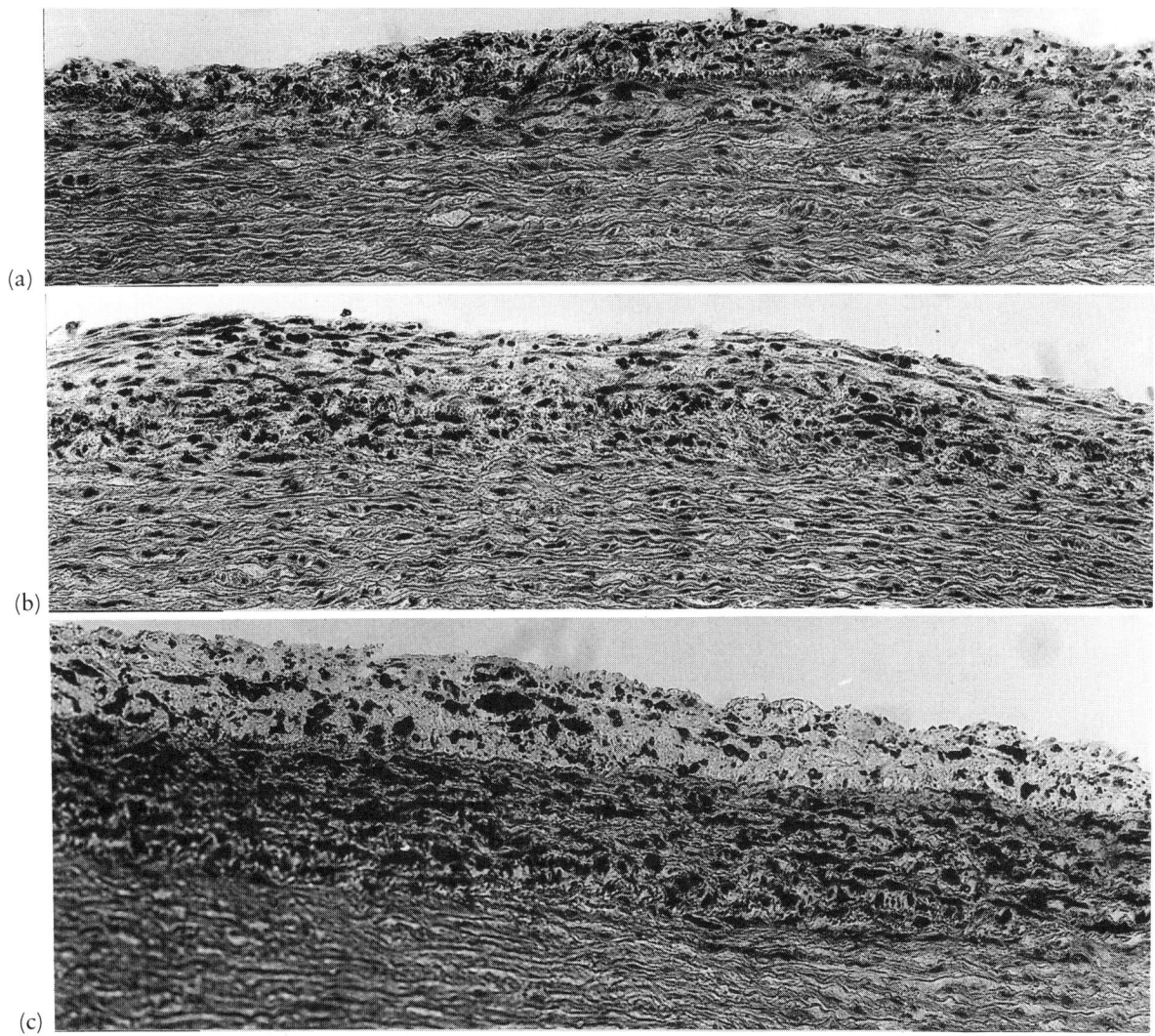

Figure 6.11 Frozen sections of aortic intima showing progression of lipid deposition. Dark-staining lipid is present in smooth muscle cells and probably some monocytes in the thin intima of (a) and (b) and particularly (c). There is increasing involvement of the innermost media most prominently in (c). Diffuse extracellular lipid deposition although present is most noticeable in (b) and (c) but cannot be distinguished in the photomicrographs. (Haematoxylin and fat stains.)

layer of fibromuscular tissue with little elastica sometimes covers grossly acellular hyalinized plaques. Superficial erosion with fibrin infiltration or mural thrombosis and eventually deep ulcerations with excavation of debris and extravasation of red cells deep in the wall are late complications of end-stage disease. Thick mural thrombi overlying zones of ulceration usually exhibit little organization. The underlying media becomes irregularly thinned and replaced by atheromatous tissue and perivascular fibrous tissue about vasa vasorum which in the media often produce extensive interruptions of the medial lamellar units. Calcific granules, metachromasia and diffuse interstitial lipid infiltration may be demonstrated in the media. Accumulation of lipophages and cholesterol clefts in the aortic media is infrequent.

The vasa vasorum in the adventitia may be more numerous than usual but generally show little evidence of diffuse hyperplastic sclerosis. Though perivascular lymphocytes and plasma cells are not infrequent, adventitial infiltration with lipophages is rare.

An aneurysm may develop as a lateral diverticulum by expansion of the mural remnants in the floor of a localized zone of ulceration (Figure 10.8), in the floor of a tear through most of the media (Figure 10.7) or as a diffuse fusiform dilatation often over the lower 10–15 cm of the abdominal aorta. Advanced atherosclerosis with ulceration and mural thrombus may line portions of the expanding sac and histologically only residual remnants of the media will be demonstrable, a Verhoeff's elastic stain facilitating identification.

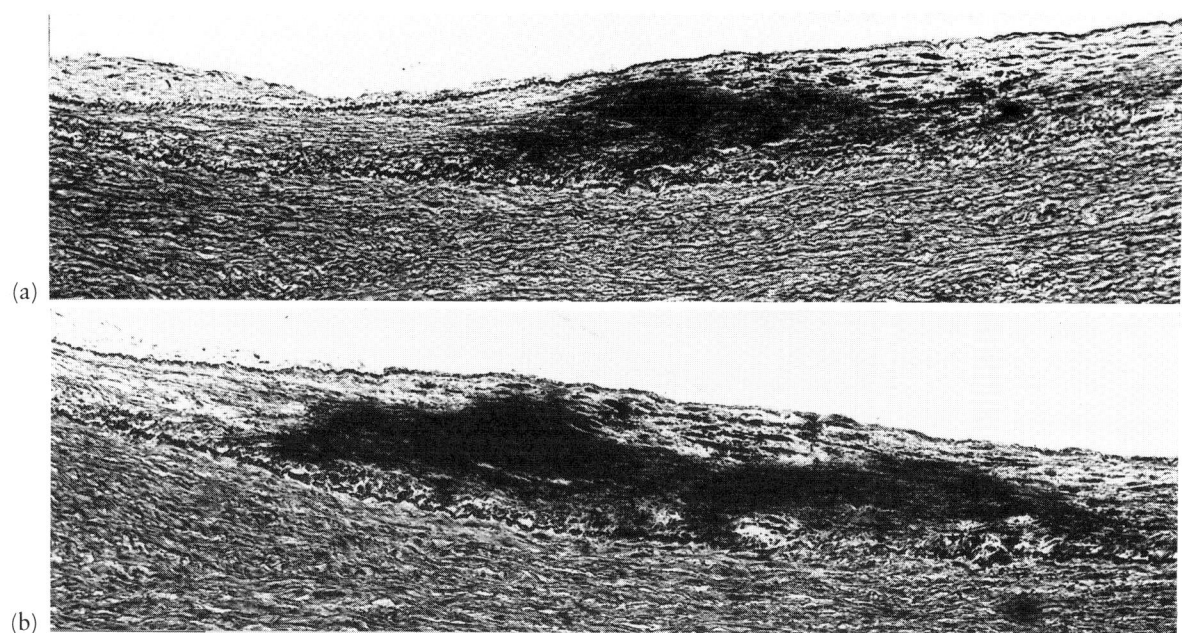

Figure 6.12 Lower magnification of aortic intima showing localized heavier accumulation of lipid in the intima. Cellular lipid is present representing the focal dense-staining deposits in the intima. There is much diffuse extracellular lipid in the intima. Note the loose intimal proliferation to the left in (a). (Haematoxylin and fat stain.)

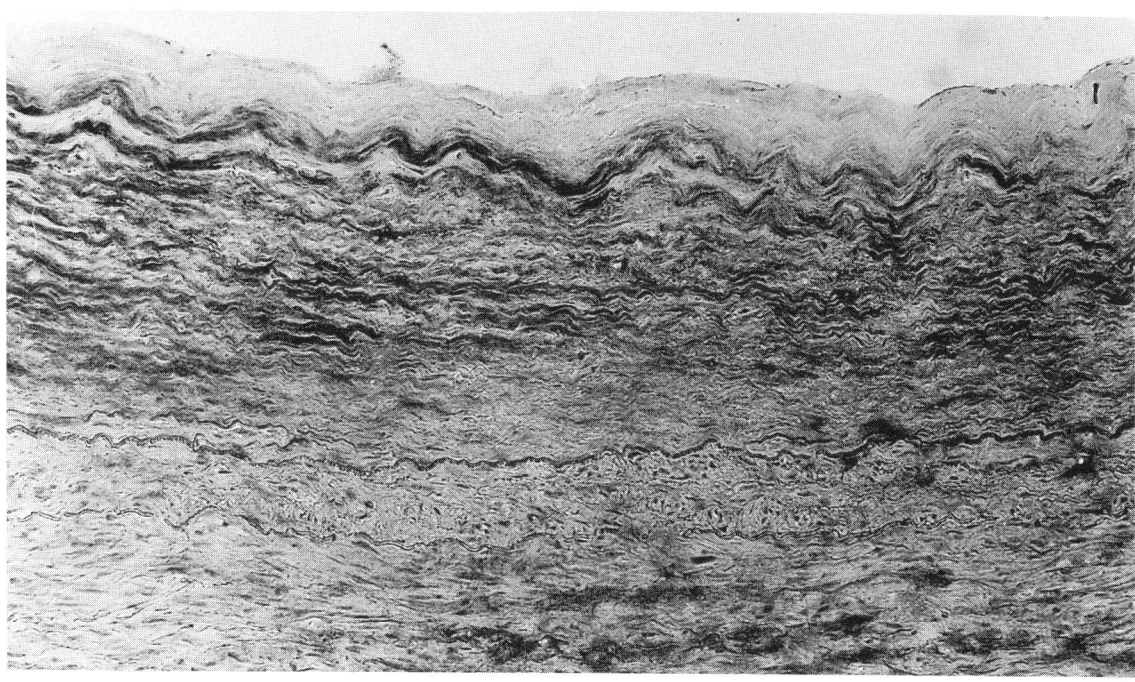

Figure 6.13 Frozen section of aorta demonstrating diffuse extracellular lipid deposition in the thick intima and underlying media. Lipid in the intima outlines wavy elastic tissue and matrix fibrous tissue. (Haematoxylin and fat stain.)

6.2.2 CEREBRAL ATHEROSCLEROSIS

Because of their thin transparent walls, the severity of atherosclerosis of cerebral arteries can be reasonably well assessed without opening the lumen or transecting the vessels serially as in extracranial arteries. The earliest macroscopic change is the development of white or opaque areas caused by intimal thickening at the facial or dorsal regions of branching sites. It is more diffuse at the upper end of the basilar artery and in the

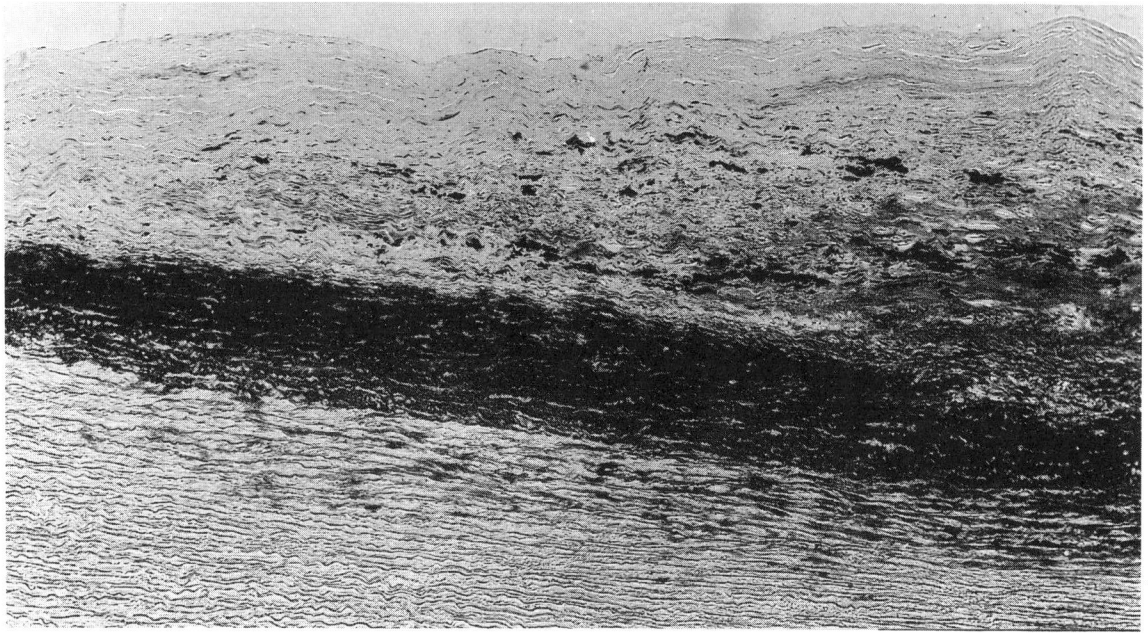

Figure 6.14 Moderately advanced atherosclerosis with very thick intima and heavy extracellular lipid accumulation at the side of a plaque. Intracellular lipid is present in the intima which is thicker where lipid is most extensive. Note lipid in the media. (Haematoxylin and fat stain.)

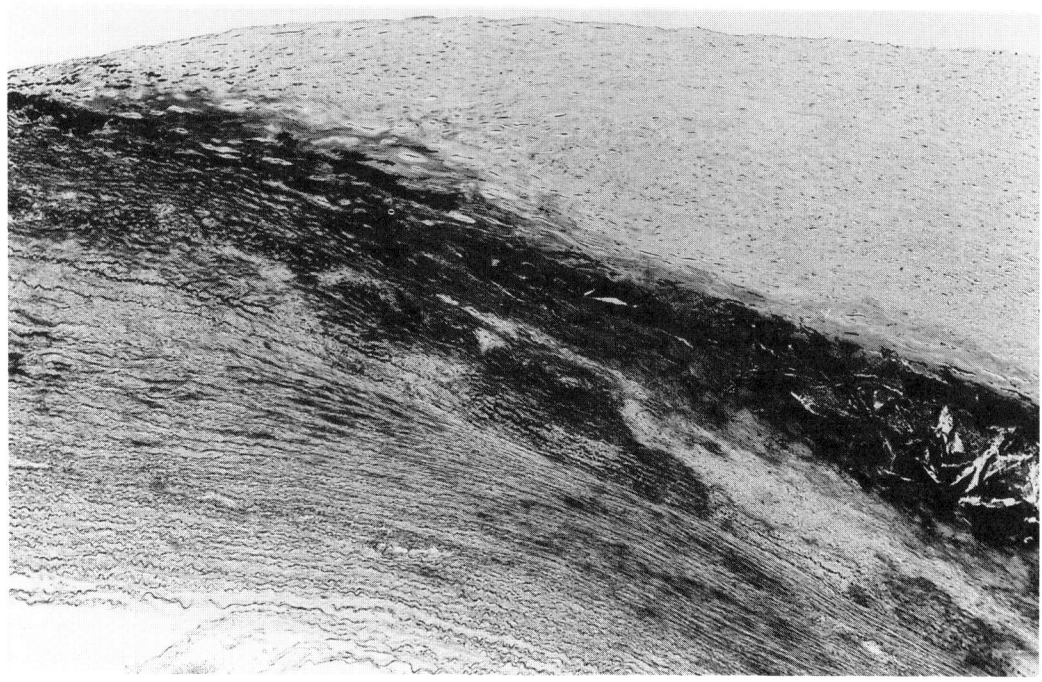

Figure 6.15 Edge of more advanced atherosclerotic plaque than in Figure 6.14. Note similarity to that of Figure 6.14. Matrix is breaking down and cholesterol crystals are appearing at the side of a developing 'atheroma' with a much thickened fibrocellular layer overlying it (in the innermost intima). There is much lipid in the media which is thinned. (Haematoxylin and fat stain.)

vertebral arteries especially after their entry through the dura mater where there is often a fusiform dilatation.

At a more advanced stage distinctly yellowish thickenings are visible at forks, at the lower end of the basilar artery, and in the curvature of the internal carotid artery. Gross staining for fat will reveal at a somewhat earlier stage fat that is often referred to as fatty streaks but these are essentially lipid deposits in

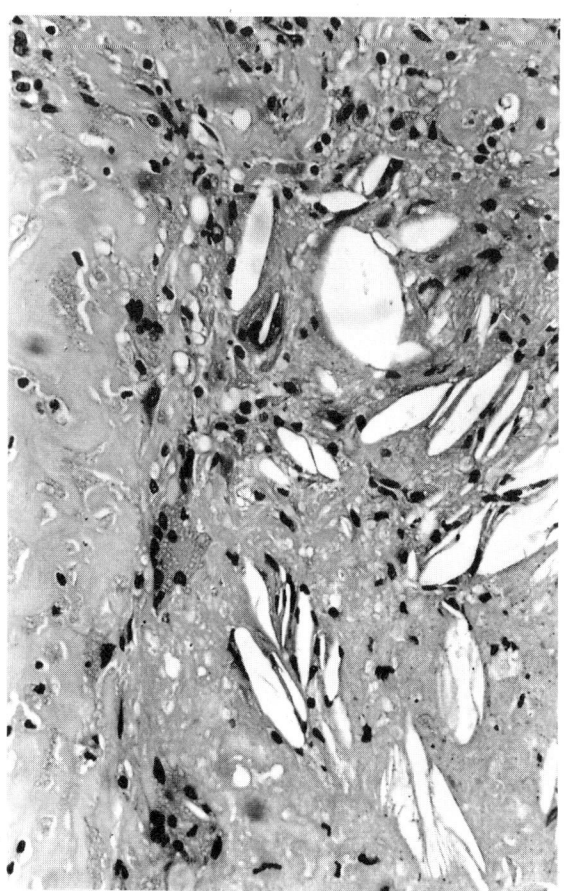

Figure 6.16 Atherosclerotic intima with foreign body giant cells about cholesterol clefts together with monocytes and possibly a few lymphocytes. Note hyaline material to the left. (Haematoxylin and eosin.)

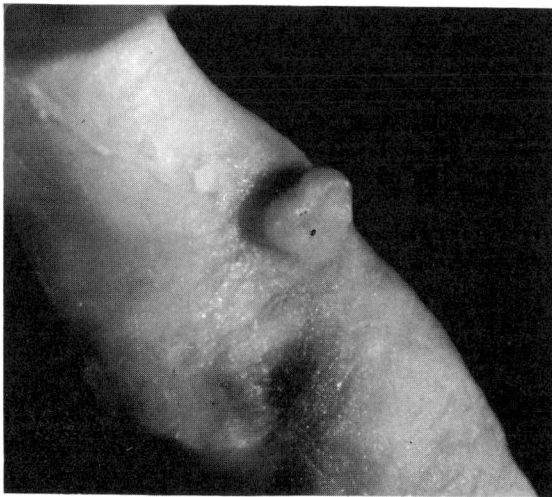

Figure 6.17 Small pultaceous nodule on surface of a cerebral artery due to herniation of caseous debris into adventitia from intima and media. Such lesions could be readily mistaken for aneurysms. (Reproduced with permission from Stehbens [19].)

intimal thickenings related to branching sites, unions or curvatures or to the extensions of such intimal proliferations.

Eccentric thickenings are particularly likely in the stems of the first part of the middle cerebral artery and the anterior cerebral artery as extensions of the lateral thickenings at the internal carotid bifurcation. Small yellow atherosclerotic thickenings are sometimes seen at the commencement of small branches.

The large basal arteries are particularly affected and with increased severity the atherosclerosis in these vessels becomes confluent and small lesions appear in the peripheral leptomeningeal arteries. The atherosclerotic arteries become more rigid and knobbly with yellow or white thickened walls or brown coloration due to siderotic pigmentation. As the atherosclerotic walls thicken, newly formed prominent vasa vasorum course over and in the adventitia. The walls tend to split or fracture when transected and the external diameter, particularly of large vessels, increases. Disparity in size between large and small vessels is enhanced. Vessels may be displaced from their usual course with increasing tortuosity. This is particularly important when a vertebral and the basilar artery form an S-shaped configuration with the opposite smaller vertebral artery joining the tortuosity near the lower end of the pons. When this tortuosity and ectasia are very pronounced, the condition is referred to as dolichoectasia. Such a configuration with displacement can lead to pressure on cranial nerves. Calcification rarely reaches the severity of that in coronary arteries.

When the arteries exhibit severe atherosclerosis, the internal carotid arteries may have fusiform dilatations whilst the vertebrobasilar arteries may be grossly enlarged with one or more dome-shaped expansions but larger aneurysmal sacs are not uncommon (Figure 10.17, p. 377). The basilar artery may exhibit a fusiform dilatation which can progress to a large spherical sac compressing the pons. Small aneurysms are not to be confused with small pultaceous nodules in the large arteries due to herniation of caseous debris into the adventitia (Figure 6.17). Because of their thin walls atherothrombotic emboli are often detectable without opening the arteries which are likely to be distended to their physiological size rather than collapsed. If the walls are thickened and opaque, serial transverse sectioning will be needed to find thrombotic occlusions sited most often in the internal carotid, middle cerebral, vertebral and basilar arteries. Localized stenotic lesions as in the coronary arteries are infrequent.

(a) Microscopy

Intimal proliferation similar to that in the aorta also develops at branching sites in cerebral arteries. It occurs not diffusely about bifurcations but initially as localized

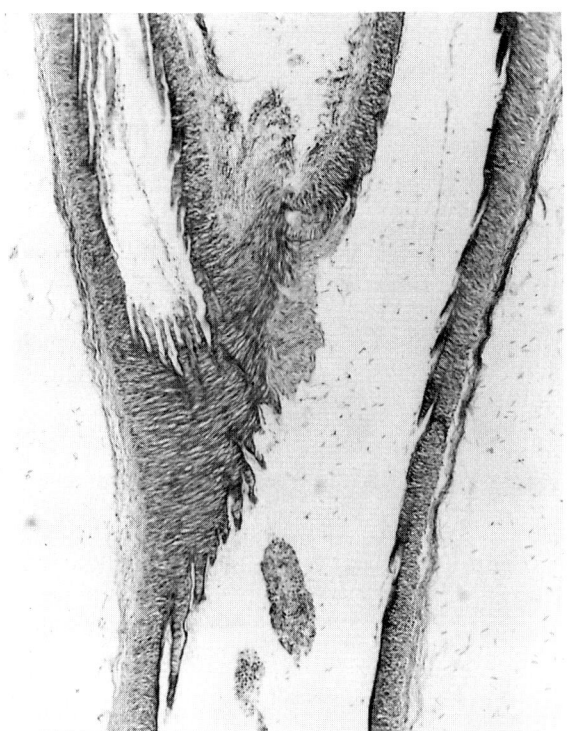

Figure 6.18 Fork of a middle cerebral artery of a neonate. Note the absence of intimal thickening except at the facial pad which is at one end of the flow divider. The muscle is less dense than in the media. (Phosphotungstic acid haematoxylin.) (Reproduced with permission from Stehbens [21].)

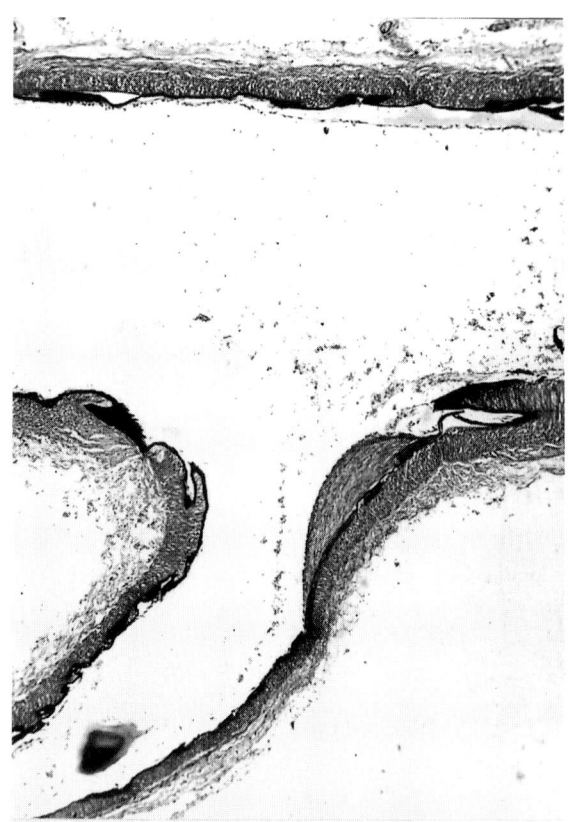

Figure 6.19 Longitudinal section through a lateral branch of a neonatal middle cerebral artery. Flow is from right to left. Note the intimal thickening (lateral pad) just inside lateral branch where flow separation is to be expected. No intimal thickening at apex or on wall of parent stem opposite the ostium. (Verhoeff's elastic stain.) (Reproduced with permission from Stehbens [18].)

intimal thickenings (pads or cushions) at specific anatomical sites about the forks (see Figure 1.3 for nomenclature). At about 26 weeks *in utero*, the internal elastic lamina at the extremities of the flow divider (face and dorsum) are thin, very lacy and pale staining. It is in this region that intimal proliferation develops (Figure 6.18) and consists predominantly of longitudinally arranged smooth muscle cells with multiple fibrillary elastic laminae and little demonstrable collagen. Metachromasia is not prominent but cell density is less than in the more compact media [18].

Similar thickening develops at the lateral angles, not over the bend but in the daughter branches commencing where the lateral wall of the parent stem diverges or curves into the branch (Figure 6.19). This location is where engineers expect boundary-layer separation to occur. The facial and dorsal thickenings progressively extend towards the apex or crotch to involve the entire flow divider. The apical pad is symmetrically located over the crest, unlike that over the flow dividers of small aortic branches. The internal elastic lamina beneath these localized intimal thickenings usually displays thinning, pale staining, some fragmentation or a very lacy appearance (Figure 6.20). Over the apex the elastic lamina is often interrupted and at times one end of the lamina may be reflected as if by recoil (Figure 6.21). These thickenings can be observed at smaller branching sites and progressively thicken and ultimately coalesce (Figure 6.20). More distinct elastic laminae form particularly under the endothelium and merge with the original lamina at the edges of the pad but often disappear near the thickest section of the intima. There may be a second such lamina somewhat deeper in the intima imparting an appearance of fraying of the elastic lamina. Fibrillary elastica is still present in the intercellular matrix.

In neonates these intimal thickenings are always present and in infancy continue to thicken and extend. The lateral pads at the bifurcation of the internal carotid arteries extend peripherally along the lateral aspect of the branches (Figure 10.34, p. 389) whilst the opposite wall of the daughter branches may appear virtually unaffected for some time. Apical thickening is frequently less prominent than facial, dorsal and lateral proliferation. Intimal proliferation at lateral angles

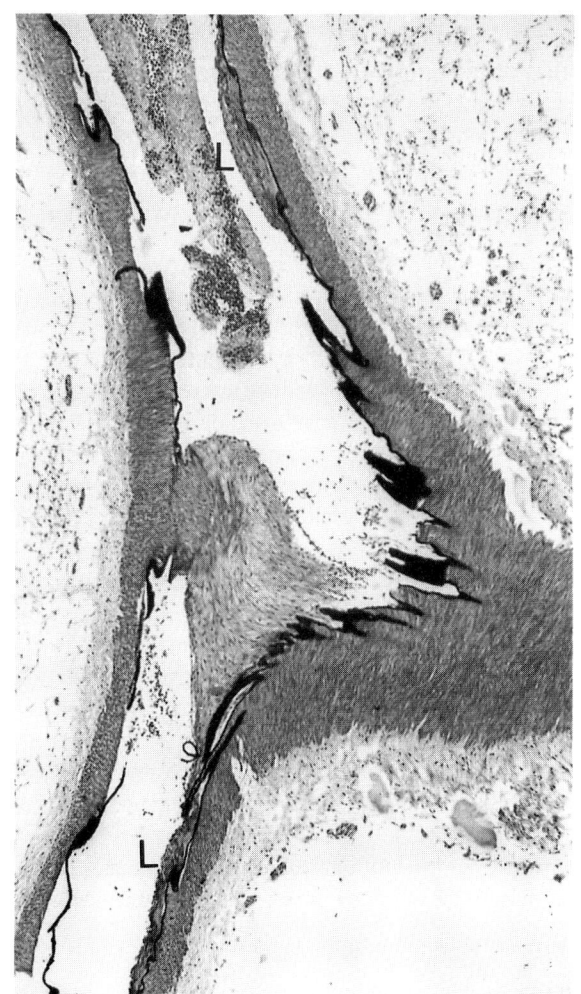

Figure 6.20 Longitudinal section through bifurcation of internal carotid artery of an infant displaying the facial pad and two lateral pads with elastosis at L. Flow is from right to left. Intimal pads are coalescing. (Verhoeff's elastic stain.) (Reproduced with permission from Stehbens [18].)

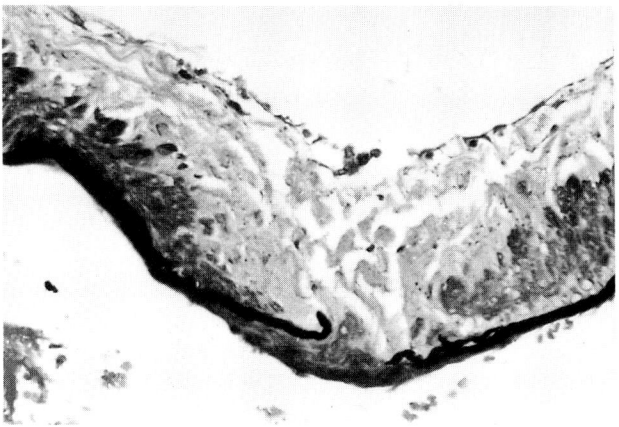

Figure 6.21 Apex of a cerebral arterial fork with disrupted internal elastic lamina. The end of the lamina on the left is doubled back as if by recoil as occurs with abrupt tears of the lamina. (Verhoeff's elastic stain and eosin.) (Reproduced with permission from Stehbens [20].)

tends to be more pronounced when the angle is acute rather than obtuse, and there is but one lateral pad when a lateral branch arises from the main stem which does not deviate from its original axis (Figure 6.19).

Intimal proliferation also occurs at the origin of small cerebral arteries and the localization appears to be similar to that at major branching sites. When a cerebral artery divides only to reunite at a variable distance downstream to produce a fenestra or if the lumen has been partitioned by a septum or traversed by a chord, intimal proliferation is greater on the downstream aspect than on the leading edge. When the septum or chord is eccentrically located in the lumen, the intimal thickening is also asymmetrical in location. Similarly intimal proliferation at the apex of the vertebrobasilar junction is considerably thicker than at the apex of arterial forks [21]. Proliferation can be observed in the stem of the internal carotid artery on the lesser curvature of the intracranial segment as the artery arches upwards, forwards and laterally towards its bifurcation. This thickening terminates prior to the bifurcation and is not continuous with that of the lateral angle of the fork.

Thickenings in the coronary and mesenteric arteries are of similar appearance and Jaffé et al. [22] reported that localization in coronary arteries was similar to that of cerebral vessels. Though referred to as pads or cushions it seems preferable to refer to them as intimal proliferation or thickening until their role in atherosclerosis is generally accepted. The cerebral arteries were not perfusion fixed under pressure and therefore it was not possible to determine the extent to which they projected into the lumen, but from Levene's work on coronary arteries [23] it is likely they did not significantly encroach on the lumen at least at the lateral angles in infancy.

In older children, the elastic lamina is more prominent and the intimal proliferation at forks more pronounced and fibrotic. The lateral thickenings extend peripherally and there may be evidence of a more diffuse thickening by involvement of the intima elsewhere. In older subjects, the original areas of proliferation, though confluent, are more stratified by accessory elastic laminae but cellularity is decreased. There is metachromasia of both intima and media. The medial muscle exhibits progressive intercellular fibrosis and hyalinization, especially subintimally, and there may be pronounced medial thinning. The internal elastic lamina may show beading and is less convoluted, whilst there may be greying of the intima with elastic stains. The intima progressively thickens and becomes hyalinized with loss and fragmentation of elastic tissue and the appearance of foam cells and cholesterol clefts which may extend even into the media. Lipophages are not numerous and giant cells are rare and seen mostly in gross atherosclerosis. The disease is usually most pronounced at facial and dorsal aspects of the fork and in lateral thickenings and their peripheral extensions. The media will be thinned beneath the lateral thickening and is usually discontinuous as if by enlargement of the raphe. The apical zones are usually thinner than at other sites about the fork.

The important feature of this intimal proliferation is its consistent occurrence, localization and progression to overt atherosclerosis without any sharp line of demarcation. The progression of atherosclerosis is from the intima ultimately to involve the media and the adventitia which may even exhibit some hyalinization and loss of elastic fibrils in its innermost part. With progressive thickening of the intima, vascularization of the wall develops and sinusoidal vasa vasorum may be seen even macroscopically in the adventitia. The atherosclerotic intima becomes relatively acellular and lipophages never become as abundant as in the cholesterol-fed rabbit. Ultimately atheromatous material may herniate into the adventitia (Figure 6.17) where it becomes surrounded by macrophages, a response contrasting with the usual paucity of phagocytic activity in the atherosclerotic intima and media. Rupture into the lumen due to intimal tears will be followed by secondary thrombosis and atheroembolism. Moreover the stenosing lesions so common in the coronary arteries are infrequent and so is round cell infiltration in the adventitia. Calcific lesions common in coronary arteries are less frequent in cerebral arteries being mostly in severely atherosclerotic and often ectatic internal carotid, vertebral and basilar arteries.

Blumenthal *et al.* [24] documented the progressive intimal thickening of cerebral arteries with age, the increase being most pronounced in larger vessels where mural tension is highest and least in the smaller cerebral arteries which at times become overtly atherosclerotic.

(b) Electron microscopy

Intimal thickenings at bifurcations in lower animals [25,26] are similar histologically and in localization to those occurring in man, although lateral pads are not present at all branching sites. Ultrastructure of the intimal thickening over the flow divider at the major renal arterial forks of rabbits [27] revealed some endothelial cells with bundles of microfibrils mostly basal in location and with irregular periodic densities. These probably correspond to so-called endothelial stress fibres displayed by fluorescence microscopy [28] and participate in interendothelial cell adhesion and attachment to subendothelial connective tissues. There was partial separation of endothelial cell junctions. Numerous areas along the basal surface of the endothelium were 'bare' or unrelated to either basement membrane or other matrix components. In addition to multiple elastic laminae, collagen, proteoglycans and smooth muscle cells there were degenerate cells, aggregates of granulovesicular cell debris (matrix vesicles) and redundant basement membrane material unrelated to cells. Some basement membranes were irregularly thickened and duplicated and at times had partially separated from the muscle cells. An occasional

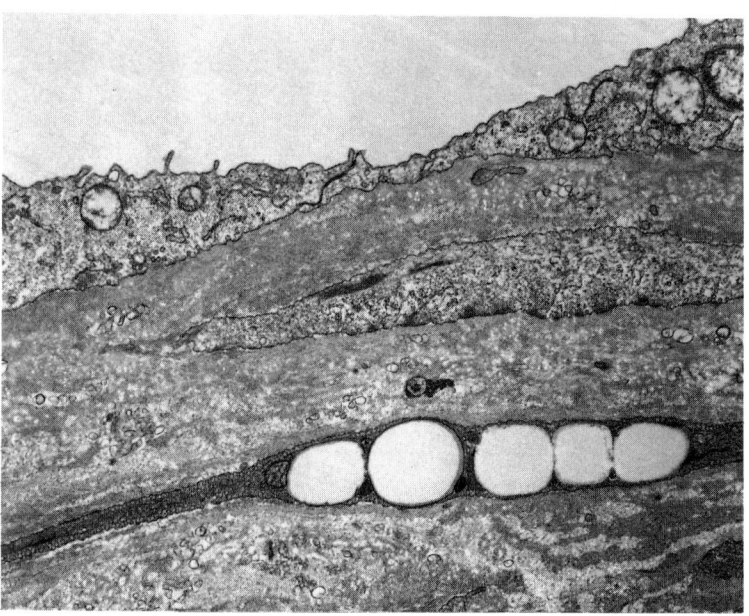

Figure 6.22 Electron micrograph of atherosclerotic cerebral artery obtained post mortem. There is a thick wall of basement membrane material beneath the endothelium. Two attenuated smooth muscle cells can be seen, one containing lysosomal lipid vacuoles and the other with little microfibrillary material. Note the paucity of collagen but much irregular basement membrane material about the cells and a few membranous vesicles in the matrix.

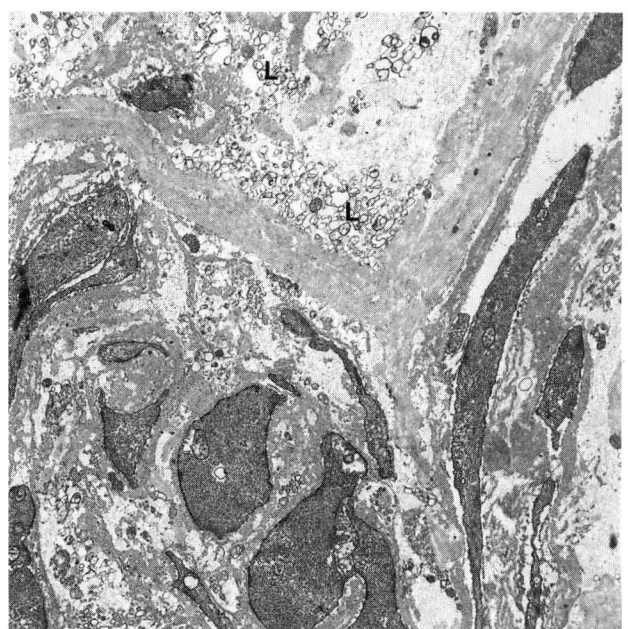

Figure 6.23 Electron micrograph of atherosclerotic cerebral artery showing irregular arrangement and separation of smooth muscle cells with abundant grey dystrophic basement membrane material and patchy separation from the smooth muscle cell plasma membrane. Note the cell debris (matrix vesicles) mostly at bottom left and transformation of matrix vesicles into lipid (L).

undifferentiated cell was observed beneath the endothelium together with some dense possibly calcified matrix vesicles, calcospherites and increased interstitial space.

An ultrastructural study of cerebral arteries and aneurysms from humans [29,30] has revealed similar findings with cellular debris present even in infancy and childhood in addition to the destruction and loss of the internal elastic lamina. With progressive age and intimal thickening the basement membranes of endothelial (Figure 6.22) and smooth muscle cells become increasingly thickened, laminated, reticulated and often separated from the related cells (Figure 6.23). This grossly abnormal basement membrane has been regarded as dystrophic, possibly indicative of loss of cohesion of intimal matrix, and appears to constitute a large proportion of the interstitial matrix. Some dense amorphous material is at times observed between the muscle cells and the separated basement membrane material.

Smooth muscle cells often display grossly abnormal shapes with indentation, branching and elongated attenuated extensions about which there is frequently a myriad of small variable-sized vesicles in and about the dystrophic basement membrane. Some muscle cells are degenerate and an occasional cell contains lysosomal lipid granules (Figure 6.22). Cellular debris progressively increases and is often present in considerable quantities even in a thin intima and in the innermost part of the media, generally closely related to the internal elastic lamina. Extracellular lipid histologically corresponds to the transformation of the granulovesicular cell debris to aggregates of larger membrane-bound electron-translucent vesicles [31] (Figure 6.23). Some membranes become multilaminated and simultaneously with these changes the matrix vesicles disappear. Ultimately large regions of the matrix consist of these fat-laden vacuoles, some of which appear to form from similar debris of disintegrated smooth muscle cells. Lipophages and macrophages about cholesterol crystals are observed in more advanced changes.

Collagen fibrils, not as prevalent in the sclerotic intima as one might expect, are often haphazardly arranged [29,30]. They tend to be short, bent and variable in size and shape [32]. At this stage there is relative depletion of elastic tissue in the intima.

6.2.3 CORONARY ATHEROSCLEROSIS

Investigation of coronary and other distributing arteries of similar calibre is more difficult than the study of cerebral arteries which are easier to inspect and dissect and their frozen sections are less contaminated by perivascular fat. The development of atherosclerosis is essentially as described in the cerebral arteries, the intimal thickening developing about the coronary ostia and at coronary branching sites with extensions peripherally downstream. Macroscopic lipid stains reveal superficial lipid at arterial branching sites and also at times foci of fat in zones of intimal thickening elsewhere. Whilst fatty streaks have been reported in coronary and other arteries even into middle age and in the elderly, neither linear streaks nor linear arrangement of fatty dots has been demonstrated. It is wiser to restrict the appellation 'fatty streaks' to the distinctive aortic lesions. Fat-containing lesions (irrespective of size) in other arteries are atherosclerotic but at a stage preceding fibrous plaques due to proliferation of fibromusculoelastic tissue in the inner intima. Some severely stenotic lesions may contain relatively little lipid, especially in the young, and other lesions contain a veritable pool of atheromatous debris deep in the wall with a greatly attenuated media externally.

The disease is most pronounced proximally in the vessels of large calibre and less pronounced distally with accentuation at branching sites. The proximal segment of the anterior descending branch of the left coronary is the site most severely affected, no doubt due to its location just distal to the largest bifurcation in the coronary circulation. Severity is also affected by the relative sizes of the arteries, being greatest in the left coronary with left coronary dominance and more severe in the right with right coronary dominance.

That the disease is more severe in males than in females has been confirmed [33]. The coronary arteries are larger in males and the heart weight is greater. It is also tenable that the coronary arteries are larger and the disease more severe in very large muscular subjects than in individuals of small, lean stature, other things being equal. This concept has not been rigorously investigated, but if true it could explain some controversial racial and national differences in atherosclerosis severity.

The examination of coronary arteries of young male military personnel killed during wars [34,36] has revealed the existence of quite severe lesions and even extreme stenosis at a young age. There is very severe involvement in coronary and cerebral arteries in young victims of about 20 years of age with aortic coarctation [37]. Macroscopic atherosclerotic lesions have been reported in 90% of males in the third decade and in all subjects over 40 years [38] and fibrous plaques in all males over 40 years and all females over 50 years of age [39]. White et al. [40] reported pronounced coronary atherosclerosis in most men over 50 years of age and one coronary artery has been found to have more than 70% lumen reduction in 66% of non-cardiac atherosclerotic patients, and in 39% of 'normal' victims of accidental death without other significant disease [41]. At least one coronary artery exhibiting 25–100% narrowing was found in 74% of adult autopsies [42]. The remarkable severity of coronary atherosclerosis in adult populations of Western countries is not generally appreciated. Angiographically, a so-called normal coronary artery may be associated with quite severe eccentric lesions and unless an artery is pressure-fixed the collapsed artery at autopsy may simulate very severe stenosis. The calibre of the lumen angiographically is the result of a tendency to ectasia and progressive intimal proliferation and does not reveal the severity of the disease. Whilst some authors emphasize the need for pressure-fixation of arteries, the relationship of eccentric plaques to the lumen during vasoconstriction and phases of the cardiac cycle may be quite different.

The coronary arteries evince a propensity to stenose and for considerable calcification of the atherosclerotic plaques. Tears and ulceration of the walls are now recognized as being responsible for mural and occlusive thrombosis. Blood may wash out atheromatous debris as well as infiltrating the adjoining arterial wall of the crevice or ulcer crater with blood and fibrin.

The severity of coronary atherosclerosis, as judged by the prevalence of stenoses, is greatest in hearts with the largest myocardial ischaemic lesions [33]. The frequency with which an occlusive coronary artery thrombus is found in association with myocardial infarction varies within wide limits in the literature. At times merely a severe stenotic lesion has been found and on other occasions a mural thrombus, whilst in some none of these lesions has been reported as present. A mural thrombus can be readily overlooked at autopsy but still be a source of extensive embolization and diminished through-flow. The frequency of occlusive thrombi tends to vary with the diligence with which they are sought. The pathological verification of clinical presentations is made difficult by the silence of many episodes and the presence or otherwise of many other factors that may influence the development of thrombus, collateral flow, coronary blood flow, cardiac function, haemodynamics and blood pressure. The acute transmural infarct is more likely to be associated with thrombotic occlusion of a main artery. The patchy subendothelial infarction is a consequence of a stenotic lesion, disturbed cardiac function and coronary blood flow. Moreover, there are non-atherosclerotic causes of myocardial ischaemia and infarction [43].

A single occlusive lesion or localized atherosclerosis is infrequent, the more common finding being severe atherosclerosis with multiple narrowings of varying degree. Likewise when coronary atherosclerosis is severe, a similar severity can be expected in the aorta, cerebral and peripheral arteries. Those dying of coronary atherosclerosis and its complications (demonstrated at autopsy) usually exhibit a more severe grade of disease than those succumbing to other disorders but considerable overlap exists. However, large variability exists in the severity of coronary atherosclerosis in subjects dying from CHD.

The coronary arteries progressively increase in diameter with age and this ectasia may be accentuated by connective tissue diseases such as Marfan's syndrome and also by arteriovenous shunts and pulmonary origin of a coronary artery resulting in a left-to-right arterial shunt. The calibre of the coronary arteries correlates with the degree of tortuosity and cardiac weight [44] but in recent years attention has been focused on some cases with prominent ectasia [45]. If the mechanical and hereditary aspects of the connective tissues in atherosclerosis are considered, it is understandable that in some subjects ectasia rather than stenosis might predominate. This ectasia should not be considered as an adaptive response on the part of the arteries to compensate for stenosing intimal proliferation, for such cause and effect should not be assumed. In practice both the stenosing proliferative response and the ectasia are prone to thrombotic occlusion [45].

In the healing phase of a myocardial infarction, a dense subendocardial mesh of parallel walled delicate vessels develops. Of moderately large calibre they run circumferentially around the ventricular wall and after a few months of healing and organization become less prominent. This small vessel density, increasing in frequency with age, is of a different nature but appears to correlate with increasing heart weight [33].

The intimal thickening in coronary arteries is essentially similar histologically and in localization about forks to that of the cerebral arteries given that coronary arteries have not been examined by serial sections [22]. There is intimal proliferation with loss of the internal elastic lamina in the proximal portion and epicardial aspect of the distal portion of the left stem at birth. By 1 to 3 years of age the entire stem has intimal thickening [13].

In the anterior descending branch of the left coronary artery intimal proliferation develops at the lateral angle, referred to as eccentric intimal thickening [46], which extends from its thickest region (often as thick as the media) near the origin of the artery, up to 1 cm distally. Apart from intimal thickening over the flow divider there may be some diffuse proliferation. Indeed at birth more of the intima exhibits thickening than remains intact. Within three years diffuse intimal proliferation covers the remaining intima of the proximal portion of the branch [13].

In the left circumflex branch intimal thickenings are related to branching sites and in infancy most of the intima displays intimal proliferation up to a thickness of one third of the wall with either an absent or fragmented internal elastic lamina.

The right coronary artery rapidly changes from an elastic artery at its origin to a muscular artery. At birth it exhibits intimal thickenings at orifices of branches. By one year of age intimal proliferation may be as thick as the media with diffuse intimal thickening continuing to extend, and in the adolescent and young adult intimal proliferation becomes the main structural component of the proximal segment [13]. As with other arteries these intimal changes become attenuated and less advanced peripherally.

The initial intimal thickenings at branchings and bifurcations have a predilection for lipid infiltration and atherosclerotic lesions [13,46]. Early lipid deposition has been found in 45% of infants in the first eight months of life with more substantial lipid deposition occurring about puberty [46]. Jaffé et al. [22] found a higher incidence of intimal fat in coronary arteries of neonates and it is likely that serial frozen sections with appropriate fat stains would have demonstrated lipid more frequently.

Meyer et al. [13] found intimal thickening was greatest in the trunk of the left coronary from whence it extended to the anterior descending branch of the left coronary artery. Whilst gaps or transverse tears developed in the internal elastic lamina, they found no calcific deposits in the elastic lamina.

Ehrich et al. [47] contended that the intimal proliferation in the coronary arteries, focal at birth, becomes more diffuse by the second decade. With intimal proliferation more pronounced in the left coronary than the right, the changes progressively extend further peripherally into smaller branches. They attempted to distinguish distinct layers within the intima but, as in the aorta, these are so variable and inconstant that no recent attempts have been made to differentiate the specific morphological layers. They, like many others, regarded the fetal and neonatal proliferation as a phase of the continuous progression to overt atherosclerosis.

Dock [48] asserted that intimal proliferations were thicker in male infants than in females but his histological sections were random. Three-dimensional assessment of the proliferations at comparable bifurcations in the two sexes using serial histological sectioning would be impractical for a significant number of infants. However, a relevant observation in coronary arteries of infants by Levene [23] was the presence of medial thinning beneath the intimal proliferation which suggests that in accordance with the concept of Thoma [49], the intimal proliferation may indeed be compensatory. During the slow silent development, the intimal surface remains smooth within both the aorta and distributing arteries and macroscopically the wall appears unchanged. It is not surprising that histologists in the past regarded these thickenings as an integral part of the arterial wall especially since they were ubiquitous. The intimal thickening does not parallel aging [50] and in uterine arteries of sows, it is affected by work load since it was found to increase with parity [11].

The progression of the disease is essentially similar to aortic and cerebral atherosclerosis except for the greater propensity for coronary thrombosis, stenotic lesions and pronounced calcification.

The coronary arteries are unique in that they course over a moving and contracting muscle and when the ventricular mass atrophies as occurs in old age and debilitating diseases, the coronary arteries become quite tortuous. The ill-effects of such tortuosity have not received much attention but the lesions are probably analogous to those described in experimental models of bends and augmented flow [51,52].

6.2.4 OTHER SPLANCHNIC ARTERIES

Atherosclerosis affects other splanchnic arteries especially close to their origin from the aorta. Atheroembolism is common but usually subclinical. The splenic artery is particularly prone to severe atherosclerosis with ectasia and tortuosity. Thrombosis may involve the major arteries especially the trunk of the superior mesenteric artery but even this is rare and more peripheral involvement occurs in the presence of good collateral circulation. Stenosis or thrombosis of the inferior mesenteric artery may occur but usually collateral circulation is sufficient to avoid disastrous consequences: small peripheral occlusions would be more frequent. Atherosclerosis mostly affects the origins of the renal arteries.

6.2.5 ATHEROSCLEROSIS OF THE CAROTID AND VERTEBRAL ARTERIES IN THE NECK

The carotid and vertebral arteries are of major importance in cerebrovascular disease. Intramural haemorrhage and ulceration are more frequent in extracranial segments than in intracranial segments. The most severe atherosclerosis of these supply vessels to the brain occurs in the carotid sinus at the origin of the internal carotid artery. The localization of lipid macroscopically has been detailed by Meyer et al. [13] but this method of determining early lipid deposition is unsatisfactory. This is a major bifurcation with a fusiform dilatation superimposed on the commencement of the internal carotid and, as could be anticipated, atherosclerosis is pronounced on the lateral wall of the sinus since two conditions predisposing to atherogenesis are present. There is considerable intimal thickening within the sinus and lipid may be found within the first decade. Haemodynamically this arterial fork and sinus are unique, as explained; however, the velocity of flow through the internal carotid angiographically is faster than that through the external carotid arterial tree, probably because of differences in peripheral resistance. It remains to be seen how much this unusual haemodynamic arrangement contributes to the cervical bruit, severe atherosclerosis in the proximal internal carotid artery and the tortuosity of the artery in its cervical segment.

Severe atherosclerosis develops from the intimal proliferation present in infancy, calcification and ulceration with thrombosis being frequent. Dilatation of the sinus comes with advancing age [53] and is likely to aggravate the situation. Angiograms demonstrate atherosclerotic and thrombotic plaques as filling defects or the irregular contours of ulceration and confirm the frequency of atherosclerotic involvement. Mural thrombosis with embolism and also thrombotic occlusion are common in the carotid sinus.

In an extensive pathological study fatty streaks and fibrous plaques were found to have the same pattern of distribution within each artery at all ages independently of geographic location. The early lesions had the same localization as advanced lesions supporting the view that the latter were derived from fatty streaks [54]. The origins of the common carotid arteries are usually not severely affected. The stem, the remainder of the cervical segment and the petrous portion of the internal carotid artery are less severely involved. The cavernous segment tends to be severely affected. The carotid siphon displays intimal thickenings at regions of boundary layer separation on the lesser curvatures of the bends and these progress to overt atherosclerosis (Figure 6.24). The greater curvatures develop thinning and calcification from infancy onwards. Early calcific deposits are related to transversely orientated tears of the internal elastic

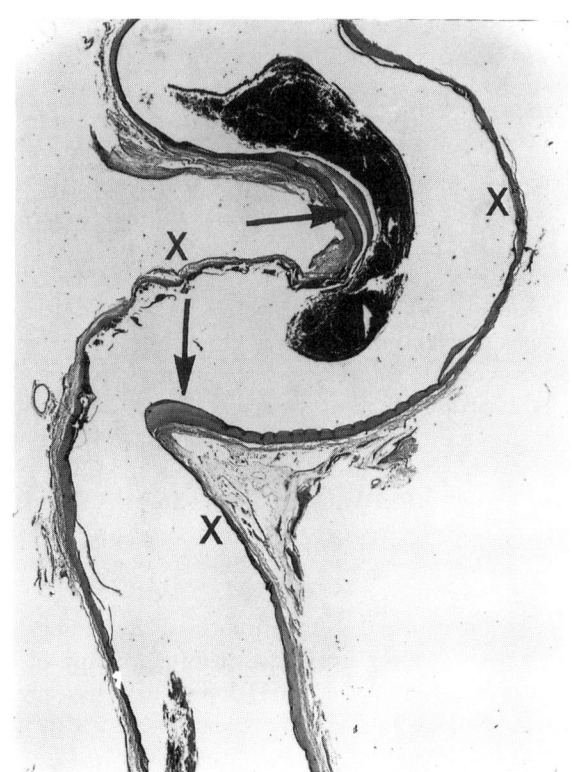

Figure 6.24 Longitudinal section through the carotid siphon of the internal carotid artery showing intimal thickening and atherosclerosis in regions of boundary layer separation (arrows) and mural thinning (X) where blood flow is likely to impinge on the vessel wall. (Verhoeff's elastic stain.) (Reproduced with permission from Stehbens [21].)

lamina. They develop earliest and are most pronounced on the sharpest flexure (4th bend) [13]. In older subjects the greater curvatures may exhibit severe mural thinning. Cavernous aneurysms angiographically appear to be expansions from the greater flexure much the same as occurs with tortuosities of the afferent arteries of experimental arteriovenous fistulae.

The acuteness of the flexures in the carotid siphon varies from individual to individual and appears to vary with age. It has been suggested that the tortuosity dampens the pulse pressure and if so the arteries do not go unscathed. Calcification of the walls increases with age and hypertension. Whether it exerts any protective advantage against further dilatation remains to be clarified.

The origin of the vertebral artery is particularly susceptible to severe atherosclerosis with calcification, stenosis, ulceration and thrombotic occlusion. Meyer [55] reported that atherosclerosis affects the vertebral artery in the neck in a segmental manner, with atherosclerotic plaques tending to involve the slightly wider or ectatic segments between the foramina of the transverse processes of the cervical vertebrae. The bony support where the artery traverses the foramina seemingly provides some protective effect. The intracranial segment of the vertebral arteries commonly develops severe atherosclerosis.

6.2.6 PERIPHERAL VASCULAR DISEASE

The arterial circulation of the lower limbs is subjected to the complications of atherosclerosis and also to atheroembolism from the descending aorta. Whilst branches of the aorta often receive such emboli, the external iliac and femoral arteries are in the direct line of flow and therefore probably receive more emboli than other branches together. Only the extensive collateral flow in the lower limbs circumvents more frequent vascular catastrophes. Whilst much of the debris and attached thrombus appears to undergo rapid clearance, cholesterol crystals and probably intimal fragments may lead to permanent occlusions which seem to be clinically silent more often than not.

Rodda [56] reported total or near total occlusion in one or more of the main arteries of one leg in 42% of 50 adult persons at autopsy and Lindbom [57] reported that occlusions of large lower limb arteries were twice as common as coronary occlusions even though silent. When symptoms or signs of ischaemia were present, but not sufficient to warrant surgical interference, 52% of 1196 such patients had angiographic evidence of progression on follow up (average of 2.5 years) [58]. The progression, more frequent in subjects over 50 years and with manifest diabetes, was more pronounced in the proximal two thirds of the femoral artery than the distal third. Progression is remarkably slow and occurs more often in major vessels proximal to an occlusion and rarely distally.

When atherosclerosis is severe in the abdominal aorta, severe involvement of the iliac arteries can be expected. Surprisingly Mitchell and Schwartz [33] found the internal iliac arteries had a higher prevalence of stenotic lesions (thrombotic or atherosclerotic) than the external iliac arteries in both male and female. Iliac arteries are more severely affected than the carotid arteries except for the carotid sinus. Iliac arteries, however, have much more arterial surface of involvement. To know the effect of multiple pregnancies on the internal iliac arteries would be enlightening. The effect of the flexion of the thigh and knee must be considerable but has not been investigated. However, the atherosclerotic changes in these vessels will be similar to those elsewhere but with greatest severity of involvement in the pelvis and thigh.

Peripheral vascular disease with severe ischaemia and gangrene are well established complications of severe atherosclerosis but its pathology is infrequently examined and its clinical diagnosis is fraught with considerable inexactitude. For this reason it is not used by epidemiologists as a surrogate monitor of the severity of atherosclerosis. Death in these subjects is frequently due to a stroke or CHD.

6.2.7 PULMONARY ARTERIES

Intimal proliferation occurs in the pulmonary elastic arteries from infancy with changes similar to but less severe than those in the aorta. Small, raised lipid-containing flecks or mounds up to 3 or 4 mm in diameter are not uncommon in elderly subjects. More severe degrees of atherosclerosis and medial calcification are quite rare. These pathological changes have not been adequately localized though their topography is expected to be similar to that in the systemic circulation [11].

The muscular arteries exhibit progressive intimal thickening with age and at times this may be 20% of the internal diameter. It may be concentric but eccentric thickenings can be recognized near branching sites even in random sections. Eccentric thickenings could be mistaken for organization of emboli but organization of thrombus does not produce a musculoelastic thickening.

Degenerative changes, more advanced in the large elastic arteries under the stress of prolonged hypertension, are similar to those occurring in the aorta but less severe because even in hypertension the pressure is still low when compared to aortic pressure.

Atherosclerosis in pulmonary arteries is accentuated by pulmonary hypertension with the severity never as gross as in the aorta. Ulceration or mural thrombus can occur but calcification is rare. Lipid-free intimal proliferation is increased and medial thinning may be apparent. Accurate topographical localization at forks has not been attempted. Hyalinization and fibrosis of the wall are less severe than in the aorta. Ectasia may be observed but aneurysms and stenotic lesions (in the absence of mural thrombus) are rare.

There is little evidence of correlation between the severity of atherosclerosis in the pulmonary arteries and the aorta, but it is uncommon for pathologists to dissect the pulmonary arteries into the secondary and tertiary branches of each artery where atherosclerosis is most severe [59]. The distribution is reminiscent of the increased severity of atherosclerosis in the distal aorta and iliofemoral arteries. Heath et al. [59] found no macroscopic atherosclerosis in pulmonary valvular stenosis except in two subjects in whom the stenosis was not severe. There were pulmonary hypertension and augmented pulmonary blood flow, both of which increase the severity of atherosclerosis: 'The presence of atheroma in the systemic arteries without atheroma in the pulmonary arteries proves that the patients had the propensity to develop atheroma if the conditions of blood pressure and flow associated with its development were present' [59].

6.2.8 UMBILICAL ARTERIES

At term the morphology of the human umbilical arteries has always been recognized as unusual in that they have no internal elastic lamina and relatively little elastic tissue but pronounced intimal proliferation. Tortuosity is common and even aneurysms have been observed.

Vascular degeneration ultrastructurally is pronounced in the arteries distally in the cord [60] and within a few days of birth lipid droplets are present in both the artery and vein. Within a month after birth, lipid containing macrophages and smooth muscle cells are found ultrastructurally. Smooth muscle cells are atypical in shape and similar to those in atherosclerosis. In late infancy degenerative changes are even more pronounced and resemble atherosclerosis. It is uncertain whether basement membrane changes and matrix vesicles are present. Detailed study of the arteries during intrauterine life is wanting.

6.2.9 THE EARLY LESIONS OF ATHEROSCLEROSIS

There is no agreement amongst pathologists or investigators regarding the early lesions of atherosclerosis, the pathogenesis of the disease or even the definition of atherosclerosis. To some atherosclerosis commences with the initial appearance of lipid in the blood vessel wall and if this is the case, then lipid is first found in the aorta during fetal life [13] and is certainly present in every aorta by the age of three years. There is nothing sacrosanct about this belief but if a pathological lesion is consistently present before lipid appears, it is reasonable to suggest that the lesion is an integral part or a precursor of the atherosclerosis. There is ample evidence to regard the intimal pads at arterial forks both in humans and in lower animals in this light. This author believes the intimal pads or cushions which develop in the aorta prior to 15 weeks and commence in the cerebral arteries about 26 weeks are very early stages of atherosclerosis.

(a) The proliferative lesion

This consists of musculoelastic intimal thickening about arterial forks, junctions and curvatures in particular, although preceded by some changes in the internal elastic lamina at least in the cerebral arteries of human fetuses. This intimal proliferation is a site of predilection for lipid deposition [13].

(b) Tears in the internal elastic lamina

Lipid is also deposited in humans in the media beneath gaps or tears in the internal elastic lamina and overt atherosclerosis can develop where elastic tears develop.

In infants the tears with calcification are accentuated in the iliac artery feeding a single umbilical artery and in the enlarged common iliac artery overt atherosclerosis develops within 18 months to 4 years [13,14]. The intimal proliferation that develops over the tears is said to have an increased affinity for lipid deposition [13].

These transversely orientated tears have subsequently been demonstrated experimentally to be the earliest histological manifestation of mural atrophy seen in the afferent artery of arteriovenous fistulae [61,62] on the lesser curvature of bends [51] and about experimental arterial forks where berry aneurysms develop [63]. They may also be related to some mixed atrophic and proliferative lesions. In such lesions overt atherosclerosis develops after some time in the afferent artery close to the fistula and in berry aneurysms.

Intimal proliferation can be preceded by thinning and disappearance or tears of the internal elastic lamina and as such can be regarded as an early change, inevitably the result of subtle physicochemical alterations beyond our present knowledge. It would be premature to regard the elastic changes as the initial lesions since there are other constituents in the vessel wall and the failure of one may be the culmination of deleterious alterations in other cellular and non-cellular mural constituents. It is convenient at present to regard the intimal proliferation at forks, curvatures and junctions and the transversely orientated tears as the two early changes of atherosclerosis since:

1. they are readily discernible histologically;
2. they occur at specific sites initially;
3. they are associated with degenerative changes;
4. they are sites with a predilection for lipid deposition;
5. they extend and progress to the recognized complications of atherosclerosis.

To differentiate intimal proliferation at arterial forks in fetuses and neonates from that observable more diffusely or as an extension of pads or cushions at forks or curvatures in older subjects [15,46] is unwarranted. This is particularly the case since these same thickenings all progress to overt atherosclerosis. Detailed study of the intimal proliferations at an earlier stage of development by longitudinal serial sections rather than step transverse sections would reveal their relationship in the coronary arteries to be the same as that in the cerebral arteries [18,21].

Gelatinous lesions or oedematous elevations of the aortic intima have been alleged to be early lesions of atherosclerosis [64,65], containing little or no lipid and apparently difficult to see. Currently there is little to support this concept and no distinguishing features histologically or ultrastructurally. Their detection may depend on illumination which gives the aorta a semitranslucent appearance. These 'lesions' may merely correspond to some non-lipid containing intimal thickening similar to fatty streaks. They do not warrant classification as an initial or early lesion.

6.2.10 COMPLICATIONS OF ATHEROSCLEROSIS

Complications are morbid changes arising during the natural history of a disease that modify its course, usually adversely [66]. In atherosclerosis the complications include:

- tortuosity, ectasia and aneurysmal dilatation
- rupture, intimal tears and ulceration
- thrombo-embolic phenomena
- stenosing intimal proliferation.

These complications, manifested clinically by way of haemorrhage, ischaemia or less often pressure effects, have been attributed to a loss of tensile strength of the vessel wall particularly the inner portion [67]. Any theory of the aetiology of atherosclerosis should explain the complications of the disease. Their interrelationship is indicated in Figure 6.25 with the underlying mechanism being an acquired mural weakness or loss of tensile strength and the principal clinical manifestations of the complications being ischaemia, haemorrhage and pressure effects.

(a) Ectasia and aneurysmal dilatation

Progressive ectasia of the aorta, coronary and cerebral arteries occurs with age [47,68,69]. Accentuation of this phenomenon may occur with connective tissue disorders or arteriovenous shunts. Two types of atherosclerosis, one involving ectasia and the other leading to stenotic lesions have been thought to exist, but dilatation and narrowing occur together with either feature dominating in any one individual. More detail is required about ectasia which is seen in a pronounced form in the afferent artery of arteriovenous shunts. Experimentally such ectasia is associated with the development of tears in the internal elastic lamina (within two to five days postoperatively) followed by progressive mural thinning with tears and loss of medial elastic tissue and disappearance of muscle [52,70]. This may be associated with increased length of the arterial segment, tortuosity and aneurysmal dilatation. Such changes can occur in the absence of overt lipid-rich lesions of atherosclerosis. Intimal proliferation with changes similar to atherosclerosis may be superimposed near the experimental shunt. Given this is an extreme instance occurring at an accelerated rate, a more slowly progressive lesion can manifest similar changes.

Ectasia and tortuosity are characteristically seen in collateral vessels and are a prominent feature of aortic coarctation. Pronounced ectasia is often associated with aneurysmal dilatation that may be fusiform, saccular or even serpentine.

Ectasia is more than physiological vasodilatation and serves no useful purpose. On present evidence the yield of the vessel wall is associated with destructive changes in the mural constituents and an acquired weakening of the wall. Dissecting aneurysm often occurring in ectatic vessels is likewise associated with reduced tensile strength and is usually not considered to be atherosclerotic although infrequently it can commence in an atherosclerotic plaque. Under physiological conditions the arterial pressure is inadequate to produce dilatation whether ectasia or a frank aneurysm and consequently

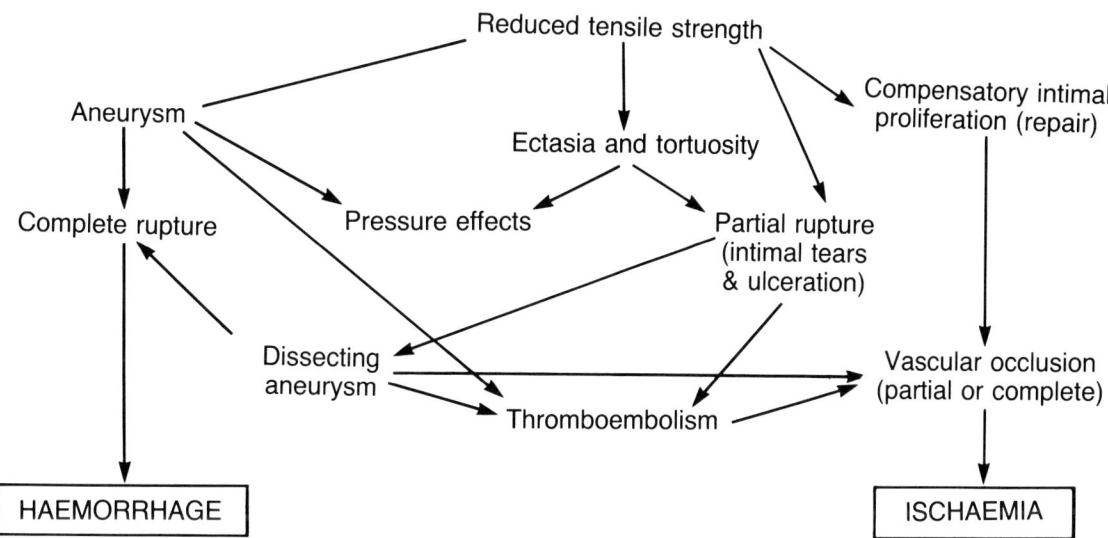

Figure 6.25 Interrelationship of complications of atherosclerosis which can be attributed to reduced tensile strength of mural connective tissue. (Reproduced with permission from Stehbens [67].)

such changes must be due to a weakness or diminished tensile strength of the wall.

(b) Tortuosities

There are instances when arteries pursue a tortuous course naturally. The aorta arches fairly abruptly such that blood ejected into the ascending segment rapidly reverses the direction of flow as it passes around the arch. The stresses to which the arch of the aorta is subjected by this configuration are considerable and in some individuals, especially hypertensives, the radius of curvature may be enlarged – the so-called unfolding of the aorta.

The vertebral arteries in the neck follow a circuitous route and the internal carotid artery exhibits a sigmoid tortuosity at the base of the skull (carotid siphon), although in early fetal life it is straight. In the adult the configuration of the carotid siphon varies from individual to individual and the sharpness of the angulation at the curvatures is quite variable, sometimes amounting to actual kinking. The originally straight leptomeningeal vessels assume a more sinuous course with further development of the cerebral cortical convolutions and sulci. During normal body movements, arteries of the limbs may be bent sharply upon themselves (as in the fetal position), lesser curvatures being frequent even in the normal anatomical position and also when arteries curve to provide blood to viscera. Whilst some arteries become tortuous as they adapt to changing anatomy during embryogenesis and development, this does not exempt them from the consequences of the associated haemodynamic stresses. Other vessels acquire tortuosity, the best known being the superficial temporal artery in man. Such tortuosities exhibit stress changes secondarily [52] and these may further accentuate the tortuosity.

Tortuosity resembles the sinuous or meandering course assumed by rivers and streams possibly because water in a channel seems to have a natural propensity to flow in a spiral direction [11,71]. The water-hammer effect of the pulse, pulsatile flow and the impedance to flow provided by branchings may, in the long term, contribute to lengthening of an arterial segment due to loss of elasticity and yield of mural connective tissues. This contention is supported by the frequency of hypertension and arteriosclerosis in patients with tortuous carotid vessels in the neck [72] and their greater prevalence in middle age and the elderly as well as the association with severe atherosclerosis. Such arteries would of necessity assume some curvature or tortuosity when they increase in length between two relatively fixed points with tortuosity becoming more prominent as the result of secondary changes resulting from the curvatures.

A classification of elongations and redundancy of arterial segments is as follows:

1. Tortuosity is any S or C-shaped elongation or undulation in the course of a vessel.
2. Coiling is an elongation or redundancy resulting in an exaggerated S-shaped curve or in a circular configuration.
3. Kinking is a sharp angulation possibly associated with some degree of stenosis in the affected system.

This classification is not ideal because it denotes the type of configuration without indicating the degree of deformity necessary for comparative studies. The configuration is not often confined to two dimensions and the curvatures are neither equal nor of regular periodicity. The abdominal aorta often exhibits some degree of tortuosity when severely atherosclerotic but usually being mild, this is frequently overlooked. In large aneurysmal sacs containing much thrombus, the channel as seen angiographically can exhibit a tortuous course.

Much attention has been focused on tortuosity of the internal carotid arteries in the neck, assumed by some to be a congenital configuration due to persistence of a curvature at the junction of the third aortic arch and dorsal aorta from which the artery has developed [73,74]. This hypothesis is difficult to substantiate without detailed investigation of the biological and physical properties of the arteries. Tortuosity is frequent in the carotid and vertebral arteries and is particularly common in the splenic artery. Such tortuosities are pronounced in Marfan's syndrome.

Tortuosity is a manifestation of arteriosclerosis of small peripheral arteries and arteriolosclerosis. Long intracerebral arteries commonly exhibit tortuosity and all such cases seem to be due to lengthening of the vessels as the vessel wall yields. It has been observed in the chronic vascular changes about chronic peptic ulceration and designated endarteritis obliterans [75]. Many small intracerebral vessels also acquire a helical or tortuous course (Figure 6.26) and this can probably be

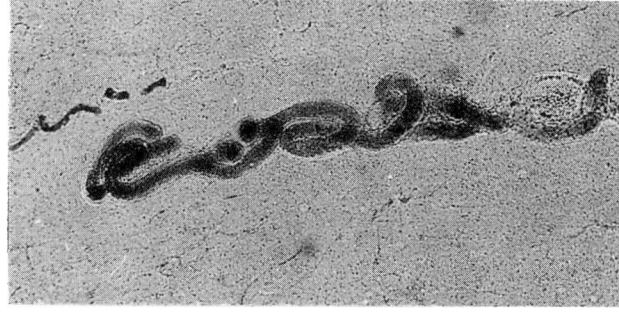

Figure 6.26 Small intracerebral vein displaying extreme tortuosity. (Fuchsin.)

attributed to degenerative changes with age in the mural connective tissues as occurs in larger vessels. Also common in phlebosclerosis and varicose veins, tortuosity is seen in its most extreme forms in the collateral circulation associated with aortic coarctation and arteriovenous fistulae.

The helical twisting of the umbilical cord is believed to be due to the helical course of the umbilical arteries which may be the result of haemodynamic stresses rather than by design to obviate snarling or kinking of the vessels.

Ertugrul [76] reported the case of a 10-year-old girl with generalized gross tortuosity and lengthening of the aorta and all major arteries, aneurysm of the ascending aorta, aortic regurgitation and telangiectasia of the cheeks as well as very prominent arterial pulsations. Histologically, arterial elastic tissue degeneration was pronounced and the intima was considerably thickened. Such pathology is probably indicative of an unrecognized metabolic connective tissue disorder.

A longitudinal section through the carotid siphon (Figure 6.24) reveals an intimal atherosclerotic proliferation related to the lesser curvatures where boundary layer separation occurs. Over the greater curvatures there is thinning and calcification. These regions are analogous respectively to the regions of sedimentary deposits and areas of scouring seen at curvatures in meandering streams. It does not follow that similar events will occur at arterial bends but it is likely that the stresses on the vessel wall will be similar.

Imparato *et al.* [77] reported intimal proliferation including lipid deposition on the lesser curvatures of experimental arterial bends in dogs. No lipid was illustrated suggesting that the quantity must have been minimal and no mention was made of the greater curvatures.

Transplanting a segment of the common carotid artery to the contralateral common carotid (end-to-end anastomosis) results in bending and twisting of the elongated vessel with each pulse. The transplanted artery can be fashioned into a U-bend by tying the tie sutures together [51,52]. If the bend is kinked, pulsatility of the main bend is accentuated. Initially at the greater curvatures, transversely orientated tears develop in the internal elastic lamina. They commence within five days and progress to mural thinning and atrophy with loss of elastic tissue and muscle. At regions of boundary layer separation on the lesser curvatures, intimal proliferation develops and lipid is deposited in sheep. Some intimal proliferation including lipid may appear eventually on the greater curvature but the wall remains thinned. These lesions were referred to as atrophic and proliferative lesions of atherosclerosis [52]. Meyer *et al.* [13] reported transversely orientated tears of the internal elastic lamina on the greater curvature of bends in the carotid siphon and splenic artery of children. Calcification of the elastic lamina characteristically occurred at the edges of the tears and intimal proliferation was found at the lesser curvatures at the sites indicated. The experimental reproduction of these two types of lesion confirms they are the result of hydrodynamic stresses. There is no reason to suggest that either is an adaptive lesion of benefit to the subject. These lesions could develop secondarily to spontaneously occurring tortuosities thereby aggravating the distortion and the degenerative changes responsible for the tortuosity.

(c) Rupture, intimal tears and ulceration

Direct spontaneous rupture of large atherosclerotic arteries is extremely rare [78] although it may occur in experimental lathyrism and copper deficiency. It can arise in small arteries where it is beyond our ability to study but in general, rupture is usually preceded by aneurysmal dilatation or dissecting aneurysm. Intimal tears and ulceration are remarkably common in atherosclerosis, being in reality partial ruptures and usually associated with some degree of dissection. The close relationship between dissections and thrombosis has been recognized in cerebrovascular pathology [21] but also occurs in the extracranial circulation.

Arterial rupture should not occur under normal physiological conditions since internal pressures from 35 to 56 times normal arterial pressure are required to rupture arteries [79]. Similar pressures are necessary to rupture the aorta [80] and are higher than those ever encountered spontaneously *in vivo*. The walls of distributing arteries weaken with age [81] and atherosclerotic artery fragility is encountered surgically [82]. The occurrence of tears therefore indicates the existence of some underlying weakness of the vessel wall, which if of normal strength, would not undergo such dissolution in the absence of trauma or some other destructive lesion. This acquired weakness has been recognized by surgeons and physiologists and is testable at autopsy as portions of the aortic intima at times readily peel off manually. Pathological fractures of bone are the result of an underlying lesion (e.g. tumour or osteoporosis) reducing the strength of the bone. The stress fractures of bones, tendons and ligaments of athletes, sportsmen, joggers and marching soldiers have been regarded as analogous to the intimal tears of arteries as they too are of necessity due to an underlying acquired weakness or loss of tensile strength of the tissues due to repetitive stress. Intramural haemorrhage from damaged vasa vasorum could occur when atheromatous debris ruptures through medial remnants into the adventitia or into the inner part of the intima due to cleavage between layers of the weakened atherosclerotic wall with damage to vasa vasorum. Such an event could be precipitated by

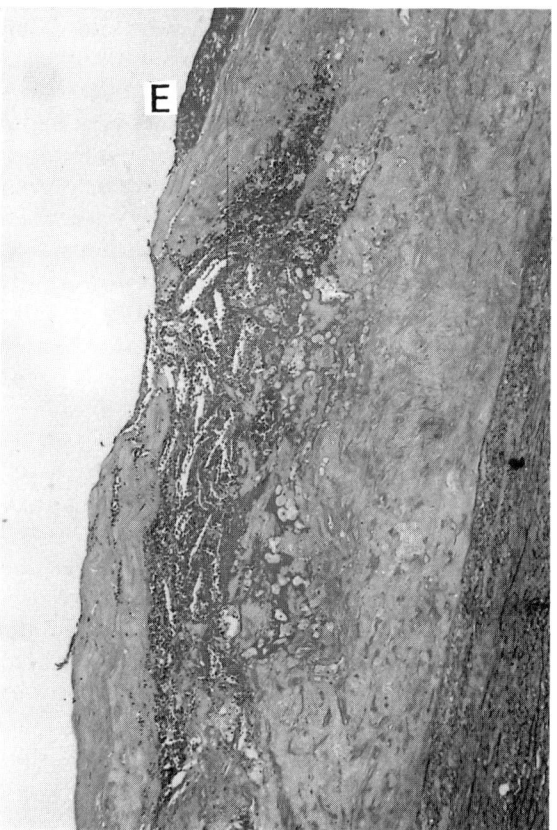

Figure 6.27 Small tear through superficial intimal tissue with extravasation of blood into atheromatous debris extending well beyond the tear. Note a subendothelial extravasation of blood at E. (Haematoxylin and eosin.)

augmented shear stress on the inner part of the intima. However, when there is significant extravasation of blood into an atheromatous cavity, it is more likely to be associated with ulceration or tearing of the overlying intima (Figure 6.27). Intramural fibrin could arise from mild damage with increased endothelial permeability of the intima or of vasa vasorum, a process referred to as insudation of plasma which may well account for much of the intramural fibrin seen in atherosclerosis.

Histologically, atherosclerosis progressively affects the vessel wall from within outwards and no layer escapes. Consequently there is need to investigate the biochemical and physical characteristics of the inner and outer parts of the affected wall. If the entire wall were affected to the same extent, direct rupture of the full thickness of the wall would occur rather than partial rupture (tearing or ulceration) with or without intramural dissection or a frank dissecting aneurysm. This is supported by the following observations:

1. Small regions of a severely atherosclerotic intima may be peeled off relatively easily at times whereas other regions, difficult to separate, necessitate cutting.
2. An external impact on the vessel wall may lacerate the intima but not the other coats, suggesting lesser tensile strength of the atherosclerotic intima [83].
3. Actual measurements of tensile strength have revealed increased fragility of the intima [84] and variation over the intimal surface and less strength over ruptured or torn plaques than unruptured plaques or the neighbouring wall [85]. The plaques were mostly torn at this margin with the neighbouring intima and less frequently over the fibrous cap. The fibromuscular caps required less stress for rupture than neighbouring intima [85–87].
4. Endarterectomy is performed for severe ulcerated atherosclerosis of a thick-walled, hard and stiff arterial wall with thrombotic occlusion. Yet following endarterectomy, the residual vessel wall consists of adventitia with or without medial remnants and is thin, soft and more pliant. The tension in the wall is increased but the endarterectomized segment of artery, though it heals and develops atherosclerosis, can continue to function as a patent arterial conduit for ten years or more.

These facts indicate that the atherosclerotic intima has less tensile strength than the more durable outer residual portion of the wall.

Architectural changes in the wall indicative of reduced vascular tensile strength or loss of cohesion are:

1. fragmentation and extensive loss of elastic tissue;
2. dystrophic and irregular disposition of basement membrane material;
3. separation of basement membrane from endothelial and smooth muscle cells;
4. plasma membrane fragility, vesiculogranular degeneration and necrosis of smooth muscle cells;
5. disintegration and irregular shaped collagen fibrils normally associated with fragility in connective tissue disorders [29,30,32,89].

(d) Thromboembolic phenomena

The principle function of a platelet is to prevent haemorrhage and therefore when a blood vessel or an aneurysm wall tears or ulcerates spontaneously, platelets adhere to the foreign or thrombogenic surface to produce a thrombus. In the development of thrombus, small platelet–leucocyte aggregates will be washed downstream only to be replaced by further platelets, leucocytes and entrapped red cells. When a larger mural thrombus forms, larger thrombi may be shed with fragments of intima, as in aortic ulceration. If the underlying intima contains atheromatous debris with little cohesion to surrounding mural tissue, the caseous debris to which platelets will adhere will be washed out giving rise to atheromatous embolism. Thrombus may then line the excavated atheromatous cavity and blood may infiltrate or dissect the undermined intimal edges to a varying degree.

All experimental evidence indicates that platelets and platelet aggregates adhere only to severely damaged endothelium or to subendothelial tissues when the endothelium is discontinuous [89,90]. Thrombus is therefore a secondary complication. Mural thrombi, whether covering the ulcerated, torn or eroded atherosclerotic wall, or covering a partial tear of an aneurysmal sac wall, can also give rise to emboli and transient or more serious ischaemic infarcts of the heart or brain. Usually when mural thrombus is visible macroscopically, the disruption of the underlying wall is more than mere endothelial denudation. In the aorta the thrombus is rarely sufficient to obstruct or occlude blood flow. When seen it is usually in the lower abdominal aorta with or without occlusion of the common iliac arteries. In smaller arteries or small veins, thrombus is more likely to become occlusive and in this way thrombosis *in situ* or emboli can result in serious obstruction to blood flow and ischaemia especially of the heart, brain and lower limbs. The underlying pathological lesion is a disrupted blood vessel wall due to an acquired weakness of mural connective tissues. Whether or not death follows such obstruction depends on many other factors and at times the ischaemia may be clinically silent.

(e) Stenosing intimal proliferation

Stenosis and occlusion of the vessel can be secondary to thrombosis but the extent to which organization of the thrombus contributes to intimal proliferation has not been determined. Some atherosclerotic lesions, particularly in coronary arteries, appear to be due to a stenosing intimal proliferation consisting of fibromusculoelastic tissue, proteoglycans and lipid accumulation with a varying degree of hyalinization and calcification. They can cause ischaemia. There may be relatively little or no lipid deposition, this being a recognized feature of atherosclerosis. Recent evidence suggests that in the anastomosed vein of an arteriovenous shunt, the degree of intimal proliferation can be two or three times the thickness of the venous wall. In a smaller vein such as is used for renal dialysis, this would lead to relatively rapid stenosis without inevitably the gross hyalinization and other degenerative changes of a more slowly developing atherosclerotic lesion. Thus the nature of the outcome in therapeutic arteriovenous shunts and venous bypass grafts may depend on vein diameter, physicochemical characteristics of the wall and prevailing haemodynamics. Biological repair is usually associated initially with over-proliferation of tissue but when the irritant or injurious agent is persistent, excessive proliferation of tissue results. This may be the underlying mechanism of some stenosing lesions which are also seen in therapeutic arteriovenous shunts and venous bypass grafts. The analogous situation is seen in skin and bone due to chronic repetitive stress, when gross overproduction of tissue is the response to a persistent stimulus [21].

When an atherosclerotic artery reaches a certain degree of stenosis, concentrically arranged subendothelial connective tissue is laid down and appears to narrow the lumen still further irrespective of the estimated shear stress which some observers consider all important. This phenomenon is also seen in small peripheral arteries.

(f) Calcification

Calcification is often considered a complication but there is no evidence that it is detrimental *per se*. It should be regarded as a manifestation of atherosclerosis as is lipid accumulation.

(g) Miscellaneous secondary complications

There are additional secondary complications that are not immediately life-threatening but can have serious consequences nevertheless.

Stenosis at origin of arterial branches and ischaemia

Stenosis of the renal artery at its origin is a well recognized entity and when pronounced is held responsible for some instances of hypertension and even severe renal ischaemia with reduction in size and impaired function [91]. Similar constriction may be due to external compression by tendinous extension of the diaphragm or psoas major muscle or other non-atherosclerotic occlusive lesions.

Stenosis of the ostia of the coronary arteries occurs in atherosclerosis but has also been attributed to syphilis and is particularly frequent in familial hypercholesterolaemia. Angiographically it is commonly seen at the origin of the vertebral artery from the subclavian and other branches of the aorta [7].

Hypertension

As indicated atherosclerosis of the renal artery either at its origin or in the stem can cause hypertension and has been said to be the commonest cause of renovascular hypertension. It is also possible that recurrent atheroemboli to the kidney can cause hypertension as demonstrated by Moore [92]. There is also the possibility that progressive sclerosis of the arterial tree with loss of its normal elastic properties accounts for the progressive elevation of systolic and pulse pressures. However, increased peripheral resistance and diminished run off due to a reduced vascular bed and stenosis or occlusion of many non-critical branches in the distal aorta and lower limbs, could also contribute to the elevation of the diastolic blood pressure. In this way the hypertension is of mechanical origin. It is also a complication of endarterectomy but the pathogenesis is obscure.

6.2.11 LOCALIZATION OF ATHEROSCLEROSIS

Atherosclerosis is often defined as a focal disease of medium and large arteries but this is misleading. It has a predilection for certain foci but in advanced stages of the disease virtually the entire aortic surface may be involved. It is important to consider sites of predilection for severe involvement because localizing factors can account for this enhanced severity.

(a) General topography

Atherosclerosis is more severe in the systemic arterial circulation in which the pressure is higher than in pulmonary arteries and is least severe in veins in which both pressure and blood velocity are lowest.

Within the systemic circulation there is variation in severity from vascular bed to vascular bed even within the same individual. Severe disease in lower limb arteries is relatively common whereas in the upper limbs severe atherosclerosis with gangrene and intermittent claudication would be most unusual. Atheroembolism may contribute to disease of lower limb arteries and the extensive collateral arcades might mask the severity of atherosclerosis in the mesenteric arteries but such factors cannot wholly explain the disparity in severity of involvement. Vessels of comparable diameter to the coronary and cerebral arteries would inevitably cause more clinical disease if the severity of their involvement was comparable. Such variation requires explanation if blood lipid levels are of prime importance. It is also unlikely that mural constituents of the vessel walls are responsible.

Within a circulatory bed the severity of atherosclerosis is proportional to the calibre of the vessel. This can probably be explained on the basis of mural tension which is directly proportional to the vessel diameter (law of Laplace) and the Reynolds number which is proportional to the diameter and velocity and which determines whether or not flow disturbances occur within a particular vessel.

In the limbs, the severity is said to be augmented by usage and there is reduced severity in a paralysed limb [93,94]. In right-handed individuals the severity in the radial artery is said to be increased and *vice versa* in the left-handed [95]. These observations, appearing to be anecdotal, require confirmation but are consistent with recent experimental evidence [70].

Hypertension aggravates the severity of atherosclerosis in each of the systemic, pulmonary and venous systems. The systolic pressure has been positively correlated with the severity of coronary and particularly cerebral atherosclerosis. The effect of pressure is also revealed in pulmonary sequestration in which a segment of the lung is supplied by an anomalous systemic artery which often manifests as severe premature atherosclerosis [96]. In aortic coarctation, aortic, coronary and cerebral atherosclerosis are of augmented severity in the young [37] and the disease is of diminished severity beyond the coarctation. It is also acknowledged that hypotension indicates the likelihood of longevity presumably due to a reduced incidence of death from cardiovascular disease. Hypertension must be regarded as an aggravating factor.

The disease affects all coats of the vessel wall, with the intima being most severely affected and the adventitia least severely suggesting that the intima has greater exposure to the aetiological factor [97].

It has been alleged [33] that the severity of aortic atherosclerosis is reduced in subjects with long-standing aortic valvular stenosis presumably due to a dampening of the systolic and pulse pressures. This, also appearing to be anecdotal, requires scientific confirmation. Dampening of the pulse pressure is associated with reduction in atherosclerosis severity beyond an aortic coarctation and an occlusion of a major artery in the lower limb is associated with progression of the arteries proximally on arteriographic follow-up but rarely is the progression distal [98]. These observations further support the role of vibrations in the atherogenesis.

(b) Factors localizing lesions to specific sites

Atherosclerosis is more severe in the distal aorta, iliac and femoral arteries than in the proximal aorta, a distribution that has been attributed to the augmented systolic and pulse pressures distally, due to pulse wave reflection and a summation effect [11]. There is the possibility of a boundary-layer effect along the posterior wall of the abdominal aorta as it curves slightly with the lumbar vertebral bodies, but the dominant effect on the posterior walls would be that of the ostia of the segmental branches.

Atherosclerosis has a predilection for fusiform dilatations such as the carotid sinus and the slightly expanded or ectatic segments of the vertebral arteries unsupported by the bone of the transverse processes of cervical vertebrae [55]. The greater involvement of the affected zones has been attributed to the greater systolic pulsatility and disturbed blood flow as in an aneurysm.

Atherosclerosis, as confirmed experimentally [99], appears to run an accelerated course in berry aneurysms [21].

Lesser severity of atherosclerosis of arteries with external mechanical support is seen in those segments of the vertebral arteries traversing the foramina in the transverse processes of cervical vertebrae [55] and in those segments of the anterior descending branch of the left coronary artery covered by a muscular bridge. Such mechanical support appears to afford some degree of protection, which would probably be of advantage to venous bypass grafts.

Atherosclerosis develops at an accelerated rate in the anastomosed veins of arteriovenous shunts for renal dialysis [101] and in the afferent artery of chronic femoral arteriovenous fistulae [102]. These observations have been confirmed experimentally [70,103].

Veins used for venous bypass grafts develop severe atherosclerosis within 18 months to 10 years, whereas the internal thoracic (internal mammary) artery is much more resilient, has a longer survival time and is no doubt less susceptible to atherosclerosis than veins, being architecturally designed to withstand arterial haemodynamics.

Atherosclerosis is prone to occur about the orifices of branches, at junctions and on the lesser curvature of bends. Accentuation of the disease at such sites has led to incrimination of non-specific haemodynamic stresses which have been regarded as localizing factors. Texon [104] alleged that the disease also occurs at sites of taper but no supportive evidence has been provided. Convergent flow tends to promote flow stability and such a configuration would be foreign to the arterial system except under pathological conditions.

Having a single umbilical artery predisposes the homolateral common iliac artery to premature atherosclerosis in infancy in accordance with the additional blood flow and augmented stress [13,14].

Arteries and veins are composed of the same cellular and non-cellular connective tissues but differ architecturally. Yet veins, which are believed to be relatively immune to atherosclerosis because of their mild or minimal involvement, develop accelerated severe disease when used in arteriovenous shunts or as bypass grafts. Architecturally they are not designed to withstand arterial haemodynamics or the stresses of a shunt. Their pathological changes must be attributed to haemodynamic stresses rather than circulating humoral factors because, if left intact like other veins elsewhere in those subjects, they would have shown only minimal involvement during the remaining years of life.

Such observations emphasize the importance of local haemodynamic factors in the pathogenesis of atherosclerosis. The importance of haemodynamic stresses has been recognized for many decades. Currently it is still acknowledged but their assigned role is usually considered to be as a localizing factor even though recent experimental evidence suggests a more dominant role [70,105].

6.2.12 SIGNIFICANCE OF INTIMAL PROLIFERATION IN INFANCY

Histologically, the arterial intima forms in the fetus as a single layer of endothelial cells superimposed on a distinct internal elastic lamina with no demonstrable intervening tissue. As indicated, areas of intimal thickening form in late fetal life about the orifices of aortic branches and at forks in distributing arteries. This intimal proliferation, commencing at specific sites about the ostia and also at junctions and curvatures, is musculoelastic together with collagen, fibrillary elastica and proteoglycans. In elastic arteries it may be difficult to distinguish from the media initially because both consist of alternate layers of smooth muscle and elastic tissue.

The nature of this intimal proliferation or thickening, though controversial, is crucial to understanding the aetiology and pathogenesis of atherosclerosis. Since these intimal proliferations progressively thicken and extend during postnatal development, it has been assumed that they constitute an integral part of the vessel wall especially as they consist of the same cellular and non-cellular constituents of the wall. It has also been assumed that they represent an adaption to changes in haemodynamics [15] and enlargement of the vessel during maturation. However, these changes do not cease at physical maturation but continue throughout life, progressively changing and merging imperceptibly with overt atherosclerosis, varying in degree from vascular bed to vascular bed, site to site and individual to individual. The early degenerative changes in the intimal thickenings histologically and ultrastructurally have been ignored with interpretations of their occurrence doubtless influenced by current belief in the validity of the lipid hypothesis. There has also been some reluctance to accept that a pathological change could be universal at such an early age.

Vascular repair following all kinds of injury is associated with smooth muscle cells in the intima but such sites of injury behave differently from thickenings at arterial forks; the muscle is not longitudinally orientated and they have not been shown to undergo the same ultrastructural degenerative changes. The longitudinal arrangement of the muscle cells and the localization of the initial thickenings (pads, cushions) are inconsistent with a sphincteric action or any other mechanism of controlling blood flow. Nerves have not been found in the early thickenings so it is unlikely they subserve a sensory function. The concept that the intimal thickening at arterial forks is the end result of the incorporation of haemodynamically induced platelet thrombi into the vessel wall with subsequent organization, is not supported by histological examination of serial sections of a large number of arterial forks in humans and lower animals [11,21,89]. There is no evidence of endothelial discontinuity in human infants or lower animals, and fibrin has not been demonstrated at such an early stage of development.

The presence of similar intimal musculoelastic thickenings in the thoracic duct, in the heart, particularly the left atrium with mitral valve dysfunction, and in lower animals must all be explained.

Intimal proliferation in arteries of infants is inconsistent with this concept of its being an adaptive change to growth and increasing hydrodynamic stresses associated with increasing flow and blood pressure during growth [15]. Adaptation implies an inherent biological or physiological ability to respond to altered environmental conditions and can occur by natural selection. An individual may adapt by physiological or behavioural changes that are not genetic but to suggest that these intimal proliferations about forks, curvatures and bends are merely adaptive to the continued physiological stresses that were responsible for the development and differentiation of mural connective tissues in the first place is questionable. The conditions can hardly be regarded as altered and are merely the physiological changes associated with growth and development both *in utero* and in postnatal life as is the increase in vessel calibre and thickness of the wall. The intimal changes are initiated *in utero* and continue throughout life. The environment of blood vessels is unchanged except for demands of growth and maturation as in all tissues. The onset of pathological changes during fetal life may be difficult for some to accept but facts have to be faced.

Bone responds to augmented stress by thickening and arteries might be expected to respond by enlargement of the artery, thickening of the artery, thickening of the elastic laminae, muscle proliferation and laying down of more collagen with the same basic architecture. This occurs in many arteries during growth and maturation. For example, the architecture of the major pulmonary arteries is that of the aortic type in high altitudes and the external iliac artery is elastic in type when supplying a single umbilical artery whilst the contralateral artery is thin and muscular in type. Yet, intimal proliferation with longitudinally arranged rather than circumferentially arranged muscle, the loss or disruption of a previously intact internal elastic lamina, medial thinning or atrophy and vesiculogranular degeneration of smooth muscle cells in the fetus and neonate are all inconsistent with the scientific concept of physiological adaptation. The concept of 'remodelling' of the vessel wall is not applicable to this situation. Remodelling following repair of a fractured bone is the response of repair tissues to the unusual stresses occasioned by the fracture with poor alignment and is indeed an integral stage of repair and occasioned by new unphysiological stresses. The intimal proliferation at forks with its attendant changes is more consistent with compensatory repair tissue due to yield by the thinned wall or altered internal elastic lamina which some authors regard as being haemodynamically induced [11,13,103,106].

The continued enlargement and extension of these thickenings, combined with progressive fibrosis, hyalinization, loss of elastica, increased calcification and even arteriectasis well after maturity, have been regarded as arteriosclerosis and distinct from atherosclerosis despite the fact that they are also manifestations of atherosclerosis. The presence of lipid deposition in any quantity is not the sole indicator of atherosclerosis but merely one of its many manifestations and not the earliest. The arbitrary separation of intimal proliferation and atherosclerosis in this way [15] and the assumption that two distinct diseases exist without clear and concise definitions of each and the means by which they are to be differentiated, is unacceptable. This is particularly so since lipid deposition in a thickened intima is universal in the aorta and coronary arteries within the first three years of life [13,22,107].

It is now widely acknowledged that musculoelastic intimal proliferation is an early stage of atherosclerosis and as such has become the basis of the 'intimal injury hypothesis' [12]. However, those who have sought to localize the earliest evidence of musculoelastic thickening of the intima [11,13,18,105], have recognized its predilection to localization at sites of branchings, curvatures and junctions which are also sites where severe atherosclerosis develops. If they are not an integral stage of atherosclerosis they must at least be precursors. The interrelationship being so close, differentiation between them becomes a matter of semantics and serves no useful purpose.

The reasons for regarding them essentially as one disease are the following:

1. The intimal proliferation in the fetus and neonate is localized to areas where atherosclerosis will develop to a severe degree and the distribution in the aorta, distributing arteries and the pulmonary arteries closely parallels the distribution of overt atherosclerosis in later life [11,18,99].
2. The loss of elastica and the presence of muscle-cell degeneration and basement-membrane changes in the early intimal thickening of neonates are early and milder changes of those that constitute essential changes of atherosclerosis at such sites [11,29].
3. Intimal proliferation, like atherosclerosis progresses throughout life but most developmental processes are established by maturity.
4. Both changes are aggravated by hypertension.
5. The lesions of coronary arteries in infants and children are identical to the early non-lipid phase of atherosclerosis in adults [11] and tend to be thickest in infants from a population with a high CHD mortality [108].
6. The intimal thickening is particularly prominent in

lower animals that are prone to atherosclerosis [109].
7. Intimal thickenings in infants, sheep and birds are sites of predilection for spontaneous lipid deposition [11,22,26].
8. It is unlikely that an internal elastic lamina would form only to fragment and disintegrate as part of an adaptive response. It is more likely to be a degenerative change such as precedes and is associated with intimal proliferation. Intimal proliferation and lipid deposition may also be superimposed on the transversely orientated tears in the internal elastic artery [13,70,105].
9. Intimal proliferation can be produced experimentally at forks, unions and curvatures and histologically resembles that naturally occurring in humans and other animals [52,63,105].
10. Intimal proliferation also develops as the initial lesion of atherosclerosis in the anastomosed veins of arteriovenous fistulae [103], venous bypass grafts [11] and berry aneurysms in man [21]. It is the initial lesion in several experimental haemodynamic models of atherosclerosis-like lesions in herbivores [70,99,103,105,110].
11. Similar thickening occurs in human veins (phlebosclerosis) and increases with age. It is also increased by hypertension, and may be associated with lipid deposition.
12. Intimal thickening in infant coronary arteries has been reported to be thicker in males than females as is consistent with the more severe coronary atherosclerosis in men than women [48]. Furthermore Wilens [111] states that intimal thickening is more pronounced in males than females for every decade.

Intimal thickening cannot be logically differentiated from atherosclerosis and must be related to the same pathological mechanisms that ultimately lead to the formation of atherosclerosis. Indeed the initial intimal thickening similar to that at arterial forks can be produced experimentally by hydrodynamic means and in some models progresses to atherosclerosis, and the intimal thickenings naturally occurring at arterial forks in stock-fed rabbits can be induced to progress to advanced atherosclerosis experimentally also by augmented hydromechanical stress [70,105]. Such experimental evidence is consistent with the specific requirements for causality in atherogenesis [5].

6.2.13 LOCALIZATION OF INTIMAL PROLIFERATION

The predilection of atherosclerosis for arterial forks has been explained on the basis of augmented haemodynamic stresses occurring at bifurcations but there is no agreement on the nature of the stresses responsible.

Since lipid is often regarded as the hallmark of atherosclerosis and spontaneous lipid deposition always occurs within a thickened intima, the localization of intimal thickening is all important. This holds particularly for the sites of initiation of such fibromusculoelastic proliferation. As indicated these are the flow divider and beyond the lateral angles.

The proliferation at the flow divider appears to have two different distributions. In cerebral arterial bifurcations in which lateral pads or thickenings are prominent, the proliferation is fairly well restricted to the flow divider. In the aortic bifurcation of the rabbit and probably of humans, the lateral thickenings are relatively limited or absent and the proliferation extends distally along the adjoining walls of the daughter branches for a variable distance. This proliferation occurs at an area believed to be subjected to high shear stress. The proliferation in the daughter branches beyond the lateral angles occurs in regions of low shear stress where boundary layer separation would be expected to occur. Any explanation for such occurrence must explain the particular involvement of both sites and how and why the changes develop into atherosclerosis and its complications.

The localization has been analysed in detail elsewhere [11] but in essence the following explanation seems the most plausible and is based on the concept of structural or engineering fatigue of the vessel wall which Halsted [112] and later Holman [113] considered responsible for the development of post-stenotic dilatation in aortic coarctation. In 1958 it was postulated [106] that the intimal proliferation at arterial forks was due to unremitting high frequency vibrations associated with disturbed flow and pulse pressure and that atherosclerosis was the ultimate effect of the same haemodynamic stresses (fatigue hypothesis).

With expansion of the cross-sectional area at the fork [6], the central flux of blood acts in the capacity of a jet with boundary layer separation laterally beyond where the lateral wall of the stem curves into the daughter branch. The ampulla-like increase in cross-sectional area often amounts to 30% or even more prior to actual division of the lumen and thus acts as an eccentric lateral diffuser [6], the angle of divergence probably determining whether or not separation occurs rather than the area ratio. The degree and rate of lateral expansion seems to be greater with wide-angled forks than with narrow bifurcation angles. The mechanical effect of the vibrations associated with the eddying on the collagen and elastin results in molecular fragmentation and weakening of the wall with compensatory intimal proliferation. This too is subjected to the same haemodynamic stresses which are maximal near the fork and dampened distally. However, distal extension of the compensatory thickening is merely a matter of time. The central flux of blood is analogous to a jet which produces vortex shedding from the flow divider, vortices alternating on either side of the apex. In narrow bifurcations and depending on the nature of secondary branchings from the primary branches, separation may be minimal and in very unequal branchings the vortices will be of unequal magnitude with the greater mechanical effect being in the larger branch or in the continuation of the parent stem beyond the origin of a small side branch. It is possible that such disturbances occur more readily in the marginal plasma zone which may be wider in the fast-flowing arterial system or in association with anaemia or a low haematocrit. The central red cell mass has a dampening effect by virtue of its viscoelastic properties.

An important effect on the apex and adjoining surfaces of the daughter branches would be the waterhammer effect of the systolic pulse which seems to be a major contributing factor in both the production of tears in the internal elastic lamina and the atrophic change that leads to berry aneurysm formation [70].

6.2.14 TEARS IN THE INTERNAL ELASTIC LAMINA

In the study of calcification in the human carotid siphon, early calcific deposits either as punctate or linear deposits occur in all children from 1 year to 16 years of age [114] particularly on the outer curvature of the most prominent flexure of the siphon (i.e. above and laterally to the origin of the ophthalmic artery). When calcification is more advanced, deposits are also found at similar locations on other curvatures more proximally at the edges of transversely orientated interruptions or tears in the internal elastic lamina but the calcification extends further into the remnants of the internal elastic laminae.

The common and internal iliac arteries are subjected to the stresses associated with the umbilical blood flow during fetal growth and development. The internal iliac arteries are substantially larger (nearly twice the circumference) than the external iliac arteries and are elastic arteries, whereas the external iliac arteries are muscular in type. Calcification similar to that in the carotid siphon develops along the lateral wall of the common iliac artery and on the dorsomedial wall of the internal iliac artery which corresponds to the outer or greater curvature of the ilioumbilical arch. The calcification again commences in the margins of tears in the internal elastic lamina with the formation of parallel transversely orientated linear calcifications, and with occasional longitudinal or oblique spindle-shaped connecting tears [13]. The calcification extends into the internal elastic lamina but spares the intervening gap. The secondary elastic laminae in the intima do not tend to calcify. The medial walls of the common iliac artery are not affected since the internal elastic lamina in the neonate is mostly deficient under the intimal proliferation which straddles the aortic bifurcation with extension distally along the medial aspect of the common iliac arteries [13]. They may also occur distally at a later time in the external iliac and femoral arteries.

A single umbilical artery occurs in 0.73% of births [13,14]. The internal elastic lamina is lost from the lateral half of the common iliac artery. The common and internal iliac arteries on the side of the single umbilical artery are elastic in type and thin and muscular on the contralateral side, as if the haemodynamic stresses associated with placental circulation were such as to stimulate production of an elastic architecture. Atherosclerotic changes were described in two infants in the common iliac arteries ipsilateral to the single umbilical artery at 18 months and four years of age. No generalized disease was found and in view of this restricted localization a general metabolic disorder seems unlikely. Meyer et al. [13] attributed the intimal proliferation superimposed on the elastic tearing and calcification as an accommodation to the diminished blood flow after cessation of the placental circulation.

Meyer et al. [13] described transverse rippling on the luminal surface of excised and retracted large muscular arteries by the end of the first decade as being due to the presence of transversely orientated elastic tears producing narrow ridges and spindle-shaped hollows which can be accentuated by blood or india ink on the endothelial surface. This is most pronounced in large limb arteries of adolescents and young adults. When perfusion fixed, only large spindle-shaped depressions are seen which correspond to the large gaps in the internal elastic lamina. This rippling may be interrupted by intimal proliferation related to orifices of branches regarded by Robertson [115] as stress zones. The rippling becomes masked by progressive diffuse intimal proliferation. However, the pattern of tears with calcification initially at the edges only but extending later into the residual elastic lamina may be related to the circular rings of calcification that characterize Mönckeberg's sclerosis.

Tears in the internal elastic lamina of the anastomosed artery in experimental arteriovenous fistulae have been demonstrated by scanning electron microscopy within two days postoperatively in muscular arteries and generally by about five days in the elastic common carotid arteries [61,62]. The elastic tissue tears increase in frequency with time postoperatively such that in some regions of chronic fistulae, the internal elastic lamina is so fragmented that much of it appears functionally ineffective. The same must apply to many vessels with extensive tearing in the human. This is also the type of tear of the internal elastic lamina that initiates dissecting aneurysms of cerebral arteries [21]. Haemodynamic stresses have been implicated in similar spontaneous tears in the internal elastic lamina in the caudal and renal arteries of rats [116,117]. Tears in the rat caudal artery may be secondary to bending of the tail, since similar tears develop on the greater curvature of bends in human arteries [13] and also in experimentally fashioned U-bends in rabbits [51,52]. A propensity for stroke in spontaneously hypertensive rats was reported to be associated with frequent, early tears in the caudal artery. It was enhanced in a specific breed of rat, and also by the administration of a lathyrogenic agent [117]. This suggests that the propensity for elastic tears may be affected by hypertension, genetics and connective tissue disorders.

Similar elastic tears have been observed in experimentally fashioned arterial forks and opposite a longitudinal arteriotomy wound. Whilst it is natural that tears may be attributed to elastase activity, their very specific location in the fetus and neonate in the naturally occurring ilioumbilical arch [13] and experimental arterial bends [51,52] and in experimental arterial forks [63], suggests otherwise. This concept is supported by the absence of demonstrable elastase activity in the affected artery and also the dissimilarity of the tears to an internal elastic lamina incubated with elastase [118]. It has been suggested the tears are due to haemodynamically induced loss of tensile strength as is the case in post-stenotic dilatation, dissecting aneurysm, intimal tears and ulceration in atherosclerosis. The experimentally induced tears appear to be the result of the augmented haemodynamic stress but to regard them as adaptive in nature is inconsistent with their association with calcification, lipid deposition, mural atrophy, aneurysm formation and atherosclerosis [13,14]. These elastic tears have been regarded as the earliest demonstrable change in the atrophic lesion. Not only is the internal elastic lamina affected, but several elastic laminae in the media may also manifest tears and the underlying muscle in the media may be lost resulting in complete medial atrophy [52].

It has been alleged that these large tears or gaps in the internal elastic lamina [13] are adaptive in nature because the vessels are unable to continue to enlarge during growth and maturation due to limited distensibility even during intrauterine life. Such a concept ignores the specific location of these tears, and their absence in many other vessels until later in life. Moreover, they develop before there is significant alteration in calibre. They are also closely linked with haemodynamic stress even in the fetus and infant and occur first and most severely at the sharpest flexure of the carotid siphon.

The tears in the internal elastic lamina of humans appear long before the membrane edges exhibit calcification. Why calcification occurs in such fragmented elastic laminae is uncertain but possibly their altered physicochemical structure renders the elastin a more suitable substrate for mineralization than is otherwise the case. These defects commence appearing at 12–16 weeks of gestation [13] and similar arteries and even the aorta and pulmonary artery could be grossly affected in like manner. These latter vessels demonstrate they can continue to enlarge and the internal elastic lamina adjusts to the increase in calibre and length of the vessels as the infant grows. To attribute these changes to physiological adaptation is unreasonable. Yet the localization is attributed to haemodynamic stresses at those sites and it is difficult to see how such extensive loss of elastic tissue can be advantageous. Other tissues and organs have to adapt to such growth including the skin, skull and other vessels without their developing such defects. To allege such accommodation is necessary because of limited ability to distend and grow is conjectural and contrary to the present evidence.

The transverse wrinkling of the aortic surface in children and adults (Figure 6.2) may be indicative of the continued stress to which the arterial wall is subjected in infancy and in adult life. It is probably distinct from the tears in the elastic lamina. It is significant that relatively loose intimal proliferation has developed in the successive troughs as if in response to eddy currents as has been suggested for the pathogenesis of intimal proliferation at arterial forks [11].

The loss and fragmentation of the internal elastic lamina in the apical region of arterial forks sometimes with bending back of the edge as if by recoil (Figure 6.21) suggests that these elastic changes may be analogous to those at curvatures where the flux of blood impinges on the vessel wall. This is supported by tears occurring adjacent to the apical sutures in experimental arterial forks [63]. Moreover, lipid occurs in these areas of thinning in man. Whilst these elastic tears may proceed to atrophy, they can also develop a variable degree of intimal thickening with or without lipid.

6.2.15 INTIMAL PROLIFERATION AND ATHEROSCLEROSIS IN LOWER ANIMALS

Intimal proliferation has been demonstrated in the cerebral arteries of a number of species by serial histological sectioning and its localization and morphology are similar to those in humans though it usually is not so severe. In sheep [26], serial frozen sections revealed lipid entirely restricted to the intimal thickenings (pads) around forks (Figure 6.28). In general the intimal proliferation was not as advanced as in humans but more severe lesions were observed in an old horse and severe atherosclerosis in a chimpanzee (Figure 6.29) [20].

Extracranial arteries of lower animals have received limited study. The intimal proliferation at the first renal artery bifurcation is over the flow divider and tends to be thicker at the apex than in cerebral arteries [25]. Lateral thickenings were absent or minimal. These thickenings are sites of predilection for dietary-induced lipid deposition [25]. The localization of thickenings at

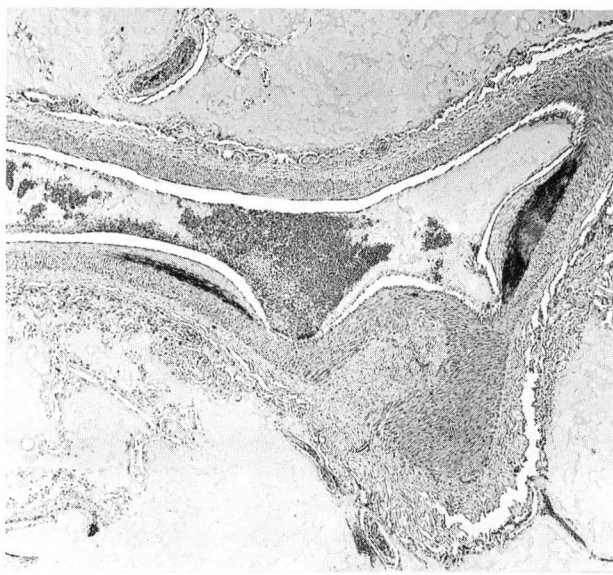

Figure 6.28 Frozen longitudinal section through a wide-angled cerebral arterial fork from a sheep displaying dark-staining lipid deep in the lateral pads. Flow is from below upwards. (Haematoxylin and fat stain.)

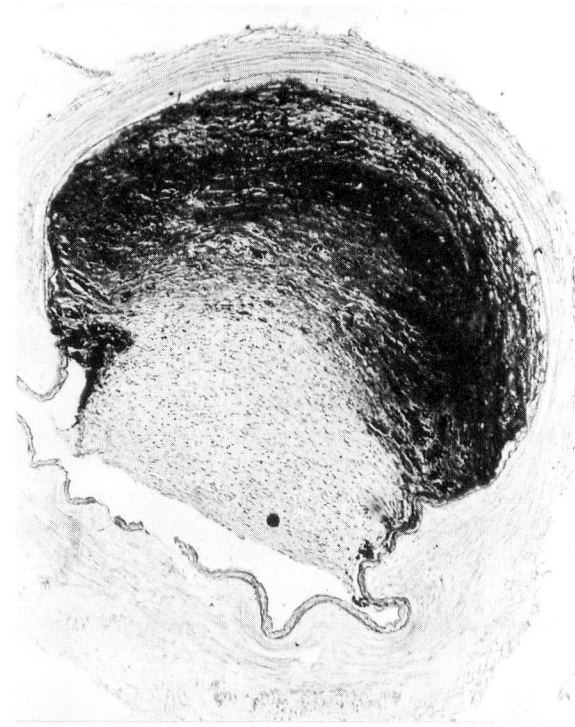

Figure 6.29 Frozen histological section of a middle cerebral artery from a female chimpanzee displaying a large plaque on one side of the vessel. The dark material deep in the intimal plaque is lipid. Note that the opposite wall has no thickening. The gaps in the internal elastic lamina are artefacts. (Haematoxylin and fat stain.) (Reproduced with permission from Stehbens [119].)

aortic branches is essentially similar although lateral thickenings if present are small. The apical thickening is considerably more extensive in the larger branch of asymmetrical bifurcations. In the rabbit the extended thickening from the apex along the dorsal surface of the aorta appears to be roughly triangular viewed *en face* and is the zone susceptible to dietary-induced lipid deposition.

Ultrastructure of intimal proliferation at the first major renal artery bifurcation in the rabbit revealed a deficient internal elastic lamina and degenerate and necrotic smooth muscle cells, granulovesicular cell debris derived from endothelium but predominantly from muscle, and discontinuous, multilaminated and redundant basement membranes about endothelial and muscle cells. Evidence of calcification was minimal. Though such intimal proliferation has been regarded as a 'normal' integral part of the arterial wall and is similar to that occurring in humans, it exhibits similar degenerative changes to those seen in intimal thickenings in human infants but not as severe as in overt atherosclerosis [27]. However, experimental production of a femoral fistula induced intimal thickenings at forks of afferent arteries to progress rapidly to overt atherosclerosis, thus indicating the important relationship of this intimal proliferation to atherogenesis [70].

The 'intimal injury hypothesis' [12] is acknowledgement of the early pathogenetic role of intimal proliferation in atherogenesis. If this is accepted then the intimal thickenings at arterial forks in lower animals are also atherosclerotic and it is the enlargement, extension and progression of these intimal thickenings that leads to the development of overt atherosclerosis in lower animals. The occurrence of atherosclerosis in lower animals including herbivores is not widely known and certainly is overlooked in deliberations on the aetiology of atherosclerosis. The occurrence of severe spontaneous atherosclerosis has been recognized in chimpanzees, gorillas and parrots for many years. It is also found in a milder form in a wide array of animals if sought. Due regard must be given to their lesser longevity and to the smaller calibre of vessels in many species, for such factors no doubt contribute to the reduced severity.

The occurrence of atherosclerosis in lower animals must be taken into account in experimental atherosclerosis because it indicates that reproduction of true atherosclerosis in an experimental animal has applicability to human disease and also that the experimental procedure might either aggravate or superimpose another disease such as a fat storage phenomenon on pre-existing atherosclerosis. For this reason care must be taken in interpreting the results of experimental procedures and in interpreting causality [5].

6.2.16 ENDOTHELIUM

The endothelium of the rabbit aorta consists of a single layer of flattened, elongated tear-shaped cells with oval nuclei [120]. The long axes of the cells and of the nuclei are usually arranged parallel to the direction of blood flow. This pattern, believed to prevail in most blood vessels, may be altered under certain circumstances and endothelial cells are not as elongated in veins. Along the crest of the flow divider in rabbits, endothelial cells are usually polygonal and at times there may be some unusual shaped cells with two or more nuclei. This pattern, similar to that in other animals, is thought to prevail in humans at least early in life.

This endothelial layer separates the blood from the artery wall and other tissues and was once believed to act virtually as a functionally inert semipermeable membrane. It is now known to provide a non-thrombogenic surface to the blood, the cells of which can produce quite an array of important pharmacological agents, vasoactive growth factors as well as fibrinolysin and basement membrane [121]. The endothelial cells are adherent to one another and to the underlying connective tissues and basement membrane when present [122], thus contributing to the cohesion of the constituents of the blood vessel walls. Myofibrillar bundles probably correspond to stress fibres in their cytoplasm no doubt participating in endothelial adhesion to their neighbours and subendothelial tissues [27].

Consistent with the imbibition concept of atherogenesis, the endothelium has been long considered as playing a pivotal role in the disease, either as the result of increased permeability, cell denudation or impaired antithrombogenic activity. It is wrong to suggest that any one cell (endothelial cell, monocyte or smooth muscle) is responsible for this disease which affects all the mural connective tissues both cellular and non-cellular even though the changes may be subtle and insidious.

Endothelial cells normally have a low turnover rate [123] compared to epithelium of the skin [124] or the intestinal tract [125]. Their usual life span, estimated to vary from 100 to 180 days, is only 60 to 120 days at arterial forks [126]. This is consistent with augmented mitotic activity in both the endothelium and medial muscle around aortic ostia [126–128]. There is no correlation with endothelial turnover and age in lower animals [128].

The augmented turnover of endothelial cells about orifices of branches occurs without denudation and even small injuries are rapidly endothelialized [129]. Whilst shear stress is often invoked as the cause of such cellular loss and other manifestations of atherosclerosis, pulsatile shear stresses much higher than previously held responsible do not denude the endothelial cells [130]. Davies et al. [131] have found that under conditions of unsteady flow similar to that observed in turbulent boundary layers, the mitotic activity increases considerably, which is consistent with a mechanical causation of such high turnover rates associated with spatial turbulent scales as small as individual cell dimensions [132]. Moreover, the shear stresses are very small compared with the pulse pressure.

Multinucleated and bizarre shaped giant cells are frequent in endothelial repair following experimental injury [133,134]. The augmented mitotic activity and giant cells at ostia of branches may reflect a similar response. They have also been observed in the human aorta with age [135]. It is unlikely that they are age-related since this atypical endothelial pattern does not occur uniformly throughout the vascular system nor in the pulmonary artery. It occurs where atherosclerosis is usually advanced as in the aorta and is now recognized as a manifestation of this disease rather than aging [136]. Similar changes have been observed in the region of the jet lesion of experimental arteriovenous shunts in rabbits [123] and random Häutchen preparations from the anastomosed veins of chronic (carotid-jugular) arteriovenous fistulae in sheep revealed a more extensive involvement similar to that of the human atherosclerotic aortic endothelium. Increased mitotic activity has also been demonstrated proximal to an experimental coarctation of the aorta [128].

Endothelial cells in atherosclerosis frequently exhibit increased organelle content as is consistent with augmented metabolic activity [137]. In the coronary arteries monocyte adhesion and penetration together with some endothelial cell loss and microthrombi were observed in advanced disease [138]. Endothelial denudation is also a manifestation of advanced disease.

Following a single experimental injury the abnormal endothelial pattern reverts to normal and the atypical pattern in atherosclerosis may indicate merely greater cellular turnover consequent upon the augmented stresses to which the endothelial cells are subjected. With increased intimal fragility in advanced atherosclerosis there may be impaired cohesion and adherence of endothelial cells. Also indicated is a persistent low-grade 'injury', for the cells would otherwise resume a conventional appearance. The low-grade injurious factor could well be haemodynamic stress [11] responsible for continuous augmented turnover of endothelial cells and smooth muscle cells of the intimal proliferation at branch sites.

Endothelial disruption occurs secondarily to transverse tears in the internal elastic lamina [139,140] but these are transient and initiate intense endothelial replication within the confines of the tear but not overlying the residual elastic remnants. It is possible that the replication may be stimulated by some elastin degradation product or perhaps more likely by alterations in the physical stresses acting on the endothelial cells. Curiously there is very little smooth muscle cell proliferation apparent despite the endothelial activity.

Proliferating endothelial cells are known to have enhanced permeability and this may correlate with the augmented mitotic activity about aortic ostia as the Evans blue technique demonstrates in the rabbit though what pertains in humans is unknown. However, increased permeability does not signify that nutrients filtering through to the extravascular tissue spaces and lymphatics will of necessity accumulate in the wall and thus lead to atherosclerosis. If this were the case, the topographical localization of atherosclerosis would differ from that prevailing in humans.

Of late, emphasis has been placed variously on the role of endothelial permeability in atherogenesis and on the production of various factors concerned with growth, mitogenic activity, endothelial relaxation, coagulation and shear stress. In addition endothelium-derived relaxant factor helps regulate muscular tone and endothelins have vasoconstrictor properties. Atherosclerosis is a chronic disease and it is inappropriate to assume causality or a pivotal role for any mediator or pharmacological activity demonstrated in short-term experiments and it is premature to speculate on the causal or major pathogenetic roles for cytokines, peptides, etc., that continue to appear in the literature. The control of the behaviour and functional activity of endothelial cells is probably a finely tuned balance of many pharmacokinetic activities of which we know relatively little at the present time.

Hyperlipoproteinaemia has been considered to be injurious to endothelium in the intimal injury hypothesis [12] but any endothelial disruption or increased permeability associated with that hyperlipaemic state is attributable to monocytic or lipophage penetration. There is also evidence that even endothelial denudation does not favour intimal proliferation [141]. It is unlikely that under physiological conditions normal metabolites damage endothelium or smooth muscle cells but if present in excessive quantities, massive storage may interfere with function. The effect of vibrational stress on endothelial cells [132] may be aggravated by lipid storage in lysosomes.

Beneath the endothelium a basement membrane develops when the intima thickens. Progressively with the development of the disease the basement membrane becomes many times thicker exhibiting a finely multilaminated appearance of relatively uniform thickness. It may incorporate small quantities of cell debris or a few collagen fibrils with areas of separation from the basal surface of the endothelium. It is not known whether this atypical basement membrane is the result of disturbed endothelial function or a concomitant change of atherogenesis.

6.2.17 SMOOTH MUSCLE CELL

The smooth muscle cell is the principal cell type in the media of all arteries and veins and also in intimal proliferation. It produces basement membrane, collagen, elastin, glycoproteins and proteoglycans. It can be phagocytic and the maintenance of vascular tone has been considered its main function but equally important is its role in producing the extracellular connective tissue proteins in response to injury and haemodynamic stress and in response to pathological changes in the vessel wall. Any consideration of its role in intimal thickening and atherosclerosis should take into account its role in endocardial thickening which may be an analogous but less severe phenomenon.

Smooth muscle cells in the vessel wall and in tissue culture exhibit different morphological appearances according to their functional state. They have been referred to as contractile and synthetic phenotypes. In the contractile state the cells, surrounded by a basement membrane, contain abundant myofibrils with relative paucity of centrally located organelles. When appropriately stimulated, muscle cells appear to decrease their content of myofibrils and to increase their content of rough endoplasmic reticulum and Golgi complex, thus assuming the synthetic state with little basement membrane. This physiological response to the need for replication and synthesis of extracellular matrix is similar to the response of endothelial cells and was originally referred to as 'undifferentiated' or 'dedifferentiated' muscle cells [142]. To regard these as different phenotypes seems to be a misuse of the term, for the cell is merely altered to increase its synthetic activity which it can seemingly accomplish at a lower rate of metabolic activity under normal circumstances in its so-called contractile form. It is acknowledged that these two states are interchangeable and not being permanent nor specific phenotypic manifestations of inherited morphological characteristics, they cannot be regarded as two distinct phenotypes any more than a pregnant woman is of a different phenotype when in the non-parous state.

Intimal smooth muscle cells proliferate in response to injury of many types and are considered responsible for the production of the extracellular matrix. Such intimal proliferation has been observed to follow morphological changes in the internal elastic lamina at bifurcations of cerebral arteries in a 26-week fetus. The elastic lamina usually shows evidence of disintegration beneath this proliferation, thought to be compensatory reparative intimal thickening; medial thinning has been observed beneath similar intimal thickenings in coronary arteries of infants [23]. Muscle cells in the intima are arranged longitudinally unlike their alignment following trauma. Ross [12], like many other authors, regarded this fibromusculoelastic intimal proliferation as a key event in the development of atherosclerosis as it precedes lipid deposition. He has also alleged that proliferation of intimal smooth muscle cells is the *sine qua non* of advanced atherosclerosis [143]. Others consider that lipid fulfils that role. However, the assumptions are erroneous pathologically for no one constituent of an atherosclerotic lesion can be considered as pathognomonic of atherosclerosis. The diagnosis depends on the method of inception, its morphology and the pathogenesis of the development of lesions and complications. Other diseases of the wall may have intimal proliferation without their being atherosclerotic.

In intimal thickening, the smooth muscle cell has been assumed to migrate from the media but it is difficult to accept that such a cell, invested by a distinct basement membrane with its attachments and anchorage to other cells and connective tissues in the matrix, can migrate. It is possible that isolated muscle cells may exist in the intima from fetal life or there may be migration in the synthetic phase but as yet migration across or through the internal elastic lamina has not been proven.

Stimulation of smooth muscle cells to proliferate by growth factors especially platelet-derived growth factor (PDGF) is an integral aspect of the 'intimal injury hypothesis'. However, the finding of one or other mediator in the whole process of atherogenesis cannot be as crucial in the aetiology and pathogenesis of the disease as the hypothesis suggests, for it is non-specific in its effect and only one of many mediators and pharmacological agents participating at every stage of atherogenesis. It is now known that the smooth muscle cell secretes other growth regulatory substances that can stimulate the muscle cells themselves as well as other cells in the neighbourhood [143]. This greatly diminishes the importance of the intimal injury hypothesis. Moreover, it must always be kept in mind just how slow under normal circumstances the progressive development of the lesions really is.

It has been said that lipid does not accumulate in smooth muscle cells in atherosclerosis as is observed in the cholesterol-fed animal, the Watanabe hypercholesterolaemic rabbit and familial hypercholesterolaemia (FH) [144]. This is not so, because lipid occurs in muscle cells of the fatty streak but is usually not prominent in advanced atherosclerosis and is not the dominant feature as in fat-storage lesions of the above disorders. In atherosclerosis the lesion is usually much less cellular. The lipid droplets are usually observed in lysosomes at the poles of the nuclei with myofibrils adjacent to the plasma membrane.

Lysosomes in vascular smooth muscle cells are capable of accumulating and hydrolysing ingested lipid [145, 146]. The smooth muscle cell can pinocytose lipoproteins and like most other cell types, has also been shown to phagocytose larger particles [147]. The early lipid in intimal smooth muscle cells may be the result of phagocytosis of matrix vesicles and there is evidence that this occurs [88,148]. Since 20% of the dry weight of a cell consists of lipid, the lysosomal digestion of such cellular debris could account for the intracellular lipid seen in the fatty streak and in the fetal intima [13]. It has been thought that intimal foam cells were derived from smooth muscle cells but it is now acknowledged that most foam cells by far are monocytic in origin. There has not been adequate differentiation of the role of these two cell types in lipid accumulation in atherogenesis. With the progressive accumulation of matrix vesicles, fat-containing matrix vesicles or debris, and the ensuing appearance of increasing amounts of extracellular fat, monocytes accumulate and dominate phagocytic activity.

Lipid-containing smooth muscle cells are not a prominent feature in advanced atherosclerosis. They are a feature of intimal proliferation in the early lesion and of the innermost media in more advanced lesions but not of extravascular smooth muscle cells. In FH, lipid within intimal smooth muscle cells is particularly pronounced at the site of the lesions and also in muscle cells in the neighbouring media, to such an extent that the cells are so distended as to appear hydropic in non-frozen sections. Yet despite extreme hypercholesterolaemia, only some smooth muscle cells are so affected in the blood vessels and no extravascular muscle cells are involved suggesting that some alteration is necessary to induce the above susceptibility.

In view of the degeneration and disintegration of endothelial and smooth muscle cells and even red cells occasioned by haemodynamic vibrational stress, it is likely that lipid-laden cells, especially large foam cells, will be even more susceptible to such degenerative change and necrosis. The presence of aggregates of lipid-laden cells may be mechanically disadvantageous in the absence of a protective matrix and mutual attachments.

In atherogenesis smooth muscle cells in the intima often become attenuated or assume atypical branching profiles in electron micrographs and their functional competence at that stage must be questioned. These changes in the smooth muscle cells are not observed in smooth muscle cells elsewhere in the body, nor in veins unless induced to do so surgically by the production of a venous bypass, an arteriovenous fistula or an aneurysm. These changes are associated with progressive thickening and reduplication of the basement membrane and large reticulated or redundant folds of basement membrane material [29,30,105]. This characteristic dystrophic accumulation of basement membrane material has been largely ignored. It follows the contour of the muscle cell often with separation from the muscle cell over variable lengths of plasma membrane. Though the intima may be firm and will cut like an unripe pear as if very fibrous, the quantity of cross-striated collagen fibrils is surprisingly low and much of the hyaline intima appears to consist of dystrophic basement membrane. There is much type IV collagen in the basement membrane together with glycoproteins and proteoglycans and it would seem that rather than the quantitative changes in these constituents, the qualitative alterations may be responsible for the abundant dystrophic accumulation. Often embedded in the basement membrane material or even between it and the muscle cell is granulovesicular cell debris.

6.2.18 ANGIOCYTIC MATRIX VESICLES (CELL DEBRIS) AND LIPID ACCUMULATION

Small membrane-bound dense granules or vesicles of lesser density accumulate in the intimal matrix. They may be found in the neonatal cerebral arteries in intimal proliferation and are related to smooth muscle cells. They progressively accumulate about individual muscle cells, along the internal elastic lamina, in the media where they are less numerous and in small quantities about adventitial fibrocytes. They appear to originate primarily from smooth muscle cells, and to a lesser extent, endothelial cells. The vesicular bodies appear to be shed from the plasma membranes of muscle cells often in large numbers whilst the cell itself appears to remain viable. Budding or a reverse pinocytosis may account for some but it seems more likely that the plasma membrane becomes fragile. Fractured plasma membranes have been observed in experimental rabbit aneurysms, possibly with leakage of cytoplasm but vesicles and plasma membrane fragments of different length can be found nearby or in the basement membrane material and matrix [88]. The same mechanism may pertain in human atherosclerosis and yet they have been virtually neglected in atherosclerosis research. In some instances, whole muscle cells disintegrate into a myriad of membrane-bound vesicles and debris. Some vesicles are extremely dense and are believed to be calcified [149] whilst others may contain fine dark apatite crystals. Calcospherites also appear but are not numerous.

Shedding of membranous material by living cells is not uncommon and shedding membrane-bound lipid droplets is the mode of apocrine secretion. As a reverse form of pinocytosis, many types of animal vesicles are budded off as membrane-bound vesicles from host cells, e.g. in the oocyst of *Plasmodium* [150] and in the periparasitic vacuoles of *Lankesterella hylae* [151]. It is pertinent that ultrasonic vibrations induce budding of cell fragments and spherical particles are characteristically associated with fatigue propagation in metal.

Similar vesicles are known to occur in cartilage, bone and dentine and have been labelled matrix vesicles which constitute a nidus for calcification. Chondrocytic matrix vesicles are believed to be lysosomal and form by budding. Their contents are uniformly dense and probably different from angiocytic matrix vesicles which appear to be merely debris, the result of granulovesicular degeneration. Matrix vesicles have been observed in the aortae of aging rats [152], the arteries of hypertensive animals [153,154], intimal thickenings at the main bifurcation of rabbit renal arteries [27], human cerebral arteries and berry aneurysms [29–31], arteriovenous fistulae [103] and experimental aneurysms [155]. They occur in intimal pads at arterial forks in neonates where they are unlikely to be the result of age *per se*. Their ready production in large quantities in haemodynamically stressed blood vessel walls suggests they result from such stresses [11].

Angiocytic matrix vesicles have also been considered to be lysosomal by virtue of their positive reaction for acid phosphatase and β-N-acetylglucosaminidase [156,157] and to be possibly responsible for abnormal collagen fibrils in blood vessel walls. Whilst some may be lysosomal by virtue of disintegration of smooth muscle cells, there is little doubt that most of the vesicular and membranous fragments are merely cell debris [11,88].

The concept of fragility of plasma membranes with the production of matrix vesicles or cell debris is consistent with the greater endothelial and smooth muscle cell turnover at branching sites. These regions are prone to medial thinning, the accumulation of matrix vesicles and atherosclerosis. The development of such vesicular structures and cell debris is also enhanced by hypertension and experimental conditions in which there are severe flow disturbances associated with intense vibratory activity (aneurysms and arteriovenous fistulae). Such observations are consistent with the findings that:

1. endothelial cells are more prone to disintegration by vibrations than shear stress [131];
2. the life span of erythrocytes (with haemolysis) is shortened in the presence of mitral stenosis and an arteriovenous fistula while closure of the fistula is associated with lengthening of the life span;
3. there is a mild haemolytic anaemia associated with hypertension, severe exercise and the marathon;
4. the explanation of the essential complications of atherosclerosis deriving from the basis of loss of tensile strength of the vessel wall is plausible.

The ends of mechanically disrupted red cell plasma membrane fragments are known to reunite to form vesicles, sometimes these are inside-out vesicles and others are right-side out [158]. Such a phenomenon may occur with smooth muscle cell membrane fragments and account for the differing behaviour of the vesicles which exist in a well oxygenated tissue fluid. In atherosclerosis these vesicles progressively accumulate in massive quantities but fail to undergo phagocytosis. Nowhere else in the body is there such an accumulation in the apparent absence of adequate phagocytic activity and resolution despite smooth muscle cells being found in

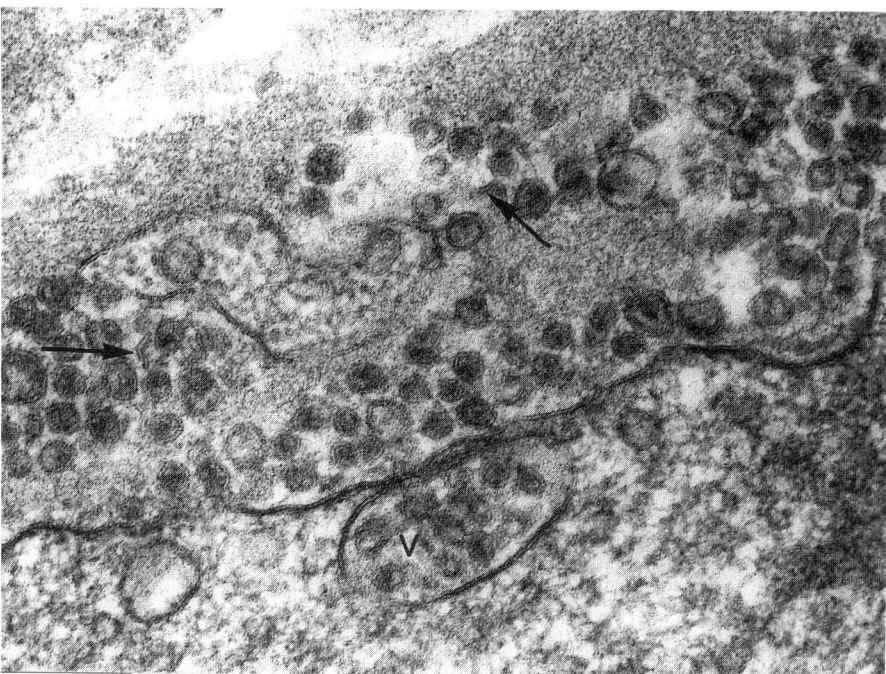

Figure 6.30 Matrix vesicles are membrane-bound blebs of cytoplasm in the intimal matrix. A smooth muscle cell below contains a vacuole (V) with matrix vesicles within suggesting phagocytosis. Note fragments of plasma membrane (arrows).

many sites and organs. Their concentration in the intima and to a lesser extent in the media and adventitia is consistent with the concept that phagocytosis in the inner part of the arterial wall is inadequate and becomes progressively more so. In experimental rabbit aneurysms these vesicles have been found in vacuoles within smooth muscle cells and also in plasma membrane pits or invaginations as if in the process of being phagocytosed [88]. Though not a prominent feature, this may account for some intralysosomal lipid in smooth muscle cells in the aortae of young humans and some early lipid deposition in haemodynamically induced lipid accumulation in rabbits (Figure 6.30) [70]. Inevitably with further disintegration of muscle cells the debris continues to accumulate and monocytic infiltration through the endothelium leads to phagocytosis of debris and lipid in the interstitial matrix.

Injection of lipid from the vessel wall into experimental animals immediately stimulates an active cellular response and phagocytosis of the lipid debris. A similar event occurs in man when atheromatous debris herniates into the adventitia only to become surrounded by a wall of lipophages and yet lipid and debris accumulate in massive quantities within the atherosclerotic intima with relatively little response. Even some intimal cells which appear to contain lipid and would normally be interpreted as a lipophage have been found ultrastructurally to be cells that have disintegrated into vesicles containing lipid while still within the investing basement membrane material. This diminished phagocytic activity contrasts with the clearance of lipid and cell debris in thrombosed atherosclerotic arteries and of atheromatous emboli from the circulation, the exception being cholesterol crystals.

The source of lipid in the intima and media has long been unexplained but for decades pathologists have taught students that unphagocytosed cell debris has an affinity for lipid and mineralization. This is seen in many chronic inflammatory disorders such as tuberculosis, old unorganized infarcts (Figure 12.11, p. 449) or haematomas; hypercholesterolaemia and hypercalcaemia are not essential. The abundance of cell debris in the vessel wall has been ignored for the last twenty years but in atherosclerosis of cerebral arteries the appearance of lipid histologically corresponds with the transformation of matrix vesicles to enlarged membrane-bound vesicles with electron translucent contents [29,31]. These enlarge and form conglomerates simultaneously with the disappearance of matrix vesicles from that area (Figure 6.31). It has been postulated that the non-specific affinity of this cell debris for lipid, possibly due to continued but uncontrolled activity or function of the cytoplasmic fragments, is the mechanism by which lipid accumulates in the interstitium of the blood vessel wall [31]. A similar phenomenon was described for the anastomosed vein of experimental arteriovenous fistulae in sheep [159].

In the imbibition theory of atherosclerosis, the so-called loosening of the ground substance is allegedly the site of lipid imbibition or infiltration. It occurs at orifices

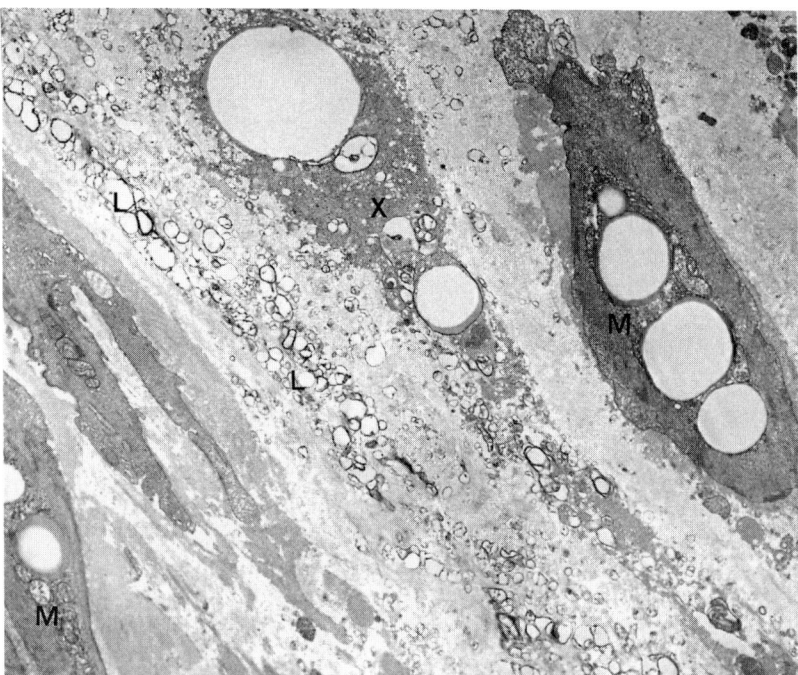

Figure 6.31 Atherosclerotic intima of human middle cerebral artery displaying lysosomal lipid in smooth muscle cells (M), much extracellular lipid (L) and the necrotic remnants of a smooth muscle cell (X) in which some debris is accumulating lipid.

of aortic branches, but such areas of increased intercellular space are zones where there is much cellular debris, presumably where muscle cells have undergone granulovesicular degeneration. The lipid hypothesis does not adequately explain this phenomenon which occurs in herbivorous animals (rabbits and sheep) with serum cholesterol levels below 100 mg/dl as well as ubiquitously in human infants without any suggestion of hyperlipidaemia. This concept is also consistent with the view that lipid accumulation is a late manifestation of atherosclerosis. Moreover isolation of lipid from atherosclerotic intima has revealed spherical particles that appear to correspond to these structures [160]. Chondrocytic matrix vesicles have an affinity for calcification in particular but also accumulate lipid [161]. Yet isolated matrix vesicles have no capacity for synthesis of lipids [162]. Why some angiocytic vesicles accumulate predominantly lipid and others become mineralized is unknown but could depend on the source of the membranes. With further disintegration of the matrix of the vessel wall and loss of cohesion of the mural connective tissues, it is not surprising that muscle cells continue to disintegrate. Monocytes, lipophages and giant cells with no protective coat of basement membrane must also undergo granulovesicular degeneration. Consequently intracellular lipid adds to the atheromatous debris, a vicious cycle becoming established. Lipid clearance from the vessel wall is then even less likely given the slow, inexorable progression of the disease. The need for postulating a metabolic disorder of lipids has not become established [163].

The deposition of neutral fat, phospholipid and cholesterol occurs in chronic inflammatory areas and degenerated tissues and appears to be a non-specific reaction to cell debris which has similarities to the lipid accumulation in atherosclerosis. Experimental bacterial pneumonitis in cholesterol-fed rabbits is characterized by preferential lipid deposition in large quantities in the inflammatory zone. The lesions are similar to the endogenous lipid pneumonia of man and to other xanthomatous reactions [164,165] but hyperlipidaemia is not essential for the development of atherosclerosis in rabbits or humans. In the rabbit, hypercholesterolaemia accentuates the lipid accumulation. In humans, it is uncertain whether or not hypercholesterolaemia augments the lipid accumulation in cell debris. It is not valid to extrapolate from rabbits to humans because the former are notorious for their inability to cope with cholesterol whereas humans cope exceedingly well. In homozygous familial hypercholesterolaemia, the lipid accumulation does not appear to have a predilection for intimal thickenings at arterial forks for some intimal pads (or cushions) were unaffected in the fatal case of a young boy [166]. Even if hypercholesterolaemia in humans accentuates lipid accumulation of atherosclerosis, which is yet to be demonstrated, it would act primarily as an aggravating factor with lipid storage superimposed on atherosclerosis.

6.2.19 LOCALIZATION OF EVANS BLUE

Evans blue (T-1824) forms a dye–protein complex with serum albumin and is often used as an intravital stain or marker of regions of increased endothelial permeability. When used in experimental animals its distribution in aortae is similar to that of dietary-induced lipid deposition as it occurs about the ostia of the aortic branches, on the lesser curvature of the aorta and about the sinuses of Valsalva [167]. The staining is a faint bluish tinge not being as well defined as the macroscopic staining of lipid deposits in the rabbit. Histologically, an occasional leucocyte has been found beneath or closely related to the endothelium and a platelet or small quantity of fibrin on the surface. Somer and Schwartz [168] demonstrated that the maximal uptake of isotope-labelled cholesterol about the fork correlated well with Evans blue staining. This localization suggests the possibility of haemodynamically induced alterations to endothelium and endothelial cell turnover is unduly high in such regions. In experimental coarctation of the aorta the dye uptake was increased proximal to the coarctation and decreased distally except for the jet lesion [169] suggesting that hypertension has a positive effect. What happens in humans is uncertain but in experimental arteriovenous fistulae and saccular aneurysms the dye uptake was augmented where proliferative lesions resembling human atherosclerosis occurred [170].

6.2.20 MATRIX PROTEINS (IN THE BLOOD VESSEL WALL)

In major blood vessels of mature animals, the turnover rate of collagen and elastin, the two major fibrous proteins basically responsible for the strength of the blood vessel walls, is low. Together with the cellular constituents, proteoglycans and other proteins in lesser quantity, they provide for the physiological requirements of blood vessels. The viscoelastic properties dampen the continuous and repetitive stresses to which the vessels are subjected.

(a) Elastin

Progressive degeneration and loss of elastic tissue is offset early in life by elastic tissue proliferation in compensatory intimal thickening but by middle age there is progressive, severe loss of elastic tissue histologically. Little is known of its qualitative changes. This is particularly pronounced in aneurysmal dilatation whether in the post-stenotic area, in a fusiform or berry aneurysm or even in an experimental aneurysmal sac formed by the autogenous venous pouch technique. One of the most interesting recent observations is the readiness with which transversely orientated splits in the arterial internal elastic lamina can be induced experimentally within two to five days postoperatively merely by producing an arteriovenous fistula or a sharp curvature [51,61,62]. The evidence is that these are mechanically rather than enzymatically produced [118] although the latter cannot be totally excluded. The possibility of demonstrating biochemical or physicochemical changes in the elastic lamina prior to or even at the time of the tear due to elastic tissue fragility seems remote at the present time. The thinning and the lacy appearance or even disruption of the internal elastic lamina that is thought to precede or occur concomitantly with intimal proliferation at arterial forks [18], though a slower less abrupt change in the lamina, is still a manifestation of loss of tensile strength.

The formation of lysyl-derived crosslinks following elastin synthesis makes the elastin relatively insoluble and resistant to most proteases [171]. Such elastin is usually only solubilized after cleavage of peptide bonds by either chemical or enzymatic procedures [172]. The elastic tissue in the anastomosed veins of experimental arteriovenous fistulae exhibits increased saline solubility as the result of the degradation of the mature elastin, because the soluble fragments extracted in this way contain the pyridinium cross-links desmosine and isodesmosine [173,174]. These degradative changes in the elastin have been linked with gross vibrational activity of the wall associated with the arteriovenous shunt, this being the first example of haemodynamically induced saline solubility of vascular elastin. It has also been reported that saline-soluble elastin can be extracted from the human aorta and pulmonary arteries [175]. Since most of the saline-soluble degradation products of elastin *in vivo* may be washed away, only small quantities are available for study and elastin-derived peptides circulating in the blood are higher in atherosclerosis than control subjects [176]. However, an *in vitro* model needs to be developed whereby a saline suspension of arterial elastin can be subjected to highly disturbed flow for a protracted period of time. Such a model has the potential for determining the mechanism of flow-induced elastin molecular degradation (as with polymers), the vulnerable regions in the elastin molecule, the repetitive physical forces that are most effective in degrading the elastin and also ultimately a possible means of grading the degradative process *in vivo*, and of increasing its resilience.

Since the internal elastic lamina is fenestrated and usually exhibits loss, disruption or fragmentation in association with intimal proliferation, it is not plausible that the lamina is a barrier to macromolecules causing their retention in the intima with the subsequent development of atherosclerosis.

(b) Collagen

Collagen is the other major structural component of the blood vessel wall and the crossbanded fibrils of types I and III provide the major contribution to the tensile strength of the wall. Type I preponderates and type III progressively increases, though it declines slightly in advancing years. The increase of type IV collagen (a major component of basement membrane) correlates with the known increase in dystrophic basement membrane material so prominent in atherosclerosis ultrastructurally [29,30]. The distribution of types I and III varies with location within the vessel wall [171] and is affected by the progressive development of atherosclerosis that is such a feature of the human vascular system. There are lesser quantities of types V, VI and VIII but their significance is unknown, except that synthesis of type V in other tissues is associated with scar formation [178].

A problem that exists in any study of these fibrous proteins is that plaque content is usually compared with 'uninvolved' or 'non-lesion' areas of the intima, whereas histologically in the adult the entire intimal surface is affected to a varying degree.

The individual collagen fibrils in blood vessels do not represent a specific collagen type and in general adventitial fibrils, produced by fibroblasts presumably, are larger than those of the intima and media produced by smooth muscle cells. The mean fibril diameter in arteries of humans and other animals increases across the arterial wall from the intima to the adventitia with a strong inverse correlation between diameter and the total amount of glycosaminoglycans [179]. In general an increase in collagen fibril diameter parallels the increase in the potential density of intrafibrillar covalent crosslinks. Consequently the large fibrils are considered to have greater tensile strength than fibrils of small diameter [180]. If tissue is designed to be elastic and to withstand creep, then a reduction in collagen fibril diameter will effectively increase the surface area per unit mass of fibrils and thus enhance the probability of interfibrillar non-covalent crosslinks between collagen fibrils and other matrix components [180]. However, the mean fibril diameter is not the only parameter reflecting tensile strength.

In a variety of inherited connective tissue disorders in humans and other animals, abnormal fibrils that are non-circular in cross-section are found ultrastructurally. These fibrils of abnormal shape are associated with increased saline solubility of collagen and reduced tensile strength of the tissue. This is seen particularly in the Ehlers–Danlos syndrome type IV which is associated with profound acquired fragility of blood vessels not apparent at birth. It would seem that such vascular collagen is more susceptible to the stresses of arterial blood flow than is the case in other subjects.

Dystrophic arrangement of collagen fibrils has been observed in the atherosclerotic intima of human cerebral arteries [29] and abnormally shaped fibrils have been described in a variety of small blood vessels from rats and humans and in diabetic angiopathy and varicose veins [157,181]. These changes have been considered as possibly due to lysosomal enzymes associated with matrix vesicles [157,181] since the combination has been regarded as medial dysplasia but a mechanical explanation for the occurrence of both seems more plausible.

Similar abnormally shaped collagen fibrils have been observed in the intima of experimental aneurysms of rabbits and sheep, and in the veins of experimental arteriovenous fistulae in sheep, conditions that are associated with proliferative lesions, similar histologically and ultrastructurally to human atherosclerosis [166,182]. Collagen fibrils in intimal proliferation exhibit greater variability being in general smaller than in controls but in addition there are fibrils that appear to be disintegrating, or coalescing with adjacent fibrils to form quite large bizarre shapes (Figure 6.32). Similar changes have also been demonstrated in human atherosclerotic intima. When in association with other degenerative changes in the intima, it is likely that they too are degenerative and non-specific, produced by haemodynamic stresses and possibly indicative of loss of tensile strength. The concept is consistent with reports of increased saline solubility of collagen in human atherosclerosis [175] and in the anastomosed veins of arteriovenous fistulae in sheep [183]. These acquired dystrophic changes in collagen and the elastic tissue degenerative changes could well contribute to the intimal fragility responsible for intimal tears, ulceration and aneurysm formation. The probability is that these ultrastructural changes may be quite advanced and more subtle biochemical changes should be sought at an earlier stage especially about the forks in fetal and neonatal arteries.

The inter-relationship of inherited connective tissue disorders and atherosclerosis requires serious consideration in view of:

1. the frequency of ectasia, tortuosity, aneurysms, dissecting aneurysms and arteriovenous fistulae in metabolic connective tissue diseases;
2. the close relationship of dissecting aneurysms of small arteries with thrombosis;
3. the genetic association with elastic tissue tears and their aggravation by lathyrism [116,117];
4. the association of the complications of atherosclerosis with acquired mural weakness.

In the past and the present the greatest emphasis in atherogenesis has been on the 'athero-' and cholesterol rather than on the 'sclerosis' and non-cellular connective tissue proteins. Concentrated study of the physico-

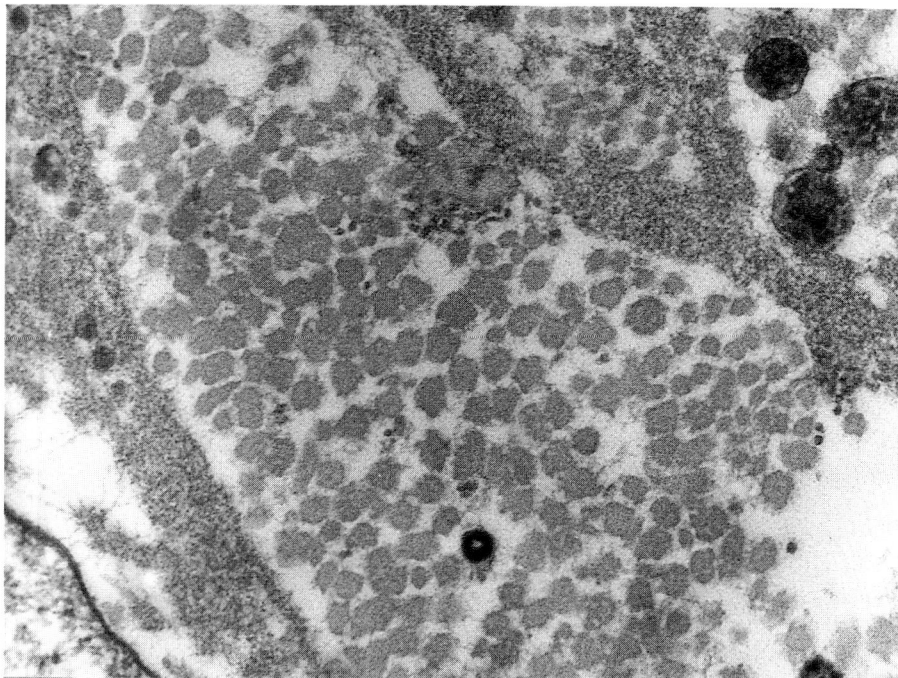

Figure 6.32 Electron micrograph of collagen fibrils from the intimal tissue of an experimental aneurysm in a rabbit. Note the variation in size and shape of collagen fibrils and the bizarre shapes in cross section. (Reproduced with permission from Stehbens and Martin [32].)

chemical nature of all the non-cellular constituents of the vessel wall and their qualitative and structural changes rather than merely quantitative alterations are long overdue.

(c) Proteoglycans

Proteoglycans are important constituents of the interstitial matrix and play a vital role in maintaining the structural integrity of normal blood vessels. They are thought to be concerned with the regulation of fibre formation and orientation during growth and repair, besides contributing to the important viscoelastic properties of the arterial wall. There are compositional alterations in atherosclerosis and much importance has been placed on the changes in polysaccharide components of proteoglycans (glycosaminoglycans) although findings have been conflicting. The evidence suggests that there is an elevation in glycosaminoglycans in the early proliferative stages but with a decline below normal values in severe atherosclerosis associated with extensive fibrosis and hyalinization. This is consistent with the paucity of metachromatic staining histologically in advanced acellular and hyalinized fibrotic lesions, whereas in the well established developmental lesions metachromasia is increased in the intima and at times especially in the media. However, there is little metachromatic staining in the very early intimal proliferation.

The findings in regard to individual glycosaminoglycans are less clear. There appears to be an increase of dermatan sulphate with increasing severity of atherosclerosis. Chondroitin-6-sulphate increases in the early stages but like heparan sulphate and hyaluronic acid declines in severe disease. Differences in the literature probably reflect the problems of defining stages of atherosclerosis and of appreciating the extensive involvement of the aortic intima even though it may be relatively smooth macroscopically. Increase in glycosaminoglycans has been reported in experimental aneurysms and veins of arteriovenous shunts [184], lesions exhibiting proliferative changes similar to atherosclerosis.

Whilst the emphasis on elastin, collagen and proteoglycans has been mostly with quantitative changes, the potentially more important qualitative changes require detailed study. The possibility of molecular scission due to repetitive stresses especially when under considerable tension warrants serious consideration, because as indicated above it may be the mechanism of elastin and collagen degradation. More recently defined protein constituents of the vessel wall (nidogen, laminin, fibronectin, etc.) no doubt also contribute to the cohesion of the mural constituents and their functional integrity is all important. There is little doubt that important cell–matrix interactions exist for the mutual benefit of individual constituents and the viscoelastic properties and strength of the wall as a whole with the smooth muscle cell being responsible for maintenance of wall tension as well as for the production of most of the extracellular matrix and its regulation.

6.2.21 INFLAMMATORY CELLS

Interest in the monocyte stemmed from the finding that early in dietary-induced hypercholesterolaemia in rabbits and rats, monocytes were found adhering to the endothelium and were held responsible for the intense foam cell infiltration of the intima that rapidly followed. In human atherosclerosis the monocyte has been accepted as the source of the lipid-laden macrophages (foam cells or lipophages) [185]. Subsequently monocytes, like many other cells, have been scrutinized for their biological activity, now being known to produce quite an array of pharmacologically active agents [185,186], including growth factors (platelet-derived growth factor, fibroblast growth factor, transforming growth factor-α), an angiogenic factor, an inhibitor of cell proliferation, interleukin-1, colony-stimulating factor-1, cachectin and several enzymes consistent with their macrophagocytic activity. They also give rise to foreign body giant cells which often surround or engulf cholesterol crystals. However, it is difficult to accept that monocytes by virtue of their presence in the intima and their many functional activities might be responsible for injuring endothelial and smooth muscle cells, the production of toxic oxidation products of lipids [185], contributing to caseation, destruction of collagen and elastin with aneurysm formation [186] and even for the initiation of intimal tears and ulceration [87]. The many functions of monocytes are intriguing but how they fit into the biological complexity of the control of cell and tissue functions within the vessel wall is beyond present-day knowledge and understanding. Assuming a causal role is unwarranted but assuming that a macrophage is pathogenic and will actively contribute to the development of the complications of atherosclerosis is biologically implausible and requires strong scientific evidence before it can be considered seriously. Whether enzymes are released in an active form on the death of macrophages or whether the enzymes are inactivated is uncertain but cannot be assumed.

Having confirmed that the plaque cap was weakened, requiring less stress for rupture than the neighbouring intima, Lendon *et al.* [87] demonstrated that the macrophage population was greater in the vicinity of the tear. Cause and effect was assumed and the weakening was attributed at least in part to enzymatic activity of the monocytes without causal evidence [86,87]. The possibility of the plaque cap being at a mechanical disadvantage has long been suggested [23] but the most likely cause of the mural weakness remains engineering fatigue.

Macrophages are found in many pathological conditions requiring repair and resolution of cell debris, but they are not attributed a causal role in infarction and chronic inflammatory or degenerative diseases. Monocytes are essentially scavenger cells and ultrastructural examination of human arteries has revealed plenty of cell debris requiring phagocytosis and clearance throughout life. Their inability to remove all such accumulated debris and their possible contribution to the cell debris when they too undergo vesiculogranular degeneration indicates a need to explain the underlying adverse environmental conditions and mechanism of cell disintegration, the enhanced turnover of endothelial and smooth muscle cells and the deficient phagocytic activity in the vessel wall.

Lymphocytes and plasma cells have long been known to accumulate in the intima in association with macrophages and possibly occasional giant cells as well as about adventitial vasa vasorum in advanced atherosclerosis. The lymphocytes have been identified as T cells with either cell type predominating from time to time. The pharmacokinetic activity of lymphocytes and plasma cells has been extensively investigated but the reason for their occurrence in atherosclerosis is unknown. They may be attracted to degenerative products of necrotic cells or degradation products of matrix proteins including elastin. Such substances might be antigenic but the presence of lymphocytes and plasma cells in response does not make atherosclerosis an inflammatory disorder. There is no evidence that these cells play any role in the early intimal proliferation or in the generation of tears of the internal elastic lamina. Their participation is essentially in advanced lesions, when they occur predominantly about vasa vasorum with no evidence of vasculitis of the adventitial vessels. Moreover, haemosiderin-laden macrophages may also aggregate about vasa vasorum if there has been extensive haemorrhage. Perivascular accumulation of these cells is non-specific and seen about the periphery of old organizing infarcts (Figure 12.11). As Parums [186] said, these inflammatory cells participate in the pathogenesis but not the aetiology of atherosclerosis.

6.2.22 PLATELETS AND GROWTH FACTORS

The prime function of platelets or thrombocytes is to be protective against haemorrhage when there is a deficit in the vessel wall and all the experimental evidence available indicates that they rarely adhere to normal endothelium [89,90]. Severe endothelial injury or a complete disruption of the non-thrombogenic endothelial layer as in intimal tears, ulceration or actual rupture is required for the production of a mural thrombus. It was thought that the platelet was pivotal in the initiation of musculo-elastic intimal proliferation (intimal injury hypothesis [188]) but discontinuities of the endothelium are now recognized as being late manifestations of atherosclerosis except possibly for tears of the internal elastic lamina.

The role of platelets in early atherogenesis is discussed elsewhere but the platelet is a source of growth factors, regulation of which no doubt is important in vascular repair, intimal proliferation and atherosclerosis.

Platelets are a source of a mitogen, the platelet-derived growth factor (PDGF) which is almost ubiquitous and capable of being produced by endothelium, monocytes and even smooth muscle cells. PDGF is also a chemoattractant for smooth muscle cells. Both monocytes and endothelial cells can produce transforming growth factor-β which can inhibit proliferation, induce cell differentiation and stimulate collagen and proteoglycan synthesis [143,185]. Though there may well be other agents participating in the cellular and matrix activity in the vessel wall, it is essential to remember these are but mediators of physiological and pathological processes of the vessel wall. To attribute a causal role in the aetiology is unwise. To suggest that inappropriate production of growth factors by endothelial cells, smooth muscle cells or monocytes [189] may be responsible for intimal proliferation is untenable in view of the independent development of atherosclerosis in different parts of the vascular system and the ubiquitous nature of such intimal proliferation in the animal kingdom.

6.2.23 VASA VASORUM

A prominent feature of vasa vasorum is their proliferation and extension into the thickened atherosclerotic wall even if none existed previously as in the cerebral arteries. Some venous vessels are often sinusoidal and may be seen macroscopically in the adventitia. If the wall is sufficiently thickened vessels penetrate into the intima as will occur in any proliferating tissue. Both undue emphasis on and a speculative role for these vessels in atherogenesis are unwarranted without evidence. Some such vessels may be damaged when the wall tears or splits as may occur in a weakened multilaminated structure causing haemorrhage but it is unlikely that such haemorrhage will be sufficient or under adequate pressure to cause obstruction of the parent lumen or a dissecting aneurysm.

6.2.24 ASSESSMENT OF SEVERITY OF ATHEROSCLEROSIS

Currently in epidemiology attempts are made at assessing progression or 'regression' of atherosclerosis to test the efficacy of some lipid-reducing substance. This has been widely tried angiographically but the silhouette reveals little about the qualitative or even quantitative changes in the arterial wall. More sophisticated echo ultrasonographic methods are now being used to measure the wall thickness or parts thereof and the lumen diameter. There are substantial errors in these techniques and when applied to small segments of vessels of small or medium calibre, it is being optimistic to suggest that such limited morphometric measurements can accurately assess progression of atherosclerosis in the arterial circulation as a whole or that they indicate the likelihood of intimal ulceration or tears and the formation of secondary thrombosis with or without occlusion and tertiary ischaemia.

The possibility is that the serum level of some degradation product of collagen or elastin or another matrix protein may be an indicator of the likelihood of an intimal tear occurring but this would still remain overall a crude indicator of progression rather than applying specifically to one site alone.

Morphological assessment or grading of the severity of atherosclerosis at autopsy is fraught with difficulties and is crude with variation in severity of grades difficult to assess after 60 years such that the suggestion has been made that the disease tends to stabilize in later life except in the cerebral circulation where it continues to progress [190].

Gross morphometric assessment of the area of intimal lipid staining is subject to variables including the limited penetrability of lipid stains through a fibrotic intima, and variations in the calibre and intimal area of the aorta or other vessels. Such measurements are concerned with crude estimates of the lipid content of the artery which does not necessarily correlate with the tendency to intimal tears etc., or to aneurysmal dilatation. To extrapolate to the aetiology of atherosclerosis from such studies is misleading.

It is important in the evolution of knowledge of atherogenesis to appreciate the limitations of these techniques and their overall significance. Neither should cause and effect be assumed as is common in epidemiological studies.

6.2.25 ASSOCIATED DISORDERS

The relationship of atherosclerosis to sex, senility and a variety of disorders and diseases must be considered as it may help to elucidate unanswered questions in atherogenesis.

(a) Sex

Atherosclerosis in pathological studies is similar in males and females but the development or progression of the disease in females tends to lag behind the male by about ten years. After the menopause there is said to be little difference but distinguishing between varying grades of end-stage disease is difficult and of limited value [190]. Whilst the obvious explanation resorted to is hormonal differences, it is well to remember physical differences in stature, body build, muscular development, physical activity and strength, all of which account for variation in vascular work load. The male heart and the diameter of coronary arteries are greater than those of the female and this being true for many other arteries, can affect atherogenesis.

There are unusual effects of blood vessels in females including spider naevi and arteriovenous shunts [11,191] and symptoms in Ehlers–Danlos syndrome are allegedly worse during menstruation [192]. Whether or not steroid hormones aggravate the laxity of connective tissues or impair healing is not known but if there is an effect, its elucidation would be of interest.

(b) Genetics

In considering this topic, the genetics of familial hypercholesterolaemia (FH) is usually discussed but this genetic disease applies to only a small minority of the population and clinically and pathologically is quite distinct. The same applies to hyperlipoproteinaemia type III. Whilst coronary heart disease (CHD) is unfortunately used synonymously with atherosclerosis, genetic factors in CHD may apply to atherosclerosis but may also be implicated in many secondary or tertiary factors that influence the likelihood of an intimal tear, the secondary thromboembolic phenomena and the tertiary cardiac and haemodynamic factors that ultimately help to determine clinical CHD and its outcome.

It is important to determine the role of genetic factors in atherosclerosis, particularly whether or not there is an inherited predisposition to the development of severe atherosclerosis and what factors influence its pathogenesis. In epidemiology, national and racial differences have been attributed to environmental rather than genetic factors, although a history of CHD is said to be an important risk factor. However, the validity of such data and interpretations of results is questionable [163] and indeed adequate differentiation between inherited genetic traits and environmental factors is not always possible.

Genetic factors appear to determine blood cholesterol, blood pressure, blood sugar levels, body build and obesity. FH is unduly represented in CHD clinically [161]. A genetic relationship exists in hypertension but it is much more difficult to determine a genetic influence with the severity of atherosclerosis. In so far as each person's biochemistry is probably individualistic like their DNA fingerprints and sebaceous secretions, genetic factors are probably determinants of protein, carbohydrate and lipid metabolism which ultimately determine the susceptibility and responses of the tissues in atherogenesis. Some indirect evidence exists in the association of thromboembolic disorders including coronary occlusion and myocardial infarction with blood group A. By contrast, subjects with group O allegedly have some measure of protection against myocardial infarction [194]. When, however, the relationship of blood groups to thrombosis was studied, no such relationship existed [195]. Nevertheless it seems on theoretical grounds that genetics must play a major but multigenic role in atherogenesis. It has been suggested that this is particularly likely in respect of connective tissue proteins and their resilience to stress [11]. The possibility of *formes frustes* of the connective tissue disturbances is a field not yet explored but the enhanced disintegration of elastic tissue in copper-deficient swine [196] and in experimental lathyrism [117] supports this view. By the application of molecular genetics lipid storage diseases can be produced in transgenic mice. Such models may be of value in the long term for subjects with FH or other lipid dystrophies with a propensity for CHD but are unlikely to offer much promise for the more than 99% of the population that does not possess such genetic defects of lipid metabolism or in elucidating the pathogenesis of vascular fragility underlying thromboembolism and aneurysmal dilatation.

(c) Hypertension

Hypertension is a clinical finding and not a specific disease and essential hypertension means only that the cause of the elevated blood pressure is unknown. Actuarial figures indicate that hypotension is associated with longevity, and elevation of blood pressure above the mean for sex and age with increased mortality. Epidemiologically it is recognized as being associated with an increased incidence of CHD and pathologically it has long been recognized as aggravating the severity of atherosclerosis whether it is in the systemic, pulmonary or venous circulation. It was once said that approximately 20 years of hypertension are necessary before the vascular effects of hypertension are manifest and it is therefore of interest that subjects with untreated aortic coarctation have a lifespan of little more than 20 years. Victims of this disorder develop severe atherosclerosis of the coronary and cerebral arteries in particular, and aneurysms of the proximal aorta and cerebral arteries (both fusiform and of the berry type) [37] are prevalent.

Atherosclerosis increases in severity with age but systolic, diastolic and pulse pressures also increase with age. Extractable lipid in coronary, cerebral and femoral arteries was related to the blood pressure levels [197] and a correlation between raised aortic lesions and the diastolic blood pressure has been found [198]. Much stress is given to the accentuation of lipid deposition in arteries of cholesterol-fed rabbits by hypertension. Emphasis recently has been on the systolic and pulse pressures but the diastolic pressure is also important. No sharp line of demarcation exists between normotension and hypertension and pressures increase with age particularly the systolic and pulse pressures. The accentuation of the pulse pressure in the abdominal aorta and large arteries of the lower limbs is associated with accentuation of the disease and the onset of hypertension is often preceded by a labile blood pressure. The effects of bouts of hypertension may be cumulative. Experimentally the synthesis of matrix fibrous proteins and proteoglycans is accentuated. Ross [185] recorded monocyte adherence and monocyte-derived macrophages in the intima in hypertensive rabbits in the absence of hypercholesterolaemia but this response may be associated with increased production of matrix vesicles or cell debris known to be increased by hypertension.

(d) Diabetes mellitus

Diabetes mellitus has an aggravating effect on atherosclerosis [199] and consequently diabetics have a high incidence of myocardial infarction, cerebrovascular insufficiency and severe peripheral vascular disease often with gangrene of the lower limbs. This association is often thought to be associated with hypercholesterolaemia which is less profound than in pre-insulin days when vascular and extravascular lipid storage was frequent [200]. Clinically, however, diabetes mellitus is commonly seen in association with hypertension and obesity. The fact that this chronic metabolic disorder affects lipid, carbohydrate and protein metabolism in every cell in the body, makes it unsurprising that a degenerative disease such as atherosclerosis is accentuated. The susceptibility to bacterial and mycotic infection is also manifest in this serious metabolic disorder and the thickened and multilaminated basement membranes in the microvasculature even in young prediabetics are similar to the early atherosclerotic changes in arteries. Weakness of the vessel wall is manifested in the retinal vessels since aneurysms of the retinal vasculature are common. The association therefore of diabetes mellitus with atherosclerosis may lie in metabolic susceptibility rather than blood lipid levels [201].

(e) Emotional stress

Coronary heart disease has often been attributed to a type A personality, seen in the conscientious individuals working unremittingly and under pressure and distinct from the converse, type B pattern. Friedman et al. [202] found that type A subjects succumbed to CHD six times more frequently than those of type B personality and that irrespective of the cause of death, coronary atherosclerosis was more severe in type A. However, type A subjects also had a slightly higher incidence of hyperlipoproteinaemia and hypertension [203]. Such observations are consistent with the long-held belief in a 'coronary personality' but the population cannot be divided into two personality types and there is difficulty in measuring emotional stress over a lifetime. Equally difficult would be measuring individual response to stress, which is probably determined genetically at least in part. Stress can also be environmental and familial. The quality of data from such studies would be too unreliable for scientific purposes. On theoretical grounds one might expect prolonged and recurrent emotional stress to affect atherosclerosis via the vasomotor system and its secondary haemodynamic effects but this remains conjectural at present although plausible.

(f) Immunological aspects

Perivascular round cell infiltration about vasa vasorum in advanced atherosclerosis may suggest an immunological reaction but as indicated this is a non-specific reaction and the result rather than the cause of the lesion.

It has been repeatedly demonstrated that trauma or injury of divers types predisposes the site of injury to dietary-induced lipid deposition. Immunologically induced injury of the vessel wall also enhances dietary-induced lipid deposition whether due to serum sickness or repeated administration of a foreign protein [204,205]. The vascular inflammatory lesions in serum sickness in rabbits occurred particularly at sites of branching and in the aortic arch (mostly in the aorta and large arteries) and corresponded to regions known to exhibit increased endothelial permeability to protein-bound dyes [206]. Since the localization of the immunologically mediated inflammatory lesions is dependent on increased permeability of the endothelium to the circulating antigen–antibody complexes, it is not surprising that lipid accumulation is enhanced at such sites. However, the inflammatory lesions in serum sickness also occur in veins but no lipid deposition is reported in the veins, suggesting that arterial haemodynamics governs immunologically enhanced lipid deposition in arteries. Moreover, such experimental evidence is not consistent with modified Koch's postulates for the experimental reproduction of atherosclerosis [144,207]. It must be concluded that the dietary-induced lipid deposition which is not atherosclerosis is either superimposed on or acts as a marker of immunological damage and that an inflammatory reaction is not a localizing factor or an early stage of atherosclerosis. Such experiments in cholesterol over-fed animals are not pertinent to atherosclerosis [5].

In transplantation, chronic rejection produces an obliterative intimal thickening of the arteries, degeneration of the media and even aneurysmal dilatation [208]. Lipid may be present such as in the coronary arteries but histologically the intimal change is unlike that of atherosclerosis. Similar obliterative proliferation of the intima of coronary arteries occurs in cardiac transplantation. Rapid development of severe 'atherosclerosis' of the coronary arteries and the mitral valve and a segment of the aorta was reported in a transplanted heart less than two years postoperatively [209]. Histologically the arteries revealed the presence of numerous plasma cells and lymphocytes with much lipid and little collagen. The recipient had hyperlipaemia which was held responsible for the unusual amount of lipid in the rejection changes and was regarded as typical of young adults with FH [210]. This subject probably had a lipid storage disorder and an immune reaction superimposed on atherosclerosis.

In general it is to be expected that the pathological changes of atherosclerosis are likely to be aggravated by a superimposed disease and the rejection phenomena in blood vessels should be regarded as such rather than merely as atherosclerosis. At present there is no sound evidence that immunological factors play an aetiological role in atherosclerosis although they may modify the course of atherosclerosis in individual cases.

(g) Virus-induced atherosclerosis

The introduction of the monocausal hypothesis by Benditt and Benditt [211] raised the possibility of the smooth muscle proliferation being due to a viral-induced mutant. This concept is now regarded as a transient digression but in the multicausal concept of atherogenesis in which many risk factors are believed to be unidentified, the possibility of a viral infection acting alone or in synergy with other factors has been entertained [212].

Infection of hypercholesterolaemic chickens with Marek's disease is not a valid model for human atherosclerosis [213]. Evidence of infection by cytomegalovirus has been considered to play a role [214] and this is common in subjects with acquired immune deficiency disease who frequently develop myocardial infarction and may have coronary lesions secondary to drug abusage. Currently little is known of viral arteritis which may be more common than is currently recognized but as with immunological damage to blood vessels, it is an aggravating factor and a second disease superimposed on the ongoing development of atherosclerosis. The detailed pathology and pathogenesis of ubiquitous atherosclerosis, its topography and complications cannot be explained by an infective process.

(h) Connective tissue disorders

In the development of complications of atherosclerosis it is apparent that connective tissue disorders associated with fragility of varying degrees could exert an adverse effect on the development of intimal tears, ulcerations, ectasia and aneurysms. A propensity to elastic tissue fragility could enhance the development of tears in the internal elastic lamina and accentuate elastic tissue degeneration and loss throughout the pathogenesis of the disease. The functional state of the vascular connective tissues is crucial in atherogenesis. It does not follow that lipid accumulation in the wall would be increased simultaneously for as explained earlier, the initial lipid accumulation appears to be related to matrix vesicle generation, whereas the fragility of the connective tissue disorders would affect the fibrous proteins (collagen and elastin particularly) and not the cellular elements of the wall.

In florid connective tissue disorders, ectasia, aneurysms, dissecting aneurysms and rupture may occur early in life. It is likely that there are *formes frustes* or varying grades of functional impairment due to subtle individual variation in connective tissue biochemistry. On the other hand there could be acquired deficiencies in the connective tissue such as copper deficiency, ascorbic acid deficiency, excess molybdenum intake and even those from drugs such as D-penicillamine. Diets obviating such detrimental effects would be beneficial.

(i) Homocystinuria

This inherited metabolic disorder is characterized by homocystine in the urine and systemic abnormalities of connective tissues. It is transmitted as an autosomal recessive and due to deficiency of cystathionine synthetase which synthesizes cystathionine from homocysteine and serine. The enzyme is normally present in the liver and brain but its absence or a low level of activity results in mental retardation, psychiatric disturbances, seizures, ectopia lentis, myopia, multiple skeletal deformities and a propensity for bone fractures. Some subjects have features of Marfan's syndrome [215].

Almost every artery and vein becomes severely narrowed by intimal proliferation and possibly thrombotic occlusion. The coronary and cerebral arteries are often involved and the aorta may be affected. Renal artery involvement may lead to hypertension which aggravates the lesions that are regarded as atherosclerotic or arteriosclerotic [215–217]. Detailed histological and ultrastructural studies of the vascular lesions are lacking but ectasia, aneurysms, mural calcifications, venous thromboses and varicose leg ulcers are frequent. The lesions do not appear to be rich in lipid and caseous lesions have not been illustrated. The pathogenesis of vascular lesions is not clear, but interference with collagen crosslinking is possibly involved and it is not surprising that in such a widespread metabolic disorder atherosclerosis is aggravated. It is likely, therefore, that the 'arteriosclerosis-like' changes are due to loss of tensile strength of collagen. Endothelial cells have been found circulating in the blood [218]. Intimal tears or endothelial denudation may lead to thrombotic events and there appears to be a platelet abnormality.

Rinehart and Greenberg [219] reported intimal proliferation in arteries of rhesus monkeys with experimental pyridoxine deficiency. The intimal thickening was similar to that in humans with accentuation of intimal thickenings at arterial forks. Elevation of endothelium was observed and the authors suggested that there must be some loss of cohesion of connective tissues. Patients with homocystinuria have responded favourably to pyridoxine (vitamin B_6) suggesting some relationship of collagen crosslinking to intimal proliferation may occur in other disorders with variation according to where the defect arises in the metabolic pathway.

Levene and Murray [220] have suggested that vitamin B_6 deficiency may be important in atherogenesis because lysyl oxidase, a copper-dependent enzyme responsible for crosslinking both collagen and elastin, is believed to be vitamin B_6 dependent. Such deficiency could interfere with normal functional integrity of collagen and elastin.

(j) Copper deficiency

This can result in neural and skeletal abnormalities, but in recent years cardiac and vascular fragility have been demonstrated in both pigs and chicks [221]. The mechanical weakness has been attributed to deficiency in crosslinking of collagen and to a lesser extent of elastin because of a deficiency of the copper-containing enzyme, lysyl oxidase. Deficient crosslinking of collagen and elastin is also manifest in lathyrism and therefore it is likely that lysyl oxidase may be inhibited by β-aminoproprionitrile (BAPN). Deficient intramolecular and intermolecular crosslinking of collagen follows administration of D-penicillamine and the resultant lesions are similar to osteolathyrism which can be ameliorated by administration of copper. Any factor causing mural weakness may potentiate the development of the complications of atherosclerosis. However, this potentially fruitful avenue of research has not been pursued.

(k) Menkes' kinky hair disease

Menkes' syndrome or kinky hair disease is an X-linked recessively inherited disorder resembling copper deficiency with no known cure. Victims usually die at an early age from functional copper deficiency and low activity of copper-dependent enzymes. The arteries exhibit precocious degenerative changes with elongation, tortuosity, aneurysmal dilatations, rupture, stenoses and areas of intimal proliferation and thrombosis. Elastic tissue degeneration is severe. The generalized nature of the connective tissue disorder is also indicated by the occurrence of emphysema, bladder diverticula and bone fractures. As in the case of homocystinuria, there has been inadequate investigation of the blood vessel wall, its ultrastructure, physicochemical characteristics and functional status especially of the connective tissues.

(l) Vitamin C

Symptoms of copper deficiency occur in sheep on pastures treated with excess molybdenum. The resulting molybdenosis manifests itself as a functional copper deficiency. Theoretically eating much mutton from sheep suffering from molybdenosis could enhance the development of atherosclerosis in humans. Sheep with molybdenosis develop subperiosteal haemorrhage and pathological fractures which are also manifestations of scurvy and it has been established that vitamin C is involved in collagen metabolism. Levene [222] reported a relationship between ascorbic acid and collagen crosslink stability indicating a possible benefit in atherosclerosis of an adequate vitamin C intake rather than the subnormal vitamin C level found in many hospitalized elderly cardiac, and even otherwise apparently well nourished subjects [223].

The serum cholesterol level is reduced in young 'healthy' individuals following vitamin C administration but in older subjects no consistent pattern was found [224]. In subjects with a history of the complications of atherosclerosis, its administration was associated with an elevation of serum cholesterol, allegedly due to the mobilization of arterial cholesterol for transport and disposal [225]. Irrespective of the effect of vitamin C on blood cholesterol, its relationship to atherosclerosis requires further investigation, particularly since scurvy is associated with vascular fragility, dilatation of small blood vessels, subperiosteal haemorrhages and an undoubted participation in collagen metabolism. This vitamin could well play a vital role in atherosclerosis and a latent deficiency may have a detrimental effect on atherogenesis. A relationship has been postulated between vitamin C and homocystinuria [226]. Furthermore its administration reduces the incidence of fractures in osteogenesis imperfecta, a disease considered to be due to defective collagen crosslinking [227].

(m) Imbalance of rare elements

Klevay [228] considered copper deficiency the most important contributor to CHD. Zinc deficiency is believed to interfere with intermolecular covalent crosslinking and selenium metabolism has also been incriminated in atherogenesis. Whilst they do not play a causal role, the possibility exists that in some individuals an imbalance of trace elements may be involved in its pathogenesis, but their role is uncertain.

(n) Effect of aging or senescence

The term 'aging' indicates changes occurring as a consequence of biological decline in functional activity (senescence) in the years after maturation and maximum reproductive activity. It encompasses changes accruing during the natural lifespan and biological decline. In man there is difficulty in determining which changes should be attributed specifically to senescence for many lesions associated with old age may be the cumulative effects of noxious agents or pathological lesions peculiar to that life period.

Many changes occur in blood vessels during life and become increasingly severe with age [11] but they are not necessarily features of senescence or indicative of any process of natural decline. Arteriosclerosis has been used to denote the progressive fibrosis or hardening of the arteries due in part to the relentless thickening of the intima and to a lesser extent to medial fibrosis. Longstanding controversy continues over the differentiation of arteriosclerosis in this sense and atherosclerosis, with no satisfactory means of differentiating between the two such that many authors have regarded them as synonymous.

Biochemical studies have revealed an increase in several constituents with age. For example the arteries exhibit a progressive increase in water content [230] and calcium. The intensity of calcium deposition is greater in the abdominal segment than in the thoracic and parallels the severity of atherosclerosis. The pulmonary artery exhibits less alteration with age [231]. The severity of calcific and elastic changes in arteries of the lower limbs has been correlated with atherosclerosis severity and mural tension [232]. Lansing [233] alleged the increase in calcification preceded the lipid deposition of atherosclerosis. These variations in calcification together with the heavy deposition in coronary arteries and lesser calcification of cerebral vessels suggest the relationship is with atherosclerosis rather than senescence.

The total lipid content of the vessel wall increases progressively with age as do cholesterol, phospholipids, lecithin and neutral fat but again such changes are related to the severity of atherosclerosis [234]. Histochemical changes also occur with age [109] and atherosclerosis severity increases with age. Biochemical changes associated with progressive atherosclerosis may mask the true changes of senescence.

When investigators refer to a normal aorta, they usually mean the neighbouring segment devoid of gross atherosclerosis but in all probability when assessed histologically or biochemically it is not free of disease either. The changes in connective tissue proteins, proteoglycans and even alterations in aortic elasticity or other physical characteristics [11] are likely to be the consequences of atherosclerosis at least in part. Comparison with the pulmonary arteries, veins and even extravascular connective tissues may reveal differences that preclude age effects. On the other hand atherosclerosis has been regarded as a disease of aging – the senescence theory of its aetiology. Individual variability, the unequal change within vessels and discrepancies in severity from vascular bed to vascular bed indicate that the changes are not aging phenomena and gradually the senescence theory has been discredited, the more telling argument being that atherosclerosis would be diffuse and uniform if merely an aging phenomenon. In recent years, the haemodynamic production of atherosclerosis and its complications in experimental animals and its development at an accelerated rate in coronary venous bypass grafts and therapeutic arteriovenous shunts indicate the disease is not due to senescence *per se*. Age is but a time factor and the disease progresses at different rates within individuals and from individual to individual. There are no changes in the blood vessel wall that are recognized as being due to senescence alone.

In two syndromes victims suffer from severe atherosclerosis and premature senility: progeria and Werner's syndrome.

(o) Progeria

Progeria (Hutchinson–Gilford syndrome) is a rare disease in which premature senility occurs in childhood. The subjects appear normal at birth but by one year of age, severe growth retardation becomes manifest typically with alopecia, loss of subcutaneous fat, muscular atrophy, a small face, beaked nose, receding chin, large cranium, exophthalmos, prominent scalp veins, sexual infantilism, a senile stance and arthritic deformities [235]. The skin appears aged, pigmented age spots are present and the voice is thin and high pitched. There is no evidence of mental retardation, nor of the tumours, cataracts and osteoporosis which are frequent manifestations of aging [236]. The disease is of low incidence in families and, as both members of monozygotic twins are affected, it is suggested that it is of genetic origin and at times due to a dominant trait [236,237], though it has been considered inherited as an autosomal recessive trait.

The average age of death is 12 years. Over 80% of deaths are due to CHD or congestive cardiac failure [236] which can occur as early as five years. The subjects are said to exhibit advanced aortic and coronary atherosclerosis. The cardiac valves may be calcified and atherosclerotic but insufficient pathological detail has been provided and illustrated. At least one case had a carotid artery aneurysm. Advanced arteriosclerosis has been recorded [238] and also hemiplegia. Though suspected, no endocrine disturbance has been established. The serum cholesterol is said to be elevated [239] but the prevalence and degree of elevation are unknown.

Osteoarthritis and atherosclerosis are both premature and severe. It seems likely that amongst other things there is also some connective tissue abnormality present in progeria and both diseases have features in common. The connective tissues of blood vessels and joints succumb to physiological stresses very early. Fibroblasts from progeric children exhibit diminished cell growth, mitotic activity, DNA synthesis and cloning efficiency [240]. As the disease appears to be more than merely a genetic defect of aging, much additional detail about the blood vessels and connective tissues is required. There is increased urinary excretion of hyaluronic acid and cultured cells have a high rate of synthesis of hyaluronic acid in both progeria and Werner's syndrome [236]: the significance of these observations is unknown. It is likely that these two diseases have reduced connective tissue endurance or response to physiological stresses, though this would not explain all their clinical manifestations.

Metageria, a rare syndrome intermediate between progeria and Werner's syndrome, is also associated with premature, severe atherosclerosis and diabetes mellitus.

(p) Werner's syndrome

This syndrome exhibits some features of premature aging and is due to an inherited autosomal recessive trait. A Libyan family with nine affected members has been reported [241]. It is rare with onset in the second decade. It is characterized by short stature, premature graying and whitening of the hair, alopecia, cataract formation, a sclerodermatous appearance of the skin, a high-pitched voice, peripheral muscular atrophy, poor wound-healing, chronic leg and ankle ulcers, hypogonadism or gonadal atrophy, soft-tissue calcification, osteoporosis and a high incidence of diabetes mellitus and other endocrine disturbances [236]. The heart is usually hypertrophied due to hypertension and there is a propensity for widespread premature vascular degeneration with vascular and cardiac calcification. Sclerosis of small renal arteries and arterioles was found in a 29-year-old male [242] but detail of the vascular pathology was limited. Premature atherosclerosis and arteriosclerosis have been alleged but since patients are usually hypertensive and death occurs in the fourth or fifth decade (409), atherosclerosis is inevitable. Widespread vascular calcification indicates that detailed analysis of the pathology of blood vessels and connective tissues is required. About 10% of afflicted subjects exhibit a predisposition to mesenchymal tumours particularly sarcomas and meningiomas [236,237].

6.3 Aetiology of atherosclerosis

The intention here is not to debate in detail the various theories proposed to explain the aetiology and pathogenesis of atherosclerosis but to present the main tenets of each hypothesis indicating briefly weaknesses, inconsistencies and the nature of the supporting evidence. Despite enormous expenditure of man hours, funds and experimental animals, there is no unanimity of opinion on the aetiology and pathogenesis which remain a rather bitter controversy.

6.3.1 LIPID HYPOTHESIS

The accumulation of caseous material and extensive calcification in advanced atherosclerosis have long intrigued pathologists and when the administration of large amounts of egg yolk or cholesterol to rabbits resulted in hypercholesterolaemia and lipid accumulation in the blood vessel wall, the lesions were regarded as atherosclerotic [243]. Interest in experimental calcification declined as the emphasis on lipids grew and anecdotal reports of severe atherosclerosis occurring in diseases with hypercholesterolaemia especially FH gave the theory further impetus [244]. For more than thirty years the lipid hypothesis has dominated practically all thinking and research into the aetiology of atherosclerosis which now accounts for almost half the total mortality in technologically advanced countries.

For the protagonists of the lipid hypothesis, the accumulation of histologically demonstrable lipid in the blood vessel wall, although only one of the manifestations, became the *sine qua non* of atherosclerosis. Some have suggested that cholesterol is the cause of atherosclerosis just as definitely as the tubercle bacillus is the cause of tuberculosis. Others have considered the disease to be a lipid metabolic disturbance manifested by an inability of the arterial wall to either adequately dispose of or metabolize lipid accumulated in the wall.

The theory essentially maintains that a high saturated fat/cholesterol diet causes an undue elevation of serum cholesterol or low density lipoprotein (LDL) levels which in turn enhances the development and progression of atherosclerosis and causes a high incidence of CHD, aided at times by several risk factors. Thus dietary saturated fat is considered the major environmental agent responsible for elevated serum lipids and severe atherosclerosis. This is now widely accepted and research has essentially focused on lipid metabolism in the belief that the source of the lipid and cholesterol in the atherosclerotic lesion must ultimately come from the blood and that blood lipid levels are affected by the diet.

The imbibition theory maintained that loosening of the connective tissues in the intima preceded imbibition or infiltration of lipid in such zones. Since hypercholesterolaemia in the rabbit and other experimental animals with or without induced hypothyroidism caused lipid-containing lesions in arteries and similar lesions occur in human FH, an elevated serum cholesterol level has been considered an important causative factor in humans. It became apparent that CHD occurred in a wide spectrum of the population, many of whom were not hyperlipidaemic according to the standard biochemical method of determining the normal reference range. Reasoning that the cholesterol level is abnormal if CHD develops, some have declared that there is no upper discrimination value [245] and that blood cholesterol is atherogenic at all blood levels.

Over the years, the accumulation of lipid in the blood vessel wall has been attributed variously to hypercholesterolaemia, altered permeability of the endothelium (which has even been assigned an unsubstantiated trapdoor effect), impenetrability of the internal elastic lamina, an affinity of proteoglycans for lipids, a metabolic disturbance of lipid metabolism in the intimal smooth muscle cells, or some impediment to removal or drainage. It has been accepted that accumulation of lipid in the wall leads to monocyte invasion with the production of foam cells and a fibrous tissue reaction. No specific local factor in the wall has been acknowledged as responsible for lipid accumulation except for augmented endothelial permeability about branching sites and augmented haemodynamic stress at bifurcations regarded by most investigators as a localizing factor. Caro and colleagues [246,247] attributed the localizing factor to low shear stress and Fry [248,249] believes high shear stress is responsible. Indeed, both high and low shear stress areas are affected and ultimately the entire wall. Subsequently there has been much emphasis on shear stress but the topography of the disease is inconsistent with these hypotheses [246–249].

The lipid hypothesis greatly stimulated lipid research and ultimately led to the discovery of defective low density lipoprotein (LDL) receptors in FH [250]. The association of homozygous FH with CHD is regarded as the strongest clinical evidence in support of a relationship between plasma cholesterol concentration and CHD.

Type III hyperlipoproteinaemia, diabetes mellitus, the nephrotic syndrome, hypothyroidism and obstructive jaundice have also been considered to provide evidence for the lipid hypothesis [244]. Secondary hyperlipoproteinaemias are being less emphasized in recent years, there being no scientific evidence for a detrimental effect on atherosclerosis.

Protagonists of the lipid theory appreciate that dietary fat or cholesterol and hypercholesterolaemia fail to explain all the features of atherosclerosis. For this reason an essential feature of the lipid hypothesis is the concept that all diseases have multiple causes and that atherosclerosis is due to a variable mix of causes in any one person. Epidemiologists prefer to use risk factor rather than cause but still use the terms interchangeably and thus for the most part atherosclerosis is regarded as due to a number of causes or risk factors acting concomitantly or synergistically. The risk factors however are for CHD and not atherosclerosis and currently almost 300 risk factors have been acknowledged [251].

In recent years investigators acknowledged a need to explain the pathogenesis of atherosclerosis in terms of major risk factors for CHD. This will be a difficult task because the role of hypercholesterolaemia remains controversial and the roles of hypertension and diabetes mellitus have not been explained except for a possible relationship to hypercholesterolaemia. Smoking is considered a strong risk factor for CHD but this does not indicate a cause and effect relationship. Inherited psychosocial stresses and personality type appear to be important in atherogenesis with haemodynamic responses to these stresses secondarily influencing disease development.

After studying twins Lundman [252] concluded from postexercise electrocardiography that smoking probably had little or no effect on CHD and that a significant genetic component was evident. Monozygotic twin studies have revealed a strong hereditary input and the possibility that CHD in smokers may be largely due to constitutional differences between smokers and non-smokers rather than to smoking *per se* [253,254].

The role of smoking in CHD and atherosclerosis, if any, is obscure. Evidence suggests that it may block amino acid crosslinking of elastin and thereby reduce its tensile strength [255] but that action is *in vitro*. Alternatively active pharmacological agents absorbed from smoke may enhance cardiac irritability in patients with moderate to severe coronary atherosclerosis and thereby precipitate sudden fatal dysrhythmia. The possibility of some smoking products inducing an immunological reaction cannot be excluded but it can only be an aggravating factor. There is no conclusive evidence of a deleterious effect specifically on atherosclerosis and smoking is not an accepted risk factor for cerebrovascular disease.

The basic evidence for support of the lipid hypothesis rests on the cholesterol-fed animal, FH and associated disorders and epidemiological evidence.

(a) The cholesterol-fed animal

It has been stated that an increased intake of cholesterol and fat is an absolute prerequisite for the experimental production of severe atherosclerosis [256] and the lipid-containing lesions resulting from overloading the animal with cholesterol and fat are regarded as atherosclerotic.

Atherosclerosis presents a varied picture but the overall appearance, including the pathogenesis of the lesions, determines whether or not experimental lesions are truly atherosclerotic. The presence of fat or calcium or any other known individual constituent does not justify the diagnosis of atherosclerosis. In the rabbit, extreme hypercholesterolaemia develops preceding the lipid deposition in the blood vessels which has a predilection for the intimal proliferation of arterial forks.

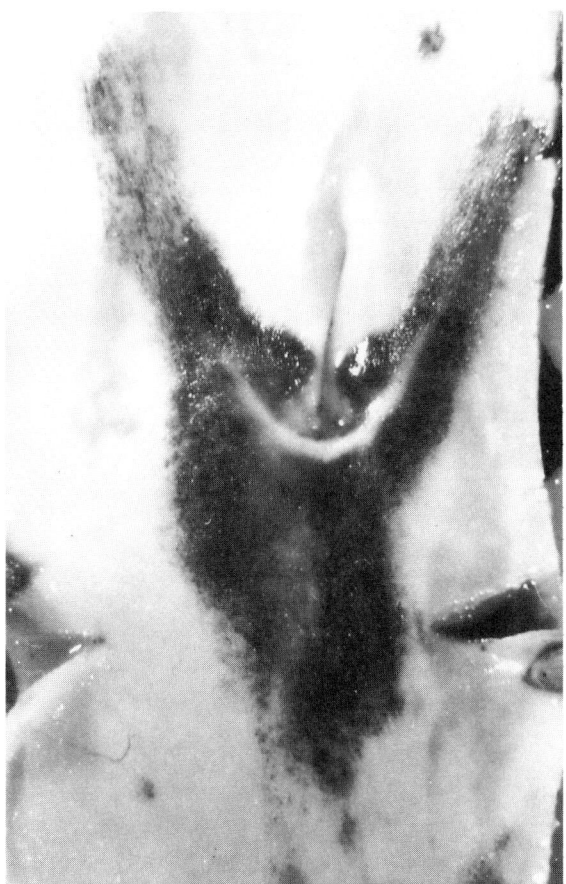

Figure 6.33 Origin of a large branch from abdominal aorta of a cholesterol over-fed rabbit showing fat accumulation and temporary sparing of the flow divider. Flow is from above down. (Reproduced with permission from Stehbens [25].)

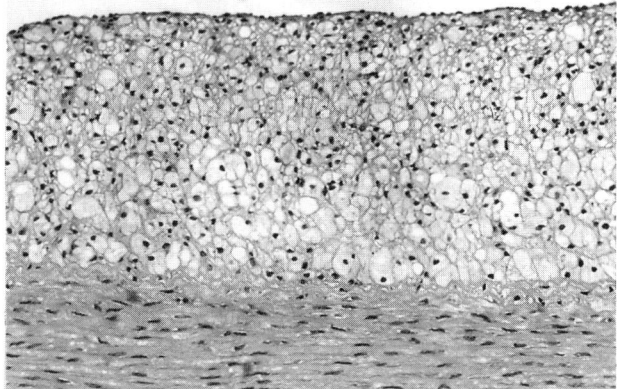

Figure 6.34 Section from an aorta from a cholesterol-fed rabbit showing the intimal thickening due to massive infiltration by lipid-laden macrophages. Note absence of interstitial tissue. (Haematoxylin and eosin.)

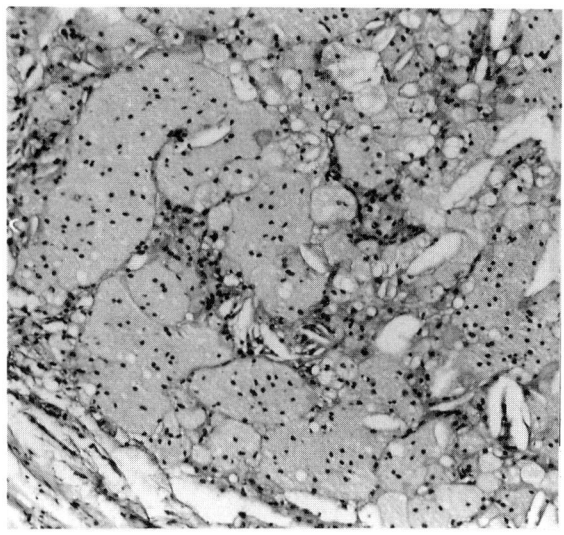

Figure 6.35 Massive multinucleated giant foam cells from intima of a cholesterol-fed rabbit. (Haematoxylin and eosin.)

The lipid accumulations extend and become more prominent forming triangular patches distal to the branch ostia of the aorta but initially sparing the flow dividers (Figure 6.33). The early foam cell lesions of the aorta have been alleged, incorrectly, to be similar to human fatty streaks. Eventually the entire aortic surface may be involved and whilst lipid accumulates initially at the extremities of the intimal thickenings at forks or elsewhere, the intimal thickening is a massive infiltration of lipid-laden macrophages (Figure 6.34) derived from monocytes with little evidence of medial destruction or thinning. At times the intima contains multinucleated foam cells (Figure 6.35). Ultrastructurally there is lipid infiltration of the intimal thickening with separation of pre-existing tissues and without the pathogenetic changes in the smooth muscle cells, basement membranes, matrix vesicles, etc., that characterize true atherosclerosis (Figure 6.36). There are no abnormally shaped smooth muscle cells though they contain large lipid droplets at the poles of the nuclei and no dystrophic basement membrane material. The lesions are essentially xanthomatous and the fibrous or sclerotic element is minimal rather than the reverse as it is in man [257]. Even Anitschkow [258] acknowledged several differences from human atherosclerosis such that characteristics of the human disease are not reproduced in the experimental rabbit.

When cholesterol feeding is intermittent or of low dosage, the vascular lesions may be more fibrotic. This is understandable since haemodynamic stress is known to alter the endothelium, fashion subendothelial connective tissues into shapes consistent with flow patterns, cause tears of the internal elastic lamina, medial atrophy, tortuosity, ectasia and aneurysm formation. Even new vascular surfaces, whether a prosthesis or medial tissue (exposed by a dissecting aneurysm or endarterectomy) will develop fibromusculoelastic tissue constituting a neo-intima. It is therefore not surprising that an intimal

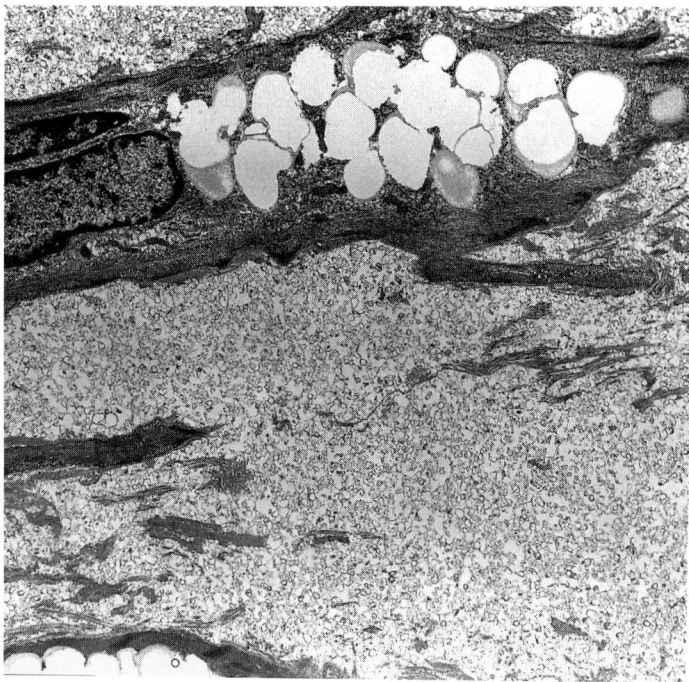

Figure 6.36 Electron micrograph of intimal thickening at main renal arterial bifurcation from a cholesterol-fed rabbit. There are lysosomal lipid vacuoles in two smooth muscle cells which are of normal shape and have no thickened basement membranes. The intimal thickening is infiltrated by fat with separation of pre-existing tissues. Matrix vesicles are not increased. (Reproduced with permission from Stehbens and Ludatscher [423].)

mass of lipid-laden macrophages as in Figure 6.34 without even intercellular adhesions and ostensibly unprotected by elastic tissue, basement membranes and proteoglycans would be susceptible to haemodynamic stress. This does not make the lesion atherosclerotic. In the florid state of overload the rabbits progressively waste away and die with a haemolytic anaemia without such fibrous reaction. The topography of the lesions is not that of atherosclerosis and the animals do not display the complications of atherosclerosis (intimal tears, ulcerations, mural thrombosis, tortuosity and aneurysms) but all have widespread extravascular xanthomatosis and at times circulating lipophages [144,207].

Other animal species have not been investigated as thoroughly as the time-honoured, convenient rabbit but review of dietary-induced lesions in other animals reveals that there is sufficient evidence to indicate a basic similarity of response. Many of the animals spontaneously develop milder atherosclerosis than that in humans, and other diseases (arteritis) can account for occasional complications. This has understandably led to claims that the dietary-induced lesions more closely resemble human atherosclerosis than the rabbit lesions.

These dietary-induced lesions have been reviewed elsewhere in more detail [144,207] with many investigators coming to different conclusions. Numerous investigators are seemingly unaware of the extent of the differences from human atherosclerosis or that experimental reproduction of the disease must comply with specific criteria modified from Koch's postulates before the lesions can be regarded as atherosclerotic [5]. Essentially, the sequential pathological changes in the vessel wall have to be similar to those occurring spontaneously in man and the experimental procedure must reproduce or be closely comparable to conditions existing in man. The dietary-induced lesions have the hallmarks of a lipid storage disorder and indeed Hueper produced similar storage disorders by administering large molecular weight polysaccharides to rabbits [75]. Carey [259], admitting the experimental hypercholesterolaemic animal models failed to reproduce the human disease, contended that a model is chosen for experimental procedures because it expresses one or more aspects of the disease similar to those occurring in humans. However, if the aim is to reproduce the disease which is the final proof of causality [5], it must be similar in all respects including the pathogenesis and the development of primary complications, otherwise incorrect deductions will be made because the implicit assumption then is that the pathogenesis of the characteristics to be studied is the same in both disorders when it is not.

Death from atherosclerosis is rare in lower animals but spontaneous lipid deposition in these animals resembles human atherosclerosis and is quite unlike the foam cell lesions that characterize the cholesterol-induced lesions (Figures 6.34, 6.35). In a study of spontaneous atherosclerosis in captive wild animals, Vastesaeger [260] considered diet to be unimportant.

(b) Familial hypercholesterolaemia (FH)

This is a relatively common, well recognized entity that in the past has been known by a variety of names emphasizing its familial occurrence, hypercholesterolaemia and xanthomatosis. It is characterized by an elevated plasma cholesterol carried in the low density lipoprotein (LDL) due to a mutant gene at the LDL receptor locus which results in a virtual absence of LDL receptors or receptors with an inability to bind and take up LDL for the use of the cells [261,264]. It is genetically determined by an autosomal dominant gene; homozygotes, occurring about one per million of the population, exhibit the purest form of the disease with blood cholesterol levels ranging from 600 to 1200 mg/dl and sometimes higher. Heterozygotes have one defective gene and their cells bind or take up LDL at about half the normal rate. Their blood cholesterol levels range from 280 to 550 mg/dl and they constitute approximately 0.2% of the population. Their prevalence is greater in South Africa and Syria possibly due to consanguinity. Blood triglyceride levels are usually normal in heterozygotes and slightly elevated in homozygotes. There is variation in the severity of the metabolic effects but most homozygotes die before 30 years of age, often from CHD or congestive cardiac failure. One homozygote died of a myocardial infarction at 18 months [262]. Heterozygotes have been known to live to the eighth decade but the mean age of death is 55 years for males and 64 years for females. Approximately 50% of male heterozygotes and a smaller percentage of female heterozygotes suffer CHD by the age of 50.

Clinically these subjects are distinct from the rest of the population with hypercholesterolaemia at birth and yellow-orange cutaneous xanthomatous lesions present at birth or by the age of four years. Many xanthomata are quite disfiguring and may interfere with normal function of the hands and feet. Arcus corneae, tendon xanthomata and migratory polyarthritis (56%) develop and some patients have hypertrichosis. These clinical features alone are sufficient to question the validity of including such subjects in general poulation samples.

The LDL receptor defect blocks the intake of LDL by the cells and consequently the serum LDL and cholesterol levels rise, the rate of synthesis being normal but LDL catabolism is defective [263]. With such high blood cholesterol levels, it is not surprising that lipid storage occurs although humans have little ability to sequester significant quantities of cholesterol in tissues other than in the aorta and its branches.

When there is an interruption in a metabolic pathway concerned with the synthesis, utilization or excretion of

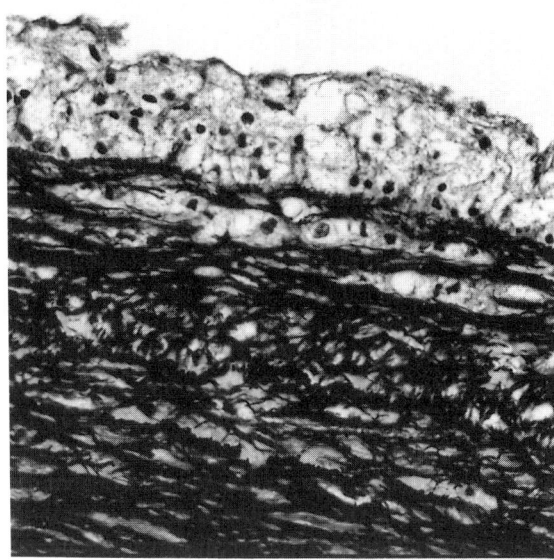

Figure 6.37 Early foam cell lesion in the aorta of a young boy with homozygous familial hypercholesterolaemia. (Verhoeff's elastic stain and eosin.) (Reproduced with permission from Stehbens and Martin [166].)

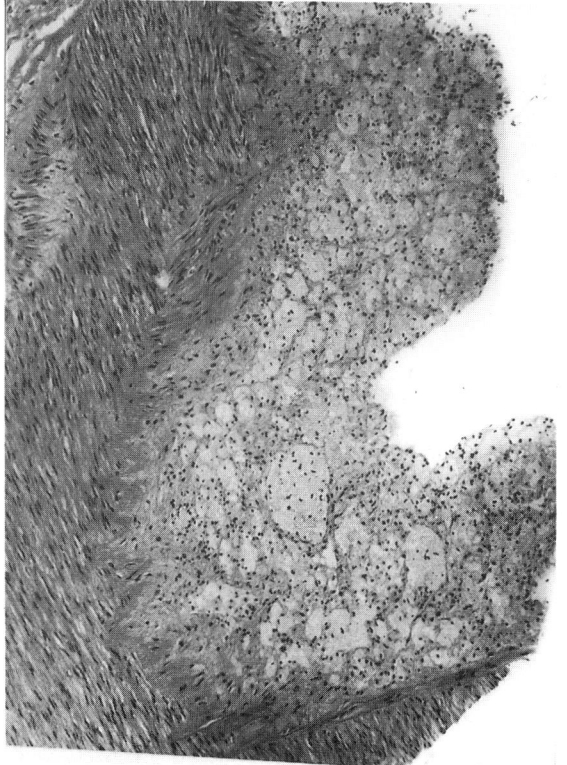

Figure 6.38 Intimal foam cell lesion in a coronary artery (homozygous FH) similar to early lesions of cholesterol-fed rabbits. (Haematoxylin and eosin.) (Reproduced with permission from Stehbens and Martin [166].)

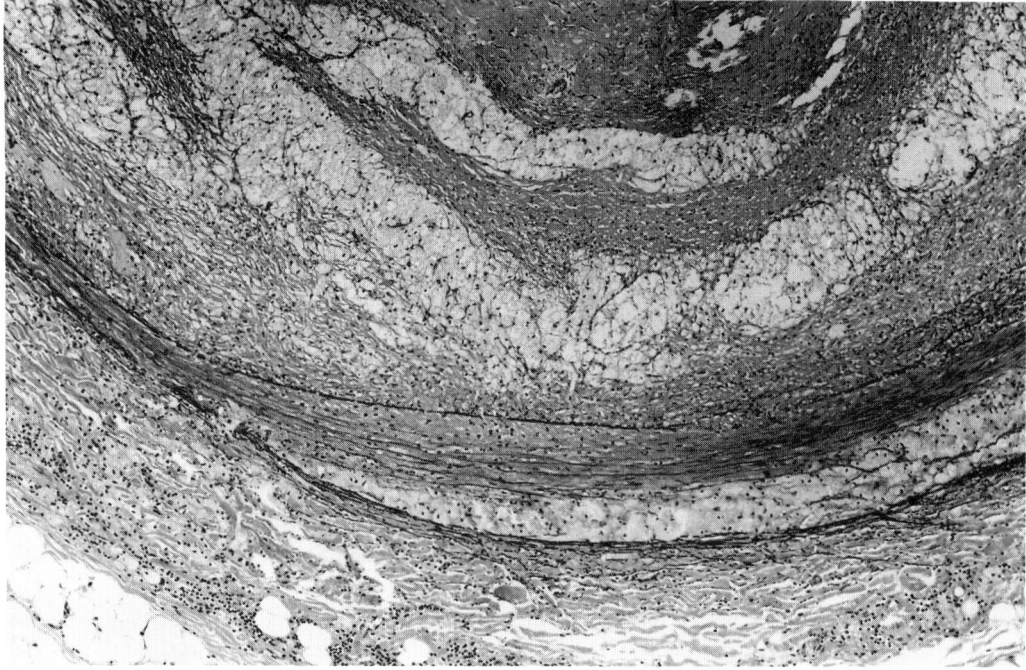

Figure 6.39 Section of coronary artery (homozygous FH) exhibiting gross intimal thickening with large accumulations of foam cells in the intima and media, thinning of the media and peppering of the adventitia with monocytes and foam cells. (Verhoeff's elastic stain and eosin.)

a metabolite due to some inherited defect, it is common for a metabolite to accumulate in excessive quantities and become stored in the reticuloendothelial system and other tissues particularly those concerned with its utilization. FH is such a disease and the pronounced hypercholesterolaemia results in lipid storage as in rabbits overloaded with cholesterol or large molecular weight polysaccharides. These disorders must be regarded as storage diseases and the lipid storage in the blood vessels of homozygotes with FH commences *in utero*. Initially the vascular lesions are essentially xanthomatous (Figures 6.37, 6.38) as is recognized in the literature with the aortic involvement referred to as xanthelasma or xanthomatosis of the aorta [166,200]. Aortic valve involvement is similar. Large foam cell accumulations in the intima may place the wall at a mechanical disadvantage and certainly cohesion between foam cells would be low. There would be stress concentration at such sites of foam cell accumulation because the viscoelastic properties of the vessel wall would be unable to absorb the pulse and vibrational stresses uniformly. Fat-laden smooth muscle cells would not respond to such stresses adequately. Endothelial stress would be severe due to a lack of subendothelial connective tissue anchorage. In view of the degenerative changes that haemodynamic stress can induce in a normal arterial wall, a foam cell lesion would not be resilient and the development of secondary fibrosis is understandable (Figure 6.39). A deficiency or absence of LDL receptors may conceivably affect more than the cholesterol metabolic pathway and secondarily affect other smooth muscle cell functions in maintaining vascular tone and the integrity and synthesis of the intercellular protein matrix. A mild dietary hypercholesterolaemia has been reported to impair arterial repair in monkeys [265] which may hold true for this lipid storage disease too. The frequency of uricaemia, aortic valvular disease, migratory polyarthritis, hypertrichosis and an elevated erythrocyte sedimentation rate suggests that other secondary metabolic complications are present and that aggravation of atherosclerosis may occur apart from the complications secondary to a thick fibroxanthomatous intima. In other words the lipid storage in the vessel wall in this disease is superimposed on naturally occurring atherosclerosis. The aortic valve cusps infiltrated with irregular xanthomatous deposits would also exhibit an accentuation of natural wear and tear on the valve cusps eventually leading to a fibrosed incompetent valve in addition to stenosis in most homozygotes and heterozygotes [166,200]

Many authors have indicated that the vascular lesions of FH differ from atherosclerosis [200,266,267]. In early publications on homozygous FH, the vascular lesions were xanthomatous and in some were likened to those of the cholesterol-fed rabbit [200]. In later reports this feature was not so pronounced, the possibility being that modification of the lesion may have occurred due to therapy, just as cessation of cholesterol feeding in rabbits

Table 6.1 Differences between homozygous familial hypercholesterolemia (FH) and atherosclerosis in humans

Characteristics	Homozygous FH	Atherosclerosis
Frequency	One in one million	Ubiquitous in *Homo sapiens*
Inheritance	Autosomal dominant gene	No specific genetic inheritance
Age of clinical disability	18 months to 30 years	Rare before the sixth decade
Heart		
Aortic valve	Stenosis 55%, ejection murmur 87%; spongy, yellow, xanthomatous deposits, ultimately becoming fibrotic and calcified; possible widening of commissures and valvular incompetence	No association
Mitral valve	Raised, yellow xanthomatous infiltration; incompetence 9.5%	Ordinarily not significantly affected, only fibrotic thickening and diffuse interstitial lipid especially of anterior leaflet
Pulmonary valve	Xanthomatous patches	No association
Ischemia, myocardial infarction and sequelae	Usual outcome	Common
Endocardial deposits	Left ventricle, atrium, chordae tendineae	Rare
Cerebrovascular disease	Rare if ever	Common concomitant
Peripheral vascular disease	Nil	Common concomitant
Aorta		
Distribution	Severe proximally	Severe distally
Aneurysm	Nil	Common
Ectasia, tortuosity	Nil	Usual
Morphology	Yellow-orange, discrete, raised sessile lesions (described as xanthelasmatous or xanthomatous)	Pale, not discrete, merges with adjoining fibrotic intima
Xanthomata	May be nodular or even tumor-like mass and can cause supravalvular aortic stenosis or obliterate sinuses of Valsalva; also involves ostia of coronary arteries	No association
Early lesion	Xanthomatosis	Interstitial lipid deep in intima
Late lesion	Eventually fibrotic but plentiful foam cells; calcification not pronounced	Sclerotic and atheromatous; fibrin insudation common; calcification often extensive
Ulcers, tears, thrombi	Infrequent superficial erosion with mural thrombosis	Usual outcome in endstage disease Fibrin insudation common. Extensive mural thrombosis frequent
Foam cells	Initially almost exclusively xanthomatous; later extensive infiltration in intima and moderate infiltration of media and to lesser extent the adventitia	Less frequently in the intima, rarely in adventitia
Stenosis of coronary ostia	Common	Not significant
Cellularity	Advanced lesions quite cellular; monocytes and lipophages	Advanced lesions peculiarly acellular and hyaline, occasional giant cells; haemosiderin-laden macrophages and some round cells
Smooth muscle cells	Extensive (bipolar) lipid vacuolation in intima and media	Lipid vacuolation (bipolar) in fatty streaks but not prominent feature in advanced disease
Media	Thinned beneath plaques and extensively disrupted in a patchy fashion with crowding of residual elastic laminae	Elastic tissue fragmentation Thinning common
Adventitia	Thickened and fibrotic beneath plaque, perivascular foam cells	May have haemosiderin-laden macrophages
Adventitial round cells	More likely to be macrophages	Often perivascular, common in advanced lesions
Vasa vasorum	Proliferation with perivascular fibrosis and foam cell accumulation, with severe interruption of elastic lamellae within the media; those in adventitia may be surrounded by lipophages and some round cell infiltration	Proliferation with some perivascular fibrosis and interruption of elastic tissue but not pronounced

Table 6.1 *Continued*

Characteristics	Homozygous FH	Atherosclerosis
Degenerative changes	Commonly exhibit endarteritis obliterans (arteriosclerosis) of small arteries associated with plaques; elsewhere unaffected	No significant change
Coronary arteries	Severely affected, patchy involvement. Initially xanthomatous; advanced lesion cellular, usually some medial thinning and foam cell infiltration; foam cell accumulations appear to be independent of intimal proliferation at branching sites; advanced lesions focal with minimal conventional diffuse changes elsewhere and in small vessels	Severe, diffuse involvement; initially fibromuscular elastic intimal proliferation commencing about branching sites. Advanced lesions diffuse and in presence of severe small vessel disease
Calcification	Infrequent or mild	Often extensive
Ectasia	Only one instance (may be due to post-stenotic effect)	Usual
Ulceration, thrombosis	Rare	Common
Smooth muscle cells	Fat vacuoles at poles of nuclei of muscle cells prominent in intimal proliferation and subjacent media	Seen in early lesion but not prominent in advanced disease. Intimal smooth muscle cells thin, attenuated, malshapen. Also lipofuscin
Adventitia	Proliferation of vasa vasorum and can have extensive foam cell infiltration	Proliferation of vasa vasorum. Foam cells rare, only seen when atheromatous debris herniates into adventitia
Interstitial lipid	Mostly in advanced stages	Abundant
Intracellular lipid	Foam cells abundant	Foam cells relatively sparse
Intimal tears, ulceration and thrombosis	Very infrequent	Common
Stenotic intimal lesions	Usual	Common
Xanthomatous lesions in pulmonary arteries	May be extensive in absence of pulmonary hypertension but less severe than in systemic circulation	Infrequent in absence of pulmonary hypertension
Veins	No reported involvement	Very mild, aggravated by venous hypertension
Small vessel disease		
Arteriosclerosis or diffuse hyperplastic sclerosis	Only associated with xanthomatous aortic lesions and in splenic arterioles	Usual and proportional to the severity of atherosclerosis in large vessels
Intimal xanthomatous change	May occlude small vessels	Nil
Vascular lesions – general		
Similarity to tendon xanthomata	Yes	No
Predominant cell type	Macrophage–foam cell	Smooth muscle cell
Cellularity	Pronounced	Pronounced acellularity
Xanthomata	Correlation of severity of extravascular xanthomata and vascular lesions	No association
Similarity to cholesterol-fed rabbit	Yes	No
Similarity to WHHL rabbit	Yes	No
Extravascular xanthomata		
Cutaneous and tendon	Usual – may interfere with manual dexterity and use of feet	No association
Visceral	Common but variable	No association
Miscellaneous		
Hypercholesterolaemia	Gross elevation	Can occur at any level
Migratory polyarthritis	56% – large peripheral joints	No association
Uricaemia	Increased in approximately one third	No special association
Elevated erythrocyte sedimentation rate	Common	No association
Hypertension	No specific association	Aggravated severity

* Reproduced with permission from Stehbens [163] and Stehbens and Martin [166].

accentuates the fibrotic element and reduction in the foam cell population. Faber [268] asserted that heart attacks in patients with xanthomatosis and hypercholesterolaemia were due to xanthomatous deposits in the intima, but that those subjects with secondary hypercholesterolaemia had fewer foam cells in the lesions. The many differences between homozygous FH and atherosclerosis have been reviewed elsewhere [166,200] but some are tabulated in Table 6.1. A pathological diagnosis must be made on the overall picture not on the presence of lipid in the arterial wall or a selected portion of one lesion.

There is need for detailed ultrastructural information on the pathogenesis of the lesions but few homozygotes are available for study. Correlation of detailed histological, electron microscopic and biochemical data is needed with the different chromosomal aberrations that are known to exist. In our present state of knowledge the pathological changes must be regarded as a mixture of lipid storage and atherosclerosis and not merely as one end of a spectrum of changes in atherosclerosis. It is quite likely that pathologists in the past, being unaware of serum cholesterol levels, have unwittingly grouped the vascular lesions of homozygotes and heterozygotes as variants of atherosclerosis. The pre-eminent fact is that pathological differences are considerable and cannot be ignored. If the vascular lesions are truly advanced atherosclerosis, the absence of aortic aneurysms (not even one instance has been reported) and of concomitant cerebrovascular and peripheral vascular disease requires explanation.

Myocardial ischaemia and infarction in FH are mostly caused by stenosis of the coronary ostia or of the artery proper by xanthomatous lesions rather than by thrombotic occlusion due to intimal tears and ulcerations. However, superficial erosions have been reported in recent years and myocardial fibrosis, infarction, atherosclerotic stenoses, intimal tears and mural thrombi may all occur in the homozygous age range and the secondary vascular effects of some recent therapeutic agents are unknown. Nevertheless the pathogenesis of CHD is usually due to stenosing lesions in the coronary arteries, possibly aggravated by red cell agglutination accompanying the elevated erythrocyte sedimentation rate. For such reasons it has been recommended that FH should be excluded from epidemiological studies of CHD [163]. Angina pectoris, myocardial infarction and sudden death are cardinal features of myocardial ischaemia but their occurrence does not make the arterial lesions atherosclerotic. Understandably a foam cell lesion subjected to prolonged aortic haemodynamic stress can be associated with endothelial denudation and secondary thrombosis but the deep tears and ulcerations are not prevalent as in atherosclerosis [166].

Heterozygotes are more numerous and their longer survival permits more advanced atherosclerotic changes to become associated with or superimposed on lipid storage. These are mixed lesions. Again hypercholesterolaemia is present at birth and there appears to be at least some overlap in serum cholesterol levels with those accepted as being in the 'normal' range. In a review of the pathological data available from heterozygotes the conclusion was reached that basic similarities to those of homozygotes existed but due to the longer survival, and a lesser degree of lipid storage, the superimposed atherosclerosis was more manifest [200]. It appears that CHD is the result of arterial stenotic lesions of the arteries rather than thrombotic occlusion. Other complications of atherosclerosis are comparatively rare and occur late in life. The aortic lesions are more severe proximally than distally [269] and aortic aneurysms rare or non-existent.

Any disease in which there is a metabolic disorder affecting every cell in the body is likely to reflect impaired resistance to a chronic degenerative disease such as atherosclerosis. Smooth muscle cells heavily laden with fat may well have impaired ability to regenerate, repair and to synthesize and maintain the connective tissue matrix. It is, therefore, possible that the development of atherosclerosis may be enhanced or aggravated by FH. However, unlike the cholesterol-fed rabbit there is no obvious predilection for lipid accumulation in ostial intimal thickenings in coronary or cerebral arteries and no exaggerated degenerative changes were observed in the intimal thickenings and bifurcations [166]. The lipid storage could enhance encroachment on the lumen by means of a space-occupying effect. The storage may interfere with the viscoelastic properties of the vessel wall or there may be an adverse connective tissue dysfunction independent of lipid storage. It would seem, however, that the disease is associated with augmented 'wear and tear' degenerative changes involving the blood vessels, cardiac valves and joints for these are features of other metabolic storage diseases [200].

Such views are not widely accepted but time will be the arbiter. The need for a qualitative and quantitative study of the vascular lesions of FH and ubiquitous atherosclerosis by experienced vascular pathologists is conceded but on current evidence they are two distinct diseases. The former is associated with a specific genetic defect and the other is not.

Considerable emphasis in FH and indeed in atherogenesis has been on smooth muscle cell lipid metabolism and the accumulation of lipid, yet smooth muscle cells occur in many anatomical sites other than the walls of blood vessels without similar involvement in hypercholesterolaemia. Even within blood vessels there are different propensities from site to site and vascular bed to vascular bed. This would suggest that vascular smooth muscle cells may differ from those elsewhere or some local factor must be governing the distribution of arterial involvement. In the cholesterol-fed rabbit, lipid accumulation has been shown to be governed by haemodynamics [270–272] but as yet this has not been demonstrated in man or in the animal counterpart the Watanabe heritable hyperlipidaemic rabbit.

(c) Familial type III hyperlipoproteinaemia

This has similarities to FH but is rare. The incidence of vascular diseases is therefore difficult to assess [272]. Most subjects are detected clinically between 40 and 70 years of age and would be expected to have manifestations of atherosclerosis. They too have xanthomatosis with subcutaneous and visceral lipid infiltration. Almost half have uricaemia and abnormal glucose tolerance test results [200].

The most detailed pathology report concerned a 57-year-old woman with recurrent myocardial infarction [273,274], diabetes mellitus, cholesterolosis of the gall bladder, numerous ceroid-containing foam cells in the spleen and bone marrow and subendothelial xanthomatous deposits in the left atrium. Foam cell infiltrations of coronary arteries were pronounced and several vessels were occluded by foam cells. A brother was similarly affected with xanthomatous coronary and peripheral vascular disease. It was even stated that the arteries were severely narrowed by foam cell deposits rather than exhibiting the usual complicated plaques of atherosclerosis [273]. These general findings have been supported by other reports indicating the lipid storage nature of the disease and the similarity of the vascular lesions to those of cholesterol-fed rabbits [275–277]. Non-rheumatic aortic stenosis and mitral incompetence have been noted even in a 9-year old boy [277]. For the same reasons as in FH, these vascular lesions cannot be considered to be purely atherosclerotic. There is also need for a qualitative and quantitative comparative study of vascular lesions with atherosclerosis of normolipidaemic individuals.

(d) Other familial lipid metabolic disorders

The number of cases studied is too small for statistical analysis of the severity of atherosclerosis and the appraisal of individual cases is not necessarily beyond question. Type IIB exhibits an increase in prebetalipoprotein or very low density lipoprotein (VLDL) as well as LDL. In type IV hyperlipoproteinaemia, there is mild to moderate increase in serum cholesterol and LDL levels frequently associated with several common metabolic and nutritional disorders involving middle-aged and elderly patients who are expected to suffer from advancing atherosclerosis.

Subjects with familial apolipoprotein B-100 deficiency display a striking similarity to FH clinically and biochemically [278] and it may well be that other inherited lipid metabolic disorders may be associated with lipid storage in man. Recently severe hypercholesterolaemia with foam cell lesions in mouse blood vessels has been reported in apolipoprotein E deficiency, one occurring spontaneously [279], the other induced by homologous recombination in embryonic stem cells [280]. Such models may help elucidate analogous human fat storage diseases but have doubtful relevance to human atherosclerosis. Lipid storage disorders such as these preclude their inclusion in epidemiological studies of CHD in man if the natural history and elucidation of the cause of atherosclerosis is the aim of the study.

When the pathological features of vascular disease are determined for each genetically derived familial hyperlipoproteinaemia, it will be possible to deduce whether or not mild degrees of hyperlipoproteinaemia have an effect on atherosclerosis *per se* or increase lipid storage in the atherosclerotic arterial intima.

(e) Watanabe heritable hyperlipidaemic rabbit

The Watanabe heritable hyperlipidaemic (WHHL) rabbit is a spontaneous animal model of FH with an absence of LDL receptors in cell membranes [281]. The rabbits differ from humans with FH in that affected rabbits also have hypertriglyceridaemia [261]. Lipid occurs in the aorta of newborn rabbits and the lesions are basically similar to those of the dietary-induced hypercholesterolaemic rabbit. There is lipid accumulation in endothelial cells as in the cholesterol-fed rabbit but not in atherosclerosis. Large lesions exhibiting fibrosis and occasional microthrombi have been observed. Cutaneous and tendon xanthomata were prevalent with the visceral xanthomatosis mild and the severity of changes variable. Despite similarities to dietary-induced vascular changes in rabbits and FH, the lesions have been cursorily regarded as atherosclerotic.

Within two to three years these rabbits develop severe stenosis of the origin of the left coronary artery another point of similarity to FH. Severe stenosis of coronary arteries during their course also arises and results in myocardial fibrosis. However, no evidence of atherosclerotic ulceration, intimal tears and dissection with thrombotic occlusion was found. The WHHL rabbit may be a useful rabbit model of an inherited lipid storage disorder involving blood vessels but the vascular lesions cannot be regarded as atherosclerotic. Similar lipid storage disorders occur in other animal species.

(f) Other hypercholesterolaemic conditions in atherogenesis

Diabetes mellitus

Subjects with diabetes mellitus exhibit unusually severe atherosclerosis, the most convincing evidence being provided by the International Atherosclerosis Project [282] which revealed greater severity in the aorta and coronary arteries than in non-diabetics. The lipid infiltration of the renal arterioles is pronounced and there is also microangiopathy in diabetics. The epidemiological evidence is considered to be strongly supportive but these diabetic patients are frequently obese and hypertensive although the 'atherogenic' effect of diabetes has been attributed to the associated hypercholesterolaemia. It has been alleged that diabetes predisposes to atherosclerosis independently of hyperlipaemia and hypertension [283].

In pre-insulin days, when given a high-fat diet therapeutically, some diabetics developed profound hypercholesterolaemia (exceeding 1300 mg/dl), associated with a creamy plasma and widespread xanthomatosis which was sometimes familial. Xanthomata, identical to other xanthomata, occurred in the skin, and viscera and foam cells were to be found in the spleen, liver, lungs and lymph nodes [284,285].

In a 33-year-old diabetic woman who died of myocardial infarction, raised yellow plaques were reported below the aortic ring and surrounding the coronary ostia with numerous similar plaques in the coronary arteries and severe stenoses. The intima of coronary arteries was markedly thickened due to collections of vacuolated fat-containing cells similar to the splenic xanthomata. The aortic intima and even vasa vasorum contained many foam cells. Even the walls of lymphatic vessels in such patients exhibited large patches of xanthoma cells [286]. The xanthomatous nature of the coronary artery intimal thickening was confirmed by other authors [284]. Foam cells also occurred in the endocardium and aortic and mitral valve leaflets. These soft bright yellow arterial lesions were specifically described as consisting of closely packed xanthoma cells and the underlying elastica was unchanged. Some aortic endothelial cells were foamy, as in the cholesterol-fed rabbit. Hepatic and Kupffer cells were laden with lipid and the splenic pulp replaced by foam cells. The obvious similarity to the cholesterol-fed rabbit was acknowledged and the lesions were regarded as lipid storage phenomena [284]. The xanthomatous and intense foam cell infiltration of tissues of diabetics has disappeared with insulin therapy although the present-day relationship of diabetes and atherosclerosis is probably influenced by pre-insulin pathology. The pathology of diabetic atherosclerosis in modern times is considered to be that of the conventional disease and the extreme hyperlipidaemia is no longer encountered although it is conceivable that diabetes mellitus may coexist with FH. Even so, in diabetes with a metabolic disturbance of protein, carbohydrate and fat affecting all cells, it is not surprising that the body's defence against bacterial and mycotic infections is impaired and that diabetes has an adverse effect on a degenerative disease such as atherosclerosis.

Chronic obstructive jaundice

Modern surgery usually prevents chronic obstructive jaundice and consequently widespread xanthomatosis in this condition is little known and rare. Fagge [287] reported widespread cutaneous xanthomata in a woman of unstated age with chronic jaundice, a coarse nodular cirrhosis and fatal haematemesis. Xanthomatous lesions were found in tendons, larynx, trachea, left atrium, aorta, and the pulmonary, carotid, subclavian and innominate arteries. Their similarity to dermal xanthomata was emphasized and they were referred to as xanthelasmata of arteries and the skin lesions as atheroma. Moreover the rarity of aortic ulceration in such patients was noted. Other authors have drawn attention to the similarity of intimal lesions sometimes consisting of giant xanthoma cells in the arteries of such patients to the widespread extravascular xanthomatosis [288].

Primary biliary cirrhosis is a rare but specific disease without extrahepatic biliary obstruction or secondary infection of the biliary duct system. After months or even years a few patients develop generalized xanthomatosis of the skin, referred to as xanthomatous biliary cirrhosis [288]. There is no familial tendency nor history of familial premature heart disease and tendon xanthomata are lacking. The size and extent of the lesions correlated with the degree of hypercholesterolaemia. These reports are mostly anecdotal and other patients with generalized cutaneous xanthomata and profound hyperlipidaemia did not have augmented atherosclerosis. Extreme hypercholesterolaemia is rare in biliary cirrhosis and there is no recent scientific comparison of the arterial lesions in subjects with biliary cirrhosis and matched controls. Anecdotal reports of the association in the old literature may be examples of a coexistent FH. Fredrickson [289] considered the frequency and severity of biliary cirrhosis of past days were different from those encountered in recent decades. Nevertheless the literature of this condition, whatever its exact diagnosis, supports the concept that the vascular lesions were a lipid storage phenomenon rather than being truly atherosclerotic.

Myxoedema

The 'myxoedema heart' is at times accompanied by angina pectoris without severe coronary atherosclerosis [290]. The hypercholesterolaemia of untreated myxoedema can be as high as that of patients with homozygous FH and can be associated with xanthomatosis. Again this is not a phenomenon of modern medicine and study of the qualitative and quantitative changes in the vascular pathology of chronic untreated myxoedema is not possible.

In view of the age of most myxoedematous patients

and the associated hypertension, adequate control material is essential and no significance can be given to anecdotal subjective estimations or isolated case reports. The vascular changes in hypothyroidism and diabetes mellitus have been likened to those of FH and the cholesterol-fed rabbit. On the other hand from a review of 150 hypothyroid patients the associated hypercholesterolaemia did not appear to affect the severity of atherosclerosis [291] which could have been attributed to hypertension or renal disease. Thannhauser [267] considered that rare patients with xanthomatosis may have had a familial dyslipidaemia such as FH prior to the development of hypothyroidism which in itself has diminished in frequency.

Hypothyroidism facilitates lipid deposition in blood vessels in experimental hypercholesterolaemia (dogs and rats) but the evidence that hypercholesterolaemia of myxoedema aggravates atherosclerosis cannot withstand critical scientific analysis [200].

Nephrotic syndrome

Hypercholesterolaemia is recognized in the nephrotic syndrome but the presence of xanthomata is exceptional. The allegation that there is an increased frequency of CHD in this syndrome is perpetuated in the literature without substantiating scientific evidence. Oppenheimer and Fishberg [284] considered the xanthomatous vascular lesions in nephrosis as well as those of diabetes mellitus and obstructive jaundice to be identical in morphology and distribution to those observed in cholesterol-fed rabbits. Little support is provided by the occurrence of golden yellow patches on the aortic and mitral valves, the endocardium, and in arteries, or extravascular fat deposits (without adequate histology) in isolated cases of lipid nephrosis in young children, one of whom had a blood cholesterol level of 100 mg/dl [292,293].

Insufficient numbers of untreated subjects prevent adequate study of this association, the misconception about which may have been due to a coexistent dyslipidaemia as with myxoedema. At present there is no evidence that the nephrotic syndrome aggravates atherosclerosis.

There is insufficient pathological evidence to support the concept that the hypercholesterolaemia associated with diabetes mellitus, chronic obstructive jaundice, myxoedema and the nephrotic syndrome causes severe premature atherosclerosis. When extreme hypercholesterolaemia is present for whatever reason, the vascular lesions have the characteristics of a lipid storage phenomenon similar to that in FH.

(g) **Other heritable metabolic diseases**

Other inherited metabolic disorders affect blood vessels and often cardiac valves. They exhibit tissue storage of a metabolite (often in blood vessels) with widespread cellular and connective tissue dysfunction because the generalized metabolic disorder will affect some viscera more than others depending on the defective metabolic pathway. It would appear that some aggravate naturally occurring degenerative diseases involving blood vessels, cardiac valves and joints [200]. However, there has not been adequate pathological analysis of the blood vessels in these diseases and on the present evidence the metabolic disorders are superimposed on naturally occurring atherosclerosis. In general the effect is deleterious and the pathological changes are essentially mixed lesions.

Fabry's disease is associated with deposition of glycosphingolipid in the cellular constituents of blood vessels, cardiac valves and most tissues. The subjects also suffer from aneurysms, varicosities, cardiac valvular disease, angina, vascular thrombosis and ischaemia and infarction of the heart and brain [294,295].

Homocystinuria is associated with abnormal collagen and elastin metabolism and possibly platelet dysfunction. There is pronounced intimal proliferation with fibrosis and elastic degeneration, luminal narrowing, thromboembolic occlusion of large and small blood vessels, and disturbance of the eye, skin and locomotor system. Ischaemic lesions of the heart and brain are also prevalent and may be fatal [296]. However, it cannot be said at present that the disease is identical to atherosclerosis.

The **mucopolysaccharidoses** are a group of genetic metabolic disorders manifested by excessive deposition of acid mucopolysaccharides in organs and tissues and excretion of large quantities of these substances in the urine. The clinical manifestations are generally severe and include skeletal deformities, joint stiffness and limitation of movement, hepatosplenomegaly, corneal opacities, hirsutism, cardiac valvular disease and neurological and mental deterioration [297]. In **Hurler, Scheie** and **Morquio's syndromes**, aortic regurgitation may occur. In Hurler syndrome there may be nodular thickening of the valve cusps and stenosis may occur with the same order of involvement as in rheumatic heart disease, indicating the combined influence of haemodynamic stress and the metabolic disturbance. The coronary arteries are preferentially affected and the metabolic disturbance appears to aggravate the intimal proliferation normally observed in these vessels [298,299]. The subjects may have angina pectoris. Mucopolysaccharides are deposited in intimal and smooth muscle cells in extensively distended lysosomes. This results in greatly increased fibrosis and elastic tissue proliferation, particularly in the aorta and coronary arteries, leading to severe luminal narrowing, a condition referred to as pseudoatheromatosis or mucopolysaccharide atheromatosis [299]. An alternative term, thesaurosclerosis, has been suggested for these lysosomal storage disorders involving metabolite storage and sclerosis of arteries which have been regarded as analogous to 'cholesterol storage' [300]. A similar overproduction of collagen may account for the associated joint stiffness.

Gross narrowing of coronary arteries occurs in gargoylism (Hurler's syndrome), the main arteries and branches being affected and the media thinned. The aorta exhibits pronounced intimal thickening with lipid deposition in addition to inclusion-laden smooth muscle cells. Even small vessels like the lenticulostriate arteries of the brain may be narrowed. Ultrastructurally, the smooth muscle cells of the arterial wall contain clear vacuoles and it has been suggested that the accumulation of a non-degradable substrate within the lysosomes of smooth muscle cells may be the initial event in storage and removal of the metabolite [301]. It is not surprising that a parallel has been drawn between these disorders and the lipid storage of the cholesterol-fed animal [300].

Ochronosis is a rare disorder of tyrosine metabolism most commonly associated with alkaptonuria, cardiovascular abnormalities and chronic degenerative joint disease [302,303]. Some subjects live a normal lifespan and consequently atherosclerosis and myocardial ischaemia are to be expected. However, other manifestations reveal a similarity to metabolic storage diseases involving the cardiovascular system including FH:

1. Cardiac valvular disease occurs with pigmentation and calcification particularly of the aortic valve, sometimes requiring an aortic valve prosthesis.
2. Atherosclerosis occurs with extensive pigmentation of the aorta and coronary arteries associated with calcification.
3. Most develop CHD.
4. Severe joint disease is usual (hips, knees and spine).

These metabolic storage disorders are superimposed on atherosclerosis and thereby modify the natural course of the disease. The possibility is that pathologists in earlier years may have likened the foam cell lesions of arteries in FH and the rare cases of extreme hypercholesterolaemia in pre-insulin diabetes mellitus and obstructive jaundice to human atherosclerosis in subjects with unrecognized familial acquired dyslipidaemia and grouped them as but variants in the spectrum of changes seen in atherosclerosis. The pathological evidence for augmented atherosclerosis caused by hypercholesterolaemia in these diseases is poorly substantiated. FH has hallmarks of a metabolic storage disease and may adversely affect atherogenesis by means of:

1. fat storage and a space-occupying effect in the vessel wall;
2. aggravation of atherogenesis by interference with general metabolic and reparative functions of endothelial and smooth muscle cells;
3. a secondary haemodynamically induced degenerative effect on intimal foam cell masses;
4. a totally independent propensity to vascular degeneration and atherosclerosis [166]. It cannot be assumed that hypercholesterolaemia or other storage diseases are all causes of atherosclerosis nor that the combined lesions are purely atherosclerotic.

6.3.2 THE PATHOLOGICAL AND EXPERIMENTAL EVIDENCE

The following observations from human pathology are inconsistent with the lipid hypothesis and cannot be explained on the basis of a circulating humoral agent (e.g. cholesterol, LDL).

1. There is variation in severity from vascular bed to vascular bed in the individual and even the differential predilection of arteries according to size, e.g. pronounced difference in severity of atherosclerosis in the aorta and the adjoining wall of its segmental branches [7].
2. Atherosclerosis of advanced degree may be in apposition with uninvolved intima in the same arterial segment as seen in both longitudinal and transverse histological sections (Figures 6.29; 10.34, pp. 208 and 389).
3. Surgeons induce severe accelerated atherosclerosis in venous bypass grafts in which the vein is subjected to arterial haemodynamics and also in the anastomosed veins of therapeutic arteriovenous shunts for renal dialysis. Yet these veins if left intact like other veins elsewhere would remain minimally affected for the remaining years of life. The vein wall accumulates lipids at all blood levels of cholesterol or LDL. The crucial factor is not the dietary lipid or serum lipid levels, but the augmented haemodynamic stresses to which the vessels are subjected [304]. The internal mammary (thoracic) artery lasts longer as a bypass graft indicating that the vein in reality is more susceptible to atherosclerosis than arteries yet under ordinary circumstances veins exhibit minimal involvement.
4. External support of an artery seems to afford the vessel some measure of protection [105].
5. The augmented flow in the common iliac artery in children with only one umbilical artery initiates premature development of atherosclerosis in that artery [13].
6. Anecdotal evidence suggests that usage aggravates the severity [94]. This is supported by experimental evidence.
7. The consistent and specific localization of intimal thickenings about forks, unions and curvatures suggests a strong haemodynamic influence and is not consistent with a causative humoral factor.

The above factors are inconsistent with the hypothesis that a circulating humoral agent such as hypercholesterolaemia or high lipoproteinaemia type II is the principal cause of atherosclerosis in humans. The concept that cholesterol is noxious at all blood levels, as has been claimed, is really implausible since cholesterol is an essential ingredient of every cell in the body. It is necessary for plasma membrane stability, fluidity and strength. It is a precursor of vitamin D, steroid hormones and of bile salts which are necessary for fat absorption. It constitutes up to 17% of the dry weight of the brain and at least 80% of cholesterol is manufactured by the body, with synthesis increasing if absorption declines and vice versa. Moreover to suggest that LDL is 'bad' and high density lipoprotein (HDL) is 'good' is inappropriate since LDL is the principal mode of transport for cholesterol to the tissues. It is understandable, however, that when there is a block in a metabolic pathway of any metabolite that a deficiency or an excessive accumulation of that metabolite will ensue both of which conditions can be deleterious.

In FH there is a total or partial functional deficiency in LDL membrane receptors and consequently LDL accumulates in excessive quantities. This, however, applies only to the minority of the population and rather than FH providing the strongest evidence that hypercholesterolaemia causes atherosclerosis, it provides little support on pathological grounds as indicated. In view of the above it is appropriate that investigators in atherogenesis review the evidence underlying their beliefs and hypotheses.

A crucial problem of research in atherogenesis is that of relating experimental animal lesions to those that occur in man. Caution is always necessary in extrapolating from animal experiments to humans even though atherosclerosis is not species-specific. In the last century tuberculosis was considered to have many causes both bacterial and non-bacterial prior to Koch's formulation of his postulates and the demonstration of the tubercle bacillus as the cause of the disease. In the belief that cholesterol is the *sine qua non* of atherosclerosis, cholesterol has been alleged to comply with Koch's postulates which are for bacteria alone [305,306].

Koch's postulates which contributed substantially to the evolution of scientific knowledge of infectious diseases, are inapplicable to chronic non-infectious, degenerative diseases such as atherosclerosis. Whilst there have been suggestions that atherosclerosis may be an inflammatory or infectious disease, or even due to a virus, these views lack scientific evidence and plausibility. In experimental atherogenesis compliance with appropriately modified postulates is essential to preclude spurious causes from consideration. The crux of such postulates is that the experimental procedure must reproduce the disease and its complications and their pathogenesis and experimental conditions must be analogous to those prevailing in man [11]. Since atherosclerosis consists of multiple lesions which develop independently of one another but ultimately coalesce, reproduction of the disease in a localized segment of a blood vessel in susceptible animals under conditions similar to those prevailing in man would comply with the spirit of Koch's postulates [5].

The irreconcilable morphological and topographical differences from atherosclerosis, the extravascular accompanying pathological lesions and the notable absence of the complications of atherosclerosis indicate that the dietary-induced lesions in experimental animals are not truly atherosclerotic but rather poor approximations although they have been widely accepted.

6.3.3 REGRESSION OF THE PATHOLOGY OF ATHEROSCLEROSIS

The concept of regression of atherosclerosis is intimately concerned with the lipid hypothesis. It has been alleged that regression of experimental atherosclerosis occurs and can be achieved by cessation of cholesterol feeding. This raises the first problem: is the lesion truly atherosclerotic? Though cholesterol-overfeeding is widely acknowledged as atherosclerotic there is sufficient evidence to question the validity of this allegation [144,207]. Anitschkow [258] acknowledged that the rabbit lesions had an abundance of lipophages, an absence of hyalinization of the plaque, relatively little sclerosis and no ulceration. The evidence is that the fat storage can be reversed at least in part and depletion of lipophages that constitute the major space-occupying component of these dietary-induced lesions will reduce intimal encroachment on the lumen. The duration of the intimal fat-storage and secondary consequences thereof may influence the quantity of residual fibrosis. Even increase in collagen and elastin in the intimal matrix has been recognized [307]. The fate of the frequent calcification that occurs during 'regression' is uncertain. In cholesterol over-fed animals the degree of reversal of effect has been exaggerated and not studied in the very long term. It is not possible to exclude the possibility of damage to the wall by such an experimental procedure. To assume that other components of the thickened intima in these rabbits will also disappear is being optimistic but the use of a model closer to atherosclerosis would provide more reliable results.

In the human it is recognized that severe destructive arterial lesions due to trauma or infection undergo repair but there is no restitution of normal architecture. In view of the grossly disturbed architecture and degenerative changes that occur in atherosclerosis proper, on pathological grounds it must be concluded that if regression is truly possible all that could be expected would be repair, thrombolysis or organization of thrombus, clearance of lipid over a period of time and the possible formation of a neo-intima in places, smoothing out irregularities. There are no greater grounds for believing that atherosclerosis can really regress than that the effects of Kawasaki's disease which apparently accounts for some instances of adult coronary artery disease [308] will regress.

The evidence is that lipid can be cleared quickly in atheroembolism but phagocytosis of lipid in atherosclerosis is very limited even in normolipidaemic subjects. Cholesterol crystals will be difficult to dispose of and calcification is more likely to increase in an old fibrotic scar. If on the other hand FH is being considered, reduction of blood cholesterol levels may reduce the space-occupying capacity of the fat storage phenomenon but to suggest that it will also reverse the concomitant atherosclerotic process is debatable and doubtful. It is also inappropriate to extrapolate from FH to the population at large as so often occurs in epidemiology. In conventional atherosclerosis the bulk of the lesion is not fat and in vibrating tool disease regression does not occur. The limited reversibility of the changes in collagen and elastin is in part due to the slow turnover of these proteins but probably also due to the cumulative effect of haemodynamic stress. Repair is possible and is regularly seen pathologically but repair tissue too is not immune to such stresses. To suppress smooth muscle replication is potentially hazardous, since the evidence is that such proliferation is reparative, replacing its loss from destructive forces and granulovesicular degeneration apart from the role in synthesis and maintenance of non-cellular connective tissue matrix.

Removal of some intimal fat can and probably does occur even in normolipidaemic subjects. The question is, however, can the medial atrophy be reversed and what of the cell debris, the disrupted internal elastic lamina, the dystrophic basement membrane material and the collagen fibril degeneration? There is no evidence at present that this process can be reversed. On the contrary it appears to be relentlessly and insidiously progressive. Nevertheless it may be possible to retard the rate of progression and avoidance of deleterious aggravating factors is desirable when they are known (e.g. hypertension and possibly deficiency of copper, vitamin B_6 or vitamin C).

The best models to assess regression would be arteriovenous fistulae in which atherosclerosis and severe destruction of the vessel wall occurs in both arteries and veins. Closure of the arteriovenous fistulae in humans has been said to induce reduction in the lumen of some vessels angiographically. Structural changes that occur are undetermined but aneurysms may appear years after closure of the shunt suggesting that the crucial physicochemical changes are cumulative.

6.3.4 EPIDEMIOLOGICAL EVIDENCE

The epidemiology of atherosclerosis is essentially the epidemiology of CHD. Since it is not possible to assess satisfactorily the severity of atherosclerosis during life, the current school of epidemiology uses CHD as a surrogate for atherosclerosis, comparing the incidence of various characteristics of subjects with CHD with those of non-coronary heart disease subjects. These characteristics are referred to as risk factors.

Specific epidemiological criteria have been established for risk factors though these are not met by the current major risk factors. General acceptance of a factor as having a causal role depends essentially on covariance with the incidence of CHD. More than 280 risk factors have now been so labelled, many of little or no consequence such as baldness, premature grey hair, wifely love, snoring, etc. Such statistical correlations do not prove a cause and effect relationship since these correlations provide only indirect evidence of possible involvement in the development of CHD and some can be the consequences of CHD (e.g. angina). The major risk factors are generally accepted as hypercholesterolaemia, hypertension, smoking, obesity, diabetes mellitus and a sedentary life style.

CHD was almost unknown at the turn of the century and yet by the middle of the century the antibiotic era had commenced and CHD became the major cause of death in technologically advanced countries. This increase in CHD mortality rates is repeatedly referred to as an epidemic which many regard as spurious [309]. There can be no epidemic of ubiquitous atherosclerosis only variation in severity. At the turn of the century the pathology of coronary occlusion and myocardial infarction had not been elucidated and deaths were variously ascribed to senility, acute, fatty or fibrous myocarditis, myocardial degeneration, angina and endocarditis. Moreover the life expectancy was only about 47 years in the USA in the early 1900s but since then longevity has substantially increased and the population has almost tripled. Since most deaths attributed to CHD occur after the age of 65 years and very few before 50 years, a great increase in deaths from CHD would be expected in an aging and expanding population especially as knowledge of its pathology and diagnostic criteria became better known only after 1926. National mortality rates for CHD in the USA peaked about 1968, and then the rate declined. This occurred in several other countries and the rise and fall of CHD mortality rates convinced epidemiologists that environmental factors were responsible for the rise and fall and that CHD was essentially preventable.

This modern school of epidemiology maintains that all diseases have multiple causes and prefers to use risk factor rather than cause, but in practice risk factors for CHD are used interchangeably with the causes of atherosclerosis. Whilst epidemiological methods were of considerable value with acute and subacute infectious diseases, they are of limited value in chronic degenerative diseases like atherosclerosis [310]. Nevertheless, belief in the lipid hypothesis was given considerable support by many pathologists who maintained that a high cholesterol diet induced atherosclerosis in experimental animals and that premature CHD and severe atherosclerosis occurred in both homozygotes and heterozygotes with very high serum cholesterol levels. Without the pathological and experimental support, epidemiological assertions would have warranted little credence.

In the 1950s Keys [311] reported an almost linear relationship between the national mortality rates for CHD and the fat available for consumption in six selected countries. This was supported by the low serum cholesterol levels, low animal fat intake, low incidence of CHD and less severe atherosclerosis in third world countries in Africa than in affluent Western populations. Following lipid depletion in rabbits and the alleged resumption of a normal histological vascular architecture in cholesterol-fed monkeys [312] after cessation of a high cholesterol diet, many regression studies were conducted on humans. Sometimes they were dietary, sometimes multiple risk reduction regimens and at times many cholesterol-lowering drugs were administered. Again clinical or fatal CHD was the end-point in such trials and many cardiologists, epidemiologists and clinical biochemists found them convincing. Legitimate criticisms were levelled at the methodology of clinical trials and yet others were convinced of their validity and benefit though the lives that were to be saved have still to be demonstrated. There is also concern over the apparent high mortality from cancer and violence amongst those with low blood cholesterol levels.

Further regression studies using angiographic and ultrasonography have been reported with allegedly favourable results and further attempts at refining the assessment of atherosclerosis in arterial segments are in progress. These results, reviewed by consensus conferences in many countries, are generally regarded as overwhelming proof of the validity of the lipid hypothesis which theorizes that a diet high in cholesterol and animal saturated fats elevates serum cholesterol and low density lipoprotein levels, in turn inducing severe premature atherosclerosis and a high incidence of CHD.

Many reports have indicated that the incidence of CHD increases with the serum cholesterol or LDL levels and there is usually, but not invariably, an inverse relationship with serum high density lipoprotein (HDL) levels. Hence HDL is regarded as 'good cholesterol'. The realization that CHD occurs in subjects with serum cholesterol levels below the upper discrimination value has led to reconsideration of the customary statistical standards for serum cholesterol in the community. It is now stated that serum cholesterol levels are too high if CHD occurs and since CHD (and certainly atherosclerosis) occurs at all blood levels, population-wide reduction in dietary intake of cholesterol and saturated animal fats is recommended by national Heart Associations or Foundations and CHD epidemiologists.

Although the lipid theory and its variants currently dominate the field of atherogenesis, certain weaknesses in the hypothesis have been indicated in the text and Smith has documented many inconsistencies and much bias in epidemiological evidence [313,314]. Methodological problems must be overcome before an adequate assessment of regression of atherosclerosis can be achieved in living subjects [315]. There is growing concern regarding the possible hazard of *trans* fatty acids and the deleterious effect of low blood cholesterol levels [163]. For critical appraisal of the regression and of the lipid hypothesis the reader is referred to other publications [163,313,314] which deal with the topic in more detail.

6.3.5 LIPID AUTOXIDATION THEORY

Normal oxygen utilization in mammalian tissue requires an enzymatically controlled four-electron reduction to form water. If oxygen accepts less than four electrons it forms highly reactive free radicals with one or more unpaired electrons. These oxyradicals can produce chemical damage to intact tissue as well as unsaturated fats, cholesterol, LDL and some proteins. Under normal circumstances only small amounts of these products are produced and are rapidly quenched by antioxidant activity.

It has been hypothesized that hypoxia due to intimal thickening with increased diffusion differences, increased demand for oxygen, inadequate vascularity and abnormal tissues reducing the oxygen diffusion rates may all encourage or accelerate oxyradical production and oxidative modification of cholesterol, LDL, tissue lipids and cellular constituents of the vessel wall. Crawford and Blankenhorn [316] have postulated that minor deviations from normal arterial wall anatomy and function can lead to oxyradical damage and accentuate atherogenesis. This of course would be difficult to prove or disprove and remains conjectural with evidence of localization of oxyradicals provided from cholesterol-fed animals. This is not to deny the arterial wall necrosis that can be produced by oxidation products of cholesterol but if hypoxia is so important in this hypothesis, atherosclerosis should be more severe in the pulmonary arterial tree and veins. Aggravation in the systemic circulation should be pronounced in cyanotic patients due to cardiac or pulmonary disease but no such evidence is available. The hypothesis also presupposes an absence or deficiency of antioxidants. The possibility is that the form of tissue damage or the ill effects of lipid peroxides may occur in atherogenesis and especially perhaps in advanced disease with a grossly thickened intima in which case it is but an aggravating factor and not causal. To suggest that it can be causal is inconsistent with current knowledge of the pathogenesis of this ubiquitous disease, its initiation *in utero*, its topography, experimental production and its production in humans by means of therapeutic arteriovenous shunts and venous bypass grafts. The hypothesis is reminiscent of the old theory of anoxia in a very thickened intima and it is important to determine the cause of the intimal thickening. Autoxidation products of cholesterol have been considered to aggravate the vascular effects of a high cholesterol diet in rabbits and consequently the angiotoxicity of oxygenated sterols has been considered to play a possible role in atherogenesis [317,318]. Not all oxygenated sterols are angiotoxic and some have been implicated as inhibitors of cholesterol biosynthesis and in regulation of sterol metabolism. Lipid peroxidation may occur in foods prior to ingestion and may be formed during cooking. The polyunsaturated fatty acids are very susceptible and the most susceptible oils are those rich in essential fatty acids but the significance for nutrition is likely to be minimal.

It is thought that lipid accumulation in atherosclerosis is primarily due to the uptake of LDL by phagocytosis. Yet when the cell cholesterol level increases, the activity of LDL receptors is decreased, leading to the belief that some other mechanism accounts for the cholesterol and lipid accumulation in the cells of the arterial wall such as monocytes. Therefore it has been assumed that LDL must be modified possibly by autoxidation to render it palatable to monocytes to enable them to become foam cells. Consequently considerable interest has been engendered in the possible effects of autoxidation modifications in atherosclerosis and being immunogenic they have been detected in serum and atherosclerotic tissue [319]. Recent evidence has fostered the belief that such modification of LDL may lead to its unregulated uptake by macrophages through a specific receptor in the acetyl LDL or scavenger receptor [320,321]. Witzum [322] believes oxidative modification of LDL in the intima may be responsible for chemotaxis of monocytes and may be a prerequisite for LDL uptake and accumulation of cellular cholesterol ester in the intima. Intervention studies in the LDL receptor-deficient Watanabe hereditary hypercholesterolaemic (WHHL) rabbit using probucol as an antioxidant have reduced the lipid uptake and development of foam cell lesions. Such experiments are of more relevance to lipid storage diseases than to atherosclerosis. Nevertheless autoxidation modification of LDL is thought to play a significant role in progression of coronary atherosclerosis in middle-aged males [319,323] and recommendations for prophylactic increase in the intake of antioxidants have followed.

These concepts assume cause and effect, ignore the fact that progressive accumulation in the vessel wall of cell debris with its known affinity for lipid precedes lipid accumulation and assume that foam cells are deleterious, whereas the more logical approach is to seek the basic reason for their presence in atherosclerosis. The more plausible explanation is that monocytes enter the intima to phagocytose cell debris (matrix vesicles). Since the matrix vesicles progressively accumulate in abundance, their phagocytosis by smooth muscle cells becomes inadequate and with continued granulovesicular degeneration of the muscle cells monocytes enter the intima in large numbers. As the debris continues to accumulate, there is little value in inhibiting phagocytic activity of monocytes and delaying clearance of cell debris.

For the most part studies of the underlying mechanisms involved in these oxygenated sterols are dependent on tissue culture rather than *in vivo* and it is unlikely that such an uncontrolled mechanism would occur only in arteries at specific sites and not in other tissues as well. LDL is an essential metabolite of cells and the possibility is that their modification may result from the atherosclerotic process rather than be causal as has been assumed.

The half-life and effective concentration of these autoxidation products are unknown. To suggest that they play a dominant pathogenic role is speculative and overlooks the protective role of the immune system and the antioxidant defence system [324] involving thiols, carotenoids, tocopherols and vitamins E, C and A [325]. The defence of living eukaryotic cells against these oxidation products is complex and it remains to be proven that they play a significant and specific role in atherogenesis. Their presence in minimally affected blood vessels and other tissues, their non-specific cytotoxicity and the lack of relevance to many other features of atherosclerosis fail to support the allegedly dominant role in atherogenesis. It cannot be denied they may play a role but it must be contributory or aggravating and not causal.

6.3.6 THROMBOGENIC THEORY OF ATHEROGENESIS

One of the major theories of atherogenesis, the thrombogenic hypothesis, was first postulated by von Rokitansky who suggested that atherosclerosis was due to encrustation of the arterial wall with material derived from the flowing blood [326]. This concept was revived in the 1940s by Duguid [327,328] who thought red thrombus was particularly likely to undergo fatty degeneration. Many atherosclerotic plaques and particularly eccentric lesions encroach on the lumen and with histological evidence of lamination, such plaques were considered the end result of organization of successive layers of mural thrombus but interpretation is not proof.

The available evidence indicates that thrombosis is secondary to intimal discontinuity in human and experimental pathology [11]. Moreover, endothelium *in vivo* and *in vitro* presents a non-thrombogenic surface to which platelets seldom adhere. Thrombosis is the secondary phenomenon and the cause of the intimal discontinuity must be primary. The distribution of thrombi differs from that of atherosclerosis and lipid is ordinarily removed rapidly from organizing mural thrombi and even from atheroemboli except for cholesterol crystals. Eccentric atherosclerotic plaques can be explained other than by incorporation of a mural thrombus which can contribute to mural thickening and encroachment on the lumen. The question is to what extent? The concept does not explain the pathogenesis of all the structural and biochemical changes in atherosclerosis nor the pathogenesis of the complications. Modifications of this hypothesis have been proposed (section 3.12). The most recent and popular variant is the 'intimal injury hypothesis'.

6.3.7 INTIMAL INJURY HYPOTHESIS

This hypothesis originated early this century when authors spoke of mechanical irritation, wear and tear, etc. Duff [329,330] invoked some invisible injury as being responsible for the localization of lipid in the vessel wall in spontaneous human atherosclerosis and in the vascular lesions of the cholesterol-fed rabbit. It was recognized earlier that physical injury localized dietary-induced lipid deposition at the site of trauma [258] and in subsequent years every conceivable vascular insult including immunological injury has had a similar effect. As such the cause of the hypothetical injury must be primary and the intimal injury the consequence thereof and not the cause of atherosclerosis. The defects in this concept were:

1. the pathogenesis and the vascular lesions were dissimilar to atherosclerosis;
2. the criteria for causality did not comply with appropriately modified Koch's postulates;
3. the lesions were self-limiting and non-progressive;
4. given time to heal the site of trauma ceased to have affinity for lipid [331];
5. methyl cellulose also accumulates at sites of trauma [332].

Injury presupposes an exogenous insult and an event of short duration but not a spontaneous occurrence under physiological conditions. Mechanical trauma is unlikely except at the aortic valve cusps or superficial veins which are not sites of severe atherosclerosis. Underlying this concept of injury is the search for a localizing factor or some local tissue factor in the wall responsible for making the vessel susceptible or receptive to lipid accumulation. It also became acknowledged that trauma could damage the endothelium and incorporate platelets, fibrin or thrombus into the vessel wall as is consistent with the thrombogenic theory and also that endothelial denudation or freshly regenerated endothelium would be a portal of entry permitting the influx of plasma into the vessel wall including LDL and thus cholesterol. Another plausible characteristic of trauma was its ability to induce intimal proliferation of smooth muscle cells even though it produces a self-limiting process of repair and regeneration with little or no intimal thickening. Yet repetitive injury might repeat all of these phenomena and sequelae. Consequently mechanical factors were thought to determine the site of lipid deposition in cholesterol-fed rabbits, or cholesterol was considered an effective marker of structural damage otherwise obscure [333]. Since lesions occurred so frequently and consistently at arterial branching sites, haemodynamics (hypertension with increased shear stress) was also invoked as an injurious agent because it was allegedly able to 'localize' atherosclerotic lesions. With the continued emphasis on hypercholesterolaemia in atherogenesis, hyperlipoproteinaemia was invoked as an injurious agent [334]. On the other hand Clowes et al. [335] found hyperlipoproteinaemia in the rat did not produce chronic endothelial injury, nor the development of proliferative intimal fibrous plaques, and did not enhance or induce persistence of established smooth muscle cell lesions or inhibit regression of trauma-induced intimal proliferation.

Inevitably repetitive intimal injury was invoked as the initiating lesion in atherogenesis and one or many factors acting synergistically were said to result in hypothetical injuries, where denuded endothelium permitted platelets to adhere to subendothelial tissues with the release of a mitogenic agent, the platelet-derived growth factors (PDGF). This specifically induced medial smooth muscle cells to proliferate and invade the intima at the same time as intimal proliferation was exposed to the noxious effects of serum lipoproteins. Thus the initial lesion was established but intimal muscle in response to trauma is not longitudinally orientated [336] as is intimal proliferation at forks and bends. PDGF allegedly stimulates intimal thickening and preceded lipid deposition [188,334]. Endothelial repair and regression allegedly took place if the event was not repeated and the balance between regression and progression was adversely affected by risk factors. With recurrent episodes, the lesion progressed until the lumen was sufficiently occluded to permit thrombosis.

The hypothetical endothelial denudation has not been confirmed and there is no evidence in the fetus and infants of such events in the intimal thickenings at arterial forks where most atherosclerotic lesions commence. Endothelial denudation in man is a late phenomenon [138]. Subsequently the hypothesis was substantially modified [12] and it was suggested that platelet damage (with release of pharmacological agents including PDGF) mediated by haemodynamic stresses, might be responsible for more subtle endothelial injury, increased permeability and setting in motion the pathogenesis of atherogenesis [12,188]. A similar train of events was also proposed earlier by Jørgensen *et al.* [337]. However, eddy currents must be widespread and not confined to large systemic arteries and there is no *in vivo* evidence that aggregated platelets alter the endothelium functionally or predispose endothelial cells to sticking of blood cells. Otherwise thrombosis would be a widespread self-propagating disorder from which there would be no recovery and this would be incompatible with life [105]. Moreover, in haemodynamically induced tears of the internal elastic lamina, endothelial disruption and thrombosis are followed by atrophy rather than muscle proliferation which is limited at least for a prolonged period of time.

This hypothesis is not a theory of the aetiology of atherosclerosis. Rather it is a theory that such a mitogenic factor is but one possible mediator of smooth muscle replication in intimal proliferation. Whilst little is known of the humoral control of smooth muscle proliferation, it is more likely to be a complex interplay of chemical mediators, activators, antagonists and co-factors rather than being due merely to one platelet derived growth factor.

In view of the remarkable ease with which endothelium is damaged with the consequent formation of (reversible) platelet–leucocyte thromboemboli, it is biologically implausible for the latter to initiate intimal proliferation and atherosclerosis. For if this were so atherosclerosis would be most pronounced in superficial veins in which there is no significant progressive lesion demonstrable irrespective of blood lipids. Moreover, this hypothesis does not explain the gamut of changes in atherogenesis, the atrophic lesions nor the complications. Thus it is not a theory of atherogenesis but a theory pertinent to only one non-pathognomonic step or mediator in the pathogenesis of the disease and even then PDGF is not produced by platelets alone, nor is it specific in its mitogenic activity. The intimal injury hypothesis is a speculative amalgamation into a unified theory of several hypotheses of pathogenetic factors. Since none of these factors progresses to atherosclerosis, the intimal injury hypothesis basically suffers from the flaws of its individual parts [89].

The most important aspects of this theory are:

1. it is a belated acceptance of the concept that musculoelastic intimal proliferation is an early and pre-lipid stage of atherosclerosis;
2. PDGF has been a strong stimulus to the development of knowledge of this and other growth factors and related pharmacological agents.

6.3.8 MONOCLONAL HYPOTHESIS

Benditt and Benditt [211] alleged that atherosclerotic fibrous plaques are derived from a single clone of cells and suggested that smooth muscle cell proliferation in atherosclerosis was monoclonal growth possibly caused by chemical mutagens, viruses or both. They examined the atherosclerotic aortic intima of four heterozygous females for the X-linked glucose-6-phosphate dehydrogenase isoenzymes and found that the plaques, even from the one individual, contained muscle cells which were either predominantly of type A or type B, with some of mixed populations. Samples from the media or thin intima revealed for the most part a mixed population of smooth muscle cells. The relatively monoclonal nature of some plaques was interpreted as indicating a neoplastic type of proliferation. Benditt [338] excluded the possibility of a selective advantage of one cell type over the other by the consistent presence of lesions composed of each cell type.

Subsequently Pearson *et al.* [399,340] essentially confirmed these findings and found that some fatty streaks were also monoclonal suggesting that they were forerunners of fibrous plaques. It is more likely that the intimal proliferation arose from a limited population of sparsely distributed smooth muscle cells in the non-thickened intima where the internal elastic lamina acts as a relative barrier inhibiting the extension of medial muscle into the intima [11]. Furthermore growth of the two cell types in X-linked mosaicism is known to be skewed quite often and Benditt's observation may be no more than this. The latter possibilities appear to be plausible explanations of the findings particularly since the plaques were not strictly speaking truly monoclonal in nature and some were distinctly mixed [338]. Certainly the findings do not warrant Benditt's postulation that the intimal proliferation of atherosclerosis was of neoplastic nature, possibly caused by some viral or chemical mutation [211]. Thomas *et al.* [341] indicated that two other alternatives exist to explain Benditt's alleged monoclonal origin of intimal cells. One of the glucose-6-phosphate dehydrogenase alleles may be linked to other genes on the X chromosome that affords preferential survival in the pathological conditions prevailing in atherosclerosis. As a consequence, cells with one allele may be more able to survive and grow than cells possessing the other allele, and this characteristic may be unrelated to A-ness or B-ness. The other alternative relates to clonal heterogeneity of cell growth potential with a continual selection of those cells capable of producing the largest number of progeny. Continued subculture *in vitro* has been found to result in predominance of one cell type at the expense of another with the eventual appearance of monotypism in the culture [342]. Thomas *et al.* [341] rightly asserted that these alternative explanations must be shown to be invalid before any acceptance of monoclonal origin as the explanation of Benditt's observed relative cellular monotypism of atherosclerotic plaques.

The current trend is to regard intimal fibromuscular

proliferation as an early phase of atherosclerosis, and the aortic intima is known to be thickened in humans, with some areas thicker than others. To differentiate plaques from non-plaque areas in the aorta is but an exercise in comparing the cell characteristics of varying stages of the one disease process, a not uncommon practice. Benditt [338] found that the aortic intimal proliferation of middle-aged and elderly people was composed of mixed cell populations. He then inferred that plaques are atherosclerotic and that the preceding intimal thickening is merely an aging process rather than being two stages of the same disorder. Referring to a 'non-plaque area' as 'non-involved' by atherosclerosis is not consistent with the facts.

Benditt [338,343] regarded atherosclerosis as consisting of three stages: the first is the initiation stage during which a cell in the artery wall (site unspecified) undergoes mutation; then when conditions exist such as to promote the expression of the selective proliferative advantage conferred by the mutation, proliferation proceeds to form a plaque; his third stage consists of the degeneration of the proliferated cells with ulceration, etc. Such a concept ignores the fact that atherosclerosis is not a focal disease but one that eventually involves the entire intimal surface of the aorta and larger arteries although certain areas tend to be affected earlier and more severely than others. Moreover, it fails to explain the ubiquitous nature of atherosclerosis in man and in the animal kingdom or the consistent topography of the disease. The cellular degeneration in Benditt's stage three is unexplained. It is unlikely to account for all the complications of the disease and the physicochemical changes occurring in the connective tissues. It is inconceivable that mutations would occur so often, so consistently and in such a regular distribution in each and every individual and animal that develops atherosclerosis even by a hypothetical mutagen or virus.

Even if Benditt's mutagenic concept were valid, the cause of the mutation still has to be the primary cause of the disease. Yet, it has already been demonstrated that the intimal proliferation which proceeds to advanced atherosclerosis with the full range of complications can be produced in several different experimental models, and is induced regularly in man in the coronary venous bypass grafts and therapeutic arteriovenous fistulae. Moreover, Benditt has assumed that there is aortic intimal proliferation due to aging and further proliferation of mutant cells leading to atherosclerotic plaques. Differentiation of these two phases has not been made, and there is much evidence that they are but manifestations of one disease. Jores' contention [344] still holds that one of the most important problems to be solved in atherosclerosis is to determine the nature of the intimal proliferation that precedes the deposition of lipid.

6.3.9 UNIFYING HYPOTHESIS

Benditt and Schwartz [345] proposed a 'unifying hypothesis' in which intimal proliferation of smooth muscle cells develops due to trapping of the muscle cells in the intima during embryogenesis or as the result of mutation and migration of muscle cells. This first step was to account for the monoclonality of the plaques. The second step was the accumulation of lipid depending on the properties of the smooth muscle cells or the connective tissue rendering the sites prone to lipid accumulation. Lipid insudation then caused cell injury which led to the accumulation of macrophages and platelets and these in turn released growth factors as proposed in the 'reaction to injury' hypothesis, thus further stimulating smooth muscle cell proliferation. The monocytes played the central role in lipid accumulation thus accounting for the lipophages. As the lesion progressed, endothelial injury might lead to loss of anticoagulant properties of the wall and so mural thrombosis resulted in occulusion of the lumen as well as providing more PDGF. This attempt at unifying several hypotheses without evidence does not explain the topography, the pathogenesis or the complications of the disease. Furthermore, altered haemodynamics in blood vessels can induce intimal proliferation where none previously existed and can also induce intimal proliferation at arterial forks in herbivorous rabbits to progress to overt atherosclerosis thus making most of their hypothesis unnecessary.

6.3.10 MECHANICAL OR HAEMODYNAMIC HYPOTHESIS

Physiological or pathological haemodynamic stresses have long been considered to play a role in the pathogenesis of atherosclerosis because of the consistent localization of atherosclerotic lesions. This is further strengthened by the precise localization of the fibromusculoelastic intimal thickenings at forks, junctions and curvatures and this intimal muscle proliferation is now widely accepted as a crucial early intimal lesion progressing to atherosclerosis. However, haemodynamics has almost universally been regarded merely as a localizing factor.

Localization of atherosclerosis in past decades has been studied primarily by staining specimens for fat in the gross and often in middle-aged or even the elderly. This is an inappropriate technique since the lipid stains have limited penetrability in a sclerotic thickened intima and consequently controversy has continued as to whether the disease occurs in high (flow divider) [248, 249] or low (lateral pads, lesser curvature of bends) [246,247] shear-stress areas, whereas it commences in both and eventually the entire aortic surface is affected as is the case in other segments of large distributing arteries. No adequate explanation is provided for the loss of cohesion, mural weakness and aneurysmal dilatation nor other manifestations of atherosclerosis by this 'shear-stress' hypothesis which ignores the fact that shear stresses are repetitive and therefore vibrations.

A number of different mechanical concepts have been considered to play a role.

(a) Wear and tear

This usually denotes the cumulative damage sustained during everyday usage, and though invoked in a general manner, the term is inappropriate and unscientific. As applied to clothing it is the cumulative effect of abrasions and tears which has no counterpart in the circulation in pathological terms since there is no vascular trauma.

(b) Trauma

Mechanical injury has frequently been incriminated but exogenous trauma cannot be responsible and does not explain the specific localization. Trauma to an artery induces musculoelastic intimal thickening but this does not progress to atherosclerosis. Nevertheless, some sort of injury has been thought to participate and Duff [329,330] concluded that in both atherosclerosis and dietary-induced lipid deposition in experimental animals, some hypothetical injury was responsible for making the arteries susceptible to lipid accumulation. Almost every conceivable type of injury including immunological injury has been used to damage segments of arteries and the administration of a high-cholesterol diet resulted in lipid deposition at the site of injury but not about a phlebotomy wound. This suggests that it is not trauma alone that is responsible for the predilection for dietary-induced lipid deposition which disappears with healing. If an artery is injured and then allowed to heal, it loses this affinity for dietary-induced lipid deposition [331] leading Duguid and Robertson [333] to conclude that cholesterol feeding is merely an effective marker of structural damage. If this were the case, then the intimal proliferation at arterial forks must be a site of continual damage for it exhibits persistent predilection for dietary-induced lipid deposition.

The intimal injury hypothesis is a perpetuation of this theme but the injury is hypothetical. Yet it must be agreed that there is a local tissue factor that predisposes the tissue at specific sites to such lipid accumulation. The evidence is that this localizing factor is haemodynamic stress associated with blood flow. In the cholesterol-fed rabbit, veins exhibit relatively little susceptibility to lipid deposition. However, in an experimental arteriovenous fistula, the anastomosed veins exhibit greater propensity for lipid deposition than the traumatized artery and vein, or the artery feeding the fistula [270]. Such experiments suggest that haemodynamic stress localizes and also governs the lipid accumulation in dietary-induced lipid deposition or cholesterolosis.

Several early authors believed that there was some mechanical irritation or flow-induced injury to the intima accounting for the imbibition of lipid into the loosened intimal tissues and Aschoff [346] invoked tugging by branches. Thoma [49] invoked a primary medial weakness (angiomalacia) with dilatation, which led to compensatory intimal thickening to maintain the cross-sectional area to its original dimensions. This was followed by anoxia and secondary degenerative changes. A drag effect on the intimal surface has been invoked and so have intimal irritation [94], intimal herniation into the interstices of the fenestrae in the internal elastic lamina, a pulsatile suction or drag effect [104,347] and shear stresses, but these theories do not explain the localization or the pathogenesis. The deposition of platelets in extracorporeal shunts led to the combination of the thrombogenic and haemodynamic concepts. This ignored the thrombogenic surface in the shunt and silting of platelets did not explain the localization or the pathogenesis [89]. Intimal pads or cushions at lateral angles were attributed to boundary layer separation [11] and increased permeability and secondary thrombosis was suggested at such sites. High and low shear stresses have been invoked but the evidence on which these views were founded was fallacious as explained earlier.

Keller [348] invoked a mass transport phenomenon to explain the distribution of atherosclerosis. The concept was based on the erroneous assumption that plaques were all localized at sites of boundary layer separation or low shear regions where relative stagnation would permit concentration of large lipoproteins thus facilitating hypothetical chemical reactions which produce an atherosclerotic plaque. Caro et al. [246,247] subsequently postulated that the distribution of early atherosclerotic lesions was determined by mass transport of cholesterol into and out of the vessel wall in accordance with changes in shear stress in the diffusion boundary layer. They alleged that cholesterol synthesized in the vessel wall could be carried away more readily in high velocity and high shear regions whereas in low shear, low velocity areas lipid would accumulate. Like so many hypotheses, this theory is concerned principally with lipid accumulation in the vessel wall and does not explain the initial intimal proliferation, the topography, pathogenesis or complications of atherosclerosis.

Considerable emphasis of late has been given to low shear stress as the principal mechanical factor in atherogenesis, usually in conjunction with the lipid hypothesis. Glagov and colleagues [349] emphasized dilatation of the artery to compensate for intimal proliferation thus maintaining a relatively stable shear stress calculated from the perfusion fixed dimensions of the arterial segment. Without knowledge of the blood velocity, such calculations are of limited value. This hypothesis is but a modern version of that proposed by Thoma that the intima thickened to maintain a constant diameter. Whilst the flowing blood would tend to maintain a circular streamlined lumen, this is not always the case and is not true at bifurcations. Angiography displays the atherosclerotic artery in silhouette with considerable irregularity in longitudinal profile. More important are the qualitative changes or functional adequacy of the mural tissues which are more likely to be adversely affected by pulsatile shear stresses, the pulse pressure and other vibrations generated in the flowing blood.

Thoma regarded the thickening as reparative due to yield of the media caused by angiomalacia but it is inappropriate to assign to the wall the ability to proliferate, to maintain a 'constant' shear stress. Cyclic stretching stimulates matrix synthesis *in vivo* [350] and vibrational stress stimulates endothelial replication. It is likely that variations in luminal contour would induce flow changes and the associated unstable stress patterns associated with flow separation could induce proliferation as a local cellular response [350].

A more detailed critique of these mechanical concepts has been published elsewhere [11].

6.3.11 FATIGUE HYPOTHESIS

In 1958, the theory was proposed that atherosclerosis was caused by haemodynamically induced fatigue of the blood vessel wall due to vibrations generated in the flowing blood together with the pulse pressure [106]. Atherosclerosis was thus defined as the degenerative and compensatory reparative changes in the blood vessel walls that are the direct consequence of haemodynamically induced fatigue [11]. The complications of atherosclerosis are the consequences of mechanical failure of the mural constituents. Although other lesions may induce some of the manifestations of atherosclerosis, they do not reproduce the characteristic manifestations of overt atherosclerosis, its pathogenesis or complications despite the fact that manifestations of atherosclerosis may be superimposed or possibly even act synergistically at times [11]. This concept of atherosclerosis explains the complications of atherosclerosis which are due to mechanical failure of the cellular and non-cellular constituents of the vessel wall. The lipid accumulation is due to a non-specific affinity for lipid in the matrix vesicles or granulovesicular cell debris and calcification likewise, although it may also be associated with collagen and elastin. This affinity for lipid is seen so widely in many degenerative diseases and explains lipid accumulation at all serum levels of cholesterol and LDL without having to regard all subjects with CHD as hypercholesterolaemic. It also explains the reproduction of atherosclerosis in herbivorous animals, in venous bypass grafts and its accelerated development in the anastomosed veins of arteriovenous fistulae.

In the engineering sense, fatigue has been known for over a century and occurs in biological materials such as timber and rubber apart from metals etc. Sound vibrations cause permanent nerve deafness and fatigue has been acknowledged as being responsible for stress fractures of bones and tendons in soldiers, athletes, sportspersons and for the post-stenotic dilatation and post-stenotic dissecting aneurysms. Typically fatigue fractures or tears are abrupt with a sharp surface such as those in the internal elastic lamina or a dissecting aneurysm quite distinct from the appearance due to a single load application.

Unfortunately most know little of fatigue or mechanical failure and some features [352] are as follows:

1. The fracture occurs when the stress amplitude is less than either the static fracture stress or the elastic limit. Failure occurs suddenly under normal operational loads, no extraordinary stress being required.
2. Cracks propagate without macroscopic deformation.
3. At a consistent level of stress amplitude, failure is dependent on a certain number of stress cycles rather than the total time under load. Under these circumstances age is but a time factor. An increase or decrease in the number of stresses required to induce failure indicates greater or lesser fatigue strength or endurance limit respectively.
4. An increase in tension or superimposing a constant stress or static load on the material increases the amplitude but not the frequency, thus accelerating the onset of fatigue by reducing the number of cycles necessary to cause failure. This phenomenon explains the role of hypertension in atherosclerosis because it increases mural tension.
5. There may be variation in amplitude and frequency but the effect is cumulative.

Temperature, water content and composition may all affect fatigue and once a minute crack or defect appears in the surface, stress concentration enhances the onset of fatigue at that site. Most materials are susceptible to fatigue. Vibrational stress inhibits embryonic growth in the mouse [353] and can cause chromosomal aberrations in cultured human lymphocytes. Such phenomena may result in impaired reparative processes if the vibrational frequency and amplitude are appropriate.

Vibrations are known to affect tissues in certain segments of the body as in vibrating tool disease, in which diffuse intimal proliferation with hyalinization, medial fibrosis and narrowing of the lumen occur in the small arteries sometimes with tortuosity and thrombotic occlusion [354]. Patients with mild symptoms similar to Raynaud's syndrome exhibit medial hypertrophy, which also occurs in the veins of arteriovenous fistulae and in hypertensive arteriolosclerosis. Skin atrophy and ulceration have accompanied this phenomenon and the atrophy may indicate poor repair or impaired replication. Dilatation of the cervix can be induced by vibrations and in the frequency range of 1 to 400 Hz, vibrations inhibit smooth muscle contraction [355] possibly by a direct effect on the actin–myosin cross-links. These vibrational effects could have a deleterious effect on atherosclerosis, aneurysms and arteriovenous fistulae and the more advanced the disease the greater could be their effect.

For additional information the reader is referred elsewhere [11] but there is important experimental evidence that requires consideration in any vascular disease where secondary haemodynamic effects on blood vessel walls may occur.

6.3.12 HAEMODYNAMIC MODELS

(a) Carotid–jugular arteriovenous fistulae

These fistulae were fashioned between the common carotid artery and the external jugular vein of stock-fed sheep with sham operations performed on the contralateral vessels [103]. The anastomosed vein was thereby subjected to severe haemodynamic vibrational stress and underwent irregular aneurysmal dilatation with intimal proliferation similar to severe phlebosclerosis of man. It progressed to extensive fibrosis, hyalinization, elastic tissue proliferation and degeneration, calcification, lipid deposition, intimal tears, dissection and mural thrombosis and intramural fibrin deposits similar to those occurring in man.

Short-term anastomoses of the renal artery to the inferior vena cava in dogs [356] produced fibrous intimal proliferation in the aorta above and below the origin of the left renal artery, the proximal and distal portions of the left renal artery and the inferior vena cava opposite the anastomoses (probably a jet lesion). The location of the changes in the aorta suggest that augmented flow into the renal artery is associated with intimal proliferation. This experiment requires follow up.

The human counterpart to this animal model of atherosclerosis is the arteriovenous shunt created therapeutically for haemodialysis in patients with chronic renal failure. In the venous segment atherosclerosis develops at an accelerated rate with thrombotic occlusion, stenosing lesions and aneurysms. The afferent artery of arteriovenous fistulae in sheep undergoes mural thinning, elongation, tortuosity and eventually aneurysmal dilatation [101]. There is profound loss of elastic tissue and muscle and in the human counterpart (the traumatic arteriovenous fistulae), aneurysmal dilatation is observed in the afferent artery [102].

(b) Experimental aneurysms

The observation that berry aneurysms often had visible atherosclerosis when the disease was minimal in the parent artery [21], even though the aneurysms are known to develop mostly in the middle aged or elderly, indicates the disease runs an accelerated course. Therefore, experimental aneurysms (berry, fusiform and lateral saccular) were fashioned using autogenous venous grafts in stock-fed rabbits [99,110]. Over one to four years, dilatation, mural thrombosis and atherosclerosis, histologically similar to the human disease, developed to a variable degree in the rabbits maintained on a stock diet.

Electron microscopy of the anastomosed veins of the sheep fistulae [159] and of the rabbit aneurysms [155] revealed the characteristic changes of human atherosclerosis [29,30]. In the intimal thickening which consists initially of multiple loosely arranged musculoelastic lamellae, there is progressive accumulation of cell debris or matrix vesicles and degeneration of smooth muscle cells. Some muscle cells become long and attenuated, others are irregularly branched. Associated with this is an increase in multilaminated basement membrane material beneath endothelial and smooth muscle cells, but there is also dystrophic arrangement of the basement membrane since thick multilaminated strands unrelated to cells and also reticulated patterns are observed. Partial separation of interendothelial cell spaces and of basement membranes from both endothelial cells and smooth muscle cells may be indicative of loss of cohesion of the vessel wall. Dystrophic changes in the collagen fibres, increased saline solubility of both collagen and elastin and evidence of fragility of the smooth muscle plasma membrane are also consistent with loss of cohesion and tensile strength.

(c) Tortuosities and U-bends

Atherosclerosis has been known to occur at arterial curvatures and a large zone is seen on the lesser curvature of the aortic arch and downstream of the ductus arteriosus in the fetus [13]. It is regularly observed in the splenic artery [104] and on the lesser curvature of the right coronary artery [357]. It is prominent in the carotid siphon (Figure 6.24) where intimal proliferation occurs just beyond the commencement of the lesser curvature of bends (i.e. in regions of boundary layer separation). Such regions progress to atherosclerosis and have a larger surface area of involvement when the flexure is sharp [13,358]. Disturbed flow has been demonstrated in such regions in glass models of similar curvatures [359].

Several authors have studied experimental tortuosities or bends and proliferative lesions have been observed in the region of the lesser curvature. Lipid deposition was reported but was not illustrated so presumably was minimal in amount [77,360]. U-bends have been fashioned on the common carotid artery of stockfed rabbits and sheep by transplanting the opposite common carotid end-to-end by microvascular surgery to the transected host carotid artery and pulling the sutures together to form a loop [52]. This was to test the effect of a curvature, since in the carotid siphon a proliferative lesion of atherosclerosis develops on the lesser curvature with atrophy and calcification on the greater curvature. In the experimental U-bend, intimal proliferation was found at comparable areas beyond the lesser curvature in rabbits and tears of the elastic lamina and extreme atrophy occurred on the greater curvatures with virtually no intimal thickening. Lipid was observed in the proliferative lesions of sheep [52].

(d) Half-ring bypass graft with stenosis

Matsuda *et al.* [361] fashioned a half-ring bypass on the rat carotid artery with a graft from the contralateral common carotid artery and a stenosis on the host carotid half-way between the two anastomotic sites. This unusual configuration produced intimal proliferation at lateral angles, on curvatures where boundary-layer separation would be expected and beyond the stenosis where turbulence would be expected. These experiments confirmed that intimal proliferation at the sites indicated is haemodynamically induced and that an inherent, special physiological or functional role for the intimal thickening is unlikely.

(e) Nephrectomy

Unilateral nephrectomy causes a substantial increase in the prevalence of spontaneous transverse tears of the internal elastic lamina in the remaining renal artery no doubt caused by the augmented flow to the hypertrophied intact kidney. These tears are accentuated by hypertension and associated with lengthening of the artery. Augmented flow and associated blood pressure changes are responsible for these early manifestations of atrophic lesions [362]. Also significant is that spontaneous tears in rat renal arteries which normally increase with age and hypertension do not progress in the presence of a stenosis of the rat tail artery proximally, suggesting that these tears are due to the pulse pressures principally.

(f) Experimental arterial forks

In experimental arterial forks fashioned by anastomosing the distal end of a transected common carotid artery to the contralateral artery in rabbits, transversely orientated tears of the internal elastic lamina developed in the arterial wall on one or other side of the neo-apex where the flux of blood impinges. Intimal proliferation developed in the proximal aspect of the transposed artery analogous to a lateral pad or cushion, indicating that intimal pads and elastic damage in arterial forks of the fetus and infant could be haemodynamically induced [63].

Scanning electron microscopy revealed that the transversely orientated tears in the internal elastic lamina on the greater curvature of bends, in the afferent arteries of carotid and femoral arteriovenous fistulae and in experimental forks appeared initially within a few days postoperatively sometimes with endothelial disruption and mural thrombosis. The tears increased in number and extent and intercommunicating tears resulted in conversion of the lamina to isolated remnants that appeared to be functionally ineffective. Fibrillary elastic tissue and some intimal thickening developed in the gaps in the long-term experiments, seemingly attempts to repair and compensate as occurs in human infants [13]. The evidence was that these elastic tears are the precursors of atrophic lesions. They are analogous to those occurring in infants, in dissecting aneurysms of cerebral arteries and to those in other animals in which they vary with breed and can be accentuated by lathyrism [117].

(g) Femoral arteriovenous fistulae

These have been produced in stock-fed rabbits by microvascular surgery. Tears in the internal elastic lamina were prominent in the abdominal aorta and homolateral iliofemoral arteries of rabbits with fistulae but were only occasional and sporadic in contralateral vessels and control animals. Intimal proliferation at branching sites proximal to the fistulae exhibited varying degrees of enlargement, extension and progression to overt atherosclerosis with lipid accumulation, fibrin deposition and mild calcification. The intimal thickenings at arterial forks can therefore be produced experimentally and can be induced to progress to overt atherosclerosis which also occurred along the posterior wall of the abdominal aorta and diffusely in the femoral artery and vein near the fistula [70]. Such findings suggest that atherosclerosis, rather than being a dietary or metabolic fat disorder, can be the consequence of haemodynamic stress as is the case in humans with venous bypass grafts and arteriovenous shunts for renal haemodialysis. However, in view of the greatly augmented flow in the aorta and iliofemoral arteries proximal to the fistula, together with the accompanying pressure changes, the results also support the concept that enhanced atherogenesis accompanies increased usage and that haemodynamic stress is much more than a localizing factor. The nature of the haemodynamic stress involved may be argued but currently vibrational stress and the resultant fatigue are the most plausible explanation. Shear stresses are variable and pulsatile and, producing vibrations, contribute to the development of fatigue.

(h) Hypercholesterolaemia and altered haemodynamics

Since haemodynamics is usually considered to be merely a localizing factor, the combined changes of haemodynamic stress and hypercholesterolaemia in rabbits were investigated by feeding cholesterol to rabbits with experimental arteriovenous fistulae and aneurysms [270,271]. The anastomosed veins of arteriovenous fistulae and the venous pouch aneurysms exhibited pronounced predilection for lipid deposition, more so than the traumatized artery and contralateral vein although the jet lesion exhibited some degree of sparing. These findings suggest that haemodynamic stresses localize lipid accumulation [270,271]. This was also reported in experimental curvatures [77]. Histologically, however, cholesterol feeding superimposed lipid storage on the haemodynamically induced changes in the blood vessel wall which was often honeycombed with lipid-laden macrophages (Figure 6.40). In other words the lesions are combined lesions although the lipophages may well be more vulnerable to the augmented stresses in these models than those habitually pertaining in the arteries.

The possibility exists that hyperlipoproteinaemia in humans may enhance lipid deposition in atherosclerosis as in arteriovenous shunts or aneurysms and consequently increase the space-occupying effect of lipid with further encroachment on the lumen. In FH where there is interference with lipid metabolism of every cell in the body, chronic diseases such as atherosclerosis may be enhanced as in diabetes mellitus. As yet there is no evidence to support such a contention nor is there strong evidence that the venous bypass graft in humans has a predilection for lipid deposition in FH. Currently there is no evidence that hypercholesterolaemia accelerates the haemodynamically induced degenerative changes and their progression to true atherosclerosis in these experimental models or in humans.

6.3.13 THERAPEUTIC MODELS

Closely related to experimental haemodynamic models in lower animals are the surgical procedures used clinically in the therapy and management of patients. With the widespread use of vascular surgery in the past few decades there are examples in humans not unlike the above experimental procedures.

(a) Venous bypass grafts

This is the surgical procedure that has occasioned most interest not merely for its therapeutic value but because veins have often been erroneously considered to be relatively immune to atherosclerosis. The lesson to be learnt is that failure to develop severe atherosclerosis does not mean the vein is immune but that it has not necessarily been exposed to the causative factor or to the same degree of stress. Veins can be spared more readily than arteries and so autologous veins are more readily available for bypass grafting. The introduction of a venous bypass graft is associated with a variable degree of inflammatory reaction and oedema in the vein and the deposition of a layer of thrombus on the areas of denuded endothelium in the first postoperative week. Occlusive thrombosis may occur early and depends on the degree of damage to the vessel assuming that the veins were reversed to permit flow. What happens to the valves has not been studied. The veins never become 'arterialized' (histologically) although macroscopically the vessel thickens due to initial hypertrophy of muscle with fibrosis in the media and fibromuscular intimal thickening. Elastic tissue proliferation occurs but the internal elastic lamina disappears and degenerative changes are progressive. Eventually the phlebosclerotic changes progress to luminal narrowing, fibrosis, hyalinization, calcification, loss of muscle and extracellular and intracellular lipid accumulation. Severe

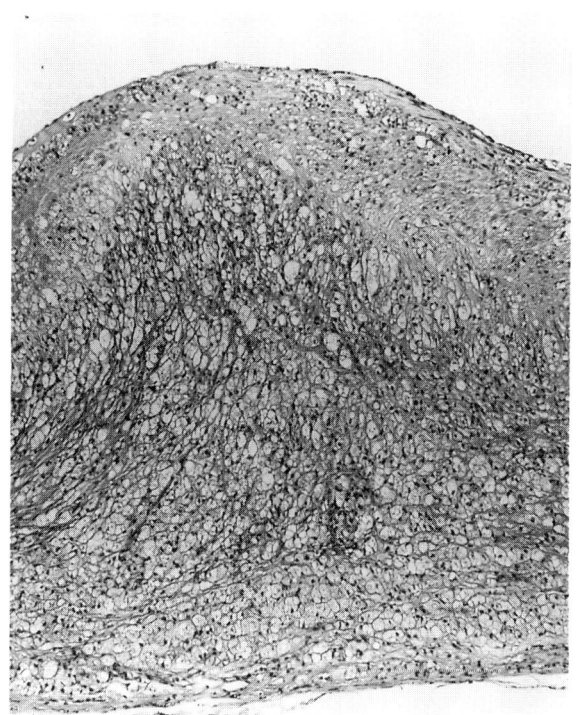

Figure 6.40 Segment of experimental aneurysm wall (rabbit) demonstrating complete loss of normal venous architecture but the wall is honeycombed with foam cells as in a fat storage disease. The animal had been on a cholesterol-rich diet postoperatively. (Haematoxylin and eosin.)

narrowing of the lumen may occur relatively early with little lipid deposition and other grafts more closely resemble conventional atherosclerosis after more protracted development with ulceration and thrombosis and occasionally aneurysmal dilatation [363,364]. Overt atherosclerosis did not occur within 12 months in the series reported by Lie *et al.* [363].

Severe narrowing may occur within 18 months and the histological features clearly resemble phlebosclerosis of varicose veins. The development of atherosclerosis in these bypass grafts has caused controversy as some authors deny its relevance to the disease of arteries. The severity under ordinary circumstances tends to be considerably milder than that observed in bypass grafts, the difference being a matter of degree.

The course is accelerated due to the severe haemodynamic stress as veins are not architecturally designed to withstand the stresses of arterial blood flow. The atherosclerosis cannot be attributed to diet or any circulating humoral agent be it cholesterol or LDL [63] since other veins and even the bypass grafts themselves, if left intact and *in situ*, would have continued to exhibit minimal or mild change for the remaining years of life.

Lie *et al.* [363] reported more severe intimal changes and atherosclerosis in hyperlipidaemic than in normolipidaemic subjects. This indicates the possibility that hypercholesterolaemia may increase the lipid content of haemodynamically stressed bypass grafts as it does in experimental venous graft aneurysms and also in venous bypass grafts in experimental animals [271]. However, qualitative assessment of the vascular changes is needed in subjects with FH compared to controls but atherosclerosis also occurred in normolipidaemic subjects.

Ultrastructurally the mural changes are likely to be identical to those in atherosclerosis in arteries [29] and in experimental aneurysms in rabbits [155].

Concern has been expressed regarding the rapidity with which these degenerative changes occur and the frequency of stenotic lesions. The factors that are likely to affect the outcome and life of the graft are:

1. **Surgical trauma.** Surgeons must appreciate the delicate nature of the blood vessel wall and the need to avoid drying.
2. **Reflex angle.** The recurrent course of coronary bypass grafts with a supravalvular attachment may be disadvantageous haemodynamically.
3. **Vessel wall.** Inherited physicochemical characteristics of the connective tissues and the thickness of the venous wall (lower limb veins preferable) contribute to the outcome. Some external support may be advantagous.
4. **Suturing.** Surgical skill and care in fashioning the anastomosis might be improved by using a stereomicroscope. A stenosis at the anastomotic site must be avoided otherwise the vessel may occlude at the anastomosis or a post-stenotic dilatation may occur. Even a bruit may be present.
5. **Distal circulation.** The state of the distal circulation is important and a good 'flow through' beneficial but increased peripheral resistance with a poor run-off would be haemodynamically detrimental to the graft.
6. **Graft calibre (disproportion).** An unusually capacious graft would be analogous to a dolichoectatic vessel and the increased mural tension is likely to accelerate the degenerative changes.
7. **Infection.** As with any cardiovascular surgery, infection must be avoided at all cost.

The introduction of the internal mammary (thoracic) artery as a bypass has led to superior results [365,366] as would be expected since the elastic artery is architecturally designed to be more resilient. The improved surgical success of these arterial grafts does not mean that the arteries are immune to atherosclerosis. The changes they exhibit will be similar to those of any artery elsewhere but the coronary haemodynamics is unique. Several of the factors that influence venous grafts will also affect arterial grafts.

Sako and Varco [367] fashioned autologous pericardium as an aortic graft in dogs and dilatation and atherosclerosis developed in animals in the long term. Rupture occurred but the combination of vein and external pericardial support was more resilient than either alone, indicating the importance of the physical strength of the graft in its patency rate and survival.

A venous patch graft will exhibit similar changes to the venous bypass graft and the possibility of aneurysmal dilatation is very real.

(b) Arteriovenous fistulae

The therapeutic use of an arteriovenous shunt has a long history and is in common use for renal dialysis in subjects with renal failure. The anastomosis may be end-to-end or end-to-side but the vein becomes distended and progressively passes through the stage of ectasia. Aneurysmal dilatation may occur and the wall of the vein thickens, retains the architecture of a vein and progressively develops phlebosclerosis and atherosclerosis. The lumen becomes irregularly narrowed and may undergo thrombosis [101]. In this respect the anastomosed vein, being much smaller than the external jugular vein of a carotid–jugular fistula, behaves differently and is less inclined to become grossly aneurysmal.

The inescapable fact is that the structural and pathological changes must be due to the augmented haemodynamic stresses to which the vein is subjected and like the venous bypass graft, the atherosclerosis cannot logically be due to dietary fat or circulating lipids.

No detailed study has been made of the afferent artery in these therapeutic fistulae but from experimental work [70] it is expected that both atrophic and proliferative lesions of atherosclerosis will rapidly develop.

This model also confirms that the haemodynamic consequences of these flow disturbances are not species-specific and consequently the experimental results are applicable to humans. These models also indicate that veins are more susceptible to atherosclerosis than arteries.

6.3.14 ATHEROSCLEROSIS AND MISCELLANEOUS FACTORS

(a) Exercise and atherosclerosis

It is advocated widely that exercise protects the heart, reduces the blood cholesterol level and is beneficial for atherosclerosis [368,369]. Jogging and marathons are commonly promoted by heart foundations and associations. In the train of this fad has been a substantial increase in orthopaedic problems with spontaneous fractures of bones of the leg and foot, ruptured tendons and torn ligaments. Yet it is still assumed that the heart and blood vessels are immune to the physical laws of nature.

The commonest cause of death in joggers and marathon runners (usually 20–59 years old) is coronary heart disease (73%) and in another 11% it is unknown [370]. For that age group, the incidence is unusually high. Another 1% die of gastrointestinal haemorrhage which is likely to be due to haemodynamic destruction of platelets, just as the same stresses cause haemolytic anaemia and contribute to the production of matrix vesicles in the blood vessel wall. Recent experimental evidence in which overt atherosclerosis is induced by augmented flow and the associated pressure changes [70], casts serious doubt on the alleged benefits derived from such excessive exertion. It is incongruous that the intimal proliferation with its attendant degenerative changes ultrastructurally in the aorta and large arteries of infants is regarded as physiological adaptation in response to increasing physiological haemodynamic stresses [15] and yet all are encouraged to waste time and effort in jogging and marathon running allegedly for fun and to avoid severe atherosclerosis and CHD when the stresses are so much greater.

In the case of bone the stresses associated with a graded increase in exercise induce further bone deposition to suit its mechanical requirements whilst endowing optimum strength and stiffness [371]. However, stress fractures in female athletes are largely independent of bone mineral density [372]. Disuse on the other hand results in bone thinning and osteoporosis. Similar effects have been observed in other components of the musculoskeletal system. Hypertrophy of muscle and the capacity to sustain a greater workload are achieved by training which also increases the tensile strength of tendons and ligaments. In other words the stress load required to rupture the tissue in a single application is increased. In football players, cricketers and athletes, rupture of tendons and torn ligaments occurs under much lesser stress loads and the effect of training on repetitive stresses that result in mechanical fatigue with failure of the connective tissues has not been tested. It is known that there is a turnover of collagen and bone even though it may be slow. The onset of graduated exercise delays the onset of fatigue in practice as seen in marching soldiers but whether this is merely by strengthening the bone and increasing its tensile strength or whether there is a genuine increase in fatigue endurance is not known.

Physical training is known to improve the efficiency of the athlete's heart. It is likely that there may also be an increase in the quantity of stress fibres in endothelial cells and some hypertrophy of smooth muscle cells or of the media as a whole. Theoretically there could be thickening of elastic laminae and additional collagen synthesis (as in hypertension) with appropriate changes in the other matrix proteins to strengthen the arterial wall, whilst maintaining the basic architecture. Such physiological adaptation may increase the tensile strength of the arterial wall which normally should be much greater than any stress load achieved under physiological conditions. However, once again it is not known whether exercise increases the fatigue endurance of the blood vessel wall. This is the crucial question not whether exercise has an effect on blood coagulation factors. What is known is that under physiological conditions, a post-stenotic dilatation can develop beyond a stenosis, ulcerations and intimal tears develop in atherosclerosis due to intimal fragility and even in the fetus and neonate, microtears or microfractures are frequent in arteries at sites of special repetitive stresses. These same transversely orientated tears or microfractures can be produced within a few days by subjecting a segment of artery to special flow conditions to which it is unaccustomed. The intimal thickenings also can be produced haemodynamically in segments of arteries by flow conditions comparable to those prevailing at forks and curvatures. Proliferative changes in the fetus or infant where there is loss of elastica or medial thinning is analogous to reparative external scaffolding or an external callus formation as in bone. It is not repair of the original damage.

Blood vessels are living structures and there is some solubilization of elastin and collagen under stress and normally even in human atherosclerosis [175] suggesting a turnover of matrix proteins as well as endothelial and smooth muscle cells. However, the degenerative changes that develop depend on genetic factors, the biochemistry of mural constituents, cardiovascular haemodynamics, the use and abuse of the body and its tissues, adequacy of nutrients, the periodic presence of noxious agents, the topography of the vascular tree and postnatal and postmaturity changes to the topography and the vessel walls secondary to other pathological conditions. At the present time the repetitive stresses of the pulse pressure and its progressive increase with age, the pulsatile blood velocity and the vortex shedding at forks, bends and junctions progressively exert their inexorable effects on the wall (compensated for in part by reparative processes), ultimately resulting in mechanical failure as the complications of atherosclerosis become manifest. Reduction in vascular workload would promote healing but currently the evidence is that the vibrational stresses are cumulative and exercise must contribute to the cumulative effect.

(b) Atherosclerosis and vascular rejection in organ transplantation

In the transplantation of organs, blood vessels undergo graft vascular disease which in its florid state is an immunological arteritis, and in its slower form with immunosuppressive therapy there is stenosing intimal proliferation sometimes caused by graft arteriosclerosis.

Macroscopically, the arteries are noticeably prominent with thick pale walls possibly with some lipid accumulation and a severely narrowed lumen. The internal elastic lamina may be intact or fragmented and the stenosing intimal proliferation is atypical, loose cellular tissue affecting the larger arteries in particular and extending peripherally to involve myocardial vessels and arterioles. There is a variable cellular infiltration of the adventitia. It is uncertain whether the cause is cell-mediated or immunological damage superimposed on pre-existing intimal proliferation and a variable degree of overt atherosclerosis.

In effect the donor arteries will have pre-existing atherosclerosis and anoxia of varying degrees. Superimposed on these changes there will be an immunological rejection phenomenon of variable intensity but associated with degenerative changes and even necrosis of smooth muscle cells with or without thrombosis. The arterial haemodynamic stresses which are not inconsiderable are likely to have a much more deleterious effect on impaired or ailing endothelial or smooth muscle cells than on homologous cells. The vascular changes in the heterologous grafted blood vessels will exhibit haemodynamically induced degenerative changes superimposed on pre-existing atherosclerosis and newly acquired immunological arteritis due to rejection. Additional factors such as FH may accelerate lipid accumulation and the possibility of a superadded opportunistic infection must also be taken into account. There seems to be not much more that can be learnt at present regarding atherogenesis in this particular model but it is inappropriate to label the changes as 'atherosclerosis'.

(c) Atherosclerosis and malignant tumours

It has been alleged for many years that subjects dying from malignant tumours had less severe aortic and coronary atherosclerosis. For the most part this has been anecdotal but some pathological studies have been conducted including a multicentre study of subjects aged 40–79 years [376]. In general subjects with malignant disease had little atherosclerosis except for males with lung or prostatic carcinoma. Men with lung carcinoma were found to have unusually severe atherosclerosis. Such studies are difficult to evaluate for there are many factors that could influence the methodology and the results. Sternby [376] concluded that there was no real evidence of a negative influence on atherosclerosis. Constitutional factors and the duration of the illness could complicate the results which were quantitative rather than qualitative. This subject is likely to remain controversial but cause and effect should not be assumed.

6.4 Medial degeneration of the aorta (medionecrosis)

Erdheim's medionecrosis has long been considered a specific disease but this must be questioned. Whilst much emphasis in atherosclerosis has been focused on the intima, relatively little has been directed at the media.

Progressively during life the aortic media displays varying changes particularly fragmentation of the medial elastic tissue laminae. The introduction of scanning electron microscopy to study the three-dimensional architecture of arterial elastic tissue cleansed of other medial constituents has drawn attention to the almost honeycomb appearance of the mural elastin. Tears not only of the elastic lamellae but also of the interconnecting fibres, bands or partitions though perceived, are difficult to recognize histologically. However, elastic stains reveal varying degrees of fragmentation which do not correlate well with the degree of intimal thickening. The latter seems to be related to medial thinning.

Fragmentation, loss of continuity of laminae and at times even an appearance of coarse granularity of the laminae suggest varying patterns of degeneration (Figure 10.11, p. 364). The extreme degradation of multiple elastic laminae is associated with extensive patchy loss of elastic tissue with accumulation of mucopolysaccharides. This has been referred to as mucocystic degeneration or medionecrosis. No doubt in such areas there may be necrosis and vesiculogranular degeneration of smooth muscle cells, but histologically the appearance is not that of conventional necrosis. The phenomenon occurs particularly in Marfan's disease but also in aortic coarctation, hypertension and in association with aortic valvular incompetence or stenosis. This pattern may occur at an unusually rapid rate due to the prevailing connective tissue disorder or the severity of the haemodynamic stress (post-stenotic). It has frequently been recognized in subjects with dissecting aneurysms of the aorta though they can occur with or without this pattern of medial degeneration which can be replicated in the anastomosed veins of arteriovenous fistulae. It has also been reported from time to time in large arteries, elastic or transitional in type. In severe degrees of fragmentation of elastic lamellae the assumption is that the elastic laminae are of reduced functional quality but in general morphology does not correlate well with functional integrity. Despite these observations it is difficult to assess the changes in the interconnecting elastic tissue fibres or bands which must play an important role in the pathogenesis of dissecting aneurysms. More detailed three-dimensional ultrastructural studies of medial elastic laminae in atherosclerosis and with age are needed.

6.5 Diseases of small blood vessels

Several degenerative diseases of small blood vessels have much in common with atherosclerosis. They are generally regarded as separate and distinct diseases and haemodynamics plays a role in their topography and variation in severity. At present they are considered separate from atherosclerosis: in time the relationship may be accepted.

6.5.1 ARTERIOSCLEROSIS (DIFFUSE HYPERPLASTIC SCLEROSIS)

It seems appropriate for the present to use the term arteriosclerosis not in its generic sense but to indicate the proliferative disease of small peripheral arteries, variously referred to as intimal elastosis or diffuse hyperplastic sclerosis, for the most part generally ignored in textbooks. The intimal thickening is relatively diffuse, though with accentuation at forks. The internal elastic lamina is degenerate, thin and interrupted, usually with thinning and fibrosis of the media (Figure 6.41). Thin and multiple poorly stained elastic laminae develop within the loose fibromuscular intimal tissue (Figure 6.42). Progressively there is increasing fibrosis

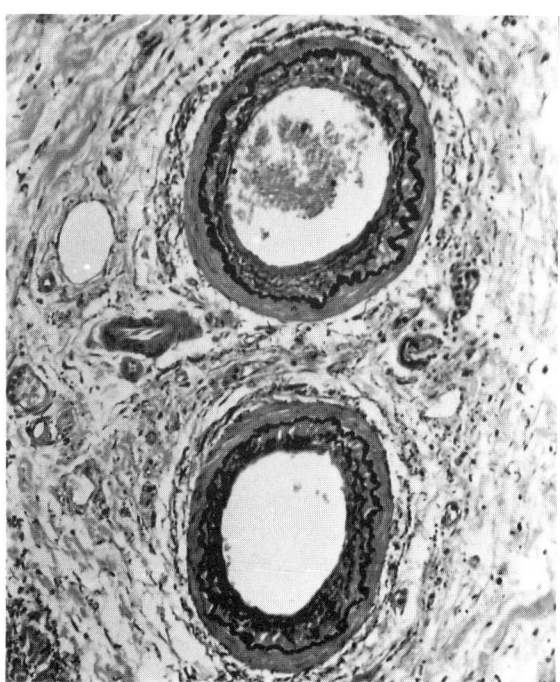

Figure 6.41 Two small arteriosclerotic parenchymal arteries with concentric musculoelastic intimal thickening and medial thinning. (Verhoeff's elastic stain and eosin.)

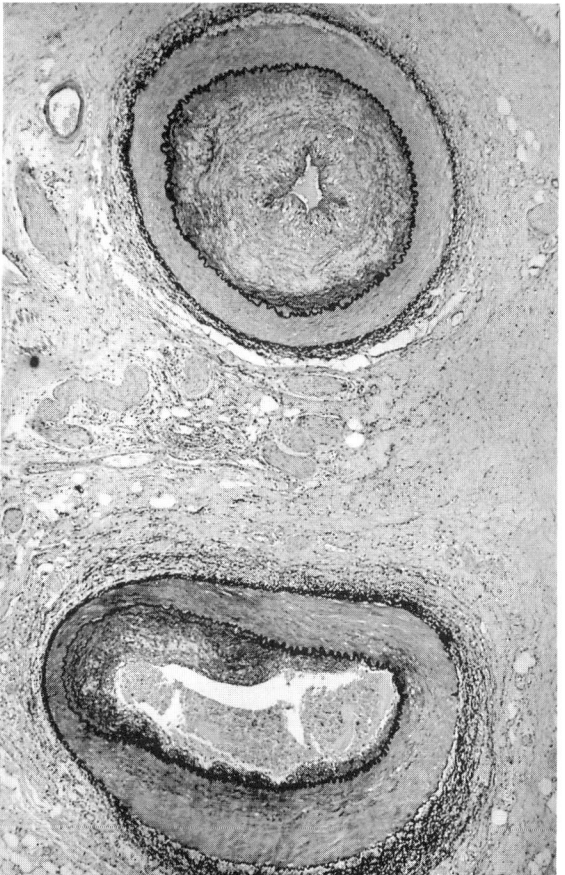

Figure 6.42 Two peripheral arteries larger than in Figure 6.43, with severe stenosis and concentric intimal thickening in the upper vessel and eccentric musculoelastic intimal thickening in the lower vessel which also has underlying medial thinning. (Verhoeff's elastic stain and eosin.)

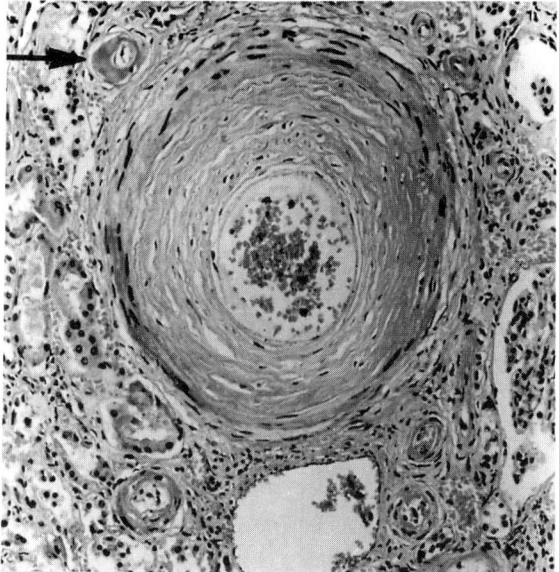

Figure 6.43 Moderately severe concentric intimal thickening of small peripheral artery. Note the thick concentric fibrous thickening of the wall with little residual media. Note hyaline arteriole (arteriolosclerosis) at top left (arrow). (Haematoxylin and eosin.)

and hyalinization of the intima and media with depletion of elastin. The lumen may be narrowed and terminally this is usually concentric (Figure 6.43). Some tortuosity may develop. Cholesterol clefts and calcification are occasionally observed. In vessels of this calibre the rarely performed frozen sections reveal the presence of diffuse extracellular lipid staining and not infrequently may outline the deficient internal elastic lamina. Lipophages may be present, usually in small numbers and occasionally in aggregates. Lipid in smooth muscle cells is not a feature. In small intracerebral arteries it is often referred to as lipohyalinosis and is associated with complete destruction of the normal architecture. Whether or not arteriectasis occurs in vessels of this calibre is unknown but in severe degrees of arteriosclerosis of cerebral arteries miliary aneurysms (miliary aneurysms of Charcôt and Bouchard) develop in old age, particularly in hypertensives (section 12.17.1(c)). The predilection of these miliary aneurysms for the cerebral circulation is consequent upon the thin walls of cerebral arteries, absence of perivascular fibrous support and possibly haemodynamic peculiarities associated with low peripheral resistance and high velocity cerebral blood flow. Ectasia and small aneurysms may occur in the extracerebral circulation but have not been reported except for retinal aneurysms in diabetes.

Arteriosclerosis of small vessels is known to increases in severity with age as with atherosclerosis. Hypertension increases the severity of the changes especially when prolonged. These thickened vessels are prominent on the cut surface of the kidneys and often pout, suggesting changes in their physical characteristics.

The outstanding feature is the histological similarity of these changes to the proliferative changes of atherosclerosis when account is taken of the lesser severity and smaller calibre of the peripheral distributing arteries. Accentuation in intimal thickness occurs over the flow divider but elsewhere tends to be relatively concentric. The presence of lipid and calcific deposits requires explanation if they are considered to be non-atherosclerotic. Arteriosclerosis of these small arteries is pronounced when atherosclerosis of large arteries is severe as if the former is a peripheral extension of the latter.

Similar changes have been observed in small arteries in the vicinity of experimental arteriovenous fistulae although no lipid was present. Ultrastructurally the arteriosclerotic arteries exhibit changes essentially similar to those of atherosclerosis with dystrophic basement membranes and matrix vesicles in addition to disruption of the internal elastic lamina, medial atrophy and fibromuscular proliferation.

Sometimes these changes are referred to as senile arteriosclerosis but they are not specifically a change of senescence and are of augmented severity in hypertensive individuals.

In pregnancy the spiral arteries of the placental bed progressively enlarge and develop tortuosity with replacement of musculoelastic tissue by fibrinoid material and fibrosis. The intima is thickened and the internal elastic lamina for the most part destroyed. As pregnancy advances, these vascular changes extend proximally into the radial arteries until even the basal arteries exhibit muscular hyperplasia and loss of elastica. Veins are less affected and at least some regression of these changes is said to occur in the puerperium [374]. In elderly females sclerotic vascular changes in the ovary are often regarded as involutional changes or disuse atrophy which is probably a misnomer. The similarity to arteriosclerosis and atherosclerosis suggests the changes are degenerative in nature as evidenced by calcification and lipid deposition and probably the end result of an augmented haemodynamic load associated with the repetitive strain of pregnancies. This concept is consistent with the observation that intimal thickening in the uterine arteries of sows is proportional to their parity [11].

These arteriosclerotic changes occur in small epicardial arteries as peripheral extensions of the atherosclerotic changes in larger coronary arteries and they are not observed to any great extent within the myocardium. They are particularly prominent in renal arteries and also in the splenic, pancreatic and adrenal vessels. They are not a prominent feature in small arteries of the stomach, intestines, liver, muscle or skin. In the lung they mostly occur in pulmonary hypertension in addition to the angiomatoid, plexiform and dilatation lesions of collateral vessels in obstructive pulmonary hypertension. In the brain they are often pronounced, occurring particularly in the deep perforating arteries of the cerebrum. Stenotic narrowing develops and is seen particularly in the renal and splenic circulations. Lipid stains are rarely performed but the frequency of lipid in these vessels is surprisingly frequent, much more so than the occurrence of intimal lipophages. Calcific stippling, found occasionally in routine autopsy material, is often overlooked.

Rats subjected to severe prolonged emotional stress for periods up to ten days were found to develop necrosis of smooth muscle cells and even matrix vesicles in the wall of small gastric arteries [375]. Vessels elsewhere were not examined and it is likely these lesions were due to a hypertensive response to acute severe stress.

6.5.2 HYALINE ARTERIOLOSCLEROSIS

Arterioles exhibit cellular thickening of their walls and this may represent medial hypertrophy which is generally considered to occur as the initial response to hypertension. The average ratio of wall thickness to the lumen diameter in the arterioles from the pectoral muscles has been found to be 1:2 in normotensives and only 1:1.4 in hypertensives [376]. The presence of degenerative changes is the most important feature, the muscle cells being replaced by a relatively homogeneous acellular hyaline material, a condition referred to as hyaline arteriolosclerosis (Figure 6.43). The wall is considerably thickened although the lumen becomes narrowed and sometimes eccentrically located. Concentric arrangement of the connective tissue, which at times appears to be periarteriolar, may present a mild onion-layer appearance.

The hyaline material has been thought to be precipitated proteins from the blood, but in reality it consists of basement membrane material primarily in the intima but also in the media [337] with cellular debris (matrix vesicles) and a loss of smooth muscle cells. The presence of fibrin indicates some insudation of plasma rather than a thrombogenic aetiology. Lipid is often present (Figure 6.44) and histochemically cholesterol is present as in atherosclerosis [378]. The wall is thickened and the lumen narrowed sufficiently to result in sclerosis of glomeruli. Arterioles like the small arteries display tortuosity.

In normotensive subjects under 20 years of age, a minor degree of arteriolosclerosis is found in the spleen in 31% and in the pancreas in 7%. It increases in prevalence with each decade especially in the spleen and is exceptional in the adrenals and liver under 40 years. The incidence and severity, however, are greatly augmented in all vessels in the presence of longstanding hypertension [379]. Bell [380] reported the frequent

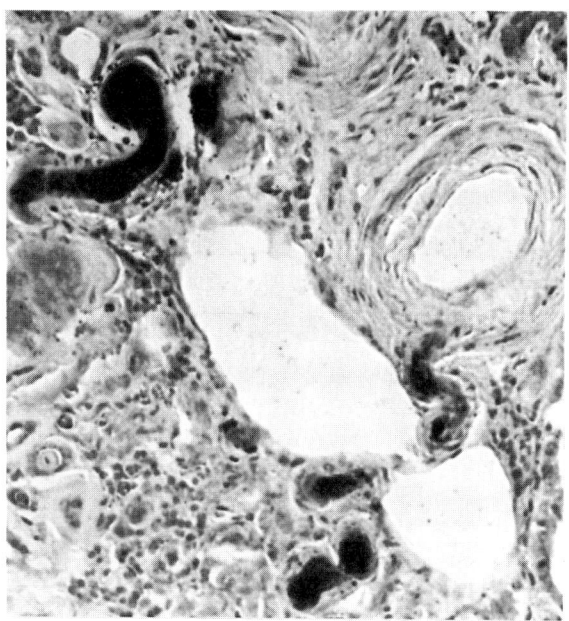

Figure 6.44 Frozen section of kidney demonstrating heavy lipid deposition in hyaline arteriolosclerosis of several arterioles. (Haematoxylin and Fett rot stain for fat.)

occurrence of subendothelial hyaline in older normotensive subjects, for it is rare before 40 years but occurs in 23.7% of those over 70 years. Severity, increasing with age even in the absence of hypertension, is greatly augmented in prevalence and degree in hypertensives. It is neither pathognomonic nor an essential feature of longstanding hypertension.

Hyaline arteriolosclerosis occurs primarily in the kidney, spleen, pancreas, adrenal glands and less often in the liver and intestines. It is not common in the skin, skeletal muscle or heart and is most infrequent in the thyroid and pituitary. Cerebral arteriolosclerosis is found primarily in aged hypertensives and rarely in the spinal cord. The presence of visceral hyaline arteriolosclerosis (other than in the spleen) is often regarded as presumptive evidence of hypertension at autopsy but this diagnosis requires additional evidence of hyperpiesis. The severity appears to be aggravated by diabetes mellitus.

In the kidney, hyaline arteriolosclerosis is found particularly at the corticomedullary junction near the arcuate arteries. The remarkable frequency of hyaline arteriolosclerosis in the spleen, even in normotensives, suggests some peculiarity of splenic blood flow is responsible for the degenerative changes. The lesser severity and predisposition for these vascular changes in some organs and the rarity or even absence in the heart supports the concept that haemodynamic stress must play an important, if not governing, role in their development. Moreover, severe arteriosclerosis of small peripheral arteries can be observed in the presence of arteriolosclerosis. Additional support is provided by the sparing of the vasculature in the kidney beyond a Goldblatt clamp on a renal artery because arterioles of the contralateral kidney exposed to the full impact of the hypertension develop arteriolosclerosis.

6.5.3 MALIGNANT HYPERTENSION

The characteristic feature of malignant hypertension or the malignant phase of hypertension is 'fibrinoid necrosis' of the walls of arterioles and small arteries (Figure 6.45). This is characterized by disruption of the vessel wall and endothelium with infiltration of the wall with fibrin, red cells and some leucocytes. This is accompanied by thrombosis which may occlude the lumen and extension of fibrin and blood into the glomeruli causing its disruption with haemorrhage into the capsular space. Pyknotic nuclei and cell debris, derived from cells in the vessel wall whether leucocytes or smooth muscle cells, have led to the concept of fibrinoid necrosis but in reality the cause is likely to be a mechanical failure of the vessel wall with the rapidity and severity of the rise in blood pressure being particularly important. Matrix vesicles, multiple laminae of thickened basement membranes and even lipid are to be found. These lesions in the kidney may produce small infarcts and severe reduction of blood flow through glomeruli results in renal failure.

In some small arteries and arterioles there is narrowing of the lumen by atypical thickening of the intima mixed with cell debris. In others concentric proliferation of mural connective tissues produces a pronounced onion-layer appearance with narrowing of the lumen particularly in the interlobular arteries of the kidney (Figure 6.46). This may be associated with fibrin, red

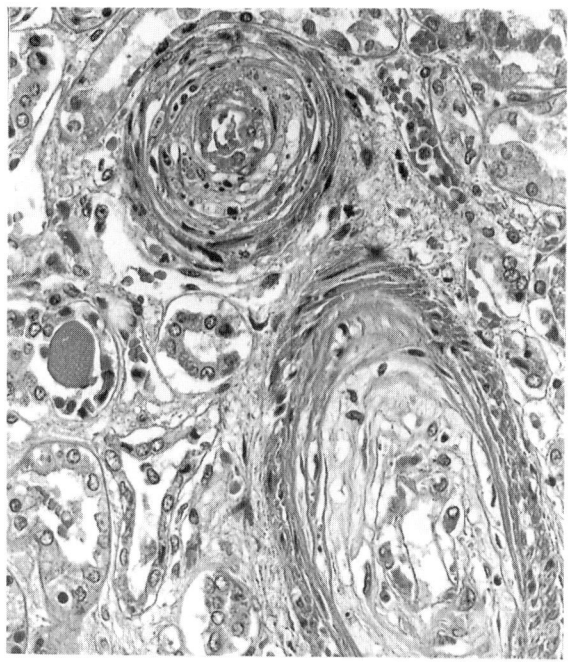

Figure 6.46 Two small renal arteries with concentric onion-layering of stenosing intimal proliferation. The upper vessel has some fibrin infiltration of the inner part of the wall from a patient with malignant hypertension. The lower vessel is cut obliquely. (Haematoxylin and eosin.)

cell and leucocyte infiltration of the wall and mural thrombosis.

The changes that complicate malignant hypertension are particularly severe in the kidney and have a similar distribution to the so-called benign arteriolosclerosis. They are, therefore, observed in the adrenals and pancreas, liver, intestines, etc. Retinal arteries also exhibit haemorrhages and infarcts with areas of oedema and exudate.

These pathological changes appear to be due to mechanical failure and loss of tensile strength of rapid onset [11]. This concept is supported by the production of similar mechanical disruption of small vessels in the rat by suddenly and artificially increasing the intravascular pressure [381]. The presence of immunoglobulins in the wall of disrupted arterioles and arteries is indicative not of an immunopathologic response as has been suggested [382] but of a breach in the wall. Fibrinoid necrosis has been reported to occur postoperatively in vessels below the coarctation of the aorta following its repair and it would appear that the sudden and unaccustomed exposure to the high pulse pressures is responsible [383].

Capillary glomerular aneurysms have been described in both human and experimental malignant hypertension [384]. In experimental malignant hypertension in the rat, multiple aneurysms of mesenteric arteries are common and resemble a polyarteritis nodosa but this does not occur in humans.

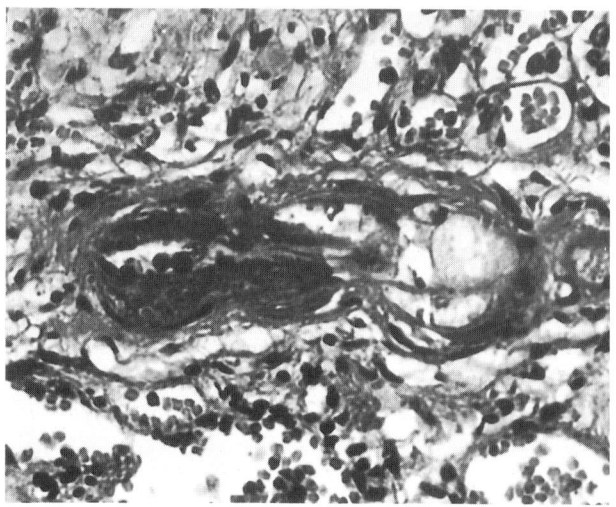

Figure 6.45 Oblique section through an arteriole heavily infiltrated with fibrin (staining darkly) and with a severely narrowed lumen. (Phosphotungstic and haematoxylin.)

These changes are not pathognomonic. They are similar to those of malignant hypertension and found in other conditions such as renal allograft rejection, the haemolytic-uraemic syndrome, the decidual vessels in toxaemia of pregnancy [385–387] and high dosage X-irradiation [388]. Malignant hypertension can also develop in progressive systemic sclerosis (generalized scleroderma).

Hypertensive encephalopathy in severe or malignant hypertension has been attributed to vasospasm of pial vessels on the surface of the brain possibly associated with fibrinoid vascular lesions due to mechanical disruption of the small peripheral resistance vessels caused by the high blood pressure. The focal oedema is due to increased permeability of the vessels. These concepts were supported by Byrom's investigations of hypertension in rats with cranial windows [384,389]. Experimentally the epileptiform fits cease following reduction in the blood pressure.

6.6 Miscellaneous degenerative changes

6.6.1 ENDARTERITIS OBLITERANS

Endarteritis obliterans, as the name implies, indicates an obliterating proliferative intimal thickening in arteries in the vicinity of chronic inflammatory lesions and has been regarded as a protective mechanism against irritants.

When blood vessels about chronic gastric ulcers were studied, the vascular changes were found to be identical to those of arteriosclerosis [75]; they exhibited concentric musculoelastic proliferation with accentuation at branching sites, medial sclerosis and atrophy, tortuosity and lipid deposition. Onion-layering as in severe hypertension and even lipid deposition in arterioles was observed. The changes were essentially similar to the milder arteriosclerosis of more distal vessels in the stomach wall and differed in degree not in kind. An artery that has caused serious bleeding may project slightly from the floor of the ulcer crater and be plugged by thrombus. Thrombosis is the protective mechanism against erosion and haemorrhage, not arteriosclerosis. Similar changes are found in vessels feeding chronic inflammatory sites although close to active tuberculous lesions, blood vessels may be incorporated in the inflammatory response, cellular infiltration and caseation. Under these circumstances a very loose non-concentric intimal proliferation is observed partially occluding the lumen. Such lesions should be regarded as tuberculous arteritis.

Vasodilatation and increased blood flow are cardinal features of inflammation. In acute leptomeningitis, this augmented blood flow is demonstrable angiographically and associated with an audible bruit on auscultation. In the chronic state the augmented flow can be associated with the above arteriosclerotic changes, which do not appear to be protective or to the advantage of the individual. In the past the diagnosis of endarteritis obliterans has too often depended on site rather than morphology.

Associated with some chronic peptic ulcers, arteriovenous shunts have been reported and also vascular ectasias, venous lakes, glomerular and cherry vascular formations in the lesser curvature of the stomach and of the skin. These were considered to be manifestations of an ulcer diathesis. The vessels illustrated suggested phlebosclerosis of veins and some arteriosclerosis and recanalization of thrombosed arteries but no specific evidence of an arteriovenous shunt [390]. There has been no support for these concepts and some vascular abnormalities may be independent of the peptic ulceration.

6.6.2 ATHEROSIS

This has been regarded as a proliferative endarteritis occurring in small decidual arteries of the placenta towards the end of pregnancy and accentuated by hypertension. It is even more pronounced in toxaemia of pregnancy and exhibits infiltration of the arterial wall with fibrin, extracellular lipid, monocytic infiltration and foam cells with severe narrowing of the lumen and placental infarcts [386,387,391]. It is likely that the fibrin infiltration is associated with intimal disruption as in malignant hypertension. The localization of these vascular lesions specifically to one vascular bed indicates that haemodynamic factors are related to their development. These changes, though occurring in small peripheral vessels, have many of the features of atherosclerosis and since placental flow is particularly rapid with a water hammer pulse, the conditions are reminiscent of those associated with a femoral arteriovenous fistula. These vascular lesions have been referred to as cholesterol arteriosclerosis but their rapid progression in vessels of such small calibre has deterred authors from assigning them to atherosclerosis. They appear to be augmented and accelerated degenerative changes associated with haemodynamic stresses of pregnancy in the presence of hypertension. It cannot be assumed that the greatly augmented flow during pregnancy [391], sufficient to produce a bruit, will have no effect on the vessel walls especially in view of recent experimental evidence [70].

These vascular changes also occur in diabetes mellitus and in association with intrauterine growth retardation of the fetus. The possibility that there may be an immunological component to the pathogenesis [392] has been entertained and likened to acute arterial homograft rejection, the latter having a greater intensity of leucocyte infiltration.

6.6.3 CAPILLARY FIBROSIS

Capillary fibrosis is associated with an increase in reticulin in the walls of cerebral capillaries and is said to be a feature of hypertensive cerebrovascular disease [21]. Capillary fibrosis has been considered a degenerative change in other vascular beds in old literature. In all probability it corresponds ultrastructurally to thickening and multilamination of the basement membrane about vessels in the microvasculature which increases with age and is accentuated by hypertension, diabetes mellitus and chronic venous insufficiency. Such changes, while not thoroughly investigated ultrastructurally and histochemically, could be similar to those related to endothelium in larger blood vessels. The predominant collagen in this basement membrane is type IV.

In diabetes mellitus the multilaminated basement membranes are indicative of increased cellular turnover and precede clinically overt diabetes. Associated with functional changes such as loss of normal vascular tone, they are suggestive of a not-so-subtle metabolic disturbance that also affects arterioles and medium-sized arteries and may occur in larger vessels accounting for the aggravating effect on atherogenesis. This so-called diabetic microangiopathy is more severe when diabetes commences early in life and the affected retinal vessels frequently develop microaneurysms. All tissues are not involved to the same degree [393].

Thinning of capillary basement membranes in muscle has been reported in subjects with myotonic dystrophy [394]. The significance of this observation is not known.

6.7 Phlebosclerosis

Just as the term arteriosclerosis was introduced to indicate hardening of the arteries, so phlebosclerosis was introduced to indicate fibrotic thickening and hardening of the veins. It has been given other names such as venofibrosis, endophlebosclerosis and venous atherosclerosis. The nature of these changes is controversial and histologically intimal proliferation is the initial and predominant alteration. Aspects of phlebosclerosis are reminiscent of atherosclerosis. It grows more severe with age although it is not a disease of senescence because of its variation in severity according to the vascular bed and is aggravated by venous hypertension. On occasions it also affects young people as well, and has been observed in the inferior vena cava and portal vein of a 23-day-old infant with congenital heart disease [395]. There is little doubt that it is ubiquitous but it has remained subclinical and has mostly been regarded as an age phenomenon. Veins usually do not feature highly in the routine autopsy unless there is evidence of thrombosis, inflammation or invasion by tumour.

The intimal thickenings consist of diffuse, flat musculoelastic proliferation with interstitial matrix and proteoglycans. They are at times protuberant and this may be exaggerated by the plane of section or localized thickening may appear protuberant with the vein in a collapsed state [396]. The smooth muscle cells are longitudinally arranged as in the arterial intima and can be visibly degenerate [396]. The medial muscle may display distinct hypertrophy but this appears to be an early phase. Ultimately there is degeneration and fibrous replacement. A few new thick elastic laminae may form in the intima, these usually being deficient and interrupted. The internal elastic lamina is frayed, disrupted and deficient and the proliferation is thicker and protuberant at sites of union with tributaries or at the site of branching, occurring over the crescentic edge in the crotch of the union or branching site. Intimal thickenings are found particularly on the venous walls adjacent to an artery and are most extensive with considerable loss of elastica, fibrosis and hyalinization in varicose veins.

Multinucleated giant endothelial cells with an irregular pattern similar to those over atherosclerotic plaques are frequent in the jugular, subclavian and brachial veins but less frequent in those of the lower limb. They occur predominantly over intimal thickenings, close to thrombi and in venous sinuses. They increase in proportion to age and atherosclerosis [396] and this is yet another similarity to atherosclerosis of arteries.

In early reports there was little emphasis on the presence of lipid deposition and calcification and it has been generally considered that 'significant amounts' do not occur. Progressive fibrosis occurs with age and hypertension, whether systemic, portal or pulmonary. Calcification is found from time to time as is lipid deposition [397]. The large lipid deposits and atheromatous degeneration as seen in arteries do not ordinarily occur but a plaque (Schilling's patch) in the inferior vena cava immediately proximal to the union of the common iliac veins is a common finding. Even an atheromatous ulcer has been observed in the portal vein in a subject with chronic portal hypertension [397].

Mild degrees of intimal proliferation are probably overlooked and regarded as an integral part of the vessel wall. However, the thickening is also affected by haemodynamic stresses, for example:

1. Thickenings are most pronounced at unions and bifurcations [396].
2. Phlebosclerosis is less severe in the pulmonary circulation than in the systemic circulation, indicating again that the blood pressure is an important determinant of the severity of the disease. The severity is said to be least in coronary veins where pressure is correspondingly least [398].
3. Schilling's patch is present in 77% of routine

hospital autopsies [399]. Most contain lipid and calcium phosphate deposits are frequent and the wider the angle of union of the common iliac veins, the more severe the lesion [94].

4. Phlebosclerotic plaques and diffuse changes are most prominent in the largest veins. They are also severe in the veins of the lower limbs where the hydrostatic pressure is highest exceeding that in the head, neck and upper limbs.
5. The thickness and severity of degenerative changes are aggravated in the systemic circulation (including the inferior vena cava) by chronic venous congestion, in the portal and splenic veins in portal hypertension and in the pulmonary veins in pulmonary hypertension [94,398–401].
6. It is of increased severity in varicose veins [402].
7. Similar phlebosclerotic changes are found in the jugular veins of carotid–jugular arteriovenous fistulae used therapeutically.

Such observations strongly support the concept that phlebosclerosis [398,403] is closely related to haemodynamic stress in relation to its localization and severity. In this regard the similarity of this relationship to that with atherosclerosis is more than coincidental.

Authors have alleged that lipid is not found in phlebosclerosis but Geiringer [404] found lipid in 25% of adults studied and careful research has demonstrated lipid in 60% of 160 intimal plaques in the inferior vena cava [399]. The changes have been accepted by many authors as atherosclerosis or atheroma [11,103,404]. If, however, these changes are not accepted as atherosclerotic in nature, then scientific reasons for such a negative view, the means of differentiation and an explanation for their presence must be forthcoming. As yet these have not been provided and the occurrence of these changes is independent of alteration in cholesterol and lipid metabolism [405].

To many, the presence of lipid in the vessel wall is the pathognomonic indicator of atherosclerosis. If this is the case, then phlebosclerosis is but a mild form of atherosclerosis. Ectasia, tortuosity and aneurysmal dilatation even with rupture and haemorrhage commonly occur in association with varicose veins and venous thrombosis is prevalent with or without varicosities.

Short [396] found thrombi occurred predominantly on areas of intimal proliferation, in the valve sinuses and at the junction with tributaries or anastomotic veins (more often in the posterior tibial vein rather than veins in the soleus). Moreover, thromboembolic phenomena are recognized to be most prevalent in countries in which coronary heart disease and severe atherosclerosis are common.

The accumulation of matrix vesicles and bizarre-shaped collagen fibrils in cross-section are two ultrastructural features observed in veins of elderly subjects and in varicose veins [156,157,181]. These are also manifestations of human atherosclerosis. However, that phlebosclerosis is analogous to atherosclerosis in arteries is strongly supported by the development of overt atherosclerosis at an accelerated rate in venous bypass grafts irrespective of site and the experimental production initially of phlebosclerosis identical to that in humans and its progression to overt atherosclerosis in arteriovenous shunts and venous graft aneurysms in herbivorous animals [99,103,110]. Ordinarily since veins do no exhibit advanced atherosclerosis, they might be considered to be relatively immune despite their similar exposure to risk factors for CHD and atherosclerosis. Yet when subjected to augmented stresses of arterial haemodynamics, they develop atherosclerosis at an accelerated rate indicating that veins by virtue of their architectural differences are more susceptible to atherogenesis than arteries.

In arteriovenous shunts performed for renal dialysis in subjects with chronic renal failure, the veins develop phlebosclerosis which progresses to overt atherosclerosis and its complications [101]. The obvious, unavoidable conclusion is that phlebosclerosis is atherosclerosis which usually occurs in milder form than in arteries but when veins are subjected to augmented haemodynamic stresses, overt atherosclerosis becomes manifest irrespective of species and diet.

6.7.1 HYPERCHOLESTEROLAEMIA AND VEINS

It is incongruous that with all the emphasis on hypercholesterolaemia in human atherosclerosis, lipid accumulation in veins is mild by comparison with that in arteries and that there has been no mention of venous involvement in familial hypercholesterolaemia. However, when veins of experimental animals are subjected to severe vibrational stress (arteriovenous fistulae, venous-pouch aneurysms), they develop severe phlebosclerosis or atherosclerosis. In association with hypercholesterolaemia, lipid is preferentially deposited in the haemodynamically stressed venous wall which becomes honeycombed with lipophages (Figure 6.40). From the study by Lie et al. [363] it is likely that lipid has a predilection for phlebosclerosis in human venous bypass grafts.

The nature of phlebosclerosis has been of little concern to pathologists because it has not been a cause of significant morbidity but with the advent of the venous bypass graft interest has increased. Whilst associations with CHD risk factors have been invoked, the above observations and the minimal venous atherosclerosis elsewhere in the body of those subjects with either venous bypass grafts or arteriovenous shunts precludes any significant role for such risk factors in the pathogenesis of phlebosclerosis or venous atherosclerosis. The evidence favours the thesis that phlebosclerosis is only an early manifestation of atherosclerosis, a contention supported by the similarity of pathogenesis, the fact that one can progress insidiously to the other, as well as the absence of logical scientific criteria to distinguish between the two. The two disorders vary in degree but not in kind. Schilling's patch has been considered the consequence of mechanical stress [398] and Stehbens [11,103] included phlebosclerosis as an integral part of atherosclerosis and as such attributed it to mechanical fatigue, the severity being consistent with the much lower flow rates, pulsatility and intravascular pressures.

6.8 Lymphangiosclerosis

The thoracic duct is lined by ovoid endothelial cells and possesses an internal elastic lamina and a media containing bundles of smooth muscle cells separated by collagen and elastica. The adventitia is composed primarily of collagen. Musculoelastic intimal proliferation is common and increases in severity with age together with medial fibrosis [406,407] and not surprisingly the changes have been likened to those of phlebosclerosis. It is accentuated in association with increased lymph flow in cirrhosis and is aggravated by chronic venous congestion. Of particular interest is the finding of lipid deposition in 99% of ducts examined for lipid even though of mild degree [406]. Other similarities to atherosclerosis are the occurrence of calcification and aneurysms [408,409]. Such observations, detracting from the thrombogenic theory of atherogenesis, indicate the need for more detailed study including electron microscopy and the hydrodynamics of lymph flow.

6.9 Vascular calcification

Calcification is common in large arteries in atherosclerosis, aneurysms and less frequently in veins and arteriovenous communications and occasionally in what appears to be an old scarred artery. The mineral content increases with age in the aorta and coronary arteries and calcification is less evident in cerebral atherosclerosis. It is seen in small peripheral parenchymal arteries, usually along the internal elastic lamina or elsewhere in the intima in routine sections from time to time but the significance is unknown and no attempt has been made to correlate such findings with mineralization of large arteries. Some consider this as part of atherosclerosis whilst others regard it as a manifestation of 'senile arteriosclerosis'.

Lansing [233] placed much emphasis on the progressive increase in calcium salts with age and was of the opinion that the increase in calcium content of medial elastic tissue preceded the formation of atherosclerotic plaques. Though possibly true, the early lesion occurs at a much earlier age. Calcification in the pulmonary arteries is also age-dependent but it is of milder degree and progresses more slowly than in the aorta suggesting that the lower blood pressure and less severe haemodynamic stress in the pulmonary circulation are responsible.

Small calcific deposits, most often in the intima or of the internal elastic lamina, are observed in routine histological material in autopsies and regarded as a manifestation of the degenerative changes affecting all arteries.

In the USA concern has been expressed about the possibility of excess vitamin D intake from vitamin D-fortified milk [410] since administration of this vitamin to rabbits produces extensive arterial calcification and gross irregularity of the arterial walls [411]. The possibility of ingestion of toxic doses deserves investigation, the need for the addition of vitamin D to milk in this day and age being questionable.

Experimental vitamin D-induced calcification produces a specific localization about arterial forks and at sites initially spared in dietary-induced lipid deposition [411]. The calcification has a predilection for the afferent artery of experimental arteriovenous shunts but not for the walls of experimental saccular aneurysms or the anastomosed veins of arteriovenous fistulae where an abundance of matrix vesicles develops rapidly. Since matrix vesicles are believed to be a nidus for calcification this finding, at variance with anticipated results, may indicate that vitamin D-induced calcification is quite distinct from that associated with the proliferative lesions of atherosclerosis.

For calcification of intracerebral vessels see section 12.20.5.

6.9.1 MÖNCKEBERG'S SCLEROSIS

This is a degenerative disease characterized by calcification within the media of medium-sized arteries particularly in the lower limbs in subjects over 50 years and often with diabetes mellitus. It is much less frequent in the upper limbs and visceral arteries. Characteristically there are circumferentially arranged bars or rings of calcification sometimes branched and becoming confluent with adjoining calcific deposits and ultimately forming rigid tubes which have been likened to a goose trachea.

It has been considered quite distinct from atherosclerosis and Mönckeberg's sclerosis is rare under 50 years of age. As atherosclerosis is ubiquitous, it is inevitable that the two conditions coexist and complete differentiation will not always be clear. In some arteries there may be extensive calcification in the media (Figure 6.47) in the presence of calcification also of the internal elastic lamina (which is within the definition of the intima) and of the innermost media. In other cases

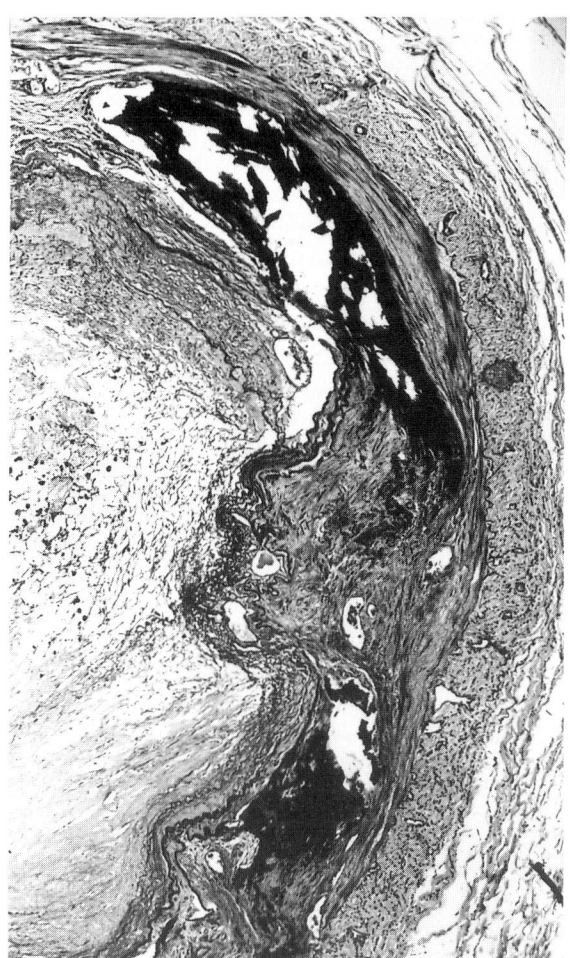

Figure 6.47 Extensive medial calcification in an artery (Mönckeberg's sclerosis). Note disturbed architecture of the media, the extensive elastosis in the intima, organization of an old thrombus in the lumen and numerous collateral vasae vasorum in the adventitia. (Verhoeff's elastic stain and eosin.)

calcification may be mid-media in location. Actual localization is not as important at this stage as explaining the aetiology of the disease and why the calcification is so extreme.

Initially calcium salts are deposited as fine granules and may be within matrix vesicles, as calcospherites or within elastic laminae. The deposits become confluent and large areas of calcification may at times proceed to actual ossification with bone marrow elements both red and yellow.

The aetiology is uncertain but similar calcification can be produced in rabbits by repeated injections of adrenalin. It has been regarded as an extreme example of the calcific deposits that increase in severity with age. It is possible that some metabolic disturbance of calcium exists but the disease is not so common that large numbers of patients can be examined for metabolic disturbances. However, the transverse tears in the internal elastic lamina associated with calcification of their margin in infancy and youth [13] cause a curious labyrinth of transversely orientated railroad tracks when stained in the gross with silver nitrate simulating the topography of Mönckeberg's sclerosis. Since calcification extends into the remnants of the elastic lamina, the Mönckeberg pattern of calcification would result. The calcification is in the internal elastic lamina and is not mid-medial. If these elastic tears are early manifestations of Mönkeberg's sclerosis the degree of calcification requires explanation. It can be associated with ischaemic changes attributable to concomitant atherosclerosis with thrombosis but apart from producing an interesting radiological appearance, it is not known for any specific clinical complication.

6.9.2 IDIOPATHIC ARTERIAL CALCIFICATION OF INFANCY

This is a rare disease in which the biochemical defect is unknown [412,413]. In some cases it is transmitted as a recessive genetic disease and can be familial. It becomes manifest early in life. The child fails to thrive and does not survive more than a few months. Extensive calcification of the coronary arteries accompanies pronounced intimal proliferation with stenotic lesions. The arteries are tortuous and the aorta may or may not be affected. Early changes involve the internal elastic lamina with pronounced medial thinning. Other arteries may be affected but the coronary arteries are almost always severely involved. The histological changes do not resemble atherosclerosis and there is no evidence that the disease is associated with hypervitaminosis D. The possibility is that a disorder of elastic tissue [414] may be the cause and there are similarities to pseudoxanthoma elasticum but also there are similarities to the calcification associated with tears of the internal elastic lamina [13].

Barson et al. [415] reported extensive arterial calcification in a newborn infant from a mother with systemic lupus erythematosus and lupus nephritis. Calcification was extensive in the internal elastic lamina with medial thinning, little intimal proliferation but thrombi in the renal arteries. Other cases occur with widespread arterial and sometimes cardiac valvular calcification without obvious disease in the mother [416] and some have onset clinically in adulthood [417]. Extensive tortuosity and distortion of anatomy may occur. Determining the cause of these rare disorders depends on thorough autopsies, tissues from early cases and an international registry for filing of data and material from many cases.

6.10 Miscellaneous diseases

6.10.1 STENOTIC INTIMAL PROLIFERATION IN CYCLISTS

Competition cyclists complaining of acute unilateral claudication at the time of maximal strain were found to have significant decrease in the ankle systolic pressure. Symptoms occurred when the thigh was acutely flexed on the pelvis and several subjects had a systolic murmur in the iliac fossa. Arteriography revealed sinuous lengthening of the external iliac artery and a moderate stenosis due to loose intimal proliferation of muscle, elastic tissue and collagen which was believed to be possibly of haemodynamic origin but not caused by atherosclerosis or fibrous dysplasia. Though the suggestion was that this syndrome was a new type of arterial degeneration [418], this seems doubtful. More information is required about the relationship of the stenosis to the inguinal ligament. The case has some points of similarity to those associated with the use of crutches and aneurysm formation.

6.10.2 DIFFUSE TORTUOSITY IN CHILDREN

Extreme degrees of tortuosity can be seen in old age but when it occurs in the very young involving many large arteries and their branches, inevitably a disturbance of connective tissue metabolism must be suspected. Such cases as a 10-year-old girl with involvement of the aorta and all its main branches [76] and extreme tortuosity of systemic and pulmonary arteries in a boy of 17 months leading to a fatal outcome are examples. Secondary changes must have occurred in these tortuosities, i.e. tears in the elastic laminae and intimal proliferation on the lesser curvatures of bends, quite apart from severe kinking with obstruction to flow. The tortuosity and secondary intimal changes with or without an aneurysm are secondary manifestations of the primary disorder which derives from the genetically determined connective tissue disorder.

6.10.3 ADVENTITIAL CYSTIC DEGENERATION

This is a rare disease most often affecting the popliteal artery in middle-aged men rather than women. The pathology consists of a cyst-like space in the arterial adventitia lined by cells similar to the mesothelium of the synovium and containing mucoid material as if a ganglion. The ultrastructure of the wall is consistent with this view and at times there is a communication with the knee joint [419]. This would suggest that the artery is secondarily involved by virtue of its proximity. The cyst can compress the arterial lumen compromising flow and so causes intermittent claudication. Compression of the artery produces a characteristic curved indentation of the lumen on angiography (the 'scimitar sign') and the dilatation during exercise accentuates the functional impediment to flow. Occlusion with thrombosis may ensue.

There is no reason to believe the lesion primarily arises from the media. It has also been observed in iliac, femoral, radial and ulnar arteries and very rarely in veins [420]. In a recent case involving the lesser saphenous vein, the pseudocystic structure enveloped the collapsed and compressed vein and appeared multiloculated. The contents consist of mucoprotein or mucopolysaccharides with a significant amount of hydroxyproline.

The aetiology is unknown. Trauma is believed to play a role. Similar mucoid cystic structures occur elsewhere unrelated to blood vessels and can be difficult to eradicate.

6.10.4 AMYLOIDOSIS AND LARGE ARTERIES

Accumulation of amyloid in and related to small vessels in secondary amyloidosis is a well recognized phenomenon and the disorder is not primarily a disease of blood vessels. However, in recent years there has been increasing recognition of amyloid deposits in many organs and also blood vessels of the elderly with or without Alzheimer's disease. In the cerebral arteries it has been linked with a specific type of intracerebral haemorrhage and dementia (section 12.17.2(b)).

In a study of 100 individuals over 60 years of age, there was little difference in results in the aorta between those over or under 80 years but a substantial increase in the prevalence of amyloid in cerebral arteries in those over 80 years [421]. Amyloid was found in two thirds of the aortae, both in the thoracic and abdominal segments and most frequently in the inner layers of the media between the laminae. In the presence of a plaque the amyloid was deep to the plaque at the border with the atrophied media and also in hyaline tissue. The deposits were not extensive and their relationship to atherosclerosis is difficult to evaluate. The amyloid is seemingly more closely related to old age than to atherosclerosis.

References

1. Osler, W. (1901) *The Principles and Practice of Medicine*, 4th edn, Young J. Pentland, Edinburgh, pp. 770–6.
2. Long, E.R. (1965) *A History of Pathology*, Dover Publ., New York, p. 4.
3. Hellwig, C.A. (1942) Atheromatosis of the mitral valve. *Am. Heart J.*, **24**, 41–9.
4. Roberts, W.C. and Buja, L.M. (1972) The frequency and significance of coronary arterial thrombi and other observations in fatal acute myocardial infarction. *Am. J. Med.*, **52**, 425–43.
5. Stehbens, W.E. (1992) Causality in medical science with reference to coronary heart disease and atherosclerosis. *Perspect. Biol. Med.*, **36**, 97–119.
6. Stehbens, W.E. (1974) Changes in the cross-sectional area of the arterial fork. *Angiology*, **25**, 561–75.
7. Cluroe, A.D., Fitzjohn, T.P. and Stehbens, W.E. (1992) Combined pathological and radiological study of the effect of atherosclerosis on the ostia of segmental branches of the abdominal aorta. *Pathology*, **24**, 140–5.

8. Vikhert, A.M. and Zhdanov, V.S. (1989) Role of rhythmic structures of aortic intima in the development of atherosclerosis. *Zentbl. Allg. Path. Anat.*, **135**, 607–17.
9. Meyer, M.W.R. and Meyer, W.W. (1992) Funktionelle Strukturen der Aorta als Prädilektionsort frühester atherosklerotischer Veränderungen (Aortic functional structures – a predilection site of earliest atherosclerotic lesions). *Zentbl. Path.*, **138**, 61–5.
10. Tanimura, A., Cho, T., Saito, Y. et al. (1986) Role of 'wave lines' (Doerr: Wellenlinie) of aorta in atherosclerosis. *Angiology*, **37**, 272–80.
11. Stehbens, W.E. (1979) *Hemodynamics and the Blood Vessel Wall*, C.C. Thomas, Springfield.
12. Ross, R. (1986) The pathogenesis of atherosclerosis – an update. *New Engl. J. Med.*, **314**, 488–99.
13. Meyer, W.W., Walsh, S.Z. and Lind, J. (1980) Functional morphology of arteries during fetal and post-natal development, in *Structure and Function of the Circulation*, (eds C.J. Schwartz, N.T. Werthessen, and S. Wolf), Plenum Press, New York, pp. 95–379.
14. Meyer, W.W. and Lind, J. (1974) Iliac arteries in children with a single umbilical artery. Structure, calcifications, and early atherosclerotic lesions. *Arch. Dis. Child.*, **49**, 671–9.
15. Stary, H.C., Blankenhorn, D.H., Chandler, A.B. et al. (1992) A definition of the intima of human arteries and of its atherosclerosis-prone regions. *Arterioscl. Thromb.*, **12**, 120–34.
16. Woolf, N. and Crawford, T. (1960) Fatty streaks in the aortic intima studied by an immune-histochemical technique. *J. Pathol.*, **80**, 405–8.
17. Smith, E.B. and Slater, R. (1972) Lipid and lipoproteins in ageing aortic intima. *Proc. Roy. Soc. Med.*, **65**, 675–7.
18. Stehbens, W.E. (1960) Focal intimal proliferation in the cerebral arteries. *Am. J. Pathol.*, **36**, 289–301.
19. Stehbens, W.E. (1963) Aneurysms and anatomical variations of cerebral arteries. *Arch. Pathol.*, **75**, 45–64.
20. Stehbens, W.E. (1981) Arterial structure at branches and bifurcations with reference to physiological and pathological processes, including aneurysm formation, in *Structure and Function of the Circulation*, vol. 2, (eds C.J. Schwartz, N.T. Werthessen and S. Wolf), Plenum Pub. Co., New York, pp. 667–94.
21. Stehbens, W.E. (1972) *Pathology of the Cerebral Blood Vessels*, C.V. Mosby, St Louis.
22. Jaffé, D., Hartroft, S., Manning, M. et al. (1971) Coronary arteries in newborn children. *Acta Paediat. Scand.*, (suppl. 219), 3–28.
23. Levene, C.I. (1956) The pathogenesis of atheroma of the coronary arteries. *J. Pathol. Bacteriol.*, **72**, 83–86.
24. Blumenthal, H.T., Handler, F.P. and Blache, J.O. (1954) The histogenesis of arteriosclerosis of the larger cerebral arteries, with an analysis of the importance of mechanical factors. *Am. J. Med.*, **17**, 337–47.
25. Stehbens, W.E. (1963) The renal artery in normal and cholesterol-fed rabbits. *Am. J. Pathol.*, **43**, 969–85.
26. Stehbens, W.E. (1965) Intimal proliferation and spontaneous lipid deposition in the cerebral arteries of sheep and steers. *J. Atheroscl. Res.*, **5**, 556–8.
27. Stehbens, W.E. and Ludatscher, R.M. (1973) Ultrastructure of the renal arterial bifurcation of rabbits. *Expl Mol. Pathol.*, **18**, 50–67.
28. Gotlieb, A.I. (1990) The endothelial cytoskeleton: organization in normal and regenerating endothelium. *Toxicol. Pathol.*, **18**, 603–17.
29. Stehbens, W.E. (1975) Cerebral atherosclerosis. *Arch. Pathol.*, **99**, 582–91.
30. Stehbens, W.E. (1975) Ultrastructure of aneurysms. *Arch. Neurol.*, **32**, 798–807.
31. Stehbens, W.E. (1975) The role of lipid in the pathogenesis of atherosclerosis. *Lancet*, **1**, 724–1.
32. Stehbens, W.E. and Martin, B.J. (1993) Ultrastructural alterations of collagen fibrils in blood vessel walls. *Connect. Tiss. Res.*, **29**, 319–31.
33. Mitchell, J.R.A. and Schwartz, C.J. (1965) *Arterial Disease*, Blackwell, Oxford.
34. Catherman, R.L., Davidson, W.H. and Townsend, F.M. (1962) Coronary artery disease in military flying personnel. *Aerospace Med.*, **33**, 1318–27.
35. Enos, W.E., Holman, R.H. and Bayer, J. (1953) Coronary disease among United States soldiers killed in action in Korea. *J. Am. Med. Ass.*, **152**, 1090–3.
36. McNamara, J.J., Molot, M.A., Stremple, J.F. et al. (1971) Coronary artery disease in combat casualties in Vietnam. *J. Am. Med. Ass.*, **216**, 1185–7.
37. Stehbens, W.E. (1962) Cerebral aneurysm and congenital abnormalities. *Aust. Ann. Med.*, **11**, 102–12.
38. Strong, J.P. and McGill, H.C. (1962) The natural history of coronary atherosclerosis. *Am. J. Pathol.*, **40**, 37–49.
39. Strong, J.P. and McGill, H.C. (1963) The natural history of aortic atherosclerosis: relationship to race, sex, and coronary lesions in New Orleans. *Exp. Mol. Pathol.*, **2** (suppl. 1), 15–27.
40. White, N.K., Edwards, J.E. and Dry, T.J. (1950) The relationship of the degree of coronary atherosclerosis with age, in men. *Circulation*, **1**, 645–54.
41. Baroldi, G. (1978) Coronary stenosis: ischemic or non-ischemic factor? *Am. Heart J.*, **96**, 139–43.
42. Spiekerman, R.E., Brandenburg, J.T., Achor, R.W.P. et al. (1960) Incidence of coronary artery disease at necropsy in a community of 30,000. *Circulation*, **22**, 816–17.
43. Cheitlin, M.D. and Virmani, R. (1989) Myocardial infarction in the absence of coronary atherosclerotic disease, in *Nonatherosclerotic Ischemic Heart Disease*, (eds R. Virmani and M.B. Forman), Raven Press, New York, pp. 1–30.
44. Hutchins, G.M., Bulkley, B.H., Miner, M.M. et al. (1977) Correlation of age and heart weight with tortuosity and caliber of normal human coronary arteries. *Am. Heart J.*, **94**, 196–202.
45. Swanton, R.H., Thomas, M.L., Coltart, D.J. et al. (1978) Coronary artery ectasia – a variant of occlusive coronary arteriosclerosis. *Br. Heart J.*, **40**, 393–400.
46. Stary, H.C. (1989) Evolution and progression of atherosclerotic lesions in coronary arteries of children and young adults. *Arteriosclerosis*, **9**, (suppl. 1), 1-19–1-32.
47. Ehrich, W., de la Chapelle, C. and Cohn, A.E. (1931) Anatomical ontogony B. Man. I. A study of the coronary arteries. *Am. J. Anat.*, **49**, 241–82.
48. Dock, W. (1946) The predilection of atherosclerosis for the coronary arteries. *J. Am. Med. Ass.*, **131**, 875–8.
49. Thoma, R. (1921) Über die Intima der Arterien. *Virchows Arch. Path. Anat.*, **230**, 1–45.
50. Velican, C. (1968) Studies on intimal connective tissue of human arteries. *Acta Anat.*, **71**, 519–41.
51. Greenhill, N.S. and Stehbens, W.E. (1985) Haemodynamically-induced intimal tears in experimental U-shaped arterial loops as seen by scanning electron microscopy. *Br. J. Exp. Pathol.*, **66**, 577–84.
52. Stehbens, W.E. (1986) Experimental arterial loops and arterial atrophy. *Exp. Mol. Pathol.*, **44**, 177–89.
53. Peterson, R.E. and Livingston, K.E. (1960) Development and distribution of gross atherosclerotic lesions at cervical carotid bifurcation. *Neurology*, **10**, 955–9.
54. Solberg, L.A. and Eggen, D.A. (1971) Localization and sequence of development of atherosclerotic lesions in the carotid and vertebral arteries. *Circulation*, **43**, 711–24.
55. Meyer, W.W. (1964) Über die rhythmische Lokalisation der atherosklerotischen Herde im cervicalen Abschnitt der Vertebralarterie. *Beitr. Path. Anat.*, **130**, 24–39.
56. Rodda, R.A. (1950) Arteriosclerosis in the lower limbs: a pathological study of fifty cases with no ischaemia. University of Otago, Dunedin, Doctorate of Medicine Thesis.
57. Lindbom, Å. (1950) Arteriosclerosis and arterial thrombosis in the lower limb. A roentgenological study. *Acta Radiol.*, (suppl. 80), 1–80.
58. Kuthan, F., Burkhalter, A., Baitsch, R. et al. (1971) Development of occlusive arterial disease in lower limbs. *Arch. Surg.*, **103**, 545–7.
59. Heath, D., Wood, E.H., Du Shane, J.W. et al. (1960) The relation of age and blood pressure in the pulmonary arteries and thoracic aorta in congenital heart disease. *Lab. Invest.*, **9**, 259–72.
60. Takagi, T., Toda, T., Leszczynski, D. et al. (1984) Ultrastructure of aging human umbilical artery and vein, *Acta Anat.*, **119**, 73–79.
61. Greenhill, N.S. and Stehbens, W.E. (1983) Scanning electron-microscopic study of experimentally induced tears in rabbit arteries. *Atherosclerosis*, **49**, 119–26.
62. Greenhill, N.S. and Stehbens, W.E. (1987) Scanning electron mocroscopic investigation of the afferent arteries of experimental femoral arteriovenous fistulae in rabbits. *Pathology*, **19**, 22–7.
63. Stehbens, W.E., Martin, B.J. and Delahunt, B. (1991) Light and scanning electron microscopic changes observed in experimental arterial forks of rabbits. *J. Exp. Pathol.*, **72**, 183–93.
64. Smith, E.B. and Smith R.H. (1976) Early changes in aortic intima. *Atheroscl. Res.*, **1**, 119–36.
65. Haust, M.D. (1971) The morphogenesis and fate of potential and early atherosclerotic lesions in man. *Human Pathol.*, **2**, 1–29.
66. Stehbens, W.E. (1981) The complications of spontaneous and experimental atherosclerosis, in *Festschrift for F.C. Courtice*, (ed. D. Garlic), School of Physiology and Pharmacology, Univ. of N.S.W., Sydney, pp. 151–8.
67. Stehbens, W.E. (1983) Fluid dynamic approaches to atherosclerosis, in *Fluid Dynamics as a Localizing Factor for Atherosclerosis*, (eds G. Schlettler, R.M. Nerem. H. Schmid-Shönbein et al.) Springer-Verlag, Berlin, pp. 3–7.
68. Cleland, J.B. (1936) Increase in diameter of the aorta with age. *Med. J. Aust.*, **1**, 818–20.
69. Godinov, V.M. (1929) The arterial system of the brain. *Am. J. Physiol. Anthropol.*, **13**, 359–88.
70. Stehbens, W.E. (1992) Experimental induction of atherosclerosis associated with femoral arteriovenous fistulae in rabbits on a stock diet. *Atherosclerosis*, **95**, 127–35.
71. Stehbens, W.E. (1975) Flow in glass models of arterial bifurcations and berry aneurysms at low Reynolds numbers. *Quart. J. Physiol.*, **60**, 181–92.
72. Parkinson, J., Bedford, D.E. and Almond, S. (1939) The kinked carotid artery that simulates aneurysm. *Br. Heart J.*, **1**, 345–61.
73. Cairney, J. (1924) Tortuosity of the cervical segment of the internal carotid artery. *J. Anat.*, **59**, 87–96.

74. Lie, T.A. (1968) *Congenital Anomalies of the Carotid Arteries*, Excerpta Medica Foundation, Amsterdam.
75. Stehbens, W.E. (1964) Vascular changes in chronic peptic ulcer. *Arch. Pathol.*, 78, 584–90.
76. Ertugrul, A. (1967) Diffuse tortuosity and lengthening of the arteries. *Circulation*, 36, 400–7.
77. Imparato, A.M., Lord, J.W., Texon, M. *et al.* (1961) Experimental atherosclerosis produced by alteration of blood vessel configuration. *Surg. Forum*, 12, 245–7.
78. Rodríguez, H.F. and Rivera, E. (1961) Spontaneous rupture of the thoracic aorta through an atheromatous plaque. *Ann. Int. Med.*, 54, 307–13.
79. Gréhant, N. and Quinquaud, H. (1885) Mesure de la pression nécessaire pour déterminer la rupture des vaisseaux sanguins. *J. Anat. Physiol., Paris*, 21, 287–97.
80. Klotz, O. and Simpson, W. (1932) Spontaneous rupture of the aorta. *Am. J. Med. Sci.*, 184, 455–73.
81. Learoyd, B.M. and Taylor, M.G. (1966) Alterations with age in the viscoelastic properties of human arterial walls. *Circulation Res.*, 18, 278–92.
82. De Palma, R.C. and Clowes, A.W. (1978) Interventions in atherosclerosis: a review for surgeons. *Surgery*, 84, 175–89.
83. Le Veen, H.H., Diaz, C. and Christoudies, G. (1973) The postendarterctomy intimal flap. *Arch. Surg.*, 107, 664–8.
84. Johnson, W.T.M., Salenga, G., Lee, G. *et al.* (1986) Arterial intimal embrittlement. A possible factor in atherogenesis. *Atherosclerosis*, 59, 161–71.
85. Richardson, P.D., Davies, M.J. and Born, G.V.R. (1989) Influence of plaque configuration and stress distribution on fissuring of coronary atherosclerotic plaques. *Lancet*, 2, 941–4.
86. Burleigh, M.C., Briggs, A.D., Lendon, C.L. *et al.* (1992) Collagen type I and III, collagen content, GAGs and mechanical strength of human atherosclerotic plaque caps: span-wise variations. *Atherosclerosis*, 96, 71–81.
87. Lendon, C.L., Davies, M.J. and Born, G.V.R. *et al.* (1991) Atherosclerotic plaque caps are locally weakened when macrophage density is increased. *Atherosclerosis*, 87, 87–90.
88. Rogers, K.M. and Stehbens, W.E. (1986) The morphology of matrix vesicles produced in experimental arterial aneurysms of rabbits. *Pathology*, 18, 64–71.
89. Stehbens, W.E. (1992) The role of thrombosis and variants of the thrombogenic theory in the etiology and pathogenesis of atherosclerosis. *Prog. Cardiovasc. Dis.*, 34, 325–46.
90. Stehbens, W.E. (1972) Platelet behaviour in the microcirculation: interaction with other formed elements and endothelium. *Thrombos. Diathes. Hemorrh.*, (suppl. 51), 177–82.
91. Cairns, H.S. (1992) Atherosclerotic renal artery stenosis. *Lancet*, 340, 298–9.
92. Moore, S. and Mersereau, W.A. Micro-embolic renal ischemia and hypertension. *Can. Med. Ass. J.*, 92, 221–4.
93. MacCallum, W.G. (1922) Arteriosclerosis. *Physiol. Rev.*, 2, 70–91.
94. Moschcowitz, E. (1929) The cause of arteriosclerosis. *Am. J. Med. Sci.*, 178, 244–67.
95. Hueper, W.C. (1944, 1945) Arteriosclerosis. *Arch. Pathol.*, 38, 162–81, 245–85, 350–64; 39, 51–61, 117–31, 187–216.
96. Khalil, K.G. and Kilman, J.W. (1975) Pulmonary sequestration. *J. Thorac. Cardiovasc. Surg.*, 70, 928–37.
97. Stehbens, W.E. (1987) Localization of atherosclerotic lesions in relation to haemodynamics, in *Atherosclerosis, Biology and Clinical Science*, (ed. A.G. Olssen), Churchill Livingstone, Edinburgh, pp. 175–82.
98. Warren, R., Gomez, R.L., Marston, J.A. *et al.* (1964) Femoropopliteal arteriosclerosis obliterans – arteriographic patterns and rates of progression. *Surgery*, 55, 135–43.
99. Stehbens, W.E. (1981) Chronic vascular changes in the walls of experimental berry aneurysms of the aortic bifurcation in rabbits. *Stroke*, 12, 643–7.
100. Geiringer, E. (1951) The mural coronary. *Am. Heart J.*, 41, 359–68.
101. Stehbens, W.E. and Karmody, A.M. (1975) Venous atherosclerosis associated with arteriovenous fistulas for hemodialysis. *Arch. Surg.*, 110, 176–80.
102. Eisenbrey, A.B. (1913) Arteriovenous aneurysm of the superficial femoral vessels. *J. Am. Med. Ass.*, 61, 2155–7.
103. Stehbens, W.E. (1974) Haemodynamic production of lipid deposition, intimal tears, mural dissection and thrombosis in the blood vessel wall. *Proc. Roy. Soc. (London) Ser. B*, 185, 357–73.
104. Texon, M. (1989) The cholesterol-heart disease hypothesis (critique) – time to change course? *Bull. N.Y. Acad. Med.*, 65, 836–41.
105. Stehbens, W.E. (1990) The lipid hypothesis and the role of hemodynamics in atherogenesis. *Prog. Cardiovasc. Dis.*, 33, 119–36.
106. Stehbens, W.E. (1958) *Intracranial Arterial Aneurysms and Atherosclerosis*, Thesis University of Sydney.
107. Holman, R.L., McGill, H.C., Strong, J.P. *et al.* (1960) Arteriosclerosis – the lesion. *Am. J. Clin. Nutr.*, 8, 85–94.
108. Pesonen, E., Norio, R. and Sarna, S. (1975) Thickenings in the coronary arteries in infancy as an indication of genetic factors in coronary heart disease. *Circulation*, 51, 218–25.
109. Adams, C.M.W. (1967) *Vascular Histochemistry*, Year Book 1967, Chicago.
110. Stehbens, W.E. (1981) Chronic changes in experimental saccular and fusiform aneurysms in rabbits. *Arch. Pathol.*, 105, 603–7.
111. Wilens, S.L. (1951) The nature of diffuse intimal thickening of arteries. *Am. J. Pathol.*, 27, 825–39.
112. Halsted, W.S. (1918) Cylindrical dilatation of the common carotid artery following partial occlusion of the innominate and ligation of the subclavian. *Surg. Gynec. Obstet.*, 27, 547–54.
113. Holman, E. (1954) The obscure physiology of poststenotic dilatation: its relation to the development of aneurysms. *J. Thorac. Surg.*, 28, 109–33.
114. Meyer, W.W. and Lind, J. (1972) Calcifications of the carotid siphon – a common finding in infancy and childhood. *Arch. Dis. Childh.*, 47, 355–63.
115. Robertson, J.H. (1960) Stress zones in foetal arteries. *J. Clin. Pathol.*, 13, 133–9.
116. Coutard, M. and Osborne-Pelligrin, M.J. (1982) Spontaneous lesions in the rat caudal artery. *Atherosclerosis*, 44, 245–60.
117. Coutard, M. and Osborne-Pelligrin, M. (1991) Rupture of the internal elastic lamina and vascular fragility in stroke-prone spontaneously hypertensive rats. *Stroke*, 22, 510–15.
118. Martin, B.J., Stehbens, W.E., Davis, P.F. *et al.* (1989) Scanning electron microscopic study of hemodynamically induced tears in the internal elastic lamina of rabbit arteries. *Pathology*, 21, 207–12.
119. Stehbens, W.E. (1963) Cerebral aneurysms of animals other than man. *J. Pathol. Bacteriol.*, 86, 161–8.
120. Silkworth, J.B. and Stehbens, W.E. (1975) The shape of endothelial cells in *en face* preparations of rabbit blood vessels. *Angiology*, 26, 474–87.
121. Jaffé, E.A. (1987) Cell biology of endothelial cells. *Human Pathol.*, 18, 234–9.
122. Stehbens, W.E. (1966) The basal attachment of endothelial cells. *J. Ultrastruct. Res.*, 15, 389–99.
123. Fallon, J.T. and Stehbens, W.E. (1972) Venous endothelium of experimental arteriovenous fistulas in rabbits. *Circ. Res.*, 31, 546–66.
124. Laurence, E.B. and Hansen, E.R. (1971) An *in vivo* study of epidermal chalone and stress hormones on mitosis in tongue epithelium and ear epidermis of the mouse. *Virchows Archiv.*, 9, 271–9.
125. Post, J. and Hoffman, J. (1969) *In vivo* replication of normal and tumor cells: relation in cancer chemotherapy, in *Human Tumor Cell Kinetics*, (ed. S. Perry), National Cancer Institute Monograph 30, Bethesda, pp. 209–24.
126. Wright, H.P. (1970) Endothelial turnover. *Thromb. Diath. Haemorrh.*, (suppl. 40), 79–84.
127. Florentin, R.A., Nam, S.C., Lee, K.T. *et al.* (1969) Increased mitotic activity in aortas of swine. *Arch. Pathol.*, 88, 463–9.
128. Wright, H.P. (1972) Mitosis patterns in aortic endothelium. *Atherosclerosis*, 15, 93–100.
129. Schwartz, S.M., Gajdusek, C.M. and Selden, S.C. (1981) Vascular wall graft control: the role of the endothelium. *Arteriosclerosis*, 1, 107–26.
130. Langille, B.L. (1984) Integrity of arterial endothelium following acute exposure to high shear stress. *Biorheology*, 21, 333–46.
131. Davies, P.F., Remuzzi, A., Gordon, E.J. *et al.* (1986) Turbulent fluid shear stress induces vascular endothelial cell turnover *in vitro*. *Proc. Natl. Acad. Sci.*, 83, 2114–17.
132. Dewey, C.F., Davies, P.F. and Gimbrone, M.A. (1988) Turbulence, disturbed flow, and vascular endothelium, in *Role of Blood Flow in Atherogenesis*, (eds Y. Yoshida, C. Caro, S. Glagov *et al.*), Springer-Verlag, Tokyo, pp. 201–4.
133. Poole, J.C.F., Sanders, A.G. and Florey, H.W. (1958) Regeneration of aortic endothelium. *J. Pathol. Bacteriol.*, 75, 133–43.
134. Stehbens, W.E. (1965) Reaction of venous endothelium to injury. *Lab. Invest.*, 14, 449–59.
135. Cotton, R. and Wartman, W.B. (1961) Endothelial patterns in human arteries. *Arch. Pathol.*, 71, 3–12.
136. Tokunaga, O., Fan, J. and Watanabe, T. (1989) Atherosclerosis and age-related multinucleated variant endothelial cells in primary culture from human aorta. *Am. J. Pathol.*, 135, 967–76.
137. Bürrig, K.-F. (1991) The endothelium of advanced arteriosclerotic plaques in humans. *Arterioscl. Thromb.*, 11, 1678–89.
138. Davies, M.J., Woolf, N., Rowles, P.M. *et al.* (1988) Morphology of the endothelium over atherosclerotic plaques in human coronary arteries. *Br. Heart J.*, 60, 459–64.
139. Jones, G.J., Martin, B.J. and Stehbens, W.E. (1992) Endothelium and elastic tears in the afferent arteries of experimental arteriovenous fistulae in rabbits. *Int. J. Exp. Pathol.*, 73, 405–16.
140. Jones, G.J., Martin, B.J. and Stehbens, W.E. (1993) Endothelium in the aorta and ilio-femoral arteries proximal to femoral arteriovenous fistulae in rabbits. *Pathology*, 25, 277–81.
141. Minick, C.R., Stemerman, M.B. and Insull, N. (1979) Role of endothelium and hypercholesterolemia in intimal thickening and lipid accumulation. *Am. J. Pathol.*, 95, 131–58.

142. Fritz, K.E., Jarmolych, J. and Daoud, A.S. (1970) Association of DNA synthesis and apparent dedifferentiational aortic smooth muscle cells *in vitro*. *Exp. Mol. Pathol.*, **12**, 354–62.
143. Ross, R. (1992) The pathogenesis of atherosclerosis, in *Heart Disease. A Textbook of Cardiovascular Medicine*, 4th edn, (ed. E. Braunwald), W.B. Saunders, Philadelphia, pp. 1106–24.
144. Stehbens, W.E. (1986) An appraisal of cholesterol-feeding in experimental atherogenesis. *Prog. Cardiovasc. Dis.*, **29**, 107–28.
145. Jerome, W.G., Minor, L.K., Glick, J.M. *et al.* (1991) Lysosomal lipid accumulation in vascular smooth muscle cells. *Exp. Mol. Pathol.*, **54**, 144–58.
146. Minor, L.K., Mahlberg, F.H., Jerome, W.G. *et al.* (1991) Lysosomal hydrolysis of lipids in a cell culture model of smooth muscle cells. *Exp. Mol. Pathol.*, **54**, 159–71.
147. Garfield, R.E., Chacko, S. and Blose, S. (1975) Phagocytosis by muscle cells. *Lab. Invest.*, **33**, 418–27.
148. Joris, I. and Majno, G. (1974) Cellular breakdown within the arterial wall. An ultrastructural study of the coronary artery in young and aging rats. *Virchows Arch. A Path. Anat. Histol.*, **364**, 111–27.
149. Greenhill, N.S., Presland, M.R., Rogers, K.M. *et al.* (1985) X-ray microanalysis of mineralized matrix vesicles of experimental saccular aneurysms. *Exp. Mol. Pathol.*, **43**, 220–32.
150. Stehbens, W.E. and Schmidt, K. (1968) Ultrastructural observations on four species of sporozoa. *J. Parasit.*, **54**, 699–710.
151. Stehbens, W.E. (1966) The Ultrastructure of Lankesterella hylae. *J. Protozool.*, **13**, 63–73.
152. Cliff, W.J. (1970) The aortic tunica intima in ageing rats. *Exp. Mol. Pathol.*, **13**, 172–89.
153. Aikawa, M. and Koletsky, S. (1970) Arteriosclerosis of the mesenteric arteries of rats with renal hypertension. *Am. J. Pathol.*, **61**, 293–322.
154. Salgado, E.D. (1970) Medial aortic lesions in rats with metacortical hypertension. *Am. J. Pathol.*, **58**, 305–27.
155. Stehbens, W.E. (1985) The ultrastructure of experimental aneurysms in rabbits. *Pathology*, **17**, 87–95.
156. Sejdewitz, V. and Staubesand, J. (1988) Immunocytochemical demonstration of lysosomal matrix vesicles in the arterial wall of the rat. *Histochemistry*, **88**, 463–7.
157. Staubesand, J. and Fischer, N. (1979) Collagen dysplasia and matrix vesicles. Researches with the electron microscope into the problem of so-called 'weakness of the vessel wall'. *Pathol. Res. Pract.*, **165**, 374–91.
158. Alberts, B., Bray, D., Lewis, J. *et al.* (1989) *Molecular Biology of the Cell*, 2nd edn, Garland Publ. Inc., New York, pp. 275–340.
159. Stehbens, W.E. (1974) The ultrastructure of the anastomosed vein of experimental arteriovenous fistulae in sheep. *Am. J. Pathol.*, **76**, 377–400.
160. Insull, W., Hata, Y., Meakin, J.D. *et al.* (1971) Morphology of lipid rich organelles in tissues of man and rat, in *Proc. Fourth Annual Scanning Electron Microscope Symposium Part 1*, pp. 337–44.
161. Anderson, H.C. (1976) Matrix vesicle calcification. *Fed. Proc.*, **35**, 105–8.
162. Wuthier, R.E. (1976) Lipids of matrix vesicles. *Fed. Proc.*, **35**, 117–21.
163. Stehbens, W.E. (1993) *The Lipid Hypothesis of Atherogenesis*, R.G. Landes Co., Austin.
164. Waddell, W.R., Sniffen, R.C. and Whytehead, L.L. (1954) The etiology of chronic interstitial pneumonias associated with lipid deposition. *J. Thorac. Cardiovasc. Surg.*, **28**, 134–44.
165. Waddell, W.R., Sniffen, R.C. and Whytehead, L.L. (1954) Influence of blood lipid levels on inflammatory response in lung and muscle. *Am. J. Pathol.*, **30**, 757–69.
166. Stehbens, W.E. and Martin, M. (1991) The vascular pathology of familial hypercholesterolemia. *Pathology*, **23**, 54–61.
167. Packham, M.A., Rowsell, H.C., Jørgensen, L. *et al.* (1967) Localized protein accumulation in the wall of the aorta. *Exp. Mol. Pathol.*, **64**, 214–32.
168. Somer, J.B. and Schwartz, C.J. (1971) Focal ³H-cholesterol uptake in the pig aorta. *Atherosclerosis*, **13**, 293–304.
169. Caplan, B.A. and Schwartz, C.J. (1973) Increased endothelial cell turnover in areas of *in vivo* Evans blue uptake in the pig aorta. *Atherosclerosis*, **17**, 401–17.
170. Stehbens, W.E. (1978) Endothelial permeability in experimental aneurysms and arteriovenous fistulae in rabbits as demonstrated by the uptake of Evans blue. *Atherosclerosis*, **30**, 343–9.
171. Gunja-Smith, Z. and Boucek, R.J. (1981) Desmosines in human urine. Amounts in early development and in Marfan's syndrome. *Biochem. J.*, **193**, 915–18.
172. Han, K.K., Davril, M., Henin-Pizieux, O. *et al.* (1980) Structural investigations of cross-linking zones in elastin. *Front. Matrix Biol.*, **8**, 104–29.
174. Davis, P.F. and Stehbens, W.E. (1986) The biochemical composition of haemodynamically-stressed vascular tissue. Part 2. The concentrations of protein and connective tissue components in the salt extracts of experimental arteriovenous fistulae. *Atherosclerosis*, **60**, 55–59.
175. Ooi, K., Lacy, M.P., Davis, P.F. *et al.* (1991) Salt-soluble collagen and elastin in the human aorta and pulmonary artery. *Exp. Mol. Pathol.*, **55**, 25–9.
176. Baydanoff, S., Nicoloff, G. and Alexiev, C. (1987) Age-related changes in the level of circulating elastin-derived peptides in serum from normal and atherosclerotic subjects. *Atherosclerosis*, **66**, 163–8.
177. Howard, P.S. and Macarak, E.J. (1989) Localization of collagen types in regional segments of the fetal bovine aorta. *Lab. Invest.*, **61**, 548–55.
178. Mayne, R. (1986) Collagenous proteins of blood vessels. *Arteriosclerosis*, **8**, 585–93.
179. Merrilees, M.J., Tieng, K.M. and Scott, H.L. (1987) Changes in collagen fibril diameters across artery walls including a correlation with glycosaminoglycan content. *Connect. Tissue Res.*, **16**, 237–57.
180. Parry, D.A.D., Barnes, G.R.G. and Cray, A.S. (1978) A comparison of the size distribution of collagen fibrils in connective tissues as a function of age and a possible relation between fibril size distribution and mechanical properties. *Proc. Roy. Soc. Lond B*, **203**, 305–21.
181. Staubesand, J. and Fischer, N. (1980) The ultrastructural characteristics of abnormal collagen fibrils in various organs. *Connect. Tissue Res.*, **7**, 213–17.
182. Martin, B.J., Leppien, B. and Stehbens, W.E. (1993) Changes in collagen fibril morphology in experimental aneurysms and arteriovenous fistulae in sheep. *Int. J. Exp. Pathol.*, **74**, 267–74.
183. Smith, R.A., Stehbens, W.E. and Weber, P. (1976) Hemodynamically-induced increase in soluble collagen in the anastomosed veins of experimental arteriovenous fistulae. *Atherosclerosis*, **23**, 429–36.
184. Rogers, K.M., Merrilees, M.J. and Stehbens, W.E. (1985) The glycosaminoglycan content of blood vessel walls with experimental aneurysms and arteriovenous fistulae. *Atherosclerosis*, **58**, 139–48.
185. Ross, R. (1992) Atherosclerosis, in *Oxford Textbook of Pathology*, vol. IIa, (eds J.O'D. McGee, P.G. Isaacson, N.A. Wright *et al.*), Oxford University Press, Oxford, pp. 798–812.
186. Parums, D.V. (1992) Aortic atherosclerosis: pathogenesis and local complications, in *Oxford Textbook of Pathology*, vol. IIa, (eds J.O'D. McGee, P.G. Isaacson, N.A. Wright *et al.*), Oxford University Press, Oxford, pp. 812–22.
187. Stehbens, W.E. (1963) Contentious features of coronary occlusion and atherosclerosis. *Bull. Postgrad. Com. Med. Univ. Sydney*, **19**, 216–5.
188. Ross, R. and Glomset, J.A. (1976) The pathogenesis of atherosclerosis. *New Engl. J. Med.*, **295**, 369–77, 420–5.
189. Di Corleto, P.E. and Fox, P.L. (1987) Endothelial cell production of growth factors – a possible role in vascular graft failure, in *Vascular Diseases. Current Research and Clinical Applications*, (eds D.E. Strandness, P. Didisheim, A.W. Clowes *et al.*), Grune & Stratton Inc., Orlando, pp. 197–207.
190. Weber, G., Bianciardi, G., Bussani, R. *et al.* (1988) Atherosclerosis and aging. *Arch. Pathol. Lab. Med.*, **112**, 1066–70.
191. Robinson, J.L., Hall, C.S. and Sedzimir, C.B. (1974) Arteriovenous malformations, aneurysms and pregnancy. *J. Neurosurg.*, **41**, 63–70.
192. Barabas, A.P. (1968) Types of Ehlers–Danlos syndrome. *Br. Med. J.*, **3**, 253–6.
193. Allan, T.M. (1962) Blood groups and heart disease. *Br. Med. J.*, **2**, 255–6.
194. Allan, T.M. (1970) Incidence of blood-group B in myocardial infarction. *Lancet*, **2**, 49–50.
195. Allan, T.M. (1973) ABO blood groups and atherosclerosis. *Atherosclerosis*, **18**, 347–51.
196. Waisman, J., Cancilla, P.A. and Coulson, W.F. (1969) Cardiovascular studies on copper deficient swine. XIII. The effect of chronic copper deficiency on the cardiovascular system of minature pigs. *Lab. Invest.*, **21**, 548–54.
197. Paterson, J.C., Mills, J. and Lockwood, C.H. (1960) The role of hypertension in the progression of atherosclerosis. *Canad. Med. Ass. J.*, **82**, 65–70.
198. Mitchell, J.R.A., Schwartz, C.J. and Zinger, A. (1964) Relationship between aortic plaques and age, sex, and blood pressure. *Br. Med. J.*, **1**, 205–9.
199. Marble, A. (1967) Angiopathy in diabetes: an unsolved problem. *Diabetes*, **16**, 825–38.
200. Stehbens, W.E. and Wierzbicki, E. (1988) The relationship of hypercholesterolemia to atherosclerosis with particular emphasis on familial hypercholesterolemia, diabetes mellitus, obstructive jaundice, myxedema and the nephrotic syndrome. *Prog. Cardiovasc. Dis.*, **30**, 289–306.
201. Stehbens, W.E. (1990) The epidemiological relationship of hypercholesterolemia, hypertension, diabetes mellitus and obesity to coronary heart disease. *J. Clin. Epidemiol.*, **43**, 733–41.
202. Friedman, M., Rosenman, R.H., Straus, R. *et al.* (1968) The relationship of behaviour pattern A to the state of the coronary vasculature. *Am. J. Med.*, **44**, 525–37.
203. Rosenman, R.W. (1967) Emotional patterns in the development of cardiovascular disease. *J. Am. Coll. Health Assoc.*, **15**, 211–14.
204. Lamberson, H.V. and Fritz, K.E. (1974) Immunological enhancement of atherogenesis in rabbits. *Arch. Pathol.*, **98**, 9–16.
205. Minick, C.R. and Murphy, G.E. (1973) Experimental induction of athero-arteriosclerosis by the synergy of allergic injury to arteries and lipid-rich diet. II. Effect of repeatedly injected foreign protein in rabbits fed a lipid-rich, cholesterol-poor diet. *Am. J. Pathol.*, **73**, 265–300.
206. Kniker, W.T. and Cochrane, C.G. (1968) The localization of circulating

immune complexes in experimental serum sickness. The role of vasoactive amines and hydrodynamic forces. *J. Exp. Med.*, **127**, 119–36.
207. Stehbens, W.E. (1986) Vascular complications in experimental atherosclerosis. *Prog. Cardiovasc. Dis.*, **29**, 221–37.
208. Darmady, E.M., Offer, J.M. and Stranack, F. (1964) Study of renal vessels by microdissection in human transplantation. *Br. Med. J.*, **2**, 976–8.
209. Thomson, J.G. (1969) Production of severe atheroma in a transplanted human heart. *Lancet*, **2**, 1088–92.
210. Robb-Smith, A.H.T. (1969) Atheroma in a transplanted heart. *Lancet*, **2**, 1248.
211. Benditt, E.P. and Benditt, J.M. (1973) Evidence for a monoclonal origin of human atherosclerotic plaques. *Proc. Natl Acad. Sci. USA*, **70**, 1753–6.
212. Hajjar, K.A., Gavish, D., Breslow, J.L. et al. (1989) Lipoprotein (a) modulation of endothelial cell surface fibrinolysis and its potential role in atherosclerosis. *Nature*, **339**, 303–5.
213. Hajjar, D.P., Fabricant, C.G., Minick, C.R. et al. (1986) Virus-induced atherosclerosis. Herpes virus infection alters aortic cholesterol metabolism and accumulation. *Am. J. Pathol.*, **122**, 62–70.
214. Hendrix, M.G.R., Daemen, M. and Bruggeman, C.A. (1991) Cytomegalovirus nucleic acid distribution within the human vascular tree. *Am. J. Pathol.*, **138**, 563–7.
215. Gibson, J.B., Carson, N.A.J. and Neill, D.W. (1964) Pathological findings in homocystinuria. *J. Clin. Pathol.*, **17**, 427–37.
216. McCully, K.S. (1969) Vascular pathology of homocysteinemia: implications for the pathogenesis of arteriosclerosis. *Am. J. Pathol.*, **56**, 111–28.
217. McCully, K.S. and Wilson, R.B. (1975) Homocysteine theory of arteriosclerosis. *Atherosclerosis*, **22**, 215–27.
218. Harker, L.A., Slichter, S.J., Scott, C.R. et al. (1974) Homocystinemia. *New Engl. J. Med.*, **291**, 537–43.
219. Rinehart, J.F. and Greenberg, L.D. (1949) Arteriosclerotic lesions in pyridoxine-deficient monkeys. *Am. J. Pathol.*, **25**, 481–91.
220. Levene, C.I. and Murray, J.C. (1977) The aetiological role of maternal vitamin B deficiency in the development of atherosclerosis. *Lancet*, **1**, 628–30.
221. Carnes, W.H. (1968) Copper and connective tissue metabolism. *Int. Rev. Connect. Tissue Res.*, **4**, 197–232.
222. Levene, C.I. (1975) Ascorbic acid and collagen synthesis in cultured fibroblasts. *Ann. N.Y. Acad. Sci. USA*, **258**, 288–304.
223. Taylor, G. (1972) Vitamin-C deficiency. *Lancet*, **2**, 1363.
224. Spittle, C.R. (1971) Atherosclerosis and vitamin C. *Lancet*, **2**, 1280–1.
225. Spittle, C.R. (1974) The action of vitamin C on blood vessels. *Am. Heart J.*, **88**, 387–8.
226. McCarthy, K.S. (1971) Homocysteine metabolism in scurvy, growth and arteriosclerosis. *Nature*, **231**, 391–2.
227. Winterfeldt, E.A., Eyring, E.J. and Vivian, V.M. (1970) Ascorbic-acid treatment for osteogenesis imperfecta. *Lancet*, **1**, 1347–8.
228. Klevay, L.M. (1987) Ischemic heart disease. A major obstacle to becoming old. *Clin. Geriat. Med.*, **3**, 361–72.
229. McClain, P.E., Wiley, E.R., Beecher, G.R. et al. (1973) Influence of zinc deficiency on synthesis and cross-linking of rat skin collagen. *Biochim. Biophys. Acta*, **304**, 457–65.
230. Abramson, D.I. and Turman, G.A. (1961) Ageing changes in blood vessels, in *Structural Aspects of Aging*, (eds G.H. Bourne and E.M.H. Wilson), Hafner, New York, pp. 45–59.
231. Gray, S.H., Handler, F.P., Blache, J.O. et al. (1953) Aging processes of aorta and pulmonary artery in negro and white races. *Arch. Pathol.*, **56**, 238–53.
232. Pariera, M.D., Handler, F.P. and Blumenthal, H.T. (1953) Aging processes in the arterial and venous systems of the lower extremities. *Circulation*, **8**, 36–43.
233. Lansing, A.I. (1952) The role of elastic tissue in the formation of the arteriosclerotic lesion. *Ann. Int. Med.*, **36**, 39–49.
234. Wahl, P. and Sanwald, R. (1969) Angiochemistry, in *Atherosclerosis*, (eds F.G. Schettler and G.J. Boyd), Elsevier, Amsterdam, pp. 141–68.
235. Atkins, L. (1954) Progeria. Report of a case with post-mortem findings. *New Engl. J. Med.*, **250**, 1065–9.
236. Russel, R.L. (1987) Evidence for and against the theory of developmentally programmed aging, in *Modern Biological Theories of Aging*, (eds H.R. Warner, R.N. Butler, R.L. Sprott et al.), Raven Press, New York, pp. 35–61.
237. Brown, W.T. (1985) Genetics of human aging. *Rev. Biol. Res. Aging*, **2**, 105–14.
238. Gabr, M., Hashem, N., Hashem, M. et al. (1960) Progeria: a pathologic study. *J. Pediat.*, **57**, 70–7.
239. Reichel, W., Garcia-Bunnel, R. and Dilallo, J. (1971) Progeria and Werner's syndrome as models for the study of normal human aging. *J. Am. Geriat. Soc.*, **19**, 369–75.
240. Vaisrub, S. (1973) Nature's experiment in unnatural aging. *J. Am. Med. Ass.*, **226**, 1565.
241. Radhakrishnan, R., Maloo, J.C., Thacker, A.K. et al. (1991) Werner's syndrome: a Libyan family with nine affected members. *Ann. Saudi Med.*, **11**, 712–15.
242. Ishii, T. and Hosoda, Y. (1975) Werner's syndrome: autopsy report of one case, with a review of pathologic findings reported in the literature. *J. Am. Geriat. Soc.*, **23**, 145–54.
243. Anitschkow, N. and Chalatow, S. (1913) On experimental cholesterin steatosis and its significance in the origin of some pathological processes. *Zentbl. Allg. Path. Path. Anat.*, **24**, 1–9. (Transl. by Pelias, M.Z. (1983) *Arteriosclerosis*, **3**, 178–82.)
244. Page, I.H. and Stamler, J. (1968) Diet and coronary heart disease. *Mod. Concepts Cardiovasc. Dis.*, **37**, 119–23.
245. Scott, R.S., Lintott, C.J., Bremer, J. et al. (1987) Hyperlipidaemia and the prevention of coronary heart disease. *N.Z. Med. J.*, **100**, 717–19.
246. Caro, C.G., Fitz-Gerald, J.M. and Schroter, R.C. (1969) Arterial wall shear and distribution of early atheroma in man. *Nature*, **223**, 1159–61.
247. Caro, C.G., Fitzgerald, J.M., Schroter, R.C. (1971) Atheroma and arterial wall shear. Observation, correlation and proposal of a shear dependent mass transfer mechanism for atherogenesis. *Proc. Roy. Soc. London (Biol.)*, **117**, 109–59.
248. Fry, D.L. (1968) Certain histological and chemical responses of the vascular interface to acutely induced mechanical stress in the aorta of the dog. *Circulation Res.*, **24**, 93–108.
249. Fry, D.L. (1969) Certain chemorheologic considerations regarding the blood vascular interface with particular reference to coronary artery disease. *Circulation*, **39**, IV-38; **40**, IV-59.
250. Brown, M.S. and Goldstein, J.L. (1986) A receptor-mediated pathway for cholesterol homeostasis. *Science*, **232**, 34–47.
251. Hopkins, P.N. and Williams, R.R. (1986) Identification and relative weight of cardiovascular risk factors. *Cardiol. Clin.*, **4**, 3–31.
252. Lundman, T. (1966) Smoking in relation to coronary heart disease and lung function in twins. *Acta Med. Scand.*, (suppl. 455), 1–75.
253. Biörck, G. (1975) *Contrasting Concepts of Ischaemic Heart Disease*, Almqvist & Wiksell International, Stockholm.
254. Corday, E. and Corday, S.R. (1975) Prevention of heart disease by control of risk factors: the time has come to face the facts. *Am. J. Cardiol.*, **35**, 330–3.
255. Laurent, P., Janoff, A. and Kagan, H.M. (1983) Cigarette smoke blocks cross-linking of elastin in vitro. *Ann. Rev. Resp. Dis.*, **127**, 189–92.
256. International Society of Cardiology (1973) *Myocardial Infarction: How to Prevent: Summary of a Meeting of the Council on Rehabilitation*, The Council, Brussels.
257. Groogogeat, Y. and Lenegre, J. (1965) Pathologie comparée l'athérosclérose spontanée et expérimentale. *Acta Cardiol.*, (suppl. 11), 15–32.
258. Anitschkow, N.N. (1967) A history of experimentation on arterial atherosclerosis in animals, in *Cowdry's Arteriosclerosis*, 2nd edn, (ed. H.T. Blumenthal), C.C. Thomas, Springfield, pp. 21–44.
259. Carey, K.D. (1978) Nonhuman primate models of atherosclerosis, in *Atherosclerosis: Its Pediatric Aspects*, (ed. W.B. Strong), Grune & Stratton, New York, pp. 41–83.
260. Vastesaegar, M.M. (1968) The contribution of comparative atherosclerosis to the understanding of human atherosclerosis. *J. Atheroscl. Res.*, **8**, 377–80.
261. Goldstein, J.L. and Brown, M.S. (1983) Familial hypercholesterolemia, in *The Metabolic Basis of Inherited Disease*, 5th edn, (eds J.B. Stanbury, J.B. Wyngaarden, D.S. Fredrickson et al.), McGraw Hill, New York, pp. 672–712.
262. McCleary, J.E., Brunsting, L.A. and Kennedy, R.L.J. (1959) Primary xanthoma tuberosum in children with classification of xanthomas. *Pediatrics*, **23**, 67–75.
263. Myant, N.B. (1991) *Cholesterol Metabolism, LDL, and the LDL Receptor*. Academic Press, San Diego.
264. Goldstein, J.L. and Brown, M.S. (1975) Familial hypercholesterolemia. A genetic regulatory defect in cholesterol metabolism. *Am. J. Med.*, **58**, 147–50.
265. Taylor, C.B. (1954) The reaction of arteries to injury by physical agents with a discussion of arterial repair and its relationship to atherosclerosis. *Symposium on Atherosclerosis*, Publication 338, Nat. Acad. of Sciences, Washington, pp. 74–90.
266. Watanabe, T., Tanaka, K. and Yanai, N. (1968) Essential familial hypercholesterolemic xanthomatosis – an autopsy case with special reference to the pathogenesis of its cardiovascular lipidosis. *Acta Pathol., Jap.*, **18**, 319–31.
267. Thannhauser, S.J. (1950) Xanthomatoses. *J. Mt Sinai Hosp.* **17**, 79–97.
268. Faber, M. (1944) Primary and secondary xanthomatosis. *Acta Med. Scand.*, **118**, 436–51.
269. Roberts, W.C., Ferrans, V.J., Levy, R.I. et al. (1973) Cardiovascular pathology in hyperlipoproteinemia. Anatomic observations in 42 necropsy patients with normal and abnormal serum lipoprotein patterns. *Am. J. Cardiol.*, **31**, 557–70.
270. Stehbens, W.E. (1973) Experimental arteriovenous fistulae in normal and cholesterol-fed rabbits. *Pathology*, **5**, 311–24.
271. Stehbens, W.E. (1981) Predilection of experimental arterial aneurysms for dietary-induced lipid deposition. *Pathology*, **13**, 735–47.
272. Morganroth, J., Levy, R.I. and Fredrickson, D.S. (1975) The biochemical, clinical, and genetic factors of type III hyperlipoproteinemia. *Ann. Int.*

Med., **82**, 158–74.
273. Roberts, W.C., Levy, R.I. and Fredrickson, D.S. (1969) Necropsy observations in familial type III hyperlipoproteinemia. *Circulation*, **40**, (suppl. 3), 172.
274. Roberts, W.C., Levy, R.I. and Fredrickson D.S. (1970) Hyperlipoproteinemia. A review of the five types with first report of necropsy findings in type 3. *Arch. Pathol.*, **90**, 46–56.
275. Cabin, H.S., Schwartz, D.E., Virmani, R. *et al.* (1981) Type III hyperlipoproteinemia: quantification, distribution, and nature of atherosclerotic coronary arterial narrowing in five necropsy patients. *Am. Heart J.*, **102**, 830–5.
276. Gown, A.M., Hazzard, W.R. and Benditt, E.P. (1982) Type III hyperlipoproteinemia and atherosclerosis: a case report and re-evaluation. *Human Pathology*, **13**, 506–10.
277. Sanguinette, M. and Picchio, F. (1971) Valvulopatia mitro-aortica ed infarti miocardici multipli in un caso di xantomatosi ipercolesterolemica. *Minerva Medica*, **62**, 2420–30.
278. Schuster, H., Rauh, G., Kormann, B. *et al.* (1990) Familial defective apolipoprotein B-100. Comparison with familial hypercholesterolemia in 18 cases detected in Munich. *Arteriosclerosis*, **10**, 577–81.
279. Zhang, S.H., Reddich, R.L., Piedrahita, J.A. *et al.* (1992) Spontaneous hypercholesterolemia and arterial lesions in mice lacking apolipoprotein E. *Science*, **258**, 468–71.
280. Plump, A.S., Smith, J.D., Hayek, T. *et al.* (1992) Severe hypercholesterolemia and atherosclerosis in apolipoprotein E-deficient mice created by homologous recombination in ES cells. *Cell*, **71**, 343–53.
281. Buja, L.M., Kita, T., Goldstein, J.L. *et al.* (1983) Cellular pathology of progressive atherosclerosis in a WHHL rabbit, an animal model of familial hypercholesterolemia. *Arteriosclerosis*, **3**, 87–101.
282. Robertson, W.B. and Strong, J.P. (1968) Atherosclerosis in persons with hypertension and diabetes. *Lab. Invest.*, **18**, 538–51.
283. Owerbach, D., Johansen, K., Billesbolle, P. *et al.* (1982) Possible association between DNA sequences flanking the insulin gene and atherosclerosis. *Lancet*, **2**, 1291–3.
284. Oppenheimer, B.S. and Fishberg, A.M. (1925) Lipemia and the reticuloendothelial apparatus. *Arch. Int. Med.*, **36**, 667–81.
285. Thannhauser, S.J. and Schmidt, G. (1946) Lipins and lipidosis. *Physiol. Rev.*, **26**, 275–318.
286. Thannhauser, S.J. and Magendantz, H. (1937–8) The different clinical features of xanthomatous diseases: a clinical physiological study of 22 cases. *Ann. Int. Med.*, **2**, 1662–746.
287. Fagge, C.H. (1873) General xanthelasma or vitiligoidea. *Pathol. Soc. London*, **24**, 242–50.
288. Weidman, F.D. and Boston, L.N. (1937) Generalized xanthoma tuberosum with xanthomatous changes in fresh scar of an intercurrent zoster. *Arch. Int. Med.*, **59**, 793–822.
289. Fredrickson, D.S. (1971) Mutants, hyperlipoproteinaemia, and coronary artery disease. *Br. Med. J.*, **2**, 187–92.
290. Vanhaelst, L. and Bastenie, P.A. (1968) Heart and coronary artery disease in hypothyroidism. *Am. Heart J.*, **76**, 845–8.
291. Blumgart, H.L., Freedberg, A.S. and Kurland, G.S. (1953) Hypercholesterolemia, myxedema and atherosclerosis. *Am. J. Med.*, **14**, 665–73.
292. Schwartz, H. and Kohn, J.L. (1935) Lipid nephrosis. A clinical and pathological study based on fifteen years' observation with special reference to prognosis. *Am. J. Dis. Child.*, **49**, 579–93.
293. Gilbert, G.G. (1941) Clinical lipoid nephrosis. *Arch. Int. Med.*, **68**, 591–8.
294. Desnick, R.J. and Sweeley, C.C. (1983) Fabry's disease: α- galactosidase A deficiency, in *The Metabolic Basis of Inherited Disease*, 5th edn, (eds, J.B. Stanbury, J.B. Wyngaarden, D.S. Fredrickson. *et al.*), McGraw Hill, New York, pp. 906–44.
295. Becker, A.E., Schoorl, R., Balk, A.G. *et al.* (1975) Cardiac manifestations of Fabry's disease. *Am. J. Cardiol.*, **36**, 829–25.
296. Mudd, S.H. and Levy, H.L. (1983) Disorders of transsulfuration, in *The Metabolic Basis of Inherited Disease*, 5th edn (eds J.B. Stanbury, J.B. Wyngaarden, D.S. Fredrickson, *et al.*), McGraw Hill, New York, pp. 522–9.
297. McKusick, V.A. (1972) *Heritable Disorders of Connective Tissue*, 4th edn, C.V. Mosby, St Louis.
298. Renteria, V.G. Ferrans, V.J. and Roberts, W.C. (1976) The heart in Hurler syndrome. Gross, histologic and ultrastructural observations in five necropsy cases. *Am. J. Cardiol.*, **38**, 487–501.
299. McKusick, V.A. and Neufeld, E.F. (1983) The mucopolysaccharide storage diseases, in *The Metabolic Basis of Inherited Disease*, 5th edn (eds J.B. Stanbury, J.B. Wyngaarden, D.S. Fredrickson *et al.*), McGraw Hill, New York, pp. 751–77.
300. Factor, S.M., Biempica, L. and Goldfischer, S. (1978) Coronary intimal sclerosis in Morquio's syndrome. *Virchows Arch.*, **379**, 1–10.
301. Goldfischer, S., Coltoff-Schiller, B., Biempica, L. *et al.* (1975) Lysosomes and the sclerotic arterial lesion in Hurler's disease. *Human Pathol.*, **6**, 633–7.
302. Abreo, K., Abreo, F., Zimmerman, S.W. *et al.* (1983) Clinicopathologic conference: a fifty-year-old man with skin pigmentation, arthritis, chronic renal failure and methemoglobinemia. *Am. J. Med.*, **14**, 97–114.
303. Kenny, D., Ptacin, M.J., Bamrah, V.S. *et al.* (1990) Cardiovascular ochronosis: a case report and review of the medical literature. *Cardiology*, **77**, 477–83.
304. Stehbens, W.E. (1992) The role of blood flow in atherogenesis and the dietary cholesterol-fat hypothesis, in *Cholesterol and Coronary Heart Disease: The Great Debate*, (eds P. Gold, S. Grover and D.A.K. Ronceri), Parthenon Publishing Group, Carnforth, pp. 101–7.
305. Dock, W. (1974) Atherosclerosis. Why do we pretend the pathogenesis is mysterious? *Circulation*, **50**, 647–9.
306. Stamler, J. and Shekelle, R. (1988) Dietary cholesterol and human coronary heart disease. *Arch. Pathol. Lab. Med.*, **112**, 1032–40.
307. Weber, G., Fabbrini, P., Resi, L. *et al.* (1986) Ultrastructural aspects of cynomolgus atherosclerotic carotid artery lesions on cholestyramine 'regression' treatment. *Vessels Appl. Pathol.*, **4**, 225–32.
308. Kato, H., Inoue, O., Kawasaki, T. *et al.* (1992) Adult coronary artery disease probably due to childhood Kawasaki disease. *Lancet*, **340**, 1127–9.
309. Stehbens, W.E. (1987) An appraisal of the epidemic rise of coronary heart disease and its decline. *Lancet*, **1**, 606–11.
310. Stehbens, W.E. (1991) Limitations of the epidemiological method in coronary heart disease. *Int. J. Epidemiol.*, **20**, 818–20.
311. Keys, A. (1953) Atherosclerosis: a problem in newer public health. *J. Mt Sinai Hosp.*, **20**, 118–39.
312. Armstrong, M.L., Warner, E.D. and Connor, W.E. (1970) Regression of coronary atheromatosis in rhesus monkeys. *Circ. Res.*, **27**, 59–67.
313. Smith, R.L. (1988) *Diet, Blood Cholesterol and Coronary Heart Disease: A Relationship in Search of Evidence*, Vector Enterprises, Santa Monica.
314. Smith, R.L. (1991) *Diet, Blood Cholesterol and Coronary Heart Disease: A Relationship in Search of Evidence*, vol. 2. Vector Enterprises, Santa Monica.
315. Stehbens, W.E. (1991) Reduction of serum cholesterol levels and regression of atherosclerosis. *Pathology*, **32**, 45–53.
316. Crawford, D.W. and Blankenhorn, D.H. (1991) Arterial wall oxygenation, oxyradicals, and atherosclerosis. *Atherosclerosis*, **89**, 97–108.
317. Imai, H., Werthessen, N.T., Subramanyam, V. *et al.* (1980) Angiotoxicity of oxygenated sterols and possible precursors. *Science*, **207**, 651–3.
318. Peng, S.-K., Taylor, C.B., Tham, P. *et al.* (1978) Effect of auto-oxidation products from cholesterol on aortic smooth muscle cells. *Arch. Pathol.*, **102**, 57–61.
319. Salonen, J.T., Ylä-herttuala, S., Yamamoto, R. *et al.* (1992) Autoantibody against oxidized LDL and progression of carotid atherosclerosis. *Lancet*, **339**, 883–6.
320. Steinberg, D., Parthesarathy, S., Carew, T.E. *et al.* (1989) Beyond cholesterol. Modifications of low-density lipoprotein that increase its atherogenicity. *New Engl. J. Med.*, **320**, 915–24.
321. Hoff, H.F., O'Neil, J., Chisholm, G.M. *et al.* (1989) Modification of low density lipoprotein with 4-hydroxynonel induces uptake by macrophages. *Arteriosclerosis*, **9**, 538–49.
322. Witztum, J.L. (1993) Role of oxidized low density lipoprotein in atherogenesis. *Br. Heart J.*, **69** (suppl.), S12–8.
323. Regnström, J., Nilsson, J., Tornvall, P. *et al.* (1992) Susceptibility to low-density lipoprotein oxidation and coronary atherosclerosis in man. *Lancet*, **339**, 1183–6.
324. DiMascio, P., Murphy, M.E. and Sies, H. (1991) Antioxidant defense systems: the role of carotenoids, tocopherols and thiols. *Am. J. Clin. Nutr.*, **53**, 194S–200S.
325. Diplock, A.T. (1991) Antioxidant nutrients and disease prevention: an overview. *Am. J. Clin. Nutr.*, **53**, 189S–93S.
326. von Rokitansky, C. (1825) *Handbuch der Pathologischen Anatomie*, (trans. by G.E. Day), Sydenham, London.
327. Duguid, J.B. (1946) Thrombosis as a factor in the pathogenesis of coronary atherosclerosis. *J. Pathol. Bacteriol.*, **58**, 207–12.
328. Duguid, J.B. (1948) Thrombosis as a factor in the pathogenesis of aortic atherosclerosis. *J. Pathol. Bacteriol.*, **60**, 57–61.
329. Duff, G.L. (1935) Experimental cholesterol arteriosclerosis and its relationship to human arteriosclerosis. *Arch. Pathol.*, **20**, 81–123, 259–305.
330. Duff, G.L. (1936) The nature of experimental cholesterol arteriosclerosis in the rabbit. *Arch. Pathol.*, **22**, 161–82.
331. Friedman, M. and Byers, S.O. (1965) Immunity of the mature thromboatherosclerotic plaque to hyercholesteraemia. *Br. J. Exp. Pathol.*, **46**, 539–44.
332. Waters, L.L. and Duff, R.S. (1952) The role of arterial injury in the localization of methyl cellulose. *Am. J. Pathol.*, **28**, 527.
333. Duguid, J.B. and Robertsion, W.B. (1957) Mechanical factors in atherosclerosis. *Lancet*, **1**, 1205–9.
334. Ross, R. and Harker, L. (1976) Hyperlipidemia and atherosclerosis. Chronic hyperlipidemia initiates and maintains lesions by endothelial cell desquamation and lipid accumulation. *Science*, **191**, 1094–1100.
335. Clowes, A.W., Ryan, G.B. and Breslow, J.L. *et al.* (1976) Absence of enhanced intimal thickening in the response of the carotid arterial wall to endothelial injury in hypercholesterolemic rats. *Lab. Invest.*, **35**, 6–17.
336. Stemerman, M.B. (1973) Thrombogenesis of the rabbit arterial plaque. *Am. J. Pathol.*, **73**, 7–26.

337. Jørgensen, L., Packham, M.A. Rowsell, H.C. et al. (1972) Deposition of formed elements of blood in the intima and signs of intimal injury in the aorta of rabbit, pig, and man. *Lab. Invest.*, **27**, 341–50.
338. Benditt, E.P. (1977) The origin of atherosclerosis. *Scient. Am.*, **236**, 74–85.
339. Pearson, T.A., Wang, A., Solez, K. et al. (1975) Clonal characteristics of fibrous plaques and fatty streaks from human aortas. *Am. J. Pathol.*, **81**, 379–88.
340. Pearson, T.A., Dillman, J.M., Solez, K. et al. (1980) Evidence for two populations of fatty streaks with different roles in the atherogenic process. *Lancet*, **2**, 496–8.
341. Thomas, W.A., Reiner, J.M., Florentin, R.A. et al. (1977) Arterial smooth muscle cells in atherogenesis: births, deaths and clonal phenomena, in *Atherosclerosis IV*, (eds G. Schettler, Y. Goto, Y. Hate et al.), Springer Verlag, Berlin, pp. 16–23.
342. Davidson, R.G., Nitowsky, H.M. and Childs, B. (1963) Demonstration of two populations of cells in the human female heterozygous for glucose-6 phosphate dehydrogenase variants. *Proc. Natl Acad. Sci.*, **50**, 481–5.
343. Benditt, E.P. (1978) The monoclonal theory of atherogenesis. *Atheroscl. Res.*, **3**, 77–85.
344. Jores, L. (1924) Arterien, in *Handbuch der speziellen pathologischen Anatomie und Histologie*, vol. 2, (eds F. Henke, O. Lubarsch), Springer, Berlin, pp. 608–786.
345. Benditt, E.P. and Schwartz, S.M. (1988) Blood vessels, in *Pathology*, (eds E. Rubin, J.L. Farber), J.B. Lippincott, Philadelphia, p. 461.
346. Aschoff, L. (1924) *Lectures on Pathology*, Hoeber, New York.
347. Rodbard, S. (1956) Vascular modifications induced by flow. *Am. Heart J.*, **51**, 926–42.
348. Keller, K.H. (1969) Mass transport phenomena in biological systems, in *Biomaterials*, (eds L. Stark, G. Agarawal), Plenum, New York, pp. 103–18.
349. Glagov, S., Zarins, C., Giddens, D.P. et al. (1988) Hemodynamics and atherosclerosis. *Arch. Pathol. Lab. Med.*, **112**, 1018–31.
350. Leung, D.Y.M., Glagov, S. and Mathews, M.B. (1976) Cyclic stretching stimulates synthesis of matrix components by arterial smooth muscle cells in vitro. *Science*, **191**, 475–7.
351. Fry, D.L. (1973) Responses of the arterial wall to certain physical factors, in *Atherogenesis: Initiating Factors. Ciba Foundation Symposium 12*, Elsevier, Amsterdam, pp. 93–125.
352. Yokobori, T. (1965) *The Strength, Fracture and Fatigue of Metals*, (Transl. by Matsuo, T. and Inoue, M.) P. Noordhoff, Groningen.
353. Bantle, J.A. (1971) Effects of mechanical vibrations on the growth and development of mouse embryos. *Aerospace Med.*, **42**, 1087–91.
354. Walton, K.W. (1974) The pathology of Raynaud's phenomen of occupational orgin, in *The Vibration Syndrome*, (ed. W. Taylor), Academic Press, London, pp. 109–19.
355. Ljung, B. and Sivertsson, R. (1980) The inhibitory response of vascular smooth muscle to vibrations, in *Vascular Neuroeffector Mechanisms*, (eds J.A. Bevan, T. Godraind, R.A. Maxwell et al.), Raven Press, New York, pp. 207–12.
356. Imparato, A.M., Baumann, G., Pearson, T. et al. (1974) Electron microscopic studies of experimentally produced fibromuscular arterial lesions. *Surg. Gynec. Obstet.*, **139**, 497–504.
357. Fox, B. and Seed, W.A. (1981) Location of early atheroma in the human coronary arteries. *J. Biomech. Eng.*, **103**, 208–12.
358. Sakata, N. and Takebayashi, S. (1988) Localization of atherosclerotic lesions in the curving sites of human internal carotid arteries. *Biorheology*, **25**, 567–78.
359. Stehbens, W.E., Fee, C.J., Stehbens, G.R. (1987) Flow in glass models simulating arterial tortuosities under steady flow conditions. *Q. J. Exp. Physiol.*, **72**, 201–14.
360. Texon, M., Imparato, A.M. and Lord, J.W. (1960) The hemodynamic concept of atherosclerosis. *Arch. Surg.*, **80**, 47–53.
361. Matsuda, I., Niimi, H., Moritake, K. et al. (1978) The role of hemodynamic factors in arterial wall thickening in the rat. *Atherosclerosis*, **29**, 363–71.
362. Osborne-Pellegrin, M.J. and Coutard, M. (1985) Effect of contralateral nephrectomy alone or in association with hypertension on rat renal artery lesions. *Atherosclerosis*, **57**, 267–80.
363. Lie, J.T., Laurie, G.M. and Morris, G.C. (1977) Aortocoronary bypass saphenous vein graft atherosclerosis. *Am. J. Cardiol.*, **40**, 906–14.
364. Downs, A.R. (1971) Repair of late vein graft occlusions. *Arch. Surg.*, **103**, 639–43.
365. Singh, R.N., Sosa, J.A. and Green, G.E. (1983) Internal mammary artery versus saphenous vein graft. Comparative performance in patients with combined revascularisation. *Br. Heart J.*, **50**, 48–58.
366. Lytle, B.W., Loop, F.D., Cosgrove, D.M. et al. (1985) Long-term (5 to 10 years) serial studies of internal mammary artery and saphenous vein coronary bypass grafts. *J. Thorac. Cardiovasc. Surg.*, **89**, 248–58.
367. Sako, Y. and Varco, R.L. (1962) Ten-year observation on autologous pericardial and venous grafts in the thoracic aorta. *Surgery*, **51**, 465–70.
368. Cooper, K.H., Pollock, M.L., Martin, R.P. et al. (1976) Physical fitness levels vs selected coronary risk factors. *J. Am. Med. Ass.*, **236**, 166–9.
369. Eichner, E.R. (1983) Exercise and heart disease. Epidemiology of the 'exercise hypothesis'. *Am. J. Med.*, **75**, 1008–23.
370. Virmani, R. and Rabinowitz, M. (1987) Cardiac pathology and sports medicine. *Human Pathol.*, **18**, 493–501.
371. Evans, G. and Egan, J. (1988) Catching up the orthopods. Mechanical forces matter in tissues other than bone. *Br. Med. J.*, **297**, 936.
372. Carbon, R., Sambrook, P.N., Deakin, V. et al. (1990) Bone density of élite female athletes with stress fractures. *Med. J. Aust.*, **153**, 373–6.
373. Sternby, N.H. (1976) Atherosclerosis and malignant tumours. *Bull. Wld. Hlth. Org.*, **53**, 555–61.
374. Brosens, I., Robertson, W.B. and Dixon, H.G. (1967) The physiological reponse of the vessels of the placental bed to normal pregnancy. *J. Pathol. Bacteriol.*, **93**, 569–79.
375. Shiraishi, M., Matsuo, K. and Takebayashi, S. (1983) Sequential ultrastructural changes of arteries in rats induced by restrained stress. *Acta Pathol. Jap.*, **33**, 265–73.
376. Kernohan, J.W., Anderson, E.W. and Keith, N.M. (1929) The arterioles in cases of hypertension. *Arch. Int. Med.*, **44**, 395–423.
377. Wiener, J., Spiro, D. and Lattes, R.G. (1965) The cellular pathology of experimental hypertension. *Am. J. Pathol.*, **47**, 457–85.
378. Baker, R.D. and Selikoff, E. (1952) The cholesterol of hyaline arteriosclerosis. *Am. J. Pathol.*, **28**, 573–81.
379. Smith, J.P. (1956) Hyaline arteriolosclerosis in spleen, pancreas and other viscera. *J. Pathol. Bacteriol.*, **72**, 643–56.
380. Bell, E.T. (1951) The pathological anatomy in primary hypertension, in *Hypertension*, (eds E.T. Bell and B.J. Clawson), Minnesota Press, Minneapolis, pp. 183–98.
381. Wolfgarten, M. and Magarey, F.R. (1959) Vascular fibrinoid necrosis in hypertension, *J. Pathol. Bacteriol.*, **77**, 597–603.
382. Burkholder, P.M. (1965) Malignant nephrosclerosis. *Arch. Pathol.*, **80**, 583–9.
383. Singleton, A.O., McGinnis, L.M.S. and Eason, H.R. (1959) Arteritis following correction of coarctation. *Surgery*, **45**, 665–73.
384. Byrom, F.B. (1969) *The Hypertensive Vascular Crisis. An Experimental Study*, Heinemann, London.
385. Sinclair, R.A., Antonovych, T.T. and Mostofi, F.K. (1976) Renal proliferative arteriopathies and associated glomerular changes. A light and electron micrographic study. *Human Pathol.*, **7**, 565–88.
386. Robertson, W.B., Brosens, I. and Dixon, H.G. (1967) The placental response of the vessels to the placental bed to hypertensive pregnancy. *J. Pathol. Bacteriol.*, **93**, 581–92.
387. Zeek, P.M. and Assali, N.S. (1950) Vascular changes in the decidua associated with eclamptogenic toxemia of pregnancy. *Am. J. Clin. Pathol.*, **20**, 1099–109.
388. Lindhop, G. (1985) Blood vessels and lymphatics, in *Muir's Textbook of Pathology*, 12th edn, (ed. J.R. Anderson), Edward Arnold, London, pp. 14.1–14.14.
389. Byrom, F.B. (1969) Vascular lesions in malignant hypertension. *Lancet*, **2**, 495.
390. Gius, J.A., Boyle, D.E., Congdon, R.H. et al. (1965) The blood vessels of the stomach in patients with peptic ulcer. *Bibl. Anat.*, **7**, 564–71.
391. Robertson, W.B., Brosens, I. and Dixon, G. (1975) Uteroplacental vascular pathology. *Europ. J. Obstet. Gynec. Reprod. Biol.*, **5**, 47–65.
392. Labarrere, C.A. (1988) Review article. Acute atherosis. A histopathological hallmark of immune aggression? *Placenta*, **9**, 95–108.
393. Stary, H.C. (1966) Disease of small blood vessels in diabetes mellitus. *Am. J. Med. Sci.*, **252**, 357–73.
394. Olson, N.D., Nuttall, F.Q., Sinha, A. et al. (1979) Thin muscle capillary basement membrane in myotoxic dystrophy. *Diabetes*, **28**, 686–9.
395. Moschowitz, E. and Strauss, L. (1964) Studies in phlebosclerosis of the inferior vena cava and portal vein in an infant 23 days old. *Arch. Pathol.*, **77**, 445–9.
396. Short, R.D.H. (1954) Orientation of structure and of thrombi in the deep veins of the leg in man. *J. Pathol. Bacteriol.*, **68**, 41–54.
397. Learmonth, J. (1951) On certain aspects of portal hypertension. *Edinburgh Med. J.*, **58**, 1–16.
398. Scotti, T.M. (1968) Diseases of veins, in *Pathology of the Heart and Blood Vessels*, 3rd edn, (ed. S.E. Gould), C.C. Thomas, Springfield, pp. 1006–40.
399. Stuart, M. and Magarey, F.R. (1960) The great veins in venous hypertension. *J. Pathol. Bacteriol.*, **79**, 319–23.
400. Moschcowitz, E. (1959) Pathogenesis of phlebosclerosis. *Arch. Pathol.*, **68**, 180–4.
401. Moschcowitz, E. (1962) Studies in phlebosclerosis. IV. Phlebosclerosis of the pulmonary veins. *Am. J. Cardiol.*, **10**, 836–9.
402. McClusky, R.T. and Wilens, S.L. (1952) The infrequency of lipid deposition in sclerotic veins. *Am. J. Pathol.*, **29**, 71–83.
403. Li, P.-L. (1940) Adaptation in veins to increased intravenous pressure with special reference to the portal system and inferior vena cava. *J. Pathol. Bacteriol.*, **50**, 121–36.
404. Geiringer, E. (1949) Venous atheroma. *Arch. Pathol.*, **48**, 401–20.
405. Lev, M. and Saphir, O. (1952) Endophlebohypertrophy and phlebosclerosis. *Am. J. Pathol.*, **28**, 401–11.
406. Rabinovitz, A.J. and Saphir, O. (1965) The thoracic duct. Significance of age-related changes of lipid in the wall. *Circulation*, **31**, 899–905.

407. Borchard, F., Borchard, H. and Huth, F. (1972) Beitrag zur lymphvaskulären Sklerose des Ductus thoracicus. Morphometrische Untersunchungen von 88 Fällen. *Beitr. Pathol.*, **146**, 145–61.
408. Kelbling, S. (1937) Über Aneurysmenbildung des Ductus thoracicus mit Atherosklerose. *Frank. Z. Path.*, **50**, 34–41.
409. Oberndorfer, D.R. (1925) Atherosklerose des Ductus thoracicus. *Zentbl. Allg. Path.*, **36**, 225.
410. Taylor, C.B. and Peng, S.-K. (1980) Vitamin D – its excessive use in the USA, in *Nutritional Elements and Clinical Biochemistry*, (eds M.A. Brewster and H.K. Naito), Plenum, New York, pp. 131–8.
411. Stehbens, W.E. (1988) Localization of experimental calcification in rabbit blood vessels with particular reference to haemodynamics. *Angiology*, **39**, 597–608.
412. Field, M.H. (1947) Medial calcification of arteries of infants. *Arch. Pathol.*, **42**, 607–18.
413. Traisman, H.S., Limpiris, N.N. and Traisman, A.S. (1956) Myocardial infarction due to calcification of the arteries in an infant. *Am. J. Dis. Child.*, **91**, 34–7.
414. Carles, D., Serville, F., Dubecq, J.P. *et al.* (1992) Idiopathic arterial calcification in a stillborn complicated by pleural hemorrhage and hydrops fetalis. *Arch. Pathol. Lab. Med.*, **116**, 293–5.
415. Barson, A.J., Campbell, R.H.A. Langley, F.A. *et al.* (1976) Idiopathic arterial calcification of infancy without intimal proliferation. *Virchows Arch. A. Path. Anat. Histol.*, **372**, 167–73.
416. Liu, C.T., Singer, D.B. and Frates, R. (1980) Idiopathic arterial calcification in infancy. *Arch. Pathol. Lab. Med.*, **104**, 589–91.
417. Mori, A., Yamaguchi, K., Fukushima, H. *et al.* (1992) Extensive arterial calcification of unknown etiology in a 29-year-old male. *Heart Vessels*, **7**, 211–4.
418. Rousselet, M.-C., Saint-Andre, J.-P. L'Hoste, P. *et al.* (1990) Stenotic intimal thickening of the external iliac artery in competition cyclists. *Hum. Pathol.*, **21**, 524–9.
419. Leu, H.J., Lagiader, J. and Odermatt, B. (1984) Pathogenesis of the so-called cystic adventitial degeneration of peripheral blood vessels. *Virchows Arch. Path. Anat.*, **404**, 289–300.
420. Lie, J.T., Jensen, P.L. and Smith, R.E. (1991) Adventitial cystic disease of the lesser saphenous vein. *Arch. Pathol. Lab. Med.*, **115**, 946–8.
421. Wright, J.R. and Calkins, E. (1974) Relationship of amyloid deposits in the human aorta to aortic atherosclerosis. *Lab. Invest.*, **30**, 767–73.
422. Stehbens, W.E. (1988) Atherosclerosis – its cause and nature. *Spec. Sci. Tech.*, **11**, 89–99.
423. Stehbens, W.E. and Ludatscher, R.M. (1983) The susceptibility of renal arterial forks in rabbits to dietary-induced lipid deposition *Pathology*, **15**, 475–85.

7 BIOCHEMISTRY AND CELL BIOLOGY OF ATHEROGENESIS

Henry F. Hoff

This chapter focuses on the role that plasma lipoproteins play in the pathogenesis and development of the atherosclerotic lesion. Published data are reviewed on the localization of low density lipoproteins (LDL), the major cholesterol-carrying lipoprotein in plasma, in both human atherosclerotic lesions with different grades of severity and in animals at different stages of the development of atherosclerosis. Additional morphologic evidence for the accumulation of very low density lipoproteins (VLDL), intermediate density lipoproteins (IDL), high density lipoproteins (HDL) and lipoprotein(a) (Lp(a)) are also given. I then present quantitative data to document the amounts of these lipoproteins that accumulate in arteries with different degrees of atherosclerosis in humans and in animals. Published evidence for the mechanisms responsible for the retention of certain lipoproteins is also provided. Structural and chemical characteristics of lipoproteins in atherosclerotic lesions are discussed with emphasis on the modifications that could lead to the development of lesions. Finally, evidence is provided on the interactions of these lipoproteins, as well as model systems for these modified lipoproteins, with vascular cells, primarily tissue macrophages. These studies address how these lipoproteins are recognized by specific receptors and describe their uptake and intracellular processing mechanisms.

Substantial evidence to be discussed in more detail in this chapter includes the fact that plasma LDL, Lp(a) and, to a lesser degree VLDL, accumulate in the arterial intima. LDL is derived primarily from the catabolism of VLDL [1], which in turn is synthesized in the liver [2]. Blood monocytes infiltrate the intima at specific anatomic sites in large arteries [3,4] and internalize the accumulated lipoproteins, leading to lipid loading of these cells [5], forming the foam cell (Figure 7.1a)[6], the hallmark of the early fatty streak lesion [7]. Some intimal smooth muscle cells also become lipid-laden (Figure 7.1(b)) [8].

The lipid-filled inclusion can take the form of roundish droplets (Figure 7.2(a)) or electron-dense organelles (Figure 7.2(b)) when such foam cells are viewed by electron microscopy. Many of these foam cells lyse, extruding the lipid-rich inclusions into the extracellular space [9]. This lysis is probably the derivation of the lipid-rich necrotic core of the lesion which is filled with lipid droplets of various sizes and cholesterol monohydrate crystals embedded in a matrix of collagen [10] (Figure 7.3). Proliferation of intimal smooth muscle cells and deposition of collagen synthesized by these cells leads to the development of a fibrous cap between the lumen and the necrotic core [11]. When the fibrous cap is enlarged where it encroaches on the vessel lumen, ischemia of end-organs can result. However, recent findings indicate that unstable angina, leading to myocardial infarction [12] is more often the result of rupture of a thin fibrous cap [13], presumably eroded by the rapid enlargement of the lipid-rich necrotic core. Such a rupture results in intravascular clot formation which leads to an occluding thrombus [14].

7.1 LDL localization in arteries

7.1.1 LOCALIZATION OF LDL IN HUMAN ARTERIES WITH ATHEROSCLEROTIC INVOLVEMENT

One of the key characteristics linking LDL with the atherosclerotic process is its localization in atherosclerotic lesions. We studied the localization pattern of LDL in the grossly normal portion of arteries, in fatty streaks and in advanced atherosclerotic lesions with distinct necrotic cores and fibrous caps, in the human aorta, coronary and carotid arteries [15–21]. We used affinity chromatography-purified antibodies to Apo-B, the protein portion of LDL [1], which were then conjugated to fluorescein isothiocyanate. LDL was localized diffusely throughout the intima of the grossly normal aorta, but not in the tunica media [20]. This localization of LDL corresponded to that of lipid following oil red O-staining.

Vascular Pathology. Edited by W.E. Stehbens and J.T. Lie. Published in 1995 by Chapman & Hall, London. ISBN 0 412 48640 7

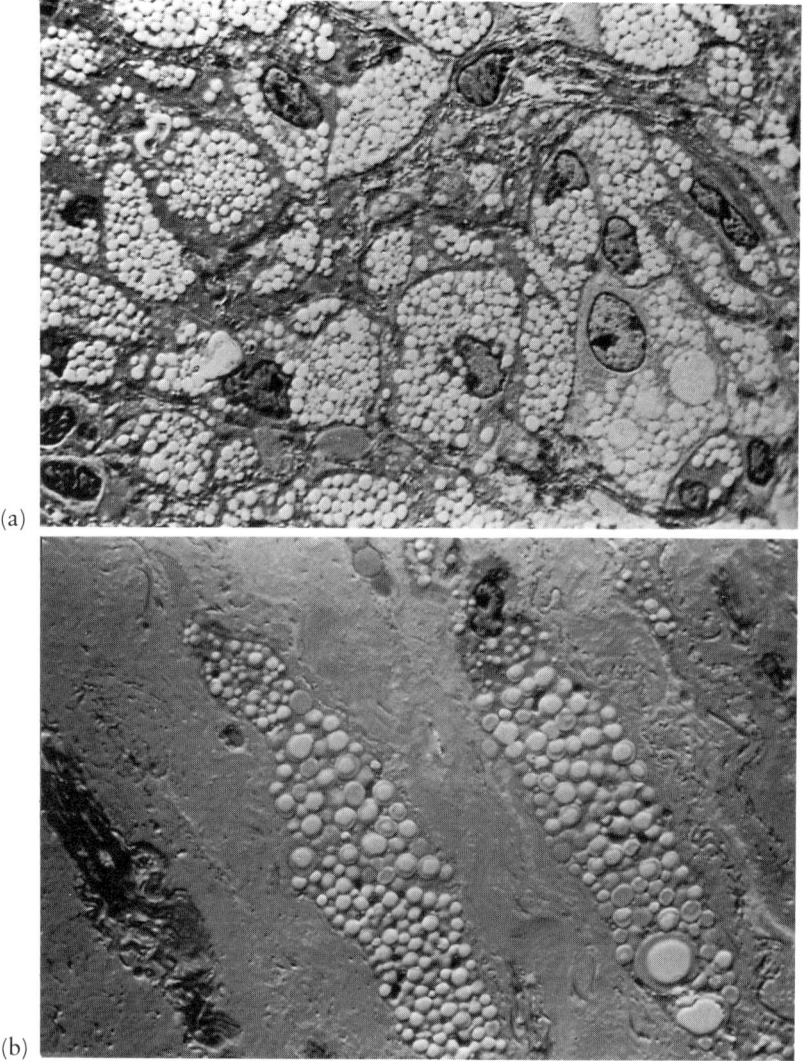

Figure 7.1 Light micrographs using interference contrast microscopy of a fatty streak lesion from a human cerebral artery. (a) Close packing of round foam cells. (b) Two spindle-shaped, lipid-laden foam cells believed to be derived from smooth muscle cells. (Reproduced with permission from Hoff [226].)

In fatty streak lesions, LDL is localized in the extracellular space between foam cells (Plate 2(a)), both within groups of elastic fibrils as well as along such fibers [16–18] (Plate 2(a)). On some occasions, especially in patients with type II hyperlipoproteinemia, LDL is also localized in foam cells [16]. LDL is only localized in the tunica media under fatty streaks of a middle cerebral artery in regions around fenestrations in the internal elastic membrane (Plate 2(b)) [18].

In advanced atherosclerotic lesions LDL is localized predominantly in the necrotic core of such plaques in the coronary artery (Plate 2(c)) [16]. Similar patterns are found in the aorta and carotid arteries. Only the area occupied by cholesterol crystals is clearly negative for LDL (Plate 2(d)) [18,19]. The accumulation of LDL is directly associated with lipid shown by oil red O-staining and with acid glycosaminoglycans (GAG) shown by alcian blue staining [16–18]. LDL is localized predominantly in the necrotic core surrounding cholesterol monohydrate crystals [21].

In the fibrous cap above such necrotic cores of human lesions, LDL is localized to some but not all bands of collagen fibers (Plate 2(e)) and to some elastic fibers [16]. In some regions, LDL surround spindle-shaped cells in the intima that are believed to be smooth muscle cells. However, regions close to such cells are devoid of LDL [21]. These areas stain positively with the PAS stain which probably represent basement membranes. When fibrous caps of an abdominal aorta of human lesions were also stained for fibrinogen or fibrin, a colocalization of LDL (Plate 2(e)) and fibrinogen (Plate 2(f)) was found in cell-free regions [16]. These patterns are similar to those reported by others in human lesions [22–25].

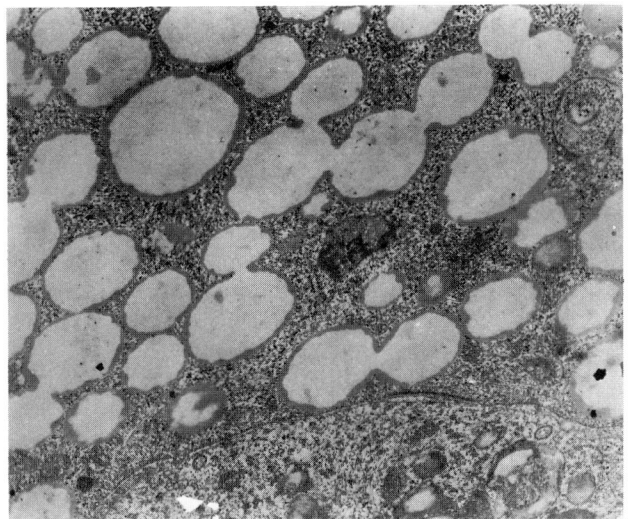

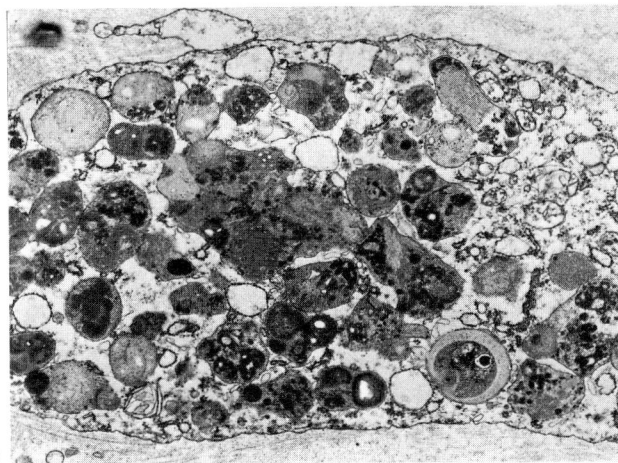

Figure 7.2 Electron micrographs of lipid-filled foam cells in a fatty streak lesion from a human cerebral artery. (a) The presence of intracellular amorphous cholesteryl oleate-rich droplets whose centers have been removed by the tissue preparations. (b) Presence of intracellular inclusions containing material of different electron densities.

7.1.2 LIGHT MICROSCOPIC LOCALIZATION OF LDL IN ATHEROSCLEROTIC LESIONS OF ANIMAL MODELS

We have also documented the localization of LDL in atherosclerotic lesions in the coronary arteries of cynomolgus monkeys on a hypercholesterolemic diet [26,27] and in the aorta [28] and coronary arteries [29] of hypercholesterolemic swine. Although the localization patterns were similar to those in human arteries, improved technical procedures provided higher resolution of LDL localization. This resolution was achieved by performing the immunostaining on sections of tissue that had been embedded in paraffin (monkey arteries) or in plastic (swine arteries). In addition, counterstains improved identification of cellular structures.

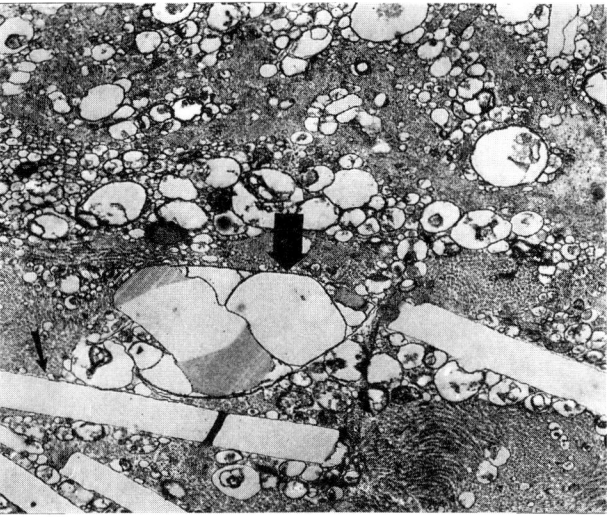

Figure 7.3 Electron micrograph of the necrotic core of a fibrous plaque lesion. Note the cholesterol crystals (small arrow) and the extracellular lipid droplets (large arrow) embedded in a matrix of collagen.

LDL in coronary arteries of the hypercholesterolemic cynomolgus monkey was, like in humans, localized predominately in the tunica intima [26]. However, some regions of the tunica media were positive for LDL, perhaps as a result of the presence of fenestrations in the internal elastic membrane. As in human lesions, quite striking was the almost one-to-one association of LDL (Plate 2(g)) and GAG revealed by alcian blue staining (Plate 2(h)). Some regions of the necrotic core showed a diffuse distribution of LDL. The LDL-negative regions appear to be sites of macrophage-derived foam cells. Indeed, in all sections of coronary arteries from hypercholesterolemic (H) monkeys, cellular sites were consistently negative (Plates 2(i), 2(j)). At higher magnification we found that the localization of LDL surrounding spindle-shaped cells in the fibromuscular cap of coronary lesions of these monkeys was highly focal (Plates 2(i), 2(j)). Some necrotic areas between spindle-shaped cells were positive for LDL (Plate 2(i)). In some regions LDL was localized along wavy bands, possibly representing elastic fibers. In other regions a narrow LDL-negative zone was seen between the LDL-positive zone and the cell surface (Plate 2(j)). Similar localization patterns have been reported by several other groups in lesions of animal models [30,31].

As in humans, the grossly normal aortic intima of H swine showed a diffuse localization of LDL (Plate 2(k)) with only a few foam cells being negative. Also, as in human lesions, LDL in fatty streaks was found in the narrow spaces between macrophage-derived foam cells in the aorta of H swine (Plate 2(l)) [28]. Proximal segments of coronary arteries such as the two orifices were characterized by the presence of diffuse intimal thickening from 20 to 100 µm [29]. Focal intimal thickenings or intimal cushions were also found at branch points in more distal regions. Such areas, especially the intimal cushions, were characterized by smooth muscle cells packed together in a dense array [29]. An edematous acellular zone rich in alcian blue-positive material believed to be GAG, was found between the endothelium and the smooth muscle cells. Elastica was usually fragmented or reduplicated in such regions. Swine on both hypercholesterolemic (H) and normolipemic (N) diets showed these intimal thickenings. Apo-B localization in the coronary arteries was confined to those edematous zones just described but was far more prevalent in H swine than in N swine when cholesterol levels in the former were in the 500 mg/dl range [29]. The topographic distribution of Apo-B localization in cross-sections of the intima of coronary arteries increased with time on the diet. The edematous zones that were positive for Apo-B were also the sites at which intimal foam cells could be seen and were the sites at which fatty streaks developed later on the diet [29]. Thus, the localization pattern of LDL in atherosclerotic lesions from animal models did not differ greatly from those in human lesions, confirming that atherosclerotic lesions induced by hypercholesterolemia resemble human lesions from normocholesterolemics.

7.1.3 ULTRASTRUCTURAL LOCALIZATION OF LDL IN HUMAN LESIONS

We have also studied the localization of Apo-B on the electron microscopic level in human intracranial arteries [32] and in the human aorta and coronary arteries [33] using an immunoperoxidase technique. In these studies unembedded sections of human arteries that had been briefly fixed with paraformaldehyde, were incubated with affinity-purified anti-Apo-B to which peroxidase had been conjugated. The reaction product depicting peroxidase was then formed with diaminobenzidine, and the tissue was further processed for electron microscopy. We found in the aorta, the coronary arteries and in intracranial arteries that spherical structures of the sizes of LDL and VLDL, as well as somewhat larger spheres, were positive for Apo-B on their surfaces (Figure 7.4(a)) [32,33]. Apo-B was localized primarily in the necrotic core of plaques but was also associated with collagen and elastic fibers (Figure 7.4(b)). Some regions of the necrotic core contained closely packed spheres in the size range of LDL (Figure 7.5(a)). This packing resembled regions that we found in the necrotic core of a type-II hyperlipoproteinemic patient, in which close packing of spheres, some in the size range of LDL, could be discerned even without immunostaining for Apo-B [34]. Thus, these ultrastructural observations confirmed and extended those obtained using immunofluorescence techniques and suggested that most of the Apo-B was

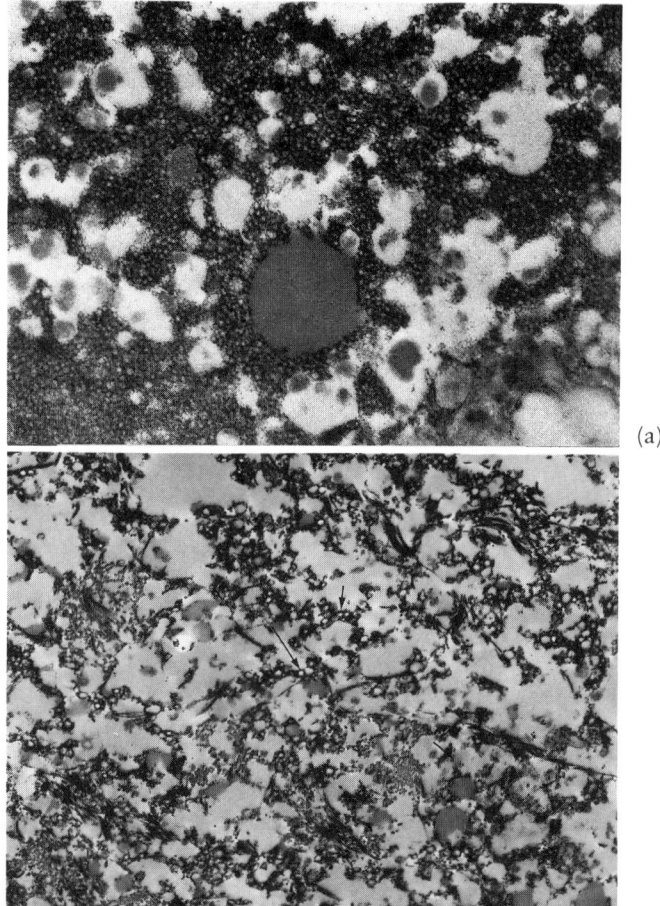

Figure 7.4 Electron micrographs of the necrotic core of an advanced atherosclerotic lesion in a human coronary artery following immunocytochemical staining of Apo-B by an immunoperoxidase technique. Spheres of about 20–30 nm diameters whose surface demonstrates the presence of reaction product depicting Apo-B can be seen (a) closely stacked together in an area also demonstrating the presence of large lipid droplets or (b) associated with elastica fibers (small arrows). (Reproduced with permission from Hoff and Gaubatz [32].)

probably associated with intact LDL particles that had insudated into the arterial intima.

7.1.4 LOCALIZATION OF OTHER LIPOPROTEINS AND APOPROTEINS IN ATHEROSCLEROTIC LESIONS FROM HUMANS AND ANIMAL MODELS

Studies on the transport of VLDL and LDL into arteries after the ingestion of radiolabeled lipoproteins by animals showed that, whereas extensive entry of LDL occurred [35], little entry of VLDL was found [36]. However, the permeability of the endothelium covering the lesions is believed to be greater than that of the endothelium over normal arteries [37]. As such, VLDL could conceivably enter into lesions.

We have used FITC-labeled antibodies to Apo-C_{III} to identify the localization of VLDL in human atherosclerotic lesions. In studies on atherosclerotic lesions in the human aorta, we identified Apo-C_{III} in regions of the necrotic core [17]. Although Apo-C_{III} co-associated with Apo-B in such regions, the topographical distribution in cross-section of Apo-B exceeded that of Apo-C_{III}. Whether this distribution was the result of differences in antibody titer or due to differences in sites responsible for binding of LDL and VLDL still needs to be determined. In one study, we also found that Apo-A_I was localized to the same areas of necrotic cores of plaques as Apo-C_{III} [17]. This similarity suggests that HDL might also show an affinity for such sites. Another group found that Apo-A was usually found at the same sites in human lesions as Apo-B [38]. Apo-E was also localized to the extracellular space of atherosclerotic lesions, with a distribution not dissimilar to the locations of Apo-B [39,40]. This localization could represent VLDL or HDL to which Apo-E is attached. Alternatively, it could represent Apo-E secreted by tissue macrophages, because these cells secrete Apo-E under culture conditions [41].

Lp(a) is a plasma lipoprotein with physical and chemical characteristics similar to LDL [42,43]. However, it possesses a unique protein called apo(a) which is highly glycosylated [42,43]. Lp(a) is an independent risk factor for coronary heart disease [44–46] and for stenosis of vein grafts [47]. Because of the structural homology between apo(a) and plasminogen [48,49], it has been suggested that Lp(a) might be antifibrinolytic [50]. In fact, under *in vitro* conditions Lp(a) competes with plasminogen for binding sites on monocytes [51] and endothelial cells [52] and sites on fibrin(ogen) [53].

Several groups have investigated the localization pattern of Lp(a) in lesions [54–57]. Because Lp(a) contains both apo(a) and Apo-B, antibodies to anti-Lp(a) contain both anti-apo(a) and anti-Apo-B. However, anti-Apo-B can be quantitatively removed from anti-apo(a) by applying the anti-Lp(a) antibody to affinity chromatography on a Sepharose LDL column [58]. The localization pattern in human lesions for apo(a) appears to be the same as that of Apo-B as shown over 20 years ago by Walton and co-workers [54], and confirmed recently by Rath *et al.* [55]. Apo(a) also co-localized with fibrinogen [56]. This is not a surprising result, given the tendency of Lp(a) to interact with fibrin(ogen) under *in vitro* conditions [50,53]. This interaction of Lp(a) with fibrinogen could, in large part, be responsible for the accumulation of Lp(a) in lesions. Recently, apo(a) has also been shown to be localized in atherosclerotic lesions from cynomolgus monkeys [57]. Further discussion on Lp(a) in lesions can be found in sections 7.2 and 7.3.

7.1.5 POTENTIAL UNDERLYING MECHANISMS FOR SPECIFIC LOCALIZATION OF LDL IN ARTERIES

Our results, as well as those of others, suggest that LDL accumulates primarily in the grossly normal tunica intima of large arteries, which is thickened in most large human arteries in adults [11]. This accumulation may be caused by a barrier function of the internal elastic membrane, as suggested by Smith and Staples [59], in which this membrane prevents the further ingress of LDL in the tunica media. Indeed, in the middle cerebral artery this elastic membrane is quite thick and LDL is only localized in the tunica media at regions in which the internal elastic membrane is fenestrated (Plate 1(a)). Smith and Staples have also proposed that high intimal accumulations of LDL are the result of size exclusion, that is, assuming that the extracellular space of the grossly normal intima functions as a molecular sieve [59]. Thus, small molecules would readily penetrate the matrix of the intima, whereas large ones could not enter it at all.

The most compelling explanation for LDL accumulation in the intima of large human arteries is that retention is caused by specific interactions of LDL with tissue components. In the grossly normal intima in humans, LDL is associated with GAG (Figure 7.5(a)). Such an association between LDL and GAG isolated from aortas has been demonstrated under *in vitro* conditions [60–65]. The association was even stronger when the GAGs were still in the form of a proteoglycan (PG) [65] suggesting that the steric configuration of the GAG 'branches' in the PG 'tree' enhanced the interaction with LDL. Changes in the structure and chemical composition of PG isolated from lesions relative to those isolated from normal arteries may also lead to enhanced interaction with LDL [66]. Further evidence for the probable association of LDL and GAG in the arterial intima was provided by studies showing that such complexes could be isolated from fatty streak lesions from humans [67] and from hypercholesterolemic rabbits [68]. Thus, LDL accumulation in fatty streaks is also the result of specific interaction with PGs found between foam cells (Figure 7.5(b)).

Recently, using immunocytochemical techniques, Galis *et al.* found a distribution of intimal proteoglycans that co-localized with LDL in injury lesions of rabbit aortas using electron microscopy [69]. These observations confirm and extend our original observations using alcian blue staining [16], that suggest an association of LDL with GAG in intimal proteoglycans. The more extensive localization in plaques compared to grossly normal intima could be the result of more abundant synthesis and deposition of proteoglycans or of chemical modifications in plaque proteoglycans [66]. A consistent finding was the association of LDL, lipid

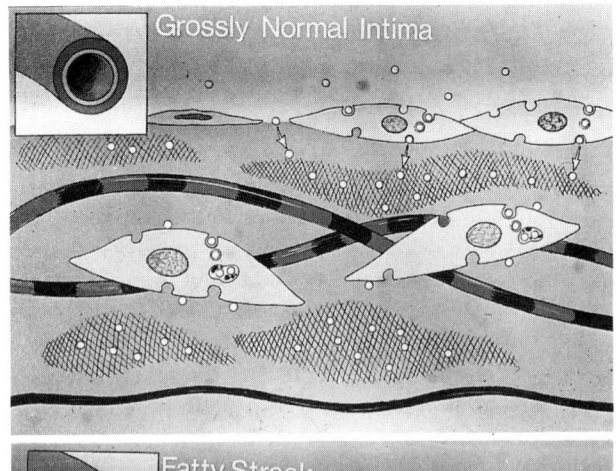
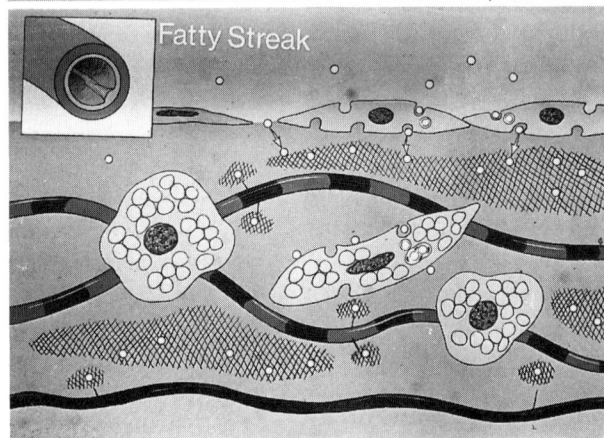
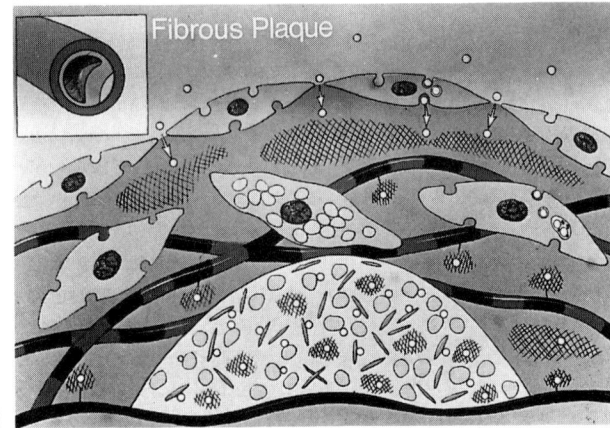

Figure 7.5 Deposition of LDL (spheres) in (a) the grossly normal intima indicated by the interactions of LDL with glycosaminoglycans in intimal proteoglycans (cross-hatched area); (b) in fatty streak lesions in which lipid-laden cells are formed by the uptake of LDL accumulating in the extracellular space bound to proteoglycans; (c) in fibrous plaques in which LDL is also associated with proteoglycans bound to elastica in the fibrous cap and to extracellular lipid in the necrotic core.

and glycosaminoglycans in the necrotic core of human atherosclerotic lesions (Figure 7.5(c)) [16,18]. This association suggests that the proteoglycans are fairly uniformly dispersed in the 'sea of lipid', consisting of intact LDL particles, cholesteryl ester droplets, and cholesterol monohydrate crystals [10]. Whether this association means that LDL is localized in the necrotic core because of its interaction with glycosaminoglycans in these regions, or because of direct interaction with neutral lipid, still needs to be addressed.

Another connective tissue element that appears to interact directly with LDL is elastic membrane (Figure 7.5(b)), which consists of elastin and glycoproteins. Perifibrous lipid is associated with elastica in arteries [70]. Earlier Kramsch et al. had found a direct interaction between LDL and such elastic tissue *in vitro* [71] that was confirmed in a recent report [72].

A third connective tissue element that appears to interact with LDL is collagen (Figure 7.5(c)). Specific modifications to collagen, or more likely their association with other macromolecules such as proteoglycans, appear to be responsible for this interaction with LDL. This association could explain why some bands of collagen fibers immunostain positively for LDL, whereas adjacent bands immunostain negatively [16,18]. We have interpreted the observation of collagen bands not immunostaining for LDL to represent regions of low permeability to LDL influx, perhaps as a result of greater crosslinking of collagen fibers in these bands [15]. Alternatively, the synthesis and accumulation of collagen may vary, thereby varying its affinity for LDL at different stages in the development of the lesion. For instance, the localization of LDL and collagen bands deeper in the fibrous caps, but not to collagen bands closer to the lumen (Plate 1(e)), could represent sclerosis at an earlier stage of lesion development, producing collagen bands of different composition than at later times. The layering pattern of collagen bands in the acellular caps of advanced atherosclerotic lesions is a common observation in human lesions [16,18].

7.2 Lipoprotein quantification in arteries

7.2.1 QUANTIFICATION OF LDL IN HUMAN ARTERIES

Several groups have published data on the accumulation of LDL in human arteries from grossly normal regions and from regions with different degrees of involvement. Extraction of LDL from arteries has been performed by squeezing tissue fluid out with a press [73] or by homogenizing tissue [74,75]. A rigorous but time-consuming way is to extract LDL from arteries with a buffer, isolate the LDL by ultracentrifugation and gel filtration, and then quantify the isolated LDL gravimetrically or chemically [76]. However, most LDL quantification methods use some form of immunochemical procedure directly on crude extracts, some after using a variety of different extraction procedures. One technique used to quantify LDL in arteries is to electrophorese LDL directly out of pieces of artery into a gel containing anti-LDL [77] and to estimate the amount of LDL from the resulting rocket height or area under the rocket in an electroimmunoassay EIA [78]. Smith and Slater [77] employed this approach in a series of studies that quantified LDL in small tissue samples with defined gross pathologies, such as fatty streaks, gelatinous lesions, and fatty fibrous plaques.

We have quantified LDL in low-speed supernatant fractions of homogenates of arterial tissue obtained at autopsy by applying such fractions to an electroimmunoassay (EIA) using anti-LDL [79,80]. Control studies showed that the homogenization procedure did not destroy Apo-B immunoreactivity when LDL was homogenized with tissue not containing endogenous Apo-B. The Apo-B extracted from arterial tissue was immunochemically identical to LDL in plasma. In one study homogenates from grossly normal intima in aortas from 40 subjects were found to contain a mean ($\pm$ SD) value of $5.4 \pm 4.0\,\mu g$ of Apo-B/mg tissue dry weight with a range of $0.3-18.5\,\mu g$ [79]. No immunoreactive Apo-B could be detected in the adjacent tunica media. A slight but significant positive correlation was found between Apo-B content and subject age, especially after 40 years of age [79]. That this Apo-B represented intact LDL was suggested from the results that almost all of the Apo-B immunoreactivity in such supernatant fractions from intimal homogenates was detected in the 1.006–1.063 density range, that is, LDL and IDL density ranges. This density fraction contained spheres with diameters of 20–25 nm, both characteristics of LDL and IDL [79].

In another study, we determined the concentration of LDL in the intima of grossly normal human arteries obtained at autopsy by measuring the total amount of Apo-B accumulated in a known volume of tissue. A mean ($\pm$ SEM) value of 1.0 ± 1.0 mg Apo-B/cm^3 of tissue (range 0.2–2.6) was obtained in 15 subjects [81]. Because the volume occupied by intimal smooth muscle cells was about 20%, this concentration of LDL was probably an underestimate. In fact, such a calculation also does not consider the volume occupied by connective tissue. The mean concentration of Apo-B in the non-atherosclerotic intima is in the range of plasma Apo-B concentrations and exceeds the anticipated concentrations of a plasma macromolecule in a tissue in which no retention mechanism is operative by 10-fold [82], as well as the concentrations of LDL in the lymph [83]. We further found that samples of lung, spleen, kidney, brain, myocardium and skeletal muscle all had values that were about 10% of plasma concentrations [81]. Human serum albumin was found to have a concentration in the arterial intima of 12.5 mg/cm^3 of tissue, or 25% of plasma concentrations.

These results clearly indicate that a retention mechanism must be responsible for the preferential accumulation of LDL in the intima of the normal human aorta. As discussed, one mechanism responsible for this accumulation is probably the specific interaction between LDL and intimal proteoglycans [60–66]. Smith and colleagues [59,77], using a different technique (extraction of LDL directly from samples of grossly normal intima), obtained similar high concentrations of LDL in the tunica intima of the grossly normal human aorta. In fact, when they separated the intima into the luminal half and abluminal half, the luminal half contained concentrations of LDL twice that found in plasma [59]. Tissue albumin concentrations were similar to ours. Recently Linden et al. [84] using a similar technique on intima samples obtained at surgery, found appreciably lower values than those found by Smith and colleagues [59,85]. It is uncertain whether this apparent discrepancy is the result of potential post-mortem artifacts obtained from autopsy samples or of other technical reasons.

We found that the Apo-B content per unit dry weight in grossly normal intima significantly and positively correlated with the corresponding plasma cholesterol concentrations [80]. Smith and Slater [86] and Onitiri et al. [87] likewise found a positive correlation using this procedure in which LDL is electrophoresed from intact tissue. Thus, the accumulation of LDL in the grossly normal intima appears to be dictated by two factors, the plasma-tissue LDL concentration gradient and the specific interaction of LDL with intimal components. A statistically significant negative correlation was found between Apo-B in grossly normal aorta intima and the tissue DNA content [88]. Because the tissue DNA reflects the cellularity of the intima (i.e. smooth muscle cells) these data are consistent with the concept that the greater the cell density, as reflected by the DNA content per unit mass, the greater the degradation of accumulated LDL.

When we attempted to quantify Apo-B in fatty-streak lesions and advanced fatty fibrous plaques, we noted that the residual tissue still contained Apo-B, as assessed by immunofluorescence [80]. Smith et al. [89] as well as Bradby et al. [90] found that when pieces of arterial tissue were directly electrophoresed into an EIA, the residual tissue still contained some Apo-B. In a group of studies, we used Triton X-100 to remove Apo-B from the residual tissue after first extracting homogenates of the tissue with a conventional buffer [91]. We compared the amounts of Apo-B in buffer and Triton-extracted fractions in fatty-streak lesions and adjacent grossly normal intima from 18 separate aortas from individuals with a mean age of 34 years [92]. Although 95% of the extracted Apo-B from grossly normal intima was buffer-extracted Apo-B, only about 25% of the total tissue Apo-B was found in this fraction from fatty streaks, the remainder was found in the Triton-extracted fraction (Table 7.1). We have used the term 'loosely bound' and 'tightly bound Apo-B' for the buffer-extracted and Triton-extracted fractions, respectively [91]. A paired t-

Table 7.1 Buffer- and Triton®-extracted Apo-B in aortic fatty streaks and adjacent grossly normal intima

Aortic region	Buffer-extracted Apo-B (mean ± SEM)	Percent of total	Triton®-extracted Apo-B (mean ± SEM)	Percent of total
Grossly normal intima	6.5 ± 0.9	95	0.4 ± 0.2	6
Fatty streaks	4.7 ± 0.5 $P < 0.05$*	75	1.9 ± 0.4 $P < 0.0005$*	29

* In paired t-test, differences between grossly normal intima and fatty streaks were statistically significant at the levels indicated.
Reproduced with permission from Hoff [92].

Table 7.2 Comparison of the mean buffer- and mean Triton®-extracted Apo-B values in fatty streaks and fibrous plaques

			Mean Apo-B value (µg/mg tissue dry weight) ± SEM	
Lesion	Mean age ± SEM	Number of cases	Buffer-extracted	Triton®-extracted
Fatty streak	34 ± 3	18	4.67 ± 0.51*	1.88 ± 0.39†
Fibrous plaque	56 ± 4	23	3.18 ± 0.41*	3.78 ± 0.31†

* Statistically significant difference using non-paired t-test: $P < 0.025$.
† Statistically significant difference using non-paired t-test: $P < 0.0005$.
Reproduced with permission from Hoff [92].

test showed the difference between the loosely and tightly bound fraction in normal intima and adjacent fatty streaks to be statistically significant (Table 7.1). The total Apo-B, expressed per unit tissue weight, was similar in normal intima and fatty streaks. Smith *et al.* [89] found that fatty streaks had a lower Apo-B content, but their technique was probably recovering only that fraction that was equivalent to the loosely bound fraction, which, in our study [92], was also lower in fatty streaks than in normal intima. Based on the immuno-fluorescence patterns of Apo-B localization in fatty streaks [16], lower amounts of Apo-B probably reflect a lower volume of extracellular space that can be occupied by LDL.

In a separate study we compared the buffer-extracted and Triton-extracted fraction in the 18 fatty streaks described above and in 23 fibrous plaques from separate individuals [92]. As seen in Table 7.2, Triton was required to remove about 50% of the total extracted Apo-B from plaques. As with fatty streaks, the total amount of Apo-B in plaques per unit weight was similar to that in normal intima, presumably as a result of dilution by regions not containing Apo-B (Plate 1(c)). These data suggest that as one progresses from normal intima to fatty streaks to fibrous plaques, a greater portion of the LDL in the arterial intima appears to be tightly bound. This greater portion presumably reflects increases in the components that have an affinity for LDL, such as plaque GAG and extracellular lipid. When fibrous plaques were dissected into their fibrotic caps and

Table 7.3 Buffer- and Triton®-extracted Apo-B from fibrotic and necrotic regions of human aortic plaques (mean ± SEM)

Lesion area	Buffer-extracted Apo-B	Triton®-extracted Apo-B
Fibrotic cap	4.85 ± 0.25	2.70 ± 0.14
Necrotic core	1.63 ± 0.05	4.69 ± 0.18

Reproduced with permission from Hoff [93].

necrotic cores, the caps had higher buffer-extractable Apo-B values, and lower Triton-extractable values than the cores (Table 7.3) [93]. Although the intima of grossly normal aortas from individuals of 39 years or older had buffer-extracted Apo-B values that were significantly higher than those from individuals under 39 years of age, the Triton-extracted Apo-B values did not differ significantly between the two groups [94]. This comparison suggests that the Triton-extracted Apo-B content is influenced more by the degree of atherosclerotic involvement than by age.

When histograms were generated for buffer- and Triton-extracted Apo-B in the grossly normal intima, fatty streaks and fibrous plaques, as well as in their individual caps and core regions, a statistically significant stepwise increase was found only for the Triton-extractable fraction (Figure 7.6). These results are consistent with immunofluorescence studies that showed most of the widespread localization of LDL to be in the

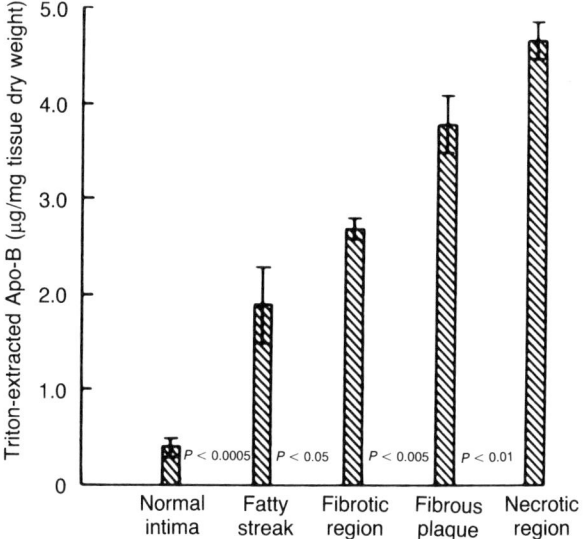

Figure 7.6 Mean ± SE of Triton-extracted Apo-B contents show significant increases from grossly normal intima to fatty streak to the fibrotic regions of fibrous plaques to the total fibrous plaque to the necrotic core of the fibrous plaques.

necrotic core. The intermediate values of the fatty streak between those of grossly normal intima and fibrous plaques provide circumstantial evidence that the fatty streak is, indeed, an intermediate stage in the development of the fibrous plaque.

When the total cholesterol content of grossly normal intima, fatty streaks and fibrous plaques was compared with their corresponding LDL-cholesterol content, calculated from the Apo-B content, about half of the cholesterol in normal intima could be in the form of LDL, whereas only 10% of the cholesterol in fatty streaks and only 5% of the cholesterol in fibrous plaques could be in the form of intact LDL [94]. It was anticipated that the Apo-B content in grossly normal intima would correlate positively with the tissue cholesterol content; this was, indeed, found (Figure 7.7(a)). Because the amount of tightly bound Apo-B was small, this positive correlation also held for total extracted Apo-B (Figure 7.7(b)).

Smith *et al.* found that the Apo-B in the residual tissue of plaques could be released by incubating the tissue with plasmin [89]. They obtained a distribution of loosely and tightly bound Apo-B in normal intima, fatty

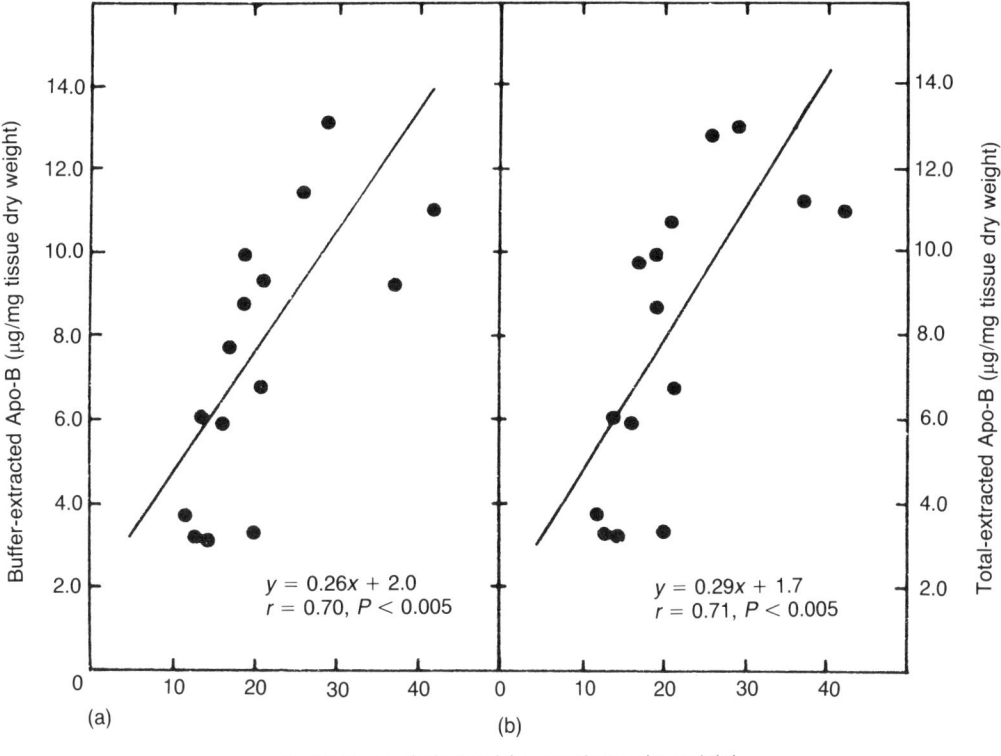

Figure 7.7 (a) Correlation of buffer-extracted Apo-B with total tissue cholesterol in the grossly normal intima. A statistically significant positive correlation was obtained. (b) Correlation of total-extracted Apo-B (buffer-plus Triton-extracted Apo-B) with total tissue cholesterol. A statistically significant positive correlation was also found. (Reproduced with permission from Hoff *et al.* [92].)

streaks and fibrous plaques that was consistent with our studies. They found, as we did, that the necrotic core regions had higher tightly bound Apo-B values than the fibrotic regions [89]. Regions containing immunochemically identifiable fibrin, in particular, were higher in Apo-B content [95,96]. We also found a positive correlation between the Triton-extractable Apo-B content in the necrotic core of fibrous plaques and the tissue cholesterol content [94]. Smith et al. [85] also found a positive correlation between tightly bound LDL and cholesterol present in the residual tissue after sequential extraction by electrophoresis.

The tightly bound fraction of Apo-B in plaques can also be extracted by digesting the residual tissue with proteases, such as collagenases or elastases [97], as Smith et al. [89] had found using plasmin. Although the amount of Apo-B extracted with elastase was only about one-half that obtained by extraction with Triton [97], the elastase-released LDL could be subjected to subsequent chemical characterization, in contrast to the detergent-released lipoprotein. In fact, particles in the size range of LDL could be seen after negative staining and electron microscopy of such digests. We used this technique for quantifying Apo-B in smaller samples of tissues such as obtained in experimental animals (discussed below).

7.2.2 QUANTIFICATION OF LDL IN LESIONS OF EXPERIMENTAL ANIMALS

The hypercholesterolemic cynomolgus monkey is an excellent model for studying the progression and the regression of atherosclerosis [98]. Because diet-induced increases in plasma cholesterol in this model are caused by increases in plasma LDL levels [98], we measured the loosely and tightly bound Apo-B fractions in the aorta of animals placed on a hypercholesterolemic (H) diet for 24 and 30 months [99]. Using the technique originally employed by Smith and Slater [77], we defined the loosely bound fraction as the Apo-B released from tissue minces after the EIA gel as measured by the height of the resulting rockets [99]. The remaining tissue was then digested with elastase, reapplied directly into the EIA gel, and the amount released, as measured from the height of the resulting rockets, represented the tightly bound fraction. Mean levels of Apo-B released per unit surface area, greatly increased in both fractions between the 24-month H-monkeys and control animals (Table 7.4). Likewise, Apo-B fractions increased between the 24-month and the 30-month intervals [99]. Thus, accumulation of LDL in atherosclerotic lesions of the aorta correlated with time on the H-diet, as well as with the size of the lesions as estimated by lesion cross-sectional area.

In one study with cynomolgus monkeys we attempted to obtain information on possible reduction in LDL levels during lesion regression, which occurs when monkeys are taken off of the H-diet [100]. However, because all the vessel samples had been fixed and embedded, we attempted to estimate Apo-B accumulation from the topographic distribution in cross-section of Apo-B localization using an immunoperoxidase technique. The study focused on the coronary artery, which, because of its size, had not been used extensively in studies on LDL accumulation in lesions. Cynomolgus monkeys were placed on an H-diet for 18 months and subsequently on a normolipemic diet for 6 and 12 months. When the distribution of Apo-B was determined at a site of the left anterior descending (LAD) branch of the left coronary artery within 4 mm from the origin (the site containing the largest lesion), the cross-sectional area decreased from 22% of the total cross-sectional area to 7% after 6 months and to 2% after 12 months (Table 7.5). Thus, even though this approach at quantification has not been rigorously validated, it suggests that the distribution and probably the amount of LDL decreases in lesions during regression. This technique has the added advantage of being able to estimate LDL accumulation in fixed and embedded tissue prepared years earlier.

We have also quantified LDL in the aorta and coronary arteries of the H-swine using the technique of direct insertion of tissue minces into the EIA and digestion with elastase [29,101]. In one study we documented the loosely and tightly bound Apo-B contents in Evans blue-positive and negative regions [102] of the aortic arch of normolipemic (N-swine) functioning as controls and H-swine maintained on the H-diet for up to 30 weeks [101]. Although the Evans blue-positive regions of the aortic arch are the sites at which fatty streak lesions first develop, i.e. they are lesion-prone sites [102], in N-swine, Apo-B content per unit area in Evans blue-positive and negative sites did not differ [101]. However, after only 6 weeks on the H-diet, the Evans blue-positive sites showed an increased Apo-B content relative to Evans blue-negative regions [101]. As anticipated, the Apo-B content of the Evans blue-positive areas increased with time on the H-diet. However, once raised lesions were observed in both the Evans blue-positive and negative regions, no differences in Apo-B levels were found. At later times lesions were also found in the abdominal aorta. Significant differences in Apo-B content were found between lesioned and lesion-free areas. The Apo-B content in lesions was higher at 30 weeks compared to 15 weeks on the H-diet. When the relative distributions of Apo-B in loosely and tightly bound fractions were compared in grossly normal Evans blue-positive regions of the aortic arch and in raised lesions from the arch or abdominal aorta, the tightly bound fraction increased as it had in humans and H-monkeys.

We also employed this technique on the coronary

Table 7.4 Mean Apo-B accumulation in the aortic arch of cynomolgus monkeys fed atherogenic and control diets

Number animals	Time on diet (months)	Diet	Total plasma cholesterol (mg/dl)	HDL cholesterol (mg/dl)	Cross-sectional intimal area (mm²)		Apo-B (mean ± SEM)			
							Loosely bound		Tightly bound	
					TA	AA	Tissue wet weight (ng/mg)	Surface area (ng/mm²)	Tissue wet weight (ng/mg)	Surface area (ng/mm²)
4	24	Control	118 ± 4	49 ± 3	0.1 ± 0.6	0.1 ± 0.1	7 ± 3	8 ± 3	0	0
7	24	Test	667 ± 37	28 ± 2	3.8 ± 0.9	2.9 ± 0.5	26 ± 6	31 ± 7	26 ± 10	25 ± 10
2	30	Control	119	54	0.4	0.4	6	7	0	0
4	30	Test	741 ± 72	29 ± 3	5.4 ± 0.7	3.2 ± 0.4	76 ± 15	75 ± 8	75 ± 8	76 ± 9

TA = thoracic aorta; AA = abdominal aorta.

Table 7.5 Reduction in estimated LDL content of LAD in cynomolgus monkeys during regression

Groups*	Following 18 months on progression diet		Following subsequent regression diet		Mean arterial cross-sectional area (mm²)	Mean intimal cross-sectional area (mm²)	Mean % of cross-sectional area occupied by reaction product depicting LDL
	Total plasma cholesterol (mg/dl)	Plasma HDL cholesterol (mg/dl)	Total plasma cholesterol (mm²)	Plasma HDL cholesterol (mm²)			
Group I (n = 8)	713 ± 169†	28 ± 11†	—	—	1.77 ± 0.86	1.46 ± 0.77	21.7 ± 4.7
Group II (n = 7)	861 ± 211	27 ± 8	224 ± 51†	38 ± 10†	1.64 ± 0.53	1.48 ± 0.47	6.9 ± 5.5
Group III (n = 9)	713 ± 132	32 ± 6	227 ± 47	50 ± 8	1.44 ± 0.64	1.19 ± 0.71	2.3 ± 1.3

All results are expressed as mean ± SD.
* Group I = 18 months H-diet; group II = 18 months H-diet, 6 months normolipemic diet; group III = 18 months H-diet, 12 months normolipemic diet.
† Average of determinations made 60 days apart during the 18-month progression time interval and the 6- and 12-month regression time intervals.
In the Wilcoxon signed-rank test, the mean percent cross-sectional area occupied by Apo-B immunoreactivity (LDL) in group I was significantly greater than that in group II ($P = 0.0032$) and group III ($P = 0.0006$). Mean percent cross-sectional area occupied by Apo-B (LDL) in group II was also significantly greater than that in group III ($P = 0.03$).

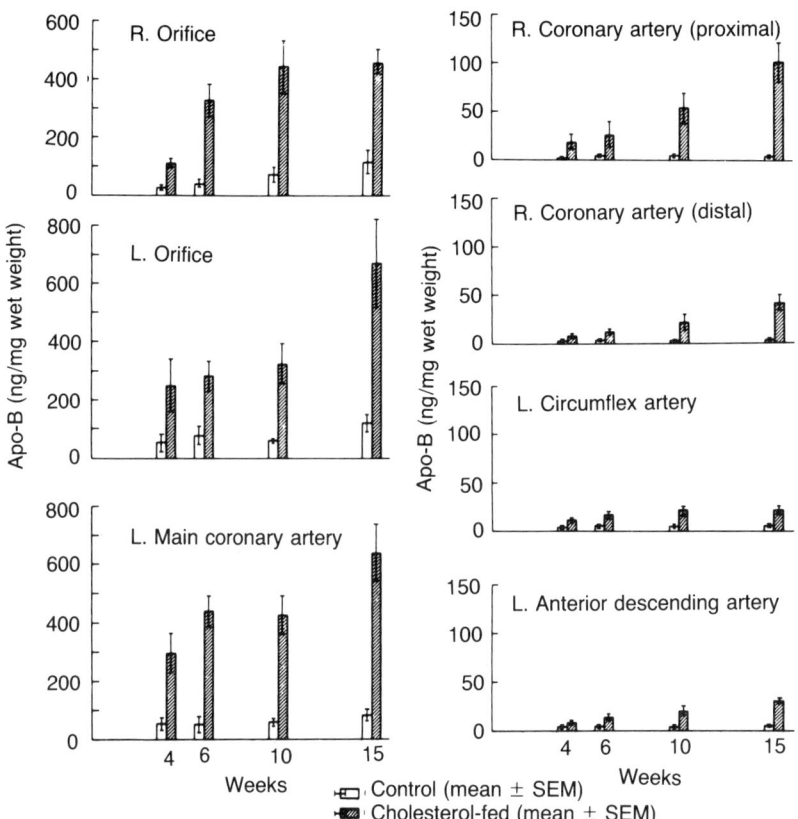

Figure 7.8 Accumulation of Apo-B (ng/mg tissue wet weight) in seven segments of the coronary arteries of cholesterol-fed and control swine at time intervals of 4, 6, 10 and 15 weeks on each diet. (R = right; L = left; x = total tissue cholesterol; y = buffer or total extracted Apo-B; r = coefficient of regression. (Reproduced with permission from Hoff et al. [101].)

arteries of H-swine, focusing our attention to the lesion-prone sites at which Apo-B was localized [29]. Our intent was to assess whether LDL preferentially accumulated at specific anatomical sites that were predisposed to atherosclerosis. The accumulation of Apo-B, measured per unit surface area, was determined in seven separate segments of coronary arteries of swine fed the H-diet or N-diet for 4–15 weeks [29]. Apo-B accumulation was consistently greater in segments from H-swine than from N-swine and was greater in proximal than in distal segments (non-branch points) of coronary arteries (Figure 7.8). This accumulation of Apo-B generally increased with time on the H-diet. Even after only 4 weeks lesions from swine on the H-diet had Apo-B values greater than corresponding ones on the N-diet. Foam cells first appeared after 6 weeks on the H-diet at the sites of initial Apo-B accumulation. The anatomic sites of Apo-B (LDL) accumulation, i.e. in the edematous, alcian blue-positive regions in diffuse and focal areas of intimal thickening, did not differ in H- and N-swine. We suggest that LDL preferentially accumulates at such sites when plasma levels are increased as a result of the H-diet, because they are sites of retention by specific tissue components. As indicated earlier, these sites are rich in GAG. In a separate study we found a direct association between Apo-B accumulation and specific chondroitin sulfates in the aortic arch of H-swine [103]. Because foam cells inevitably appear at these anatomic sites, but only after LDL accumulation, our data suggest that early lesion development is a function of events occurring before the induction of hypercholesterolemia, presumably hemodynamically induced injury.

7.2.3 SPATIAL DISTRIBUTION AND ACCUMULATION OF LDL IN ANIMAL MODELS AND HUMANS

We have developed an immunotransfer procedure that can determine both the spatial distribution of LDL (immunoreactive Apo-B) along the intima and media of large arteries, such as the aorta, and can quantify LDL along the entire surface of the aorta [104]. Aortas opened longitudinally along their ventral aspect were positioned so that their intimal side abutted against a gel containing glyoxyl agarose, to which anti-LDL had been covalently coupled. LDL was electrophoresed out of the aorta into the agarose gel where it was immunofixed

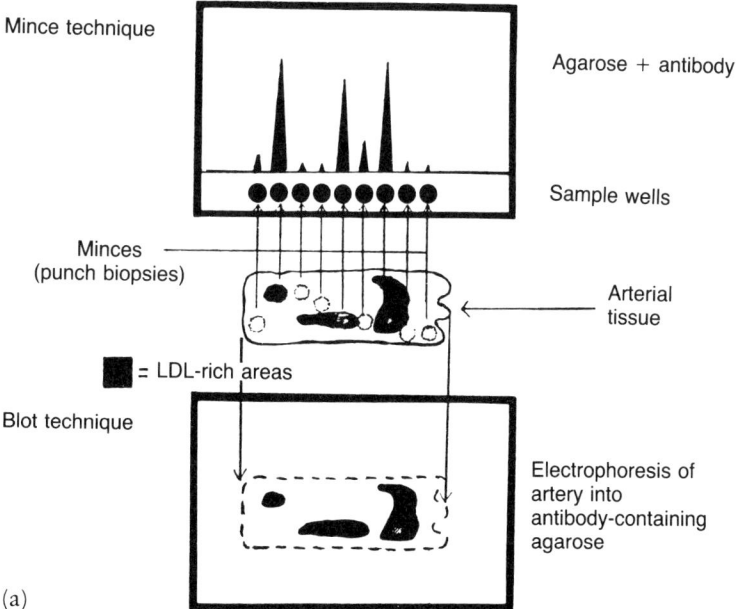

Figure 7.9(a) Comparison of LDL quantification by electroimmunoassay (rockets) in plug of arteries and spatial distribution of LDL along the arterial intima by electrotransfer.

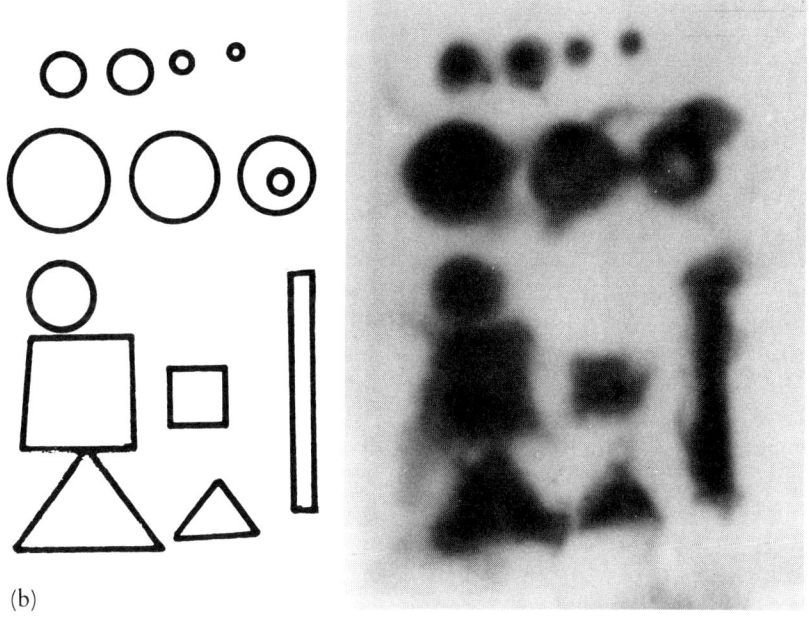

Figure 7.9(b) Same spatial distribution of ^{125}I-LDL applied to wells in an agarose gel and on an autoradiogram depicting the LDL immunofixed in a glyoxyl agarose gel.

[104]. This distribution was then made visible first by incubating the gel with ^{125}I-anti-LDL, which bound to free epitopes on the immunofixed LDL, and then by subjecting the washed and dried gel to autoradiography (Figure 7.9(a)). The spatial distribution of LDL in the artery was shown to be accurately transferred to the gel (Figure 7.10(b)), and the procedure was shown to be specific for LDL [104]. Application of increasing concentrations of LDL to wells in a gel substituting for tissue resulted in a dose-dependent increase in the autoradiographic grain density.

If such standards were applied to gels adjacent to tissue samples, the amounts of LDL in the tissue could be quantified from the standard curve of grain density versus LDL concentration. The distribution of LDL along the abdominal aortas of 10- and 31-week-old normolipemic swine was determined by converting autoradiographic grain densities to isopleths of LDL

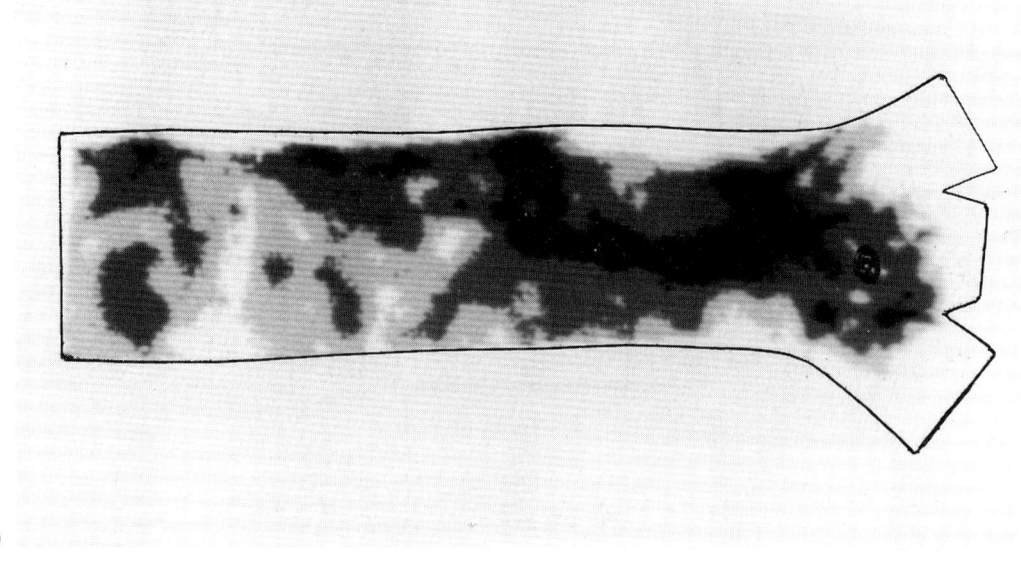

(c)

Figure 7.9(c) Computer-assisted image of the density distribution of an autoradiogram depicting LDL in the intima/media of the terminal abdominal aorta of a 10-week-old normolipemic swine. Superimposed isopleths of LDL concentrations along the aortic surface generated by four ranges of concentrations. (Figures 7.9(a–c) reproduced with permission of Hoff et al. [104].)

concentrations by computer-assisted image analysis (Figure 7.10(c)). These distribution were focal and ranged between 10 ng and 225 ng of Apo-B/mm² of intima surface area. This procedure lends itself not only to studies relating lipoprotein accumulation to atherogenesis but also to any studies dealing with tissue accumulation of any macromolecules.

We have also used this electrophoretic transfer procedure to document the accumulation of LDL in human arteries [105]. We wished to determine whether LDL-rich anatomic sites were regions of intimal thickening. We therefore determined the topographic distribution of LDL-rich sites at the iliac bifurcation of grossly normal abdominal aortas and adjacent common iliac arteries in six subjects ranging in age from 16 to 36 years [105]. We transferred LDL by electrophoresis from the tissue into an agarose gel containing anti-LDL and then stained the immunofixed LDL in the gel for lipid, after establishing a stoichiometric relationship between lipid staining and immunochemically determined Apo-B in LDL. We determined that the cutoff between LDL-rich and LDL-poor zones was 37 ng Apo-B/mm² intimal surface area. Measures of intimal thickening showed that sections of LDL-rich zones were three times thicker than LDL-poor zones. These data are consistent with studies in animal models indicating that sites of diffuse or focal intimal thickening are regions in which LDL first accumulates [29]. These are usually the sites at which the fatty streaks first appear [106].

7.2.4 ACCUMULATION OF HDL IN HUMAN ARTERIES

We quantified the accumulation of HDL, estimated by the amounts of Apo-A$_I$, the major protein of HDL [1], in homogenates of both grossly normal aortic intima and in advanced atherosclerotic aortic lesions [107,108]. Using an RIA for Apo-A$_I$, we found that grossly normal intimas ($n = 12$) contained a mean ($\pm$ SEM) buffer-extractable Apo-A$_I$ content of 0.7 $\pm$ 0.1 µg/mg tissue dry weight with a range of 0.1–1.2 µg/mg [107]. The corresponding mean $\pm$ SEM buffer-extractable Apo-B content from these intimas was 3.5 $\pm$ 0.5 µg/mg tissue dry weight with a range of 0.9–5.7 µg/mg. The mean Apo-B to Apo-A$_I$ ratio was 6.6 (range 1.8–23.6). In a later study, Ylä-Herttuala et al. confirmed such levels of Apo-A$_I$ in human lesions [109]. We found only negligible tightly bound Apo-A$_I$ in the residual tissue of grossly normal aortic intima. In atherosclerotic lesions ($n = 19$) the mean ($\pm$ SEM) buffer-extracted Apo-A$_I$ content was 0.6 $\pm$ 0.4 µg/mg tissue dry weight (range = 0.2–1.9 µg/mg) whereas the corresponding mean ($\pm$ SEM) buffer-extracted Apo-B content was 3.1 $\pm$ 0.6 µg/mg (range 0.4–10.2 µg/mg) [108]. The mean Apo-B to Apo-A$_I$ ratio was 5.7. Also, no measurable Triton-extractable Apo-A$_I$ was found in the residual tissue after initial buffer extraction. The tunica media underlying these intimas gave negligible values for Apo-A$_I$. Assuming that Apo-A$_I$ reflects the accumulation of HDL in the arterial intima, our results suggest that on a weight basis, plaques do not accumulate more HDL than do grossly normal regions. Secondly, there is no tight binding of HDL to lesions, in contrast to LDL. Thirdly, the concentration of HDL is 10% of that usually found in plasma, which is a value expected for a plasma-derived macromolecule in the interstitial space of tissue, if no specific retention mechanism were operative, in contrast to the case for LDL. However, the weak localization pattern of Apo-A_I in immunofluorescence studies [17,38] could indicate a slight retention by some tissue components.

From the quantitative studies on Apo-A_I accumulation in arteries, we conclude that the concentration of HDL probably depends on the plasma concentration. This relationship could help explain the putative anti-atherogenic effect of HDL, i.e. it is a negative risk factor for coronary heart disease [110]. If HDL can remove cholesteryl esters from foam cells, as proposed in the reverse cholesterol concept [111], the higher the interstitial HDL concentrations, the greater the potential removal. Recently, it was shown that infusing high concentrations of HDL into experimental animals reduced diet-induced atherosclerosis [110]. Furthermore, transgenic mice in which the Apo-A_I gene had been removed showed increased atherosclerosis induced by high cholesterol diets [112]. We will discuss the different forms Apo-A_I that were found in lesions in section 7.3.5.

7.2.5 ACCUMULATION OF Lp(a) IN HUMAN ARTERIES

As indicated earlier, much attention has been devoted to the structure and function of Lp(a) in light of the numerous publications indicating that Lp(a) is an independent risk factor for CHD [44–47] and the structural homology of the protein unique for Lp(a), apo(a) with plasminogen [48,49], which is believed to be responsible for several antifibrinolytic properties of apo(a) [50–53]. We quantified the accumulation of apo(a) in human arteries with atherosclerotic involvement obtained at surgery using an RIA employing anti-apo(a) [58]. We extracted tissue with a phosphate-buffered saline (PBS) overnight at 4°C without homogenization, because preliminary studies showed that homogenization of tissue destroyed apo(a) immunoreactivity. When the apo(a) content of grossly normal tissue was assessed, negligible levels were found. However, substantial levels of apo(a) were found in plaque [58]. When the residual tissue was assessed for the presence of apo(a) by immunoperoxidase after PBS extraction, significant reaction product was found. Among a number of detergents and dissociating agents, 6 M GuHCl was the most effective in removing residual apo[a] from PBS-extracted tissue. We defined the PBS-extracted apo(a) fraction as loosely bound and the GuHCl extracted fraction as tightly bound [58]. We also measured the Apo-B content in these two fractions with a separate RIA. The apo(a) content (ng/g tissue wet weight) was less than 10% that of the corresponding Apo-B content as measured in iliac and femoral atherosclerotic lesions from 26 cases (Table 7.6). This finding was not too surprising in that plasma apo(a) levels are only about 5% that of Apo-B levels. Somewhat unexpected was that only about 18% of the total plaque apo(a) content could be extracted with PBS (the remainder with GuHCl), whereas 68% of the total plaque Apo-B content could be extracted with PBS (Table 7.6). The relative difference in amounts in the two fractions suggests that apo(a), depicting Lp(a), is bound tighter in human atherosclerotic lesions than is LDL, depicted by Apo-B. We also found that both the loosely bound fraction and the tightly bound fraction, and therefore the total apo(a), correlated positively with plasma apo(a) contents (Figure 7.10).

When normalized for equal plasma concentrations, Lp(a) appears to bind to an even greater extent than LDL in human atherosclerotic lesions. Similar observations were made by Cushing et al. [113] using minces of tissue inserted into the EIA as first described by Smith and Slater [77]. Rath et al. [55] also found these associations using extraction procedures similar to ours but with different absolute amounts. The tight binding we found for Lp(a) in lesions could be the result of the strong interactions of Lp(a) with connective tissue elements such as GAGs [114]. It could also be the result of the specific binding of Lp(a) with fibrin, as suggested by Smith and Cochran [115] who showed that plasmin

Table 7.6 Apo(a) and Apo-B in plasma and plaques

		Plaque apolipoprotein content			
	Plasma apolipoprotein concentration (mg/dl)	Loosely bound µg/g tissue wet wt	(%)	Tightly bound µg/g tissue wet wt	(%)
Apo(a)	4.3 ± 4.5*	3.6 ± 4.5	(17.5)	17.0 ± 17.0	(82.5)
Apo-B	95.2 ± 43.1	215.0 ± 116.0	(68.3)	99.6 ± 66.9	(31.7)

* Mean ± SD of 26 cases studied.

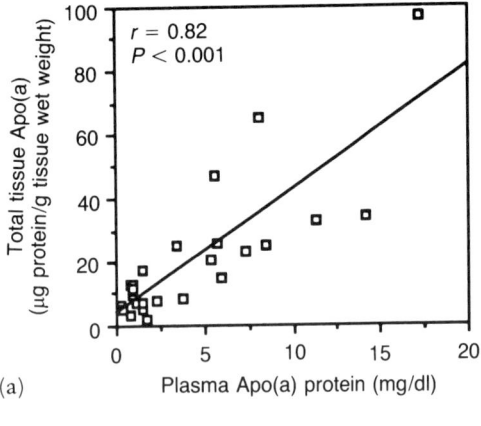
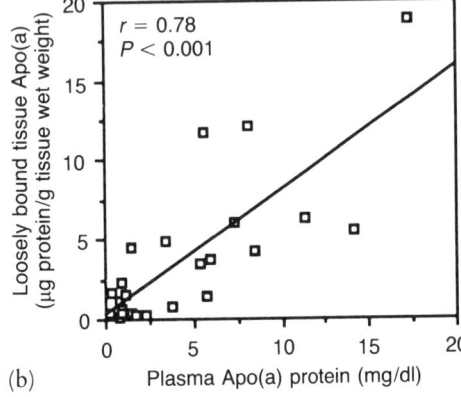
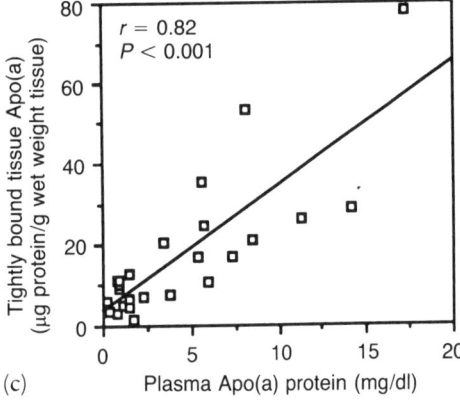

Figure 7.10 Correlation of plasma apo(a) with total (a), loosely bound (b), and tightly bound (c) apo(a) in 26 cases studied. (Reproduced with permission from Pepin *et al.* [58].)

digestion of lesions resulted in the co-release of Lp(a) and fibrinogen and/or fibrin. Several studies have shown that Lp(a) interacts avidly with fibrin(ogen) under *in vitro* conditions [50,53]. This interpretation is consistent with results showing an association of Lp(a) with fibrinogen and fibrin in lesions [56]. Finally, the tight binding of Lp(a) in lesions may be the result of aggregation of Lp(a) induced by Ca^{2+} via crossbridges. Such complexes can form at physiological Ca^{2+} concentrations [116].

7.3 Physicochemical characterization of lipoproteins in arteries

7.3.1 CHARACTERIZATION OF LDL IN HUMAN ARTERIES

Having quantified the accumulation of Apo-B in the human aorta with grossly normal anatomy and with atherosclerotic involvement, we sought to determine whether the Apo-B was in the form of intact LDL and whether such LDL had undergone any structural or chemical modification while residing in the arterial intima. Initially, we isolated a lipoprotein fraction by ultracentrifugation in the 1.006–1.063 density range from both homogenates of grossly normal intima and from plaques [117]. Over 90% of the Apo-B immunoactivity in such homogenates could be isolated in this density fraction. In the grossly normal intima Apo-B was associated with particles in the size range of plasma LDL, and the 1.006–1.063 density fraction had the same lipid composition as LDL. Ylä-Herttuala *et al.* further separated such a fraction from grossly normal intima into <1.012 and 1.021–1.046 density fractions (IDL and LDL, respectively) and found that particles in the former were larger than in the latter [118]. However, the 1.006–1.063 fraction from plaque homogenates in our study demonstrated size heterogeneity, as well as an altered lipid composition, characterized by a decrease in cholesteryl esters and an increase in unesterified cholesterol relative to plasma LDL [117]. It is unlikely that the homogenization procedure caused these changes, because non-homogenized saline extracts of the same plaques gave the same chemical composition. Furthermore, when ^{125}I-labeled LDL was added to tissue minces and the mixture was homogenized, most of the label was recovered in the 1.006–1.063 density fraction [117]. Because the 1.006–1.063 density fraction contained no anisotropic material, it is unlikely that this fraction contained any of the anisotropic cholesterol monohydrate crystals from the necrotic core. In addition to Apo-B, the 1.006–1.063 density fraction derived from plaques contained albumin as indicated by sodium dodecyl sulfate-polyacrylamide gel electrophoresis (SDS-PAGE). The cholesteryl ester moiety from the 1.006–1.063 density fraction from both grossly normal intima and plaques showed a reduced linoleate and arachidonate content relative to LDL. Finally, the 1.006–1.063 density fraction, from both normal intima and plaque showed an increased electrophoretic mobility relative to LDL [117]. Hollander *et al.* [119] also isolated an LDL-like fraction by subjecting non-homogenized saline extracts of human lesions to ultracentrifugation. They detected the presence of other proteins in such samples. Ylä-Herttuala et al. found that an LDL-like fraction isolated from grossly normal intima [118] had an increased electronegative charge.

Given the size heterogeneity of the 1.006–1.063 density fraction of plaques, as well as the presence of albumin, we considered the possibility that other material in plaques, such as cell debris or cholesteryl ester-rich particles derived from the necrotic core of plaques, would be present in this density range. Such contamination could lead to erroneous physical and chemical characteristics. However, if such contaminants were larger than LDL, we should be able to separate the larger particles from the LDL and IDL-sized particles by gel exclusion chromatography. Hollander et al. [119] had also used combinations of ultracentrifugation and gel filtration to isolate fractions in the <1.006 density range and the 1.006–1.063 density range from 1 M NaCl extracts of plaques which they termed arterial VLDL and LDL, respectively.

We modified our original procedure [120] to isolate an LDL-like population from extracts of arterial intima by combinations of ultracentrifugation and gel filtration, as shown in the flow diagram in Figure 7.11. When we subjected the 1.006–1.063 density fraction from homogenates of grossly normal intima to gel filtration, most of the cholesterol and all of the immunoreactive Apo-B essentially co-eluted with the plasma LDL [120]. However, when the 1.006–1.063 density fraction from plaque homogenates was subjected to gel filtration, most of the cholesterol was found in the void volume fraction, although much of the immunoreactive Apo-B was confined to the retained fraction that co-eluted with plasma LDL (Figure 7.12). During immunoelectrophoresis the void volume fraction remained at the origin, probably because of the large size of the particles, as was also shown by electron microscopy after negative staining [120]. However, the LDL-sized fraction demonstrated the increased electrophoretic migration observed for the 1.006–1.063 density fraction (Figure 7.13). When the LDL-sized fraction was subjected to SDS-PAGE, only Apo-B_{100} was observed, whereas serum albumin was associated with the larger particles found

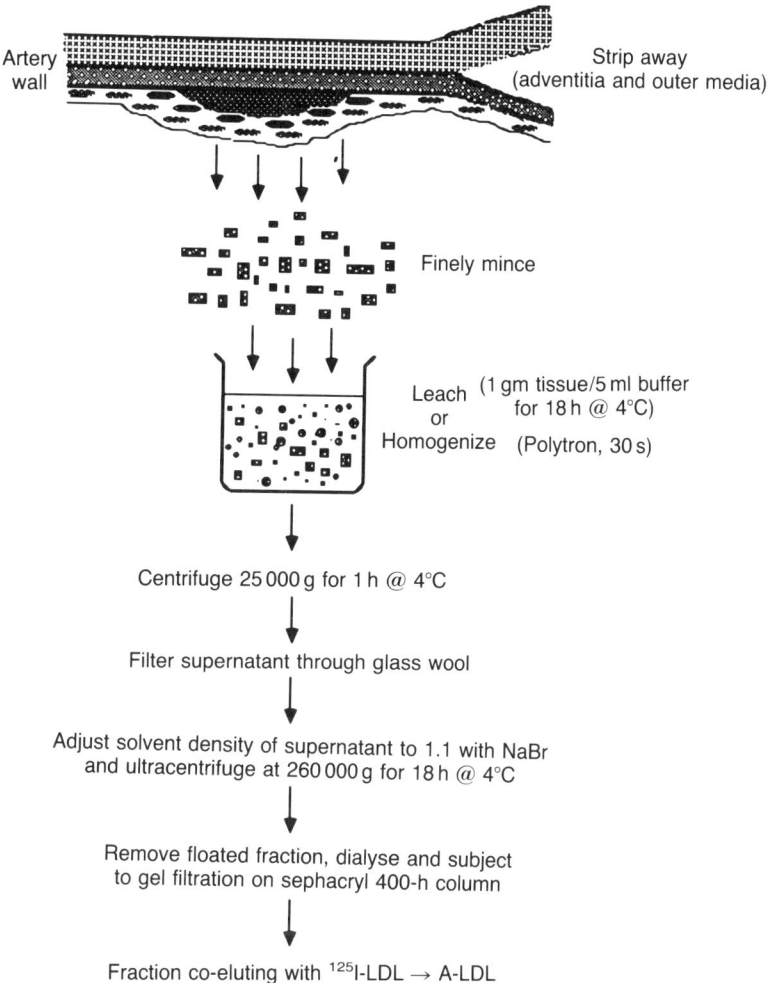

Figure 7.11 Isolation of lesion-derived LDL or A-LDL from human atherosclerotic lesions. (Reproduced with permission from Hoff et al. [180].)

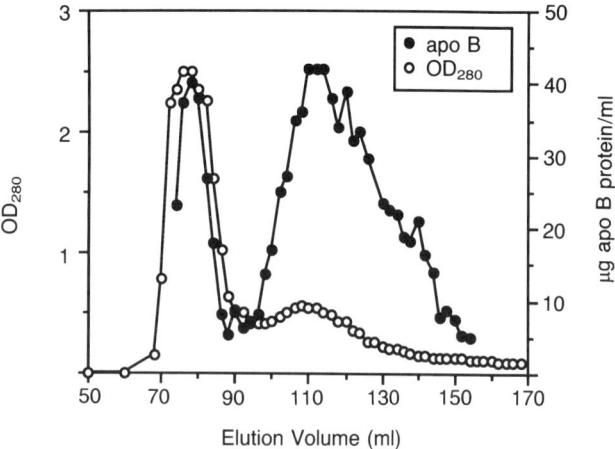

Figure 7.12 Elution profile of a d<1.10 density fraction from a non-homogenized extract of human aortic lesion on a gel filtration column. Immunoreactive Apo-B is found both in the void volume fraction (elution volume position = 75 ml) and in a retained fraction co-eluting with plasma LDL (peak tube at elution volume = 112 ml). Apo-B was measured by RIA.

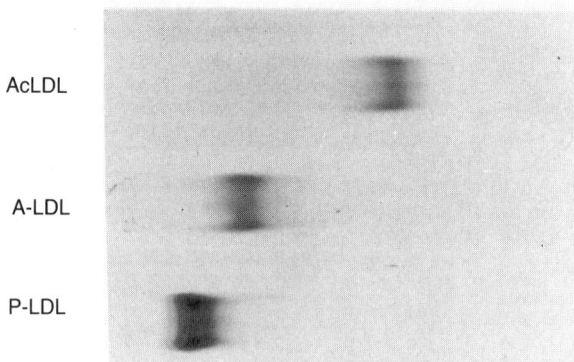

Figure 7.13 Agarose electrophoresis (1%) of plasma (P-)LDL, lesion-derived LDL (A-LDL), and acetyl LDL (AcLDL) following staining with oil red-O demonstrating the increased mobility of A-LDL relative to P-LDL.

in the void volume fraction [120]. When the lipid composition of the LDL-sized fraction and void-volume fraction of the 1.006–1.063 fraction from plaque homogenates was assessed, the LDL-sized fraction resembled the composition of LDL, whereas the void volume fraction showed an increase in the unesterified cholesterol-to-cholesteryl ester ratio relative to that in LDL. It is likely that the void volume contained an unesterified cholesterol-rich lipoprotein fraction that is free of immunoreactive Apo-B. Large unesterified cholesterol-rich particles in lesions have been characterized and will be described in section 7.6.3.

When the fatty acid composition of the cholesteryl ester fraction was determined in the LDL-sized and void volume fractions of the 1.006–1.063 density fraction from both homogenates of plaques and grossly normal intima, the linoleate and arachidonate composition was significantly reduced compared to that of LDL [120]. This reduction was accompanied by a relative increase in palmitate, stearate and oleate. A similar pattern was detected in the triglyceride fraction. A reduced linoleate content was also detected in the 1.006–1.019 fraction of saline extracts of grossly normal aortic intima by another group [118]. When we analyzed the void volume fraction, it mimicked the original 1.006–1.063 fraction, containing a high linoleate content, consistent with the observation that the void-volume contained most of the lipid in the 1.006–1.063 fraction [120]. It is unlikely that this result represented oxidation of the LDL-sized fraction after extraction, because the larger-sized particles did not show such a decrease in linoleate and arachidonate [120], two unsaturated fatty acids that are more prone to oxidation [121]. An increase in sphingomyelin and a decrease in lecithin was found in such a fraction by another group [122,123]. In further studies we showed that the LDL-sized fraction had a mean hydrated density that was slightly lower and much more heterogeneous than that of LDL [124]. In addition, no changes in the amino acid composition were found between lesion-isolated LDL and plasma LDL.

We considered the possibility that the increase in negative charge of the LDL-sized particles isolated from both grossly normal intima and plaque was caused by the specific binding of sulfated GAG. Several studies have reported the isolation of LDL–GAG complexes from saline extracts of human fatty-streak lesions [67], fibrous plaques [125], and rabbit fatty-streak lesions [68]. However, even after incubation of the aorta-extracted LDL with chondroitinase ABC, which degrades chondroitin sulfates, and would presumably digest away these GAG if present in the particle, the increase in electrophoretic mobility remained unchanged [120]. It is likely that LDL–GAG complexes dissociated during our extraction and isolation procedures at high salt concentrations. Thus, the increased electrophoretic mobility must be the result of changes other than binding of GAG. It could represent the preferential accumulation of a subclass of plasma LDL with an increased sialic acid content. Isoelectric focusing indicates that plasma LDL consists of numerous subclasses with different surface charges due to heterogeneity in their sialic acid contents [126,127]. Sialic acid-enriched LDL could form Ca^{2+} induced crossbridges with GAG-containing proteoglycans in the arterial intima. However, so far no definitive data have shown that LDL accumulating in the arterial intima is enriched in sialic acids.

7.3.2 CHARACTERISTICS OF OXIDIZED LDL

Several groups have shown that LDL can be induced to undergo oxidation by incubation with endothelial cells

[128], smooth muscle cells [129] or macrophages [130], or with oxygen in the presence of Cu^{2+} [131,132]. Because some of the physical and chemical characteristics of oxidized LDL included increases in electrophoretic mobility and reductions in linoleate and arachidonate content [132], we and others sought to determine whether LDL extracted from normal intima and from atherosclerotic lesions has other properties shared by oxidized LDL. The discussion in this and the next section is limited to the physical and chemical properties. In section 7.4.4 the sharing of functional properties of lesion-extracted LDL and oxidized LDL is discussed. However, before addressing such similarities, it is necessary to overview the physical and chemical modifications that LDL undergoes after oxidation.

Oxidation of LDL consists of a complex series of events leading to multiple changes in the composition of its lipid and protein constituents [132–134]. Initial modifications are the free radical-induced formation of hydroperoxides in the unsaturated fatty acids of esterified lipids, of hydroperoxy- and oxysterols, and scission of the protein portion of LDL, Apo-B_{100} [132]. Most of the fragmented Apo-B still remains with the LDL particle. Lipid hydroperoxides cleave rapidly to form a variety of products, such as reactive aldehydes, including malondialdehyde (MDA), and 4-hydroxynonenal (HNE) [133], which can react with Apo-B_{100} to form Schiff-base adducts with lysine residues on Apo-B_{100} [132]. This blockage of the positively charged lysine residues is responsible for the increased negative charge of oxidized LDL. HNE can also form thiol linkages with proteins [134,135].

When LDL is extensively oxidized, particle aggregation also occurs, especially when oxidation occurs at

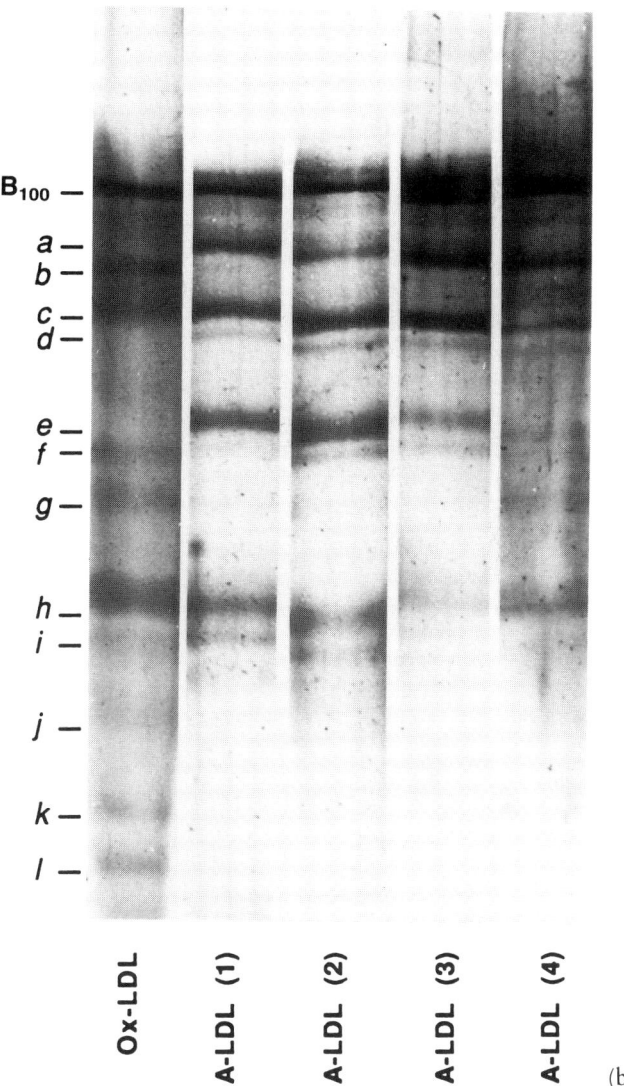

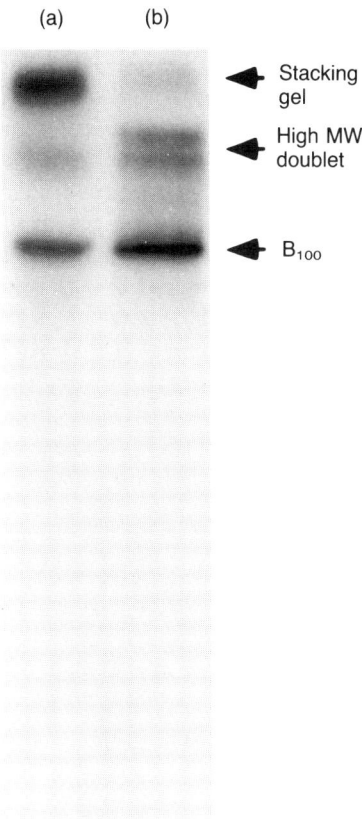

Figure 7.14(a) Autoradiogram of sodium dodecyl sulfate polyacrylamide (3–12%) gel electrophoresis (SDS-PAGE) of ^{125}I-LDL modified with both 20 mM malondialdehyde (MDA) and 6 mM 4-hydroxynonenal (HNE) (panel a) and with HNE alone (panel b). Most of the label is found in the stacking gel in (a), whereas a high molecular weight (MW) doublet is observed in (b). (Reproduced with permission from Hoff and O'Neil [140].)

Figure 7.14(b) SDS-PAGE (3–8%) of LDL oxidized with Cu^{2+} for 8 h (ox-LDL) and four separate samples of A-LDL following silver staining. Numerous fragments of Apo-B are of the same molecular weight in the different samples of A-LDL and in ox-LDL.

high concentrations of LDL [136]. This aggregation appears to be caused primarily by interparticle cross-bridging induced by such reactive aldehydes as HNE [137]. We have found that Apo-B_{100} crosslinking occurs in LDL modified directly with HNE (Figure 7.14(a)) [137], as well as in Cu^{2+} oxidized LDL (Figure 7.14(b)) [136], as indicated by the inability of delipidated Apo-B to enter into a 3–12% SDS-PAGE gel. Interestingly, when LDL was modified concurrently with HNE and MDA, particle aggregation did not take place, presumably because no, or very little, interparticle cross-linking had occurred [138]. This lack of crosslinking is evidenced by the far greater migration of Apo-B from LDL modified by both HNE and MDA into a 3–12% acrylamide gel during SDS-PAGE than of Apo-B from LDL modified only with HNE (Figure 7.14(a)).

7.3.3 LDL EXTRACTED FROM HUMAN ATHEROSCLEROTIC LESIONS IS OXIDIZED

One characteristic found by us [139,140] and others [141,142] in LDL extracted from human lesions is fragmentation of Apo-B_{100} (Figure 7.14(b)). We had not detected such fragmentation in lesion-extracted LDL previously, because we stained SDS-PAGE gels with Coomassie Blue which was not sensitive enough to detect the minor fragments [120]. However, after staining with silver or after immunoblotting for Apo-B using an affinity-purified polyclonal antibody to LDL, we readily detected multiple bands [139,140]. In an earlier study in which LDL was extracted by homogenizing the tissue, we actually found little intact Apo-B_{100} remaining [139]. However, when milder extraction was performed with saline without homogenization, more Apo-B_{100} was still present [140]. When similar procedures were performed on LDL extracted from grossly normal intima, fragmentation was much less than in LDL isolated from plaque [142]. Although others have reported that such free radical-induced scission of Apo-B_{100} gives randomly-sized fragments [143], we found fragments of similar, if not identical size in samples of LDL oxidized by Cu^{2+} [136] and for different samples of lesion-extracted LDL. In fact, many of the fragments were of the same size in Cu^{2+} oxidized LDL and in lesion-extracted LDL (Figure 7.14(b)) [140]. The observation of Apo-B_{100} fragmentation was also made in samples of LDL extracted from lesions derived from Watanabe heritable hypercholesterolemic (WHHL) rabbits [144].

As indicated above, a consistent finding in both oxidized LDL and lesion-extracted LDL was an increased particle electrophoretic mobility (Figure 7.B) [120,140]. When ^{125}I-LDL was injected into individuals undergoing endarterectomy, the ^{125}I-LDL that had accumulated in lesions removed at surgery also showed this increased negative charge [145]. Interestingly, no fragmentation of this ^{125}I-LDL was found. As in oxidized LDL, the increased negative charge on the particle is caused by the blockage of the positively charged lysine residues on Apo-B_{100} by reactive aldehydes formed during the decomposition of the hydroperoxides formed during oxidation [132], to create Schiff-base adducts. These adducts can be identified by their specific fluorescence properties [134]. At an excitation (ex) wave length of 360 nm, oxidized LDL gives a maximum emission (em) fluorescence at 430 nm [134]. When the fluorescence properties of LDL extracted from human lesions were compared to LDL oxidized with 5 μM Cu^{2+} for 8 hours, both gave essentially identical fluorescence properties (Figure 7.15) [140]. Monoclonal antibodies have been generated using LDL modified with MDA that recognizes MDA-protein adducts

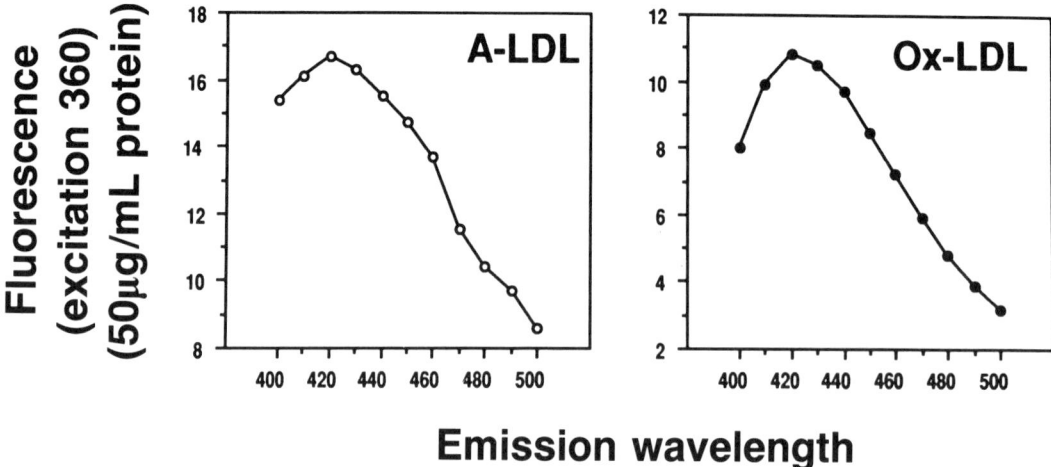

Figure 7.15 Emission spectra of LDL extracted from human atherosclerotic lesions (A-LDL) and oxidized LDL (ox-LDL) between 400 and 500 nm at an excitation wavelength of 360 nm. (Reproduced with permission from Hoff and O'Neil [140].)

[146,147] and using LDL modified with HNE that recognizes HNE-protein adducts [146].

Both the anti-MDA-LDL [146,147] and the anti-HNE-LDL [146] have been used to immunostain the extracellular space of advanced atherosclerotic lesions, suggesting the presence of such epitopes in proteins associated with the interstitial space. To show that these epitopes were present on LDL in lesions, such LDL isolated by density gradient ultracentrifugation to isolate a 1.019–1.063 density fraction was subjected to SDS-PAGE and immunoblotted with monoclonal antibodies directed at epitopes on LDL, MDA-modified LDL and HNE-modified LDL [141]. Apo-B_{100}, as well as fragments of Apo-B in the lesion-extracted LDL, was positive for all three epitopes [141], indicating that this LDL had been modified by these aldehydes. Because such modification is characteristic for oxidation [132–134], these data are consistent with the fact that some LDL particles isolated from lesions were oxidized.

We have extended these observations by showing a concentration-dependent increase in binding of both lesion-extracted LDL and LDL oxidized with 5 μM Cu^{2+} for 8 hours to anti-MDA-LDL using a slot-blot assay (Figure 7.16) [140]. Unmodified plasma LDL showed no binding. Thus, there is compelling immunochemical evidence indicating that some LDL particles accumulating in human atherosclerotic lesions had undergone oxidation. Recently, in unpublished observations, we found that lesion-extracted LDL can be further separated by ion exchange chromatography into subpopulations of LDL particles with greater and lesser degrees of oxidation.

Oxidation of lesion-extracted LDL has also been found in WHHL rabbits by measuring increases in thiobarbituric acid-reactive substances [144] as well as increase in lysolecithin in lesion-extracted LDL. Lysolecithin is released during oxidation by the activation of phospholipase A2 [148]. Several groups have detected an increase in the cholesterol to protein ratio in both oxidized LDL [132] and in lesion-extracted LDL [140,141]. This increase is probably caused by some removal of Apo-B_{100} after fragmentation. A shift from unesterified to esterified cholesterol has also been detected in both lesion-extracted LDL and in oxidized LDL [132,141]. Oxidation of LDL isolated from grossly normal human aortas, if present at all, appears to be much lower than in LDL isolated from lesions, as assessed by antibodies recognizing oxidized LDL [142]. Other characteristics of LDL oxidation such as electrophoretic mobility are also lower than in lesion-extracted LDL [142].

7.3.4 CHEMICAL AND PHYSICAL CHARACTERIZATION OF Lp(a) IN HUMAN LESIONS

We previously quantified the apo(a) content of human atherosclerotic lesions obtained at surgery [58]. We had operationally divided the extracted apo(a) into loosely and tightly bound apo(a), as shown earlier for Apo-B_{100}, based on the observation that only a fraction of the total apo(a) could be extracted with phosphate-buffered saline [58]. The remainder could be extracted with GuHCl. We had assumed that the apo(a) in the saline and the GuHCl extracts were in the form of intact Lp(a), but the data proving this similarity were limited to similar migrations of each fraction and plasma Lp(a) on agarose electrophoresis. In fact, the apo(a) in the tissue migrated somewhat faster [58]. To evaluate whether the apo(a) in both fractions was in the form of intact Lp(a) we first subjected the PBS extract to ultracentrifugation to isolate a <1.10 density fraction, and then subjected this fraction to gel filtration [149]. Immunoreactive apo(a) eluted slightly ahead of plasma Lp(a), and was equally divided between the retained fractions and the void volume fraction.

The roughly Lp(a) sized fraction isolated from plaque also contained immunoreactive Apo-B [149]. When these particles were further fractionated by density gradient ultracentrifugation into a 1.06–1.08 density range, this subpopulation was essentially free of any LDL-like particles. It possessed the increased electrophoretic mobility of apo(a) in the crude extract, an apo(a) to Apo-B ratio of roughly 1, consistent with

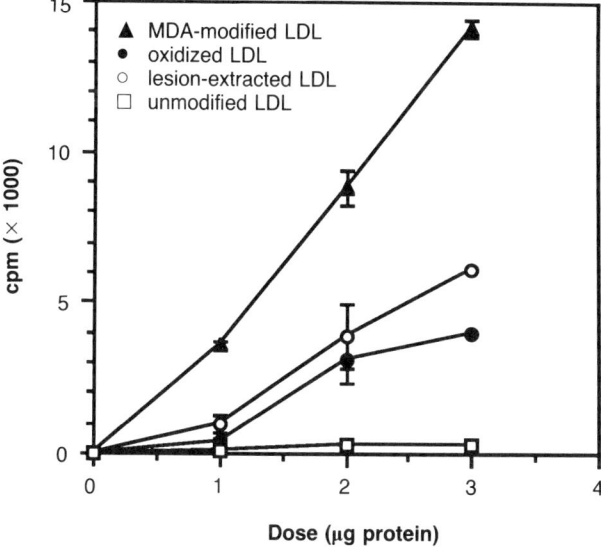

Figure 7.16 Dose response of binding of modified LDL to a monoclomal antibody recognizing an epitope on MDA-modified LDL using a slot blot assay on nitrocellulose sheets. Reactivity estimated by the obtained slopes was highest for MDA-modified LDL, followed by equal reactivity for oxidized LDL and lesion-extracted LDL. Unmodified LDL showed no reactivity. (Reproduced with permission from Hoff and O'Neil [140].)

intact plasma Lp(a), and a density in the range of plasma Lp(a) [149]. However, we also showed that lesion-extracted Lp(a) had higher conjugated diene levels and increased fluorescence at 360 ex/430 em [134]. These parameters, together with the increased electrophoretic mobility, suggested that some of the plaque-extracted Lp(a) had oxidized, as we and others had shown for some of the plaque-extracted LDL [140,141]. Rath et al. [55] also detected immunoreactive apo(a) in plaque extracts in the 1.06–1.08 density fraction. Because the plaque and corresponding plasma Lp(a) showed the same isoform pattern [55,149], there did not appear to be specific retention of one isoform over another in plaques. Although the characterization data just described were obtained from autopsy cases, comparison of the electrophoretic mobilities of apo(a) from plaque extracts obtained at autopsy or at surgery showed similar increases in electrophoretic mobility in agarose electrophoresis, indirectly suggesting that the described changes were unlikely to result from post-mortem modifications.

The apo(a) in the void volume-fraction, which was as great as in the Lp(a) sized fraction, also contained Apo-B, as shown by immunoblots of non-reducing PAGE gels [149]. Fibrinogen and/or fibrin was also detected immunochemically in this fraction. However, it was not definitively shown that fibrin[ogen] was directly associated with particles containing apo(a). We speculate that much of the apo(a)-containing material represents aggregated forms of modified Lp(a), perhaps oxidized. Oxidized Lp(a), like oxidized LDL [136], probably undergoes aggregation, perhaps due to covalent interactions between Apo-B and apo(a) on both molecules on the same or separated particles. MDA induces covalent binding between apo(a) and Apo-B in Lp(a) [150]. We have shown that Lp(a) can be induced to aggregate in the presence of physiologic concentrations of Ca^{2+} [116]. Whether any of the aggregates containing apo(a) represent such Ca^{2+}-induced aggregates of Lp(a) still needs to be determined.

When crude PBS extracts of plaques obtained at autopsy were subjected to SDS-PAGE and immunoblotted for apo(a), a far greater degree of degradation of apo(a) was found in plaque extracts than in corresponding post-mortem plasma [149]. When such samples were subjected to ultracentrifugation at density of 1.21, the fragments of apo(a) were associated with the >1.21 density fraction, suggesting that the fragments had been dissociated from the particle [151]. Whether this dissociation is the result of proteolytic digestion of Lp(a) in lesions or of free radical-induced scission of apo(a) during oxidation remains to be determined. Unexpectedly, this lipid-free immunoreactive apo(a) was primarily associated with material in the molecular weight range of IgG [151]. Whether this association represents a tendency of apo(a) fragments to bind to IgG or is caused by some other mechanisms still needs to be determined.

Because the GuHCl extracts of tissue previously extracted with PBS probably represented a form of apo(a) that readily associated with other plaque components or with itself, we concluded that any further fractionation of this extract should be performed in the presence of such a dissociating agent as GuHCl. Indeed, removing the GuHCl by dialysis resulted in aggregation of the apo(a) in this extract. When the GuHCl was subjected to gel filtration in the presence of 6 M GuHCl, substantial immunoreactive apo(a) was found in a retained fraction eluted just slightly after plasma Lp(a) [149]. Thus, under dissociative conditions, a particle roughly in the size range of Lp(a) containing apo(a) immunoreactivity could be identified in this tightly bound apo(a) fraction. Even after removal of the GuHCl by dialysis, a fraction containing both apo(a) and Apo-B immunoreactivity could be isolated by affinity chromatography on a Sepharose anti-Apo-B affinity column [149]. Particles in the size range of Lp(a) could also be observed in this fraction. Thus, intact, but perhaps chemically modified Lp(a), is likely also present in the tightly bound fraction of apo(a) in plaque. Whether this tight binding is caused by self-aggregation as a result of oxidation or tight binding to other plaque components, still needs to be determined. Interactions of Lp(a) with other lipoproteins, such as LDL [152], with fibrin(ogen) [53], and with GAG [114] have been reported.

7.3.5 CHEMICAL AND PHYSICAL CHARACTERIZATION OF APO-A-I IN HUMAN ARTERIES

We quantified Apo-A-I in the grossly normal intima and in plaques from human aortas obtained at autopsy as an indicator of the accumulation of HDL [107,108]. To assess whether the Apo-A-I was within an intact HDL particle, we initially subjected homogenates of plaques, grossly normal intima, and plasma to ultracentrifugation at density of 1.21. Whereas greater than 90% of the Apo-A-I immunoreactivity in plasma and in normal intima was in the d<1.21 density fraction, only 50% was in this fraction in plaque extracts [108]. When samples were further divided by ultracentrifugation into d>1.21, d1.063–1.21, and d<1.063 density fractions, about 20% of the total Apo-A-I immunoreactivity in plaques was also found in the d<1.063 density fraction, and only a little over 30% in the HDL density range d1.063–1.21 [108]. By contrast, most of the immunoreactive Apo-A-I from plasma and normal intima remained in the 1.063 to 1.21 density fraction. Because nonhomogenized samples of plaques gave a similar distribution, it is unlikely that this shift in density distribution in plaques is the result of artifactual binding of Apo-A-I to particles in a lower-density fraction.

In contrast to the uniform size of particles in the plasma d1.063 to 1.21 (HDL) density fractions, particles in the plaque d1.063 to 1.21 fraction were quite heterogeneous as shown by electron microscopy after negative staining [108]. However, when this fraction was subjected to gel filtration, most of the Apo-A-I was found in the size range of plasma HDL. Removal of the larger particles devoid of immunoreactive Apo-A-I in the void volume fraction markedly reduced the size heterogeneity as seen by electron microscopy. The HDL-sized fraction showed the presence on SDS-PAGE of only one band of the same size as Apo-A-I [108]. On electrophoresis, the plaque HDL migrated slightly faster than plasma HDL, possibly as a result of oxidation. Similar results were obtained when the plaque 1.063 to 1.21 density fraction was subjected to affinity chromatography on a Sepharose anti-Apo-A-I column. When the relative lipid compositions of plaque HDL and plasma HDL were compared, plaque HDL was enriched in unesterified cholesterol and depleted in esterified cholesterol relative to plasma HDL [108]. Little difference in triglyceride or phospholipid contents was found. This result suggests that some tissue unesterified cholesterol might have attached to HDL particles in lesions. It could also mean that HDL cholesteryl esters may have been hydrolyzed.

Apo-A-I was also detected in the d>1.21 density fraction [108]. This fraction contained variable amounts of phospholipid, but no detectable cholesterol. On two dimensional electrophoresis, this fraction showed one high but weakly staining peak that migrated slower than HDL. This fraction was unlikely the result of post-mortem artifacts, because no differences were found between its amounts in post- and ante-mortem plasma. It was also not the result of the homogenization extraction procedure, because the same results were obtained with and without homogenization. We cannot, at present, rule out an enhanced sloughing during ultracentrifugation of Apo-A-I from HDL particles in plaques relative to Apo-A-I in plasma HDL. Possibly, such sloughing is enhanced by chemical or physical modifications to the particle while residing in lesions. It still needs to be determined whether this fraction plays some role in reverse cholesterol transport, that is, from peripheral tissue such as from arteries to the liver [153].

7.4 Functional characteristics of lipoproteins in human arteries

7.4.1 OXIDIZED LDL: FUNCTIONAL PROPERTIES OF MONOMERIC PARTICLES

One of the modifications that LDL appears to undergo in the arterial intima is oxidation, presumably by free radicals released from different cells in the arterial intima such as endothelium [128], smooth muscle cells [129], and monocyte-derived macrophages [130]. Oxidized LDL possesses a number of functional properties. This discussion will be limited to only those that are directly relevant to the atherosclerotic process.

One of the initial events in atherogenesis is the binding of blood monocytes to the endothelial lining at lesion-prone anatomic sites of the vasculature and their subsequent recruitment into the intima to become tissue macrophages [3,4]. Mildly oxidized LDL under culture conditions, upregulates a receptor on endothelial cells that is responsible for the specific binding of blood monocytes to the endothelium [154]. Mildly oxidized LDL also induces the endothelium to synthesize monocyte chemotactic protein-1 (MCP-1) [155], a potent chemoattractant for blood monocytes [156]. Lysolecithin, formed from lecithin by the action of phospholipase A2 during oxidation [148], is also chemotactic for monocytes [157]. Finally, mildly oxidized LDL stimulates endothelial cells to produce monocyte colony-stimulating factor (M-CSF), which is responsible for the development and maturation of macrophages [158].

A second key step in the development of early atherosclerotic lesions is the formation of lipid-laden macrophages or foam cells [5] as described in the introduction to this chapter. Plasma LDL is recognized by the LDL receptor on monocyte–macrophages [159], but their internalization leads to a down-regulation of the LDL receptor, thereby preventing further uptake of LDL [159]. However, if LDL undergoes oxidation, this form of LDL is recognized by the scavenger receptor on macrophages [132], as well as possibly by other receptors [160,161]. Because these receptors are not downregulated by the internalized cholesterol from the LDL, uptake continues unabated until the cell is filled with internalized lipoprotein [162]. Much of this lipoprotein is degraded, and the liberated, unesterified cholesterol is re-esterified with oleate to form cholesteryl oleate inclusions [162].

An additional functional property of oxidized LDL is cytotoxicity to cells [163]. The active agent(s) appears to be an oxidized sterol [164], reactive aldehydes such as HNE [165,166] or both. Another component of oxidized LDL lipids, presumably an oxidized sterol, is specifically toxic for proliferating cells [167]. Thus, oxidation of LDL could induce of a number of key events in atherogenesis.

7.4.2 OXIDIZED LDL: FUNCTIONAL CHARACTERISTICS OF AGGREGATED PARTICLES

As indicated earlier in this chapter, aggregation is a characteristic of extensively oxidized LDL, especially if oxidation occurs at high LDL concentrations [136]. We separated the soluble (primarily monomeric particles as

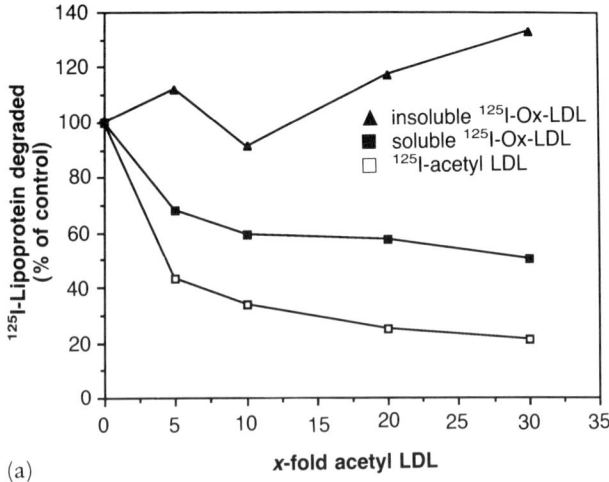

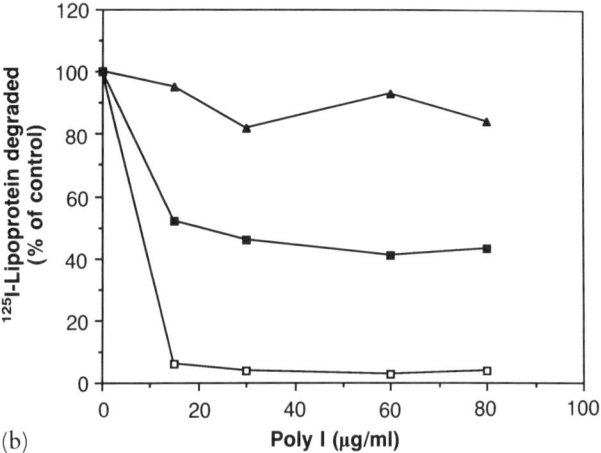

Figure 7.17 Inhibition of the degradation in MPM of the soluble and insoluble fractions of ^{125}I-ox-LDL and ^{125}I-acetyl LDL by polyinosinic acid (a) and unlabeled acetyl LDL (b). Labeled lipoproteins were incubated with MPM at a final concentration of 5 µg/ml in incubation media in the absence or presence of increasing amounts of competitor. (Reproduced with permission from Hoff et al. [136].)

assessed by electron microscopy) and insoluble portions of ^{125}I-labeled extensively oxidized LDL by centrifugation, and incubated each separately with macrophages in culture at identical concentrations. In general, the uptake and degradation of the insoluble fraction was higher than the corresponding soluble fraction [136]. This increased uptake may be the result of the fact that uptake of the insoluble fraction was via phagocytosis, in contrast to uptake of the soluble fraction, based on competition studies with cytocholasin D [136], an inhibitor of phagocytosis [168]. We found that neither excess unlabeled acetyl LDL (Figure 7.17(a)) nor polyinosinic acid (Figure 7.17(b)), two ligands for the scavenger receptor on macrophages [162], inhibited the degradation in macrophages of ^{125}I-insoluble oxidized LDL [136]. By contrast, both inhibited the degradation of ^{125}I-soluble oxidized LDL by about 50%. This result suggests that the receptor interactions of the two forms of oxidized LDL with macrophages appear to differ. In a separate study, unlabeled soluble oxidized LDL was a good inhibitor for the degradation in macrophages of ^{125}I-insoluble oxidized LDL [136].

As indicated earlier, we used LDL modified at high concentrations with HNE as a model for insoluble oxidized LDL [137], because particle aggregation was extensive in both [136,137]. Such aggregation appears to be the result, in large part, of intermolecular cross-bridging of the Apo-B molecules by such bifunctional aldehydes as HNE [137]. When macrophages were incubated with HNE-modified LDL for 48 hours, the cells were filled with oil red O-positive droplets (Figure 7.18(a)) [137]. The same result was obtained when macrophages were incubated with insoluble oxidized LDL [169]. Macrophages incubated for the same interval with plasma LDL showed no inclusions (Figure 7.18(b)). Uptake and degradation of ^{125}I-labeled HNE-LDL was linear over the 48 hours [137]. This degradation could not be inhibited by excess unlabeled acetyl LDL, suggesting that the scavenger receptor was not operative. However, it is conceivable that the aggregated HNE-LDL binds to multiple receptors, thereby increasing the affinity of such aggregates with a given receptor to degrees that preclude the ability of unlabeled ligands to compete adequately for the aggregated ligand. Thus, the question of recognition of both HNE-LDL and insoluble oxidized LDL by specific receptors is as yet unexplained.

In a separate electron microscopy study, we observed that colloidal gold-labeled HNE-LDL aggregates were frequently associated with clathrin-coated pits on the surface of macrophages (Figure 7.19(a),(b)) similar to the binding of gold-labeled LDL (Figure 7.19(c)) [170]. The LDL receptor and the scavenger receptor have been reported to be associated with such clathrin-coated pits [171]. However, another group found that the scavenger receptor was not always associated with clathrin-coated pits [172]. As with insoluble oxidized LDL, aggregated HNE-LDL is internalized by phagocytosis, because uptake and degradation are inhibited by cytochalasin D [137]. This uptake mechanism is consistent with the morphological observations of gold-labeled HNE-LDL being engulfed by the pseudopodia of macrophages, leading to internalization of the aggregate (Figure 7.20(a),(b)). That no uptake by macrophages of HNE-modified LDL was observed after co-incubation of gold-labeled HNE-LDL and cytochalasin D [170], is again consistent with uptake occurring via phagocytosis. Further processing of the HNE-LDL by macrophages was shown by the condensation of gold particles (increases in number of particles per unit of surface area) between the phagosomes containing internalized

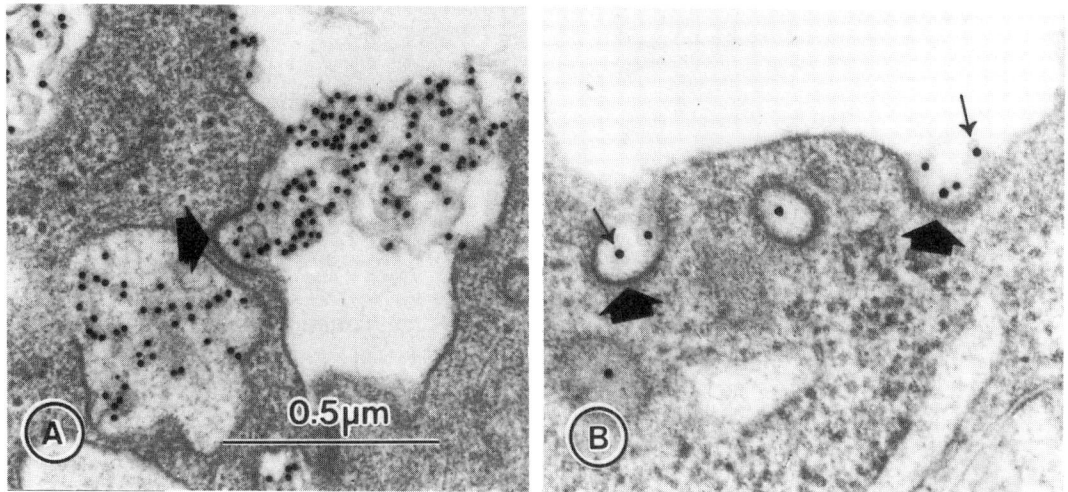

Figure 7.18 Light micrographs of oil red-O-stained mouse peritoneal macrophages (MPM). Cells plated on coverslips were incubated with LDL induced to aggregate by modifying with 4-hydroxynonenal (HNE) (a) or with unmodified LDL (b) at a final concentration of 40 μg for 48 h at 37°C. (Reproduced with permission from Hoff et al. [137].)

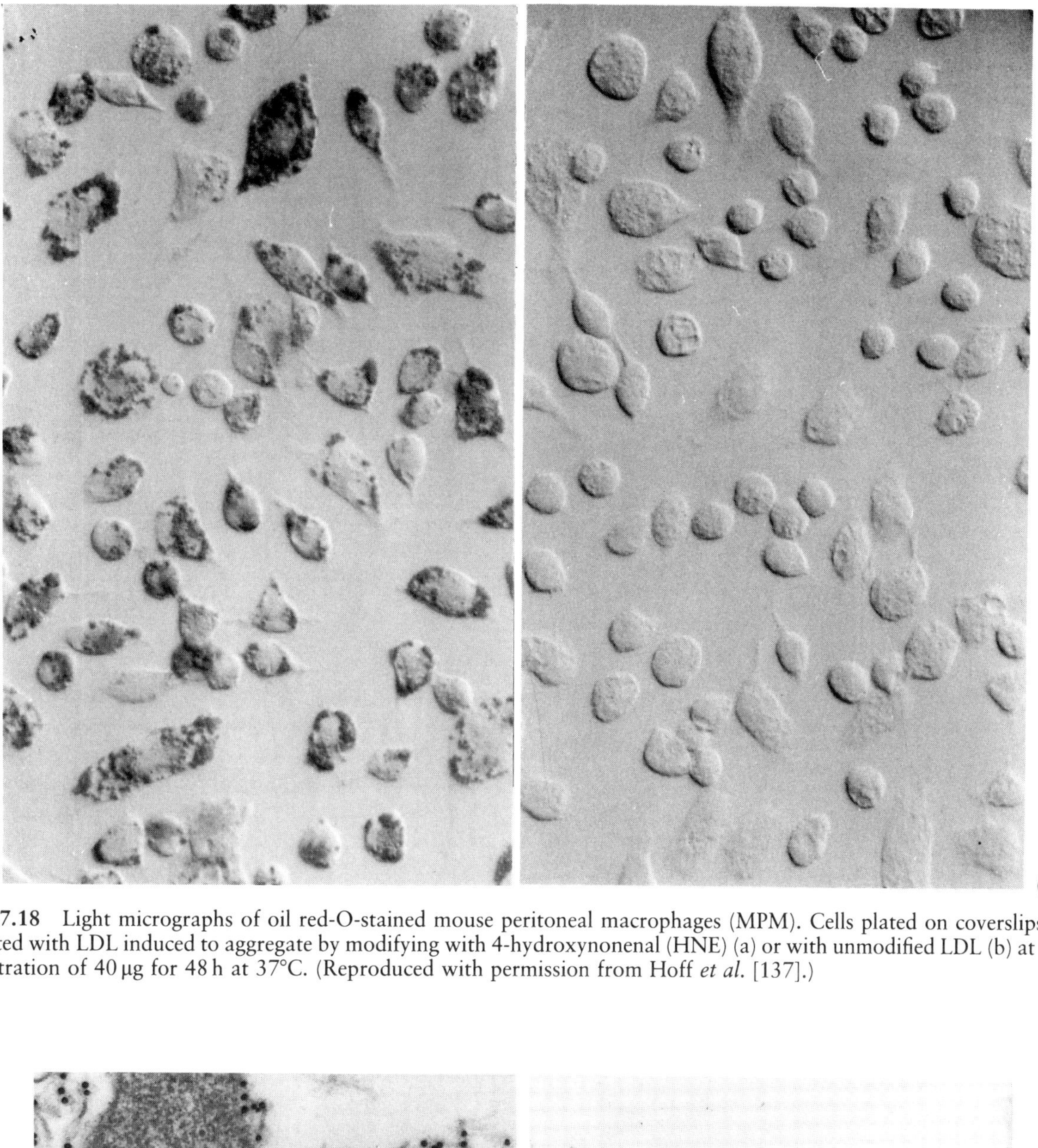

Figure 7.19 Electron micrograph of cultured MPM incubated with colloidal gold-labeled HNE-modified LDL (a) or colloidal gold-labeled LDL (b) for 4 h at 37°C illustrating the association of coated pits (large arrows) with gold particles. In (b) small circles with low electron density representing LDL particle (small arrows) can be observed surrounding the 18 nm diameter electron-dense gold particles. (Reproduced with permission from Hoff and Cole [170].)

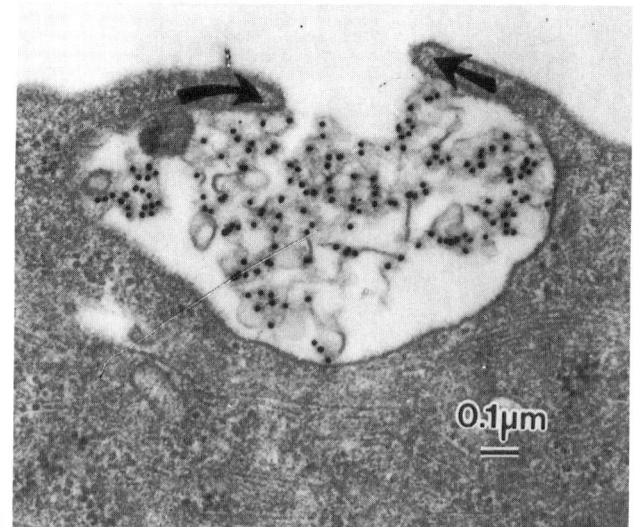

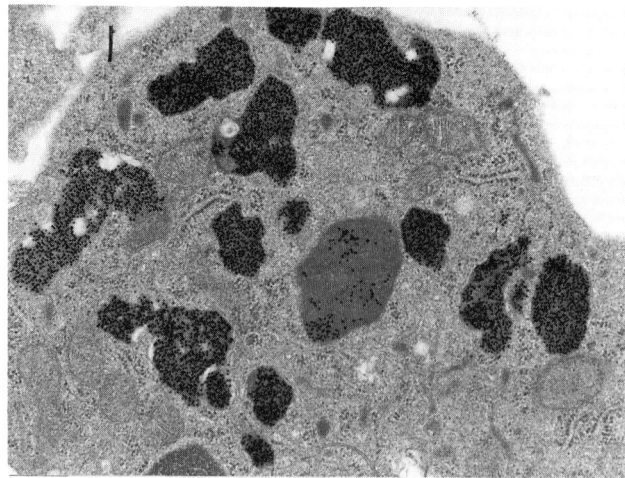

Figure 7.21 Electron micrograph demonstrating organelles with increasing numbers of colloidal gold per unit area believed to represent different time intervals of processing of the HNE-modified LDL. Arrow depicts highly condensed gold particles in lysosomes. (Reproduced with permission from Hoff and Cole [170].)

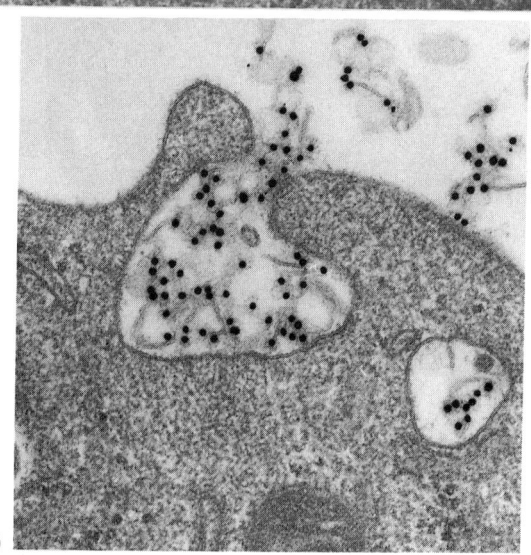

Figure 7.20 Electron micrographs of MPM incubated with gold-labeled HNE-modified LDL for 4 h at 37°C illustrating phagocytosis of the aggregated material. Pseudopods surrounding (a) and engulfing (b) the surface-bound material can be seen. (Reproduced with permission from Hoff and Cole [170].)

HNE-LDL and organelles believed to be acid phosphatase-positive lysosomes (Figure 7.21).

7.4.3 OXIDIZED LDL: ROLE IN ATHEROGENESIS

In vivo evidence for a significant role of oxidized LDL in the atherosclerotic process comes from several sources. One is data showing that administration of antioxidants can inhibit the atherosclerotic process in experimental animals. Several groups have found that the potent antioxidant, probucol, inhibited the development of atherosclerotic lesions in the WHHL rabbit [173–175], as well as in the cholesterol-fed New Zealand white rabbit [176]. Other antioxidants such as vitamin E have also been shown to reduce lesion development in primates [177]. The formation of foam cells was reduced after oral administration of antioxidants, which decreased the uptake and accumulation of labeled LDL into lesion foam cells after their injection into rabbits [173]. Recently, epidemiological data have shown that administering antioxidants to humans can reduce cardiovascular disease [178,179], probably by inhibiting atherosclerosis of the coronary arteries.

7.4.4 LESION-EXTRACTED OXIDIZED LDL: FUNCTIONAL PROPERTIES

The second major line of evidence linking oxidized LDL to atherosclerosis is the observation described earlier in more detail, that LDL accumulating in atherosclerotic lesions from humans and animal models had undergone oxidation [140,141]. Not described before is the evidence showing that LDL extracted from human atherosclerotic lesions is taken up more avidly by mouse peritoneal macrophages in culture than plasma LDL [140,141]. In initial studies uptake by macrophages over periods of 48 hours led to large increases in cholesteryl ester accumulation and to oil red O-positive droplets, similar to those found in foam cells [139]. When LDL extracted from plaque homogenates by combinations of ultracentrifugation and gel filtration were incubated with mouse peritoneal macrophages in culture, uptake was not inhibited by acetyl LDL [124]. Based on these findings, we concluded that uptake of lesion-extracted LDL was not mediated by the scavenger receptor. However, we later observed that some of the samples had undergone aggregation between the time of gel

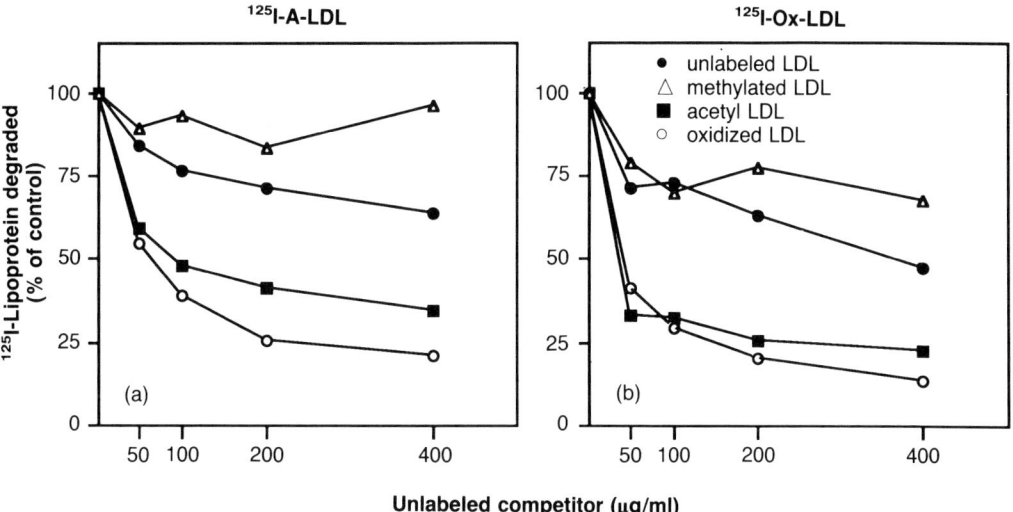

Figure 7.22 Degradation by MPM of ^{125}I-A-LDL (a) and ^{125}I-ox-LDL (b) in the absence and presence of increasing amounts of unlabeled LDL, methylated LDL, acetyl LDL and ox-LDL. MPM were incubated for 4.5 h at 37°C with 20 μg protein/ml of labeled lipoproteins in the absence and presence of unlabeled competitors. (Reproduced with permission from Hoff and O'Neil [140].)

filtration in which LDL-sized particles were isolated, and the time of incubation with macrophages. Extended storage of such lesion-extracted LDL (more than two weeks), and concentration steps induced particle aggregation even in the presence of protease inhibitors [180].

In our initial studies characterizing lesion-extracted LDL, we had shown that when plasma LDL was co-isolated with lesion-extracted LDL, it did not show any enhanced interaction with macrophages [139]. However, LDL accumulated and modified in lesions is possibly more susceptible to aggregation than is plasma LDL. To avoid the possibility that the homogenization procedure would exacerbate this effect, we modified our extraction procedure (Figure 7.11), which consisted of extracting tissue minces at 4°C overnight with PBS containing a cocktail of antioxidants, protease inhibitors, and antibacterial agents, but avoiding homogenization. We reassessed whether the scavenger or the LDL receptor was responsible for the internalization of lesion-extracted LDL by macrophages. Based on biochemical characteristics described previously in this chapter, oxidation appeared to be a major type of modification. To assess recognition by the scavenger receptor, we incubated primary cultures of mouse peritoneal macrophages with radiolabeled lesion-extracted LDL, defined as ^{125}I-A-LDL [140]. We found that unlabeled acetyl LDL was effective in partially inhibiting the uptake and degradation of ^{125}I-A-LDL by macrophages (Figure 7.22(a)). Unlabeled LDL induced a modest inhibition, but only at a 20-fold concentration. That this inhibition was specific comes from data showing that methylated LDL, which is not recognized by the LDL receptor [159], did not inhibit ^{125}I-A-LDL degradation [140]. If a typical sample of A-LDL contains oxidized particles, unlabeled Cu^{2+} oxidized LDL should also inhibit the degradation of ^{125}I-A-LDL. In fact, we found than unlabeled oxidized LDL was even more effective in inhibiting the degradation of ^{125}I-A-LDL than unlabeled acetyl LDL (Figure 7.22(a)). In the same study, unlabeled oxidized LDL and unlabeled acetyl LDL effectively inhibited the degradation of ^{125}I-oxidized LDL (Figure 7.22(b)). In a separate study we found that unlabeled A-LDL also inhibited the degradation of ^{125}I-oxidized LDL.

When ^{125}I-A-LDL was incubated with secondary cultures of rabbit aortic smooth muscle cells that express the LDL receptor but not the scavenger receptor, A-LDL was internalized by these cells to a lower degree than corresponding amounts of labeled plasma LDL [181]. The internalization of A-LDL by these cells was mediated by the LDL receptor, assessed by both the ability of excess unlabeled LDL to inhibit degradation of ^{125}I-A-LDL and to inhibit stimulation of cholesterol esterification [181]. In contrast to the situation in macrophages in which aggregated A-LDL resulted in higher uptake and degradation as a result of phagocytosis [140], the opposite was true in smooth muscle cells. These cells showed a poorer uptake and degradation of A-LDL that was induced to aggregate by concentrating [180] than did monomeric A-LDL [181]. Other forms of aggregated, modified LDL such as insoluble oxidized LDL and HNE-LDL, likewise, showed minimal uptake by smooth muscle cells. Thus, because the aggregated forms of A-LDL showed little uptake, the form that was taken up by smooth muscle cells appeared to be essentially unmodified LDL. Because such LDL induces down-regulation of the LDL receptor after longer incubation times [159], cholesterol accumula-

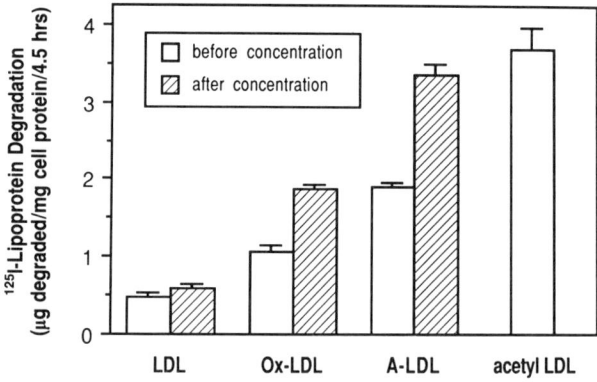

Figure 7.23 Degradation by MPM of ^{125}I-LDL, ^{125}I-ox-LDL and ^{125}I-A-LDL before and after 20-fold concentration steps. Lipoproteins were added to the incubation medium at a final concentration of 20 μg/ml and incubations performed for 4.5 h at 37°C. (Reproduced with permission from Hoff and O'Neil [140].)

studies we showed that aggregated forms of LDL showed greater uptake and subsequent degradation in macrophages than did monomeric forms, as a result of phagocytosis [136,137]. Based on these results, we anticipated that implementing a concentration step on A-LDL or oxidized LDL, which induces aggregation of about 20% of the particles, would result in greater uptake than corresponding unconcentrated and, therefore monomeric A-LDL particles when incubated with macrophages at equal concentrations. In fact, this assumption was confirmed (Figure 7.23) [140]. By contrast, plasma LDL, which did not aggregate after an equivalent degree of concentration, also showed no increased uptake by macrophages.

Steinbrecher and Lougheed characterized LDL extracted from human lesions, but with less involvement, as well as from grossly normal regions [142]. Oxidation of LDL in lesions was less extensive than in our studies [142]. Apo-B fragmentation was present, but recognition by monoclonal antibodies to epitopes on oxidized LDL was minimal. Macrophage uptake was not extensive and was scavenger-receptor negative. LDL from grossly normal intima showed no evidence of oxidation. The increase in uptake and cholesterol esterification correlated with the amount of cholesterol in the void volume after gel filtration, consistent with phagocytosis of aggregates.

tion did not increase when smooth muscle cells were incubated with A-LDL [181]. If these mechanisms were operative *in vivo*, they would suggest that A-LDL is not responsible for inducing the lipid loading of smooth muscle cells that occurs during atherosclerosis [8].

We wanted to assess whether the lability of A-LDL to aggregate was the result of oxidative changes. We, therefore, subjected both A-LDL and moderately oxidized LDL (8 h incubation with 5 μM Cu^{2+}) to a 20-fold concentration step and asked whether both would undergo particle aggregation. Both samples showed an increase in aggregation of about 20% [140]. In other

Collectively, these studies indicate that A-LDL appears to be internalized by macrophages through three possible mechanisms (Figure 7.24). One is by the LDL receptor, which appears to play only a minor role in inducing lipid loading of macrophages, because of

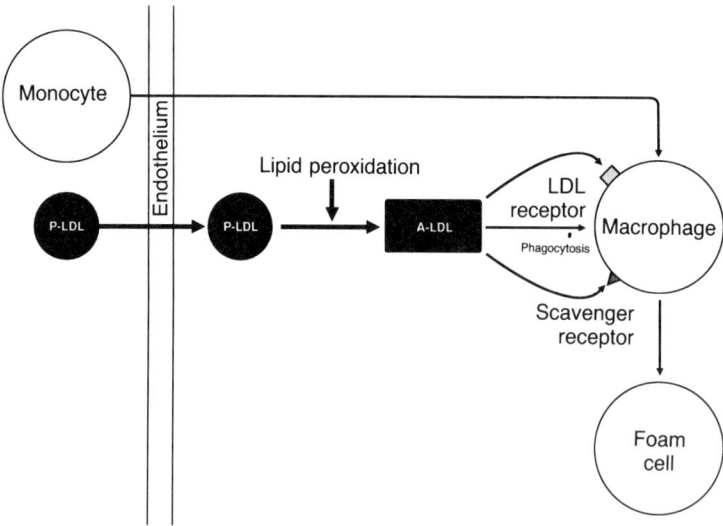

Figure 7.24 Depiction of one mechanism by which LDL (P-LDL) that accumulates in atherosclerotic lesions may become modified by lipid peroxidation to become A-LDL. This can lead to uptake by macrophages by two mechanisms in addition to the LDL receptor. These are via the scavenger receptor and via phagocytosis. Since these two uptake mechanisms are not downregulated by intracellular cholesterol, uptake remains uncontrolled and macrophages become lipid-laden, i.e. foam cells are formed.

the cholesterol-induced down-regulation of the LDL receptor [159]. We believe that a given sample of A-LDL would contain variable amounts of unmodified LDL.

A second uptake mechanism for more extensively modified forms of A-LDL is by the scavenger receptor [132,162] as well as other putative receptors recognizing oxidatively modified LDL [160,161]. Because of the lack of down-regulation of this receptor [162], monomeric A-LDL entering this route could induce lipid loading of macrophages and could be partly responsible for foam cell formations in fatty streak lesions [7]. The amounts extractable from advanced lesions are presumably underestimates of the amounts of oxidized LDL originally in the lesions because tissue macrophages would likely have internalized them. The presence of epitopes characteristic of oxidized LDL in lipid-filled macrophages in lesions is consistent with such internalization.

The third uptake mechanism we believe to be operative in inducing lipid loading of macrophages is the phagocytosis of aggregated oxidized LDL (Figure 7.24). The immunocytochemical data showing LDL closely pressed together in lesions (Figures 7.4(a),(b)) [32,33] suggest that LDL aggregates are present in lesions. We will discuss the uptake of other forms of aggregated or fused LDL in section 7.6.2. Whether this phagocytosis requires initial binding to a surface receptor such as the scavenger receptor, still needs to be determined.

7.4.5 OXIDIZED LDL: DEFICIENT PROCESSING IN MACROPHAGES

Several lines of evidence suggest that oxidized LDL is poorly processed in primary cultures of macrophages. A group of studies showed that the percent of ^{125}I-oxidized LDL internalized by macrophages that was degraded to trichloracetic acid-soluble label (TCA) is far lower than corresponding values for labeled acetyl LDL [132,160,182,183]. The comparison was made with acetyl LDL because both are partially recognized by the scavenger receptor [132,160]. Another study identified the presence of the poorly extractable lipid called ceroid in macrophages after long-term incubations of macrophages with oxidized LDL [184]. If ceroid represents the left-over products of poorly digested oxidized LDL, its presence would indicate that oxidized LDL is poorly degraded. As discussed earlier in this chapter, macrophage-derived foam cells in atherosclerotic lesions immunostain with monoclonal antibodies that recognize epitopes unique to oxidized LDL [185], to MDA–lysine adducts [146,147], and to HNE–lysine adducts [146]. This fact suggests that the protein moiety of internalized oxidized LDL is still not completely degraded and appears to represent the accumulation of undegraded oxidized LDL. Transmission electron micrographs of foam cells in lesions reveal organelles filled with electron-dense material [34], that contained ceroid [186]. This electron-dense material may represent unprocessed internalized lipoprotein [169].

As indicated earlier, extensively oxidized LDL undergoes particle aggregation, in large part as a result of crosslinking of Apo-B in separate particles by bifunctional aldehydes, such as HNE [136,137], formed during the decomposition of linoleate hydroperoxide [134]. We asked whether any difference would be found in the degradation in macrophages of the soluble portion and the insoluble portion of LDL oxidized with Cu^{2+} for 24 hours (supernatant and pellet fraction, respectively, after low-speed centrifugation). The soluble portion consisted primarily of monomeric particles [136]. When the percent of internalized oxidized LDL that became degraded was compared between the soluble and insoluble fractions applied at equal concentrations, a greater percent of the soluble fraction became degraded. Thus, particle aggregation or crosslinking of proteins appeared to lead to poor lysosomal degradation [169]. We established immunochemically the presence of undegraded Apo-B in cultured macrophages after incubation for 24 hours with insoluble oxidized LDL (Figure 7.25(a)). By contrast, incubation of macrophages for the same time with acetyl LDL did not lead to any intracellular accumulation of undegraded Apo-B (Figure 7.25(b)).

To assess whether crosslinking of Apo-B was responsible for the poorer protein degradation in macrophages of insoluble oxidized LDL relative to soluble oxidized LDL, we incubated macrophages with insoluble HNE-modified LDL. Because we [169] as well as others [183] found that such HNE-modified LDL was more poorly degraded than acetyl LDL, it is highly likely that such protein crosslinking affected subsequent lysosomal degradation. Particle aggregation may require that the uptake mechanism by macrophages be phagocytosis, and that fusion of phagosomes with lysosomes [187] is not as efficient as the corresponding fusion of endosomes that have internalized soluble forms of oxidized LDL. To address this question, we induced particle aggregation in unmodified LDL, in acetyl LDL, and in soluble oxidized LDL by vortexing, as described earlier [188], and asked whether the aggregated forms were more poorly degraded in macrophages than their corresponding monomeric forms. In each case we found that the aggregated form was more poorly degraded than the corresponding soluble form (unpublished observations). Thus it is possible that the uptake mechanism, in addition to the modification of the substrate by crosslinking, may lead to poorer protein degradation, probably the result of intracellular routing away from lysosomes.

To assess the potential *in vivo* relevance of these observations, we asked whether lesion-extracted LDL

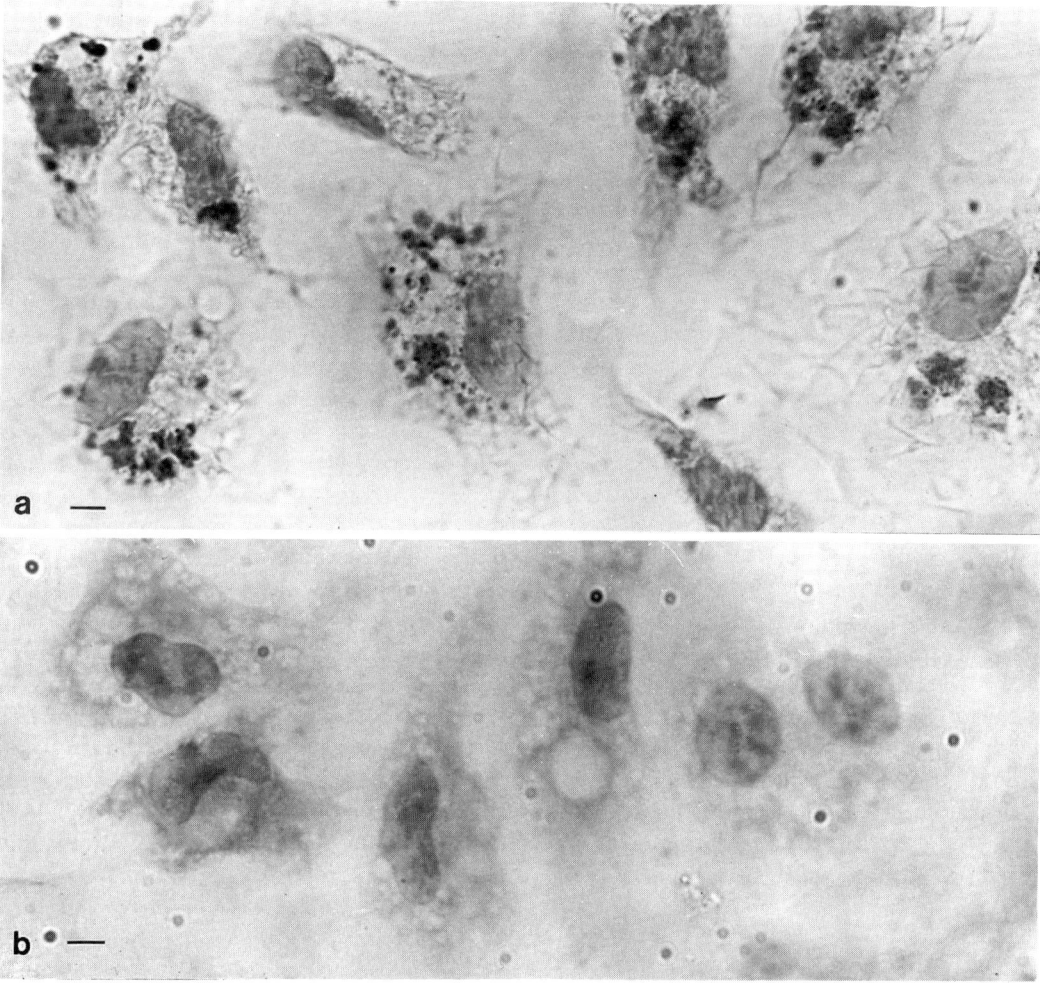

Figure 7.25 Light micrographs of MPM immunostained for Apo-B using an immunoperoxidase technique following incubation for 24 h with 20 µg/ml of (a) ox-LDL or (b) acetyl LDL, showing reaction product only in the former. (Reproduced with permission from Hoff et al. [169].)

when induced to aggregate by concentrating [180], would be degraded more poorly in macrophages than its monomeric counterpart. Again, we found that the aggregated form showed much poorer degradation of internalized lipoprotein than its monomeric counterpart [169]. Thus, ceroid formation in macrophages [184] may be more extensive after the uptake of insoluble than of soluble forms of lesion-extracted LDL, previously shown to be oxidized [140].

Because binding and uptake mechanisms for soluble and insoluble forms of oxidized LDL appear to differ [136], we also assessed degradation in macrophages after incubating cells with labeled lipoprotein, changing the medium, and then determining the degree of degradation of internalized lipoprotein. Thus, any influence of differences in binding and uptake mechanisms could be minimized. However, as in our previous studies, the percent of internalized lipoprotein that was still degraded after 18 to 24 hours, remained lowest for insoluble oxidized LDL, intermediate for soluble oxidized LDL and highest for acetyl LDL [169]. Interestingly, vortex-aggregated LDL showed almost as low a degradation as insoluble oxidized LDL.

Several groups have studied the cell-free degradation of oxidized LDL, of LDL, and of acetyl LDL by extracts of macrophages [183,189] or by mixtures of cathepsin B and D, two lysosomal proteases [132,169,183]. Each group, including our own, showed that when incubation was extended for periods exceeding 24 hours, the percentage of applied lipoprotein that was degraded was greater for LDL and acetyl LDL than for oxidized LDL [169,183,189]. This result confirmed data obtained in macrophages and indicated that the reduced degradation of Apo-B_{100} in oxidized LDL by lysosomal proteases was probably the result of chemical modification of Apo-B_{100} during oxidation.

We have extended their observations by showing that insoluble oxidized LDL was degraded more poorly by mixtures of cathepsin B and D than soluble oxidized LDL, i.e. the percentage of ^{125}I-lipoprotein that was degraded to TCA-soluble products after an incubation of 33 hours was lower for insoluble oxidized LDL than for soluble oxidized LDL [169]. Another group showed that more extensively oxidized LDL was more poorly degraded by macrophage extracts than less oxidized LDL [183]. This group also found that aggregated HNE-modified LDL was more poorly degraded by such extracts than LDL modified with lower concentrations of HNE that yielded a soluble product [183]. Because particle aggregation by HNE is induced by crosslinking Apo-B_{100} on separate particles [137], these data suggest that crosslinked Apo-B_{100} is not as amenable to degradation by lysosomal proteases as unmodified LDL. When we incubated vortex-aggregated LDL with mixtures of cathepsin B and D at pH 5.0, it was as readily degraded as LDL or acetyl LDL [169]. Thus, particle aggregation without intermolecular crosslinking had no effect on the ability of these enzymes to degrade Apo-B_{100} in a cell-free system. The discrepancy between the intracellular and cell-free results could be the result of separate routing of phagosomes containing aggregated ligands to lysosomes, resulting in poor degradation of aggregated lipoproteins relative to monomeric ones. It would be important to establish the mechanism responsible for such different routing.

Although hydrolysis of cholesteryl esters from oxidized LDL may also be deficient in macrophages [132,190], this deficiency has not been unequivocally proven. Stimulation of cholesterol esterification is decreased by oxidized LDL relative to an equivalent uptake by acetyl LDL [190]. However, it is uncertain whether components of oxidized LDL, such as oxidized sterols, inhibit the key enzyme in this stimulation of ACAT [162], or whether the unesterified cholesterol is accessible to this enzyme. It is important to determine whether hydrolysis of cholesteryl esters in oxidized LDL is deficient, as was shown for the degradation of Apo-B_{100}. If this deficiency is determined, it would be important to define the underlying reasons. Is it hydroperoxide formation of fatty acids or cholesterol moieties that impede the action of an acid cholesterol hydrolase?

7.5 Physical and functional properties of other lipoproteins

Figure 7.26 illustrates the large number of cholesterol-containing lipoproteins, in addition to oxidized LDL, that induce or are speculated to induce lipid loading of macrophages (foam cell formation). In this section the structural and functional properties of several of these lipoproteins are summarized, including functions other than the lipid loading of macrophages. When LDL enters the arterial intima, it can undergo a wide number of modifications as discussed below.

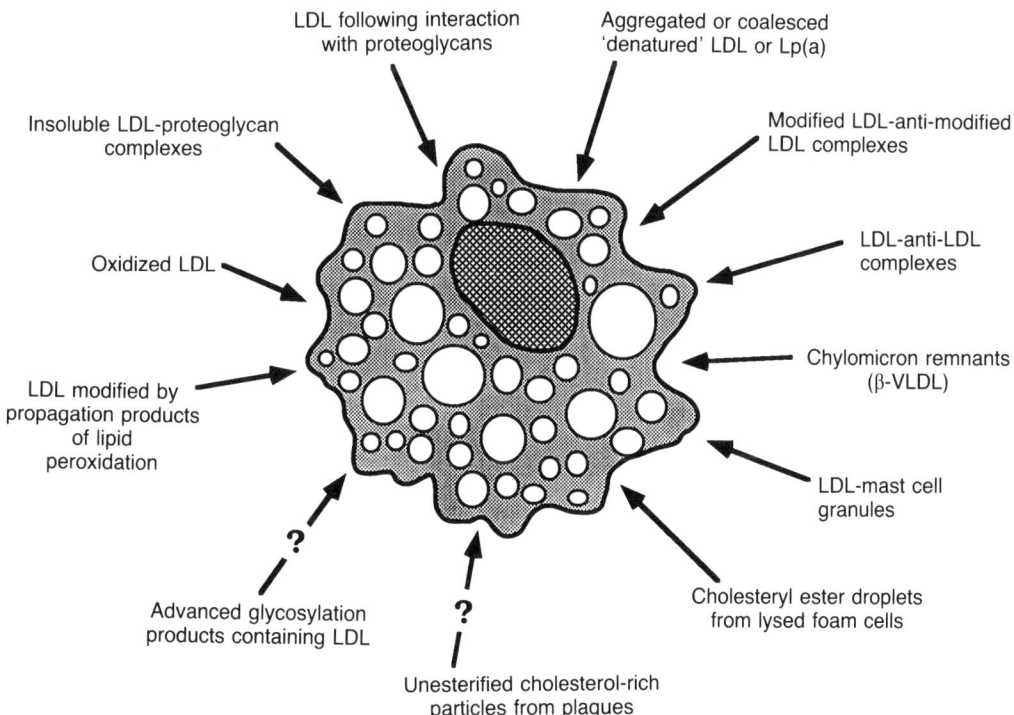

Figure 7.26 Foam cell formation showing the large number of cholesterol-rich substrates that can be taken up by tissue macrophages leading their formation. (Reproduced with permission from Hoff et al. [238].)

7.5.1 LDL MODIFIED BY PRODUCTS OF LIPID PEROXIDATION

LDL can be modified directly with products of lipid peroxidation, including hydroperoxides [191] and their decomposition products, such as a number of reactive aldehydes [192] in addition to HNE [135,166,193]. Some of these products are probably the active ingredients in cigarette smoke, which can modify LDL and increase its uptake by macrophages [194]. Soluble forms of LDL modified with these products are internalized by macrophages via the scavenger receptor [192]. When LDL at low concentrations is modified with HNE, it is also recognized by the scavenger receptor [136]. When LDL was modified concurrently with HNE and MDA, two of the most predominant aldehydes formed during the decomposition of linoleate hydroperoxide [121], the modified LDL remains monomeric [138], even when concentrations of LDL and HNE resulted in almost complete aggregation of LDL [137]. It appears that the MDA prevents the intermolecular crosslinking induced by HNE, possibly by competing for specific amino acid side chains. LDL modified by both HNE and MDA is also recognized by the scavenger receptor [138].

When LDL was incubated with extracts of human atherosclerotic plaque obtained at surgery, enhanced uptake relative to unmodified LDL was found in macrophages, as measured both by the degradation of ^{125}I-LDL and by the stimulation of cholesterol esterification [195]. Because the same modifications also occurred to LDL during incubation with non-homogenized extracts of arterial plaque, the component interacting with LDL was probably not an artifact created during the homogenization procedure. LDL that had been separated from plaque components by affinity chromatography was also internalized by macrophages, suggesting that the modification induced by the extracts occurred directly on the LDL particle and was not the result of facilitated uptake induced by some plaque component. Moreover, it suggests that the modification did not continue over the incubation period with macrophages. The modification of LDL appears to be specific for arterial tissue, because plaques, and to a lesser extent grossly normal intima, were the only tissues studied that demonstrated enhanced stimulation of cholesterol esterification, i.e. no increase with liver, muscle or skin extracts [195]. When delipidated Apo-B from tissue-treated ^{125}I-LDL was subjected to SDS-PAGE, autoradiograms revealed, in addition to the Apo-B$_{100}$ band characteristic of Apo-B, a doublet of higher molecular weight than Apo-B$_{100}$ and a band just entering the gel, both at the expense of the Apo-B$_{100}$ band. No lower molecular weight bands indicative of Apo-B degradation were seen. This result suggested that free radical-induced oxidation of LDL was not responsible for this modification.

No increase in electrophoretic mobility during agarose electrophoresis or increases in thiobarbituric acid-reactive substances (TBARS) were detected when LDL was incubated with extracts in the presence of butylated hydroxytoluene (BHT), a potent free radical scavenger [132]. However, BHT could not inhibit the uptake of plaque extract-modified LDL by macrophages, suggesting that the change in LDL responsible for this enhanced cellular recognition was not free radical-induced oxidation of LDL. However, interaction of LDL directly with products formed during the decomposition phase of lipid peroxidation, such as the aldehydes HNE and MDA, hexanal and 2,4,-heptadienal [121], could be responsible for the enhanced uptake. This possibility is consistent with the observation that LDL modified with MDA or with HNE forms high molecular weight doublets (Figure 7.14(a)) [138], as seen for LDL incubated with plaque extracts [195]. Such aldehydes are conceivably sequestered in lipid droplets or membrane debris in the necrotic cores of plaques.

Although the above explanation is currently the most plausible for this modification of LDL, there are others. One is that specific interactions of LDL with GAG in plaque protoglycans leads to enhanced uptake by macrophages [196] as will be discussed in more detail below. Another possibility is that LDL might react with glycosylated connective tissue components [197], which are then recognized by macrophages. Glycosylated LDL is recognized by a unique receptor on macrophages, facilitating its uptake [198]. Yet a third explanation is that Apo-E, secreted from macrophages [41] in the tissue, bind to LDL and induce recognition by a receptor with high affinity for Apo-E, such as the LDL receptor [199] or the LDL receptor-related protein (LRP) [200]. As indicated later, Apo-E has been identified by us on LDL-sized and larger structures isolated from atherosclerotic lesions.

7.5.2 LDL-ARTERIAL PROTEOGLYCAN COMPLEXES SHOW ENHANCED UPTAKE BY MACROPHAGES

As indicated earlier one of the key interactions LDL undergoes in the arterial intima is complexing with GAG in intimal PGs [60,66], as suggested by association in morphologic studies [16,18] and the isolation of complexes of LDL and PGs from lesions [67,68,125]. Complexes of LDL with arterial PGs can promote cholesteryl ester accumulation in macrophages *in vitro* [196,201–204]. Some complexes are described as being soluble when added to the incubation medium [196]. Others are clearly large aggregates that are taken up by phagocytosis [201–204]. This uptake is especially true of complexes of LDL with heparin and fibronectin [202]. Fibronectin is responsible for the binding [and subsequent phagocytosis] by macrophages of large complexes of LDL with heparin and fibronectin [204]. Fibronectin binds to specific sites on heparin [204] that, in turn, binds specifically to LDL [205], providing a mechanism by which LDL can be carried 'piggy-back' into the cell.

Soluble complexes of LDL and PGs stimulated cholesterol esterification in a dose-dependent, saturable manner, resulting in accumulation of cholesteryl esters [196]. Such stimulation of cholesterol esterification was linear over a 32-hour incubation period. Because cytochalasin D inhibited this stimulation by 6–16%, it is unlikely that uptake of these complexes is mediated by phagocytosis and that the complexes are highly aggregated. Such complexes of ^{125}I-LDL and PG are apparently recognized by the scavenger receptor on macrophages, because both polyinosinic acid and acetyl LDL inhibit uptake and degradation by 37% and 52%, respectively [196]. Moreover, excess amounts of complex inhibit the degradation of ^{125}I-acetyl LDL. The recognition of such complexes by the scavenger receptor could be the result of oxidation of the LDL in these studies. Because competition by excess acetyl LDL was not complete, LDL-PG complexes probably bind to a separate receptor in addition to the scavenger receptor. Since excess unlabeled LDL also did not block the degradation in macrophages of ^{125}I-LPL-PG complexes, uptake of these complexes is not likely mediated by the LDL receptor. Furthermore, complexes of PG with methylated LDL were taken up, as well as LDL-PG complexes [196]. Methylated LDL is not recognized by the LDL-receptor [159], which is further evidence for the lack of recognition of such complexes by the LDL receptor on macrophages.

Recently, LDL that had interacted with arterial PG, was shown to be internalized more avidly by human monocyte-macrophages than control LDL [206,207]. LDL was first mixed with PG to form insoluble complexes. These complexes were then dissociated with high salt and the LDL was separated from the PG. The uptake appeared to be mediated by the LDL receptor, based on competition studies with LDL [206,207]. The increased interaction with the LDL receptor appeared to be caused by the exposure of normally hidden arginine and lysine groups in Apo-B_{100} after interaction with PG. This group also showed that the formation of LDL-PG complexes changed the lipid organization of the lipoprotein particle as shown by low-angle X-ray scattering and differential scanning calorimetry [208]. They also showed modifications to the conformation of polar segments of Apo-B_{100}, which reduces the thermal stability in the LDL particle [208]. Because basic regions of Apo-B_{100} were exposed after interaction with PGs, such LDL was more sensitive to tryptic digestion [208]. In addition, such LDL is more sensitive to oxidation [208]. This sensitivity suggests the possibility that when LDL is retained in the arterial intima by being bound to intimal protoglycans, it can be oxidized more readily than when in a free form. A similar observation was made when LDL was modified with MDA when coupled to heparin [209].

7.5.3 LDL-IMMUNE COMPLEXES: PHAGOCYTOSIS BY MACROPHAGES

Several laboratories have found that immune complexes of LDL formed *in vitro*, are rapidly internalized by macrophages and can lead to lipid loading of such cells [210–212]. Initially it was unclear whether uptake would be mediated by the Fc receptor recognizing this portion of the antibody to LDL or by the LDL receptor. Aggregates of LDL induced by vortexing still bind to the LDL receptor [188], even though uptake is mediated by phagocytosis. Recent studies by Lopes-Virella and colleagues [211,212] using competition experiments have clearly shown that the Fc receptor is responsible for uptake of immune complexes. In fact, uptake of LDL in such complexes is greater than when monomeric LDL is chemically modified, as by acetylation, probably because the LDL complex is internalized by phagocytosis.

The concept of immune complexes of LDL in the circulation has been advocated for a number of years [213]. Likewise, the presence of IgG in atherosclerotic lesions has been well documented [214,215]. The fact that some of these IgG were antibodies directed at LDL and that immune complexes of LDL were present in lesions was also established [216]. Witztum and coworkers [216] proposed that immune complexes of modified LDL exist both in the circulation and in atherosclerotic lesions. Evidence has been presented for non-enzymatic glycation of Apo-B in LDL from diabetics, as well as for the presence of immune complexes of glycated LDL [217]. Likewise, a recent report indicates the presence of immune complexes of oxidized LDL in the circulation [218]. The level of these complexes is correlated with cardiovascular disease [218]. An LDL-like fraction isolated from WHHL rabbits immunostained positively for both epitopes unique for oxidized protein adducts, such as MDA-lysines and HNE-lysines, as well as IgG [141]. Whether these immune complexes represent filtration and trapping of such complexes derived from the circulation or the formation of immune complexes within lesions, still needs to be determined. Uptake of LDL immune complexes appears to have additional functions beyond lipid loading of cells. They have been shown to up-regulate the LDL receptor on human monocyte-macrophages, in contrast to the down-regulation induced by unmodified LDL [212]. Uptake of LDL immune complexes increases the secretion of TNFα, a cytokine that may implement lysis of cells in lesions [212].

7.5.4 LDL MODIFIED BY SECRETORY GRANULES OF MAST CELLS: ENHANCED UPTAKE

Recently, the enhanced uptake of LDL by macrophages was verified by still another complexing mechanism related to that of arterial PGs. Serosal mast cells contain secretory granules composed of a heparin-PG matrix in which neutral proteases are embedded [219]. When mast cells are stimulated, these electron-dense granules exocytose and form two pools of granules, one still associated with the parent mast cells and one free in the extracellular space [219]. When mast cells are incubated with macrophages in the presence of LDL, the LDL binds to the heparin-PG in the exocytosed granules. The neutral proteases in the granules extruded into the extracellular space degrade Apo-B_{100} in the bound LDL. This degradation leads to the fusion of LDL particles on the surface of the granules. These granules are then phagocytosed by the macrophages. The uptake does not appear to be mediated by the LDL receptor. However, much more uptake occurs than when LDL is in a monomeric form. The internalized, fused LDL is rapidly degraded in macrophage lysosomes, and the liberated unesterified cholesterol is re-esterified to form cholesteryl oleate, membrane-free inclusions [219]. By contrast, LDL bound to granules still associated with mast cells does not undergo proteolysis. When these LDL-granule complexes were re-internalized by mast cells, they were poorly degraded by lysosomes. This inability to degrade LDL appears to be a characteristic of mast cells. The fused LDL particles formed by the action of granule proteases resemble the extracellular lipid droplets found in atherosclerotic lesions [10]. They are discussed more extensively below. Collectively, these experiments with mast cells suggest that some LDL in atherosclerotic lesions fuse in regions in which granulated mast cells are present.

7.6 Large lipid-rich particles isolated from atherosclerotic lesions — structure and function

As indicated earlier, a large fraction of the volume of advanced fatty fibrous atherosclerotic lesions consists of large lipid-containing particles rich in cholesteryl esters, unesterified cholesterol or both. Typically Apo-B_{100}-containing particles comprise only about 5% of the total cholesterol in such lesions [93]. Thus, even though essentially all of the lesion cholesterol is assumed to be derived from accumulating plasma LDL, it is clear that most of the cholesterol represents metabolized LDL. The most frequently cited mechanism for the derivation of the cholesteryl ester-rich droplets in the extracellular space is the lysis of foam cells and the extrusion of cholesteryl oleate-rich droplets into the extracellular space [6]. However, because advanced lesions are enriched in cholesteryl linoleate, an alternative mechanism for the derivation of these large structures, needs to be identified, one of which is direct modification of LDL in the extracellular space [10].

7.6.1 STRUCTURES AND DERIVATION OF CHOLESTERYL ESTER-RICH PARTICLES IN LESIONS

Several different models have been used to induce fusion of LDL particles to form larger structures. When LDL is modified directly (at high LDL concentrations) with such reactive aldehydes as HNE, aggregation of monomeric particles occurs [137]. However, frequently, larger structures also form [137]. Modification of LDL with phospholipase C also induces the fusion of LDL into larger particles [220], probably by modifying the phospholipids on the particle surface. The interaction of LDL with sphingomyelinase induces similar structural changes [221]. Guyton and co-workers [222] have used vortexing of LDL as a model of the structural modifications just reported. A variety of structures were seen by electron microscopy; the predominant form was large lipid-rich droplets, similar to the major particles in atherosclerotic lesions. Collectively, these results suggest that LDL may undergo a variety of modifications that affect its surface configuration and that induce not only the aggregation of monomeric particles as seen after extensive oxidation [136], and the direct modification with HNE [137], but also particle fusion.

7.6.2 MECHANISM OF UPTAKE OF CHOLESTERYL ESTER-RICH PARTICLES ISOLATED FROM LESIONS OR FORMED *IN VITRO*

Fused LDL particles are readily internalized by macrophages in culture, predominantly by phagocytosis [220], although the possibility of uptake of cholesteryl ester droplets devoid of protein by a fusion mechanism, has to be considered. For instance, when cultured smooth muscle cells were incubated with an 'oil layer' of cholesteryl ester droplets by inverting onto the surface of tissue culture plates, uptake of these droplets was rapid and extensive [223]. Although it was speculated that uptake was mediated by phagocytosis, no evidence (such as inhibition by cytochalasin D) was provided.

One key question is whether the uptake, presumably via phagocytosis, is receptor-mediated. In one of our initial studies on the interaction of lesion-derived lipid particles and macrophages in culture, we found that a large cholesteryl ester-rich fraction (void volume of an agarose A-50 column) extracted from human advanced lesions, stimulated cholesterol esterification in macrophages in a dose-dependent fashion, reaching saturation at high concentrations [224]. By contrast, these particles

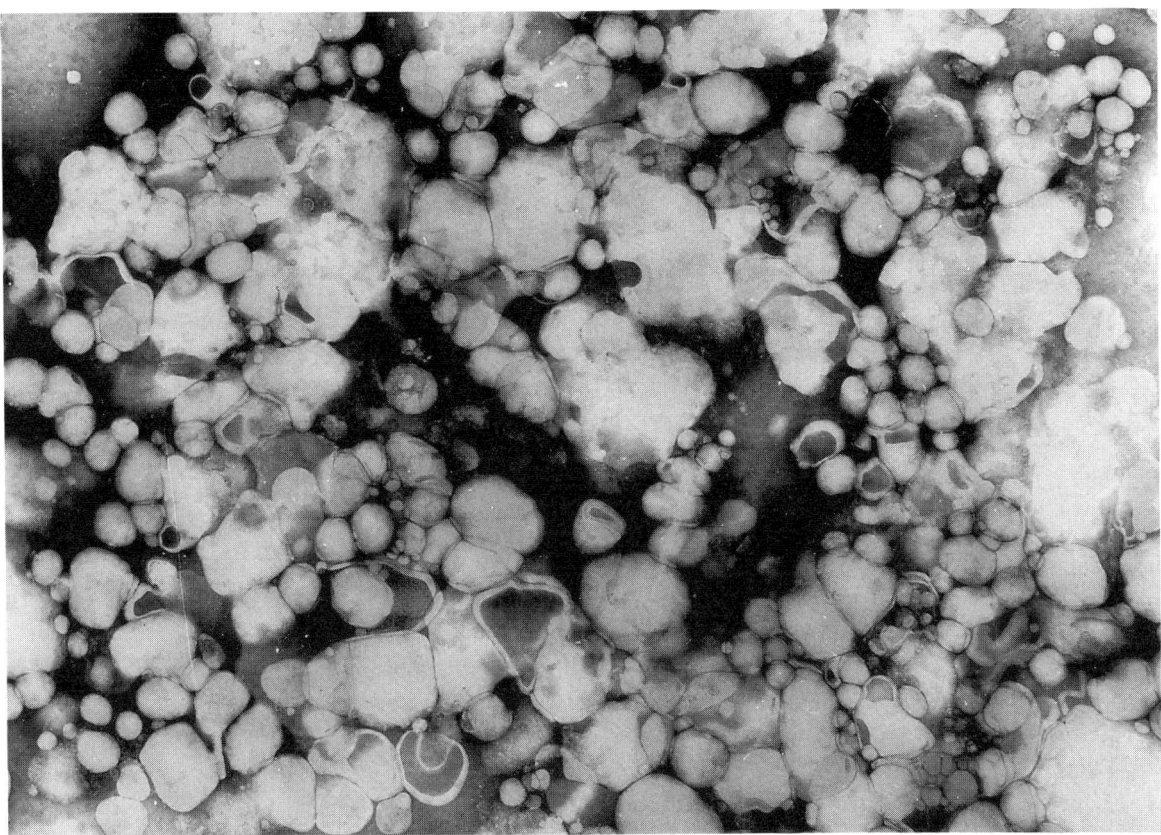

Figure 7.27 Electron micrograph of a negatively stained sample of large lipoproteins isolated from human atherosclerotic plaque homogenates. (Reproduced with permission from Hoff and Clevidence [225].)

showed little stimulation in fibroblasts. Lipid-rich extracts from other organs, such as liver or adrenal glands, also failed to stimulate cholesterol esterification. Uptake of such particles was linear over time [224]. Stimulation of cholesterol esterification required hydrolysis of the internalized particle in lysosomes, because lysosomal inhibitors prevented esterification. Receptor recognition was assessed by incubating macrophages with labeled plaque extractsmodified LDL in the presence of competitors for the scavenger receptor, polyinosinic acid and fucoidin. Both competitors inhibited stimulation of the lesion extract fractions almost as much as stimulation by acetyl LDL. However, because the extract fraction inhibited the degradation of ^{125}I-acetyl LDL by only 15%, it is still questionable whether uptake of these particles was mediated by the scavenger receptor. Interestingly, pre-incubation of this fraction with pronase greatly inhibited the stimulation of cholesterol esterification in macrophages [224].

These data suggest that a protein on the surface of the particle is involved in the uptake mechanism, presumably by binding to a specific receptor. However, the reduced stimulation of cholesterol esterification in macrophages by lipoproteins after digestion with pronase, is possibly the result of fewer particles adhering to the cell layer and interacting with these cells. The decrease in buoyant density of these cholesteryl ester-rich lipoproteins after enzymatic digestion, rather than the proteins associated with these particles functioning as ligands for binding to cell surface receptors, could be responsible for this reduced esterification.

In a later study we again isolated such a fraction either by homogenization or by leaching from plaque minces and isolated samples with similar structural properties [225]. Electron microscopy of negative stained samples of such fractions revealed the presence of large structures heterogeneous in size and shape (Figure 7.27). They resemble the structures in the d<1.006 density fraction of plaque extracts viewed by scanning electron microscopy and described by Hollander et al. [119]. These authors also showed pock-marked spheres resembling the fusion products observed after vortexing LDL [222].

When macrophages were incubated for 24 hours with these large cholesteryl ester-rich structures, they formed numerous inclusions with electron-dense material in addition to cholesteryl oleate droplets (Figure 7.28) [225]. These structures resembled the electron-dense material observed in foam cells of fatty streak lesions [226] and of cultured macrophages after long-term

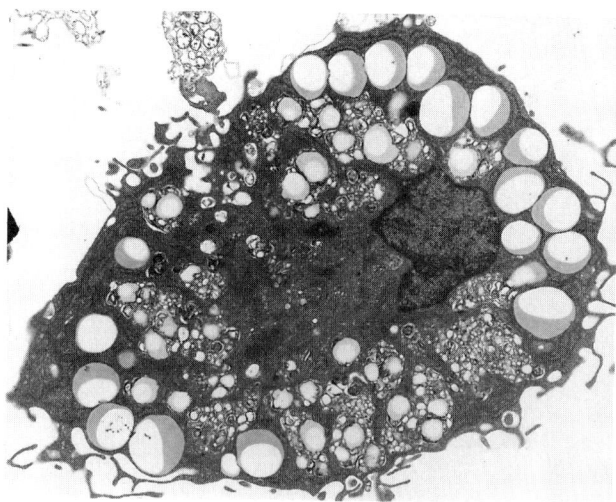

Figure 7.28 Electron migrograph of MPM incubated for 48 h with large lipoproteins isolated from human atherosclerotic plaques. The cell contains two type of inclusions, an amorphous droplet (with white centers depicting lipid extracted during tissue processing) and vacuoles containing vesicular structures presumed to be partially-processed lipoproteins in lysosomes. (Reproduced with permission from Hoff *et al.* [238].)

incubation with oxidized LDL [184]. Because macrophages were incubated continuously with the large lipoproteins for 24 hours, we cannot assess whether this accumulation is a transient pile-up of unprocessed lipoprotein as a result of phagocytosis or represents a more permanent lack of processing, as in the case of oxidized LDL [181–183].

We re-addressed the question of whether specific proteins associated with large cholesteryl ester-rich particles were responsible for binding to specific receptors on macrophages. By immunoblotting techniques, we detected the presence of Apo-B_{100}, Apo-E, albumin and fibronectin on these particles [225]. However, after several ultracentrifugation flotations of the particles, the albumin and fibronectin were removed, leaving only Apo-B_{100} and Apo-E. Apo-E may be responsible for the initial binding of these particles to the macrophage surface before phagocytosis, lipoproteins containing Apo-E have been shown to bind to the LDL receptor with higher affinity than lipoproteins with only Apo-B_{100} [199]. β-VLDL is elevated in rabbits or dogs fed a hypercholesterolemic diet [227]. Such lipoproteins containing both Apo-B and Apo-E bind with higher affinity to the LDL receptor than lipoproteins containing only Apo-B [227]. Apo-E has been reported to be associated with LDL-like particles extracted from grossly normal intima [118]. In preliminary studies, we found that Apo-E is associated with particles in the size range of LDL and larger particles. Lesion-extracted LDL uptake and degradation by macrophages can be inhibited by excess amounts of lipoproteins that contain Apo-E, such as HDL, presumably via the LDL receptor. Apo-E in lipoproteins extracted from lesions may be derived from tissue macrophages. Apo-E is distributed in the extracellular space of plaques [38–40] and does not interact with plasma LDL. It will be of interest to establish the mechanism responsible for the enhanced binding of Apo-E to LDL and other cholesteryl ester-rich particles in lesions. Figure 7.29 summarizes potential mechanisms by which lipid loading of macrophages can be induced. These include LDL oxidation, LDL degradation by hydrolytic enzymes and subsequent fusion, LDL aggregation by oxidation or LDL complexing with connective tissue elements, and cholesteryl ester droplets released from foam cells. Apo-E secreted from foam cells binds to different structures, facilitating uptake by other macrophages.

7.6.3 UNESTERIFIED CHOLESTEROL-RICH PARTICLES ISOLATED FROM LESIONS

In addition to the cholesteryl ester-rich droplets extracted from lesions and believed to be derived from lysed foam cells or from LDL that has undergone fusion, two groups have reported the characteristics of an unesterified cholesterol-rich particle isolated from lesions [228–231]. Originally such particles were identified in lesions by staining with filipin [228]. They appear in the extracellular space of the intima after initiating an atherogenic diet in rabbits [230]. One group found an association between Apo-B and unesterified cholesterol in such early lesions [231]. Chao *et al.* [229] isolated and characterized such particles by combinations of gel filtration and density gradient ultracentrifugation from lesions in both human and rabbit aortas. Particles were isolated in a 1.02–1.08 density range with a peak density of 1.036 and molar ratio of unesterified cholesterol to phospholipid of about 2.5:1. About 80% of the cholesterol was in an unesterified cholesterol form, and particle diameters were between 70 and 300 nm. The particles consisted of unilamilar and multilamilar structures. The predominant phospholipid in the particle was sphingomyelin. Mora *et al.* [231] isolated unesterified cholesterol rich particles from rabbit aorta after initiating an atherogenic diet that possessed many of the characteristics of the particles isolated by Chao *et al.* [229]. Initially Mora *et al.* reported that unesterified cholesterol-rich particles possessed Apo-B immunoreactivity [230]. However, subsequently, when subjecting the samples to an anti-Apo-B sepharose affinity column, they were able to separate LDL-like material that contained all of the Apo-B from the larger particles which consisted of liposomes of various sizes [231]. Unique to their study was the observation that these particles appeared after only two weeks on the atherogenic diet, and the observation that albumin was

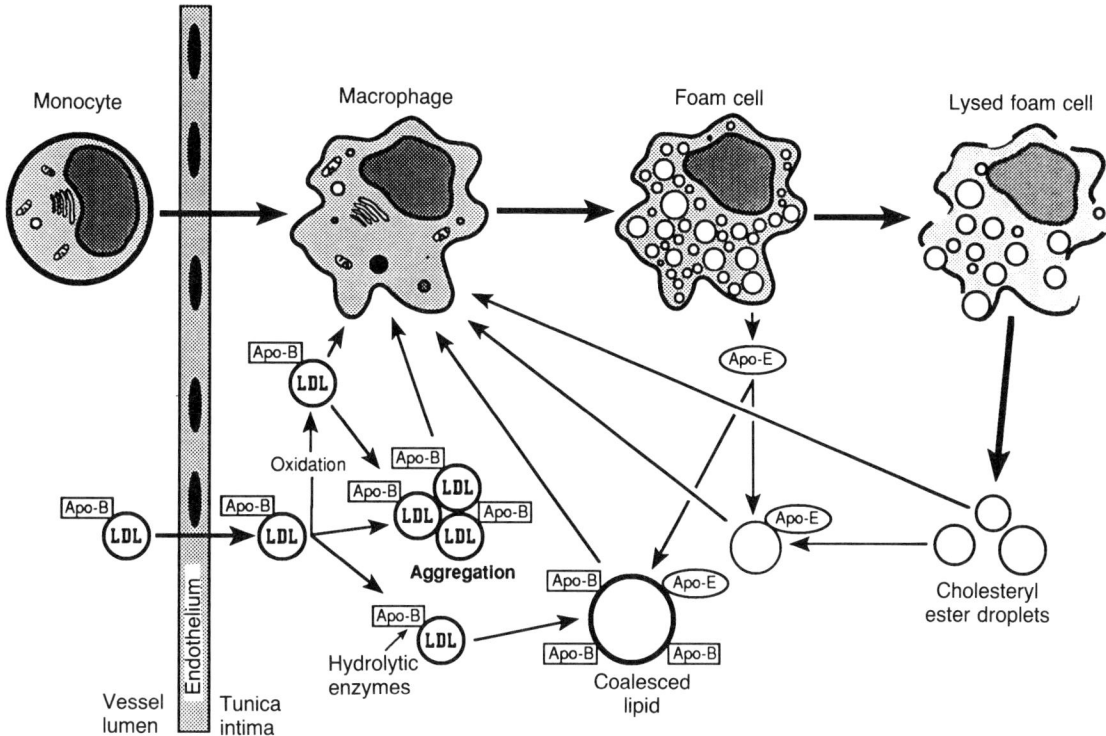

Figure 7.29 Different cholesterol-containing fractions present in the tunica intima of an atherosclerotic plaque and how each contributes to the formation of additional foam cells and therefore the further development of atherosclerotic lesions. (Reproduced with permission from Hoff et al. [238].)

associated with these particles. Because this albumin could not be removed and was not detectable immunochemically until after disruption of the liposomes by dissociating agents, these investigators concluded that the albumin was in the center of the liposomes [231].

The rapidity of development of such structures brings to mind a recent study using freeze etching and electron microscopy in which larger structures, that were either aggregated lipoproteins or fused lipoproteins, were observed in the subendothelial space of rabbits shortly after inducing hypercholesterolemia [232]. In a later study this group observed the appearance of structures resembling fused lipoproteins in the subendothelial space just a few hours after infusion of LDL into rabbits [233].

The question of the derivation of these structures is an intriguing one. Chao et al. [229] suggested that they may be derived from the efflux of cholesterol from macrophages, because such cells secreted multilamellar structures that are rich in unesterified cholesterol [234]. Another possibility is the release of lysosomes enriched in unesterified cholesterol after lysis of foam cells in rabbit lesions. After phagocytosis of cholesteryl oleate droplets by macrophages, there is a transient accumulation of unesterified cholesterol in lysosomes [235]. A third possibility recently addressed by this group is that these large unesterified cholesterol-rich particles may be formed by the hydrolysis of LDL by neutral cholesterol hydrolase [236]. Only if the LDL was initially degraded with proteases, such as trypsin, or subjected to oxidation (in which Apo-B_{100} is also fragmented by free radical-induced scission [143]), would cholesterol hydrolase significantly degrade LDL. These results are particularly exciting in that they suggest that the unilamellar or multilamellar structures, found as early as two weeks after feeding in an animal model, could be created by the combinations of proteolytic degradation and cholesteryl ester hydrolysis or oxidation of LDL and cholesteryl ester hydrolysis. It will be important to establish whether LDL can be oxidized or degraded by proteases after such short time intervals and whether neutral cholesterol hydrolases are present in the extracellular space at the early time intervals.

These large unesterified cholesterol-rich particles appear to have functional properties in addition to inducing lipid loading of macrophages. A complement-activating lipid particle of 100–500 nm diameter was isolated from human aortic atherosclerotic lesions [237]. This particle, isolated from saline extracts by density gradient ultracentrifugation and gel filtration, had an unesterified cholesterol-to-total cholesterol ratio of 0.58 and an unesterified cholesterol-to-phospholipid ratio of 1.2. This lipid activated the alternative pathway of complement in a dose-dependent manner.

7.7 Conclusions

This overview of lipoproteins and atherogenesis has attempted to collate the extensive information on this subject into a form that will be understandable for those not directly involved with research in this area. It also represents a somewhat personal view of this subject, since I have been directly involved within this research for more than twenty years. I have shown that lipoproteins containing Apo-B preferentially accumulate in the intima of large arteries, as a result of specific interactions with such connective tissue elements as proteoglycans. These lipoproteins, especially LDL, undergo structural and chemical modifications. A primary modification is oxidation, which changes several functional properties, one of which is enhanced uptake by tissue macrophages derived from circulating monocytes, either by the scavenger receptor if monomeric or by phagocytosis if aggregated. This enhanced uptake leads to lipid loading of these cells (foam cells), which is characteristic of fatty streak lesions. In addition to oxidation and complex formation with proteoglycans, accumulating LDL can undergo complexing with antibodies to form immune complexes and can undergo fusion after enzymatic degradation. Large cholesteryl ester-rich particles appear in the extracellular space, derived from the lysis of foam cells and the extrusion of cholesteryl oleate droplets. These complexes of LDL with other tissue elements, unesterified cholesterol-rich particles or cholesteryl ester-rich particles, are all rapidly internalized by macrophages to induce lipid loading of these cells and possibly also by smooth muscle cells at later stages in the development of atherosclerotic lesions.

References

1. Gotto Jr, A.M., Pownall, H.J. and Havel, R.J. (1986) Introduction to the plasma lipoproteins. *Methods Enzymol.*, **128**, 3–41.
2. Havel, R.J. (1984) The formation of LDL: mechanisms and regulation. *J. Lipid Res.*, **25**, 1570–6.
3. Gerrity, R.G. (1981) The role of the monocyte in atherogenesis. I. Transition of blood-borne monocytes into foam cells in fatty lesions. *Am. J. Pathol.*, **103**, 181–90.
4. Faggiotto, A. and Ross, R. (1984) Studies of hypercholesterolemia in the nonhuman primate: II. Fatty streak conversion to fibrous plaque. *Arteriosclerosis*, **4**, 341–56.
5. Schaffner, T., Taylor, K., Bartucci, E.J. et al. (1980) Arterial foam cells with distinctive immunomorphologic and histochemical features of macrophages. *Am. J. Pathol.*, **100**, 57–80.
6. Geer, J.C. (1965) Fine structure of human aortic intimal thickening and fatty streaks. *Lab. Invest.*, **12**, 1764–83.
7. McGill Jr, H.C. (1968) Fatty streaks in the coronary arteries and aorta. *Lab. Invest.*, **18**, 560–70.
8. Geer, J.C. and Haust, M.D. (1972) Smooth muscle cells in atherosclerosis, in *Monographs on Atherosclerosis*, vol. 2, (eds O.J. Pollak, H.S. Simms and J.E. Kirk) Karger, Basel, pp. 1–140.
9. Portman, O.W. (1970) Arterial composition and metabolism: esterified fatty acids and cholesterol. *Adv. Lipid. Res.*, **8**, 41–114.
10. Bocan, T.M.A., Schifani, T.A. and Guyton, J.R. (1986) Ultrastructure of the human aortic fibrolipid lesion: formation of the atherosclerotic lipid-rich core. *Am. J. Pathol.*, **123**, 413–24.
11. Ross, R. (1986) The pathogenesis of atherosclerosis: an update. *New Engl. J. Med.*, **314**, 488–500.
12. Ambrose, J.A., Tannenbaum, M.A., Alexopoulos, D. et al. (1988) Angiographic progression of coronary artery disease and the development of myocardial infarction. *J. Am. Coll. Cardiol.*, **12**, 56–62.
13. Fuster, V., Badimon, L., Badimon, J.J. and Chesebro, J.H. (1992) The pathogenesis of coronary artery disease and the acute coronary syndromes: Parts 1 and 2. *New Engl. J. Med.*, **326**, 242–50; 310–8.
14. Constantinides, P. (1966) Plaque fissures in human coronary thrombosis. *J. Atheroscl. Res.*, **6**, 1–17.
15. Hoff, H.F., Jackson, R.L., Mao, J.T. and Gotto, A.M. (1974) Localization of low density lipoproteins in arterial lesions from normolipemics employing a purified fluorescent labeled antibody. *Biochim. Biophys. Acta*, **351**, 407–15.
16. Hoff, H.F., Lie, J.T., Titus, J.L. et al. (1975) Lipoproteins in atherosclerotic lesions. Localization by immunofluorescence and apo-low density lipoproteins in human atherosclerotic arteries from normal and hyperlipoproteinemics. *Arch. Pathol.*, **99**, 253–8.
17. Hoff, H.F., Heideman, C.L., Jackson, R.L. et al. (1975) The localization patterns of plasma apo-lipoproteins in human atherosclerotic lesions. *Circ. Res.*, **37**, 72–9.
18. Hoff, H.F., Heideman, C.L. and Gaubatz, J.W. (1975) Apo-low density lipoprotein localization in intracranial and extracranial atherosclerotic lesions from human normolipoproteinemics and hyperlipoproteinemics. *Arch. Neurol.*, **32**, 600–5.
19. Hoff, H.F., Heideman, C.L., Noon, J.P. and Meyer, J.S. (1975) Localization of apolipoproteins in human carotid artery plaques. *Stroke*, **6**, 531–4.
20. Hoff, H.F., Heideman, C.L., Gaubatz, J.W. et al. (1977) Quantitation of apolipoprotein B (apoB) in grossly normal human aorta. *Circ. Res.*, **40**, 56–63.
21. Hoff, H.F., Ruggles, B.M. and Bond, M.G. (1980) A technique for localizing LDL by immunofluorescence in formalin-fixed and paraffin-embedded atherosclerotic lesions. *Artery*, **6**, 328–39.
22. Kao, V.C. and Wissler, R.W. (1965) A study of the immunohistochemical localization of serum lipoproteins and other plasma proteins in human atherosclerotic lesions. *Exp. Mol. Pathol.*, **4**, 465–79.
23. Walton, K.W. and Williamson, N. (1968) Histological and immunofluorescent studies on the human atheromatous plaque. *J. Atherscl. Res.*, **8**, 599–624.
24. Woolf, N. and Pilkington, T.R. (1965) The immunohistochemical demonstration of lipoproteins in vessel walls. *J. Pathol. Bacteriol.*, **90**, 459–63.
25. Yomantas, S., Elner, V.M., Schaffner, T. and Wissler, R.W. (1984) Immunohistochemical localization of apolipoprotein B in human atherosclerotic lesions. *Arch. Pathol. Lab. Med.*, **108**, 374–8.
26. Hoff, H.F. and Bond, M.G. (1984) LDL localization in advanced atherosclerotic plaques of coronary arteries of cynomolgous monkeys. *Artery*, **12**, 104–16.
27. Hoff, H.F., Yamauchi, Y. and Bond, M.G. (1985) Reduction in tissue LDL accumulation during coronary artery regression in cynomolgus macaques. *Atherosclerosis*, **56**, 51–60.
28. Feldman, D.L., Hoff, H.F. and Gerrity, R.G. (1984) Immunohistochemical localization of apoB in aortas from hyperlipemic swine. Preferential accumulation in lesion-prone areas. *Arch. Pathol. Lab. Med.*, **108**, 817–22.
29. Yamauchi, Y. and Hoff, H.F. (1984) Apolipoprotein B accumulation and development of foam cell lesions in coronary arteries of hypercholesterolemic swine. *Lab. Invest.*, **51**, 325–32.
30. Davis, H.R. and Wissler, R.W. (1984) Apoprotein B quantification in rhesus and cynomolgus monkey atherosclerotic lesions. *Atherosclerosis*, **50**, 241–52.
31. Rosenfeld, M.E., Palinski, W., Ylä-Herttuala, S. et al. (1990) Distribution of oxidation specific lipid-protein adducts and apolipoprotein B in atherosclerotic lesions of varying severity from WHHL rabbits. *Arteriosclerosis*, **10**, 336–49.
32. Hoff, H.F. and Gaubatz, J.W. (1976) Ultrastructural localization of plasma lipoproteins in human intracranial arteries. *Virchows Arch. Path. Anat. Physiol.*, **369**, 111–22.
33. Hoff, H.F. and Gaubatz, J.W. (1977) Ultrastructural localization of apolipoprotein B in human aortic and coronary atherosclerotic plaques. *Exp. Mol. Pathol.*, **26**, 214–17.
34. Hoff, H.F. (1973) Human intracranial atherosclerosis. II. A histochemical and ultrastructural study of atheromatous plaques. *Virchows Arch. Path. Anat. Physiol.*, **361**, 97–108.
35. Duncan, Jr, L.E., Buck, K. and Lynch, A. (1963) Lipoprotein movement through canine aortic wall. *Science*, **142**, 972–3.
36. Stender, S. and Zilversmit, D.B. (1981) Transfer of plasma lipoprotein components and of plasma proteins into aortas of cholesterol-fed rabbits. Molecular size as a determinant of plasma lipoprotein influx. *Arteriosclerosis*, **1**, 38–49.
37. Davies, M.J., Woolf, N., Rowles, P.M. and Pepper, J. (1988) Morphology of the endothelium over atherosclerotic plaques in human conary arteries. *Br. Heart J.*, **60**, 459–64.
38. Bocan, T.M.A., Brown, S.A. and Guyton, J.R. (1988) Human aortic fibrolipid lesions: immunochemical localization of apolipoprotein B and

apolipoprotein A. *Arterioslcerosis*, **8**, 499–508.
39. Babaev, V.R., Dergunov, A.D., Chenchik, A.A. et al. (1990) Localization of apolipoprotein E in normal and atherosclerotic human aorta. *Atherosclerosis*, **85**, 239–47.
40. Murase, T., Oka, T., Yamada, N. et al. (1986) Immunohistochemical localization of apolipoprotein E in atherosclerotic lesions of the aorta and coronary arteries. *Atherosclerosis*, **60**, 1–6.
41. Basu, S.K., Brown, M.S., Ho, Y.K. et al. (1981) Mouse macrophages synthesize and secrete a protein resembling apo E. *Proc. Natl Acad. Sci. USA*, **78**, 7545–9.
42. Utermann, G. (1989) The mysteries of lipoprotein(a). *Science*, **246**, 904–10.
43. Scanu, A. and Fless, G.M. (1990) Lipoprotein(a). Heterogeneity and biological relevance. *J. Clin. Invest.*, **85**, 1709–15.
44. Armstrong, V.W., Cremer, P., Eberle, P. et al. (1986) The association between serum Lp(a) concentrations and angiographically assessed coronary atherosclerosis. Dependence on serum LDL levels. *Atherosclerosis*, **62**, 249–57.
45. Dahlen, G.H., Guyton, J.R., Attar, M. et al. (1986) Association of levels of lipoprotein Lp(a), plasma lipids, and other lipoproteins with coronary artery disease documented by angiography. *Circulation*, **74**, 758–65.
46. Cressman, M.O., O'Neil, J., Heyka, R.J. et al. (1992) Lp(a) levels are predicters of accelerated atherosclerosis in patients maintained on chronic hemodialysis. *Circulation*, **86**, 475–582.
47. Hoff, H.F., Beck, G.J., Skibinski, C.I. et al. (1988) Serum Lp(a) levels are a predictor of vein graft stenosis following coronary artery bypass surgery in humans. *Circulation*, **77**, 1238–44.
48. Eaton, D.L., Fless, G.M., Kohr, W.J. et al. (1987) Partial amino acid sequence of apolipoprotein(a) shows that it is homologous to plasminogen. *Proc. Natl Acad. Sci. USA*, **84**, 3224–8.
49. McLean, J.W., Tomlinson, J.E., Kuang, W.-J. et al. (1987) cDNA sequence of human apolipoprotein(a) is homologous to plasminogen. *Nature*, **300**, 132–7.
50. Loscalzo, J., Weinfeld, M., Fless, G. and Scanu, A.M. (1990) Lipoprotein(a), fibrin binding and plasminogen activation. *Arteriosclerosis*, **10**, 240–5.
51. Gonzalez-Gronow, M., Edelberg, J.M. and Pizzo, S.Y. (1989) Further characterization of the cellular plasminogen binding site: evidence that plasminogen 2 and lipoprotein(a) compete for the same site. *Biochemistry*, **28**, 2374–7.
52. Hajjar, K.A. (1991) The endothelial cell tissue plasminogen activator receptor. Specific interaction with plasminogen. *J. Biol. Chem.*, **266**, 21962–70.
53. Harpel, P.C., Gordon, B.R. and Parker, T.S. (1989) Plasmin catalyzes binding of lipoprotein(a) to immobilized fibrinogen and fibrin. *Proc. Natl Acad. Sci. USA*, **86**, 3847–51.
54. Walton, K.W., Hitchens, J., Magnani, A.L. and Khan, M. (1974) A study of methods of identification and estimation of Lp(a) lipoprotein and of its significance in health, hyperlipidaemia and atherosclerosis. *Atherosclerosis*, **20**, 323–46.
55. Rath, M., Niendorf, A., Reblin, T. et al. (1988) Detection and quantification of lipoprotein(a) in the arterial wall of 107 coronary bypass patients. *Arteriosclerosis*, **9**, 579–92.
56. Niendorf, A., Rath, M., Wolf, K. et al. (1990) Morphological detection and quantification of lipoprotein(a) deposition in atheromatous lesions of human aorta and coronary arteries. *Virchows Arch. [A]*, **417**, 105–11.
57. Nachman, R.L., Gavish, D., Azrolan, N. and Clarkson, T.B. (1991) Lipoprotein(a) in diet-induced atherosclerosis in nonhuman primates. *Atheroscl. Thromb.*, **11**, 32–38.
58. Pepin, J., O'Neil, J. and Hoff, H.F. (1991) Quantification of apo(a) and apo B in human atherosclerotic lesions. *J. Lipid Res.*, **33**, 317–28.
59. Smith, E.B. and Staples, E.M. (1980) Distribution of plasma proteins across the human aortic wall. Barrier functions of endothelium and internal elastic lamina. *Atherosclerosis*, **37**, 579–90.
60. Wight, T. (1989) Cell biology of arterial proteoglycans. *Arteriosclerosis*, **9**, 1–20.
61. Camejo, G. (1982) The interaction of lipids and lipoproteins with the intercellular matrix of arterial tissue: its possible role in atherogenesis. *Adv. Lipid Res.*, **19**, 1–53.
62. Wagner, W.D., Edwards, I.J., St Clair, R.W. and Baraka, J. (1989) Low density lipoprotein interaction with artery-derived proteoglycan: the influence of LDL particle size and the relationship to athersclerosis susceptibility. *Atherosclerosis*, **75**, 49–59.
63. Iverius, P.H. (1972) The interaction between human plasma lipoproteins and connective tissue glycosaminoglycans. *J. Biol. Chem.*, **247**, 2607–13.
64. Mourao, P.A.S. and Bracamonte, C.A. (1984) The binding of human aortic gycosaminoglycans and proteoglycans to plasma low density lipoproteins. *Atherosclerosis*, **50**, 133–46.
65. Vijayagopal, P., Srinivasan, S.R., Radhakrishnamurthy, B. and Berenson, G.S. (1981) Interaction of serum lipoproteins and a proteoglycan from bovine aorta. *J. Biol. Chem.*, **256**, 8234–41.
66. Steele, R.H., Wagner, W.D., Rowe, H.A. and Edwards, I.J. (1987) Artery wall derived proteoglycan-plasma lipoprotein interaction: lipoprotein binding properties of extracted proteoglycans. *Atherosclerosis*, **65**, 51–62.
67. Srinivasan, S.R., Dolan, P., Radhakrishnamurthy, B. and Berenson, G.S. (1972) Isolation of lipoprotein-acid mucopolysaccharide complexes from fatty streaks of human aortas. *Atherosclerosis*, **16**, 95–104.
68. Mawhinney, T.P., Augustyn, J.M. and Fritz, K.E. (1978) Glycosaminoglycan–lipoprotein complexes from aortas of hypercholesterolemic rabbits. *Atherosclerosis*, **31**, 155–67.
69. Galis, Z.S., Misbahuddin, Z.A. and Moore, S. (1993) Co-localization of aortic apolipoprotein B and chondroitin sulfate in an injury model of atherosclerosis. *Am. J. Path.*, **142**, 1432–8.
70. Guyton, J.R., Bocan, T.M. and Schifani, T.A. (1985) Quantitative ultrastructural analysis of perifibrous lipid and its association with elastin in nonatherosclerotic human aorta. *Arteriosclerosis*, **5**, 644–52.
71. Kramsch, D.M. and Hollander, W. (1973) The interaction of serum and arterial lipoproteins with elastin of the arterial intima and its role in lipid accumulation in atherosclerotic plaques. *J. Clin. Invest.*, **52**, 236–47.
72. Podet, E.J., Shaffer, D.R., Gianturco, S.H. et al. (1991) Interaction of low density lipoproteins with human aortic elastin. *Arteriosc. Thromb.*, **11**, 116–22.
73. Klimov, A.N., Denisenko, A.D. and Magracheva, E.Y. (1974) Preparations of tissue fluid of the vessel wall and determination of its lipoproteins. *Atherosclerosis*, **19**, 243–51.
74. Gerö, S., Gergely, J., Jakab, L. et al. (1961) Comparative immunoelectrophoretic studies on homogenates of aorta pulmonary arteries and inferior vena cava of atherosclerotic individuals. *J. Atheroscl. Res.*, **1**, 88–91.
75. Hanig, M., Shainoff, J.R. and Lowy, A.D. (1956) Flotation lipoproteins extracted from human atherosclerotic aortas. *Science*, **124**, 176–7.
76. Hollander, W. (1976) Unified concept on the role of acid mucopolysaccharides and connective tissue proteins in the accumulation of lipids, lipoproteins and calcium in the atherosclerotic plaque. *Expl Mol. Path.*, **25**, 106–20.
77. Smith, E.B. and Slater, R.S. (1970) The chemical and immunological assay of low-density lipoproteins extracted from human aortic intima. *Artherosclerosis*, **11**, 417.
78. Laurell, C.B. (1972) Electroimmunoassay. *Scand. J. Lab. Invest.*, **29**, (suppl. 124), 21–37.
79. Hoff, H.F., Heideman, C.L., Gaubatz, J.W. et al. (1977) Quantitation of apolipoprotein B (apoB) in grossly normal human aorta. *Circ. Res.*, **40**, 56–63.
80. Hoff, H.F., Heideman, C.L., Gotto Jr, A.M. and Gaubatz, J.W. (1977) Apolipoprotein (apoB) retention in the grossly normal and atherosclerotic human aorta. *Circ. Res.*, **41**, 684–90.
81. Hoff, H.F., Gaubatz, J.W. and Gotto, A.M. (1979) ApoB concentration in the normal human aorta. *Biochim. Biophys. Res. Comm.*, **85**, 1424–30.
82. Hong, J., Pflug, J. and Reichl, D. (1984) Comparison of apoprotein B of low density lipoproteins of human interstitial fluid and plasma. *Biochem. J.*, **222**, 49–55.
83. Reichl, D., Myant, N.B. and Pflug, J.J. (1977) Concentration of lipoproteins containing apolipoprotein B in human peripheral lymph. *Biochim. Biophys. Acta*, **489**, 98–105.
84. Lindén, T., Bondjers, G., Fager, G. et al. (1989) Apolipoprotein B in human aortic biopsies in relation to serum lipids and lipoproteins. *Atherosclerosis*, **77**, 159–66.
85. Smith, E.B. and Staples, E.M. (1982) Plasma protein concentrations in interstitial fluid from human aortas. *Proc. Roy. Soc. Lond. B.*, **217**, 59–75.
86. Smith, E.B. and Slater, R.S. (1972) Relationship between low density lipoproteins in aortic intima and serum lipid levels. *Lancet*, **I**, 463–9.
87. Onitiri, A.C., Lewis, B., Bentall, H. et al. (1976) Lipoprotein concentrations in serum and in biopsy samples of arterial intima. A quantitative comparison. *Atherosclerosis*, **23**, 513–19.
88. Hoff, H.F., Heideman, C.L. and Gaubatz, J.W. (1977) Relationship between retention of buffer-extracted apoB and components of the human aortic intima. *Artery*, **3**, 379–94.
89. Smith, E.B., Massie, I.B. and Alexander, K.M. (1976) The release of an immobilized lipoprotein fraction from atherosclerotic lesions by incubation with plasmin. *Atherosclerosis*, **25**, 71–84.
90. Bradby, G.H.V., Walton, K.W. and Watts, R. (1979) The binding of total low density lipoproteins in human arterial intima affected and unaffected by atherosclerosis. *Atherosclerosis*, **32**, 403–22.
91. Hoff, H.F., Heideman, C.L., Gaubatz, J.W. et al. (1978) Detergent extraction of tightly-bound apoB from extracts of normal and aortic intima and plaques. *Expl Mol. Pathol.*, **28**, 290–300.
92. Hoff, H.F., Heideman, C.L., Gaubatz, J.W. et al. (1978) Quantitation of apoB in human aortic fatty streaks: a comparison with grossly normal intima and fibrous plaques. *Atherosclerosis*, **30**, 263–72.
93. Hoff, H.F., Heideman, C.L., Gaubatz, J.W. et al. (1978) Correlation of apolipoprotein B retention with the structure of atherosclerotic plaques from human aortas. *Lab. Invest.*, **38**, 560–7.
94. Hoff, H.F., Karagas, M., Heideman, C.L. et al. (1979) Correlation in the human aorta of apoB fractions with tissue cholesterol and collagen

content. *Atherosclerosis*, **32**, 259–68.
95. Smith, E.B., Alexander, K.M. and Massie, I.B. (1976) Insoluble 'fibrin' in human aortic intima. Quantitative studies on the relationship between insoluble 'fibrin', soluble fibrinogen and low density lipoprotein. *Atherosclerosis*, **23**, 19–39.
96. Smith, E.B., Keen, G.A. and Grant, A. (1990) Factors influencing the accumulation in fibrous plaques of lipid derived from low density lipoprotein. I. Relation between fibrin and immobilization of apo B-containing lipoprotein. *Atherosclerosis*, **884**, 165–71.
97. Hoff, H.F. and Gaubatz, J.W. (1979) Residual apoB in aortic plaques: comparison of amounts extracted with hydrolytic enzymes and with Triton X-100. *Artery*, **6**, 89–107.
98. St Clair, R.W. (1983) Atherosclerosis regression in animal models – current concepts of cellular and biochemical mechanisms. *Prog. Cardiovasc. Dis.*, **26**, 109–32.
99. Hoff, H.F. and Bond, M.G. (1982) Accumulation of lipoproteins containing apoB in the aorta of cholesterol-fed cynomolgous monkeys. *Atherosclerosis*, **43**, 329–39.
100. Hoff, H.F., Yamauchi, Y. and Bond, M.G. (1985) Reduction in tissue LDL accumulation during coronary artery regression in cynomolgus macaques. *Atherosclerosis*, **56**, 51–60.
101. Hoff, H.F., Gerrity, R.G., Naito, H.K. and Dusek, D.M. (1983) Quantitation of apolipoprotein B in aortas of hypercholesterolemic swine. *Lab. Invest.*, **48**, 492–504.
102. Gerrity, R.G., Richardson, M., Somer, J.B. *et al.* (1977) Endothelial cell morphology in areas of *in vivo* Evans blue uptake in the aorta of young pigs. II. Ultrastructure of the intima in areas of differing permeability to proteins. *Am. J. Pathol.*, **89**, 313–34.
103. Hoff, H.F. and Wagner, W. (1986) ApoB accumulation in the aortic arch in hypercholesterolemic swine is associated with alterations in tissue sulfated glycosaminoglycan composition. *Atherosclerosis*, **61**, 231–36.
104. Hoff, H.F., Dusek, D. and Lynn, M. (1986) Spacial distribution and accumulation of low density lipoproteins in the abdominal aorta of swine: determination by a novel electrotransfer procedure. *Lab. Invest.*, **55**, 377–86.
105. Spring, P.M. and Hoff, H.F. (1989) LDL accumulation in the grossly normal human iliac bifurcation and common iliac arteries. *Expl Mol. Pathol.*, **51**, 179–85.
106. Stary, H.C. (1983) Macrophages in coronary artery and aortic intima and in atherosclerotic lesions of children and young adults up to age 29, in *6th International Symposium on Atherosclerosis V*. (eds F.G. Schettler, A.M. Gotto, G. Middlehoff *et al.*), Springer-Verlag, New York, pp. 462–6.
107. Heideman, C.L. and Hoff, H.F. (1980) Quantitation of buffer-soluble apo A-I in the human aorta by electroimmunoassay. *Artery*, **6**, 354–67.
108. Heideman, C.L. and Hoff, H.F. (1982) Lipoproteins containing apo A-I extracted from human aortas. *Biochim. Biophys. Acta*, **711**, 431–44.
109. Ylä-Herttuala, S., Solakivi, T., Hirvonen, J. *et al.* (1987) Glycosaminoglycans and apolipoproteins B and A-1 in human aortas. *Arteriosclerosis*, **7**, 333–40.
110. Badimon, J.J., Badimon, L. and Fuster, V. (1990) Regression of atherosclerotic lesions by high density lipoprotein plasma fraction in the cholesterol-fed rabbit. *J. Clin. Invest.*, **85**, 1234–41.
111. Rothblat, G.H., Mahlberg, F., Johnson, W.J. and Phillips, M.C. (1992) Apolipoproteins, membrane cholesterol domains, and the regulation of cholesterol efflux. *J. Lipid Res.*, **33**, 1091–8.
112. Rubin, E.M., Krauss, R.M., Spangler, E.A. *et al.* (1991) Inhibition of early atherogenesis in transgenic mice by human apoliproprotein A-I. *Nature*, **353**, 265–7.
113. Cushing, G.L., Gaubatz, J.W., Burdick, B.J. *et al.* (1989) Quantitation and localization of apolipoproteins (a) and B in coronary artery bypass vein grafts resected at re-operation. *Arteriosclerosis*, **9**, 593–603.
114. Bihari-Varga, M., Gruber, E., Rotheneder, M. *et al.* (1988) Interaction of lipoprotein(a) [Lp(a)] and low density lipoprotein with glycosaminoglycans from human aorta. *Arteriosclerosis*, **8**, 851–7.
115. Smith, E.B. and Cochran, S. (1990) Factors influencing the accumulation in fibrous plaques of lipid derived from low density lipoprotein. II. Preferential immobilization of lipoprotein(a) Lp(a). *Atherosclerosis*, **84**, 173–81.
116. Yashiro, A., O'Neil, J. and Hoff, H.F. (1993) Insoluble complex formation of lipoprotein(a) with low density lipoprotein in the presence of calcium ions. *J. Biol. Chem.*, **268**, 4709–15.
117. Hoff, H.F., Bradley, W.A., Heideman, C.L. *et al.* (1979) Characterization of an LDL-like particle in the human aorta from grossly normal and atherosclerotic regions. *Biochim. Biophys. Acta*, **573**, 361–74.
118. Ylä-Herttuala, S., Jaakkola, O., Ehnholm, C. *et al.* (1988) Characterization of two lipoproteins containing apolipoproteins B and E from lesion-free human aortic intima. *J. Lipid Res.*, **29**, 563–72.
119. Hollander, W., Paddock, J. and Colombo, M. (1979) Lipoproteins in human atherosclerotic vessels. I. Biochemical properties of arterial low density lipoproteins, very low density lipoproteins, and high density lipoproteins. *Expl Mol. Pathol.*, **30**, 144–71.
120. Hoff, H.F. and Gaubatz, J.W. (1982) Isolation, purification, and characterization of a lipoprotein containing apoB from the human aorta. *Atherosclerosis*, **42**, 273–97.
121. Esterbauer, H., Gebicki, J., Puhl, H. and Jürgens, G. (1992) The role of lipid peroxidation and antioxidants in oxidative modification of LDL. *Free Rad. Biol. Med.*, **13**, 341–90.
122. Tailleux, A., Torpier, G., Caron, B. *et al.* (1993) Immunological properties of apoB-containing lipoprotein particles in human atherosclerotic arteries. *J. Lipid Res.*, **34**, 719–28.
123. Camejo, G., Hurt, E. and Romano, M. (1985) Properties of lipoprotein complexes isolated by affinity and chromatography from human aorta. *Biomed. Biochim. Acta*, **44**, 389–401.
124. Morton, R.E., West, G.A. and Hoff, H.F. (1986) A low density lipoprotein-sized particle isolated from human atherosclerotic lesions is recognized by a non-scavenger receptor mechanism on macrophages. *J. Lipid Res.*, **27**, 1124–34.
125. Srinivasan, S.R., Dolan, P., Radhakrishnamurthy, B. *et al.* (1975) Lipoprotein-acid mucopolysaccharide complexes of human atherosclerotic lesions. *Biochim. Biophys. Acta*, **388**, 58–70.
126. Camejo, G., Mateu, L., Lalaguna, F. *et al.* (1976) Structural individuality of human serum LDL associated with a differential affinity for a macromolecular component of the arterial wall. *Artery*, **2**, 79–97.
127. Camejo, G., López, A., López, F. and Quiñones, J. (1985) Interaction of low density lipoproteins with arterial proteoglycans. The role of charge and sialic acid content. *Atherosclerosis*, **55**, 93–105.
128. Morel, D.W., DiCorleto, P.E. and Chisolm, G.M. (1984) Endothelial and smooth muscle cells alter low density lipoprotein in vitro by free radical oxidation. *Arteriosclerosis*, **3**, 215–22.
129. Heinecke, J.W., Baker, L., Rosen H. and Chait, A. (1986) A superoxide-mediated modification of low density lipoprotein by arterial smooth muscle cells. *J. Clin. Invest.*, **77**, 757–61.
130. Cathcart, M.K., Morel, D.W. and Chisolm III, G.M. (1985) Monocytes and neutrophils oxidize low density lipoproteins making it cytotoxic. *J. Leukocyte Biol.*, **38**, 341–50.
131. Steinbrecher, U.P. (1987) Oxidation of human low density lipoprotein results in derivatization of lysine residues of apolipoprotein B by lipid peroxide decomposition products. *J. Biol. Chem.*, **262**, 3603–8.
132. Steinbrecher, U.P., Zhang, H. and Lougheed, M. (1990) Role of oxidatively modified LDL in atherosclerosis. *Free Rad. Biol. Med.*, **9**, 155–68.
133. Jürgens, G., Hoff, H.F., Chisolm, G.M. and Esterbauer, H. (1987) Modification of human low density lipoproteins by oxidation: characterization and patholphysiological implications. *Chem. Phys. Lipid*, **45**, 315–36.
134. Esterbauer, H., Schaur, R.J. and Zollner, H. (1991) Chemistry and biochemistry of 4-hydroxynonenal, malondialdehyde and related aldehydes. *Free Rad. Biol. Med.*, **11**, 81–128.
135. Uchida, K. and Stadtman, E.R. (1992) Selective cleavage of thioether linkage in proteins modified with 4-hydroxynonenal. *Proc. Natl Acad. Sci. USA*, **89**, 5611–15.
136. Hoff, H.F., Whitaker, T.E. and O'Neil, J. (1992) Oxidation of LDL leads to particle aggregation and altered macrophage recognition. *J. Biol. Chem.*, **267**, 602–9.
137. Hoff, H.F., O'Neil, J., Chisolm, G.M. *et al.* (1989) Modification of LDL with 4-hydroxynonenal induces uptake of LDL by macrophages. *Arteriosclerosis*, **9**, 538–49.
138. Hoff, H.F. and O'Neil, J.A. (1993) Modification of LDL with 4-hydroxynonenal and malondialdehyde as a model for soluble oxidized LDL. *J. Lipid Res.*, **34**, 1209–17.
139. Clevidence, B.A., Morton, R.E., West, G. *et al.* (1984) Cholesterol esterification in macrophages: stimulation by lipoproteins containing apoB isolated from human aortic plaques. *Arteriosclerosis*, **4**, 196–207.
140. Hoff, H.F. and O'Neil, J. (1991) Lesion-derived low-density lipoprotein and oxidized low density lipoprotein share a lability for aggregation, leading to enhanced macrophage degradation. *Arterioscl. Thromb.*, **3**, 1209–22.
141. Ylä-Herttuala, S., Palinski, W., Rosenfeld, M.E. *et al.* (1989) Evidence for the presence of oxidatively modified low density lipoprotein in atherosclerotic lesions of rabbit and man. *J. Clin. Invest.*, **84**, 1086–95.
142. Steinbrecher, U.P. and Lougheed, M. (1992) Scavenger receptor-independent stimulation of cholesteryl esterification in macrophages by low density lipoprotein extracted from human aortic intima. *Arterioscl. Thromb.*, **12**, 608–25.
143. Fong, L.G., Pathasarathy, S., Witztum, J.L. and Steinberg, D. (1987) Nonenzymatic oxidative cleavage of peptide bonds in apoprotein B-100. *J. Lipid Res.*, **28**, 1466–77.
144. Daugherty, A., Zweifel, B.S., Sobel, B.E. and Schonfeld, G. (1988) Isolation of low density lipoprotein from atherosclerotic vascular tissue of Watanabe heritable hyperlipidemic rabbits. *Arteriosclerosis*, **8**, 768–77.
145. Shaikh, M., Martini, S., Quiney, J.R. *et al.* (1988) Modified plasma-derived lipoproteins in human atherosclerotic plaques. *Atherosclerosis*, **69**, 165–72.
146. Palinski, W., Ylä-Herttuala, S., Rosenfeld, M.E. *et al.* (1990) Antisera and monoclonal antibodies specific for epitopes generated during oxidative modification of low density lipoprotein. *Arteriosclerosis*, **10**, 325–35.
147. Haberland, M.E., Fong, D. and Cheng, L. (1988) Malondialdehyde-altered protein occurs in atheroma of Watanabe heritable hyperlipidemic

rabbits. *Science*, **241**, 215–17.
148. Parthasarathy, S., Steinbrecher, U.P., Barnett, J. *et al.* (1985) Essential role of phospholipase A_2 activity in endothelial cell-induced modification of low density lipoprotein. *Proc. Natl Acad. Sci. USA*, **82**, 3000–4.
149. Hoff, H.F., O'Neil, J. and Yashiro, A. (1993) Partial characterization of Lp(a) extracted from human atherosclerotic lesions. *J. Lipid Res.*, **34**, 789–98.
150. Haberland, M.E., Fless, G.M., Scanu, A.M. and Fogelman, A.M. (1991) Malondialdehyde modification of lipoprotein(a) produces avid uptake by human monocyte-macrophages. *J. Biol. Chem.*, **267**, 4143–51.
151. Hoff, H.F., O'Neil, J. and Yashiro, A. (1994) Lipid-free apo(a) in human atherosclerotic lesions. *Chem. Phys. Lipids*, **67**, 419–28.
152. Trieu, V.N., Zioncheck, T.F., Lawn, R.M. and McConathy, W.J. (1991) Interaction of apolipoprotein(a) with apolipoprotein B-containing lipoproteins. *J. Biol. Chem.*, **266**, 5480–5.
153. Reichl, D. and Miller, N.E. (1986) The anatomy and physiology of reverse cholesterol transport. *Clin. Science*, **70**, 221–31.
154. Berliner, J.A., Territo, M.C., Sevanian, A. *et al.* (1990) Minimally modified low density lipoprotein stimulates monocyte endothelial interactions. *J. Clin. Invest.*, **85**, 1260–6.
155. Cushing, S.D., Berliner, J.A., Valente, A.J. *et al.* (1990) Minimally modified low density lipoprotein induces monocyte chemotactic protein 1 in human endothelial cells and smooth muscle cells. *Proc. Natl Acad. Sci. USA*, **87**, 5134–8.
156. Valente, A.J., Rozek, M.M., Sprague, E.A. and Schwartz, C.J. (1992) Mechanisms in intimal monocyte-macrophage recruitment. *Circulation*, **86**, (suppl. III), 20–25.
157. Quinn, M.T., Parthasarathy, S. and Steinberg, D. (1988) Lysophosphatidylcholine: a chemotactic factor for human monocytes and its potential role in atherogenesis. *Proc. Natl Acad. Sci. USA*, **85**, 2805–9.
158. Rajavashisth, T.B., Andalibi, A., Territo, M.C. *et al.* (1990) Modified low density lipoproteins induce endothelial cell expression of granulocyte and macrophage colony stimulating factors. *Nature*, **344**, 254–7.
159. Goldstein, J.L. and Brown, M.S. (1993) Low-density lipoprotein pathway and its relation to atherosclerosis. *Ann. Rev. Biochem.*, **46**, 897–930.
160. Sparrow, C.P., Parthasarathy, S. and Steinberg, D. (1989) A macrophage receptor that recognizes oxidized low density lipoprotein but not acetylated low density lipoprotein. *J. Biol. Chem.*, **264**, 2599–604.
161. Arai, H., Kita, T., Yokode, M. *et al.* (1989) Multiple receptors for modified low density lipoproteins in mouse peritoneal macrophages: different uptake mechanisms for acetylated and oxidized low density lipoproteins. *Biochem. Biophys. Res. Comm.*, **159**, 1375–82.
162. Brown, M.S. and Goldstein, J.L. (1983) Lipoprotein metabolism in the macrophage: implications for cholesterol deposition in atherosclerosis. *Ann. Rev. Biochem.*, **52**, 223–61.
163. Morel, D.W., Hessler, J.R. and Chisolm, G.M. (1983) Low density lipoprotein cytotoxicity induced by free radical peroxidation of lipid. *J. Lipid Res.*, **24**, 1070–6.
164. Sevanian, A. and Hochstein, P. (1985) Mechanisms and consequences of lipid peroxidation in biological systems. *Lipid Peroxidation*, **5**, 365–90.
165. Hoff, H.F., Chisolm, G.M., Morel, D.W. *et al.* (1988) Chemical and functional changes in LDL following modification by 4-hydroxynonenal, in *Oxy-radicals in Molecular Biology and Pathology*, (eds P.A. Cerutti, I. Fredovich and J.M. McCord). Alan R. Liss, Inc., NY, pp. 459–72.
166. Benedetti, A., Comporti, M. and Esterbauer, H. (1980) Identification of 4-hydroxynonenal as a cytotoxic product originating from the peroxidation of liver microsomal lipids. *Biochim. Biophys. Acta.*, **620**, 281–96.
167. Kosugi, K., Morel, D.W., DiCorleto, P.E. and Chisolm, G.M. (1987) Toxicity of oxidized low density lipoproteins to culture fibroblasts is selective for the S phase of the cell cycle. *J. Cell. Physiol.*, **102**, 119–27.
168. Cooper, J.A. (1987) Effects of cytochalasin and phalloidin on actin. *J. Cell Biol.*, **105**, 1473–8.
169. Hoff, H.F., Zyromski, N., Armstrong, D. and O'Neil, J.A. (1993) Aggregated oxidized LDL is poorly processed in mouse peritoneal macrophages. *J. Lipid Res.*, **34**, 1919–29.
170. Hoff, H.F. and Cole, T.B. (1990) Macrophage uptake of LDL modified by 4-hydroxynonenal: an ultrastructural study. *Lab. Invest.*, **64**, 254–64.
171. Anderson, R.G.W. (1986) Methods for visualization of the LDL pathway in cultured human fibroblasts. *Methods Enzymol.*, **129**, 201–6.
172. Robenek, H., Schmitz, G. and Assmann, G. (1984) Topography and dynamics of receptors for acetylated and malondialdehyde-modified low-density lipoprotein in the plasma membrane of mouse peritoneal macrophages as visualized by colloidal gold in conjunction with surface replicas. *J. Histochem. Cytochem.*, **32**, 1017–27.
173. Carew, T.E., Schwenke, D.C. and Steinberg, D. (1987) Antiatherogenic effect of probucol unrelated to its hypocholesterolemic effect: evidence that antioxidants in vivo can selectively inhibit low density lipoprotein degradation in macrophage-rich fatty streaks and slow the progression of atherosclerosis in the Watanabe heritable hyperlipidemic rabbit. *Proc. Natl Acad. Sci. USA*, **84**, 7725–9.
174. Mao, S.J.T., Yates, M.T., Parker, R.A. *et al.* (1991) Attenuation of atherosclerosis in a modified strain of hypercholesterolemic Watanabe rabbits using a probucol analog (MDL 29, 311) that does not lower serum cholesterol. *Arterioscl. Thromb.*, **11**, 1266–75.

175. Kita, T., Nagano, Y., Yokode, M. *et al.* (1987) Probucol prevents the progression of atherosclerosis in Watanabe heritable hyperlipidemic rabbit, an animal model for familial hypercholesterolemia. *Proc. Natl Acad. Sci. USA*, **84**, 5928–31.
176. Daugherty, A., Zweifel, B.S. and Schonfeld, G. (1989) Probucol attenuates the development of aortic atherosclerosis in cholesterol-fed rabbits. *Br. J. Pharmacol.*, **98**, 612–18.
177. Verlangieri, A.J. and Bush, M.J. (1992) Effects of d-α-tocopherol supplementation on experimentally induced primate atherosclerosis. *Amer. Coll. Nutr.*, **11**, 131–8.
178. Gey, E., Puska, P., Jordan, P. and Moser, U.K. (1991) Inverse correlation between plasma vitamin E and mortality from ischemic heart disease in cross cultural epidemiology. *Am. J. Clin. Nutr.*, **53**, 3268–43.
179. Riemersma, R.A., Wood, D.A., Macintyre, C.C.A. *et al.* (1991) Risk of angina pectoris and plasma concentrations of vitamins A, C and E and carotene. *Lancet*, **337**, 1–5.
180. Hoff, H.F., O'Neil, J. and Cole, T.B. (1991) Macrophage degradation of LDL extracted from human aortic plaque: effect of isolation procedures on the interaction of LDL extracted from human aortic plaques with macrophages in culture. *Expl Mol. Pathol.*, **54**, 72–86.
181. Hoff, H.F., Pepin, J. and Morton, R.E. (1991) Modified low density lipoprotein isolated from atherosclerotic lesions does not cause lipid accumulation in aortic smooth muscle cells. *J. Lipid Res.*, **32**, 115–24.
182. Lougheed, M., Zhang, H. and Steinbrecher, U.P. (1991) Oxidized low density lipoprotein is resistant to cathepsins and accumulates within macrophages. *J. Biol. Chem.*, **266**, 14519–25.
183. Jessup, W., Mander, E.L. and Dean, R.T. (1992) The intracellular storage and turnover of apolipoprotein B of oxidized LDL in macrophages. *Biochim. Biophys. Acta*, **1126**, 167–77.
184. Ball, R.Y., Bindman, J.P., Carpenter, K.L.H. and Mitchinson, M.J. (1986) Oxidized low density lipoprotein induces ceroid accumulation by murine peritoneal macrophages in vitro. *Atherosclerosis*, **60**, 173–81.
185. Boyd, H.C., Gown, A.M., Wolfbauer, G. and Chait, A. (1989) Direct evidence for a protein recognized by a monoclonal antibody against oxidatively modified LDL in atherosclerotic lesions from a Watanabe heritable hyperlipidemic rabbit. *Am. J. Pathol.*, **135**, 815–25.
186. Mitchinson, M.J. (1982) Insoluble lipids in human atherosclerotic plaques. *Atheosclerosis*, **45**, 11–15.
187. Gruenberg, J. and Howell, K.E. (1989) Membrane traffic in endocytosis: insights from cell-free assays. *Ann. Rev. Cell. Biol.*, **5**, 453–81.
188. Khoo, J.C., Miller, E., McLoughlin, P. Steinberg, D. (1988) Enhanced macrophage uptake of low density lipoprotein after self-aggregation. *Arteriosclerosis*, **8**, 348–58.
189. Roma, P., Bernini, F., Fogliatto, R. *et al.* (1992) Defective catabolism of oxidized LDL by J774 murine macrophages. *J. Lipid Res.*, **33**, 819–29.
190. Zhang, H., Basra, H.J.K. and Steinbrecher, U.P. (1990) Effects of oxidatively modified LDL on cholesterol esterification in cultured macrophages. *J. Lipid Res.*, **31**, 1361–9.
191. Fruebis, J., Parthasarathy, S. and Steinberg, D. (1992) Evidence for a concerted reaction between lipid hydroperoxides and polypeptides. *Proc. Natl Acad. Sci. USA*, **89**, 10588–92.
192. Steinbrecher, U.P., Lougheed, M., Kwan, W.-C. and Dirks, M. (1989) Recognition of oxidized low density lipoprotein by the scavenger receptor of macrophages results from derivatization of apolipoprotein B by products of fatty acid peroxidation. *J. Biol. Chem.*, **264**, 15216–23.
193. Uchida, K. and Stadtman, E.R. (1993) Covalent attachment of 4-hydroxynonenal to glyceraldehyde-3-phosphate dehydrogenase. A possible involvement of intra- and intermolecular cross-linking reaction. *J. Biol. Chem.*, **268**, 6388–93.
194. Kita, T., Yokode, M., Arai, H. *et al.* (1993) Cigarette smoke, LDL and cholesteryl ester accumulation in macrophages. Implications for atherosclerosis. *Ann. N.Y. Acad. Sci.*, **686**, 91–8.
195. Hoff, H.F. and O'Neil, J. (1988) Extracts of human atherosclerotic lesions can modify LDL leading to enhanced uptake by macrophages. *Atherosclerosis*, **70**, 9–41.
196. Vijayagopal, P., Srinivasan, S.R., Xu, J. (1993) Lipoprotein-proteoglycan complexes induce continued cholesteryl ester accumulation in foam cells from rabbit atherosclerotic lesions. *J. Clin. Invest.*, **91**, 1011–18.
197. Brownlee, M., Vlassara, H. and Cerami, A. (1985) A nonenzymatic glycosylation product on collagen covalently traps low density lipoprotein. *Diabetes*, **34**, 938–41.
198. Vlassara, H. (1992) Receptor-mediated interactions of advanced glycosylation end products with cellular components within diabetic tissues. *Diabetes*, **41**, 52–56.
199. Koo, C., Wernette-Hammond, M.E. and Innerarity, T.L. (1986) Uptake of canine β-very low density lipoproteins by mouse peritoneal macrophages is mediated by a low density lipoprotein receptor. *J. Biol. Chem.*, **261**, 11194–201.
200. Kowal, R.C., Herz, J., Weisgraber, K.H. *et al.* (1990) Opposing effects of apolipoproteins E and C on lipoprotein binding to low density lipoprotein receptor-related protein. *J. Biol. Chem.*, **265**, 10771–9.
201. Vijayagopal, P., Srinivasan, S.R., Jones, K.M. *et al.* (1985) Complexes of low density lipoproteins and arterial proteoglycan aggregates promote cholesteryl ester accumulation in mouse macrophages. *Biochim. Biophys.*

Acta, 837, 251–61.
202. Falcone, D.J., Mateo, N., Shio, H. et al. (1984) Lipoprotein-heparin-fibronectin-denatured collagen complexes enhance cholesteryl ester accumulation in macrophages. J. Cell. Biol., 99, 1266–74.
203. Ylä-Herttuala, S., Jaakola, O., Solakivi, T. et al. (1986) The effect of proteoglycans, collagen and lysyl oxidase on the metabolism of low density lipoprotein by macrophages. Atherosclerosis, 62, 73–80.
204. Falcone, D.J. and Salisbury, B.G.J. (1988) Fibronectin stimulates macrophage uptake of low density lipoprotein-heparin-collagen complexes. Arteriosclerosis, 8, 263–73.
205. Burstein, M. and Scholnick, H.R. (1973) Lipoprotein-polyanion-metal interactions. Adv. Lipid Res., 11, 67–108.
206. Camejo, G., Hurt, E., Wiklund, O. et al. (1991) Modifications of low density lipoprotein induced by arterial proteoglycans and chondroitin-6-sulfate. Biochim. Biophys. Acta, 1096, 253–61.
207. Hurt, E., Bondjers, G. and Camejo, G. (1990) Interaction of LDL with human arterial proteoglycans stimulates its uptake by human monocyte-derived macrophages. J. Lipid Res., 31, 443–54.
208. Hurt-Camejo, E., Camejo, G., Rosengren, B. et al. (1992) Effect of arterial proteoglycans and glycosaminoglycans on low density lipoprotein oxidation and its uptake by human macrophages and arterial smooth muscle cells. Arteriosci. Thromb., 12, 569–83.
209. Haberland, M.E., Olch, C.L. and Fogelman, A.M. (1984) Role of lysines in mediating interaction of modified low density lipoproteins with the scavenger receptor of human monocyte macrophages. J. Biol. Chem., 259, 11305–11.
210. Klimov, A.N., Denisenko, A.D., Popov, A.V. et al. (1985) Lipoprotein-antibody immune complexes: the catabolism and role in foam cell formation. Atherosclerosis, 58, 1–15.
211. Lopes-Virella, M.F., Griffith, R.L., Shunk, K.A. and Virella, G.T. (1991) Enhanced uptake and impaired intracellular metabolism of low density lipoprotein complexed with anti-low density lipoprotein antibodies. Arterioscl. Thromb., 11, 1356–67.
212. Griffith, R.L., Virella, G.T., Stevenson, H.C. and Lopes-Virella, M.F. (1988) Low density lipoprotein metabolism by human macrophages activated with low density lipoprotein immune complexes: a possible mechanism of foam cell formation. J. Expl Med., 168, 1041–59.
213. Orekhov, A.N., Tertov, V.V., Kabakov, A.E. et al. (1991) Autoantibodies against modified low density lipoprotein. Nonlipid factor of blood plasma that stimulates foam cell formation. Arterioscl. Thromb., 11, 316–26.
214. Hollander, W., Colombo, M.A., Kirkpatrick, B. and Paddock, J. (1979) Soluble proteins in the human atherosclerotic plaque: with special reference to immunoglobulins, C_3-complement component, α1-antitrypsin and α1-macroglobulin. Atherosclerosis, 34, 391–405.
215. Parums, O. and Mitchinson, M.J. (1981) Demonstration of immunoglobulin in the neighbourhood of advanced atherosclerotic plaques. Atherosclerosis, 38, 211–16.
216. Witztum, J.L. and Steinberg, D. (1991) Role of oxidized low density lipoprotein in atherogenesis. J. Clin. Invest., 88, 1785–92.
217. Witztum, J.L., Steinbrecher, U.P., Kasaniemi, Y.A. and Fisher, M. (1984) Autoantibodies to glucosylated proteins in the plasma of patients with diabetes mellitus. Proc. Natl Acad. Sci. USA, 81, 3204–8.
218. Salonen, J.T., Ylä-Herttuala, S., Yamamoto, R. et al. (1992) Autoantibody against oxidized LDL and progression of carotid atherosclerosis. Lancet, 339, 883–7.
219. Kokkonen, J.O. and Kovanen, P.T. (1990) The metabolism of low density lipoproteins by rat serosal mast cells. Eur. Heart J., 11, 134–46.
220. Heinecke, J.W., Suits, A.G., Aviram, M. and Chait, A. (1991) Phagocytosis of lipase-aggregated low density lipoprotein promotes macrophage foam cell formation. Sequential morphological and biochemical events. Arterioscl. Thromb., 11, 1643–51.
221. Xu, X.-X. and Tabas, I. (1991) Sphingomyelinase enhances low density lipoprotein uptake and ability to induce cholesteryl ester accumulation in macrophages. J. Biol. Chem., 266, 24849–58.
222. Guyton, J.R., Klemp, K.F. and Mims, M.P. (1991) Altered ultrastructural morphology of self-aggregated low density lipoproteins: coalescence of lipid domains forming droplets and vesicles. J. Lipid Res., 32, 953–62.
223. Wolfbauer, G., Glick, J.M., Minor, L.K. et al. (1986) Development of the smooth muscle foam cell: Uptake of macrophage lipid inclusions. Proc. Natl Acad. Sci. USA, 83, 7760–4.
224. Goldstein, J.L., Hoff, H.F., Ho, Y.K. et al. (1981) Stimulation of cholesteryl ester synthesis in macrophages by extracts of atherosclerotic human aortas and complexes of albumin/cholesteryl esters. Arteriosclerosis, 1, 210–26.
225. Hoff, H.F. and Clevidence, B.A. (1987) Uptake by mouse peritoneal macrophages of large cholesteryl ester-rich particles isolated from human atherosclerotic lesions. Expl Mol. Pathol., 46, 331–44.
226. Hoff, H.F. (1972) Human intracranial atherosclerosis: a histochemical and ultrastructural study of gross fatty streak lesions. Am. J. Pathol., 69, 421–30.
227. Fainaru, M., Mahley, R.W., Hamilton, R.L. and Innerarity, T.L. (1982) Structural and metabolic heterogeneity of β-very low density lipoproteins from cholesterol-fed dogs and from humans with Type III hyperlipoproteinemia. J. Lipid Res., 23, 702–14.
228. Kruth, H.S. (1985) Subendothelial accumulation of unesterified cholesterol. An early event in atherosclerotic lesion development. Atherosclerosis, 57, 337–41.
229. Chao, F.-F., Blanchette-Mackie, E.J., Chen, Y.-J. et al. (1990) Characterization of two unique cholesterol-rich lipid particles isolated from human atherosclerotic lesions. Am. J. Pathol., 136, 169–79.
230. Mora, R., Lupu, F. and Simionescu, N. (1989) Cytochemical localization of β-lipoproteins and their components in successive stages of hyperlipidemic atherogenesis of rabbit aorta. Atherosclerosis, 79, 183–95.
231. Mora, R., Simionescu, M. and Simionescu, N. (1990) Purification and partial characterization of extracellular liposomes isolated from the hyperlipidemic rabbit aorta. J. Lipid Res, 31, 1793–807.
232. Frank, J.S. and Fogelman, A.M. (1990) Ultrastructure of the intima in WHHL and cholesterol-fed rabbit aortas prepared by ultra-rapid freezing and freeze-etching. J. Lipid Res., 30, 967–78.
233. Nievelstein, P.F., Fogelman, A.M., Mottino, G. et al. (1991) Lipid accumulation in rabbit aortic intima 2 hours after bolus infusion of low density lipoprotein: a deep-etch and immunolocalization study of ultrarapidly frozen tissue. Arterioscl. Thromb., 11, 1795–805.
234. Robenek, H. and Schmitz, G. (1988) Ca^{++} antagonists and ACAT inhibitors promote cholesterol efflux from macrophages by different mechanisms. II. Characterization of intracellular morphologic changes. Arteriosclerosis, 8, 57–67.
235. Tangirala, R.K., Mahlberg, F.H., Glick, J.M. et al. (1993) Lysosomal accumulation of unesterified cholesterol in model macrophage foam cells. J. Biol. Chem., 268, 9653–60.
236. Chao, F.F., Blanchette-Mackie, E.J., Tertov, V.V. et al. (1991) Hydrolysis of cholesteryl ester in low density lipoprotein converts this lipoprotein to a liposome. J. Biol. Chem., 267, 4992–8.
237. Seifert, P.S., Hugo, F., Tranum-Jensen, J. et al. (1990) Isolation and characterization of a complement-activating lipid extracted from human atherosclerotic lesions. J. Expl Med., 172, 547–57.
238. Hoff, H.F., O'Neil, J., Papin, J.M. and Cole, T.B. (1990) Macrophage uptake of cholesterol-containing particles derived from LDL and isolated from atherosclerotic lesions. Eur. Heart J., 11, 105–15.

8 HISTOCHEMISTRY AND IMMUNOCHEMISTRY OF VASCULAR DISEASE

Dinah V. Parums

8.1 Histochemistry of vascular disease

Histochemical techniques are of special value in vascular pathology. They include those that demonstrate not only vascular cellular morphology but also demonstrate the integrity of elastic fibres, normal and abnormal connective tissue, micro-organisms, the integrity of basement membranes, soluble and insoluble lipids, fibrin, depositions such as calcium, amyloid and endogenous pigments such as iron and lipofuscin and inflammatory cell populations.

The methodologies for performing these techniques may be consulted in standard texts such as Pearse [1] or Bancroft and Cook [2]. In this chapter, some aspects of histochemistry that are of special relevance to vascular pathology will be covered. Some histochemical topics of relevance to the immunohistochemistry of vascular disease will be mentioned again in section 8.2.

8.1.1 HISTOCHEMICAL METHODS FOR LIGHT MICROSCOPY OF VASCULAR DISEASE

(a) Haematoxylin and eosin (H&E)

Tissue morphology in vascular pathology may be best assessed after H&E staining as described by Cole [3].

Method
After dewaxing, paraffin sections are placed in the following: 30% haematoxylin for 5 min, tap water for 5 min, 1% acid alcohol for 5–10 s, water for 5 min, Scott's solution for a few seconds, 0.5% eosin for 10 s and water for 5 min; they are finally dehydrated through alcohols, cleared in xylene and mounted in distrine dibutyl phthalate xylene (DPX) mountant. H&E staining results in blue nuclei, pink cytoplasm, deep pink muscle fibres, pale pink collagen, orange red blood cells and deep pink fibrin.

(b) Elastic van Gieson (EVG)

EVG staining is used to assess the degree of fibrosis and elastin within tissue sections [4] (Plate 3).

Method
After dewaxing, paraffin sections are placed in the following: 0.5% acidified potassium permanganate for 5 min, water to rinse, 2% oxalic acid to bleach, 95% industrial grade alcohol and then Miller's stain for 2–3 h. Slides are rinsed in 95% industrial grade alcohol, next in water and then counterstained with van Gieson for 3 min. Stained sections are dehydrated through graded alcohols, cleared in xylene, and mounted in DPX mountant. EVG stains elastin blue/black, collagen red and red blood cells yellow.

8.1.2 LIPID HISTOCHEMISTRY

The use of histochemical techniques to interpret histological structural changes in chemical terms was pioneered over 150 years ago by botanists who used iodine to detect starch granules [1]. It was not until 1936, when Lison first published *Histochemie Animale*, that histochemistry was first recognized as an established science [5]. Until that time, biologists and pathologists had to assess microscopical preparations morphologically.

The word **lipid** has been defined by Lovern (1955) as 'a derivative of fatty acids and their metabolites' [6]. The major lipid classes consist of fatty acids linked to alcohols, such as glycerol, by ester bonds or to bases, by amide bonds. Some contain, in addition, organic bases, phosphoric acid and sugars. The term **fat** is generally applied to triglycerides and the word 'oil' to fats that are liquid [1]. In histochemical terms, the most useful distinction is that between hydrophobic and hydrophilic lipids, which determines their predilection for organic solvents or aqueous reagents.

Ceroid has been classified only by its solubility and staining characteristics [7]. It is classified as a lipopigment – a sudanophilic substance which is insoluble in lipid solvents and is acid-fast. Ceroid is found in most advanced human atherosclerotic plaques [8], both extracellularly and within macrophages, both in granule and 'ring' forms. Both the extracellular and intracellular ceroid possess a characteristic laminated or 'fingerprint' appearance under electron microscopy with a periodicity of 8–14 nm.

Ceroid will fluoresce apple green under UV excitation (Plate 4) and this is one method of detecting its presence in a vessel. This property should also be borne in mind when using immunofluorescence techniques in the study of vascular disease.

An alternative definition of a lipopigment has been proposed by Dowson [9] as 'a constituent of tissue which exhibits yellow autofluorescence'. The characteristic autofluorescence emission spectrum from ceroid has been distinguished from that of lipofuscin and these two lipopigments are thought to differ in composition [9].

Ceroid is sudanophilic, which indicates that hydrophobic sudan dyes can dissolve in it. In contrast to most other sudanophilic substances, ceroid is resistant to lipid extraction by the solvents used in the preparation of paraffin sections. It may be visualized in routinely processed tissue sections which have been treated with ethanol and xylene by the use of lipid stains such as oil red-O (ORO).

(a) Oil-red-O method (ORO) [10]

Atheroma contains soluble lipid in the form of cholesterol and insoluble lipid in the form of ceroid. Indeed, insoluble lipid or ceroid is the hallmark of the advanced plaque. In order to determine the presence of atheroma as distinct from organized thrombus within a vessel, of atheroemboli, and to grade any atherosclerotic lesion, a reliable lipid stain is recommended. We have found ORO to be reliable for the detection of soluble lipid in frozen sections and for insoluble lipid in formalin-fixed, paraffin-embedded material (Plate 5).

Method

0.5 g of ORO is dissolved in 200 ml of isopropyl alcohol and warmed in a 56°C water bath for 1 h as the stock solution. The working solution is prepared prior to use by adding 4 parts of distilled water to 6 parts of stock solution. This is filtered prior to use. Sections are rinsed in water, followed by rinse in 60% isopropyl alcohol prior to staining with the working solution for 10 min. Sections are then washed briefly in 60% isopropyl alcohol and thoroughly in water prior to counterstaining with Carazzi's haematoxylin for 2 min. Sections are washed and mounted in glycerol-gelatin. Unsaturated, hydrophobic lipids stain red.

(b) Nile blue sulphate method (NBS) [11]

Method

10 ml of 1% H_2SO_4 is added to 200 ml of 1% Nile blue sulphate (Sigma) and boiled under reflux for 1 h. This solution is cooled and filtered and the pH adjusted to 2.0. Sections are stained with Nile blue sulphate solution at 37°C for 30 min prior to differentiation in 1% acetic acid for 2 min. Sections are washed well and mounted in glycerol-gelatin. Phospholipids and free fatty acids stain blue.

(c) Periodic acid–Schiff (PAS) [12]

Method

Schiff's reagent is prepared by adding 1 g of basic fuchsin to 200 ml of boiling distilled water. On cooling, 2 g of sodium metabisulphite is added followed by 2 ml of concentrated HCl and 2 g of charcoal. The mixture is filtered and stored in the dark at 4°C. Sections are taken to water and treated with periodic acid solution for 5 min, rinsed and treated with Schiff's reagent for 15 min. Sections are washed in tap water for 10 min, counterstained with haematoxylin, dehydrated and mounted in DPX. Diastase digestion could be incorporated into the technique to digest glycogen. PAS-positive material, such as ceroid, stains magenta (Plate 6).

(d) Modified Ziehl–Neelsen (MZN) [1]

Method

Carbol fuchsin solution is prepared by dissolving 1 g of fuchsin (Sigma) in 10 ml of ethanol; 5 g of phenol is then dissolved in 100 ml of distilled water, the two solutions mixed and the whole is filtered. Sections are taken to water and stained in filtered carbol fuchsin solution for 3 h at 56°C, washed well in water and differentiated in 1% acid-alcohol for 3 min. Sections are washed and counterstained by incubation in 0.2% aqueous methylene blue for 1 min prior to washing. Sections are dehydrated and differentiated in alcohol. Lipopigments are stained bright magenta.

8.1.3 LECTIN HISTOCHEMISTRY

Lectins, from the Latin word *legere*, to choose, are sugar-binding proteins or glycoproteins of non-immune origin, which agglutinate cells and/or precipitate glycoconjugates having saccharides of appropriate complementarity. They bear at least two recognition sites which bind non-covalently to specific carbohydrate residues without modifying these residues chemically.

Lectins were discovered in 1888 by Stillmark [13], who reported that extracts of castor beans (*Ricinus communis*) agglutinated human and some other animal erythrocytes. Since then, numerous lectins have been identified, purified and characterized from diverse sources including plants, bacteria, fungi, invertebrates and vertebrates. Lectins have been utilized extensively to isolate glycoproteins and polysaccharides and as tools to investigate the sugar residues of the cell surface coat or glycocalyx. In histopathology, they have been used as histochemical markers to identify a variety of cell types in histologic sections.

Lectins have specific affinities for different cell types in lymphoid tissues [14]. It has been reported that Concanavalin A (Con A), *Phaseolus vulgaris* agglutinin (PhA) and wheat germ agglutinin (WGA) show strong cytoplasmic staining for macrophages in formalin-fixed, paraffin-embedded sections of reactive lymph nodes [14]. *Ulex europaeus* agglutinin (UEA) has been shown to be a useful marker for vascular endothelium [15] and peanut agglutinin (PNA) is known to bind to germinal centre lymphocytes of B cell origin [16].

8.2 Immunocytochemistry of vascular disease

The concept of using labelled antibodies to localize antigens in histological tissue sections was pioneered by Coons *et al.* in 1941 [17] who used fluorescein-labelled antibodies. Since then, the concept has been modified and expanded and today, immunolabelling techniques have enabled the localization of cells and tissues with improved diversity, sensitivity and specificity of staining reactions.

Of the many types of label available to denote the site of antibody binding, fluorescence and enzyme-conjugated antibodies have been most widely used for light microscopy. Although the immunofluorescence method is simple and requires no inhibition of endogenous enzyme or incubation in substrate, the technique suffers from the disadvantage that the preparations are not permanent because the fluorescence label eventually fades. Another difficulty encountered when the complex topographical relationship of cells is studied in the atherosclerotic artery with this label is that the background details are difficult to appreciate. In contrast, the use of immunoenzyme techniques allow both the label and the tissue architecture to be visualized and allows for combinations of histochemical and immunohistochemical staining. For these reasons, immunoenzyme localization seems most appropriate for the study of vascular disease.

Antibodies can be raised to a wide range of molecular entities: cell structural components, cell products (cytokines, enzymes, immunoglobulins) and cell surface receptors. Most antibodies are raised against components and products of normal cells, but some are directed against antigens derived from malignant cells.

8.2.1 FACTORS GOVERNING THE CHOICE OF IMMUNOHISTOCHEMICAL METHOD

Many immunohistochemical methods are available, so many that one could easily become confused and swamped by the apparent complexity of the situation [18]. How should the tissues be obtained, fixed and processed? Which antibodies should be used? Which immunodetection system should be used? Whilst this diversity may be of benefit for scientific study, the constraints imposed within a diagnostic setting means that only a small number of possibilities can be considered. The following are the major criteria upon which the choice of techniques for routine diagnostic applications is made:

1. **Sensitivity** A sensitive technique will reveal small amounts of antigen with minimal background staining. This depends upon the avidity, affinity and titre of the primary antibodies and the sensitivity of the detection system. Although it is desirable to obtain sufficient sensitivity to ensure an accurate diagnosis, this must be balanced against the effect upon the cost and the length of time taken to perform the technique.
2. **Reliability and reproducibility** For daily use, consistency of results is more important than exquisite sensitivity which may be time-consuming and inconsistent. Thus, a method which is simple to operate in terms of the number of steps involved and in the simplicity of the reagents employed, gives fewer opportunities for error.
3. **Cost** Immunohistochemical methods can be expensive in terms of operator time, reagents and equipment. However, a careful choice at the outset can reduce these costs without compromising the final result.
4. **Versatility** Any method needs to be applicable to all types of tissue and tissue preparation.
5. **Applicability to automation and batch staining.**
6. **Safety.**

8.2.2 TISSUE PREPARATION

The mainstay of the diagnostic pathology laboratory is the formalin-fixed block of tissue, processed to paraffin wax, sectioned and mounted upon glass slides. It is a system which has been used for many decades, reflecting the histopathologist's need to provide a diagnosis based largely upon morphological criteria. It will undoubtedly remain the mainstay for years to come, it is a system with considerable limitations.

The procedures necessary to produce the wax block and the subsequent sections can have deleterious effects upon many of the tissue components which one wishes to demonstrate. Loss, diffusion, reduction, chemical alteration or masking of antigen may occur making demonstration difficult if not impossible. It is important to appreciate that the range of antigens which can be demonstrated in paraffin-processed tissue is restricted when compared to that achieved in frozen sections. The decision whether to fix material or arrange for some to be frozen depends critically on which antigens one wishes to demonstrate.

(a) Reception of specimens

Tissues should be dealt with promptly by freezing or fixation to retain maximum tissue antigenicity without compromising the morphology or allowing autolysis to occur and to avoid antigen loss and diffusion.

Satisfactory studies can also be performed on tissues taken at autopsy with the freshest tissue generally giving the best results.

(b) Section quality

The basic requirement of any method using tissue sections is to produce high quality, flat, thin sections mounted upon clean slides. Scored, inappropriately thick or compressed sections do not make for easy interpretation, are more likely to be removed during the immunostaining procedure and give inconsistent results.

(c) Section adhesives

The duration of some methods may increase the chances of the section being removed from the slide. Where problems are likely to occur, a number of adhesives can be employed without interfering with the subsequent procedures. We routinely employ gelatine–chrome-alum-coated slides for all work involving cryostat and freeze-dried sections and for paraffin-processed sections, particularly those containing atheroma, which may readily detach. This latter category also includes tissues that have been subject to acid decalcification or which have been suboptimally processed.

A procedure for the coating of slides with gelatine–chrome–alum is described in *Protocol 1* below. Gelatin coatings may not be sufficient to ensure adequate adhesion when sections have to be pretreated with various proteolytic enzymes, in which case stronger adhesives such as poly-L-lysine or one of a number of commercially available adhesives may be used.

Protocol 1 (Gelatin–chrome–alum coating of slides [18])

1. Dissolve 2.5 g gelatin in 500 ml distilled water by heating to 50°C with continuous stirring.
2. When dissolved, add 0.25 g chrome–alum and mix well.
3. Cool to room temperature and store at 4°C.
4. Before use, heat the solid to 60°C and filter the resultant liquid into a Coplin jar or other staining tank.
5. Dip the clean slides into the solution, carefully avoiding contamination of bench surfaces. Load the slides into racks and place in a 60°C incubator for at least 1 h to dry. When cool, slides can be placed in boxes and stored at room temperature.

(d) Frozen sections

Cryostat sections of frozen tissues offer the best opportunity for the demonstration of the broadest spectrum of antigens. However, this can only be achieved if those tissues have been collected and handled appropriately at the outset, and once sectioned, fixed in such a way that good antigen preservation and tissue morphology are achieved. A suitable procedure is given in *Protocol 2* below.

Tissue selection, freezing and storage

Tissues selected for frozen section studies ideally need to be of a size no larger than 10 × 10 × 5 mm, labelled appropriately and snap-frozen in liquid nitrogen. It may, in some circumstances, be advantageous to use isopentane cooled by liquid nitrogen to hasten the freezing process. Once frozen, tissue should be stored in liquid nitrogen or in a −70°C freezer and when required for sectioning, their temperature should not be permitted to rise above −20°C. It should also be noted that long-term storage of tissue blocks at low temperatures has a dessicating effect and so the storage system should take this into consideration.

Sectioning

For most work, sections should be cut at 4–6 μm. They are then covered and left to air-dry for a minimum of 30 min at room temperature and up to 24 h at 4°C. When sections are not required for immunostaining within 24 h, slides should be wrapped back-to-back and sealed in aluminium foil and stored at −20°C.

Fixation

Absolute acetone, used either at room temperature or at 4°C is used. Sections are immersed for 10 min and then allowed to air-dry. Antibodies or blocking agents are applied directly to the dry section and thereafter, the section must not be allowed to dry.

Protocol 2 (Preparation of frozen sections for immunocytochemistry)

1. Cut 5 μm cryostat sections from snap-frozen tissue blocks and air-dry. If sections are not required for immunostaining within 24 h, wrap the slides in foil, label them and store at −20°C. When needed, remove them from the freezer, allowing them to reach room temperature before unwrapping, and proceed.
2. Label the slides with the name of antibody to be applied.
3. Fix the slides for 10 min in acetone at room temperature.
4. Allow to air dry. Antibody is applied directly to the dry section.

(e) Paraffin sections

Each of the steps involved in producing paraffin sections may cause the loss of tissue antigens. A useful number and range of antigens are detectable following routine histological processing schedules, but there are certain points to bear in mind to ensure that the chances of obtaining good staining are optimized.

Fixation

Most conventional histological fixatives are formulated for good morphological preservation, with formalin-based solutions being the most widely used. These reagents affect antigenic preservation and this problem increases with extended exposure to the fixative. It might seem advantageous therefore to make use of alternative fixatives. However, there are as yet no other reagents that have achieved the reliability of formalin for routine histopathology, but of these, Bouins, periodate–lysine–paraformaldehyde (PLP) and PLP-dichromate are the most widely advocated.

Formalin is believed to destroy some antigens completely, while many others are masked by the fixation. One way of extending the range of antigens available for demonstration on formalin-fixed, paraffin-processed tissue is to utilize a method with enhanced sensitivity so that low levels of antigen can be demonstrated. Another method is to pretreat the sections prior to immunostaining with a proteolytic enzyme. Before embarking upon this regimen it is worth considering the mechanism by which formalin preserves tissues. In short, methylene bridges are formed between amino groups. This cross-linking between proteins may then mask sites available for antibody binding and it is their removal that needs to be addressed.

Proteolytic enzymic digestion

A number of enzymes have been used for this purpose:

- trypsin
- pepsin
- pronase
- protease
- proteinase K.

Section drying

Antigens may be denatured by excessive or prolonged heating. For most work, drying for 8–24 h at 37°C is usually satisfactory. If a rapid result is required, 15–60 min at 60°C may be used. Particularly sensitive antigens may benefit from drying at room temperature.

Storage of blocks

Blocks processed to paraffin wax are conveniently stored at room temperature which appears to have little or no affect on most formalin-resistant antigens.

Decalcification

The presence of calcium salts in tissue, particularly in atherosclerotic arteries and the aorta, presents an obstacle to the collection of good sections. Hence it is desirable to remove them following tissue fixation. A wide range of solutions is available for this purpose with considerable variation in their effect upon antigenic preservation. In general, chelating agents offer preservation of the greatest spectrum of antigens although some acids if used for brief periods can be used and still give scope for immunohistochemical studies.

Microwave technique

Recent interest has centred on the use of microwaves to reveal or retrieve antigens lost by standard processing procedures. Using this technique, shown in *Protocol 3* below, we have been able to demonstrate tissue antigens of relevance to cardiovascular pathology (Table 8.1), like Ki67, hitherto not detected by any antibody on tissues prepared by conventional means. This method also allows for improved demonstration of antigens that were only variably or weakly expressed, such as smooth muscle actin, HLA-DR and desmin. For certain antigens such as CD31, von Willebrand factor (vWF), HLA-DR and CD68 the technique replaces the use of proteolytic enzyme digestion regimens.

Protocol 3 (Microwave method)

1. Dewax and rehydrate sections. If a technique incorporating a peroxidase label is used, block endogenous enzyme activity as usual.
2. Wash in distilled water.
3. Place slides in a glass rack in a Pyrex dish and immerse in sufficient of any one of the following solutions to cover the slides:
   - 0.01 M sodium citrate, $Na_3C_6H_5O_7 2H_2O$ (2.94 g/l)
   - 0.01 M sodium bicarbonate, $NaHCO_3$ (0.84 g/l)
   - 0.01 M HCl/sodium citrate buffer, pH 6.0 (33 ml 0.01 M sodium citrate + 17 ml 0.01 M HCl.

   Cover the dish with microwave-proof clingfilm. Puncture to allow the steam to escape.
4. Microwave for 5 min at full power. Check fluid level and top up as necessary. Microwave for a further 5 min at full power. Remove from oven and allow to stand for 10–15 min in the hot solution.
5. Wash in distilled water and then in buffer. Proceed with immunohistochemical technique.

8.2.3 ANTIBODIES USED IN VASCULAR PATHOLOGY

There is a wide range of antibodies to human tissue antigens currently available for immunohistochemical investigation. Many of these have been shown to have an important role in diagnosis and newly characterized ones are being introduced continuously.

Immunohistochemical analysis depends on the expression of different proteins on functionally distinct populations of cells [19]. Antibodies specific for unique epitopes on marker molecules can be used to identify the presence and distribution of cells and tissue components. Many of these marker molecules have been classified as 'cluster of differentiation' (CD) molecules, named for the 'cluster' of antibodies which recognize a specific molecule [20]. This has helped to standardize the antibody markers and has facilitated comparison of studies from different laboratories. These molecules are often important in cell function, in promoting cell–cell interactions or in transducing signals that lead to cell activation, proliferation and differentiation [20].

Table 8.1 Monoclonal antibodies used in immunophenotyping

Antibody clone	CD designation	Main specificity/cell association	Reference
3D4	CD3	T cells, TCR-associated	22
T3-10	CD4	T helper/inducer cells, some Mø	23
Tü102	CD8	T cytotoxic/suppressor cells	23
UCHL1*	CD45R0	T primed/memory cells, some Mø	24
SS2/36	CD10	B cells, CALLA, GC	25
HD37	CD19	Pan B cells (not plasma cells)	26
L26*	CD20	B cell subpopulation	27
mb-1	–	B cell, IgM-associated	28
RFD6	–	RER, plasma cells	29
21A5	CD21	C3d-R, mature B cells, FDC, GC	30
4KB128	CD22	Mature B cells	31
bcl-2-100	–	B & T cell, apoptotic involvement, not in GC	32
R4/23	–	FDC (high density), low density on B cells	33
4KB51	–	Mantle zone cells	34
EBM/11	CD68	Most Mø, monocytes	35
KP1*	CD68	Most Mø, monocytes	36
PD7/26*	CD45RB	Leukocyte common antigen	37
JC70*	CD31	PECAM, endothelial cells, some T, B, Mø	38
F8/86*	–	Factor VIII, most endothelial cells, von Willebrand factor	39
Ki-67	–	Proliferation-associated nuclear antigen for cells in G1, S, G2 and M (not G0) of cycle	40
PC10	–	PCNA, cyclin – proliferating cells in G1 and S phase of cell cyles	41
Y2/51	CD61	Platelet glycoprotein IIIa	42
13D5	E-selectin	Activated endothelial cells	43
14C11	ICAM-1	Activated endothelial cells, macrophages and lymphocytes	44
4B2	VCAM-1	Activated endothelial cells, macrophages and follicular dendritic cells	45
CIV22		Type IV collagen on basement membrane	46
1A4		α-smooth muscle actin for smooth muscle cells	39
TAL.1B5	–	MHC Class II, HLA-DR α chain	47

* MAb that bind antigens on formalin-fixed paraffin embedded tissue.
Abbreviations: FDC = follicular dendritic cell; GC = germinal centre; Mø = macrophage; NK = natural killer; PECAM = platelet endothelial cell adhesion molecule; RER = rough endoplasmic reticulum; TCR = T cell receptor; C3b-R = complement receptor C3b.

Inflammatory reactions can vary widely and immunohistochemistry can help to differentiate and classify these inflammatory processes, providing insight into the mechanisms of inflammation. Cells involved in chronic inflammation include T and B lymphocytes, macrophages and endothelial cells; their distribution, frequency and cell associations may reflect the level of disease activity, and can be studied through immunohistochemistry.

Cells can be divided into phenotypical as well as functional subsets using monoclonal antibodies specific for markers whose expression varies depending on the cell type and state of differentiation [20]. Lymphocytes, for example, can be divided into T (CD3) or B cells (CD19/22), and T cells can be divided into helper/inducer (CD4) and cytotoxic/suppressor (CD8) populations and further into primed/memory cells (CD45R0) or naive cells (CD45RA). Mature B cells include CD19, 20 and 22 populations, while plasma cells can be recognized with monoclonal antibodies specific for rough endoplasmic reticulum (RFD6). Macrophages have also been shown to be a heterogeneous population of cells, not only in size, shape and localization, but also by the differential expression of cell markers such as CD68 (EBM 11, KP1).

Table 8.1 lists the antibodies currently used in the Department of Histopathology, Royal Postgraduate Medical School, Hammersmith Hospital, for diagnostic and research purposes, in the study of vascular disease [21]. The use of many of these antibodies is discussed in Chapter 9.

As examples, Plates 7 and 8 illustrate the use of a monoclonal antibody, KP1 (CD68) which localizes to macrophages and may be of use in detecting macrophage populations in early atherosclerotic plaques (Plate 7) and in granulomatous inflammatory diseases such as giant cell (temporal) arteritis (Plate 8).

(a) Identification of vascular endothelial cells

Vascular endothelial cells play an important role in coagulation, inflammation, immunity, regulation of vascular tone and in a wide variety of synthetic and metabolic functions. Endothelial cells also play a pivotal role in immunological diseases, angiogenesis in tumours, transplantation rejection, atherogenesis and placentation. Their role in health and disease is therefore of interest to histopathologists and for this reason it is important to be able to recognize these cells in routine tissue sections. Morphologically, endothelial cells can be difficult to distinguish from other cell types and although a variety of markers is available to the diagnostic histopathologist, all have serious limitations.

Vascular endothelial cells can give rise to both benign and malignant tumours. Angiosarcomas, although rare, pose a diagnostic problem for the histopathologist as they are tumours with varying morphological patterns. Vascular differentiation may be absent and they may be mistaken for other soft tissue sarcomas or for undifferentiated carcinomas. Staining of these tumours with antibodies to FVIII-related antigen (FVIII-Rag) has been disappointing with reports of lack of staining and of cross reactions with carcinomas [38]. *Ulex europaeus* agglutinin lectin shows variable staining of angiosarcoma cells and is not endothelial cell-specific, binding to squamous cell carcinomas and synovial sarcomas as well as to neoplasms arising from colonic epithelium [38].

A new monoclonal antibody has been raised to CD31 (JC70) [38] which has been found to be more reliable than current endothelial markers [48] (Plates 9 and 10).

(b) Antibody screening

For each newly acquired antibody, there is a need to assess its reactivity. Points of note are:

1. the stated specificity of the antibody: the use of multiblocks of frozen or paraffin processed tissue, can be a great assistance here;
2. establishing an appropriate working dilution for the immunodetection system to be used;
3. tissue fixation and processing, including the use of proteolytic agents.

(c) Storage and handling of antibodies

For commercial antibodies the data sheets should provide details of the best way to store antibodies to retain their activity. Do not necessarily assume that storage at 4°C is appropriate in every case since some are better preserved at −20°C. If this is the case, following initial assessment of the antibody, aliquot the antibody into convenient volumes before storage. Whilst storage at 4°C may be detrimental, repeated freezing and thawing usually leads to even more rapid deterioration of reagents.

8.2.4 IMMUNOLABELLING SYSTEMS IN VASCULAR PATHOLOGY

The evolution and development of systems available to label the site of antibody–antigen interaction reflects the need to increase the overall sensitivity of the visualization procedure and to improve the versatility of the techniques.

These aims may be achieved by using an alternative, more readily visualized label or by developing the immunodetection system in such a way that for every antigen site, a greater amount of label can be bound.

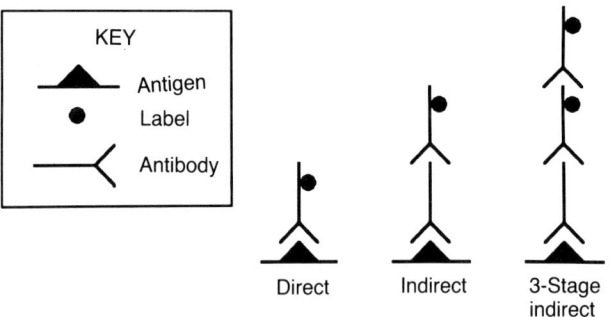

Figure 8.1 Direct and indirect techniques.

(a) Choice of immunodetection system

The simplest method is to conjugate a label directly to the antibody or antibodies against a given antigen. This conjugate is then applied to the tissue section in a single step, the **direct** technique. Whilst simple, this is not particularly sensitive and does not allow the antisera to be used in other methods.

To improve this, an **indirect** technique can be employed. Here the tissue section is incubated with an unlabelled primary antibody, followed by a secondary antibody conjugated with the label of choice, raised against the species of the primary antisera. This allows a single labelled antibody to be used with a large number of primary antibodies provided they are raised in the same species. Since in the secondary antisera a number of antibodies will bind to the primary antibody there is an increase in sensitivity (Figure 8.1).

Sensitivity can be enhanced by applying a third step, a labelled antibody raised against the species in which the second antiserum has been raised. This is the **three-stage** or **enhanced indirect** technique (Figure 8.1).

Other approaches to immunolabelling systems have been devised, some of which are in regular use, while other have rather more specialized use in research applications. However, a number of these techniques have particular value for diagnostic pathology.

Peroxidase – anti peroxidase (PAP), alkaline phosphatase – anti-alkaline phosphatase (APAAP) [49]

These two techniques make use of a soluble immune complex which is formed from the natural affinity between an enzyme label and an antibody against that enzyme. It is important that the antibody used in the complex must be raised in the same species as the primary antibody to enable a second antibody (referred to as the link or bridging antibody) to bind the two together. The link antibody must be used in excess such that after combining with the primary antibody, the second Fab portion is free to bind to the antibody which forms the immune complex (Figure 8.2).

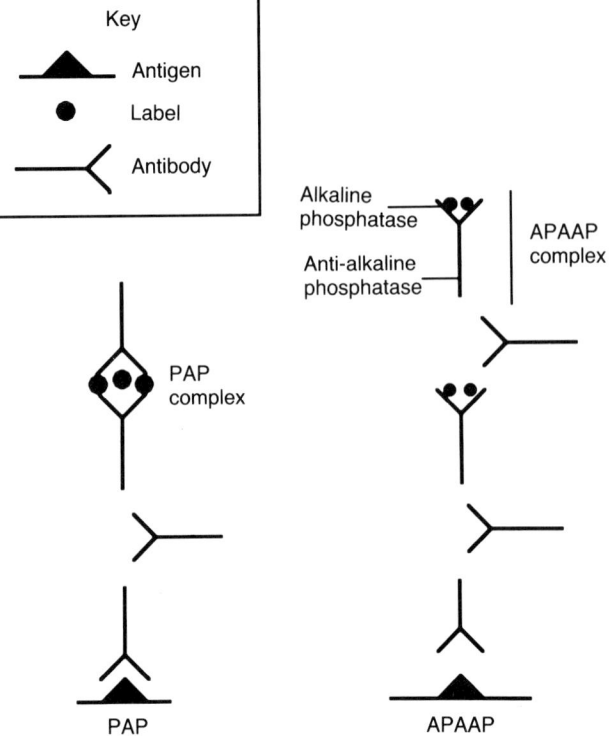

Figure 8.2 PAP and APAAP techniques.

Avidin – biotin and streptavidin – biotin systems (ABC systems) [52]

These methods make use of the natural affinity of avidin and streptavidin for the small protein, biotin, with up to four molecules of biotin binding to each avidin molecule. This affinity is commonly incorporated in immunocytochemistry systems in one of two ways. The final step is either labelled avidin, or a complex formed between labelled biotin and avidin. Both methods require a link antibody, raised against the species in which the primary antibody has been raised, and which has been covalently bound to biotin (Figure 8.3).

Both methods are sensitive and are usually used with enzyme labels. Streptavidin methods are said to represent an improvement over avidin, since streptavidin has an isoelectric point close to neutral which minimizes non-specific binding to charged groups in tissue. Because streptavidin is a protein rather than a glycoprotein, there is no binding with tissue lectins or endogenous oxidizing agents such as ceroid.

(b) Choice of label

The binding that takes place between antigen and antibody needs a label to make it visible. A number have been proposed, each with their own advantages and

Fluorescein isothiocyanate (FITC)

Fluorescent dyes are not widely used in diagnostic pathology mainly because of the lack of permanent preparation, the need for fluorescence microscopy, the problems of autofluorescence of oxidized lipids and elastin and the difficulty of correlating antigen expression with morphology. However, because of their optical sensitivity and ease of use, this label is often employed as part of a direct or indirect system for the detection of immunoglobulin.

Horseradish peroxidase (HRP)

The conjugation to antibodies and other reagents of the enzyme horseradish peroxidase (HRP) is the most widely used of the immunolabelling systems available. Although HRP itself is invisible, it can be readily visualized by a number of simple histochemical procedures using H_2O_2 as substrate with the following colorimetric reagents:

- 3,3′-diaminobenzidine (DAB)
- 3-amino-9-ethylcarbazole
- 4-chloro-1-naphthol
- *p*-phenylenediamine pyrocatechol (Hanker–Yates reagent)
- tetramethyl benzidine
- homovanillic acid
- naphthol pyronine.

Of these, DAB gives a reaction product which is insoluble in organic solvents allowing the slides to be mounted in a synthetic medium to give a permanent preparation.

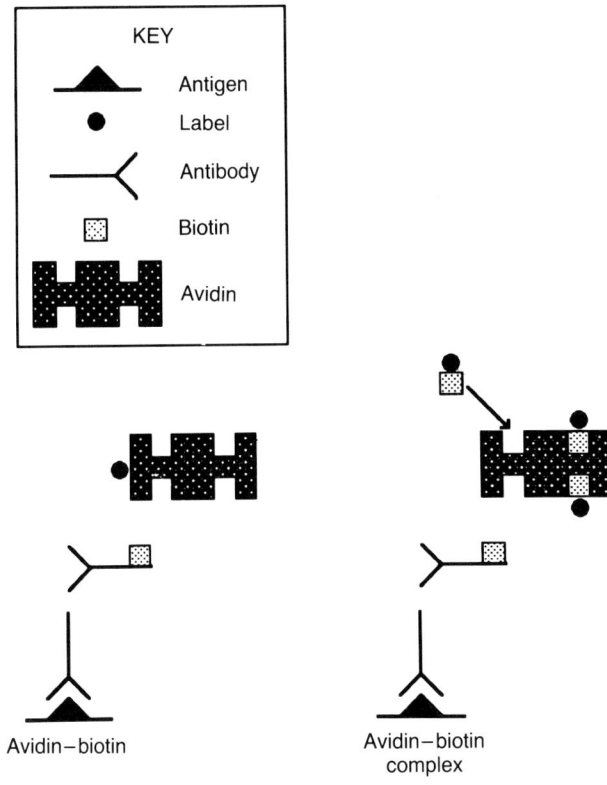

Figure 8.3 Avidin–biotin techniques.

disadvantages for use in the diagnostic laboratory (Table 8.2). Three have enjoyed wide usage for some years while a fourth has gained some acceptance in more recent times.

Table 8.2 Labels for immunohistochemistry

Type of label	Advantages	Disadvantages	Examples
Fluorescent dye	• Optically sensitive • Methods are quick to perform	• Requires specialized microscopical equipment • Non-permanent • Difficult to relate to tissue morphology	• Fluorescein isothiocyanate • Rhodamine • Phycoerythrin • Texas red
Enzyme	• Permanent • No requirement for special microscopy • Versatile	• Endogenous enzymes	• Horseradish peroxidase • Alkaline phosphatase • Glucose oxidase • β-galactosidase • Cytochrome oxidase
Metal	• Sensitive	• Expensive reagents • Silver intensification is a capricious technique	• Colloidal gold • Silver
Metalloprotein	Mainly applicable to electron microscopy		• Ferritin
Radioisotopes	Mainly used in research applications		• ^{131}I • ^{35}S • ^{32}P • ^{14}C

This accounts for the popular and widespread use of this chromogen. The reaction product with DAB can be intensified or its colour changed using various salts of heavy metals. This may increase the sensitivity of the method and also have applications in double labelling techniques [49,50].

Alkaline phosphatase (ALP)

Although less widely used than HRP in immunocytochemistry, alkaline phosphatase has an important place in the repertoire of immunohistochemical methods [18]. From a practical viewpoint there is no need to block endogenous enzyme activity prior to incubation with antisera as this may be achieved by the addition of levamisole at a rate of 1–5 mM, to the substrate medium.

Problems with the use of this enzyme are that the substrate solutions are more complex than those for DAB and that the stained sections need to be mounted in aqueous media. To give a blue reaction, useful in double labelling techniques, substitute Fast Blue BB for Fast Red TR.

Gold

The use of gold particles as a label for immunocytochemistry in light microscopy is relatively new. Whilst the technique has remained primarily within the domain of the electron microscopist and in many research establishments, it has found favour within a number of diagnostic laboratories.

Immuno-gold (IG) labelling alone is not a particularly sensitive method for the visualization of tissue antigens. To increase the sensitivity, sections or cells may be post-incubated with a silver colloid solution with the gold labels acting as nuclei for the deposition of silver (IGSS). This gives a stable, black product and is potentially a highly sensitive technique [51].

(c) **Methods of choice for vascular pathology**

Each technique has its own advantages and disadvantages, with no single technique optimized for every application [21]. A number of immunolabelling systems need to be used to provide the best results.

Three commonly used methods are given in *Protocols 4–6* [18].

Protocol 4 (HRP conjugated avidin–biotin complex (ABC) [50] using polyclonal (rabbit) antisera)

1. **Paraffin sections only** Block endogenous peroxidase enzyme activity with either 0.6% hydrogen peroxide in 80% methanol for 20 min or 3% hydrogen peroxide in distilled water for 10 min.
2. Wash well in running tap water, in distilled water and then in TBS.
3. Incubate for 15 min in 20% normal swine serum (NSS) in TBS.
4. Remove excess serum/buffer from the slide, apply the primary antibody, optimally diluted in 20% NSS in TBS, and incubate for 30 min.
5. Wash with two changes of TBS over 10 min.
6. Remove excess buffer, apply biotinylated swine anti-rabbit Ig (e.g. DAKO E353, UK) optimally diluted in TBS, and incubate for 30 min.
7. Wash with two changes of TBS over 10 min.
8. Remove excess buffer, apply preformed HRP-conjugated ABC (e.g. DAKO K355), and incubate for 30 min.
9. Wash with two changes of TBS over 10 min.
10. Develop sections by incubation in hydrogen peroxide/0.05% DAB in TBS, or other substrate for 3–5 min.
11. Wash well in running tap water.
12. Counterstain with haematoxylin, differentiate and blue in Scott's sub-tap water as necessary.
13. Dehydrate, clear and mount in DPX.

This technique can be modified to utilize monoclonal murine antibodies by using:

- normal rabbit serum in step 3
- the antibody diluted in rabbit serum in step 4
- biotinylated rabbit anti-mouse Ig in step 6.

Protocol 5 (Alkaline phosphatase–anti-alkaline phosphatase (APAAP) method [49] using monoclonal (mouse) antibodies)

The method below incorporates one additional cycle of reagents in the detection system (steps 7–10). To increase the overall sensitivity of the method it may be desirable to repeat this cycle an additional one or two times.

1. Apply the primary antibody, optimally diluted in TBS, and incubate for 25 min at room temperature.
2. Wash, over 5 min, in two changes of TBS.
3. Apply rabbit anti-mouse (e.g. DAKO Z259), optimally diluted in TBS, and incubate for 25 min.
4. Wash for 2 min in TBS.
5. Apply preformed APAAP complexes optimally diluted in TBS and incubate for 25 min.
6. Wash for 2 min in TBS.
7. Apply rabbit anti-mouse (as in step 3) for 10 min.
8. Wash for 2 min in TBS.
9. Apply APAAP complexes (as in step 5) for 10 min.
10. Wash for 2 min in TBS.
11. Incubate the slides for 10–15 min in freshly prepared substrate solution.
12. Wash in buffer and then distilled water.

13. Counterstain lightly with haematoxylin blue in Scott's sub-tap water.
14. Mount in aqueous medium.

Protocol 6 (Three-stage indirect immunoperoxidase technique for use with monoclonal (mouse) primary antibodies)

1. **Paraffin sections only** Block endogenous peroxidase enzyme activity with 0.6% hydrogen peroxide in 80% methanol for 20 min or 3% hydrogen peroxide in distilled water for 10 min.
2. Wash well in running tap water and then distilled water.
3. Wash in TBS, pH 7.6.
4. Drain the slides of excess buffer, apply the primary antibody, suitably diluted in TBS, and incubate for 30 min.
5. Wash in three changes of TBS of 5 min each.
6. Remove excess buffer, apply HRP-conjugated rabbit anti-mouse immunoglobulin (e.g. DAKO P260) optimally diluted in 10% normal human serum in TBS and incubate for 30 min.
7. Wash in three changes of TBS of 5 min each.
8. Remove excess buffer, apply HRP-conjugated swine anti-rabbit immunoglobulin (e.g. DAKO P217) optimally diluted in 10% normal human serum in TBS and incubate for 30 min.
9. Wash in three changes of TBS of 5 min each.
10. Incubate sections in DAB/H_2O_2 or other substrate for up to 5 min.
11. Wash well in running tap water.
12. Counterstain with haematoxylin, differentiating as required.
13. Dehydrate in graded alcohols, clear in xylene and mount in DPX.

8.2.5 CONTROLS

Each immunocytochemical test requires some form of parallel check or control procedure. Negative results must be shown to be due to the absence of antigen and not faulty technique. Similarly, a positive result must be due to specific binding by antibody and not some other extraneous factor. Controls over reagents, tissues and the procedures employed need to be incorporated [18].

(a) Reagent controls

When a new antibody is received into a department, the only checks necessary are to optimize its working dilution (and on fixed and embedded sections to assess the use of proteolytic digestion) on known positive material and to check for non-specific staining on tissues that do not express the antigen. Only if problems of crossreactivity become evident should there be a need to perform additional absorption controls.

(b) Procedural controls

These serve to ensure that immunostaining protocols are followed correctly and that reagents remain active. These controls have two formats.

Tissue controls

One must be sure that the working antibody retains the activity for which it is intended. Therefore, for each primary antibody within a batch of staining, include a section of tissue which is known to be positive for the antigen of interest. That tissue section should have been fixed and processed in an identical fashion to the test section and be treated in the same way as the test throughout the staining procedure. When selecting a positive control, use tissue with low to moderate amounts of antigen present, rather than ones with abnormally heavy deposits.

For many antigens it may not even be necessary to include a known positive tissue control. Factor VIII-related antigen, vimentin etc. are found in every tissue section and so act as built-in controls for the antibodies directed against them.

Primary antibody control

The efficacy of primary antibodies may be controlled by substitution by a non-immune reagent in a parallel section. A number of possible options for substitution exist:

- by primary antibody that has been absorbed by its antigen;
- by another, irrelevant antibody;
- with non-immune serum from the same species in which the primary antibody was raised;
- by omission of primary antibody.

The first option is the most specific but due to the high cost of pure antigen is rarely performed in routine laboratories; the second is often achieved by virtue of using a panel of reagents for diagnosis; the third or fourth option can be incorporated as necessary.

8.2.6 EQUIPMENT AND REAGENTS

When the best approach to immunohistochemistry has been selected and tissues prepared for study accordingly, immunostaining can be started. Although many of the practical details regarding individual procedures have been given some consideration, there are a number of general points that require discussion.

Immunohistochemistry can be performed using equipment which is readily available in the laboratory. If a department is able to prepare paraffin sections and has access to a cryostat, the following items will also be required:

- liquid nitrogen store or −70°C deep freeze.
- −20°C deep freeze
- 4°C refrigerator
- incubation chamber
- micropipetting system, 5 μl–1 ml.
- staining tanks/Coplin jars/slide racks
- primary and control antibodies
- secondary and tertiary antisera and reagents
- normal (blocking) sera
- reagents for buffers and substrates
- counterstains and mountants.

8.2.7 SPECIAL PROBLEMS ENCOUNTERED IN VASCULAR PATHOLOGY

(a) Improving staining

The considerable recent improvement in our understanding of immunocytochemistry, the improvement in the quality of reagents and the better advice available through the marketing companies has led to a reduction in some of the problems of old. Difficulties do still arise, mainly in three areas:

- poor morphology;
- weak or no staining;
- heavy background staining.

Apart from introducing new antibodies and detection systems, there are a number of ways in which the quality of staining can be improved. The aim is to obtain at least one of the following:

- more intense staining;
- decreased cost by using more dilute reagents;
- decrease in the time taken to perform the method.

This can be realized by paying due care and attention to each of the stages of the method used, so as to retain optimal preservation of antigen and morphology:

- correct proteolytic enzyme;
- suitable strategy for the blocking of endogenous enzymes;
- correct dilution of antibodies;
- correct preparation of substrates and enhancements;

(b) Special stains and counterstains

A counterstain is usually applied to assist the localization of antigens within the tissue. Haematoxylin is most commonly used although where a substrate is used that gives an alcohol-soluble reaction product, aqueous haematoxylins (e.g. Mayer's) should be employed. When the reaction product is blue, methyl green or neutral red may be used although these are not very satisfactory when aqueous mountants are used.

Counterstains, of which Evans' Blue is the most widely used, may be used in conjunction with fluorescent labels.

It may be possible to perform histochemical reactions or more complex special stains, e.g. trichromes, on the same sections. These require a colour contrast with the immunostaining and depend on each procedure not having a deleterious effect on the other.

(c) Tissue pigments and their removal

Whilst antibodies may exhibit crossreactivity or bind non-specifically to tissue constituents, there are a number of pigments that occur in tissue sections which may detract from the interpretation of results. Iron salts, lipofuscin, carbon and ceroid may, in certain circumstances, be a problem as may deposits which remain following treatment in formalin or mercuric chloride based fixatives. There are several strategies available for dealing with these situations.

Removal of pigment

The prime consideration of any method used in the removal of tissue pigment is that it must not interfere with tissue antigenicity. This limits the available options but some pigments can be satisfactorily dealt with.

1. **Formalin pigment.** The classic histological approach to this problem is by immersion in alcoholic picric acid for 10 min followed by washing in water. This protocol can be used prior to immunostaining although it may have a deleterious effect upon antigens. However, the techniques used for blocking of endogenous peroxidase enzyme in immunoperoxidase techniques also serve to remove formalin pigment and so additional procedures may not be needed.
2. **Mercury pigment.** This can be removed either prior to immunostaining, or with immunoperoxidase techniques prior to counterstaining, by immersion in alcoholic iodine for 5 min followed by decolourization in 5% sodium thiosulphate.
3. **Melanin.** Deposits of melanin can be removed by a 5-min immersion in 0.25% potassium permanganate followed by decolourization in 2% oxalic acid. This may have an adverse effect on some antigens so appropriate controls, i.e. known positive tissue controls which have been similarly treated, must be stained in parallel. The technique may also result in increased section loss and adhesives are advocated.

Alternative substrate

Most pigments are brown-black and are therefore easily confused with DAB, for example. The use of other substrates for use with HRP systems or alternative labels (e.g. alkaline phosphatase) may overcome any confusion.

Comparison with negative control

The pigments will be present in a negative control section of the same tissue block and so comparison of control and test section should allow the distinction of pigment and the immunocytochemical reaction.

Histochemical demonstration of pigment

In some circumstances, it may be possible to demonstrate the pigment by the use of a histochemical procedure in a contrasting colour to enable a clear distinction to be made.

(d) Reduction of non-specific staining

In sections, antibodies may bind non-specifically to reactive or charged groups so making assessment of staining difficult. This reactivity can be reduced by blocking with protein solutions such as non-immune serum, bovine serum albumin (BSA) or fetal calf serum (FCS). These may be added to the antibody diluent and also employed alone prior to incubation with antisera.

Non-specific staining may also result from unwanted antibodies in the antisera and it may be possible to remove these by adsorbing the antiserum with powdered or homogenized extract of tissue such as brain or liver.

Binding of protein to free aldehyde groups can occur. Pre-blocking with sodium borohydride will alleviate this problem.

(e) Assessing a negative result

An antibody designated as suitable for use on fixed, paraffin processed tissue, particularly a monoclonal antibody, may be found not to work despite all other reagents in the method being shown to be active.

The first step to check is that the fixation and processing regimen has been appropriate for the preservation of the antigen; attention should also be paid to any proteolytic enzyme treatment that may be required. If staining remains unsatisfactory, test the antibody on acetone-fixed sections of frozen tissue. If negative, repeat with a different detection system and, if that situation remains, check the antibody expiry date and storage conditions and if this is not an explanation, consult the suppliers [18]. If the frozen section test is positive, process the block of tissue used, or one similar, to paraffin wax. If that is positive the original test block probably did not contain the antigen. If the new block is negative, fixative and/or processing is at fault, the protocol may have to be amended to obtain satisfactory antigen demonstration.

If a technique has been performed and the positive and negative controls give the expected result but the test is negative, there are a number of possible causes:

- no antigen is present
- antigen is present at levels too low to be detected by the method employed, showing the benefit of using a highly sensitive technique at the outset.
- test tissue has been over-fixed or poorly processed and sectioned; this can easily be overcome by ensuring that the positive tissue control has identical characteristics to the test.

Most of the problems encountered are due to operator error. This underlines the general principle that a complete familiarization with the techniques used is essential before any method is started and that the procedures should be strictly adhered to at all times. In particular, before starting to use a new antibody or detection system obtained from a commercial source, be aware of the limitations of that reagent. To these ends, thorough familiarization with details given in the accompanying data sheets and also in any publications describing the reagent is vital.

8.2.8 COMBINATION TECHNIQUES

The demonstration of two or more antigens in the same tissue section can be achieved in a number of ways:

(a) Sequential staining

The tissue section is stained to demonstrate a particular antigen and the result photographed. The antigen–antibody complex is then eluted, or the substrate decolourized using potassium permanganate, before a second antibody is applied to demonstrate the second antigen of interest.

(b) Simultaneous staining

The most effective approach to double labelling is to demonstrate and visualize two or more antigens at the same time. This can be achieved in two ways:

1. by applying one antibody and detection system, to demonstrate the label appropriately and then to follow with a sequence to demonstrate a second antigen;
2. by mixing both sets of reagents and using in a single staining sequence, if antibodies from different species are used.

The method may be carried out using:

- two or three fluorescent labels (usually used as directly conjugated antibodies);
- a single enzyme label for the demonstration of the two antigens but each visualized with a different substrate;
- a pair of enzyme labels [52] (Plate 9);
- a combination of enzyme and immunofluorescence [53] (Plate 10).

It is important that there is no crossreactivity between the different components of the system used. Ideally, primary antibodies need to be raised in different species with no additional crossreactivity between the reagents in the two detection systems.

Care is needed to select the right substrate in order to obtain a good contrast in colour of reaction products. Also, depending upon the antigens under investigation, antibody dilutions may need to be adjusted to get a good balance of staining whereby one reaction is not masked with the other.

Our preference is to utilize the sequential double labelling technique, despite it being a longer method, with the use of two different enzyme labels [54] irrespective of the species in which the antibody is raised. Provided adequate controls are performed to check for crossreactivity it is possible to utilize primary antibodies from the same species.

This review has been written to provide guidance to the vascular pathologist in choosing the most appropriate of the modern histochemical and immunohistochemical pathways for diagnosis and research. Should further protocols be required then the reader is advised to consult the histochemical [1] and immunohistochemical texts [54,55]. It is clear that there are now no barriers to what the vascular pathologist may accomplish at the light microscopy level.

Acknowledgements

The author would like to thank Andrew Heryet and the staff of the Department of Cellular Pathology, John Radcliffe Hospital Oxford and Susan Van Noorden and the staff of the Department of Histopathology, Royal Postgraduate Medical School, Hammersmith Hospital, for the laboratory protocols included in this review.

References

1. Pearse, A.G.E. (1968) *Histochemistry, Theoretical and Applied*, 2nd edn, Churchill Livingstone, Edinburgh.
2. Bancroft, J.D. and Cook, H.C. (1984) *Manual of Histological Techniques*, Churchill Livingstone, London.
3. Cole, E.C. (1943) Studies in haematoxylin stains. *Stain Tech.*, **18**, 125–9.
4. Miller, P.J. (1971) An elastin stain. *Med. Lab. Tech.*, **28**, 148–9.
5. Lison, L. (1936) *Histochemie Animale*, 1st edn, Gautier, Villars, Paris.
6. Lovern, J.A. (1955) *The Chemistry of Lipids of Biological Significance*, Methuen, London.
7. Hartroft, W.S. and Porta, E.A. (1965) Ceroid. *Am. J. Med. Sci.*, **250**, 324–5.
8. Mitchinson, M.J. (1982) Insoluble lipids in human atherosclerotic plaques. *Atherosclerosis*, **45**, 11–15.
9. Dowson, J.H. and Harris, S.J. (1981) Quantitative studies of the autofluorescence derived from neuronal lipofuscin. *J. Microscopie*, **123**, 249–58.
10. Lillie, R.D. and Ashburn, L.L. (1943) Supersaturated solutions of fat stains in dilute isopropanol for demonstration of acute fatty degeneration not shown by Herxheimer's technique. *Arch. Pathol.*, **36**, 432–5.
11. Smith, J.L. (1908) On the simultaneous staining of neutral fat and fatty acids by oxazine dyes. *J. Pathol. Bacteriol.*, **12**, 1–8.
12. Schiff, U. (1866) Eine neue Reihe organischer Diamine. *Justus Liebigs Ann. Chem.*, **140**, 92.
13. Stillmark, H. (1888) Uber Rizin, ein giftiger Ferment aus dem Samen von *Ricinus communis L.* und einigen anderen Euphorbiaceen. Inaug. Dis. Dorpat.
14. Hsu, S.-M. and Ree, H.J. (1983) Histochemical studies on lectin binding in reactive lymphoid tissue. *J. Histochem. Cytochem.*, **31**, 538–41.
15. Holthofer, H., Virtanen, M.D., Kainiemi, L. et al. (1982) *Ulex europeus* I lectin as a marker for vascular endothelium in human tissues. *Lab. Invest.*, **47**, 60–66.
16. Rose, M.L., Habeshaw, J.A., Kennedy, R. et al. (1981) Binding of peanut lectin to germinal centre cells; a marker for B cell subsets of follicular lymphoma. *Br. J.Canc.*, **44**, 68–74.
17. Coons, A.A., Creech, H.J. and Jones, R.N. (1941) Immunological properties of an antibody containing a fluorescent group. *Proc. Soc. Expl Biol. Med.*, **47**, 200–2.
18. Heryet, A.R. and Gatter, K.C. (1993) Immunocytochemistry for light microscopy, in *Diagnostic Molecular Biology: a Practical Approach*, (eds. S. Herrington and J.O'D. McGee), Oxford University Press, Oxford, p. 7.
19. Milstein, C. and Cuello, A.C. (1983) Hybrid hybridomas and their use in immunohistochemistry. *Nature*, **305**, 537–8.
20. Knapp, W., Dörken, B., Gilks, W.R. et al. (eds) (1989) *Leukocyte Typing IV. White Cell Differentiation Antigens*. Oxford University Press, Oxford.
21. Parums, D.V., Heryet, A.R. and Gatter, K.C. (1994) The role of immunocytochemistry in cardiovascular pathology. *Cardiovasc. Pathol.* (in submission)
22. Kung, P.C., Goldstein, G., Reinherz, E.L. and Schlossman, S.F. (1979) Monoclonal antibodies defining distinctive human T cell surface antigens. *Science*, **206**, 347–9.
23. Erber, W.N., Pinching, A.J. and Mason, D.Y. (1984) Immunocytochemical detection of T and B cell populations in routine blood smears. *Lancet*, **1**, 1042–5.
24. Smith, S.H., Brown, M.H., Rowe, D. et al. (1986) Functional subsets of human helper-inducer cells defined by a new monoclonal antibody, UCHL1. *Immunology*, **58**, 63–70.
25. Stein, H., Gerdes, J. and Mason, D.Y. (1982) The normal and malignant germinal centre. *Clin. Haematol.*, **11**, 531–59.
26. Pezzutto, A., Dorken, B., Feller, A. et al. (1986) HD37 monoclonal antibody; a useful reagent for further characterization of 'non T, non B' lymphoid malignancies, in *Leukocyte Typing II*, Springer Verlag, New York 391–402.
27. Ishii, Y., Takami, T., Yuasa, H. et al. (1984) Two distinct antigen systems in human B lymphocytes; identification of cell surface and intracellular antigens using monoclonal antibodies. *Clin. Expl Immunol.*, **58**, 183–92.
28. Mason, D.Y., Cordell, J.L., Tse, A.G.D. et al. (1991) The IgM-associated protein mb-1 as a marker of normal and neoplastic B cells. *J. Immunol.*, **147**, 2474–82.
29. Ling, N.R., MacLennan, I.C.M. and Mason, D.Y. (1987) B cell and plasma cell antigens; new and previously defined clusters, in *Leukocyte Typing III. White Cell Differentiation Antigens*, (ed. A. McMichael et al.), Oxford University Press, Oxford, pp. 302–35.
30. Petzer, A.L., Schulz, T.F., Eigentler, A. et al. (1988) Structure and functional analysis of CR2/EBV receptor by means of monoclonal antibodies and limited tryptic digestion. *Immunology*, **63**, 47–53.
31. Stein, H., Gerdes, J. and Mason, D.Y. (1982) The normal and malignant germinal centre. *Clin. Haematol.*, **11**, 531–59.
32. Pezzella, F., Tse, A.G.D., Cordell, J. et al. (1990) Expression of the bcl-2 oncogene protein is not specific for the 14;18 transloaction. *Am. J. Pathol.*, **137**, 225–32.
33. Naiem, M., Gerdes, J., Adulaziz, Z. et al. (1983) Production of a monoclonal antibody reactive with human dendritic reticulum cells and its use in the immunohistologic analysis of lymphoid tissue. *J. Clin. Pathol.*, **36**, 167–75.
34. Pulford, K.A.F., Falini, B., Heryet, A. et al. (1987) A new monoclonal anti-B cell antibody for routine diagnosis of lymphoid tissue biopsies, in *Leukocyte Typing III. White Cell Differentiation Antigens*, (ed. A. McMichael et al.), Oxford University Press, Oxford, p. 828.
35. Kelly, P.M.A., Bliss, E., Morton, J.A. et al. (1988) Monoclonal antibody EBM/11: high cellular specificity for human macrophages. *J. Clin. Pathol.*, **41**, 510–5.
36. Pulford, K.A.F., Rigney, E.M., Micklem, K.J. et al. (1989) KP1 – a new monoclonal antibody that detects a monocyte/macrophage associated

antigen in routinely processed tissue sections. *J. Clin. Pathol.*, **42**, 414–21.
37. Warnke, R.A., Gatter, K.C., Falini, B. *et al.* (1983) Diagnosis of human lymphoma with monoclonal antileukocyte antibodies. *New Engl. J. Med.*, **309**, 1275–81.
38. Parums, D.V., Cordell, J.L., Micklem, K. *et al.* (1990) JC70: a new monoclonal antibody that detects vascular endothelium associated antigen on routinely processed tissue sections. *J. Clin. Pathol.*, **43**, 752–7.
39. Naiem, M., Gerdes, J., Adulaziz, Z. *et al.* (1982) The value of immunohistological screening in the production of monoclonal antibodies. *J. Immunol. Meth.*, **50**, 145–60.
40. Gerdes, J., Schwab, U., Lemke, H. and Stein, H. (1983) Production of a mouse monoclonal antibody reactive with a human nuclear antigen associated with cell proliferation. *Int. J. Cancer*, **31**, 13–20.
41. Waseem, N.H. and Lane, D.P. (1990) Monoclonal antibody analysis of the proliferating cell nuclear antigen (PCNA). Structural conservation and the detection of a nucleolar form. *J. Cell. Sci.*, **96**, 121–30.
42. Gatter, K.C., Cordell, J.L., Hurley, H. *et al.* (1988) The immunohistological detection of platelets, megakaryocytes and thrombi in routinely processed specimens. *Histopathology*, **13**, 257–67.
43. Wellicome, S.M., Thornhill, M.H., Pitzalis, C. *et al.* (1990) A monoclonal antibody that detects a novel antigen on endothelial cells that is induced by tumour necrosis factor IL-1 or lipopolysaccharide. *J. Immunol.*, **144**, 2558–65.
44. Dustin, M.L., Rothlein, R., Bhan, A.K. *et al.* (1986) Induction by IL 1 and interferon-g: tissue distribution, biochemistry, and function of a natural adherence molecule (ICAM-1). *J. Immunol.*, **137**, 245–54.
45. Elices, M.J., Osborn, L., Takada, Y. *et al.* (1990) VCAM-1 on activated endothelium interacts with the leukocyte integrin VLA-4 at a site distinct from the VLA-4/fibronectin binding site. *Cell*, **60**, 577–84.
46. Odermatt, B.F., Lang, A.B., Ruttner, J.R. *et al.* (1984) Monoclonal antibodies to human type IV collagen: useful reagents to demonstrate the heterodimeric nature of the molecule. *Proc. Natl Acad. Sci. USA*, **81**, 7343–7.
47. Epenetos, A.A., Borrow, L.G., Adams, T.E. *et al.* (1985) A monoclonal antibody that detects HLA-DR region antigen in routinely fixed, wax embedded sections of normal and neoplastic lymphoid tissue. *J. Clin. Pathol.*, **38**, 12–17.
48. Page, C., Rose, M., Yacoub, M. and Pigott, R. (1992) Antigenic heterogeneity of vascular endothelium. *Am. J. Pathol.*, **141**, 673–83.
49. Cordell, J.L., Falini, B., Erber, W.N. *et al.* (1984) Immunoenzymatic labeling of monoclonal antibodies using immune complexes of alkaline phosphatase and monoclonal anti-alkaline phosphatase (APAAP complexes). *J. Histochem. Cytochem.*, **32**, 219–29.
50. Hsu, S-M and Fanger, H. (1981) Use of avidin-biotin-peroxidase complex (ABC) in immunoperoxidase techniques. *J. Histochem. Cytochem.*, **29**, 577–80.
51. Holgate, C., Jackson, P., Cowan, P. and Bird, C. (1983) Immunogold-silver staining: a new method of immunostaining with advanced sensitivity. *J. Histochem. Cytochem.*, **31**, 938–44.
52. Mason, D.Y., Abdulaziz, A., Falini, B. and Stein, H. (1983) Single and double immunoenzymatic techniques for labeling tissue sections with monoclonal antibodies. *Ann. N.Y. Acad. Sci.*, **238**, 1073–9.
53. Ramshaw, A.L. and Parums, D.V. (1992) Combined immunohistochemical and immunofluorescence method to determine the phenotype of proliferating cell populations. *J. Clin. Pathol.*, **45**, 1015–17.
54. Krausz, T., Schofield, J.B., Van Noorden, S. *et al.* (1993) Application of immunocytochemistry to fine needle aspirates, in *Fine Needle Aspiration Cytopathology*, (ed. J.A. Young), Blackwell Scientific Publications, London, p. 310.
55. Polak, J. and Van Noorden, S. (eds) (1986) *Immunocytochemistry. Practical Applications in Pathology and Biology*, 2nd edn, Wright PSG, Bristol.

9 INFLAMMATION AND ATHEROSCLEROSIS

Dinah V. Parums

9.1 Inflammation and atherogenesis

Cardiovascular disease remains the chief cause of death in the USA and Western Europe, and atherosclerosis, the principal cause of myocardial and cerebral infarction, accounts for the majority of these deaths.

One of the problems in the study of the nature of human atherosclerosis lies in the lack of unanimity about the definition of the histopathological structure of the lesion [1]. The term 'atheroma' was commonly used by the Greek writers [2] and again by von Haller in 1735 [3] to describe the yellow, intimal plaques or nodules containing 'gruel-like' material. Virchow [4] was not completely satisfied with this name and believed that these intimal nodules not only contained fat but also proliferating cells. Virchow thought these cells were inflammatory and adopted the name '**endarteriitis chronica sive nodosa**'. This name never became popular because others doubted its inflammatory nature.

Turnbull [5] defined **atheroma** as follows: 'Atheroma is a degeneration which affects, and is almost confined to, the intima. It is found in both the elastic and muscular arteries, but is commoner in the large elastic vessels. The degeneration is characterized by the accumulation of debris, which is at first fatty and is later frequently impregnated by calcium.'

Atherosclerosis was introduced by Marchand in 1904 [6] and was popularized by Aschoff [7]. The World Health Organization [8] gives the definition of atherosclerosis as 'a variable combination of changes of the intima of arteries consisting of focal accumulations of lipid, complex carbohydrates, blood and blood products, fibrous deposits and calcium deposits associated with medial changes' (Figure 9.1).

We see atherosclerosis in terms of the clinical horizon or the clinical sequelae of its local complications, most commonly as ischaemia and infarction. In this chapter, the role of inflammation in atherogenesis and as a local complication of advanced atherosclerosis, namely chronic periaortitis and periarteritis, will be considered.

9.1.1 CHARACTERIZATION OF INFLAMMATORY CELLS IN ATHEROSCLEROSIS

(a) Intimal inflammation

In the 19th century, Virchow noted the inflammatory nature of the atheromatous plaques and suggested that chronic inflammation in the intima might be of importance in atherogenesis [4]. Later, morphological evaluations suggested the presence of macrophages in lesions [9]. This has since been confirmed by immunohistochemistry, which shows that lipid-laden foam cells in fatty streaks and in fibrofatty plaques are predominantly macrophage rather than smooth muscle cell in origin [10,11,12] (Figure 9.2). These findings have shifted the emphasis of research from smooth muscle cells to the inflammatory component of the plaque [13].

Immunohistochemical investigations have shown that numerous T lymphocytes are present in the early and advanced plaque [14–19]. CD4-positive T helper-associated and CD8-positive T cytotoxic/suppressor-associated lymphocytes have been detected in the plaque in varying ratios [17,18]. Jonasson et al. [14] demonstrated the distribution and compartmentalization of cells in specific regions of the atherosclerotic plaque in surgical carotid arteries. They showed that there were 20% T cells, most abundant in the fibrous cap, 60% macrophages, particularly in the lipid core shoulder region, and less than 1% B cells. In contrast, non-atheromatous arteries showed little or no inflammation [14]. T lymphocytes and macrophages are present in the intima of early human aortic and coronary lesions. T cells could be important both as a source of chemotactic factors for monocytes and in the regulation of macrophage lipoprotein uptake.

Foam cell necrosis is the hallmark of fibrofatty plaques, with a necrotic core of lipids and proteins surrounded by cellular degeneration. The fibrofatty plaque is composed of a necrotic core covered by a fibrous cap of smooth muscle cells, some macrophages

---

Vascular Pathology. Edited by W.E. Stehbens and J.T. Lie. Published in 1995 by Chapman & Hall, London. ISBN 0 412 48640 7

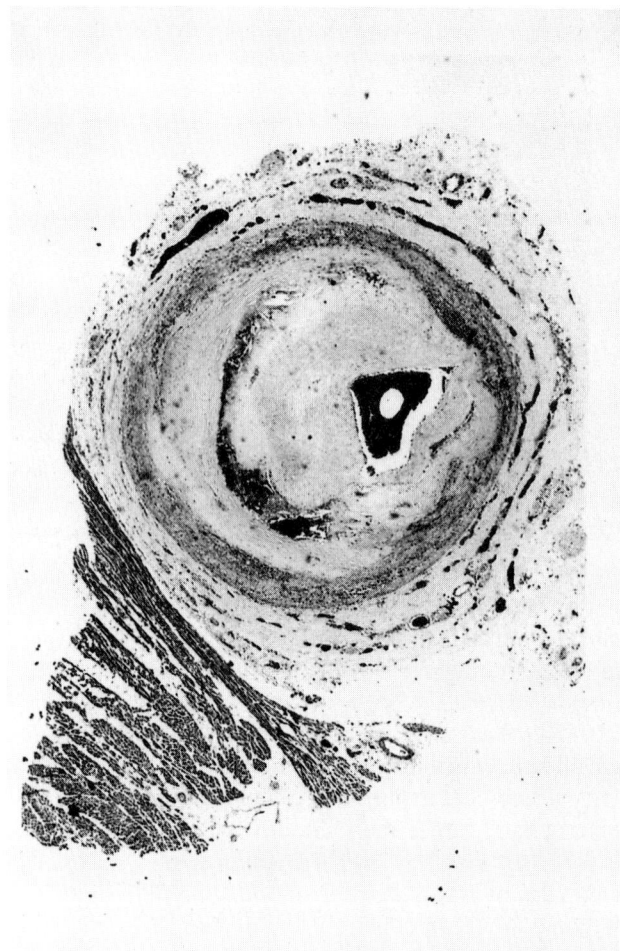

Figure 9.1 Light micrograph of a human coronary artery showing almost complete occlusion of the vessel lumen with atheroma and organized thrombus. Note the angular cholesterol clefts in the atheroma and the dark haemorrhage in the middle of the atheromatous plaque. (Haematoxylin & Eosin.)

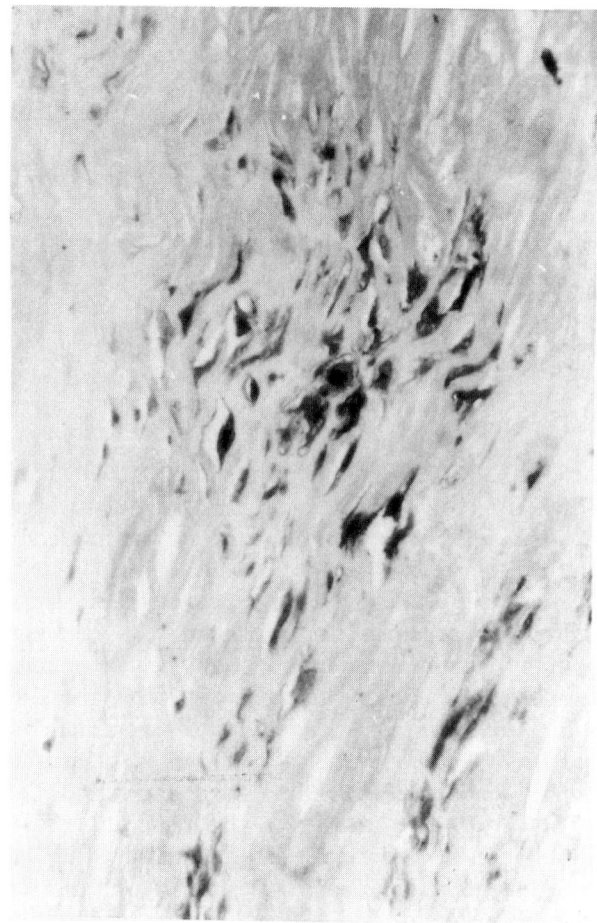

Figure 9.2 This light micrograph shows the base of an advanced atherosclerotic plaque stained with a mouse monoclonal antibody to human macrophages (KP1, CD68), using the indirect immunoperoxidase technique and a dark brown staining substrate. Note the abundance of both spindle shaped and foamy macrophages in the lesion.

and dense connective tissue lined by endothelium. Smooth muscle cells, which have migrated from the media to the intima, are proliferating and are present beneath and above the necrotic core. Foam cells are predominant in the shoulder region of the core [20]. These progressive atherosclerotic lesions are preferentially located to arterial branches, apparently due to haemodynamic stress at these points, and are particularly common and most severe in the abdominal aorta and coronary arteries.

The development of atherosclerosis initially involves intimal accumulation of inflammatory cells and lipids from the plasma, and the proliferation and migration of smooth muscle cells from the underlying media into the intima. In addition, there is collagen, elastin and proteoglycan deposition, modification of low density lipoproteins, and development of lipid-laden macrophage-derived foam cells in the plaque. As atherosclerosis progresses there is endothelial disruption, medial thinning, neovascularization, fibrosis of the plaque, calcification, thrombosis, and chronic inflammation and fibrosis of the media and adventitia [21,22,23]. These are the features of the advanced or complicated human atherosclerotic plaque.

Until recently, much of the research on atherosclerosis has emphasized lipid/cholesterol metabolism, atherosclerotic risk factors and morphological studies. With a growing realization that the plaque is not merely a mass of inert lipid, but that atherosclerosis is a highly cellular and dynamic process, more attention has been paid to the pathogenesis of this disease. This has revealed the cellular nature of atherosclerotic lesions, as well as an active inflammatory component in the disease [20,24].

(b) Activation of inflammatory cells

The presence of inflammatory cells does not in itself prove their role in atherogenesis. It has become increasingly clear, however, that cellular activation and maturation is an integral part of plaque development. Not only are monocytes thought to develop into macrophages in the plaque, but other signs of activation such as MHC class II, interleukin-2 receptor, cytokines and adhesion molecule expression have been detected in atherosclerotic lesions [18,24].

Hansson and colleagues [16,17] using immunohistochemical techniques, have detected T lymphocytes and macrophages in atherosclerotic plaques from carotid endarterectomy specimens, but noted that B lymphocytes and natural killer (NK) cells were absent. Macrophages comprised approximately 50% of the cells of the atheromatous plaque. They noted that T cells, macrophages and smooth muscle cells were capable of expressing HLA-DR antigen. They also noted that T cells expressed interleukin-2 (IL-2) receptor and were associated with interferon-γ (IFN-γ) secretion. They suggested, that T cell–smooth muscle cell interactions occur during atherogenesis.

MHC class II antigens have been detected on smooth muscle cells adjacent to lymphocytes and on many T cells in the plaque [24]. Immunohistochemical detection of IL-2 receptors on T cells in the plaque further emphasized the active nature of the inflammatory response [17,18]. The same research has also suggested that there may be a specific immune response associated with the development of atherosclerosis. Hansson proposed that antigens in the plaque are presented in association with MHC class II molecules on smooth muscle cells and on macrophages, resulting in a local activation of T cells and their subsequent modulatory function on other cells in the plaque [17].

(c) Cellular immune mechanisms

The exact role of cellular immune response in atherosclerosis still needs clarification. A protective function has been demonstrated in animal models, where arterial balloon catheterized injury, coupled with induced T-cell depletion (caused by monoclonal antibodies or removal of the thymus), has resulted in the development of larger lesions [25]. Furthermore, injection of the cytokine IFN-γ into animals inhibits smooth muscle proliferation and results in smaller lesions [25]. Since T cells are the prime producers of this cytokine, Hansson has hypothesized that T cells modulate smooth muscle cell proliferation during vascular repair. It has also been shown that IFN-γ can inhibit the expression of scavenger receptors and subsequent development of foam cells [26].

It is possible that intimal macrophages may play a protective role against the cytotoxic effects of oxidized LDL, at least in early lesions. Macrophages are thought to play an initial role in clearing accumulated lipids and may even be responsible for plaque regression, although there is no evidence proving that macrophages leave the lesion via the intimal endothelium.

It is likely that both macrophages and T cells contribute to lesion progression. Since both T cells and macrophages produce cytokines, the increase in their number and activation in relation to the size of lesion would seem to indicate that they perpetuate the development of atherosclerosis [20]. Macrophages may also contribute to plaque development by oxidizing LDL and by causing plaque necrosis [13].

Cardiac transplant rejection results in accelerated atherosclerosis in the coronary arteries. Researchers have hypothesized that this may be an immune-mediated complication of rejection which mimics typical atherosclerosis [27–29]. While there are many differences between transplant 'atherosclerosis' and the slowly progressive atherosclerosis, they both involve the proliferation of smooth muscle cells and an accumulation of lipid-laden macrophages and T cells. Ross has speculated that low-grade endothelialitis, echoed in transplant rejection, plays a role in the development of atherosclerosis [29].

(d) Humoral immune mechanisms

Atherosclerotic plaques contain deposits of immunoglobulins that are not present in non-atherosclerotic lesions [19]. Complement factors have been found with a similar tissue distribution, suggesting that local complement activation may occur in the plaque [19,30].

Serum sickness has been repeatedly correlated with development or aggravation of the atherosclerotic process [31] and anti-endothelial auto-antibodies have been shown to correlate with peripheral vascular disease [32]. Several micro-organisms, particularly herpes viruses, have been implicated in the pathogenesis of atherosclerosis [33]. The local response to these pathogens is likely to be both cell-mediated and antibody-based.

Antibodies to modified lipoproteins have been described, by various workers, in association with complications of atherosclerosis [34]. How these antibodies may be implicated in the aetiology of human atherosclerosis remains controversial.

9.1.2 CYTOKINES AND ATHEROSCLEROSIS

The initiation and propagation of the immune response depends not only on interactions between cell surface molecules but also on humoral factors. Cells of the immune system may be viewed as endocrine cells which, when activated, produce large amounts of hormone-like substances called interleukins or cytokines. These molecules have been shown to affect growth and gene expression in vascular cells (Table 9.1).

Monocytes and macrophages, when activated, produce several factors that are important for inflammatory

Table 9.1 Cytokines of the immune system

Cytokine	Source
IL-1	Monocyte/macrophage, endothelial cells, NK cells, smooth muscle cells
IL-2	T cells, NK cells
IL-3	T cells
IL-4	T cells, NK cells
IL-5	T cells
IL-6	Many cell types
IFN-α	Leucocytes
IFN-γ	T cells, NK cells
Tumour necrosis factor (TNFα)	Monocyte/macrophage, smooth muscle cells, NK cells
Lymphotoxin (TNFβ)	T cells
Platelet-derived growth factor (PDGF)	Monocyte/macrophage, endothelial cells, smooth muscle cells, megakaryocyte/platelet

and immune responses. They also produce growth promoters, the best known of which is PDGF [35]. Interleukin-1 (IL-1) is probably the best characterized interleukin. The vascular effects of IL-1 on endothelial cells include:

- induction of procoagulant activity;
- induction of reorganization of endothelial monolayers;
- stimulation of adhesion of granulocytes, lymphocytes and monocytes;
- stimulation of proliferation
- increase in vascular permeability
- induction of IL-1 release by positive feedback.

Its effects on smooth muscle cells include:

- stimulation of proliferation;
- induction of PDGF secretion;
- induction of IL-1 release by positive feedback.

The activated macrophage also produces a 17-kD protein called tumour necrosis factor (TNF) or cachectin. The vascular effects of TNF-α on endothelial cells include:

- induction of procoagulant activity;
- induction of reorganization of endothelial monolayers;
- stimulation of adhesion of granulocytes, lymphocytes and monocytes;
- inhibition of proliferation *in vitro*;
- induction of angiogenesis;
- induction of MHC gene expression.

Its effects on smooth muscle cells include:

- induction of Class I MHC genes;
- modulation of IFN-γ-induced Class II MHC genes.

Since the lymphocyte makes a structurally related substance, lymphotoxin, the macrophage product is often identified as TNF-α. TNF-α can also be produced by vascular smooth muscle cells. It induces vascular and inflammatory responses similar to those of IL-1 but may also cause tumour cell cytotoxicity and cachexia in malignant disease.

The activated T lymphocyte is a rich source of many biologically active proteins, the best characterized of which is IFN-γ. IFN-γ has three major effects; it induces expression of MHC genes; inhibits cell proliferation; and induces antiviral activity. In addition, it affects expression of a variety of genes in many different cell types including macrophages and vascular cells. The vascular effects of IFN-γ on endothelial cells include:

- induction of reorganization of endothelial monolayers;
- induction of new surface proteins associated with autoimmune responses;
- inhibition of proliferation;
- increase in vascular permeability;
- inhibition of PDGF and IL-1 expression;
- induction of Class I MHC gene expression;
- induction of Class II MHC gene expression.

Its effects on smooth muscle cells include:

- induction of Class I MHC gene expression;
- induction of Class II MHC gene expression;
- inhibition of proliferation.

Plaque macrophages and T cells have been shown to produce specific cytokines that, by influencing cell proliferation and lipid accumulation, seem to be important for lesion progression. Macrophages also synthesize platelet-derived growth factor (PDGF) which may cause proliferation of smooth muscle cells [29]. Interferon-γ, which is known to induce cellular expression of MHC class II and which is synthesized by activated T cells, was detected by immunohistochemistry in and around a few lymphocytes in the atherosclerotic plaque [17]. Monocyte chemoattractant protein-1 (MCP-1) has also been detected in human plaques, in smooth muscle cells and in macrophages by *in situ* hybridization, and in endothelial cells and macrophages by immunohistochemistry [36]. MCP-1 is thought to attract monocytes to the site of the atherosclerotic plaque. In addition, the expression of MCP-1 can be induced *in vitro* by minimally oxidized LDL in endothelial cells and macrophages. MCP-1 and oxidized LDL may, in fact, result in a self-perpetuating process in atheroma: MCP-1 influences macrophage accumulation, macrophages oxidize LDL, oxidized LDL stimulates further MCP-1 synthesis and so on. To date, other cytokines, including macrophage colony-stimulating factor, tumour necrosis factor-α (TNF-α), interleukin-1 (IL-1), transforming growth factor-β (TGF-β) and heparin-epidermal growth factor (h-EGF), have also been identified in atherosclerotic lesions [32,35,36].

9.1.3 ADHESION MOLECULES AND ATHEROSCLEROSIS

Adhesion molecules are fundamental in regulating inflammation. They are required for initial leukocyte adhesion to endothelial cells, for specific cellular recruitment into inflammatory tissue sites, for cell–cell interaction and signalling, and for lymphoid organization [37].

E-selectin (formerly, endothelial leukocyte adhesion molecule-1 (ELAM-1)), intercellular adhesion molecule-1 (ICAM-1) and vascular cell adhesion molecule-1 (VCAM-1) can be upregulated by cytokines during activation, and synthesized *de novo* during inflammation [38–40]. E-selectin was originally identified as a neutrophil adhesion molecule and was thought to be primarily a mediator of acute inflammatory adhesion [38–41]. It also plays a role in adhesion of memory T cells *in vitro*, and homing *in vivo* in skin inflammation [42,43]. The cell type which binds to E-selectin may be dependent on the local microenvironment under the influence of various cytokines [44,45]. ICAM-1 has been shown to be upregulated in inflammatory responses although it is also present in non-inflamed tissue [46]. ICAM-1's co-receptor includes leukocyte function antigen-1 (LFA-1, α1β2 integrin), which is constitutively expressed on all leukocytes, although it can also be upregulated [38,47]. The ability of LFA-1 to bind ICAM-1, however, also depends upon qualitative changes resulting from its molecular conformation within the cell membrane [48]. VCAM-1 (also known as INCAM-110) primarily regulates mononuclear cell adhesion, and its co-receptor, very late activation antigen-4 (VLA-4, α4β1 integrin), is expressed by these cells [49,50].

A greater understanding of adhesion molecules is revealing their immense complexity and importance in inflammatory processes. Much of our current knowledge of the structure and functions of these molecules derives from *in vitro* work using binding assays, antibody-blocking studies and expression cloning, while the use of monoclonal antibodies in immunohistochemistry has helped to reveal the *in situ* spatial and temporal adhesion molecule expression patterns and has helped in understanding their potential roles *in vivo*.

The expression of activation-dependent adhesion molecules is also likely to be important in the progression of atherosclerotic inflammation [44]. One of the first morphological changes in the disease involves monocyte adherence to the endothelium, followed by an intimal involvement of inflammatory cells in the development of atherosclerosis. Adherence of monocytes and lymphocytes to the endothelium requires specific adhesion molecules; their induction may be crucial in determining not only the initiation but also the progression and clinical consequences of inflammation [51]. Adhesion molecules have recently been investigated in early atherosclerosis in both animal models and in human tissue, but the adhesion process in the slowly progressive human atheromatous lesions is as yet unclear [52,53].

It has recently been shown that E-selectin and ICAM-1 are expressed by intimal endothelial cells in normal coronary arteries and overlying aortic fatty streaks; that as aortic atherosclerosis develops, ICAM-1 expression is associated with intimal lymphocyte and macrophage populations (Plate 9) and that E-selectin and VCAM-1 expression in the aortic adventitia increases with the severity of the atheromatous plaque and with the development of adventitial inflammatory cell infiltrates [54] (Plate 10). Gimbrone *et al.* [55] have suggested the importance of adhesion molecules in the early recruitment of mononuclear cells in atherosclerosis, and athero-ELAM (the rabbit equivalent of VCAM-1) has been shown to be expressed on rabbit intimal endothelial cells during atherogenesis. Moreover, VCAM-1 expression appears to precede macrophage migration in the rabbit model [52]. Poston *et al.* [53] however, have reported ICAM-1 expression, but not VCAM-1 or E-selectin, on intimal endothelium overlying fatty streaks and fibrofatty plaques on human post-mortem samples suggesting its possible role in the recruitment of monocytes into the plaque. However, the role of adhesion molecules in early human atherosclerosis remains to be fully elucidated [51].

9.2 Macrophages, oxidized lipids and atherosclerosis

9.2.1 MACROPHAGES AND ATHEROSCLEROSIS

A role for blood-borne mononuclear cells in atherogenesis was first suggested by work on diet-induced lesions in

334 INFLAMMATION AND ATHEROSCLEROSIS

rabbits [9]. Electron microscopy of spontaneous human atherosclerosis supported this [55,56] as have cell marker studies [57] and, more recently, using immunohistochemistry with monoclonal antibodies [10–12] (Figure 9.2). Thus it has been shown that lipid-laden 'foam cells' in early and advanced atherosclerotic plaques are monocyte-derived macrophages rather than smooth muscle cells.

Macrophages participate in the immune response by presenting foreign antigen to T lymphocytes. The macrophage does this by internalizing antigen by endocytosis. There then follows partial degradation of the antigen within the macrophage lysozomes followed by transfer of antigen fragments to the macrophage cell surface. The antigen fragments associate with polymorphic cell surface MHC proteins and the antigen receptor of the T lymphocyte then binds to this macromolecular complex on the macrophage surface.

Monocytes have been shown to preferentially bind to injured endothelium. This is partially due to an interaction between the Fc receptor of the monocyte and IgG which is absorbed onto cytoskeletal intermediate filaments. The binding of IgG also activates the complement cascade which in turn generates anaphylatoxin C5a, an important chemoattractant for monocytes and granulocytes. Another mechanism for recruitment of monocytes to the vessel is via endothelial expression of specific leukocyte adhesive proteins.

Current theories of atherogenesis take into account haemodynamic forces, endothelial damage, platelet function, thrombosis, smooth muscle cell migration and proliferation, cholesterol levels, lipoprotein infiltration and modification, viral infection, senescence and inflammation. It seems likely that all these factors can participate in the development of atherosclerosis and that it is a combination of these and other as yet unknown factors which may determine the extent and severity of plaque development and clinical sequelae.

9.2.2 MODIFICATION OF LOW DENSITY LIPOPROTEIN BY MACROPHAGES

The recognition that foam cells in human atherosclerotic plaques are macrophages lends new importance to studies on lipoprotein uptake.

Cholesterol is transported around the body mainly in the form of low density lipoprotein (LDL). Most cell types, including macrophages and smooth muscle cells, take up exogenous cholesterol from LDL for which they have high affinity receptors. In times of cholesterol excess, these receptors are down-regulated and thus the cell is prevented from becoming overloaded. In homozygotes with familial hypercholesterolaemia, these receptors are defective and plasma LDL levels are abnormally high [58–60]. In this disease, macrophages in a variety of tissues become filled with lipid droplets. The most likely mechanisms to account for this phenomenon are uptake of LDL by a low-affinity, non-receptor-mediated, non-saturable pathway related to LDL concentration or by uptake of modified forms of LDL via a 'scavenger receptor pathway'. These scavenger receptors for modified LDL are present in macrophages and endo-

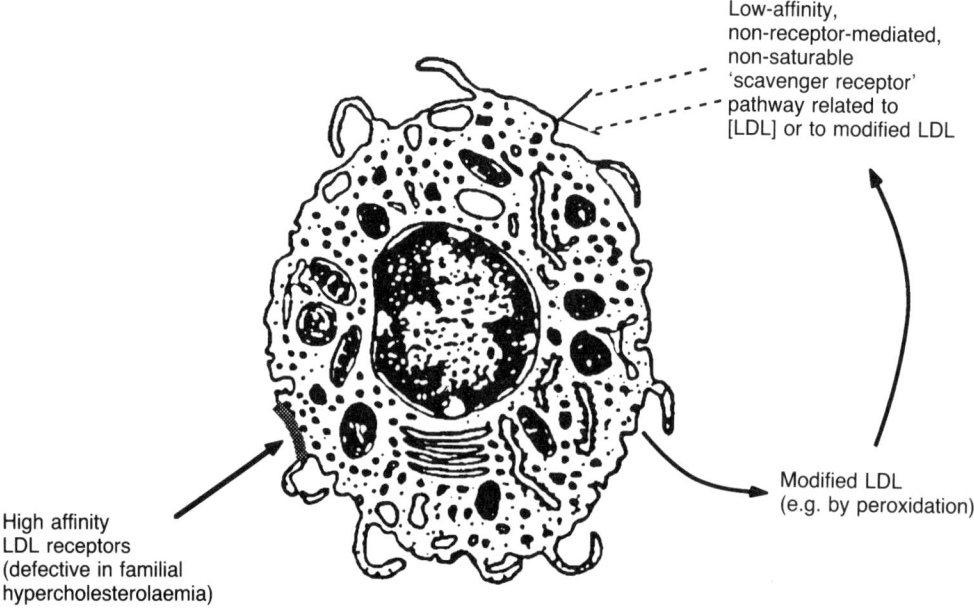

Figure 9.3 Role of macrophages in the uptake and modification of low density lipoprotein.

thelial cells but not in other cells. The scavenger receptors for modified LDL are not down-regulated by high cellular cholesterol levels. This leads to the development of the bloated, lipid-laden macrophage foam cell (Figure 9.3).

LDL which has been chemically modified, for example by acetylation or oxidation, is taken up more readily by macrophages *in vitro* and cleared from the bloodstream *in vivo* than 'native' or unmodified LDL [60,61]. It has been shown that LDL extracted from aortic wall is taken up more avidly by mouse peritoneal macrophages than is native LDL [62,63] and so is LDL from inflammatory fluid [64].

Intimal influx and accumulation of LDL begins at the earliest stages of atherosclerosis. LDL, in the form of ceroid, is also present in abundance in advanced atheroma [65]. Most cells take up LDL via high affinity LDL receptors, which are down-regulated when the cellular cholesterol content is adequate. Macrophages (the cells implicated in the formation of plaque foam cells) *in vitro* are only able to take up native LDL slowly [58]. They are, however, more readily able to take up modified forms of LDL, and this led to the proposal that these lipoproteins were taken up by a scavenger mechanism [58,66]. Scavenger receptors have been detected on macrophages in human atheroma and they avidly take up modified forms of LDL, permitting cellular ingestion and degradation of these lipoproteins and serving to clear potentially damaging molecules.

9.2.3 OXIDIZED LIPIDS AND ATHEROSCLEROSIS

There is increasing evidence that oxidative modification of low density lipoprotein plays an important role in atherogenesis. *In vitro* macrophages and endothelial cells can oxidize LDL, and this modified LDL is readily taken up by macrophages via the scavenger pathway to form lipid-ladem foam cells [63,66,67]. In addition, LDL isolated from atherosclerotic lesions resembles this experimentally oxidized LDL [67].

Antibodies that recognize oxidized LDL but not native LDL have been shown to react with atherosclerotic lesions. Human serum contains antibodies to oxidized LDL but not to native LDL and these antibodies have been correlated to the progression of carotid atherosclerosis [28,34] and to the progression of chronic periaortitis.

Further indirect evidence supporting a role for oxidized LDL is provided by the observation that antioxidant therapy decreases progression of atherosclerosis in animal models [68]. Finally, oxidized LDL acquires various properties not found in native LDL which are consistent with plaque progression. Oxidized LDL is a chemoattractant for monocytes and inhibits macrophage motility. This might explain high macrophage counts in the plaque that increase in relation to plaque LDL. Oxidized LDL also has cytotoxic properties which cause endothelial cell injury *in vitro*, and which would explain the necrotic core formation in fibrofatty plaques. In addition, oxidized LDL can induce the synthesis and release of chemotactic substances such as cytokines, which are thought to lead to further plaque development.

In the arterial intima, this role of the macrophage may be crucial to the development of the atherosclerotic plaque. Macrophages are known to release harmful enzymes when they die [69] and they also secrete substances which cause cell proliferation [70]. In addition, oxidized lipids have been shown to damage enzymes and membranes, to cause necrosis [71] and to decrease prostacyclin production [72]. One other result of LDL modification is that it may be rendered antigenic [73]. It is therefore possible that auto-allergy to this modified LDL is a factor in the development or the pathogenesis of atherosclerosis.

9.2.4 CEROID

Ceroid is commonly seen in both early and advanced atherosclerotic plaques, both extracellularly and within macrophages, particularly at the necrotic base [65] (Figure 9.4). Ceroid may be regarded as the insoluble end-product of oxidation of LDL in the macrophage and is thought to consist of polymerized products of oxidized lipoproteins. It can be made artificially in the laboratory by oxidizing low density lipoprotein (LDL) [63]. Immunoglobulin-secreting plasma cells in the aortic adventitial infiltrate occur in chronic periaortitis; this has been interpreted as evidence that chronic periaortitis is due to an auto-allergic reaction to a component of the atherosclerotic plaque [34,74].

The possibility that ceroid, which is produced by macrophages in atheroma, might be antigenic was first suspected when human immunoglobulin was found to localize to ceroid in atherosclerotic plaques from patients with chronic periaortitis [75]. Circulating antibodies to oxidized LDL and ceroid are present in patients with atherosclerosis and chronic periaortitis [34].

9.2.5 THE MACROPHAGE HYPOTHESIS

The 'response to injury hypothesis' [20] is based on the view that haemodynamic injury to the arterial wall leads to endothelial denudation, followed by platelet adhesion and degranulation, which in turn results in the release of platelet-derived growth factor (PDGF) causing proliferation of smooth muscle cells. This, along with the accumulation of intracellular and extracellular lipid, basal necrosis and laying down of collagen and connective tissue matrix led to the development of the lesion.

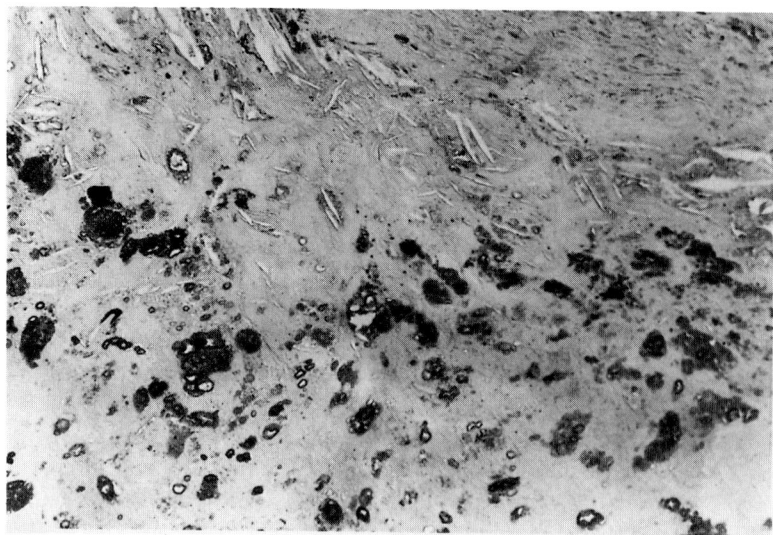

Figure 9.4 This light micrograph shows a routinely processed section of an advanced human atherosclerotic plaque which has been stained with a dark red lipid stain, oil red-O. Note the cholesterol clefts in the upper portion of the photograph. These are sites where soluble cholesterol crystals have dissolved out of the section during routine processing. The dark red staining granules and ring forms which remain represent the insoluble lipid, ceroid which is elaborated in the atheroma by macrophages.

Inherent in this view is the conviction that most, if not all of the cells in the lesion, particularly the lipid-laden foam cells, are derived from smooth muscle cells.

It is now apparent that foam cells which are present in fatty streaks and at the edges of most advanced plaques, are macrophages and that macrophages are found in the necrotic base of the advanced atherosclerotic plaque. Smooth muscle cells are present in diffuse intimal thickening and are increased in number in larger lesions.

The 'macrophage hypothesis' can be seen as a unifying concept which may shed some light on the mechanisms of atherogenesis but may also permit some understanding of how atherosclerosis causes human disease.

In terms of the development of the clinical complications of atherosclerosis, the most important role of the macrophage includes their interactions with lipoproteins; secretion of monokines which recruit and modulate the behaviour of other cells; release of enzymes; release of oxygen radicals and their ability to modify lipoprotein, rendering it toxic, immunogenic and more amenable to the scavenger receptor pathway. Their role thus includes:

- secretion of IL-1, IL-6, TNFα, PDGF;
- secretion of growth factors for smooth muscle cells;
- transport of LDL into the intima;
- secretion of cytokines which are chemoattractant for leucocytes;
- secretion of cytokines which are chemoattractant for monocytes;
- secretion of angiogenic factors;
- oxidation of LDL;
- secretion of factors which induce phenotypic modulation of smooth muscle cells, from a contractile to a secretory form;
- secretion of neutral proteases which degrade collagen and elastin;
- production of oxygen free radicals;
- production of ceroid;
- antigen presentation to B cells and T helper cells.

9.3 Chronic inflammation and advanced atherosclerosis

9.3.1 INFLAMMATION AND ADVANCED ATHEROSCLEROSIS; SUBCLINICAL CHRONIC PERIAORTITIS

In 1915, Allbutt described atherosclerosis as 'a very chronic inflammation' and noted the 'round cell growth' in the adventitia [76]. Brief mention of these cellular aggregates, associated with advanced atherosclerotic plaques, have since been made by other workers who have interpreted them variously [22,23].

While inflammation in early atherosclerosis appears confined to the intima, as the lesion progresses and the media thins, inflammation begins to involve the entire wall beneath the atherosclerotic plaque, leading eventually to inflammatory changes in the adventitia and media [21] (Figures 9.5, 9.6). The inflammatory cells consist of lymphocytes and plasma cells (Figure 9.7), macrophages and abundant new vessels with high endo-

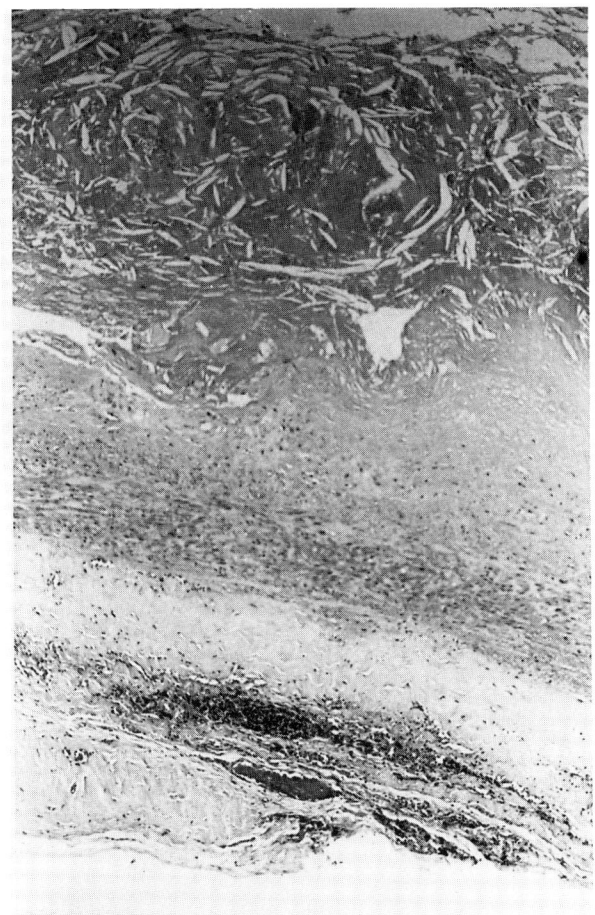

Figure 9.5 Abdominal aorta showing atheroma 'nibbling' through and disrupting the media (top) and focal aggregates of chronic inflammatory cells in the adventitia (bottom). This is subclinical chronic periaortitis and the macroscopic appearance of the aorta is shown in Figure 9.10. (H&E.)

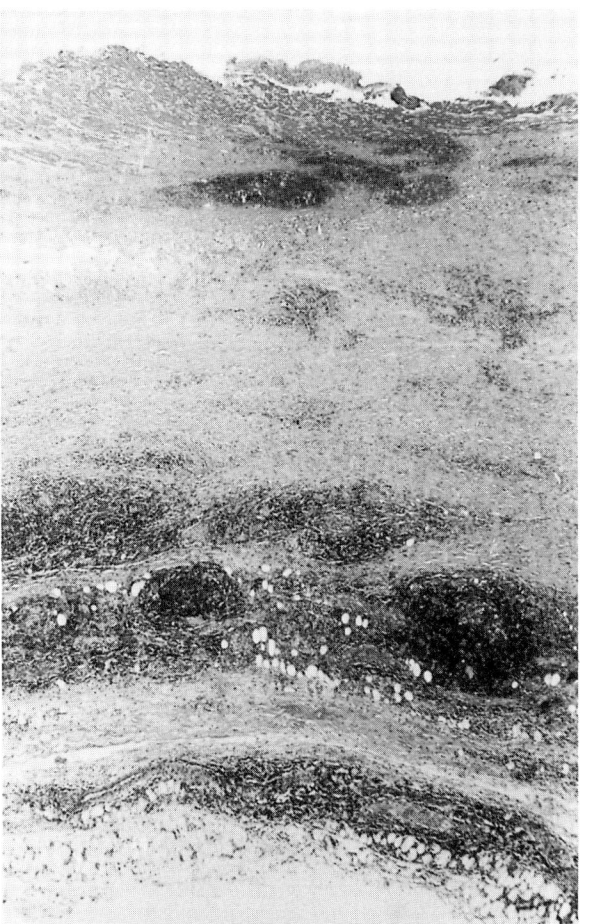

Figure 9.6 Abdominal aorta showing replacement of the media. There is more severe adventitial chronic inflammation producing a visibly thickenened aortic wall (8 mm). Note the lymphoid follicle formation in the adventitia (bottom). This case was called an 'inflammatory aneurysm' by the surgeon resecting the aortic aneurysm, who noticed the thickened wall. (H&E.)

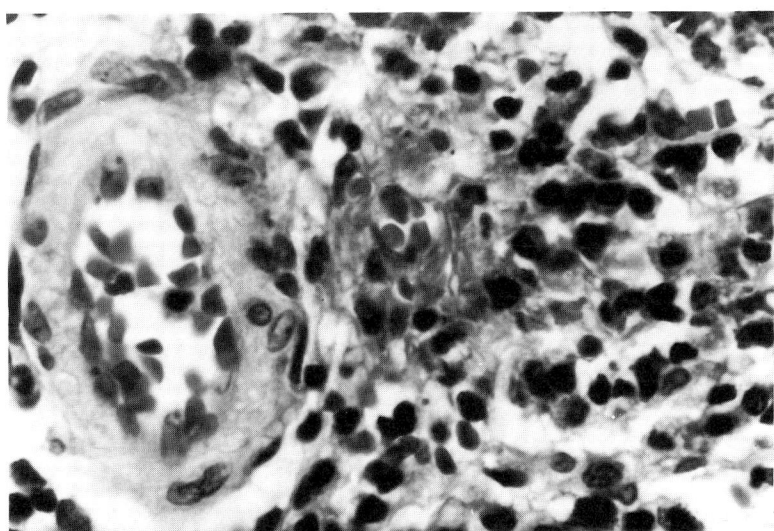

Figure 9.7 Chronic inflammatory cells in subclinical chronic periaortitis consist of lymphocytes, plasma cells and macrophages, seen here clustered around the vasa vasorum in the adventitia. (H&E.)

thelial cells. Dense cellular aggregates are seen and lymphoid follicles are common.

Lymphocytes and macrophages in the intima of atherosclerotic arteries have been described by light and electron microscopy. In 1979, Joris and colleagues, in an electron microscopic study in the rat, observed the infiltration of blood-borne mononuclear cells into the intima and proposed that this was in response to a chemical message, perhaps an antigen, originating from the media [78].

In 1962, Schwartz and Mitchell suggested that arterial adventitial infiltrates of small lymphocytes correlated with the severity of the intimal atheromatous lesion and not with the anatomical site of the plaque nor with the patient's age or sex [21]. Furthermore, these workers described the predominance of lymphocytes and plasma cells in the adventitia and media. They pointed out that in other conditions in which adventitial cellular changes occur, including polyarteritis nodosa, giant cell arteritis and disseminated lupus erythematosus, the cellular pattern was different to that found associated with the advanced atherosclerotic plaque. They suggested that these changes were involved in the pathogenesis rather than the aetiology of atherosclerosis and were due to some 'change in immunological tolerance' to a component of the plaque itself.

In 1981, it was noted that while advanced plaques with intact media showed very little adventitial inflammation, those with medial thinning and disruption were invariably associated with more severe adventitial infiltrates [74]. It has since become clear that advanced plaques are seldom without adventitial inflammation once the media has been disrupted [23,74,75].

In a review of the histology of atherosclerotic aortas and arteries, 92% showed some degree of inflammation [23]. Medial thinning and well formed aggregates of adventitial lymphoid cells were present in 49% [23]. Therefore subclinical chronic periaortitis and periarteritis is a common histological finding, seen on routine autopsy histology. The critical degree of aortic thickening which determines whether or not the surgeon notices the inflammation and where clinical complications begin to arise appears to be 0.5 cm. [23].

9.3.2 CLINICAL CHRONIC PERIAORTITIS

In 1890, in his first volume of *Archives of Surgery*, Hutchinson made a comment that 'in elderly patients, arteries are liable to a spreading inflammation which glues the artery to its sheath'. He noted that inflammation was the hallmark of atheroma which differentiated it from 'senile change' or 'fatty degeneration' [77].

Lymphocytic inflammation of the arterial adventitia is most often found in the abdominal aorta, a region affected by severe atherosclerosis and the commonest site of aneurysm formation [22,78] (Figure 9.8). The

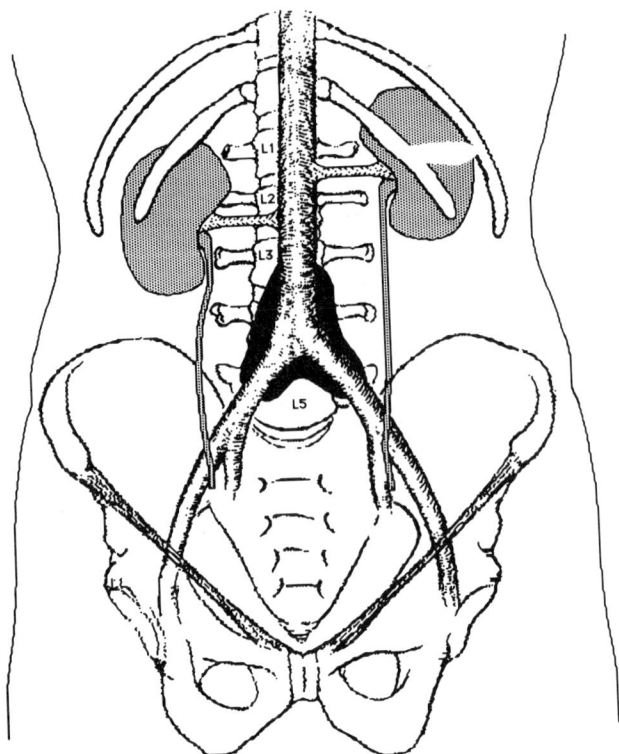

Figure 9.8 Common site for atherosclerotic aortic aneurysm and for clinical chronic periaortitis. Human aorta and its anatomical relations are shown. The lower abdominal aorta above the aortic bifurcation is the site where atherosclerosis is most severe. This is also the site where the local complications of atherosclerosis are most severe. These local complications include stenosis of the aortic lumen, calcification, thrombosis, aneurysm formation and chronic inflammation (chronic periaortitis).

inflammation can be severe enough to affect the entire aorta, resulting in adhesion and obstruction of adjacent structures such as the ureters, duodenum or the inferior vena cava [79]. These complications have been reported as a variety of disease entities termed 'idiopathic retroperitoneal fibrosis', 'peri-aneurysmal retroperitoneal fibrosis', 'mediastinal fibrosis', and 'inflammatory aneurysm'. All of these disorders show periaortic inflammation associated with advanced atherosclerosis and medial disruption and are histologically identical, with similar chronic inflammatory cell types [22,23] (Figure 9.9). They differ only in degree and site of inflammation and fibrosis, presence or absence of aneurysm, and whether there is secondary involvement of nearby organs [22,23].

The incidence of clinical chronic periaortitis may be of the order of 0.4%. Like 'idiopathic retroperitoneal fibrosis', 'inflammatory aneurysms' show advanced atherosclerosis, inflammation and a variable degree of adventitial fibrosis [22,23]. Both feature periaortic inflammation which can extend into the peritoneum and

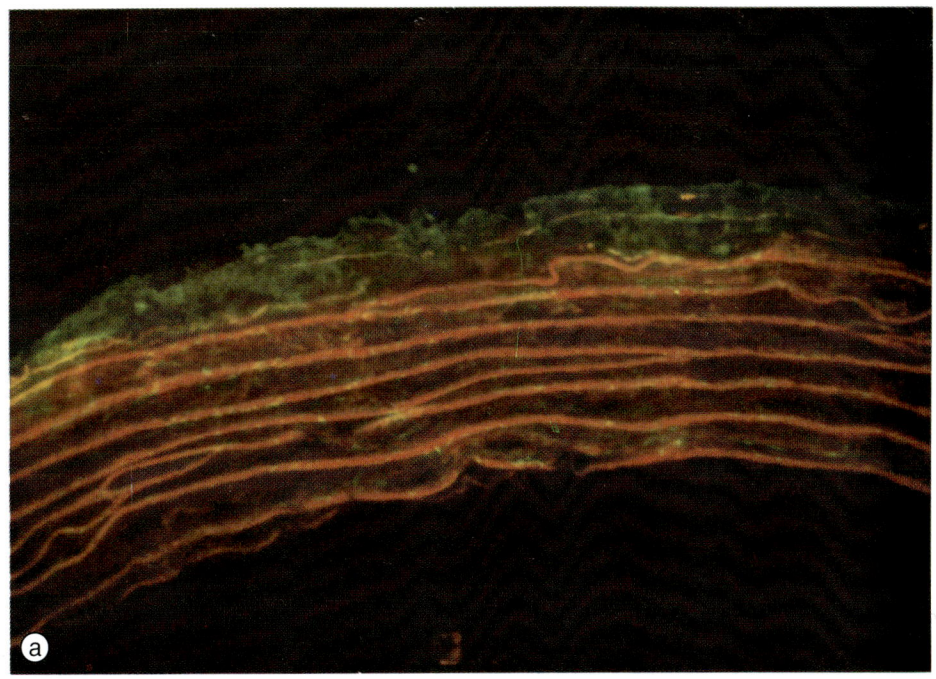

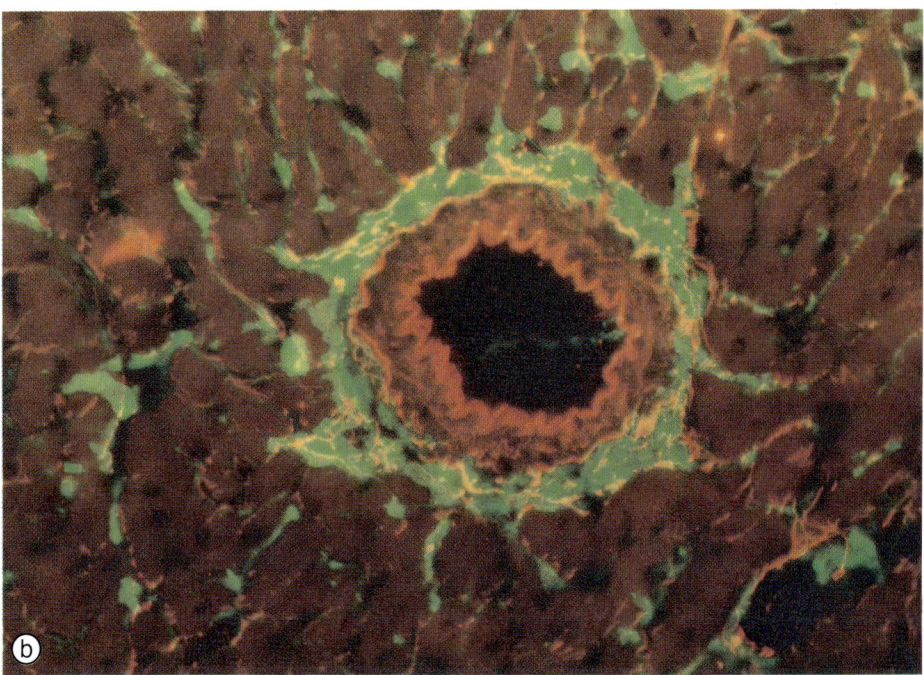

Plate 1 Double antibody staining showing (a) the location of elastin (red) in relation to collagen type III (green) in rat coronary artery and (b) elastin staining of the elastic laminae (red) with collagen type I staining (green) mainly in the adventitial layer (top).

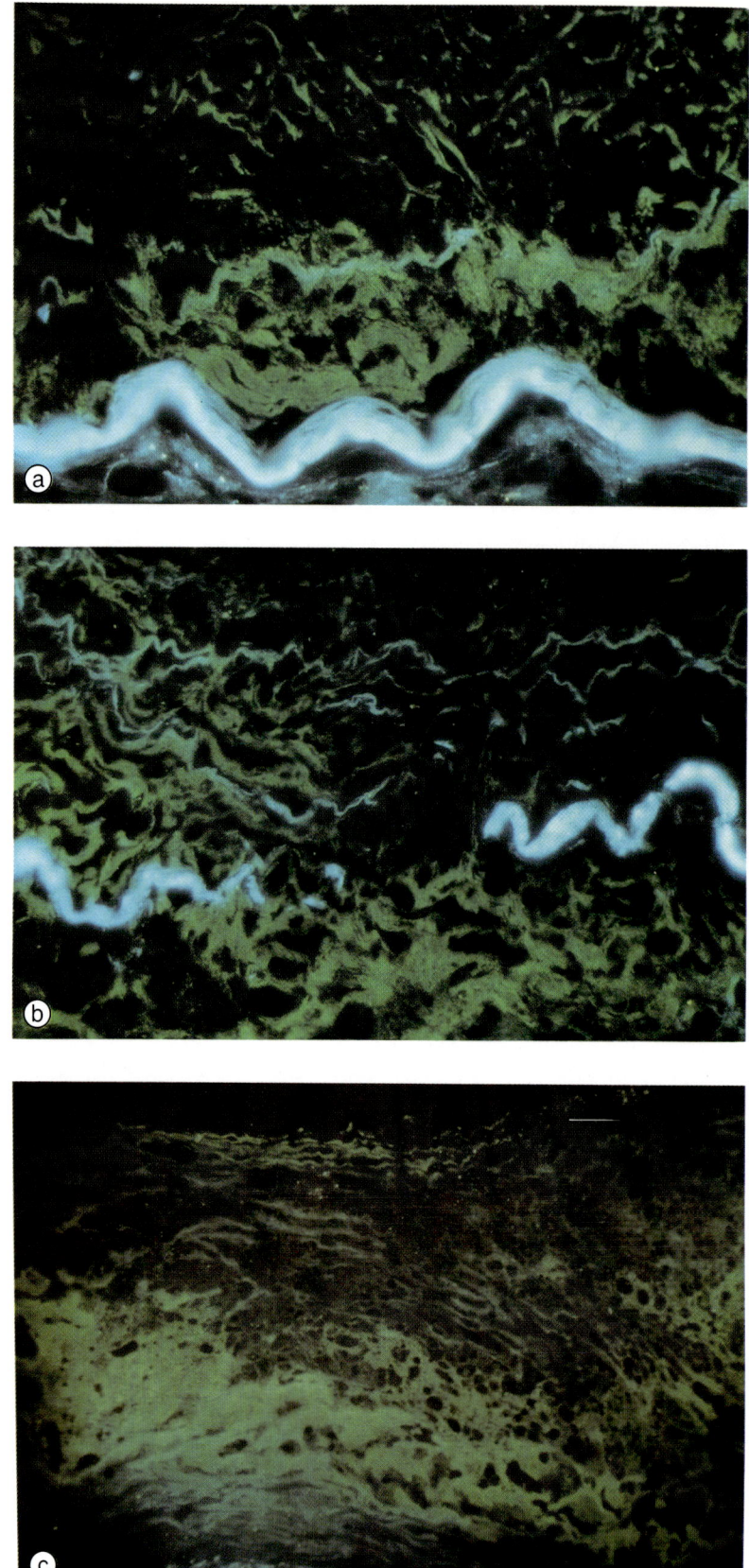

Plate 2 (a) Fatty streak lesion in a human cerebral artery; localization of Apo-B (green) immunofluorescence between elastic lamellae but on the intimal side of the thick internal elastic membrane (white). (b) Area adjacent to that seen in (a) but showing a fenestration in the internal elastic membrane and Apo-B (green) on the medial side. (c) Fibrous plaque in a human coronary artery; localization of Apo-B (green) by immunofluorescence in the necrotic core and associated with some collagen fibers in the fibrous cap close to the lumen (top of micrograph).

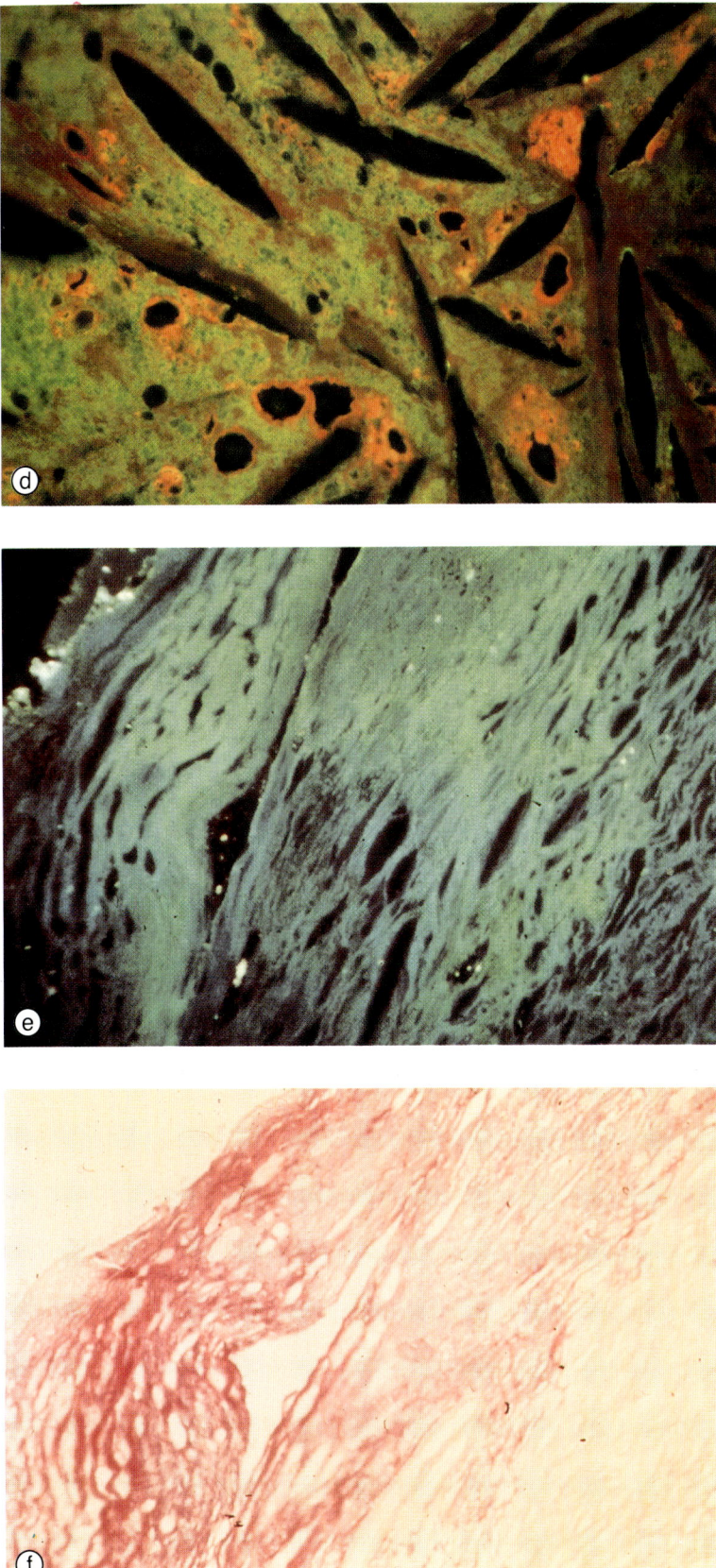

Plate 2 *contd* (d) Necrotic core of a fibrous plaque from a human aortic lesion; localization of Apo-B (green) by immunofluorescence as a diffuse distribution throughout the necrotic core with the exception of areas occupied by cholesterol monohydrate crystals, capillaries and regions originally occupied by lipid droplets. (e) Fibrous plaque in a human ab-dominal aorta, localization of Apo-B by immunofluorescence in the fibrotic cap. (f) Serial section of (d); localization of fibrin (pink) by the PTAH stain illustrating the same distribution as Apo-B.

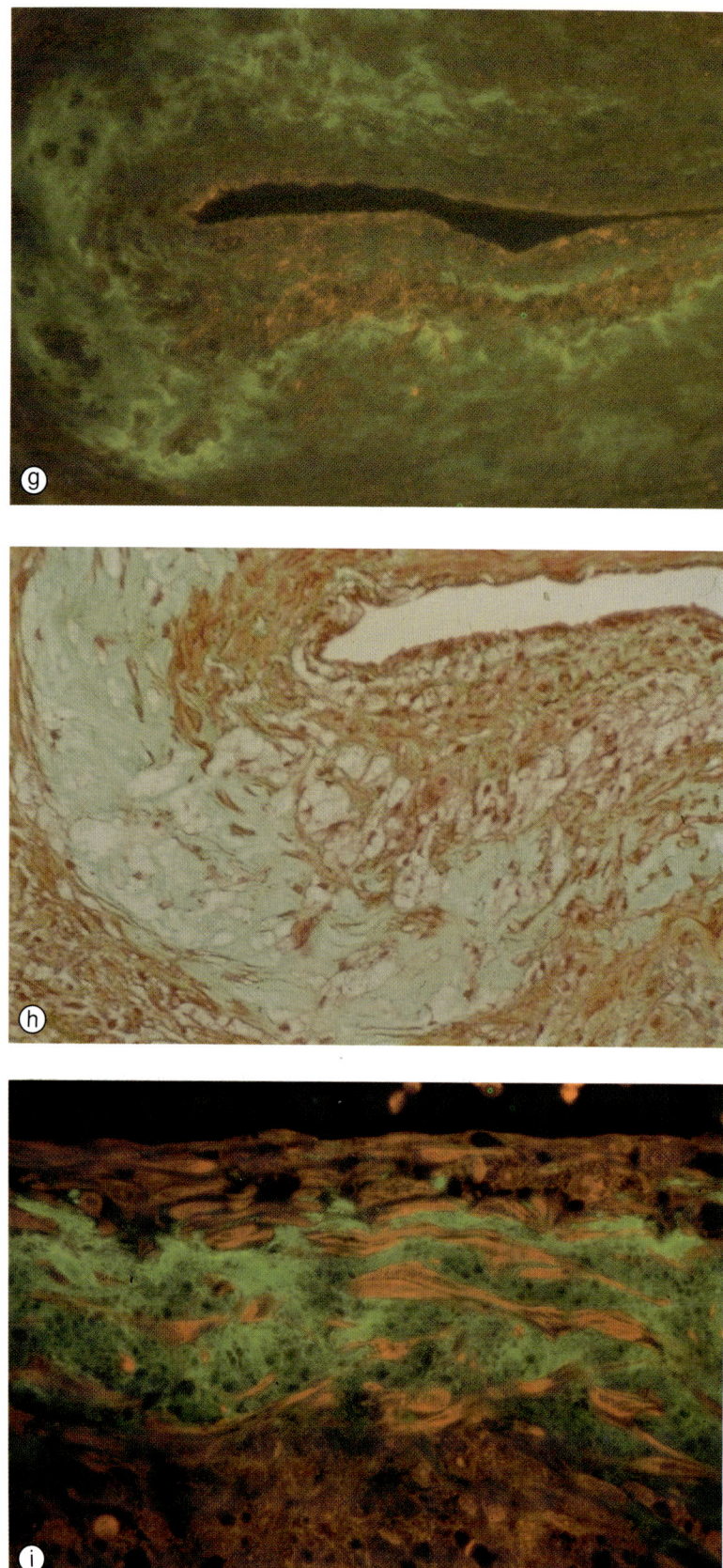

Plate 2 *contd*   (g) Lesion in the left circumflex coronary artery from a hypercholesterolemic cynomolgus monkey. Localization of Apo-B (green) by immunofluorescence in the extracellular space between intimal smooth muscle cells (orange) and in areas of necrosis. (h) Serial section of (d) but stained with Movat's pentachrome stain illustrating that the Apo-B-positive regions are positive for alcian blue suggesting the colocalization of Apo-B and GAG. (i) Lesion in the left circumflex coronary artery from a hypercholesterolemic cynomolgus monkey. Localization of Apo-B (green) by immunofluorescence between smooth muscle cells (orange).

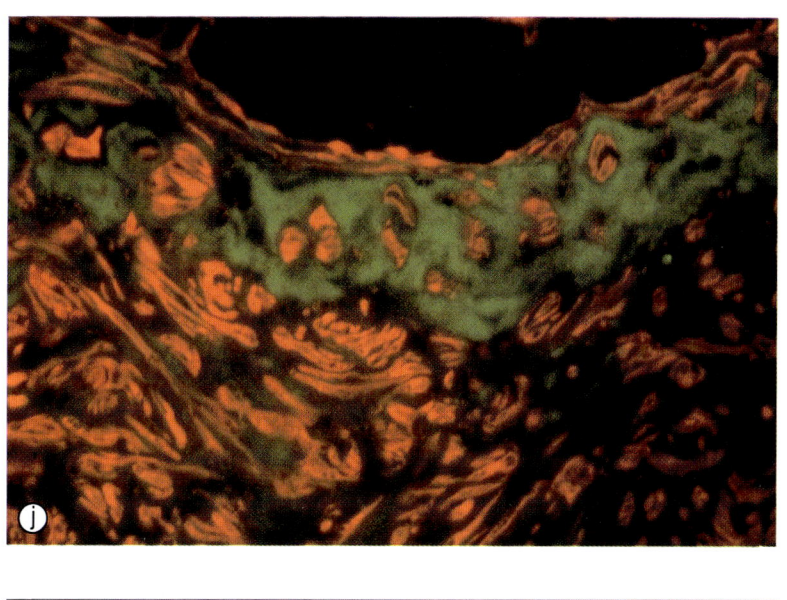

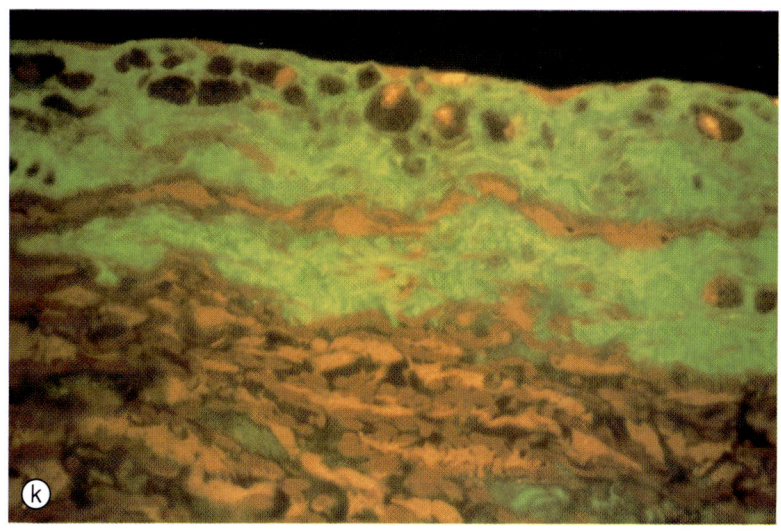

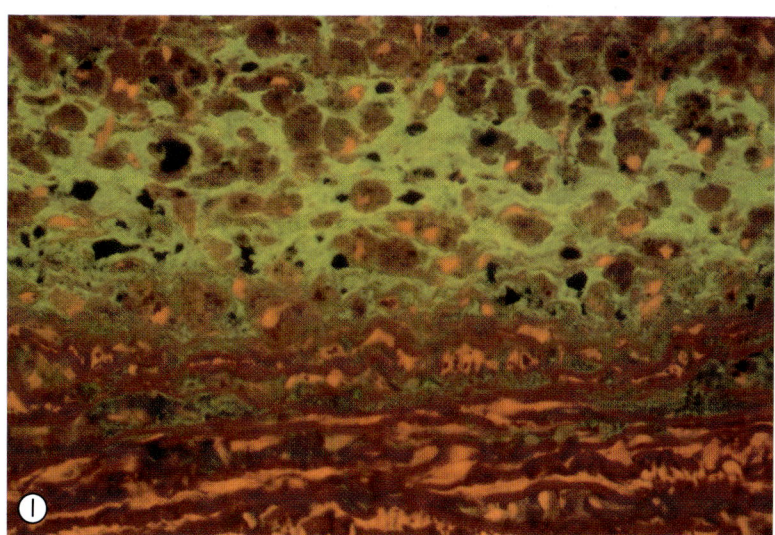

Plate 2 contd (j) Lesion in the right cornary artery from a hypercholesterolemic cynomologus monkey. Localization of Apo-B (green) by immunofluorescence in the fibrous cap of an advanced lesion. Note that a small but discrete distance separates the Apo-B-positive sites from the surface of smooth muscle cells (orange). (k) Grossly normal region of the aorta from a hypercholesterolemic swine. Localization of Apo-B (green) almost solely to the tunica intima and to the spaces between intimal smooth muscle cells (orange). (l) Fatty streak lesion in the aorta from a hypercholesterolemic mouse. Localization of Apo-B (green) in the narrow spaces between foam cells (brown) in the intima. (a) and (b) reproduced with permission from *Archives of Neurology*; (c), (e), (f), (k) and (l) reproduced with permission from *Archives of Pathology*; (g), (h), (i) and (d) reproduced with permission from *Artery*.)

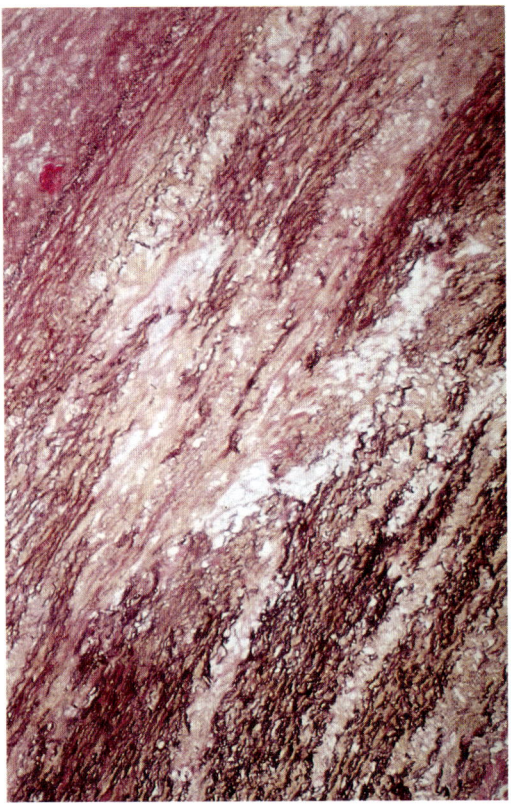

Plate 3 EVG stain in a section of aortic tissue demonstrating cystic medial necrosis with severe elastopathy in a case of Marfan's syndrome (collagen red; elastic fibres black)

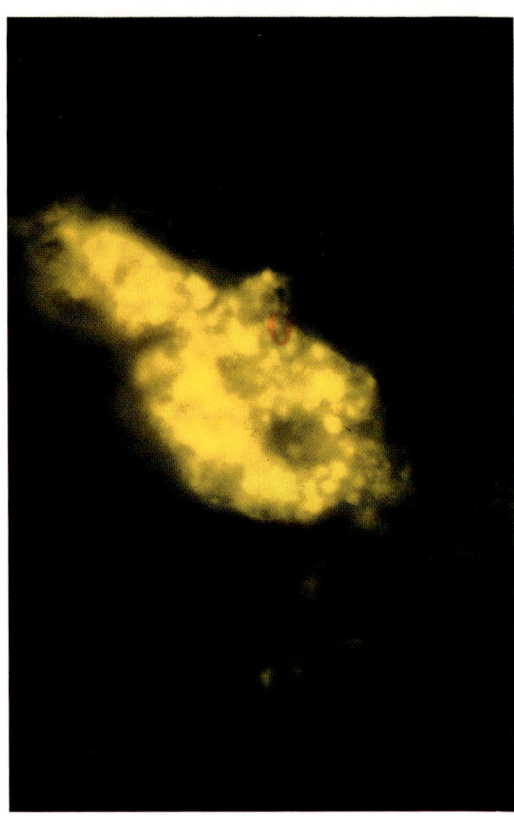

Plate 4 High power view of a ceroid-containing macrophage in the base of an atheromatous plaque, viewed under UV light, showing apple green autofluorescence.

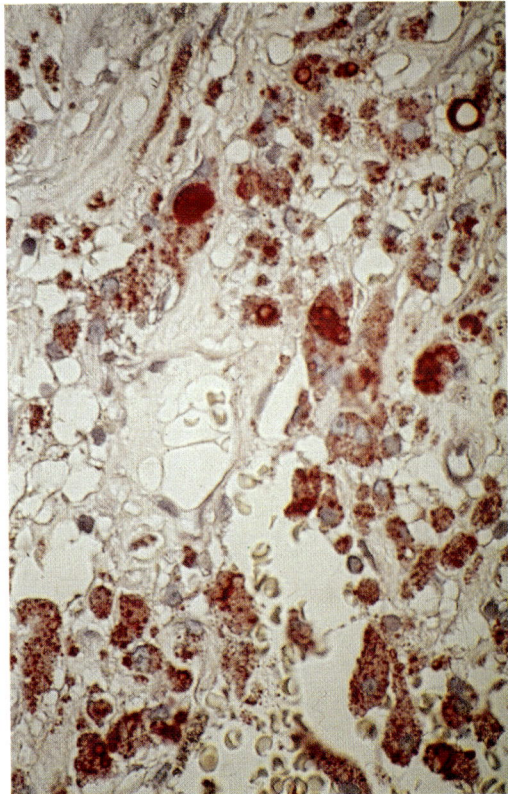

Plate 5 High power view of the base of an atheromatous plaque in a routinely fixed, paraffin-embedded tissue section, showing insoluble ceroid granules and ring forms stained red with ORO.

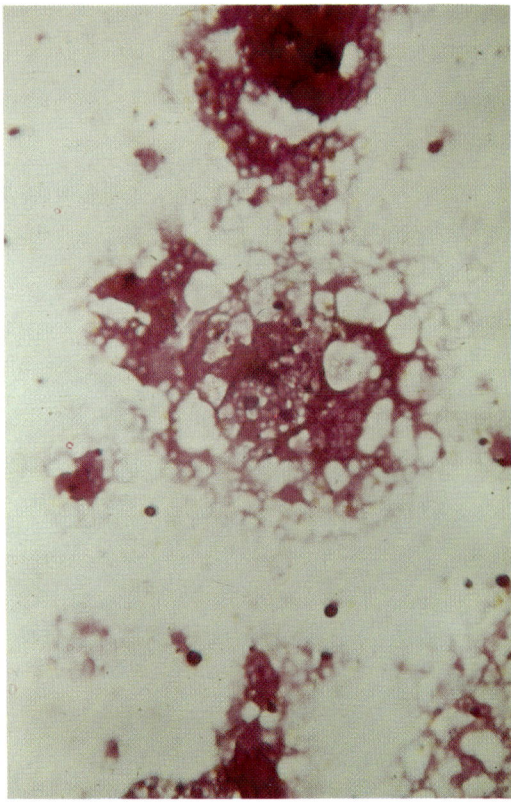

Plate 6 Cell smear of ceroid extracted from an atheromatous plaque stained magenta with PAS.

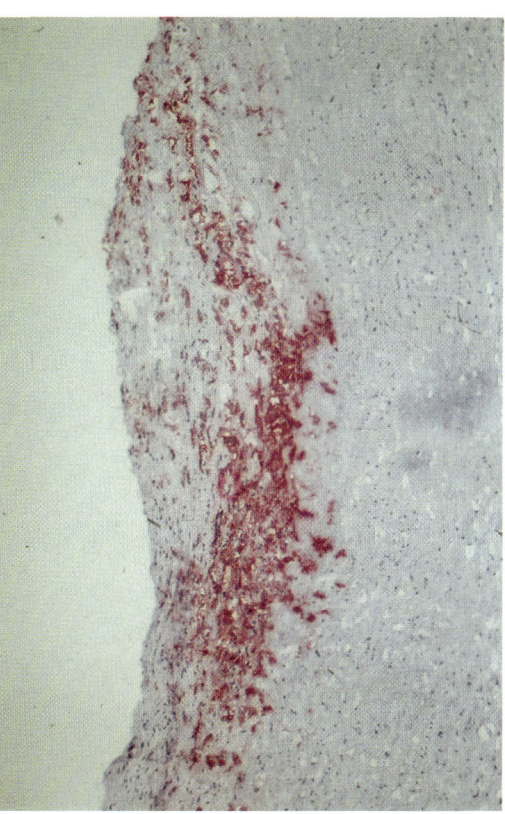

Plate 7 Monoclonal antibody KP1 stains macrophage populations in the intima of a coronary artery containing an early atherosclerotic plaque (APAAP with Fast Red).

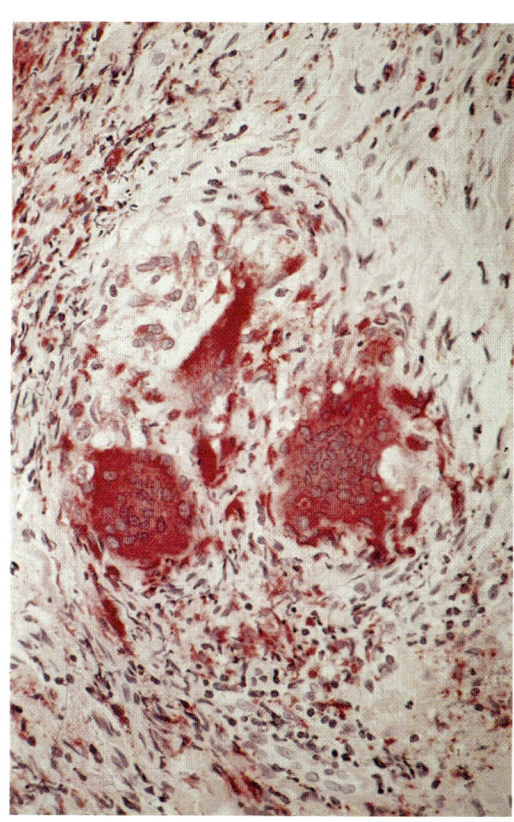

Plate 8 High power view of a giant cell granuloma in a temporal artery from a case of temporal arteritis stained with monoclonal antibody KP1 (APAAP with Fast Red).

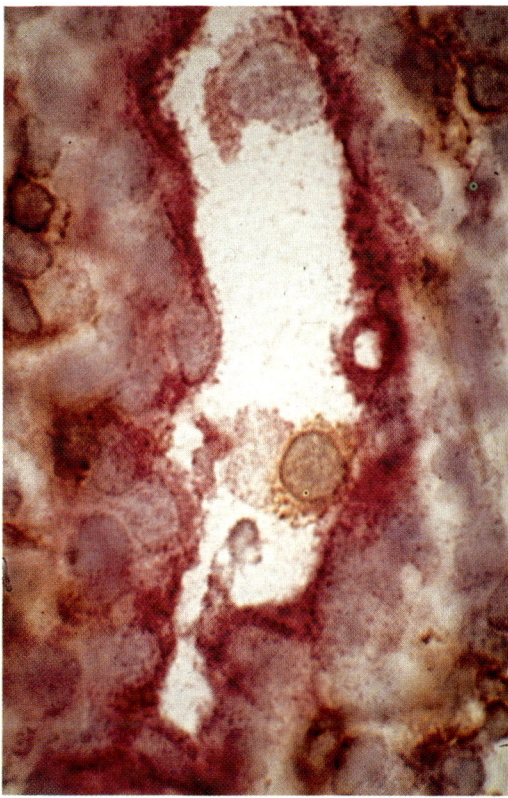

Plate 9 High power view of the inflamed adventitia in case of chronic periaortitis showing double immunostaining for endothelial cells with CD31 (red) and T suppressor lymphocytes with CD8 (brown) using a combination of APAAP and indirect immunoperoxidase techniques.

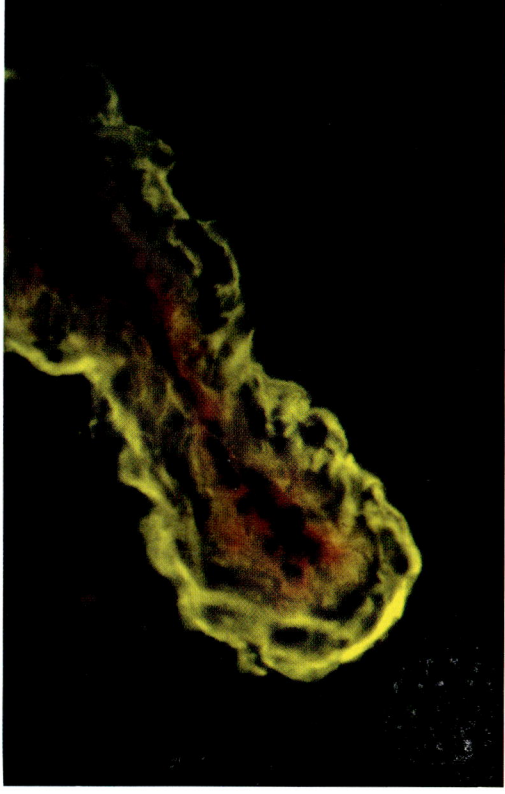

Plate 10 High power view of a vasa vasorum showing double immunofluorescence and immunohistochemical staining for endothelial cells with CD31 (red) and Type IV collagen (CIV22) (green) using a combination of APAAP and immunofluorescence techniques.

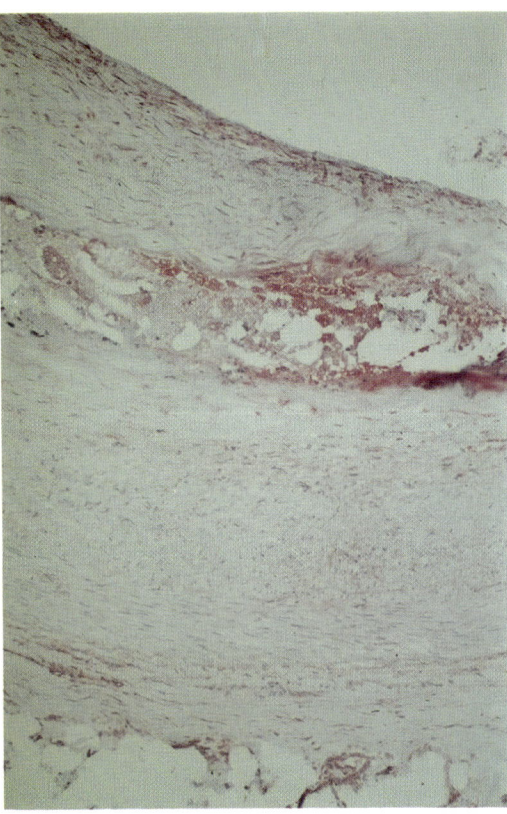

Plate 11 Low power view of a fibrofatty plaque showing ICAM-1 staining in the intima (top of photograph), in the macrophage-rich areas of atheroma beneath the fibrous cap and on the adventitial vasa vasorum (bottom of photograph). (Immunohistochemistry using APAAP and Fast Red.)

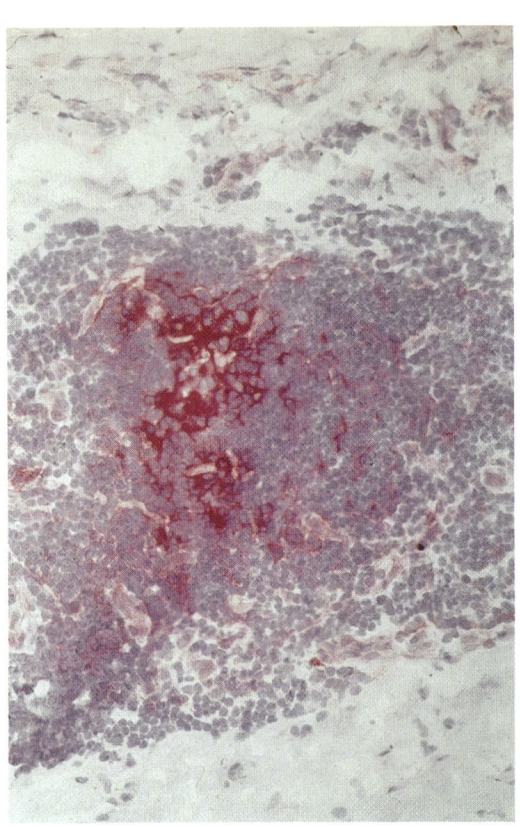

Plate 12 Intense VCAM-1 staining of aortic adventitial lymphoid aggregate associated with advanced intimal lesion (not shown). (Immunohistochemistry using APAAP and Fast Red.)

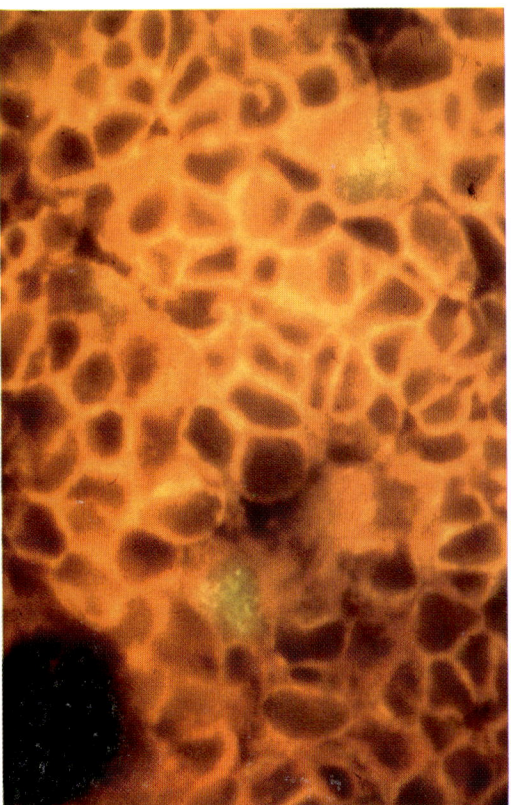

Plate 13 High power view of the inflamed aortic adventitia in a case of chronic periaortitis showing CD4-positive T helper cells (red/orange) some of which show green Ki-67-positive nuclei. (Double immunohistochemistry with APAAP and Fast Red and immunofluorescence with fluorescein.)

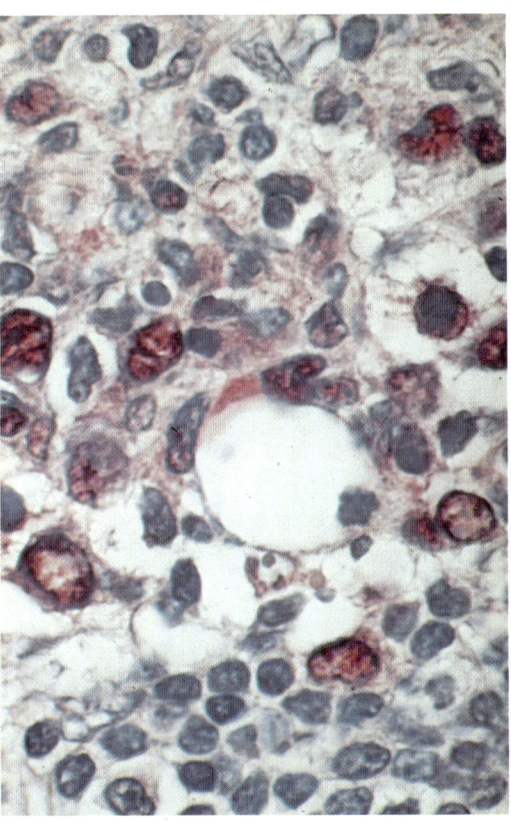

Plate 14 High power view of the inflamed aortic adventitia in a case of chronic periaortitis showing PCNA-positive proliferating cells within a germinal centre.

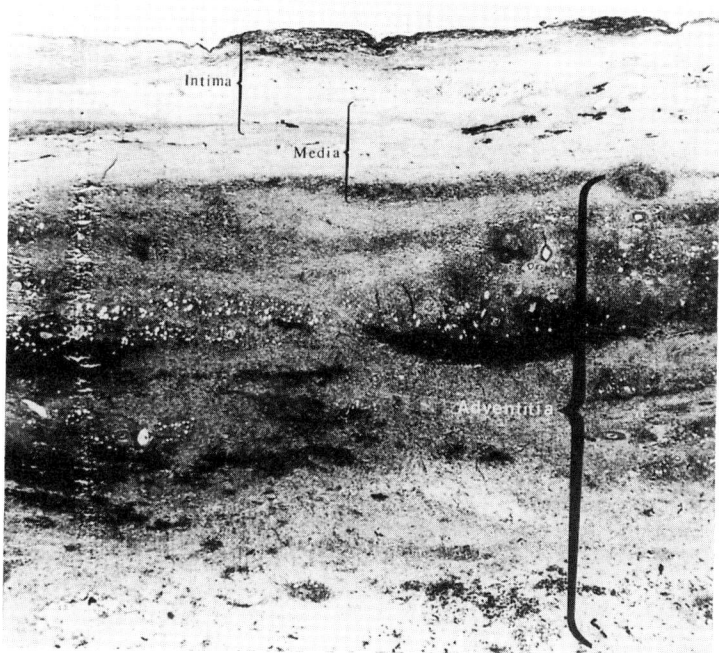

Figure 9.9 Low power scanning view of the wall of the aorta in a case of clinical chronic periaortitis showing the atheromatous intima, the thinned media and the thickened adventitia (10 mm). The outer limit of the fibrosis extends below the outer edge of the photomicrograph. (H&E.) (Scale 1 cm = 1 mm.) (Reproduced with permission from Parums [23].)

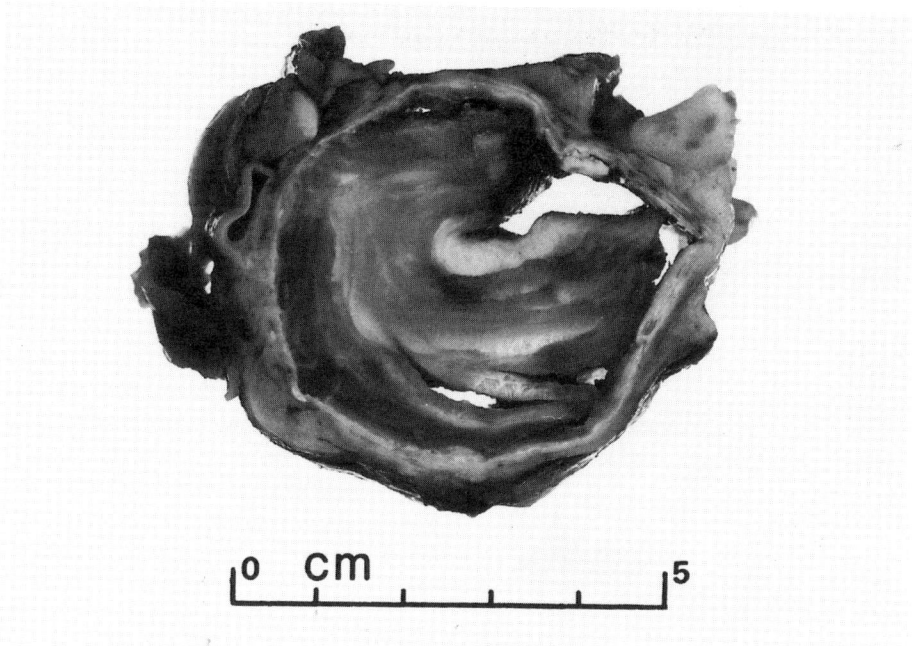

Figure 9.10 Macroscopic photograph of a transected atherosclerotic abdominal aortic aneurysm showing intimal atherosclerosis and laminated thrombus. The aortic wall was not noted to be thickened macroscopically but histology showed the features of subclinical chronic periaortitis, namely advanced atherosclerosis, medial thinning and adventitial chronic inflammation and is shown in Figure 9.5.

entrap ureters or other neighbouring structures (Figure 9.9). The age, gender and symptoms of those afflicted are also similar in both diseases, and they both are sensitive to steroids [79–81].

(a) 'Inflammatory aneurysm' – chronic periaortitis in the dilated aorta

Abdominal aortic aneurysms are most commonly associated with advanced atherosclerosis. The aneurysm is secondary to thinning of the aortic media, probably due to the atherosclerosis (Figure 9.10).

Occasionally, the surgeon sees an abdominal aortic aneurysm encased in fibrous tissue which extends into the retroperitoneum (Figure 9.11). For some time, surgeons and pathologists have tended to classify these abdominal aortic aneurysms as either 'atherosclerotic' or 'inflammatory'. These so-called 'inflammatory aneurysms' of the aorta have a reported incidence of 2.5–10% of all aortic aneurysms [81,82].

Walker introduced the term 'inflammatory aneurysm' in 1972 to describe abdominal aortic aneurysm with macroscopically evident fibrosis, thickening of the wall and dense adhesions to nearby structures [82]. These accounted for 10% of the aneurysms he studied, and it was suggested that these 'inflammatory aneurysms' were a different clinical entity from other atherosclerotic aneurysms, perhaps due to an immune response to blood products leaking through the weakened aneurysm wall [82].

In a thirty year review of 2816 abdominal aortic aneurysms undergoing elective surgical repair, Pennell and colleagues [81] reported an incidence of 4.5% of inflammatory aneurysms. The mean age of presentation was 64.2 years which compares with 65.5 years in this present study. They found that back and abdominal pain were the most common presenting symptoms in addition to weight loss; 50% were hypertensive at presentation. ESR was significantly raised above that of the atherosclerotic group ($P < 0.001$). These workers also reported a family history of aortic aneurysm in 7.6%, peripheral vascular disease in 26.6% and ischaemic heart disease in 39.4%. Mean aortic diameter was 78 mm and mean aortic wall thickness was 13 mm, which are greater diameters than those observed in aneurysms in the present study. They observed that the histological findings of medial degeneration, adventitial thickening and infiltration with lymphocytes and plasma cells were 'identical to those of idiopathic retroperitoneal fibrosis' except than in the latter the aorta is undilated.

To add to the confusion, the term 'peri-aneurysmal retroperitoneal fibrosis' has been used to describe the condition in which ureteric blockage has occurred as a result of fibrosis around atherosclerotic aneurysms of the abdominal aorta [80]. Pennell and colleagues [81] reported ureteral involvement in 23% of patients with 'inflammatory aneurysms'. The inflammatory infiltrate is the same as that seen in both 'idiopathic retroperitoneal fibrosis' and 'inflammatory aneurysms'; there is a raised ESR and the disease is sensitive to corticosteroids.

Thus it has been claimed that 'inflammatory aneurysms' are distinct from 'atherosclerotic aneurysms', and that in the former the aneurysm may be caused by inflammation rather than by atherosclerosis [82,83]. Others, however, have shown that 'inflammatory aneurysms' differ only in the extent of chronic inflammation and fibrosis from 'atherosclerotic aneurysms', and claim that the former are really a consequence of atherosclerosis [22,23]. Rose and Dent [84] showed that inflammation and fibrosis were present in virtually all aneurysms sectioned and that both types of aneurysm are associated with advanced atherosclerosis. Mitchinson [22] reported that a minority of aneurysms show more severe peri-aneurysmal inflammation and fibrosis, but no consistent criterion exists for distinguishing these aneurysms from others, and there is no evidence to support a separate aetiology. Furthermore, the frequency of 'inflammatory aneurysm' reported in the literature is variable, ranging from 2.5 to 10% of abdominal aortic aneurysms, with wall thickness from 5 to 50 mm [81]. While patients with extensive fibrosis suffer higher morbidity and mortality than those with other atherosclerotic aneurysms [85], there are no clear criteria for the diagnosis of distinct disorders.

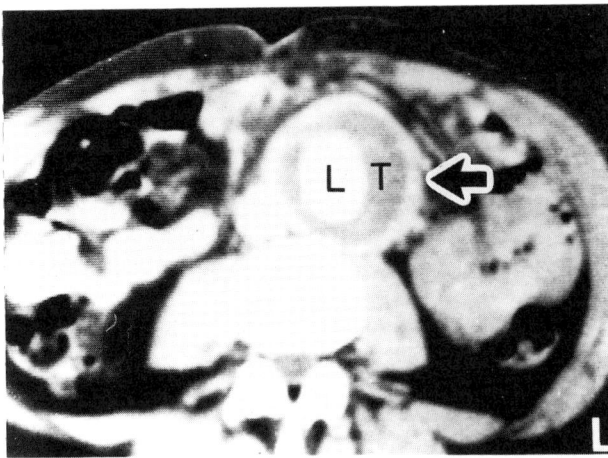

Figure 9.11 This is a contrast enhanced abdominal CT scan from a case of 'inflammatory aneurysm' which shows a dense, periaortic mass measuring 8 mm in thickness (arrow). The histology is shown in Figure 9.6. The aorta is 55 mm in diameter. The lumen (L) is opacified but not the thrombus (T) within the sac. Note the relation of the inflammatory tissue peripheral to the flecks of calcium present in the right lateral portion of the aortic wall.

Causes of inflammation associated with aortic aneurysm formation including Takayasu's and giant cell aortitis

Inflammation of the aorta, 'aortitis', has been recognized as an entity since the late 16th century when aortic aneurysm was known to be associated with syphilis. From the 15th century until the beginning of this century, syphilis was widespread in many countries and was probably the commonest cause of aortitis. Today, there are numerous but rare causes of aortitis which can lead to aneurysm formation. Infectious causes include:

- Syphilis
- Bacteria, e.g. *Staphylococcus, Pseudomonas, Pneumococcus, Salmonella, E. coli*
- Tuberculosis
- Fungi.

Non-infectious causes include:

- Giant cell aortitis
- Takayasu's aortitis
- Polyarteritis nodosa
- Rheumatoid arthritis
- Rheumatic fever
- Ankylosing spondylitis
- Relapsing polychondritis
- Behçet's disease
- Infantile polyarteritis or Kawasaki disease
- Systemic lupus erythematosus
- Sarcoidosis
- Cardiac myxoma embolus
- Churg–Strauss syndrome
- Wegener's granulomatosis.

Although chronic periaortitis is the commonest form of aortic inflammation and is seen around advanced atherosclerotic plaques, other inflammatory diseases affecting the aorta include polyarteritis nodosa, Kawasaki's disease, giant-cell aortitis, systemic lupus erythematosus, Takayasu's aortitis and syphilis [21,22]. The adventitial inflammation associated with atherosclerotic plaques can, however, be clearly distinguished from these other inflammatory disorders of the arteries, showing different adventitial changes, cell types, distribution and sites [22].

Takayasu's arteritis (non-specific aortoarteritis) was first described by Savory in 1856 [86] and is variously known as 'pulseless disease', 'young female arteritis', 'idiopathic aortitis', 'non-specific aortoarteritis' and 'aortic arch syndrome'. The disease occurs predominantly in women (female:male ratio 8:1). The age of onset is between 10 and 20 years although cases in infancy and late middle age have been reported. In half of cases, onset is associated with systemic symptoms such as fever, malaise, weight loss and joint pain. The process can involve the aortic arch and its branches, the thoracic, descending and abdominal aorta and the pulmonary arteries (subclavian arteries in 85%; descending thoracic aorta 67%; renal arteries 62%; carotid arteries 44%; aortic arch 27% and coronary arteries 30%) [87,88]. It is not associated with atherosclerosis but is thought to have an immune aetiology, possibly to mycobacterial antigens, and can be associated with arterial or aortic aneurysm. In the early stages, there is focal and segmental infiltration of the adventitia and media by lymphocytes and plasma cells. Eventually, all layers of the aorta are involved and destroyed with resultant intimal proliferation, fibrosis, obliteration of the vasa vasorum and variable chronic inflammatory infiltrate. The vessel lumen may become obliterated by a combination of fibrosis and thrombosis. Periaortic adhesions and fibrosis may occur [89].

The distribution of arterial and aortic lesions and the histopathology may be identical in giant cell and Takayasu's aortitis. However, in giant cell aortitis, the most intense inflammation tends to be located at the region of the internal elastic lamina and outer media whereas in Takayasu's disease the lesions are most prominent in the adventitia and outer part of the aortic wall. Intimal thickening and narrowing of the aortic lumen occurs in both conditions and aortic dilatation is seen in both conditions but only Takayasu's disease can produce aortic arch narrowing or coarctation [89].

Takayasu's disease begins usually during the first four decades of life but the onset of giant cell aortitis is rare or virtually unknown before 50 years. Giant cell aortitis appears more commonly in Caucasians, whereas Takayasu's disease is more frequently seen in people of Oriental and Indian ancestry [89].

(b) 'Idiopathic retroperitoneal fibrosis' – chronic periaortitis in the undilated aorta

'Idiopathic retroperitoneal fibrosis' (IRF) was first described by Albarran in 1905 [90] but is best known by the name of Ormond who described it in 1948 [91]. Typically, it is a disease of middle-aged to elderly males who develop chronic inflammation and fibrosis around the lower abdominal aorta. This inflammatory process tends to drag neighbouring hollow structures towards the mid-line. The disease usually presents as a urological problem with obstruction of one or both ureters, often resulting in hydronephrosis.

IRF is associated with weight loss, malaise and raised erythrocyte sedimentation rate (ESR) [92]. Brooks and colleagues [93], from a study of 12 patients who had abdominal CT scans before and after biopsy diagnosis of 'idiopathic retroperitoneal fibrosis', found that all showed decrease in size of the periaortic mass at follow-up, even though two of these patients had not been treated with steroids. These investigators suggested that the mass in chronic periaortitis shrinks as part of its natural history. The variable proportions of cells and

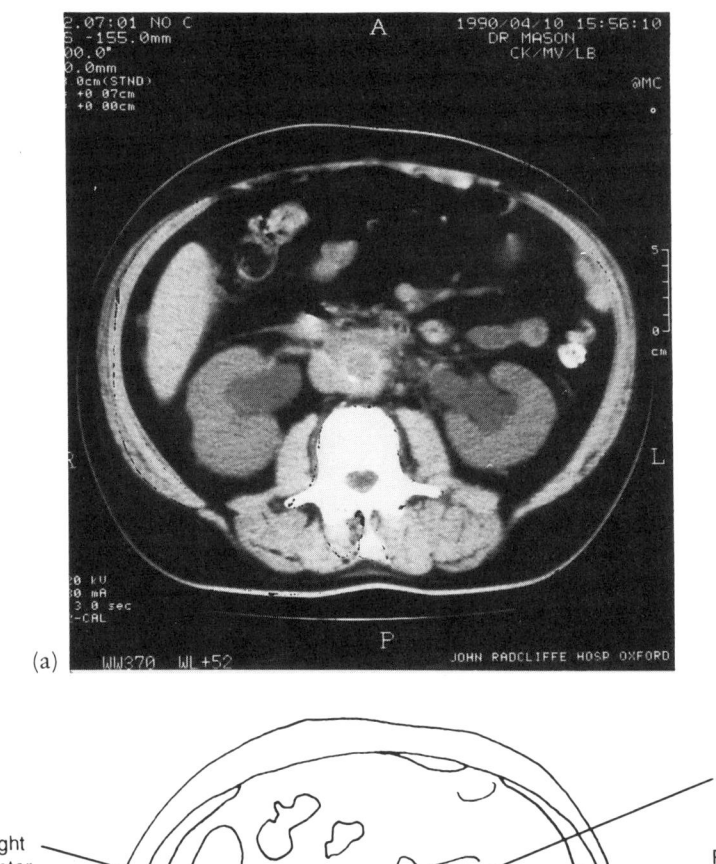
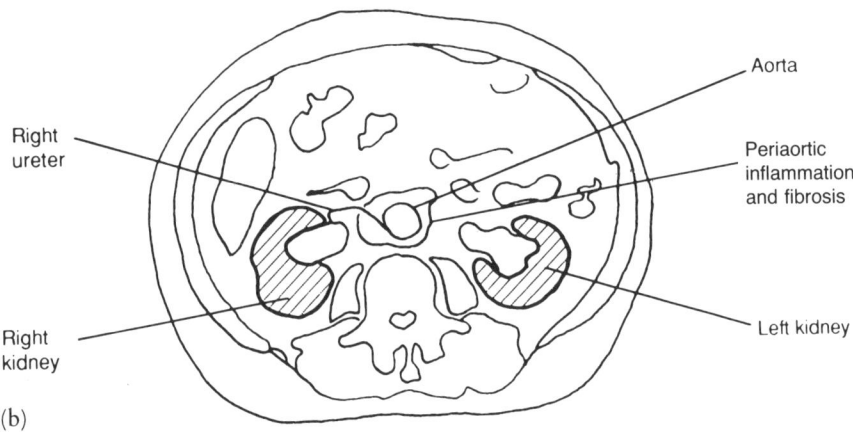

Figure 9.12(a) and (b) Abdominal CT scan from a case of 'idiopathic retroperitoneal fibrosis' showing calcified atheroma lining the aorta. The aorta was surrounded by a cuff of soft tissue which has engulfed the ureters resulting in bilateral hydronephrosis. The aorta was not increased in diameter.

fibrous tissue seen histologically in chronic periaortitis suggests that in its early stages the tissue is highly cellular and contains immature fibroblasts and later evolves into predominantly fibrous tissue, contracting as it does so. This would account for the 'dragging' of mobile structures, like the ureters, medially towards the aorta.

The periaortic distribution of the IRF first emerged from necropsy studies [78] (Figure 9.12(a),(b)) and has been confirmed by computed tomography (CT) [94]. The presentation is associated with a raised erythrocyte sedimentation rate (ESR) and there is often a dramatic response to steroids [78–80]. Histology reveals advanced aortic atherosclerosis with medial disruption and adventitial infiltrates of lymphocytes and plasma cells [95,96]. Characterization of the inflammatory cell populations using immunhistochemistry shows this to be a predominantly B lymphocyte inflammatory response with similar T cell and B cell populations as those seen in a spectrum of inflammation associated with atherosclerotic abdominal aortic aneurysms [97–99].

In a review describing 60 patients with 'idiopathic retroperitoneal fibrosis', Baker and colleagues [92] noted that the mean age of presentation was 56 years and that the commonest presenting symptoms were flank pain, abdominal pain and weight loss. They found that these patients presented with a mean diastolic blood pressure of 93.0 mmHg, normochromic, normocytic anaemia and a raised ESR. These findings are consistent with those of the present study. These investigators agree that CT appearances show the essentially periaortic nature of the mass and support the concept of chronic periaortitis.

As early as 1972, Mitchinson proposed that the inflammation seen in IRF may be due to 'leakage of atherosclerotic material into the adventitia'. He suggested the examination of serum from these patients to search for circulating antibodies to components of the plaque such as lipoproteins [95].

Idiopathic mediastinal fibrosis

A similar chronic inflammatory process occurs much less commonly around the thoracic aorta. This is known as 'idiopathic mediastinal fibrosis' (IMF). The histopathological findings in IMF are identical to those in IRF and the two conditions may occur in contiguity through the diaphragm.

Other causes of fibrosis in the retroperitoneum

The term 'idiopathic retroperitoneal fibrosis' is misleading because it allows the incorporation of eccentric causes of fibrosis in the retroperitoneum, such as malignant neoplasm, endometriosis and diverticulitis into the category of what is a periaortic disease. Non-malignant causes can include:

- Diverticulitis
- Endometriosis
- Infection
- Post-irradiation
- Crohn's disease
- Inflammatory pseudotumour
- Idiopathic retractile (sclerosing) mesenteritis
- Intra-abdominal (mesenteric) desmoid
- Fibromatoses of infancy and childhood
- Paraganglioma
- Gardner's syndrome
- Drugs such as methysergide, hydralazine, ergotamine.

Malignant causes include:

- Sarcoma
- Lymphoma
- Myeloma
- Metastatic carcinoma.

(c) **Chronic periarteritis**

The presence of adventitial and medial lymphocytes associated with atherosclerosis in coronary arteries was first reported early this century [76]. Since then, inflammation and fibrosis has frequently been described around coronary arteries in association with advanced human atherosclerotic plaques [100–106]. In 1956, it was suggested that this inflammation represents a low-grade reaction to atherosclerosis or to thrombus [102].

Inflammation and fibrosis is frequently seen around coronary arteries in association with advanced atherosclerotic plaques. In this situation, the triad of atherosclerosis, medial thinning and adventitial inflammation is termed 'chronic periarteritis' [22]. The association of 'inflammatory aneurysm' and coronary arteritis has also been described in a number of patients [104,105].

Stratford *et al.* [106] characterized the nature of the inflammatory infiltrate in coronary arteries with atherosclerosis: 46% showed adventitial infiltrates, with an equal number of B and T lymphocytes and a lower proportion of macrophages detected by immunohistochemistry. This led these workers to suggest that the inflammation developed as a secondary feature of the atheromatous lesion.

9.3.3 CHARACTERIZATION OF INFLAMMATORY CELLS IN CHRONIC PERIAORTITIS

(a) **Lymphocyte populations**

Monoclonal antibodies have been used to study the nature of the inflammatory cell infiltrates in surgical biopsy material from cases of clinical chronic periaortitis [98,99].

In each sample, organized lymphoid tissue was observed; this was a predominantly plasmacytic response. The infiltrate was composed of approximately 10% macrophages (EBM11 positive), 55% B cells (CD19/22 positive), 35% T cells (CD3 positive) with T helper lymphocytes (Th) (CD4 positive) and T suppressor lymphocytes (Tc/s) (CD8 positive) in a ratio of between 3 and 4 to 1. These cells were organized into secondary follicles with germinal centres. The predominance of CD4 over CD8 positive cells was as would be expected in a B cell response to local extracellular antigen, requiring T cell help. No polymorphonuclear cells or natural killer (NK) cells were observed.

(b) **Activation and proliferation markers**

Extensive MHC class II expression has been detected in the inflamed aortic wall. B cells and macrophages abundantly express this antigen, as do many of the T cells, endothelial cells and non-lymphoid cells.

The most direct evidence for an ongoing immune response, however, is the high level of lymphocyte proliferation using the two markers, Ki-67 (Plate 13) and PC10 (Plate 14), whose antigens are only present during proliferation. High levels of proliferation were especially noted in the most severely inflamed cases described as subclinical chronic periaortitis indicating a possible eventual progression to the clinically relevant disorders.

This proliferation may be a response to local growth factors released by the chronic inflammatory cells and may contribute to aortic wall thickening. Tissue cell proliferation occurs from the earliest stages of atherosclerosis, and smooth muscle cell proliferation in particular is thought to play a critical role in the pathogenesis of atherosclerosis. The number of proliferating cells correlated with the degree of inflammation. These proliferating cells are found predominantly around the germinal centre within the secondary follicles. They can comprise up to 10% of the lymphocytes. Monoclonal antibodies to the IL-2 receptor revealed a small proportion of the cells, again mostly around germinal centres, to be activated [107].

The expression of MHC Class II antigen was also observed using monoclonal antibodies to the HLA DR antigen: 60–80% of the cells in the inflamed tissue expressed this antigen [99,107]. The antigen was expressed by macrophages, B cells, endothelial cells, smooth muscle cells and by many of the T cells. This abundant expression indicates a highly immunologically activated site. The MHC Class II molecule is important in antigen presentation and is required for recognition of antigen by T helper cells and for the subsequent initiation of an immune response. It is, however, unclear if all of these cells are acting as antigen-presenting cells. This abundant, or perhaps aberrant, expression is also seen in other chronic inflammation reactions, as well as in most autoimmune diseases; it may indicate a loss of immunological control.

(c) Aortic associated lymphoid tissue (AALT)

Lymphoid follicles are found in peripheral lymphoid organs such as lymph nodes, spleen and tonsil, in mucosal associated lymphoid tissue (MALT) such as in the bronchus (BALT) and in the gut (GALT), and at sites of chronic antigen presentation such as in Hashimoto's thyroiditis and rheumatoid arthritis.

Lymphoid follicles containing germinal centres are observed in over 50% of cases of clinical chronic periaortitis (Figure 9.13) and are present in association with advanced atherosclerosis [108].

High endothelial cells, with occasional lymphocytes adhering to the luminal surface, are evident in the periphery of these lymphoid follicles. Plasma cells are abundant and are predominantly present in the periphery of secondary follicles. Tangible body macrophages are observed. Cases referred to as 'inflammatory aneurysm' show extensive fibrosis but fewer lymphoid follicles. In agreement with immunohistochemical analyses of secondary lymphoid follicles in peripheral lymphoid organs, secondary lymphoid follicle staining in chronic periaortitis demonstrated that the inflammatory cells were in different stages of maturation [99,108].

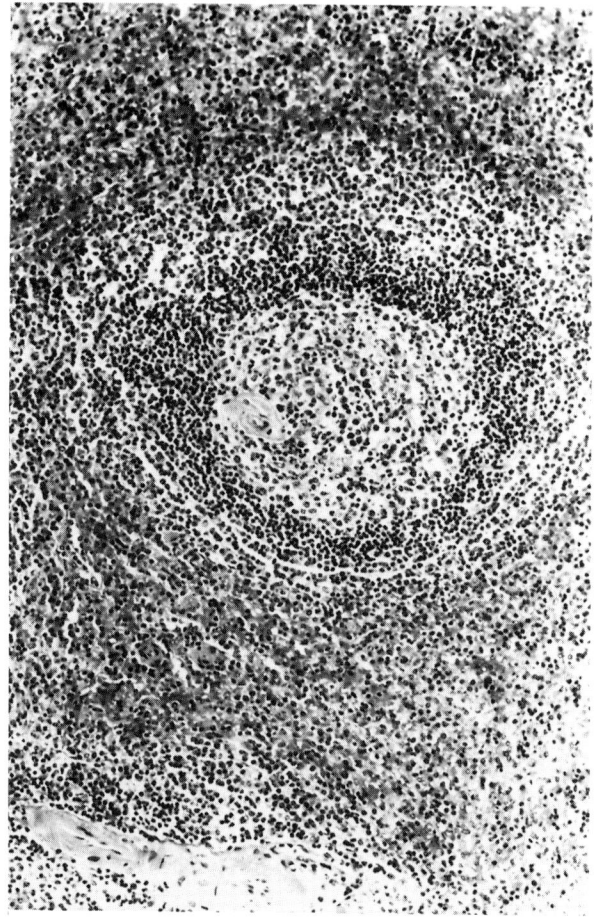

Figure 9.13 The adventitia in clinical chronic periaortitis contains a dense chronic inflammatory cell infiltrate which may form lymphoid follicles. (H&E.)

This supports the presence of active germinal centres in this inflammatory reaction.

These are not periaortic lymph nodes adhering to the fibrous tissue but may be part of an extended immune response trying to deal with the persistent antigens within the aortic tissue. This could be a similar reaction to what occurs in the development of MALT and in the development of lymph node-like tissue in the thyroid gland of Hashimoto's thyroiditis. It is proposed, therefore, that chronic periaortitis, secondary to atherosclerosis, has the potential to form aortic associated lymphoid tissue or AALT.

9.3.4 CYTOKINES AND CHRONIC PERIAORTITIS

The expression of both cytokine-specific messenger RNA (mRNA) and cytokine-specific protein can be extremely transient. They are often present at very low levels, are short lived and are often produced by only a small number of cells in the total population.

In order to determine the presence and relative abun-

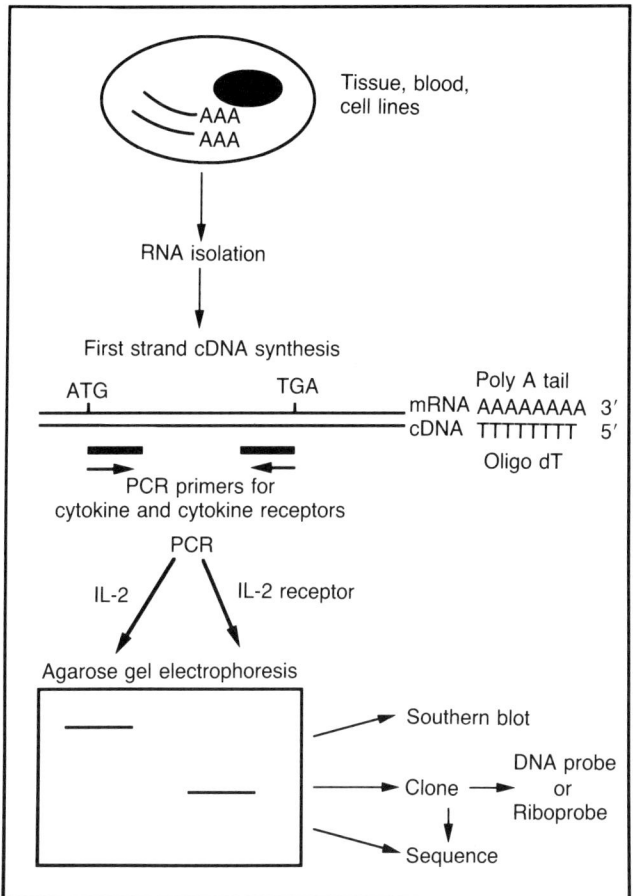

Figure 9.14 Polymerase chain reaction (after reverse transcription) for detection of cytokine mRNA in cells isolated from inflamed atherosclerotic aorta.

dance of cytokines, the protein product may be measured by Western blot analysis, by immunohistochemistry and by soluble immunoassays such as the reverse haemolytic plaque assay (RHPA) or the enzyme-linked immunosorbant assay (ELISA). Cytokine mRNA can be detected by Northern blotting, by RNA dot and slot blotting, by RNAase protection assays, by *in situ* hybridization or by the polymerase chain reaction (PCR) following reverse transcription (Figure 9.14).

Because protein assays for cytokines are often difficult to reproduce due to the unstable nature of the cytokine product, it is often preferable to study mRNA expression, which in many instances is a reflection of the protein product [109]. Of the techniques for measuring cytokines, PCR is the most reproducible as well as being extremely sensitive, requiring only small amounts of cellular RNA.

PCR-assisted mRNA analysis permitted a rapid, highly sensitive and reproducible, semi-quantitative initial screening of RNA samples for the presence of cytokines (Figure 9.14). The *in vivo* presence of cytokine and cytokine receptor mRNA transcripts has been investigated for six cases of inflamed atherosclerotic aortic tissue [110].

TNF-α was not detected in chronic periaortitis by this method, but the other pro-inflammatory cytokines, IL-1α and IFN-γ were detected in all six cases. IL-2, IL-4 and the IL-2 receptor were also detected [110].

None of these cytokines was expressed in the normal aortic wall. Cytokine research indicates that chronic periaortitis shows persistent and relatively stable features required for the maintenance of the disease process.

These mediators are thought to control the intimal inflammation as well as the altered functions of smooth muscle cells. While cytokines are clearly important in the inflammatory component of plaque formation, they must also be playing a role in chronic periaortitis where the inflammation is much more intense than that present in the intima.

9.3.5 ADHESION MOLECULES AND CHRONIC PERIAORTITIS

The activation inducible adhesion molecules, E-selectin, ICAM-1 and VCAM-1, are all expressed in the chronically inflamed aortic adventitial tissue, although to a varying degree [54].

ICAM-1, and especially VCAM-1 correlates strongly with the adventitial mononuclear cell infiltrate suggesting its importance in the development of this B cell dominant chronic inflammatory response. These adhesion molecules are expressed in a similar pattern (albeit to different extents) from the mildest inflammation to the most extreme forms of chronic periaortitis with severe fibrosis [111]. This suggests a role for these adhesion molecules in the perpetuation and development of this chronic inflammatory response.

VCAM-1's presence on non-vascular cells in the centre of most lymphoid aggregates (from the smallest to the largest) and its strongest expression in germinal centres also suggests a role in lymphoid follicle formation, especially in germinal centre development and thus in B cell maturation. The strong germinal centre expression of the ligand of VCAM-1, VLA-4, is consistent with this hypothesis. These results support other work showing its importance in germinal centres. Frozen section binding studies have shown that VLA-4 and VCAM-1 are required for activated human B cells to bind to germinal centres [50]. Adhesion of B cells to follicular dendritic cells requires both ICAM-1/LFA-1 and VCAM-1/VLA-4.

E-selectin is consistently expressed across a spectrum of inflammation in the aortic wall [111]. Its lesser expression in the absence of inflammation, however, does suggest that E-selectin is up-regulated during the onset of the inflammation.

Pro-inflammatory cytokines have been shown to induce the expression of ICAM-1, E-selectin and VCAM-

1 *in vitro* and *in vivo* [45,112]. IL-4 can also induce VCAM-1 while inhibiting the expression of E-selectin [45]. This may explain the differential pattern of expression of VCAM-1 and E-selectin within the inflamed aortic wall as cytokines can act very locally.

9.4 Chronic periaortitis as a local complication of atherosclerosis

9.4.1 HISTOPATHOLOGY

In the normal adult aorta, the media represents about 60–70% of the total aortic wall thickness. The intima and adventitia occupy about 15–20% each. The atherosclerotic aorta displays intimal thickening by 50–100%. In chronic periaortitis, there is similar intimal proliferation, the media is markedly attenuated and there is profound thickening of the adventitia. The total aortic wall thickness may be increased several fold (Figure 9.15).

As to the question of whether the inflammation is the cause or a consequence of the atheroma, it is likely that the latter is the case, for the following reasons. Inflammation is not seen in the adventitia of arteries and aortas unless there is advanced atherosclerosis. Advanced atherosclerotic plaques are seen which show no evidence of adventitial inflammation.

9.4.2 CLINICAL FINDINGS

Patients with subclinical chronic periaortitis and periarteritis, as determined by histology, show a spectrum of adventitial inflammation which is unrelated to age, sex or anatomical site but which relates to the presence of advanced atherosclerosis and medial thinning and is consequent upon the presence of advanced atherosclerosis.

Significant differences between patients with subclinical and clinical chronic periaortitis are the raised ESR (mean 18.25 mm/h vs 66.25 mm/h), raised creatinine (mean 91.06 μmol/l vs 214.25 μmol/l) and increased adventitial thickness (mean 2.2 mm vs 10.6 mm) in the latter group [23].

The only significant differences between the cases of 'inflammatory aneurysm' and 'idiopathic retroperitoneal fibrosis' is the increase in aortic diameter in the former (mean 55.1 mm vs 20.13 mm respectively) [23].

9.4.3 COMPUTED TOMOGRAPHY (CT)

CT has an established role in the preoperative diagnosis of chronic periaortitis, by demonstrating the periaortic

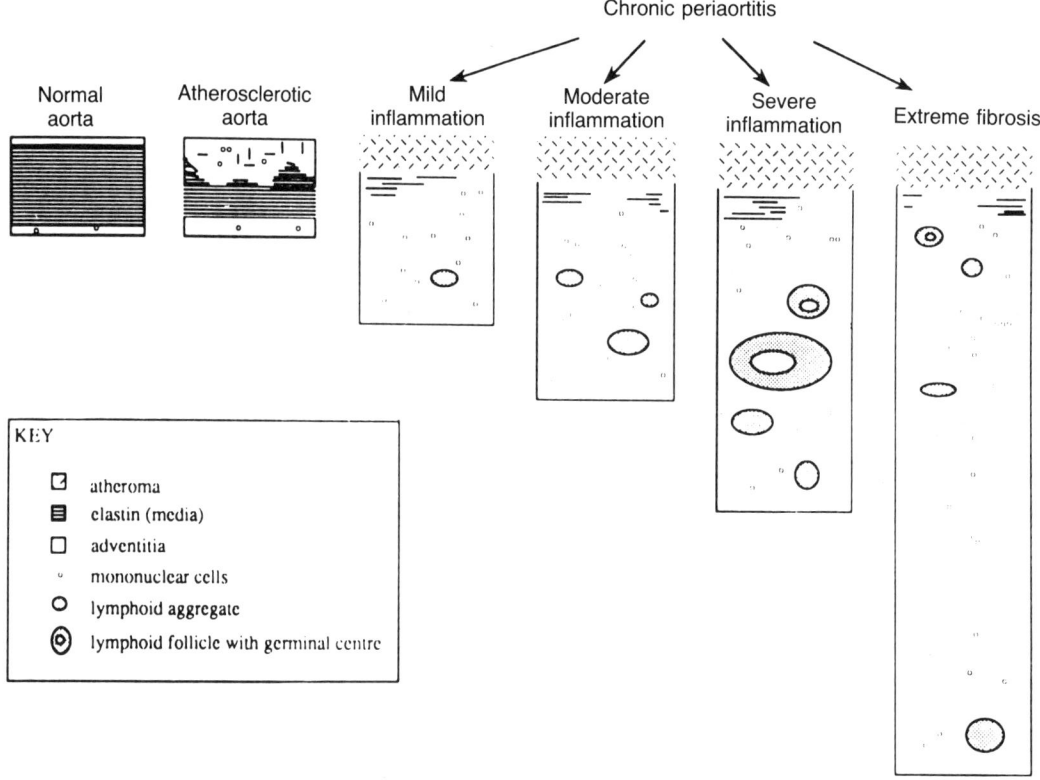

Figure 9.15 Relative proportions of the intima, media and adventitia in the nomal aorta, in subclinical chronic periaortitis and in clinical chronic periaortitis. In the latter condition, it is the adventitial inflammation and fibrosis which leads to the clinical effects such as obstruction of the ureter and back pain.

mass [93]. Other isolated case reports have shown shrinkage of the periaortic mass in response to steroid therapy in 'idiopathic retroperitoneal fibrosis' [113] and in 'inflammatory aneurysm' [114]. The successful use of long-term steroid therapy supports the view that chronic periaortitis is not a disease of infectious origin but of immune origin.

9.4.4 SYSTEMIC FIBROTIC DISORDERS

Finally, the core of textbook chronic periaortitis, or rather 'idiopathic retroperitoneal fibrosis' and 'inflammatory aneurysm', is surrounded by a substantial and mysterious fringe of clinical associations which are ill-defined and which vary in both their severity and characteristics, examples being pulmonary hyalinizing granuloma, lymphomatoid granulomatosis, Reidel's thyroiditis [115], sclerosing cholangitis [116] and pseudotumour of the orbit. Comings and colleagues [117] grouped all of these fibrotic diseases under the heading 'multifocal fibrosclerosis'.

Recent large studies of IRF [91] and 'inflammatory aneurysms' [81] have not confirmed these associations.

9.4.5 DIET AND DRUGS

The view that in atherosclerosis the macrophage is doing harm to the arterial wall is supported by the inhibition of experimental atherosclerosis by a variety of anti-inflammatory drugs [118]. Oxidized lipids elaborated by macrophages are thought to have a cytotoxic and biologically active role.

The role of oxidized lipids derives support from the human epidemiological studies linking vitamin E or selenium deficiency with enhanced risk of the complications of atherosclerosis [119]. Furthermore, a number of reports have suggested a beneficial effect of antioxidants in experimental atherosclerosis [120]. It is possible that the widely canvassed anti-atherogenic effects of the fatty acids of fish oils may be related to their reported inhibition of the oxidative inflammatory activity of phagocytes [121].

If lipid oxidation is important in atherogenesis and the progression of the lesion with its associated clinical sequelae, intervention in the process should be aimed at sites where most of the oxidation occurs. From the research presented in this chapter, it is apparent that the macrophage foam cell is the likely culprit in the production of oxidized lipids. However, there are other possible candidates.

Some foods such as dehydrated milk and eggs are susceptible to oxidation on storage and on cooking and some of the oxidation products can be absorbed from the blood [122]. Oxidation might also occur in the blood where lipid peroxides are thought to be more common in patients with hyperlipidaemia and atherosclerosis [123].

As yet, the role of these dietary factors in chronic periaortitis has not been investigated. If this disease is secondary to atherosclerosis, they should be involved in the prevention of the development of this inflammatory process.

Retroperitoneal fibrosis has been associated with the use of methysergide. Methysergide is an indole derivative with a strong structural similarity to serotonin. It is used in the treatment of migraine. Its mechanism of action is uncertain but in the context of IRF it is suggested that it damages the vessel wall by provoking vasospasm by simulating the peripheral effects of serotonin [94,95]. It is notable that IRF in patients treated with methysergide is often accompanied by fibrosis at other sites.

The benefits of corticosteroid therapy for IRF are well known. The rapidity of response seen in patients with ureteric obstruction supports the view that the ureter is not blocked by fibrosis but rather by oedema and inflammation. This is confirmed histologically. It is not known whether oedema and inflammation obstruct the ureter directly or indirectly, by interfering with nerve or blood supply. Despite the value of steroid therapy, almost all surgeons still regard ureterolysis as the first line of management.

9.4.6 COMPARISONS WITH AUTOIMMUNE DISEASES

Chronic periaortitis is thought to have an autoallergic cause. The allergen is believed to be a component of ceroid, likely to be oxidized LDL, elaborated in the human atheroma. This allergen is sequestered from the immune response unless the media is breached. The atheromatous plaque may therefore act as an immunologically 'privileged site'.

The inflammation seen in chronic periaortitis is thus clearly an ongoing immune response and seems to have the potential to progress to local clinical complications resulting from the extensive fibrosis of the aortic wall. It is difficult to imagine that such intense immune activity is without aetiological significance, showing as it does many similarities with other chronic inflammatory reactions including autoimmune disorders such as rheumatoid arthritis and thyroiditis.

Key features of human autoimmune disease appear to include the chronicity of the reaction, the mononuclear cell population (often in the absence of an acute inflammation), increased vascularity, the presence of high endothelial cells, lymphoid follicle formation with germinal centres (AALT), extensive local MHC class II expression, expression of IL-2 receptors, and abundant expression of adhesion molecules and cytokines. That all of these features are found in chronic periaortitis suggests parallels with diseases recognized as having a chronic inflammatory/autoimmune aetiology.

It may be, however, that the immune response in chronic periaortitis is not due to a loss in tolerance, as proposed for rheumatoid arthritis and Hashimoto's thyroiditis, but is an immune response to a changed, potentially toxic, self-protein such as modified LDL. While antibodies to oxidized LDL are present in the blood of many adults, in advanced atheroma modified LDL is both persistent and abundant, and the immune system appears unable to clear it. As in rheumatoid arthritis and thyroiditis, however, the maintenance of the chronic inflammation in chronic periaortitis is probably due to the continual interaction between a number of immunological components: specific lymphocytes, antigen-presenting cells, surface receptors and cytokines act together in an attempt to clear the persistent immunogen. Moreover, this active chronic inflammation, like that in rheumatoid arthritis, seems to contribute to the progression of the disease.

While the severity of inflammation in chronic periaortitis is not related to the age of the patient, it may be related to the length of time of antigen exposure or to the onset of tissue vascularization. The early atherosclerotic plaque may represent a site of relative immunological privilege, permitting cell entrance through the intimal endothelium but preventing their exit. These cells, trapped in the plaque, may not be able to promote a full-blown immune response until the media is breached or new vessels form in advanced or complicated plaques, allowing communication with nearby lymph nodes. This model is supported by the correlation between tissue vascularization, medial thinning and adventitial inflammation demonstrated in this study. Chronic periaortitis may, indeed, represent the end-stage of the immune response, directed at antigens elaborated in the atherosclerotic plaque during atherogenesis.

Antibodies to oxidized LDL are present in the serum of patients with atherosclerosis and of elderly patients; these antibodies are present in increased titres in patients with chronic periaortitis [34] and immunoglobulin has been localized to ceroid in the atherosclerotic plaque [74,75]. Oxidized LDL has been shown to be as effective as IL-1 at inducing endothelial cell adhesion and this adhesion can be inhibited by antioxidants [124]. Thus LDL, modified by exposure to monocytes or endothelial cells in the arterial wall, may increase the adhesive properties of the endothelium. Whatever the initiating mechanism may be for atherogenesis, this hypothesis provides an explanation for how atherosclerosis and indeed, chronic periaortitis, may progress, become a self-perpetuating process and ultimately result in clinically significant disease. The properties that determine the severity of chronic periaortitis in any individual will lie at the level of the endothelial cell adhesion and antigen presentation as in any advanced atherosclerotic plaque, modified, antigenic lipoproteins are always present in abundance [125].

9.4.7 PRESENT THEORIES OF PATHOGENESIS

Immunohistochemical staining revealed a predominance of B lymphocytes in chronic periaortitis. Since B cells usually respond to specific antigen, this finding suggests the presence of an exogenous antigenic stimulus such as modified LDL, abundant in the plaque and known to be immunogenic. Many of the B cells are in fact proliferating *in situ*, again suggesting that there may be specific antigen recognition and clonal expansion of these cells. The presence of many plasma cells in the periphery of lymphoid aggregates indicates successful selection in the germinal centres of antigen-specific immunoglobulin-secreting cells.

The B cell infiltration correlates to the expression of VCAM-1, an adhesion molecule which has been implicated both in lymphocyte recruitment and in germinal centre formation. Moderate VCAM-1 expression was detected in vessels and strong VCAM-1 expression was detected on follicular dendritic cells in the centre of B cell aggregates.

CD4-positive T helper-associated lymphocytes are found surrounding B cells. As these cells are required for antigen-specific B cell stimulation and differentiation into effector and memory cells, they clearly play an important role in driving this inflammatory response. Identification of occasional proliferating T helper cells also indicates that these cells have been primed and are responding in an antigen-specific manner, consistent with the presence of T memory cells in the tissue. The presence of non-proliferating, diffuse, CD8-positive T cells within the lymphoid follicles is also consistent with B cell response to an extracellular antigen, where these T cells may be functioning in a regulatory capacity rather than a cytotoxic one.

Macrophages are present in virtually all immune responses and their presence as well as their heterogeneity in chronic periaortitis is consistent with their role in antigen presentation to T cells, in phagocytosis of germinal centre apoptotic cells, in fibrosis, and in cytokine synthesis and secretion. IL-1, which is secreted by macrophages upon stimulation by T cells during antigen presentation, is abundant in the inflamed aortic wall, as detected by PCR-assisted amplification of RNA and by RNA hybridization.

MHC class II molecule is a surface receptor normally expressed by macrophages and B cells but induced on various cell types during inflammation. It is required for antigen presentation and recognition by T helper cells, leading to the subsequent initiation and progression of a specific cell-mediated immune response. The expression of MHC class II on cells in the inflamed aortic wall thus indicates their potential antigen-presenting capacity; the apparent co-expression of ICAM-1, also required for T cell response to antigen presentation, strongly supports this. These findings are also consistent with the detection in chronic periaortitis of IFN-γ, a cytokine known to induce the expression of these surface receptors.

Clearly the advanced human atherosclerotic aortic wall is a common site for chronic inflammation, involving fibrosis and an organized distribution of B and T lymphocytes, of macrophages and of dendritic cells, with abundant cytokine and adhesion molecule expression. Cell types, their organization and the presence of germinal centres support the presence of a specific immune response in chronic periaortitis. The consistent presence of cytokines reveals the relatively stable immunological features required for the maintenance and progression of chronic inflammation.

9.4.8 TERMINOLOGY

The term 'idiopathic retroperitoneal fibrosis' perpetuates the image of a disease of unknown cause, arising from somewhere in the retroperitoneum. However, the typical form of this condition always has a periaortic origin and fibrosis is a variable component of the inflammation seen.

The term 'inflammatory aneurysm' is another inaccuracy. It perpetuates the image of aneurysm secondary to an inflammatory process. While this may be the mechanism of mycotic aneurysm, which is very rare, the present study has shown that both medial thinning, giving rise to aneurysmal dilatation, and adventitial inflammation are sequelae of atherosclerosis. It is evident from this study that virtually all atherosclerotic abdominal aortic aneurysms are chronically inflamed to some degree. These findings support the hypothesis that chronic periaortitis is a common local complication of advanced atherosclerosis, and that aneurysms can not be separated into either 'inflammatory' or 'atherosclerotic' types.

The term 'chronic periaortitis' is recommended to refer to the spectrum of subclinical or clinical adventitial inflammation associated with advanced atherosclerosis and medial thinning in dilated and undilated aortas. It has the advantage of pathological accuracy. It is likely that vascular surgeons and urologists will continue to use the terminology with which they are familiar [126]. However, this concept of chronic periaortitis as a local complication of advanced atherosclerosis is finding increasing support from pathologists, radiologists and even surgeons [23,85,94].

9.4.9 FUTURE RESEARCH

The development of a human monoclonal antibody specific for oxidized LDL might prove to be a clinically important area of future research in chronic periaortitis. The extensive B cell infiltrate in chronic periaortitis would facilitate the development of such an antibody. Aortic tissue-derived B cells may be transformed in culture with Epstein–Barr virus, followed by fusion to a mouse myeloma fusion partner. Such an antibody could be used to image human atheroma *in vivo*. This would be of particular value given that atherosclerosis is still difficult to assess by non-invasive techniques. It could also be used to confirm the presence of oxidized LDL in the tissue wall. Activated endothelium in the new vessels in the adventitia and in the base of the atheroma may also be targets for imaging atherosclerosis using labelled antibodies. The most likely target would be E-selectin, which is strongly expressed by activated endothelium associated with advanced atherosclerosis.

Inflammation in human atherosclerosis is of importance in the genesis and progression of atherosclerosis and, as this chapter has concluded, chronic inflammation is also a local complication of atherosclerosis which may give rise to clinical sequelae of its own.

It remains to be seen whether or not the inflammatory process occurring in the intima in atherogenesis and in the adventitia in chronic periaortitis are part of the same process, occurring in two different microenvironments or whether they are distinct. In either case, understanding the mechanisms of cytokine and cell interactions in chronic periaortitis may lead to therapeutic strategies for the diagnosis or treatment of the inflammatory process associated with atherogenesis and with the development of chronic periaortitis.

References

1. Pickering, G. (1963) Arteriosclerosis and atherosclerosis; the need for clear thinking. *Am. J. Med.*, **34**, 7–18.
2. Long, E.R. (1993) in *Arteriosclerosis*, (ed. E.V. Cowdry), MacMillan, New York, p. 28
3. Von Haller, A. (1735) *Opuscula Pathologica*. Bousquet, Lausanne.
4. Virchow, R. (1862) Gesammelte Abhandlunger z. Wizsentschaftlichen Medicin, in *Phlogose und thrombose in Gefässystem*. Max Hirsch, Berlin, p. 458.
5. Turnbull, H.M. (1915) Alterations in arterial structure and their relation to syphilis. *Quart. J. Med.*, **8**, 210–13.
6. Marchand, F. (1904) Über Arteriosklerose (Atherosklerose). *Verhandl. Kongr. Inn. Med.*, **21**, 23–27.
7. Aschoff, L. (1933) in *Arteriosclerosis*, (ed. E.V. Cowdry), MacMillan, New York, p. 6.
8. World Health Organization (1958) Report of a study group: Classification of atherosclerotic lesions. *WHO Tech. Rep. Series*, **143**.
9. Anitschow, E. (1933) Experimental arteriosclerosis in animals, in *Arteriosclerosis*, (ed. E.V. Cowdry), MacMillan, New York, pp. 271–322.
10. Aqel, N.M., Ball, R.Y., Waldmann, H. and Mitchinson, M.J. (1984) Monocytic origin of foam cells in human atherosclerotic plaques. *Atherosclerosis*, **53**, 265–71.
11. Aqel, N.M., Ball, R.Y., Waldmann, H. and Mitchinson, M.J. (1985) Identification of macrophage and smooth muscle cells in human atherosclerosis using monoclonal antibodies. *J. Pathol.*, **146**, 197–204.
12. Klurfield, D.M. (1985) Identification of foam cells in human atherosclerotic lesions as macrophages using monoclonal antibodies. *Arch. Pathol.*, **109**, 445–9.
13. Mitchinson, M.J. and Ball, R.Y. (1987) Macrophages and atherogenesis. *Lancet*, **ii**, 146–8.
14. Jonasson, L., Holm, J., Skalli, O. *et al.* (1986) Regional accumulations of T cells, macrophages, and smooth muscle cells in the human atherosclerotic plaque. *Arteriosclerosis*, **6**, 131–8.
15. Gown, A.M., Tsukada, T. and Ross, R. (1986) Human atherosclerosis II.

Immunocytochemical analysis of the cellular composition of human atherosclerotic lesions. *Am. J. Pathol.*, 125, 191–207.
16. Hansson, G.K., Jonasson, L., Lojsted, B. *et al.* (1988) Localisation of T lymphocytes and macrophages in fibrous and complicated plaques. *Atherosclerosis*, 72, 135–40.
17. Hansson, G.K., Holm, J. and Jonasson, L. (1989) Detection of activated T lymphocytes in the human atherosclerotic plaque. *Am. J. Pathol.*, 135, 169–75.
18. Van der Wahl, A.C., Das, P.K., Van de Berg, D.B. *et al.* (1989) Atherosclerotic lesions in humans. In-situ immunophenotypic analysis suggesting an immune mediated respone. *Lab. Invest.*, 61, 166–70.
19. Hansson, G.K., Holm, J. and Kral, J.G. (1984) Accumulation of IgG and complement factor C3 in human arterial endothelium and atherosclerotic lesions. *Acta Pathol. Microbiol. Immunol. Scand.*, 92A, 429–35.
20. Ross, R. (1986) The pathogenesis of atherosclerosis – an update. *New Engl J. Med.*, 314, 488–500.
21. Schwartz, C.J. and Mitchell, J.R.A. (1962) Cellular infiltration of the human arterial adventitia associated with atheromatous plaques. *Circulation*, 2, 73–8.
22. Mitchinson, M.J. (1984) Chronic periaoritits and periarteritis. *Histopathology*, 8, 589–600.
23. Parums, D.V. (1990) The spectrum of chronic periaortitis. *Histopathology*, 16, 423–31.
24. Jonasson, L., Holm, J., Skalli, O. *et al.* (1985) Expression of Class II transplantation antigen on vascular smooth muscle cells in human atherosclerosis. *J. Clin. Pathol.*, 76, 125–31.
25. Hansson, G.K., Holm, J., Holm, S. *et al.* (1991) T lymphocytes in inhibit the vascular response to injury. *Proc. Natl Acad. Sci. USA*, 88, 10530–4.
26. Geng, Y. and Hansson, G.K. (1992) Interferon-γ inhibits scavenger receptor expression and foam cell formation in human monocyte-derived macrophages. *J. Clin. Invest.*, 89, 1322–30.
27. Uys, C.J. and Rose, A.G. (1984) Pathologic findings in long term cardiac transplants. *Arch. Pathol. Lab. Med.*, 108, 112–6.
28. Salonen, J.T., Yla-Herttuala, S., Yamamoto, R. *et al.* (1992) Autoantibody against oxidized LDL and progression of carotid atherosclerosis. *Lancet*, 339, 883–7.
29. Ross, R. (1990) The mechanisms of atherosclerosis – a review. *Adv. Nephrol.*, 19, 79–86.
30. Pang, A.S., Katz, A. and Minta, J.O. (1979) C3 deposition in cholesterol-induced atherosclerosis in rabbits: a possible etiologic role for complement in atherogenesis. *J. Immun.*, 123, 1117–23.
31. Minick, C.R. and Murphy, G.E. (1973) Experimental induction of arteriosclerosis by the synergy of allergic injury to arteries and lipid-rich diet. II Effect of repeatedly injected foreign protein in rabbits fed a lipid-rich, cholesterol-poor diet. *Am. J. Pathol.*, 73, 265–300.
32. Cerilli, J., Brasile, L. and Karmody, A. (1985) Role of the vascular endothelial cell antigen system in the aetiology of atherosclerosis. *Ann. Surg.*, 202, 329–34.
33. Benditt, E.P., Barrett, T. and McDougal, J.M. (1983) Viruses in the aetiology of atherosclerosis. *Proc. Natl Acad. Sci. USA*, 80, 6386–9.
34. Parums, D.V., Brown, D.L. and Mitchinson, M.J. (1990) Serum antibodies to oxidized low density lipoprotein and ceroid in chronic periaortitis. *Arch. Pathol. Lab. Med.*, 114, 383–7.
35. Shimokado, K., Raines, E.W., Madtes, D.K. *et al.* (1985) A significant part of the macrophage-derived growth factor consists of at least two forms of PDGF. *Cell*, 43, 277–86.
36. Takeya, M., Yoshimura, T., Leonard, E.J. and Takahashi, K. (1993) Detection of monocyte chemoattractant protein-1 in human atherosclerotic lesions by an anti-monocyte chemoattractant protein-1 monoclonal antibody. *Hum. Pathol.*, 24, 534–9.
37. Springer, T.A. (1990) Adhesion receptors of the immune system. *Nature*, 346, 425–34.
38. Simmons, D., Makgoba, M.W. and Seed, B. (1988) ICAM, an adhesion ligand of LFA-1, is homologous to the neural cell adhesion molecule NCAM. *Nature*, 331, 624–7.
39. Bevilacqua, M.P., Stengelin, S., Gimbrone Jr, M.A. and Seed, B. (1989) Endothelial leukocyte activation adhesion molecule 1: an inducible receptor for neutrophils related to complement regulatory proteins and lectins. *Science*, 243, 1160–5.
40. Osborn, L., Hesslon, C., Tizard, R. *et al.* (1989) Direct expression cloning of vascular cell adhesion molecule 1, a cytokine-induced endothelial protein that binds to lymphocytes. *Cell*, 59, 1203–11.
41. Munro, J.M., Pober, J.S. and Cotran, R.S. (1991) Recruitment of neutrophils in the local endotoxin response: association with de novo endothelial expression of endothelial leukocyte adhesion molecule-1. *Lab. Invest.*, 64, 295–9.
42. Picker, L.J., Kishimoto, T.K., Smith, C.W. *et al.* (1991) ELAM-1 is an adhesion molecule for skin-homing T cells. *Nature*, 349, 796–9.
43. Shimizu, Y., Shaw, S., Graber, N. *et al.* (1991) Activation-independent binding of human memory T cells to adhesion molecule ELAM-1. *Nature*, 349, 799–802.
44. Gimbrone, M.A., Obin, M.S., Brock, A.F. *et al.* (1989) Endothelial interleukin-8: a novel inhibitor of leukocyte-endothelial interactions. *Science*, 246, 1601–3.
45. Thornhill, M.H., Wellicome, S.M., Mahiouz, D.L. *et al.* (1991) Tumor necrosis factor combines with IL-4 or IFN-γ to selectively enhance endothelial cell adhesiveness for T cells. The contribution of vascular cell adhesion molecule-1-dependent and independent binding mechanisms. *J. Immun.*, 146, 592–8.
46. Dustin, M.L., Rothlein, R., Bhan, A.K. *et al.* (1986) Induction by IL 1 and interferon-γ: tissue distribution, biochemistry, and function of a natural adherence molecule (ICAM-1). *J. Immun.*, 137, 245–54.
47. Smith, M.E.F. and Thomas, J.A. (1990) Cellular expression of lymphocyte function associated antigens and intercellular adhesion molecule-1 in normal tissue. *J. Clin. Pathol.*, 43, 893–900.
48. Rothlein, R. and Springer, T.A. (1986) The requirement for lymphocyte function-associated antigen 1 in homotypic leukocyte adhesion stimulated by phorbol ester. *J. Expl Med.*, 163, 1132–49.
49. Elices, M.J., Osborn, L., Takada, Y. *et al.* (1990) VCAM-1 on activated endothelium interacts with the leukocyte integrin VLA-4 at a site distinct from the VLA-4/fibronectin binding site. *Cell*, 60, 577–84.
50. Freedman, A.S., Munro, J.M., Rice, G.E. *et al.* (1990) Adhesion of human B cells to germinal centres *in vitro* involves VLA-4 and INCAM-110. *Science*, 249, 1030–3.
51. Berman, J.W. and Calderon, T.M. (1992) The role of endothelial cell adhesion molecules in the development of atherosclerosis. *Cardiovasc. Pathol.*, 1, 17–28.
52. Cybulsky, M.I. and Gimbrone, M.A. (1991) Endothelial expression of a mononuclear leukocyte adhesion molecule during atherogenesis. *Science*, 251, 788–91.
53. Poston, R.N., Haskard, D.O., Coucher, J.R. *et al.* (1992) Expression of intercellular adhesion molecule-1 in atherosclerotic plaques. *Am. J. Pathol.*, 140, 665–73.
54. Wood, K.W., Cadogan, M.D., Ramshaw, A.L. and Parums, D.V. (1993) The distribution of adhesion molecules in human atherosclerosis. *Histopathology*, 22, 437–44.
55. Gimbrone, M.A., Bevilacqua, M.P. and Cybulsky, M.I. (1990) Endothelial-dependent mechanisms of leukocyte adhesion in inflammation and atherosclerosis. *Ann. N.Y. Acad. Sci.*, 598, 77–85.
56. Haust, M.D. (1971) The morphogenesis and fate of potential atherosclerotic lesions in man. *Hum. Pathol.*, 2, 1–29.
57. Scaffner, T., Taylor, K., Bartucci, E.J. *et al.* (1980) Arterial foam cells with distinctive immunomorphological and histochemical features of macrophages. *Am. J. Pathol.*, 100, 57–80.
58. Goldstein, J.L., Ho, Y.K., Basu, S.K. and Brown, M.S. (1979) Binding site on macrophages that mediate uptake and degradation of acetylated LDL producing massive cholesterol deposition. *Proc. Natl Acad. Sci. USA*, 76, 333–7.
59. Fogelman, A.M., Seager, J., Haberland, M.E. *et al.* (1982) Lymphocyte-conditioned medium protects human monocyte-macrophage from cholesteryl ester accumulation. *Proc. Natl Acad. Sci. USA*, 79, 922–6.
60. Mahley, R.W., Innerarity, T.L., Weisgraber, K.H. and Oh, S.Y. (1979) Altered metabolism (in vitro and in vivo) of plasma lipoproteins after selective chemical modification of lysine residues of the apo-proteins. *J. Clin. Invest.*, 64, 743–50.
61. Van der Schroeff, J.G., Havekes, L., Emeis, J.J. *et al.* (1983) Morphological studies on the binding of low density lipoprotein and acetylated low density lipoprotein to the plasma membrane of cultured lymphocytes. *Exp. Cell. Res.*, 145, 95–103.
62. Clevidence, B.A., Morton, R.E., West, G. *et al.* (1984) Cholesterol esterification in macrophages; stimulated by lipoproteins containing apo-B isolated from human aortas. *Arteriosclerosis*, 4, 196–207.
63. Ball, R.Y., Bindman, J.P., Carpenter, K.L.H. and Mitchinson, M.J. (1986) Oxidised low density lipoprotein induces ceroid accumulation by murine peritoneal macrophages in vitro. *Atherosclerosis*, 60, 173–81.
64. Raymond, T.L. and Reynolds, S.A. (1983) Lipoproteins of the extravascular space; alterations in low density lipoproteins of interstitial inflammatory fluid. *J. Lipid Res.*, 24, 113–18.
65. Mitchinson, M.J., Hothersall, D.C., Brooks, P.N. and DeBurbure, C.Y. (1985) The distribution of ceroid in human atherosclerosis. *J. Pathol.*, 145, 177–83.
66. Brown, M.S. and Goldstein, J.L. (1983) Lipoprotein metabolism in the macrophage; implications for cholesterol deposition in atherosclerosis. *Ann. Rev. Biochem.*, 52, 223–61.
67. Yla-Hettuala, S., Plinski, W., Rosenfeld, M.R. *et al.* (1989) Evidence for the presence of oxidatively modified low density lipoprotein in atherosclerotic lesions of rabbit and man. *J. Clin. Invest.*, 79, 1086–95.
68. Carew, T.E. (1989) The role of biologically modified low density lipoprotein in atherosclerosis. *Am. J. Cardiol.*, 63, 18–22.
69. Cookson, F.B. (1971) The origin of foam cells in atherosclerosis. *Br. J. Expl Pathol.*, 52, 62–69.
70. Ziats, N.P. and Robertson, A.L. (1981) Effects of peripheral blood monocytes on human vascular cell proliferation. *Atherosclerosis*, 38, 401–10.
71. Logani, M.K. and Davies, R.E. (1980) Lipid oxidation; biological effects and anti-oxidants – a review. *Lipids*, 15, 485–95.
72. Moncada, S., Gryglewski, R.J., Bunting, S. and Vane, J.R. (1976) A lipid peroxide inhibits the enzyme in blood vessel microsomes that generates from prostaglandin endoperoxides the substance (prostaglandin X) which

prevents platelet aggregation. *Prostaglandins*, **12**, 715–20.
73. Steinbrecher, U.P., Fischer, M., Witztum, J.L. and Curtiss, L.K. (1984) Immunogenicity of homologous low density lipoprotein after methylation, ethylation, acetylation, and carbamylation; generation of antibodies specific for derivatised lysine. *J. Lipid Res.*, **25**, 1109–16.
74. Parums, D. and Mitchinson, M.J. (1981) Demonstration of immunoglobulin in the neighbourhood of advanced atherosclerotic plaques. *Atherosclerosis*, **38**, 211–16.
75. Parums, D.V., Chadwick, D.R. and Mitchinson, M.J. (1986) The localisation of immunoglobulin in chronic periaortitis. *Atherosclerosis*, **61**, 117–23.
76. Allbutt, C.T. (1915) *Diseases of the Arteries*, vol. 1, MacMillan, London.
77. Hutchinson, J. (1890) On the diseases of the arteries. *Arch. Surg.*, **1**, 84–86.
78. Mitchinson, M.J. (1972) Aortic disease in idiopathic retroperitoneal fibrosis. *J. Clin. Pathol.*, **25**, 287–93.
79. Mitchinson, M.J. (1970) The pathology of idiopathic retroperitoneal fibrosis. *J. Clin. Pathol.*, **23**, 681–9.
80. Clyne, C.A.C. and Abercrombie, G.F. (1977) Perianeurysmal retroperitoneal fibrosis; two cases responding to steroids. *Br. J. Urol.*, **49**, 463–72.
81. Pennell, R.C., Hollier, L.H., Lie, J.T. *et al.* (1985) Inflammatory abdominal aortic aneurysms: a thirty year review. *J. Vasc. Surg.*, **2**, 859–69.
82. Walker, D.I., Bloor, K., Williams, G. and Gillie, I. (1972) Inflammatory aneurysms of the abdominal aorta. *Br. J. Surg.*, **59**, 609–14.
83. Bloor, K. and Humphreys, W.V. (1979) Aneurysms of the abdominal aorta. *Br. J. Hosp. Med.*, **21**, 568–83.
84. Rose, A.G. and Dent, D.M. (1981) Inflammatory variant of abdominal atherosclerotic aneurysm. *Arch. Pathol. Lab. Med.*, **105**, 409–13.
85. Baskerville, P.A., Blakeney, C.G., Young, A.E. and Browse, N.L. (1983) The diagnosis and treatment of peri-aortic fibrosis (inflammatory aneurysms). *Br. J. Surg.*, **70**, 381–5.
86. Savory, W.S. (1856) Case of a young woman in whom the main arteries of both extremities and of the left side of the neck were throughout completely obliterated. *Med. Chir. Trans. Lond.*, **39**, 205.
87. Lupi, H.E., Sanchez, T.G., Marcuschamer, J. *et al.* (1977) Takayasu's arteritis: clinical study of 107 cases. *Am. Heart. J.*, **93**, 94.
88. Sen, K.P. (1968) Obstructive disease of the aorta and its branches. *Indian J. Surg.*, **30**, 289–327.
89. Lie, J.T. (1991) Takayasu arteritis in *Systemic Vasculitides*, (eds A. Churg and J. Churg), Igaku Shoin, New York, pp. 159–79.
90. Albarran, J. (1905) Rétention renale par periureterité; liberation externe de l'uretere. *Assoc. France Urol.*, **9**, 511–17.
91. Ormond, J.K. (1948) Bilateral ureteral obstruction due to envelopment and compression by an inflammatory retroperitoneal process. *J. Urol.*, **59**, 1072–9.
92. Baker, L.R.I., Mallinson, W.J.W., Gregory, M.C. *et al.* (1988) Idiopathic retroperitoneal fibrosis; a retrospective analysis of sixty cases. *J. Urol.*, **60**, 497–503.
93. Brooks, A.P., Reznek, R.H., Webb, J.A. and Baker, L.R.I. (1987) Computed tomography in the follow up of retroperitoneal fibrosis. *Clin. Radiol.*, **38**, 597–601.
94. Dixon, A.K., Mitchinson, M.J. and Sherwood T. (1984) Computed tomographic observations in peri-aortitis; a hypothesis. *Clin. Radiol.*, **35**, 39–42.
95. Mitchinson, M.J. (1972) Some clinical aspects of idiopathic retroperitoneal fibrosis *Br. J. Surg.*, **59**, 58–60.
96. Mitchinson, M.J. (1986) Retroperitoneal fibrosis revisited. *Arch. Pathol. Lab. Med.*, **110**, 784–6.
97. Parums, D.V., Choudhury, R., Shields, S.A. and Davies, A.H. (1991) Characterization of inflammatory cells associated with 'idiopathic retroperitoneal fibrosis'. *Br. J. Urol.*, **67**, 564–8.
98. Parums, D.V. and Ramshaw, A.L. (1990) Immunohistochemical characterization of inflammatory cells in biopsies from abdominal aortic aneurysms. *J. Pathol.*, **160**, 160A.
99. Ramshaw, A.L. and Parums, D.V. (1990) Immunohistochemical characterization of inflammatory cells associated with advanced atherosclerosis. *Histopathology*, **17**, 5430–552.
100. Gerlis, L.M. (1956) The significance of adventitial infiltrations in coronary atherosclerosis. *Br. Heart J.*, **18**, 166–72.
101. Horn, H. and Finkelstein, L.E. (1940) Arteriosclerosis of the coronary arteries and the mechanism of their occlusion. *Am. Heart J.*, **19**, 655–9.
102. Morgan, A.D. (1956) *The Pathogenesis of Coronary Occlusion*. Blackwell Publications, Oxford.
103. Pereira, M.C., Filho, A.A., Lastoria, S. and Franco, M. (1981) Inflammatory aneurysm of the abdominal aorta with coronary arteritis. *Arch. Pathol. Lab. Med.*, **105**, 678–9.
104. Mitchinson, M.J., Wight, D.G.D., Arno, J. and Milstein, B.B. (1984) Chronic coronary periarteritis in two patients with chronic periaortitis. *J. Clin. Pathol.*, **37**, 32–36.
105. Cohle, S.D. and Lie, J.T. (1988) Inflammatory aneurysm of the aorta, aortitis and coronary arteritis. *Arch. Pathol. Lab. Med.*, **112**, 1121–5.
106. Stratford, N., Britton, K. and Gallagher, P. (1986) Inflammatory infiltrates in human coronary atherosclerosis. *Atherosclerosis*, **59**, 271–6.
107. Ramshaw, A.L. and Parums, D.V. (1991) Inflammatory cells in chronic periaortitis are activated and proliferating. *J. Pathol.*, **163**, 12A
108. Ramshaw, A.L., Roskell, D.E. and Parums, D.V. (1992) Characterization of aortic associated lymphoid tissue (AALT) in advanced atherosclerosis. *J. Pathol.*, **169**, 179A.
109. Brenner, C.A., Tam, A.W., Nelson, P.A. *et al.* (1989) Message amplification phenotyping (MAPPing): a technique to simultaneously measure multiple mRNAs from small numbers of cells. *Biotechniques*, **7**, 1096–103.
110. Ramshaw, A.L., Roskell, D.E., Parums, D.V. (1994) Cytokine gene expression in aortic adventitial inflammation associated with advanced atherosclerosis (chronic periaortitis). *J. Clin. Pathol.*, **47**, 721–7.
111. Ramshaw, A.L. and Parums, D.V. (1993) The distribution of adhesion molecules in chronic periaortitis. *Histopathology*, **24**, 23–32.
112. Cotran, R.S., Gimbrone Jr, M.A., Bevilacqua, M.P. *et al.* (1986) Induction and detection of a human endothelial activation antigen *in vivo*. *J. Expl Med.*, **164**, 661–6.
113. Larrieu, A.J., Weiner, I., Abston, S. and Warren, M.M. (1980) Retroperitoneal fibrosis. *Surg. Gynaec. Obstet.*, **150**, 699–702.
114. Feldberg, M.A.M. and Hene, R.J. (1983) Perianeurysmal fibrosis and its response to corticosteroid treatment; a computerized tomography follow up in 1 case. *J. Urol.*, **130**, 1163–4.
115. Turner-Warwick, R., Nabarro, J.D.N. and Doniach, D. (1966) Riedel's thyroiditis and retroperitoneal fibrosis. *Proc. Roy. Soc. Med.*, **59**, 596–8.
116. Bartholomew, L.G., Cain, J.C. and Woolner, L.B. (1963) Sclerosing cholangitis. *New Engl. J. Med.*, **269**, 8–12.
117. Comings, D.E., Skubi, K.B. and Eyes, J. (1967) Familial multifocal fibrosclerosis. *Ann. Intern. Med.*, **66**, 884–92.
118. Bailey, J.M. and Butler, J. (1985) Anti-inflammatory drugs in experimental atherosclerosis. Part 6 (combination therapy with steroid and non-steroid agents). *Atherosclerosis*, **54**, 205–12.
119. Ellis, N.I.A., Lloyd, B., Lloyd, R.S. and Clayton, B.E. (1984) Selenium and vitamin E in relation to risk factors for coronary heart disease. *J. Clin. Path.*, **37**, 220–60.
120. Parthasarathy, S.P., Young, S.G., Witztum, J.L. *et al.* (1986) Probucol inhibits oxidative modification of LDL. *J. Clin. Invest.*, **77**, 641–4.
121. Leslie, C.A., Gonnermann, W.A., Ullman, M.D. *et al.* (1985) Dietary fish oil modulates macrophage fatty acids and decreases arthritis susceptibility in mice. *J. Expl Med.*, **162**, 1336–49.
122. Taylor, C.B., Peng, S.-K., Werthessen, N.T. *et al.* (1979) Spontaneously occurring angiotoxic derivatives of cholesterol. *Am. J. Clin. Nutr.*, **32**, 40–57.
123. Goto, Y. (1982) Lipid peroxides as a cause of vascular diseases, in *Lipid Peroxides in Biology and Medicine*, (ed. K. Yagi), Academic Press, New York, pp. 295–303.
124. Frostegard, J., Haegerstrand, A., Gidlund, M. and Nilsson, J. (1991) Biologically modified LDL increases the adhesive properties of endothelial cells. *Atherosclerosis*, **90**, 119–26.
125. Mitchinson, M.J. (1982) Insoluble lipids in human atherosclerotic plaques. *Atherosclerosis*, **45**, 11–15.
126. Lie, J.T. (1992) Inflammatory aneurysm of the aorta or chronic periaortitis: a nosological quandry. *Cardiovasc. Pathol.*, **1**, 75–77.

10 ANEURYSMS

William E. Stehbens

10.1 Definitions

Aneurysm is derived from the Greek *aneurysma*, from *ana* meaning *across* and *eurys* meaning *broad*. It thus denotes a widening or dilatation and unless otherwise indicated, is used to refer exclusively to aneurysms of arteries. Aneurysm generally alludes to an arterial dilatation, although cardiac and venous aneurysms occur and microcirculatory vessels may be so affected. It is sometimes used loosely and incorrectly in reference to gross dilatation of the left atrium in chronic mitral stenosis. When referring to aneurysms of veins or the heart the distinction should be specifically indicated.

Aneurysms, first defined and described by Galen [1], are persistent localized dilatations of the vessel wall classified according to their aetiology and sometimes shape or anatomical site. **True aneurysms** are formed by the yielding of constituents of the vessel wall which of necessity exhibits profound histological and structural changes (Figure 10.1). A **false aneurysm** in contradistinction results from partial or complete mural disruption and the pulsatile haematoma thus formed from the extravasated blood is walled off by perivascular tissues and fibrinous coagulum producing a tamponade effect to stanch bleeding and to retain functional continuity with the lumen of the parent vessel. Since small traumatic aneurysms displayed angiographically may subsequently undergo thrombotic occlusion, it is more likely that a functional communication with the parent artery persists from the time of trauma and extravasation of blood. A false aneurysm may also form following vascular surgery due to separation or dehiscence of the suture line shortly after surgery. Aneurysmal dilatation of scar tissue along the proximal suture line of the aorta and a prosthesis months or years after surgery should rightfully be regarded as a true aneurysm due to stress concentration at the site, associated with differences in the physical characteristics of the wall and prosthesis.

Arteriectasis (Figure 10.2) is a generalized diffuse dilatation over a considerable length of the artery and is not to be confused with aneurysmal dilatation which may occur concomitantly. Some degree of ectasia is known to occur throughout life in the aorta, coronary and cerebral arteries but this does not make it a physiological process. Such vessels are particularly prone to severe atherosclerosis and display progressive degenerative changes. A cylindroid aneurysm involves a defined length of the artery. A longer length of vessel is involved than with a fusiform aneurysm and it is not as diffuse as ectasia. Severe arteriectasis associated with tortuosity has been referred to as a serpentine aneurysm and differentiation between pronounced ectasia and diffuse aneurysmal dilatation is not always possible as they are but variations in severity. However, such lesions being infrequent, the difficulty seldom arises. Dilatation of collateral vessels under the stimulus of the increased demand of anoxic tissues for blood is akin to arteriectasis and such vessels are prone to tortuosity and aneurysmal dilatation. Arteriectasis may also lead to a post-stenotic effect beyond the passage of an artery (e.g. the vertebral artery) through a bony foramen (cervical vertebra) or through a fibrous aperture such as the dura mater. Such strictures prevent expansion causing disparity in calibre of the artery and the post-stenotic effect would result in further dilatation.

In an attempt to standardize reporting of aneurysms, Johnston *et al.* [2] specified that an aneurysm should have at least a 50% increase in diameter compared to the expected normal diameter of the artery with reference to normal diameters for that artery based on population statistics. Since the diameter will vary with age, sex, body build, etc., the comparison should be with the adjoining undilated segment rather than that of a hypothetical norm of the population at large. Johnston *et al.* [2], defined **arteriomegaly** as a diffuse enlargement involving 'several arterial segments' with an increase in diameter greater than 50% of the expected normal diameter, and ectasia as a diffuse dilatation less than 50% of the normal value. Such a classification ignores the importance of comparing the degree and extent of the dilatation in the individual and does not take into account berry aneurysms of the cerebral arteries. A localized evagination with an increase in diameter of less than 50% can still be an (early) aneurysm and associated with altered haemodynamics.

A **fusiform aneurysm**, as its name implies, is a

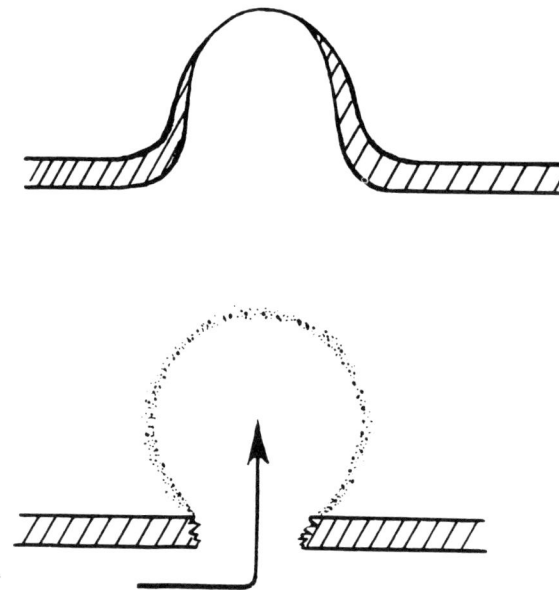

Figure 10.1 Diagram of a true aneurysm (above) formed by dilatation and attenuation of the wall of the parent artery and a false aneurysm (below) formed by rupture or tearing of the parent artery with the sac wall formed by fibrinous coagulum and compressed surrounding tissues. The thrombus lining the false sac then becomes organized.

fusiform dilatation of the whole blood vessel wall for a short distance depicting the shape and localized extent of the dilatation. By continued expansion it may form a large globoid or spherical dilatation with the proximal artery entering the sac and the distal arterial segment emerging as if an efferent vessel. Saccular is the term usually applied to a sac arising from only part of the vessel wall. The phenomenon is sometimes referred to as a lateral saccular aneurysm to distinguish it from berry aneurysms which are saccular but arise from the apical region or crotch of bifurcations.

Miliary aneurysm (or **microaneurysm**) is a term introduced by Charcôt and Bouchard in reference to microaneurysms of intracerebral arteries related to cerebral haemorrhage (Chapter 12). At times the term has unfortunately been applied to the larger berry aneurysms (Figure 10.2) of the large basal arteries of the brain but should be restricted to the small intracerebral lesions described by Charcôt and Bouchard.

Dissecting aneurysm has been defined as 'a lesion produced by penetration of the circulating blood into the substance of the wall of a vessel with subsequent extension of the diffused blood for a varying distance between its layers' [3].

An **arteriovenous communication** or aneurysm results from a pathological communication between an artery and a neighbouring vein. Diffuse and localized aneurysmal dilatations of the vessels frequently accompany the pathological communication. When the

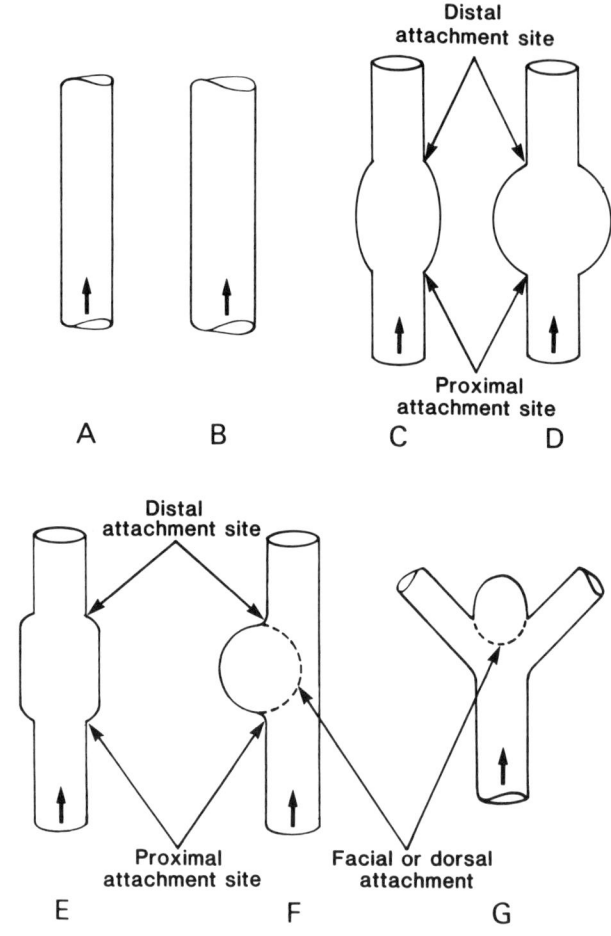

Figure 10.2 Types of dilatation in contrast to the normal artery (A) and the diffuse dilatation of arteriectasis (B). A fusiform aneurysm (C) can by enlargement progressively assume a spherical shape (D). Below is a cylindrical aneurysm (E), a localized dilatation from the side of an arterial stem (lateral aneurysm) (F) and the conventional berry type (G) arising from the crotch of a fork. Note the broad base of origin or attachment to the parent stem.

communication or anastomosis is relatively small either between adjoining vessels or from the internal carotid artery into the surrounding cavernous sinus, **arteriovenous fistula** is the term often used. Arteriovenous aneurysm is not the most appropriate term for the pathological changes associated with an arteriovenous shunt. Fistula or arteriovenous communication should be applied more often because many of the associated features are secondary manifestations of the arteriovenous shunt. Arteriovenous anomaly or maldevelopment is inappropriate because it presupposes a developmental error, whereas the true aetiology is uncertain and the pathogenesis ill-understood. It is wiser not to make such an assumption until there is scientific evidence in support. Inappropriate terminology is misleading and often habitually perpetuated despite the contrary evidence.

Irrespective of their morphological features or anatomical location, aneurysms are (most appropriately) classified primarily according to their aetiology with the exception of dissecting aneurysms and arteriovenous aneurysms, such terms indicating a specific type of lesion.

Aneurysms may form as the result of an inflammatory reaction associated with destruction of the vessel wall which then dilates and ruptures although the lesion may be so rapidly destructive as to rupture without the preceding dilatation occurring. Those that form as the result of a bacterial arteritis possibly of embolic origin are often referred to as mycotic, septic-embolic or embolomycotic. They should be referred to as bacterial aneurysms which may result from embolism or direct spread from an adjoining lesion. Mycotic aneurysm should rightfully be restricted to those of fungal origin. These **infective aneurysms**, once treated satisfactorily with antibiotics, may persist, in which case they may progress and the wall will then develop a neointima. On the other hand occlusive thrombosis or healing possibly with some calcification of a much thickened wall can result. An elastic stain may help to elucidate the previous destructive nature of the lesion, remnants of residual elastic lamina being found in unusual locations and distribution.

In the absence of trauma or an inflammatory lesion, large blood vessels rarely rupture without preceding aneurysmal dilatation or mural dissection. Cerebral arteries have been alleged to rupture directly but it is more than likely that the aneurysm was small or damaged, particularly if fixed before dissection because prolonged fixation hardens the haematoma making dissection difficult. There have been few cases of direct aortic rupture. Some prior dilatation is generally present [4,5].

10.1.1 ARTERIECTASIS

During infancy and childhood arteries enlarge according to individual physiological demands as the body grows to maturity. However, measurements of the aorta and coronary and cerebral arteries indicate that in general there is a progressive enlargement in calibre throughout life, even after physical maturity [6,8]. This is accompanied by general loss of elasticity and increase in length with development of tortuosity. The increase in calibre results in increased mural stress (Laplace's Law) and augmentation of the effects of haemodynamic stress. When arteriectasis is pronounced, the calibre of the vessel becomes irregular and aneurysmal dilatations develop. This is seen in the aorta, the wall of which may be flaccid at autopsy with multiple aneurysms and mural thrombi. Cylindroid and serpentine aneurysms denote varying stages of this process. Dissecting aneurysms may also complicate severe ectasia.

Ectasia of the ascending aorta is commonly seen in subjects with aortic valvular incompetence secondary to syphilis, bicuspid aortic valves, aortic valvular stenosis and in Marfan's syndrome. In the latter the dilatation involves the aortic ring and secondary aortic incompetence results. Aortic dilatation in the aged has been associated with an aortic systolic ejection murmur which probably is not innocent as some authors assume [9].

The afferent artery to an arteriovenous shunt becomes ectatic as the blood flow progressively increases and may progress to irregular dilatation, tortuosity and aneurysmal dilatation [10]. Collateral vessels also undergo ectasia and characteristically tortuosity and possibly even aneurysmal dilatation.

10.1.2 PHLEBECTASIA

Phlebectasia is a state of ectasia of veins but the term is not commonly used. Ectatic veins are usually tortuous and of irregular calibre being therefore generally regarded as varicosities. Hence ectasia precedes the varicose state. A number of unusually dilated veins within the brain parenchyma is referred to as a venous angioma and some such veins may also be tortuous. Their true nature is ill-understood, but they could be manifestations of an arteriovenous shunt. Idiopathic ectasia of the jugular vein in children [11] may also be associated with an undisclosed arteriovenous shunt. The anastomosed veins of arteriovenous fistulae (experimental, therapeutic or traumatic) develop ectasia, tortuosity and irregular aneurysmal dilatation as the duration of the fistula lengthens. However an end-to-end anastomosis may also develop severe intimal proliferation and irregular narrowing in addition to saccular aneurysms [12].

10.1.3 TELANGIECTASIA

Telangiectasis is a localized region of small ectatic vessels which histologically may exhibit multiple fusiform and saccular aneurysmal dilatations (Chapter 14).

10.2 Aneurysms of the aorta

The aorta is generally regarded as the most common site for aneurysms; they are of quite diverse nature and often dramatic because of their large size and massive haemorrhage on rupture.

10.2.1 SYPHILITIC ANEURYSMS

Syphilis, once considered the most frequent cause of aortic aneurysms, has declined in incidence with the advent of the antibiotic era and syphilitic aneurysms are now, and hopefully will remain, rare or unknown. In the past it is likely that syphilitic aneurysms were overdiagnosed. Aneurysms, especially if saccular, in the proximal aorta were usually classified as syphilitic but in early years there were limitations to the validity of serological testing. It is likely that severely atherosclerotic aortas with aneurysms in the presence of intimal wrinkling, elastic disruption in the media and perivascular round cell infiltration about vasa vasorum were at times unjustifiably classified as syphilitic, when such changes occur in atherosclerosis.

Aortic involvement occurred in the tertiary stage and was most pronounced and at times restricted to the ascending aorta and arch, often stopping dramatically at the level of the ligamentum arteriosum. It was frequently associated with aortic valvular disease with thickening and shortening of the valve cusps and widening of the commissures, aortic incompetence, left ventricular hypertrophy and often dilatation, a jet lesion on the septum beneath the valve and variable ectasia of the proximal aorta. The aortic surface was puckered and wrinkled with intimal thickening and often stenosis of the coronary ostia.

Microscopically endarteritis and periarteritis were features of all stages of syphilis. In the tertiary stage the aorta at times exhibited gross destruction of medial elastic tissue resulting in irregular scarring with intense round cell infiltration in the media and adventitia. Frank gummatous inflammatory change was said to occur with endothelioid cells, lymphocytes, plasma cells, a rare Langhans giant cell, necrosis with the outlines of pre-existing inflammatory tissues visible and pronounced narrowing of vasa vasorum with perivascular round cell infiltration. Miliary gummas were said to occur. It was not noted for intimal tears and thrombosis. In view of the age of these victims, atherosclerosis would have been superimposed and, as with any such disease, may well have been accentuated by the underlying syphilis with irregularity of the intimal surface and altered physical characteristics of the wall. Much of the fibrous tissue was relatively avascular and hyaline.

The ectasia often progressed to a frank fusiform aneurysm and saccular aneurysms, sometimes of large size, developed causing displacement of surrounding structures, pressure effects on the recurrent laryngeal nerve, lungs and mediastinal structures, and pressure erosion of vertebrae (Figure 1.1, p. 2) (even leading to paraplegia), sternum and ribs. Such aneurysms sometimes presented in the neck or through the upper anterior chest wall and eventually ruptured through the skin with dramatic, horrifying results. Internal rupture of aneurysms of the ascending aorta may occur into the pericardial sac, the mediastinum, pleural cavity and superior vena cava. The mural thrombus can give rise to emboli.

The aortic valvular incompetence together with some dilatation of the aortic ring as part of the syphilitic process results in a water-hammer or Corrigan's pulse, characterized by a steep, sudden incline of the pulse contour and a greatly increased pulse pressure with an abrupt decline to a low diastolic pressure level. The effect of this Corrigan's pulse on the proximal aorta, which serves as a windkessel or pressure reservoir, has not been thoroughly investigated but the water-hammer effect must contribute significantly to the mural damage and aneurysm formation since it is a very destructive force. Considerable destruction of elastic tissue and muscle can be the consequence of severe haemodynamic stress [10,13] and aortic incompetence *per se* is often associated with ectasia and dissecting aneurysm of the ascending aorta [14,15].

Rheumatoid spondylitis and arthritis are at times associated with aortitis remarkably similar to that of syphilis, including the characteristic involvement of the aortic valves with thickening and shortening of the cusps and widening of the commissures. This incompetence is also asociated with an aortitis proximally that closely resembles syphilitic aortitis [16,17]. It occurs mostly with spondylitis and in males commencing some 10 years or more after the onset of the arthritis. The similarity of these changes to those of syphilis raises questions as to the underlying pathogenesis of the aortic changes in both diseases. It does not appear to be associated with rheumatic fever [18]. The apparent absence of aortic aneurysm may indicate only lesser severity because ectasia of the ascending aorta may be present [17]. One subject had an aneurysm of the aortic sinus [16]. Gross destruction of medial elastic tissue can occur in the apparent absence of syphilis and rheumatoid arthritis. Whether there is a common underlying factor or the syphilis coexisted with the few cases of rheumatoid spondylitis reported to have aortic incompetence and panaortitis is uncertain. Marquis *et al.* [17] reported negative serological reactions for syphilis in their cases and suggested the name idiopathic medial aortopathy and arteriopathy for the extensive destruction of the media. The fact that similar changes may occur also in Reiter's syndrome [19] and scleroderma led them to suggest a possible autoimmune process. They were of the opinion that the changes are also seen in a wide variety of diseases including rheumatic fever and rheumatoid arthritis. The uncertainty and non-specificity of these aortic changes [17] indicate the real need for a registry of unusual pathological lesions of the vascular system.

D-Penicillamine is a potent remission-inducing drug used in rheumatoid arthritis but it is also lathyrogenic [20]. It inhibits the biosynthesis of collagen crosslinks which may be of value in symptomatic clinical improvement but its effect on the functional integrity of the blood vessel wall requires investigation. By interfering with collagen crosslinks (of great importance to the tensile strength of collagen) it may contribute to serious degenerative changes in the aorta and large vessels. Whether or not it contributes to the degenerative changes here described in rheumatoid arthritis deserves consideration.

10.2.2 TUBERCULOUS ANEURYSMS

Tuberculous aortitis was an infrequent complication of para-aortic tuberculous lymphadenitis developed by direct spread. It was a disorder of the pre-antibiotic era but once present and unchecked, aortic aneurysm developed and frequently ruptured. Many of the non-aneurysmal aortas also ruptured [21]. With the resurgence of tuberculosis in this era of autoimmune deficiency syndrome (AIDS) and antibiotic resistance, such lesions may be seen again.

10.2.3 ATHEROSCLEROTIC ANEURYSMS OF THE AORTA

The peak incidence of aortic atherosclerotic aneurysms is in the seventh decade with males being affected more often than females. There is a slight predominance in hypertensives as distinct from normotensives and the high pressure should also accelerate the natural history of the disease. The frequency of thoracic aortic aneurysms has declined substantially this century and abdominal lesions are by far the commonest. An increase in the incidence of abdominal aortic aneurysms has been reported in recent years in many Western population groups in both autopsy studies and in symptomatic aneurysms [22,23]. This has been attributed to improved diagnostic capabilities and also to the aging population despite the much publicized alleged reduction in both coronary and cerebrovascular disease.

In abdominal aortic aneurysms both smoking and hypertension have been incriminated but particularly genetic factors. X-linked inheritance has been claimed, whereas in other studies autosomal and polygenic inheritance has been alleged [22]. Collin and Walton [24] found a much higher incidence of abdominal aortic aneurysm on ultrasonography amongst brothers of subjects with aortic abdominal aneurysms than in the general population, leading them to suggest it is a familial disease. Instances have been reported [25,26] in identical twins, but the aorta was not the only site involved. Other examples of familial concentration have been reported [27], including association of aneurysms with Marfan's syndrome, Ehlers–Danlos syndrome and type III collagen deficiency. It is difficult to conceive of a genetic defect specifically for an abdominal aortic aneurysm or for any other specific site. The possible genetic mechanism would be for an inherited connective tissue disorder, a disease affecting smooth muscle function or an inherited tendency for a specific type of arterial haemodynamic stress which has now been recognized as being of paramount importance in several types of aneurysmal dilatation. The most well recognized group in the connective tissue disorders of which there are likely to be some undiscovered or *formes frustes* includes Marfan's and Ehlers–Danlos syndromes and perhaps cutis laxa. Copper deficiency has been suggested [28] and refuted [29]. These disorders then become predisposing factors because of the altered connective tissue properties that render the vessel walls less resilient. Constitutional traits may be equally or even more important in determining the haemodynamics that predisposes to aneurysmal dilatation. Hypertension aggravates the situation independently of any other inheritance.

These aneurysms, fusiform or saccular but generally the former (80%), are most often situated in the abdominal segment distally, as is consistent with the augmented severity of atherosclerosis in that aortic segment (Figures 10.3, 10.4). Multiple aneurysms are common and the common iliac arteries may also be ectatic or aneurysmal often with widening of the bifurcation angle and some displacement (Figures 10.5, 10.6). On occasions the whole aorta is severely ectatic and multiple saccular aneurysms containing thrombus may develop in the aorta and other arteries.

The aneurysms develop slowly and insidiously with a diffuse ectasia of the infrarenal segment of the aorta often with elongation and tortuosity. Elongation has been considered an invariable precursor of fusiform

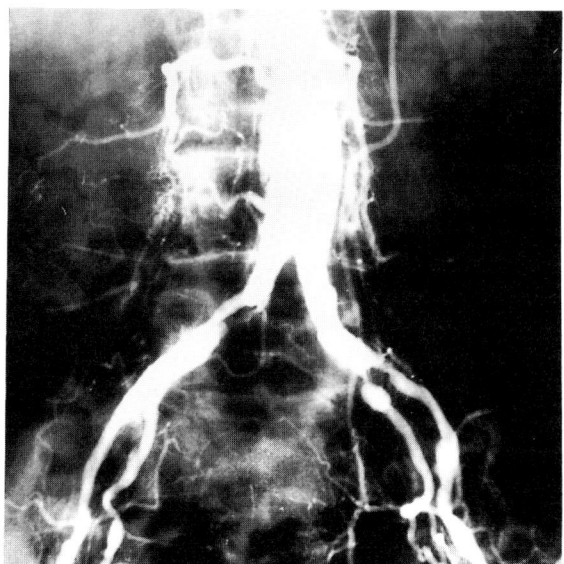

Figure 10.3 Angiogram showing slight fusiform aneurysm at dilatation of the abdominal aorta in association with severe atherosclerosis of the iliofemoral arteries with stenoses, tortuosity and irregular displacement. (By courtesy of Mr P.R. Meech.)

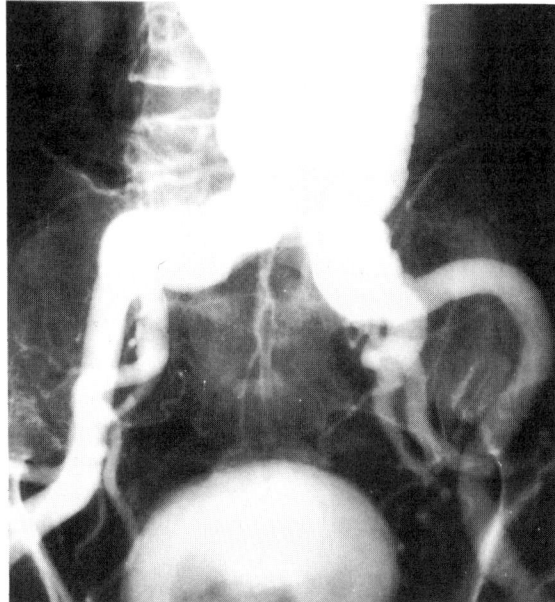

Figure 10.4 Angiogram of a large aortic aneurysm with irregular dilatation and displacement of the common iliac arteries. Note the widened aortic bifurcation angle and the irregular course of the other iliac arteries. (By courtesy of Mr W.C. Shirer.)

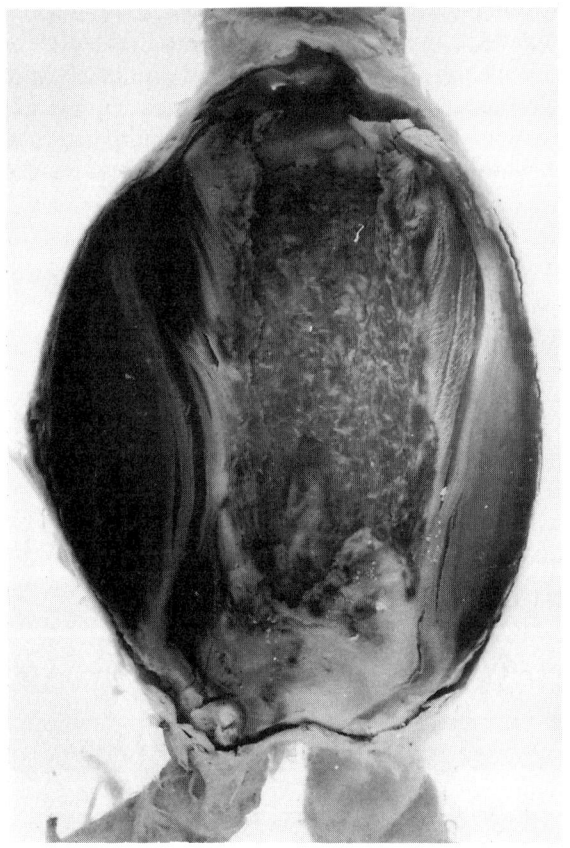

Figure 10.5 Fusiform aortic aneurysm opened to demonstrate the laminated thrombus and the ragged surface of the central functional lumen. (Reproduced with permission from Stehbens [337].)

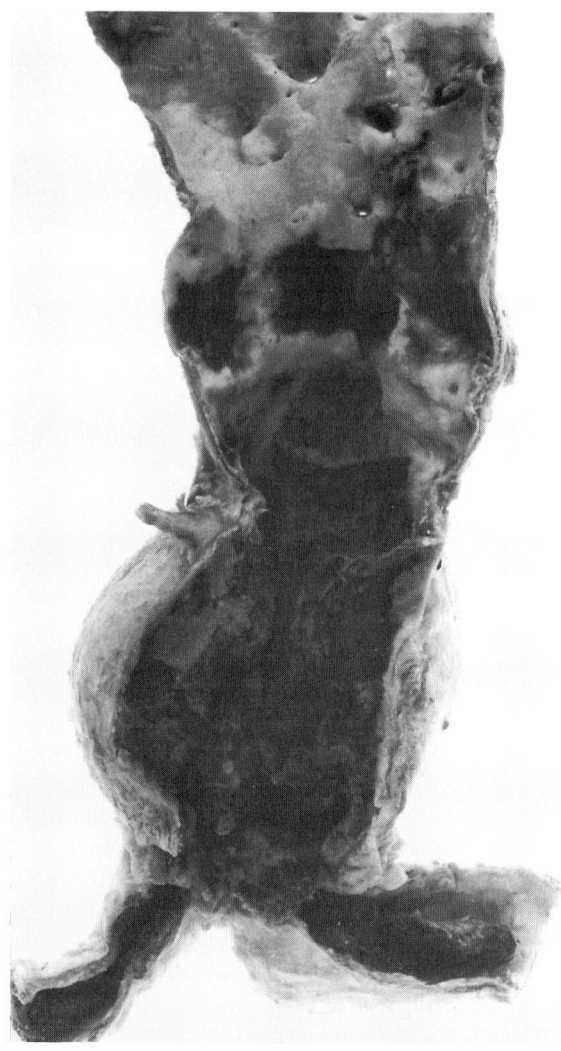

Figure 10.6 Atherosclerotic abdominal aortic aneurysm containing occlusive thrombus. The left common iliac artery is aneurysmal and grossly angulated increasing the angle of bifurcation. Note multiple thrombi in the aorta above the aneurysm.

aneurysms [30] but it is more likely to be concomitant with ectasia. Progressively the dilatation becomes fusiform with yielding of the wall over a considerable distance, perhaps with areas of atherosclerotic ulceration and mural thrombus. Normally the length is roughly one third longer than the width but the dilatation may be more elongated and can become spherical. Much of the media will have been lost and only remnants of the residual media may be detected with an elastic tissue stain.

The loss of medial lamellae in association with intimal thickening does not indicate that the latter destroys the former by inducing ischaemia. Vasa vasorum are capable of invading the intima and experimental evidence indicates that extensive destruction of medial tissue can occur in the absence of intimal proliferation [10,13].

Abdominal aortic aneurysms run a more protracted course than previously believed and modern ultrasonic techniques enable the increase in size to be monitored and facilitate detection at an earlier stage of development. Small aneurysms usually enlarge by about 0.21 cm per year but this can be greater [31] especially with larger aneurysms [32]. In 92 patients with aneurysms less than 6 cm in diameter, 39% died within two years and of 46 with aneurysms larger than 6 cm, 72% were dead within two years but not all were due to aneurysmal rupture [33]. In an autopsy study of 473 subjects with abdominal aortic aneurysms, death was due to rupture in 118 (25%), and rupture was responsible in 9.5% when the aneurysms were less than 4 cm in diameter and in 60.5% of those with aneurysms 10 cm or more in diameter [34]. No definite aneurysm should be regarded as safe from rupture, even those under 4 cm in diameter [35] although it has been suggested that those with a diameter less than the width of the body of the third lumbar vertebra are not likely to rupture [35]. Risk of haemorrhage increases with size of aneurysm, rate of increase in girth and the presence of hypertension. Those that increase in diameter by more than 1 cm per year whilst being regularly monitored by ultrasonography and have a diameter over 6 cm wide are at particular risk of rupture [36].

The floor of an ulcerated atherosclerotic plaque with undermined edges may progressively yield initially to form a small dome-shaped dilatation which can ultimately become distinctly saccular. Such lesions (Figures 10.7, 10.8) were first considered to be involved by Coates and Auld [37]. The abrupt termination of the elastic tissue is suggestive of a medial tear and there may be little residual media in the floor of the ulcer (Figure 10.8). Such lesions no doubt were responsible for the prolonged controversy prior to this century as to whether aortic aneurysms were true or false [1]. They could account for some lateral saccular aneurysms of the aorta.

Rupture of the aneurysm is often through a tear of 2–3 cm mostly at the site of maximum width. The aneurysmal wall is severely atherosclerotic macroscopically and microscopically with almost invariably some mural thrombus, and atherosclerosis runs a more rapid course within aneurysms [38,39]. There is a variable degree of calcification in the sac wall. With large aneurysms thrombus may totally line the wall and the blood channel may run an irregular course through the thrombus, the inner surface of which is often red and friable (Figure 10.5) and not inspissated as is usual with laminated thrombus. There may be total occlusion of the abdominal aortic aneurysm (Figure 10.6) or possibly of just one common iliac artery. Embolism must be of frequent occurrence and contribute to the peripheral arterial occlusive disease of the legs more often than imagined. Ectasia, tortuosity or aneurysmal dilatation of the common iliac arteries are common accompaniments.

A third of the patients with a diagnosed abdominal aortic aneurysm are likely to die within one year, 80% within five years and most within ten years. When symptoms referable to the aneurysm appear, 60–80% may die within the first year mostly from rupture [40]. However, such aneurysms may run a more protracted course, one patient being known to have survived 24 years [41]. Survival and prognosis depend essentially on aneurysm size when first encountered and the rapidity with which it enlarges. The cause of the rupture has

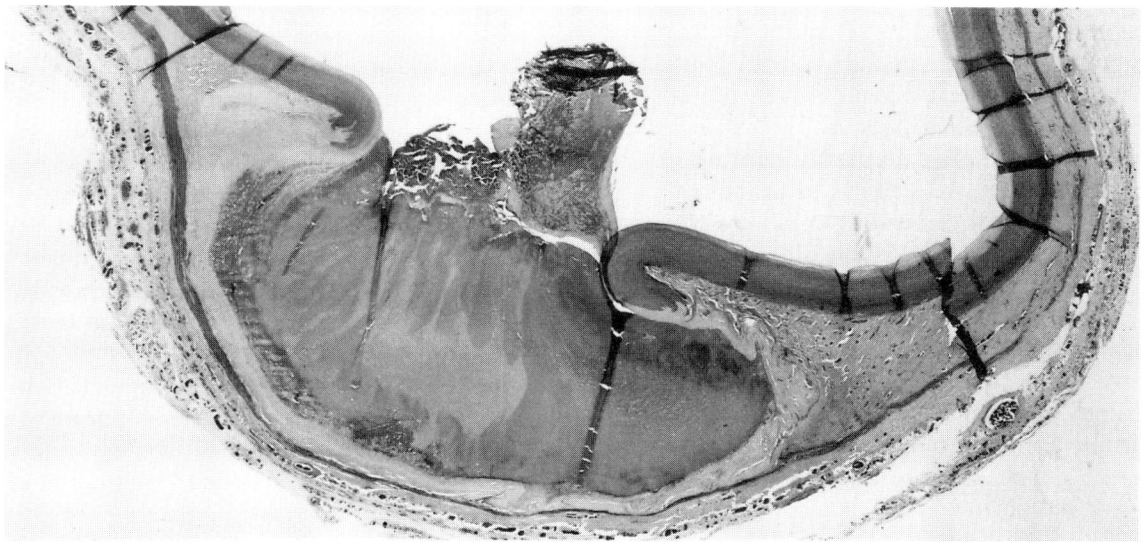

Figure 10.7 Low magnification of a tear through the aortic media with some undermining and dissection of the wall at the edges of the tear. The cavity contains thrombus, excavation of which could lead to a localized saccular aneurysm. (Weigert's elastic tissue stain.)

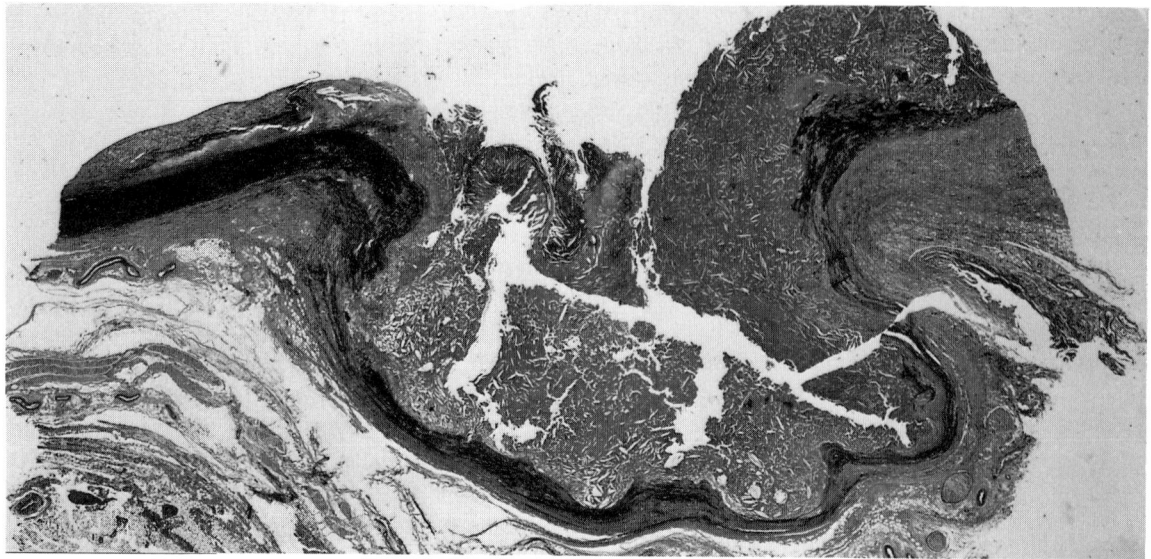

Figure 10.8 Section through an ulcerated atherosclerotic aortic wall with aneurysmal bulging from the adventitial surface. (Weigert's elastic tissue stain.)

frequently been attributed to progressively increased tension in the wall due to the law of Laplace. While progressive increase in mural tension is a factor, the weakness of the wall must ultimately be due to the haemodynamic forces and mechanical failure of the wall that were responsible for the tear, ulceration or dilatation in the first place. Small 'blebs' on the aneurysmal wall have been considered by Hunter et al. [42] as the cause of some aneurysmal ruptures and a similar lesion has been attributed to lupus erythematosus [43].

Patel [44] has reported the apparent tamponade effect of an organized periaortic aneurysmal haematoma limited by outer aortic adventitial tissue or mesentery. Such a chronic lesion must be infrequent but the limitation of bleeding by this acute tamponade effect may be the means of sealing small initial leaks. On rupture these fusiform abdominal aneurysms are likely to bleed into the retroperitoneal space, and less frequently into the peritoneal cavity, pelvis, a viscus or the inferior vena cava producing an arteriovenous shunt. Erosion of the spinal column is a slow insidious process (Figure 1.1, p. 2) and more frequent than with thoracic aneurysms. Colonic infarction is a serious fatal complication of ruptured abdominal aortic aneurysms and has been attributed to low cardiac output at operation and the administration of α-adrenergic vasopressor agents [42].

The complications of atherosclerotic aneurysms in the thorax are similar to those associated with syphilitic aneurysms although they do not appear to develop to the enormous dimensions of thoracic aneurysms reported in the first half of this century. This may be due to a difference in aetiology or otherwise to improvements in their diagnosis and management.

The commonest site in the thoracic aorta is the ascending segment. It usually commences as a diffuse fusiform dilatation in association with some elongation and ectasia of the aorta. This may occur with a normal aortic valve ring and valve, but aortic valvular stenosis, aortic valvular incompetence and bicuspid aortic valve predispose to these aneurysms. Hypertension possibly with a bicuspid aortic valve and some incompetence contributes to their occurrence in coarctation of the aorta. When long lengths of the thoracic aorta are ectatic, tortuosity is usually pronounced. Saccular aneurysms of the thoracic aorta may also affect the descending thoracic segment. They may be multiple. Rupture is most often into the pleural cavity and mediastinum, less often into the lung or oesophagus.

Marfan's syndrome predisposes to saccular aortic aneurysms although more frequently they are dissecting or fusiform in type. Dilatation of the aortic ring with some valvular incompetence may occur. This is often associated with ectasia or aneurysmal dilatation of the ascending aorta. They have the characteristic ocular and musculoskeletal abnormalities and cardiovascular complications become significant from the second decade onwards.

It has been suggested that patients with unusually large arteries due to greater body size are prone to aortic aneurysm and that some subjects possibly with a connective tissue disorder develop large arteries and aneurysms [46]. The term arteriomegaly used for such vessels has also been applied to the large arteries of acromegalics.

With current surgical therapy of aortic saccular, fusiform or dissecting aneurysms, surgical intervention allows longer survival. The progression of other pre-existing aneurysms or the development of new lesions frequently causes late postoperative death. This is particularly likely in subjects with grossly ectatic aneurysms, or Marfan's syndrome or a healed dissecting aneurysm [47] and led to the recommendation for annual monitoring of the aorta postoperatively.

There has been controversy of late about aortic aneurysms and those of the abdominal aorta in particular. A denial of the role of atherosclerosis has resulted because of the lack of correlation with coronary heart disease risk factors and the inability to explain the dilatation. McGee et al. [48] concluded from their biochemical analysis that there was a similar synthetic response in both occlusive disease and aneurysmal dilatation but that proteolytic activity might determine the clinical course of the disease. It has been argued that the aneurysms may be distinct from atherosclerosis and connective tissue disorders, i.e. collagen type III deficiency or copper deficiency might be responsible, but these hypotheses have not been supported [49]. In a study of aortic aneurysms and aortic atherosclerosis, Reed et al. [50] concluded that the determinants were the same for both although this has not met with unanimous agreement [51].

Increased proteolytic and elastolytic activity has been found in abdominal aortic aneurysms [52,53] but it does not follow that the aneurysms are due to such enzymatic activity. Their presence does not necessarily indicate activity and post-stenotic aneurysms should be used as a control. Neither does the presence of such enzymes indicate causality and care must be taken before attributing a causal role to any chemical mediator without strong scientific evidence. Confounding the results of leucocytic enzymatic activity by inclusion of thrombus in the aneurysm wall must be excluded. The gross histological destruction of the aortic wall that occurs in atherosclerosis cannot be ignored and the presence of such dilatation signifying mural weakness suggests that mechanical factors may well underlie the atherosclerotic aneurysms as occurs with post-stenotic aneurysms, those associated with arteriovenous fistulae and dissecting aneurysms.

It was recently observed that abdominal aortic aneurysms were unduly represented in subjects who had lost a leg by amputation during the war. The pattern emerged that the abdominal aortic aneurysm formed with a tortuous bend (convexity) to the side of the amputation and widening of the external iliac artery on the contralateral (patent) side (Figure 10.9) [54]. The higher the amputation the greater the haemodynamic changes. The amputation caused an asymmetrical reduction of iliac artery calibre and blood flow. This observation is consistent with the haemodynamic concept of atherosclerosis and the production of similar tortuosity, atrophic and proliferative lesions of athero-

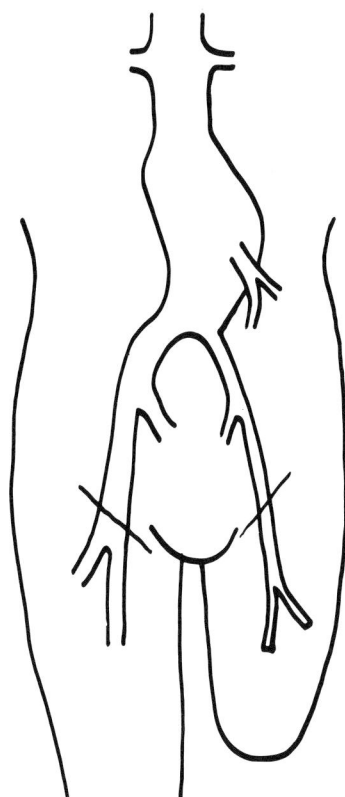

Figure 10.9 Tortuosity and aneurysmal dilatation that is prone to develop years after above-knee amputation of the left leg. The direction of the curvatures is reversed in the right leg amputation (Redrawn with permission from Vollmar et al. [54].)

sclerosis and aneurysm formation in arteries proximal to an experimental arteriovenous fistula [10]. These experimental findings indicate that both proliferative atherosclerosis and aneurysm formation can be produced by grossly augmented flow with associated alterations in blood pressure. It also raises the possibility that vascular disease or indeed an arteriovenous shunt in one limb could thereby accentuate the degenerative changes in the abdominal aorta with a propensity for abdominal aortic aneurysm. Just as hereditary factors and connective tissue disorders can adversely affect the development of early atrophic changes in arterial walls which are precursors of aneurysm formation, so could such changes aggravate the haemodynamic production of aortic aneurysms in man.

Aortic aneurysms in young adults are most likely to be associated with a connective tissue disorder, coarctation of the aorta, trauma, infection and inflammatory diseases (Takayasu and Kawasaki diseases) and severe hypertension. This is also true for children and complications of umbilical catheterization have recently become a distinct clinical entity. Critically ill neonates subjected to long-term umbilical artery catheterization, if they develop infections, are prone to bacterial aortitis at sites of intimal trauma to the thoracic and abdominal aorta, the iliac arteries or even multiple sites. The catheter is often the source of infection, usually staphylococcal. Thrombus forms at the site of injury or there may be a false aneurysm. Infection produces a destructive aortitis and an aneurysm which may either rupture early or progressively enlarge following antibiotic therapy only to present clinically a few months or years later [55]. Risk increases with the duration of catheterization.

10.2.4 INFLAMMATORY ABDOMINAL AORTIC ANEURYSM

Subjects with systemic lupus erythematosus have been reported with dissecting aneurysms of the aorta and extracranial vertebral arteries, (fungal) mycotic aneurysms, angiitic coronary artery aneurysms, and aneurysms of cerebral arteries which may be due to transmural angiitis or berry aneurysms. The effects of drug therapy may affect the pathogenesis of each of these lesions. Inflammatory aneurysm of the abdominal aorta with the aortic wall embedded in retroperitoneal fibrosis extending around the inferior vena cava also [56] is a hazard. A similar fibrosis has been observed about the coronary arteries in a case of inflammatory aneurysm [56].

Abdominal aortic aneurysms with similar retroperitoneal fibrosis occur in the absence of systemic lupus erythematosus and controversy surrounds their differentiation from atherosclerotic aortic aneurysms. The presence of chronic inflammatory cells is well recognized in the intima and especially in the adventitia of advanced atherosclerotic disease but their role is unknown. Such changes are related to chronic degenerative diseases and even bland infarcts which cannot be regarded as primarily inflammatory diseases although inflammation is part of the process of repair and organization. Some authors regard the inflammatory aneurysms as distinct from atherosclerotic aneurysms and others as the extremes of a spectrum. The controversy will be elucidated by determining the aetiology of chronic periaortitis and retroperitoneal fibrosis.

10.2.5 SPONTANEOUS AORTIC RUPTURE

This is an exceedingly rare condition in the absence of some aneurysmal dilatation or a dissecting aneurysm. Few instances have been reported [4,5] but the incidence could be higher. Its rarity suggests that loss of tensile strength of the mural connective tissues is indicative of a weakness of the inner part of the wall and only slow yield of the outer part. The tear of a dissecting aneurysm is in reality a partial rupture. The histological features of the aorta are similar and exhibit severe degenerative change. Copper deficiency experimentally can cause large rents in the aortic wall but spontaneous aortic rupture can also occur in humans on long-term steroid therapy [57]. Two such cases were associated with transmural tears, a false aneurysm in one and a periaortic haematoma in the other. Arteries may tear like wet tissue paper indicating the remarkable vascular fragility in the Ehlers–Danlos syndrome. The fragility was attributed to impaired reparative processes that no doubt are continuous throughout life at a subtle level of activity.

10.2.6 POST-STENOTIC DILATATION

Post-stenotic dilatation is classically seen in aortic coarctation (Figure 10.10) and is a fascinating phenomenon. In a series of experiments Halsted [58] demonstrated that dilatation of the arterial wall distal to a ligature constricting the lumen to one third or one quarter of its original dimension, caused 'whirlpool-like play of blood in the relatively dead pocket just below the constriction'. He postulated that the post-stenotic dilatation was the consequence of this disturbed blood flow and this phenomenon explained the subclavian aneurysms associated with cervical ribs and aneurysms distal to coarctation of the aorta [58]. Holman reported the phenomenon beyond aortic and pulmonary valve stenoses and could reproduce the phenomenon at will in experimental animals and in rubber tubing [59,60]. He

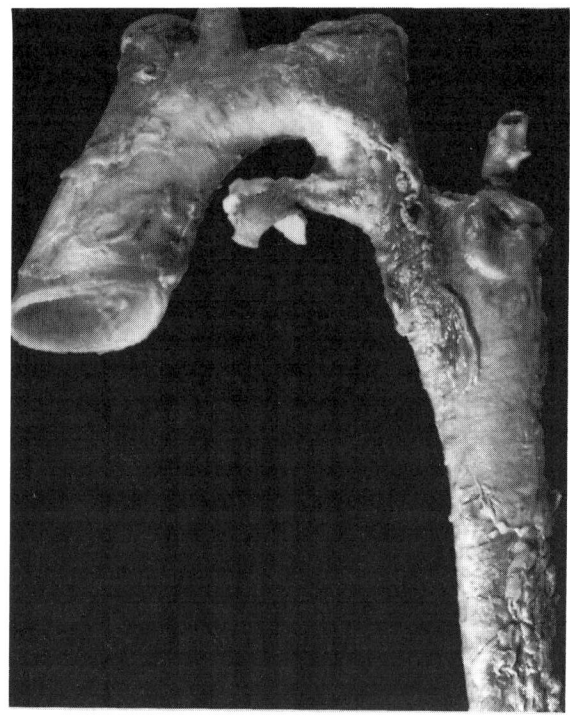

Figure 10.10 Coarctation of the aorta at the site of insertion of the ligamentum arteriosum. Note the fusiform dilatation and collapsed saccular pouch below the coarctation.

explained the phenomenon as being due to mechanical or engineering fatigue of the vessel wall or rubber tubing due to their vibration induced by the high velocity jet flow into the expanded artery beyond the stenosis. Holman and his colleagues also demonstrated that a vibrating spatula or rod within a water-filled segment of rubber tubing closed at each end also caused dilatation maximal at the zone of maximum vibrations. Increase of pressure within the tubing hastened development of the dilatation and rupture [61]. The concept of engineering fatigue was further supported by the experimental studies of Roach [62]. The dilatation develops when the thrill and bruit beyond the stenosis is maximal, and profound degenerative changes occur in the elastic tissue with some fibrosis and intimal thickening. A jet lesion develops at the site of impact of the jet flow but atherosclerosis may develop within the post-stenotic zone. Human arteries dilate more readily with higher frequencies and increasing age of the subjects but this may be the consequence of the degree of atherosclerosis already developed prior to testing *in vitro*. Roach [62] believes that specific frequencies are required for specific arteries and this may be due to resonance with amplification at certain frequencies, the resonant modes being determined by mural stress, arterial geometry and the acoustical environment. The evidence is that the mural effect of the poststenotic flow is cumulative and irreversible, because surgical correction of coarctation of the aorta may be followed some years later by aneurysmal dilatation of the poststenotic zone.

The morphological changes in mural constituents underlying these post-stenotic dilatations have not been studied in detail but the evidence available indicates that severe accelerated degenerative changes occur [63,64] with severe elastic tissue degeneration from childhood and increased intimal proliferation. A jet lesion with wrinkling and roughening of the intima occurs distal to the stenosis and is similar to those of grossly disturbed flow and jet lesions in experimental aneurysms and arteriovenous shunts. The morphological, biochemical and biophysical responses, though varying in rapidity of development and severity, are probably similar.

This post-stenotic dilatation is a non-specific phenomenon which has wide applicability to human pathology and its frequent occurrence in coarctation of the aorta suggests that other aneurysms associated with the condition may also be acquired and not due to congenital weakness of the arterial wall as was once assumed. It also indicates that vibratory activity of lesser frequency and amplitude may likewise cause similar degenerative changes over a longer time frame.

With further enlargement of the post-stenotic dilatation the mural tension is increased thereby further augmenting the effect of disturbed flow within the sac. The pulsatility of the dilatation is also augmented even though dampened by the stenosis. However, in conventional fusiform and saccular aneurysms this increased pulsatility exerts a most serious effect on the wall. Irrespective of the reason for the initial aneurysmal dilatation, whether inflammatory, traumatic or degenerative, this hydrodynamic effect is essentially similar to that in the poststenotic dilatation. The course may be slower due to the less intensive flow disturbance.

10.2.7 DISSECTING ANEURYSM OF THE AORTA

The aorta is by far the most frequent site for dissecting aneurysm, and in most instances, apart from ectasia consistent with age and hypertension, there is no aneurysmal dilatation. It is merely an acute aortic dissection two to three times more frequent in males than females and most often occurring over the age of 60 years. These subjects usually have long-standing hypertension which may account for a higher incidence amongst American negroes. Normotension may be present in subjects under 40 years of age with evidence of Marfan's syndrome or some connective tissue disorder. It has also been recorded in subjects with systemic lupus erythematosus and the effect of the hypertension and chemotherapy must be taken into account when considering the pathogenesis. Subjects with aortic valvular disease are of an intermediate age group. There is generally said to be an unduly high incidence of dissecting aneurysms in pregnancy [65]. They have been reported frequently in turkeys with as yet no satisfactory explanation though they could have been exposed to an unidentified lathyrogenic substance or there may be a genetic connective tissue disorder.

The aorta is frequently ectatic or exhibits incipient aneurysmal dilatation. There are three important pathological features of dissecting aneurysms (portal of entry, dissection and rupture). Firstly there is the initial tear (Figure 10.11), usually a linear, transversely orientated, fairly sharp-edged laceration (2–3 cm in length) looking at times like an artefact consequent upon an incision. The tear may even be circumferential [66]. It occurs a few centimetres above the aortic valve cusps but may be within 10 cm. Less frequently the portal of entry is found in the vicinity of the insertion of the ligamentum arteriosum. Rare tears are longitudinally orientated and may be branched. There is usually no obvious lesion to account for the tear which extends deep into the media for a varying distance. The entrance less often is through an atheromatous plaque or ulcer more likely in the abdominal aorta than further proximally. A healed tear (Figure 10.11(b)) with no significant dissection but with separated margins is a rare finding at autopsy. An occasional subject may have no intimal tear but one must be sceptical about such reports.

Having gained entry the blood splits the aortic wall (Figure 10.12) for a varying distance proximally, distally and circumferentially close to the junction of the

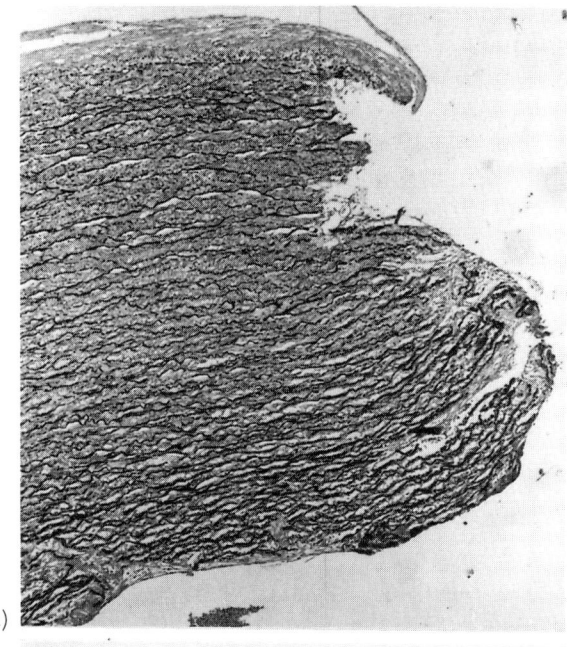

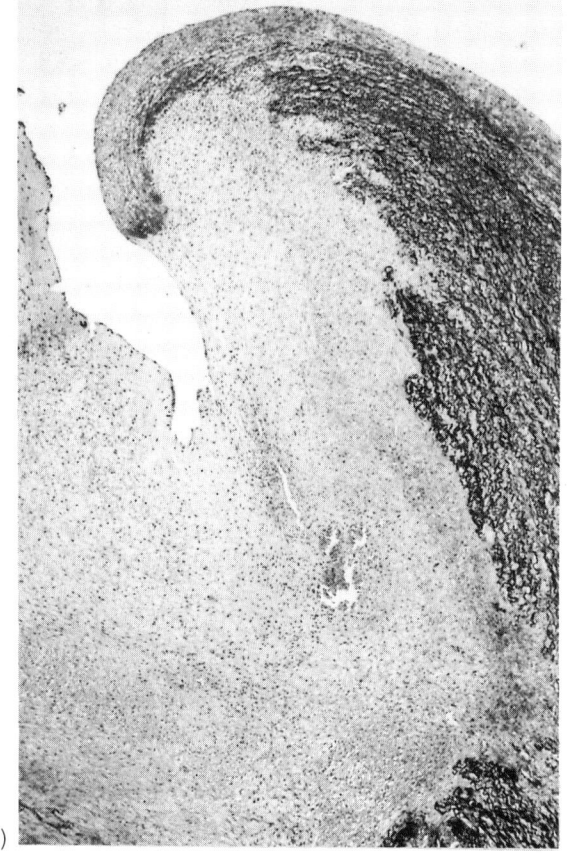

Figure 10.11 Fairly abrupt edge of the tear of a dissecting aneurysm with a small amount of adherent thrombus matter (a) and in (b) the edge of an old tear has healed with fibrocellular proliferation and no significant dissection. (Verhoeff's elastic stain and eosin.)

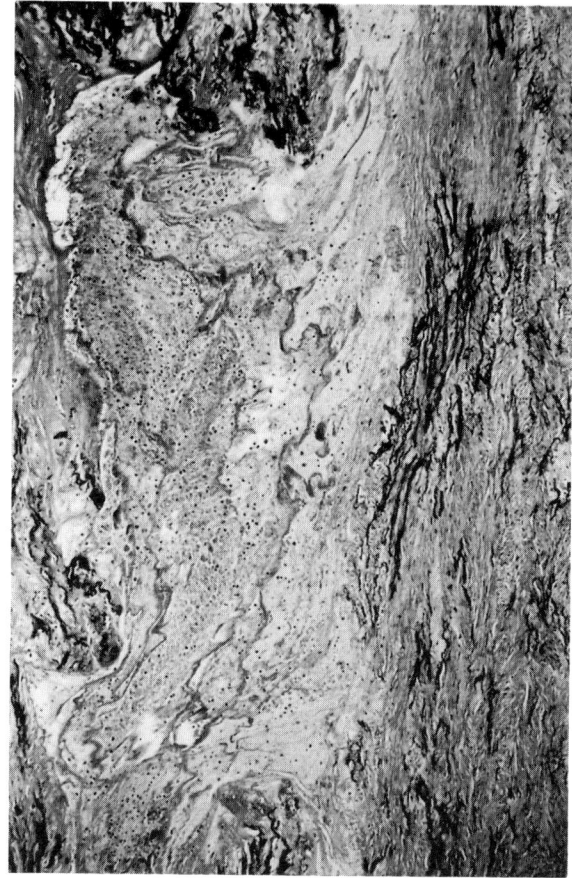

Figure 10.12 Aorta from a subject with dissecting aneurysm showing intramural blood clot or thrombus and the ragged edge along the plane of cleavage. Note the large areas of the aortic wall devoid of elastic tissue (to the right) as commonly occurs in this disorder. (Verhoeff's elastic stain and eosin.)

middle and outer third of the media (Figure 10.13). The pulsatile blood flow is no doubt important in the dissection with the direction of the applied forces being disadvantageous to the aortic wall. Retrograde spread with external rupture into the pericardial sac results in haemopericardium and cardiac tamponade. Distally it can extend to the abdominal aorta and even to the bifurcation and iliac arteries, unless it ruptures internally through a re-entry tear or externally to produce massive haemorrhage. It may extend into branches such as the great branches from the arch. The dissection may completely encircle the aorta or its branches. It may not involve the entire circumference in which case the inner layer may encroach on the true lumen and possibly come into apposition with the opposite wall thus occluding the artery.

In larger branches the dissection is close to the junction of the media with the adventitia. Small branches traversing the dissected wall may be stretched, attenuated or compressed according to the degree of separation of the two layers with reduction of blood

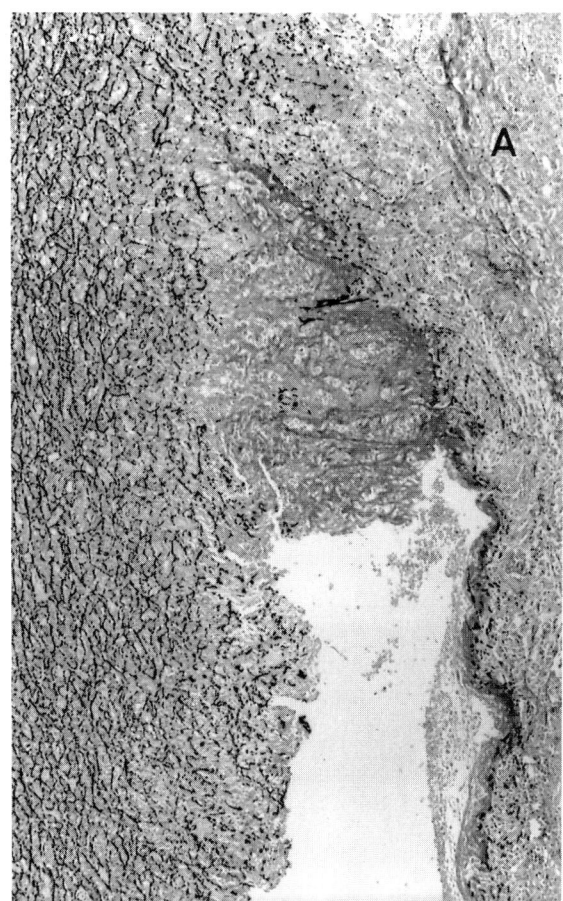

Figure 10.13 End of the plane of cleavage of a dissecting aneurysm in the deep media. Note the thrombus and the proximity to the adventitia (A). Compare with Figures 10.11 and 10.12 for variation in elastic tissue degeneration. (Verhoeff's elastic stain.)

flow through the branch. Rupture of the vessel may occur with reconstitution of flow from the false lumen into the branch or occlusion by thrombosis. Ischaemia results from occlusion of aortic branches or embolism. Paraplegia may result from occlusion of the large anterior spinal artery of Adamkiewicz.

The blood in the newly formed lumen will clot and the degree of separation is variable. Consumption coagulopathy has been noted [67]. Re-entry distally in the aorta or in a branch relieves obstruction but thrombus forms on the inner surfaces of the false lumen (Figure 10.13) and provides emboli for the distal circulation. Re-entry into the aorta distally permits survival for a varying period of time and reduces the likelihood of external rupture but the emboli in association with shock and hypotension can cause foci of infarction.

The De Bakey classification divides dissections into three types [68]:

- Type I dissection originates with a tear in the ascending aorta and involves the entire length.
- The rare type II is limited to the ascending aorta and often associated with some dilatation of the aorta, aortic valvular incompetence and congestive cardiac failure.
- Type III commences distal to the origin of the left subclavian artery and spares the ascending aorta and arch.

A more recent classification [68] divides the subjects into only two types. Type A includes all cases where the ascending aorta is involved and is more than twice as frequent as type B in which the portal of entry and the aortic dissection are beyond the left subclavian artery. Type A subjects are somewhat younger, hypertension is not so common and mortality is usually due to rupture into the pericardial sac. Type B subjects are older with a higher incidence of hypertension and severe atherosclerosis.

Dissection appears to be a gradual process with shifting pain but can be symptomless. External rupture and fatal haemorrhage cause death in about 95% of subjects within a few days. Rupture into the pericardial sac is the most frequent site of fatal haemorrhage with cardiac tamponade and is more likely when the tear is located in the ascending aorta or arch. There is occasional rupture into the right atrium. The left pleural cavity is a frequent site of haemorrhage [69], which may also occur into the mediastinum, the sheath of the pulmonary arterial trunk causing compression, or into the retroperitoneum. On occasions a false aneurysm may form and subsequently rupture. The haematoma may cause acute stenosis of the ascending aorta as can occur in the common carotid or brachiocephalic arteries. A few patients survive for several years following a re-entry tear with the false lumen becoming endothelialized. A neo-intima develops and ultimately atherosclerosis if survival is long enough. Mural thrombosis and aneurysm formation may develop in the false channel.

Small healed tears are at times found incidentally at autopsy and it is likely that such tears are more frequent than currently recognized. Delayed rupture of spontaneous tears of the ascending aorta may occur [70] and also recurrent dissection [71]. The junction of the middle and outer thirds of the media is regarded as the watershed between supply externally from the vasa vasorum and the inner part of the wall from the lumen. The depth of the tear may be important but the major factor probably is the cohesion of the mural connective tissues and their overall loss of tensile strength, the tears no doubt exhibiting greater fragility in the inner part of the wall. In the large extracranial branches the dissection is mostly between media and adventitia and in the cerebral arteries usually between the intima and media (i.e. external to the internal elastic lamina). It has been alleged that dissecting aneurysm can occur without a tear but this seems hardly possible.

Histologically the initial tear is an abrupt separation of multiple medial lamellar units often without any dramatic histological alteration and not a ragged irregular tear of successive elastic laminae. The dissection occurs in the depth of the tear and small fragments of elastic laminae may project into the false passage (Figure 10.12) in which there can be a variable thickness of extravasated blood and fibrinous deposit.

Dissecting aneurysms of the aorta are usualy ascribed to Erdheim's cystic medial necrosis, in which there is irregular patchy loss of elastic laminae and the intervening muscle and matrix are replaced by an accumulation of mucopolysaccharides. There is no cystic change. The metachromatic staining is due to the presence of chondroitin sulphate C in these 'lakes' or spaces devoid of elastica. There is no true necrosis in such regions histologically and ultrastructurally it would be surprising if there was not a significant increase in granulovesicular degradation of the medial smooth muscle cells. However, in adult life the medial elastic laminae exhibit variable but often considerable fragmentation diffusely throughout the media and many dissecting aneurysms are seen without so-called Erdheim's cystic medial necrosis (and *vice versa*) which is so often a feature in the aortas of subjects with chronic hypertension (including coarctation of the aorta) and Marfan's syndrome. To account for the mural weakness there must be a widespread loss of cohesion of the cellular and non-cellular connective tissue components together with tears, degeneration and loss of elastic tissue. Kita *et al.* [72] found the major features of aortae with dissecting aneurysm were greater elastic tissue fragmentation and less fibrosis. By scanning electron microscopy Nakashima *et al.* [73] observed an increase in interlaminar connecting elastic fibres in hypertensives with a decrease in the outer media, whilst in aortic dissection there was irregularity and loss of interconnecting fibres especially in the outer media (Figure 10.14). Histologically, fragmentation of the medial elastic laminae is common (Figure 10.13). In general it is not possible to correlate the tensile strength of the tissue with its histological appearance, there being no specific histological feature that can be regarded as pathognomonic of dissecting aneurysm.

Survival is accompanied by tissue response to the damage and haemorrhage with the formation of a neointima in the false passage. Small linear infarcts of the aortic media may occur characterized by necrosis of smooth muscle cells with preservation of elastic laminae. Sometimes a dissection associated with minimal separation can undergo healing with organization and the intervening space is devoid of elastic tissue.

Gore and Seiwert [74] emphasized the prevalence of 'congenital' anomalies in subjects under 40 years of age with dissecting aneurysm including Marfan's syndrome in which there is less durable connective tissues especially in the cardiovascular and musculoskeletal systems. Other significant associations are aortic coarctation, bicuspid aortic valves and patent ductus arteriosus. Aortic coarctation is associated with chronic hypertension and often with bicuspid aortic valves. There

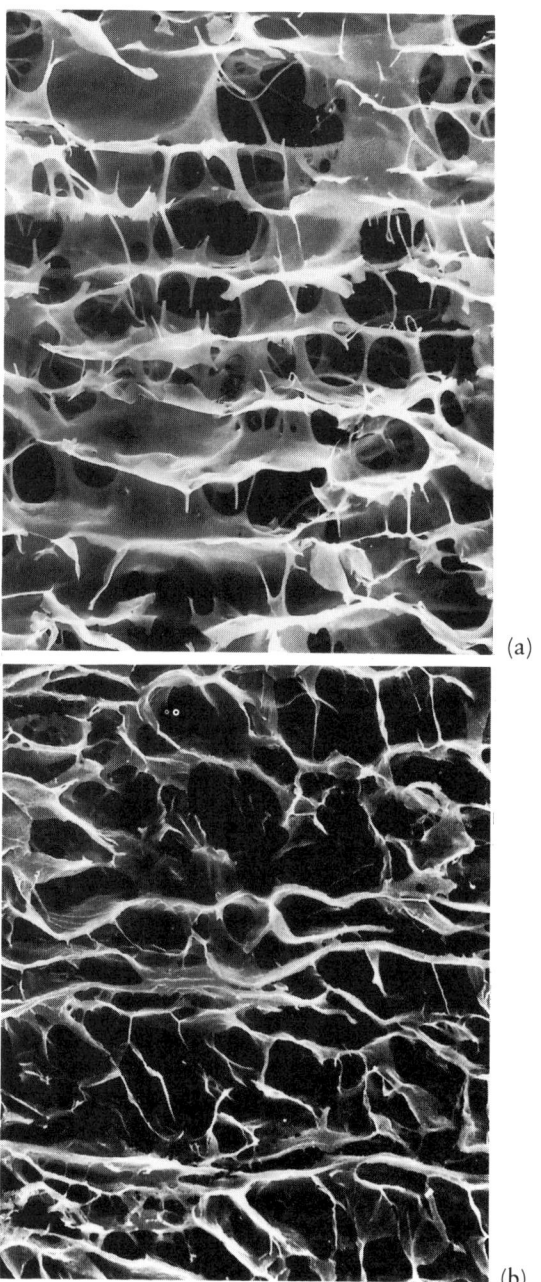

Figure 10.14 (a) Three-dimensional architecture of control aortic media showing multiple elastic laminae with interconnecting elastic fibres and bands. (b) The elastic laminae from the outer media of a subject with dissecting aneurysm are less distinct being fragmented and the interconnecting fibres are less in evidence. (c) A lower magnification of the media from a subject with 'cystic medial necrosis' showing gross disruption of the medial laminae and their interconnections. (Reproduced with permission from Nakashima *et al.* [73].)

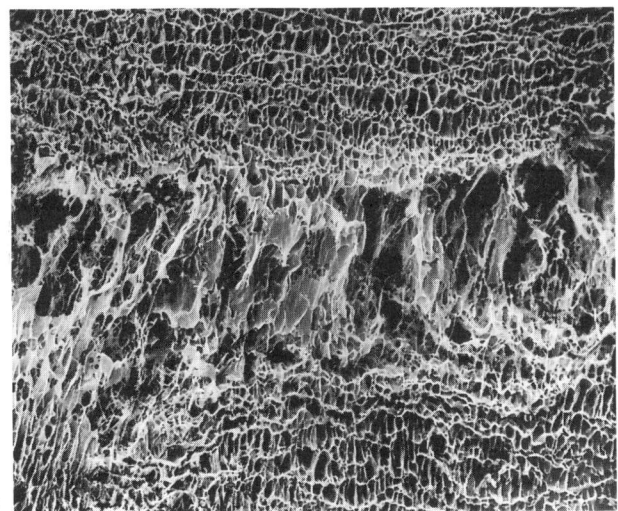

(c)

Figure 10.14 *Continued*

seems to be no reason for bicuspid aortic valves *per se* to cause dissecting aneurysms. Apart from a susceptibility to bacterial endocarditis, such valves often become thickened, fibrotic and incompetent. It is possible that the water-hammer effect of the pulse predisposes to medial elastic degeneration, ectasia and dissecting aneurysm. The patent ductus arteriosus may also have a water-hammer pulse acting in a similar manner.

A family has been reported [75] with several members over two generations having aortic dissecting aneurysms without Marfan's syndrome or an obvious type III collagen abnormality.

Braunstein [76] emphasized the role of hypertension in dissecting aneurysm and the preceding aortic dilatation both of which would increase the mural tension in the aortic wall. Dilatation of the ascending aorta is common in aortic coarctation, Marfan's syndrome and aortic stenosis. Dissecting aneurysms of the aorta may also be due to giant cell arteritis [77]. They have been associated with prolonged steroid therapy [78] as for systemic lupus erythematosus and generalized fibromuscular dysplasia [79].

Animals fed a lathyrogenic substance or a copper-deficient diet develop dissecting aneurysms similar to those of Marfan's syndrome and there may be some antedecedent aortic dilatation. A lesser quantity of a lathyrogen produces intimal tears, disruption and disappearance of elastic laminae, fibrous proliferation about the tears and fusiform aortic aneurysms [80,81]. Copper deficiency can be even more severe with the aorta exhibiting longitudinal rents in the wall without dissection.

There is a general lack of knowledge of the degenerative changes in the media. Elastic tissue fragmentation and loss is a progressive change that occurs in all subjects at varying rates. It can be produced in the elastic common carotid artery of rabbits following production of a carotid–jugular fistula and the elastic loss can be extreme [82].

Turri *et al.* [83] found 50% of subjects with pure aortic valvular incompetence had aortic root dilatation, a precursor of aortic tears and dissection. The finding that dissecting aneurysms can occur beyond aortic valvular incompetence is further evidence that the dissections are mechanically induced by haemodynamic stress [84] with hypertension and connective tissue diseases being predisposing factors. Even further support is provided by the occurrence of similar mural tears with limited dissection of the wall in the anastomosed veins of experimental arteriovenous fistulae in sheep [85].

Considerable heterogeneity occurs in histopathological and biochemical parameters in control subjects and in those with ectasia of the aortic ring (including Marfan's syndrome). Fibrosis and loss of cellularity increase with fragmentation and loss of elastic tissue. Correlation between the histological and biochemical changes has been found to be strong but correlation with the degree of ectasia and the biochemistry was poor, and it was concluded that the elastin content biochemically was not necessarily indicative of elastin fragmentation [86]. There was, however, considerable overlap with the findings in the control subjects. Such observations do not necessarily reveal the quality and physical characteristics of the elastic laminae.

There is a predisposition to dissecting aneurysm in subjects with aortic valvular stenosis. The dissection commences in the post-stenotic zone complicating a severely ectatic or mild aneurysmal dilatation of the ascending aorta [14,15,87]. Dissecting aneurysm may also commence in the poststenotic region beyond an aortic coarctation suggesting that haemodynamics plays an important role in the pathogenesis. The intimal tears and dissection beyond the stenoses were regarded as non-specific manifestations of post-stenotic haemodynamic stress. It could be further tested by inducing long-term aortic valvular incompetence or aortic valvular stenosis in experimental animals. Intravascular pressure never reaches more than a fraction of the pressure required to tear the aorta experimentally [88]. In most subjects with dissecting aneurysm, being over 40 years of age and usually hypertensive, degenerative changes in the aortic media are universal and Gore [89] regards such degeneration as the *conditio sine qua non* of the disease. The pathogenesis of dissecting aneurysms has been much debated and basic mechanics underlying the dissection have not been explained. The important conclusions to be reached are that:

1. the initial requirements are a loss of tensile strength of the arterial wall sufficient to permit tearing (entry, re-entry and external rupture) as seen in haemodynamic stresses associated with hypertension, post-

stenotic dilatation, aortic valvular incompetence with a water-hammer effect and inherited or acquired connective tissue disorder associated with reduced durability of the mural connective tissues;
2. an appropriate access of a pulsatile stream of blood through the tear to the plane of cleavage;
3. loss of cohesion of the vessel wall as the result of medial degenerative changes [84] (Figure 10.14).

Intimal tears and dissecting aneurysms, though not usually regarded as a manifestation of atherosclerosis, have been considered as such and due to a more rapidly progressive degeneration of the wall than the intimal ulceration, plaque formation and aneurysmal dilatation [84]. Not infrequently there is atherosclerotic aneurysmal dilatation either in the ascending aorta or in the abdominal aorta in association with aortic dissection [90]. In chronic dissecting aneurysms extensive aneurysmal dilatation may involve the outer wall of the false passage or there may be an independent abdominal aortic aneurysm. These subjects usually manifest severe, even fatal vascular disease and its complications at other sites.

Blunt abdominal injuries, most often due to motor vehicle accidents (seat belts or steering wheel injuries), can precipitate dissecting aneurysm in subjects with severely atherosclerotic aortae. The injury fractures, lacerates or disrupts the full thickness of the wall [91].

A few instances of dissection of the aorta in association with cocaine abuse have been reported. In one instance the ascending aorta was dilated and there was concomitant coronary artery dissection. These are usually hypertensive subjects in the fourth or fifth decades [92].

10.2.8 ANEURYSMS OF THE AORTIC SINUSES (OF VALSALVA)

These uncommon aneurysms have been attributed to bacterial endocarditis, syphilis, dissecting aneurysm, atherosclerosis and congenital factors. When not inflammatory they have tended to be regarded as congenital in nature often for want of a better explanation, but these too are frequently complicated by infection which on occasion has been tuberculous. Normally the sinuses bulge slightly and the aneurysms mostly involve the floor (apex or fundus of the sinus) and the cusp. Though classified as congenital when there is no obvious cause, they are probably not present at birth. There is need for a detailed histological study of the sinuses with advancing age and consideration of the stresses to which they are subjected. These aneurysms may be associated with a bicuspid aortic valve and dissecting aneurysm of the aorta. The sinuses can also be incorporated into an aneurysm of the ascending aorta. A recent histological report of four unruptured aneurysms of the non-coronary sinus revealed extensive elastic tissue loss from the aortic wall [93] and Marfan's syndrome can readily predispose to such lesions.

These aneurysms are almost entirely intracardiac as they enlarge. They may extend into the cardiac chambers or encroach on the pulmonary valve, the atrioventricular valve, the conducting bundle or pulmonary and coronary arteries [94,95]. Most involve the right coronary sinus or the right part of the non-coronary sinus and are thought to be due to blood pressure effects on a hypothetical congenital weakness of the wall. The aneurysms are usually single but involvement of three valve sinuses in a man of 81 years was reported as congenital [96]. The sacs which may grow to a considerable size, are usually less than 4 cm in diameter with an oval opening up to 1.5 cm in width. They also lead to aortic valvular incompetence by deforming the aortic ring or rupture into a low-pressure chamber, usually the right atrium, ventricle or the pulmonary artery causing a left-to-right shunt. They may also rupture into the pericardial sac, the pleural cavity or the pulmonary artery.

Ehlers–Danlos syndrome has been reported in association with aortic valvular incompetence and aortic sinus dilatations [97] which suggests that haemodynamics combines with a connective tissue disorder to produce the aneurysms. The lack of aneurysmal involvement of the corresponding sinuses of the pulmonary artery and valve is indicative that haemodynamic stresses play an important role in their pathogenesis.

10.3 Pulmonary artery aneurysms

Non-dissecting aneurysms of the pulmonary trunk or proximal pulmonary arteries are rare as would be expected in a low-pressure circulation. Pulmonary artery aneurysms in the absence of arteriovenous aneurysms were, in the past, attributed to syphilis when involving the trunk or major branches and tuberculosis when involving the branches related to pulmonary fibrocaseous tuberculosis (Rasmussen's aneurysms). These diseases no longer constitute major causes. Congenital heart disease with bacterial endocarditis can lead to mycotic or bacterial aneurysms due to embolic seeding but these too are infrequent. In this age of intravenous drug usage a complicating endocarditis can produce a similar event [98].

Medionecrosis as in the aorta has been incriminated and these structural changes appear to be only an accentuation of naturally occurring degenerative changes particularly likely to occur with hypertension and Marfan's disease. Severe degenerative changes will also occur with an arteriovenous fistula. Isolated cases have been reported. They may be bilateral producing hilar shadows on X-ray [99]. Mostly prolonged pulmonary hypertension will be a predisposing factor and the trunk is the common site. Cardiopulmonary lesions associated with the hypertension are present. Multiple aneurysms have been reported in subjects with persistent recurrent thromboses and probably pulmonary emboli and secondary hypertension [100].

Whilst most cases will be attributed to atherosclerosis or a degenerative change in the arteries, the degree of involvement will not be as pronounced as in the systemic circulation. Congenital defects or an idiopathic classification have been used as explanations of some lesions. Such cases should be referred to an experienced vascular pathologist.

There may be rupture into the mediastinum or a bronchus. Large aneurysms with mural thrombus can be a source of peripheral pulmonary embolism.

Aneurysms may complicate pulmonary valvular stenosis, in which case they are of the post-stenotic variety and may develop a dissecting aneurysm. They can complicate long standing pulmonary hypertension where the underlying disease is atherosclerosis, the pulmonary trunk being most often affected. Peripheral aneurysms, sometimes multiple, may occur but as these are distinctly unusual, a non-degenerative cause should be sought. There is also a need to study the effect of lobectomy and pneumonectomy on the remaining pulmonary arteries and on the pathogenesis of pulmonary aneurysms.

Dissecting aneurysms of the pulmonary artery are rare. Most subjects have pulmonary hypertension and are younger than those with aortic dissection [101]. It also occurs with Marfan's syndrome, pulmonary valvular stenosis, patent ductus arteriosus and congenital heart disease usually with a left-to-right shunt. The features are essentially similar to those in aortic dissection but the degree of dissection is much less. The tears are not necessarily transverse and usually involve the trunk with rupture externally, either the full thickness or partially with variable dissection [102]. The pulmonary trunk may be dilated and haemorrhagic externally with a variable degree of dissection. Healed tears may be found and histologically pronounced degenerative changes are present in the pulmonary trunk and arteries including 'mucoid medial degeneration'. A mural tear with limited dissection in a subject with primary pulmonary hypertension may be the nidus for a substantial mural thrombus *in situ* in the pulmonary trunk.

10.4 Extracranial carotid and vertebral arterial aneurysms

Aneurysmal dilatation may form secondarily in vein patch grafts of the cervical carotid arteries, but aneurysms of these arteries are more often traumatic, bacterial or dissecting in nature. They may follow endarterectomy and angiography. Inadvertent injection into the wall of the carotid artery for angiography has resulted in dissecting aneurysm and arterial occlusion whilst drug usage may initiate an acute arteritis and bacterial aneurysms.

Spontaneous carotid aneurysms in the neck are rare, usually atherosclerotic and can be bilateral. They usually involve the region of the carotid sinus of the internal carotid artery. The internal carotid and common carotid aneurysms are of about equal frequency with the latter usually due to trauma. The external carotid artery is much less frequently involved. Aneurysms of the extracranial segment of the internal carotid artery may present as a firm pulsatile mass protruding internally either into the tonsillar fossa or parapharyngeal region or externally about the angle of the mandible [103]. Some patients present with neurological symptoms and signs and a bruit may be due to an associated stenotic lesion in the neck. Internal bleeding is infrequent. Large sacs containing thrombus can be a source of emboli and transient or more serious ischaemic attacks. They may be simulated by loops or severe kinks complicating extreme tortuosity since they too can appear as firm pulsatile swellings in the neck or parapharyngeal region.

Extreme tortuosity may lead to aneurysmal dilatation of the greater curvature of a bend, probably more likely with a sharp flexure. Fibromuscular dysplasia may predispose to aneurysm formation as can Marfan's syndrome and pseudoxanthoma elasticum. Congenital defects of the wall as an explanation of some aneurysms should be treated with scepticism.

Aneurysms of the extracranial segment of the vertebral arteries are uncommon but usually due to trauma. They may be traumatic, saccular or dissecting aneurysms or arteriovenous fistulae. Iatrogenic lesions have occurred when intra-arterial angiographic injections were made directly into vertebral arteries. The behaviour of such lesions would be similar to those elsewhere but could lead to thrombotic occlusion with propagation of the thrombus.

Spontaneous aneurysm may occur in the presence of Marfan's syndrome, Ehlers–Danlos syndrome or progeria and more recently aneurysms and arteriovenous communications involving vertebral arteries have been reported in association with von Recklinghausen's neurofibromatosis type I [104]. In this there appears to be a milder generalized connective tissue disorder than the above well recognized inherited connective tissue disorders: these subjects are prone to easy bruising, increased skin elasticity and joint mobility in addition to a propensity for aneurysms, arteriovenous fistulae, occlusions and rupture of medium-sized arteries which could be the consequence of trauma. Alternatively, aneurysms may be secondary to occlusion of other arteries or arteriovenous fistulae.

10.5 Aneurysms of the subclavian artery

In subjects with a complete cervical rib, there is an upward extension of the thorax. The subclavian artery then arches high into the base of the neck, being readily palpable above the clavicle. It becomes compressed between the cervical rib and the tendinous attachment of the anterior scalene muscle, possibly accentuated by drooping of the shoulders. Dilatation of the subclavian artery distally then ensues as a post-stenotic phenomenon. Halsted [58] was first to interconnect these two phenomena, providing proof by experimental production of post-stenotic aneurysms.

Neurological symptoms are usually not manifest until early adult life and are caused by traction on the brachial plexus by drooping shoulders, it is thought, if the rib is incomplete. Complete cervical rib is more prone to produce vascular complications with frank aneurysmal dilatation [105]. Mural tears with mural thrombosis develop or an occlusive thrombosis can ensue. Emboli to the hands are frequent. About twenty years elapse between the development of post-stenotic dilatation and the complications of frank aneurysmal dilatation. This supports the hypothesis that:

1. the poststenotic dilatation progresses to aneurysm formation with persistence of these same haemodynamic stresses;
2. thrombosis is the consequence of mural weakness and tearing.

Removal of the cervical rib results in no angiographic change in the mild post-stenotic dilatation even after nine years. This suggests that the haemodynamic stresses associated with a mild post-stenotic dilatation are probably less severe on the wall than if the constriction had not been relieved. However, longer follow-up is desirable. Frankly atherosclerotic aneurysms of the first portion of the subclavian artery are decidedly rare though more likely in elderly hypertensive subjects. The aneurysm has also been attributed to medionecrosis [106] but this is merely severe degenerative change in the media.

The aneurysms are fusiform in shape and mural calcification may be visible radiologically. If of any size, rupture may occur into the pleural cavity, mediastinum, cervical tissues and even into the oesophagus or trachea. Thromboembolic phenomena are frequent as indicated.

Aneurysmal dilatation of the origin of an aberrant right subclavian artery which takes origin from the descending aspect of the aortic arch, passes behind the oesophagus which it displaces anteriorly and often obstructs [107]. It may be mistaken for an aortic arch or innominate artery aneurysm and is usually atherosclerotic. It can co-exist with an aortic aneurysm [108].

Aneurysm of the left subclavian artery may be involved in coarctation and dissecting aneurysms of the aorta. Bacterial aneurysms are rare.

10.6 Aneurysms of the iliac and femoral arteries

Atherosclerotic aneurysms of the common iliac artery are of frequent occurrence as they so often accompany abdominal aortic aneurysms (Figures 10.4 and 10.6), which, being proximal and larger, are more likely to be symptomatic. It is for this reason that bifurcation grafts are so commonly used. The iliac arteries are often ectatic, tortuous, aneurysmal and grossly displaced with considerable alteration in the aortic angle of bifurcation. They are often multiple and rarely enlarge to a massive size without an aortic aneurysm. Markowitz and Norman [109] said there was a small group of women who during or after pregnancy developed iliac artery aneurysms but such instances must be rare. These aneurysms could rupture into the bowel especially in the presence of diverticulitis raising the possibility of an infectious origin.

Atherosclerotic aneurysms of the femoral arteries are even more infrequent than isolated iliac artery lesions. However, apart from bacterial aneurysms due to local or haematogenous spread and inherited connective tissue disorders, traumatic aneurysms can occur and especially those associated with a traumatic arteriovenous fistula which often involves the upper thigh. The aneurysmal dilatation even postoperatively may extend back to the aorta.

The recent observations of Vollmar et al. [54] on the haemodynamic induction of aortic aneurysms in leg amputees also included undue dilatation of the iliofemoral arteries on the patent side (Figure 10.9) and this imbalance of blood flow into the two limbs due to ligation or pathological stenoses could and does predispose to iliofemoral aneurysms.

False aneurysms of the femoral arteries in drug addicts due to repeated femoral arterial injections with or without infection pose a new medical and social problem [110].

10.7 Popliteal aneurysms

Aneurysms of the popliteal artery are infrequent and most often due to atherosclerosis. Some may be traumatic and others mycotic. In view of the frequency of arteriovenous communications in association with varicose veins, popliteal aneurysms may be associated with such cryptic shunts. They are more frequent in males than females and most are in the sixth and seventh decades. More than half of the subjects have hypertension [111]. Diabetes mellitus and coronary heart disease are frequent.

The aneurysms are usually fusiform in shape developing over a considerable length of the artery and commencing as a localized zone of ectasia which progressively expands. They are frequently bilateral (up to 45%) [112] and often associated with aneurysms proximally.

Localization of aneurysms to this site has been attributed to excessive bending and extension of the knee in cavalry officers due to prolonged horse riding and in previous years in postboys due to bicycle riding. When the knee is acutely flexed the popliteal artery is almost bent back on itself and severe disturbance of flow would be expected. Recent experimental evidence indicates extensive tears and fragmentation of the internal elastic develop within days in U-shaped bends fashioned in elastic arteries and are eventually followed by severe mural atrophy [113,114]. In chronic experiments intimal proliferation with lipid deposition occurs beyond the lesser curvature until eventually intimal proliferation with lipid deposition also involves the greater curvature. Progression of these changes can lead to aneurysmal dilatation. Aneurysms are, however, far from common at the elbows but the arteries are smaller. Whether or not the pulse pressure is also higher as it is in the iliofemoral arteries is uncertain.

Gedge et al. [115] attributed popliteal aneurysms to a post-stenotic phenomenon, the artery being constricted either where it passes through the hiatus of the adductor magnus tendon or distal to the arcuate ligament uniting the head of the fibula with the posterior ligaments of the knee joint. This may well be a contributing factor but the actual constriction must be demonstrated and the possibility exists that relative constriction and a post-stenotic effect may be secondary to ectasia which would be inhibited by the adductor magnus tendon and arcuate ligament.

Most aneurysms arise distal to the adductor foramen though some involve the femoral artery and many also involve branches of the popliteal artery [116]. In recent years attention has been drawn to the popliteal artery entrapment syndrome in which the artery runs medially around or through the medial head of the gastrocnemius muscle, or the artery in its normal location is crossed dorsally by a lateral insertion of the medial head of that muscle. Variations exist but the end result can be intermittent ischaemia and claudication even in young athletes [117]. Post-stenotic aneurysms are considered to be frequent accompaniments of these anatomical variations [118].

Mural thrombosis is common within the aneurysm and the blood may take a tortuous course through the thrombus. The thrombotic walls of this passage can provide a rich source of emboli to the leg and foot. These aneurysms can rupture and by further expansion cause erosion of the popliteal surface of the femur, pressure on the posterior tibial nerve, and if large enough, produce a generalized pressure effect in the popliteal fossa resulting in impaired venous return and oedema. They can also cause ischemia of the leg and foot due to thrombosis of the popliteal artery and multiple emboli leading to eventual amputation possibly obviated by early grafting.

10.8 Aneurysms of the splanchnic arteries

Aneurysms are found on the splanchnic arteries supplying the viscera of the thorax and abdomen. Their rarity is evidenced by the infrequency of spontaneous haemorrhage in the thorax and abdomen (abdominal apoplexy) after excluding aneurysms of the aorta and cardiac rupture. However, their prevalence clinically is increasing with improved diagnostic techniques and selective arteriography. Hypertension plays a prominent role [119].

Trauma may be responsible in rare instances but the vessels are so deep-seated that penetrating wounds would be required. Septic emboli associated with bacterial endocarditis is more common. Other varieties of non-infectious arteritis may so disrupt the arterial wall that aneurysmal dilatation will follow and haemorrhage may occur. Splanchnic arteries are highly susceptible to polyarteritis nodosa and the small calibre of the involved arteries is such that thrombosis with minor infections is more likely than serious haemorrhage.

Syphilis must have been a rare cause of splanchnic aneurysms. Positive serological tests for syphilis do not make the aneurysm luetic and verification of their authenticity is now not possible, nor are they likely to be encountered.

Aneurysms of the splanchnic vessels can complicate fibromuscular dysplasia, which is probably overdiagnosed. The associated hypertension and the post-stenotic effect could contribute to aneurysm formation but a connective tissue disorder should be excluded in this disease. Most aneurysms are degenerative in nature with incidence likely to increase in aging populations.

Dissecting aneurysms occur from time to time but are rare. The dissection will be near the outer media or clearly between the media and adventitia. Little information is available regarding the nature of the initial tear, but recent experimental work indicates that under certain conditions profound destruction of the elastic tissue even to the adventitia can be induced haemodynamically.

Whenever an unexplained aneurysm occurs especially in a young subject, the possibility of an infectious origin, an associated arteriovenous shunt or a connective tissue disorder, particularly if the aneurysms are numerous, must be considered. In the past, unexplained aneurysms, especially in young subjects, were assumed to be congenital in nature but such facile assumptions without evidence are inappropriate in science.

10.8.1 CORONARY ARTERY ANEURYSM

Whilst progressive increase in the diameter of the coronary arteries occurs with age, abnormal dilatations, whether ectasia or aneurysmal, are rare. In 30 patients with coronary arterial ectasia detected by angiography, sometimes the irregular and diffuse dilatation of one or more vessels was found to be up to seven times the branch diameter, dilatation being most pronounced in the proximal segments. The arteries were usually severely atherosclerotic, with calcification. The subjects did not differ significantly from other subjects with obstructive coronary disease in sex, age, prevalence of angina, metabolic disorders or short-term prognosis [120,121]. A later study of 978 subjects with coronary artery aneurysms revealed that they did not form a distinct group from those with severe atherosclerosis [122] which is likely, therefore, to be a cause of their lesions. Long-term prognosis is poor with the likelihood of myocardial infarction, although rupture of an aneurysm is another possibility [120].

Most coronary aneurysms are atherosclerotic being either fusiform or saccular. Males are more commonly affected than females. There is frequently tortuosity and ectasia and if these are pronounced, especially if other systemic arteries have aneurysms, a connective tissue disorder or vascular shunt should be excluded. Multiplicity is common and concomitant aneurysms of the aorta are frequent. Daoud et al. [123] reviewed 89 cases in 1963, but they are being encountered more frequently with use of angiography. Most of their aneurysms were atherosclerotic and a congenital origin was alleged in 18% even though almost half the subjects were aged between 60 and 85 years.

Berry type aneurysms occur in the splanchnic arteries including the coronary circulation but are distinctly rare. It is reasonable to assume that the haemodynamic mechanisms responsible for those in the cerebral circulation are also responsible for those in the splanchnic circulation. The difference in frequency is due to the architectural differences between cerebral and extra-cranial arteries.

Some aneurysms become quite large (6 cm) [124]. Diffuse ectasia with aneurysmal enlargement, as in Figure 10.15, can be atherosclerotic but connective tissue disorders and a vascular shunt should be excluded. Those associated with a bruit and extreme tortuosity are likely to be associated with an arteriovenous shunt. A woman with Osler–Weber–Rendu disease with two large pulmonary arteriovenous fistulae, a basilar aneurysm and pontine telangiectasia had left coronary artery ectasia and aneurysm [126]. The combination is unusual and raises the question of whether there was also a cardiac arteriovenous shunt.

When a coronary artery communicates with a cardiac chamber, the pulmonary arterial trunk or vein,

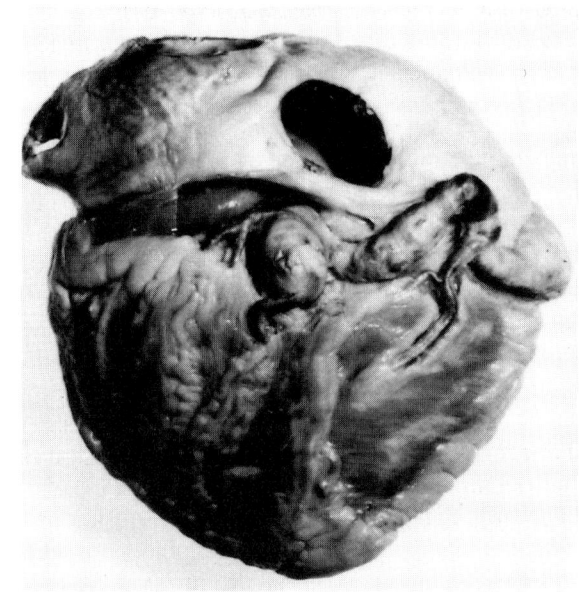

Figure 10.15 Diffuse ectasia and aneurysmal dilatation of a coronary artery such as this can be atherosclerotic but connective tissue disorders and a vascular shunt require exclusion. (Reproduced with permission from Daoud et al. [123].)

there is grossly increased blood flow as in the case of an arteriovenous shunt, which also induces premature severe atherosclerosis [10]. The mural atrophy that would occur could readily lead to aneurysms even in young subjects and a congenital aetiology could be invoked incorrectly. Such could be the reason for an accompanying bruit.

Coronary artery aneurysms can rupture, irrespective of their cause, and produce haemopericardium and cardiac tamponade although its development would be slower. Alternatively it is common for these aneurysms to be incidental findings at autopsy with death resulting from other cardiovascular lesions, including a ruptured aortic aneurysm [123]. Infective and dissecting aneurysms are dealt with in sections 10.12 and 10.14 respectively.

Dissecting aneurysm of the coronary arteries is rare and is most often found in the anterior descending branch of the left coronary. Dissection of the wall occurs deep in the media or external to the media and has been linked with pregnancy [127] and the use of contraceptive pills. There has been difficulty in understanding the nature of these lesions in the absence of trauma or a connective tissue disorder but ultimately they must be due to loss of tensile strength consequent upon degeneration of the mural connective tissues. Hypertension is not a prominent factor and a few cases are due to Marfan's syndrome.

Coronary venous bypass grafts constitute a different entity, because the transplanted veins are more susceptible to atherosclerosis and therefore develop accelerated severe atherosclerosis due to the augmented haemodynamic stresses of arterial flow for which they are not architecturally designed. A number of grafts develop aneurysms [128] and iatrogenic aneurysms complicate angioplasty [129].

10.8.2 SPLENIC ARTERY ANEURYSMS

The splenic artery has a long unbranched course in loose areolar tissue along the upper border of the pancreas and is noted for its remarkable tortuosity and the severity of atherosclerosis. These facts point to a peculiarity of the splenic circulation such that the augmented haemodynamic stresses account for the severe atherosclerosis and tortuosity of the trunk. Splenic artery aneurysms make up about 58% of all splanchnic artery aneurysms [130,131] and mostly involve the main trunk, although some occur in the hilum. Any berry aneurysm should be considered as an acquired lesion. Splenic aneurysms are more frequent in females and may reach giant proportions. They occur mostly in the distal part of the artery. Most are atherosclerotic and the tortuosity may contribute to aneurysm formation as in the carotid siphon.

Rupture of splenic aneurysms has often been reported during pregnancy and a particular propensity for rupture during gestation has been reported repeatedly. Pregnancy imposes additional stresses on the circulation especially during labour quite apart from possible hormonal influences. Splenic artery aneurysms are unduly frequent in hepatic cirrhosis, portal hypertension and splenomegaly. Increased splenic arterial blood flow and arteriectasis would be contributing factors in their pathogenesis [131]. There is a remarkably high incidence of splenic aneurysms in liver transplant recipients and they have a strong propensity for rupture [132,133].

The aneurysms may be multiple and found on the convexities of the tortuosities. They have also been reported in association with cerebral and aortic aneurysms, fibromuscular dysplasia [130,134], Marfan's disease [130], bacterial endocarditis and arteritis.

Dissecting aneurysm of the splenic artery is rare [135] and as in other extracranial medium-sized arteries, the dissection is close to the adventitia. The mortality is high as it is for ruptured saccular or fusiform splenic aneurysms.

10.8.3 RENAL ARTERY ANEURYSMS

Non-traumatic and non-inflammatory renal aneurysms are of several types. Atherosclerotic stenosis of the origin of the renal artery is not only a cause of hypertension but can be associated with a post-stenotic aneurysm of the main artery. Fibromuscular dysplasia in younger subjects affecting the renal artery may also cause a post-stenotic aneurysm with medial destruction and the associated haemorrhage aggravating the situation. Most renal aneurysms are saccular and few will be post-stenotic in type, although fibromuscular dysplasia has been recorded in about 50% of subjects [136].

Stanley et al. [136] reported that 75% of saccular aneurysms occurred at primary or secondary renal artery bifurcations. Berry aneurysms also involve the renal artery bifurcation being more likely to be found incidentally at autopsy or on angiography but they are known to rupture. Schwartz and White [137] found 15 subjects with saccular aneurysms of the renal arteries in 154 unselected autopsies. They were mostly berry aneurysms and multiple in five subjects. This high incidence has not been confirmed, small aneurysms being so easily overlooked at autopsy.

Rupture is rare. Calcified renal aneurysms are thought to have a low rate of rupture [138]. Hypertension has been reported as unduly frequent in association with renal arterial aneurysms and the thrombus within the sac has been assumed to be responsible for secondary renal hypertension [139], possibly the result of recurrent embolism. Alternatively the hypertension is primary and predisposes to aneurysmal dilatation.

The pathological changes in the renal arteries following unilateral nephrectomy in humans and experimental aneurysms would be of interest to determine the effect of augmented physiological flow on the major bifurcations and arterioles. Aneurysms have been reported in solitary hypertrophied kidneys [140,141]. Rupture of an aneurysm in a transplanted kidney during pregnancy is on record [142]. Renal artery aneurysms also develop in the presence of Ehlers–Danlos syndrome and proximal to arteriovenous communication in the kidney [143].

10.8.4 MISCELLANEOUS SPLANCHNIC ANEURYSMS

Non-inflammatory aneurysms are rare in other splanchnic vessels, atherosclerotic and berry aneurysms [144] being the two main types encountered. Causes of these aneurysms are similar to those of other splanchnic arteries. Their true frequency is difficult to estimate and unruptured aneurysms are overlooked at autopsy unless sought in a deliberate, methodical manner.

Hepatic aneurysms may rupture into the biliary tract with melaena and jaundice or into the peritoneal cavity. Aneurysms of the coeliac, gastric, gastroepiploic, pancreaticoduodenal, mesenteric, jejunal, iliac and colic arteries occur but only complications will indicate their presence. Rupture is the likely complication and results in haemorrhage into a viscus, the peritoneal cavity or retroperitoneum. Recurrent silent leakage into a viscus is a cause of severe anaemia and the aneurysms may be multiple [144].

Occasionally a dissecting aneurysm occurs and may be misdiagnosed if it is found at autopsy. Bacterial aneurysms occur sporadically but are unlikely to be discovered unless they cause symptoms. The presence of a bruit is more suggestive of an arteriovenous shunt than an aneurysm which can, however, be secondary to the shunt.

10.8.5 UMBILICAL ARTERY ANEURYSMS

Aneurysms of the umbilical arteries occur very infrequently. One instance involved a fetus with no other abnormality except a single umbilical artery and cardiomegaly. The patent aneurysm was 4.6 cm in its largest dimension with medial thinning, intimal calcification and much mural thrombosis. Death at 36 weeks *in utero* was attributed to asphyxia caused by compression of the umbilical vein and the cardiomegaly may have been due to hypertension. These aneurysms are consistent with the contention that the histological features of the umbilical artery including paucity of elastic tissue represent degenerative changes in this age group. Another fetus with a fusiform aneurysm but with two umbilical arteries died of hypoxia due to compression of the umbilical vein and the other artery within the confined space of the cord [145].

10.9 Complications of aneurysms

Not only is the aneurysmal dilatation indicative of a pathological weakness of the arterial wall but so is its progressive enlargement and eventual rupture. These are of course offset by physiological attempts at reparative thickening and reinforcement of the wall.

10.9.1 RUPTURE OF ANEURYSMS

The evidence available is that aneurysms enlarge relentlessly until complications occur. The rate of enlargement varies, as is seen even in the behaviour of experimental autogenous vein graft aneurysms in sheep. Individual haemodynamics and biochemistry account for differences in progression. The rate of growth is probably slower than was once believed and can only be determined after detailed, long-term observation of the natural history and by monitoring the size of many aneurysms by non-invasive means.

Spontaneous rupture is the most common and most feared of all complications. Characteristically there are premonitory leaks prior to severe, if not fatal haemorrhage. Apart from augmented pulsatility these warning leaks provide the primary means of clinical diagnosis. When rupture occurs all anatomical structures in the neighbourhood may be involved. However, minor leaks due to yielding of the sac wall will initiate thrombosis which may be followed by organization and endothelialization. With continued enlargement of the sac and increasing tension on the wall, progressive yielding of the wall may lead to recurrent tearing and leakage or fatal bleeding. Secondary nodules as seen in cerebral aneurysms have been demonstrated to be false sacs following leakage. Such secondary dilatations may rupture before they can be reinforced.

Enlargement of the sac is not always uniform. There is a tendency to form a spherical sac, but probably this occurs mostly where the flux of blood impacts on the sac wall. Consequently older areas of the aneurysm containing laminated thrombus may become pushed backwards from the basal attachment thus initiating the development of unusually shaped aneurysms.

Lipid accumulation with cholesterol clefts may occur in the outer parts of the thrombus with at times some mineralization. These phenomena are seen mostly in the sac wall of enlarging aneurysms. The walls are relatively acellular with vasa vasorum about the outer surface together with perivascular round cell infiltration and siderophages.

Haemorrhage from ruptured aneurysms may be rapidly fatal with extravasation of blood into the loose surrounding tissues or into a body cavity, viscus, vein or through the skin with a fatal deluge. Some aneurysms are less likely to rupture than others, and generally the size of the sac is an important criterion. No doubt the critical size is related to the ratio of the largest dimension to the calibre of the vessel and possibly the area of attachment. Of large aortic aneurysms (7–12 cm in their largest diameter) 82% had ruptured compared to only 4% of those measuring 3–6 cm [146]. The rate of development seems to be an important factor particularly if symptoms are present.

Harrow and Sloane [138] reported that rupture had not occurred in 69 radiologically calcified saccular aneurysms of the renal artery, whereas 24 of 100 non-calcified renal aneurysms had ruptured. They suggested that mural calcification was protective. This may be so but their review of splenic aneurysms was inconclusive. Radiologically calcified cerebral aneurysms are considered unlikely to rupture but they usually exhibit little calcification which in aortic aneurysms does not ensure safety from fatal rupture.

Hypertension is generally regarded as an aggravating factor which on theoretical grounds is difficult to deny. An increase in pressure due to physical effort, lifting, etc., as with cerebral aneurysms, may precipitate rupture of an already weakened wall. Likewise mild or severe trauma may precipitate rupture although the injury may be fortuitous. Little is known of the stress and strain to which blood vessels may be subjected at the moment of impact but since blunt injuries can at times lacerate arteries, the tearing of an aneurysm wall is certainly conceivable with otherwise non-fatal injuries.

(a) Pregnancy

Aneurysmal rupture of small peripheral arteries has long been considered to occur with undue frequency during pregnancy mostly in the third trimester. Isolated cases are often reported and rupture of cerebral aneurysms and subarachnoid haemorrhage have been considered likely to be adversely affected by the haemodynamic changes of pregnancy. The stress of labour is not the precipitating factor since the maximum incidence occurs between the 26th and 36th weeks [146,147] and the mortality is not significantly different from that of the non-gravid state. The mean age of the women so affected is 30 years [147], which is 20 years less than for aneurysms at autopsy in a general hospital [7]. There is no detailed statistical analysis of the evidence to prove conclusively one way or the other, the review by Barrett et al. [148] being non-committal. The effect of multiple pregnancies has not been studied.

Barrett et al. [148] concluded that the great majority of pregnancy-related ruptures of aortic aneurysms have been dissecting in type. There appears to be an increase with age but not necessarily with parity and about 50% are hypertensive. The usual predisposing disorders (aortic coarctation, Marfan's syndrome, aortic valvular disease) are seen in these patients and many have electrocardiographic evidence of myocardial ischaemia [148]. The prognosis of aortic dissecting aneurysm in pregnancy is poor.

Rupture of splenic artery aneurysms exhibits a propensity for females and it is generally considered that rupture during pregnancy is not fortuitous [149]. It was estimated some years ago that of all recorded cases, 11% occurred in pregnant women [150]. More recently Barrett et al. [148] emphasized the rarity of non-inflammatory aneurysms in women of child-bearing age, yet half of all ruptured arterial aneurysms in women under 40 years of age are pregnancy-related. Up to 20% of all ruptured splenic artery aneurysms occur in pregnancy and 69% rupture in the third trimester, 12% in the first two trimesters, 13% in labour and 6% in the puerperium. Multiparous women are said to be particularly prone to splenic aneurysm rupture [148,149]. Unfortunately these aneurysms are silent until rupture and perhaps mild abdominal symptoms are overlooked or misdiagnosed during pregnancy. The result is enhanced mortality for both mother (64%) and fetus (72.2%) [151].

Saccular aneurysms of the renal artery are said to be prone to rupture during pregnancy [138,150] but satisfactory statistical analysis is lacking. Literature reviews of selective case reporting provide false statistics. In pregnancy-related coronary artery aneurysms, all were dissecting aneurysms involving the left anterior descending coronary artery and most were postpartum [148]. Pregnancy-related rupture of four cases of ovarian artery aneurysm and a predisposition of multiparous women for ovarian artery aneurysms has been alleged [148]. These aneurysms are too infrequent to provide reliable statistics and the same may be said for aneurysms of uterine arteries and other rare splanchnic arterial aneurysms.

Currently, hormonal effects on the cellular and non-cellular connective tissues of blood vessels are uncertain but indirect evidence would suggest a strong possibility of some influence:

1. There is a predominance of cerebral and splenic aneurysms in females.
2. There is a tendency for vascular disturbances to occur during pregnancy (varices, cutaneous spider naevi, relapse and remission of symptoms related to spinal angiomas).
3. There is a recognized effect of pregnancy on pelvic connective tissues.
4. There is the influence of menstruation or aneurysmal headache and spontaneous bleeding in the Ehlers–Danlos syndrome.
5. There is lesser development of reparative intimal proliferation in females [152].
6. There is impaired reparative growth of connective tissues under the influence of steroids [84]. It is also possible that steroids could affect the tensile strength of vascular connective tissue since antiovulatory progestogens induce aortic rupture in hamsters [153].

(b) Haemodynamic stress

Ample experimental evidence has accumulated to indicate that haemodynamic stresses can be responsible for ectasia, post-stenotic dilatation, dissecting aneurysm, berry aneurysms and gross mural atrophy. These changes are associated with severe elastic destruction and loss, muscle degeneration and collagen changes, all of which must adversely affect the tensile strength of the vessel wall. The haemodynamics of aneurysm has been discussed elsewhere [84] but experimental venous-graft aneurysms develop accelerated atherosclerosis and may progress to rupture. More interesting is the observation that collagen fibrils in the aneurysmal wall undergo shape changes indicative of fibril degeneration [154]. These changes have in the past been associated with hereditary connective tissue disorders and loss of tensile strength of collagen. The findings together with elastic tissue depletion are likely to be morphological manifestations of loss of tensile strength of the wall and could help explain the progressive dilatation and ultimate rupture of the aneurysms. Further enlargement accentuates the haemodynamic stresses and the vicious cycle may then lead to recurrent haemorrhage. Rupture leads to the formation of a false sac or the aneurysm may become occluded by thrombus which will become organized and replaced by fibrous tissue. It too may stretch and tear again.

(c) Progressive enlargement and thrombosis

Rupture of an aneurysm usually occurs at the fundus or at the site of the jet lesion and thrombus is initially deposited at the site of leakage. Formation of the characteristic laminated thrombus in an aneurysm requires recurrent intermittent yielding of the wall and the deposition of new layers of thrombus. This deposition must occur on the outer side rather than on the inner surface because old layers of thrombus do not appear to stretch with the wall and when leakage occurs, it does so deep to the laminated thrombus. There is no evidence that it burrows through laminated thrombus. Moreover, there is usually little effective organization of the thrombus. Further reinforcement of the wall must occur before organization can be completed. The thrombus when chronic no doubt becomes inspissated, inelastic and possibly shrinks. These factors in combination seem to result in dissection between the sac wall and the thrombus with either rupture or deposition of another layer and successive layers of clot or thrombus. The pathogenesis of this laminated thrombus requires *in vivo* confirmation.

The above relentless cycle leading to enlargement results in pressure effects, both local and general. For an aneurysm at any site local pressure effects on the surrounding anatomical sites must be considered. Organization of blood and fibrin may result in adhesion of the sac wall to adjoining anatomical structures which may be affected by the pulsatile mural stresses resulting in fibrosis and impaired function quite apart from direct pressure. The typical erosion of vertebral bodies and the lesser effect on the intervertebral discs are well known. The erosion of the skin or walls of viscera is not due merely to pressure and displacement with the blood bursting through the skin by force. It must also be due to a weakening of the surrounding fibrous tissues. This is seen well in the rupture of a varicose vein through the skin in the absence of trauma. Such phenomena are more consistent with a vibrational effect on the tissues than shear stresses or pressure effects.

General pressure effects occur when an enlarging aneurysmal sac lies within a relatively confined space leading to increased pressure such as within the skull, spinal canal, pelvis, popliteal fossa or even the umbilical cord. The aneurysm in effect acts as a space-occupying lesion producing generalized pressure effects.

(d) Mural thrombosis and organization

An explanation for the limited organization of mural thrombus over some years despite slow relentless growth has been offered. It would appear that the presence of the laminated thrombus within the sac does not reduce the tension in the sac wall nor protect it from the haemodynamic vibrational stresses induced at the entrance and in its functional lumen. It is possible that vibrational stress may impair repair processes but there is need for further information on the propagation and dampening of the vibrations in the thrombus and connective tissues.

It has been maintained that there is retrograde propagation of the thrombus from the sac to the parent vessel but it is difficult to conceive of this happening very often in a saccular aneurysm. It is more likely to occur in a small vessel aneurysm such as those of Charcot and Bouchard or in small false aneurysms of leptomeningeal vessels. Those that thrombose and occlude the parent artery may not all be saccular. Occasionally thrombus within a large fusiform abdominal aortic aneurysm may thrombose but this probably results when much thrombus within the sac is not firm and laminated (Figure 10.6). The flow channel has a circuitous route through recently formed soft friable red thrombus which can lead to embolism distally but a large embolus can occlude the aneurysm or a common iliac artery.

A very rare event is the organization of a berry aneurysm found incidentally at autopsy several years after a subarachnoid haemorrhage (Figure 10.16). Whilst these events are infrequent, there was still a small diverticulum in the neck of the aneurysm. This may have

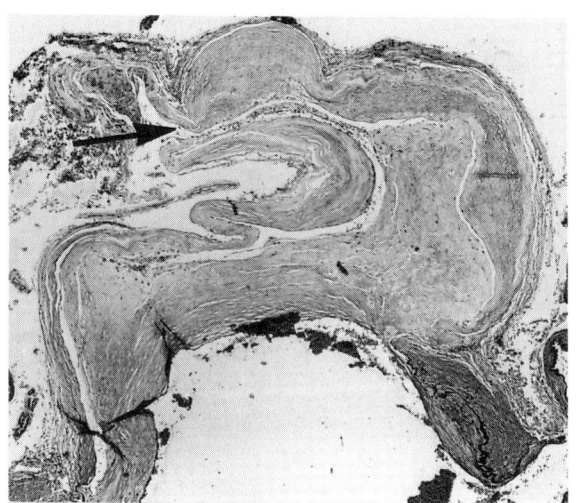

Figure 10.16 Cerebral berry aneurysm thought to have ruptured 44 years before. Sac is collapsed and site of old rupture is indicated by an arrow. The sac wall can still be recognized. Lumen is filled with acellular hyaline tissue, the result of organization of thrombus. Siderophages were present in the adventitia about the rupture site. A small residual lumen is present below. (Verhoeff's elastic stain and eosin.) (Reproduced with permission from Stehbens [204].)

been dormant but as there was no evidence of enlargement, it could well be classified as an example of self-cure [7].

Ligation of the cervical segment of the internal carotid artery was once a common form of therapy for ruptured cerebral aneurysms. Initially when such ligation was customary, the pulse and systolic pressures were dampened. It is known that in some instances the aneurysm seals itself off but grows only to present years later as a large space-occupying lesion. The possibility also exists that ligation may have precipitated a further aneurysm elsewhere in the cerebral circulaion or caused a contralateral second aneurysm to rupture [155].

Embolism from an aneurysm is well recognized with subclavian, popliteal and aortic poststenotic aneurysms. It is seemingly more common than is generally recognized in the case of large aortic aneurysms. More recently berry aneurysms in the cerebral circulation have been incriminated in some transient ischaemic attacks.

(e) Infections

Superadded infection may occur in aneurysms on rare occasions. It has been reported in abdominal aortic aneurysms following bacteraemia but must be very rare in small vessels. An important function of platelets is their ability to adhere to foreign surfaces, including some bacteria which they can sequestrate in platelet–leucocyte thrombi [156]. They may adhere to mural thrombi in aneurysmal sacs where the larger surface available in aortic aneurysms reflects the greater frequency of this event in aortic aneurysms. The possibility also exists that a similar pathogenetic infective process may involve an ulcerated atherosclerotic lesion in the abdominal aorta causing an infective aneurysm. The organisms incriminated have been both haemolytic and non-haemolytic streptococci, *Staphylococcus aureus*, *Salmonella*, *Streptococcus pneumoniae* and gram-negative bacteria including *Escherichia coli*.

Secondary infection of the thrombus would augment embolism and enhance septicaemia and the possibility of endocarditis. It could spread to the adjacent arterial wall, perianeurysmal tissues and precipitate rupture. The possibility of a fungal infection in an immunosuppressed subject following cardiovascular surgery and renal or cardiac transplantation is real.

10.10 Aneurysms of the cerebral circulation

Abnormal arterial dilatations more commonly involve the cerebral arteries than other vessels of similar calibre doubtless due to the unique structure of these vessels. A branch of neurosurgery has developed during the last forty years concerned with their management and much new knowledge of their aetiology and pathogenesis has evolved.

10.10.1 ARTERIECTASIS

After physical maturation has been attained the cerebral arteries are known to continue increasing in girth with age. This ectasia is likely to be greater in larger arteries than in smaller vessels, thereby augmenting differences in calibre that may exist early in life. However, arteriectasis is applied to large cerebral arteries which have enlarged relatively uniformly beyond the size normally seen at autopsy. Severe atherosclerosis is usually present and associated tortuosity is likely. Vertebral and basilar arteries are commonly affected. Since the two vertebral arteries are generally unequal in calibre, the larger vertebral often forms an S-shaped tortuosity with the basilar artery and since the walls are firm and sclerotic, the displaced arterial segments may produce pressure symptoms by compressing cranial nerves overlying the pons and medulla. A more extreme degree of this ectatic state is a cylindroid aneurysm usually affecting the vertebrobasilar arteries, sometimes with extreme tortuosity. Dome-shaped or saccular aneurysms may be superimposed on these atherosclerotic vessels (Figure 10.17).

Arteriectasis also affects the fourth or terminal segment of the internal carotid artery although angiographically there appears to be some proportional diminution in the size of the segment, possibly because the cavernous segment becomes ectatic more readily due to the effect of the curvatures or flexures of the cavernous sinus. However, ectasia of the terminal segment

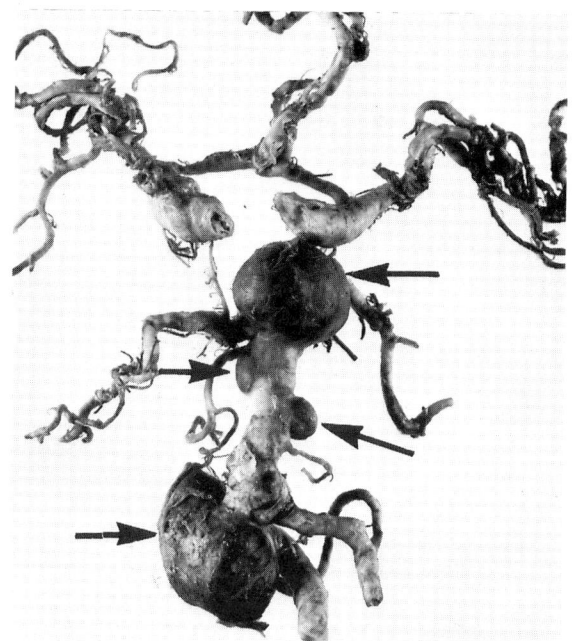

Figure 10.17 Circle of Willis with severe atherosclerosis and ectasia of the vertebral and basilar arteries. Two large saccular aneurysms and two sessile aneurysms are indicated by arrows. Note the voluminous internal carotid arteries.

merges with fusiform aneurysmal dilatation of this segment at times with considerable thinning of the wall.

Dolichoectasia (dolichomega artery) is a term infrequently used for grossly elongated and ectatic vertebral and basilar arteries. The degree of dilatation is more than that customarily seen in cerebral arteries and verges on diffuse aneurysmal dilatation. These dilatations are merely due to advanced atherosclerosis with diffuse ectasia. A wide external diameter may suggest severe ectasia although the lumen may exhibit stenoses. The condition is associated with a high incidence of abdominal aortic aneurysm [157].

10.10.2 CAROTID ANEURYSMS OF THE CAVERNOUS SEGMENT

This rare aneurysm occurs mostly in females [7]. It has to be of considerable size before it becomes obvious being more readily detected in the earlier stages of development by angiography which reveals progression from ectasia to a serpentine or fusiform dilatation of the artery and then a diffuse expansion of the greater curvature of the distal flexure of the carotid sinus. It can also involve the horizontal segment [158]. Though rarely of any consequential size, it can expand and become more spherical presenting at autopsy as a globoid mass or saccular aneurysm to the one side or both sides of the pituitary fossa if bilateral. By enlargement, such aneurysms take up progressively more of the middle cranial fossa, stripping up the dura mater as they slowly grow. They can become massive with calcification of the wall and erosion of the skull. In a youth of 16 years, White and Adams [159] recorded a large aneurysm that expanded distally to involve the intracranial segment of the internal carotid and middle cerebral artery. These aneurysms have been classified into three groups according to whether they cause pressure symptoms in the anterior, middle or posterior zones of the cavernous sinus [160]. Pressure effects on the pituitary gland may develop. Rupture is infrequent but a cause of spontaneous carotid cavernous arteriovenous fistulae, an event occurring predominantly in females and in every decade though mostly from the third to the ninth. The cavernous sinus can be obliterated and rupture may occur into the cranial cavity with subarachnoid haemorrhage, or into the temporal lobe, although this is rare. It can bulge into the sphenoid sinus and cause epistaxis. Ligation of one carotid artery in the neck in a subject with bilateral cavernous aneurysms resulted in a contralateral carotid cavernous fistula possibly precipitated by the increased haemodynamic stress consequent upon augmented flow in the contralateral vessel [161].

There has been much conjecture regarding the aetiology of these aneurysms ranging from the perpetual reiteration of hypothetical congenital weaknesses to the persistence of a primitive trigeminal artery aneurysm; nor is there evidence that they are related to the origin of vestigial branches of the cavernous segment of the internal carotid artery. Their mode of development can be explained on the basis of recent experimental evidence. In experimentally fashioned U-bends in the common carotid artery, sharp flexures such as can occur in the carotid sinus and appear to become more acute with age, can be associated with greatly augmented pulsatility of the greater curvature [113,114]. In this area transversely orientated tears of the internal elastic lamina develop within days and progressively the muscle and elastic tissue disappear resulting in thin fibrous tissue with endothelium and a few elastic remnants. This mural atrophy is known to be the forerunner of aneurysmal dilatation and is the explanation of the pathogenesis of these aneurysms. However, compensatory intimal proliferation may be superimposed on the atrophic changes and aneurysmal dilatation is not inevitable. The possibility of its development is enhanced by hypertension or a connective tissue disorder associated with reduced endurance, augmented flow due to an arteriovenous shunt and a very acute carotid flexure for whatever reason. These aggravating factors explain the wide variation in age. For example, very large diffuse bilateral aneurysmal dilatations of the petrous and intracavernous segments of the internal carotid artery in children under 10 years of age are most unusual [162,163] and indicate the possibility of an underlying connective tissue disorder. It is inappropriate to assume they are congenital without evidence. Aneurysms of these segments of the internal carotid artery also occur in older individuals. They are often mistaken for glomus tumours and many are due to erosive middle ear, pharyngeal or tonsillar infection, mastoid surgery, skull fractures or other trauma. Some are distinctly atherosclerotic.

10.10.3 FUSIFORM ANEURYSM

Fusiform aneurysms of the terminal segment of the internal carotid artery are rarely of consequential size (Figure 10.17). Their maximum diameter is at the level of the origin of the posterior communicating artery. Some giant aneurysms of the internal carotid artery may originate from fusiform dilatations but their dimensions make dissection and identification of arterial origin difficult.

Large fusiform aneurysms are more commonly found involving the basilar artery, affecting part or whole of the stem (Figures 10.18 and 10.19). These aneurysms are the result of atherosclerosis and loss of elasticity. Hydrodynamic studies of glass models of such junctions reveal extraordinary flow disturbances in the stem especially with wide angles of union [164]. Such aneurysms may progressively expand to form quite a large

ANEURYSMS OF THE CEREBRAL CIRCULATION 379

sac resulting in compression of the pons and possibly cranial nerves particularly if there is any lateral displacement due to tortuosity. Large aneurysms can become spherical in time with the parent artery entering proximally and emerging distally as an efferent artery. Rupture is rare but can occur [165]. There may be associated ischaemic changes in the brain due to the severity of the atherosclerosis or from thromboemboli. The modes of presentation are predominantly due to compression or ischaemia.

Small fusiform aneurysms are to be found low on the intracranial segments of the vertebral arteries after their emergence from the dura mater. They may be bilateral and even cylindrical or saccular dilatations may be observed. They have been found in 10.8% of 185 circles of Willis from adult brains [166]. Histologically there is intimal thickening and sclerosis with medial thinning and much less elastica but not necessarily gross overt atherosclerosis. Vasa vasorum are often prominent and indicative of the mural thickening. They have been regarded as post-stenotic in type.

10.10.4 SACCULAR ARTERIAL ANEURYSM

Non-inflammatory saccular aneurysms are of two main types, those arising from the stem of an artery, and those arising in the fork of bifurcations. Statistics on saccular aneurysms usually pertain to a combination of these two types but early in the century often pertained to all macroscopically visible aneurysms.

(a) Saccular aneurysms unrelated to forks

These are far less common than berry-type aneurysms being found almost invariably with some atherosclerosis. They occur on the stems of the vertebral, basilar (Figure 10.17) and internal carotid arteries (cavernous and intracranial segments). They tend to arise in older individuals than do berry aneurysms but due to their infrequency, the age distribution has not been adequately determined.

They are frequently multiple and usually have rigid sclerotic walls with prominent vasa vasorum and variable siderotic pigmentation. The arteries may be tortuous, ectatic and of irregular contour. The sacs, often more than 1 cm in diameter, rarely rupture but progressively enlarge and may become space-occupying lesions causing nerve compression. Otherwise they are found fortuitously at autopsy. This type is regarded as atherosclerotic in nature, and due to an acquired local weakness of the wall (accentuated by tortuosity) or progressive excavation of an atherosclerotic ulcer with dilatation of the underlying mural remnants.

Fusiform aneurysms and saccular aneurysms unrelated to forks generally arise as the result of severe overt atherosclerosis. Histological examination of the parent

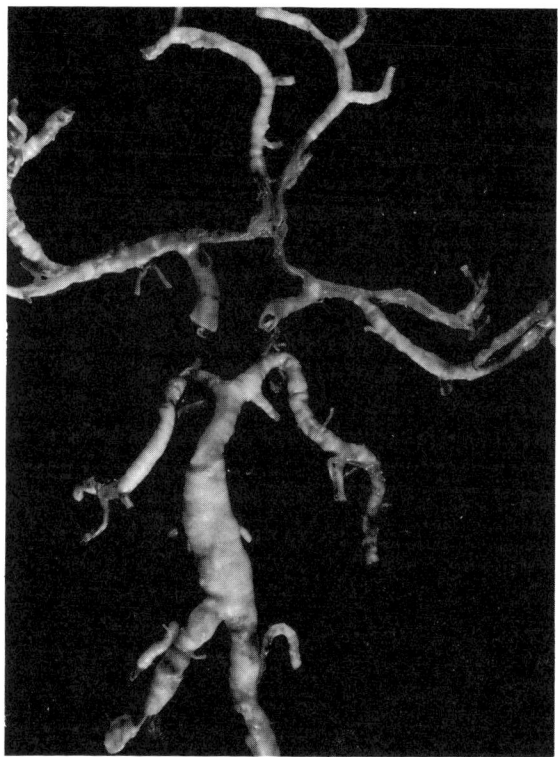

Figure 10.18 Fusiform aneurysm of basilar artery of an atherosclerotic circle of Willis. Note the irregular contour of the arteries. (Reproduced from Stehbens [7].)

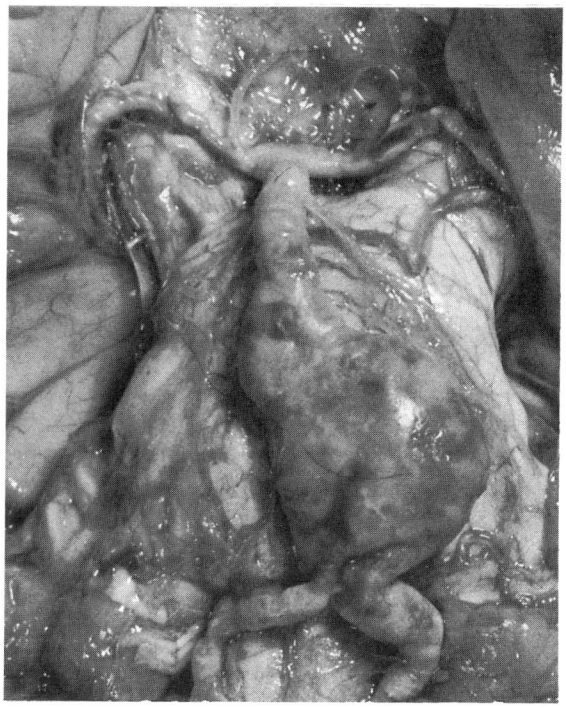

Figure 10.19 Large bulbous fusiform aneurysm of the basilar artery. Note irregular calibre of the left vertebral artery. (Reproduced from Stehbens [7].)

artery confirms this. The sac arises from a broad base and exhibits profound loss of elastic tissue, much fibrosis and a variable accumulation of lipid and calcification. Round cell infiltration is likely in the adventitia and vasa vasorum may be prominent. Siderophages in the wall indicate either leakage or biological attempts at organization of the mural thrombus. Elastic tissue stains may indicate how the aneurysm formed but if the sac is large, most elastin will have been lost.

In tortuous arteries there may be atrophic thinning of the wall on the outer aspect of the curvature and aneurysmal dilatation may be present without gross overt atherosclerosis. Sclerotic changes can develop secondarily.

(b) Aneurysms at arterial forks (berry aneurysms)

Berry aneurysms were so named because they often resembled small berries on a stalk and were often multiple. The term is inappropriate but has been used specifically for this type of aneurysm for many years for want of a better more explicit medical term. Controversy over their aetiology has continued since the last century when they were regarded as congenital aneurysms and are still often assumed to be so.

In 1859 Gull [167] contended the aneurysmal pouch looked 'as transparent and normal in appearance as the rest of the vessel giving the impression that it might have been some original deformity'. This implied a congenital maldevelopment of cerebral aneurysms which at that time were thought to constitute a disease of young people. All cerebral aneurysms were grouped together and bacterial or mycotic aneurysms occurring in young people were more frequent. At the turn of the century the aneurysms were labelled congenital and lesions of unknown aetiology occurring in young people are commonly assumed to be of such origin.

At the turn of the century the average life span was only 46 years and berry aneurysms occur predominantly in those over 40 years of age when degenerative diseases prevail. Their anecdotal association with polycystic kidneys, aortic coarctation and other 'congenital abnormalities' was interpreted as co-existence of congenital abnormalities. The occurrence of multiple aneurysms and their association with variations of the circle of Willis were considered in the same light. Forbus [168] labelled the medial raphes at arterial forks 'congenital defects', assuming without evidence that they were sites of weakness and therefore examples of maldevelopment rather than adventitial wedges of reinforcement acting as raphes. Forbus postulated that the wall was weak and that with elastic tissue degeneration, the wall yielded to the blood pressure and the alleged defect became evaginated. This correlated with the absence of media in the advanced aneurysm without thought being given to the discrepancy in the size of the 'defect' and that of the aneurysm. Considerable alteration of the arterial wall must occur if any segment balloons out to the size of even a medium-sized aneurysm. The absence of berry aneurysms in neonates and infants led to the amended concept that they were acquired but due to a congenital weakness of the wall and it is understandable that Forbus' paper [168] consolidated this opinion. The increase in population and longevity (more than 25 years) this century resulted in an increased prevalence of aneurysms and inevitably anecdotal reports of familial occurrence, sometimes in twins. This fostered the congenital theory as did reports of aneurysms on the arteries feeding intracranial arteriovenous shunts, which have also been assumed to be developmental anomalies. The presence of only mild atherosclerosis at times and the absence of gross atherosclerosis as occurs in abdominal aortic aneurysms delayed acceptance of the degenerative theory by some clinicians and pathologists. Erroneous beliefs die hard and tend to be perpetuated since once in the literature, they gain the magical potency of the written word and continue unquestioned. Later the supportive evidence was demonstrated to be spurious [7,169,170] and an acquired pathological origin is now accepted.

This is one of the commonest aneurysms in humans, perhaps even more common than those of the aorta, their frequency at autopsy depending on the diligence with which they are sought. For this reason autopsy incidence is not a reliable indication of prevalence in the community and comparisons between countries are unreliable. There is a slight predominance of female involvement with most aneurysms occurring between 40 and 70 years of age, peak incidence being about 50 years. They are not congenital and are exceedingly rare in the first decade. Most aneurysms found at that age are inflammatory or associated with an arteriovenous shunt.

In view of their frequency it is not surprising that instances of familial occurrence will be detected in the community especially since hypertension is familial and likely to predispose to aneurysm formation, Dalgaard [171] suggested that cerebral aneurysms were autosomal dominant. Carroll and Haddon [172], who made a study of persons under 35 years of age dying with a cerebral aneurysm, found no familial aggregation. Analysis of patients with aneurysms and their relatives led to the conclusion that the evidence was inadequate to determine a familial aggregation [173,174].

Lozano et al. [175] concluded from the literature that familial aneurysms had ruptured earlier than in non-familial cases and the sacs were somewhat smaller. They also reported that familial aneurysms were more likely to occur at identical or mirror sites than in non-familial cases. This view may be biased due to the enhanced tendency for such aneurysms to be reported and more detailed analysis of the circles of Willis would be required than is usually recorded. Since circles of Willis are not identical in monozygous twins, it is difficult to accept that anecdotal reports of identical locations or mirror image location of aneurysms in siblings or even in twins is significant.

Aneurysms have been reported in the families of 6.7% of aneurysm patients although only 0.4% of their siblings were affected [176]. Many other authors have reported on families with several affected members in two or three generations, sometimes with consanguineous marriages [175,177,178]. Whilst some have stated that no firm conclusion may be reached regarding inheritance, it has also been suggested that aneurysms are transmitted as an autosomal dominant trait with limited penetrance [179] or as a multifactorial trait with variable phenotypic expression [180].

In a study of genetic markers in 45 patients with cerebral aneurysms, typing of 18 different antigens was performed [181]. An association was found with three genetic markers and the authors suggested that the genes involved in aneurysm development may be on chromosome 6. However, in view of the small number of subjects, some associations are likely to be found but are not necessarily of biological significance. Moreover it is not certain that the aneurysms were all of the berry type. The C3-F gene was tested for an association with cerebral aneurysms but no association found [182]. HLA antigens and complement types in patients with cerebral aneurysms were investigated and only HLA-DR2 had any association with a small group of patients [183] but this is a tenuous relationship with assumed biological significance.

A number of subjects with Ehlers–Danlos syndrome (type IV) has been reported with cerebral aneurysms [7]. These subjects in the type IV syndrome are unable to synthesize type III collagen, a normal constituent of blood vessels. Subsequently several patients deficient in type III collagen were reported with cerebral aneurysms, but without other manifestations of Ehlers–Danlos syndrome [184]. This is in dispute [185,186] but even so such an observation gives no support to the congenital theory since the aneurysm would be a secondary manifestation and a collagen deficiency is not essential for the development of aneurysms. The collagen deficiency would be a predisposing factor in some subjects, just as lathyrism predisposes to but is not essential for the development of experimental aneurysms. Moreover, the partial deficiency of type III collagen occurs only sporadically and not in familial cases.

In a review ter Berg et al. [177] admitted that a large part of the familial occurrence can be explained by fortuitous aggregation. It is possible that *formes frustes* of inherited connective tissue disorders may predispose to these lesions as will hypertension. However, on the present basis of experimental production of atherosclerosis, mural atrophy and aneurysm production [10,113,169,187] the evidence strongly supports haemodynamically induced fatigue as the underlying mechanism and it is known that there is genetic predisposition to early mural atrophy and also to mechanical fatigue biologically even in timber. It is also likely that this genetic predisposition is multifactorial with many pathogenetic mechanisms contributing to the final common pathway but not specifically to the development of berry aneurysms.

(c) **Pathology**

Most of these aneurysms are less than 1 cm in their largest diameter appearing initially as little more than a filling out of the apical angle, often translucent and very thin-walled (Figure 10.20). The redundant wall may be better appreciated by perfusion of the vessels and viewing the forks with a stereomicroscope. Such aneurysms arise in the apical angle of bifurcations (Figure 10.21) or at the adjoining surface of one or other daughter branch. In some forks the sac arises towards the facial or dorsal aspect of the fork. Occasionally sacs arise from both facial and dorsal aspects of the fork (Figure 10.22) but two distinct aneurysms from the one fork is a rare phenomenon. Berry aneurysms also originate from the apex of a fenestration of an arterial stem (Figure 10.23) but not from the junction of the divided lumen nor from the lateral angles of forks.

The aneurysms enlarge forming small sessile or dome-shaped dilatations but even in the early stages of their development this area of attachment is broad based compared to the diameter of the parent vessel (Figure 10.24). They are neither polypoid nor pedunculated and as they grow their basal attachment enlarges seemingly by taking up some of the adjacent wall (Figure 10.25). The early aneurysmal wall is thin and flimsy but pro-

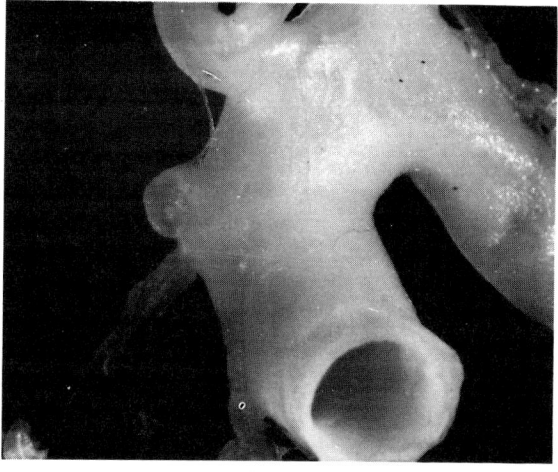

Figure 10.20 Small thin-walled transparent aneurysm arising at the origin of the anterior choroidal artery. (Reproduced with permission from Stehbens [166].)

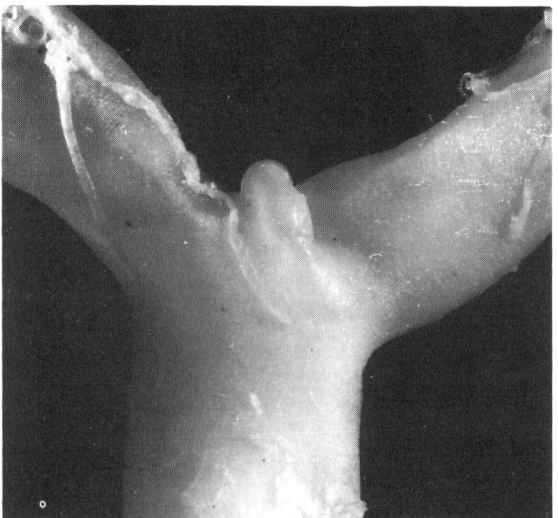

Figure 10.21 Early aneurysm of the middle cerebral artery presenting as a redundant fold of the wall. (Reproduced from Stehbens [7].)

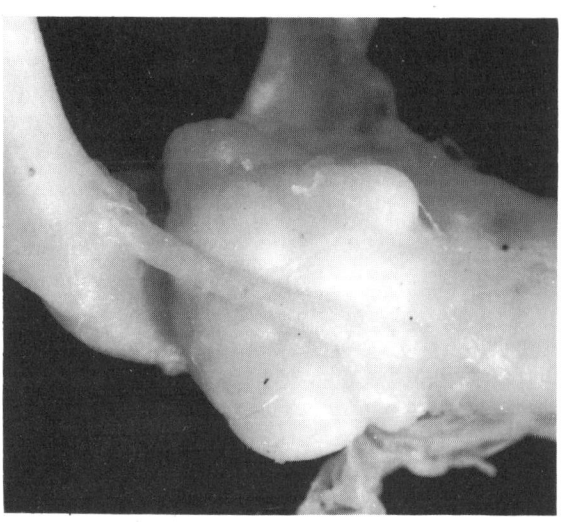

Figure 10.23 Aneurysm arising from the fork formed by an artery and a small branch that subsequently rejoins the parent artery. (Reproduced from Stehbens [7].)

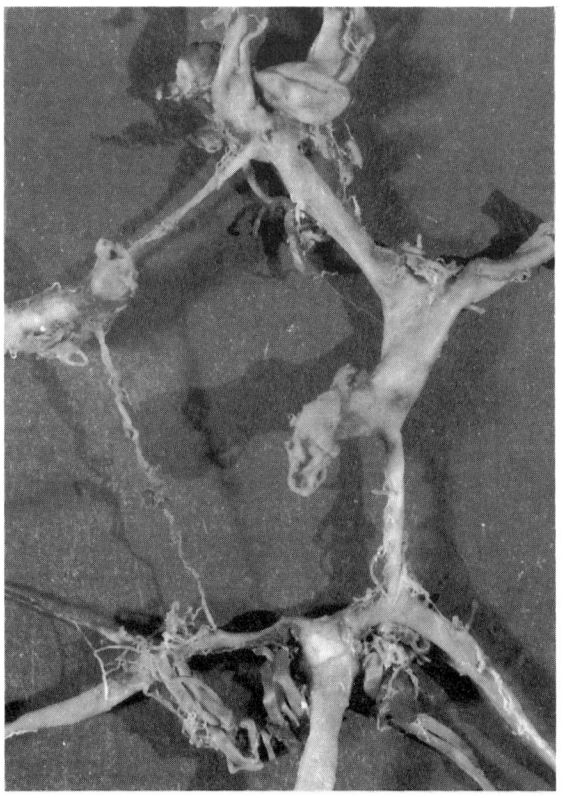

Figure 10.22 Circle of Willis displaying a tenuous right posterior communicating artery and two aneurysms arising from the anterior communicating artery which is really a fork mostly supplied by the proximal segment of the left anterior cerebral artery. The right internal carotid artery continues on into the middle cerebral artery. (Reproduced with permission from Stehbens [166].)

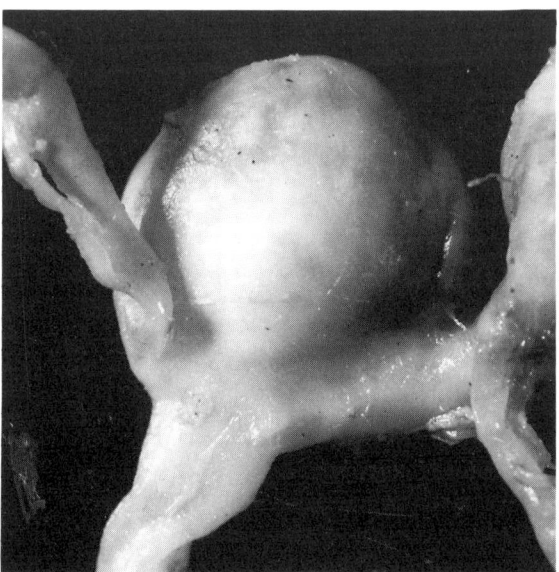

Figure 10.24 Unruptured aneurysm arising from a broad area at a fork of the middle cerebral artery. This aneurysm indicates the neurosurgical difficulty in clipping the aneurysm without obstructing flow and without leaving a residual cul de sac from which the aneurysmal sac can grow. (Reproduced with permission from Stehbens [166].)

gressively thickens. Overt atherosclerosis is present in the walls of larger aneurysms. The presence of this type of intimal tissue with adventitia and the absence of an intervening media lent support to the congenital or maldevelopmental hypothesis. In reality in the very early preaneurysmal changes, the media that is present becomes progressively lost and attenuated. Atherosclerotic plaques are sometimes more prominent in the aneurysm sac than in the parent arteries.

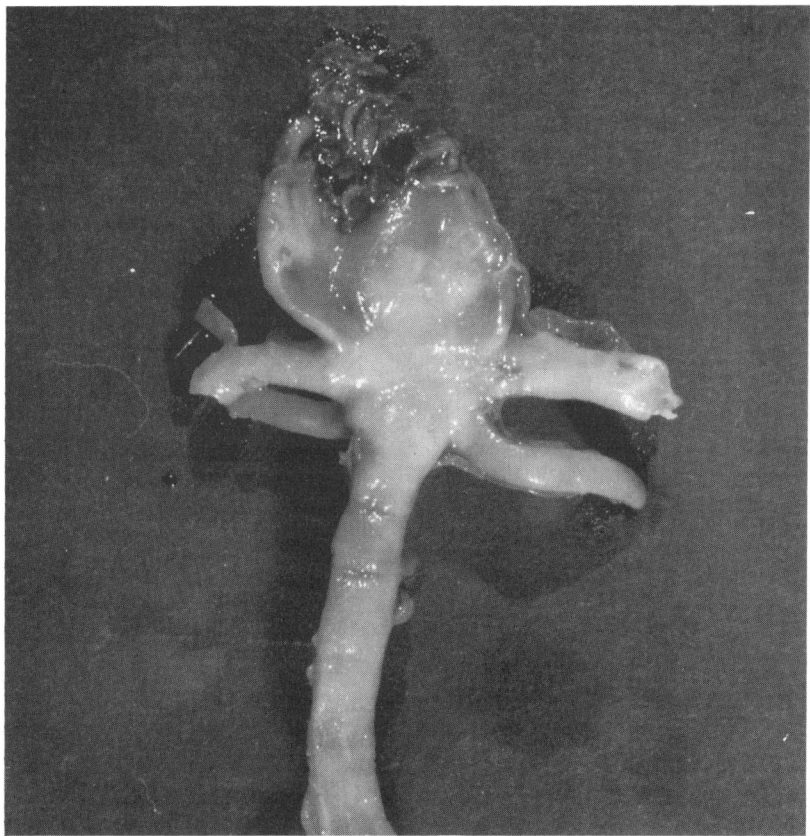

Figure 10.25 Aneurysm arising from the basilar bifurcation that ruptured directly into the third ventricle. Note the broad base. (Reproduced with permission from Stehbens [166].)

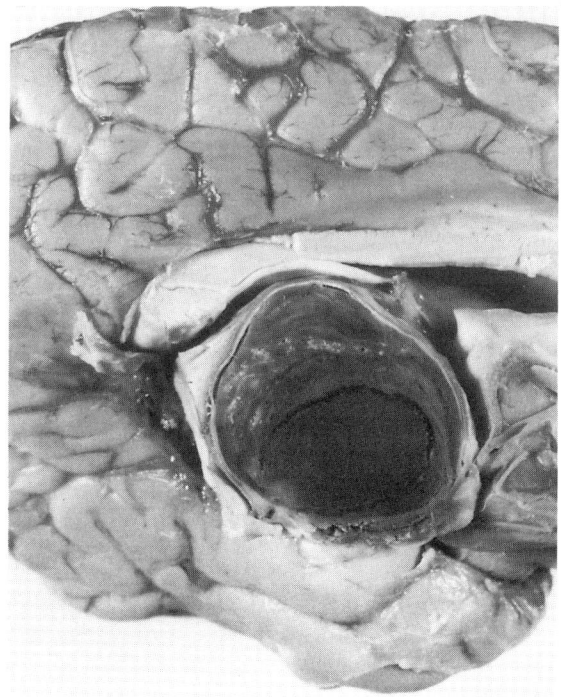

Figure 10.26 Aneurysm from the basilar bifurcation containing laminated thrombus and extending into the ventricular system beneath the corpus callosum. Note the dark clotted blood in the functional lumen.

If the sac grows above 1 cm without rupturing, atherosclerosis is prominent. Those larger than 2.5 cm are referred to as giant aneurysms (Figure 10.26). They can grow to 9 cm in diameter forming large space-occupying lesions that are difficult to manage. Mostly they are related to the internal carotid, the basilar or vertebral arteries and much less often the middle cerebral arteries. Giant aneurysms contain laminated thrombus with little evidence of organization and the blood angiographically may take a tortuous course through the thrombus. The wall is very fibrous with atherosclerosis and a variable degree of calcification though usually much less than splenic or renal aneurysms.

The ultimate shape and behaviour of an aneurysm after its formation is dependent on many factors with little information available from its external configuration and shape of the functional lumen.

Rupture, when it occurs, is at the fundus (Figure 10.25) and rerely at the sides or neck. Rupture may result in the formation of a false sac at the fundus (Figure 10.27) and larger aneurysmal sacs may have more than one dome-shaped swelling. On serial sectioning these have proven to be false sacs. Mural thrombus will develop at the site of leakage or rupture often

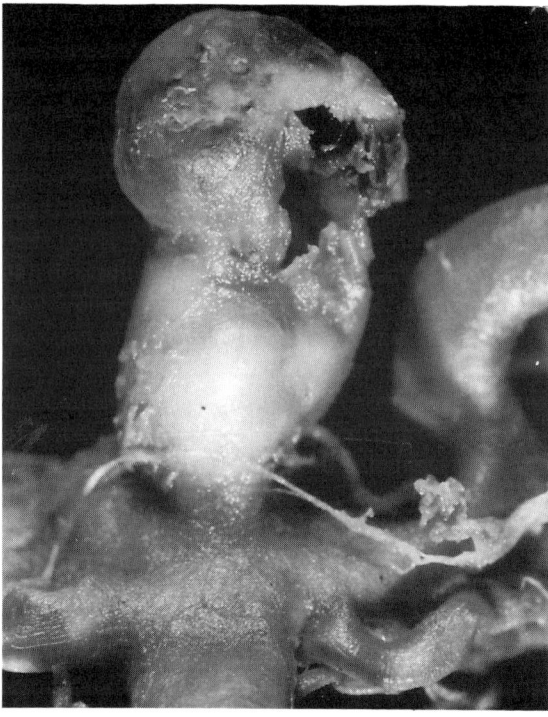

Figure 10.27 Basilar bifurcation aneurysm with opaque wall due to atherosclerosis. The distal half is a false aneurysm that has ruptured (Reproduced from Stehbens [7].)

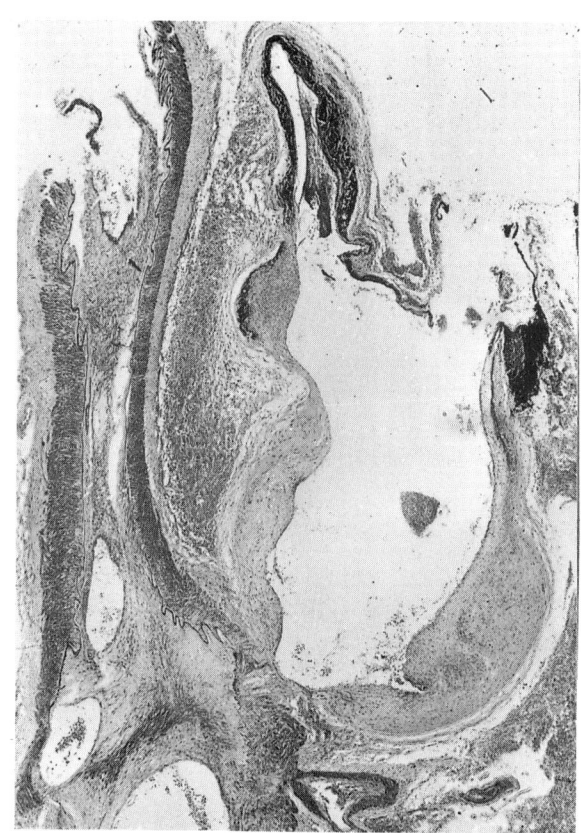

Figure 10.28 Low magnification of a ruptured berry aneurysm with irregularly thick walls at the sides (plaques) and thinning near the fundus at the top where rupture has occurred. The dark staining material at the fundus is fibrin which is attached to and infiltrating the margins of the aperture. The parent artery exhibits considerable intimal thickening. (Phosphotungstic acid and haematoxylin.) (Reproduced from Stehbens [7].)

with some haemorrhagic extravasation or fibrin infiltration of the wall at the margins of the tear (Figure 10.28). The external surface may adhere to rust-coloured meninges, nerves, blood clot, neighbouring vessel or brain following leakage and organization. The sac can be embedded in brain substance to a variable extent.

Older patients tend to have larger aneurysms [188, 189] confirmed by angiography but age does not preclude the presence of small sacs. Aneurysms do not run the rapid course that was the previous perception suggested by the disastrous outcome once the aneurysm ruptured. The rate of enlargement varies and sudden growth may be due to rupture with the formation of a false sac. Angiography reveals that the rate of enlargement is slow and complications are not likely if the sac is less than 5 mm. The larger the aneurysm, the more rapid growth is likely to be and leakage and rupture can be expected when the aneurysm is between 5 and 10 mm.

The assertion that an aneurysm can be avulsed at the time of rupture leaving a ragged hole in the artery wall is probably false and due to lack of serial sectioning or due to dissection after prolonged fixation in which case the blood becomes inspissated, the lesion being extremely difficult to dissect. The sac is probably then removed with the clot.

Unruptured aneurysms can be found at autopsy with surprising frequency if sought assiduously and expertly and the smaller the sac the less likely is the aneurysm to be found. A rusty zone or nodule on the surface of the wall indicates previous minimal leakage and angiographic evidence indicates these aneurysms can be expected to enlarge.

Some aneurysms have been observed to diminish over time and even to disappear [190] but reappearance has been recorded [191]. Pathological follow-up is necessary in such cases.

Aneurysms are frequently multiple and berry aneurysms are no exception, occurring in up to 20–30% of subjects. More than two or three are unusual but as many as seven have been found and eight in a female chimpanzee [192]. Up to 12 have been reported [193] and such large numbers, especially if the subjects are younger than usual, suggest the possibility of a connective tissue disorder. Hypertension has also been reported to enhance the tendency to multiplicity [194]. However, no particular aetiological significance should be attributed to multiple cerebral aneurysms which are commonly associated with degenerative diseases nor can they be used to support a maldevelopmental hypothesis, e.g. bilateral popliteal aneurysms occur in up to 56% of affected subjects [112].

Berry aneurysms occur primarily at the origin of the large and to a lesser extent small branches of the major arteries and in or close to the circle of Willis. They rarely occur peripherally on more distal leptomeningeal or cortical arteries and never on the penetrating or parenchymal arteries. At least 80–85% of berry aneurysms arise from the anterior half (internal carotid circulation) of the circle of Willis and its branches and the remaining 15–20% occur posteriorly on the vertebrobasilar circulation probably because major arterial bifurcations are more numerous anteriorly than posteriorly. Whether there is another flow factor involved in this predisposition anteriorly is not known.

The commonest site has been regarded as the middle cerebral artery bifurcation (within 2–3 cm from its origin) in pathological material, and either the internal carotid bifurcation or the anterior communicating artery in clinical material. Small aneurysms at the bifurcation or at the origin of successive small branches from the middle cerebral artery are readily missed clinically. This probably accounts for the discrepancy [7].

Intracranial aneurysms of the internal carotid artery occur primarily at the terminal bifurcation or at the origin of the posterior communicating artery. Aneurysms of the stem of the internal carotid artery may be damaged during removal of the brain and the true relationship to the origin of the ophthalmic branch may be lost. Some arise from the apical region of the ophthalmic artery but others, arising more distally, are not true berry aneurysms. Aneurysms in the foramen lacerum or the carotid canal are very rare and can cause severe pain, unilateral cranial nerve lesions, bone erosion and bleeding into the ear or nose or both but are usually due to trauma or infection. Those arising from the origin of the posterior communicating artery, often commencing as a funnel-shaped or steer-horn dilatation (Figure 10.29), are distinctly more frequent than those at the origin of the anterior choroidal artery apparently because of the much smaller size of the latter.

Aneurysms of the middle cerebral artery arise from the apical angle of a major bifurcation or trifurcation usually within 2–4 cm of its origin. Aneurysms may arise at the origin of three successive large branches of the proximal stem but those commencing more than 5 cm from the origin should be suspected of being inflammatory in nature. Aneurysms may be symmetrically located on the internal carotid and middle cerebral artery, even occasionally in twins but the anatomy of the circle of Willis is individualistic and such an occurrence is no doubt coincidental. The anterior communicating artery is a common site with the sac arising in the angle formed by one anterior cerebral

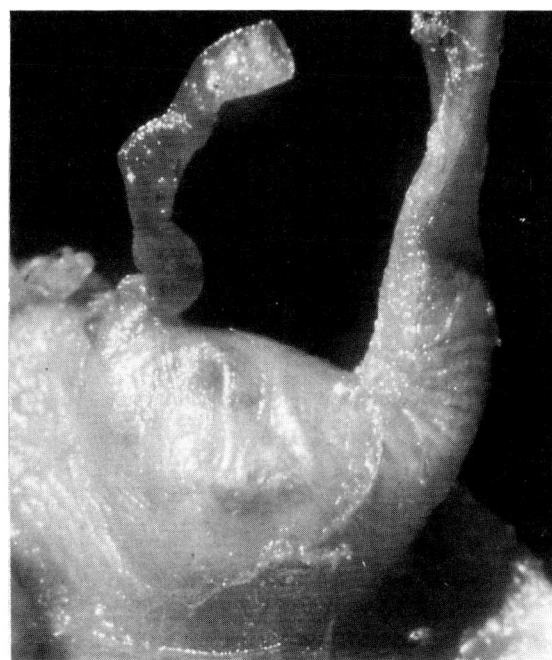

Figure 10.29 Steer-horn dilatation at origin of a posterior communicating artery from the internal carotid artery. Note the wall which is thinned and histologically exhibited mural atrophy. (Reproduced from Stehbens [7].)

artery (Figure 10.22) and the anterior communicating artery, which is usually shunting blood to the opposite side or to branches of the anterior communicating artery [7,166]. The proximal segments of the anterior cerebral arteries are frequently unequal in calibre and the aneurysm develops in the fork of the larger artery which shunts blood to the contralateral distal anterior cerebral via the anterior communicating artery. For an aneurysm to arise from the side of the smaller proximal anterior cerebral artery would be most unusual. Aneurysms are infrequently located in forks of the distal ramifications of the anterior cerebral artery but when present are most often close to the genu of the corpus callosum at the origin of the frontopolar or callosomarginal arteries [195].

Berry aneurysms of the vertebrobasilar system are much less frequent than those on the carotid systems as might be expected given the paucity of large arterial forks. Most arise from the basilar bifurcation and grow to sizeable proportions usually directed upwards to the floor of the third ventricle where they can obstruct the ventricular system even with a posterior extension into the mid-brain [196]. Aneurysms arise at the origin of the posterior or anterior inferior cerebellar arteries or from the internal auditory artery and even between a superior cerebellar and the ipsilateral posterior cerebral artery. Aneurysms, however, can arise from the origin of any vessel if proximal to an arteriovenous shunt. Some aneurysms originate from the apex of the basilar artery or from the dorsal aspect of the ampulla which gives rise to the two superior cerebellar and two posterior cerebral arteries. This has been attributed to the enhanced mural tension that must exist at that site [7,170], and possibly because the base of the aneurysm may progressively take up more of the basilar stem so that the sac eventually lies above and posterior to the bifurcation. Some aneurysms allegedly arise from the lateral angles, or the junction of the posterior cerebral and posterior communicating arteries but are demonstrated in drawings rather than photographs. Berry aneurysms characteristically arise from regions of the arterial wall where the flux of blood impinges on the vessel wall and not from other regions but displacement of the stem or branches, for whatever reason, with change in alignment or imbalance of flow, may enhance aneurysm formation.

At least 90% will be found at one or more of the following sites:

- bifurcation of the internal carotid artery
- carotid origin of the posterior communicating or anterior choroidal arteries
- at branches of the middle cerebral artery within 4 cm of its origin
- anterior communicating artery
- the basilar artery bifurcation.

There is an unexplained slight preponderance of aneurysms on the right side and genuine berry aneurysms can occur on distal leptomeningeal vessels but it is well to remember that any aneurysm that is of unusual location or atypical in any way or in the very young must be examined histologically in detail. The failure to provide adequate histology and expert review of the pathology of some bizarre aneurysms described in the literature accounts for incorrect deductions regarding aetiology and the pathogenesis of aneurysms in general. Peripheral aneurysms are more likely to be inflammatory or even traumatic in origin whilst in the presence of an arteriovenous shunt, an aneurysm may develop on an enlarged artery or vein in the most unusual locations. Diffuse aneurysmal dilatation may indicate previous arteritis. Large aneurysms within the brain or involving the choroid plexus are likely to be associated with an arteriovenous shunt. Aneurysms of meningeal arteries are extremely rare probably because of their size and reinforcement by dural fibrous tissue but they can be traumatic in origin.

Fenestrations of the vertebral or basilar artery are commonly recognizable macroscopically and may be central or off centre. They vary in length of duplication of the artery and are also found in the anterior or middle cerebral arteries. They are of no great importance or significance except that they provide an additional bifurcation from which an aneurysm may arise (Figure 10.23) doing so at the proximal and not the distal end.

Aneurysms at these sites have led to the allegation that these are sites of congenital weakness, but without proof [197]. Such an unwarranted assumption ignores the high frequency of subdivisions of the lumen by partitions or cords of different size, mostly about the anterior communicating artery, whereas the vertebrobasilar arteries would be the most frequent site with aneurysms. No evidence has been provided to indicate that aneurysms have any special predilection for development at such sites. Moreover these duplications are more common in lower animals, e.g. sheep [7], in which cerebral aneurysms have not been found. Partial thrombosis of one side of a fenestration can give the false appearance of an aneurysm angiographically [198].

Aneurysms have been reported in association with persistent trigeminal and persistent hypoglossal arteries. Controversy surrounds the significance of these carotid–basilar anastomoses and their true prevalence, even in minute form, is unknown. Individual case reports of an aneurysm in association with persistence of one of these vessels does not prove an association with developmental errors. Atherosclerosis is severe in many of these subjects who tend to suffer from other cerebral lesions including tumours but statistically at present there is no evidence that there is an undue propensity in these patients to develop cerebral aneurysms. If, on the other hand, severe stenosis or thrombotic occlusion resulted in greatly augmented collateral flow through such a persistent carotid–basilar artery, an aneurysm might arise due to the change in haemodynamic stresses at one of the arterial forks so affected.

Aneurysms in children under five years of age, apart from being exceedingly uncommon, have a different distribution occurring particularly on the peripheral branches of the middle and anterior cerebral arteries, often grow to a giant size and are usually not true berry aneurysms. Their peripheral location on these arteries and the age group suggests they may be of traumatic origin, inflammatory or associated with an arteriovenous shunt [199].

The intima of the parent artery at the entrance to a small berry aneurysm is invariably thickened (Figure 10.30) even if slightly so and the internal elastic lamina is likely to exhibit some fragmentation with elastic fibrils in the intimal thickening. The media may end abruptly with or without some fibrosis and attenuation or may be reflected into the neck for a short distance. Evidence of atherosclerosis by way of lipophages, is usually present in the intimal proliferation about the fork. The aneurysmal sac may consist of a thin layer of fibrous tissue and endothelium (Figure 10.31) with few or no remnants of adventitial elastic fibrils remaining or there may be some musculoelastic intimal proliferation closely resembling that at the forks of neonates. The small sacs are usually very thin without evidence of rupture. The aneurysm wall thickens as it grows and

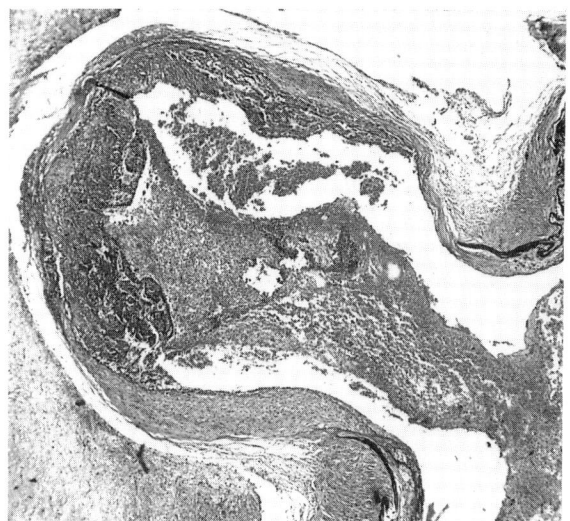

Figure 10.30 Berry aneurysm exhibiting intimal thickening and fairly abrupt termination of the media at the entrance to the sac which has ruptured at the fundus but is sealed with thrombus. (Verhoeff's elastic stain.) (Reproduced from Stehbens [7].)

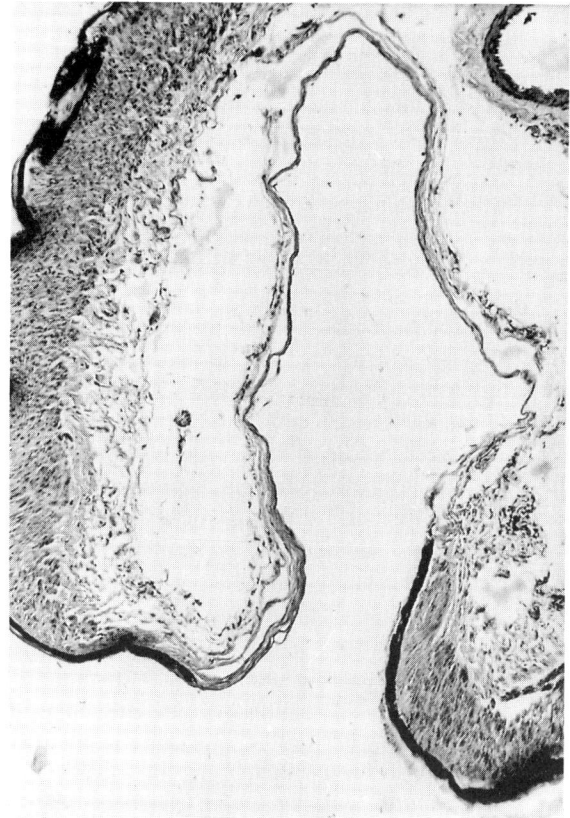

Figure 10.31 Small unruptured berry aneurysm with a remarkably thin wall consisting of endothelium and a thin layer of fibrous tissue (attenuated adventitia). Note the evagination on the left does not involve all the medial raphe. (Verhoeff's elastic stain and eosin.) (Reproduced from Stehbens [7].)

where there is active intimal type proliferation, there may even be a thin secondary elastic lamina with metachromasia.

Larger sacs may have a thin wall at the neck where the wall is apposed to the adventitia of the branch. Intimal proliferation develops at the sides of the sac and the fundus is more often fibrous and thinner but elastic tissue is difficult to find. Only remnants remain indicating that there is elastic tissue proliferation early, although not in larger aneurysms. A few round cells may be present near the neck and vasa vasorum are absent. The internal elastic lamina and the media terminate relatively abruptly at the neck even though the aneurysm must have enlarged and involved more of the parent arterial wall. Atherosclerosis becomes prominent and plaques are found indistinguishable from those in the parent artery except for the absence of elastin and even remnants of the original media. There may be more intimal proliferation at the neck in the adjacent daughter branch and degenerative changes in the parent artery are usually pronounced.

Calcification is little in evidence in cerebral aneurysms and some unruptured aneurysms exhibit mural thrombus or part of the wall may consist of fibrin (incipient rupture). Organization of mural thrombus is little in evidence although there may be lipid-stippling, lipophages, cholesterol clefts and calcification at the edge of the thrombus. The giant aneurysms with laminated thrombus have extensive fibrosis in their walls and some calcification, lipid, siderophages and vasa vasorum with adhesions unless stripped during dissection. Ossification is rare and no extensive xanthomatous infiltrations have been observed.

Aneurysms from patients with coarctation of the aorta or polycystic disease of the kidneys do not differ from those in patients without such congenital disorders.

The fundus remains thinner and more fibrous and when rupture has occurred, the wall tapers to the rupture site with fibrin tags and thrombus adherent to the edge and patchy fibrin infiltration in the adjacent wall, particularly on the inner aspect (Figure 10.28). The mural thrombus is secondary to the tear, there being no evidence that fibrinoid necrosis precipitates rupture. With progressive but intermittent enlargement of the sac associated with some induration and inspissation of the thrombus, it is likely that dissection and extravasation of blood occurs between the old thrombus and the sac wall with coagulation and repetition of this phenomenon. This would account for the limited organization of mural thrombi in aneurysms.

Experimental aneurysms including the berry-type have been produced in rabbits by microvascular surgery using a segment of vein as a graft. These sacs develop intimal thickening with destruction of the media and loss of most elastic tissue, and this progresses to atherosclerosis ultrastructurally identical to the human disease [38,39]. This has been attributed to the high frequency vibrations and increased pulsatility that occur in human cerebral aneurysms [84,200,201] and may be used eventually as a diagnostic tool. Such observations support the haemodynamic theory of atherogenesis [85,202] and also explain why on occasions atherosclerosis is more severe within a berry aneurysm than in the parent artery [7] indicating an accelerated course of the disease.

Nyström [203] reported two unruptured aneurysms that were completely calcified but provided no detail. Three additional sacs were said to be filled with atheromatous masses, a feature not previously described and also not illustrated. Such masses were more likely due to herniation of atheromatous debris through the adventitia forming a small soft pultaceous nodule walled by lipophages [166,204].

Hegedüs [205] reported the absence of reticular fibres in sporadic areas immediately deep to the internal elastic lamina of two subjects with dissecting aneurysms of the cerebral arteries. Previously he demonstrated a reduction in medial reticular fibres in subjects with cerebral aneurysms [206] and assumed a causal relationship alleging that such deficiency may indicate an intrinsic predisposition to cerebral aneurysms and arterial dissection. However, these changes could just as readily be acquired. His studies did not indicate that the aneurysm patients form a distinct group from birth, but Chyatte *et al.* [207] confirmed the observation and admitted the changes could be manifestations of cerebral 'aneurysm disease' rather than an inherent mural deficiency. In view of the non-specific development of cerebral aneurysms [187] and of early atrophic lesions experimentally under haemodynamic stress [170], it is unwise to speculate on intrinsic mural deficiencies without stronger evidence.

(d) Ultrastructure

The ultrastructure of cerebral aneurysms reveals a picture similar to that of atherosclerosis of the cerebral arteries except for the absence of elastin and even medial remnants [208,209]. The early aneurysmal changes exhibit similar severe cellular degenerative changes and loss of elastic tissue, thus substantiating the degenerative nature of these early lesions rather than intimating an origin from a developmental defect.

(e) Initiation and development

Berry aneurysms were long assumed to be congenital abnormalities due to maldevelopment of the arterial wall with either an inborn defect or the persistence of some undifferentiated vestigial vessel, supposedly an area of weakness, gradually yielding to produce an aneurysm. They are not congenital despite the search to prove them so [7]. There is no evidence of the hypothetical weakness and why vestigial vessels should cause aneurysms in the human cerebral circulation in particular has never been explained. Evidence purportedly in support of such speculations has not withstood modern scientific scrutiny [7].

They occur infrequently in splanchnic arteries, there being a special propensity for the cerebral arterial tree. This has been attributed to their thinner walls macroscopically and microscopically, less elastic tissue which is concentrated in the internal elastic lamina, a thin media and only scanty fibrillary elastic tissue in the thin adventitia, there being no distinct external elastic lamina (Figure 1.6, p. 11) [7]. The reduced peripheral resistance in cerebral arteries with their more rapid blood flow may be associated with an augmented pulse pressure and reflected waves could accentuate this.

These architectural peculiarities of cerebrospinal arteries are not confined to humans alone although non-inflammatory and non-parasitic aneurysms are rare in lower animals. A few instances of authentic berry aneurysms in chimpanzees have been reported [192,210] and early aneurysmal change in a gorilla. Why berry aneurysm are virtually confined to humans in whom they are prevalent is no doubt due to:

- human longevity
- the large brain and large size of human cerebral arteries
- the greater severity of atherosclerosis than in lower animals
- possibly, a higher incidence of hypertension.

Forbus [168] attributed aneurysms to so-called medial defects consisting of an adventitial wedge extending wholly or partially through the media to the intima. These medial defects, found in cerebral arteries of all ages, were assumed to represent defects in the wall. They are in reality merely raphes between the medial musculature of the two branches (apical raphe) or of a branch and the parent stem (lateral angle raphe) exerting vasoconstrictive forces in virtually opposite directions. They occur at the apex and also at the lateral angle and are ubiquitous in the cerebral, systemic and pulmonary circulations of humans and all lower animals so far investigated [7]. They increase in frequency with age, their biological distribution is at complete variance with the distribution of aneurysms biologically and there is no scientific evidence that they are areas of weakness [7,211]. They cannot be considered causal or even predisposing to aneurysm formation. If and when involved in the aneurysmal sacs, the event is fortuitous.

Three early aneurysmal changes have been described and occur predominantly in middle age except for an association with aortic coarctation [7,204].

ANEURYSMS OF THE CEREBRAL CIRCULATION 389

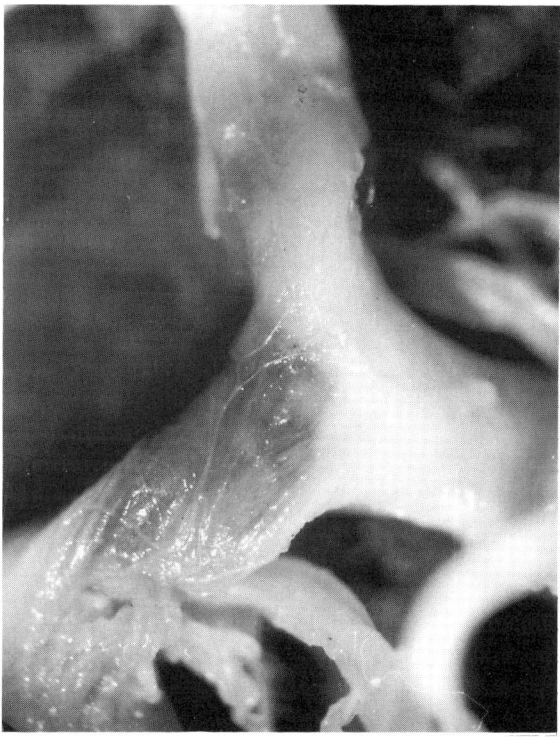

Figure 10.32 An area of thinning of a cerebal arterial fork. The affected wall is transparent in contrast to the opacity of the thicker wall elsewhere. (Reproduced from Stehbens [7].)

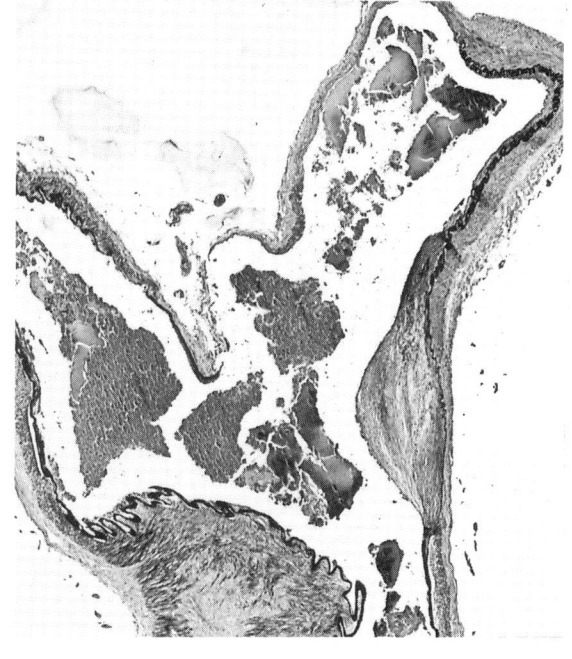

Figure 10.34 Fork exhibiting more extensive mural thinning of media and adventitia than in Figure 10.33. Note loss of elastic tissue, muscle and fibrous tissue along the distal aspect of the daughter branch. The media is still visible along much of the wall except at the bulge. Note the lateral pad and its extension along the proximal or lateral aspect of the branch. (Verhoeff's elastic stain and eosin.) (Reproduced with permission from Stehbens [204].)

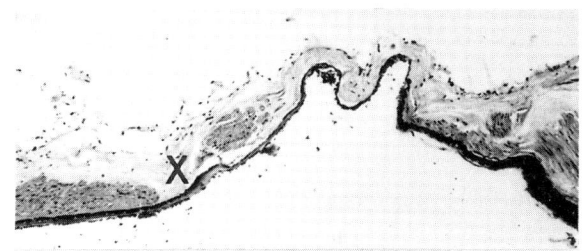

Figure 10.33 Area of mural thinning in a cerebral arterial fork. Note that the loss of medial muscle and the early aneurysm do not involve the apex (X). (Verhoeff's elastic stain and eosin.)

1. **Areas of thinning** may be seen macroscopically within the apical angle, the thinness of the wall contrasting with the thicker, more opaque, adjacent wall (Figure 10.32). Histologically, these are regions of severe mural atrophy (Figure 10.33) with loss and fragmentation of the internal elastic lamina, attenuation, fibrosis and disappearance of the media and thinning of the adventitia with loss of its elastic fibrils (Figure 10.34). These areas of thinning or mural atrophy are found adjacent to the apical raphe which when involved must be fortuitous or a secondary event. Ultrastructurally, these early aneurysmal changes are associated with paucity or absence of elastica, thickening, lamination, redundancy and separation of basement membranes and abundant muscle debris. In some instances lipid is present at the sides, but not in the regions of maximum thinning [208]. These changes occur in human atherosclerosis and have been produced experimentally by haemodynamic means [13,209].

2. **Steer-horn or funnel-shaped dilatations** which occur predominantly at the origin of the posterior communicating artery [7,204] (Figure 10.29) are sometimes called infundibular dilatations [212]. Serial histological sections reveal that these too are areas of medial atrophy (Figure 10.35) but the dilatation is more diffuse possibly because it usually occurs at a somewhat smaller branch.

3. **Micro-evaginations** were found by serial histological sections in the apical region of cerebral arterial forks or adjacent to the apex but did not extend beyond the adventitia. There is fragmentation and variable loss of the internal elastic lamina and some exhibit slight intimal thickening (Figure 10.36). One evagination with a disrupted wall contained a microthrombus over the defect [7]. They may constitute an earlier stage than mural thinning and with pressure fixation may result in blunting or flattening of the

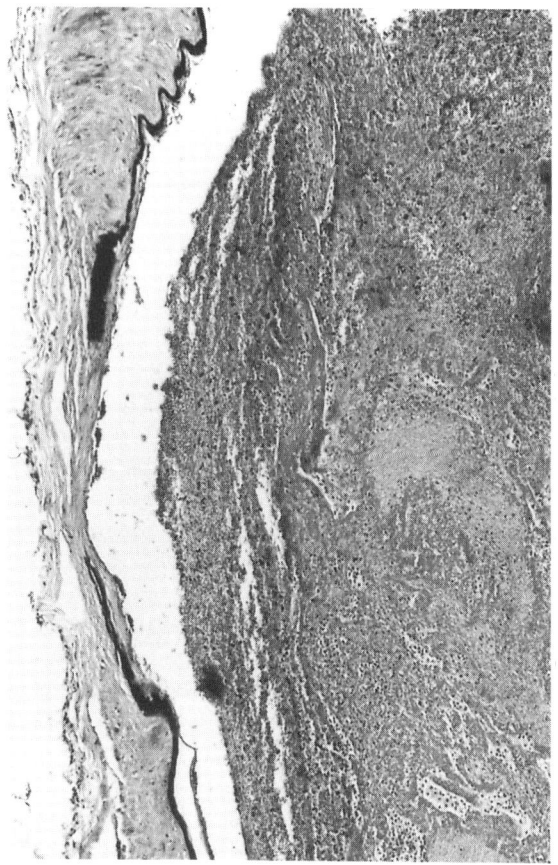

Figure 10.35 Diffuse mural thinning with medial fibrosis and loss of muscle. Note the abrupt termination of upper end of internal elastic lamina reminiscent of those produced experimentally. (Verhoeff's elastic stain and eosin.)

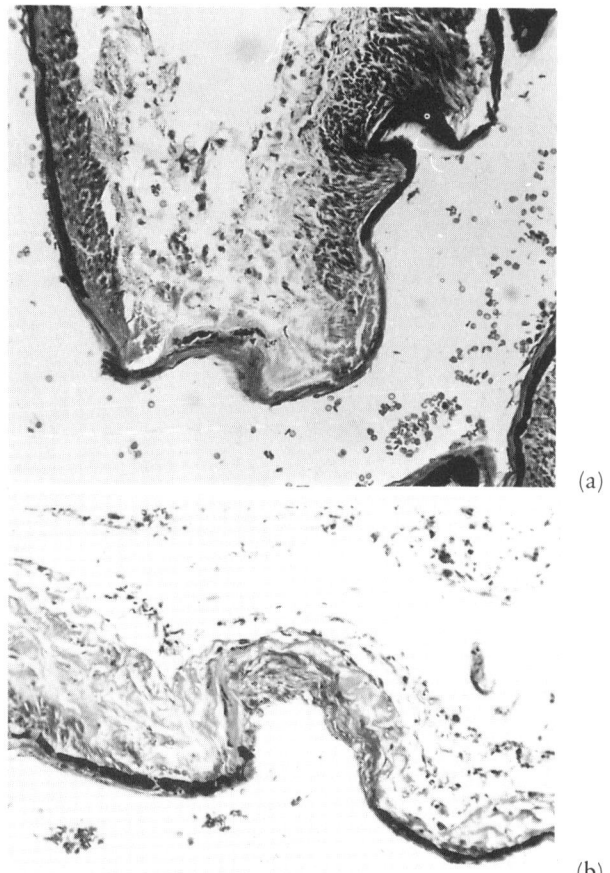

Figure 10.36 Apices of cerebral arterial forks showing: (a) flattening of the apex with evagination into only part of the medial raphe and fragmentation and loss of the elastic lamina; (b) evagination into only part of the apical medial raphe. Note the fragmentation of the elastic lamina and early intimal proliferation within the micro-evagination which would not protrude beyond the adventitia. (Verhoeff's elastic stain and eosin.) ((a) Reproduced from Stehbens [7]; (b) reproduced with permission from Stehbens [170].)

apex which would serve only to aggravate the haemodynamic disturbance at the site. Involvement of only part of the raphe suggests that some change in part of the raphe must be responsible for the evagination rather than the raphe being a site of inherent weakness.

Study of mural atrophy and aneurysms reveals the media is usually lost prior to significant dilatation and it is surprising how thin the wall can be even in the presence of aneurysmal dilatation without evidence of rupture or leakage (Figure 10.31). Intimal type proliferation subsequently occurs and is probably compensatory proliferation to reinforce the wall. The absence of media in the developed aneurysm is not indicative of congenital absence of the media as suggested by Forbus [168], but an acquired degenerative change that can be produced experimentally in a U-shaped curvature in rabbits and in the afferent arteries of arteriovenous fistulae [10,113]. Moreover, the attachment area or base of the aneurysms is far greater than the dimensions of the medial raphes (Figure 10.25) from which the sacs allegedly develop. The subsequent degenerative changes that occur in cerebral aneurysms [208] are similar even ultrastructurally to those of experimental venous-pouch aneurysms developed in rabbits by microvascular surgery [38,39]. These observations indicate that the degenerative changes in human berry aneurysms develop merely in response to hydrodynamic stresses to which the wall is subjected. The media is rapidly thinned and may completely disappear with the elastin fragmented, sparse and depleted in much of the wall. Any residual media incorporated in the wall of human berry aneurysms is consequently not likely to persist for long and, therefore, the absence of media in naturally occurring aneurysms in humans lends no support to a congenital hypothesis or developmental origin due to an absence of media as in medial raphes. The absence of the media is an acquired change which can be reproduced experimentally by haemodynamic means [10,113] (Figure 10.37).

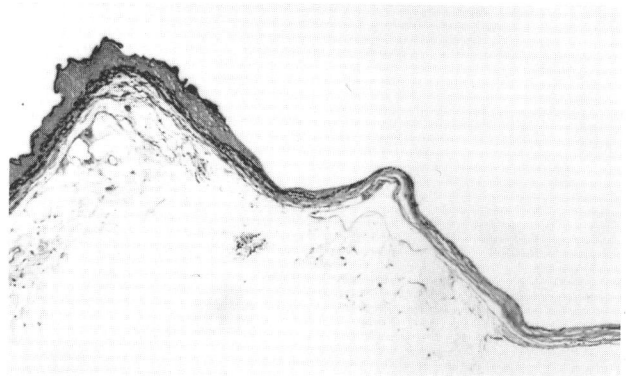

Figure 10.37 Section from a rabbit femoral artery proximal to an arteriovenous fistula [10] showing gross destruction of the normal architecture with only residual adventitial remnants to the right. Note the fragmented internal elastic lamina. (Verhoeff's elastic tissue stain and eosin).

10.10.5 COMPLICATIONS

(a) Rupture

Rupture is the most feared complication and is to be regarded as the terminal event in their natural history. Berry aneurysms are more likely to rupture than other varieties of degenerative cerebral aneurysm. Small premonitory leaks often herald a severe incapacitating or fatal haemorrhage and provide a clue to diagnosis. Most sacs rupture when between 5 and 10 mm in diameter and those over 2.5 cm without laminated mural thrombus are particularly prone to rupture. The thrombus itself would most likely have been initiated by partial rupture (tearing of the wall). Such large aneurysms act as space-occupying lesions. When multiple aneurysms are present, it is likely that the largest sac will rupture, especially if the sac is multilocular, since nodular dilatations are mostly false sacs. If two aneurysms are present on the one artery it is likely to be the larger proximal sac that has ruptured. Rupture can occur during angiography and only rarely do two aneurysms rupture simultaneously whether both are intracranial or one is extracranial [196].

The sac wall is frequently thin at the neck and yet rupture almost invariably occurs at the fundus. Early aneurysms with flimsy walls must be weak but do not rupture. They rupture when larger and with thicker walls so that the tensile strength of the tissue cannot be determined on morphological grounds either quantitatively or qualitatively at present. Some additional change in the wall is responsible for the tearing and rupture. The mechanism of rupture is likely to be intimately related to the initial cause of the aneurysmal dilatation.

Hypertension is associated with increased mural tension, a higher pulse pressure, and pulsatility and, therefore, an enhanced propensity for rupture. An increase in blood pressure associated with exertion and emotional stress even though transient, may contribute to the cumulative stress. Some aneurysms rupture during sleep as well as during physical effort, jogging, defaecation, coitus, coughing or parturition [7,213]. Severe physical exertion has been incriminated and so has head injury but little is known of the stresses and strains to which major arteries are subjected during cranial injuries. Whatever the alleged precipitating factor may be, the aneurysmal sac has to be fragile and close to rupture.

Type III collagen deficiency has been incriminated in some subjects [184,214] and is apparently related to Ehlers–Danlos syndrome type IV which is known to be associated with an acquired fragility of the blood vessel wall and a propensity for carotid cavernous aneurysms, cerebral dissecting aneurysms and other cerebral aneurysms [214]. This has been disputed [185,186] but even so some members of an extended family suffer from type III collagen deficiency and others have normal type III collagen levels although both groups may develop cerebrovascular lesions. The likelihood is that it is the more rapid failure of the collagen fibrils under repetitive stress that is responsible for the aneurysm than necessarily an absence of type III collagen. In experimental venous pouch aneurysms that can develop the complications of spontaneous aneurysms, the intimal proliferation within the sacs contains many of the abnormally shaped collagen fibrils associated with Ehlers–Danlos syndrome and similar diseases and is thought to indicate collagen and vascular fragility [154,215]. The development of abnormally shaped collagen fibrils and fibril disintegration are non-specific phenomena indicative of molecular fragmentation. They may also be manifestations of the acquired mural weakness and loss of cohesion leading to progressive aneurysmal growth and eventual rupture. The findings of Pope and his colleagues [184,214] do not mean that all aneurysms are due to deficiency of type III collagen but that a connective tissue disorder, whether a mutant type III collagen deficiency, Ehlers–Danlos syndrome type IV, Marfan's syndrome or some other connective tissue disorder, may predispose to aneurysm formation much the same as lathyrism facilitates development of experimental cerebral aneurysms [187]. Rupture of the aneurysm is not the consequence of aneurysmal enlargement and tension outstripping the ability of the wall to proliferate and reinforce itself because remarkably thin walls do not rupture. Size and mural tension contribute by accelerating the onset of fatigue. Each aneurysm has a wall of variable thickness and correlation is poor between wall thickness and rupture which results from mural weakness due to mechanical failure of the connective tissues [84,169].

The evidence for rupture of splenic aneurysms during pregnancy is more convincing than for cerebral aneurysms. However, in the presence of an aneurysm that could rupture, the strain of labour is an additional stress that is probably best avoided. The mortality rates in pregnant women are not significantly different from those of non-pregnant women.

(b) Haemorrhage

The aneurysms are mostly situated within the subarachnoid space and by virtue of the preference of berry aneurysms for the anterior half of the circle of Willis, subarachnoid haemorrhage will be mostly basal, extending between the hemispheres anteriorly into the interpeduncular fossa, into one or both Sylvian fissures and extending over the convexities of the frontal and pariental lobes according to the site of haemorrhage and its severity. A small haemorrhage will be relatively localized to the site of the aneurysm. The blood initiates a haemogenic meningitis with some local cortical oedema (preceded by a potassium ion shift [216]). A large localized haematoma between the frontal lobes or in the Sylvian fissure can act as a space-occupying lesion but fatal haemorrhage is usually not restricted to the subarachnoid space alone. Massive subarachnoid haemorrhage by producing cerebral tamponade can be fatal.

Organization of the blood clot may result in adhesions of the aneurysmal sac to the pia mater so that a recurrent haemorrhage may extend directly into the brain tissue especially if the sac is embedded in the cortex. As a consequence the haemorrhage may cause an intracerebral haematoma and intraventricular haemorrhage as well. Aneurysms at the bifurcation of the internal carotid artery embedded in the cortex may rupture into the anterior horn of the lateral ventricle and cause subarachnoid haemorrhage primarily or wholly in the cisterna magna and about the hindbrain, although siderotic staining elsewhere may suggest previous bleeding from an aneurysm. Likewise aneurysms of the anterior communicating artery may rupture into the third ventricle or either anterior horn of the lateral ventricles to produce a massive intraventricular haemorrhage with little cerebral damage. Those at the basilar bifurcation often grow into or rupture into the third ventricle causing a similar posterior fossa subarachnoid haemorrhage and unless the search for an aneurysm is thorough, an unexplained intravascular haemorrhage may be the diagnosis.

Recurrent subarachnoid haemorrhage may result in extensive adhesions, obliteration of the subarachnoid space but rarely hydrocephalus. Recurrent aneurysmal bleeding is known to cause superficial siderosis (or haemosiderosis) of the central nervous system but this is not specific for aneurysmal haemorrhage [7,217].

Massive intracerebral and/or intraventricular haemorrhage occurs in up to 70% of fatal cases of

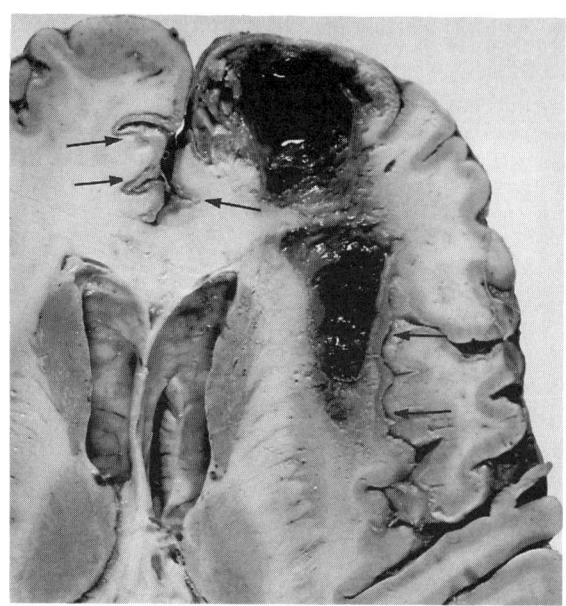

Figure 10.38 Frontal lobe haematoma from a ruptured aneurysm of the internal carotid bifurcation. Note the cortical softenings (arrows). (Reproduced from Stehbens [7].)

ruptured berry aneurysms (Figure 10.38). Sites of involvement are given in Table 10.1. Large intracerebral haematomas are more likely to be fatal than a rupture with minimal cerebral involvement. Secondary pontine haemorrhage is not uncommon. Intraventricular extension of the haemorrhage is not invariable and massive bleeding into the ventricular system can cause death within a few hours, no doubt due to blood clot obstructing the aqueduct leading to internal haemocephalus. This can lead to tears in the walls of the lateral ventricles [218] and pressure effects on pontine, medullary and cerebellar structures. Subependymal haemorrhage in the lateral ventricles, about the aqueduct and in the anterior hypothalamus have been described [219]. Subdural haemorrhage with ruptured cerebral aneurysms has been reported with variable frequency (up to 20%) but blood in the subdural space is usually small in quantity and seldom sufficient to be clinically significant or to present as a primary subdural haematoma. The blood would be expected to come from the internal carotid, vertebral or basilar arteries but the aneurysm rarely lies exclusively in the subdural space. More than half have been alleged to have originated from the middle or the anterior communicating arteries and tears in the arachnoid are difficult to demonstrate at autopsy. The possibility is that some subdural haemorrhages may be traumatic due to a fall at the time of loss of consciousness.

Some aneurysms from the petrous segment of the internal carotid artery may bleed into the ear and re-

Table 10.1 Tabulation of sites of intracerebral haemorrhage and intraventricular extension from ruptured aneurysms

Site of aneurysm	Intracerebral haemorrhage	Extension into ventricular system
Internal carotid artery at origin of posterior communicating artery	Temportal lobe damaging hippocampal gyrus, uncus, dentate gyrus	Temporal horn of lateral ventricle
Internal carotid bifurcation	Frontal lobe	Anterior horn of lateral ventricle
Anterior communicating artery	One or both frontal lobes; may extend posteriorly to the external capsule	Anterior horn of lateral ventricle; may rupture through the thin lamina terminalis into the third ventricle
Middle cerebral artery	Frontal or temporal lobes, into the insula to involve external capsule, basal ganglia	Lateral ventricle
Vertebral artery	Minimal parenchymal damage	–
Basilar bifurcation	Floor of third ventricle	Third ventricle

current epistaxis may occur with a cavernous sinus aneurysm bleeding into the sphenoid sinus. Such aneurysms are rare and the possibility of an atypical aetiology (infectious) must be considered whenever there is haemorrhage at an unusual site.

(c) Perianeurysmal gliosis

This is likely to occur when the sac lies within a depression or pocket in the brain parenchyma. Brain tissue does not take kindly to pulsations and there may also be some round cell infiltration and siderophages if leakage has occurred previously.

(d) Ischaemic lesions

Ischaemic cerebral lesions, from cortical ischaemia (Figure 10.38) to massive infarction and sometimes multiple sites, are implicated in 45–75% of fatal aneurysmal ruptures [220–222]. Small early haemorrhagic cortical infarctions are readily overlooked but must be sought. Crompton [220,221] found significant infarction (i.e. at least one third of the cortical distribution of one of the major cerebral arteries or ganglionic necrosis of 5 mm or more) in 75% of his 159 subjects dying at least 24 hours after the onset. Infarctions were mostly pale and generally involved the cortex alone. They were sometimes laminar not involving the full thickness of the cortex suggesting relative ischaemia. They were more frequent in females than males. The underlying mechanism is controversial and the lesions have been presumed to be due to vasospasm, displacement and attenuation of branches due to local pressure effects associated with the expanding haematoma, tearing or damage to small perforating branches, and reduced regional cerebral blood flow. The latter correlates well with the clinical severity of the neurological deficit. Other factors that may be involved are atherosclerosis, hypotension and small posterior communicating arteries limiting the collateral flow but local tamponade must be an important factor for consideration. The cortical ischaemic lesions are not confined to the vessels on which the aneurysm is situated. Whilst thrombi may be found in a very few cases, it is generally accepted that thrombotic occlusion is not responsible.

Other ischaemic lesions can be present due to general pressure effects on major arteries such as partial or intermittent compression of the posterior cerebral arteries against the tentorium cerebelli in cases of transtentorial herniation or compression of branches of the anterior cerebral artery against the falx cerebri when there is a substantial shift to the opposite side beneath the falx. There may also be smaller ischaemic lesions involving the hypothalamus or the pituitary [7].

(e) Embolism and transient ischaemic attacks

These are not well recognized complications of cerebral aneurysms. The aneurysm is likely to be relatively large with mural thrombus. Transient ischaemic attacks or other embolic phenomena can be the mode of presentation even when an aneurysm is unsuspected [223,224] but other sources of emboli should be excluded.

(f) Miscellaneous complications of ruptured aneurysms

The most important secondary effects of rupture are the pressure effects, essentially those from a rapidly raised supratentorial pressure contributing to secondary necrosis or haemorrhage in the pons and cerebral peduncles, compression of the posterior cerebral arteries against the tentorium cerebelli and the anterior cerebral artery against the falx cerebri, herniation of the uncus and hippocampal gyrus into the incisura tentori, compression of the aqueduct of Sylvius with secondary hydrocephalus or haemocephalus, compression of the oculomotor nerve, pressure and indentation of the contralateral cerebral peduncle (Kernohan's notch), herniation of the hind-brain into the foramen magnum with cerebellar–tonsillar compression and possibly necrosis, brain-stem compression and herniation of the cerebral cortex (often of the motor area) into the pacchionian bodies.

Degeneration of the granular layer of the cerebellum is a little known complication of a ruptured aneurysm [219,225], together with Purkinje cell necrosis. These changes are probably anoxic and terminal.

Severe subarachnoid haemorrhage may also be associated with intraocular (subhyaloid) haemorrhage, albuminuria, glycosuria, neurogenic ulceration in the upper gastrointestinal tract and cardiac ischaemic changes [7].

(g) Sequelae to aneurysmal rupture

Following aneurysmal rupture, thrombus adheres to the sides of the perforation with some fibrin infiltration or extravasation of blood in the edges of the tear. Thrombotic sealing is frequent and occurs more readily if the breach is only a partial rupture. A clotting-accelerating factor in the cerebrospinal fluid [226] will promote clotting of blood to reinforce the thrombotic plug.

Ruptured aneurysms have their highest rate of rebleeding on the first day and about 50% will rebleed during the six months after the haemorrhage. Thereafter, the rate drops to at least 3% per year [227]. Rebleeding is frequently fatal. False sacs may rupture or be reinforced by organization of the wall and further thrombosis. The progression of laminated thrombus in the enlarging sac is similar for these aneurysms and those at other sites.

It is possible for a small aneurysm to be virtually filled with thrombus and for organization to occur as in Figure 10.16. Such an occurrence is probably rare. Two such aneurysms were encountered and in each a small residual lumen persisted. Such a sac may be dormant but in view of the survival period, could have been regarded as an example of self-cure. Recent experience has revealed that aneurysmal sacs partially filled with balloons but bearing a small residual lumen near the neck may be followed by dilatation of the small residual lumen with rupture [228].

Some years earlier, ligation of the internal carotid artery in the neck was a favoured therapeutic measure for some aneurysms the purpose being to enhance thrombosis and healing by dampening the blood pressure. This manoeuvre is of uncertain benefit [229]. In some patients there was recurrent haemorrhage from the original aneurysm or a second unsuspected aneurysm. There were also reports of aneurysms on the opposite side rupturing or appearing. The procedure also resulted in aneurysms continuing to enlarge and presenting years later as space-occupying lesions [7]. In view of the demonstrated risk of aneurysm formation due to imbalance of flow at forks on the collateral circulation [187], this procedure requires careful monitoring.

There have been reports of aneurysms spontaneously disappearing angiographically and some of reappearance [230]. Thrombosis may occur spontaneously in some and the thrombus may undergo lysis and excavation with reconstitution of the patency. Other aneurysms progressively enlarge producing pressure effects locally and generally. Local pressure effects are most often nerve compression especially the third and sixth cranial nerves but any of the cranial nerves from the optic on can be compressed. Sometimes there is haemorrhage into a nerve trunk.

Giant aneurysm, classified as such when more than 2.5 cm in diameter, can grow up to 9 cm and more, producing symptoms and signs of a space-occupying lesion. These large aneurysms have a particularly high incidence of nerve palsy but it is likely that their propensity for haemorrhage is reduced. They also are more often associated with pituitary dysfunction due to pressure. Careful dissection is required to determine their true vessel of origin.

Skull changes due to chronically elevated intracranial pressure can occur but otherwise erosion of the anterior clinoid process, expansion of the sella turcica and unilateral enlargement of the optic foramen and superior orbital fissure may be observed radiologically.

Aneurysmal sacs may exhibit calcification and there may also be shift of the pineal gland or displacement of the choroid plexus.

(h) Prognosis

Berry aneurysms have been notorious for a heavy death toll and serious incapacitating sequelae amongst the survivors. At least 50% would be expected to perish but with recent surgical and neuroradiological therapeutic manoeuvres, the prognosis is believed to have improved substantially and no doubt will continue to do so. The giant aneurysms are difficult to manage and the pressure effects themselves can cause considerable disability. However, in view of the frequency of multiplicity of aneurysms the prognosis depends not only on the aneurysm so treated but also on the possibility of another sac that may be already forming.

10.10.6 ASSOCIATED CONDITIONS

The aetiology of berry aneurysms has been cause for much controversy and a number of anatomical and pathological conditions believed to be unduly prevalent in subjects with these aneurysms have often been regarded as suggestive of a congenital or developmental hypothesis.

(a) Anatomical variation of the circle of Willis

Anatomical variations of the cerebral arteries are often regarded as congenital abnormalities and Padget [231] alleged that in cerebral aneurysms such variations were more frequent in those with cerebral aneurysms than in controls, suggesting that this association was indicative of an underlying mural weakness or defective development of the arteries. Stehbens [7,166] concluded that:

1. anatomical variations of the circle of Willis are not congenital abnormalities, nor do they indicate the presence of some underlying hypothetical arterial weakness which might be responsible for the development of aneurysms;
2. the anatomy of the circle of Willis and its branches is as individualistic as a fingerprint as in other animals and other vascular beds which are not associated with similar aneurysms;
3. the variations are of little consequence except for the role they play as collaterals and for their effect on haemodynamic stress;
4. Padget's evidence was invalid [7,166].

Some variations develop because of convenience or a mechanical advantage and interference with the primordial vascular plexus will cause cessation of flow through some channels and compensatory enlargement of alternative channels. The adaptability of the vascular system to changing circumstances is one of the most remarkable features of embryogenesis and angiogenesis, and this applies to the extracranial and the intracranial circulations. To suggest that variations in cerebral arterial topography predispose directly to the development of cerebral aneurysms other than by haemodynamic means is unwarranted, unsubstantiated speculation [7].

The normal circle of Willis is a complete anastomotic polygon and variability of the respective sizes is normal. The classic pattern depicted in textbooks is unrealistic and idealized and the prime function of the circle of Willis is its potential for provision of collateral flow. These views do not preclude the possibility that some variation may predispose to aneurysms or make it unlikely for one to develop at a specific fork.

It has been noted that pronounced inequality of the proximal segments of the anterior cerebral arteries is common when there is an aneurysm on the anterior communicating artery, which then serves as a shunt to equalize flow in the distal segments (Figure 10.22). The haemodynamics of the shunt appears to be the important feature rather than any hypothetical mural weakness for which there is no evidence [166]. No aneurysm has yet been observed at the bifurcation of the basilar artery when the bulk of the blood to the posterior cerebral arteries is derived from the internal carotid arteries. This suggests that reduced stress at such a fork is a factor in the absence of aneurysms at that site.

Of 11 circles of Willis with an aneurysm on one or two internal carotid arteries, the sac was present on the larger vessel seven times, on the smaller twice and bilaterally twice. Such numbers, though too small for statistical analysis, indicate a trend and intimate the importance of the role of haemodynamics in aneurysm formation.

Kayembe *et al*. [232] found a tendency for correlation in cases with asymmetry of the posterior communicating arteries and aneurysms on the internal carotid artery with the posterior communicating artery. Other instances have been reported, such as:

- pulseless disease with occlusion of the right common carotid artery and left subclavian arteries with two aneurysms on the left internal carotid and a basilar bifurcation aneurysm [233];
- basilar bifurcation aneurysm following unilateral or bilateral carotid occlusion [234];
- basilar bifurcation aneurysm and left common carotid artery occlusion, with the basilar supplying both the left internal and external carotid arteries [235];
- occlusion of the middle cerebral artery supplied by the ipsilateral anterior cerebral artery with three aneurysms on the leptomeningeal collateral vessels [236];
- agenesis of the left internal carotid artery and aneurysm of the right middle cerebral artery [237];
- aneurysms on collateral vessels compensating for occlusion of cerebral arteries in seven patients [238].

These observations are further supported by the aneurysms occurring on collateral vessels in moyamoya disease and experimental aneurysm production by common carotid artery ligation in rats and monkeys [187].

(b) Hypertension

Cerebral aneurysms and the ill-effects of hypertension occur mostly in later life when degenerative vascular changes are most manifest. Most authors consider hypertension to be unduly frequent with cerebral aneurysms (and subarachnoid haemorrhage) [7]. This view is not unanimous but a trend is apparent and on theoretical grounds hypertension would certainly aggravate aneurysmal dilatation. Its incidence in those with multiple cerebral aneurysms is higher than in those with a single sac [239]. They have occurred in association with phaeochromocytoma and in general have been regarded as part of the hypertensive complex.

(c) Congenital abnormalities

The coexistence of congenital abnormalities and berry aneurysms is the main argument used in substantiation of the congenital theory of their aetiology. A statistical analysis found the association was not significant and when specific anomalies were considered, their association with aneurysms was not less than the frequency of the anomaly in the population [64]. The only three 'congenital' abnormalities regarded as commonly associated with aneurysms are aortic coarctation, polycystic disease of the kidneys and arteriovenous aneurysms.

(d) Coarctation of the aorta

Aortic coarctation and polycystic kidneys are the only two 'congenital diseases' usually associated with prolonged hypertension and both have an unduly high incidence of cerebral aneurysms. The age incidence of those with coarctation is not the middle-aged group but usually young subjects with a mean age of about 21–24 years [7,64]. Moreover, coarctation of the aorta is associated with severe coronary and cerebral atherosclerosis and other aneurysms usually regarded as degenerative or acquired including post-stenotic aneurysms. Coarctation and polycystic disease no doubt predispose to cerebral aneurysms because of the prolonged hypertension. Even after surgical repair of the coarctation there may be persistent hypertension and the post-stenotic aneurysm may appear postoperatively. False aneurysms at the surgical site and also degenerative aortic aneurysm may develop. Cerebrovascular disease both haemorrhagic and non-haemorrhagic may occur in patients followed up postoperatively and some will be aneurysmal [240]. The possibility is that pre-existing or newly developed cerebral aneurysms may be responsible because pre-aneurysmal lesions have been found even in young subjects with coarctation [204]. However, sudden death in these subjects may be due to one of many possible cardiovascular and cerebrovascular disorders. Many of these subjects have other cardiac defects and Taussig [241] considered that those with aortic valvular insufficiency and coarctation are particularly prone to rupture of the aorta and cerebrovascular accidents. From 10 to 12% of subjects with coarctation die of intracranial haemorrhage, mostly of aneurysmal origin. This is the only cardiac disease that has been associated with berry aneurysms, there being only one case in which a cerebral aneurysm occurred in association with a patent ductus arteriosus [242]. The infantile type of coarctation has been associated only once with cerebral aneurysm [243]. Cerebral aneurysms have also been associated with abdominal coarctation of the aorta [7].

(e) Polycystic disease of the kidneys

Autosomal dominant polycystic disease of the kidneys is associated with hypertension in about 75% of those coming to autopsy and is almost invariably present in those with berry aneurysms. These subjects usually have severe atherosclerosis and may also have aortic aneurysms [7]. The propensity for cerebral aneurysm probably lies in the fact that they have long-standing hypertension from a young age when hypertension is neither suspected nor sought. The incidence of cerebral aneurysm in patients with polycystic disease of the kidneys and a family history of cerebral aneurysm has been estimated as close to 40% [244]. It has been suggested that there may be a predisposition to cerebral aneurysms independently of polycystic disease [245]. The experimental evidence confirms the importance of hypertension in berry aneurysm formation [187]. These subjects with polycystic disease of the kidneys may also suffer primary intracerebral haemorrhage [7].

(f) Cerebral arteriovenous communications

Arteriovenous communications (or malformations) are of undetermined aetiology and many may well be acquired due to trauma rather than to developmental anomalies as is usually assumed. The evidence in humans is that cerebral aneurysms have a particular propensity for the arteries feeding an arteriovenous shunt [7,170]. The malignant nature of these parasitic arteriovenous shunts is often not appreciated nor is how they drain or steal blood from neighbouring arteries by collateral vessels that enlarge. Ectasia and tortuosity with mural thinning characteristically occur in the artery feeding an arteriovenous shunt which may induce a considerable increase in blood flow through the feeding arteries, a greatly increased cardiac output and even a Corrigan's pulse. Whilst berry aneurysms form on the afferent arteries, non-berry aneurysmal dilatations may develop in the tortuous veins and collateral arteries involved in the shunt. The extensive degenerative changes even with aneurysm formation and atherosclerosis have been produced experimentally in herbivorous animals [10,13]. The mural thinning and atrophy that precede berry aneurysm formation readily occur in experimental arteriovenous fistulae [10].

There is now considerable evidence to support the thesis that berry aneurysms associated with arteriovenous communications are acquired lesions and the consequence of haemodynamic stress but the need still exists to follow the natural history of experimental cerebral arteriovenous shunts (in chimpanzees preferably) to document the progressive enlargement, aneurysm formation and involvement of other vessels and in addition to study the regression of both the atrophic and proliferative lesions of atherosclerosis.

(g) Fibromuscular dysplasia (hyperplasia)

Cerebral aneurysms have been reported in several patients with fibromuscular dysplasia of extracranial arteries [246,247] which commonly causes renal artery stenosis and hypertension mostly in females. The true nature of this disorder is unknown but the co-existence of hypertension, sometimes even in the malignant phase, together with profound elastic tissue destruction, gross thinning of the media and proliferative stenotic lesions suggests a complex disorder that may stem from an underlying connective tissue disorder. The vascular lesions may be widespread with deformation of the lumen angiographically (corrugated or 'string-of-beads' appearance) and involve the carotid and vertebral arteries in the neck with transient ischaemic attacks and occasionally occlusive thrombosis. Even post-stenotic dilatations and bruits may occur.

Mettinger [248] suggested that cerebral aneurysms occur in as many as 50% of cases of fibromuscular dysplasia. However, it is of concern that most clinical diagnoses are based on angiographic appearances rather than the vascular pathology. The cerebral aneurysm of one such case was clearly not a conventional berry aneurysm due to the high cellularity (polymorphs and giant cells) of the wall [249].

The string-of-beads appearance and increased tortuosity of the cervical internal carotid artery and vertebral arteries is distinctive but the histology is not always convincing [250]. It has been suggested that the morphology of the affected arteries is similar to that associated with methocel administration in the arterial wall and may be due to an acquired connective tissue disorder [7]. Most of the vascular complications reported are renal artery stenoses, cerebral aneurysms and a few cases of arteriovenous communications.

The association of this disorder with cerebral aneurysm has not been analysed statistically nor studied histologically nor has its true nature been elucidated. Some associations may be fortuitous [251]. There is however a need to investigate the functional and biochemical nature of the connective tissues and until more is known of the disease and its association with cerebral aneurysms, it is unwise to speculate on the aetiological relationship with cerebral aneurysms. The association could be due to the hypertension and the associated destructive vascular changes in the vessel well [7].

(h) Hereditary connective tissue disorders

Collagen and elastin are the two fibrous proteins primarily responsible for the tensile strength of the vessel wall and hereditary metabolic disorders of connective tissues understandably may predispose to aneurysms.

Ehlers–Danlos syndrome (hyperelastosis cutis)

This is a heterogeneous group of inherited metabolic collagen disorders of which type IV manifests a deficiency of type III collagen, arterial fragility, aneurysms of peripheral arteries, vascular fragility, varicose veins, a propensity to haemorrhage from minor injuries, dissecting aneurysm of the aorta, spontaneous carotid cavernous arteriovenous fistulae and rupture of the intestines apart from other manifestations of the disease. The aneurysms and vascular disorders are often multiple and likely to affect the victims at a younger age than most cerebral aneurysms. It is interesting that the varicose veins in this syndrome are associated with arteriovenous communications [226].

Abnormal collagen shaped fibrils and fraying are found in the skin and blood vessels of this disease by electron microscopy. Such changes are observed in many inherited connective tissue disorders in humans and lower animals and are associated with connective tissue fragility. The changes are non-specific and probably acquired since they have also been observed in a variety of blood vessels from lower animals and humans [252] and more recently in the walls of experimental aneurysms and arteriovenous fistulae and cerebral atherosclerosis in man [154,215]. These changes are likely to be the effect of prolonged and severe physical stress and manifestations of the acquired connective tissue fragility which occurs prematurely in connective tissue disorders.

The occurrence of premature degeneration of the collagen fibrils in Ehlers–Danlos syndrome is consistent with the delayed onset of the effects of connective tissue disorders (i.e. fragility). The vessels are liable to disintegrate on handling. This tissue state, if it had existed from the fetal stage, would be incompatible with even the trauma of birth.

The probability is that there may be *formes frustes* of this and other connective tissue disorders as yet to be identified and defined. Pope *et al.* [184,214] assert that some subjects with cerebral aneurysms have a deficiency of type III collagen but without the other manifestations of the syndrome. Since type III collagen appears to be prominent in early intimal repair, its deficiency may predispose to aneurysm formation though this finding does not indicate that all or even most of these aneurysms are due to such a connective tissue disorder. The deficiency of type III collagen in cerebral aneurysms is controversial [185,186]. Nevertheless some cerebral aneurysms, whether familial, single or multiple could be associated with as yet undisclosed connective tissue disorders which are aggravating factors rather than primarily causative. The aneurysm is non-specific, does not require a connective tissue disorder to contribute to its pathogenesis and cannot therefore be regarded as requiring some congenital mural weakness for its aetiology.

Marfan's syndrome

This syndrome is recognized as predisposing to dilatation of the aortic ring with valvular incompetence, ectasia of the ascending aorta, elongation, tortuosity and kinking of the aorta and dissecting aortic aneurysm. It is also associated with saccular and fusiform aneurysms of the aorta and aneurysms of other extracranial arteries. Giant cerebral aneurysms have been reported [253] and in another subject, pre-aneurysmal changes similar to those occurring in non-Marfan subjects were found [254] confirming the concept that the pathogenesis of berry aneurysms is the same. It is likely that this association is more frequent than has been recognized to date and that aneurysms should be sought in these subjects.

Pseudoxanthoma elasticum

The underlying defect is thought to reside in elastin and degenerative changes occur with pronounced premature arterial calcification and thrombosis with infarction. Hypertension no doubt contributes to the premature arterial degeneration which is associated with myocardial infarction and fibrosis and also aneurysms, aortic dilatation, widespread arterial calcification and occlusions and even phlebectasia, all of which are consistent with loss of tensile strength of the connective tissues. Cerebral aneurysms and carotid cavernous fistula have been reported [255–257] in this rare disease. A ruptured aneurysm of a tortuous anterior spinal artery participating in collateral circulation occurred in another afflicted subject [258].

(i) Multiple progressive intracranial arterial occlusions (moyamoya disease)

This disease, first described in and occurring principally in Japanese, occurs mostly in the those under 21 years of age. Subarachnoid haemorrhage is the commonest initial clinical manifestation in those over 21 years of age. The syndrome is associated most often with bilateral occlusion of the internal carotid arteries at the level of the atlas, but sometimes at the level of the fourth cervical vertebra. Less frequently the occlusion is unilateral. The occlusions may have been the result of an arteritis [7] with carotid occlusion early in life in view of the young age of the subjects. Angiographically there is an angiomatous vascular network of dilated collateral vessels at the base of the brain and in the pial circulation. The vascular network appears to be a massive collateral circulation and has been likened to a rete mirabile or even an arteriovenous aneurysm. It compensates for the arterial occlusions and consists of transdural communications from the external carotid arteries to branches of the internal carotid arteries and enlarged perforating vessels of the anterior choroidal and posterior cerebral arteries.

Histologically these vessels exhibit lipohyalinosis, occluded and recanalized vessels, fibrin infiltration in the wall, severe fibrosis, thrombosis and miliary aneurysm which could be responsible for the fatal haemorrhage although berry aneurysms of the circle of Willis also occur in these subjects [259,260]. Even a large lenticulostriate aneurysm has been reported [261]. Ultrastructurally the moyamoya vessels exhibit severe degenerative changes similar to those of 'hypertensive patients who died with massive intracerebral haemorrhage' and to those described in human atherosclerotic intima [208,209], i.e. intimal thickening, degeneration and atrophy of smooth muscle cells, muscle cell debris (matrix vesicles), redundant basement membrane, medial thinning and necrotic muscle cells. Some vessels have been occluded. Little lipid was thought to have been present [262].

Tortuosity and ectasia are characteristic of collateral vessels which are prone to bleed either by direct rupture or from a large saccular or berry aneurysm, collateral vessels having a propensity to rupture [7]. The occlusion, no matter the cause, appears to be the primary event and the collateral vessels are secondary with aneurysms resulting from the haemodynamic stresses associated with the augmented flow.

(j) Miscellaneous associated disorders

Due to the frequency of berry aneurysms in humans, it is inevitable that they occur coincidentally with many diseases. Such associations often lead to publication of the finding and the significance of such an isolated association is usually doubtful. Some, however, warrant further study and a pathogenetic association could be significant.

There is ample evidence that a considerable arteriovenous shunt is associated with **tumours**, meningiomas in particular and cerebral aneurysms have been reported in a number of cases [7,263]. Arteriovenous shunts also occur with glioblastoma multiforme (astrocytoma types III and IV), haemangioblastomas, papillomas of the choroid plexus and even metastatic carcinoma but aneurysms have been reported primarily with meningioma. The feeding arteries and veins of the tumour as well as the artery with the aneurysm should be investigated and compared with the known vascular changes arising in experimental arteriovenous shunts.

An intracranial lipoma with a saccular cerebral aneurysm [264] or a fusiform dilatation of associated vessels in a few patients cannot be used to postulate vascular maldevelopment. Considerable information on the vascular pathology is required rather than an angiogram and the possibility of an arteriovenous shunt in association with the tumour as is the case with meningioma must be considered before any speculation is warranted.

Diffuse ectasia of all cerebral arteries and bilateral giant cavernous aneurysms in acromegaly [265] may be associated with **growth hormonal effects** on arteries. Sutton *et al.* [266] reported fusiform dilatation of the carotid artery (29% incidence) developing after radical surgery of childhood craniopharyngiomas, there being no evidence of augmented flow associated with an arteriovenous shunt in these lesions of low metabolic rate. The authors attributed the vascular lesions to surgical manipulation of the artery.

Tuberous sclerosis is rare with many manifestations including angiomyolipoma in the kidneys and aneurysmal formation in the interlobar arteries [267]. A few cases have been reported with cerebral aneurysms with or without polycystic kidneys which also may occur in tuberous sclerosis. The association of tuberous sclerosis and cerebral aneurysm in five young patients is too tenuous to suggest an arterial dysplasia as the underlying origin of cerebral aneurysms although there may be a connective tissue disorder responsible since these associations are in young subjects [268].

Phaeochromocytoma with multiple cerebral aneurysms is an unusual combination in a 13-year-old boy [269] and must be regarded as an anecdotal experience although the intermittent hypertension may have contributed to the lesions.

Cerebral aneurysms have been reported in subjects with **sickle cell anaemia** which is associated with subarachnoid haemorrhage from time to time. An unduly frequent association has been alleged between sickle-cell anaemia and cerebral aneurysms [270]. The few case reports on record do not support this contention which requires further supportive evidence, nor is there evidence of grossly increased frequency amongst the Negro population of Africa [271]. The association may be fortuitous and there seems to be no corresponding association when other types of anaemia are under consideration.

Systemic lupus erythematosus is known to have a predilection for the cardiovascular system with hypertension being found in such patients. Aneurysms of cerebral arteries have been reported. Whilst some may be associated with autoimmune arteritis and even fungal arteritis, in several instances there is no specific evidence of an arteritis as the underlying pathological mechanism [272]. Hypertension may be contributory and the prolonged steroid therapy a further risk.

A history of orbital pain or **headache**, distinct from that of subarachnoid haemorrhage, is common in patients with cerebral aneurysms [188]. The headaches are frequently considered to be associated with vascular or vasomotor changes. The pain may be due to migraine or to pressure or stretching of a nerve by an aneurysm or even to stretching of the artery or sac itself. However, such concepts are speculative. Migraine has been considered a frequent precursor of cerebral aneurysmal dilatation and ophthalmoplegic migraine, once a known entity, is rarely heard of in modern times. Usually the oculomotor nerve is affected and this could be due to aneurysmal pressure by a sac in the internal carotid artery. The effect of vasomotor changes in migraine is unknown.

10.10.7 AETIOLOGY OF BERRY ANEURYSMS

The congenital theory of these aneurysms evolved from assumptions and circumstantial evidence which fail to withstand scientific analysis. Features such as multiplicity and familial occurrence are equally supportive of a degenerative aetiology. Both theories (congenital and degenerative) have been analysed elsewhere [7,170,196]. The pathology and pathogenesis reviewed here are consistent with the haemodynamic development of berry aneurysms. Essentially, the early aneurysmal changes are examples of mural atrophy. This has been reproduced experimentally in the afferent artery of arteriovenous fistulae [10,82,85] and at the greater curvature of experimental U-bends [113] where the flux of blood impinges on the vessel wall. The earliest manifestation of such changes is abrupt tears in the internal elastic lamina. The tears are also features of the apical region of arterial forks (Figures 6.18 (p. 188), 10.35, 10.36) and adjacent to the neo-apex of experimentally fashioned arterial forks [273]. They have been classified as atrophic lesions of atherosclerosis.

Hashimoto, Hazama and colleagues [187,274] successfully produced aneurysms of cerebral arteries by ligating the common carotid artery in the neck of hypertensive lathyritic rats and subsequently in monkeys. The aneurysms developed at arterial forks where there was imbalance of flow due to participation in the collateral flow to the opposite side with and without hypertension and lathyrism, both of which served only to enhance their development. Some aneurysms were fusiform but others, typically berry in type, were preceded by mural atrophy. The congenital theory, unfortunately, persists despite scientific evidence to the contrary. The ultimate proof of causality remains, as always, the experimental production of the disease.

Ligation of the common or internal carotid artery in man has often been performed therapeutically. Although there has not been adequate follow-up, anecdotal evidence suggests that some aneurysms present years later as space-occupying lesions. From the above investigations it is possible that aneurysms may develop in vessels participating in the collateral flow secondarily to ligation or thrombotic occlusion of the internal carotid or vertebral arteries as indicated in section 10.10.6(a). This concept is further supported by the development of aneurysms in moyamoya disease. It is also possible that an increased or decreased run-off from a branch might lead to similar imbalance of flow at the fork sufficient to contribute to the atrophy. Hypertension and connective tissue disorders would enhance this tendency. There is need to determine those haemodynamic parameters most likely to induce the precursor atrophic lesions of atherosclerosis.

Whilst many authors still consider some congenital abnormality underlies the development of cerebral aneurysms, detailed review of the evidence referred to in this chapter and elsewhere [7,170] provides no basis for a congenital developmental error. The recent experimental reproduction of atrophic changes that precede overt aneurysms [10] and the experimental production of aneurysms [187] support the haemodynamic fatigue hypothesis of their production. Such experiments constitute the ultimate proof of causality.

After the formation of aneurysms in man, intimal proliferation develops when often initially there was none or it was insignificant. To examine the effect of aneurysmal haemodynamics on the sac wall, three types of venous pouch aneurysm (berry, fusiform and lateral saccular) were fashioned by microvascular surgery in rabbits. In each instance intimal proliferation occurred, elastic tissue and medial degeneration were pronounced and overt atherosclerosis histologically and ultrastructurally identical to the human disease developed [38,39], indicating that most of the mural changes in the walls of berry aneurysms are secondary events.

It must be concluded that cerebral berry aneurysms are acquired degenerative lesions intimately related aetiologically to haemodynamic stresses at arterial forks. Those degenerative changes are in effect nonspecific complications of mechanical failure of the mural connective tissues. The association with an inherited connective tissue disorder in which the tensile strength of the arterial wall is seriously diminished usually after a lag period of up to 20 years, indicates that the aneurysms can be secondary complications of a primary connective tissue disease. It does not follow that all subjects with berry aneurysms have connective tissue disorders which, like hypertension, have an aggravating effect on the pathogenesis of berry aneurysms, but not being essential they cannot, therefore, be causal.

10.10.8 ANEURYSMS OF THE SPINAL ARTERIES

Aneurysms of the spinal arteries are uncommon, no doubt because of their small calibre and infrequency of severe atherosclerosis even though their physiological environment and histology are similar to those of the cerebral vessels. Mycotic and traumatic aneurysms could occur but are not likely to be found due to the infrequency of examination of the spinal canal at autopsy. Most spinal aneurysms have occurred in patients with aortic coarctation or arteries feeding spinal arteriovenous aneurysms.

Enlarged anterior spinal arteries in coarctation participate in the collateral circulation and may exhibit considerable tortuosity. The complications include the anterior spinal artery syndrome (due to spinal artery thrombosis), compression myelitis and saccular aneurysms. Progressive spinal cord compression untreated can lead to a complete transverse cord lesion and also to subarachnoid haemorrhage in addition to paraplegia and sensory loss [7].

Syphilis has been incriminated in the past rightly or wrongly and as well as other inflammatory aneurysms with haemorrhage and ischaemic changes, arteriovenous aneurysm should be sought in other cases.

10.11 Traumatic aneurysms of peripheral arteries

Traumatic aneurysms are rarely encountered clinically and have been classified into false, dissecting and mixed varieties. Dissecting aneurysms are discussed under that heading. The injury is thought to severely damage the arterial wall and either the remnants may yield or a haematoma, limited by thrombus and compressed surrounding tissues, restricts further bleeding by a tamponade effect but maintains continuity with the arterial lumen, as indicated earlier. Some traumatic aneurysms may be due to perforating injuries but blunt trauma can be responsible. When involving small vessels, thrombotic occlusion and disappearance of the aneurysm is more likely than with traumatic lesions of large arteries.

The wall initially consists primarily of fibrin intermixed with perivascular matrix but this will in time become endothelialized with the formation of a neo-intima. An appropriate elastic stain can assist in delineating the original wall and the extent of the injury.

In the systemic circulation, the venae comitantes are also likely to be injured simultaneously thereby producing an arteriovenous shunt and if this is small, there may be no bruit or thrill detectable initially. In the cerebral circulation skull fractures are likely to tear or seriously injure the cavernous segment of the internal carotid artery causing a carotid cavernous fistula or one involving the small peripheral leptomeningeal arteries. Most traumatic cerebral aneurysms are due to closed head injuries (62%). These small aneurysms range in size from a few millimetres to 2 cm and are mostly globular in shape. By virtue of the small calibre of the traumatized artery, thrombotic occlusion is likely but those that persist constitute a serious hazard since the wall initially consists only of partially organized thrombus. Sizeable traumatic aneurysms of large cerebral arteries are probably much less likely to thrombose and so may bleed or undergo repair. The associated mortality of the rupture of traumatic aneurysms exceeds 50% [275,276].

Cerebral traumatic aneurysms may complicate surgical procedures (11%) and about 27% are caused by perforating injuries [277]. Subjects with connective tissue disorders would be more prone to traumatic aneurysms and arteries other than the superficial leptomeningeal branches could be injured by abrasion against the skull or compressed against the margins of the falx cerebri, tentorium cerebelli or the sphenoid bone.

The possibility that rupture or leakage of pre-existing aneurysms may be precipitated by relatively minor head injuries is controversial. Determining the relationship of trauma to aneurysms with bleeding depends partially on the history and also on the nature of the aneurysm. There is no evidence that trauma has ever produced a berry aneurysm although it could precipitate bleeding when rupture is imminent. Trauma may be sustained on falling after losing consciousness and aneurysms of other types are usually distinctive. Assessment of individual cases depends on detailed study of the evidence. This does not preclude the possibility of some injury damaging a large basal artery with the production of a silent traumatic aneurysm detected some years later but this scenario is conjecture.

10.12 Mycotic (septic embolic) aneurysms

There are many types of inflammatory aneurysms, both of infectious and non-infectious origin but mycotic or septic embolic aneurysm applies to an aneurysm due to septic embolism, usually from bacterial endocarditis. A few aneurysms develop as the result of direct spread of infection to the artery from neighbouring tissues but most are of embolic origin. The term mycotic should apply only to those of fungal origin. Unfortunately it is in current usage as indicative of those due to septic (bacterial) emboli. A change in terminology is overdue. These aneurysms are usually complications of intravascular infections, mostly secondary to bacterial endocarditis and less often from infections outside the heart such as those in a patent ductus arteriosus or aortic coarctation. More frequent as complications in the pre-antibiotic era, they still constitute an important class of aneurysms due to the increase in cardiovascular surgery, vascular prostheses and drug abusage.

Bacterial aneurysms in general most often involve the aorta with splanchnic vessels next, followed by the cerebral circulation and the limbs [7]. Not all of these will be of embolic or mesenteric origin and some may appear *de novo* from subclinical infections or in association with a severe pulmonary inflammatory lesion with septicaemia.

Most of these aneurysms complicate bacterial endocarditis and direct spread from aortic valvular endocarditis involves the sinuses of Valsalva with secondary involvement of coronary arteries which is a serious lesion, inoperable in the past. Metastatic involvement of the aorta distally, or of the iliac arteries or distally in the limbs with or without a preceding atherosclerotic aneurysm, is each a well recognized complication, as are sources of embolic lesions to the distal vessels of the limbs. Infected aortoiliac aneurysms are said to be increasing in prevalence probably because of aging populations and the organisms reported in fatal cases include *Salmonella* spp., *Bacteroides fragilis*, *Staphylococcus aureus* and *Pseudomonas aeruginosa* [278].

Bacterial aneurysms may involve the pulmonary trunk by direct spread from pulmonary valvular endocarditis or *de novo*, presumably due to unrecognized transient bacteraemia, but mycotic aneurysms, sometimes multiple, may develop in large or small pulmonary arteries due to septic emboli from infective thrombophlebitis. Pulmonary hypertension, either primary or secondary to multiple thromboemboli or a congenital left-to-right shunt is frequent in these subjects.

The splanchnic involvement includes the renal, splenic, coronary, mesenteric and gastric arteries primarily. However, in view of the large cerebral blood flow, cerebral mycotic aneurysms are more common than any aneurysms of the individual splanchnic arteries, and constitute up to about 20% of all bacterial aneurysms. Whether or not haemorrhage from rupture is more prevalent is difficult to know but surgical intervention is more feasible with non-cerebral vessels than with the leptomeningeal branches of the cerebral arteries.

Cerebral mycotic aneurysms are usually less than 1 cm in diameter. They may reach 3 cm however, or involve one or multiple lengths of the leptomeningeal arteries appearing as multiple fusiform aneurysms. Multiplicity often involving different vascular beds varies from 14 to 50%. They are usually peripherally located on small pial vessels most often branches of the middle cerebral arteries. They can be bilateral and are atypical of degenerative aneurysms (Figure 10.39) being haemorrhagic with rough fibrinous material on the adventitial surface. The aneurysm may contain friable

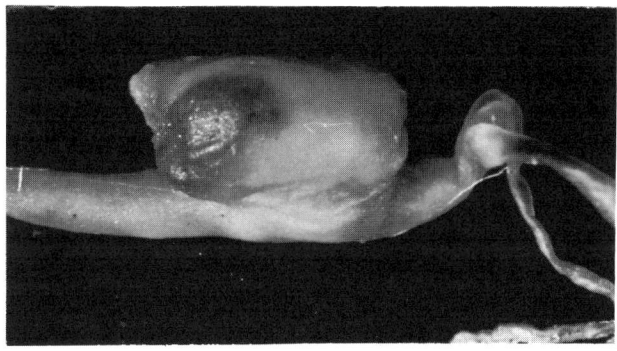

Figure 10.39 Irregularly shaped bacterial aneurysm arising from a cerebellar artery. Note the discoloured wall.

or even purulent thrombus in the sac occluding most if not all of the lumen. Evidence of leakage may be apparent.

Rupture of a cerebral bacterial aneurysm may be the mode of presentation but even so recurrent leakage precedes the final rupture. Aneurysms of other arteries may be associated with an occlusive but painful lesion as the inflammation involves surrounding tissues and the aneurysm is often larger than intracranial lesions possibly because of the thicker walls. It is more likely that the endocarditis will make its presence felt clinically in the first instance, but they may occur *de novo*. The peak age incidence is from 10 to 30 years as is consistent with bacterial endocarditis but they can involve all ages.

The causative organisms in association with subacute bacterial endocarditis are most likely to be *Streptococcus viridans*, and less often *Streptococcus faecalis* or anaerobic streptococci. In acute endocarditis which may be terminal or a complication of an overwhelming infection, the important causative organisms are *Staphylococcus aureus*, *Staphylococcus epidermis*, *Streptococcus pneumoniae*, *Streptococcus pyogenes*, *Haemophilus influenzae* and less often the gonococcus, *Pseudomonas* or even fungi (*Candida* spp. or *Aspergilla* spp.). Uncommon organisms are being reported with increasing frequency.

Predisposing disorders are rheumatic and congenital heart disease, cardiac valvular surgery, insertion of prostheses and intravenous drug abusage. Infectious aneurysms may also occur in meningitis in immunocompromised patients receiving chemotherapy [279].

The pathogenesis of mycotic aneurysms has not been studied experimentally in detail and it is assumed that the friable emboli of all sizes are shed and in only some will an embolus induce an arteritis, or bacteria may gain entrance through an endothelial discontinuity, possibly even adherent to one or a few platelets. Once the arteritis is established destruction will initiate thrombosis. The thrombus may not be sufficient to prevent dilatation and rupture because it too will be invaded by the bacteria. Molinari *et al.* [280] reported that aneurysms usually occurred proximal to bacteria-infected foreign body emboli experimentally, raising the possibility that the arterial pulse may have contributed to aneurysmal dilatation of the arteritic wall. A septic embolus, initiating the arteritis, may migrate distally extending the area of arteritis. Histologically the destruction of the wall can be extreme (Figure 10.40) with extensive loss of the internal elastic lamina especially in the presence of leucocytic elastolytic activity. Yielding of the wall with leakage may be partly offset by protective thrombus but the arterial wall will yield, with haemorrhage a risk at any time. The wall may be so weak that haemorrhage occurs without prior dilatation. The contour of the wall may suggest aneurysmal dilatation but histologically the lumen is filled with septic thrombus merging with remnants of the arteritic wall. The possibility of bacteria lodging in vasa vasorum is plausible but there are none in cerebral arteries prior to their development in atherosclerosis. Secondary infection of an atherosclerotic ulcer is a possibility but not likely in the aorta before middle age. Inflammatory changes in the surrounding tissues will vary in severity and extent with small neighbouring vessels liable to be secondarily involved.

The use of antibiotics with these lesions essentially controls the bacteria allowing healing to occur. However, rupture may occur during the healing phase [281] (Figure 10.41). The end result may be an occluded thrombosed vessel with gross destruction of the wall. Appropriate elastic tissue stains facilitate appraisal. Bacterial colonies seemingly become the nidus for calcification which can occur quite early. The problems for the patient and clinician then revolve about the degree of tissue damage in the neighbourhood and in the area of supply, and the residual aneurysm or aneurysms when the vessel is patent, dilated and severely damaged.

Infections of pre-existing aortic aneurysms have been discussed but little is known about bacterial or fungal seeding of pre-existing aneurysms on more peripheral arteries. This must be rare but there have been two cases in which saccular berry aneurysms were believed to have been infected secondarily from a bacterial endocarditis [282].

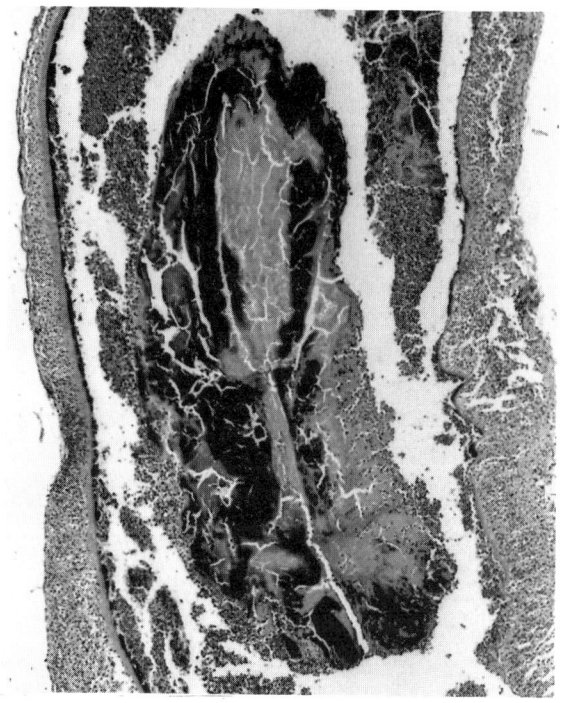

Figure 10.40 Bacterial aneurysm of a cerebral artery. Note the intense inflammatory cell infiltration and architectural destruction of the arterial wall. Bacterial colonies are black. (Haematoxylin and eosin.) (Reproduced from Stehbens [7].)

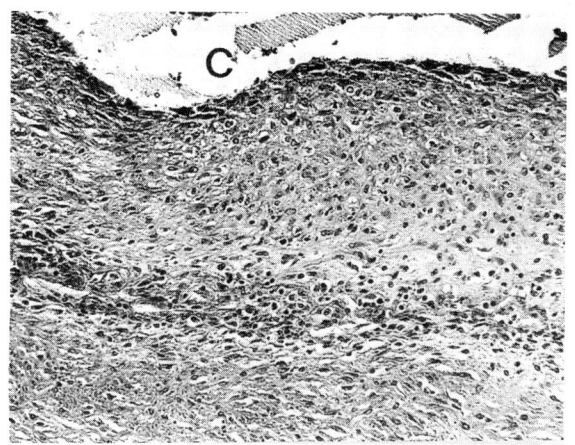

Figure 10.41 Part of the wall of a cerebral aneurysm that ruptured 2 weeks after commencement of antibiotic therapy. No evidence of the structure of an arterial intima was present and the cellular infiltration of the wall is pleomorphic, occurring prior to complete resolution of the infection and healing. The cavity of the aneurysm (C) is above and there is fibrous tissue externally (below). (Haematoxylin and eosin.)

When considering aneurysms secondary to septic emboli, it must be stressed that with the exception of neoplasms, there is no evidence that bland non-septic emboli cause aneurysmal dilatations.

Necrotizing angiitis has been reported as the cause of aneurysms in drug abusers [283] and the possibility of co-existing infection in such cases is real.

10.12.1 FUNGAL (MYCOTIC) ANEURYSMS

These aneurysms should rightfully be regarded as mycotic aneurysms. Fungi are rarely the cause of embolic aneurysms. Rhinocerebral mucormycosis is due to an infection by saprophytic fungi of the class *Phycomycetes*. These fungi have a predilection for invasion of a growth along the arterial walls causing thrombotic and haemorrhagic lesions. Only an occasional lesion is aneurysmal. These fungi frequently cause pulmonary mucormycosis and embolic spread to the brain rather than endocarditis being the source of metastasis. Other causes may be *Candida* spp., *Aspergillus* spp., *Penicillium* spp. [279, 284] and *Nocardia asteroides*. These result in fatal haemorrhage. Fungal infections are particularly associated with diabetes mellitus and prolonged antibiotic and immunosuppressive therapy with steroids.

10.12.2 PARASITIC ANEURYSMS

Parasitic aneurysms are more common in horses and cattle than in humans. However, arterial destruction, aneurysm formation, haemorrhage and even thrombosis have been attributed on rare occasions to *Angiostrongylus cantonensis*. *Gnathostoma* spp. is responsible in some regions of Thailand for 14–30% of deaths attributed to cerebral haemorrhage. The vascular lesions are said to be caused by meandering nematodes, and multiple small aneurysms similar to traumatic aneurysms develop on small peripheral arteries causing multiple parenchymal haemorrhages [285].

Granulomatous encephalitis and arteritis caused by free-living amoebas of the genera *Naegleria* and *Acanthamoeba* are extremely rare in the central nervous system but the arteries may be invaded causing fibrinoid necrosis of the walls, thrombosis, aneurysms and haemorrhage [286].

10.13 Neoplastic (oncotic) aneurysms

Aneurysmal dilatation of small arteries may be due to metastatic tumour invasion of their walls and this, though rare, is most commonly observed with cardiac myxoma. These myxomas occur most frequently in the left atrium (75%) and emboli to peripheral systemic arteries may be multiple. In 50% of cases cerebral arteries are involved mostly affecting the middle cerebral arteries at times bilaterally. The vertebrobasilar arteries are affected less often and similar aneurysms involve extracranial arteries. They produce multiple occlusions, stenoses and irregular dilatations.

Cardiac myxomas are of two types. The very rare familial variety mostly involving young men (mean age 24 years) is often multicentric and associated with multiple skin lesions (pigmentation, naevi, myxoma), and other tumours of the adrenal, pituitary and testes, and myxoid mammary fibroadenoma [287,288]. The non-familial type is mainly a disorder of middle-aged women (mean age is 51 years) and is usually a solitary myxoma of the left atrium.

The aneurysms are irregularly fusiform or lobulated grey-white swellings not more than 5 mm wide but can be up to 25 mm in their largest diameter usually along small peripheral arteries often near the sites of branch-

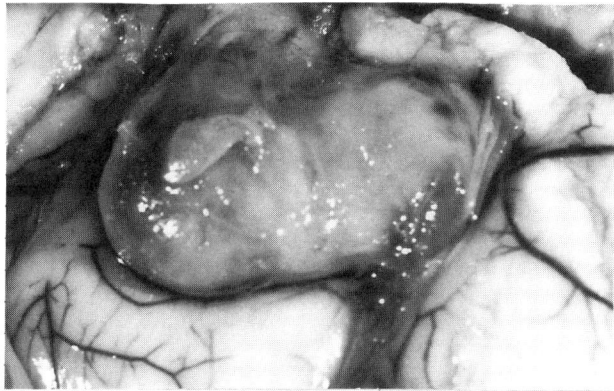

Figure 10.42 Aneurysm of a leptomeningeal artery caused by embolism from a cardiac myxoma (Reproduced with permission from New *et al.* [338].)

ing (Figure 10.42). The myxomatous tissue infiltrates and destroys the architecture producing stenoses and irregular dilatation. The matrix is myxoid containing abundant mucopolysaccharides with stellate or polygonal cells with scant eosinophilic cytoplasm and occasionally multiple nuclei. Connective tissue proliferation in the arterial wall causes thickening and may be secondary to the tumour or to the augmented haemodynamic stresses consequent upon destruction of mural tissues. There is a mild inflammatory response. Diagnosis depends on the presence of the cardiac myxomas with multiple embolic phenomena. Cerebral complications may be the first manifestation of a silent myxoma and are responsible for the deaths of at least a third of subjects with a myxoma in the left atrium or ventricle [288]. These myxoma cells exhibit co-expression of epithelial, mesenchymal and neuroendocrine antigens on immunohistochemical study [289].

Metastatic uterine choriocarcinoma can produce aneurysms in women during the reproductive period and may cause haemorrhagic occlusive lesions or aneurysmal dilatations. Clinically ischaemic lesions occur and subarachnoid haemorrhage is common [196, 290]. Chemotherapy with surgical resection has been successful [290].

The possibility is that oncotic aneurysms may be more common than is currently recognized if angiography was performed in such subjects. However, compression and thrombotic occlusion of the lumen seem to be more frequent.

10.14 Dissecting aneurysms of peripheral arteries

Dissecting aneurysms of peripheral arteries are uncommon, the most frequent being those involving the cerebral arteries followed by those of the brachiocephalic (innominate) or carotid arteries in the neck. They also occur in the arteries of the limb.

10.14.1 DISSECTING ANEURYSMS OF CERVICAL ARTERIES

Dissection of the arteries of the neck may be extensions of an aortic dissecting aneurysm. Those confined to the cervical arteries alone are of two types. Spontaneously occurring dissecting aneurysms of the carotid and vertebral arteries are rare arising mostly in middle age. They may be multiple. Isolated cases may be post-stenotic [291] or associated with Marfan's syndrome [292]. Hypertension is not a prominent feature and the dissection, like all dissections in peripheral extracranial arteries, is usually at the junction of the media and adventitia. Some degenerative changes in the arteries display metachromasia with loss of muscle and elastica and have been likened to medionecrosis of the aorta, but few pathologists are sufficiently *au fait* with the degenerative changes frequently seen in these arteries to assess the extent of departure from the normal. The medial degenerative changes are those usually associated with atherosclerosis in its broad sense. The lesions behave in much the same manner as those of the aorta except that complete occlusion of the vessel is more frequently due to thrombosis.

The second variety is due to trauma such as that due to inadvertent intramural injection when performing carotid angiography. Premature medial degenerative changes would enhance the likelihood of the dissection which can be minor. The dissection is sometimes sub-intimal and produces a flap-like valve but more often it is deeper. Dissecting aneurysms may also be due to indirect non-penetrating injuries to the neck and the arteries may be unduly brittle or fragile. Vertebral artery dissection may be initiated by subluxation of the cervical spine [293]. These dissecting aneurysms can obstruct blood flow to the brain by occluding the original channel or may thrombose. Haemorrhage from such lesions is unusual.

Schievink *et al.* [294,295] drew attention to the combination of spontaneous cervical artery dissection with intracranial aneurysm and a familial occurrence in four families. Since the pathology of these cases is unavailable, it is likely that the underlying disease is non-specific, degenerative and typical of such lesions possibly with a predisposition to premature mechanical failure and acquired weakness of the connective tissues which may at times be inherited. Only in this sense can it be regarded as an arteriopathy. Similarly bilateral involvement [296] or multiple lesions throughout the body must be regarded in the same light and with further knowledge of inherited connective tissues, techniques for assessing collagen and elastin durability will be developed.

10.14.2 DISSECTING ANEURYSMS OF SPLANCHNIC ARTERIES

These are rare lesions and the dissection is usually close to the junction of media and adventitia in middle-aged individuals. The extent of the dissection is limited and likely to be associated with occlusion or a superadded thrombotic occlusion with which it may be confused (Figures 10.43 and 10.44).

Those involving the coronary arteries are more often found in females [297] and more than one third in a literature review occurred in the puerperium, most often in the anterior descending branch of the left coronary. Some have been assumed to be due to congenital defects because of the difficulty in explaining their pathogenesis.

Dissecting aneurysms have also been found in the renal gastric, splenic, hepatic, coeliac and mesenteric arteries [298–301]. They may be associated with

DISSECTING ANEURYSMS OF PERIPHERAL ARTERIES 405

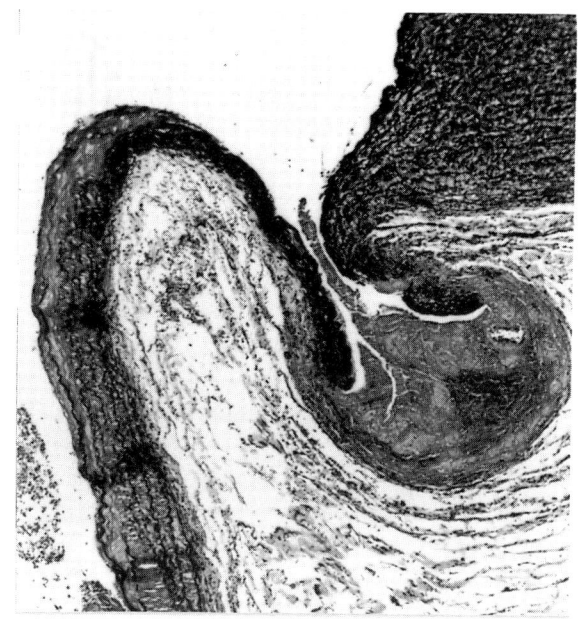

Figure 10.43 Tear of an intercostal artery at its origin immediately beyond an aortic coarctation. The dissection is limited but is at the junction of the media and adventitia with superadded thrombosis. (Verhoeff's elastic stain and eosin.)

Marfan's syndrome and hypertension is not as frequent as with aortic dissection. These lesions also have limited dissection and may be mistaken for arterial thrombosis (Figure 10.44), haemorrhage being rare.

Multiple dissecting aneurysms of peripheral distributing arteries in a woman of 52 years have been reported [302]. The multiplicity of lesions occurring within such a short time span suggests rapid onset of failure, possibly due to a connective tissue defect but abuse of pressor drugs must also be considered.

10.14.3 DISSECTING ANEURYSMS OF CEREBRAL ARTERIES

The brain and cord may suffer ischaemic effects from dissecting aneurysms of the aorta or cervical arteries, not only from arteries obstructed by the dissection but also from thromboembolism.

Primary dissecting aneurysms of cerebral arteries have been recognized with increasing frequency, the dissection being subintimal, i.e. between the internal elastic lamina and the media (Figure 10.45). The tears appear to be transverse. The dissection is of variable extent

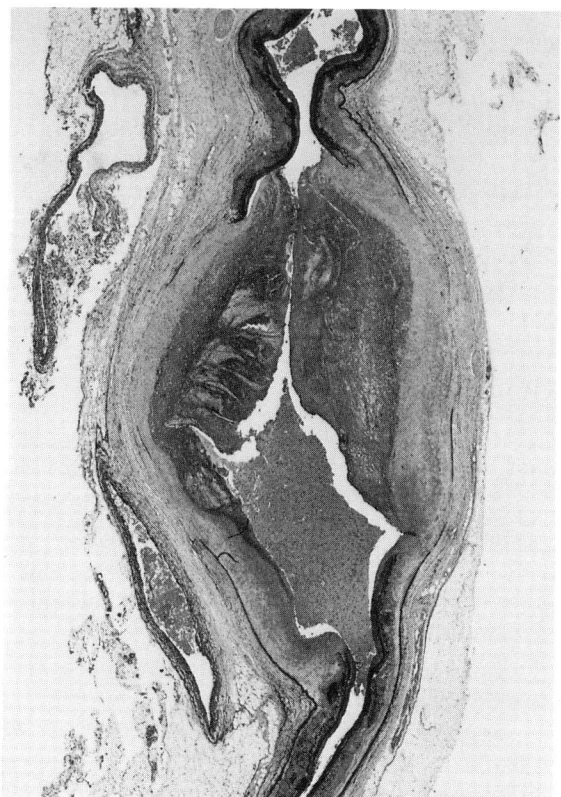

Figure 10.44 Longitudinal section with chronic dissection close to the adventitia of an extracranial artery. Healing has occurred leaving a spindle-shaped swelling of the artery and the mural thrombus is almost occlusive. Note abrupt tear of the intima and most of the media. (Verhoeff's elastic stain and eosin.)

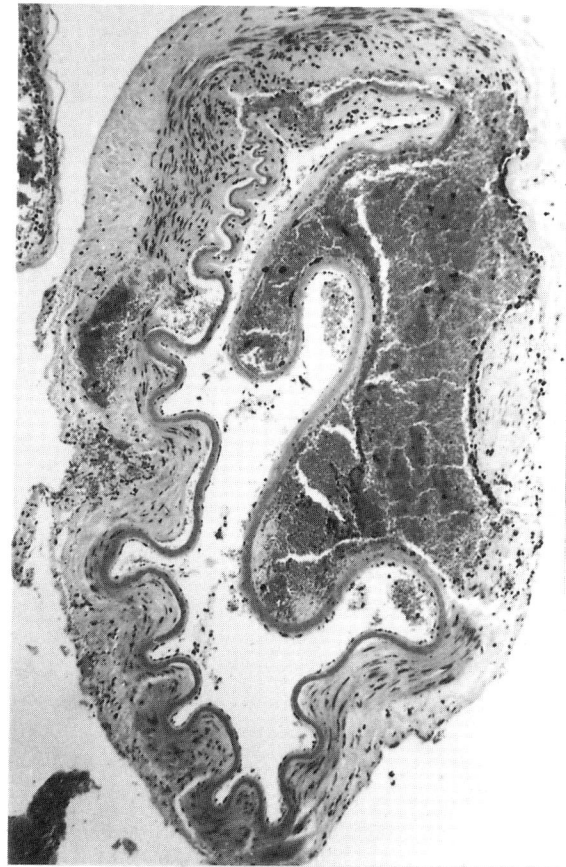

Figure 10.45 Acute dissecting aneurysm of a small branch of the middle cerebral artery with subintimal haematoma and secondary tearing of the media. (Haematoxylin and eosin.) (Reproduced with permission from Stehbens [196].)

and rupture may be external with subarachnoid haemorrhage possibly combined with ischaemia due to luminal obstruction. There may also be a re-entry tear distally with survival as in the case studied by Norman and Urich [303]. Limited dissection can be associated with thrombotic occlusion and unless adequate histological study of the lesion is undertaken (preferably in a longitudinal plane of section), the true nature of the lesion may not be recognized. Such lesions can be mistaken for simple arterial thrombosis (Figure 3.9) and there is obvious overlap between these lesions. Dissections in middle and old age have been reported in association with extreme ectasia and tortuosity (dolichoectasia) [304].

These dissecting aneurysms occur mostly in the second, third and fourth decades with a mean age of 27 years although the range is from six months to 70 years [7,196]. There is a preponderance of males and as yet such aneurysms are unrelated to pregnancy except for one patient who had a dissection 15 days post partum. The arteries display relatively little atherosclerosis and the affected segment is distended, discoloured and resembles a recent thrombus. If there has been external rupture, there may be an extensive subarachnoid haemorrhage with much blood clot adherent to the arterial segment dissected. Fixation of periarterial haematoma for some length of time will make dissection and recognition of the lesion more difficult. The wall may appear to be haemorrhagic and even somewhat dilated. The associated infarct will be pale but there can also be combined intracerebral and subarachnoid haemorrhage. After healing, the affected segment will be narrower and more opaque than usual.

In the case reported by Norman and Urich [303], flow had been re-established and a septum divided the artery into two channels, curiously without new elastic tissue proliferation or the musculoelastic neo-intima that would be expected. More distally the elastic lamina was compressed and incorporated in the wall to one side of the artery (Figure 10.46).

The wall in the region of the dissection may exhibit some dilatation and even become aneurysmal with mural thrombosis but this is unusual. In one case there was an associated traumatic aneurysm [305]. An associated necrotizing arteritis has been observed in a 15-year-old boy who had been on intravenous pressor drugs and such lesions could become increasingly common with an increase in drug abusage.

The middle cerebral artery is the vessel most frequently involved and the dissection may also involve the internal carotid and anterior cerebral arteries. The basilar artery and terminal segment of the vertebral artery or even the commencement of the posterior cerebral artery are also commonly affected. Bilateral dissections have also been reported [306]. Serial sectioning may be required to determine the full extent of the

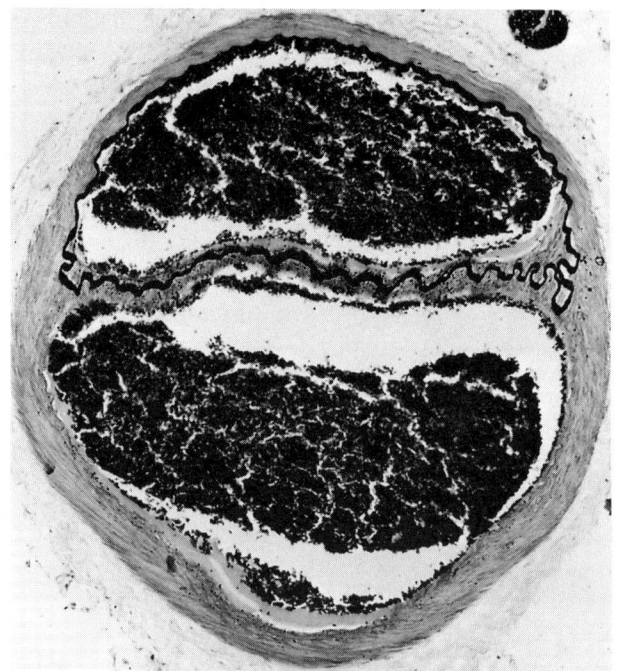
(a)

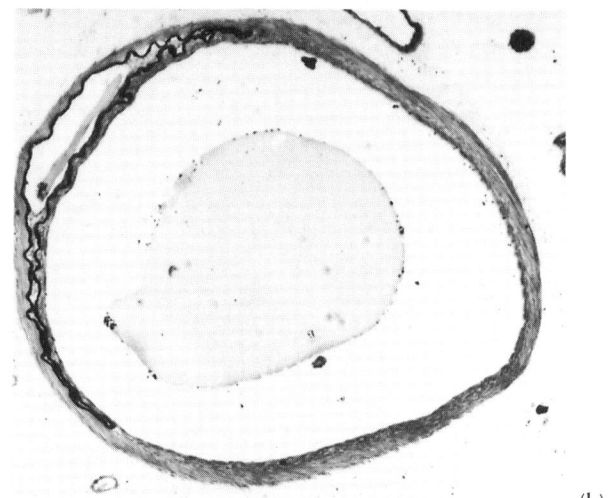
(b)

Figure 10.46 Chronic dissecting aneurysm of the middle cerebral artery with re-entry of the false passage into the original lumen. (a) There is a septum dividing the lumen into a true lumen and a false lumen. (b) The true lumen of a branch is almost obliterated. Specimen obtained years after the original dissection in infancy [303]. Note the virtual absence of new elastic tissue or intima. (Verhoeff's elastic stain and eosin.) (By courtesy of Dr H. Urich.)

tears which are remarkably similar to those involving the internal elastic lamina in the atrophic lesions produced haemodynamically [114].

Cerebral dissecting aneurysms can occur spontaneously or without undue physical effort, but the single most common precipitating factor is trauma, often blunt but sometimes following neurosurgery. The skull is rarely fractured. Many tears occur spontaneously without trauma, suggesting that the stresses associated with head injuries may precipitate tearing of an internal elastic lamina that is already unduly fragile. This tearing of the inner part of the wall is consistent with the concept of the inner part displaying greater fragility than the outer half.

There has been much debate regarding the underlying cause of dissecting aneurysms of cerebral arteries from syphilis to atherosclerosis. Recent experimental studies indicate that such tears can be readily produced by augmented haemodynamic stress and that elastase activity is unlikely to be the underlying mechanism [309]. Mechanical failure seems more likely. Similar tears occur spontaneously in lower animals, are widespread in human infants and are aggravated by hypertension and lathyrism in rats. This suggests that hypertension and inherited connective tissue disorders are likely to predispose to these lesions in humans and also probably to destructive lesions of the media such as drug-induced necrotizing arteritis [196].

10.15 Aneurysms of the microcirculation

10.15.1 MICROANEURYSMS OF THE RETINA

Small dilatations of retinal capillaries and of major thoroughfare channels may be associated with or develop from small capillary U-shaped loops in subjects with diabetes mellitus in particular. Some vessels are merely ectatic. They are also seen in old age, glaucoma, and retinal vasculitis and are prominent in macroglobulinaemia. They occur particularly on vessels emerging from the optic disc [308] and are considered to be diverticula of the capillary basement membrane [309]. Some contain PAS-positive material and lipid [84,310]. There may be leucocytes and increased endothelial cellularity [309]. Fluorescein angiography has revealed they are more numerous than seen clinically and are often perfused only intermittently with nonperfused capillaries in the neighbourhood. These microaneurysms have been found to form and disappear with subsequent formation of new lesions. Pituitary ablation appears to reduce the rate of new aneurysms whilst increasing the rate of disappearance [311]. There is little tendency to rupture but minor haemorrhage may occur.

The nature of these retinal microaneurysms is uncertain. They appear to be associated with increased capillary pressure since they may be induced experimentally by photocoagulation of tributaries of the retinal vein and they occur spontaneously when the central retinal vein is thrombosed. They complicate experimental diabetes in rats and at least some can be prevented by insulin therapy [312]. The tensile strength of the capillaries must be reduced as it is with aneurysms of larger vessels and with the aggravation by diabetes mellitus and increased intravascular pressure, haemodynamic stresses appear to play a role. It is noteworthy that insulin reduces, but does not abolish, these aneurysms and this may also be true of the capillary basement membrane changes elsewhere in diabetics.

Retinal capillary microaneurysms also occur secondarily to retinal vasculitis in which there is considerable retinal periphlebitis with increased capillary pressure [313]. Such aneurysms are consistent with the above pathogenesis. In a recent case retinal aneurysms underwent gradual resolution over seven years [314].

10.15.2 MICROANEURYSM OF SKIN CAPILLARIES

Small saccular aneurysmal dilatations occur at or near the apex of capillary loops in the nailfolds of control subjects. They are more common in patients with progressive systemic sclerosis and related disorders [315]. They may be more frequent in such patients with microangiopathy but since they arise in control subjects, their occurrence is only aggravated by such diseases. They may be related to the retinal microaneurysms but their histology and ultrastructure require detailed study especially during their initiation and development.

10.16 Venous aneurysms

Varicose veins must be regarded as the venous equivalent of grossly tortuous and ectatic arteries. Both phenomena are attributed to weakness of the vessel wall and each can progress to frank aneurysmal dilatation. Many of the large varicose veins should be regarded as aneurysmal since their diameters are often several times that of the original vessel and the dilatations are also localized as in haemorrhoids. Moreover they are prone to both haemorrhage and thrombosis.

Apart from varicose veins, the most common cause of venous aneurysms is an arteriovenous shunt. In arteriovenous shunts the vein can become grossly and irregularly dilated even at some distance from the site of the shunt. Like aneurysms elsewhere they tend to cause pressure effects and are associated with intimal tears, mural thrombosis and haemorrhage following complete rupture. Massive venous aneurysms are seen in aneurysms of the great vein of Galen which is also associated with arteriovenous shunts, the cause being obscure [7].

A solitary vein may be affected as in an aneurysm of the superior vena cava reported by Bell et al. [316]. In this instance trauma was suspected to be the cause. Portal venous aneurysms or those of a tributary, usually in association with trauma, acute pancreatitis or portal hypertension can also be solitary [317]. Even with arteriovenous shunts the aneurysmal dilatation may affect predominantly one vein or a dural sinus such as with aneurysms of the vein of Galen.

Some venous lesions are of considerable size and remain unexplained. They are readily assumed to be congenital anomalies but are more likely to be due to an arteriovenous shunt difficult or even impossible to find. Improved technology in the future may confirm such speculation. Some vena caval aneurysmal dilatations defy explanation [318], e.g. the saccular aneurysm of the superior vena cava described by Hidriegi *et al.* [319]. This 7 cm diameter venous pouch had a fibrous wall and only a small pedicle connecting it with the vena cava. In view of the low pressure in veins, it is difficult to imagine that trauma or inflammation alone could be responsible for venous dilatation of such magnitude without thrombosis. Degenerative changes as in an arteriovenous shunt can induce mural weakness and allow dilatation and should be observable histologically at least in some part of the sac wall.

Small aneurysmal dilatations of superficial veins may be found clinically from time to time in the arm, chest and leg. Large veins such as the external jugular, popliteal and long saphenous veins can also be involved [320]. Histologically phlebosclerotic changes should be anticipated in the wall and can explain associated thromboembolic phenomena that may ensue. They occur primarily in the middle aged and peculiarities of the associated haemodynamics should be sought. In view of the low blood pressure associated with these lesions progression is likely to be slow and insidious. When rapid, it is even more likely that an arteriovenous shunt is involved or again some metabolic connective tissue disorder may aggravate the dilatation.

The probability is that vessels involved in an arteriovenous shunt can thrombose thereby reducing the shunt but leaving behind enlarged ectatic or aneurysmal vessels which persist in a dilated state.

10.16.1 THERAPEUTIC VENOUS ANEURYSMS

Distinct saccular aneurysms are also prone to develop in veins used for venous bypass grafts and in the anastomosed veins of therapeutic arteriovenous shunts maintained for renal dialysis [12]. The changes in these latter veins are similar histologically and ultrastructurally to atherosclerosis.

Venous patches are often used to repair artery walls during some surgical procedures and this segment of vein develops degenerative changes and atherosclerosis. Occasionally a patch may rupture several days postoperatively. The source of the vein may be an important factor in the outcome, those from the lower leg being marginally more likely to rupture than saphenous patches from the groin [321]. It is always possible that rupture may be associated with an occult infection. Aneurysmal dilatation of such patches is also a possibility.

Seven aneurysms developed in a series of 756 glutaraldehyde-stabilized umbilical vein grafts implanted over 7.5 years [322]. The earliest appeared at 31 months and mechanical fatigue together with alteration of crosslinks and immunological factors were thought to be responsible. Dilatation of both the graft and the investing polyester mesh was sometimes associated with mural thrombus and in some instances rupture with haemorrhage and false aneurysm formation. Angiography demonstrated gross irregularity of the lumen in several, an indication of atherosclerosis which was demonstrable histologically.

10.17 Thoracic duct aneurysms

A little known and perhaps more exotic aneurysm is that involving the thoracic duct in association with lymphangiosclerosis [323,324]. Such aneurysms and the pathogenesis of sclerotic changes in the large lymphatic vessels require detailed pathological and hydrodynamic investigation.

10.18 False aneurysms

It is estimated that 4–6% of patients with grafting operations on the aorta or more peripheral arteries develop anastomotic false aneurysms [325]. These false aneurysms may form at the site of any arterial anastomosis, usually a therapeutic procedure because of a pathological process chiefly atherosclerosis. Not surprisingly some sutures cut through the fragile and even normal tissue subjected to the considerable stresses of arterial blood flow. Other factors such as failure of sutures or grafts can be responsible, as can hypertension. Such events may permit the formation of a false aneurysm which, in due course, may rupture particularly when rapidly formed. Some early false aneurysms can be caused by occult infections. Other aneurysms, perhaps not recognized for years, become manifest by occlusion of an artery, ischaemia or a pulsatile swelling and commonly lead to haemorrhage.

Aneurysms especially at the proximal end of an aortic prosthesis for atherosclerotic aneurysm can occur at any time. Those that are early postoperatively are more likely to be false or pseudoaneurysms but those that develop over a considerable period of time should not be so classified. They occur in an atherosclerotic wall at a site of increased stress because of differences in compliance between the artery wall and the prosthesis. Some aneurysms have formed through the prosthesis due to failure of the synthetic graft.

10.19 Iatrogenic aneurysms

Pence *et al.* [326] reported aneurysms 9–20 years after treatment in three of eight survivors from a series of patients treated with external beam craniospinal irradiation and intrathecal gold for medulloblastoma. The three aneurysms involved the posterior cerebral arteries.

They had ruptured and were associated with extensive atherosclerosis throughout the circle of Willis. They were not berry aneurysms and no additional detail was provided. The aneurysms and 'atherosclerosis' of the circles of Willis needed further study presumably since the subjects all died of subarachnoid haemorrhage at a very early age.

10.20 Miscellaneous and unusual aneurysms

Aneurysmal dilatation may occur in vessels of any calibre given sufficient time and any concomitant disease process capable of weakening the mural connective tissues such as in the vessels of telangiectases and retinal capillaries. In addition to the lesions already discussed other lesions warrant attention. Some are associated with or likely to be associated with a metabolic connective tissue disorder.

Cerebral aneurysms in infants are rare and as indicated, are usually traumatic, inflammatory or associated with an arteriovenous shunt. Any person presenting with a large number of aneurysms should be suspected of having a connective tissue disorder and any aneurysm, especially atypical lesions, should be referred to an experienced vascular pathologist. For example, in a recent case multiple small peduncular aneurysms arose from the stems of small branches of one middle cerebral artery. The walls were unusually thick and cellular and there were remnants of the media and the fragmented internal elastic lamina [327]. The true cause of such lesions is uncertain and they are not atherosclerotic.

Neurofibromatosis is of two types. Type I is the classic or peripheral type (von Recklinghausen's disease) and type II is the acoustic or central type with bilateral 8th nerve schwannomas and other nervous system tumours but without vascular disorders. Type I neurofibromatosis is associated with stenoses, occlusion, rupture and aneurysms or arteriovenous fistulae of medium- or small-sized arteries. Most of the aneurysms and arteriovenous fistulae have involved extracranial arteries [328,329]. The nature of these vascular lesions is not clear apart from elastic tissue degeneration, concentric smooth muscle proliferation and medial thinning [330]. The skin and joint laxity, easy bruising and the association with aneurysms and arteriovenous fistulae are all suggestive of a mild inherited connective tissue disorder. There is no evidence that the lesions are secondary in any way to adventitial neurofibromas.

Two aneurysms on unusual locations (cavernous carotid segment and a posterior inferior cerebellar artery) were found on a dwarf with the **3-M syndrome** at 8.5 years of age [331]. Joint hypermobility and the frequency of joint dislocations in the 3-M syndrome are compatible with a metabolic connective tissue disorder.

Kahn *et al.* [332] reported cerebral berry aneurysms in three young boys with an unusual genetically transmitted syndrome typified by characteristic facies, pulmonary emphysema, cirrhosis and bilateral symmetrical cerebral calcifications. Insufficient information is available to explain the pathology but the emphysema and berry aneurysms at such an early age suggest that the metabolic disturbances encompassed connective tissues.

Osteogenesis imperfecta is recognized as an inherited connective tissue disorder but a distinctive pathology of the vascular system is not often a feature. Dilatation of the aortic root and aortic valvular insufficiency have been reported. In one subject there was a saccular aneurysmal pouch on the anterior leaflet of the mitral valve together with aortic valvular insufficiency and a torn valve cusp.

The nature of **progeria** is unknown, but the victims are prone to degenerative vascular disease, including coronary heart disease. It is not surprising, therefore, that a 22-year-old progeric woman was reported with bilateral carotid artery aneurysms although the pathology of the vessels was not available [333].

10.20.1 ACID MALTASE DEFICIENCY

The lysosomal enzyme acid maltase (alpha-1-glucosidase) is deficient in the three types (infantile, juvenile and adult varieties) of type II glycogen storage disease (Pompe's disease). Blood vessels are not frequently involved. Glycogen is found in the cytoplasm, autophagic vacuoles or lysosomes with cellular degeneration and necrosis of cerebral artery smooth muscle cells and pericytes of smaller vessels. Small amounts of enzyme activity in the juvenile and adult no doubt explain this longer survival. The extensive involvement of the vascular smooth muscle cells interferes with connective tissue production and function. Fusiform aneurysms of the basilar artery have been found in a few victims [334,335] and associated with late adult onset of the deficiency. In a 40-year-old male hypertensive, there was 'arteriosclerosis' of the basal arteries of the brain and multiple small aneurysms in the brain parenchyma (mostly in the cerebellum) similar to the microaneurysms of Charcôt and Bouchard [336]. Other small arteries exhibited hyalinosis often with perivascular accumulation of haemosiderin-laden macrophages. Changes consistent with atherosclerosis and also evidence of severe smooth muscle cell degeneration and necrosis in the media were observed in larger arteries. A 29-year-old died from rupture of a giant fusiform basilar artery aneurysm [335].

References

1. Stehbens, W.E. (1985) History of aneurysms. *Med. Hist.*, **11**, 274–80.
2. Johnston, K.W., Rutherford, R.B., Telson, M.D. *et al.* (1991) Suggested standards for reporting on arterial aneurysms. *J. Vasc. Surg.*, **13**, 452–8.

3. Shennan, T. (1934) Dissecting aneurysms. *Med. Res. Council Spec. Report Ser.*, no. 193.
4. Klotz, O. and Simpson, W. (1932) Spontaneous rupture of the aorta. *Am. J. Med. Sci.*, **184**, 455–73.
5. Copping, G.A. (1953) Spontaneous rupture of abdominal aorta. *J. Am. Med. Ass.*, **151**, 374–6.
6. Cleland, J.B. (1936) Increase in diameter of the aorta with age. *Med. J. Aust.*, **1**, 818–20.
7. Stehbens, W.E. (1972) *Pathology of the Cerebral Blood Vessels.* C.V. Mosby, St Louis.
8. Ehrich, W., de la Chapelle, C. and Cohn, A.E. (1931) Anatomical ontogeny B. Man. I. A study of the coronary arteries. *Am. J. Anat.*, **49**, 241–82.
9. Vittal, S.B., Luisada, A.A. and Rao, D.B. (1976) Importance of aortic dilatation in the genesis of the innocent systolic ejection murmur of the aged. *J. Am. Geriat. Soc.*, **24**, 366–70.
10. Stehbens, W.E. (1992) Experimental induction of atherosclerosis associated with femoral arteriovenous fistulae in rabbits on a stock diet. *Atherosclerosis*, **95**, 127–35.
11. Gordon, D.H., Rose, J.S., Kottmeier, P. et al. (1976) Jugular venous ectasia in children. *Radiology* **118**, 147–9.
12. Stehbens, W.E. and Karmody, A.M. (1975) Venous atherosclerosis associated with arteriovenous fistulas for hemodialysis. *Arch. Surg.*, **110**, 176–80.
13. Stehbens, W.E. (1990) The lipid hypothesis and the role of hemodynamics in atherogenesis. *Prog. Cardiovasc. Dis.*, **33**, 119–36.
14. McKusick, V.A., Logue, R.B. and Bahnson, H.T. (1957) Association of aortic valvular disease and cystic medial necrosis of the ascending aorta. *Circulation*, **16**, 188–94.
15. Heath, D., Edwards, J.E. and Smith, L.A. (1958) The rheologic significance of medial necrosis and dissecting aneurysm of the ascending aorta in association with calcific aortic stenosis. *Proc. Staff Meetings Mayo Clin.*, **33**, 228–34.
16. Clark, W.S., Kulka, J.P. and Bauer, W. (1957) Rheumatoid aortitis with aortic regurgitation. *Am. J. Med.*, **22**, 580–92.
17. Marquis, Y., Richardson, J.B., Ritchie, A.C. et al. (1968) Idiopathic medial aortopathy and arteriopathy. *Am. J. Med.*, **44**, 939–54.
18. Toone, E.C., Pierce, E.C. and Henniger, G.R. (1959) Aortitis and aortic regurgitation associated with rheumatoid spondylitis. *Am. J. Med.*, **26**, 255–63.
19. Paulus, H.E., Pearson, C.M. and Pitts, W. (1972) Aortic insufficiency in five patients with Reiter's syndrome. *Am. J. Med.*, **53**, 464–72.
20. Junker, P. and Lorenzen, I. (1983) Reversibility of D-penicillamine induced collagen alterations in rat skin and granulation tissue. *Biochem. Pharmacol.*, **32**, 1753–7.
21. Volini, F.I., Olfield, R.C., Thompson, J.R. et al. (1962) Tuberculosis of the aorta. *J. Am. Med. Ass.*, **181**, 78–83.
22. Reilly, J.M. and Tilson, M.D. (1989) Incidence and etiology of abdominal aortic aneurysms. *Surg. Clinics N. Amer.*, **69**, 705–11.
23. Norman, P.E., Castleden, W.M. and Hockey, R.L. (1991) Prevalence of abdominal aortic aneurysms in Western Australia. *Br. J. Surg.*, **78**, 1118–21.
24. Collin, J. and Walton, J. (1989) Is abdominal aortic aneurysm familial? *Br. Med. J.*, **229**, 493.
25. Tilson, M.D. and Seashore, M.R. (1984) Fifty families with abdominal aortic aneurysms in two or more first-order relatives. *Am. J. Surg.*, **147**, 551–3.
26. Borkett-Jones, H.J., Stewart, G. and Chilvers, A.S. (1988) Abdominal aortic aneurysms in identical twins. *J. Roy. Soc. Med.*, **81**, 471–2.
27. Loosemore, T.M., Child, A.H. and Dormandy, J.A. (1988) Familial abdominal aortic aneurysms. *J. Roy. Soc. Med.*, **81**, 472–3.
28. Tilson, M.D. (1982) Decreased hepatic copper levels. A possible chemical marker for the pathogenesis of aortic aneurysms in man. *Arch. Surg.*, **117**, 1212–3.
29. Senapti, A., Carlson, L.K., Fletcher, C.D.M. et al. (1985) Is tissue copper deficiency associated with aortic aneurysms? *Br. J. Surg.*, **72**, 352–3.
30. Blakemore, A.H. (1947) The clinical behavior of arteriosclerotic aneurysm of the abdominal aorta: a rational surgical therapy. *Ann. Surg.*, **126**, 195–207.
31. Nevitt, M.P., Ballard, D.J. and Hallett, J.W. (1989) Prognosis of abdominal aortic aneurysms. *New Engl. J. Med.*, **321**, 1009–14.
32. Zöllner, N., Zoller, W.G., Spengel. F. et al. (1991) The spontaneous course of small abdominal aortic aneurysms. Aneurysmal growth rates and life expectancy. *Klin. Wochenschr.*, **69**, 633–9.
33. Szilagyi, D.E., Elliott, J.P. and Smith, R.F. (1972) Clinical fate of the patient with asymptomatic abdominal aortic aneurysm and unfit for surgical treatment. *Arch. Surg.*, **104**, 600–6.
34. Darling, R.C., Messina, C.R., Brewster, D.C. et al. (1977) Autopsy study of unoperated abdominal aortic aneurysms. The case for early resection. *Circulation*, **56** (suppl. 2), II-161–4.
35. Ouriel, K., Green, R.M., Donayre, C. et al. (1992) An evaluation of new methods of expressing aortic aneurysm size: relationship to rupture. *J. Vasc. Surg.*, **15**, 12–20.
36. Scott, R.A.P., Ashton, H.A. and Kay, D.N. (1991) Abdominal aortic aneurysm in 4237 screened patients: prevalence, development and management over 6 years. *Br. J. Surg.*, **78**, 1122–5.
37. Coats, J. and Auld, A.G. (1893) Preliminary communication on the pathology of aneurysms, with special reference to atheroma as a cause. *Br. Med. J.*, **2**, 456–60.
38. Stehbens, W.E. (1981) Chronic vascular changes in the walls of experimental berry aneurysms of the aortic bifurcation in rabbits. *Stroke*, **12**, 643–7.
39. Stehbens, W.E. (1981) Chronic changes in experimental saccular and fusiform aneurysms in rabbits. *Arch. Pathol.*, **105**, 603–7.
40. Gore, D. (1962) Rupture of abdominal aortic aneurysm. *Lancet*, **1**, 888–90.
41. Brindley, P. and Stembridge, V.A. (1956) Aneurysm of the aorta. A clinicopathologic study of 369 necropsy cases. *Am. J. Pathol.*, **32**, 67–82.
42. Hunter, G.C., Leong, S.C., Yu, G.S.M. et al. (1989) Aortic blebs: possible site of aneurysm rupture. *J. Vasc. Surg.*, **10**, 93–9.
43. Stehbens, W.E., Delahunt, B., Shirer, W.C. et al. (1993) Aortic aneurysm in systemic lupus erythematosus. *Histopathology*, **22**, 275–7.
44. Patel, K.R. (1992) Ruptured abdominal aortic aneurysms: a new perspective. *J. Vasc. Surg.*, **16**, 661–2.
45. Meissner, M.H. and Johansen, K.H. (1992) Colon infarction after ruptured abdominal aortic aneurysm. *Arch. Surg.*, **127**, 979–85.
46. Tilson, M.D. and Dang, C. (1981) Generalized arteriomegaly. A possible predisposition to the formation of abdominal aortic aneurysms. *Arch. Surg.*, **116**, 1030–2.
47. Crawford, E.S., Coselli, J.S., Svensson, L.G. et al. (1990) Diffuse aneurysmal disease (chronic aortic dissection, Marfan, and mega aortic syndromes) and multiple aneurysms. *Ann. Surg.*, **211**, 521–37.
48. McGee, E.S., Baxter, B.T., Shively, V.P. et al. (1991) Aneurysm or occlusive disease – factors determining the clinical course of atherosclerosis of the infrarenal aorta. *Surgery*, **110**, 370–5.
49. Dobrin, P.B. (1989) Pathophysiology and pathogenesis of aortic aneurysms. *Surg. Clin. N. Am.*, **69**, 687–703.
50. Reed, D., Reed, C., Stemmerman, G. et al. (1992) Are aortic aneurysms caused by atherosclerosis? *Circulation*, **85**, 205–11.
51. Tilson, M.D. (1992) Aortic aneurysms and atherosclerosis. *Circulation*, **85**, 378–9.
52. Busuttil, R.W., Rinderbriecht, H., Flesher, A. et al. (1982) Elastase activity: the role of elastase in aortic aneurysm formation. *J. Surg. Res.*, **32**, 214–17.
53. Herron, G.S., Unemori, E., Wong, M. et al. (1991) Connective tissue proteinases and inhibitors in abdominal aortic aneurysms. *Arteriosc. Thromb.*, **11**, 1167–77.
54. Vollmar, J.F., Paes, E., Pauschinger, P. et al. (1989) Aortic aneurysms as late sequelae of above-knee amputation. *Lancet*, **2**, 834–5.
55. Cribari, C., Meadors, F.A., Crawford, E.S. et al. (1992) Thoracoabdominal aortic aneurysms associated with umbilical artery catheterization: case report and review of the literature. *J. Vasc. Surg.*, **16**, 75–86.
56. Cohle, S.D. and Lie, J.T. (1988) Inflammatory aneurysm of the aorta, aortitis, and coronary arteritis. *Arch. Pathol. Lab. Med.*, **112**, 1121–5.
57. Smith, D.C. and Hirst, A.E. (1979) Spontaneous aortic rupture associated with chronic steroid therapy for rheumatoid arthritis in two cases. *Am. J. Roentgen.*, **132**, 271–3.
58. Halsted, W.S. (1916) An experimental study of circumscribed dilation of an artery distal to a partially occluding band, and its bearing on the dilation of the subclavian artery observed in certain cases of cervical rib. *J. Expl Med.*, **24**, 271–85.
59. Holman, E. (1954) On circumscribed dilation of an artery immediately distal to a partially occluding band: poststenotic dilatation. *Surgery*, **36**, 3–24.
60. Schnoor, E.E., Ellis, E.E., Da Costa, I.A. et al. (1955) Experimental studies in poststenotic dilatation. *Stanford Med. Bull.*, **13**, 351–6.
61. Bruns, D.L., Connolly, J.E., Holman, E. et al. (1959) Experimental observations on post-stenotic dilatation. *J. Thorac. Cardiovasc. Surg.*, **38**, 662–9.
62. Roach, M.R. (1979) Hemodynamic factors in arterial stenosis and poststenotic dilatation, in *Hemodynamics and the Blood Vessel Wall*, (ed. W.E. Stehbens), C.C. Thomas, Springfield, pp. 439–64.
63. Reifenstein, G.H., Levine, S.A. and Gross, R.E. (1947) Coarctation of the aorta. *Am. Heart J.*, **33**, 146–68.
64. Stehbens, W.E. (1962) Cerebral aneurysm and congenital abnormalities. *Aust. Ann. Med.*, **11**, 102–12.
65. Schnitker, M.A. and Bayer, C.A. (1944) Dissecting aneurysm of the aorta in young individuals, particularly in association with pregnancy. With report of a case. *Ann. Intern. Med.*, **20**, 486–511.
66. Maurer, I.C. and Bernhard, A. (1992) Circumferential rupture of the ascending aorta in a fusiform aneurysm. *Surgery*, **112**, 956–9.
67. ten Cate, J.W., Timmers, H. and Becker, A.E. (1975) Coagulopathy in ruptured or dissecting aneurysms. *Am. J. Med.*, **59**, 171–6.
68. Eagle, K.A. and de Sanctis, R.W. (1992) Diseases of the aorta, in *Heart Disease*, (ed. E. Braunwald), W.B. Saunders Co., Philadelphia, 1528–57.
69. Ergin, M.A., Galla, J.D., Lansman, S. et al. (1985) Acute dissections of the aorta. *Surg. Clin. N. Amer.*, **65**, 721–41.

70. Shkrum, M.J. and Silver, M.D. (1991) A prospective study of the morphological aspects of tumor involvement of the pulmonary vessels. *Pathology*, **24**, 146–9.
71. Robinson, G., Siegelman, S., Attai, L. *et al.* (1972) Recurrent dissecting aneurysm of the aorta. *N.Y. State J. Med.*, **72**, 2328–31.
72. Kita, Y., Nakamura, K. and Itoh, H. (1990) Histologic and histometric study of the aortic media in dissecting aneurysm. Comparison with true aneurysm and age-matched controls. *Acta Pathol. Jap.*, **40**, 408–16.
73. Nakashima, Y., Shiokawa, Y. and Sueshi, K (1992) Alterations of elastic architecture in human aortic dissecting aneurysm. *Lab. Invest.*, **62**, 751–60.
74. Gore, I. and Seiwert, V.J. (1952) Dissecting aneurysm of the aorta. *Arch. Pathol.*, **53**, 121–41.
75. Nicod, P., Bloor, C., Godfrey, M. *et al.* (1989) Familial aortic dissecting aneurysm. *J. Am. Coll. Cardiol.*, **13**, 811–19.
76. Braunstein, H. (1963) Pathogenesis of dissecting aneurysm. *Circulation*, **28**, 1071–80.
77. Magarey, F.R. (1950) Dissecting aneurysm due to giant-cell aortitis. *J. Pathol. Bacteriol.*, **62**, 445–6.
78. Watts, A.E. and Dubois, E.L. (1977) Acute dissecting aneurysm of the aorta as the fatal event in systemic lupus erythematosus. *Am. Heart J.*, **93**, 378–81.
79. Gatalica, Z., Gibas, Z. and Martinez-Hernandez, A. (1992) Dissecting aortic aneurysm as a complication of generalized fibromuscular dysplasia *Hum. Pathol.*, **23**, 586–8.
80. Lalich, J.J. (1967) Aortic aneurysm in experimental lathyrism. *Arch. Pathol.*, **84**, 528–35.
81. Paik, W.C.H. and Lalich, J.J. (1970) Factors which contribute to aortic fibrous repair in rats fed β-aminopropionitrile. *Lab. Invest.*, **22**, 28–33.
82. Stehbens, W.E. (1973) Experimental arteriovenous fistulae in normal and cholesterol-fed rabbits. *Pathology*, **5**, 311–24.
83. Turri, M., Thiene, G., Bortolotti, U. *et al.* (1990) Surgical pathology of aortic valve disease. A study based on 602 specimens. *Europ. J. Cardiothorac. Surg.*, **4**, 556–60.
84. Stehbens, W.E. (1979) *Hemodynamics and the Blood Vessel Wall*, C.C. Thomas, Springfield.
85. Stehbens, W.E. (1974) Haemodynamic production of lipid deposition, intimal tears, mural dissection and thrombosis in the blood vessel wall. *Proc. Roy. Soc. (London) Ser. B*, **185**, 357–73.
86. Halme, T., Savunen, T., Aho, H. *et al.* (1985) Elastin and collagen in the aortic wall: changes in the Marfan syndrome and annuloaortic ectasia. *Exp. Mol. Pathol.*, **43**, 1–12.
87. Burchell, H.B. (1955) Aortic dissection (dissecting hematoma; dissecting aneurysm of the aorta). *Circulation*, **12**, 1068–79.
88. Sailer, S. (1942) Dissecting aneurysm of the aorta. *Arch. Pathol.*, **33**, 704–30.
89. Gore, I. (1953) Dissecting aneurysms of the aorta in persons under forty years of age. *Arch. Pathol.*, **55**, 1–13.
90. Cambria, R.P., Brewster, D.C., Moncure, A.C. *et al.* (1988) Spontaneous aortic dissection in the presence of coexistent or previously repaired atherosclerotic aortic aneurysm. *Ann. Surg.*, **208**, 619–24.
91. Yamamura, S., Okadome, K., Komori, K. *et al.* (1992) Acute abdominal aortic dissection and lower extremity ischemia after blunt trauma – case report and literature review. *Int. J. Angiol.*, **1**, 40–4.
92. Cohle, S.D. and Lie, J.T. (1992) Dissection of the aorta and coronary arteries associated with acute cocaine intoxication. *Arch. Pathol.*, **116**, 1239–41.
93. Jebara, V.A., Chauvaud, S., Portoghese, M. *et al.* (1992) Isolated extracardiac unruptured sinus of Valsalva aneurysms. *Ann. Thorac. Surg.*, **54**, 323–6.
94. Jones, A.M. and Langley, F.A. (1949) Aortic sinus aneurysms. *Br. Heart J.*, **11**, 325–41.
95. Sakakibara, S. and Konno, S. (1962) Congenital aneurysm of the sinus of Valsalva. Anatomy and classification. *Am. Heart J.*, **63**, 405–24.
96. Pomerance, A. and Davies, M.J. (1965) Congenital aneurysms of all three sinuses of Valsalva. *J. Pathol. Bacteriol.*, **89**, 607–10.
97. Takahashi, T., Koide, T., Yamaguchi, H. *et al.* (1992) Ehlers–Danlos syndrome with aortic regurgitation, dilation of the sinuses of Valalva, and abnormal dermal collagen. *Am. Heart J.*, **123**, 1709–12.
98. Bartter, T., Irwin, R.S. and Nash, G. (1988) Aneurysms of the pulmonary arteries. *Chest*, **94**, 1065–75.
99. Girgas, R., Kavuru, M.S., Miller, M. *et al.* (1992) Bilateral proximal pulmonary artery aneurysms simulating hilar adenopathy. *Chest*, **102**, 311–13.
100. Hughes, J.P. and Stovin, P.G.I. (1959) Segmental pulmonary artery aneurysms with peripheral venous thrombosis. *Br. J. Dis. Chest*, **53**, 19–27.
101. Shilkin, K.B., Low, L.P. and Chen, B.T.W. (1969) Dissecting aneurysm of the pulmonary artery. *J. Pathol.*, **98**, 25–9.
102. Walley, V.M., Virmani, R. and Silver, M.D. (1990) Pulmonary arterial dissections and ruptures: to be considered in patients with pulmonary arterial hypertension presenting with cardiogenic shock or sudden death. *Pathology*, **20**, 1–4.
103. Mokri, B., Piepgras, D.G., Sundt, T.M. *et al.* (1982) *Mayo Clin. Proc.*, **57**, 310–21.
104. Schievink, W.I. and Piepgras, D.G. (1991) Cervical vertebral artery aneurysms and arteriovenous fistulae in neurofibromatosis Type I: case reports. *Neurosurgery*, **29**, 760–5.
105. Short, D.W. (1975) The subclavian artery in 16 patients with complete cervical ribs. *J. Cardiovasc. Surg.*, **16**, 135–41.
106. Persaud, V. (1968) Subclavian artery aneurysm and idiopathic cystic medionecrosis. *Br. Heart J.*, **30**, 436–9.
107. Javid, H. and De Laria, G.A. (1983) Carotid and subclavian aneurysms, in *Aneurysms*, (eds M.D. Kerstein, P.V. Moulder and W.R. Webb), Williams & Wilkins, Baltimore, pp. 27–61.
108. Hunter, J.A., Dye, W.S., Javid, H. *et al.* (1970) Arteriosclerotic aneurysm of anomalous right subclavian artery. *J. Thorac. Cardiovasc. Surg.*, **59**, 754–8.
109. Markowitz, A.M. and Norman, J.C. (1961) Aneurysm of the iliac artery. *Ann. Surg.*, **154**, 777–87.
110. Padburg, F., Hobson, R., Lee, B. *et al.* (1992) Femoral pseudoaneurysm from drugs of abuse: ligation or reconstruction? *J. Vasc. Surg.*, **15**, 642–8.
111. Quraishy, M.S. and Giddings, A.E.B. (1992) Treatment of asymptomatic popliteal aneurysm: protection at a price. *Br. J. Surg.*, **79**, 731–2.
112. Gifford, R.W., Hines, E.A. and Janes, J.M. (1953) An analysis and follow-up study of one hundred popliteal aneurysms. *Surgery*, **33**, 284–93.
113. Stehbens, W.E. (1986) Experimental arterial loops and arterial atrophy. *Exp. Mol. Pathol.*, **44**, 177–89.
114. Greenhill, N.S. and Stehbens, W.E. (1985) Haemodynamically induced intimal tears in U-shaped arterial loops as seen by scanning electron microscopy. *Br. J. Exp. Pathol.*, **66**, 577–84.
115. Gedge, S.W., Spittel, J.A. and Ivins, J.C. (1961) Aneurysm of the distal popliteal artery and its relationship to the arcuate popliteal ligament. *Circulation*, **24**, 270–3.
116. Buda, J.A., Weber, C.J., McAllister, F.F. *et al.* (1974) The results of treatment of popliteal artery aneurysms. A follow-up study of 86 aneurysms. *J. Cardiovasc. Surg.*, **15**, 615–19.
117. Darling, R.C., Buckley, C.J., Abbott, W.M. *et al.* (1974) Intermittent claudication in young athletes: popliteal artery entrapment syndrome. *J. Trauma*, **14**, 543–52.
118. Berger, H.A. and Stegmann, T. (1992) Aneurysms in popliteal artery entrapment syndrome. *Int. J. Angiol.*, **1**, 35–9.
119. Smith, J.A., Macleish, D.G. and Collier, N.A. (1989) Aneurysm of the visceral arteries. *Aust. N.Z. J. Surg.*, **59**, 329–34.
120. Markis, J.E., Joffe, C.D., Cohn, P.F. *et al.* (1976) Clinical significance of coronary arterial ectasia. *Am. J. Cardiol.*, **37**, 217–22.
121. Aintablian, A., Hamby, R.I., Hoffman, I. *et al.* (1978) Coronary ectasia: incidence and results of coronary bypass surgery. *Am. Heart J.*, **96**, 309–15.
122. Swaye, P.S., Fisher, L.D., Litwin, P. *et al.* (1983) Aneurysmal coronary artery disease. *Circulation*, **67**, 134–8.
123. Daoud, A.S., Pankin, D., Tulgan, H. *et al.* (1963) Aneurysms of the coronary artery. *Am. J. Cardiol.*, **11**, 228–37.
124. Zonerasch, S., Zonerasch, O., Rhee, J.J. *et al.* (1975) Giant coronary artery aneurysm. *J. Am. Med. Ass.*, **231**, 179.
125. Perloff, J.K., Urschell, C.W., Roberts, W.C. *et al.* (1968) Aneurysmal dilatation of the coronary arteries in cyanotic congenital cardiac disease. *Am. J. Med.*, **45**, 802–10.
126. Tsuiki, K., Tamada, Y. and Yasui, S. (1991) Coronary artery aneurysm without stenosis in association with Osler–Weber–Rendu disease – a case report. *Angiology*, **81**, 55–8.
127. Smith, J.C. (1975) Dissecting aneurysms of coronary arteries. *Arch. Pathol.*, **99**, 117–21.
128. Forster, D.A. and Haupert, M.S. (1991) Large mediastinal mass secondary to an aortocoronary saphenous vein bypass graft aneurysm. *Ann. Thorac. Surg.*, **52**, 547–8.
129. Vassanelli, C., Turri, M., Morando, G. *et al.* (1989) Coronary arterial aneurysms after percutaneous transluminal coronary angioplasty – a not uncommon finding at elective follow-up angiography. *Int. J. Cardiol.*, **22**, 151–6.
130. Stanley, J.C., Thompson, N.W. and Fry, W.J. (1970) Splanchnic artery aneurysm. *Arch. Surg.*, **101**, 689–97.
131. Stanley, J.C. and Fry, W.J. (1974) Pathogenesis and clinical significance of splenic artery aneurysms. *Surgery*, **76**, 898–909.
132. Bronsther, O., Merhar, H., Van Thiel, D. *et al.* (1991) Splenic artery aneurysms occurring in liver transplant recipients. *Transplantation*, **52**, 723–4.
133. Ayalon, A., Wiesner, R.H., Perkins, J.D. *et al.* (1988) Splenic artery aneurysms in liver transplant patients. *Transplantation*, **45**, 386–9.
134. Lie, J.T. (1982) Arterial dysplasia and splenic artery aneurysms. *Vasc. Surg.*, **16**, 268–74.
135. Merrell, S.W. and Glovickzi, P. (1992) Splenic artery dissection: a case report and review of the literature. *J. Vasc. Surg.*, **15**, 221–5.
136. Stanley, J.C., Rhodes, E.L., Gewertz, B.L. *et al.* (1975) Renal artery aneurysms. *Arch. Surg.*, **110**, 1327–33.
137. Schwartz, C.J. and White, T.A. (1965) Aneurysm of the renal artery. *J.*

Pathol. Bacteriol., **89**, 349–56.
138. Harrow, B.R. and Sloane, J.A. (1959) Aneurysm of renal artery: report of five cases. *J. Urol.*, **81**, 35–41.
139. Milton, S.H. (1962) Aneurysm of the renal artery and hypertension. *Lancet*, **2**, 1024–6.
140. Dayton, B., Helgerson, R.B., Sollinger, H.W. *et al.* (1990) Ruptured renal artery aneurysm in a pregnant uninephric patient: successful ex vivo repair and autotransplantation. *Surgery*, **107**, 708–11.
141. Gonzales, E.T., Grimes, J.H., Seigler, H.F. *et al.* (1974) Renal artery aneurysm in a solitary kidney: successful surgical repair. *South Med. J.*, **67**, 368–70.
142. Richardson, A.J., Liddington, M., Jaskowski, A. *et al.* (1990) Pregnancy in a renal transplant recipient complicated by rupture of a transplant renal artery aneurysm. *Br. J. Surg.* **7**, 228–9.
143. Savastano, S., Feltrin, G.P., Miotto, D. *et al.* (1990) Renal aneurysm and arteriovenous fistula. Management and transcatheter embolization. *Acta Radiol.*, **31**, 73–6.
144. Hoehn, J.G., Bartholomew, L.G., Osmundson, P.J. *et al.* (1968) Aneurysm of the mesenteric artery. *Am. J. Surg.*, **115**, 832–4.
145. Fortune, D.W. and Östör, A.G. (1978) Umbilical artery aneurysm. *Am. J. Obstet. Gyn.*, **131**, 339–40.
146. Crane, C. (1955) Arteriosclerotic aneurysm of the abdominal aorta. *New Engl. J. Med.*, **253**, 954–8.
147. Pedowitz, P. and Perell, A. (1957) Aneurysms complicated by pregnancy Part II. Aneurysms of the cerebral arteries. *Am. J. Obstet. Gyn.*, **73**, 736–49.
148. Barrett, J.M., van Hooydonk, J.E. and Boehm, F.H. (1982) Pregnancy-related rupture of arterial aneurysms. *Obstet. Gyn. Survey*, **37**, 557–66.
149. Holdsworth, R.J. and Gunn, A. (1992) Ruptured splenic artery aneurysm in pregnancy. A review. *Br. J. Obstet. Gyn.*, **99**, 595–7.
150. Tapp, E. and Hickling, R.S. (1969) Renal artery rupture in a pregnant woman with neurofibromatosis. *J. Pathol.*, **97**, 398–402.
151. Algwiser, A.A. (1991) Rupture of splenic artery aneurysm during pregnancy: three case reports with a review of the literature. *Ann. Saudi Med.*, **11**, 221–4.
152. Dock, W. (1946) The predilection of atherosclerosis for coronary arteries. *J. Am. Med. Ass.*, **131**, 875–8.
153. Cobb, L.M., Bloom, H.J.G., Roe, F.J.C. *et al.* (1971) Rupture of the aorta produced in the hamster by anti-ovulatory progestogens. *Nature*, **229**, 50–1.
154. Stehbens, W.E. and Martin, B.J. (1993) Ultrastructural alterations of collagen fibrils in blood vessel walls. *Connect. Tiss. Res.*, **29**, 319–21.
155. Stehbens, W.E. (1990) The pathology and pathogenesis of intracranial berry aneurysms. *Neurol. Res.*, **12**, 29–34.
156. Stehbens, W.E., Sonnenwirth, A.C. and Kotrba, C. (1969) Microcirculatory changes in experimental bacteremia. *Expl Mol. Pathol.*, **10**, 295–311.
157. Gauter, J.C., Hauw, J.J., Awada, A. *et al.* (1988) Artères cérébrales dolichoectasiques. *Rev. Neurol. (Paris)*, **144**, 437–46.
158. Linksey, M.E., Sekhar, L.N., Hirsch, W. *et al.* (1990) Aneurysms of the intracavernous carotid artery: clinical presentation, radiographic features, and pathogenesis. *Neurosurgery*, **26**, 71–9.
159. White, J.C. and Adams, R.D. (1955) Combined supra- and infraclinoid aneurysms of internal carotid artery. *J. Neurosurg.*, **12**, 450–9.
160. Jefferson, G. (1938) On the saccular aneurysms of the internal carotid artery in the cavernous sinus. *Br. J. Surg.*, **26**, 267–302.
161. Poppen, J.L. (1951) Specific treatment of intracranial aneurysms. *J. Neurosurg.*, **8**, 75–102.
162. Guha, A., Montanera, W. and Hoffman, H.J. (1990) Congenital aneurysmal dilatation of the petrous-cavernous carotid artery and vertebral basilar junction in a child. *Neurosurgery*, **26**, 322–7.
163. Gum, G.K., Nadell, J.A., Numaguchi, Y. *et al.* (1988) Giant aneurysms of bilateral internal carotid arteries in a child. *Child's Nerv. Syst.*, **4**, 161–3.
164. Stehbens, W.E. and Stehbens, G.R. (1985) Flow in glass models simulating vascular junctions under steady flow conditions. *Q. J. Exp. Physiol.*, **70**, 515–26.
165. Shokunbi, M.T., Vinters, H.V. and Kaufmann, J.C.E. (1988) Fusiform intracranial aneurysms. Clinicopathologic features. *Surg. Neurol.*, **29**, 263–70.
166. Stehbens, W.E. (1963) Aneurysms and anatomical variation of cerebral arteries. *Arch. Pathol.*, **75**, 45–64.
167. Gull, W.M. (1859) Cases of aneurism of the cerebral vessels. *Guy's Hosp. Rep.*, **5**, 281–304.
168. Forbus, W.D. (1930) On the origin of miliary aneurysms of the superficial cerebral arteries. *Bull. Johns Hopkins Hosp.*, **47**, 239–84.
169. Stehbens, W.E. (1989) Etiology of intracranial berry aneurysms. A review. *J. Neurosurg.*, **70**, 823–31.
170. Stehbens, W.E. (1983) Etiology and pathogenesis of intracranial berry aneurysms, in *Intracranial Aneurysms*, vol. 1, (ed. J.L. Fox), Springer-Verlag, New York, pp. 358–95.
171. Dalgaard, O.Z. (1957) Bilateral polycystic disease of the kidneys. *Acta Med. Scand.*, **158** (suppl. 328), 1–255.
172. Carroll, R.E. and Haddon, N. (1964) Birth characteristics of persons dying of cerebral aneurysms. *J. Chron. Dis.*, **17**, 705–11.
173. Bannerman, R.M., Ingall, G.B. and Graf, C.J. (1970) The familial occurrence of intracranial aneurysms. *Neurology*, **20**, 283–92.
174. Endtz, L.J. (1968) Familial incidence of intracranial aneurysms. *Acta Neuropathol.*, **19**, 297–305.
175. Lozano, A.M. and Leblanc, R. (1987) Familial intracranial aneurysms. *J. Neurosurg.*, **66**, 522–8.
176. Norrgård, Ö., Angquist, K.-A., Fodstad, H. *et al.* (1987) Intracranial aneurysms and heredity. *Neurosurgery*, **20**, 236–9.
177. ter Berg, H.W.M., Dippel, D.W.J., Limburg, M. *et al.* (1992) Familial intracranial aneurysm. *Stroke*, **23**, 1024–30.
178. Shinton, R., Palsingh, J. and Williams, B. (1991) Cerebral haemorrhage and berry aneurysm: evidence from a family for a pattern of autosomal dominant inheritance. *J. Neurol. Neurosurg. Psychiat.*, **54**, 838–40.
179. Evans, T.W., Venning, M.C., Craig, F.A.S. *et al.* (1981) Dominant inheritance of intracranial berry aneurysm. *Br. Med. J.*, **283**, 824–5.
180. Halal, F., Mohr, G., Toussi, T. *et al.* (1983) Intracranial aneurysms: a report of a large pedigree. *Am. J. Med. Genet.*, **15**, 89–95.
181. Norrgård, Ö., Beckman, G., Beckman, L. *et al.* (1987) Genetic markers in patients with intracranial aneurysms. *Hum. Hered.*, **37**, 255–9.
182. Østergaard, J.R., Bruun-Petersen, G., Kristensen, B.Ø. (1986) The C3-F gene in patients with intracranial saccular aneurysms. *Acta Neurol. Scand.*, **74**, 356–9.
183. Østergaard, J.R., Brunn-Petersen, G. and Lamm, L.U. (1986) HLA antigens and complement types in patients with intracranial saccular aneurysms. *Tissue Antigens*, **28**, 176–81.
184. Pope, F.M., Nicholls, A.C., Narcisi, P. *et al.* (1981) Some patients with cerebral aneurysms are deficient in type III collagen. *Lancet*, **1**, 973–5.
185. Leblanc, R., Lozano, A.M. and van der Rest, M. (1989) Absence of collagen deficiency in familial cerebral aneurysms. *J. Neurosurg.*, **70**, 837–40.
186. Leblanc, R., Lozano, A.M., van der Rest, M. (1990) Familial cerebral aneurysms and type III collagen deficiency. *J. Neurosurg.*, **72**, 157–8.
187. Hazama, F. and Hashimoto, N. (1987) An animal model of cerebral aneurysms. *Neuropathol. Appl. Neurobiol.*, **13**, 77–90.
188. Locksley, H.B. (1966) Report on the Co-operative Study of intracranial aneurysms and subarachnoid hemorrhage. Section 5, part 2. Natural history of subarachnoid hemorrhage, intracranial aneurysms and arteriovenous malformations. *J. Neurosurg.*, **25**, 321–68.
189. Sato, O., Kobayashi, M., Kamitani, H. *et al.* (1978) Intracranial aneurysms in geriatric patients: angiographic features and angioautotomographic analyses. *Neuroradiology*, **16**, 147–9.
190. Hollin, S.A. and Gross, S.W. (1966) Changing size of an aneurysm. Report of a case. *J. Neurosurg.*, **24**, 473–5.
191. Spetzler, R.F. and Martin, N.A. (1986) A proposed grading system for arteriovenous malformations. *J. Neurosurg.*, **65**, 476–83.
192. Stehbens, W.E. (1963) Cerebral aneurysms of animals other than man. *J. Pathol. Bacteriol.*, **86**, 161–8.
193. Zacks, D.J. (1978) Multiple intracranial aneurysms. *Am. J. Roentgen.*, **130**, 180–2.
194. Andrews, R.J. and Spiegel, P.K. (1979) Intracranial aneurysms. *J. Neurosurg.*, **51**, 27–32.
195. Snyckers, F.D. and Drake, C.G. (1973) Aneurysm of the distal anterior cerebral artery. *S.A. Med. J.*, **47**, 1787–91.
196. Stehbens, W.E. (1983) The pathology of intracranial arterial aneurysms and their complications, in *Intracranial Aneurysms*, vol. 1, (ed. J.L. Fox), Springer-Verlag, New York, 272–357.
197. San-Galli, F., Leman, C., Kien, P. *et al.* (1992) Cerebral arterial fenestrations associated with intracranial saccular aneurysms. *Neurosurgery*, **30**, 279–83.
198. Kalia, K.K., Pollack, I.F. and Yonas, H. (1992) A partially thrombosed fenestrated basilar artery mimicking an aneurysm of the vertebrobasilar junction: case report. *Neurosurgery*, **30**, 276–8.
199. Stehbens, W.E. (1982) Intracranial berry aneurysms in infancy. *Surg. Neurol.*, **18**, 58–60.
200. Ferguson, G.G. (1970) Turbulence in human intracranial saccular aneurysm. *J. Neurosurg.*, **33**, 485–97.
201. Aaslid, R. and Nornes, H. (1984) Musical murmurs in human cerebral arteries after subarachnoid hemorrhage. *J. Neurosurg.*, **60**, 32–6.
202. Stehbens, W.E. (1958) Intracranial arterial aneurysms and atherosclerosis, Thesis, University of Sydney.
203. Nyström, S.H.M. (1970) On factors related to growth and rupture of intracranial aneurysms. *Acta Neuropathol.*, **16**, 64–72.
204. Stehbens, W.E. (1963) Histopathology of cerebral aneurysms. *Arch. Neurol.*, **8**, 272–85.
205. Hegedüs, K. (1985) Reticular fiber deficiency in the intracranial arteries of patients with dissecting aneurysm and review of possible pathogenesis of previously reported cases. *Eur. Arch. Psychiat. Neurol. Sci.*, **235**, 102–6.
206. Hegedüs, K. (1984) Some observations on reticular fibres in the media of the major cerebral arteries. *Surg. Neurol.*, **22**, 301–7.
207. Chyatte, D., Reilly, J. and Tilson, M.D. (1990) Morphometric analysis of reticular and elastin fibers in the cerebral arteries of patients with intracranial aneurysms. *Neurosurgery*, **26**, 939–43.

208. Stehbens, W.E. (1975) Ultrastructure of aneurysms. *Arch. Neurol.*, **32**, 798–807.
209. Stehbens, W.E. (1975) Cerebral atherosclerosis. *Arch. Pathol.*, **99**, 582–91.
210. Andrus, S.B., Portman, O.W. and Riopelle, A.J. (1968) Comparative studies of spontaneous and experimental atherosclerosis in primates. II. Lesions in chimpanzees including myocardial infarction and cerebral aneurysms. *Prog. Biochem. Pharmacol.*, **4**, 393–419.
211. Stehbens, W.E. (1959) Medial defects of the cerebral arteries of man. *J. Pathol. Bacteriol.*, **78**, 179–85.
212. Hassler, O. and Saltzman, G.F. (1959) Histologic changes in infundibular widening of the posterior communicating artery. *Acta Pathol. Microbiol. Scand.*, **46**, 305–12.
213. Locksley, H.B. (1969) Natural history of subarachnoid hemorrhage, intracranial aneurysms, and arteriovenous malformations, in *Intracranial Aneurysms and Subarachnoid Hemorrhage. A Co-operative Study*, (eds A.L. Sahs, G.E. Perret, H.B. Locksley *et al.*), Lippincott, Philadelphia, pp. 37–108.
214. Pope, F.M., Limburg, M. and Schievink, W.E. (1990) Familial cerebral aneurysms and type III collagen deficiency. *J. Neurosurg.*, **72**, 156–7.
215. Martin, B.J., Leppien, B. and Stehbens, W.E. (1993) Changes in collagen fibril morphology in experimental aneurysms and arteriovenous fistulae in sheep. *Int. J. Expl Pathol.*, **74**, 267–74.
216. Hubschmann, O.R. and Kornhauser, D. (1980) Cortical cellular response in acute subarachnoid hemorrhage. *J. Neurosurg.*, **52**, 456–62.
217. Koeppen, A.H.W. and Barron, K.D. (1971) Superficial siderosis of the central nervous system. *J. Neuropathol. Expl Neurol.*, **30**, 448–69.
218. Harris, L.S., Roessman, U. and Friede, R.L. (1968) Bursting of cerebral ventricular walls. *J. Pathol. Bacteriol.*, **96**, 33–8.
219. Tomlinson, B.E. (1959) Brain changes in ruptured intracranial aneurysm. *J. Clin. Pathol.*, **12**, 391–9.
220. Crompton, M.R. (1964) Cerebral infarction following the rupture of cerebral berry aneurysms. *Brain*, **87**, 263–80.
221. Crompton, M.R. (1964) The pathogenesis of cerebral infarction following the rupture of cerebral berry aneurysms. *Brain*, **87**, 491–510.
222. Arseni, C. and Nash, F. (1968) Cerebral ischemia in the course of ruptured aneurysms. *Eur. Neurol.*, **1**, 308–24.
223. Fisher, M., Davidson, R.I. and Marcus, E.M. (1980) Transient focal cerebral ischemia as a presenting manifestation of unruptured aneurysms. *Ann. Neurol.*, **8**, 367–72.
224. Stewart, R.M., Samson, D., Diehl, J. *et al.* (1980) Unruptured cerebral aneurysms presenting as recurrent transient neurologic deficits. *Neurology*, **30**, 47–51.
225. Crompton, M.R. (1965) Subtentorial changes following the rupture of cerebral aneurysms. *Brain*, **88**, 75–84.
226. Barabas, A. (1970) The effect of CSF on blood clotting. *Minerva Neurochirug.*, **14**, 314–23.
227. Jane, J.A., Kassell, N.F., Torner, J.C. *et al.* (1985) The natural history of aneurysms and arteriovenous malformations. *J. Neurosurg.*, **62**, 321–3.
228. Kwan, E.S.K., Heilman, C.B., Shucart, W.A. *et al.* (1991) Enlargement of basilar artery aneurysm following balloon occlusion – 'water hammer effect'. *J. Neurosurg.*, **75**, 963–8.
229. Editorial. (1987) Common carotid ligation for intracranial aneurysm. *Lancet*, **1**, 77–8.
230. Bohmfalk, G.L. and Story, J.L. (1980) Intermittent appearance of a ruptured cerebral aneurysm on sequential angiogenesis. *J. Neurosurg.*, **52**, 263–5.
231. Padget, D.H. (1944) The circle of Willis, its embryology and anatomy, in *Intracranial Arterial Aneurysms*, (ed. W.E. Dandy), Comstock, New York, pp. 67–90.
232. Kayemba, K.T., Sasahara, M. and Hazama, F. (1984) Cerebral aneurysms and variations in the circle of Willis. *Stroke*, **15**, 846–50.
233. Masuzawa, T., Kurokawa, T., Oguro, K. *et al.* (1986) Pulseless disease associated with multiple intracranial aneurysms. *Neuroradiology*, **28**, 17–22.
234. Yamanaka, C., Hirohata, T., Kiya, K. *et al.* (1987) Basilar bifurcation aneurysm associated with bilateral internal carotid occlusion. *Neuroradiology*, **29**, 84–88.
235. Sherakawa, N., Murayama, Y., Ueda, S. *et al.* (1990) A case of basilar bifurcation aneurysms associated with common carotid artery occlusion. *Neurol. Surg.*, **18**, 581–5.
236. Ezura, M. and Kagawa, S. (1991) Multiple aneurysms caused by hemodynamic stress and hypertension. *Stroke*, **22**, 1608–9.
237. Tangchai, P. and Khaoborisut, V. (1970) Agenesis of internal carotid artery associated with aneurysm of contralateral middle cerebral artery. *Neurology*, **20**, 809–12.
238. Matsuda, M., Handa, J., Saito, A. *et al.* (1983) Ruptured cerebral aneurysms associated with arterial occlusion. *Surg. Neurol.*, **20**, 4–12.
239. Kwak, R., Mizoi, K., Katakura, R. *et al.* (1979) The correlation between hypertension in past history and the incidence of cerebral aneurysms, in *Cerebral Aneurysms. Experiences with 1000 directly operated cases*, (ed. J. Susuki), Neuron Pub. Co., Tokyo, pp. 20–4.
240. Cohen, M., Fuster, V., Steele, P.M. *et al.* (1989) Coarctation of the aorta. Long-term follow-up and prediction of outcome after surgical correction. *Circulation*, **80**, 840–5.
241. Taussig, H.B. (1947) *Congenital Malformations of the Heart*, The Commonwealth Fund, New York, pp. 464–98.
242. Berthrong, M. and Sabiston, D.C. (1951) Cerebral lesions in congenital heart disease. A review of autopsies on one hundred and sixty-two cases. *Bull. Johns Hopkins Hosp.*, **89**, 384–406.
243. Hirano, A., Barron, K.D. and Zimmerman, H.M. (1959) Ruptured aneurysms of the supraclinoid portion of the internal carotid and of the middle cerebral arteries. *J. Nerv. Ment. Dis.*, **129**, 35–53.
244. Fehlings, M.G. and Gentili, F. (1991) The association between polycystic kidney disease and cerebral aneurysms. *Canad. J. Neurol. Sci.*, **18**, 505–9.
245. Lozano, A.M. and Leblanc, R. (1992) Cerebral aneurysms and polycystic kidney disease: a critical review. *Canad. J. Neurol. Sci.*, **19**, 222–7.
246. Belber, C.J. and Hoffman, R.B. (1968) The syndrome of intracranial aneurysm associated with fibromuscular hyperplasia of the renal arteries. *J. Neurosurg.*, **28**, 556–9.
247. Palubinskas, A.J., Perloff, D. and Newton, T.H. (1966) Fibromuscular hyperplasia: an arterial dysplasia of increasing clinical importance. *Am. J. Roentgen.*, **98**, 907–13.
248. Mettinger, K.L. (1982) Fibromuscular dysplasia and the brain. 11. Current concept of the disease. *Stroke*, **13**, 53–8.
249. Bolander, H., Hassler, O., Liliequist, B. *et al.* (1978) Cerebral aneurysm in an infant with fibromuscular hyperplasia of the renal arteries. *J. Neurosurg.*, **49**, 756–9.
250. Rinaldi, I., Harris, W.E., Kopp, J.E. *et al.* (1976) Intracranial fibromuscular dysplasia: report of two cases, one with autopsy verification. *Stroke*, **7**, 511–6.
251. Lie, J.T. and Kim, H.-S. (1977) Fibromuscular dysplasia of the superior mesenteric artery and coexisting cerebral berry aneurysm. *Angiology*, **28**, 256–60.
252. Staubesand, J., Schmiebusch, H., Seydewitz, V. *et al.* (1981) Matrix vesicles in the walls of arteries subjected to 'load failure', in *Matrix Vesicles*, (eds A. Ascenzi, E. Bonucci, B. de Bernard), Wichtig Editore srl, Milano, pp. 249–56.
253. Finney, H.L., Roberts, T.S. and Anderson, R.E. (1976) Giant intracranial aneurysm associated with Marfan's syndrome. *J. Neurosurg.*, **45**, 342–7.
254. Stehbens, W.E., Delahunt, B. and Hilless, A. (1989) Early berry aneurysm formation. *Surg. Neurol.*, **31**, 200–2.
255. Dixon, J.M. (1951) Angioid streaks and pseudoxanthoma elasticum with aneurysm of the internal carotid artery. *Am. J. Ophthal.*, **34**, 1322–3.
256. Scheie, H.G. and Hogan, T.F. (1957) Angioid streaks and generalized arterial disease. *Arch. Ophthal.*, **57**, 855–68.
257. Rios-Montenegro, E.N., Behrens, M.M. and Hoyt, W.F. (1972) Pseudoxanthoma elasticum. *Arch. Neurol.*, **26**, 151–5.
258. Kito, K., Kobayashi, N., Mori, N. *et al.* (1983) Ruptured aneurysm of the anterior spinal artery associated with pseudoxanthoma elasticum. *J. Neurosurg.*, **58**, 126–8.
259. Yamashita, M., Oka, K. and Tanaka, K. (1983) Histopathology of the brain vascular network in moyamoya disease. *Stroke*, **14**, 50–8.
260. Yabumoto, M., Funahashi, K., Fujii, T. *et al.* (1983) Moyamoya disease associated with intracranial aneurysms. *Surg. Neurol.*, **20**, 20–4.
261. Grabel, J.C., Levine, M., Hollis, P. *et al.* (1989) Moyamoya-like disease associated with a lenticulostriate region aneurysm. *J. Neurosurg.*, **70**, 802–3.
262. Takebayashi, S., Matsuo, K. and Kaneko, M. (1984) Ultrastructural studies of cerebral arteries and collateral vessels in moyamoya disease. *Stroke*, **15**, 728–32.
263. Bloomgarden, G.M., Byrne, T.N., Spencer, D.D. *et al.* (1987) Meningioma associated with aneurysm and subarachnoid hemorrhage: case report and review of the literature. *Neurosurgery*, **20**, 24–6.
264. Futami, K., Kimura, A. and Yamashita, J. (1992) Intracranial lipoma associated with cerebral saccular aneurysm. *J. Neurosurg.*, **77**, 640–2.
265. Weir, B. (1992) Pituitary tumors and aneurysms. *Neurosurgery*, **30**, 585–91.
266. Sutton, L.N., Gusnard, D., Bruce, D.A. *et al.* (1991) Fusiform dilatation of the carotid artery following radical surgery of childhood craniopharyngiomas. *J. Neurosurg.*, **74**, 695–700.
267. Beall, S. and Dalaney, P. (1983) Tuberous sclerosis with intracranial aneurysm. *Arch. Neurol.*, **40**, 826–7.
268. Blumenkoff, B. and Huggins, M.J. (1985) Tuberose sclerosis and multiple intracranial aneurysm. *Neurosurgery*, **17**, 797–800.
269. De Souza, T.G., Beriad, L., Shapiro, K. *et al.* (1986) Phaeochromocytoma and multiple intracerebral aneurysms. *J. Paediat.*, **118**, 947–9.
270. Oyesiku, N.M., Barrow, D.L., Eckman, J.R. *et al.* (1991) Intracranial aneurysms in sickle-cell anemia: clinical factors and pathogenesis. *J. Neurosurg.*, **75**, 356–63.
271. Ohaeghbulam, S.L. (1992) Pathogenesis of sickle-cell anemia and aneurysm. *J. Neurosurg.*, **76**, 1050.
272. Hashimoto, N., Handa, H. and Taki, W. (1986) Ruptured cerebral aneurysms in patients with systemic lupus erythematosus. *Surg. Neurol.*, **26**, 512–16.
273. Stehbens, W.E., Martin, B.J. and Delaunt, B. (1991) Light and scanning

electron microscopic changes observed in experimental arterial forks of rabbits. *Int. J. Expl Path.*, **72**, 183–93.
274. Hashimoto, N., Kim, C., Kikuchi, H. et al. (1987) Experimental induction of cerebral aneurysms in monkeys. *J. Neurosurg.*, **67**, 903–5.
275. Burton, C., Velasco, F. and Dorman, J. (1968) Traumatic aneurysm of a peripheral cerebral artery. *J. Neurosurg.*, **28**, 468–74.
276. Rumbaugh, C.L., Bergeron, R.T., Talalla, A. et al. (1970) Traumatic aneurysms of the cortical cerebral arteries. *Radiology*, **96**, 49–54.
277. Asari, S., Nakamura, S., Yamada, O. et al. (1977) Traumatic aneurysm of peripheral cerebral arteries. *J. Neurosurg.*, **46**, 795–803.
278. Reddy, D.J., Shepard, A.D., Evans, J.R. et al. (1991) Management of infected aortoiliac aneurysms. *Arch. Surg.*, **126**, 873–9.
279. Barrow, D.L. and Prats, A.R. (1990) Infectious intracranial aneurysms: comparison of groups with and without endocarditis. *Neurosurg.*, **27**, 562–73.
280. Molinari, G.F., Smith, L., Goldstein, M.N. et al. (1973) Pathogenesis of cerebral bacterial aneurysms. *Neurology*, **23**, 325–32.
281. Stehbens, W.E. and Manz, H.J. Rupture of antibiotic-treated bacterial aneurysm of an intracranial artery in a young girl. Case report. (Submitted for publication.)
282. Ray, H. and Wahal, K.M. (1957) Subarachnoid hemorrhage in subacute bacterial endocarditis. *Neurology*, **7**, 265–9.
283. Citron, B.P., Halpern, M., McCarron, M. et al. (1970) Necrotizing angiitis associated with drug abuse. *New Engl. J. Med.*, **283**, 1003–11.
284. Davidson, R.G., Nitowsky, H.M. and Childs, B. (1963) Demonstration of two populations of cells in the human female heterozygous for glucose-6-phosphate dehydrogenase variants. *Proc. Natl Acad. Sci. USA*, **50**, 481–5.
285. Nye, S.W., Tangchai, P., Sundarakiti, S. et al. (1970) Lesions in the brain in eosinophilic meningitis, *Arch. Pathol.*, **89**, 9–19.
286. Martinez, A.J., Sotelo-Avila, C., Alcalá, H. et al. (1980) Granulomatous encephalitis, intracranial arteritis, and mycotic aneurysm due to a free-living ameba. *Acta Neuropathol.*, **49**, 7–12.
287. Wold, L.E. and Lie, J.T. (1980) Cardiac myxomas. A clinicopathologic profile. *Am. J. Pathol.*, **101**, 219–34.
288. Vinters, H.V. (1991) Interaction between the heart and brain, in *Cardiovascular Pathology*, vol. 2, 2nd edn, (ed. M.D. Silver), Churchill Livingstone, New York, pp. 1029–71.
289. Curschellas, E., Toia, D. and Boener, M. (1991) Cardiac myxomas: immunohistochemical study of benign and malignant variants. *Virchows Arch. Pathol. Anat.*, **418**, 485–91.
290. Fujiwera, T., Mino, S., Nagao, S. et al. (1992) Metastatic choriocarcinoma with neoplastic aneurysms cured by aneurysm resection and chemotherapy. *J. Neurosurg.*, **76**, 148–51.
291. Anderson, R.McD. and Schecter, M.M. (1959) A case of spontaneous dissecting aneurysm of the internal carotid artery. *J. Neurol. Neurosurg. Psychiat.*, **22**, 195–201.
292. Austin, M.G. and Schaefer, R.F. (1957) Marfan's syndrome, with unusual blood vessel manifestations. *Arch. Pathol.*, **64**, 205–9.
293. Jabre, A. (1991) Subintimal dissection of the vertebral artery in subluxation of the cervical spine. *Neurosurgery*, **29**, 912–15.
294. Schievink, W.I., Mokri, B., Michels, V.V. et al. (1991) Familial association of intracranial aneurysms and cervical artery dissection. *Stroke*, **22**, 1426–30.
295. Schievink, W.I., Mokri, B. and Piepgras, D.G. (1992) Angiographic frequency of saccular intracranial aneurysms in patients with spontaneous cervical dissection. *J. Neurosurg.*, **76**, 62–6.
296. Milandre, L., Pérot, S., Salamon, G. et al. (1989) Spontaneous dissection of both extracranial internal carotid arteries. *Neuroradiology*, **31**, 435–9.
297. Malloch, J.A. (1974) Dissecting aneurysm of coronary artery. *N.Z. Med. J.*, **79**, 914–18.
298. Watson, A.J. (1956) Dissecting aneurysm of arteries other than the aorta. *J. Pathol. Bacteriol.*, **72**, 439–49.
299. Callicott, J.H. and Hoke, H.F. (1968) Dissecting aneurysm of the common hepatic artery. *Arch. Pathol.*, **85**, 681–5.
300. Guerrero, E.C. (1970) Primary dissecting aneurysm of the hepatic artery. *Arch. Pathol.*, **89**, 569–73.
301. Guthrie, W. and Maclean, H. (1972) Dissecting aneurysms of arteries other than the aorta. *J. Pathol.*, **108**, 219–35.
302. Boquist, L. and Berg, P. (1970) Multiple dissecting aneurysms in peripheral arteries. *J. Pathol.*, **100**, 145–8.
303. Norman, R.M. and Urich, H. (1957) Dissecting aneurysm of the middle cerebral artery as a cause of acute infantile hemiplegia. *J. Pathol. Bacteriol.*, **73**, 580–2.
304. Mizutani, T. and Aruga, T. (1992) 'Dolichoectatic' intracranial vertebrobasilar dissecting aneurysm. *Neurosurgery*, **31**, 765–73.
305. Paul, G.A., Shaw, C.-M. and Wray, L.M. (1980) The traumatic aneurysm of the vertebral artery. *J. Neurosurg.*, **53**, 101–5.
306. Adelman, L.S., Doe, F.D. and Sarnat, H.B. (1974) Bilateral dissecting aneurysms of the internal carotid arteries. *Acta Neuropathol.*, **29**, 93–7.
307. Martin, B.J., Stehbens, W.E., Davis, P.F. et al. (1989) Scanning electron microscopic study of hemodynamically-induced tears in the internal elastic lamina of rabbit arteries. *Pathology*, **21**, 207–12.
308. Madsen, P.H. (1966) Aneurysms on new-formed pre-papillary and pre-retinal vessels in proliferative diabetic retinopathy. *Br. J. Ophthalmol.*, **50**, 527–32.
309. Ashton, N. (1963) Studies of the retinal capillaries in relation to diabetic and other retinopathies. *Br. J. Ophthalmol.*, **47**, 521–38.
310. François, J., Neetens, A. and Trau, S. (1969) Retinal micro-aneurysmata. *Ophthalmologica*, **158**, 273–83.
311. Editorial. (1971) Microaneurysms in diabetic retinopathy. *Br. Med. J.*, **2**, 548.
312. Musacchio, I.T.L., Palermo, N., Rodriguez, R.R. (1964) Microaneurysms in the retina of diabetic rats. *Lancet*, **1**, 146.
313. Editorial. (1972) Retinal vasculitis. *Br. Med. J.*, **1**, 480–1.
314. Owens, S.L. and Gregor, Z.J. (1992) Vanishing retinal arterial aneurysm: a case report. *Br. J. Ophthalmol.*, **76**, 637–8.
315. Bollinger, A., Saesseli, B., Hoffman, V. et al. (1991) Intravital detection of skin capillary aneurysms by videomicroscopy with indocyanine green in patients with progressive systemic sclerosis and related disorders. *Circulation.*, **83**, 546–51.
316. Bell, M.J., Gutierrez, J.R., Du Bois, J.J. (1970) Aneurysm of the superior vena cava. *Radiology*, **95**, 317–18.
317. Vine, A.S., Sequeira, J.C., Widrich, W.C. et al. (1979) Portal vein aneurysm. *Am. J. Roentgenol.*, **132**, 557–60.
318. Sweeney, J.P., Turner, K. and Harris, K.A. (1990) Aneurysm of the inferior vena cava. *J. Vasc. Surg.*, **12**, 25–7.
319. Hidvegi, R.S., Modry, D.L., La Flêche, L. (1979) Congenital saccular aneurysm of the superior vena cava: radiographic features. *Am. J. Roentgen.*, **133**, 924–7.
320. Friedman, S.G., Krishnasastry, K.V., Doscher, W. et al. (1990) Primary venous aneurysms. *Surgery*, **108**, 92–5.
321. O'Hara, P.J., Hartzer, N.R., Krajewski, L.P. et al. (1992) Saphenous vein patch rupture after central endarterectomy. *J. Vasc. Surg.*, **15**, 504–9.
322. Dardik, H., Ibrahim, I.M., Sussman, B. et al. (1984) Biodegradation and aneurysm formation in umbilical vein grafts. *Ann. Surg.*, **199**, 61–8.
323. Oberndorfer, Dr. (1925) Atherosclerosis des Ductus thoracicus. *Zentbl. Allg. Path.*, **36**, 225.
324. Kelbling, S. (1937) Über Aneurysmenbildung des Ductus thoracicus mit Atherosklerose. *Frankfurt Zeitschr. Pathol.*, **50**, 34–41.
325. West, J.P., Lattes, C. and Knox, W.G. (1971) Anastomotic false aneurysms. *Arch. Surg.*, **103**, 348–50.
326. Pence, D.M., Kim, T.H. and Levitt, S.H. (1990) Aneurysm, arachnoiditis and intrathecal Au (Gold). *Int. J. Radium Oncol. Biol. Phys.*, **18**, 1001–4.
327. Cedzich, C., Schremm, J. and Röckelein, G. (1990) Multiple middle cerebral artery aneurysms in an infant. *J. Neurosurg.*, **72**, 806–9.
328. Smith, M.A.P. and White, J.A.M. (1974) Ruptured cervical aneurysm with neurofibromatosis. *S. Afr. Med. J.*, **48**, 945–6.
329. Malecha, M.J. and Rubin, R. (1992) Aneurysms of the carotid arteries associated with von Rechlinghausen's neurofibromatosis. *Pathol. Res. Pract.*, **188**, 145–7.
330. Salyer, W.R. and Salyer, D.C. (1974) The vascular lesions of neurofibromatosis. *Angiology*, **25**, 510–19.
331. Mueller, R.F., Buckler, J., Arthur, R. et al. (1992) The 3-M syndrome: risk of intracerebral aneurysm? *J. Med. Genet.*, **29**, 425–7.
332. Kahn, E., Markowitz, J., Duffy, L. et al. (1987) Berry aneurysms, cirrhosis, pulmonary emphysema, and bilateral symmetrical cerebral calcifications: a new syndrome. *Am. J. Med. Genet.*, (suppl. 3), 343–56.
333. Green, L.N. (1981) Progeria with carotid artery aneurysms. *Arch. Neurol.*, **38**, 659–61.
334. Makos, M.M., McComb, R.D., Adickes, E.D. et al. (1985) Acid maltase deficiency and basilar artery aneurysms: a report of a sibship. *Neurology*, **35**, (suppl. 1), 193–4.
335. Matsuoka, Y., Senda, Y., Hirayama, M. et al. (1988) Late-onset acid maltase deficiency associated with aneurysm. *J. Neurol.*, **235**, 371–3.
336. Kretzschmar, H.A., Wagner, H., Hübner, G. et al. (1990) Aneurysms and vacuolar degeneration of cerebral arteries in late-onset acid maltase deficiency. *J. Neurol. Sci.*, **98**, 169–83.
337. Stehbens, W.E. (1988) Atheosclerosis – its cause and nature. *Spec. Sci. Technol.*, **11**, 88–99.
338. New, P.F.J., Price, D.L. and Carter, B. (1970) Cerebral angiography in cardiac myxoma. *Radiology*, **96**, 335–45.

11 ATHEROEMBOLISM: CLINICAL AND EXPERIMENTAL ASPECTS

Bruce A. Warren

11.1 Clinical aspects

11.1.1 DETACHMENT OF EMBOLI FROM ATHEROMATOUS PLAQUES

Atherosclerosis is a disease of large arteries manifested by multiple swellings called atheromas. These swellings in the inner aspect of the walls of the arteries are composed of fibrofatty tissue. The atheroma appears to have a development phase from a fibrofatty lesion which matures to form a pultaceous central mass surrounded by fibrous tissue. The fibrous tissue which covers the atheroma and separates it from the arterial lumen can break down and allow the escape of the central mass of degenerated tissue into the bloodstream leaving an ulcer on the inner surface of the arterial wall. Figure 11.1 illustrates the appearance of the contents of an atheroma by light microscopy. Calcification can ensue in the walls of the ulcer, or in fibrous tissue surrounding the atheroma.

The release by the attrition of the fibrous cap of the atheroma of the atheromatous material into the bloodstream is the genesis of atheroembolism. It is a late phase in the pathology of the atheromatous plaque.

During experimental investigation of atheroembolism, atheromatous material was harvested from human aortas at autopsy. A good yield of pultaceous material from the central part of an atheroma was about 200 mg. Atheromas varied considerably in the nature of their central core. Some 'immature' atheromas contained within the central mass a relative excess of fibrous tissue and the material was thus not suitable for the purpose of grinding and injection of the material in the study of experimental atheroembolism.

Embolism of types other than atheroembolism may be derived from atheromatous plaques. The common variety of platelet thromboembolism may be generated by the irregular surface which is often denuded, at least in part, of endothelium. Fragments and derivatives of the collagen of the vessel wall can be released from the edges, walls and floor of atheromatous ulcers and can be the nidus of thromboembolic episodes.

11.1.2 INCIDENCE AND DISTRIBUTION OF ATHEROEMBOLISM

In studies of spontaneous atheroembolism in general series of post-mortem examination, the incidence has been as high as 4% [1] and as low as 0.79% [2]. If in the autopsy there are major complications of atherosclerosis (for example atherosclerotic occlusion of vessels) then the incidence of atheroembolism is higher: 15.8% in patients with atherosclerotic occlusion of the aorta and 31% for atherosclerotic aneurysm of the aorta which has not been treated by operation. The highest incidence (77.3%) has been found in patients who had a repair of their atherosclerotic aortic aneurysm and who died in the postoperative phase [3].

In the major studies [1–3] of the general incidence of atheroembolism, this disorder was seen only when there was severe atherosclerosis. No atheroemboli were seen when only minimal atherosclerosis was present. The indicator of possible atheroembolism was marked to advanced atherosclerosis of the aorta and it would be expected that ulcerated lesions with an ulcer bed of porridge-like consistency would be most favourable for the production of atheroembolism. These studies provide information on the incidence of atheroembolism at autopsy.

Maurizi and co-workers [1] studied 100 consecutive autopsies and found that 4% showed atheroembolism of the lower extremities. From their detailed examination of 25 autopsy cases with atheromatous emboli they came to the conclusion that embolism of the arteries of the lower limb was greater in incidence than that of the renal arteries, if this region (lower limb arteries) was examined during the autopsy procedure.

The incidence of atheroembolism was examined in 2126 post-mortem examinations conducted at Kingston Hospital, Surrey, UK by Kealy [2], over the period from 1970 to 1977. In autopsies of all patients over the age of 60 years, tissue blocks were removed and studied for atheroembolism. In this large series only 16 showed tissue evidence of atheroembolism (an incidence of 0.79%). The author considered that this was probably a

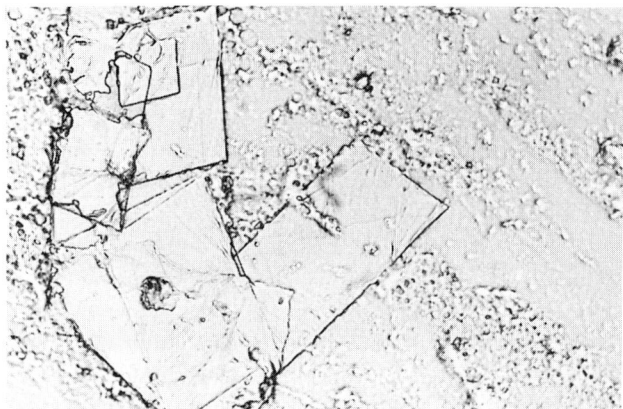

Figure 11.1 Soft centre of a human fibrolipid plaque suspended in saline and spread on a slide. Various irregular forms and occasional rhomboid forms of cholesterol crystals can be seen. Droplets of lipid material are also present.

falsely low incidence because in this retrospective series the incidence was completely dependent upon the number, size and site of the tissue blocks removed at autopsy for microscopy. The 16 autopsies which showed atheroembolism were composed of nine men and seven women and the average age was 76.7 years. In all cases there was marked to severe atherosclerosis of the aorta. Ulceration of the aortic wall with calcification was frequently present and some showed weakening and aneurysmal dilation of the aortic wall. Soft porridge-like atheromas were present in three of the aortas. Hypertension was a constant feature of this group and the erythrocyte sedimentation rate was often increased and sometimes markedly so. The most common site of atheroembolism in this series was the kidney (13 of the 16). Other organs affected in decreasing order were the spleen (7), ileum (3), liver (2), colon, brain, pancreas and prostate (1 each). Kealy found that the sizes of the involved arteries varied considerably. The arteries varied from 150 to 1100 µm in diameter with an average of 464 µm.

The appearances of the atheroembolic lesions appeared to vary depending upon the duration from the time of lodgement of the embolus. Recent lesions lacked a vascular response. In older lesions there were changes such as endarteritic thickening due to fibrosis together with multinucleated foreign body giant cells in some instances. If the kidneys were involved in this disease process gross scarring of the subcapsular surface was visible macroscopically and the kidneys were contracted. Marked ischaemic changes were noted on microscopic examination. The inter- and intralobular arteries were frequently blocked by emboli. Since all patients had suffered from hypertension the kidneys showed the atherosclerotic changes found in this disease. The actual changes due to the emboli because of this background were sometimes obscure. In two patients splenic infarcts were noted. The feeding artery at the apex of the infarct in one was seen to be plugged by an atheroembolus. In one case in which cerebral infarction occurred due to cerebral atheroembolism, a meningeal artery was found blocked by the embolus. In observations of the small and large intestine atheroemboli were noted blocking the small vessels of the submucosa. In one instance damage had proceeded to ulceration and perforation of the ileum. In the pancreas focal areas of fibrosis following atheroembolism were present.

11.1.3 CLINICAL EFFECTS OF ATHEROMATOUS EMBOLI

In 1960 a study [4] recounted the histories of three patients with chronic renal failure due to atheroembolism from severely atherosclerotic aortas. Four more patients with significant renal atheroembolism were described in another study [5]. The kidney, spleen and pancreas were the commonest organs affected. The sizes of the arteries involved were between 150° and 200 µm in diameter. In this series, the principal distinguishing elements of the lesions were the biconvex cholesterol crystal clefts and the intimal cells of the arterial wall which had proliferated to surround the crystals. No associated thrombus was detected but this would not be expected because of the age of the lesions and the fact that the thrombotic response to atheromatous material is an early effect and is extinguished by intimal proliferation and fibrosis. The various end results of atheroembolism clinically are likely to be associated with the persistence or the lysis of the secondary thrombus which occurs.

Kealy [2] found that atheroembolism (presumably persistent) may give rise to a syndrome of eosinophilia, low grade fever, anaemia and a high erythrocyte sedimentation rate. Atheroembolism should be numbered among other possible causes for this syndrome which includes vasculitis, subacute bacterial endocarditis, collagen disorders and polyarteritis. In one of Kealy's cases the patient presented with an increased immunoglobulin (IgG).

Recurrent spontaneous atheroembolism has been considered by investigators [5,6] as a frequent occurrence of severe ulcerative atherosclerosis of the aorta. Gore and Collins [6] collected 16 cases of atheroembolism in a period of a few months. There were three amputated legs and 13 autopsies. Death in the autopsied cases was due to renal failure, myocardial infarction, encephalomalacia and in one instance death occurred during an operation for the resection of an aortic aneurysm. Repeated showering by atheroemboli was found and the lesions appeared to vary in the time from lodgement.

11.1.4 EFFECTS OF IMPACTION OF PLATELET AGGREGATES AND ATHEROEMBOLISM

One study [7] distinguished between embolism due to an atheromatous plaque which becomes dislocated from the arterial wall and the more crumbly emboli comprising cholesterol crystals and other components of the central mass of the atheroma. They termed the former – the embolism of the whole plaque – atheroembolism, and the latter, cholesterol emboli. Because of the lipid solvents used in the production of standard paraffin-embedded sections, the fatty components of the contents of the atheroma are removed and are hence unstained in haematoxylin and eosin stained sections. By terming the embolism of the pultaceous material which results from rupture of the fibrous cap of an atheroma, a cholesterol embolus, the authors deny the important components of lipid and necrotic material which are also present. The term atheroemboli here is used to mean material discharged into the bloodstream from an ulcerated fibro-lipid atheromatous plaque.

Another study [8] suggested that atheromatous lesions could induce two types of emboli:

- emboli of platelet aggregates derived from the irregular and often scarred surface of the atheromatous plaque without any of the deeper contents of the plaque;
- other emboli derived from the depths of the atheroma, consisting of semisolid fragments.

The first variety of embolism is due to platelet aggregation and does not derive any unusual features from its origin from the roughened surface of an atheroma. The second variety is based on its origin from an atheroma and, indeed, contains part of the interior of that lesion.

The disease in humans can be modelled in animals by the injection of material derived from human atheromas [9,10]. These are models of the second type described [8] whereby the soft centre of the atheroma is swept into the circulation. Very occasionally the fibrous covering of a plaque can become loose and continue downstream as a major embolus, often with dire results.

Platelet embolic injury to arterial intima was reported by Lough and Moore [11]. They inserted a magnesium aluminium wire into the aorta of experimental animals above the renal arteries. This produced platelet aggregates in showers and resulted in injury to the intima of renal arterioles which were analyzed after varying time intervals of from 3 to 21 days. A platelet fibrin and red cell meshwork was produced on the surface of the arteriole. Mononuclear cells removed this, and endothelial cells multiplied and advanced into the mass to replace the monocytes. In the smooth muscle cells in association with the presence of lipid, there was vacuolization of mitochondria and fracturing of the myofilaments. Endothelial cells and macrophages were still able to be picked out as separately identifiable types of cells and no cells of intermediate type were found.

The stability of differentiation of the smooth muscle cells in the walls of arteries varies when there is foreign material and especially platelet aggregates in the lumen of an artery. When a vessel is occluded by atheromatous material the smooth muscle cells develop fibroblastic properties [10]. When platelet aggregation and adhesion occur, shape change ensues and there is a discharge of two mitogenic substances (and perhaps others) [12]. These are platelet-derived growth factor (PDGF) and epidermal growth factor. There is also another factor which has the curious property of inhibition of growth under some conditions and supporting growth under others (transforming growth factor β) [13]. Mitogenic and chemoattractant characteristics are possessed by PDGF for the smooth muscle cells of the vessel wall; β-thromboglobulin and platelet factor IV are chemoattractant for monocytes. Complicating the changes induced by platelet aggregation, adhesion and release reaction are those features induced by the atheromatous material itself. Impaction of an atheroembolus gives rise to an acute inflammation progressing to a panarteritis [14].

11.1.5 CUTANEOUS AND LOWER LIMB ATHEROEMBOLISM

Episodes of acute ischaemia of the lower limb due to emboli are usually from the left ventricle. In a series of 4635 cases of peripheral embolism, one study [15] established that 1.4% were due to atheroembolism and that the vast majority (90%) were from the heart. This is probably an underestimate because a large number of emboli are overlooked.

The development of cutaneous lesions from atheroemboli is inconstant. The earliest reports of cutaneous atheroembolism were in 1949 [16] and 1959 [17]. The latter paper records the characteristic lesions of atheroembolism in a biopsy taken from the edge of a cutaneous ulcer.

The identification of livedo reticularis as a major complication of atheroembolism has also been made [18]. Leroy [19] described a series of 65 patients whose ages ranged from 47 to 86 years, with cutaneous manifestations of atheroembolism. In this series there was a major sex bias, there being 59 men and 6 women. In one third of the cases there was an abdominal or iliac aneurysm and in the other two thirds numerous atheromas of the abdominal aorta. The common accompaniments of severe atherosclerosis may be present such as arterial hypertension, coronary arterial insufficiency, cerebrovascular accidents and atherosclerosis of the lower limbs.

In some cases the onset of cutaneous atheroembolism is announced by pain in the area. This is characteristically of a coarse stinging nature with dissemination to the base of the back and lower limbs, in the legs or sometimes only in the toes. The obliteration of a large vessel can be excluded by the absence of pallor, coldness of the part and neurological signs. In most of the cases the pulses are easily found. Other painful manifestations of cutaneous atheroembolism are diffuse muscular pain, a heaviness in the lower limbs and a scalding sensation. In some instances a polymyositis [20] is simulated because of the occurrence of a myalgia and an increase in muscle enzyme levels.

Epigastric area abdominal pain in conjunction with lower limb pain may be due to emboli in abdominal organs [21]. Abdominal pains may be associated with nausea, vomiting, diarrhoea and alimentary bleeding. At autopsy in this type of case, emboli are usually found in a number of organs such as the kidney, oesophagus, stomach, intestine, spleen, liver and pancreas. For example one case [23] has been reported of pain in the left side associated with haematuria, probably related to the renal atheroembolism found on post-mortem examination.

Pain commences with embolism, occurring as a cramping abdominal pain 3 h after arteriography [24] and after each arteriography in another report [25]. There was a parallelism between elevation of arterial hypertension and pain in the studies of Fisher et al. [18]. Pain may occur in the epigastric region the calves and the shoulders [22]. In a patient who is thought to have intermittent claudication ascribed to atherosclerosis, a sudden recrudescence of the claudication together with persistence of distal pulses should alert the physician to the possibility of atheroembolism [26].

Atheroemboli produce a variety of cutaneous lesions. At one extreme there may be little change, at the other purple toes, ulceration and a gangrenous area may develop. Lesions due to cutaneous atheroembolism which do not occur except with atherosclerosis are livedo reticularis, nodules or purpura. Livedo reticularis was found in 55% of 65 observations on cutaneous atheroembolism in one series [19]. Usually the presentation is of an inflammatory form with a reddish purple, wide-linked network. If the meshwork is unclear it may present as a violet marbling of the skin. In 64% of the livedo reticularis manifestations the characteristic appearance was found on the loins, lower abdomen and lower limbs. Restriction of the livedo occurred to the legs (27%) or to the feet (9%) in other instances. Livedo is rarely found in the upper limbs but it has been recorded on all four extremities [27] One of the characteristic features of atheroembolic livedo is that it can vary in intensity from day to day [28].

The most uncommon manifestion of cutaneous atheroembolism is dermal nodules. These were noted in 12% of 65 cases of cutaneous atheroembolism [19]. Dermal nodules appear in the erythematocyanotic meshes, i.e. after livedo has occurred, and may suggest that the condition is a form of polyarteritis nodosa. They can occur on the thigh, the leg superficial to the tibia and on the calf. The dermal nodules may be well demarcated and just under the epidermis (2–4 cm in diameter) or may be larger, poorly defined (3–12 cm in diameter) and may be associated with muscle injury.

Purpura was found in 17% of Leroy's series [19] and had a distribution similar to that of livedo, i.e. abdomen and lower limbs, buttocks and thighs, legs and feet. It may manifest as a petechial purpura [29] or a necrotic purpura. In each case cutaneous biopsy showed the characteristic lesions of atheroemboli. The purpura was not accompanied by alteration in haemostatic balance except in occasional cases, e.g. when disseminated intravascular coagulation may be present as in the report by Leroy et al. [30].

A common (41%) manifestation of atheroembolism is the occurrence of purple toes, described variously as cyanosis, acrocyanosis, toes of dark colour, purple coloration, etc. One or more toes may show the colour change [26] or only the colour of the pulp of the toes may be changed [31]. In one case [32] purple toes were reported with spotty discolouration of the plantar arch which regressed when the leg was raised. Pain often accompanies colour modification [33]. This may be sudden, cold or be associated with paraesthesia. Pain does not invariably accompany colour change and there may be absence of pain. The purple coloration occurs in a region which is affected by severe atherosclerosis and there is often persistence of peripheral pulses [31]. This purple coloration is usually reversed after surgical treatment of the generating area for the emboli.

Apart from the superficial form there may be a deeper form with gangrene requiring amputation of the affected toes [34]: 23% of cases showed ulceration and these ulcers were on the great toe, fifth toe, heel, legs or over dermal nodules. Ulceration is apparent before venous trophic changes, cessation of distal pulses and intermittent claudication [19]. Progression may occur towards gangrene requiring amputation. Although some of the ulcers may be a result of arteriopathy, others are due to atheroemboli which can be verified by histological examination of the ulcer site [14,22]. In 44% of embolic cases, gangrene sometimes evolved from purple toes [19].

Although the syndrome of pain, a sensation of coldness in the toes and intermittent claudication suggests gangrene secondary to common arteriopathy, there are certain features which are suggestive that in some cases embolic phenomena are important. The gangrene present in these instances is disproportionate to the other ischaemic changes which are present [35]. The foot and posterior tibial pulses can be found in about half of the gangrene cases of this type. The cutaneous necrosis can be sometimes quite superficial.

In a number of instances the cutaneous manifestations of atheroembolism can pass unnoticed because of the severe symptoms produced by visceral atheroembolism. The symptoms are triggered by ischaemia due to showers of atheroemboli. In order of frequency of associated visceral manifestation the affected organs were kidney (40), spleen (28), pancreas (27), gastrointestinal tract (17) and liver (15). Other organs affected were skin (32), skeletal muscle (20), brain (8) and heart (2) in 65 cases [19].

If a patient is thought to have severe atherosclerosis the three findings of sudden pain in the lower limbs, livedo reticularis and paradoxical presence of distal pulses, are together very suggestive of peripheral atheroembolism. However, the diagnosis of atheroembolism is a difficult one to make before death. In Leroy's series [19] the diagnosis was made in only 58% when cutaneous manifestations were present. This diagnosis was confirmed by skin biopsy (13 cases), muscle biopsy (13 cases), biopsy of amputated extremity (12 cases), fundoscopic examination (8 cases), renal biopsy (4 cases) and prostatic and bone marrow biopsy (1 case each). In one series of 25 [1], the diagnosis was not made in any of the cases before death.

Skin biopsy provides a means of early diagnosis of atheroembolism: 32 of 65 patients had a biopsy of the lesion present and in 13 this permitted diagnosis [19]. In 19, skin biopsy at autopsy revealed atheroembolism. The lower limbs were always the site of the skin biopsies. Muscle biopsies also achieved diagnosis in 65% of cases (13 out of 20 patients).

11.1.6 RENAL ATHEROEMBOLISM

Atheroembolism resulting in acute renal insufficiency may develop from massive embolism due to material detached by a surgical event [3,22] or arteriography [25,36]. Spontaneous atheroembolism rarely gives rise to acute renal insufficiency [29,31].

Constant showering of the kidney may, however, produce chronic renal failure. At initial presentation such patients usually have a raised urea and creatinine [19]. In one study the diastolic pressure was most elevated in patients with atheroembolism and this elevation often coincides with the commencement of the embolic process [23,34,37].

In a patient aged 60 [6] arterial hypertension regressed after nephrectomy of a kidney damaged by atheroembolism. The recurrence of hypertension two years latter heralded renal injury in the remaining kidney by atheroemboli. Atheroemboli are considered to induce or at least aggravate a pre-existing arterial hypertension. In biopsies, cholesterol crystals can sometimes be found in the afferent arterioles.

The part of the aorta predominantly affected by atherosclerosis in man is the abdominal region. In marked atherosclerosis of the aorta, well developed atheromas usually are found caudal to the origins of the renal arteries. Extension proximal to the level of the renal arteries can often evolve and ulcerated atheromas upstream can shower atheroemboli into the ostia of the renal arteries. Even caudal lesions, if there is turbulence, can achieve renal embolism.

In patients with widespread aortic atherosclerosis, renal scarring and damage commonly results from atheroembolic occlusion and subsequent fibrosis. The characteristic lesion is fibrous replacement of the lumina of small vessels with the presence of cholesterol crystals which are biconvex.

In a study of 755 renal biopsies [38] atheroemboli were found in eight men ranging in age from 49 to 72 years. The common clinical picture was recent deterioration of renal function of unknown cause. Of the eight, six were hypertensive, two showed hyperlipidaemia, one a leaking aortic aneurysm, one had carcinoma of the pancreas and one chronic glomerulonephritis. Better results were achieved when epoxy resin-embedded sections were stained with toluidine blue compared with routinely produced paraffin sections stained by haematoxylin and eosin [38]. This report was the first description of the incidence of spontaneous atheroembolism in renal biopsies in man. In indicates an incidence of approximately 1%. Aortic surgery, trauma and arteriography in patients with a severely atherosclerotic aorta can considerably increase this figure. These authors considered that if atheroemboli could be found in a random renal biopsy then the disease process had occurred in such a widespread distribution that a clinically significant degree of impairment was likely. In such a case atheroembolism would explain the occurrence of deteriorating renal function or exaggerated hypertension.

Renal biopsy is considered a useful procedure in the diagnosis of atheroembolism by most authors [38,39] despite some opposing views [34]. The appearances of an atheroembolus in a renal arteriole are shown in Figure 11.2.

Lie [40] puts forward a clinical syndrome of atheroembolism which he calls 'the unexplained renal failure–hypertension syndrome'. He points out that in the documented 221 cases of atheroembolism found in English reports up to 1987, 81% were known to be associated with renal failure, or hypertension and frequently both. The other syndromes which Lie recognized as being due to this disease were lower limb ischaemia (blue toe syndrome), abdominal pain (visceral ischaemia syndrome), unexpected heart attack (repetitive small stroke syndrome) and the pseudovasculitis syndrome.

Jones and Iannaccone [38] put forward the following suggestion as to the evolution of the lesions which they observed. Small arteries are impacted by emboli which contain esters or crystals of cholesterol with or without cellular debris derived from atheromas. Injury to the

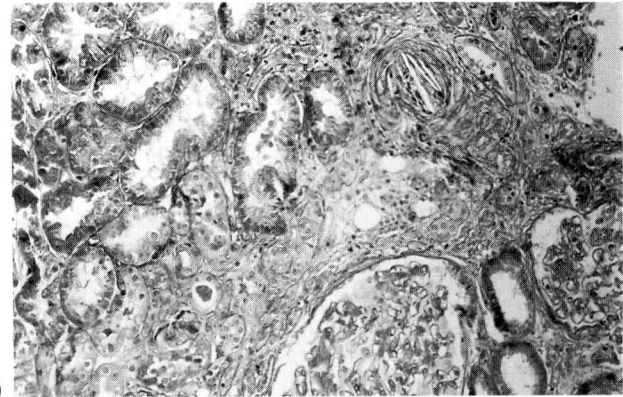
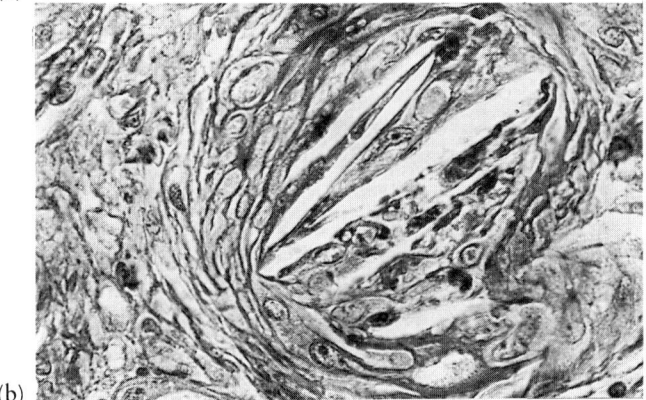

Figure 11.2 Renal biopsy specimen from a man aged 65 with malignant hypertension. It shows the typical appearance of a small artery obstructed by an atheroembolus. In the central area the typical biconvex crystals 'end-on' are seen obstructing the lumen of the vessel. A cellular reaction to the crystals has occurred. (a) Low power view showing relationship of the arteriole to neighbouring renal structures. (b) Higher power view to illustrate cellular reaction to the embolus. (Picro Mallory stain.)

endothelial lining ensues and an inflammatory response is triggered. One of the manifestations of this is vessel-wall oedema. Histiocytes surround the crystals in the next period and may fuse to form multinucleated cells occasionally. Endothelium grows over the histiocytes covering the crystals and a new lumen results which is much smaller than the original one.

Intimal cell proliferation produces collagen and basement membrane. The cholesterol crystals are by this process removed from the lumen and end up in an extraluminal position in the wall of the blood vessel. If repeated embolic episodes occur, the above process can appear at different stages. In our work on experimental renal atheroembolism [10] we reached similar conclusions as to the progression of atheroemboli in small renal arteries in the experimental situation.

Jones and Iannaccone [38] noted an osmiophilic layer on the surface of the cholesterol crystals confirming our observation and agreed that it represented partial dissolution of cholesterol. They proposed the hypothesis that enzymic activity at the cytoplasmic crystal interface resulted in a disintegration of the surface of the crystal. Because a unit membrane structure was not found at the crystal cytoplasmic interface it was deduced that the cell treated the crystal as if it were triglyceride within the cell. Hence it was not enclosed in a limiting membrane. The finely granular substance seen sometimes within the cholesterol crystal structure was believed to be due to an infiltration of plasma protein into the cholesterol crystal lattice.

11.1.7 LOWER LIMB ATHEROEMBOLISM

This subject has been dealt with in part under section 11.1.6 on cutaneous atheroembolism. Anderson and Richards [41] considered that since atheroemboli were swept into the arteries of the lower limb, muscle biopsies in this region would be of value in establishing the diagnosis of atheroembolism. Embolized arteries in skeletal muscle were found to be arteriolar in size averaging 100–200 μm in diameter. This is consistent with that reported by Uys and Watson [5] but larger than in our study in the kidney [10]. The preparation of material for studies on experimental atheroembolism involved grinding the human atheromatous material so that it would pass through a 27-gauge needle, hence it would be expected to proceed further down the arterial tree.

Kwaan et al. [42] discussed three patients with peripheral atheroembolism. These events resulted from the dislodgement of a fragment of aortic plaque and the content of atheromas. They consider that although the great majority of arterial thromboemboli are derived from mural thrombi attached to cardiac chambers a source from severely affected atherosclerotic aortas should not be forgotten. Another aspect is that both myocardial infarction and aortic atherosclerosis are common so that some individuals can suffer from both conditions. Atheroembolism should be kept in mind as a source of peripheral embolism. In their first case a diagnosis of myocardial infarction led to a deduction that the source of a peripheral embolus was from an endocardial mural thrombus. The patient re-presented six weeks after the first embolectomy with progressive pain, coldness of the right leg with discoloration of the toes on that side. There were physical findings identical with those of the first admission. Radiological investigation revealed an atheroma near the aortic bifurcation and occlusion of the right common iliac artery. On histological examination atheromatous material was identified in the embolus removed at the repeat operation. An aortoiliac endarterectomy was carried out. Gangrenous changes had occurred in the toes at the time of admission and eventually amputation was required. Atheroemboli were identified within the digital vessels of the amputated toes.

Their second case [42] involved an atheromatous plaque 3 by 5 mm which was found surrounded by thrombotic material in an embolus. The region of the bifurcation of the aorta was identified as the source. Treatment was aortoiliac endarterectomy which removed the source of the emboli. In their third case episodes of discoloration and numbness of the right toes were noted by the patient. Multiple filling defects were seen within the terminal aorta. Aortoiliac endarterectomy resulted in a complete recovery.

Proximal ulcerated atheromas were the source of lower limb arterial emboli in another series of 10 cases [43]. The author identified two clinical syndromes: in the first, embolization of cholesterol rich atheromatous debris in terminal arteries produced livedo reticularis or local digital ischaemia; in the second the clinical presentation was the result of thrombi produced by the irregularities and particularly the erosions present in the aortic wall. Emboli in this second group were larger and the clinical findings were similar to emboli of cardiac origin. Biplanar aortography was found to be most useful in reaching a diagnosis. Anticoagulation did not prevent recurrent episodes of embolism. Graft replacement of the diseased arterial segment or endarterectomy was considered the preferred treatment. Lumbar sympathectomy was found to be beneficial in patients in whom cutaneous ischaemia was persistent.

Schechter [44] examined 17 patients with atheroembolism of the lower limbs, aged from 52 to 74 years with a mean age of 61 years. The male to female ratio was 15:2. He considered that the syndrome of lower limb atheroembolism typically started suddenly with pain and subcutaneous ischaemia which showed itself as livedo reticularis in the presence of intact pedal pulses. Arteriography permitted localization of the origin of the atheroemboli either from atheromas in the aorta or an aortic aneurysm. Confirmation of atheroembolism is possible in his view by skin or muscle biopsies and the main aim of treatment is removal of the origin of the emboli and appropriate grafting or endarterectomy procedures.

11.1.8 CORONARY ATHEROEMBOLISM

Thrombosis associated with atheromatous plaques in the aorta can occur without immediate dire consequences. When the lumen of the artery is much smaller, as in the coronary and cerebral arterial system such is not the case.

The first report of coronary atheroembolism is attributed [45] to Panum [46] in 1862. Panum examined the coronary arteries of the sculptor Albert Bertel Thorvaldsen (1770–1844) who designed the Lion of Lucerne and who died suddenly. Panum described atheromatous material occluding a coronary artery and he deduced that it had originated from a ruptured atheroma.

Woolf [47] recorded the microscopic appearance of a coronary artery segment of a middle-aged man who died suddenly. The coronary artery was occluded by a hinge of tissue which allowed entry into the plaque centre. Platelet aggregates were mixed with the necrotic debris and cholesterol crystals of the atheroma. The thrombotic material then extended out and occluded the adjacent lumen. He was of the opinion that the initiating event for such a process was a crack in the fibrous cap of the atheroma in the coronary vessel. Cap damage associated with endothelial loss has resulted in low local levels of prostaglandin I_2 formation [48] and platelets will contact collagen fibres with subsequent aggregation and thrombus initiation.

Coronary artery lesions have been examined [49] in fatal cases of myocardial ischaemia. In 40% of these cases, the thrombotic occlusion of coronary arteries showed rupture of the covering of the atheroma. The soft middle portion of the atheroma discharged through the gap in the fibrous covering and the resulting thrombotic and atheromatous mix occluded the lumen. The frequency of fissures in atherosclerotic lesions underlying 20 coronary artery occlusions has also been studied [50]: cracks were found in all cases examined.

Woolf [47] advises that step serial sections may be required if fissuring of the fibrous cap of the atheroma is to be revealed and that there may be considerable anatomical complexity of thrombi and their relationship with a ruptured atheromatous plaque.

A softened centre of the plaque may have a bearing on this situation and a large basal pool size might indicate alteration from the usual constituents [51] with, in addition, a necrotizing cholesteryl ester (such as cholesteryl esters of hydroxy octadecadenoic acid) which have been located in ulcerated atheromas [52]. Crawford [53] agrees that ruptures are common but does not consider them to be always present in cases of coronary artery thrombosis. He has postulated that where rupture of the fibrous cap of an atheroma occurs, blood enters the soft centre and may dissect the intima. As the blood enters, the soft central contents of the atheroma escape into the lumen where they may be caught in thrombotic material or be swept distally as an embolus. Coagulation within the cavitated central part of the plaque now occurs and extends through the gap into the lumen progressing in some instances to complete obstruction.

Newman et al. [54] examined the records of 25–44-year-old men dying of coronary heart disease during a specific time period. A majority of men who died suddenly of coronary arterial disease showed extensive advanced disease. Occlusive thrombi were found in 32.3%. The time frame of sudden death was defined as minutes to 2 hours. A progression of softening, rupture and ulceration was suggested as the evolution of coronary mural thrombi by Strong, a member of his group [55]. Coronary arterial spasm may be induced by thromboxone A_2 elaboration by platelet aggregates. Distal atheroemboli may also contribute to continuing myocardial damage.

11.1.9 CEREBRAL ATHEROEMBOLISM

Chiari (cited by Jeynes [56]) in 1906 detailed embolism into the cerebral vasculature which resulted in a stroke. Hunt [57] considered that extracranial carotid atherosclerosis should be borne in mind in the diagnosis of cerebral lesions suspected of being due to vascular factors. Stenotic factors were held to be the causation of transient ischaemic attacks until it was put forward [58,59] that embolism would be a mechanism which more readily explained the associated features.

Among the factors marshalled for an embolic origin for transient ischaemic attacks (TIA) were that they were sudden, short and the effects focal and random, and that on occlusion of the common carotid artery TIAs stopped [56]. Other evidence included the fact that closure of a common carotid artery could be tolerated by a patient without producing TIAs.

The exact contribution of embolism in general is controversial [56]. High figures of 68% [60] and 46% [61] have been given by some authors. One report [62] found that 54% of 160 patients who were candidates for carotid endarterectomy had ulcerated atheromatous lesions. A range of figures mostly between 10 and 33% is usually cited [1,58,63–67]. A number of observers have indicated that the carotid bifurcation produces showers of atheroemboli [68–70].

The main sources of cerebral emboli are the cardiac chambers and atherosclerotic lesions of the major neck vessels. Wood and Correll [62] examined 160 endarterectomy cases and came to the following conclusions with regard to the commonest site for the origin of atheroemboli in neck vessels, the carotid bifurcation:

1. The posterior wall was the commonest area of the artery to be affected.
2. The lesions for the most part were elongated (approximately 3–4 cm) parallel to the long axis of the artery and ulceration occurred in the central part of the plaque.
3. The common and internal carotid arteries were the usual sites of plaques.
4. Bilateral lesions were found in one third of cases.

The major sites which act as the sources of cerebral atheroemboli in the neck and head are, from the commonest to the least common: the carotid bifurcation, the union of the vertebral arteries to form the basilar artery, the internal carotid siphon and the posterior cerebral artery basilar junction [71,72].

The size of the vessels where atheroemboli impact in the cerebral arterial system have been described to be between 8 and 83 μm [73], less than 100 μm [74] and between 150 and 200 μm [7].

The actual site in the brain where atheroemboli lodge varies but in one series [74] no infarcts due to atheromatous emboli were found in mid-line structures generally and not in the pons, mid-brain and medulla specifically. In the cerebellum, atheroemboli were found only in cerebellar leptomeningeal vessels. The regions most affected were the areas of supply of the distal middle cerebral and posterior cerebral arteries [74,75] and in these areas the cortical and subcortical tissues and the lesions are often multiple. In addition the internal carotid artery may be involved [76]. The emboli commonly were impacted in the leptomeningeal branches [77–81]. One review [82] of atheroembolism to the spinal cord showed that the lesions in that location are similar to those present in the brain.

The character of the damage resulting from atheroemboli is determined by a number of factors. The embolus tends to lodge in a region of narrowing, especially bifurcation. Fisher and Adams [83] stress the influence of the circle of Willis, the collateral circulation available to the part (reviewed by Baker *et al.* [84]) and the extent of the associated blood coagulation around the embolus.

11.1.10 ATHEROEMBOLISM OF THE GASTROINTESTINAL TRACT

Atheroemboli may produce embolic obstruction of arteries beneath the gastrointestinal mucosa [73]. Atheroembolism of the arteries of the gastrointestinal tract was reported in three cases [85]. All were male and their ages were 65, 65 and 74 years. In two, melaena had occurred before their last admission to hospital. Atheroembolism derived from an aorta severely affected by atherosclerosis, resulted in widespread embolism with areas of infarction. Gastrointestinal haemorrhage was the clinical sign of these underlying events. In each of these cases at autopsy atheroembolism was found to be widespread and the kidneys, pancreas, adrenals and skeletal muscles were usually involved.

In these cases the stomach and small intestine were affected and in two cases the large intestine also and in one the oesophagus. When the stomach was affected there were scattered petechiae in the mucosa of the fundus and the lesser curve. Within small submucosal arteries and arterioles cholesterol crystals were noted when frozen sections were viewed by polarized light. Microinfarcts were relatively rare. In the small intestine atheroembolism resulted in congestion of villi and, on the antimesenteric region, longitudinal petechiae. Microscopy revealed small areas of haemorrhagic necrosis which sometimes evolved into acute ulcerations. Re-epithelialized superficial mucosal ulcerations were found. Cholesterol crystals were noted in the submucosal vessels.

The nature of the damage resulting from atheroembolism depends firstly on the region of distribution of affected arteries and arterioles. Secondly a major factor is the degree of collateral circulation available (especially in the 'watershed' regions in that distribution). There is, therefore, a range of injury which varies from minimal change such as mucosal swelling and petechiae with or without superficial ulceration to major damage resulting in necrosis of the mucosa and/or full bowel wall infarction.

The clinical findings in gastrointestinal atheroembolism are varied. The findings of diffuse abdominal pain, paralytic ileus and repeated sporadic melaena are common features and some or all of these are usually present. A case of renal failure, splenic infarcts and duodenal ulceration after aortofemoral bypass and aortic ligation has been reported [86] as a result of showers of atheroemboli. From clinical and pathological evidence it was considered that the atheroemboli were gradually released following an aortofemoral bypass operation. The change in flow pattern produced by the resulting aortic blind alley exacerbated the possibility of release of emboli. A 70-year-old woman had small bowel obstruction secondary to atheromatous embolism [45]. Her initial complaint at the age of 68 years, was bilateral calf claudication for one and a half years with pain in her foot at night a recent event. Pulses below the femorals were absent. Radiologic examination of the aorta revealed localized calcification spread throughout the abdominal aorta but no aneurysmal dilatation. Increasing severity of the claudication necessitated an aortoiliac endarterectomy. This allowed her to return to her usual living style. Two years after this operation she complained of intermittent diarrhoea, sporadic vomiting, abdominal fullness and weight loss over a period of 4 months when she presented at hospital. Included in the investigations was radiologic examination of her gastrointestinal tract. This showed dilated distal jejunum. The operative findings were a narrowed thickened 4 cm length of distal ileum proximally associated with dilated loops of small bowel. Resection of the abnormal region and end-to-end anastomosis of the viable bowel were carried out. Uneventful recovery from this operation occurred. Pathologic examination of the surgical specimen showed a 17 cm length of ileum which was 8 cm in its greatest diameter. There was a 4 cm length of narrowed bowel in the middle of the length of ileum. In this region the circumference of the bowel was 2.5 cm. Superficial ulceration of 1 cm diameter was noted in the narrowed segment. Deeper to the ulcer was submucosal fibrous tissue with focal chronic inflammatory changes. Within several submucosal arteries were atheromatous emboli. Microscopy revealed in the obstructions, cholesterol crystals, multinucleated foreign body giant cells, occasional scattered groups of eosinophils and intimal fibroblastic response.

A 'subnecrotizing' ischaemia may develop as the arterial supply to the bowel is compromised by showers of atheroemboli and this may proceed to fibrous structure of the intestine and subsequent obstruction as occurred in the above case. From the information derived from experimental studies [10,87,88], an appropriate explanation of these developments would be as follows. Due to the incorporation within arterial walls of the remnants of atheroemboli, especially cholesterol crystals, and the myointimal vascular response, a silting-up effect on the vascular network ensues. This would be exacerbated by the cumulative effect of many separate showers of atheroemboli in the downstream distribution area of vessels affected by atherosclerotic lesions.

The cholesterol crystals seen by microscopy in vessel walls or in occlusive fibrous obstructions are the markers of end-stage embolism, and are the incorporated remains of the original atheroemboli. They are not due to a dystrophic process at that site.

Colonic pathology due to atheroembolism includes haemorrhage and even perforation [89]. Diagnosis can be derived by biopsy of the ischaemic ulcer. Atheroemboli may result in such damage sufficiently severe to cause perforation of the colon [90].

11.1.11 ATHEROEMBOLISM AS A SURGICAL PROBLEM

Atheroembolism is emerging as a complication in cardiac surgery [91] and interventional transluminal coronary angiography [92] as well as in arterial grafts and bypass grafts in the treatment of claudication of the lower extremities and limb threat.

In 1982 the first observations of fatal perioperative myocardial infarction following coronary artery bypass grafting (CABG) were reported in 13 cases [93]. The sites of origin were ulcerated atheromas in the aortic root near the site of the vein graft ostia in five instances. In two cases atheroemboli arose from mechanical disturbance of plaques in major epicardial arteries and in a further two the most likely origin was from coronary endarterectomy sites. The event took place during initial revascularization procedures and represents a risk of 0.22% in a series of 4095 initial CABG procedures. During repeat CABG operations a further four cases developed. This was considered to be due to dislodgement of atheroemboli during manipulation of old vein grafts in which atheromas had evolved. This represents a risk of 2.29% in 175 repeat CABGs. These authors advocate the identification of patients at risk of this phenomenon by analysis of angiograms prior to repeat CABG. Severe graft atherosclerosis should be distinguished from myointimal hyperplasia. Ligation of the vein graft at the level of the distal anastomosis should be carried out as soon as possible on reopening the chest in order to reduce the risk of atheroembolism. Atheroembolism is considered by some to be an underestimated cause of perioperative myocardial infarction [93,94].

Observations on atheroembolic perioperative infarction during repeat coronary bypass surgery in a survivor have been made [95]. Atheromas were demonstrated preoperatively in a previous bypass graft. Infarction appeared to be due to atheroembolic occlusion of a large coronary branch. The risks of atheroemboli showering from atheromas in old vein grafts is dependent upon the time from the original operation. Atherosclerosis of vein grafts takes some 5 to 10 years after operation to develop [96].

Atheroembolism from the ascending aorta has been reviewed and non-cardiac causes of death examined in patients undergoing cardiac operations [91]. As the age of patients rose the non-cardiac causes of death increased. The autopsy findings in 221 patients undergoing myocardial revascularization or valve operations between 1982 and 1989 were analysed. The mean age was 65.6 ± 9.5 years with the range from 32 to 94 years; 58.8% (130) were male. Embolic disease was identified in 69 patients (31.2%) and atheroemboli or derived lesions found in 48 patients (21.7%). Seven patients had disseminated intravascular coagulation and 14 thromboembolism. A great increase in the incidence of atheroembolism occurred in the period, from 4.5% in 1982 to 48.3% in 1989. The distribution of the lesions was brain (16.3%), spleen (10.9%), kidney (10.4%) and pancreas (6.8%); 62.5% of 48 patients exhibited multiple sites of atheroembolism. Atheroemboli were less common in patients undergoing valve procedures when compared with those undergoing coronary artery procedures (8.9%:26.1%). Severe atherosclerosis of the ascending aorta predisposed to atheroembolism. Atheroembolism occurred in only 2% of patients who had little atherosclerosis of their ascending aorta and in 37.4% of those with severe disease; 95.8% of patients with atheroemboli had severe atherosclerosis of the ascending aorta. A direct correlation existed between age, severe atherosclerosis of the ascending aorta and the occurrence of atheroemboli.

Cardiac catheterization [97], percutaneous transluminal coronary angioplasty [92], angiographic techniques [98] and laser angioplasty [99] have all been associated with atheroembolism.

Biologic tissues may be vaporized by laser energy and this has been used in clearing obstructive lesions due to atherosclerosis. Human cadaver aortas were injured by organ laser and solid phase debris analyzed. The debris from calcified plaque was the highest (79%) while that from normal aorta intima, fatty streaks and fibrous plaques were 3.2, 2.7 and 3.7% respectively.

In one study [92] it was found that although percutaneous transluminal coronary angioplasty was less invasive than repeat coronary bypass grafting, in 2.5–3% of cases it was complicated by atheroembolism. In 98 patients who had elective angioplasty, five patients had non-Q wave myocardial infarctions indicated by elevated serum creatine kinase levels. Atheroembolism was considered the most likely diagnosis in four. In the two patients who died, autopsy showed multiple atheroemboli in the distal epicardial artery supplied by the graft. Multiple infarcts, some of which antedated the procedure, were found. Older vein grafts are, therefore, prone to recurrent atheroembolism as well as angioplasty-related events. Three cases of atheroembolism following cardiac catheterization have been reported [97]. All patients were elderly and had extensive atheromatous disease. In one, histological evidence confirmed the diagnosis at autopsy and in the remaining two, clinical features of this disorder developed. Their ages were 72, 66 and 84 years. Severe hypercholesterolaemia was not a feature. There was no undue difficulty at the time of catheterization. In the autopsied case the superior mesenteric artery was occluded with a macroembolus and the mucosal arteries contained microemboli. The kidney, pancreas, spleen and liver also showed atheroemboli. As well as the original cardiac pathology, rapidly progressive renal failure was a major contributory cause of death of all three patients.

Transient eosinophils can be encountered in atheroembolism [100,101] but leukocytosis and neutrophilia may also occur [97].

One study described 47 patients who underwent selective catheterization of middle and lower thoracic intercostal and upper lumbar arteries to identify the major contribution to the anterior spinal artery [102]. This has variously been described as the artery of Adamkiewicz, the arteria radiculomedullares magna and the great radicular artery. In one patient there was significant atheroembolism and transient lower extremity paraesthesias occurred in another. These authors presented the risks of spinal cord injury during repair of various segments of atherosclerotic descending aorta and found that it was maximal in the proximal part of the descending aorta. The risk of paraplegia developing after aortic repair depends on the possibility of damage to the great radicular artery and the extent of the length of the aortic segment undergoing repair.

Problems of aortoiliac disease will occur post-renal transplantation with increasing frequency due to better survival and extended indications for renal transplantation [103]. This report describes aortoiliac reconstruction in two such patients. One had overt atheroembolism with its origin in aortoiliac occlusive disease and the other a slow rupture of an aortic aneurysm. Maintenance of perfusion of the transplant kidney was provided by a temporary axillofemoral graft.

Atheroembolism can be an important cause of the need for femoral distal reconstruction in the absence of technical problems and progressive distal atherosclerosis [104]. In 156 patients who had femoral distal bypass for lower limb ischaemia, 15 were recognized as having graft failure due to an atheroembolic event. In 10 there was early graft failure. A proximal non-occlusive atheromatous lesion may give rise to atheroembolism resulting in distal bypass graft failure.

Of patients undergoing femorofemoral bypass graft procedures for severe claudication or limb threat, 23 of 24 were impotent preoperatively in one series [105]. In 17 of these, 23 femorofemoral bypass restored erectile function.

Atheroembolism has been confirmed as an important clinical entity often but not invariably associated with severe atherosclerotic arterial disease [106–108] although some of its modes of presentation may be enigmatic [108]. The surgical management of disseminated atheroembolism presents a challenge. It has been suggested [107] that in the high-risk patient, axillobifemoral bypass with iliac ligation may be an approach to recurrent atheroemboli in the feet. Recurrent atheroembolism to viscera and renal failure are associated with poor prognosis.

11.2 Experimental aspects

11.2.1 EXPERIMENTAL MODELS OF ATHEROEMBOLISM

The pathophysiology of atheroembolism requires experimental examination to determine the qualitative and quantitative aspects of the disorder. Questions such as: What is the nature of the material released into the blood by atheroembolism? How does this react with platelets and the coagulation cascade in the blood? What happens downstream to emboli thus generated, i.e. what are immediate, intermediate and late effects of atheroembolic episodes? What are the quantitative effects of embolism on a normal and a diseased vascular bed? Are there possible therapeutic strategies which may avert severe consequences to the part affected by atheroembolism?

With these questions in mind an overall plan of investigation of renal, lower limb and cerebral atheroembolism was developed and carried out over a number of years [10,87,88,121]. The experimental plan was adapted as far as possible to mimic similar pathological events in man. The dose of the material was varied. Observed events in the experimental situation were noted and such events monitored in clinical and especially post-mortem material. The material initially used was whole human atheromatous material. In later experiments discrete components of the atheromatous material were used in a paralled manner to the whole atheromatous preparation.

Experimental atheroembolism before 1970

Experimental work on atheroembolism dates from Flory [109], who advanced a concept of the pathogenesis of atheroembolism founded on observations in humans and experimental animals. Experimental work related to atheroembolism has consisted of injecting varying amounts and concentrations of pure cholesterol, human atheromatous material and derivatives of human atheromatous material into arteries in a number of organs. Observations on the effects of such injections were made at specific regular intervals. Flory emphasized in his paper the fact that crystals found in arteries must have arrived by an embolic process. He deduced this because of the following reasons:

1. A positive correlation occurred in autopsies between the presence of cholesterol crystals in occluded vessels and the severity of atherosclerosis.
2. In non-occluded vessels of equivalent size to occluded vessels no crystals were present in the arterial wall.
3. He believed that crystals in the wall arrived in that position via the process of organization.

Otken in 1959 [9] considered that there were two qualitatively different types of embolism. Firstly a mixed form containing all of the material of the atherosclerotic plaque and secondly crystalline material only. He detected initially an inflammatory response and, with the mixed form of embolus, subsequent organization. Because he failed to find crystals one month after injection he reached the conclusion that after conversion to a soluble form they were removed. Although another report [110] also did not find crystals after one month, all other investigations have noted that crystals persist for long periods, at least several months [14].

11.2.2 THE REACTION OF PLATELETS TO THE CONTENTS OF ATHEROMA

The reactivity of human atheromatous material with blood has been studied by a number of researchers [111–113]. While Kirk [113] regarded atheromatous material to be non-thrombogenic, Conner et al. [111] examined a 2% saline suspension of human atheromatous material from various sites and in a Chandler tube (rotating tube), and found that there was reduced thrombus generation time. Byers and Friedman [112] tested gruel from an experimental model of atherosclerosis. Animals on a high cholesterol diet developed 'thrombo atherosclerotic plaques'. Material from these plaques as well as human atheromatous material and other material was assessed using a Chandler tube apparatus with the substrate being rabbit recalcified blood. Their findings were that the experimental gruel was mildly thrombogenic but that human atheromatous material, a lipid extract, fibrotic material and control times were not thrombogenic. In work of this nature it is unwise to cross species boundaries.

If atheromatous material is combined with platelet-rich plasma in a tube arranged in a circle and rotated on a turntable (Chandler tube apparatus) a thrombus is formed at the leading edge of the column of fluid in the tube. The human platelet in the unactivated state is an anuclear biconvex disc which has special properties associated with its plasmalemmal membrane. When activated the platelet disc changes shape and puts out long filiform processes [114]. Adhesion is initially by these processes but approximation of the main mass of the platelet promptly ensues. Platelet–platelet adhesion is at first reversible but may go on to irreversible aggregation and fibrin formation. This is a common response of disturbed platelets from whatever reason. Among the more characteristic features of the human platelet are those of adhering to other platelets and to foreign surfaces, i.e. surfaces not usually presented to the platelet in its circulation around the body. Following adhesion and activation there is the release of a series of amines and other substances into the local environment.

Atheromatous material in a Chandler tube is capable of inducing shape change and platelet aggregation around such material [114]. The variations in thrombogenicity of various components of the human atheromatous plaque have been studied [114] both using this method and by *in vivo* experiments. The usual methods of paraffin embedding and staining with haematoxylin and eosin for the examination of tissues for light microscopy removes cholesterol crystals and most lipids. This results in a much reduced presence of such substances. Scanning electron microscopy when used with special techniques – namely freeze drying with subsequent metal coating – can reveal cholesterol crystals and lipids to a far greater degree. The structure of cholesterol crystals in human atheromatous plaques is preserved [116].

In the experimental situation components of atheroma, particularly cholesterol crystals, are protected by this technique. They were observed in the ascending thrombus formation which took place when 0.25–0.36 g of atheromatous material was injected into the right common iliac arteries of eight rabbits. Platelets recently activated, as evinced by the nature of their pseudopodia, were seen on the tip of the ascending thrombus [116]. They possessed intertwining pseudopodia as shape changes to platelets were induced by the thrombotic events.

11.2.3 ARTERITIS DUE TO ATHEROEMBOLISM

After the injection of atheromatous material into experimental animals it eventually impacts in the blood vessels. There is a thrombotic reaction at first and depending on the amount of the material injected this may subside or it may continue. The contents of the atherosclerotic plaque irritate the vessel wall in all sizes of arteries and produce an arteritis or a panarteritis.

Otken [9] developed an experimental model of atheroembolism in rabbits. He ground human atheromatous material in a mortar to the extent that it would pass through an 18-gauge needle. The next step consisted of injecting 2.5 ml of this suspension into the left and right cardiac ventricular chambers. Injection into the left cavity was performed in three rabbits and into the right in five. A panarteritis was found to have developed 24 h after injection in the affected circulatory field. Those arteries which harboured cholesterol crystals underwent proliferative changes in their intima. In one rabbit, pure cholesterol crystals were injected; 24 h later at autopsy these were not found.

Cholesterol crystal embolism has also been studied [14] in 16 rabbits and nine dogs. In rabbits the site of injection was the main ear vein. The cholesterol crystals were noted in the small and medium-sized pulmonary arteries of the animals. At three days a panarteritis was noted which included many leucocytes and eosinophils. Cholesterol crystals tended to act as permanent foreign material.

Although partial dissolution of cholesterol crystals in the circulation may occur, Otken's suggestion that cholesterol crystals within 24 h of injection change from their crystalline form and become completely soluble is unlikely [6,10,87,88]. The platelet response and the associated lipid material may influence cholesterol crystal dissolution.

The importance of the effect of any immunological response to the heterologous proteins injected with the atheromatous material has been raised by some authors [6,9,109]. However, there is close parallelism between the observations in man, as described above and those in the experimental situation. The reaction of the arterial wall to mild injury such as the reaction of the arterial wall to a silk tie within the lumen [117] is similar to other types of damage including atheroembolism [10].

The cholesterol granuloma may be modified by phospholipid [118]. Pellets of phospholipid, talc, cholesterol and cholesterol–phospholipid mixtures were implanted in rats subcutaneously. Lesions developed and these were assessed by both histochemical and histological means. Labelling by tritium cholesterol of cholesterol and cholesterol–phospholipid mixtures was carried out and this allowed autoradiographic assessment of the effects caused by these pellets. The granuloma produced by cholesterol was able to be characterized by the appearance of lipid macrophages, giant cells, cholesterol aggregation and encapsulation by fibrous tissue. Persistence of this granuloma continued for at least 56 days. The addition of phospholipid to cholesterol changed the nature of the lesion produced and its duration. In this lesion, macrophages occurred in sheets and there was dispersion of cholesterol within them. Giant cells were unusual. Near resolution of such lesions took place within 56 days after insertion of the pellets.

The effects of implantation of free fatty acids, purified sterol, sterol esters and phosphoglycerides on connective tissue in rats have been studied [119]. Slow resorption of cholesterol-free fatty acids, saturated mono-unsaturated and *trans*-polyunsaturated cholesterol esters was noted. These agents were strongly sclerogenic. *Cis*-polyunsaturated cholesterol esters were found to be mobilized rapidly and were relatively non-sclerogenic. The fibrosis induced by triglycerides was not marked. These authors concluded that collagen deposition in the intima was not a reaction to these substances. However, free cholesterol and the more saturated fatty acid esters would be predicted on their results, to be able to induce intimal collagen deposition. Our results [10,87,88] indicate that there is slow mobilization of cholesterol crystals in mammalian arteries and that fibrosis ensues around impacted crystals and to this extent our results concur with the above findings.

11.2.4 EXPERIMENTAL RENAL ATHEROEMBOLISM

The evolution of the lesions of atheroembolism in the mammalian kidney has been studied [10]. The source of the atheromatous material was human aortas at post mortem. The soft central region of atheromas was scooped out under surgically clean conditions. Atheromatous material mixed with thrombotic material was avoided. When enucleating the material, collection was stopped as soon as the interior of the fibrous shell of the atheroma was reached. Saline was added to this yellowish material with highlights of small cholesterol crystals after weighing the material. Gentle grinding was carried out and a suspension of 1 g of material in 5 ml of saline achieved. The material was ground finely enough to pass through in this type of suspension a 27-gauge needle. Anaesthesia was induced in 25 male rabbits of 4–6 kg with Nembutal 40 mg/kg body weight and maintained with ether. The left renal artery was accessed by opening the abdominal cavity by a longitudinal incision following shaving of the animal and packing the intestines to one side. Identification of the left kidney followed and it was separated from the perirenal fat. In these experiments 0.5 ml of the atheromatous suspension was injected into the left renal artery. The abdominal wall incision was sutured in layers and 160 000 i.u. of procaine penicillin injected into a hind leg. The animals were killed at 30 min, 1, 26 and 48 h, 3, 4, 6, 7 and 15 days and 1 month after this injection by an overdose of Nembutal; specimens were taken from the anaesthetized animal at these times. Cold 3% glutaraldehyde in phosphate buffer was infused into the left renal artery. After this the animal was killed. The specimens were processed and examined by electron microscopy. Studies of the qualitative changes found in renal arteries following atheroemboli over time, allowed delineation into three major divisions: the early period from 30 min to 2 days, the intermediate from 2 to 4 days and the later period from 5 days to 1 month. The features of the start of the early period were dominated by the interaction of the atheromatous material with the circulating blood.

The atheroembolus created as indicated above was constituted by a diverse range of structures which included plasmalemmal membranes, fat droplets, myelin figures, prominent cholesterol crystals and debris of varying types. Platelet aggregates were present within and at the margins of the embolus in specimens removed 30 min post injection. Secondary thrombosis in the stationary column of blood that ensued following atheroembolic occlusion of a vessel occurred sometimes in the adjacent arteriolar segment. In the situation where the atheroembolus occluded the vessel, endothelial cells were damaged for over 75% of the vessel circumference. The remains of the damaged cells appeared to be represented in part by myelin figures. This endothelial damage brought the next layer of the wall directly into contact with the luminal contents and smooth muscle cells could impinge upon the embolus. Partial shedding of endothelial cells from their basement membrane was observed. Lesser damage included swelling of mitochondria and of the endothelial cells.

At 2 h postinjection, fibrin, fat droplets and cholesterol crystals continued to be present in the lumen of the affected vessels. Fibrin was less in the 2-h specimen than that present in the 30-min specimen. Some emboli were non-occlusive. Platelets had aggregated and formed fibrin in the lumen with, in addition, platelet adhesion to the underlying basement membrane uncovered by endothelial damage. In the damaged and rounded-up endothelial cells, dilated endoplasmic reticulum was noted. In the 6-h postinjection specimen, leucocyte emigration was present and platelets formed a layer on the bare basement membrane. Figure 11.3 illustrates endothelial damage at the embolic site.

The smooth muscle cells started to deteriorate at this time and fibrin and lipid droplets were found in the cytoplasm of some cells. Cholesterol crystals impacted in arteries and appeared forced into vessels slightly too small in lumen to accommodate them so that the rest of the wall of the vessel was made taut. The internal elastic lamina was stretched over the ends of the cholesterol crystals spanning the lumen, also pushing together the basement membrane of the endothelium and the internal elastic lamina. At a period of 12–48 h postinjection, macrophages were noted in the lumina and red cells had moved through the damaged vessel wall. Striated fibrin and platelet thrombi had formed on the basement membrane uncovered by destruction of endothelial cells. This first early phase in atheroembolism was marked by the

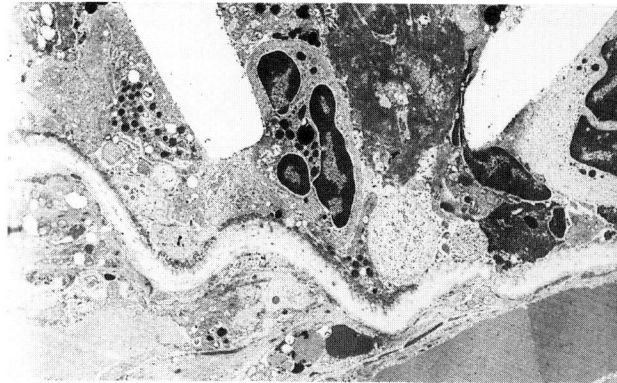

Figure 11.3 Early phase of the effects of an atheroembolus, illustrating the appearance of the embolic site 12 h postinjection. Profiles of two cholesterol crystals are present together with a leucocyte between them. The elastic lamina is bare.

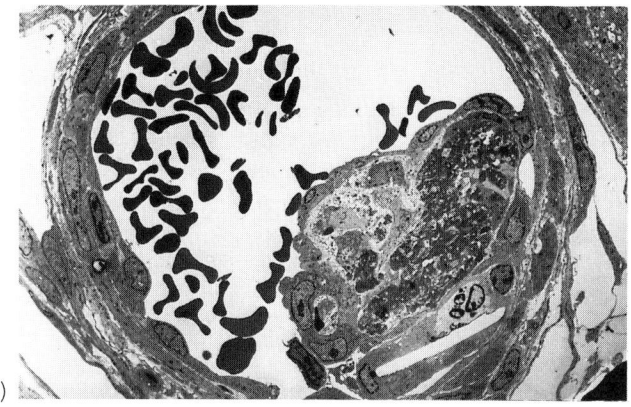

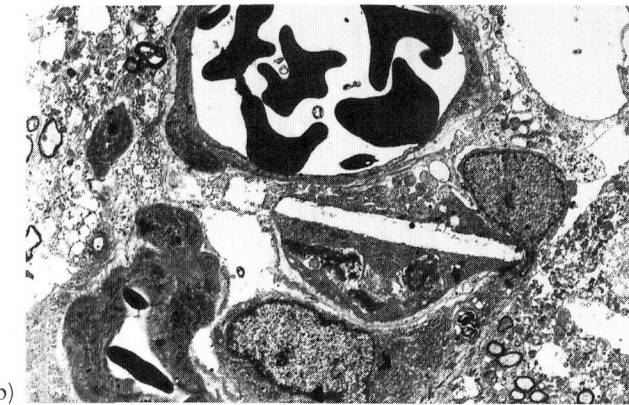

Figure 11.4 Intermediate phase in the changes that occur after impaction of an atheroembolus. (a) The embolus has retracted to one side of the vessel. Organization of the remaining fibrin is taking place and a cholesterol crystal is separated from the lumen 3 days postinjection. (b) The cholesterol crystal has become external to the vessel wall in this embolic site 3 days after injection.

induction of thrombosis with endothelial and smooth muscle injury in the environs of the atheroembolus. Cholesterol crystals, while certainly obvious as part of the atheroembolus, were noted as part of the embolus, but were not as conspicuous at this stage compared with their prominent position in the later evolution of the atheroembolus.

In the maturation of the lesion formed by the atheroembolus, the next stage is the interval from 2 to 4 days postinjection – the intermediate period. Figure 11.4 illustrates the intermediate phase. The ultimate course of the pathology of the area of the lesion is dependent upon whether the integrity of the vessel wall has been maintained through the early period. In embolic sites where the arterial wall has sustained greatest injury during the early period, distinguishing components of the vascular wall was difficult. With continued existence of at least part of the vessel wall, some developing features became evident. Leucocyte movement and passage of platelets and red cells into the injured parts of the vessel wall were noted. Obstruction of the vessel lumina at this stage was via a mixture of platelets, sludged red cells, cholesterol crystals and atheromatous debris. At 3 days in some of the emboli, fibrin and lipid had been removed from the obstructing mass. The profiles of cholesterol crystals were apparent embedded across diagonals of the vessel. The surface of the crystals was covered by condensed protein, formed at least in part by a plasma adsorbate on the crystals formed because of their foreign surface property compared with the usual surfaces presented to the blood. Platelets adhered to the flat surfaces and to the ends of the cholesterol crystals, and were flattened against the surfaces of the crystal.

The resilient nature of endothelium was evinced by the formation of flaps at or near the endothelial intercellular sites. The flap of an endothelial cell was produced by release of a portion of the cell from the basement membrane and a bridge was formed which covered the cholesterol crystal and in effect sequestrated it from the original lumen. A portion of the original sleeve of endothelium remained unaltered. A new endothelial lining was produced by the sliding of flaps of adjacent endothelial cells over the face of cholesterol crystals abutting the endothelial layer. The resolution of the atheroembolus had not proceeded as far as this in all samples of the 3-day specimens and some lumina were still filled by leucocytes, cholesterol crystals and macrophages, some of which contained small cholesterol crystals. At the step junctions between cholesterol crystal plates, osmophilic droplets were seen and may represent partial solubility of the crystals at these points. Larger cholesterol crystals evoked a multinucleated cell response.

In some 3-day preparations fibroblast-like cells were noted surrounding the crystals. Dilated endoplasmic reticulum was found in these cells and collagen strands occurred between these cells. In these vessels the lumina were almost obstructed except for a few red cells. In some instances endothelial bridges extended from the vessel wall to divide the original lumen of the vessel. In the late period (5 days onwards) the embolic site matured with eventual resolution or organization of the luminal contents. Some examples of 6-day specimens showed cholesterol crystals encircled by macrophages which often possessed myelin figures in their cytoplasm. The original limit of the vessel in a number of cases could be discerned because of the persistence of at least part of the internal elastic lamina. Because of the wall damage, red cells had leaked external to this membrane and the lumen contained a changing embolic mass. Macrophages penetrated the elastic lamina. Primitive channels lined by endothelium were present in the occluded section at this time. Platelet phagocytosis by endothelial cells was noted. Between the proliferating intimal cells could be identified further collagen fibres at this time. Progression of the evolution of changes in the embolus occurred with various significant milestones.

An apparently steady state was achieved when the original lumen was reconstructed into a number of endothelial lined channels and the cholesterol crystals had been excluded from contact with flowing blood. This was accomplished by the cholesterol crystals being surrounded by fibrous tissue and myofibroblasts. They were then within the wall of the vessel in the fibrous septae (covered by endothelium) dividing the lumina. The cholesterol crystals were the most permanent part of the atheroembolus and were found in the 1-month preparations. If the viability of the vessel wall was maintained in the early period, then, after resolution of most of the components of the atheroembolus the cholesterol crystals evoked a myofibroblastic response. In the later period remaining lipid was ingested by macrophages. The sequelae of the changes at the embolic site are shown in Figure 11.5.

11.2.5 EXPERIMENTAL CEREBRAL ATHEROEMBOLISM

Cerebral atheroembolism was studied [87] in a similar way to that described above under experimental renal atheroembolism. Atheromatous material was prepared by harvesting it from human aortas at autopsy and ground so that a suspension of 1 g/5 ml saline would go through a 27-gauge needle. In this series of experiments, 16 male rabbits 4–6 kg were anaesthetized and the neck shaved; 0.5 ml of the suspension was injected into the left common carotid artery and the wound closed. The predominant vascular distributions in the rabbit are similar to those in man. Variations from the human pattern are that a single anterior cerebral trunk is formed and the superior cerebellar arteries arise from the circle of Willis. The absence of any rete mirabile allows the pattern of progression of emboli to be akin to that of man. Within the first 12 h after injection six animals died. The animals that survived 12 h were killed at time

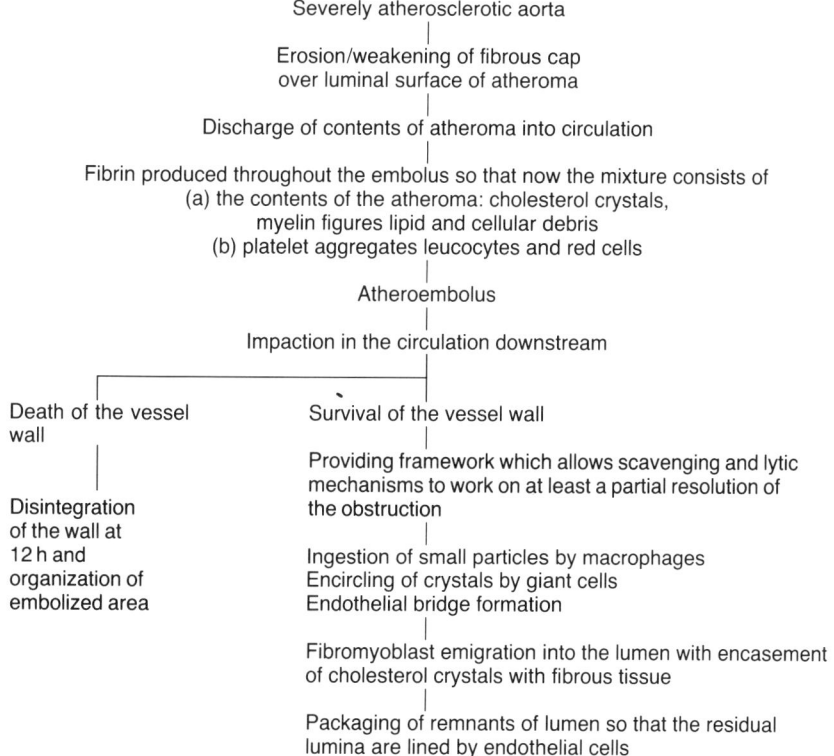

Figure 11.5 Pathogenesis of atheroembolism and its sequelae.

Table 11.1 The sequence of events at the embolic site following impaction of an atheroembolus*

Early period: 30 min to 2 days	Thrombosis and panarteritis	Ultrastructural features: mixture of atheromatous material such as cholesterol crystals, myelin figures, cellular debris with platelet aggregates and fibrin; leucocytic invasion of vessel wall may occur
Intermediate period: 2 to 4 days	Removal by lytic mechanism of thrombotic material; reforming of lumen to exclude cholesterol crystals	Endothelial cell flaps formed and these cover the cholesterol crystals; sequestration of cholesterol crystals in vessel wall and start of myofibroblast proliferation
Late period: 5 days onwards	Fibrosis around cholesterol crystals; new lumina lined by endothelial cells	Extensive myofibroblast proliferation around cholesterol crystals; formation and laying down of collagen.

* Source: Warren and Vales [10].

intervals of 1 (2 animals), 2, 3, 5, 7, 15, 25 days (2 animals) and 1 month after injection.

The basic types of reaction observed in experimental renal atheroembolism were observed in these experiments on cerebral atheroembolism. The sequence of changes at the embolic site is shown in Table 11.1. There was an initial induction of thrombosis often associated with an inflammatory response. The next stage was partial or temporary resolution of the thrombus. This was followed by a late period in which there was fibrosis around cholesterol crystals. Because they were, in this stage, incorporated into the vessel wall, they were excluded from contact with flowing blood. The death within 12 h of six of the animals in the above experiment at a dose of 0.5 ml of 200 mg/ml atheromatous material (i.e. 100 mg) prompted lowering of the dose in a subsequent series of experiments [120] to a concentration of 125 mg/ml. Human atheromatous material in suspension was injected into the left common carotid artery. Varying doses of atheromatous material were injected into 38 rabbits, namely 30 mg (three animals), 40 mg (four animals), 50 mg (five animals), 53 mg (five animals), 60 mg (four animals), 75 mg (six animals) and 80 mg (three animals). In four animals, 1 cc of saline was injected, and in another four, 80 mg of homogenated liver was the suspended substance. The animals injected with saline or liver survived without symptoms until killed some days after injection, and no infarcted cerebral lesions or cerebrovascular emboli were found. Of those given a dose of 55 mg or less of human atheromatous material, all survived except for one animal who received a dose of 50 mg. Death occurred within 7 h in all animals that had received a dose of 60 mg or more; 75% of the animals died within 2 min of the injection. In two animals which survived 7 h, one given 30 mg and the other 60 mg, neurological signs were observed: right-to-left head drift, some loss of muscle tone and a general inability to posture normally with a preference for a right-sided resting posture. Non-surviving animals possessed totally occluded segments in the circle of Willis and ipsilateral large branches from it. The vessels were congested and contained whitish material. The middle cerebral artery was the vessel most frequently occluded. This is summarized in Figure 11.6.

In animals given sublethal doses no obstructed vessels were seen at this level. The surface of the brains did not show softening in any animal. On the coronal surfaces of sliced brains two surviving animals had internal parenchymal lesions. These areas of softening appeared in the more posterior slices and were variable in size. In both surviving and non-surviving animals, parenchymal vessels exhibited similar regions of congestion and obstruction. Occluded vessels were noted scattered throughout the cortical and subcortical parenchyma

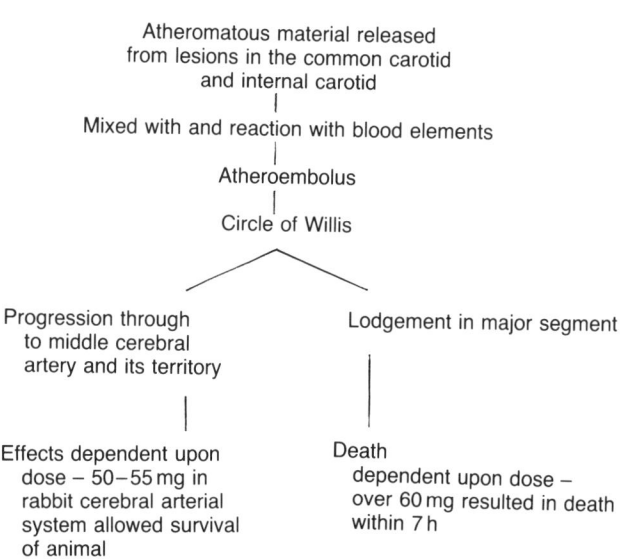

Figure 11.6 Cerebral atheroembolism.

EXPERIMENTAL ASPECTS 431

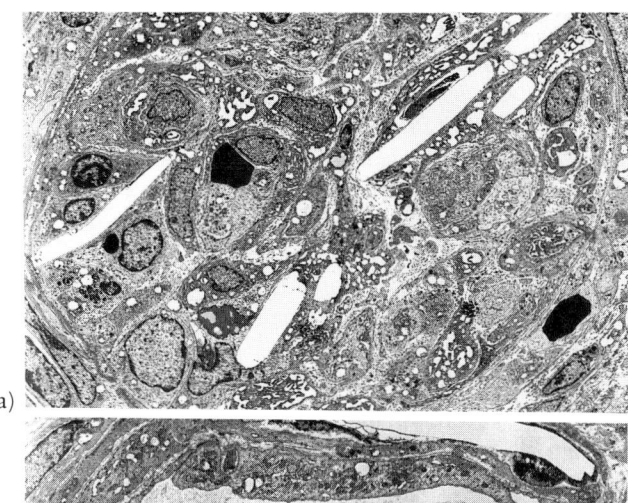

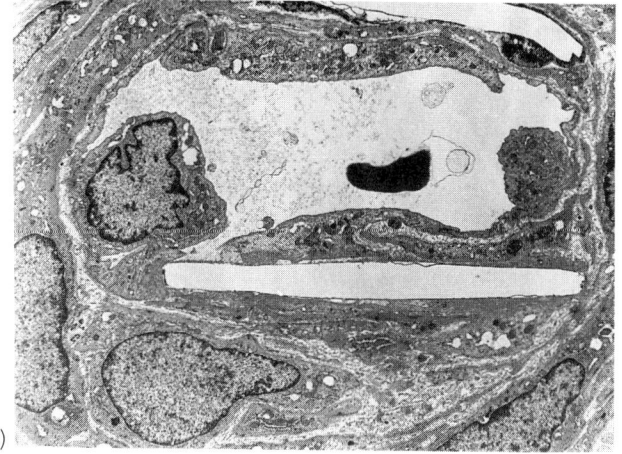

Figure 11.7 Late effects of an atheroembolus in a small vessel. (a) This vessel embolic site has resulted in complete obstruction of the lumen with only one recognizable profile of a red cell present. Five fragments of cholesterol crystals are present 6 days postinjection. (b) In this embolic site the two cholesterol crystals have moved to the walls of the vessel to leave a central lumen.

within the distribution of the ipsilateral middle cerebral artery. The late effects at the embolic sites are illustrated in Figure 11.7. In unprocessed human atheromatous material cholesterol crystals have a rhomboid shape and maximum dimensions of about 150 µm. In the processed, i.e. ground, atheromatous material, cholesterol crystals are much smaller and are of the order or 20–50 µm in maximum dimension [120].

Occluded vessels varied in size from 10 to over 800 µm in diameter and included major vessels which were components of the circle of Willis or branches from these major vascular structures. The vessels on electron microscopic examination contained cholesterol crystal spaces within an occlusive mass of lipid, cellular debris, fibrin and amorphous material mixed with elements of the blood particularly platelets. Some pericytes surrounding occluded vessels contained inclusions which were consistent with absorbed luminal contents or necrotic parenchymal material. Where the embolic event had produced infarction some vessels were surrounded by phagocytes, glial cells and pericytes. Assessment of the distribution of infarcts and occlusions in this system has been made [121]. This work [120,121] demonstrated in a mammalian cerebral arterial distribution system a threshold for the dose of atheromatous material which will produce death of the tissue associated with the target artery and confirmed earlier work on limb arteries.

11.2.6 EXPERIMENTAL LOWER LIMB ATHEROEMBOLISM

From analysis of work on experimental renal and cerebral atheroembolism [10,87] it became evident that one of the determinants in the survival of tissues following atheroembolism was the dose of the material presented to the arterial tree of the target organ. Quantitative studies on limb atheroembolism were conducted [122]. Material from human aorta was prepared as in earlier studies except that the atheromatous gruel was ground to a fine paste sufficient to allow passage through a 25-gauge needle and brought to a concentration of 0.25 g to 2 ml of sterile saline solution. In preparation for injection, anaesthetized male rabbits (3–5 kg) had the lower abdomen and hind legs shaved. Firstly the right femoral artery was located and partially isolated; 0.35–1 ml of the suspension was injected into the vessel, haemostasis secured by pressure for 3 min and then the skin sutured. The animals exhibited no distress and hopped around normally. Examination at autopsy at 13, 14, 15, 17 and 18 weeks postinjection revealed no thrombi except in the animal killed at 13 weeks in which in a small right-sided thrombus near the injection site was noted.

Following these experiments atheromatous suspension was injected into the right common iliac artery in different doses. In the anaesthetized animal an abdominal mid-line incision was made and the bladder contents aspirated to reveal the aortic bifurcation. Progressively increasing amounts of atheromatous material from 200 to 400 mg suspended in 2 ml of saline were injected. Pressure was applied to the left common iliac artery while the injection was made into the right common iliac artery. After haemostasis was secured by 3 min pressure over the puncture site, the abdomen was closed with sutures. This set of experiments contained two control animals. In one the injection consisted of 2 ml saline and in the other 250 mg of ground liver. No thrombi were found at autopsy and no alteration from normal during life was observed.

At first the natural course of events was allowed to proceed. Death within 1–3 days, usually 24 h, occurred in five animals injected with 200 mg or more of atheromatous material. Impaired movement of the right leg was noted. Autopsy revealed thrombosis of the peripheral arterial system with extension up to the aortic bifurcation and sometimes into the lower aorta. Another two animals were injected with doses of 250 mg of atheromatous material. They were killed 3 h and 5 h postinjection. In each there was thrombosis of the right common iliac artery and in the 5-h animal involvement of the aortic bifurcation had occurred as well as thrombosis of the left femoral artery.

These experiments allowed division into two groups; namely the survivors who tolerated the doses of atheromatous material injected and those in which death of the animal ensued following ascending arterial thrombosis. The watershed dose level was 200 mg. When 200 mg or more of atheromatous material was injected, the animals died from ascending secondary thrombosis at about 1.5 days postinjection on average. Death took place within hours of the ascending thrombosis reaching the aortic bifurcation and involving the lower end of the abdominal aorta.

No physical abnormalities were seen in rabbits injected with the lower levels of dose of atheromatous material even up to 18 weeks postinjection. As the doses were increased, the first effect was survival of the animal with a limp. At the highest level (over 200 mg) there was increasing immobility of one or both hind limbs. In an animal that survived for the longest period in the sector (3 days), gangrene of the toes of the right foot had developed. The vessel segment containing the ascending thrombosis revealed damaged endothelium in the region of the embolus, leucocytes migrating through the endothelium into the wall of the artery and endothelium raised from its anchoring points. Leucocytes accumulated at the level of the basement membrane.

It is postulated that there is an 'atheromatous burden' for any specific vasculature. Below this threshold level almost complete if not complete removal of the elements of the atheroembolus occurs without untoward effect. Above this level a continuing thrombosis occurs, in which case death of the tissue supplied by the target artery ensues, which may result in the death of the animal. This is illustrated in Figures 11.8 and 11.9. The variability of presentation of atheroembolism in man may depend upon the release of critical dosage levels for specific target arterial systems.

Additional study of this phenomena was carried out whereby the ascending thrombus was examined *in situ* at the leading edge [116,123]. In this ascending arterial thrombosis there is an active surface which extends in a proximal fashion against the flow of blood rather than with it as in venous thrombosis. The early stages of platelet adhesion and aggregation can be observed as the increment at the leading edge of the thrombus. Early platelet shape change is noted with extensive pseudopodial formation. Layering occurs around the atheroembolus of various blood elements including platelets, fibrin and leucocytes.

The determination of lethal doses for the cerebral and lower limb arterial system led to the further investigation of the thrombogenicity and lethality of components of

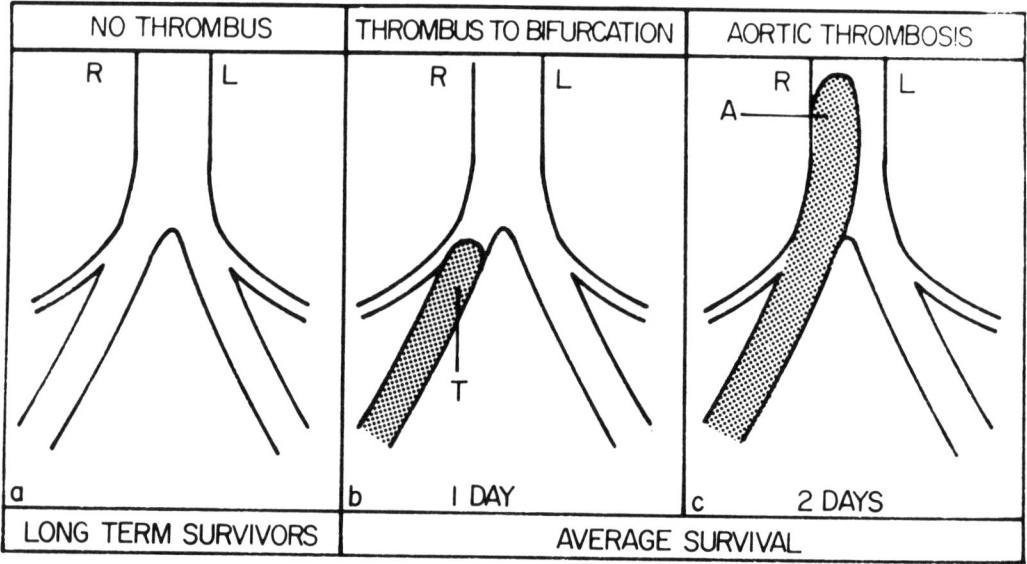

Figure 11.8 Post-mortem findings at the bifurcation of the aorta in limb experimental atheroembolism. (a) In the long-term survivors no thrombi were found (apart from a small thrombus at injection site in one animal). (b) In animals dying within 1 day of the injection of the material the thrombus (T) did not extend beyond the bifurcation. The actual head of the thrombus did not completely occlude the right common iliac artery although the following thrombus eventually did so. (c) In animals surviving for 2 days after injection of a large amount of atheromatous material, the thrombus advanced beyond the bifurcation into the main trunk of the aorta (A). Plugging of the left common iliac due to the aortic thrombus occurred on occasion. R = right; L = left. (Reproduced with permission from Warren and Lytton [122].)

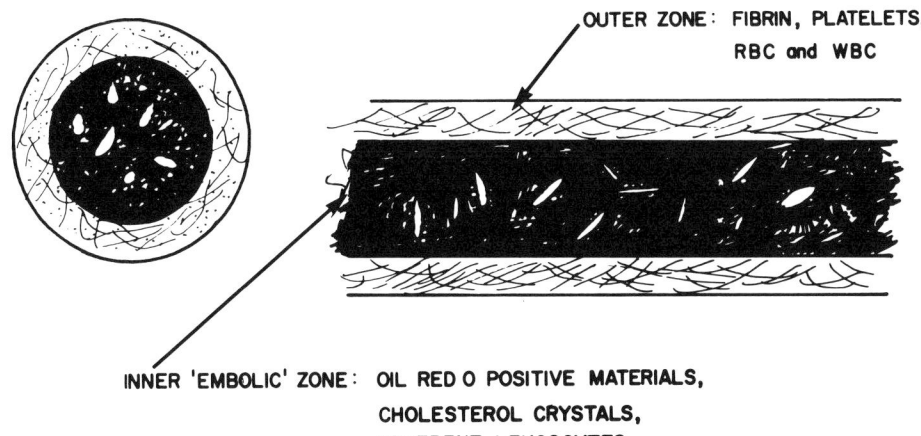

Figure 11.9 Examination by frozen section of the head of the thrombus 5 h after injection of atheromatous material in limb arteries revealed the following structure: (a) an outer zone next to the endothelium; (b) an inner 'embolic' zone. The atheroembolus was thus incorporated into a thrombus. (Reproduced with permission from Warren and Lytton [122].)

human atheromatous material [7,124]. Human atheromatous material was separated into lipid and non-lipid fractions by ether and chloroform-methyl alcohol procedures. The length, weight and volume of experimental thrombi induced by whole material and the non-lipid extract of human atheromatous material in a Chandler tube apparatus were compared. Non-lipid material produced thrombi that were significantly greater in length weight and volume. *In vivo* studies revealed that while a maximum non-lethal dose of whole material when injected into the left common carotid arteries of rabbits was between 50 and 60 mg, the amount was much less when the material was separated into non-lipid components. The respective figures were 8 mg for the non-lipid material and between 15 and 30 mg for the lipid material. The thrombogenic response to atheroemboli material is a critical step in the evolution of an occlusive extending thrombus.

References

1. Maurizi, C.P., Barker, A.E. and Trueheart, R.E. (1968) Atheromatous emboli. A postmortem study with special reference to the lower extremities. *Arch. Path.*, **86**, 528–34.
2. Kealy, W.F. (1978) Atheroembolism. *J. Clin. Path.*, **31**, 984–9.
3. Thurlbeck, W.M. and Castleman, B. (1957) Atheromatous emboli to the kidneys after aortic surgery. *New Engl. J. Med.*, **257**, 442–7.
4. Greendyke, R.M. and Akamatsu, Y. (1960) Atheromatous embolism as a cause of renal failure. *J. Urol.*, **83**, 231–7.
5. Uys, C.J. and Watson, C.E. (1963) The effects of atheromatous embolization on small arteries and arterioles. *S. Afr. Med. J.*, **37**, 69–73.
6. Gore, I. and Collins, D.P. (1960) Spontaneous atheromatous embolism: review of the literature and a report of 16 additional cases. *Am. J. Clin. Path.*, **33**, 416–26.
7. Eliot, R.S., Kanjuh, V.I. and Edwards, J.E. (1964) Atheromatous embolism. *Circulation*, **30**, 611–18.
8. Wolter, J.R. and Ryan, R.W. (1972) Atheromatous embolism of the central retinal artery. *Arch. Ophthal.*, **87**, 301–4.
9. Otken, I.B. (1959) Experimental production of atheromatous embolism. *Arch. Path.*, **68**, 685–9.
10. Warren, B.A. and Vales, O. (1973) The ultrastructure of the stages of atheroembolic occlusion of renal arteries. *Br. J. Exp. Path.*, **54**, 469–78.
11. Lough, J. and Moore, S. (1972) Platelet embolic injury: the healing process. *Expl Mol. Path.*, **17**, 132–44.
12. Ross, R. (1986) The pathogenesis of atherosclerosis: an update. *New Engl. J. Med.*, **314**, 488–500.
13. Piez, K.A. (1990) Preface. *Ann. N.Y. Acad. Sci.*, **593**, i–ii.
14. Snyder, H.E. and Shapiro, J.L. (1961) A correlative study of atheromatous embolism in human beings and experimental animals. *Surgery, St Louis.*, **49**, 195–204.
15. Wagner, R.B. and Martin, A.S. (1973) Peripheral atheroembolism confirmation of a clinical concept, with a case report and review of the literature. *Surgery*, **73**, 353–9.
16. Zak, F.G. and Elias, K. (1949) Embolization with material from atheromata. *Am. J. Med. Sci.*, **218**, 510–15.
17. Hoye, S.J., Teitelbaum, S., Gore, I. *et al.* (1959) Atheromatous embolization. A factor in peripheral gangrene. *New Engl J. Med.*, **261**, 128–31.
18. Fisher, E.R., Hellstrom, H.R. and Meyers, J.D. (1960) Disseminated atheromatous emboli. *Am. J. Med.*, **29**, 176–80.
19. Leroy, D. (1986) The cutaneous manifestations of atheroembolism, in *Atheroembolism*, (ed. B.A. Warren), CRC Press, Florida, pp. 67–91.
20. Haygood, T.A., Fessel, W.J. and Strange, D.A. (1968) Atheromatous microembolism simulating polymyositis. *J. Am. Med. Ass.*, **203**, 135–7.
21. Hory, B., Saint-Hillier, Y., Dupond, J.L. *et al.* (1977) Maladie athéroembolique avec anticorps antinucléaires simulant une périarterite noueuse. *Nouv. Presse Med.*, **6**, 2243–4.
22. Carvajal, J.A., Anderson, W.R., Weiss, L. *et al.* (1967) Atheroembolism. An etiologic factor in renal insufficiency, gastrointestinal haemorrhages and peripheral vascular diseases. *Arch. Intern. Med.*, **119**, 593–9.
23. Richards, A.M., Eliot, R.S., Kanjuh, V.I. *et al.* (1965) Cholesterol embolism. A multiple system disease masquerading as polyarteritis nodosa. *Am. J. Cardiol.*, **15**, 696–707.
24. Harrington, J.T., Sommers, S.C. and Kassirer, J.P. (1968) Atheromatous emboli with progressive renal failure. Renal arteriography as the probable inciting factor. *Ann. Intern. Med.*, **68**, 152–60.
25. Lonni, Y.G.W., Matsumsto, K.K. and Lecky, J.W. (1969) Post aortographic cholesterol (atheromatous) embolization. *Radiology*, **93**, 63–5.
26. Sayre, G.P. and Campbell, D.C. (1959) Multiple peripheral emboli in atherosclerosis of the aorta. *Arch. Intern. Med.*, **103**, 799–806.
27. Sieniewicz, D.J., Moore, S., Moir, F.D. *et al.* (1969) Atheromatous emboli to the kidneys. *Radiology*, **92**, 1231–40.
28. Rosansky, S.J. (1982) Multiple cholesterol emboli syndrome. *South. Med. J.*, **75**, 677–80.
29. Bloom, M.G., Winthrop, L.H. and Sarosi, G.A. (1972) Spontaneous cholesterol emboli renal failure. *Minn. Med.*, **55**, 1099–102.
30. Leroy, D., Michel, M., Mandard, J.C. *et al.* (1981) Association d'une coagulation intravasculaire disséminée et d'embolies cutanées de cristaux de cholestérol. *Ann. Dermatol. Venereol.*, **108**, 665–73.
31. Roujeau, J., Albahany, C., Guillaume, J. *et al.* (1965) Embolies athéromateuses diffuses avec insuffisance rénale. Etude anatomo-clinique d'un cas. *Sem. Hôp. Paris*, **41**, 1161–4.
32. Juillet, Y. and Cukier, A. (1981) Embolies de cholestérol et pseudo-périarterite noueuse. *Nouv. Presse Med.*, **10**, 177.
33. Regester, R.F. (1979) Renal failure secondary to spontaneous atheromatous microembolism. *J. Tenn. Med. Assoc.*, **73**, 328–30.

34. Retan, J.W. and Miller, R.E. (1966) Microembolic complications of atherosclerosis. *Arch. Intern. Med.*, **118**, 534–45.
35. Perdue, G.D. and Smith, R.B. (1969) Atheromatous microemboli. *Ann. Surg.*, **169**, 954–9.
36. Pollitt, J. and Lee, B.M. (1971) Renal failure from atheroembolism after translumber aortography. *J. Am. Geriat. Soc.*, **19**, 989–95.
37. Justrabo, E., Faivre, J.M., Guillermand, H. et al. (1982) Les embolies des cristaux de cholestérol. Aspects anatomo-cliniques et pathogéniques. A propos de deux observations dont un cas de pseudo-périartérite noueuse. *Sem. Hôp. Paris*, **58**, 1489–96.
38. Jones, D.B. and Iannaccone, P.M. (1975) Atheromatous emboli in renal biopsies. *Am. J. Pathol.*, **78**, 261–76.
39. Kassirer, J.P. (1969) Atheroembolic renal disease. *New Engl. J. Med.*, **280**, 812–18.
40. Lie, J.T. (1992) Cholesterol atheromatous embolism. The great masquerader revisited. *Path. Ann.*, **27** (pt 2), 17–50.
41. Anderson, W.R. and Richards, A.M. (1968) Evaluation of lower extremity muscle biopsies in the diagnosis of atheroembolism. *Arch. Path.*, **86**, 535–41.
42. Kwaan, J.H., Molen, R.V., Stemmer, E.A. et al. (1975) Peripheral embolism resulting from unsuspected atheromatous aortic plaques. *Surgery*, **78**, 589–93.
43. Kempczinski, R.F. (1979) Lower-extremity arterial emboli from ulcerating atherosclerotic plaques. *J. Am. Med. Ass.*, **241**, 807–10.
44. Schechter, D.C. (1979) Atheromatous embolization to lower limbs. *N.Y. State J. Med.*, **79**, 1180–6.
45. Mulliken, J.B. and Bartlett, M.K. (1971) Small bowel obstruction secondary to atheromatous embolism: case report and review of the literature. *Ann. Surg.*, **174**, 145–50.
46. Panum, P.L. (1862) Experimental Beiträge zur Lehre von der Embolie. *Arch. Path. Anat.*, **25**, 308–38 (cited by Mulliken and Bartlett, [45]).
47. Woolf, N. (1982) The morphology of theroscerotic lesions, in *Pathology of atherosclerosis*, (ed. N. Woolf), Butterworth Scientific, London, pp. 47–82.
48. O'Grady, J., Moncada, S. and Vane, J.R. (1982) Role of platelets and vessel wall prostaglandins in thrombosis, in *Thrombosis and Atherosclerosis* (Year Book), (eds N.U. Bang, J.L. Glover, R.W. Holden and D.A. Triplett), Medical Publishers, Chicago, pp. 323–40.
49. Bouch, D.C. and Montgomery, D.L. (1970) Cardiac lesions in fatal cases of recent myocardial ischaemia from a coronary care unit. *Br. Heart J.*, **32**, 795–803.
50. Constantinides, P. (1966) Plaque fissures in human coronary thrombosis. *J. Atheroscl. Res.*, **6**, 1–17.
51. Brooks, C.J.W., Steel, G., Gilbert, J.D. et al. (1971) Lipids of human atheroma Part 4. Characterization of a new group of polar sterol esters from human atherosclerotic plaques. *Atherosclerosis*, **13**, 223–7.
52. Harland, W.A., Gilbert, J.D., Steel, G. et al. (1971) Lipids of human atheroma Part 5. The occurrence of a new group of polar sterol esters in various stages of human atherosclerosis. *Atherosclerosis*, **13**, 239–46.
53. Crawford, T. (1977) The pathology of coronary artery occlusion, in *Pathology of Ischaemic Heart Disease*, Butterworths, London, pp. 47–70.
54. Newman III, W.P., Tracey, R.E., Strong, J.P. et al. (1982) Pathology of sudden coronary death in sudden coronary death, (eds H.M. Greenberg and E.M. Dwyer Jr), *Ann. N.Y. Acad. Sci.*, **382**, 39–49.
55. Strong, J.P. (1983) Myocardial infarction in patients with patent coronary bed – a pathologist's viewpoint, in *Proceedings of the Florence International Meeting on Myocardial Infarction*, vol. II, (ed. G.G. Neri Serneri), Excerpta Medica, Amsterdam, pp. 647–59, (quoted by Newman et al. [54]).
56. Jeynes, B.J. (1986) Cerebral atheroembolism and its relationship to thrombotic stroke, in *Atheroembolism*, (ed. B.A. Warren), CRC Press, Florida, pp. 41–65.
57. Hunt, J.R. (1914) The role of carotid arteries in the causation of vascular lesions of the brain with remarks on certain features of symptomatology. *Am. J. Med. Sci.*, **14**, 704.
58. Gunning, A.J., Pickering, G.W., Robb Smith, A.H.T. et al. (1964) Mural thrombosis of the internal carotid artery and subsequent embolism. *Q. J. Med.*, **33**, 155–95.
59. Moore, W.S. and Hall, A.D. (1970) Importance of emboli from carotid bifurcation in pathogenesis of cerebral ischaemic attacks. *Arch. Surg.*, **101**, 708–16.
60. Lhermitte, F. and Gautier, J.C. (1975) Sites of cerebral arterial occlusions, in *Modern Trends in Neurology*, vol. 6, (ed. D. Wilkins), Butterworths, London, pp. 123–40.
61. Jorgenson, L. and Torvik, A. (1966) Ischaemic cerebrovascular diseases in an autopsy series. I Prevalence, location and predisposing factors in verified thrombo-embolic occlusions and their significance in the pathogenesis of cerebral infarction. *J. Neurol. Sci.*, **3**, 490–509.
62. Wood, E.H. and Correll, J.W. (1969) Atheromatous ulceration in major neck vessels as a cause of cerebral embolism. *Acta Radiol. Diagn.*, **9**, 520–6.
63. Schwartz, C.J. and Mitchell, J.R.A. (1961) Atheroma of the carotid and vertebral arterial systems. *Br. Med. J.*, **2**, 1057–63.
64. Conley, J.E., Bernhard, V.M., Maddison, F.E. et al. (1973) Cerebral emboli and the atheromatous carotid artery. *J. Cardiovasc. Surg. Spec. Issue*, pp. 447–50.
65. Sturgill, B.C. and Netsky, M.G. (1963) Cerebral infarction by atheromatous emboli. *Arch. Pathol.*, **76**, 189–96.
66. Hollenhorst, R.W. (1961) Significance of bright plaque in retinal arterioles. *J. Am. Med. Ass.*, **178**, 23–9.
67. Ehrenfeld, W.K., Hoyt, W.F. and Wilie, E.J. (1966) Embolization and transient blindness from carotid atheroma. Surgical considerations. *Arch. Surg.*, **93**, 787–94.
68. Moossy, J. (1961) Cerebral infarction and intracranial arterial thrombosis. *Arch. Neurol.*, **14**, 119–23.
69. Houser, O.W., Sundt, T.M., Holman, C.B. et al. (1974) Atheromatous disease of the carotid artery. Consolidation of angiographic clinical and surgical findings. *J. Neurosurg.*, **41**, 321–31.
70. Fisher, C.M. (1959) Observations of the fundus oculi in transient monocular blindness. *Neurology*, **9**, 333–47.
71. Escourolle, R. and Poirier, J. (1971) II Ischaemic vascular pathology of arterial origin:infarction, In *Manual of Basic Neuropathology*, W.B. Saunders, Philadelphia, pp. 82–101.
72. Fisher, C.M. (1975) in *Modern Concepts of Cerebrovascular Disease*, (ed. J.S. Mayer), Spectrum Publishing, New York. p. 21.
73. Winter, W.J. (1957) Atheromatous emboli: a cause of cerebral infarction. *Am. Med. Ass. Arch. Pathol.*, **64**, 137–42.
74. Soloway, H.B. and Aronson, S.M. (1964) Atheromatous emboli to the central nervous system. *Arch. Neurol.*, **11**, 657–67.
75. Ross Russell, R.W. (1970) The origin and effects of cerebral emboli. *Mod. Trends Neurol.*, **5**, 178–88.
76. Fisher, M. (1951) Occlusion of the internal carotid artery. *Am. Med. Ass. Arch. Neurol. Psychiat.*, **65**, 346–77.
77. Sussman, E.B. and Porro, R.S. (1974) Pituitary apoplexy the role of atheromatous emboli. *Stroke*, **5**, 318–23.
78. David, N.J., Kintworth, G.K., Friedberg, S.J. et al. (1963) Fatal atheromatous cerebral embolism associated with bright plaques in the retinal arterioles. *Neurology*, **13**, 708–13.
79. Price, D.L. and Harris, J. (1970) Cholesterol emboli in cerebral arteries as a complication of retrograde aortic perfusion during cardiac surgery. *Neurology*, **20**, 1209–14.
80. Darling, R.C., Austen, W.G. and Linton, R.R. (1967) Arterial embolism. *Surg. Gynecol. Obstet.*, **124**, 106–14.
81. Ball, C.J. (1966) Atheromatous embolism to the brain retina and choroid. *Arch. Ophthal.*, **76**, 690–5.
82. Slavin, R.E., Gonzalez-Vitale, J.C. and Marin, O.S.M. (1975) Atheromatous emboli to the lumbo sacral spinal cord. *Stroke*, **6**, 411–16.
83. Fisher, M. and Adams, R.O. (1951) Observations on brain embolism with special reference to the mechanisms of haemorrhagic infarction. *J. Neuropathol. Expl Neurol.*, **10**, 92–3.
84. Baker, A.B., Dahl, E. and Sandler, B. (1963) Cerebrovascular disease, etiologic factors in cerebral infarction. *Neurology*, **13**, 445–54.
85. Anderson, W.R., Richards, A.M. and Weiss, L. (1967) Hemorrhage and necrosis of the stomach and bowel due to atheroembolism: a correlative study of atheromatous emboli to the gastrointestinal tract in humans and experimental animals. *Am. J. Clin. Path.*, **48**, 30–8.
86. Stout, C., Hartsuck, J.M., Howe, J. et al. (1972) Atheromatous embolism after aortofemoral bypass and aortic ligation. *Arch. Path.*, **93**, 271–5.
87. Warren, B.A. and Vales, O. (1975) Electron microscopy of the sequence of events in the atheroembolic occlusion of cerebral arteries in an animal model. *Br. J. Expl Path.*, **56**, 205–15.
88. Warren, B.A. and Vales, O. (1976) The ultrastructure of the reaction of arterial walls to cholesterol crystals in atheroembolism. *Br. J. Expl Path.*, **57**, 67–77.
89. Obriain, D.S., Jeffers, M., Kay, E.W. et al. (1991) Bleeding due to colonic atheroembolism. Diagnosis by biopsy of adenomatous polyps or ischaemic ulcer. *Am. J. Surg. Pathol.*, **15**, 1078–82.
90. Anderson, W.R. and Braverman, T. (1991) Colon perforation due to cholesterol embolism. *Hum. Pathol.*, **22**, 839–41.
91. Blauth, C.I., Cosgrove, D.M., Webb, B.W. et al. (1992) Atheroembolism from the ascending aorta. An emerging problem in cardiac surgery. *J. Thorac. Cardiovasc. Surg.*, **103**, 1104–11.
92. Trono, R., Sutton, C. and Hollman, J. (1989) Multiple myocardial infarctions associated with atheromatous emboli after PTCA of saphenous vein grafts. A clinicopathologic correlation. *Cleve. Clin. J. Med.*, **56**, 581–4.
93. Keon, W.J., Heggtveit, H.A. and Leduc, J. (1982) Perioperative myocardial infarction caused by atheroembolism. *J. Thorac. Cardiovasc. Surg.*, **84**, 849–55.
94. Heggtveit, H.A. (1984) Coronary atheroembolism. *New Engl. J. Med.*, **310**, 722.
95. Fitzgibbon, G.M. and Keon, W.J. (1987) Atheroembolic perioperative infarction during repeat coronary bypass surgery: angiographic documentation in a survivor. *Ann. Thorac. Surg.*, **43**, 218–19.
96. Grondin, C.M., Pomar, J.L., Herbert, Y. et al. (1984) Reoperation in patients with patent atherosclerotic coronary vein grafts: a difficult approach to a different disease. *J. Thorac. Cardiovasc. Surg.*, **87**, 379–85.

97. Ong, H.T., Elmsly, W.G. and Friedlander, D.H. (1991) Cholesterol atheroembolism: an increasingly frequent complication of cardiac catherisation. *Med. J. Aust.*, **154**, 412–14.
98. Palmer, F.J. and Warren, B.A. (1988) Multiple cholesterol emboli syndrome complicating angiographic techniques. *Clin. Radiol.*, **39**, 519–22.
99. Labs, J.D., Merillat, J.C. and Williams, G.M. (1988) Analysis of solid phase debris from laser angioplasty: potential risks of atheroembolism. *J. Vasc. Surg.*, **7**, 326–35.
100. Drost, H., Buis, B., Haan, D. *et al.* (1984) Cholesterol embolism as a complication of left heart catheterization. Report of seven cases. *Br. Heart J.*, **52**, 339–42.
101. Wilson, D.M., Salazer, T.L. and Farkouh, M.E. (1991) Eosinophiluria in atheroembolic renal disease. *Am. J. Med.*, **91**, 186–9.
102. Williams, G.M., Perler, B.A., Burdick, J.F. *et al.* (1991) Angiographic localization of spinal cord blood supply and its relationship to postoperative paraplegia. *J. Vasc. Surg.*, **13**, 23–33.
103. Gibbons, G.W., Madras, P.N., Wheelock, F.C. *et al.* (1982) Aortoiliac reconstruction following renal transplantation. *Surgery*, **91**, 435–7.
104. Flinn, W.R., Harris, J.P., Rudo, N.D. *et al.* (1981) Atherombolism as cause of graft failure in femoral distal reconstruction. *Surgery*, **90**, 698–706.
105. Merchant Jr, R.F. and DePalma, R.G. (1981) Effects of femorofemoral grafts on postoperative sexual function: correlation with penile pulse volume recordings. *Surgery*, **90**, 962–70.
106. Wagner, R.B. and Martin, A.S. (1973) Peripheral atheroembolism: confirmation of a clinical concept, with a case report and review of the literature. *Surgery*, **73**, 353–9.
107. Kaufman, J.L., Stark, K., Brolin, R.E. (1987) Disseminated atheroembolism from extensive degenerative atherosclerosis of the aorta. *Surgery*, **102**, 63–70.
108. Kwaan, J.H., Connolly, J.E. (1977) Peripheral atheroembolism: an enigma. *Arch. Surg.*, **112**, 987–90.
109. Flory, C.M. (1945) Arterial occlusions produced by emboli from eroded aortic atheromatous plaques. *Am. J. Path.*, **21**, 549–66.
110. Langer, E. and Spelsberg, G.A. (1959) Experimental atheromatous arterial emboli in kidney. *Beitr. Path. Anat.*, **86**, 197–210.
111. Connor, W.E., Hoak, J.C. and Warner, E.D. (1965) The role of lipids in thrombosis, in *Pathogenesis and Treatment of Thrombotic Diseases*, (ed. F.K. Duckert), F.K. Schattauer Verlag, Stuttgart, pp. 193–208.
112. Byers, S.D. and Friedman, M. (1964) Contribution of atheromatous gruel to thrombus formation. *Proc. Soc. Expl Biol. Med.*, **115**, 436–8.
113. Kirk, J.E. (1962) Thromboplastin activities of human arterial and venous tissues. *Proc. Soc. Expl Biol. Med.*, **109**, 890–2.
114. Warren, B.A., Vales, O. and Khan, S. (1975) Platelet pseudopodia and their involvement in adhesion: observations by transmission and scanning electron microscopy. *Excerpta Medica*, **357**, 43–51.
115. Jeynes, B.J. and Warren, B.A. (1981) Thrombogenicity of components of atheromatous material. *Arch. Path. Lab. Med.*, **105**, 353–7.
116. Warren, B.A., Jeynes, B.J. and Chauvin, W.J. (1978) SEM studies of atheromatous plaques in man and the interaction of blood with plaque contents in experimental animals. *Scann. Electron Microsc.*, **2**, 441–8.
117. Poole, J.C.F., Cromwell, S.B. and Benditt, E.P. (1971) Behaviour of smooth muscle cells and formation of extracellular structures in the reaction of arterial walls to injury. *Am. J. Path.*, **62**, 391–414.
118. Adams, C.W.M., Bayliss, O.B., Ibrahim, M.Z.M. and Webster Jr, M.W. (1963) Phospholipids in atherosclerosis: the modification of the cholesterol granuloma by phospholipid. *J. Path. Bact.*, **86**, 431–6.
119. Abdulla, Y.H., Adams, C.W.M. and Morgan, R.S. (1967) Connective tissue reactions to implantation of purified sterol, sterol esters, phosphoglyceride glycerides and free fatty acids. *J. Path. Bact.*, **94**, 63–71.
120. Jeynes, B.J. and Warren, B.A. (1982) Cerebral atheroembolism. An animal model. *Stroke*, **13**, 312–8.
121. Jeynes, B.J. (1986) An assessment of the extent and distribution of experimentally induced cerebral atheroembolic vascular occlusions and infarcts. *Artery*, **14**, 35–42.
122. Warren, B.A. and Lytton, D.G. (1976) The effects and morphology of atheroembolism in limb arteries, an experimental study. *Pathology*, **8**, 231–45.
123. Warren, B.A., Chauvin, W.J. and Jeynes, B.J. (1977) The induction of arterial thrombosis by injected atheromatous material. *Proc. Microsc. Soc. Can.*, **4**, 114–15.
124. Jeynes, B.J. and Warren, B.A. (1981) Thrombogenicity of components of atheromatous material. *Arch. Pathol. Lab. Med.*, **105**, 353–7.

12 CEREBROVASCULAR DISEASE

William E. Stehbens

The vascular system of the brain and spinal cord exhibits unique morphological and architectural peculiarities not seen in other organs (Chapter 1). The reasons for these differences appear to be bound up with the phenomena responsible for the unique functions of the vulnerable, highly specialized tissues of the central nervous system. From the point of view of the pathologist, the cerebral blood vessels are easier and more convenient to dissect than extracranial vessels, although each of the four major arteries of supply has an extracranial segment that must be considered in cerebrovascular pathology.

12.1 Cerebrovascular mortality and epidemiology

Cerebrovascular disease is generally regarded as the third most common cause of death in the Western world and from the age of 65 years is the second most common cause of death after heart disease. With longevity increasing its clinical importance is growing. In 1978 it was estimated that one in three persons in England and Wales [1] would develop clinical cerebrovascular disease.

Cerebrovascular disease and stroke are non-specific terms that encompass

- cerebral softening due to thrombosis superimposed on atherosclerosis or to atheroembolism;
- cerebral haemorrhage;
- subarachnoid haemorrhage.

Each is an imprecise diagnosis and could encompass lesions that are secondary and not primarily due to degenerative vascular disease. The International Classification of Diseases also includes spasm of cerebral arteries and unspecified strokes [2].

Stroke is a non-specific term indicating the abrupt onset of a neurological deficit irrespective of cause and is thus often used synonymously with cerebrovascular disease or to encompass cerebral haemorrhage and thromboembolic infarction. More often than not it refers to the sudden onset of symptoms and signs of vascular insufficiency or infarction. When the neurological deficit is severe, it is referred to as a major stroke and as a little stroke when there is a slight deficit. Though such terms lack precision and therefore ought to be avoided, they are in common usage.

The disability and high mortality attributable to vascular disease in technologically advanced populations highlight the need to determine factors that may aggravate, predispose to or cause cerebrovascular diseases with a view to preventing or ameliorating the effects. Epidemiologists rely on the incidence of clinical sequelae such as cerebrovascular disease or stroke as a surrogate marker of the severity of atherosclerosis. This practice is more inappropriate than the use of coronary heart disease (CHD) because:

1. the wide variation in age and severity of atherosclerosis in the subdivisions of cerebrovascular disease which are usually considered to have distinctly different aetiologies;
2. atherosclerosis is ubiquitous;
3. the severity of atherosclerosis tends to be less in primary intracerebral haemorrhage than with atherosclerotic infarction or embolism and least with berry aneurysms.

Another complicating factor is the apparent difference in atherosclerosis with transient ischaemic attacks between Japan and Western countries [2]. Small intracerebral arteries are more commonly affected than extracranial carotid arteries in the Japanese, suggesting different disease aetiologies. Cerebral arteritis may also be more prevalent in Asian countries [3], thus affecting the accuracy of using cerebrovascular disease as a universal surrogate monitor for atherosclerosis severity.

Cerebrovascular disease mortality rates are being increasingly used to establish a relationship with CHD risk factors and for comparisons of stroke incidence between and within countries. According to such data stroke mortality rates in the United Kingdom and the United States have been falling by some 30 to 50% in the last 30 years [4] and the decline is said to have commenced earlier in some populations [5]. These vital statistics give only crude indications of incidence and

Table 12.1 Diagnostic error for subdivisions of cerebrovascular disease*

Type of lesion	Number of cases diagnosed clinically and confirmed at autopsy	Number of cases diagnosed clinically but not confirmed at autopsy (false +ve)	Number of cases diagnosed at autopsy but undiagnosed clinically (false −ve)
Cerebral haemorrhage	257	282 (52.3)	120 (31.8)
Cerebral thrombosis and embolism	159	192 (54.7)	151 (48.7)
Subarachnoid haemorrhage	112	53 (32.1)	19 (34.5)

*Source: Heasman and Lipworth [11].
False-positive and false-negative diagnostic percentage rates are in parentheses.

mortality rates whether national or regional. They are too inaccurate for scientific use. The diagnostic error as determined by autopsy monitoring is unacceptably high [6] and Hartveit [7] estimated the accuracy rate to be about 50%. In the Framingham study approximately 40% of stroke diagnoses were incorrect and of 196 persons who died of stroke, the diagnosis was not on the death certificate in 35% [8]. A later Framingham report gave the false positive rate as 21% and the false negative rate as 40% [9] without taking into account the diagnostic error for subclassification of strokes. Kurtzke [2] estimated that deaths for subdivisions of stroke are incorrectly differentiated in 30 to 80% of cases and that the differentiation between cerebral haemorrhage and thrombosis was hazardous. There are additional problems involving the exclusion of contributory causes in monocausal death certificates, errors in coding, diagnostic fashions, errors in census data, lack of registration of deaths, non-medical certification of deaths and certifying practices [6]. It must be concluded that use of such mortality rates provides inexact, fallacious data and allows indeterminate overlap in epidemiological studies. To use pooled data for stroke by ignoring the subdivisions of stroke would be even worse. National stroke mortality rates provide fallacious estimations of the incidence of fatal strokes giving no indication of the frequency of non-fatal strokes, many of which result in permanent disability. It would also be erroneous to believe that such data can be used for scientific purposes or as the bases of population-based programmes to prevent cerebrovascular disease.

Treating all cerebrovascular diseases as one will not provide significant epidemiological findings and Kurtzke [2] concluded that no deduction could be made on the relationship of environmental factors using this data. There is no justification for Kuller's view [10] that misclassification of neurological diseases such as stroke is a minimal problem. The use of subdivisions of stroke also provides fallacious data. For example in the survey of 75 hospitals of the British National Health service, the diagnostic inaccuracy for the three main types of stroke was substantial (Table 12.1). There is variation from hospital to hospital, and with age and time. Overall weaknesses in epidemiological methodology for CHD [12] also apply to epidemiological studies of stroke.

Based on such diagnostic inaccuracy, an association of blood lipids and lipoproteins has been sought with cerebrovascular disease as with CHD even though their mortality rates have not paralleled each other this century. The evidence for a relationship has been found generally inadequate [2,10] and in 1968, a Framingham Study report indicated that a reduction in the morbidity and mortality from CHD, stroke and peripheral vascular disease by lowering blood lipids was unproven [13]. Even so diabetes mellitus, hyperlipidaemia, obesity and smoking have been considered to have much less relevance to stroke than to heart disease [14]. Seemingly this has been the reason for the greater concentration on lipids in CHD. In more recent years the interest has escalated. For individuals beyond the middle years afflicted with strokes due to atherosclerosis, serum cholesterol levels are generally normal and paradoxically the Framingham study showed an increased risk for stroke in women with low blood LDL levels [15]. Overall a significant correlation between cholesterol and stroke has not been found [16,17]. In a review of 16 prospective studies, no significant association was found in 13 although the authors believed a true association may have been missed, and no relationship was found between hyperlipidaemia and cerebral infarction in Japan [18]. Significantly no consideration was taken of the diagnostic errors inherent in such studies. Inconsistencies negate the validity of an hypothesis and the Japanese situation is such an inconsistency [10,19], which is reinforced by the decline in stroke mortality in the USA for decades prior to that in CHD [20].

An inverse association between serum cholesterol and the risk of intracerebral haemorrhage and a positive correlation for non-haemorrhagic stroke [21,22] have been reported. This indicates the serious fallacy of combining all types of stroke in epidemiological studies and the possibility that properly conducted studies and reliable investigations using appropriate and accurately measured parameters might reveal important relationships. The error inherent in misdiagnosis has been recognized [6,23] and an increase in incidence detection rates of less severe strokes coincident with the introduction of computed tomography has raised the possibility of an end to the decline in stroke [24].

A close correlation has been found between hypertension and strokes both haemorrhagic and ischaemic [2,10,25] and this is consistent with pathological and clinical experience. Hypertension is particularly associated with primary intracerebral haemorrhage but less so with aneurysmal subarachnoid haemorrhage, and hypertension and diabetes mellitus are recognized to be associated with atherosclerotic infarction. Pooling all types of stroke, primary or secondary, must mask valid relationships.

Hereditary factors have long been regarded as of importance in stroke mortality and Alter and Kluznik [26] found hypertension and heart disease were significantly frequent in relatives of stroke victims. After allowing for these two factors there was no obvious genetic tendency in stroke but this does not preclude the possibility of a genetic tendency to atherosclerosis, or another cause of stroke. In a study of twins, a five-fold increase in stroke prevalence was found among monozygotic compared to dizygotic twins [27] but whilst this is suggestive, it is far from conclusive since hypertension also is genetically dependent in many instances.

As with CHD there has been a tendency to speculate on trends in stroke mortality and the factors responsible despite Feinstein's admonition that 'no knowledgeable clinician or pathologist in the second half of the 20th century believes that single choices of death certificate diagnoses can indicate specific causes of death and that these choices can represent the actual occurrence of the specified diseases' [28].

12.2 Carotidynia

This is an obscure migraine-like syndrome associated with severe bilateral or unilateral facial and neck pain and carotid tenderness in the region of the carotid bifurcation from which the referred pain to the face and head is believed to originate [29,30]. The pain is throbbing or pulsatile in nature and sometimes associated with previous or simultaneous vascular headaches. It occurs mostly in middle-aged and elderly subjects of either sex and rarely in children. There are no bruits or consistent angiographic findings.

Emotional factors have been considered important [31] and it is not associated with an arteritis. The disorder is believed to be similar to migraine with relief provided by antimigraine therapy. Augmented and painful dilatation and pulsatility of the carotid artery has been noted and tenderness or exquisite pain. The aetiology is obscure though some localized vasomotor or even pathological distension of the carotid arteries may be responsible. There are no known certain pathological sequelae but a few cases have been associated with aneurysmal dilatation of the internal carotid artery [32].

12.3 Tortuosity, coiling, kinking and anatomical displacement

The cervical segment of the internal carotid artery often displays a variable degree of tortuosity, at times bilateral. Some tortuosity has been observed in four of 20 fetuses (five months to full term) in one of whom it was bilateral [33]. Most often seen between the ages of 40 and 70 years, it is frequently associated with severe cerebrovascular disease, aneurysms, stenotic lesions and hypertension [34]. When pronounced, it exhibits severe kinking or coiling, rendering the artery more susceptible to damage when anatomically displaced and to misdiagnosis as an aneurysm.

Maldevelopment has been postulated as the underlying reason but this is difficult to accept in the absence of any detailed investigation of the histological and physical properties of the arteries. There is reluctance to accept the possibility that degenerative changes in blood vessels can occur *in utero*, in infancy and in childhood.

Flow in at least one of the four main arteries of supply to the brain can at times be interrupted by certain positions of the head. This may be associated with osteoarthritis of the cervical spine and under such conditions impaired or obstructed flow during sleep might predispose to elongation in collaterals. The underlying pathology and changes in the physical characteristics of the arterial connective tissues require study but are probably similar to those occurring in association with bends and tortuosity in collateral vessels [35]. They are likely to be enhanced by inherited connective tissue disorders. Double loops have been reported in a subject with Marfan's syndrome and the lengthening of the arteries to permit such severe degrees of tortuosity must be considerable. The possible relationship with so-called physiological murmurs in the neck requires exploration and a frequent coexistence with aneurysms has been noted [34].

Symptoms and signs of cerebrovascular insufficiency may be associated with kinking and coiling of the internal carotid arteries especially in older subjects though it is difficult to be sure that kinking actually obstructs cerebral flow. Extreme tortuosity with kinking or buckling can involve the common carotid, brachiocephalic and subclavian arteries [36] especially in the presence of severe atherosclerosis.

Much less attention has been given to tortuosity of the extracranial segments of the vertebral arteries, which are restricted by their passage through foramina of the transverse processes of the cervical vertebrae. The cervical segment of the vertebral artery exhibits varying degrees of tortuosity with loops and kinks and even pressure erosion of the cervical vertebral body and pedicle. Extreme tortuosity may facilitate kinking or compression during movements of the head and osteophytes in cervical osteoarthritis render such tortuosities more vulnerable to pressure effects [3].

With these deformations, concern must be for the severe degenerative changes that can ensue [35], although the presence of severe atherosclerosis of other arteries to the brain, anatomic variation of the circle of Willis, variations in blood pressure, antihypertensive therapy and hypovolaemia, can make severe angulation and transient ischaemic attacks more critical [37].

Tortuosities of the intracranial segment of the vertebral arteries and the basilar artery are obviously associated with severe atherosclerosis. With the frequent inequality in size of the vertebral arteries, the dominant vertebral artery and the basilar artery frequently form an S-shaped tortuosity which is usually associated with arteriectasis and sometimes aneurysms. The lateral displacement of such enlarged and often rigid, if not calcified, vessels results in pressure and or displacement of nerves (oculomotor, trigeminal, abducent, facial and auditory). A tortuous ectatic vertebral artery may deform and compress the glossopharyngeal, vagus, accessory and hypoglossal nerves, as can the posterior inferior cerebellar artery. Medial deviation of both vertebral arteries has led to compression of the medulla oblongata in a woman with Chiari malformation [38].

The internal carotid artery is too short in its intracranial segment to exhibit tortuosity but the carotid siphon varies considerably in the sudden sharpness of its flexures. It is more likely to cause nerve compression when ectatic and aneurysmal. The other main basal arteries can be quite tortuous but tortuosity is most prominent in association with arteriovenous aneurysms.

The optic nerve and chiasma may be compressed by the internal carotid, anterior cerebral or ophthalmic arteries with some degree of optic atrophy [39]. It has been suggested that some degenerative changes in the optic nerves and tracts may be caused by ischaemia due to compression of small branches from severely atherosclerotic components of the circle of Willis.

The oculomotor nerve, by virtue of its close relationships to several arteries, is particularly often subject to compression especially by aneurysms. If the basilar bifurcation is high, the superior cerebellar artery may cause angulation of the nerve [39]. This will be by the posterior cerebral if the bifurcation is low or one of its branches may pass through the nerve (diastasis), a condition often associated with neural disturbances. The posterior communicating artery, especially when large and atherosclerotic, can compress the oculomotor nerve against the dural roof of the cavernous sinus [40]. The internal carotid artery in its cavernous segment can compress the oculomotor nerve, the three divisions of the trigeminal nerve and the abducent nerve. The trigeminal nerve may be grooved by the posterior cerebral or the superior cerebellar arteries. Such grooving of cranial nerves can be symptomless and without loss of function.

The anterior inferior cerebellar artery occasionally passes through the abducent nerve or deeply grooves it. Diplopia or convergent squint has been attributed to nerve compression by the anterior inferior cerebellar artery. A tortuous and atherosclerotic vertebral artery may also compress the abducent nerve. The facial and auditory nerves can be compressed by tortuous basilar and vertebral arteries and also the posterior inferior cerebellar artery. The internal auditory artery often arises inside the internal auditory meatus from the anterior inferior cerebellar artery and in such a confined space the auditory nerve is in jeopardy.

12.4 Vascular compression

Veins are more readily compressed than arteries because of their thinner walls and lower intravascular pressure, but the rich venous collateral circulation usually ensures adequate drainage. Occlusion of dural sinuses or major veins can be more serious especially if there is tumour invasion with secondary thrombosis. Narrowing and occlusion of arteries by intracranial tumours are not common but occur particularly with meningiomas, pituitary tumours and extradural tumours located principally at the base of the brain and involving the major arteries [41].

Vascular obstruction by pressure is prone to occur at the edges of the falx cerebri, tentorium cerebelli, foramen magnum, the rostral portion of the Sylvian fissure and the interpeduncular fossa. Grossly increased intracranial pressure can interfere with the general circulation of the brain but only flow studies can detect the extent of microvascular or parenchymal vascular stasis and compression about haematomas and other space-occupying lesions.

Compression of brain tissue against a rigid edge results in haemorrhagic necrosis in the floor of the pressure grooves [42] and these lesions become glial scars. The vessels crossing the grooves may be sharply indented or compressed. The posterior cerebral artery may be compressed against the free edge of the tentorium cerebelli as it courses around the cerebral peduncle which itself can be deeply grooved (Kernohan's notch). As herniation of the hippocampal gyrus progresses (supratentorial pressure), the site of compression shifts posteriorly until only a portion of the artery in the calcarine fissure is affected. Accordingly, the medial aspect of the occipital lobe is the area most frequently affected and the lesions may be bilateral. The necrosis is usually cortical, haemorrhagic or ischaemic with the white matter involved if the compression is complete. The arterial supply to Ammon's horn from the posterior cerebral artery runs perpendicular to the tentorial edge and is very readily compressed [42].

Branches passing through the interpeduncular fossa to the thalamus, the medial sector of the upper pons and mid-brain may be involved. The cerebral peduncles may be elongated and with progressive herniation into the interpeduncular fossa, the perforating arteries are compressed [42], at times causing ischaemia of most of the thalamus and usually with secondary vascular lesions of the mid-brain and pons.

With increased supratentorial pressure the posterior communicating artery is affected only in very severe cases. Being smaller, the anterior choroidal artery is more vulnerable but usually only pallidal branches are compressed causing necrosis in the medial part of the globus pallidus [39,42].

The anterior cerebral artery or branches may be compressed against the free edge of the falx cerebri with the angulate gyrus usually escaping involvement. Branches of the middle cerebral artery may be compressed against the sphenoid ridge. The stem is often unaffected.

With raised infratentorial pressure, cerebellar tissue herniates upwards through the tentorium compressing branches of the superior cerebellar arteries on the upper surface of the lateral lobes against the posterior rim of the foramen magnum. The tonsillar necrosis that occurs with herniation into the foramen magnum is secondary to vascular compression.

With elevated supratentorial pressure the basal vein is compressed between the mid-brain and the herniated temporal lobe. Very severe herniation may cause kinking of the great cerebral vein of Galen at its entry into the straight sinus in the falx cerebri. Both lesions will aggravate intracranial pressure by causing venous congestion and oedema. Infratentorial pressure causing cerebellar herniation upwards through the tentorium can lead to compression of the great vein of Galen against the splenium of the corpus callosum with venous obstruction to it and the basal veins.

12.5 Cerebral atherosclerosis

The cerebral arteries undergo progressive increase in calibre with age (ectasia) and there is a concomitant variable degree of tortuosity and irregularity of outline as atherosclerosis progresses. These arteries are amongst those that tend to be severely affected by atherosclerosis. The advantage of their thin walls is that atherosclerosis can be recognized from the external surface, first as white, opaque areas at branching sites and then eventually when more widespread with opacification, rigidity and irregularity of the walls. Discolouration of the adventitial surface due to haemorrhage or siderosis from breakdown of haemoglobin is a feature. Macroscopically visible vasa vasorum are to be seen when walls are thickened and require additional blood supply, there being no vasa vasorum in cerebral arteries initially.

One feature of atherosclerosis, that is recognizable in cerebral arteries macroscopically, is the presence of occasional small soft nodules on the surface of large severely atherosclerotic arteries. On one occasion a polypoid pultaceous swelling has simulated a small aneurysm [3]. Histological sectioning revealed these lesions as areas of herniation of caseous atherosclerotic debris (Figure 6.17) into the adventitia, the lipid-rich debris being surrounded by lipophages. A small atherosclerotic nodule is sometimes visible at the commencement of a small branch from a large cerebral artery and occasionally a small transversely orientated linear plaque.

Other aspects of cerebral atherosclerosis and age changes from infancy are dealt with in Chapter 6.

12.6 Murmurs

Pathological murmurs have several causes.

12.6.1 ATHEROSCLEROTIC STENOSIS

Systolic murmurs over the cervical arteries in association with severe atherosclerosis are a feature of stenotic atherosclerotic lesions of the carotid sinuses, the most common site. The bruit can be the earliest sign of carotid artery insufficiency [43] and may be transmitted up the carotid to the cranium usually being inaudible a few centimetres below the sinus. A stenosis in the carotid siphon may produce a murmur best detected over the eye [44]. Murmurs from the skull can generally be heard best over the orbit, ear or a trephine hole. Murmurs of the subclavian and vertebral arteries in the neck are less common. The presence of such a murmur is not associated necessarily with symptomatic cerebrovascular disease. Disappearance of such a murmur can signify complete or almost complete occlusion.

A hyperkinetic systolic bruit over the eye resulting from occlusion of the contralateral internal carotid artery is due to compensatory increase in flow and velocity.

12.6.2 ARTERIOVENOUS FISTULAE

A cranial bruit due to an arteriovenous shunt is distinctive and can be distressing but is not always present when flow through the fistula or shunt is low. The murmur has at times been used as an indicator of shunt recurrence. It usually emanates from the fistula but with a diffuse shunt, the bruit may be more hyperkinetic in type and not so distressing. Potter [45] estimated that bruits were present in 20–50% of lesions shown by angiography to be arteriovenous shunts.

12.6.3 INTRACRANIAL ARTERIAL ANEURYSMS

A few cerebral aneurysms have been associated with an audible bruit on auscultation and occasionally a thrill

[46]. These are not usual characteristics of aneurysms and an associated cryptic arteriovenous aneurysm may have been responsible. In recent years using electronic amplification cranial bruits have been detected emanating from berry aneurysms [47]. The bruit can be abolished by ipsilateral compression of the cervical artery of supply and there has been no correlation with the size of the sac or of the entrance.

12.6.4 TUMOURS

An arteriovenous shunt together with a bruit is sometimes associated with intracranial tumours (meningiomas, Lindau's haemangioblastoma, gliomas, acoustic neurinoma, ependymoma). Vascular tumours of the glomus jugulare can be markedly vascular and accompanied by a shunt.

Physiological murmurs of the head and neck are frequently detected and are discussed in section 1.2.4.

12.7 Cerebrovascular insufficiency

Vascular insufficiency varies from mild, transient symptoms of anoxia to those of massive, fatal encephalomalacia. The many causes are associated with an inadequate supply of blood and oxygen to an area of brain.

12.7.1 TRANSIENT ISCHAEMIC ATTACKS (TIA)

Transient stroke-like episodes (e.g. bouts of faintness, weakness, loss of consciousness or brief neurological deficit) are common in the elderly and pass within minutes or hours. The abrupt onset and total or almost complete recovery suggest a vascular disturbance. Definitions of TIA have varied. Although not sacrosanct the time limit of approximately 24 hours is often used, the essential feature being the transient duration. These episodes may presage a major ischaemic attack that is fatal or permanently disabling [48].

The fleeting nature of clinical episodes obviously leads to suggestions of vasospasm. Though not considered to be the cause, it cannot be excluded in all cases. Haemodynamic crises such as a sudden reduction of systemic blood flow and pressure in subjects with a precarious blood supply to the brain due to stenotic or occlusive lesions in the arteries of supply, may be responsible. Evidence has been provided that symptoms of vertebrobasilar ischaemia (often related to posture) may occur with anterior pituitary and adrenocortical insufficiency [49]. The vascular steal phenomenon could be responsible by shunting blood destined for the brain to extracranial parts because of increased functional demand.

Rotation or extension of the head, when associated with severe atherosclerotic tortuosity and kinking, fibromuscular hyperplasia or dysplasia of the cervical arteries [50], or cervical osteoarthritis with pressure on a vertebral artery can cause temporary reduction of flow in the absence of adequate collateral flow.

It is now accepted that, in the majority of subjects, microembolism is responsible. Microemboli consisting of platelets and atheromatous debris may be observed passing through retinal arteries during an attack of amaurosis fugax and evidence of atheroembolism may be found in the brain post mortem [51]. Russell [52] described three types of retinal emboli:

- white emboli of cardiac origin causing segmental blockage with permanent retinal damage;
- small white platelet–fibrin plugs migrating through the retinal circulation within minutes;
- small refractile plaques (atheromatous debris) partially obstructing the branches.

Hollenhorst [53] described bright yellow, orange or copper plaques believed to be atheromatous emboli in retinal arterioles. Desquamated pieces of intima may not enter retinal vessels, being more likely to enter and obstruct larger cerebral arteries. Calcareous emboli from cardiac valves have been incriminated but this would be a rare event [51]. It is also likely that silent microembolism to the brain is more frequent than patient numbers manifesting clinical symptoms or signs would indicate. The association of TIA with ulceration and mural thrombus in the carotid sinus occurs in a significant number of cases with embolism from the commencement of one of the vertebral arteries or from the subclavian artery proximal to the origin of the vertebral artery in instances of vertebrobasilar insufficiency. Severe stenosis in the cervical segment of the internal carotid artery may be associated with superficial erosion not demonstrable angiographically or some additional cardiac or blood pressure change may lead to insufficiency of blood flow.

Embolism may also originate from the aorta, the cardiac valves or mural thrombi within the left atrium or ventricle. These may account for the cases in which no source of emboli can be found clinically in the neck and though difficult to demonstrate, should be sought post mortem. Emboli from the heart have the potential to be larger and therefore the ischaemia may be of longer duration than microemboli from the carotid sinus. Although microemboli from cerebral and even extracranial aneurysms occur, they are infrequent [54,55].

Characteristically thrombi are associated with repeated fragmentation, embolism and further accretion of platelets and leucocytes so that recurrent embolism is likely. Many may be small and clinically insignificant but by a cumulative effect could impair flow or run-off. Flow through the carotid arteries is not as random as some may believe and so recurrent ischaemic events are likely within the same general area and will occur most frequently in the distribution of the middle cerebral artery. Mostly there is retardation of flow rather than permanent occlusion. A rapid mechanism for clearance of autogenous cellular and non-cellular connective tissue material and lipid from the blood stream seems to exist. The secondary haemorheological and biochemical (lipoprotein) effects that atheroembolism has on the blood and its constituents have not been investigated. It is highly likely that increased blood viscosity associated with red cell aggregation (sludging) may aggravate cerebrovascular insufficiency. Hypoglycaemia has been blamed for transient or localized neurological disturbances in diabetics with carotid stenosis, the attacks being prevented by endarterectomy [56].

Not all emboli resolve completely and small cortical ischaemic lesions could remain symptomless. Transient episodes may also occur with bacterial endocarditis although their septic nature would result in inflammatory lesions of varying severity.

Recurrent TIAs have been followed by severe cerebral infarction after a lapse of time (averaging three years) due to internal carotid or middle cerebral artery artery occlusion in up to two thirds of such patients. Localization of the infarct is usually within the same domain as the premonitory microembolism, the frequency of which can vary from only two to several per week over more than a year of observation. Some mild attacks cease spontaneously and an occasional attack precedes primary cerebral haemorrhage. These TIAs need not be followed by major cerebral infarcts, for small ulcerated lesions may heal and the finding of a thrombotic ulcer is less likely as time passes. However, the outcome is unpredictable. There is more chance of hemiparesis in a TIA involving the vertebrobasilar system being followed by a major catastrophe than would be the case in milder episodes.

Endarterectomy for such attacks is followed by healing and obviously thromboembolism initially although the microemboli should be readily resolved consisting mainly of platelets and leucocytes. Endothelialization commences within two or three days from both ends and a neo-intima develops. This neo-intima progressively develops atherosclerosis as occurs on the lining of prostheses or the false lumen of a chronic or healed dissecting aneurysm [57]. Recurrent stenotic lesions with or without ulceration and thrombosis may develop within a variable period of time postoperatively.

These subjects usually have severe widespread atherosclerosis and death may follow the complications of atherosclerosis elsewhere. Small or multiple ischaemic lesions or even haemorrhage should not be unexpected.

12.7.2 STEAL SYNDROMES

The normal pressure gradient maintaining blood flow to the brain may be disturbed under certain pathological conditions and cause diversion of blood from the brain

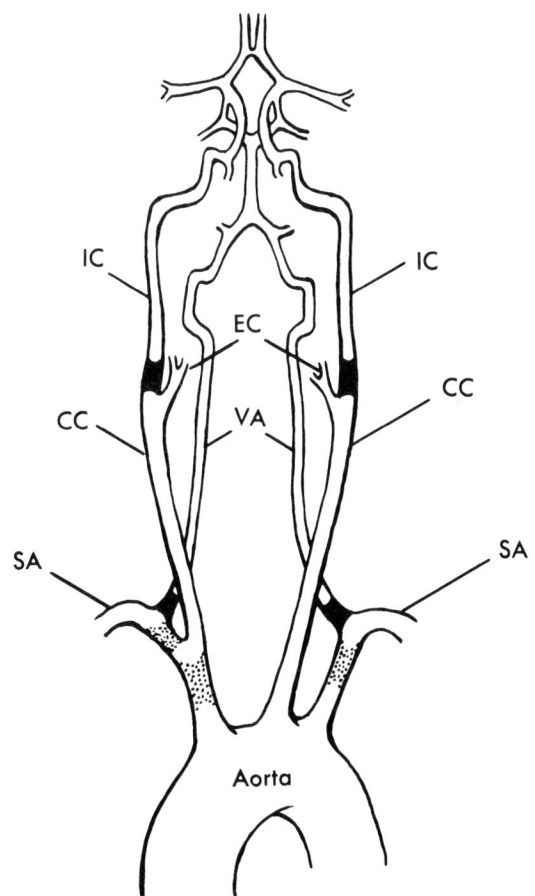

Figure 12.1 Major arteries of the neck and circle of Willis. The black segments are the extracranial sites where stenosis and occlusion are particularly likely to occur (carotid sinuses and commencement of the vertebral arteries). The stippled segments are sites of infrequent occlusion causing the common varieties of the subclavian steal syndrome. CC = common carotid artery; EC = external carotid arteries; IC = internal carotid artery; SA = subclavian artery; VA = vertebral artery. (Reproduced from Stehbens [3].)

to an alternative area of supply such as the upper limb. This, the subclavian steal syndrome or brachial–basilar insufficiency, is a clinical indicator of occlusion or severe stenosis of an artery proximal to the field of supply. Thus exercise or heavy use of the right arm may cause or aggravate vertebral artery insufficiency which can occur at rest when the right subclavian artery proximal to the origin of the vertebral artery is severely stenosed or occluded (Figure 12.1). The brachial artery 'steals' blood from the right vertebral artery depending on the anatomy of the circle of Willis and the respective sizes of the two vertebral arteries. In patients who have survived the development of this obstructive lesion, the collateral flow derived from several other sources will normally provide sufficient blood to the homolateral arm [3]. Mostly, these collateral anastomoses are small though cumulative. If the two vertebral arteries are large, their junction is a convenient anastomotic communication through which blood from the left vertebral artery supplements flow to the right arm with reversal of flow in the right vertebral artery. Such a siphoning effect can compromise the basilar artery blood flow producing vertebrobasilar insufficiency rather than intermittent claudication in the right upper limb and at times actual cerebral infarction can occur (upper spinal cord, brain stem, cerebellum, thalamus and occipital lobes).

The size of the constituent parts of the circle of Willis is of importance since the availability of collateral flow increases the possible alternatives for the steal syndrome. When the posterior communicating arteries are sufficiently large, the carotid circulation may contribute to the subclavian steal phenomenon. In 207 collected cases, 45% had cerebral symptoms alone, 40% had combined cerebral and upper limb symptoms, 10% had symptoms pertaining to the arm and the remainder had no symptoms [58]. Experimentally, systemic vasopressors increase the steal phenomenon [59].

Subclavian steal syndrome also encompasses cases in which the innominate artery is significantly stenosed or occluded. In such instances the shunt is via the homolateral carotid and vertebral arteries, but if the carotid artery is also stenosed or the collateral circulation is poor, the steal occurs via the vertebral artery alone. The homolateral vertebral artery with retrograde flow may supply the subclavian as well as the common carotid arteries.

Other variations of the steal syndrome are common with blood shunted through the circle of Willis as is sometimes observed in angiograms. When the phenomenon is bilateral (1–2%), the shunt occurs through the circle of Willis or through collaterals from the external carotid artery. An obstruction of the first part of the vertebral artery or a vertebral arteriovenous shunt may cause reversal of flow through only part of the vertebral artery. Alternatively collaterals from the external carotid may provide blood to the vertebrobasilar system beyond the occlusion. The syndrome is two or three times more frequent in males than females and the mean age is only about 49 to 52 years [58]. The artery is more often occluded than stenosed (3:1) and atherosclerosis is usually responsible. The left subclavian is involved in about 62% of cases, the right in 28% and the innominate or brachiocephalic in 10% [58]. The subclavian steal phenomenon is amenable to surgical correction by providing alternative collateral flow, although restenoses can occur.

The syndrome has causes other than atherosclerosis, such as the Blalock–Taussig procedure (anastomosis of subclavian artery to the pulmonary artery) for pulmonary stenosis or atresia [60], obstruction or severe stenosis of the subclavian artery and the aortic arch syndrome.

Other steal phenomena exist. Stenosis of the innominate (brachiocephalic) and the left subclavian arteries results in bilateral reversal of vertebral artery flow with blood siphoned from the internal carotid arteries. Occlusion of the common carotid artery with reversal of flow in the internal carotid artery and conventional flow in the external carotid has been referred to as the internal–external carotid steal or the external carotid artery steal. The face, scalp and neck are then supplied at the expense of the cerebral circulation. Even therapeutic ligation of the common carotid artery can result in vertebrobasilar insufficiency due to diversion of blood from the basilar to the internal carotid arteries. Usually in this form of vascular steal the occlusion is spontaneous, the result of atherosclerosis, and accompanied by severe occlusive disease of other major arteries to the brain. Less frequently, a combination of subclavian and external carotid artery steal exists.

12.7.3 AORTIC ARCH SYNDROME

Several diseases diminish or obliterate pulses in arteries arising from the aortic arch, hence the 'aortic arch syndrome'. In well established cases, no pulses may be palpable in the head, neck or upper limbs and collateral vessels are well developed. Trophic changes (alopecia, ulceration of the nasal septum, mouth or skin) are prone to occur. The patients experience frequent transient attacks of syncope, fatigue and vertigo. There may be permanent cerebral damage, even hemiplegia depending on the degree of ischaemia. The carotid sinus is often unduly sensitive accounting for systemic hypertension, a condition regarded as reversed aortic coarctation. Takayasu's arteritis is the most frequent cause but others include syphilitic arteritis with or without an aortic aneurysm, giant cell arteritis, chronic dissection of the aorta, and trauma or thromboembolism [61]. Superadded thrombosis will occur in such disorders.

12.8 Cerebral infarction or encephalomalacia

A cerebral infarct (or softening) is a localized area of ischaemic necrosis ranging in size from a microscopic focus to a massive area involving virtually one entire cerebral hemisphere. Less severe ischaemia produces reversible neurological dysfunction. These thromboembolic disorders account for about 62% of deaths from cerebrovascular disease. In the past cerebral infarcts have been divided into embolic and non-embolic but without the benefit of thorough autopsies differentiation is not always possible.

Most of these infarcts (92%) occur after the age of 50 years. The incidence is negligible under 35 years of age climbing steeply from about 55 years to a maximum in the seventh and eighth decades. In young children they are more likely to be due to arteritis or embolism from cardiac disease. In some of the younger adults the infarcts are due to non-atherosclerotic lesions but hypertension and diabetes mellitus are prevalent under 50 years of age. They are somewhat more frequent in males than females.

12.8.1 PATHOLOGY OF INFARCTION

Infarcts are essentially of two types, pale or haemorrhagic (red) and may be recent or old depending on their duration and stage of resolution. A pale infarct (ischaemic necrosis or anaemic infarct) is usually difficult to recognize macroscopically within the first 24 hours, after which time degenerative and reparative processes assist recognition. The earliest change is slight swelling of the infarcted cortex and white matter with an indistinct margin between the two (Figure 12.2). The tissue feels soft and is more readily washed away under running water than non-infarcted tissue but such washing is not a good procedure for histology. Fixation accentuates the difference in texture. There may be some small punctate cortical haemorrhages and extravasation of blood into the subarachnoid space. The affected cortex becomes thicker and a split often develops between the cortex and white matter (Figure 12.3) and also about the lenticular nucleus. Generalized swelling of the infarct develops with flattening of the gyri, shift of the mid-line and herniations under the falx cerebri or through the tentorium cerebelli reaching a maximum about the sixth day after which the swelling commences to subside. The hemispherical displacement to the opposite side varies from 3 to 14 mm independently of the downward displacement. At one week the infarcted area

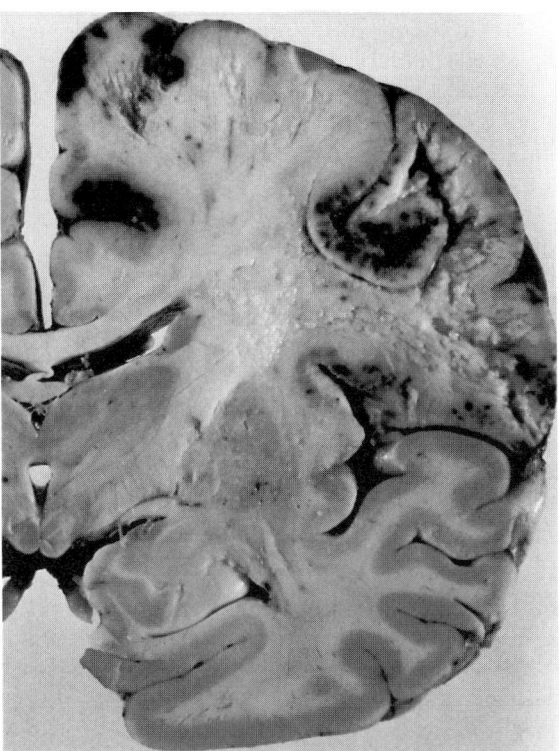

Figure 12.3 Coronal section of hemisphere displaying cerebral softening over the parietal surface involving only part of the area of supply of the middle cerebral artery and the medial cortical aspect of the hemisphere and medial 3 cm of the superior surface. Multiple haemorrhages becoming confluent within the affected cortex especially within sulci typify haemorrhagic infarction. Some underlying white matter at top right has split away from the haemorrhagic cortex.

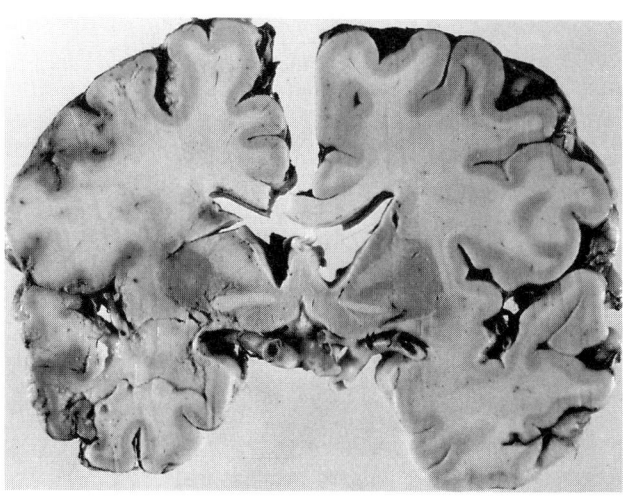

Figure 12.2 Coronal section through cerebrum with extensive recent softening in the distribution of the middle cerebral artery. Note the loss of differentiation between grey and white matter in the affected area (cortex and lenticular nucleus) and the fragility and loss of normal consistency of fixed brain tissue. There are some petechial haemorrhages and congestion of the softened grey matter. (Reproduced from Stehbens [3].)

is well demarcated and within two weeks, the softened tissue is disintegrating, crumbling and resembling cottage cheese (Figure 12.4). The process of resorption of the friable, semifluid infarct continues until resorption (which can take several months) is complete.

In old infarcts, the overlying meninges may be slightly thickened and opaque, wrinkled and depressed below the neighbouring cortex. The old infarct is replaced by a depression or space in the brain, frequently with gliosed remnants of thin and possibly pigmented cortex and white matter about the edges and fibrous tissue with blood vessels within the space. Involvement of brain adjacent to the ventricles may simulate ventricular enlargement. The borders of the space are usually well demarcated but irregular with a moth-eaten appearance (Figure 12.5).

Small infarcts are represented by small regions of cortical thinning and irregularity giving the pial surface a granular appearance and in some large infarcts unabsorbed debris becomes encapsulated but rarely proceeds to calcification.

Red or haemorrhagic infarcts (Figure 12.3) are asso-

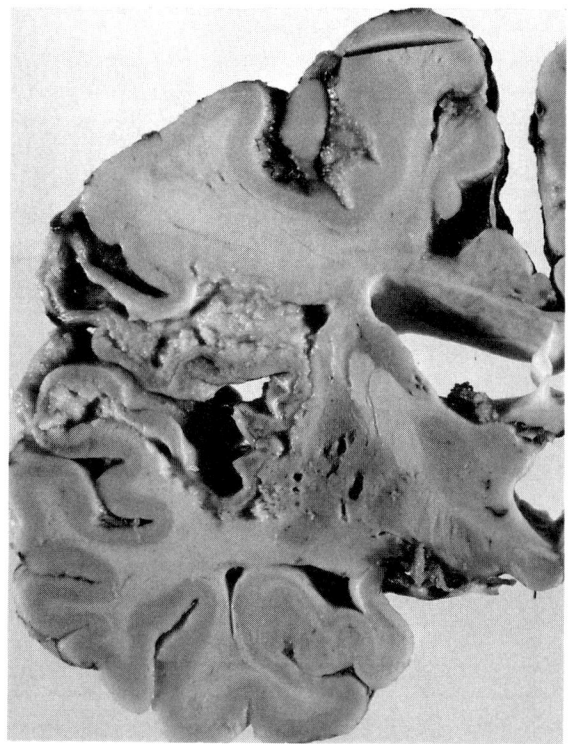

Figure 12.4 Cerebral softening in distribution of the middle cerebral artery. The infarcted tissue with the appearance of crumbling caseous material is undergoing liquefaction and phagocytosis. Note multiple small lacunar infarcts in basal ganglia.

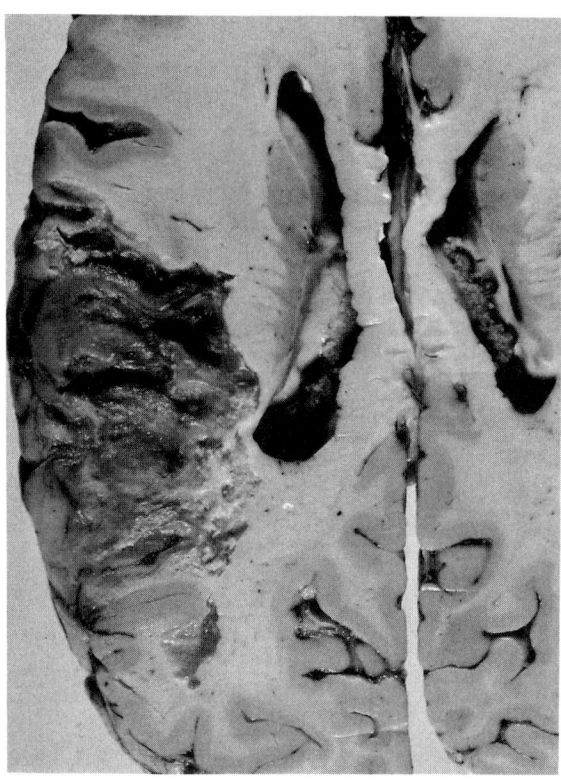

Figure 12.5 Old cerebral softening within the distribution of the middle cerebral artery. Note the spongy and moth-eaten appearance, the sharply defined edges of the infarct and the survival of subependymal tissue. (Reproduced from Stehbens [3].)

ciated with multiple small variable sized haemorrhages imparting a pink to red punctate appearance to the cortex. The haemorrhages may coalesce and the cortex then is diffusely red and haemorrhagic with some haemorrhage into the subarachnoid space. The underlying white matter usually escapes. Haemorrhagic zones may be restricted to the edges of the infarct involving the sides and depth of the sulci rather than the summit of the gyri. Red infarcts usually do not approach the severity of necrosis of pale infarcts but can be larger. In massive infarcts of the middle cerebral artery, there is haemorrhagic infarction in the basal ganglia, particularly the putamen and it is less severe in the caudate nucleus. Softenings in the brain stem are usually pale (Figures 12.6 and 12.7) with an occasional small haemorrhage.

Cerebellar infarcts involve the grey and white matter of the folia and rarely the deep white matter. They are generally pale but some exhibit haemorrhagic mottling and because of the good collateral circulation do not tend to be grossly destructive and cystic as in the cerebrum. In old cerebellar infarcts the architecture of the folia tends to persist even if shrunken.

Infarcts of the brain in the border zones between territories of supply (watershed areas) are prone to occur in cerebral arterial insufficiency, sometimes precipitated by

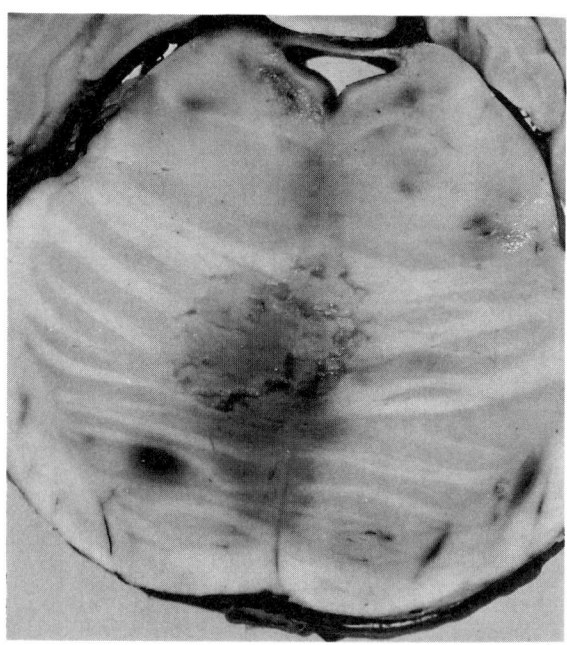

Figure 12.6 Section of pons showing central area of recent softening with some discoloration due to blood.

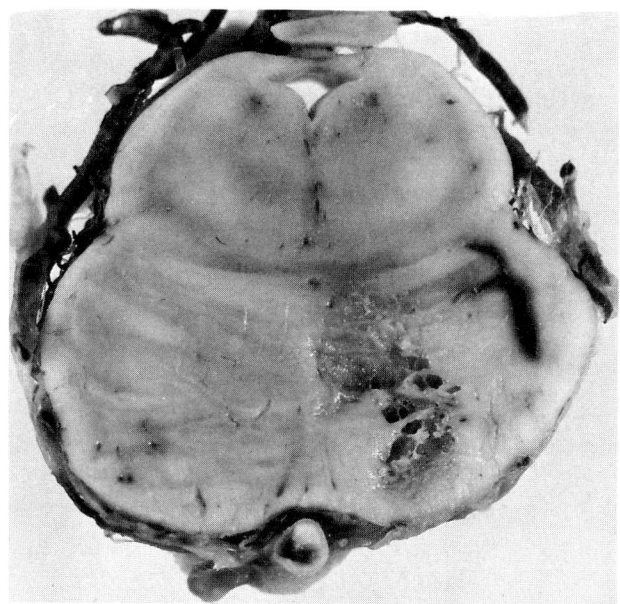

Figure 12.7 Section of pons demonstrating a localized region of old softening which has a moth-eaten appearance. (Reproduced from Stehbens [3].)

hypotension, a fall in cardiac output or severe atherosclerosis with stenoses in the cervical arteries.

Cerebral ischaemia due to arterial occlusion produces a central zone that is densely ischaemic surrounded by a less densely ischaemic penumbral zone in which cells are at risk and may remain viable or reversibly ischaemic for up to eight hours. Cells in the peripheral zone can therefore be salvaged by reperfusion or by drugs that may limit extension of the densely ischaemic zone into the peripheral penumbral region [62,63].

The principal cause of cell dysfunction and death in ischaemia is energy depletion, there being a failure to maintain adequate adenosine triphosphate (ATP) levels leading to degradation of macromolecules of vital importance to membrane and cytoskeletal integrity, proteolytic cleavage of components of the cytoskeleton and their anchorage to the cell membrane, to loss of ion homeostasis involving cellular accumulation of Ca^{2+}, Na^+ and Cl^-, with osmotically obligated water, and to the production of metabolic acids resulting in acidosis intra- and extracellularly. The rise in intracellular Ca^{2+} is due to the loss of calcium pump function because of ATP depletion and the rise in membrane permeability to calcium. This non-physiological elevation in Ca^{2+} is believed to cause cell damage by lipolytic and proteolytic activity and by alterations of protein phosphorylation which secondarily affects protein synthesis. A second key event in the ischaemic zone is the activation of anaerobic glycolysis due to lack of oxygen in association with an adequate energy source and this leads to intracellular and extracellular acidosis that jeopardizes survival of the ischaemic tissue by disrupting ion homeostasis.

There is also evidence that free radicals in the ischaemic tissue are mediators of ischaemic cell death and that they are particularly prone to affect the microvasculature adversely aided and abetted by other mediators of inflammatory reactions.

The elucidation of these biochemical changes in ischaemia will provide knowledge that may facilitate reversal of the changes and ultimately the reduction of necrosis to a minimum.

(a) Microscopic

If death follows shortly after the onset of ischaemia, no histological change is likely. Swelling of the perineuronal and perivascular astrocytic processes occur early imparting the histological appearance of oedema. The nerve cells shrink and the cytoplasm appears brick red. Within six to eight hours polymorphonuclear leucocytes are prominent in and about cortical blood vessels with variable ecchymoses. By 24 hours the cortex exhibits oedema, neurones may be undergoing karyolysis, polymorphs are more plentiful and the tissue exhibits friability. The tissue appearance is of coagulation necrosis. Polymorphs increase to a maximum in two or three days but many are necrotic and their number diminishes.

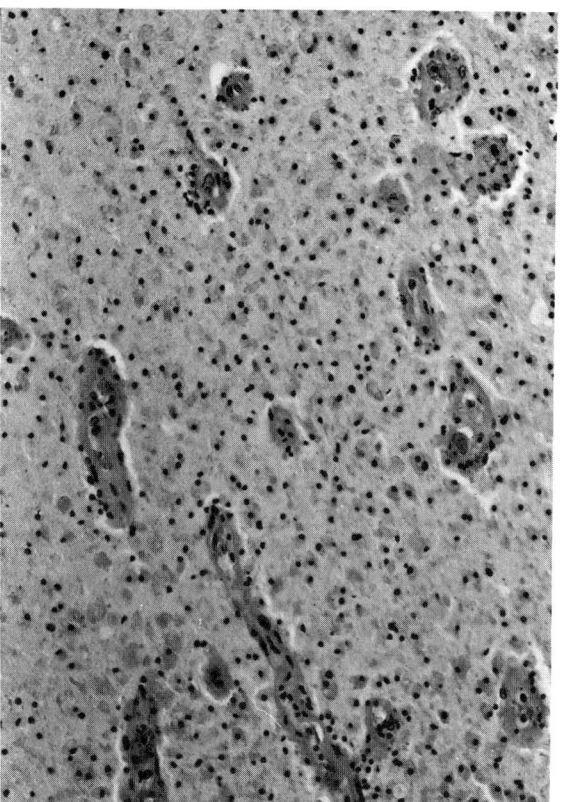

Figure 12.8 Extensive microglial infiltration of infarcted brain tissue with ghosts of necrotic cells and thickened vessel walls. (Haematoxylin and eosin.) (Reproduced from Stehbens [3].)

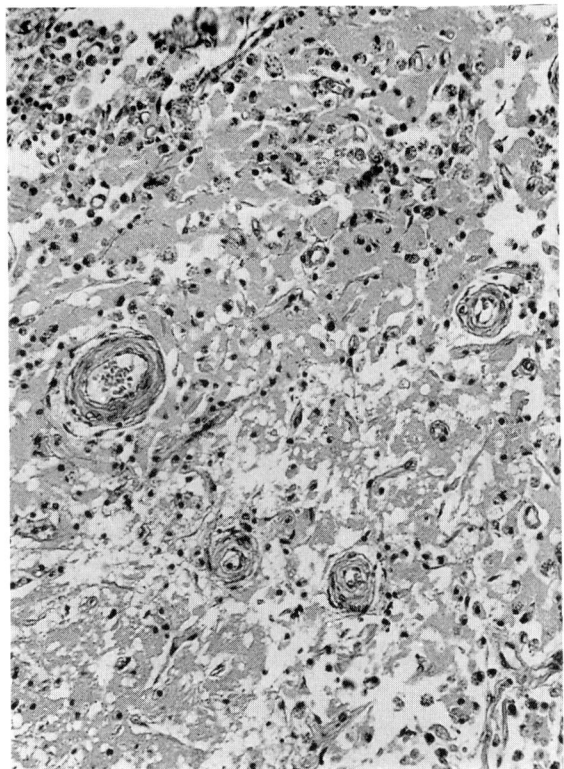

Figure 12.9 Cerebral softening with infiltration of necrotic parenchyma with microglial phagocytes. Note the small arteries with loss of normal architecture, concentrically thickened fibrous walls and narrowing of their lumina resembling diffuse hyperplastic sclerosis. (Haematoxylin and eosin.) (Reproduced from Stehbens [3].)

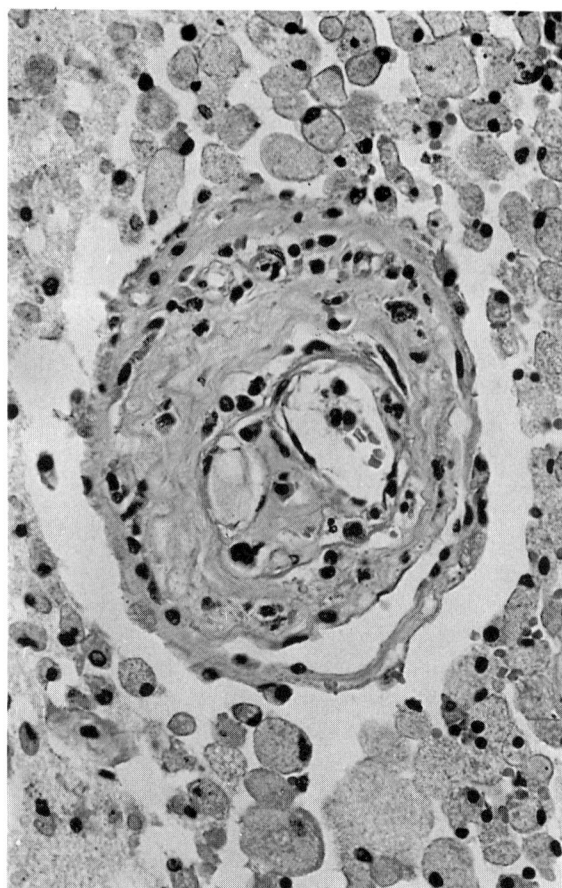

Figure 12.10 Numerous microglial cells with vacuolated cytoplasm (lipophages) or compound granular corpuscles in an infarct with an unusually thick-walled vessel which may have undergone recanalization or perivascular fibrosis. (Haematoxylin and eosin.) (Reproduced with permission from Stehbens [3].)

Transformed microglia with small dark-staining round or oval nuclei with dark eosinophilic homogeneous cytoplasm (Figure 12.8) appear at about 24 hours and increase in number and phagocytic activity (Figure 12.9). Their cytoplasm becomes foamy and they predominate at seven days replacing necrotic parenchyma. Blood vessels, some fibrous tissue, debris and many lipophages (Figure 12.10) are found between some surviving parenchyma which becomes gliosed. Progressively the lipophages disappear although in several large infarcts some tissue does not liquify but persists as necrotic debris in which there may be many cholesterol crystals (Figure 12.11). Perivascular lymphocytes are to be found in the surrounding glial tissue with numerous gemistocytic or swollen astrocytes, and sometimes there is moderate fibrosis.

In the infarcted cortex, blood vessels may be necrotic, small vessels have thickened walls (Figure 12.8), some may contain thrombus or emboli whilst others are recanalized (Figure 12.10). In healed or resolved infarcts, some vessels exhibit unusually pronounced degenerative changes (Figures 12.9 and 12.12), possibly due to the haemodynamic overload during healing rather than endarteritis obliterans.

The white matter undergoes coagulation necrosis and demyelination is detectable at 24 hours. Oligodendroglia undergo karyolysis and the infarcted zone is pale in comparison to the surrounding pink tissue. In regions bordering the infarct, the tissue is replaced by a loose spongy glial network (Figure 12.13) containing a few vessels and some lipophages, but usually the gliosis is dense surrounding the cavity resulting from colliquative necrosis and phagocytic activity. The subarachnoid space has a similar cellular response and there may be some mild meningeal fibrosis. Calcification of unresolved lipid rich debris is rare [3].

In haemorrhagic infarction, multiple haemorrhages reflect the macroscopic appearance (Figure 12.14) and haematoidin and haemosiderin are found reflecting the breakdown of the extravasated red blood cells. Haemosiderin appears within two to ten days and haematoidin by the end of the second week. Iron encrustation of shrunken nerve cells (ferrugination) occurs

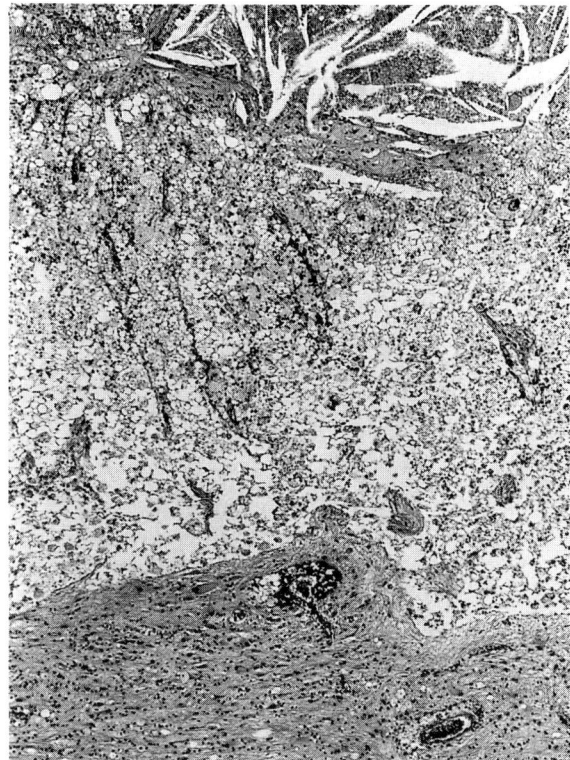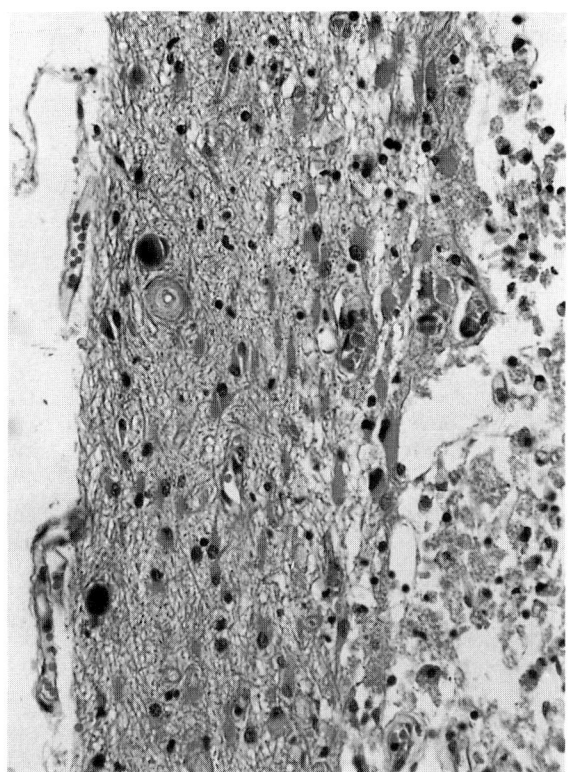

Figure 12.11 Margin of extensive cerebral softening with a central zone of fibrous trabeculae and lipophages. The necrotic brain (above) has undergone coagulation necrosis and contains numerous cholesterol crystals. The gliosed surviving parenchyma (below) has a sharp margin and perivascular lymphocytic cuffing of one blood vessel. (Haematoxylin and eosin.) (Reproduced with permission from Stehbens [3].)

Figure 12.12 Surviving strip of subpial cortex (left) with numerous gemistocytic astrocytes bordering the softening (right) which contains many microglial phagocytes. Next to one of the two corpora amylacea is an arteriole with a very narrow lumen and acellular hyaline wall (arteriolosclerosis). (Haematoxylin and eosin.) (Reproduced with permission from Stehbens [3].)

but otherwise the organization is essentially similar to that of the pale infarct.

In cerebellar infarcts, the degree of damage is less. Purkinje cells are susceptible, dying early. Their nuclei undergo karyolysis and at times the calcified cell body remains. Necrosis of the granular layer is observed and few cells remain. The molecular layer undergoes coagulation necrosis and the cells exhibit increased eosinophilia. Lipophages are mostly in the white matter and there is progressive resorption. The arborescent folia are mostly retained, though some may be destroyed and others reduced in size.

In red infarction of the cerebellum, small haemorrhages occur in the molecular and granular layers, in the white matter of the folia and in the subarachnoid space, but a blood lake forms in the plane of cleavage between the Purkinje and granular layers. Resorption follows the general pattern for the cerebrum.

(b) Distribution of infarcts

Cerebral infarcts are common at autopsy, variable in size, often multiple and incidental. The territory of the middle cerebral artery is the most frequently infarcted and accounts for more than 50% of all infarcts and supratentorial lesions are about four times more frequent than subtentorial involvement [64]. Emboli in the internal carotid artery may extend peripherally to involve the middle cerebral artery and those lodging at the bifurcation will involve the anterior cerebral artery as well. Emboli often lodge at the middle cerebral trifurcation and smaller emboli involve the trunk. Complete occlusion of the anterior cerebral artery alone is infrequent. More often the territory of one or several of its branches is occluded.

Occlusion of the posterior cerebral artery occurs in 10–15% of cerebral infarctions. Transtentorial herniation accompanied by compression of the artery against the tentorium usually causes haemorrhagic infarction.

The vertebral artery is often occluded between the arch of the atlas and the union of the two vertebrals with about one quarter at the level of the foramen magnum. Occasionally it is bilateral. An occlusion in the cerebral segment may be symptomless. Occlusion of the posterior inferior cerebellar artery (Wallenberg's syndrome or the lateral medullary syndrome) is occasionally

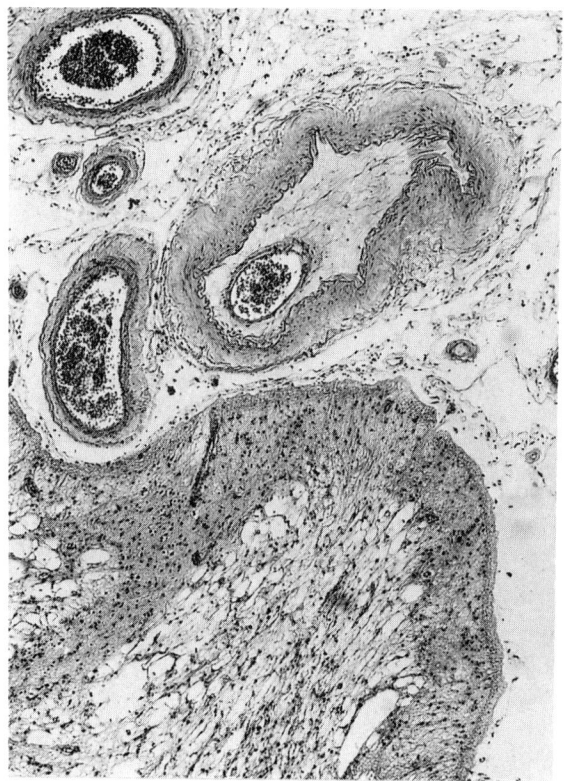

Figure 12.13 Edge of infarct showing gliosed cortex overlying spongy tissue consisting of irregularly sized spaces and astrocytes. Note the pial artery narrowed by acellular collagen, the result of recanalization of thrombus. (Haematoxylin and eosin.) (Reproduced with permission from Stehbens [3].)

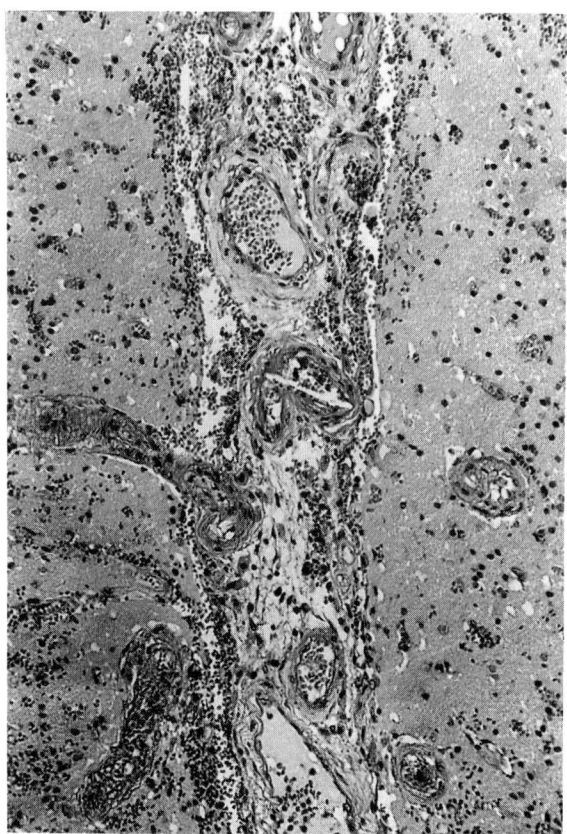

Figure 12.14 Haemorrhagic softening of recent origin with haemorrhage in the subarachnoid space of the sulcus and a cholesterol crystal within the lumen of a small pial artery indicating atheroembolism. (Haematoxylin and eosin.) (Reproduced with permission from Stehbens [3].)

caused by an obstruction of this artery though more often it is by vertebral artery occlusion.

Thrombosis of the basilar artery is more common in males than females and two thirds of cases are associated with hypertension. Atherosclerosis of the vertebrobasilar system is usually advanced and these patients often have neurological symptoms for months or years before the final illness. The occlusion may occur at any level in the artery and the thrombus may propagate into vertebral or posterior cerebral arteries. Concomitant involvement of the occipital lobes in infarction depends on the source of blood supply to the posterior cerebral arteries and alternate collateral flow. Involvement of the cerebellum is usually minimal because of its rich collateral circulation.

Infarcts associated with cerebral aneurysm are dealt with in section 10.10.5(b).

(c) Pathogenesis of cerebral ischaemia

Occlusion of a major artery of supply is not necessarily synonymous with infarction, there being many factors that influence the outcome (Chapter 3, p. 73), which is ultimately dependent on the balance of divers factors that vary from patient to patient. These factors are sufficiently numerous, variable and complex to make the clinical and pathological consequences of vascular obstruction so different in the individual response that the outcome is difficult to predict. These many factors are essentially secondary, the most common participating aetiological factor being thrombotic or embolic occlusion of the artery of supply.

In the Co-operative Stroke Study [65] in seven centres in the United States 380 patients were studied, 57.4% having a thrombosis, 26% thrombosis or embolism, 7.4% embolism and 8.4% transient ischaemic attacks. Opinions differ as to which is the more frequent but generally this is considered to be thrombosis [2]. The carotid arterial tree was involved in 74.7% and the vertebrobasilar system in 22.1% with the site being uncertain in 3.2%.

Most haemorrhagic infarcts are due to arterial embolism (apart from venous thrombosis) and the thrombotic embolus with time and fibrinolysis moves distally in the circulation, possibly even disappearing. This allows collateral blood, mainly cortical, into the necrotic tissue and vessels of the infarcted cortex and haemorrhage follows. Fisher and Adams [66] believe that arterial thrombosis has to be proximal to the circle of Willis to cause a red infarct. However, infarcts secondary to a dissecting aneurysm of the aorta may be red, pale or mixed [67].

Pale softenings are the result of complete blockage sufficiently prolonged to cause the infarction that remains uniformly ischaemic and in which the onset of necrosis progresses rapidly. Partial occlusion with defective return of the circulation and patchy functional disturbances in the area preceding the onset of necrosis of the parenchyma and vessels elicit red softening in the pathogenesis of which collateral flow is crucial. Simple ligation of the middle cerebral artery distal to the origin of the perforating branches produces pale infarction but with more proximal occlusion the infarct is in part haemorrhagic. An increase in blood pressure after ligation of the middle cerebral artery causes a haemorrhagic infarct [68], as does ligation in a hypertensive animal, but not when collateral flow is prevented by prior ligation of the anterior and posterior cerebral arteries. Low molecular weight dextrans, which ordinarily reduce massive red cell aggregation (sludging), protect against haemorrhagic tendencies and the use of anticoagulants may induce extensive haemorrhage into the infarct. In transtentorial herniation and compression of the posterior cerebral artery, red infarction is attributed to intermittent obstruction. Ultimately the haemorrhagic tendency is dependent on the availability of collateral flow after the vessels in the infarcted zone become necrotic.

The adequacy or otherwise of collateral flow determines whether or not an infarct will follow an occlusion of a vessel and its size. The collateral circulation may be pre-existing or may have developed due to progressive stenosis of the supply channel. Usually it requires a stenosis of about 90% before there is reduced flow distally but this will be intermittent depending on fluctuations in blood pressure and cardiac output from time to time. Collateral flow in the cerebral leptomeningeal vessels is usually limited and a sudden occlusion provides no time for increasing the size of collateral vessels. The circle of Willis, dependent on its anatomy, may or may not limit the infarction but on occasions may contribute to the infarction according to its anatomical configuration. Severe atherosclerosis of alternative vessels of supply may limit the ability of collaterals to compensate for an occlusion in a neighbouring vessel. For example severe stenosis of the external carotid artery in the presence of occlusion of the ipsilateral internal carotid artery limits the possible collateral flow through peripheral anastomotic channels between the intracranial and extracranial circulations.

Severe anaemia and the effects of exposure to carbon monoxide gas may contribute to infarction as can anoxaemia associated with chronic lung disease or congestive cardiac failure. A fall in blood pressure below the customary level in the presence of a precarious blood flow may also lead to cerebral ischaemia. Stokes–Adams attacks, surgical or pathological shock or induced hypotension can induce cerebral ischaemia, and postoperative hemiplegia is uncommon but well recognized. In such instances the normal blood flow is precarious and the changed functional haemodynamic status is the final blow.

Hypertension by aggravating atherosclerosis contributes to the development of cerebral infarction. Its incidence [3] varies from 47 to 75%, and the association is considered more frequent than with myocardial infarction. The correlation with lacunar softening is at least 95% and hypotensive therapy has been thought to have reduced the frequency of cerebral infarction in hypertension [69]. The blood pressure usually rises with the onset of a cerebrovascular accident such as infarction and falls gradually to normal values during convalescence. The increase is thought to be of neurogenic origin.

Cerebral infarction as a complication of cardiac disease is a common autopsy finding in general hospitals where it tends to be attributed to embolism from a mural thrombus secondary to myocardial infarction, cardiac aneurysm, auricular fibrillation and chronic valvular disease. The site of the embolus is often not found but the general coexistence of severe atherosclerosis with complications in the coronary, cerebral and peripheral arteries must not be forgotten. Ulcerated plaques have been found in the aortic arch in 26% of 239 patients with cerebrovascular disease but in only 5% of 261 subjects with other neurological diseases, suggesting that emboli derived from the aorta may be responsible for a significant number of cerebral embolic episodes [70].

Cerebral embolism is particularly frequent in bacterial endocarditis and thromboembolic cerebral lesions are common in congenital cyanotic heart disease, some being due to thrombi in veins or venous sinuses. Polycythaemia may contribute to this association as can sludging of the red blood cells [71].

In young subjects with cerebral infarction the commonest causes are cardiogenic emboli and premature atherosclerosis [72] although Petty et al. [73] reported embolic stroke following the smoking of 'crack' cocaine, the embolus allegedly being derived from cocaine-induced cardiomyopathy and left atrial thrombus. Cocaine users develop myocardial infarction which can be a source of emboli but in a recent case cocaine also caused aortic and coronary artery dissection [74]. Other ischaemic cerebral events may follow intravenous drug abuse with necrotizing arteritis and dissecting aneurysm of cerebral arteries.

Arterial thrombosis precipitating cerebral infarction

is usually due to atherosclerosis, the thrombus forming on a tear or ulceration of an atheromatous plaque due to an acquired weakness of the arterial wall. The thrombus may propagate to the next major branching but the factors influencing such propagation have not been studied in depth. It appears to be more frequent in the cerebral tree than in the coronary circulation.

The thrombus on the ulceration, whether in the carotid sinus or elsewhere, characteristically sheds emboli and this may be continuous or intermittent, silent or clinically evident. New areas of ulceration may develop and some healing is assumed but currently there is no way of observing the natural history of such lesions. Many such lesions in medium-sized distributing arteries (coronary, internal carotid artery) progress to occlusive thrombosis and it has been estimated that those that ulcerate and develop thrombosis usually have a preexistent stenosis of at least 50% and usually more than 75% [75]. The tear or ulceration may be the consequence of a poststenotic haemodynamic effect.

Intramural haemorrhage into a plaque is in reality extravasation and dissection of an ulcerated atherosclerotic plaque. Histology of endarterectomy specimens frequently exhibits areas of thrombosis, superficial erosions with superadded thrombus and evidence of healing and thrombus organization.

In the pathogenesis of cerebral infarction emphasis was for a long time on local causes but in the internal carotid arterial tree particularly, thrombotic occlusions are not nearly as frequent as in the coronary circulation. Causes of cerebral infarction are numerous but the common moderate to massive cerebral infarct is now known to be caused most often by occlusion of extracranial arteries. Fisher [48,76] emphasized the importance of multiple cerebral emboli with transient ischaemic effects as premonitory symptoms of a subsequent massive infarction due to thrombotic occlusion of the internal carotid sinus and artery. Subsequent pathological and angiographic studies have confirmed the prevalence of moderate stenosis to complete occlusion of one or more large cervical arteries in aging subjects, particularly in those with cerebrovascular disease. However, estimates of the degree of narrowing or stenosis tend to be subjective and inaccurate and often it is not clear whether the percentage of narrowing refers to the diameter or the cross-sectional area. It has been estimated that blood flow is likely to be significantly reduced only when the cross-sectional area is less than 2 mm^2 and reduction is probable when reduced to 5 mm^2 [77]. In a pathological study [78] ulceration was found in at least one of the cervical arteries supplying the brain in 14% of 93 autopsy subjects (over 35 years of age), mostly in the internal carotid arteries. Stenoses have also been found in a large percentage of autopsies in both intra- and extracranial arteries in subjects with or without cerebral infarction [75,79]. Occlusion of the cervical internal carotid artery was bilateral in six of 50 patients at autopsy and unilateral in the remainder. Embolism was responsible for a minority, but in those in whom the site of thrombosis was determined, it had commenced in the carotid sinus in 77.8%, in the siphon in 22.2% and in approximately one third the thrombus had propagated beyond the bifurcation of the internal carotid artery. In most of the remainder, it had propagated as far as the carotid siphon. Retrograde thrombosis occurred in three of the six cases of siphon thrombosis but was absent in cases of embolic occlusion of the siphon.

Stenoses and occlusion have been found to be frequent in the first inch of the vertebral artery. Some were associated with cerebellar infarction [79]. Such lesions could jeopardize impoverished carotid arterial flow and stenoses in both arterial systems leading to the use of the term caroticovertebral stenosis. In one case the vertebral arteries maintained a precarious flow in the presence of bilateral internal carotid artery occlusion. Under such conditions progression of vertebral artery disease could precipitate lesions in the carotid area of the cerebrum [79].

Controversy persists as to whether occlusion of the cervical or its intracranial arteries is the most frequent cause of ischaemic infarction of the brain. The various studies have not been comparable and difficulty exists in differentiating thrombosis *in situ* from embolism. There is a need for detailed autopsy study of these occlusive lesions but increasing difficulties have arisen from religious, ethical, ethnic and embalming restrictions on the autopsy. At present it would seem that occlusion of extracranial arteries is distinctly more common and occurs at the common carotid bifurcation and the carotid sinus in particular (Figure 12.1). Occlusions of the first inch of the vertebral artery and the cavernous segment of the internal carotid are much less frequent. Thrombosis of the intracranial segment of the internal carotid is less frequent than the cranial segment of the vertebral artery but may have been initiated in the neck.

In those under 40 years of age trauma is the most common cause of vertebral artery obstruction [80]. The vertebral artery in its extracranial course is often displaced laterally and sometimes severely distorted by osteoarthritic bony outgrowths in the region of the neurocentral joint. Lateral displacement and partial obstruction of the vertebral arteries by herniated cervical intervertebral discs is unlikely to produce complete occlusion but distally after the artery leaves the foramen of the atlas, tortuosity may be extreme such that extension or rotation of the head may induce flexion, kinking and obstruction [81]. Obstruction of the vertebral artery not only by osteophytes but also by fascial bands (deep cervical fascia) during head rotation has been suggested. Since head movements may compress the vertebral artery in the neck, there seems no reason why such repeated injuries might not at times precipitate embolism or thrombotic occlusion. This is supported by the occasional report of chiropractic manipulation of the head and neck precipitating thrombosis or embolism, with at times a fatal outcome [82,83]. The case has been reported of a boy with excessive mobility of the axis which led to transient obstruction with neurological deficit even with syncope, on forcing the head backwards [84]. Trauma can provoke such an injury, in one instance precipitating a dissecting aneurysm of the vertebral artery [85,86]. Yates [87] found adventitial haemorrhage and torn branches, and in one case thrombosis of the vertebral arteries resulted from birth injuries. External compression of the arteries with thrombosis was suggested as a cause of permanent ischaemic damage in this age group [87].

Kinking of the internal carotid artery is often associated with evidence of cerebral insufficiency leading to surgical correction at times. Rotation or certain positions of the head may cause symptoms [88,89]. In one patient arterial insufficiency and kinking of the internal carotid were associated with a bruit and palpable thrill originating from the kinking. Pressure gradients of 20–30 mmHg have been found across such a deformity and resection has been found to relieve symptoms and decrease the pressure gradient [89]. Abrupt turning of the head can lead to damage to the internal carotid because of stretching and compression by the lateral process of the atlas to which the vessel is frequently adherent [90]. Perforating, lacerating, iatrogenic and closed neck injuries, even traumatic dissecting aneurysms, may result in occlusions of the internal carotid artery or a large cerebral artery.

Head injuries can be complicated by thrombotic occlusion of the intracranial segment of the internal carotid artery, usually from severe frontal trauma associated with a fracture through the base of the skull. Small false aneurysms or dissecting aneurysms of leptomeningeal arteries due to trauma usually thrombose and it may be difficult to differentiate parenchymal trauma from the effects of small thrombotic lesions.

There are many other disorders that can be associated with thrombosis of the arteries supplying the brain including inflammatory and infectious diseases of blood vessels, haematological disorders and contraceptives, drug abuse and expanding aneurysms or tumours of the base of the skull.

(d) **Large vessel embolism**

Embolism of large arteries supplying the brain accounts for up to 40% of cerebral infarcts. Multiple lesions, especially if haemorrhagic and with a possible source, all suggest an embolic aetiology. A thrombus impacted at a branching site, not adherent to the wall and folded upon itself or if the thrombus contains material from a distant site also supports an embolic origin. Emboli are almost certainly present elsewhere in the branches of the aorta.

Mostly, embolic infarctions (peaking in the sixth decade) tend to occur in younger subjects than non-embolic infarctions (peaking in the seventh decade), but the embolic group is heterogeneous and the diseases or lesions responsible determine the age of occurrence.

Cardiac causes include bacterial endocarditis, non-bacterial thrombotic endocarditis [91], rheumatic heart disease, auricular fibrillation, myocardial infarction and its sequelae, myocarditis, surgical procedures and prostheses, endocardial fibrosis, foreign bodies and tumour emboli. The majority of large emboli results from myocardial infarction.

Emboli may also originate from the aorta and cervical arteries to the brain involved by atherosclerotic ulceration and thrombosis, aneurysms, dissecting aneurysm, arteritis and trauma. Larger emboli may occlude the cervical segment of the internal carotid and fewer are found in the cavernous or intracranial segments. Most are found in the middle cerebral artery. The anterior cerebral is only occasionally occluded. Very few emboli affect the brain stem and those in the vertebrobasilar system are inclined to lodge in the posterior cerebral arteries. Many emboli are not found because like those in the pulmonary circulation, most disappear without trace. The frequency with which they may be demonstrated angiographically is higher when the interval between the onset of symptoms and angiography is short [92]. Migration of thrombi from the internal carotid artery into the branches of the middle cerebral artery seemingly takes hours and after two or three weeks no embolus may be found. Solid emboli cause vasodilation, which appears to facilitate the passage of the embolus along the artery, and migration from the carotid occurs more quickly than disappearance from the middle cerebral artery.

Small vessel embolism to the brain is usually due to atheroembolism, although multiple small emboli also occur from bacterial endocarditis or other thrombi in the heart or large vessels proximal to the brain. Infrequently foreign bodies may embolize to the brain following cardiac surgery and ischaemic injuries from fat and air embolism [3].

(e) **Associated pathological findings**

Cerebral swelling

Like acute infarcts of the viscera, swelling of the infarcted zone occurs with imbibition of fluid raising the intracranial pressure within the first week. The increase in volume depends on the size of the infarct and when more than one major cerebral artery is obstructed, the shift of the mid-line and herniation through the tentorium and into the foramen magnum can become hazardous. If there is some additional complication such as haemorrhage, this aggravates the situation although with haemorrhagic infarcts there is often not as much frankly necrotic tissue participating. Maximum shift occurs in about six days and the swelling then tends to subside during the second week. Severe tentorial herniation commonly causes secondary mid-brain or pontine haemorrhage and less often ischaemia. Compression of the brain stem may be associated with cerebellar infarction but this is usually not as severe as with supratentorial lesions. Compression and distortion of the aqueduct may produce obstructive hydrocephalus necessitating ventricular drainage.

Secondary degeneration

With large infarcts involving the motor cortex or its fibres, secondary degeneration of corticospinal fibres will ensue with reduction in size and asymmetry of the cerebral peduncle, pons and corticospinal tracts.

Cardiovascular disease

Cardiac disability with severe coronary atherosclerosis and hypertension will be frequent concomitants of strokes but in addition by virtue of the large destructive cerebral lesion, some electrocardiographic changes are likely, similar to those with subarachnoid and aneurysmal haemorrhage and without significant CHD.

Neurogenic ulceration

Both acute and chronic gastric ulceration can complicate major strokes.

Hyaline globules of the adrenal

In approximately 15% of cerebral infarcts, round eosinophilic hyaline globes (3–30 µm diameter) are observed extracellularly and less often intracellularly in both the polygonal and chromaffin cells of the adrenal medulla [93]. Of unknown significance, they occur in a variety of diseases, especially bacterial infections.

Laboratory data

The cerebrospinal fluid is generally clear macroscopically but may have some erythrocytes microscopically or xanthochromia in haemorrhagic infarcts. The pressure, usually below 200 mm of water, can reach 400 mm and the risks of lumbar puncture in subjects with an elevated supratentorial pressure should be remembered. There may be leucocytosis peaking at about three days or the leucocyte count may be at a high normal level.

12.8.2 PROGNOSIS

The prognosis for major ischaemic strokes ultimately depends on the size and location of the infarct, other vascular disease of the brain and heart and age of the patient. Comparing the outcome from different studies depends on the classification and detail provided. In general 10–20% of subjects die during the initial stroke but not suddenly and of the survivors, about 50% die within five years. Of the survivors less than 50% will resume previous employment or work part-time, the remainder suffer varying grades of incapacitation or are bedridden. Those under 50 years of age usually have less severe grades of stroke and the mortality is higher with hypertension, recurrence, and vertebrobasilar strokes. Death other than directly from the stroke can be due to respiratory disease (mostly bronchopneumonia) and quite often coronary artery thrombosis or congestive cardiac failure. Occlusive vascular disease is prevalent in patients with chronic brain syndrome. Serious mental deterioration and dementia can be precipitated by cerebral infarctions.

12.9 Other ischaemic lesions

12.9.1 LACUNAR SOFTENINGS (ETAT LACUNAIRE)

Lacunes are deep areas of softening ranging from 0.5 mm to lesions up to 1.5 cm in diameter or length, caused by occlusion of the long perforating arteries chiefly from the middle cerebral, posterior cerebral and basilar arteries to the basal ganglia or pons. They are very frequent but are often overlooked because of their size. Their shape and size are irregular. They are old rather than recent infarcts. For this reason they frequently appear as small holes or cavities (Figure 12.4), occasionally traversed by one or two thin trabeculae and filled with clear watery liquid, hence their name. The walls of some are rusty brown or, if of more recent origin, may be haemorrhagic. Some may be small clefts in the white matter and orientated in the direction of the fibres.

Fisher [94] reported that clinically they manifest minor neurological disturbances, called lacunar strokes such as:

- a pure motor hemiplegia or hemiparesis
- a pure sensory stroke
- a syndrome combining cerebellar ataxia and weakness of the corresponding leg
- dysarthria and clumsiness of one hand due to a lacune in the upper midline of the pons.

Some lacunes are clinically silent but the clinical picture is variable because of their variation in size and position. It has been suggested that as most are asymptomatic (81%), lacunar infarcts are more heterogeneous in their clinical manifestations and the incidence of hypertension may be less than previously envisaged [95].

Sites of predilection are the lenticular nucleus especially the putamen, the thalamus, pons, central white matter, internal capsule, centrum ovale, corpus callosum and rarely the cerebellum. No lesions have been found in the cortex, cerebral peduncles, medulla or spinal cord.

In one study, of 114 persons with lacunar softenings, 71 were males and 43 females: only 8.7% were under 50 years of age, the peak incidence being the seventh decade. They may be responsible for up to 90% of hemiplegias in subjects over 60 years of age [96,97]. Although approximately one third were diabetic in one series and 46% were smokers [95], this does not necessarily indicate a causal relationship.

Lacunes histologically are small softenings and contain some connective tissue trabeculae traversing the lumen. There may be some gliosis in the walls, some residual lipophages and a variable number of siderophages depending on the haemorrhage prior to occlusion of the miliary aneurysms of Charôt and Bouchard.

Obstruction of the small perforating vessels at their origin from the major cerebral arteries does not seem to be responsible [96]. Total occlusion of the miliary aneurysms appears to be the mechanism and since many of these aneurysms are lined by thrombus possibly after slight leakage, it is not surprising that such small lesions undergo occlusive thrombosis. Fisher [97] found occluded miliary aneurysms in 45 of 50 lacunes, at times with anterograde and retrograde thrombosis and organization. In view of the close relationship of hypertension to these miliary aneurysms, the presence of lacunar softenings has been regarded as presumptive evidence of the existence of hypertension but such a deduction may exaggerate the relationship which some authors consider to exist in only 64% of patients [95].

Millikin and Futrell [98] suggested such small infarcts could result from embolic occlusion of intracerebral vessels. Fisher's explanation and the finding of sclerosed or thrombosed Charcôt Bouchard aneurysms is a plausible theory but does not exclude the possibility of emboli or thrombi occluding the same vessels. However, emboli are not so likely to enter the perforating arteries but the event could be associated with severe atherosclerosis and many of the patients will be hypertensive. Consistent with this view is the occurrence of lacunar infarction complicating cardiac and aortic arch angiography [99] which is more prevalent than when Fisher studied the lacunes. Larger infarcts may follow cardiac catheterization [100].

12.9.2 MISCELLANEOUS CAUSES OF ISCHAEMIA

(a) Circulatory arrest

The brain has pronounced susceptibility to anoxia or ischaemia and in cases of cardiac arrest of two to three minutes duration in humans, anoxic encephalopathy develops. A period of survival is essential for the structural changes in response to the anoxia to develop. The anoxia may initiate irreversible selective changes and the damage may be only to nerve cells, which vary in susceptibility. Extensive generalized convolutional atrophy is found with widening of sulci especially in the frontal, parietal and occipital regions and in the cerebellum. The cortex is thin and exhibits extensive laminar necrosis. The deep white matter may be slightly grey and the ventricles dilated. Softening of the caudate nucleus and putamen occurs in some subjects and at times the entire grey matter is necrotic.

(b) Brain-stem ischaemia and supratentorial pressure

Secondary haemorrhages are known to occur in the brain stem under conditions of rapidly increased supratentorial pressure and ischaemic changes can also arise in this location under the same conditions. It is likely that the ischaemic changes may transpire under slightly less severe conditions prior to actual rupture and haemorrhage from small branches. Other ischaemic changes resulting from brain shift secondary to expanding space-occupying lesions include compression of:

1. the posterior cerebral artery and branches by the tentorial margin (ischaemic or haemorrhagic);
2. anterior choroidal by the tentorial edge;
3. anterior cerebral by the falx cerebri;
4. middle cerebral artery by the lesser wing of the sphenoid bone;
5. cerebellar arteries by the tentorial margins or the rim of the foramen magnum [42].

(c) Puerperal hemiplegia and stroke

Sudden onset of hemiplegia in a young healthy woman during pregnancy or the puerperium though a rare event is still a cause for concern. It has been attributed to cerebral venous thrombosis but this has often been conjecture. The cause is unknown. The enhanced tendency for thrombosis has been linked with hormonal factors and the frequency of cerebral thrombotic episodes (arterial and venous) in women using oral contraceptives. As yet there is no satisfactory explanation.

(d) Multiple progressive intracranial arterial occlusions

Taveras [101] reviewed multiple progressive intracranial arterial occlusions in young adults and children. The syndrome consists of unilateral or bilateral occlusion of multiple intracranial segments of the internal carotid arteries, of the middle and anterior cerebral arteries and sometimes of the basilar and posterior cerebral arteries. The occlusions are thought, perhaps incorrectly, to be chronic.

A 30-year-old woman who died of this disorder [102] suffered night sweats, pyrexia, nightmares, progressive confusion, headache and nausea, with an elevated erythrocyte sedimentation rate and her temperature eventually rose to 106°F. This clinical picture was similar to other reported cases and is indicative of a protracted febrile illness. The occluded, stenosed arteries at autopsy were suggestive of a diffuse destructive lesion with organized thrombotic occlusion of arteries and small branches. One middle cerebral artery had a recent thrombosis with small cystic spaces in the loose intimal thickening. Older lesions displayed gross fibrosis of the media and adventitia as well as of the intima with stenoses or occlusion. A rich collateral circulation had developed.

The disease, more common in the Japanese, is associated with repetitive transitory ischaemic episodes and usually preceded by a febrile illness. Electron microscopic and immunohistochemical study of some arteries [103] has not been revealing. Most authors consider the disease to be a chronic progressive occlusive disease of the cerebral arteries because of the development of prominent collateral circulation at the base of the brain via unaffected leptomeningeal arteries, transdural anastomoses between leptomeningeal vessels and branches of the external carotid, and a very prominent network of vessels in the basal ganglia and upper brain stem, at times filling the anterior and middle cerebral arteries. This syndrome appears to be the same as that originally reported in the Japanese as 'moyamoya' disease, rete mirabile or haemangiomatous malformations at the base of the brain. The aetiology is obscure. The occlusion may commence *in utero* [104], infancy or childhood.

There is need to investigate the acute or early lesions of the cerebral arteries in detail (including electron microscopy), rather than seek a causative lesion in advanced stages or in the secondary collateral circulation. A possible viral infection has yet to be excluded. The morphology of the rete vessels is consistent with that of collateral vessels which were originally considered to be indicative of some dysplastic or haemangiomatous process. These vessels, which manifest severe degenerative changes, are prone to aneurysmal dilatation and haemorrhage. The probability is that the cause of the arterial occlusion may not always be due to this syndrome and that the rich collateral network is a non-specific change.

(e) Haematological disorders

Thromboses can be found within the cranium in polycythaemia rubra vera, not necessarily in every affected subject but multiple softenings in the brain and cord with transient paralyses and sensory disturbances are prevalent.

In patients dying of sickle cell anaemia, capillary hyperaemia and thromboses are usually pronounced and sickle cells are observable in the lumen of vessels in the subarachnoid space at the margin of haemorrhages in the depths of the sulci. Small foci of softening and areas of demyelination are prevalent in the white matter and large areas of old or recent infarction are uncommon. There may be some arteriolar thickening, siderosis of cerebral vessels and lipid globules occluding small cerebral vessels resembling fat embolism.

(f) Microcirculatory occlusions

Small microthrombi occluding vessels in the cerebral microcirculation occur in a number of diseases only some of which are primarily vascular disorders. Some are transitory occlusions and leave no permanent damage. Trauma may be responsible but also intravenous infusions may lead to leucocyte–platelet microthrombi perhaps with red cell sludging as well. Particulate matter, some fat emulsions, anaphylactic reactions, malaria, bacteraemia and disseminated intravascular coagulopathy appear to induce similar microcirculatory changes [105] which need to be studied and graded clinically. The red cell aggregation will cause increased viscosity, a raised erythrocyte sedimentation rate and sluggish blood flow none of which factors has been fully appreciated. It is also a feature of macroglobulinaemia of Waldenström in man [106] and fat embolism following injury is a recognized cause of microcirculatory occlusion in the brain. The embolism need not be the result of direct embolism but is an unexplained lipoprotein instability. Caisson disease may be associated with nitrogen bubbles and tumour emboli may reach the brain via the vertebral venous plexus.

Similar microcirculatory changes can be induced by the administration of fatty meals, the effect being more pronounced with fats containing a high percentage of saturated fatty acids [107]. The oxygen availability is reduced and convulsions can be induced in hamsters after a cream meal [108]. The significance of these findings in man is uncertain but the sludging effect with relative stasis is capable of producing severely diminished blood flow.

(g) Thrombosis of cerebral veins and dural sinuses

The incidence of these thromboses is less than early in the century due to antibiotics and better control of the fluid balance of sick patients. Thrombosis of the sigmoid sinus was a relatively frequent complication of otitis media whereas this is now a rarity. Almost 75% are under five years of age.

Marantic thrombosis occurs in wasted and debilitated children and is a terminal event in the presence of severe toxaemia, reduced blood flow and often cardiac insufficiency. Malnutrition, dehydration and infectious diseases play a major role, but local inflammatory disease rarely causes cerebral venous or sinus thrombosis nowadays. Venous thrombosis in the puerperium is likely when associated with severe vomiting and diarrhoea and occurs in many wasting diseases particularly with carcinomatosis and congenital heart disease with severe right-sided cardiac insufficiency and chronic venous congestion.

A variety of other causes [33] is complicated by these thrombotic events including trauma from accidents, birth injuries, surgery, tumour invasion, paroxysmal nocturnal haemoglobinuria and blood dyscrasias such as sickle cell anaemia, polycythemia rubra vera and leukaemia.

Local inflammatory disease, now a rare cause, must be kept in mind in subjects with acute or chronic mastoiditis which can readily spread through the bone and dura mater, possibly even by diploic veins draining to the sinus. Thrombosis of the cavernous sinus can be secondary to spread of infection by veins draining the danger zone of the face (upper lip, nose, orbital and frontal regions of the face). The superior longitudinal sinus may be thrombosed secondarily to infectious lesions in the scalp, nose and paranasal air sinuses, osteomyelitis of the skull, meningitis, encephalitis or terminally in septicaemia.

Thrombosis of cerebral veins and dural sinuses occurs in subjects with thrombotic events in the lower limbs or viscera including pulmonary embolism or in the clinical state labelled as thrombophlebitis migrans [109]. It is also possible that infection from the pelvis can spread to the dural sinuses via the vertebral venous plexus.

Currently cerebral venous thrombosis affects young women either during pregnancy or in the puerperium but is not as common as thrombosis in the deep veins of the lower limbs. Those occurring during pregnancy develop in the third trimester but most are puerperal. This is similar to femoral vein thrombosis suggesting that there is a common factor underlying the thrombotic tendency associated with pregnancy. Some thrombi develop during the first trimester following an abortion or threatened abortion but are infrequent and in the past may have been related to illegal, unhygienic abortions.

The commonest site of an intracranial venous thrombosis is the superior longitudinal sagittal sinus and it is usually nonseptic. Those associated with sepsis are most often observed in the sigmoid and straight sinus. Propagation of thrombus from the superior longitudinal sinus can extend to other sinuses and the draining tributaries. Thrombosis of cerebral veins alone is said to occur in only 10% of cases and most often in association with the posterior three fifths of the superior sagittal sinus. The opposite side is likely to be involved secondarily.

The superior longitudinal sagittal sinus, though the commonest site for non-septic thrombosis such as with pregnancy, puerperium, trauma, marasmus and cachexia, can be involved by secondary spread of infection from the scalp or nose or by secondary propagation from the transverse sinus or cortical veins. The Rolandic veins are often affected so that motor and sensory disturbances result. Thrombosis of the straight sinus or the great cerebral vein (of Galen) is likely to be associated with or caused by extension of thrombus from the superior longitudinal sagittal sinus or the transverse sinus. The transverse sinus can be thrombosed secondarily and propagation to the sigmoid with extension to the internal jugular vein is likely.

The inferior petrosal sinus may be involved by infections of the middle ear and the superior petrosal sinus by spread from the ear through the tegmen tympani or by spread from the inferior petrosal or cavernous sinus.

Cavernous sinus thrombosis is usually septic from spread of infection from the danger area of the face, or from the inferior or superior petrosal sinuses. It may be bilateral and the venous tributaries are also usually thrombosed with congestion and oedema of the orbits and proptosis. Suppurative meningitis is almost invariably present and infarction of the pituitary gland may occur secondarily.

Most thrombi have the usual macroscopic and microscopic characteristics of thrombi. Some may be partially organized or even recanalized. In cases of sepsis, the local inflammatory reaction is usually suppurative and spread of infection can be rapid via emissary and anastomotic veins. There can be suppuration within the sinus and purulent meningitis and a cerebral or cerebellar abscess may follow. Commonly thrombosis is secondary to acute or chronic mastoiditis and local inflammation in the sinus wall may occur without bacterial invasion. Rarely is there tumour in the thrombus.

There are plentiful anastomoses between the superficial cerebral veins and the sinuses and thrombotic occlusion therefore may be limited in extent. The rapidity of the occlusion is crucial as rapid occlusion does not allow collaterals to develop and often there may be no significant change in the underlying brain. In others there is haemorrhagic softening of both grey and white matter (Figure 12.15). The area of brain involved

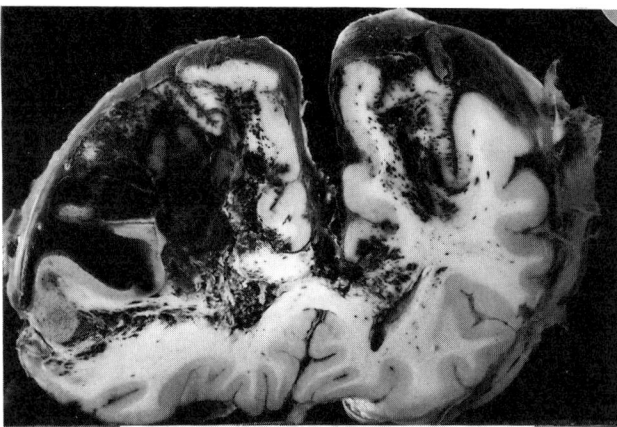

Figure 12.15 Coronal section of cerebrum with haemorrhagic infarction of both hemispheres due to superior longitudinal sagittal sinus thrombus which extended into parietal cortical veins. Note unequal size and involvement of the hemispheres, the confluence of multiple haemorrhages involving both grey and white matter and the extensive subarachnoid haemorrhage.

may be less than the drainage area of the occluded vessels according to the adequacy of the collateral circulation. The infarcts commence as multiple ecchymoses which coalesce to form a swollen haemorrhagic portion of brain with retention of pre-existing architecture. It is not fibre-splitting as in primary intracerebral haemorrhage and the edge has many small haemorrhages surrounding the main haemorrhagic zone. There is in addition much more subarachnoid bleeding than with the red infarcts associated with arterial occlusions and at times subdural extravasation of blood is present.

In extensive thrombosis of the superior longitudinal sinus and tributaries, cerebral swelling, oedema and congestion raises intracranial pressure to fatal limits before extensive haemorrhage occurs. The parenchymal lesions are bilateral but not necessarily symmetrical. The massive increase in supratentorial pressure may precipitate secondary pontine haemorrhage. The parietal lobes are infarcted most frequently although the frontal and occipital lobes are affected almost as often. The temporal lobes are seldom affected. Occlusion of the great cerebral vein of Galen results in haemorrhagic infarction in the mid-line structures in the drainage area. Consequently there is extensive bilateral softening in the basal ganglia and perhaps intraventricular haemorrhage, the cerebellum and brain stem being rarely affected.

Organization of small non-lethal zones occurs in the usual manner with opaque meninges, and xanthochromic staining over the shrunken, atrophic brownish-yellow cortex with old cystic and laminar softenings. Enlarged collateral vessels may be apparent.

12.9.3 OTITIC HYDROCEPHALUS

Otitic hydrocephalus is a term applied by Symonds [110] to a syndrome primarily affecting children with a history of acute or chronic mastoiditis with weakness or paralysis of both lateral recti muscles (sixth nerve palsy), headache and greatly increased intracranial pressure without appreciable increase of cerebrospinal fluid cells or protein. Many have thrombosis of the lateral sinus. In this benign condition bilateral optic nerve atrophy develops unless the intracranial pressure is relieved.

The occlusion of the major (right) lateral sinus or thrombosis of the left with extension to the torcular (confluence of the sinuses) and the posterior segment of the superior sagittal sinus obstructs venous drainage from most of the brain and results in internal hydrocephalus [109] which is due to increased venous pressure.

Although it is not always immediately fatal, the prognosis of thrombosis of major dural sinuses is poor in view of the cerebral infarction, haemorrhage, congestion, oedema and the intracranial hypertension. The prognosis for cortical venous thromboses depends on the extent and propagation of the thrombus. At times these lesions are small and may be mistaken for small cortical arterial softenings.

12.9.4 CEREBRAL THROMBOSIS AND ORAL CONTRACEPTIVES

Women over 35 years of age on oral contraceptives have at least a four-fold increase in incidence of stroke and thromboembolic disorders, including cerebral arterial, venous and massive venous sinus thrombosis [111]. The increase, said to be independent of smoking and blood pressure, has been attributed to a high oestrogen content. Men on oestrogen for prostatic cancer also have an increased propensity for thrombotic lesions. There is an increase in plasma antiplasmin, plasminogen, fibrinogen and platelet adhesiveness with a decrease in serum antithrombin activity. The pathogenesis is obscure and the thrombi are thought to be usually in veins. Cerebral arterial occlusions from the pulmonary veins are embolic. Thromboembolic disorders tend to be more pronounced with blood groups A, B and AB but this is not necessarily related to contraceptive use.

Various changes in blood vessels [111] have been incriminated including fibrinoid swelling of intracerebral arterioles [112] but at present the vascular lesion is unknown.

12.10 Ischaemic lesions of the spinal cord

Ischaemic lesions of the spinal cord are rare. Occlusions of the medullary portion of the anterior spinal artery are most often overshadowed by the consequences of obstruction of the vertebral and perhaps the basilar artery. Therefore occlusion of the spinal portion of the anterior spinal artery is seen more frequently and is associated with the distinct syndrome of sudden paraplegia, anaesthesia of the syringomyelic type with disturbances of urination and defecation. Occlusion of the posterior spinal artery is seen much less often.

12.10.1 PATHOGENESIS

There are various causes of spinal cord ischaemia.

(a) Trauma

Trauma may be associated with damage sufficiently severe to cause thrombosis of spinal arteries with or without vertebral dislocation and the ischaemia may extend for several segments above or below the site of cord injury. Trauma involving segmental vessels in the thorax or abdomen rather than the spine may obstruct, avulse or cause thrombosis of an intercostal or lumbar artery producing secondary effects on the cord. Injury to the great anterior medullary artery of Adamkiewicz (usually from the second left lumbar artery but varying from the 8th thoracic to the 4th lumbar), because of its being the largest anterior medullary artery, is serious and can result in ischaemia of the anterior two thirds of the cord distal to the level of its junction with the anterior spinal artery. Lack of blood supply to other anterior medullary arteries is not nearly so critical.

(b) Compression of the spinal arteries

Compression of the veins may precede compression of the anterior spinal artery but their collateral flow is rich. Arterial compression can result from any space-occupying lesions (primary or secondary tumours), osteoarthritic spurs or a herniated intervertebral disc.

(c) Postoperative complications

Intentional or accidental surgical ligation of anterior medullary arteries, especially the great anterior medullary artery can cause serious postoperative spinal cord ischaemia especially with surgery about the level of the diaphragm. Prolonged clamping of the aorta may result in similar ischaemic injuries. A mishap in performing spinal angiography occasionally leads to thrombosis of a spinal artery with infarction of the cord [113].

(d) Atherosclerosis

The spinal arteries are so small that atherosclerosis is unlikely to be directly responsible for their occlusion. The ostia of many segmental arteries especially in the distal aorta become occluded due to atherosclerotic ulceration and thrombosis [114]. Fortunately the collateral circulation seems to be adequate otherwise spinal cord ischaemia would be extremely common. Spinal cord lesions attributed in the past to atherosclerosis are in all probability examples of atheroembolism and even cases of sudden acute transverse myelitis may also be due to the same cause. Atherosclerosis or arteriosclerosis may cause relative ischaemia as might fibrinoid necrosis of any cause but such lesions, rather than involving a large segment of the cord, tend to be small.

Atherosclerosis has replaced syphilis as the most usual cause of spinal cord ischaemia and it is claimed that it can cause intermittent claudication of the cord with impoverished blood flow to the cord brought on by exertion (suggestive of a vascular steal) and transient ischaemic attacks which may be followed by frank infarction. The pathogenesis of these lesions remains obscure probably because of their infrequency. Whether ischaemia is the cause of a few rare cases of progressive disease of the spinal cord in elderly subjects with irregular cavitation of the cord and progressive atrophic paraparesis [115] is uncertain.

(e) Hypotension

Hypotension can cause ischaemia but usually in the presence of severe aortic atherosclerosis when some part of the cord has a precarious blood supply provided by collaterals.

(f) Miscellaneous causes

Ischaemia of the cord may occur in aortic coarctation, the distal part of the cord at times suffering from relative ischaemia. The symptoms and signs may be overshadowed by compression by the enlarged tortuous anterior spinal artery or rarely by an aneurysm.

Bacterial endocarditis, caisson disease, polyarteritis nodosa, syphilitic arteritis, malaria and arteriovenous shunts may all be associated with ischaemia.

12.10.2 PATHOLOGY OF THE INFARCT

Spinal cord infarction caused by these variable, often unexplained pathogenetic mechanisms is usually pale; distribution is according to the artery of supply affected. Resolution of the infarcts is basically similar to their resolution in the brain and results in a cystic or collapsed gliosed area.

The anterior two thirds of the cord are involved more frequently than the posterior third (Figure 12.16). The areas of the cord most susceptible to ischaemia are at the border zone between areas of supply by the anterior medullary arteries and the watershed area between the regions supplied by the anterior and posterior spinal arteries. The pial arterial plexus maintains the viability

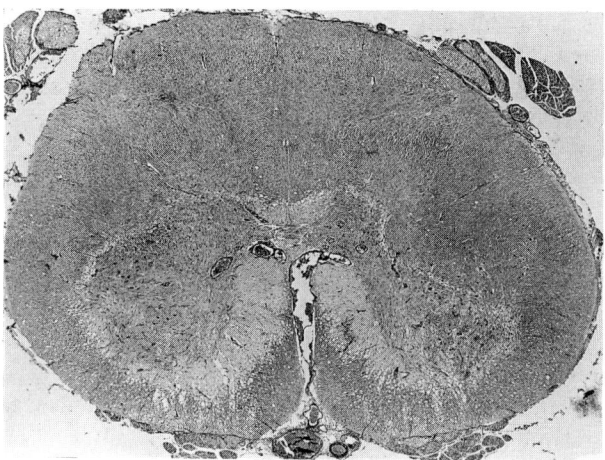

Figure 12.16 Recent butterfly-shaped infarct of the spinal cord associated with a dissecting aneurysm of the aorta. The two anterior horns, the centre and adjacent white matter are infarcted. (Haematoxylin and eosin.) (Reproduced from Stehbens [3].)

of the superficial subpial zone and the infarct, therefore, involves the anterior central portion of the cord.

12.10.3 VENOUS INFARCTION

The venous plexuses usually provide for adequate collateral flow of blood and so venous obstruction would have necessitated the involvement of many veins such as can occur in spinal thrombophlebitis. The anterior horn cells may be spared but the rest of the white matter becomes shrunken and gliosed.

12.11 Intracranial and intraspinal haemorrhage

12.11.1 INTRACRANIAL EXTRADURAL HAEMATOMA

The accumulation of blood between the dura mater and the inner table of the skull is an extradural haematoma, an uncommon event and usually the consequence of a blunt injury to the skull or a fall. The acute haematoma causes a dramatic clinical syndrome in 22%–39.5% of subjects with a skull fracture. Whilst it may occur at any age, it is found most often in the second to fifth decades. Males being subject to greater risk of trauma, the lesion is more common in males than females.

(a) **Precipitating factors**

Trauma

The most frequent cause of intracranial extradural haemorrhage is a head injury associated with a traffic accident or less frequently, a fall either accidental or suicidal in nature. It can result from a blow to the head during a fight, mugging, sport or horseplay, or in some cases from unknown injury. The trauma can be relatively slight but is usually severe. There may be no memory of a head injury possibly due to post-traumatic amnesia. The severity can be gauged from the duration of unconsciousness and from the associated injuries to the scalp, skull and brain. The susceptibility of the skull to fracture has been attributed to undue thinness or fragility of the bone. There is no scientific evidence to substantiate alleged racial differences in propensity for this type of lesion.

Extremely severe cranial injuries and depressed fractures are uncommonly associated with extradural haematomas except in children. It is also an uncommon event with penetrating wounds, no doubt because drainage of extravasated blood is likely to be adequate and cerebral damage dominates the clinical state of the patient. A mild head injury has been alleged to cause extradural haemorrhage. However, in general, the trauma is quite severe and there may be no external evidence of injury.

Ventricular decompression

Massive extradural haemorrhage is a relatively unknown complication of ventricular decompression occurring predominantly in children and young adults with internal hydrocephalus [117]. In the chronic hydrocephalic state, it is possible the dura mater becomes less firmly adherent to the calvarium and with this weak attachment, the pull on the dura mater via connecting vessels separates the dura from the bone with secondary haemorrhage from nutrient vessels to the bone. The concept of detachment following decompression via these vascular attachments is not attractive. Subdural haemorrhage may also follow decompression in hydrocephalics possibly due to avulsion of small veins traversing the subdural space but the clinical development of such an event tends to be slower than the dramatic onset of extradural haemorrhage.

Miscellaneous causes

Bleeding disorders seldom cause extradural haemorrhage. Small intradural haemorrhages are more common. There are also exceptionally rare cases associated with haemangiomas of the skull and dura [118,119], chronic suppurative otitis media or sinusitis with spread to the bone and middle meningeal artery, internal carotid artery or a dural sinus [3]. There has been a rare instance of a bilateral extradural haemorrhage occurring for no apparent reason during open-heart surgery for tetralogy of Fallot in a 10-year-old girl [120].

12.11.2 PATHOLOGICAL FINDINGS

Extradural haematomas are most often acute and consist of a saucer-shaped accumulation of typical 'redcurrant jelly' blood clot up to 10 or 12 cm in diameter and 4 or 5 cm thick. They can be larger measuring up to 900 ml in volume. Some haematomas are of insignificant size but others can range up to 400 g in weight, Fatal haematomas usually weigh over 75 g with an average of about 122 g, about twice that of the average subdural haematoma [3].

Most haematomas are acute, being less than three or four days old when treated surgically or viewed at autopsy. Survival for longer periods of time is likely if the haematoma is smaller and with a lesser neurological deficit. The acute haematoma will, with time, become black and tarry in consistency with progressively brownish coloration until it is rusty brown and semiliquid. Chronic haematomas become encapsulated with fibrous, brownish granulation tissue growing from the dura mater. Because newly formed blood vessels are more susceptible to minor injury, fresh bleeding may occur. Calcification may arise in the overlying dura mater and possibly even bone formation continuous with the calvarium at the margins of the old haematomas but this would be rare.

The classical site is in the temporal region and much less frequently they are frontal, frontoparietal, occipital or in the posterior fossa (especially in children and young adults). The base is not often involved. They are rarely bilateral but may involve both sides when over the vertex or in the posterior fossa. The old concept was that the temporal haematoma was limited from further extension by the attachment of the dura mater to the suture lines of the skull and the attachment of dural sinuses but this misconception was exposed when their distribution was mapped.

Extradural haematoma is the most common traumatic space-occupying lesion in the posterior cranial fossa and has a high mortality due to the slow progression of symptoms since it is usually of venous origin.

In the classic syndrome of extradural haematoma, the bleeding is thought to come from a branch of the middle meningeal artery in the region of the pterion, where the vessels are often enclosed in a bony tunnel or lie within a deep groove in the inner table of the calvarium. A fracture passing across their path would be expected to damage both artery and vein, venous damage being the more certain outcome. These grooves are caused mainly by the *venae comitantes* rather than the arteries and are less prominent in children than in adults. Bleeding has been said to stem from either the arteries or the veins or from lacerated large dural (lateral, superior longitudinal or sigmoid) sinuses [121]. Bleeding has been attributed to the anterior or posterior branches or even the main stem of the middle meningeal artery but derives from the anterior or posterior meningeal vessels when the haematoma is at an unusual site. There may be massive bleeding from the internal carotid artery injured at the foramen lacerum with fractures through the base of the skull [122,123]. Diploic vessels bleed through the fracture site or from separated suture lines but not to a significant degree. Emissary veins may be responsible and following surgical drainage of a haematoma, bleeding can recur from undetected injuries or from supply vessels to the bone as the haematoma is in effect subperiosteal. Even a false traumatic aneurysm or an arteriovenous fistula may be responsible for recurrent post-surgical haemorrhage. True degenerative meningeal aneurysms are exceedingly rare.

There has been controversy over the separation of the dura mater from the bone especially since bleeding is often of venous origin but a severe blow with a mallet to the side of a cadaver's head can detach dura mater with or without fracturing the skull. Separation is not successful when the head is unsupported [124]. The extent of separation is thought to be too localized to account for the large area of involvement in fracture, leading to the assumption that progressive dissection of the dura mater from the bone follows as haemorrhage continues.

If a branch of a meningeal artery is ruptured, the arterial jet has been said to act as an hydraulic ram stripping the dura mater further [125]. If the bleeding is venous, it is unlikely that further stripping will occur. The physics of this separation needs to be investigated but no doubt the ease with which the dura is stripped will vary from subject to subject. It is said to be least firmly attached in the temporal region [126]. A mild scorbutic condition may enhance this dissection since in this condition subperiosteal haemorrhages are frequent due to loss of cohesion between periosteum and bone.

As most extradural haematomas are the consequence of injury, evidence of trauma such as bruising, laceration or abrasions of the scalp is likely to be found and there may be injuries elsewhere. Subepicranial and subpericranial haematomas may produce swelling over the lesion together with a feeling of bogginess. Otorrhoea or bleeding from the nose, pharynx or ear suggests a skull fracture which is usually but not invariably present. Freytag [127] found fractures in 98.1% of 211 cases and separation of suture lines may be observed instead. The fracture may not be within the operative zone but usually intersects the meningeal vascular grooves or venous sinuses. Radiological displacement of the bones is not essential though displacement may have been significant at the time of injury. Fractures of the inner table alone have been incriminated.

The haematoma can cause considerable cerebral compression and there may be concomitant subdural haemorrhage and damage to the brain itself with secondary pressure effects. Head injuries of such severity are likely to be associated with cerebral and subarachnoid haemorrhage. Haematomas over the vertex can cause compression of the superior longitudinal sagittal sinus and retard venous return. The elevated supratentorial pressure can result in secondary pontine and mid-brain haemorrhage. The third cranial nerve may be injured and papilloedema and subhyaloid haemorrhages are possible concomitants.

Blood loss is occasionally significant from leakage through a scalp wound or accumulates under the galea aponeurotica. In very young children the haematoma may amount to a significant fraction of total blood volume.

Extradural haematomas to the posterior fossa displace and compress the cerebellum and brain stem resulting in secondary pontine haemorrhage as has been demonstrated experimentally [128]. They may also compress and obstruct the aqueduct resulting in moderate hydrocephalus, aggravating the already jeopardized cerebral circulation. Ventriculography some time after surgical removal of the haematoma has revealed mild to moderate dilatation of the ventricular system, and if asymmetry exists, the lateral ventricle opposite the side of the haematoma is the larger.

12.11.3 MORTALITY

The classical clinical syndrome is quite dramatic consisting of a fall or blow to the head followed by:

1. concussion with loss of consciousness for a variable period of time;
2. recovery with a lucid interval lasting up to several hours or days;
3. the return of coma possibly preceded by headache, drowsiness and vomiting;
4. decerebrate rigidity and death.

Variation in the clinical picture is frequent, leading to delays in diagnosis. Reduction in mortality which may be as high as 76%, depends on early recognition and treatment but the prognosis also depends on the severity of associated injuries which can include subdural haemorrhage, cerebral contusions and secondary pressure effects. The mortality is highest over 70 years and lowest in children [121].

Profuse haemorrhage will accelerate clinical evolution of this dramatic emergency, though death and severe mortality are avoidable more often than not when adequate surgical drainage is instituted early [129].

12.12 Spinal extradural haematoma

This rare entity occurs mostly in adults and requires prompt recognition to avoid serious neurological sequelae due to sudden compression of the spinal cord causing paraparesis, paraplegia or quadriplegia. The haematoma may follow severe back injuries such as spinal fractures or dislocations, blows to the back, falls or penetrating injuries (bullets or stab wounds). Birth injuries can cause spinal extradural haemorrhage but are rarely sought in neonatal autopsies [130]. A traumatic lumbar puncture may be responsible. Haemorrhage can follow a rather minor injury or fall but in non-traumatic cases, the onset of back pain with subsequent development of symptoms and signs of cord compression within an hour or a few days may be precipitated by coughing, straining, lifting or the Valsalva manoeuvre. Blood dyscrasias including anticoagulant therapy can be responsible although it may be only minor or incidental to more widespread haemorrhage. Cases have occurred in haemophilia and polycythaemia rubra vera. Extradural haemangioma is a recognized cause as are arteriovenous fistulae.

The thoracic region is most frequently involved. The haematoma extends over the length of two to three vertebrae but can extend from the skull to the lower thoracic vertebrae [3] with variable subdural and subarachnoid haemorrhage. The haematoma at autopsy will be blackish red and up to 1 cm thick with discolouration proportional to the age of the haematoma. The cerebrospinal fluid may be haemorrhagic or xanthochromic and myelography will demonstrate obstruction in the subarachnoid space. The cord may appear compressed and haemorrhagic, contused or oedematous and eventually some softening becomes apparent with cystic spaces, degeneration and gliosis. Dense vascular granulation tissue encapsulates a chronic haematoma. Long fibre tracts are more susceptible and residual paraparesis or paraplegia can occur.

Little information is available about the attachments of the dura mater to the vertebral canal, the anatomy differing from that within the skull. There is soft fatty tissue with plexiform thin-walled veins in addition to the attachments to the posterior longitudinal ligament of the vertebral column. Blood therefore permeates the extradural fat and clotting should localize the haematoma. The dura mater is readily displaced inwards towards the cord by an expanding haematoma with compression of pial vessels and the cord. The source of bleeding is believed to be venous in traumatic cases. In the absence of an arteriovenous shunt there is no evidence that the veins are varicose and to suggest undue weakness of vessels is mere speculation.

12.13 Subdural haematoma

Subdural haematoma is a localized extravasation of blood into the subdural space, which is usually only a potential cavity between the dura mater and the arachnoid mater. It is classified as acute, subacute or chronic according to the duration of the haematoma and is four times more frequent than extradural haematoma [127].

The disorder is an emergency in the acute stage and in the chronic form often tragically misdiagnosed. The preponderance of subdural haematomas in males is considered to be due to their greater activity and aggressiveness. The ratio of males to females is approximately 2:1, and 3:1 in the chronic form. There is a peak in the age distribution in the first decade primarily due to birth trauma with others being the result of accidental falls fracturing the skull during the first two years of life. Thereafter, there is a steady increase in incidence to a maximum in the sixth or seventh decade before it declines [3].

12.13.1 PRECIPITATING FACTORS

(a) Trauma

This is the most common cause of subdural haematoma in all age groups. Fatal subdural haematomas in stillborn and newborn infants arise from rupture of the great cerebral vein of Galen with extensive subdural haemorrhage extending between the cerebral hemispheres and over the surface of the brain or from superficial leptomeningeal arteries over the hemisphere, usually branches of the middle cerebral artery [131]. Bleeding in most cases has been attributed to stretching and rupture of small venous tributaries of the great cerebral vein of Galen near its junction with the straight sinus. Such haemorrhages are believed to result from a difficult labour or from moulding of the head and tearing of the tentorium or small communicating veins.

Subdural haematoma also occurs *in utero*, usually due to severe blows to the maternal abdomen in automobile accidents. Recently cases have been reported in Pacific Islander stillbirths and were thought to be due to traditional deep palpation with a view to external cephalic version for breech presentations which are regarded as undesirable [132–134]. Some had intracerebral and intraventricular haemorrhage. Two live births were associated with macrocephaly and large subdural haematomas. A high incidence of hydrocephalus in such stillbirths was also attributed to the intraventricular haemorrhage and it was thought a similar mechanism may be the cause of unexplained hydrocephalus in other nationalities [134,135].

Multiple head injuries of differing severity complicate the process of infants learning to sit, stand, walk, run and climb and subdural haematoma is an infrequent but recognized complication in this age group. Some subdural haematomas in association with evidence of multiple contusions and fractures were once thought to result from scurvy but are now believed to be examples of the 'battered baby' syndrome. Malnutrition may accompany the injuries. Many are fatal and others may result in permanent brain damage with mental retardation, an almost invariable consequence in this age group.

In later years subdural haematoma is said to occur in 9–13% of all severe head injuries stemming from accidents or violence, being considerably more common than extradural haematoma [3]. It is present in at least 50% of fatal head injuries due to blunt force in addition to those chronic cases not becoming apparent immediately after head injury. Most are due to major trauma sufficient to cause loss of consciousness but others follow less severe and at times quite trivial injury without loss of consciousness. There remains a significant number unassociated with injury although posttraumatic amnesia can be responsible for the lack of recall. A very few have been attributed to coughing but in such instances some additional undisclosed factor must predispose to haemorrhage.

Indirect trauma such as a fall on the buttocks, blast injury and even whiplash injuries [136] have been incriminated. Minor or moderate bumps or blows to the head can be incorrectly incriminated in the pathogenesis of chronic subdural haematoma and no evidence of a congenital predisposition has been established. Acute and chronic alcoholism are frequently associated with injuries and accidents but there is no evidence that alcohol *per se* predisposes to such haemorrhage, although alcoholic intoxication is involved in more than half the cases of acute haematomas. Of 102 cases of chronic haematomas 74% were alcoholics [137].

(b) Senility and mental disease

The peak incidence for acute, subacute and chronic subdural haematomas lies between 50 and 70 years, with an overall 52% occurring over 50 years and 14.5% in those over 70 years of age [3]. This contrasts with the age distribution of extradural haematoma in which the peak incidence is in the third decade, and suggests there is a propensity for subdural bleeding, most instances of which are traumatic in the elderly. This could be due to cerebral atrophy leading to increased traction and greater likelihood of damage to the vessels bridging the subdural space since in later ages the subarachnoid space will be enlarged allowing more movement of the brain within the cranial cavity.

Subdural haematomas have been considered a frequent complication of mental illness. Inmates of mental institutions may be subject to more frequent head injuries than the general population. The mental retardation or dementia may be secondary to chronic subdural haematoma or the disparity between brain size and skull capacity may be greater.

(c) Ventricular decompression and pneumoencephalography

Subdural haemorrhage is a recognized complication of ventricular decompression in hydrocephalics. Likewise pneumoencephalography has been sporadically reported as a cause of subdural haemorrhage. In all likelihood both of these procedures lead to greater traction and tearing of small veins traversing the subdural space in the arachnoid–dural attachments. Both procedures lend support for this as the explanation of the predisposition of the elderly to the disorder.

(d) Infective theory

Chronic subdural haematomas were once considered to be infective as manifested by the encapsulating granulation tissue and secondary haemorrhage primarily in the insane. The concept has now been dispelled. There is one recorded secondary infection of a chronic haematoma [138].

(e) Nutritional factors

The role of scurvy and vitamin K deficiency has probably been overestimated and as indicated scurvy is no longer considered to be a frequent cause. It could well be a contributing factor as malnutrition is a frequent accompaniment of child abuse.

(f) Blood dyscrasias

Bleeding due to blood dyscrasias is usually relatively slight in extent but occurs at multiple sites and, therefore, although significant subdural haemorrhage is not common, it can occur in thrombocytopenia, leukaemia and liver disease. Haemophilia is less likely to be a cause with modern management. Fatal subdural haematoma has been a frequent complication of anticoagulant therapy such as warfarin and is often potentiated by pharmacological agents. Increased awareness of this side-effect is mandatory. The subjects are often middle-aged or elderly, no doubt because of the frequent anticoagulant therapy for myocardial infarction [3]. The haematoma may or may not be associated with mild trauma and its presence may not be recognized for weeks or months after cessation of therapy. Haemorrhage can be present elsewhere within the cranium.

(g) Haemodialysis

Subdural haematomas have been reported following acute or chronic haemodialysis [139,140]. This has been attributed to brain shrinkage and overstretching of the subdural bridging veins with the use of hypertonic solutions. Since subdural, subarachnoid and intracerebral haemorrhage have also occurred in experimental animals, trauma does not appear to be an important factor in these subjects.

(h) Miscellaneous factors

Subdural haemorrhage has been associated with ruptured cerebral aneurysms, of both the berry and bacterial type. Usually this is supratentorial with significant bleeding only rarely though it can contribute to the raised intracranial pressure. It has been reported with primary non-traumatic intracerebral haemorrhage but an unrecognized aneurysmal haemorrhage must be excluded and it can be due to a head injury occasioned by falling, secondary to loss of consciousness. A variety of other disorders has been associated with subdural haemorrhage (such as eclampsia, arteriovenous angiomatous lesions, tumours and subcortical abscesses). Subdural haemorrhage, uncommon amongst epileptics, has been thought to complicate grand mal convulsions. Trauma sustained during a convulsion may contribute to or be responsible for the bleeding [3].

12.13.2 PATHOLOGY

The amount of subdural bleeding can vary. It is sometimes a thin diffuse coating of blood or xanthochromic staining but is usually disregarded unless there is a substantial accumulation. Minor haemorrhage may be overshadowed by more significant cerebral damage and in infancy small haematomas may be significant. They need not be as thick as in adults in whom they may be up to 4 cm deep, ranging from 50 to 200 ml in volume and up to 300 g in weight with a mean of about 125 g. The haematomas are ovoid and disc-shaped but concave on the arachnoid surface. Some chronic haematomas are more localized and like a biconvex disc with cerebral indentation due to pressure. Correlation between haematoma size and the severity of underlying brain damage or clinical status is not good. It has been estimated that when the haematoma exceeds 50 ml there is some neurological deficit or psychiatric disturbance and when over 100 ml death is likely to be due to the subdural haemorrhage [141].

On removal of the calvarium, the exposed dura mater will be tense and the acute subdural clot imparts a bluish or black colour due to the underlying redcurrant jelly clot. The haematoma is initially soft, gelatinous, moist and being under pressure, readily detached from the dura and confined to the region of trauma. It becomes drier and firmer within a few days and more adherent to the dura mater though it may also be adherent to the underlying brain if severely contused. The underlying cerebrum will be compressed with flattening of the gyri and narrowing of sulci.

Large thick haematomas can cover much of the cerebral hemisphere and elsewhere there may be a thin coating of blood with shift of the brain and compression of the gyri and the ipsilateral ventricle.

In subacute haematomas the dura mater is tense and

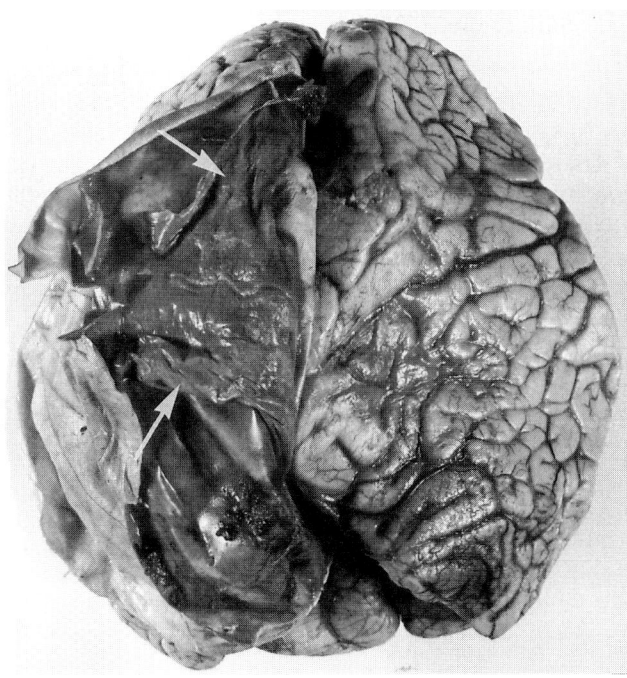

Figure 12.17 Brain dura mater from right hemisphere reflected to the left showing severe compression of the right hemisphere and discoloured inner surface of dura mater with encapsulating neomembrane (arrows) of a chronic haematoma. The rusty brown contents escaped on opening the haematoma.

brownish. The haematoma is dark brown, firm, saucer-shaped and adherent to the dura with evidence of encapsulation and organization being principally from the dura. The encapsulated chronic haematoma is firmly adherent to the dura mater and chocolate brown or even rusty in appearance with fluctuant rusty brown contents that escape on incision (Figure 12.17). The inner capsule takes about 3–4 weeks to develop. The capsule may be 1–4 mm thick, heavily pigmented and with a shiny surface facing the arachnoid, to which it may be partially adherent depending on the severity of injury and probably the degree of immobility of the brain within the skull. The pressure in the haematoma has been measured at 7 or 8 cm of water [124]. The underlying brain can be severely compressed with evidence of previous injury and haemorrhage. Calcification may occur in the capsule but ossification is rare [142]. In infants calcification or ossification may be found with asymmetry and enlargement of the skull. Such chronic changes are less likely to occur with improved ancillary aids and medical care.

Supratentorial haematomas are characteristically frontoparietal and nearer the frontal pole than the parietal. They can be quite extensive and at times may reach the floor of the anterior and middle fossae. There may be blood in the posterior fossa following a fractured skull but chronic haematomas in this site are rare.

The reason for the propensity for the frontoparietal convexity is unknown. The falx and tentorium may serve as partitions limiting spread but mid-line bleeding is more likely to result in bilateral haematomas. In adults the bleeding is bilateral in up to 30%, whereas in infants and children the incidence is higher (71%) [3] possibly because the falx cerebri is not well developed in neonates.

The haematoma undergoes organization, encapsulation and liquefaction of the contents. Histological determination of age of the haematoma is difficult because few pathologists have access to sufficient specimens for such assessment. Initially the haematoma becomes consolidated into a localized mass and as organization is from the dura mater, it is difficult to see how complete fibrotic encapsulation can occur within a few weeks as has been alleged. A mild inflammatory response can be anticipated initially and macrophages containing erythrocytes and haemosiderin will be seen within five days. Progressively the dural surface develops a neomembrane with granulation tissue, inflammatory cells, newly formed blood vessels and thickening on its inner surface with accumulation of siderophages but little evidence of lipid. Small haemorrhages may resolve without encapsulation and leave a layer of haemosiderin pigmented fibrous tissue on the inner surface of the dura.

In old haematomas the fibrous capsule becomes increasingly dense, hyaline and heavily pigmented with some round cell accumulations. The contents are liquified and vascularization is diminished but pigmentation persists for many years. The reason for late enlargement of a chronic haematoma is controversial and attributed to an osmotic effect or multiple small haemorrhages [143]. Evidence of fresh bleeding is difficult to assess. Variation in the age of the blood is not unexpected in view of the age of the victims, their frail physical and mental state and the propensity for new blood vessels to bleed on slight trauma or even with straining.

A subdural accumulation of xanthochromic or blood stained fluid (50–100 ml) without blood clots is referred to as a subdural hygroma (or hydroma). It is thought to be due to a small haemorrhage diluted by cerebrospinal fluid through an arachnoidal laceration. It appears to be related to subdural haematomas which could also be associated with such leakage at the time of injury. Their distribution and the structure of the capsule are similar to those of subdural haematomas. They occur in the posterior fossa also [145].

Bleeding is commonly believed to be due to the tearing or avulsion of poorly supported thin walled blood vessels bridging the subdural space, encountered most often in four locations:

1. lateral aspect of the frontal lobe, 1–4 cm lateral to the superior longitudinal sinus and less often over the parietal convexity;

2. the inferior surface of the temporal lobe to the tentorium and the dura of the middle cranial fossa;
3. the apex of the temporal pole to the dura over the sphenoid bone;
4. numerous aberrant subtentorial veins, involved only rarely.

There has been controversy regarding the source of bleeding as to whether it is arterial or venous in traumatic haematomas. The evidence indicates that it may stem from vein, artery or dural sinus [3]. Little is known of stresses on intracranial vessels when head injuries are sustained and these will be aggravated by cerebral atrophy which allows more movement of the brain within the skull. This increases the likelihood of damage to transdural vessels particularly veins under conditions likely to place them under stretch. With direct trauma to the brain or contrecoup injuries, artery, vein or both may bleed. The haematoma may originate from dural vessels and sinuses in tentorial tears during birth or with trauma. It is also associated with thrombotic occlusion of pial veins with massive haemorrhagic cerebral infarction and bleeding from aneurysms, arteriovenous communications, intracerebral haemorrhage and tumours. In old haematomas the source of bleeding is difficult to locate.

12.13.3 ASSOCIATED LESIONS

Since by far the commonest cause of subdural haematoma is trauma, there is likely to be other evidence of injury about the head and face in the acute and subacute phase. Fractured skull is much less frequent than with extradural haemorrhage. In fatal cases it may be over 70% whereas the incidence is much less in non-fatal cases encountered clinically especially with chronic haematomas. In fatal cases of fractured skull the incidence of subdural haematoma is about 70% and higher with comminuted fractures or those involving the vault, most dying within 24 hours. Most fractures occur on the posterior or lateral aspects of the skull and fewer involve the vault or anterior region. Haematomas are more likely to be bilateral when the skull is fractured.

Extradural bleeding may be associated with subdural haemorrhage but subarachnoid haemorrhage and cerebral contusions with or without contre coup injuries are practically the rule in acute, severe cases. Contre coup injuries are common and there may be traumatic intracerebral haemorrhage of severe degree. With the rapidly increased supratentorial pressure, secondary pontine and mid-brain haemorrhage or softening and associated pressure effects on the brain must be considered. With chronic haematomas in adults there may be thinning and even perforation of the skull [146].

Chronic subdural haematoma in infants is associated with skull enlargement and bulging of the anterior fontanelle simulating hydrocephalus with papilloedema. The calvarium may be thin and even asymmetrical due to the pressure effect of the haematoma [146]. Untreated subdural haematomas in infants in contradistinction to those in adults are often associated with hydrocephalus due to haemogenic meningitis and compression with obliteration of the subarachnoid space. Ventricular dilatation may occur with haematomas in the posterior fossa.

12.13.4 SEQUELAE

Patients may die in the acute stage from cerebral compression and associated injuries. If non-traumatic, the outcome depends on haemorrhage severity and the nature of the primary disorder. If the haemorrhage is small, spontaneous even subclinical resorption can occur. Absorption of larger quantities of blood should not be expected as:

1. the subdural space is the border zone between cerebral and systemic circulations;
2. the dura mater is comparatively avascular;
3. the arachnoid is relatively impervious;
4. little cerebrospinal fluid is absorbed from the subdural space.

Small quantities of blood can no doubt be resolved. Experimental subdural injections of blood frequently fail to produce an encapsulated haematoma. Absorption of blood must occur clinically but the conditions under which a chronic haematoma occurs are unknown. Early diagnosis and surgical evacuation are essential to avoid death or mental deterioration in subdural haematoma. Subsidence of an angiographically demonstrable subdural haematoma can occur with conservative management [147]. Patients, if they survive, may die of associated diseases or succumb to intercurrent infection or coincidental causes. Cerebral compression is the important fatal result of subdural haematoma. In the first stage, the blood displaces cerebrospinal fluid and venous blood. In the second stage the haematoma reduces the capacity of the venous drainage system and thus interferes with venous drainage causing secondary engorgement with irritative symptoms. In the third phase the intracranial pressure impairs the microcirculation leading to cerebral anaemia, most pronounced near the haematoma and causing cessation of function and paralytic symptoms in addition to general pressure effects, shifting of the brain and compression of other vascular and non-vascular structures.

Some physiological adaptation may occur in slowly enlarging lesions as with chronic haematomas, but with cerebral compression, neuronal loss and gliosis and even loss of white matter there is irreparable disabling cerebral damage and serious mental deterioration.

Even after a considerable survival time, sudden

deterioration and loss of consciousness may occur. Possibly due to some additional haemorrhage, it may also portend secondary pontine haemorrhage. The pathogenesis of the slowly progressive chronic haematoma of the aged is often associated with dementia if surgical evacuation is delayed and it often presents without a history of injury. Recurrent small haemorrhages seem to be responsible for the enlargement but the condition has not been reproduced experimentally.

12.14 Spinal subdural haematoma

This rare lesion is much less frequent than spinal extradural haemorrhage. Trauma is the usual cause and generally the haematoma is not of sufficient size to cause spinal cord compression. Acute haemorrhage may complicate bleeding states including haemophilia and spinal cord compression has followed lumbar puncture in subjects on anticoagulants. Chronic spinal haematomas are unknown.

12.15 Subarachnoid haemorrhage

The subarachnoid space is unique in that it not only surrounds the brain, spinal cord and cauda equina but contains cerebrospinal fluid that bathes all the large and even small distributing arteries and the veins whilst communicating with the ventricles and the Virchow–Robin spaces. Subarachnoid haemorrhage is not a specific disease. It merely denotes the presence of blood in the cerebrospinal fluid and clinicians must determine the source and nature of the bleeding which stems from variously:

- blood vessels within the subarachnoid space;
- parenchymal haemorrhage with blood escaping into the cerebrospinal fluid of the space directly through the cortex and dura mater or via the ventricular system;
- the choroid plexus with blood escaping via the ventricular system;
- blood within the dural space reaching the subarachnoid space through a rent in the arachnoid mater.

In reality all instances of bleeding into the space are secondary in nature, despite the prefix primary or spontaneous in reference to non-traumatic bleeding from vessels within the subarachnoid space itself. Subarachnoid haemorrhage is of two major types, traumatic and non-traumatic.

12.15.1 TRAUMATIC SUBARACHNOID HAEMORRHAGE

Trauma is the most common cause of subarachnoid haemorrhage, which is associated with a great variety of head or spinal injuries, including homicidal, suicidal, accidental, war injuries and birth injuries. It accompanies most head injuries associated with intracranial bleeding at other sites and the less severe head injuries that are a feature of the various falls and accidents consequent upon learning to sit, stand, run and play games. It is difficult to imagine any normal active child completely escaping some minor haemorrhages of this nature. For more severe haemorrhages the reader is referred to textbooks of forensic pathology and those dealing specifically with injuries to the brain and spinal cord.

12.15.2 NON-TRAUMATIC SUBARACHNOID HAEMORRHAGE

Non-traumatic subarachnoid haemorrhage is caused by a heterogeneous group of diseases but in the classification of cerebrovascular disease, primary intracerebral haemorrhage is frequently excluded even though it is usually associated with blood-stained cerebrospinal fluid. Trauma and primary intracerebral haemorrhage apart, the commonest cause is rupture of a berry aneurysm of the cerebral arteries. The history, pathology and clinical manifestations of subarachnoid and aneurysmal haemorrhage are closely interwoven and often treated almost synonymously. The causes of subarachnoid haemorrhage are multiple and clinical management depends on accurately diagnosing the disease responsible despite its now being classified as a specific entity in the International Classification of Diseases.

The peak incidence falls between 45 and 60 years and usually there is a slight predominance of females, possibly correlating with a similar incidence of cerebral aneurysms.

Some physical and emotional stress is often invoked as a precipitating factor in the onset. While such may be the case in some instances, in the Co-operative Study of Intracranial Aneurysms and Subarachnoid Haemorrhage [147], the onset in 33% of cases was during sleep. Since most people spend approximately one third of the day in sleep, this suggests the onset is a random event. Pregnancy is often invoked as a precipitating factor. The haemorrhage is usually during parturition or post partum but analysis of many cases does not suggest a significant relationship with pregnancy.

(a) **Pathology**

Analysis of large collections of cases excluding trauma and primary intracerebral haemorrhage indicates that a ruptured cerebral aneurysm is responsible for 50–70% of cases. In the past a lower incidence has often been recorded much depending on the extent and thoroughness of angiographic studies. With improving technology and diagnostic techniques the incidence of undetermined cause should progressively fall.

Bleeding is less frequent in association with bacterial or infective aneurysms but with arteritis it rarely occurs without aneurysmal dilatation. Arteriovenous shunts, haemangiomas and occlusive cerebrovascular disease including thrombosis of dural sinuses or leptomeningeal veins and secondary pontine haemorrhage are all important causes of subarachnoid haemorrhage. It rarely complicates meningitis or an abscess with secondary involvement of an artery or vein or merely infective thrombophlebitis.

Haemorrhage into or about intracranial tumours is frequent, especially glioblastoma multiforme (astrocytoma Grade IV), melanoma and choriocarcinoma, but haemorrhage has been reported in association with most types. Usually haemorrhage is into the tumour and rarely presents clinically as a subarachnoid haemorrhage.

Autoimmune and necrotizing lesions of small vessels such as in polyarteritis and systemic lupus erythematosus are infrequent causes. The latter may also be associated with haemorrhage from a berry or mycotic aneurysm.

Blood dyscrasias constitute a most important cause of subarachnoid haemorrhage and include haemophilia, aplastic or hypoplastic anaemia, leukaemia, thrombocytopenia, polycythemia rubra vera, sickle cell anaemia, splenic anaemia, pernicious anaemia, bleeding during anticoagulant therapy, hypoprothrombinaemia and Waldenström's macroglobulinaemia.

Subarachnoid haemorrhage clinically may be associated with recovery without the cause being determined. This may be attributed to the limitations of angiography in localizing small aneurysms or to some cryptic angioma or small arteriovenous shunt. However, one unexplained finding about the microaneurysms of Charcôt and Bouchard is their prevalence in the subcortical white matter of the cerebrum and their apparently silent course. Small haemorrhages occur in or near the cortex but are most infrequent although it has been suggested that they may be responsible for some subarachnoid haemorrhages of undisclosed cause [3]. Haemorrhage from subcortical microaneurysms could easily bleed into the subarachnoid space where the blood could be more readily accommodated than in the cerebral parenchyma from more deeply situated aneurysms. Lacunar infarcts would be less likely to follow thrombosis of miliary aneurysms because of the rich blood supply.

Pathologically at autopsy, the cause of fatal subarachnoid haemorrhage should be found routinely. An undetermined cause is so rare that it is usually due to inadequate examination of the arteries for aneurysms.

The distribution of blood in the non-traumatic subarachnoid haemorrhage often provides a clue to aetiology. It is important to inspect the arteries in the fresh state prior to fixation which, if prolonged, may lead to such induration of the clot as to make dissection extremely difficult. Blood anteriorly located at the base is probably due to berry aneurysms as is consistent with their localization. The haemorrhage also extends over frontal and temporal lobes. When in the posterior fossa, it is likely to be due to some posterior fossa lesion or caused by leakage from the ventricular system via the foramina of Luschka and Magendi but derives originally from an intracerebral haemorrhage. When multiple, it tends to be due to a bleeding disorder. Otherwise the blood will probably be localized close to the causative lesion.

Blood in the subarachnoid space incites a mild haemogenic meningitic reaction which may simulate meningitis with leukocytosis, pyrexia, meningismus and vomiting in association with severe headache. Some blood escapes from the subarachnoid space via the lymphatics within the first two days and thereafter the remainder is cleared by phagocytosis and organization often resulting in some residual meningeal fibrosis and pigmentation, frequent about the aneurysm. Adhesions between the sac wall and the pia mater facilitate subsequent rupture directly into brain substance and thence into the ventricular system. Meningeal fibrosis, especially if recurrent and with approximation of the pia and arachnoid due to raised intracranial pressure, can lead to hydrocephalus. Siderosis and fibrosis of arachnoid villi are said to contribute to the hydrocephalus [148].

In the process of organization and clearance of the blood clot, siderophages may be very numerous with some seen years after the original bleed. Iron encrustation of the connective tissues can at times be found especially near the aneurysm. Deposition of large quantities of iron pigment in the leptomeninges and the subpial and subependymal tissues of the brain and cord can result from repeated subarachnoid haemorrhage constituting a rare pathological entity namely, superficial siderosis of the central nervous system. This is associated with dementia, nerve deafness, cerebellar ataxia and neurological abnormalities attributed to widespread iron encrustation of the central nervous system [149]. It is seen in association with intracranial aneurysms, Sturge–Weber disease, 'venous malformations', angioma of the spinal cord and both primary (ependymoma, oligodendroglioma) and secondary tumours [3].

(b) **Associated lesions**

Albuminuria and glycosuria are frequent in patients with subarachnoid haemorrhage being attributed variously to damage to the floor of the third ventricle and increased blood sugar and dehydration of comatose patients. The mechanism is undetermined but the presence of renal disease and diabetes mellitus should be excluded.

Electrocardiographic abnormalities simulating ischaemic heart disease and even bundle-branch block may complicate cerebrovascular accidents especially subarachnoid haemorrhage. These have been attributed to physical disturbance to the circle of Willis, damage to the orbital surface of the frontal lobe, 'sympathetic storms' and anoxia. Subendocardial haemorrhages and myocytolysis have been found whilst in other cases there is no abnormality. The pathogenesis may be similar to that of neurogenic peptic ulceration in patients with stroke or brain trauma [3].

(c) **Prognosis**

Non-traumatic subarachnoid haemorrhage is a serious event and the mortality and prognosis are those of the underlying causative lesion. When no cause can be discovered, the prognosis is better but must still be guarded, there being the likelihood of an undiscovered aneurysm, neoplasm, angioma, arteriovenous shunt or a blood dyscrasia. Prolonged follow-up and a more intensive search for the underlying lesion are indicated.

The prognosis for aneurysmal subarachnoid haemorrhage has been recently given such that 50% die after a clip is placed on the aneurysm with half the survivors remaining severely disabled [150].

12.16 Spinal subarachnoid haemorrhage

Subarachnoid haemorrhage, originating in the spinal cord, is most often due to trauma both in the neonate and in postnatal life. In the neonate it is associated with injuries to the spinal cord and brain stem, and possibly occurs in association with spinal extradural or subdural haemorrhage. It can be due to traction injury.

Subarachnoid haemorrhage is very likely to be one of the manifestations of serious injuries to the back and spinal cord in childhood and adult life. The injury is usually a major feature of the presenting history and iatrogenic haemorrhage from lumbar puncture has been responsible for paraplegia. Serious bleeding from this procedure is rare [3].

Since arteries supplying the spinal cord are quite small, degenerative lesions are much less frequent than intracranially. Aneurysms are also infrequent unless associated with coarctation or an arteriovenous shunt in which case the vessels will be much enlarged, participating in collateral or augmented flow and subject to severe degenerative changes. Bacterial aneurysms could, of course, involve spinal arteries.

Arteriovenous communications, hemangiomas and telangiectases may cause spinal subarachnoid haemorrhage but in the differential diagnosis blood dyscrasias and neoplasms must not be forgotten.

Spinal subarachnoid haemorrhage is of little consequence such as that occurring usually with lumbar puncture. However, blood in the subarachnoid space can cause haemogenic meningitis with symptoms more related to the back and legs if dorsal root irritation occurs. The bleeding is more likely to be multifocal if due to blood dyscrasias except in the case of haemophilia. A localized haematoma associated with clotting can cause spinal cord compression with paraplegia. The bleeding is rarely fatal.

12.17 Intracerebral haemorrhage

Haemorrhage into brain parenchyma is best dealt with according to its cause.

12.17.1 PRIMARY INTRACEREBRAL HAEMORRHAGE

Primary intracerebral haemorrhage is a term used to indicate significant haemorrhage into the parenchyma of the encephalon and not just the cerebrum. It is nowadays considered to be due to haemorrhage from miliary or microaneurysms of Charcôt and Bouchard, and is in that sense secondary. The term primary cerebral haemorrhage has persisted since the days when it was considered to be primary, spontaneous or of unknown aetiology. It is sometimes referred to as apoplectic or hypertensive haemorrhage but primary intracerebral haemorrhage is preferable until a more appropriate designation is agreed upon. The term apoplexy is an old term and best avoided as it is sometimes also used for massive haemorrhage in extracranial sites.

Over the years primary intracerebral haemorrhage has been a common cause of death in Western countries and in 1969 Kurtzke [2] estimated it constituted approximately 16% of all cerebrovascular deaths. In 1986 the incidence was given as 4% [151] and subarachnoid haemorrhage estimated as 10%. A common cause of death in autopsy rooms of general hospitals in the 1950s, it can no longer be so regarded. Reduced prevalence has been attributed to the widespread use of antihypertensive therapy.

The mortality rates for cerebrovascular disease and its subcategories are unreliable [6] as indicated but the reduced incidence in the community is generally accepted.

The familial incidence of primary intracerebral haemorrhage is in all probability due to the familial occurrence of hypertension with which it has a strong association. It usually has a peak incidence and mean age in the sixth decade, most cases occurring between 40 and 75 years of age. Nevertheless 8.6% occur under 40 years of age. Figures of age distribution in the literature are not necessarily valid as they may also include instances of secondary haemorrhage. The diagnosis of primary intracerebral haemorrhage in the young should only be made after thorough exclusion of secondary causes. In the elderly, especially in those with senile dementia and an absence of hypertension, cerebral amyloid angiopathy should be considered and has given further credence to a familial occurrence of cerebral haemorrhage.

Hospital series usually include more males than females although there is probably little difference in the sex incidence.

It has been maintained that this disorder is particularly prone to occur in the John Bull type of individual but correlation of body types with specific cerebrovascular diseases is not a popular avenue of investigation and must take into account the diagnostic accuracy or inaccuracies of subtypes [6]. There are variations in incidence of this disorder on ethnic, geographical and sociological grounds but such data should be treated with considerable caution. In the USA differences between Caucasians and Negroes and the higher incidence amongst Negroes have been attributed to the greater prevalence of hypertension. The high incidence in Japan has been attributed to the high salt intake and associated hypertension but there is evidence that this is at least in part spurious because the condition is overdiagnosed [2,3]. Such inaccuracies highlight the need for improvement in the quality of epidemiological data and for an improved autopsy rate.

The extreme rarity of primary intracerebral haemorrhage in lower animals is of aetiological interest and correlates with the lower severity of degenerative vascular disease in most other animals.

(a) Pathology

Statistics on the pathological features of primary intracerebral haemorrhage are confusing and their interpretation is difficult because some series include secondary haemorrhages and exclude others on the basis of size. The diagnosis has come to be associated pathologically with a haemorrhage of considerable or massive proportions with the exclusion of small lesions. This aspect may account for differences in survival in clinical studies.

Small haemorrhages up to 2 or 3 cm in diameter occur almost anywhere within the brain evincing a predilection for the grey matter or the subcortical white matter. They are round or oval and circumscribed without surrounding punctate or satellite haemorrhage. Such small lesions allow recovery and healing and haemosiderin-laden macrophages (siderophages) may be present for years after. Most reports on primary intracerebral haemorrhage exclude such lesions but many may have been due to cerebral amyloid angiopathy. Of the large haemorrhages seen at autopsy,

approximately 79% occur in the cerebrum, 14% in the pons and 7% in the cerebellum.

Cerebrum

The haemorrhage occurs most often in the basal ganglia, thalamus and internal capsule. On removal of calvarium the dura mater is tense and on opening the dura mater, the cerebrum is under considerable tension with flattened gyri and shallow sulci especially over the affected side. The usual signs of raised supratentorial pressure will be obvious. Subarachnoid haemorrhage, when present, is usually mild and in the posterior fossa due to leakage of blood from the fourth ventricle. The cerebrum on the affected side is often fluctuant and visibly enlarged with compression of the contralateral hemisphere and shift of the midline.

The haematoma is a mass of recently coagulated blood (Figure 12.18) which can be readily removed from a ragged walled cavity up to 10 cm or more in diameter. There may be a few fragments of cerebral tissue or debris in the clot and the brain has the appearance of being pushed aside by the expanding haematoma, i.e. a fibre-splitting haemorrhage. Small punctate haemorrhages are present in the surrounding brain tissue. The haemorrhage commonly ruptures into

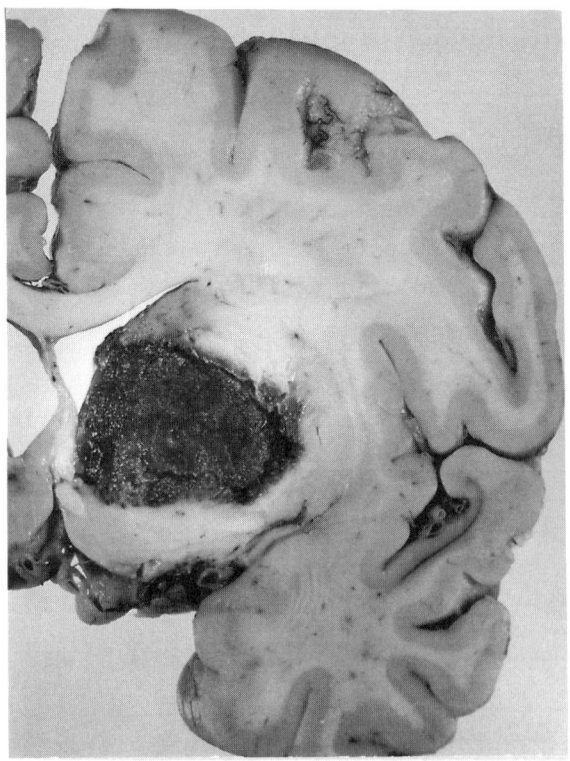

Figure 12.18 Primary intracerebral haemorrhage in the basal ganglia and internal capsule. Note proximity to the lateral ventricle.

the ventricular system which is likely to be filled with clotted blood. Infrequently rupture is through the covering cortex to produce some parietal subarachnoid haemorrhage.

The most frequent site is in the region of the basal ganglia and thalamus. These have been divided into medial and lateral ganglionic haemorrhages with the dividing line passing anteroposteriorly between the putamen laterally and the globus pallidus medially. Lateral haemorrhage occurs in the external capsule, putamen and claustrum and commonly rupture is into the ventricular system. Small haemorrhages here need not be fatal. One of the large vessels of the lateral lenticulostriate arteries coursing near the outer part of the putamen has been designated as the 'artery of cerebral haemorrhage' because of its frequent involvement.

Medial ganglionic haemorrhages involve the globus pallidus, corpus striatum and thalamus and are almost invariably fatal because only recent haemorrhages are found. Other subclassifications have been suggested but most authors only indicate the localization in general terms. The commonest site of haemorrhage varies with the author, there being difficulty in determining the origin of bleeding.

Old haemorrhages exhibit a capsule due to organization with progressive change in colour of the blood clot from 'redcurrant jelly' to rusty brown. Between the capsule of a very old haematoma, there is a thin zone of diminished consistency suggestive of a plane of cleavage. With small haemorrhages that are quite old, cause is difficult to determine. Haemorrhages of all sizes have been included in some series, giving rise to the allegation that the high mortality of this type of haemorrhage has been exaggerated.

As explained haemorrhages associated with cerebral amyloid angiopathy were included in past statistics. Their incidence has increased due to aging of Western populations and increased longevity and their relative frequency and importance will be increased because of the reduction of primary intracerebral haemorrhage due to widespread use of antihypertensive therapy. Now that they have been recognized and distinguished from haemorrhages due to Charcôt-Bouchard aneurysms, they should be separated as a distinct category.

From 7 to 32.3% of all primary intracerebral haemorrhages occur in the frontal, parietal, occipital or temporal lobes. The most frequent site varies with the author and again the validity of the figures depends on the quality of the autopsy. Haematomas in the central substance of the white matter vary considerably in size and usually lie close to cortical grey matter. Not as lethal as those involving the basal ganglia, they should not be diagnosed until secondary haemorrhages have been excluded. It is likely that not all of these are truly primary intracerebral haemorrhages. Some could be of aneurysmal origin since aneurysms are and have been frequently overlooked at autopsy or not sought assiduously. Table 10.2 may be of assistance in distinguishing between these two types of haemorrhage.

Primary pontine haemorrhage

Primary pontine haemorrhage (Figure 12.19) is thought to be more frequent than cerebellar haemorrhage with the average age of onset slightly less than for haemorrhage elsewhere. Primary pontine haemorrhage is usually considered to constitute about 10 to 16% of all primary haemorrhages. The presence of hypertension is the general rule, pontine haemorrhage being particularly likely with malignant hypertension. Goto et al. [152] classified these haemorrhages as tegmental and tegmentobasilar according to their location, volume and symptomatology deeming them to be clinically distinct.

Pontine haemorrhage tends to commence near the mid-level of the pons close to the junction of the basis pontis and the tegmentum and to be symmetrically placed and up to 5 cm in diameter. It may extend into

Table 12.2 Differentiation between aneurysmal and primary intracerebral haemorrhage in miscellaneous sites in the cerebrum.

Site of haemorrhage	Aneurysmal haemorrhage	Primary hypertensive intracerebral haemorrhage
Frontal and temporal lobes	Common	Infrequent
Parietal lobe and corona radiata	Uncommon	Frequent
Occipital lobe	Rare	Rare
External capsule	Frequent	Particularly common
Isolated haemorrhages in the thalamus or caudate nucleus	Nil	Characteristically
Caval, callosal and bilateral frontal	Most likely	Most unlikely

* Cerebral haemorrhage associated with cerebral amyloid angiopathy is not included and is grouped with secondary causes.

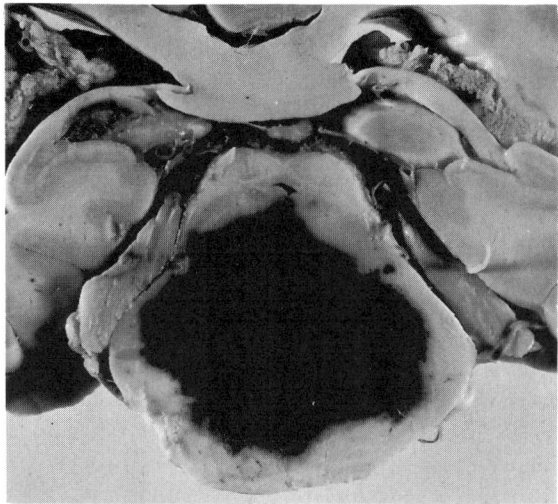

Figure 12.19 Large recent primary pontine haemorrhage. (Reproduced from Stehbens [3].)

the cerebral peduncles as far as the hypothalamus or even the thalamus and into the middle cerebellar peduncles for a short distance. It rarely ever extends into the medulla oblongata. If the haemorrhage is of moderate size, the pons may appear soft and fluctuant. Rupture is hardly ever directly into the subarachnoid space but more frequently into the fourth ventricle, the blood then escaping into the subarachnoid space of the posterior fossa.

The haemorrhage tends to run a rapid course and signs of raised intracranial pressure effects on the brain are not prominent. Primary haemorrhage into the midbrain without extension into the pons is unusual. Likewise haemorrhage into the medulla oblongata is rare and more likely to be secondary to an arteriovenous or angiomatous lesion or due to anticoagulant therapy.

Cerebellar haemorrhage

Primary cerebellar haemorrhage is the commonest cause of non-traumatic intracerebellar haemorrhage. Its frequency varies in different reports depending to some extent on the inclusion of secondary bleeding. The haematoma varies in size up to about 5 cm and usually originates in the region of the dentate nucleus on one or other side and less often in the vermis. It has been suggested that left-sided haemorrhages preponderate but to establish this a large series would be required with complete exclusion of secondary haemorrhages. The haematoma may extend into the cerebellar peduncle and occasionally into the brain stem. The blood reaches the subarachnoid space directly more often than intracerebral haemorrhage, and rupture into the fourth ventricle is less common. The haematoma may produce distortion and compression of the cerebellum and

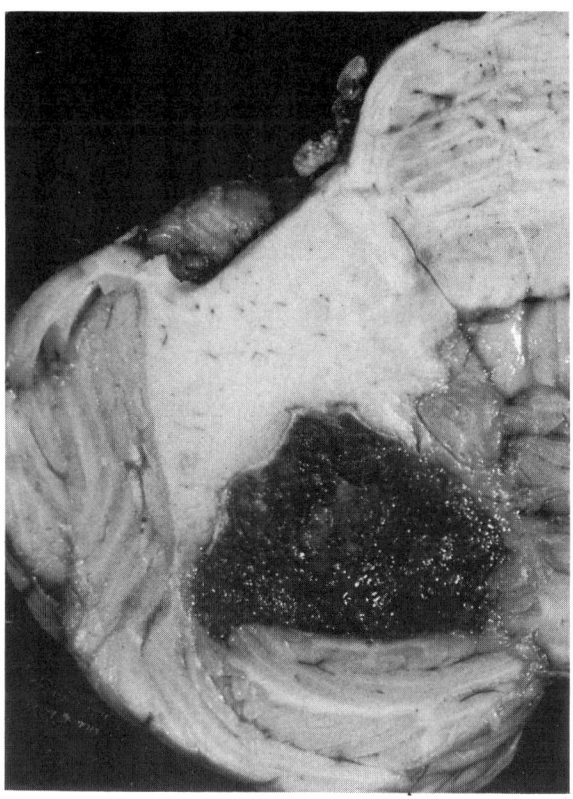

Figure 12.20 An old haematoma of the cerebellum. The contents were rust-coloured. Note the fibrous capsule surrounding the haematoma and the cleft between the capsule and white matter. (Reproduced from Stehbens [3].)

brainstem and at times transtentorial herniation of the cerebellum. The aqueduct may be occluded producing acute hydrocephalus. These events usually run a rapid course but, with the production of an encapsulated rusty brown haematoma, survival is a possibility (Figure 12.20).

Associated lesions

The frequency of extension of primary cerebral haemorrhage into the ventricular system depends on the size, location and proximity to the ventricular system but intraventricular rupture is commoner by far than direct extension into the subarachnoid space except in cerebellar haemorrhages. This results in blood stained or frank blood clot in the ventricles and blood reaching the subarachnoid space via the fourth ventricle. It is therefore usually most prominent in the posterior fossa.

Secondary pontine haemorrhage may occur and in the past was probably often precipitated by diagnostic lumbar punctures which were routine before the hazard of this procedure was recognized. Secondary pressure effects other than secondary brain-stem haemorrhage may also occur particularly with large intracerebral haematomas and considerable shift and herniation of the cerebrum.

Subdural haematoma is not a frequent association but occurs more often with cerebellar haemorrhage by direct extension. The possibility of traumatic origin of the subdural bleeding together with other signs of trauma occasioned by falling at the time of the stroke must always be taken into account. It is rare for such bleeding to be of significant degree.

In view of the frequency of hypertension in primary cerebral haemorrhage other small haemorrhages or lacunar softenings related to miliary aneurysms elsewhere may be found and also lesions secondary to severe atherosclerosis of arteries feeding the brain. The occurrence of aneurysms of the large cerebral arteries in association with hypertension and primary intracerebral haemorrhage is not unknown and can arise in subjects with polycystic renal disease.

Specific variations of the circle of Willis are not known to be associated with primary intracerebral haemorrhage or its location, although Fisher [65] believes that thalamic haemorrhages are more likely when the posterior cerebral arteries are supplied primarily from the internal carotid arteries. Consistent with this view Yates and Hutchinson [153] contend that stenotic or occlusive lesions of the large extracranial arteries to the brain may protect against primary intracerebral haemorrhage. This is a likely and plausible phenomenon.

By virtue of the close association with hypertension, primary intracerebral haemorrhage may occur with all disorders causing secondary hypertension and also the ill-effects of a long-standing hypertension. Hypertension of whatever cause predisposes to this type of haemorrhage and the higher the blood pressure the greater is the propensity. Russell [154] found pontine haemorrhage preponderated in subjects with the severe grades of hypertension and a significantly greater heart weight has been reported in subjects with hind-brain haemorrhage [155].

Microscopy

Histologically the haematoma is merely clotted blood in which a few remnants of brain tissue are embedded. The brain at the edge of the haematoma exhibits necrosis, oedema and multiple extravasations of blood, some of which are perivascular. The walls of small blood vessels may be necrotic and infiltrated with fibrin and red cells but such changes are not common. Evidence of long-standing hypertension may be observed in the small arteries such as arteriolosclerosis and diffuse hyperplastic sclerosis. Many blocks must be examined before some of the degenerative changes associated with this type of haemorrhage can be found and other possible causes of the haemorrhage excluded. Much diligence is required to find the small arteries with irregularly

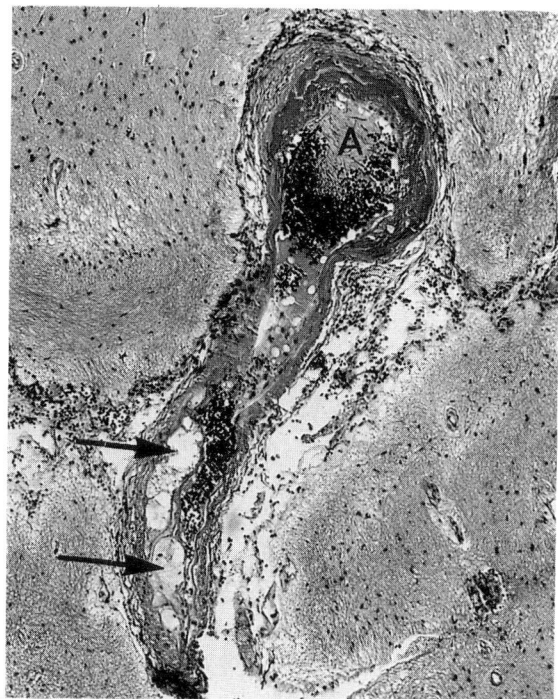

Figure 12.21 Miliary aneurysm (A) in the superficial layer of the cortex is lined with fibrin and arises from a severely atherosclerotic vessel with foam cells (arrows) in the wall. Such vascular changes are usually referred to as lipohyalinosis. There are a few round cells about the aneurysm. (Haematoxylin and eosin.) (Reproduced from Stehbens [3].)

thickened hyaline acellular walls. The wall may stain for lipid or there may be a few lipophages in paraffin sections (the so-called lipohyalinosis) (Figure 12.21). At times distinct aneurysmal enlargement of vessels will be observed, possibly with evidence of previous haemorrhage or even thrombotic occlusion. Finding the actual aneurysm responsible is almost impossible as many vessels may be torn or damaged secondarily to the haemorrhage.

If the patient survives for any length of time, the reaction to the haematoma and damage will be more advanced with oedema, leucocytic invasion and microglial infiltration progressing to organization and fibrous encapsulation surrounded by gliosis (Figure 12.20). Siderophages, haematoidin and lipid accumulation are prominent. Small haematomas shrink to a slit-like, rust-coloured cavity. Cholesterol crystals are observed within the degenerate cellular debris of long-standing incompletely organized haematomas. Iron encrustation of the connective tissue in the capsule and calcification are found in old haematomas. There is often perivascular lymphocytic infiltration, sometimes in association with fat or haemosiderin-laden macrophages in the pericapsular gliotic zone.

(b) Mortality

The prognosis of a massive primary intracerebral haemorrhage of the classical type is grim and death is usual within one to two days. Most subjects die within a week. There is a better prognosis for smaller haemorrhages although, as indicated, cerebellar and pontine haemorrhages run a relatively short course. The prognosis therefore is dependent on size and location of the haematoma. The better prognosis of these haemorrhages may be due to the smaller size or inclusion of cases due to amyloid angiopathy.

(c) Aetiology

Because of the frequent presence of premonitory symptoms it was once thought that this disorder was basically haemorrhagic infarction, a contention with which the appearance of the haematoma is inconsistent. The concept of prehaemorrhagic softening was popular for many years. Softening allegedly reduced tissue support resulting in haemorrhage into the softened parenchyma through necrotic blood vessel walls. However, the haematoma does not have the appearance of confluent multiple haemorrhages from small vessels even though capillary fragility is said to be increased in hypertension [156]. The rapidity of onset of the stroke suggests that the bleeding is arterial particularly since the haemorrhage appears to be fibre-splitting rather than a diffuse infiltration of brain parenchyma as with venous infarction.

Cerebral vessels are difficult to rupture even with pressures as high as 1520 mmHg [157]. Such abnormal pressures are not encountered under physiological conditions and post-mortem experimental evidence is always open to indefensible criticism. Nevertheless, this evidence suggests that blood vessels are weakened with age, a state accentuated by hypertension. The occurrence of this type of apoplectic haemorrhage primarily in the brain may well be explained by the thin walls and architectural differences seen in cerebral arteries. In any case there is need for investigation of vascular physical properties including tensile strength of intracranial blood vessels.

Feigin and Prose [158] observed fibrin infiltration of the walls of small intracerebral arteries. Relating it to the intracerebral haemorrhage, they considered it fibrinoid arteritis. Perivascular haemorrhage consists of multiple eccentric layers of fibrin and blood cells in the perivascular space about the blood vessel and they have been observed in this type of haemorrhage and are likely to be consequences of the haemorrhage. Rupture may be associated with some dissection of the wall and false aneurysm formation [3].

Miliary aneurysms of Charcôt and Bouchard are small, saccular, fusiform or irregular dilatations

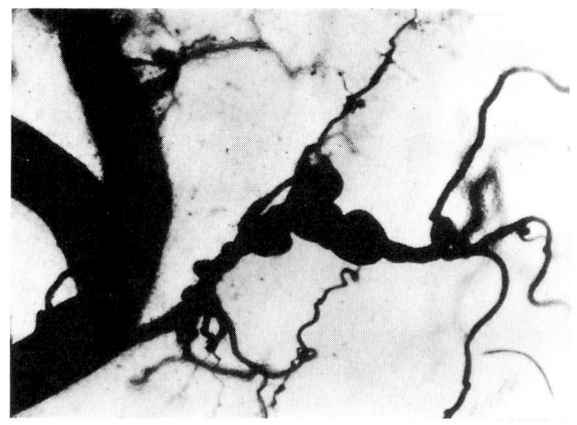

Figure 12.22 Cleared specimens prepared after post-mortem angiography displaying microaneurysms on intracerebral vessels. (Reproduced with permission from Russell [160].)

(0.2–2 mm in diameter) on the intracerebral vessels (Figure 12.21) [159]. They occur most often in the thalamus and corpora striata, with diminishing frequency in the pons, cerebral cortex, claustrum, cerebellum, cerebellar peduncles and least often in the centrum ovale. Charcôt and Bouchard popularized the thesis that they caused cerebral haemorrhage but early this century the aneurysms were considered to be false aneurysms and the effect rather than the cause. Russell [160,161] rekindled interest in these aneurysms and together with the detailed studies of Cole and Yates [162,163] established that these aneurysms were the origin of the haemorrhage. They arise sometimes at branching sites and are frequently multiple on a single vessel (Figure 12.22). For the most part confined to arteries below 250 µm, they also occur on lenticulostriate arteries with a diameter of 0.5 mm.

In a study of 200 brains [162,163], 100 from normotensive subjects and 100 from hypertensives, 46 hypertensive brains had miliary or microaneurysms but only seven normotensive brains had aneurysms. The frequency increased with age, the seven normotensive individuals all being elderly. Aneurysms were also found in 86% of hypertensive subjects with primary intracerebral haemorrhage and in 35% of hypertensive brains without haemorrhage. Aneurysmal distribution roughly corresponded with the distribution of haemorrhage into the cerebrum, pons and cerebellum except for the unexplained prevalence in the subcortical white matter of the cerebrum [3].

The fibrin infiltration of the arterial wall associated with primary intracerebral haemorrhage by Feigin and Prose [158] may be a secondary effect of the haemorrhage or may result in haemorrhage. It is not possible to attribute the haematomas to the miliary aneurysms alone and other vascular lesions could be responsible. At the present time, these aneurysms are the most likely cause. Direct rupture of the small vessels is a possibility but usually aneurysms precede this event in larger arteries much depending on the severity and rapidity of onset of the underlying arterial disease. This appears to be arteriosclerosis or diffuse hyperplastic sclerosis with degenerative changes in the arterial wall, hyalinization, loss of muscle and elastic tissue and lipid accumulation. At times lipophages are prominent with the changes sometimes being referred to as lipohyalinosis of the wall (Figure 12.21). The inner surface may be covered by thrombus with a variable degree of infiltration of the wall with fibrin, red cells and leucocytes. There may be mild round cell infiltration of the adventitia and surrounding tissue (Figure 12.21), and some siderophages indicating previous leakage and perianeurysmal gliosis (Figure 12.23). The perivascular space may be absent. Often a section through the aneurysm is mistaken for an unusually large arteriosclerotic artery and serial histological sections will be required to prove the nature of the aneurysmal dilatation. Alternatively the dilatation seen in longitudinal sections and the evidence of bleeding are highly suggestive. Attention has been drawn to the similarity of the degenerative changes in the arteries and miliary aneurysms to those of atherosclerosis [3,105].

Miliary aneurysms may leak or bleed profusely. In the case of a leakage, mural thrombus will develop on the luminal surface possibly lining the whole sac. In view of the small sac size, occlusive thrombosis is more likely than in large vessels following breach of the wall and haemorrhage [3]. This being the case, haemorrhage is prevented but a small lacunar softening with a variable amount of haemosiderin staining is likely to result. An organized thrombosed miliary aneurysm (Figure 12.23) may often be found in the vicinity of a lacunar softening.

Fisher [164] classified miliary aneurysms into three types:

- saccular aneurysms often at forks and measuring 300–1100 μm, with the parent vessel usually less than 150 μm in diameter;
- asymmetrical fusiform aneurysms;
- lipohyalinotic aneurysms associated with 'fibrinoid', arteritis and atherosclerotic changes.

The presence of fibrin, a few leucocytes and round cell infiltration does not make the aneurysms inflammatory. Charcôt and Bouchard originally believed the vascular changes were due to an arteritis, but atherosclerosis or arteriosclerosis was also considered inflammatory in the last century.

Rosenblum [165] discussed the presence of fibrin infiltration of the walls of miliary aneurysms and whether it is a primary change. The controversy centres around the term fibrinoid necrosis, which in reality signifies fibrin infiltration of the vessel wall due to its disruption which is usually mechanical as in malignant hypertension and aneurysmal rupture. In miliary aneurysms when the wall has yielded with or without leakage, fibrin infiltration of the wall ensues. Fibrinoid necrosis is not a cause of aneurysm formation nor of rupture but the consequence of incipient or previous leakage.

Challa et al. [166] consider aneurysms of Charcôt and Bouchard to be rarer than previously alleged and that in three-dimensional studies arterioles exhibit twists and coils that can be mistaken for miliary aneurysms when studied by pressure infusion as performed in previous studies. They concluded that cerebral haemorrhage has little to do with these in their view rare miliary aneurysms. However, miliary aneurysms exist and they can bleed and produce lacunar infarcts. Histological sections are not consistent with tortuosities. The finding of coils and tortuosities in the microcirculation is of considerable interest and the finding of relatively few Charcôt–Bouchard aneurysms in hypertensives may be due to antihypertensive therapy. Serial histological sections could also reveal whether or not a miliary aneurysm is authentic or merely a tortuosity.

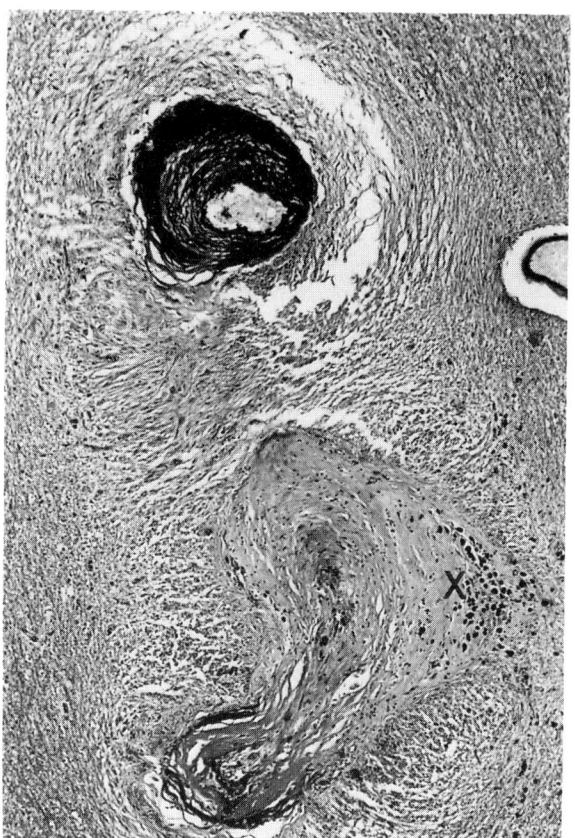

Figure 12.23 Two miliary aneurysms. The upper aneurysm contains much mural thrombus (fibrin appears black) with a small lumen possibly due to the plane of section. The lower aneurysm appears to have leaked, thrombosed and undergone organization. Siderophages present at X. (Phosphotungstic acid haematoxylin.)

The predisposition of the human brain to primary intracerebral haemorrhage and miliary aneurysms seems to be associated with the peculiarly thin walls of intracranial blood vessels, the propensity in humans to longevity, and the high incidence of prolonged hypertension and severe atherosclerosis to which the degenerative changes in intracerebral arteries are related. Unexplained and unexplored aspects are:

1. 30% of all miliary aneurysms occur in the cerebral subcortical white matter;
2. the apparent absence of such haemorrhage and miliary aneurysms in the medulla oblongata and spinal cord;
3. the prevalence of miliary aneurysms in Japanese in whom cerebral haemorrhage has been alleged to be unusually common;
4. the effect of antihypertensive therapy on existing miliary aneurysms;
5. the prevalence of miliary aneurysms in young hypertensive subjects.

12.17.2 SECONDARY INTRACEREBRAL HAEMORRHAGE

(a) Traumatic intracerebral haemorrhage

Few realize just how delicate and susceptible to injury blood vessels and endothelium are. The extent is readily seen in rabbit ear chambers subjected to very mild injury. The mildest injury precipitates thromboembolic phenomena in the microcirculation and possibly extensive stasis. The large human brain lying with little supportive connective tissue in a skull with an irregular inner surface and containing sharp-edged fibrous septa is probably contused more often than we wish to believe. It is difficult to conceive of even moderate or significant trauma to the head without some cerebral contusion and haemorrhage.

Penetrating injuries will be encountered in forensic pathology to which the reader is referred. Accidental penetrating injuries from tools and sharp objects can also cause grievous injuries with severe haemorrhage and possibly secondary infection.

Intracerebral haematomas, less common than extradural or subdural haematomas in closed head injuries, are often found under skull fractures and with other types of injury. Intracerebral haematomas without cortical contusions constitute an important though infrequent group, sometimes appearing clinically after a lucid interval. They are present in about 15% of fatal injuries, being single or multiple and occurring most often in the subfrontal and temporal regions [121]. The cerebellum is affected less frequently. Frontal haematomas are due to a blow over the occiput and rarely frontal blows, whilst temporal haematomas are due to a lateral blow to the same side of the head [167]. Mortality rates do not correlate well with haematoma site and in a study of 63 cases, approximately 40% came under hospital care within 48 hours and 10% later than two weeks. There is concern over the authenticity of a traumatic aetiology with a prolonged delay [63] and such cases must be considered individually.

Basal ganglia haematomas are deep and intracerebral and involve the corpus striatum, the globus pallidum or the thalamus. Usually the associated contusions are severe and associated with road traffic accidents. The physical principles involved in this type of haematoma are obscure [121] but almost certainly are due to shearing stresses caused by rapid acceleration and deceleration.

The delayed appearance of traumatic intracerebral haematomas is more common than previously thought and can be recognized by the use of sequential computerized tomography. These late or spät haematomas are said to be associated with a vascular injury at the time of the initial trauma with local factors (tissue pressure, vasoconstriction, thrombogenic factors, thrombosis) minimizing or preventing acute bleeding. After an interval a reduction in tissue pressure and possibly thrombolytic activity results in resumption of bleeding perhaps also through damaged capillaries [168].

The reader is referred to neuropathology texts for full discussion on the various types of traumatic haemorrhagic brain lesions including contusion, lacerations, contre coup injuries, pituitary lesions and haemorrhages in infants and newborns.

(b) Secondary non-traumatic intracerebral haemorrhages

Secondary brain stem haemorrhage

This type of haemorrhage was first described in 1911 by Attwater [169], who reported concomitant haemorrhage into the pons and mid-brain in subjects with haemorrhage into the basal ganglia particularly in the presence of extension into the ventricular system. Subsequently found to occur with any lesion causing rapidly rising supratentorial pressure, it may complicate acute extradural, subdural and subarachnoid haemorrhages, ruptured aneurysms and arteriovenous aneurysms, acute haemocephalus, massive encephalomalacia and tumours with haemorrhage. Less frequently it occurs with posterior cranial fossa lesions causing gross displacement and deformity of the pons.

Haemorrhage in the brain stem tends to be rostral and multiple, many extravasations often coalescing. In the mid-brain the haemorrhages are usually in the tegmentum about the aqueduct. An elongated mid-line haemorrhage extending anteroposteriorly in the mid-

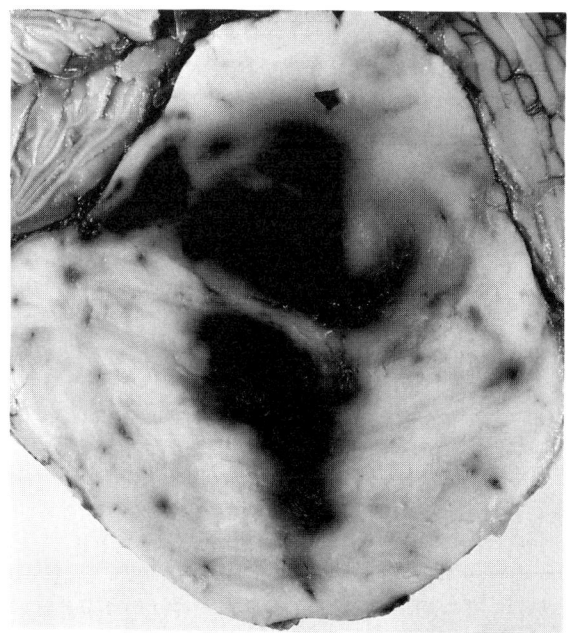

Figure 12.24 Secondary pontine haemorrhage mainly in the mid-line with some lateral spread and an appearance of confluent haemorrhages. (Reproduced from Stehbens [3].)

brain and pons (Figure 12.24) commences as multiple splinter haemorrhages about the long perforating arteries in the mid-line but can involve those more laterally placed. These haemorrhages can become confluent and be asymmetrical or extensive and involve most of the pons simulating a primary pontine haematoma. The haemorrhage usually does not extend above the tentorium and is seldom continuous with a primary supratentorial intracerebral haemorrhage. It is not known why these secondary pontine haemorrhages do not extend into the medulla. Some oedema and necrosis may accompany the haemorrhage. Survival is infrequent and accompanied by a pigmented cystic lesion in the necrotic area and a variable degree of incapacitation. Increase in differential pressure between that above and that below the tentorium such as occurs with lumbar punctures or jugular vein compression may increase the herniation and precipitate the haemorrhage.

When it was realized that these secondary haemorrhages, which occur predominantly in the pons, were associated with supratentorial rather than infratentorial lesions, Dill and Isenhour [170] produced experimentally in dogs pontine haemorrhage with a supratentorial expanding mass. Many theories attempted to account for the secondary haemorrhage. The most likely mechanism was explained by Dott and Blackwood [128,171] as follows. The upper end of the basilar artery is anchored to the tentorial edge by the posterior cerebral arteries and thereby to the circle of Willis. Downward displacement of the brain stem in transtentorial herniation causes lengthening and angulation of the penetrating branches of the basilar artery. Infarction or haemorrhage thus result from vasospasm or tearing of the branches. This analysis was supported by the important experimental work on cadavers by Johnson and Yates [128]. Downward displacement of the brain stem unduly elongates the penetrating arteries because the posterior part of the brain stem is thrust down further than the anterior portion. The result may be vasospasm or even tearing of the arteries and leakage of the injection medium when post-mortem angiography is performed on brains with secondary pontine haemorrhage (Figure 12.25). The dye, flowing back and alongside the vessels, mixes with blood extravasated ante mortem. Arterial lesions have also been observed in the anterior lobe of the cerebellum, the vascular supply of which is likewise derived from the long attenuated branches arising from the superior cerebellar arteries and subjected to considerable stress in tentorial herniation. Arteries are preferentially damaged rather than veins which are naturally more tortuous permitting considerable stretch when the brain is distorted. Johnson and Yates [128] also demonstrated that application of lateral pressure to the upper pons and midbrain during injection brought about extravasation of injection medium simulating brain-stem haemorrhage. Application of lateral pressure to the mid-brain during the injection induced extravasations of dye from torn vessels simulating actual haemorrhages restricted to this region (Figure 12.26). They believed that lateral pressure by temporo-occipital lobe herniation could flatten the mid-brain and upper pons sufficiently to increase the anteroposterior diameter by at least 1 cm. Lateral pressure alone was thought sufficient to cause arterial bleeding in some cases and in others to intensify the effects of the downward displacement. During secondary pontine haemorrhage there is disruption of vessels with periarterial haemorrhage and expansion of the adventitia and perivascular pia mater.

The development of secondary mid-brain or pontine haemorrhage in a subject with a serious supratentorial lesion is likely to be rapidly fatal and no doubt the demise of seriously ill patients was often hastened by a lumbar puncture. Rapid decompression may help survival but cannot repair existing damage. This type of haemorrhage must have been substantially diminished with greater awareness of the danger of lumbar puncture in subjects with raised intracranial pressure.

Cerebral amyloid angiopathy (congophilic angiopathy)

Amyloidosis has long been recognized as occurring infrequently in the brain and is mostly restricted to pial vessels and also advanced atherosclerotic arteries. Interest developed in amyloid deposits in cerebral blood vessels after 1972 when Gadmundsson et al. [172] drew attention to a peculiarly high frequency of cerebral

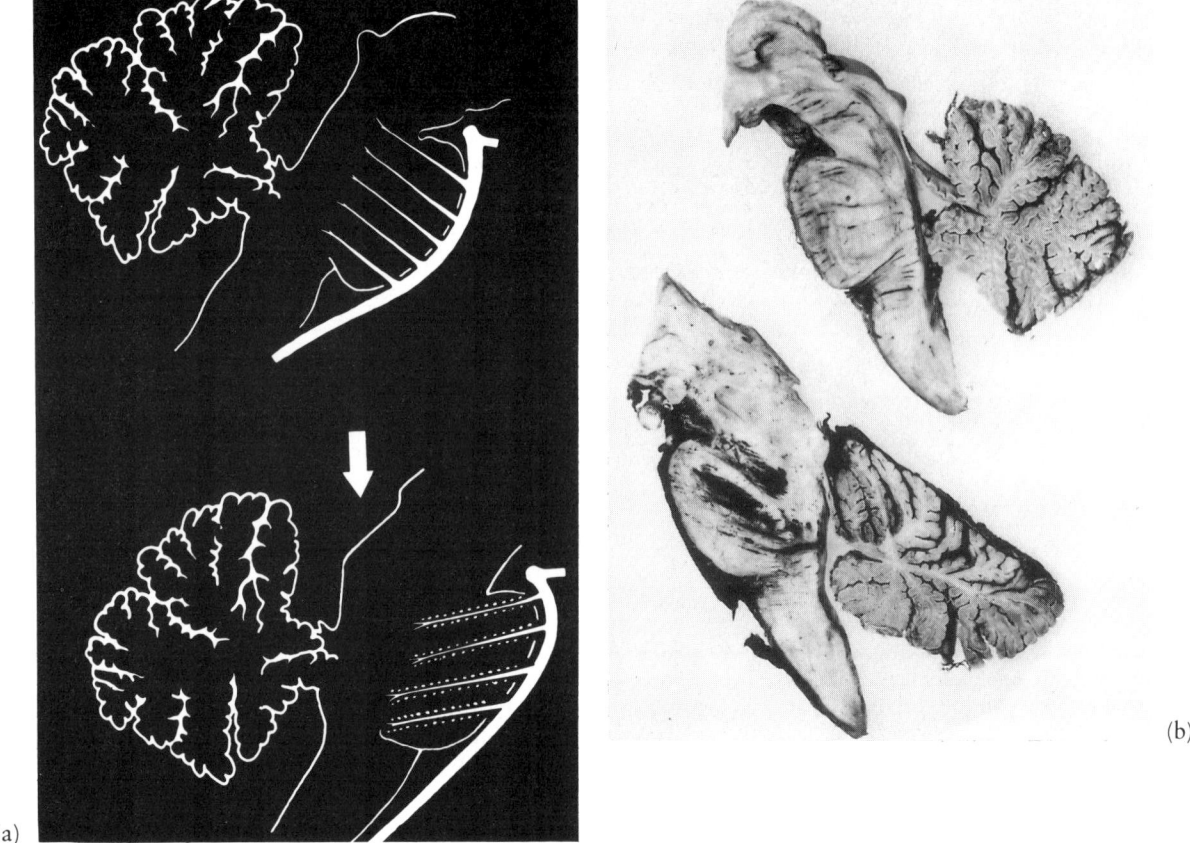

Figure 12.25 (a) Diagram to explain the elongation and downward displacement of the long penetrating pontine arteries from the basilar artery, their normal anatomy above and the distortion due to the downward pressure (arrow) below. (b) Corresponding photographs showing normal anatomy above and extravasation of dye in the pons post mortem (below) due to downward pressure on the pons with pontine distortion. (Reproduced with permission from Johnson and Yates [128].)

haemorrhage in a single family. It was considered the haemorrhages resulted from amyloid angiopathy. In all some 84 family members were thought to have died from cerebral haemorrhage attributable to amyloid angiopathy, 59% being under 40 years of age. The youngest was 15 years. Only one subject had tuberculosis and the syndrome appeared to have been transmitted by an autosomal dominant trait. Whilst amyloidosis of cerebral blood vessels has been associated with senile plaques and familial presenile dementia, in which only the smallest arteries are affected, the familial cases were associated with atherosclerosis of arteries larger than arterioles and in the absence of senile plaques or obvious signs of dementia. The absence of hypertension was noted and the haemorrhage attributed to amyloid-induced mural weakness of arterioles and small arteries.

Eleven patients belonging to two generations of a Dutch family were reported with cerebral and cerebellar haemorrhage and cerebral infarction mostly in the fifth and sixth decades [173]. The disorder was believed to have been transmitted as an autosomal dominant mode of inheritance and dementia was considered to be a manifestation of the angiopathy. Extensive amyloidosis also occurs in a rare inherited syndrome with leptomeningeal, brain and vitreous amyloid deposits [174,175]. Parenchymal involvement is rare but this group of subjects is unusual with visceral vascular amyloid also. Several cases have been reported with an autosomal dominant inheritance characterized by progressive dementia and spastic paralysis with or without cerebral haemorrhage together with amyloid angiopathy in the cord and haemorrhages and infarcts in the cerebellum and hippocampus.

Subsequently, many non-familial cases of cerebral haemorrhage have been recognized in the elderly, predominantly over the age of 70 years with incidence increasing with age. They occur sporadically in the community and at least 30% have progressive senile dementia [176]. In more than 50% there is histopathological evidence of Alzheimer's disease (senile plaques and neurofibrillary degeneration) and very rarely an association with systemic visceral amyloidosis [177].

This syndrome is associated with cerebral infarcts and

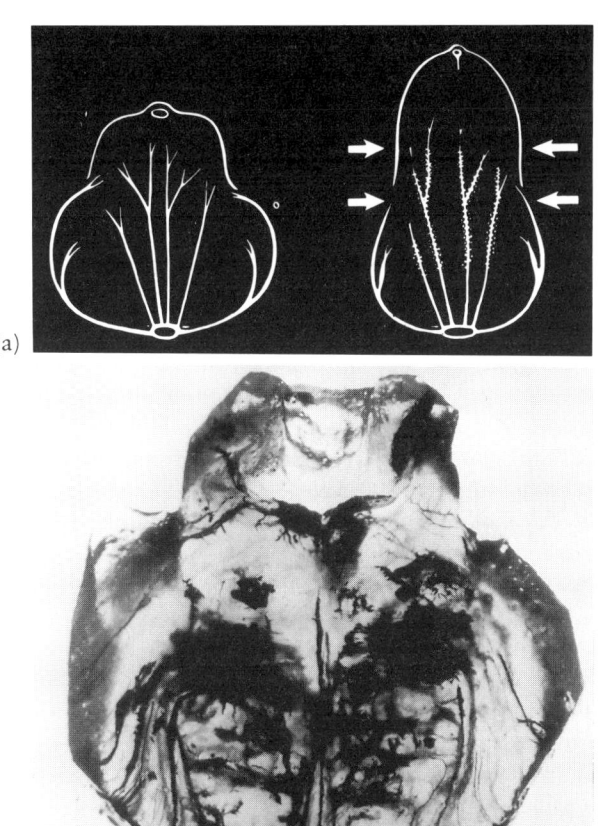

Figure 12.26 (a) Illustration of mechanism by which lateral pressure on the pons (arrows) produces gross elongation of the long penetrating arteries with extravasation (dots) of injected dye post mortem resulting from distortion of the pons. (b) Radiograph of a section of pons subjected to lateral pressure during intra-arterial sodium iodide mixture at autopsy with extravasation into the pons simulating secondary pontine haemorrhage. (Reproduced with permission from Johnson and Yates [128].)

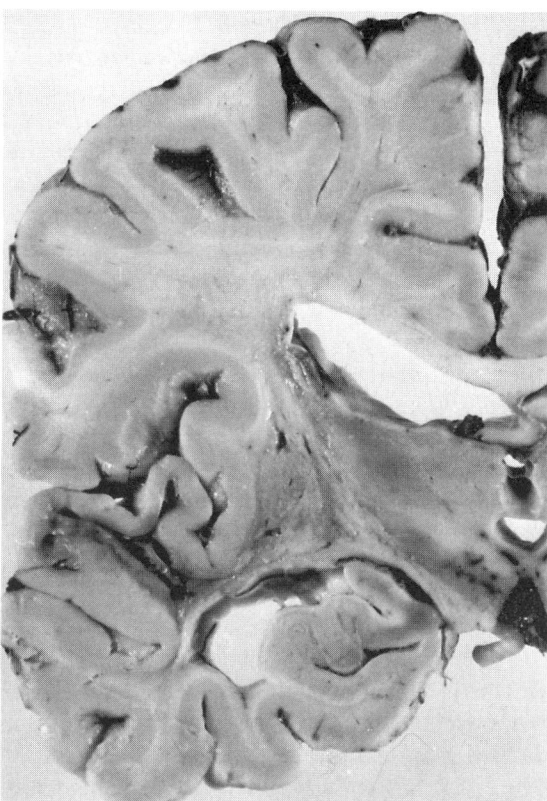

Figure 12.27 Subcortical pigmented slit-like cavity in the superior temporal gyrus and temporal operculum. Adjoining cortex is slightly reduced in width and the cavity has collapsed. This is the type of subcortical haematoma likely to occur in cerebral amyloid angiography. Note small lacunar cavities in basal ganglia. (Reproduced from Stehbens [3].)

particularly non-fatal subcortical (lobar) haemorrhage, especially in the frontal and parietal lobes and less frequently in occipital and temporal lobes [177]. Caplan [178] said in the elderly this accounted for one third of cerebral haemorrhages. They are likely to recur over months or years and at times two haemorrhages occur simultaneously. Scattered cortical and subcortical satellite haemorrhages have been encountered [179] with hypertension reported in only 20–40% of these [177] in contrast to the deep primary haemorrhages. There is no association with diabetes mellitus or paraproteinaemia [180].

The haemorrhages commonly rupture directly through the cortex into the subarachnoid space and with recovery leave pigmented subcortical spindle or slit-like spaces (Figure 12.27) often associated with multiple, small cortical infarcts. Surgical drainage is often followed by rebleeding due to impaired haemostasis. Whilst many of these haemorrhages are small and non-fatal, they can be quite massive and even bilateral [181,182].

The amyloid deposits are found in the media and adventitia of medium-sized and small cortical and leptomeningeal arteries and may extend into the perivascular tissues. The vessels exhibit severe narrowing of the lumen, thickening of the basement membrane, with loss of elastic tissue and medial muscle and rarely fibrinoid necrosis. They are seldom associated with miliary aneurysms. The amyloid has a strong affinity for Congo red and exhibits yellow green birefringence. Ultrastructurally the vessels contain unbranched randomly orientated amyloid fibrils 9–11 nm in diameter similar to those of systemic amyloid and senile plaques of Alzheimer's disease. Immunohistochemical staining using an avidin-biotin-peroxidase complex technique with a monoclonal antibody to the β/A4 protein has been found to be more sensitive [183]. The cerebrovascular amyloid has a molecular weight of 4200 daltons, and a unique amino acid composition and sequence. The amyloid from Down's syndrome and Alzheimer's disease differs by only one amino acid of the 28 known residues in the sequence [177]. β protein is derived from a precursor encoded by a gene on chromosome 21; the substitution of a single amino acid glutamine for glutamic acid at position 22 of the amyloid β protein may ultimately be responsible for the disposition of the amyloid protein within the cerebral blood vessels [184].

The precise pathogenesis of the haemorrhage in this syndrome is obscure with little evidence that the haemorrhage is due to the Charcôt–Bouchard aneurysms although they occur in the subcortical region of the cerebrum. Minor head injuries or even minor infarcts may possibly cause bleeding which persists because of the inability of vascocontrictor activity of an amyloid infiltrated arteriole or artery. This can result in extensive haemorrhage into the ventricles and subdural space [184]. However this would apply to the arteries with lipohyalinosis. Their brittle character has resulted in difficult postoperative bleeding due to inability to achieve haemostasis. It is also of interest that massive haemorrhage can complicate heavily amyloid-infiltrated vessels, particularly in the urinary bladder and gastro-intestinal tract.

The relationship of amyloid angiopathy to cerebral haemorrhage is an issue requiring more information. It has been assumed that the amyloid-affected vessels are fragile and therefore rupture and bleed but the prevalence of amyloid angiopathy in the elderly is high and the non-specificity of the deposits is of concern. Some affected vessels thrombose.

Vascular amyloid deposits are known to occur in a wide variety of neurological disorders including Alzheimer's disease, Down's syndrome, a demyelinating disease resembling multiple sclerosis, dementia associated with boxing, cerebral vasculitis and arteritis [177], X-irradiation necrosis of the brain and vessels of arteriovenous shunts [3]. A relationship to rheumatoid vasculitis has been suggested [185]. Amyloidosis also occurs, although rarely in the brain as a tumour-like mass originating within the brain or the choroid plexus [186]. Such lesions may well have commenced in blood vessels. Amyloid deposition has also been found in cerebral vessels of lower animals [187].

In a study of autopsy cases over the age of 60 years, amyloid deposition was found in 38% of subjects with cerebral haemorrhage, in 25% of those with infarction and in 32% of a control group, indicating that it is a common pathological finding in the elderly. However, the vascular involvement was found to be more closely associated with subcortical (lobar) haemorrhages than with the conventional deep haemorrhages particularly involving the basal ganglia [183]. In another series of 67 subjects over 75 years of age, who died of causes unrelated to amyloid angiopathy, 45% had microscopic findings consistent with amyloid angiopathy [188]. The severity of the age deposits is age-related and more than 50% of patients in the tenth decade have some degree of cerebral amyloid angiopathy. However, miliary aneurysms with and without hypertension also increase in prevalence with age. Cerebrovascular amyloidosis is common with and without Alzheimer's disease in which it occurs without any apparent propensity for cerebral haemorrhage. There is need for knowledge of vascular amyloid deposition in degenerative vascular disease, in atherosclerosis of large extracranial arteries and in arterioles and small arteries in the eighth decade and beyond, independent of visceral amyloidosis and paraproteinaemia. The apparent non-specificity of amyloid angiopathy is of concern and there is need to know whether its presence is actually responsible for the fragility or whether it interferes with the haemostatic properties of the vessel. The fragility of the affected vessels requires testing for there is evidence of collagen fibrillary degeneration in aging vessels, those in aneurysm walls and arteriovenous fistulae and atherosclerosis. On the other hand extensively amyloid-infiltrated blood vessels may bleed more profusely (impaired haemostasis) than unaffected vessels following minor trauma and an expanding haematoma might then initiate a vicious cycle.

It appears that there is a group of elderly subjects with this type of recurrent and not immediately fatal subcortical cerebral haemorrhage with and without small infarcts. Whether the amyloid angiopathy is causal or a coincidental finding should be determined and pathogenesis of the haemorrhages elucidated. The extensive cerebral damage both haemorrhagic and ischaemic is likely to impair cerebral function independently of Alzheimer's disease in which the amyloid angiopathy is quantitatively accentuated [177]. This does not detract from the importance of the familial incidence of non-hypertensive cerebral haemorrhage associated with cerebral amyloid angiopathy in specific families.

(c) Neoplasms

Large primary tumours of the central nervous system may bleed into their substance possibly due to the tumour outstripping the blood supply, thrombosis or neoplastic infiltration of vessels or from arteriovenous shunts associated with their vascularity. Glioblastoma multiforme (or astrocytoma grade III or IV) has the greatest propensity for haemorrhage. Sudden haemorrhage in a tumour perhaps with subarachnoid haemorrhage is an infrequent mode of presentation. It is more likely that the haemorrhage will raise the supratentorial pressure causing a fatal termination with or without secondary pontine haemorrhage. The more vascular the tumour, the greater is the chance of haemorrhage.

Metastatic tumours (haematogenous spread) to the brain may be associated with intracerebral haemorrhage, predominantly choriocarcinoma and melanoma. The former understandably invades blood vessels but the reason for haemorrhage from melanoma in the brain whether primary or secondary is difficult to understand in view of the lack of a similar propensity for haemorrhage in extracranial sites.

(d) Postendarterectomy haemorrhage

Carotid endarterectomy is a common procedure in the management and prevention of cerebrovascular ischaemia. Postoperative complications include cerebral infarction, hypertension and headache. Thromboembolic phenomena are quite understandable complications of such a procedure and the pathogenesis of the hypertension is obscure. However, correcting the impaired flow results in increased blood flow on the ipsilateral side and in the presence of hypertension, hyperperfusion and possibly cerebral embolism. Some subjects suffer seizures [189], cluster headaches, hemicrania and other head pains including carotidynia [190]. This hyperperfusion associated with hypertension may also precipitate cerebral haemorrhage [168,178,191,192], a phenomenon that Caplan [178] considers analogous to that induced by amphetamines, cocaine, exposure to extreme cold, trigeminal nerve stimulation, post-heart transplantation and post-surgical correction of congenital heart disease. Kaplan [168] considered the phenomenon may be aggravated by some prior ischaemia (reperfusion). It is reminiscent of arteriolar fibrinoid necrosis below an aortic coarctation following its surgical correction. Such phenomena require further investigation. The important features in postendarterectomy haemorrhage are:

1. significant hypertension, a fixed minor neurological deficit of at least four weeks duration and a very severe unilateral carotid stenosis pre-operatively;
2. a symptom-free interval postoperatively followed by an abrupt onset of systemic hypertension and sudden onset of progressive cerebral haemorrhage on the side of the carotid stenosis and prior cerebral infarction [193].

(e) Blood dyscrasias

Haemorrhage into the central nervous system is a serious hazard of the heterogeneous blood dyscrasias. Intracerebral haemorrhage is a frequent, serious complication of leukaemia. Like haemorrhage at other sites both intracranially and extracranially, the bleeding tends to be multiple and small to moderate in extent. There is usually evidence of haemorrhage at other sites and a single haematoma is rare. Careful evaluation to exclude primary intracerebral haemorrhage in older patients with chronic leukaemia is required. Bleeding is usually from small vessels in and about grey, round or oval leukaemic infiltrations which may compress, infiltrate and possibly cause stasis and necrosis of the vessel wall in association with thrombocytopenia. Haemorrhages are usually in the white matter causing death in up to 30% of affected patients. Such deaths are usually attributed to thrombocytopenia occurring particularly in acute lymphoblastic leukaemia or in an acute exacerbation of a chronic form. A fungal invasion of cerebral blood vessels can occur in leukaemia and be responsible for massive bleeding through an arteritic wall.

Intracerebral haemorrhage, a complication of haemophilia, is less common than subdural and subarachnoid haemorrhage and not as frequent with modern management of haemophilia. There is a longer survival than in earlier years.

In thrombocytopenia the haemorrhage is usually purpuric but at times massive. In thrombotic thrombocytopenia the haemorrhages are petechial or purpuric.

Intracerebral haemorrhage is a serious complication of anticoagulant therapy [194]. Any haemorrhage is likely to be aggravated and become quite serious, especially if into the subdural or subarachnoid space. Haemorrhage superimposed on an infarct and particularly embolic haemorrhagic infarct is a hazard. Some haemorrhages may be instances of primary intracerebral haemorrhage in hypertensive subjects and the possibility exists that a mild leak from a miliary aneurysm may become a massive haemorrhage. Bleeding, occurring during anticoagulant therapy may be due to serious underlying pathology or an unrelated lesion from which bleeding has originated.

Bleeding due to hypoprothrombinaemia from whatever cause (haemorrhagic disease of the newborn, severe hepatic diseases, vitamin K deficiency, salicylate therapy, or idiopathic (familial) hypoprothrombinaemia) may be multiple but exhibits little propensity to be purpuric in type. It tends to be massive, atypical in site quite often, and usually precipitated by trauma.

In sickle cell anaemia multiple petechial haemorrhages may occur with capillary thrombosis, and extensive haemorrhagic softenings or haemorrhages have been encountered. Aneurysms have also been reported and in view of the frequency of the anaemia amongst Negroes berry aneurysms are to be expected but whether there is a particular propensity to this type of aneurysm is yet to be determined.

Haemorrhage or haemorrhagic softening may occur in polycythemia rubra vera and there is a haemorrhagic diathesis in about two thirds of patients with

Waldenström's macroglobulinaemia. Congenital afibrinoginaemia is a rare disorder and those afflicted may suffer from recurrent intracerebral haemorrhage.

Coronary thrombolysis with streptokinase or tissue plasminogen activator in conjunction with heparin infusion has been useful therapy for acute myocardial infarction in selected subjects. It has been associated with local haemorrhagic complications and cerebral haemorrhage. For this reason thrombolytic therapy is contraindicated in patients with strokes, transient ischaemic attacks, cerebral injury, hypertension, intracranial aneurysms, arteriovenous aneurysms, amyloid angiopathy and anticoagulant therapy [184].

(f) Inflammatory and infectious disorders

Infections, both bacterial and mycotic, can lead to intracerebral haemorrhage particularly with bacterial endocarditis but rarely with meningitis. Mucormycosis, by invading blood vessel walls, can result in haemorrhage with or without aneurysmal dilatation. Small haemorrhages may occur with septicaemia and also encephalitis. Diseases such as polyarteritis nodosa, systemic lupus erythematosus and other vasculitides also cause small haemorrhages generally. Systemic lupus erythematosus can be associated with mycotic arteritis and also berry aneurysms.

(g) Miscellaneous causes

Small perivascular haemorrhages (ring haemorrhages) may be found in a variety of maladies such as fat embolism, concussion, blood dyscrasias, high altitudes, intoxication, acute haemorrhagic leucoencephalitis and malaria. The haemorrhages are confined to the white matter. The extravasation of red cells surrounds a zone of perivascular necrosis possibly with fibrin infiltration.

Heat stroke is associated with a tendency to haemorrhage because of hypoprothrombinaemia, hypofibrinogenaemia, thrombocytopenia, increased capillary permeability and endothelial damage. Petechial haemorrhages are found particularly in the walls of the third ventricle and the floor of the fourth ventricle. More extensive haemorrhage is a possibility and intravascular thrombi are found in small vessels.

Massive bleeding may occur in eclampsia, petechial haemorrhages being more common.

Spontaneous intracerebral bleeding in children and adolescents is infrequent. In the absence of hypertension and chronic vessel disease, it is most likely to be a secondary haemorrhage and cryptic angiomas and arteriovenous aneurysms should be sought. Most intracranial haemorrhages in this age group will be traumatic and extracerebral apart from contusions.

Unexplained intracerebral haemorrhage in the absence of trauma, and hypertension, especially if the subject is under 40 years of age, sets the scene for a meticulous search for an aneurysm, a cryptic angioma or arteriovenous aneurysm and for tumour.

12.18 Intraventricular haemorrhage

Intraventricular haemorrhage in the neonate is usually due to trauma with haemorrhage from the choroid plexus, the internal cerebral or one of the terminal veins and at times will be sufficient to produce a redcurrant jelly cast of the ventricular system. Smaller haemorrhages may occur as the result of prolonged anoxia with prematurity a predisposing condition.

Primary intraventricular haemorrhage in the adult is rare and most likely to come from the choroid plexus. Usually it is of a secondary nature with blood escaping from the parenchyma as the result of primary intracerebral haemorrhage or ruptured berry aneurysms. Papilloma or an arteriovenous shunt of the choroid plexus may present as subarachnoid haemorrhage and a bleeding diathesis must be excluded at all ages. Profuse bleeding may lead to tamponade with a clot or pressure effect obstructing the aqueduct and acute haemocephalus results, sometimes with tears and lacerations of the ventricular walls. Intraventricular haemorrhage is usually terminal.

12.19 Intraspinal haemorrhage

Dislocations and fractures of the spine are the commonest cause of spinal haemorrhage and as with compression, squashed cord tissue may be forced caudally or cranially along the dorsal white columns giving a typical appearance of haematomyelia. The degree of bleeding will vary but in the absence of trauma, secondary haemorrhages are responsible. Arteriovenous haemorrhages are more frequent than aneurysms although both may be present. Leukaemia and bleeding diatheses must be considered.

12.20 Miscellaneous conditions

12.20.1 HYPERTENSIVE ENCEPHALOPATHY

This is a term introduced to describe the acute or subacute cerebral episode occurring within the terminal weeks or months of severely hypertensive patients, usually those with malignant hypertension or in toxaemia of pregnancy. It is manifested by severe headache, convulsions, amaurosis, mental confusion, stupor or coma and sometimes transient neurological disturbances such as hemiplegia, monoplegia, hemianaesthesia and aphasia. Following the experimental work of Byrom [195] this state is associated with oedema, arteriolar vasoconstriction, fibrinoid necrosis of the alveolar walls, petechial haemorrhages and possibly some necrosis of the tissue supplied. These lesions are possibly confined to the watershed areas between the areas supplied by the three major cerebral arteries.

12.20.2 DRUG ABUSAGE

A number of drugs of abuse have cardiovascular effects that could contribute to strokes in normal or susceptible people. Intravenous drugs causing an acute elevation of blood pressure or persistent oral administration can be quite dangerous. Vasculitis is common with drug abusage. Acute necrotizing arteritis with dissecting aneurysm of a cerebral artery has been recorded [196]. Recently cocaine usage has reached almost epidemic proportions in the USA. Whilst crack cocaine can induce coronary lesions with myocardial infarction, and embolism to the brain can be a complication, cocaine has also been responsible for several cerebral deaths and subjects with pre-existing diabetes mellitus or hypertension are at risk. Cocaine has been incriminated in haemorrhage from cerebral aneurysms and arteriovenous shunts, intracerebral haemorrhage and subarachnoid haemorrhage as well as cerebral ischaemic infarcts [197]. Vasculitis was not specifically identified but the infarcts were considered to be cortical lesions in the distribution of the middle cerebral artery or the vertebrobasilar arteries mostly in young adults. Contaminants may contribute to the development of complications [197].

12.20.3 MIGRAINE

Migraine is one of the most common neurological disorders and varies in its clinical manifestations. It is associated with increased vasomotor reactivity and the pathogenesis of the headache and visual aura is controversial. It has been linked in the past with cerebral aneurysms and ophthalmoplegic migraine was considered a distinct entity. Since cerebral aneurysms are so common, coexistence of these two disorders would be expected and as yet there is no strong evidence to suggest a cause and effect relationship. In more recent years an association has been alleged from time to time with cerebral infarction, embolism, haemorrhage, intimal and adventitial fibrosis and dissecting aneurysms of a cerebral artery.

The initial phase of vasoconstriction is followed by vasodilatation, which provokes the migrainous headache and the vessels affected become painful, ache and throb. Some of the neurological disturbances associated with migraine including aphasia or even pareses cause concern but as yet there appears to be no scientific evidence of a causal relationship to permanent pathological lesions or clinical disability. The development of intracerebral haematomas during a migrainous headache [168,198] in four middle-aged normotensive women with late-onset migraine may be significant but the underlying pathogenesis is obscure. It is not known whether the haemodynamic changes during a migrainous episode can contribute to the development of an aneurysm, particularly when factors of a labile blood pressure and naturally occurring degenerative changes are superadded. This may be so and likewise they may contribute to their growth and eventual rupture. Vasospasm in one vascular bed may be associated with compensatory vasodilatation in an adjoining bed. There is also sufficient experimental evidence to indicate that haemodynamic stress with hyperperfusion and associated blood pressure changes can induce profound degenerative changes in arteries. This in all likelihood can be said as well for severe physical exertion and sport. More information is required on the specific changes in the blood vessels repeatedly affected in migraine and cluster headaches but this is difficult to obtain and prove. It seems that haemodynamic stresses associated with migraine, like other episodes, emotional or physical, are of contributory rather than primary aetiological importance [3].

12.20.4 VASCULAR SIDEROSIS

This is also known as pallidal siderosis or calcinosiderosis and is an autogenous iron deposition in and

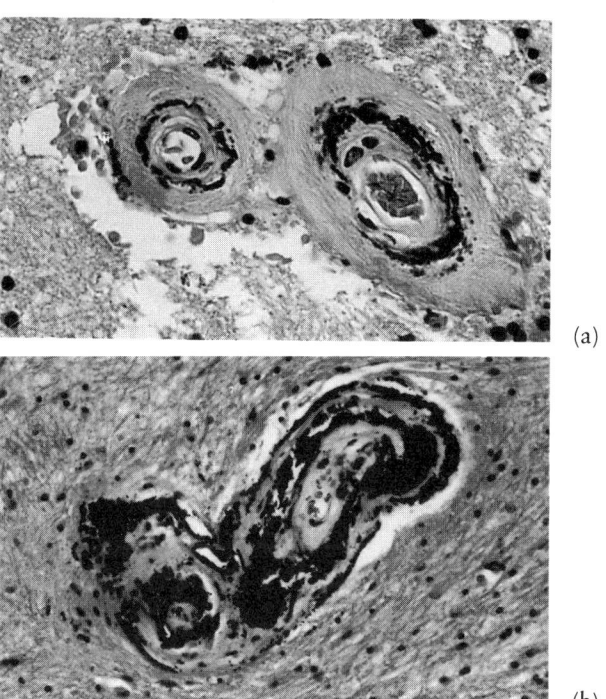

Figure 12.28 Vascular siderosis in two small stenosed arteries with luminal narrowing (a) and more extensive deposition with severe stenosis in (b). (Haematoxylin and eosin.)

about small blood vessels particularly of the globus pallidus. Its frequency in adult brains at autopsy has varied from 48 to 68.5% but is 80% in those over 70 years of age [199]. Strassman [200] asserted that it occurs regularly in those over 60 years of age but he also found it in a 7-year-old idiot. Despite the frequency, the significance is unknown.

It occurs particularly in the anterior part of the globus pallidus and in the putamen and caudate nucleus, the striatum, dentate nucleus and the substantia nigra [200] but is not restricted to these zones and can be present in oligodendrogliomas and metastatic tumours. The deposits are densely basophilic, and in about 2.5% of cases the deposits, though not all vessels, will contain calcium. Stippling commences about capillaries initially, increasing in quantity to form a sheath about the vessels affecting both arteries and veins. The siderosis also involves the intimal thickening in arteriosclerotic vessels including the elastic tissue. There is often pronounced narrowing or even stenosis of these vessels (Figure 12.28) which may be independent of the siderosis since this is principally a disease of the very elderly. In severe cases ferrugination of glial and nerve cells develops with, not infrequently, evidence of cerebrovascular disease, principally ischaemic infarcts in the cerebellum.

12.20.5 IDIOPATHIC SYMMETRICAL CALCIFICATION OF CEREBRAL VESSELS

Calcification of small cerebral arteries, veins and capillaries appears to be a response to varied pathological influences, including various forms of encephalitis and endocrine disorders (particularly hypoparathyroidism) that account for most instances [201]. Vascular calcification occurs in 28% of cases of idiopathic hypothyroidism and in 48% of cases of pseudohypoparathyroidism [202] and also in hypervitaminosis D and destructive bone lesions [203].

Some instances appearing *de novo*, are idiopathic and without a familial tendency. There is a similar calcific involvement of vessels in the Sturge–Weber syndrome. A distinct familial trend is apparent in some subjects, often in association with microcephaly and oligophrenia [201] involving two or even three siblings in a family. The subjects, mostly between 30 and 50 years of age, exhibit progressive dementia and extrapyramidal dysfunction [204].

The localization of vascular calcification is uniform, being most severe in the putamen and the central regions of the cerebellar hemispheres about the dentate nucleus. The globus pallidus, thalamus, parts of the cerebral cortex and centrum ovale are affected to a varying degree but with a bilateral distribution.

The brain is usually small with atrophic gyri and massive calcification or 'brain stones' in the basal ganglia, the cerebral white matter and the dentate nucleus. Calcium is deposited near to or in the walls of small blood vessels, often with severe narrowing or complete occlusion of the lumen which could account for the patchy perivascular gliosis. The calcium content of the concretions consists of 11 mg% of dry weight with a small quantity of iron (32 μg% of dry weight) [203] which would explain the weakly positive Prussian blue reaction at the periphery and in new deposits. Calcium occurs as phosphate and there are traces of magnesium and cystine. The aetiology is unknown.

12.20.6 SENILITY AND DEMENTIA

There has been a long-standing controversy over the role of vascular disease in senility and dementia. It seems plausible that severe cerebral atherosclerosis with sporadic involvement of small vessels together with patchy gliosis, multiple infarcts and ischaemic change can also account for reduced cerebral blood flow, diminished metabolic activity and varying grades of mental impairment. However, atherosclerosis is likely to be severe in most elderly subjects and dementia could occur concomitantly with but independently of vascular changes.

Oxygen utilization and cerebral blood flow are significantly reduced in organic dementia whatever the cause and oxygen uptake is usually inversely proportional to intellectual impairment [205].

Sokoloff [206] studied a carefully selected group of elderly subjects and concluded that reduced cerebral blood flow and metabolism are not necessarily the result of the aging processes *per se* and could be due to impaired cerebral circulation and metabolic function. Consistent with this concept is the finding of dementia four to twelve times more frequently in subjects with lacunar infarcts than in the normal population [207]. A more specific correlation between dementia and cerebral vascular disease is seen in Binswanger's disease.

12.20.7 BINSWANGER'S DISEASE

There are many descriptive synonyms for the subacute or chronic progressive arteriosclerotic encephalopathy [208]. Clinically there is slowly progressive mental deterioration with focal neurological manifestations including aphasia, hemianopia, hemipariesis and hemianaesthesia and sometimes associated apoplectiform attacks of dizziness, faintness or loss of consciousness. Cerebral atherosclerosis is usually moderate or severe but no major infarcts occur. The central white matter is firm, dull grey and reduced in volume with ventricular dilatation. There is extensive demyelination in the central white matter, état criblé and numerous small infarcts including lacunar infarcts. The cortex, subcortical arcuate fibres and convolutional white matter are relatively spared. Histologically, the changes have been attributed to severe arteriosclerosis of the long perforating arteries to the deep white matter. Cutting the hemispheres in cross-section reveals the diffuse bilateral demyelinating changes in the deep periventricular white matter. Computerized tomography and magnetic resonance imaging have also demonstrated this relatively symmetrical periventricular low density white matter which is considered characteristic [208], the rarefied areas being referred to as leukoaraiosis [209].

Most (68%) have dementia, disturbances of gait (54%) and hypertension (57%) although there is much variation in the literature. There is poor pathological correlation with the degree of dementia and Fisher [208] concluded that the hyalinized sclerotic arteries in the white matter are the hallmark of this disease. Since such vascular changes are not pathognomonic and cannot be divorced from atherosclerosis of large cerebral arteries which exhibit minimal disease in 20% of cases, the correlation is not particularly convincing especially in the absence of other characteristic vascular episodes. The arteriolar and small arterial changes may be secondary manifestations of the primary neuronal and demyelinating disorder associated with dementia. Although the vessels are most infrequently narrowed or occluded and many subjects are normotensive, the vascular ischaemia is thought to be the underlying cause of the parenchymal changes. Rather than maximum involvement being periventricular, the watershed areas might be those most severely affected if ischaemia is truly the underlying mechanism.

In our present state of knowledge it is best to consider the aetiology of Binswanger's disease as unknown rather than labelling it as an arteriosclerotic encephalopathy.

References

1. Haberman, S., Capildeo, R. and Rose, F.C. (1978) The changing mortality of cerebrovascular disease. *Q. J. Med.*, **47**, 71–88.
2. Kurtzke, J.F. (1969) *Epidemiology of Cerebrovascular Disease*, Springer-Verlag, Berlin.
3. Stehbens, W.E. (1972) *Pathology of the Cerebral Blood Vessels*, C.V. Mosby, St Louis.
4. Barer, D., Leibowitz, R., Ebrahim, S. *et al.* (1989) Vitamin C status and other nutritional indices in patients with stroke and other acute illnesses: a case-control study. *J. Clin. Epidemiol.*, **42**, 625–31.
5. Garraway, W.M., Whisnant, J.P., Furlan, A.J. *et al.* (1979) The declining incidence of stroke. *New Engl J. Med.*, **300**, 449–52.
6. Stehbens, W.E. (1991) Validity of cerebrovascular mortality rates. *Angiology*, **42**, 261–7.
7. Hartveit, F. (1977) Clinical and post-mortem assessment of the cause of death. *J. Pathol.*, **123**, 193–210.
8. Wolf, Dr (1978) Discussion. *Adv Neurol.*, **19**, 310–11.
9. Corwin, L.I., Wolf, P.A., Kannel, W.B. *et al.* (1982) Accuracy of death certification of stroke: the Framingham Study. *Stroke*, **13**, 818–21.
10. Kuller, L.H. (1978) Epidemiology of stroke. *Adv. Neurol.*, **19**, 281–311.
11. Heasman, M.A. and Lipworth, L. (1966) *Accuracy of Certification of Cause of Death*, HMSO, London.
12. Stehbens, W.E. (1993) *The Lipid Hypothesis of Atherogenesis*, R.G. Landes, Austin.
13. Dawber, T.R. and Thomas, H.E. (1968) Prophylaxis of coronary heart disease, stroke, and peripheral atherosclerosis. *Ann. N.Y. Acad. Sci.*, **149**, 1038–57.
14. Marquardsen, J. (1986) Epidemiology of strokes in Europe, in *Stroke. Pathophysiology, Diagnosis and Management*, (eds H.J.M. Barnett, B.M. Stern, J.P. Mohr *et al.*), Churchill Livingstone, New York, pp. 31–43.
15. Yatsu, F.M. (1986) Atherogenesis and stroke, in *Stroke. Pathophysiology, Diagnosis and Management*, (eds H.J.M. Barnett, B.M. Stern, J.P. Mohr *et al.*), Churchill Livingstone, New York, pp. 45–56.
16. Tell, G.S., Crouse, J.R. and Furberg, C.D. (1988) Relation between blood lipids, lipoproteins, and cerebrovascular atherosclerosis. *Stroke*, **19**, 423–30.
17. Qizilbash, N., Duffy, S.W., Warlow, C. *et al.* (1992) Lipids are risk factors for ischaemic stroke: overview and review. *Cerebrovasc. Dis.*, **2**, 127–36.
18. Tanaka, H., Hayashi, M., Date, C. *et al.* (1985) Epidemiologic studies of stroke in Shibita, a Japanese provincial city: preliminary report on risk factors for cerebral infarction. *Stroke*, **16**, 773–80.
19. Omae, T., Takeshita, M. and Hirato, Y. (1976) The Hisayama study and joint study on cerebrovascular disease in Japan, in *Cerebrovascular Diseases*, (ed. P. Scheinberg), Raven Press, New York, pp. 255–65.
20. Garraway, W.M., Whisnant, J.P. and Drury, I. (1983) The continuing decline in the incidence of stroke. *Mayo Clin. Proc.*, **58**, 520–3.
21. Yano, K., Reed, D.M. and MacLean, C.J. (1989) Serum cholesterol and hemorrhagic stroke in the Honolulu Heart Program. *Stroke*, **20**, 1460–5.
22. Iso, H., Jacobs, D.R., Wentworth, D. *et al.* (1989) Serum cholesterol levels and six-year mortality from stroke in 350,977 men screened for the Multiple Risk Factor Intervention Trial. *New Engl J. Med.*, **320**, 904–10.
23. Wylie, C.M. (1972) Epidemiology of cerebrovacular disease. *Handb. Clin. Neurol.*, **11**, 183–207.
24. Broderick, J.P., Phillips, S.J., Whisnant, J.P. *et al.* (1989) Incidence rates of stroke in the eighties: the end of the decline in stroke? *Stroke*, **20**, 577–82.
25. Kittner, S.J., White, L.R., Losonczy, K.G. *et al.* (1990) Black–white differences in stroke incidence in a national sample. *J. Am. Med. Ass.*, **264**, 1267–70.
26. Alter, M. and Kluznik, J. (1972) Genetics of cerebrovascular accidents. *Stroke*, **3**, 41–8.
27. Brass, L.M., Isaacson, J.L., Merikangas, K.P. *et al.* (1992) A study of twins in stroke. *Stroke*, **23**, 221–3.
28. Feinstein, A.R. (1985) *Clinical Epidemiology. The Architecture of Clinical Research*, W.B. Saunders, Philadelphia.
29. Murray, T.J. (1979) Carotidynia: a cause of neck and face pain. *Can. Med. Ass. J.*, **120**, 441–4.
30. Raskin, N.H. and Prusiner, S. (1977) Carotidynia. *Neurology*, **27**, 43–6.
31. Roseman, D.M. (1968) Carotidynia. *Handb. Clin. Neurol.*, **5**, 375–7.
32. Countee, R.W. (1979) Carotidynia or carotid artery aneurysm. *Neurology*, **29**, 422–3.
33. Cairney, J. (1924) Tortuosity of the cervical segment of the internal carotid artery. *J. Anat.*, **59**, 87–96.
34. Weibel, J. and Field, W.S. (1965) Tortuosity, coiling, and kinking of the internal carotid artery. I. Etiology and radiographic anatomy. *Neurology*, **15**, 7–18.
35. Stehbens, W.E. (1986) Experimental arterial loops and arterial atrophy. *Expl Mol. Pathol.*, **44**, 177–89.
36. Hsu, I. and Kistin, A.D. (1956) Buckling of the great vessels. *Arch. Int. Med.*, **98**, 712–19.
37. Vannix, R.S., Joergenson, E.J. and Carter, R. (1977) Kinking of the internal carotid artery. Clinical significance and surgical management. *Am. J. Surg.*, **134**, 82–9.
38. Kobayashi, T., Ogawa, A. and Kameyama, M. *et al.* (1992) Chiari malformation with compression of the medulla oblongata by the vertebral arteries. *J. Neurosurg.*, **77**, 307–9.
39. Sunderland, S. (1957–8) The tentorial notch and complications produced by herniations of the brain through that aperture. *Br. J. Surg.*, **45**, 422–38.
40. Scotti, G. (1974) Internal carotid origin of a posterior cerebral artery. *Arch. Neurol.*, **31**, 273–5.
41. Launay, M., Fredy, D., Merland, J.J. *et al.* (1977) Narrowing and occlusion of arteries by intracranial tumors. *Neuroradiology*, **14**, 117–26.
42. Lindenberg, R. (1955) Compression of brain arteries as pathognomonic factor for tissue necrosis and their areas of predilection. *J. Neuropathol. Expl Neurol.*, **14**, 223–43.
43. Cevasse, L.E. and Logue, R.B. (1958) Carotid artery murmurs: continuous murmur over carotid bulb – new sign of carotid artery insufficiency. *J. Am. Med. Ass.*, **167**, 2177–82.
44. Cohen, J.H. and Miller, S. (1956) Eyeball bruits. *New Engl J. Med.*, **255**, 459–64.
45. Potter, J.M. (1955) Angiomatous malformations of the brain: their nature and prognosis. *Ann. Roy. Coll. Surg. Engl.*, **16**, 227–43.
46. Campbell, E., Perese, D. and Bigelow, N.H. (1954) Excision of multisaccular supratentorial aneurysm of infratentorial origin. *J. Neurosurg.*, **11**, 422–8.
47. Ferguson, G.G. (1970) Turblence in human intracranial saccular aneurysm. *J. Neurosurg.*, **33**, 485–97.
48. Fisher, M. (1952) Transient monocular blindness associated with hemiplegia. *Arch. Ophthalmol.*, **47**, 167–203.
49. Gilroy, J. and Meyer, J.S. (1963) Pituitary insufficiency with cerebrospinal symptoms. *New Engl J. Med.*, **269**, 1115–9.

50. Rainer, W.G., Cramer, C.G., Newby, J.P. *et al.* (1968) Fibromuscular hyperplasia of the carotid artery causing positional cerebral ischemia. *Ann. Surg.*, 167, 444–6.
51. Harrison, M.J.G. (1982) Pathogenesis, in *Transient Ischemic Attacks*, (eds C. Warlow and P.J. Morris), Marcel Dekker, New York, pp. 21–46.
52. Russell, R.W.R. (1968) The source of retinal emboli. *Lancet*, 2, 789–92.
53. Hollenhorst, R.W. (1961) Significance of bright plaques in the retinal arterioles. *J. Am. Med. Ass.*, 178, 23–9.
54. Hoffman, W.P., Wilson, C.B. and Townsend, T.J. (1979) Recurrent transient ischemic attacks secondary to an embolizing saccular cerebral artery aneurysm. *J. Neurosurg.*, 51, 103–6.
55. McCollum, C.H., Wheeler, W.G., Noon, G.P. *et al.* (1970) Aneurysms of the extracranial carotid artery. Twenty-one years' experience. *Am. J. Surg.*, 137, 196–200.
56. Portnoy, H.D. (1965) Transient 'ischemic' attacks produced by carotid stenosis and hypoglycemia. *Neurology*, 15, 830–2.
57. Stehbens, W.E. (1982) Atherothrombosis of arteries to the eye and brain, in *Transient Ischemic Attacks*, (eds C. Warlow and P.J. Morris), Marcel Dekker, New York, pp. 47–63.
58. Heidrich, H. and Bayer, O. (1969) Symptomatology of the subclavian steal syndrome. *Angiology*, 20, 406–13.
59. Sammartino, W.F. and Toole, J.F. (1964) Reversed vertebral artery flow. *Arch. Neurol.*, 10, 590–4.
60. Folger, G.M. and Shah, K.D. (1965) Subclavian steal in patients with Blalock–Taussig anastomosis. *Circulation*, 31, 241–8.
61. Ross, R.S. and McKusick, V.A. (1953) Aortic arch syndromes. *Arch. Int. Med.*, 92, 701–40.
62. Siesjö, B.K. (1992) Pathophysiology and treatment of focal cerebral ischemia. Part I. Pathophysiology. *J. Neurosurg.*, 77, 169–84.
63. Siesjö, B.K. (1992) Pathophysiology and treatment of focal cerebral ischemia. Part II. Mechanisms of damage and treatment. *J. Neurosurg.*, 77, 337–54.
64. Aronson, S.M. and Aronson, B.E. (1966) Ischemic cerebral vascular disease. *N.Y. State Med. J.*, 66, 954–7.
65. Fisher, C.M. (1961) Clinical syndromes in cerebral artery occlusion, in *Pathogenesis and Treatment of Cerebrovascular Disease*, (ed. W.S. Fields), C.C. Thomas, Springfield, pp. 151–81.
66. Fisher, M. and Adams, R.D. (1951) Observations on brain embolism with special reference to the mechanism of hemorrhagic infarction. *J. Neuropathol. Expl. Neurol.*, 10, 92–4.
67. Chase, T.N., Roseman, N.P. and Price, D.L. (1968) The cerebral syndrome associated with dissecting aneurysms of the aorta. *Brain*, 94, 173–90.
68. Faris, A.A., Harden, C.A. and Poser, C.M. (1963) Pathogenesis of hemorrhagic infarction of the brain. 1. Experimental investigations of role of hypertension and of cerebral circulation. *Arch. Neurol.*, 9, 468–72.
69. Prineas, J. and Marshall, J. (1966) Hypertension and cerebral infarction. *Br. Med. J.*, 1, 14–17.
70. Amarenco, P., Duyckaerts, C., Tzourio, C. *et al.* (1992) The prevalence of ulcerated aortic plaques in the aortic arch in patients with stroke. *New Engl J. Med.*, 326, 221–5.
71. Tanahashi, N., Gotoh, F., Tomita, M. *et al.* (1989) Enhanced erythrocyte aggregability in occlusive cerebrovascular disease. *Stroke*, 20, 1202–7.
72. Bevan, H., Sharma, K. and Bradley, W. (1990) Stroke in young adults. *Stroke*, 21, 382–6.
73. Petty, G.W., Brust, J.C.M., Tatemichi, T.K. *et al.* (1990) Embolic stroke after smoking 'crack' cocaine. *Stroke*, 21, 1632–5.
74. Cohle, S.D. and Lie, J.T. (1988) Inflammatory aneurysm of the aorta, aortitis, and coronary arteritis. *Arch. Pathol. Lab. Med.*, 112, 1121–5.
75. Castaigne, R., Lhermitte, R., Gautier, J.-C. *et al.* (1970) Internal carotid artery occlusion. *Brain*, 93, 231–58.
76. Fisher, M. (1954) Occlusion of the carotid arteries. *Arch. Neurol. Psychiat.*, 72, 187–204.
77. Brice, J.G., Dowsett, D.J. and Lowe, R.D. (1964) Haemodynamic effects of carotid artery stenosis. *Lancet*, 2, 1363–6.
78. Mitchell, J.R.A. and Schwartz, C.J. (1965) *Arterial Disease*, Blackwell, Oxford.
79. Hutchinson, E.C. and Yates, P.O. (1957) Carotico-vertebral stenosis. *Lancet*, 1, 2–8.
80. Humphrey, J.G. and Newton, T.H. (1960) Internal carotid artery occlusion in young adults. *Brain*, 83, 565–78.
81. Sheehan, S., Bauer, R.B. and Meyer, J.S. (1960) Vertebral artery compression in cervical spondylosis. *Neurology*, 10, 968–86.
82. Ford, F.R. and Clark, D. (1956) Thrombosis of the basilar artery with softenings in the cerebellum and brain stem due to manipulation of the neck. *Bull. Johns Hopkins Hosp.*, 98, 37–42.
83. Tatlow, W.F.T. and Bammer, H.G. (1957) Syndrome of vertebral artery compression. *Neurology*, 7, 331–40.
84. Ford, F.R. (1952) Syncope, vertigo, and disturbances of vision resulting from intermittent obstruction of the vertebral arteries due to defect in the odontoid process and excessive mobility of the second cervical vertebra. *Bull. Johns Hopkins Hosp.*, 41, 168–73.
85. Carpenter, S. (1961) Injury of neck as cause of vertebral artery thrombosis. *J. Neurosurg.*, 18, 849–53.
86. Simeone, F.A. and Goldberg, H.L. (1968) Thrombosis of the vertebral artery from hyperextension injury to the neck. *J. Neurosurg.*, 29, 540–4.
87. Yates, P.O. (1959) Birth trauma to the vertebral arteries. *Arch. Dis. Child*, 34, 436–41.
88. Rundles, W.R. and Kimbell, F.D. (1969) The kinked carotid syndrome. *Angiology*, 20, 177–94.
89. Derrick, J.R. Carotid kinking and cerebral insufficiency. *Geriatrics*, 18, 272–5.
90. Boldrey, E., Maass, I. and Miller, E. (1956) The role of atlantoid compression in the etiology of internal carotid thrombosis. *J. Neurosurg.*, 13, 127–39.
91. Barron, K.D., Siqueira, E. and Hirano, O. (1960) Cerebral embolism caused by non-bacterial thrombotic endocarditis. *Neurology*, 10, 391–7.
92. Fieschi, C. and Bozzao, L. (1969) Transient embolic occlusion of the middle cerebral internal carotid arteries in cerebral apoplexy. *J. Neurol. Neurosurg. Psychiat.*, 32, 236–40.
93. Hart, M.N. and Cyrus, A. (1968) Hyaline globules of the adrenal medulla. *Am. J. Clin. Pathol.*, 49, 387–91.
94. Fisher, C.M. (1967) A lacunar stroke. *Neurology*, 17, 614–17.
95. Tuszynski, M.H., Petito, C.K. and Levy, D.E. (1989) Risk factors and clinical manifestations of pathologically verified lacunar infarctions. *Stroke*, 20, 990–9.
96. Fisher, C.M. (1965) Lacunes: small deep cerebral infarcts. *Neurology*, 15, 774–84.
97. Fisher, C.M. (1969) The arterial lesions underlying lacunes. *Acta Neuropathol.*, 12, 1–15.
98. Millikan, C. and Futrell, N. (1990) The fallacy of the lacune hypothesis. *Stroke*, 21, 1251–7.
99. Cacciatore, A. and Russo, L.S. Lacunar infarction as an embolic complication of cardiac and arch angiography. *Stroke*, 22, 1603–5.
100. Oliva, A. and Scherokman, B. (1988) Two cases of occipital infarction following cardiac catheterization. *Stroke*, 19, 773–5.
101. Taveras, J.M. (1969) Multiple progressive intracranial arterial occlusions: a syndrome of children and young adults. *Am. J. Roentgen.*, 106, 235–68.
102. Mastri, A.R., Silverstein, P.M., Gold, L. *et al.* (1973) Multiple progressive intracranial arterial occlusions. *Stroke*, 4, 380–6.
103. Li, B., Wang, C.-C., Zhao, Z.-Z. *et al.* (1991) A histological, ultrastructural, and immunohistochemical study of superficial temporal arteries and middle meningeal arteries in moyamoya disease. *Acta Pathol. Jap.*, 41, 521–30.
104. Prensky, A.L. and Davis, D.O. (1970) Obstruction of major cerebral arteries in early childhood without neurological signs. *Neurology*, 20, 945–53.
105. Stehbens, W.E. (1979) *Hemodynamics and the Blood Vessel Wall*, C.C. Thomas, Springfield.
106. Logothetis, J., Silverstein, P. and Coe, J. (1960) Neurologic aspects of Waldenström's macroglobulinemia. *Arch. Neurol.*, 3, 564–73.
107. Swank, R.L. (1959) Changes in blood of dogs and rabbits by high fat intake. *Am. J. Physiol.*, 196, 473–7.
108. Swank, R.L. and Nakamura, H. (1960) Convulsions in hamsters after cream meals. *Arch. Neurol.*, 3, 594–600.
109. Kalbag, R.M. and Woolf, A.Z. (1967) *Cerebral Venous Thrombosis*, Oxford University Press, London.
110. Symonds, C.P. (1956) Otitic hydrocephalus. *Neurology*, 6, 681–5.
111. Vessey, M.P., Doll, R., Fairbairn, A.S. *et al.* (1970) Postoperaive thromboembolism and the use of oral contraceptives. *Br. Med. J.*, 3, 123–6.
112. Altschuler, J.H., McLaughlin, R.A. and Neuberger, K.T. (1968) Neurological catastrophe related to oral contraceptives. *Arch. Neurol.*, 19, 264–73.
113. Editorial. (1974) Spinal stroke. *Lancet*, 2, 1299–1300.
114. Cluroe, A.D., Fitzjohn, T.P. and Stehbens, W.E. (1992) Combined pathological and radiological study of the effect of atherosclerosis on the ostia of segmental branches of the abdominal aorta. *Pathology*, 24, 140–5.
115. Jellinger, K. and Neumayer, E. (1962) Myélopathies progressives d'origine vasculaire. *Rev. Neurol.*, 106, 666–9.
116. Garland, H., Greenberg, J. and Harriman, D.G.F. (1966) Infarction of the spinal cord. *Brain*, 89, 645–62.
117. Sangupta, R.P. and Hankinson, J. (1979) An unusual case of multiple intracranial aneurysms. *Acta Neurochir.*, 45, 259–75.
118. Gallagher, J.P. and Browder, E.J. (1968) Extradural hematoma – experience with 167 patients. *J. Neurosurg.*, 29, 1–12.
119. Kessler, L.A., Lubie, L.G. and Koskoff, Y.D. (1957) Epidural hemorrhage secondary to cavernous hemangioma of the petrous portion of the temporal bone. *J. Neurosurg.*, 14, 329–31.
120. Hoffman, H.J. and Mustard, W.T. (1973) Spontaneous intracranial extradural hematoma occurring during open-heart surgery. *Can. J. Surg.*, 16, 1–2.
121. Crooks, D.A. (1991) Pathogenesis and biomechanics of traumatic intracranial haemorrhages. *Virchows Arch. A Path. Anat.*, 418, 479–83.
122. Helmer, F.A., Sukoff, M.H. and Plaut, M.R. (1968) Angiographic extravasation of contrast medium in an epidural hematoma. *J. Neurosurg.*, 29, 652–4.
123. Youmans, J.R. and Schneider, R.C. (1960) Post-traumatic intracranial

hematomas in patients with arrested hydrocephalus. *J. Neurosurg.*, **17**, 590–7.
124. Paul, M. (1955) Haemorrhage from head injuries. *Ann. Roy. Coll. Surgeons Engl.*, **17**, 69–101.
125. Ford, L.E. and McLaurin, R.L. (1963) Mechanisms of extradural hematomas. *J. Neurosurg.*, **20**, 760–9.
126. McLaurin, R.L. and Ford, L.E. (1964) Extradural hematoma. *J. Neurosurg.*, **21**, 364–71.
127. Freytag, E. (1963) Autopsy findings in hard injuries from blunt force. *Arch. Pathol.*, **75**, 402–13.
128. Johnson, R.T. and Yates, P.O. (1956) Brain stem haemorrhage in expanding supratentorial conditions. *Acta Radiol.*, **46**, 250–6.
129. Mendelow, A.D., Karmi, M.Z., Paul, K.S. *et al.* (1979) Extradural haematoma: effect of delayed treatment. *Br. Med. J.*, **1**, 1240–2.
130. Towbin, A. (1964) Spinal cord and brain stem injury at birth. *Arch. Pathol. Lab. Med.*, **77**, 620–32.
131. Potter, E.L. (1961) *Pathology of the Fetus and Infant*, 2nd edn, Year Book Medical Pub. Co., Chicago.
132. Gunn, T.R. and Becroft, D.M.O. (1984) Unexplained intracranial haemorrhages in utero: the battered fetus. *Aust. N.Z. J. Obstet. Gynaecol.*, **24**, 17–22.
133. Becroft, D.M.O. and Gunn, T.R. (1985) Intracranial haemorrhages in Pacific Island stillbirths: is traditional massage the cause? *N.Z. Med. J.*, **98**, 18–19.
134. Becroft, D.M.O. and Gunn, T.R. (1989) Prenatal cranial haemorrhage in 47 Pacific Islander infants: is traditional massage the cause? *N.Z. Med. J.*, **102**, 207–10.
135. Gunn, T.R., Mora, J.D. and Becroft, D.M.O. (1988) Congenital hydrocephalus secondary to prenatal intracranial haemorrhage. *Aust. N.Z. J. Obstet. Gynaecol.*, **28**, 197–200.
136. Van Gijn, J. and Wintzen, A.R. (1969) Whiplash injury and subdural haematoma. *Lancet*, **2**, 592.
137. Vance, P.C. (1950) Rupture of surface blood vessels on cerebral hemispheres as a cause of subdural haemorrhage. *Arch. Pathol.*, **61**, 992–1006.
138. Bucy, P.C. (1942) Subdural hematoma. *Ill. Med. J.*, **82**, 300–10.
139. Leonard, C.D., Weil, E. and Scribner, B.H. (1969) Subdural haematoma in patients undergoing haemodialysis. *Lancet*, **2**, 239–40.
140. Del Greco, F. and Krumlovsky, F. (1969) Subdural haematoma in the course of haemodialysis. *Lancet*, **2**, 1009–10.
141. Aronson, S.M. and Okazaki, H. (1963) A study of some factors modifying response of cerebral tissue to subdural hematoma. *J. Neurosurg.*, **20**, 89–93.
142. Cusick, J.F. and Bailey, O.T. (1972) Association of ossified subdural hematomas and a meningioma. *J. Neurosurg.*, **37**, 731–4.
143. Markwalder, T.-M. (1981) Chronic subdural hematomas: a review. *J. Neurosurg.*, **54**, 637–45.
144. Fisher, R.G., Kim, J.K. and Sachs, E. (1958) Complications in posterior fossa due to occipital trauma – their operability. *J. Am. Med. Ass.*, **167**, 176–82.
145. Hashimoto, N., Sakakibara, T., Yamamoto, K. *et al.* (1992) Two fluid-blood density levels in chronic subdural hematoma. *J. Neurosurg.*, **77**, 310–34.
146. Meredith, J.M. and Gish, G.R. (1952) Chronic subdural hematoma in an adult producing marked erosion and perforation of the overlying dura and skull. *J. Neurosurg.*, **9**, 639–43.
147. Locksley, H.B. (1966) Report on the Cooperative Study of Intracranial Aneurysms and Subarachnoid Hemorrhage, Section 5, Part 1. Natural history of subarachnoid hemorrhage, intracranial aneurysms, and arteriovenous malformations. *J. Neurosurg.*, **25**, 219–39.
148. Ellington, E. and Margolis, G. (1969) Block of arachnoid villus by subarachnoid hemorrhage. *Neurosurgery*, **30**, 651–7.
149. Koeppen, A.H.W. and Barron, K.D. (1971) Superficial siderosis of the central nervous system. *J. Neuropathol. Expl Neurol.*, **30**, 448–69.
150. van Gijn, J. (1992) Subdural haemorrhage. *Lancet*, **339**, 653–5.
151. Wolf, P.A., Kannel, W.B. and McGee, D.L. (1986) Prevention of stroke: risk factors, in *Stroke. Pathophysiology. Diagnosis and Management*, (eds H.J.M. Barnett, B.M. Stein, J.P. Mohr *et al.*), Churchill Livingstone, New York, pp. 967–88.
152. Goto, N., Kaneko, M., Hosaka, Y. *et al.* (1980) Primary pontine hemorrhage: clinicopathological correlations. *Stroke*, **11**, 84–90.
153. Yates, P.O. and Hutchinson, E.C. (1961) *Cerebral Infarction: The Role of Stenosis of the Extracranial Cerebral Arteries*. Medical Research Council Special Report 300, London.
154. Russell, D.S. (1954) The pathology of spontaneous intracranial haemorrhage. *Proc. Roy. Soc. Med.*, **47**, 689–704.
155. Dickinson, C.J. and Thomson, A.D. (1960) High blood-pressure and stroke: necropsy study of heart-weight and left ventricle hypertrophy. *Lancet*, **2**, 342–5.
156. Griffiths, J.Q. and Lindauer, M.A. (1944) Increased capillary fragility in hypertension: incidence, complications and treatment. *Am. Heart J.*, **28**, 758–62.
157. Lampert, H. and Müller, W. (1925–6) Bei welchem Druck kommt es zu einer Ruptur der Gehirngefässe? *Frankfurt Pathol.*, **33**, 471.
158. Feigin, I. and Prose, P. (1959) Hypertensive fibrinoid arteritis of the brain and gross cerebral hemorrhage. *Arch. Neurol.*, **11**, 98–110.
159. Charcôt, J.M. (1881) *Clinical Lectures on Senile and Chronic Diseases*, New Sydenham Society, London.
160. Russell, R.W.R. (1963) Observations on intracranial aneurysms. *Brain*, **86**, 425–42.
161. Russell, R.W.R. (1968) Pathogenesis of primary intracerebral hemorrhage, in *Cerebral Vascular Disease. Sixth Conference*, (eds J.F. Toole, R.G. Siekert and J.P. Whisnant), Grune & Stratton, New York, pp. 152–60.
162. Cole, F.M. and Yates, P.O. (1967) The occurrence and significance of intracerebral micro-aneurysms. *J. Pathol. Bacteriol.*, **93**, 393–411.
163. Cole, F.M. and Yates, P.O. (1967) Intracerebral microaneurysms and small cerebrovascular lesions. *Brain*, **90**, 759–68.
164. Fisher, C.M. (1972) Cerebral miliary aneurysms in hypertension. *Am. J. Pathol.*, **66**, 313–30.
165. Rosenblum, W.I. (1979) Miliary aneurysms and 'fibrinoid' degeneration of cerebral blood vessels. *Human Pathol.*, **8**, 133–9.
166. Challa, V.R., Moody, D.M. and Bell, M.A. (1992) The Charcôt–Bouchard aneurysm controversy: impact of a new histologic technique. *J. Neuropathol. Expl Neurol.*, **51**, 264–71.
167. Jamieson, K.G. and Yellart, J.D.N. (1972) Traumatic intracerebral hematoma. Report of 63 surgically treated cases. *J. Neurosurg.*, **37**, 528–32.
168. Caplan, L. (1988) Intracerebral hemorrhage revisited. *Neurology*, **38**, 624–7.
169. Attwater, H.L. (1911) Pontine haemorrhages. *Guy's Hosp. Rep.*, **65**, 339–89.
170. Dill, J.V. and Isenhour, CE. (1939) Etiologic factors in experimentally produced pontile hemorrhages. *Arch. Neurol. Psychiat.*, **41**, 1146–52.
171. Dott, N. and Blackwood, W. (1951) Communication to the Society of British Surgeons. Cited by Johnson and Yates [128].
172. Gadmundsson, G., Hallgrimsson, J., Jonasson, T.A. *et al.* (1972) Hereditary cerebral haemorrhage with amyloidosis. *Brain*, **95**, 387–404.
173. Watterndorff, A.R., Bots, G.Th.A.M., Went, L.N. *et al.* (1982) Familial cerebral amyloid angiopathy presenting as recurrent cerebral haemorrhage. *J. Neurol. Sci.*, **55**, 121–35.
174. Okayama, M., Goto, I., Omea, T. *et al.* (1978) Primary amyloidosis with familial vitreous opacities. *Arch. Int. Med.*, **138**, 105–11.
175. Goren, H., Steinberg, M.C. and Farboody, G.H. (1980) Familial oculoleptomeningeal amyloidosis. *Brain*, **103**, 473–95.
176. Gilles, C., Brucher, J.M., Khoubesserian, P. *et al.* (1984) Cerebral amyloid angiopathy as a cause of multiple intracerebal hemorrhages. *Neurology*, **34**, 730–5.
177. Vinters, H.V. (1987) Cerebral amyloid angiopathy. A critical review. *Stroke*, **18**, 311–24.
178. Caplan, L.R. (1992) Intracerebral haemorrhage. *Lancet*, **339**, 656–8.
179. Mandybur, T.I. and Bates, S.R.D. (1978) Fatal massive intracerebral hemorrhage complicating cerebral amyloid angiopathy. *Arch. Neurol.*, **35**, 246–8.
180. Lee, S.-S. and Stemmermann, G.N. (1978) Congophilic angiopathy and cerebral hemorrhage. *Arch. Pathol. Lab. Med.*, **102**, 317–21.
181. Okazaki, H., Reagan, T.J. and Campbell, R.J. (1979) Clinicopathological studies of primary cerebral amyloid angiopathy. *Mayo Clin. Proc.*, **54**, 22–31.
182. Kalyan-Ramam, U.P. and Kalyan-Raman, K. (1984) Cerebral amyloid angiopathy causing intracranial hemorrhage. *Ann. Neurol.*, **16**, 321–9.
183. Ishihara, T., Takahashi, M., Yokota, T. *et al.* (1991) The significance of cerebrovascular amyloid in the aetiology of superficial (lobar) cerebral haemorrhage and its incidence in the elderly population. *J. Pathol.*, **165**, 229–34.
184. Leblanc, R., Haddad, G. and Robitaille, Y. (1992) Cerebral hemorrhage from amyloid angiopathy and coronary thrombolysis. *Neurosurgery*, **31**, 586–90.
185. Mandybur, T.I. (1979) Cerebral amyloid angiopathy possible relationship to rheumatoid vasculitis. *Neurology*, **29**, 1336–40.
186. Lampert, P. (1958) Tumor forming atypical amyloidosis of the choroid plexus with invasion of the cerebral white matter. *J. Neuropathol. Expl Neurol.*, **17**, 604–11.
187. Dayan, A.D. (1971) Comparative neuropathology of ageing. Studies on the brains of 47 species of vertebrates. *Brain*, **94**, 31–42.
188. Toole, J.F. (1990) *Cerebrovascular Disorders*, 4th edn, Raven Press, New York, p. 425.
189. Kieburtz, K., Ricotta, J.J. and Moxley, R.T. (1990) Seizures following carotid endarterectomy. *Arch. Neurol.*, **47**, 568–70.
190. Messert, B. and Black, J.A. (1978) Cluster headache, hemicrania, and other head pains: morbidity of carotid endarterectomy. *Stroke*, **9**, 559–69.
191. Piepgras, D.G., Morgan, M.K., Sundt, T.M. *et al.* (1988) Intracerebral hemorrhage after carotid endarterectomy. *J. Neurosurg.*, **68**, 532–6.
192. Pomposelli, F.B., Lamparello, P.J., Riles, T.S. *et al.* (1988) Intracranial hemorrhage after carotid endarterectomy. *J. Vasc. Surg.*, **7**, 248–55.
193. Caplan, L.R., Skillman, J., Ojemann, R. *et al.* (1978) Intracranial hemorrhage following carotid endarterectomy: a hypertensive complication?

Stroke, **9**, 457–60.
194. Kase, C.S., Robinson, R.K., Stein, R.W. *et al.* (1985) Anticoagulant-related intracerebral hemorrhage. *Neurology*, **35**, 943–8.
195. Byrom, F.B. (1969) *The Hypertensive Vascular Crisis. An Experimental Study*, Heinemann, London.
196. Stehbens, W.E. (1983) The pathology of intracranial aneurysms and their complications, vol. 1, in *Intracranial Aneurysms: A Text and Atlas*, (ed. J.L. Fox), Springer-Verlag, New York, pp. 272–357.
197. Levine, S.R. and Welch, K.M.A. (1987) Cocaine and stroke. *Stroke*, **22**, 25–30.
198. Cole, A.J., Aubé, M. (1987) Late-onset migraine with intracerebral hemorrhage: a recognizable syndrome. *Neurology*, **37**, 238.
199. Slager, U.T. and Wagner, J.A. (1956) The incidence, composition, and pathological significance of intracerebral vascular deposits in basal ganglia. *J. Neuropathol. Expl Neurol.*, **15**, 417–31.
200. Strassman, R. (1949) Iron and calcium deposits in the brain; their significance. *J. Neuropathol. Expl Neurol.*, **8**, 428–35.
201. Norman, R.M. and Urich, H. (1960) The influence of a vascular factor on the distribution of symmetrical cerebral calcification. *J. Neurol. Neurosurg. Psychiat.*, **23**, 142–7.
202. Bronsky, D., Kushner, D.S., Dubin, A. *et al.* (1958) Idiopathic hypoparathyroidism and pseudohypoparathyroidism: case reports and review of the literature. *Medicine*, **37**, 317–52.
203. Adachi, M., Wellmann, K.F. and Volk, B.W. (1968) Histochemical studies on the pathogenesis of idiopathic non-arteriosclerotic cerebral calcification. *J. Neuropathol. Expl Neurol.*, **27**, 483–99.
204. Friede, R.L., Magee, K.R. and Mack, E.W. (1961) Idiopathic nonarteriosclerotic calcification of cerebral vessels. *Arch. Neurol.*, **5**, 279–86.
205. Freyhan, F.A., Woodford, R.B. and Kety, S.S. (1951) Cerebral blood flow and metabolism in psychoses of senility. *J. Nerv. Ment. Dis.*, **113**, 449–56.
206. Sokoloff, L. (1959) Circulation and metabolism of brain in relation to the process of aging, in *The Process of Aging in the Nervous System*, (eds J.E. Birren, H.A. Imus and W.F. Windle), Blackwell Scientific Publ., Oxford, pp. 113–26.
207. Loeb, C., Gandolfo, C., Croce, R. *et al.* (1992) Dementia associated with lacunar infarction. *Stroke*, **23**, 1225–9.
208. Fisher, C.M. (1989) Binswanger's encephalopathy: a review. *J. Neurol.*, **236**, 65–79.
209. Hachinski, V.C., Potter, P. and Merskey, H. (1987) Leuko-araiosus. *Arch. Neurol.*, **44**, 21–3.

13 DISEASES OF THE VEINS AND LYMPHATIC VESSELS, INCLUDING ANGIODYSPLASIA

Hans Jörg Leu and J.T. Lie

13.1 Venous malformations

Vascular malformations (angiodysplasia) are congenital disorders involving arteries, veins and sometimes capillaries and lymphatics. They are believed to develop during early embryonic life and they are of uncertain etiology. Few vascular malformations affect veins only and a number of venous malformations include arteriovenous shunts that may be demonstrated histologically but not by clinical means. The distinction between venular and capillary malformations is often blurred and many hemangiomas involve capillaries, venules, veins and arteries and may be associated with arteriovenous shunts. Even the distinction between true vascular neoplasms and hamartomas or congenital malformations may be difficult.

13.1.1 ETIOLOGY

The etiology of vascular malformations is controversial. The importance of exogenous influences during the early embryonic life, especially of viral infections [1], toxic substances, drugs and trauma, has been emphasized. Hereditary factors are at times implicated in certain types of vascular malformations [2–6] and familial occurrence has also been described occasionally [7–9]. Some systemic malformations with vascular involvement such as the Louis-Bar [10], Hippel–Lindau, Rendu–Osler, Sturge–Weber and Krabbe syndromes [2] and the so-called blue rubber bleb syndrome are clearly inherited disorders. Hereditary factors are also of major importance in lymphatic vessel malformations. Congenital hypoplasia of superficial lymph collectors (the cause of primary lymphedema) is definitely a familial disorder.

13.1.2 PATHOGENESIS

In spite of the variable clinical manifestations and gross anatomic features, the histopathology is somewhat more uniform, with changes that can be identified as agenesis, aplasia, hypoplasia, hyperplasia and dysplasia. In addition to the structural malformation, secondary degenerative alterations may develop with increasing age. All the known varieties of vascular malformations may be attributed to one or more of the above five basic categories. In the embryo, angiogenesis in the extremity occurs on days 27–29. During the second month the vascular system becomes differentiated into arteries and veins. Their finite wall structure, however, is not established before 4½ months [11]. The stage of embryonic development at which the exogenous influence occurs may determine the type and severity of the malformation. The suggestion that the later period of embryonic life is more vulnerable to exogenous influences [12] seems highly questionable. It is well known that the likelihood of developing a malformation from exposure to rubeola infection and drug toxicity decreases in late embryonic life.

13.1.3 HISTOPATHOLOGY

Although the variable gross anatomy of vascular malformations may be quite obvious, the histopathological differences are more subtle. Differences between hypoplasia and hyperplasia of the vessel wall musculature, and the amount and distribution of collagen and elastic fibers, frequently admix with secondary age-related degenerative changes such as atrophy, fibrosis and aneurysm formation. Hemorrhage due to aneurysmal rupture is a serious complication, especially in cerebral hemangiomas. In venous malformations, another common feature is the formation of thrombi and their later calcification into so-called phleboliths. In arteriovenous shunts the venous segment may show a reactive hyperplasia of the smooth muscle and elastic tissue (so-called 'arterialization' of veins). In later stages, the venous wall undergoes degenerative changes such as medial and intimal fibrosis and aneurysm formation. Dysplastic vessels are characterized by irregular development of the

Vascular Pathology. Edited by W.E. Stehbens and J.T. Lie. Published in 1995 by Chapman & Hall, London. ISBN 0 412 48640 7

Table 13.1 Classification of vascular malformations (angiodysplasias) according to the group characteristics (Hamburg classification)*

Species	Forms	
	Truncular	Extratruncular
Predominantly arterial defects	Aplasia or obstruction Dilatation	Angiomatous form
Predominantly venous defects	Aplasia or obstruction Dilatation	Infiltrating form Angiomatous form
Predominantly A–V shuntings	Deep fistulae Superficial fistulae	Infiltrating form Angiomatous form
Combined vascular defects	Arterial and venous Angiolymphatic	Angiolymphatic form Angiomatous form

*Source: Belov et al. [20].

smooth musculature, by the oblique and interwoven course of the muscle bundles in the media, rudimentary development, fragmentation, or duplication of the elastic lamellae in the vessel walls.

13.1.4 CLASSIFICATION OF VASCULAR MALFORMATIONS

Numerous attempts have been made to classify the vascular malformations [13–24] and none is satisfactory or universally accepted. Most of the suggested classifications employ a plethora of terminology with tacit assumption of embryogenesis, resulting in more confusion than clarification. Although many of the eponymic syndromes bearing proper names are generally recognized, they are often differently defined and interpreted. It is probably preferable to provide a descriptive classification of the morphological alterations of blood vessels as the diagnosis, which may be lumped (Table 13.1) [20], or split (Table 13.2) [24], according to the individual's preference.

13.1.5 TYPES OF VENOUS MALFORMATIONS

(a) Malformations of large veins

Such malformations involve agenesis, aplasia and hypoplasia of large veins as well as persistence of embryonic veins that normally undergo regression before birth. Many of these conditions are asymptomatic because functionally sufficient collaterals have been developed. Stenoses and ectasias, however, may have hemodynamic consequences such as venous stasis and/or thrombus formation.

The following malformations of large veins have been described [25]:

1. *Venae cavae* Abnormal junctions of the superior vena cava with the coronary sinus, the pulmonary vein or the portal vein with subsequent aplasia of the original trunk; anomalies of the inferior vena cava such as agenesis or aplasia with development of a collateral circulation.
2. *Pulmonary veins* Various formations of a common trunk of the superior pulmonary veins or inferior pulmonary veins; abnormal junction with the left anonymous vein, the right atrium or the superior vena cava; junction of the right pulmonary vein with the superior vena cava combined with dextroposition of the heart and hypoplasia of the right lung (scimitar syndrome).

Table 13.2 Classification of vascular malformations (angiodysplasias)

Species	Forms
Arterial malformations	Fibromuscular dysplasia Coarctation Kinking Arteriomegaly Congenital aneurysms
Arteriovenous shunts	Isolated or systemic Macro- or microshunts Arteriovenous hemangiomas
Venous malformations	Dysplasia Phleboectasia Atretic, hypoplastic or malformed valves
Venocapillary malformations/angiomas	
Venolymphatic malformations/angiomas	
Lymphatic malformations	Hypoplasia of prefascial collectors Lymphangiomas or lymphangiectasias Lymphangiomyomatosis
Miscellaneous angiodysplasias with systemic involvements	Klippel–Trenaunay syndrome Servelle–Martorell syndrome Von Hippel–Lindau syndrome Sturge–Weber–Krabbe syndrome Rendu–Osler–Weber syndrome Angioneurofibromatosis

3. *Subclavian and axillary veins* Abnormal course of the subclavian vein through the anterior scalenic space; abnormal course or development of the vena basilica, vena cephalica and vena axillaris.
4. *Pelvic and leg veins* Agenesis and duplication of the femoral and popliteal veins [26]; persistence of the femoropopliteal vein (communication between the great saphenous vein and the femoral vein); persistence of the vena marginalis lateralis [27]; aplasia of the short saphenous vein with formation of dilated and enlarged collaterals along the sural nerve [28]; junction varieties of the main superficial leg veins with the great saphenous and the femoral vein [29]; aplasia and hypoplasia of the deep leg veins and the pelvic veins (frequently combined with systemic angiodysplasias); multiple phlebectasias of the extremity veins, sometimes combined with similar alterations of intestinal, scrotal and intraosseous veins; penetration of inguinal lymph nodes by the great saphenous vein [30].

(b) **Aplasia and hypoplasia of valves in deep leg veins [31]**

The valves may be absent or rudimentary, decreased in number or merely functionally incompetent. Both genders are about equally affected [32], and the disorder may be familial [33,34]. The patients are frequently tall, slender and even of the arachnoid body type. The resulting venous reflux is often followed by the development of secondary chronic venous insufficiency (incompetence of perforating veins, stasis edema, dilation of superficial veins, trophic skin changes). The onset of symptoms is usually around puberty. Retraction, deformation and fibrosis of the valves are the typical histopathologic findings.

(c) **Venous aneurysms**

Isolated venous aneurysms are rare. Aneurysms of non-varicose veins have been described in the terminal segments of the greater and lesser saphenous veins, axillary veins, superior vena cava, jugular veins, femoral veins, popliteal veins, azygos veins, pulmonary veins and veins of the musculus soleus [35].

(d) **Diffuse phlebectasia of Bockenheimer [36]**

This generalized phlebectatic disorder involves deep, superficial and perforating veins of one or more limbs with a predilection for the upper extremities. It is characterized by progressive atrophy of the elastic and muscular wall elements. Arteriovenous shunts are believed to be absent [37]. The majority of patients are female, between 10 and 50 years of age [37]. Phlebography shows segmental ectasia, cavernous venous plexus and phleboliths. The condition is not apparent at birth; it usually manifests itself during puberty or pregnancy.

(e) **Miscellaneous types of phlebectasia**

Other types of localized phlebectasias may present as varicocele or as spinal varicosities. Rare types of more or less systemic phlebectasias have been described involving the bone [38], jejunum, oral cavity and scrotum [39] and as cystic venous angiomatosis [40].

(f) **Venous hemangiomas**

Venous hemangiomas consist of glomus-like clusters of dysplastic veins of different size and shape. They occur subcutaneously in striated muscles, orbits, the brain and, occasionally, in bones. The majority represent congenital malformations [41]. True hemangiomatous neoplasms exist. They contain no differentiated blood vessels but instead they consist of proliferating capillaries in the interstitium – so-called hemangioreticuloma of von Albertini [42].

Morphologically, hemangiomatous malformations are characterized by interwoven and obliquely arranged smooth muscle bundles with various degrees of medial and intimal fibrosis. The elastic lamellae may be absent or rudimentary and the vessel lumens may be occluded by fresh, organized or calcified thrombi (phleboliths). Secondary degenerative lesions may be superimposed. If an arteriovenous shunt exists, the venous walls may be thickened by hyperplasias of smooth muscle and elastic fibers ('arterialized' veins). Ectasia and aneurysm formation are the common sequelae.

Hemangiomas are a frequent feature of systemic vascular malformations often associated with arteriovenous communication. Arteriovenous microshunts can be confirmed only by histological examination of serial sections, and several types of arteriovenous communication may be distinguished:

- small dysplastic arteries terminating into fan-like capillaries
- angiomatoid plexus consisting of ectatic capillaries or venules
- cavernous angiomas draining directly into larger dysplastic veins [43].

Ultrastructurally the endothelial lining of hemangiomas is interrupted by denuded areas and the basement membrane is inconspicuous. Around the capillaries, Schwann cells and sheathless or sheath-containing nerve fibers frequently appear. On denuded areas of the endothelial layer, platelet aggregations may occur and a pericapillary edema exists [44]. Sclerosing hemangiomas are characterized by collagen deposition, fibrosis and obliteration of vascular lumens.

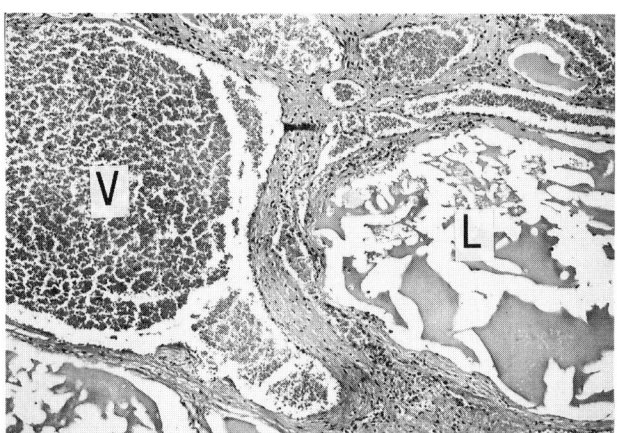

Figure 13.1 Hemangiolymphangioma, consisting of venous cavern (V) with erythrocytes and lymphatic cavern (L) with lymph and lymphocytes. (H&E.)

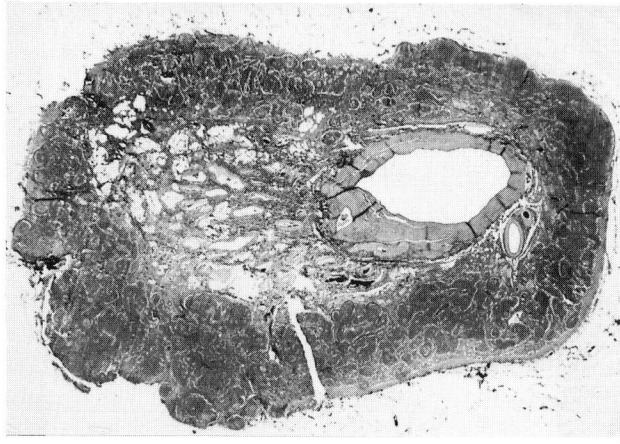

Figure 13.2 Angiodysplasia: penetration of an inguinal lymph node by the saphenous vein. (H&E.)

(g) Hemangiolymphangioma (Figure 13.1)

The structure consists of a mixture of veins, capillaries and lymphatic vessels. The latter are ectatic or cystic. Ultrastructurally lymphatic vessels may be recognized by flat endothelial cells with short, oblique intercellular spaces, absent or interrupted basement membrane and exterior attachment fibers. The vessel lumens contain lymphatic fluid with some lymphocytes.

(h) Systemic angiodysplasias of predominantly venous types

Systemic angiodysplasias are malformations derived from both mesoderm and neuroectoderm. Several major varieties are recognized (Figures 13.2–13.7).

Klippel–Trenaunay syndrome

Klippel–Trenaunay syndrome is characterized by the triad of:

- hemihypertrophy of soft tissue and bone
- varicose veins
- port-wine stains and/or hemangiomas.

The development of hemihypertrophy is believed to be due to the existence of arteriovenous microshunts in the epiphyseal area of the long bones resulting in an increased oxygen supply. Apart from elongation and enlargement of the long bones, syndactylia is a frequent feature. The port-wine stains are simple telangiectasias of cutaneous capillaries. They may be of metameric extent. The hemangiomas are of the cavernous capillary or venous type, or a combination of both. Arteriovenous shunts occur more frequently than is generally recognized. The malformations of larger veins may consist of ectasia, agenesis, aplasia or hypoplasia, persistence of embryonic veins (e.g. the vena marginalis lateralis), absence or deformity of venous valves, varicosities, and

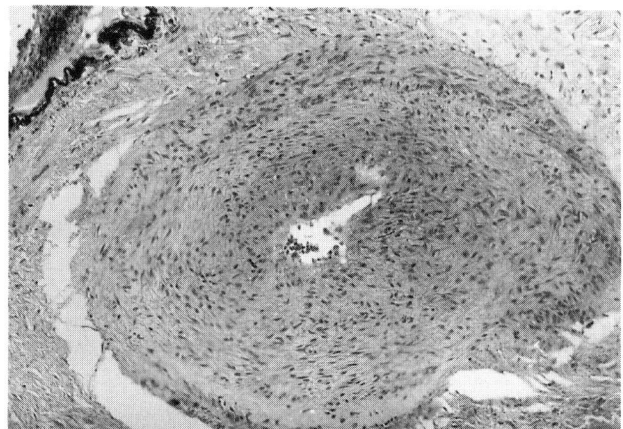

Figure 13.3 Systemic angiodysplasia, type Klippel–Trenaunay: dysplastic artery without elastic fibers or membranes. (Elastic stain.)

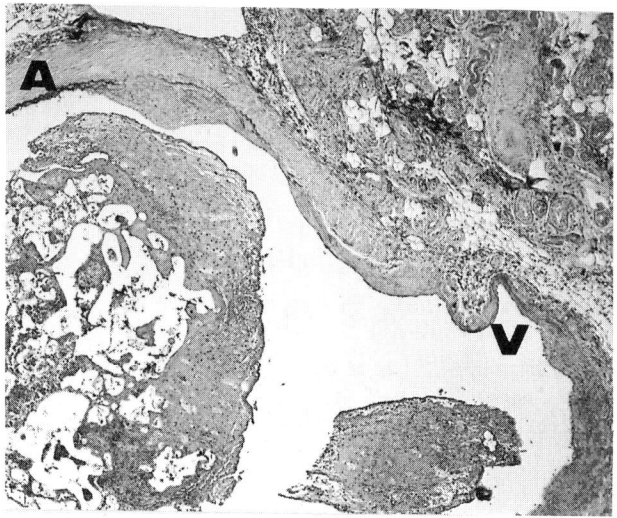

Figure 13.4 Systemic angiodysplasia, type Parkes–Weber. Direct shunt between an artery (A) and a vein (V). (Elastic stain.)

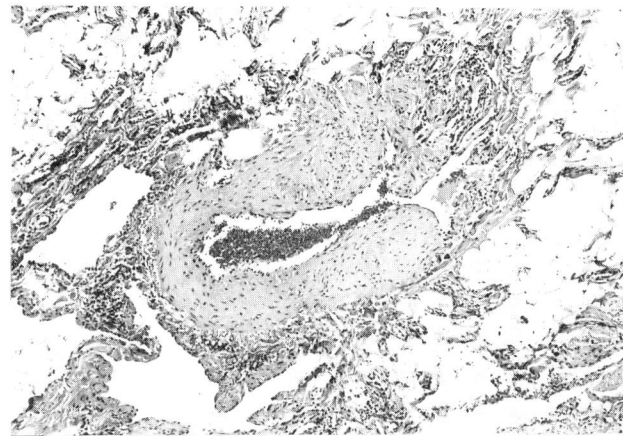

Figure 13.5 Systemic angiodysplasia, type Klippel–Trenaunay with multiple A–V microshunts. A small artery in connection with several fan-like capillaries. (H&E.)

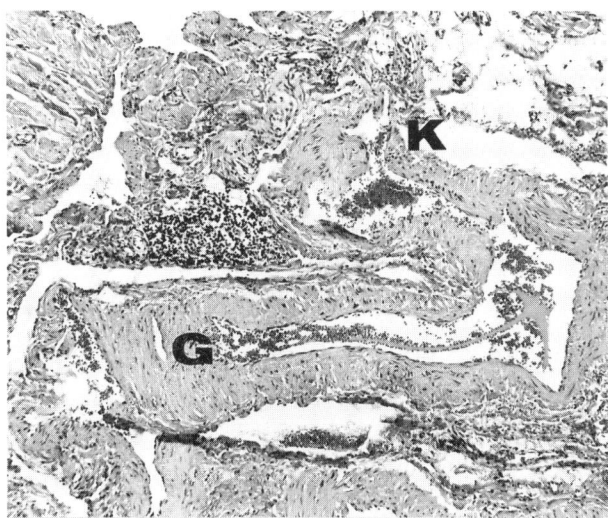

Figure 13.6 Systemic angiodysplasia, type Klippel–Trenaunay. Arterial vessel (G) in connection with cavernous spaces (K). (H&E.)

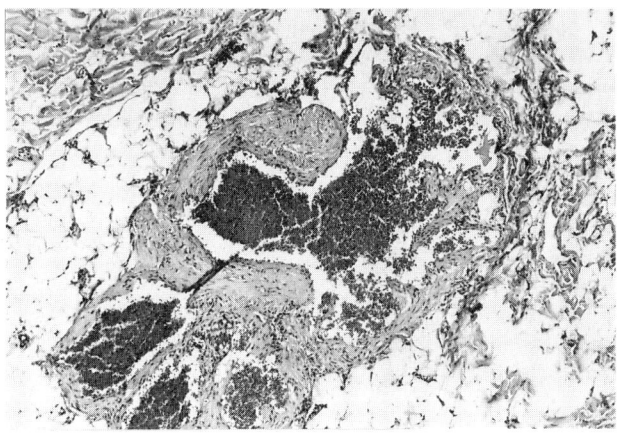

Figure 13.7 Systemic angiodysplasia, type Klippel–Trenaunay. Small artery opening into a thin-walled venous channel. (H&E.)

incompetent perforating veins [44,45]. The latter are responsible for the final development of trophic skin lesions. Anomalies of the lymphatic vessels (hypo- and hyperplasia of lymph collectors, lymphatic cysts) may occur in addition.

Parkes–Weber syndrome

This is a variant of Klippel–Trenaunay syndrome with additional large-vessel arteriovenous communications [45].

Servelle–Martorell syndrome

In this condition the hemihypertrophy is replaced by a hemihypoplasia involving skeletal and soft tissue. Venous hemangiomas are preferentially localized in the knee area including the knee joint and bones of the lower leg.

In various other systemic malformations such as the syndrome of Louis–Bar (cerebellar leptomeninx); of Sturge–Weber, Krabbe and of Hippel–Lindau (brain, retina, leptomeninx); of Maffucci (dyschondroplasia or enchondromatosis and hemangiomatosis of the upper or lower extremities), the venous hemangiomas are only a minor part of the systemic malformation.

13.2 Degenerative venous diseases

13.2.1 PHLEBOSCLEROSIS (Figures 13.8–13.11)

Phlebosclerosis is a common alteration of non-varicose and varicose veins. Both genders are equally affected. In non-varicose veins its incidence increases with age and to a variable degree. The intimal fibrosis of superficial leg veins may have begun under the age of 20. In our own experience, 60% of all subjects are affected by intimal sclerosis, with moderate to severe degrees increasing from 6% in the under-40 age group to 34% in subjects between 61 and 90 years; 33% of all subjects have a moderate to severe phlebosclerosis of the media [46]. Phlebosclerosis is found with equal prevalence in all the segments of the long saphenous vein and also in the smaller superficial vein branches. Intimal fibrosis predominates over medial and adventitial fibrosis and is more conspicuous in the superficial than in the deep leg veins. The deep leg veins may show slight degrees of intimal, medial and adventitial fibrosis, but extensive alterations are seldom observed. In deep leg veins that are adjacent to arteries with severe atherosclerosis, marked intimal proliferation may be observed, usually secondary to organized thrombus [46].

Phlebosclerosis should probably be considered as a physiological rather than pathological process because it occurs in the majority of the aging population without causing symptoms. In certain instances, phlebosclerotic

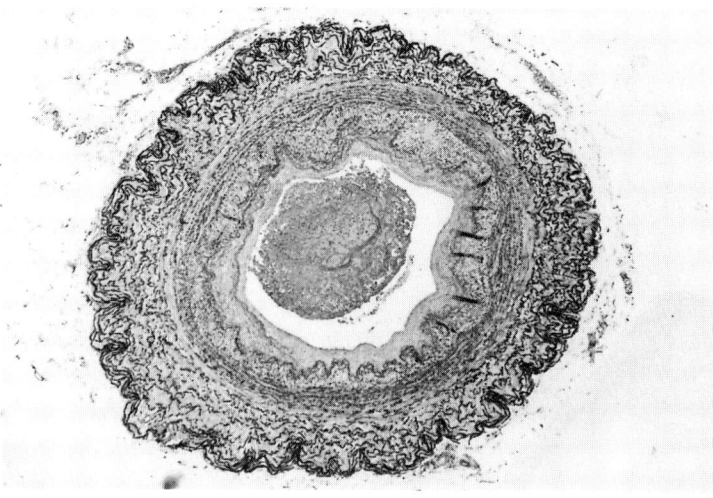

Figure 13.8 Primary intimal phlebosclerosis in a non-varicose vein. (Elastic stain.)

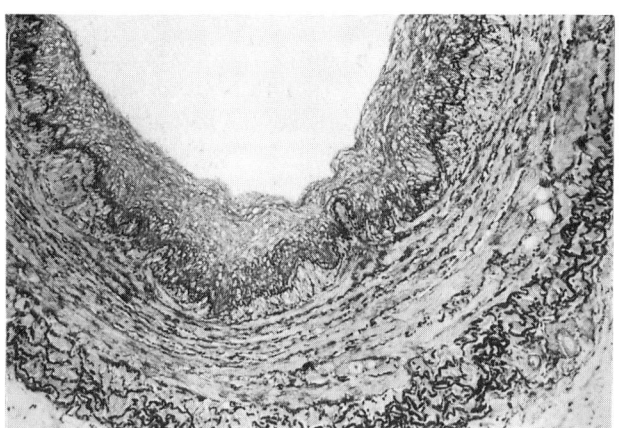

Figure 13.9 Primary intimal phlebosclerosis in an infant of 2 years. (Elastic stain.)

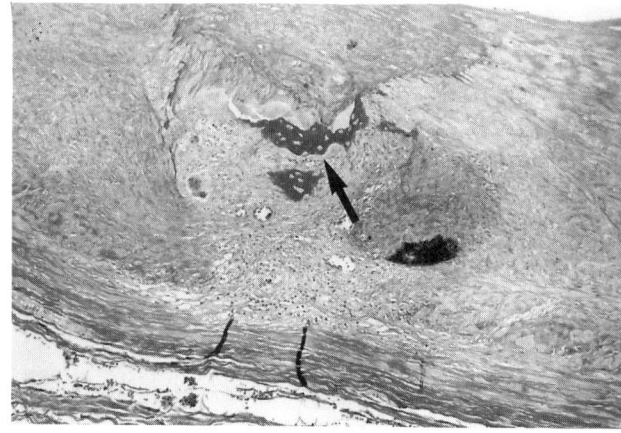

Figure 13.11 Ossification (arrowed) in the wall of a sclerotic deep lower leg vein. (Van Gieson stain.)

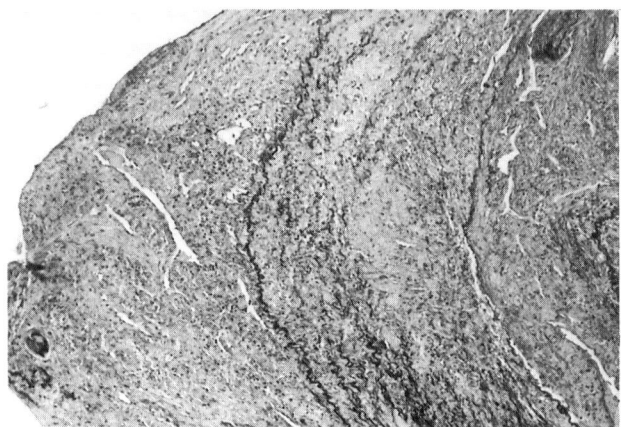

Figure 13.10 Venous spur in the left iliac vein. Intimal proliferation with neoformation of elastic fibers and intimal capillaries (organized thrombotic appositions). (Elastic stain.)

alterations may have some clinical significance. Intimal sclerosis predisposes the deep leg veins to thrombosis from the combination of endothelial injury and altered laminar flow of the blood. Fibrosis of one or more layers of the vessel wall may reduce the maximum blood storage capacity of the superficial leg veins and impede reflexive vasoconstriction.

The venous valves are usually not affected in phlebosclerosis unless they, independently, have been altered by thrombosis or are congenitally deformed. In the normal population or in patients with primary varicose veins affected by phlebosclerosis we did not detect fibrotic alterations of the venous valves [46]

Phlebosclerosis occurs commonly in varicose veins but phlebosclerosis is not a prerequisite of varicosity. Even advanced cases of varicose veins may remain relatively unaffected by phlebosclerosis. Milder degrees of varicosity with tortuosity, ectasia and alternating hypertrophy/atrophy of the smooth muscles are not more frequently affected by phlebosclerosis (intimal fibrosis in 37%, medial fibrosis in 36%) than normal veins [47]. Atrophic wall segments are often more severely affected by phlebosclerosis than segments with hypertrophic musculature. Thus, phlebosclerosis is not a cause of varicose veins, but varicosity may enhance the development of phlebosclerosis [48], and there is no direct correlation between arteriosclerosis and phlebosclerosis of the companion arteries and veins, respectively [49]. Clinically, calcification of superficial veins and the adjacent subcutaneous tissue may result in the formation of leg ulcers with limited healing capacity [50,51]. Even ossification may occur in the walls of superficial and deep leg veins with longstanding varicosity and advanced phlebosclerosis [52].

13.2.2 SECONDARY PHLEBOSCLEROSIS

Fibrous thickening of the intima and diffuse or plaque-like fibrosis of the media/adventitia are common sequelae of thrombotic events or postinflammatory repair process. This secondary fibrosis should be distinguished from primary phlebosclerosis. Intimal fibrosis of organized thrombus usually shows distinct vascularization and the postinflammatory medial scar tissue is often associated with focal destruction of the internal elastic lamella.

13.2.3 VENOUS SPUR

The term 'venous spur' refers to a half moon-shaped fibrotic intimal apposition plaque in the left common iliac vein due to external pressure by the impinging right common iliac artery [53] or the promontorium [54]. Histologically, the spur-like intimal cushion contains newly formed and duplicated elastic fibers. Similar to the situation in the so-called popliteal entrapment syndrome, impingement of the lumen causes hemodynamic alterations. Both of these factors (external pressure and hemodynamic alterations) predispose to recurrent thrombosis. This may explain the prevalence of left-sided thrombosis of the iliac and common femoral vein [53,55].

13.2.4 VARICOSE VEINS (Figures 13.12–13.18)

(a) Etiology and epidemiology

The etiology of primary varicose veins is unknown. Epidemiological investigations [56] show that age is the main risk factor: 20% of the subjects around 20 years and 80% of those around 60 years are affected by varicose veins. Race and habitual posture at work have little bearing on the incidence. Gender, hereditary factors, obesity, number of pregnancies, abortions, age

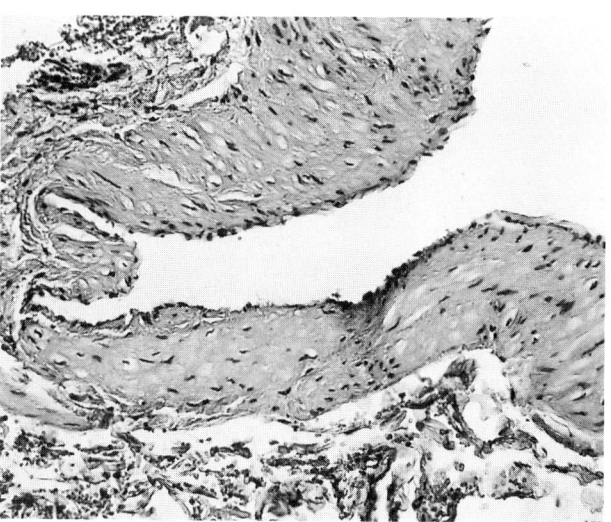

Figure 13.12 Varicose vein with alternating atrophy and hypertrophy of the media musculature. (H&E.)

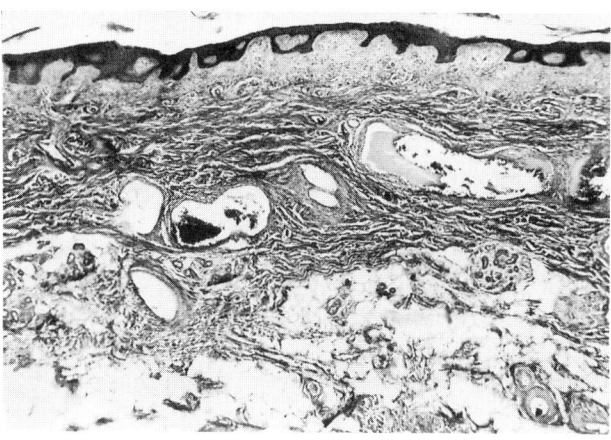

Figure 13.13 Chronic venous insufficiency: lipodermatosclerosis and dilation of superficial vein branches. (Van Gieson stain.)

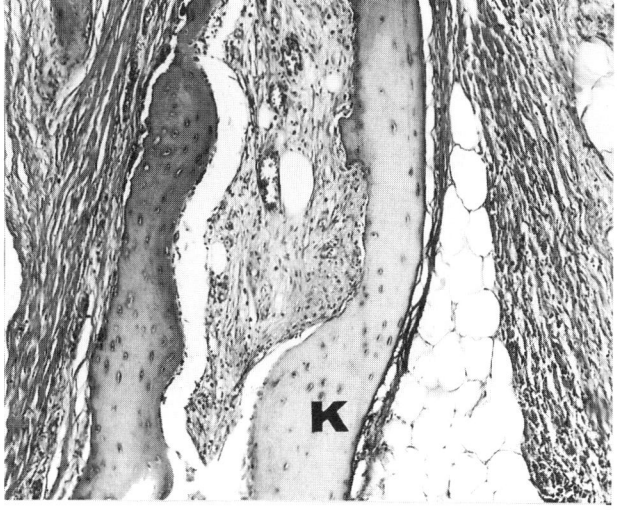

Figure 13.14 Ossification (K) in fibrous subcutaneous plaque in chronic venous insufficiency. (H&E.)

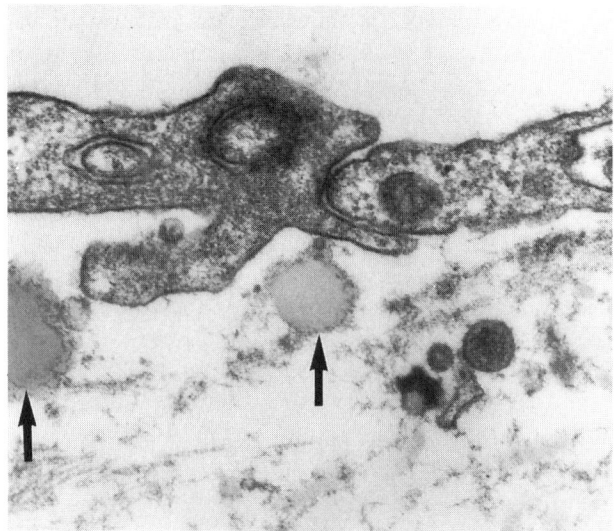

Figure 13.15 Electron micrograph of pericapillary space in chronic venous insufficiency (so-called halo) with edema and lipid droplets (arrows) but without traces of fibrin. (Phosphate-buffered glutaradehyde.)

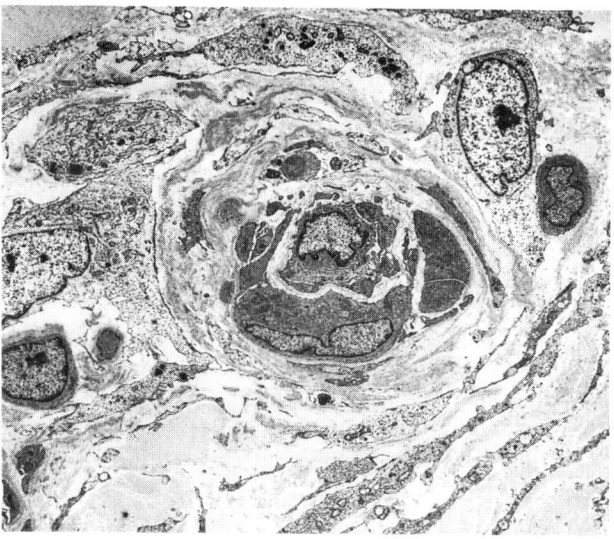

Figure 13.17 Electron micrograph of an obliterated small vessel in chronic venous insufficiency. (Phosphate-buffered glutaraldehyde.)

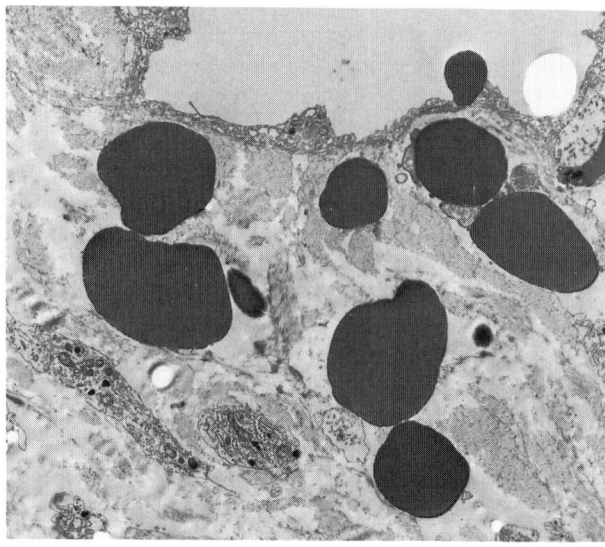

Figure 13.16 Electron micrograph of dilated capillary in chronic venous insufficiency with extravasation of erythrocytes into the edematous pericapillary space. (Phosphate-buffered glutaraldehyde.)

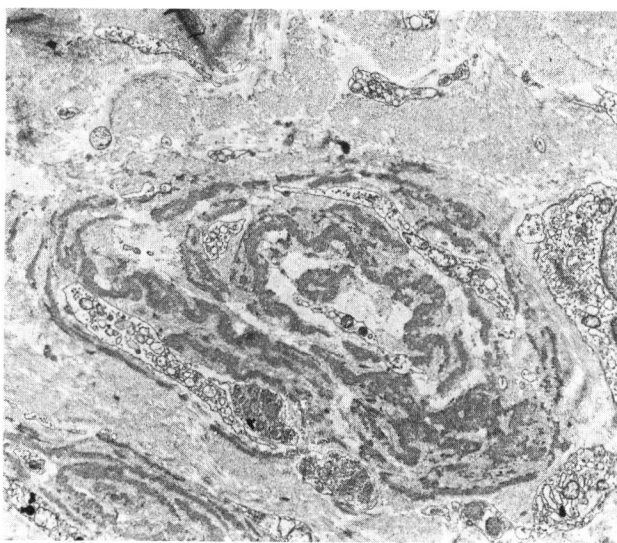

Figure 13.18 Electron micrograph of an obliterated small vessel in chronic venous insufficiency. (Phosphate-buffered glutaraldehyde.)

at menarche, tight dresses, hormonal contraceptives and the anatomically unfavorable reflux conditions in the left iliac vein are important only if two or more of these factors act in synergy. The incidence of varicosities increases at least five-fold, compared with control persons of the same age when two or more risk factors are present [56].

Phlebosclerosis is not a prerequisite of varicose veins but a secondary phenomenon following longstanding varicosity [57–62]. The venous valves are not directly involved in primary varicose veins. A decrease in number of the deep vein valves during lifetime, as believed by some authors [63,64] has not been confirmed by others [33,47,65]. Functional valvular deficiency in varicose veins is secondary to the ectasia of the muscular wall. Metabolic disturbances within the venous wall have also been cited as etiological factors of varicosity [66–68]. Ultrastructural changes of endothelial cells (necrosis and accumulation of Weibel–Palade bodies) and of smooth muscle cells (activation of smooth muscle cells, occurrence of extracellular lysosomes) have been described in varicose veins [69–73], but in all probability these alterations are secondary phenomena. The role of small, congenital arteriovenous shunts as a possible cause of varicose veins has been emphasized [74–76], but radioisotope studies [77,78] have failed to confirm the existence of such shunts.

All the observed morphological alterations such as fibrosis, atrophy of smooth muscles and elastic fibers, valve insufficiency, ectasia and tortuosity are secondary degenerative changes [48,57,58,73,79]. They are indistinguishable from primary phlebosclerosis occurring in non-varicose veins.

Primary varicose veins mainly occur in the lower extremities, i.e. in superficial large and small veins, perforating veins and deep veins of the soleus and gastrocnemius muscles. Varicose veins are unknown in animals. The erect posture with the resulting special functional task of the insufficiently protected superficial leg veins appears to be a predisposing factor of varicosities. Ectatic veins may occur at other sites (upper extremities, thoracic and abdominal wall, head, viscera (esophageal varices) and spinal cord (spinal varicosities), but these alterations are practically always due to congenital malformations or sequelae of post-thrombotic or other wall lesions.

Secondary varicose veins may be due to a variety of disorders: post-thrombotic lesions of the venous wall including the valves; congenital malformations (aplasia of deep veins, decreased number or deformity of deep vein valves, multiple A–V shunts, systemic angiodysplasias, diffuse phlebectasia of Bockenheimer, etc.); singular A–V macroshunts due to injury; hormonal influences such as pregnancy, hormonal contraception, hormone treatments; atrophy of the calf muscles (impairment of the calf muscle pump as part of the venous reflux mechanism) due to palsy, immobility, joint arthrosis and post-traumatic conditions; obstruction of the pelvic reflux by external compression (overlying artery, aneurysms of adjacent arteries, hernia, etc.) or by intramural lesions (tumors, inflammatory-related fibrosis, etc.).

A decrease of the elasticity of the skin in aged subjects has been believed to be an important factor for the development of varicose veins. Recent investigations, however, have shown that this theory is unfounded [80].

(b) Morphology of varicose veins

The early detectable alterations consist of alternating partial hypertrophy and partial atrophy of the media smooth muscles. The hypertrophy might be explained as a functional adaption in order to compensate for a loss of muscle tone. The result is an irregular wall diameter combined with ectasia and tortuosity of the vein. The venous valves are not impaired in primary varicose veins. In secondary varicosities due to post-thrombotic lesions they appear retracted and fibrotic. The elastic fibers (internal elastic lamella and fibers within the media and adventitia) may be inconspicuous and, in later stages, they appear frayed and fragmented. The intima may be normal or fibrotic. By light microscopy, the endothelial lining appears intact. Severe and longstanding varicose veins usually show extensive intimal thickening and, in rare cases, even with deposits of cholesterol/fatty acids and calcifications. The media consists of atrophic smooth muscle, replacement fibrosis and fragmentation of the elastic fibers.

Vascularized intimal cushions may be an indication of a post-thrombotic state and focal destruction of the internal elastic lamella may be a sign of a postinflammatory lesion.

Ultrastructurally, the intima of varicose veins is focally denuded of endothelium or is partially covered by necrotic endothelial cells. The endothelial cells that surround denuded areas or necrotic endothelial cells, contain increased numbers of Weibel–Palade bodies. This might indicate a defense mechanism against thrombocyte aggregations. Indications of an increased endothelial permeability (dilated intercellular spaces, increased pinocytotic activity), however, are not observed [70,72].

Morphology and pathogenesis of trophic skin alterations in chronic venous insufficiency

By chronic venous insufficiency we understand a condition of venous congestion characterized by leg edema and trophic skin lesions. It is due to insufficiency of perforators and/or deep leg veins. Varicosities of superficial veins alone do not induce trophic skin lesions because even in ectatic and tortuous superficial veins the venous reflux is sufficiently mitigated by the competent perforator system, the intact valves in the deep veins and the supporting effect of the calf muscle pump. Only when the perforating vein system alone or in combination with deep vein valve lesions becomes incompetent, are the pressure waves that occur during ambulation partly transferred from the deep into the superficial venous system. The raised intravenous pressure results in a chronic venous congestion in the cutaneous and subcutaneous microvasculature. The elevated intracapillary pressure is responsible for the occurrence of endothelial cell injury.

The morphological findings in chronic venous insufficiency are well known [81,82]. The events leading to the development of trophic skin lesions may be considered an 'injury and repair' phenomenon [81].

The majority of capillaries appear dilated with diameters varying from 50 to 120 µm in comparison with 8 (smallest capillaries) to 50 µm (small venules) [83] under normal conditions. The endothelial layer is flat with a thin, fenestrated or even partially interrupted basement membrane. Ultrastructurally the endothelial cells show an irregular luminal cell surface, with dilated intercellular spaces, formation of gaps and fenestrations, numerous micropinocytotic vesicles and increased numbers of Weibel–Palade bodies. The pericapillary space contains edematous fluid, occasional lipid droplets, erythrocytes (which may be seen passing in bizarre deformation through the dilated intercellular spaces) and erythrocyte fragments. Fibrin is not observed in the pericapillary space, neither free nor ingested by the macrophages. The edema of the pericapillary spaces merges imperceptibly into the denser surrounding tissue. It contains a mixed cellular inflammatory infiltrate consisting of macrophages, lymphocytes, plasma cells and occasional neutrophils, eosinophils and mast cells. The inflammatory infiltrate is pronounced in ulcerated areas where the necrotic tissue contains a predominance of neutrophils intermingled with plasma, fibrin, red blood cells and cellular debris. In the dermal papillae, especially around ulcer-bearing areas, capillaries may appear in glomerulus-like clusters showing elongation, tortuosity, endothelial thickening and occasional obliteration by fibrin-rich thrombi. By immunohistochemical marking of type IV collagen (main component of the basement membrane) a multilayered appearance with an ill-defined, frayed outer surface of the basement membrane may be demonstrated.

These alterations indicate the occurrence of focal infarction followed by fibrous repair. Focal infarcts may coalesce into larger necrotic areas involving the skin and subcutis (crural ulcers). The observation of 'fibrin-cuffs' around capillaries [84,85] is a sequel of tissue necrosis and not a primary alteration [81,86]. Also the so-called 'trapping' of white blood cells (accumulation of white blood cells in the extremity of patients with chronic venous insufficiency) [87,88] is a sign of tissue repair.

13.2.5 AMYLOIDOSIS OF VEINS (Figure 13.19)

Subendothelial deposits of amyloid in the veins may be observed in systemic amyloidosis. The deposits are usually found in the inner layers of the media, directly below the internal elastic lamella. They consist of hyaline circumscript masses, observed mostly in visceral and small pulmonary veins.

13.2.6 LIPOIDOSIS OF VEINS

Lipid deposits in the walls of small veins occur in cases of generalized lipoidosis [89] and do not have clinical consequences.

13.2.7 CYSTIC ADVENTITIAL DEGENERATION IN VEINS (Figure 13.20)

Although the alterations of cystic adventitial degeneration in veins (as well as those in arteries) occur within the vessel walls in the majority of cases, they represent not primary dysplasia of the blood vessels but ectopic mucinous material of a joint capsule or a bursa. They are mentioned here because they may mimic other forms of peripheral vascular disease. In veins the disorder is rare and has few clinical consequences [90–93]. The lesions (arterial and venous) are always found in the proximity of a joint. The adventitia is expanded by cysts containing a mucinous, alcian-blue positive material. The inner surface of the cysts has no cellular lining or is partly covered by one or several layers of cuboid cells with round nuclei and the ultrastructural characteristics of mesothelial cells. The cysts may be connected by a duct with an adjacent joint. Compression of the lumen by the intramural cysts predisposes to thrombosis of the affected artery or vein.

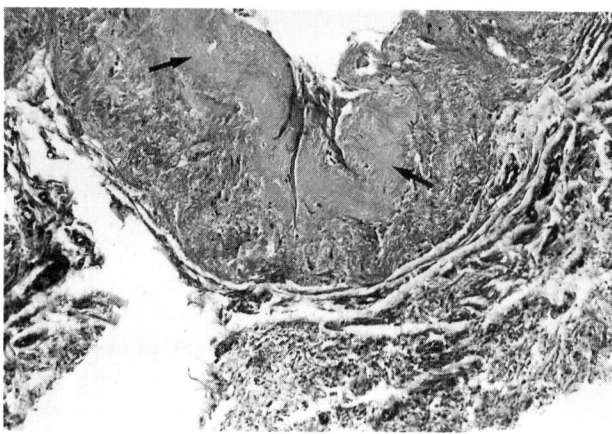

Figure 13.19 Amyloid deposits (arrows) within the wall of a vein. (H&E.)

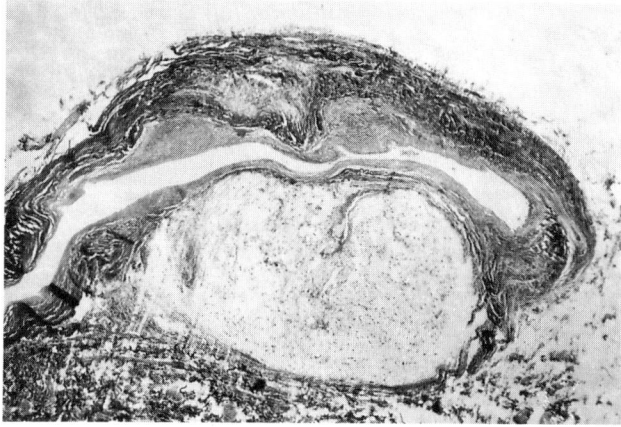

Figure 13.20 Intramural cystic adventitial degeneration (CAD) in a vein. (Van Gieson stain.)

13.3 Circulatory venous disturbances

13.3.1 THROMBOSIS (Figures 13.21–13.26)

(a) Etiology

Three basic factors (Virchow's triad) are responsible for the development of an arterial, venous or capillary thrombosis; namely, coagulation disorders, stasis and vessel wall alterations.

Coagulation disorders

A number of disorders affecting the blood components may be responsible for thrombus formation: hereditary and acquired blood dyscrasias; disorders affecting the coagulation factors only; paraneoplastic hypercoagulable state; diseases affecting number and integrity of red and white blood cells and thrombocytes; factors influencing the aggregation of thrombocytes; and the like.

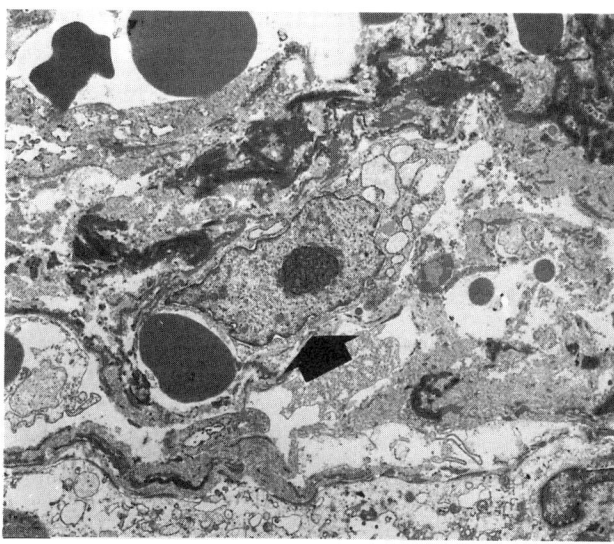

Figure 13.21 Mononuclear cells with differentiation into macrophages within a thrombus containing fibrin, cell debris and deteriorating erythrocytes. (Phosphate-buffered glutaraldehyde.)

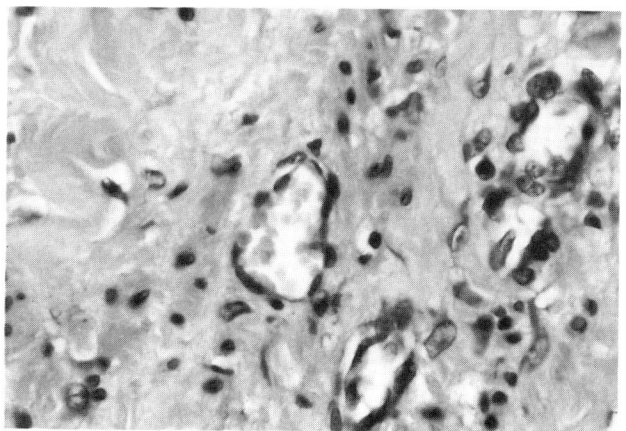

Figure 13.22 Formation of the first primitive capillary channels within the organizing thrombus. (H&E.)

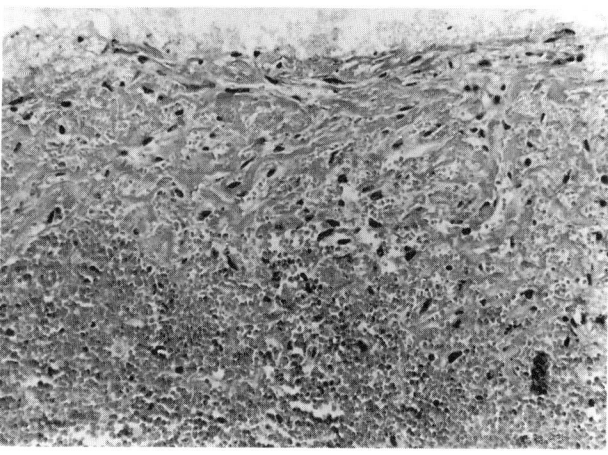

Figure 13.23 Proliferation of fibroblast-like cells in an organizing thrombus. (H&E.)

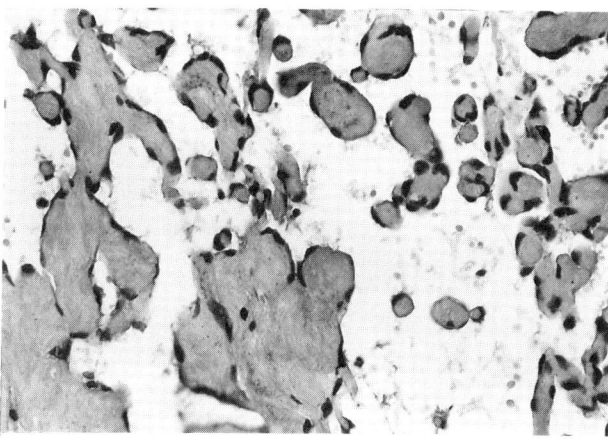

Figure 13.24 Intravascular papillary endothelial hyperplasia: papillary structures consisting of collagen tissue covered by endothelial cells. (H&E.)

Stasis

Blood stasis may be responsible for the development of thrombosis, but as a single factor in an otherwise normal homeostatic milieu, its importance has probably been overestimated. Venous stasis may be due to local alterations such as ectasia (varicose veins) or insufficiency of deep vein valves or to general disorders such as immobilization, and diseases of heart and circulation.

Vessel wall alterations

Injury to the endothelium may be caused by trauma, inflammation, immunologic and degenerative lesions,

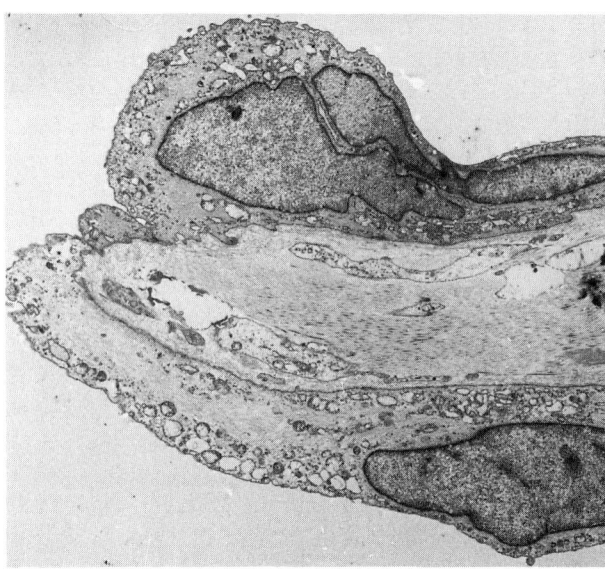

Figure 13.25 Electron micrograph of intravascular papillary endothelial hyperplasia: the endothelial cells still resemble primitive mesenchymal cells, the stromal tissue contains collagen fibers and fibroblasts. (Phosphate-buffered glutaraldehyde.)

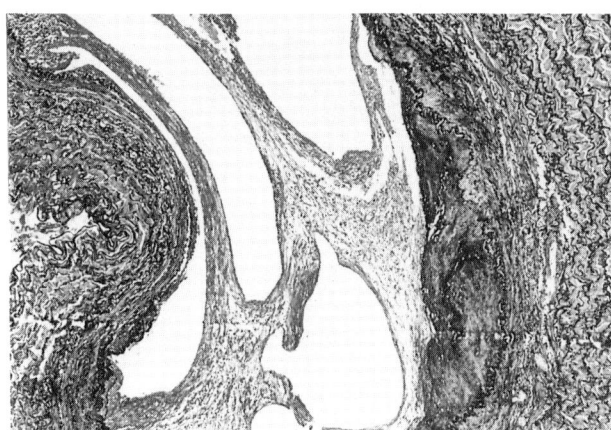

Figure 13.26 Post-thrombotic state: recanalized vein with fibrous septa between the vascular spaces. (Elastic Van Gieson stain.)

harmful effects of chemicals, drugs and hormones, and neoplasms. Alterations of the venous wall may also be induced by perivascular disorders such as scar tissue, tumors, lymphadenopathy, hernia, abscess formation and compression by ligaments or overlying arteries.

(b) Phlebothrombosis and thrombophlebitis

The often used terms 'phlebothrombosis', 'thrombophlebitis', and 'deep thrombophlebitis' are vague and ill-defined. The ordinary thrombosis is not due to a primary inflammation of the wall. The term 'phlebitis' should be reserved for primary inflammatory diseases such as septic phlebitis, migrating phlebitis, etc., accompanied by a secondary thrombosis. It should also be kept in mind that superficial, deep and visceral vein thrombosis all have a similar morphology, natural outcome and potential complications.

(c) Localization of venous thrombosis

Venous thrombi may occur anywhere. Sites of predilection are the pelvic and leg veins. Many investigations have dealt with the question, whether the majority of lower extremity thromboses originate in the iliofemoral or in the calf veins. One study [94] has shown that leg vein thrombosis begins simultaneously at several sites, namely in venous sinuses of the calf and foot and in valve pockets of the femoral vein. Others [95] have demonstrated that 70% of all leg vein thromboses are extended, involving three or four levels, and that left-sided localization predominates. In the evaluation of the statistics on the frequency and site of thrombosis, it must be borne in mind that most of the pelvic vein thrombi remain unrecognized because they do not necessarily cause symptoms and that they are seldom looked for routinely and systematically at autopsy.

(d) Incidence of venous thrombosis

The reported autopsy incidence of venous thrombosis varies from 0 to 40% [96–99], being highest in patients who died from malignancies (40%) [99]. The incidence of postoperative thrombosis has decreased markedly after the introduction of prophylactic measures such as anticoagulation, early mobilization, and compression of the legs by tight bandages or elastic hosiery.

(e) Morphology and course of venous thrombosis

The first platelet aggregates often occur adjacent to endothelial gaps or necrotic endothelial cells. They accumulate crosswise to the flow direction. After degranulation of thrombocytes and fibrin formation, white and red blood cells adhere in a coral rift pattern and form a so-called aggregation thrombus or white thrombus. A rapidly coagulating column of erythrocytes (so-called coagulation thrombus or red thrombus) may be added. Most thrombi are mixed, containing alternating white and red thrombi. The attachment point at the venous wall (thrombus head) is a white thrombus and the additional tail of the thrombus is a red thrombus. Venous thrombosis is a rather uniform process following a pattern which is identical in deep and superficial leg veins, in cerebral veins, in hepatic veins (Budd–Chiari syndrome), and also in secondary thrombosis, e.g. following inflammatory vascular diseases. The main components are always fibrin and blood cells. Between the fibrin network, erythrocytes and white blood cells are present in varying amounts. The fibrin-rich areas contain high amounts of polymorphonuclear leukocytes. Special types of thrombi include hyaline thrombi in capillaries (fibrin-rich thrombi in the renal glomeruli), debris thrombi (by cell debris due to hemolysis), and sludging of erythrocytes occurring in sickle-cell disease.

The fate and organization of thrombi

Venous thrombi are practically always organized by connective tissue. This is performed mainly by cells from the vessel wall which invade the thrombus. However, it has been shown in several *in vivo* experiments that organization also takes place when a contact between thrombus and the endothelium is prevented by insertion of a plastic tube [100–103]. This organization initiates from mononuclear blood cells which are present in every thrombus [104,105] and which multiply by mitosis [106,107], and differentiate into macrophages, endothelial cells, fibroblasts and even smooth muscle cells. The inclusion of fragmented erythrocytes in macrophages has given rise to the theory of vascular tube formation by these cells [108–110]. This seems improbable in view of the short survival time of erythrocytes outside the bloodstream [111,112]. The future endothelial cells derive from primitive mesenchymal cells (mononuclear cells included in the thrombus). This transformation has been confirmed by electron microscopy [100,101,111] including the acquisition of factor VIII and specific organelles such as Weibel–Palade bodies and other characteristics of endothelial cells (multivesicular bodies, micropinocytotic vesicles and a rudimentary basement membrane). They begin to line the crevices within the organizing thrombus matrix until a continuous endothelial layer is established. Other cells differentiate into fibroblasts, which later form collagen fibers and smooth muscle cells [100,101,111].

Estimation of the age of thrombi and emboli

The time period between the onset of blood clotting and complete organization of the thrombus varies according to the type of vessel (artery or vein), size of vessel and condition of the vessel wall (arteriosclerotic or phlebosclerotic plaques impede thrombus organization).

The stepwise organization of a thrombus follows a regular pattern with more or less fixed time intervals. This permits an approximate age determination of thrombi and emboli (Table 13.3). However, it must be remembered that polymorphonuclear leukocytes are sensitive to autolytic processes. Age determination in autopsy material and in biopsy material with inadequate fixation is therefore difficult and may give rise to misinterpretations [113]. Furthermore, it must be emphasized that not all thromboses are an abrupt event. The growth of a thrombus is step-like, with intermittent acquisition of new material and the process may last several days. Consequently, the emboli may consist of segments of different age and may even be superimposed by fresh thrombotic material which has been formed at the site where the embolus is adherent. This newest thrombotic material, if present, may indicate the actual period of embolization. If it is absent, the estimated age of the material is valid only for the original thrombus

Table 13.3 Chronology of organization of thrombi and emboli

Age	Within the thrombus	Reaction between vessel wall and thrombus
a few hours	Red and white blood cells intact; appearance of fibrin	None
1–4 days	Agglutination of erythrocytes; disappearance of thrombocytes	None
4–8 days	Beginning pyknosis of polymorphonuclear leukocytes; increasing number of mononuclear cells	Invasion of spindle-shaped cells from the intima into the thrombus
8–12 days	Increasing pyknosis of polymorphonuclear leukocytes; abundance of mononuclear cells; appearance of macrophages in the thrombus periphery	Invasion of capillaries; the first collagen fibers invading the thrombus can be identified
12–17 days	Pyknosis and karyolysis of practically all the polymorphonuclear leukocytes	Appearance of capillary sinuses (dilated capillaries) in the thrombus periphery
15–18 days	Appearance of endothelial cells covering the thrombus surface; fragmentation of the thrombus periphery with beginning endothelialization of the spaces	
18–25 days	Disappearance of the mononuclear cells; some necrotic polymorphonuclear leukocytes are still recognizable; appearance of fibroblasts and capillary channels; endothelialization of the thrombus surface	Increasing appearance of collagen fibers
25–60 days	Formation of connective tissue between the capillaries in thrombus	Enlargement and confluence of the capillary sinuses
60 days	Appearance of the first elastic fibers/fibrils	Increasing recanalization

and nothing can be deduced about the timing of embolization.

Later sequelae of the thrombus

In the course of several weeks, dependent on venous caliber, the thrombosed vessel is organized into a fibrous cord (in small veins) or becomes recanalized (in larger veins). The recanalization into a patent vascular tube develops by coalescence of sinusoidal networks into larger channels separated at first by fibrous strands. Later, this web-like pattern of fibrous tissue is resorbed and the venous lumen is more or less reconstituted. The venous wall, however, is permanently damaged. It remains thickened by fibrous scar tissue with fibrotic and, usually, deformed incompetent valves (post-thrombotic state).

The organization process is identical in deep and superficial veins. The sequelae, however, are different. A post-thrombotic state in superficial veins is unimportant, whereas in deep leg veins it leads to the development of a chronic venous congestion with subsequent trophic skin changes. Mural, non-occlusive thrombi in large veins are organized into intimal cushions which have no clinical consequences unless venous valves are included in the process.

Small veins are recanalized in three weeks [114], large veins in 6–8 months [106,115]. After two years, 85–90% of all occluded deep leg veins are recanalized [53,116]. In non-recanalized thrombi, the fibrous scar tissue may undergo calcification. In saccular aneurysms (varicose veins, cavernous hemangiomas, other vascular malformations), such round-shaped calcified thrombi are called phleboliths.

(f) Special types of thrombosis

Veno-occlusive disease of the lung

Thrombotic occlusion of multiple small pulmonary veins with subsequent development of pulmonary hypertension and right heart insufficiency of unknown etiology is known as veno-occlusive disease of the lungs. Viral infection is considered as a possible cause of this uncommon disease [117]. The histopathology typically shows fibrous occlusions of small pulmonary veins with conspicuous involvement of pulmonary venules and occasionally phlebitis and venulitis.

Budd–Chiari syndrome

This clinical entity is characterized by thrombotic occlusions of small hepatic veins with or without concomitant thrombosis of the inferior vena cava and occasionally, the superior vena cava or the portal vein. Thrombosis may be initiated by compression of the vena cava or portal vein by tumors, trauma, inflammatory liver diseases, hormonal influences or idiopathic coagulation disorders.

Phlegmasia coerulea dolens

An extensive thrombosis of many large and small extremity veins may cause a blockage of the entire venous reflux. The subsequent rise of the tissue pressure is responsible for an interruption of the arterial circulation with subsequent ischemia (so-called venous gangrene). Postoperative, post-traumatic, puerperal and neoplastic conditions have been mentioned as etiologic factors [118].

Thrombosis of upper extremity veins

Although rare, they may be caused by the thoracic outlet or costoclavicular syndrome or by occupational trauma to the axillary and/or subclavian vein (so-called effort thrombosis) [119].

Thromboses of the superior/inferior vena cava

They may be linked with neoplasia, renal vein thrombosis, Budd–Chiari syndrome, intestinal infections and venous spur in the left common iliac vein.

Thromboses of deep leg veins

These may occur after long voyages with bent knees, following jogging exercises, prolonged bed rest or immobilization.

Thrombosis of cerebral veins

This is usually due to adjacent inflammatory processes or trauma.

Thrombosis of retinal veins

This is a disorder of the older age groups probably due to local degenerative disease.

Thromboses of portal, mesenteric and splanchnic veins

These frequently accompany neoplasias or inflammatory processes of the adjacent tissue (see section 15.7 for portal hypertension.)

Multiple thromboses

These often occur in hypereosinophilic syndromes (e.g. Löeffler's disease).

Iatrogenic thrombosis

Repeated intravenous injections, as in parenteral nutrition or therapeutic infusion, sclerotherapy of varicose veins, varicocele and hemangiomas, may damage the venous endothelium with subsequent thrombotic occlusion. Modern substances of low toxicity and limited effect on the endothelial layer have made sclerotherapy a safe method in use worldwide. The resulting thrombi are believed to have a low fibrin content because the fibrin has infiltrated the media and caused a local inflammation. A tightly applied bandage compresses the vein and enhances a quick organization without risk of embolism and development of a significant perivenous inflammation.

Thrombosis secondary to inflammatory venous diseases

Secondary thrombosis may be due to any disease enhancing blood coagulation among which inflammatory wall alterations play an important role. Irrespective of the etiology (bacterial or viral infection, autoimmune diseases or irradiation injury), the morphology and stages of organization of the thrombus are identical to those in primary thrombosis. A peculiar feature, however, is characteristic of thrombosis in migrating phlebitis irrespective of etiology (idiopathic, related to Buerger's disease, Mondor's disease or collagen diseases). The peripheral areas of the thrombi contain microabscesses, consisting of necrotic polymorphonuclear leukocytes and giant cells of the Langhans type. The significance of this finding is unknown.

Disseminated intravascular coagulation (DIC)

This condition is characterized by a diffuse fibrin-rich coagulation of the blood in widespread microvascular system. It is due to a disorder of hemostasis and may be induced by a variety of diseases causing hemorrhages and/or thrombosis. The lesions are usually systemic and may affect any organ including vast areas of the skin. The mortality is high (67%). Symptoms may vary. Underlying diseases include infectious diseases, neoplasia, hemolytic anemia, cardiovascular diseases, hereditary vascular diseases (Osler's disease, syndrome of Kasabach and Merrit), cavernous hemangiomas, paraprotein disorders, amyloidosis, autoimmune diseases, vasculitides, arteriovenous shunts, trauma, surgical trauma, liver diseases, thromboembolism, neurologic disorders, and coagulation disorders [120]). The pathology findings are uniform and non-specific: capillaries and venules, occasionally also small veins and arteries are occluded by fibrin-rich thrombi. The vessel walls may be ruptured, with extravasation of erythrocytes into the surrounding tissue. Inflammatory infiltrates are often absent. The thrombi are usually of identical age. In most cases they are fresh; they may appear to be organized if death is not instantaneous. Skin lesions include hemorrhages, microinfarcts and even gangrene.

Intravascular papillary endothelial hyperplasia

First described by Masson [121], this intraluminal endothelial proliferation occurs in veins, occasionally also in cavernous hemangiomas and rarely in arteries. It is a benign pseudotumor and represents a variant of thrombus organization. Papillary thrombus fragments are covered by elongated cells with the ultrastructural characteristics of fibroblasts, which later are transformed into endothelial cells [122]. They are clearly separated from the underlying stroma by a basement membrane. The stroma contains loose or dense collagen tissue. The lesion is sometimes misinterpreted as a malignant endothelial tumor. The differential diagnosis must include true neoplasms such as intravascular hemangioendothelioma or epithelioid hemangioma.

(g) **Thrombosis associated with neoplastic disease**

Deep and superficial vein thrombosis commonly co-exist with neoplastic disease; its incidence in autopsy series may be as high as 40% according to one report [99]. Venous thromboembolism has been associated with virtually every type of malignant tumor, especially with gastrointestinal, urogenital and lung cancers. Although usually observed in advanced stages of the disease, both deep vein thrombosis and pulmonary thromboembolism may appear before the cancer becomes symptomatic and, therefore, may lead to an earlier diagnosis of cancer. According to recently reported studies, a malignant neoplasm was detected during hospital admission in 12 of 113 (10.6%) deep vein thrombosis patients [123] and cancer was diagnosed in 9 of 78 (11.5%) consecutive patients with acute pulmonary embolism [124]. In neither group were there known risk factors for deep vein thrombosis or pulmonary embolism other than an underlying neoplastic disease.

(h) **The post-thrombotic syndrome**

Thrombotic occlusions of pelvic and deep leg veins are frequently responsible for the later development of a so-called post-thrombotic syndrome. Clinically it is characterized by a chronic leg edema of varying severity and the eventual development of trophic skin alterations including crural ulcers. The latter are mostly situated at the medial ankle or supramalleolar area. This is due to the localization of so-called Cockett perforator veins which communicate the deep posterior tibial veins with the superficial posterior arch vein, a small branch of the great saphenous vein. This weak-walled small vein branch cannot withstand the high pressure waves from the deep venous system and easily becomes dilated and insufficient. The resulting venous congestion mainly concerns the ankle and supramalleolar area.

Epidemiological investigations have shown that post-thrombotic syndromes and especially crural ulcers rarely develop after isolated pelvic vein thrombosis and commonly when several segments of the deep leg veins including lower leg and popliteofemoral veins are involved [95,125–128].

Histopathology of post-thrombotic leg veins shows more or less recanalized thrombi with one or several irregularly shaped lumina. The venous valves are shrunken fibrous protuberances on the vessel wall of irregular diameter characterized by a thickened, vascularized intima with fibrotic degeneration of media and adventitia. The vasa vasorum of the media may be increased in number and are dilated. They may be surrounded by residual lymphocytic infiltrates (secondary reactive inflammation).

The skin and subcutaneous tissue at the ankle and supramalleolar area may show the same alterations as in primary chronic venous insufficiency. Additional damage to the prefascial lymphatic collectors may be responsible for the development of a superimposed chronic lymphedema.

(i) Embolism

The term embolism refers to the displacement of intravascular material in the direction of the blood flow and subsequent lodgement downstream. In systemic venous embolism the emboli finally reach the pulmonary circulation and occlude pulmonary arteries and arterioles. Passage through an open foramen ovale into the systemic arterial circulation appears not to be as rare as generally believed and accounts for 5% of the arterial emboli [129]. Embolic material may consist of thrombi, fatty particles, normal tissue, air, tumor fragments, parasites, foreign bodies, atheromatous material or amniotic fluid.

The histologic appearance of embolized and *in situ* thrombi is identical. The age determination usually considers only the age of the underlying thrombosis which may antedate the embolic displacement by many days or even weeks. The time interval between thrombus formation and embolization depends on many factors such as vessel caliber, intraluminal pressure and condition of the vessel wall, etc. In a large vein or a venous aneurysm, although the center of the thrombus may remain unorganized for a long time, the peripheral areas in contact with the vessel wall are already completely organized. These thrombi become firmly attached to the vessel wall at the first appearance of collagen fibrils around days 8–10. From that moment on, the risk of embolization decreases rapidly.

The majority of venous emboli originate from thrombi in the pelvic, femoral and popliteal veins. The embolization of thrombi in large veins may be sudden and unexpected. Parts of the thrombus may be loosened and dislodged before they become firmly attached and organized. Emboli from lower extremities without involvement of the popliteal vein are rare. According to a recent study of 5039 autopsy cases [130], 12.6% of pulmonary emboli were from thrombi in the superior vena cava and the jugular veins, whereas 59.4% originated in veins of the lower half of the body; a source could not be identified in the remaining 28% of cases.

13.4 Inflammatory venous diseases (Figures 13.27–13.29)

Inflammatory diseases in singular veins may be infection-related or due to an autoimmune reaction, occasionally also to local application of toxic substances. Systemic inflammatory venous disorders are mainly observed in

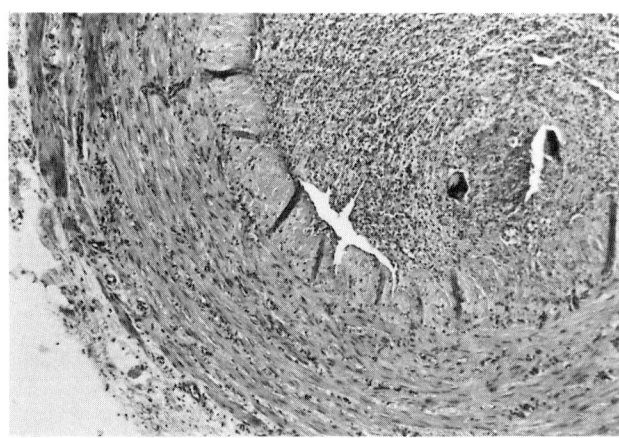

Figure 13.27 Migrating phlebitis in a superficial vein with chronic panphlebitis, thrombosis and microabscesses with giant cells at the periphery of the thrombus. (H&E.)

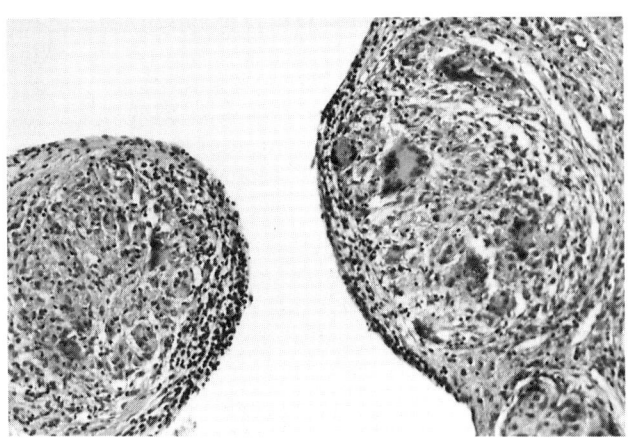

Figure 13.28 Venous intramural granulomas with giant cells in Boeck's disease (hepatic veins with subsequent Budd–Chiari syndrome). (H&E.)

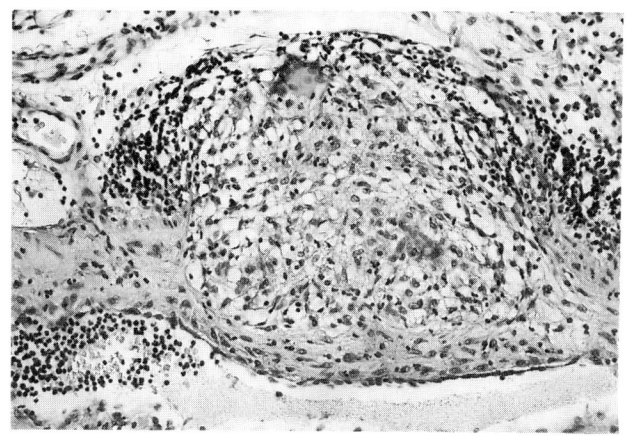

Figure 13.29 Granulomatous panphlebitis in mesenteric veins: granulomas with giant cells of the Langhans type. (H&E.)

systemic vasculitides of primary or secondary nature. The latter are discussed in the chapter on vasculitides.

13.4.1 INFECTION-RELATED PHLEBITIS

Infection-related vasculitis in general has been reported due to bacterial, fungal, mycobacterial (leprosy, tuberculosis), spirochetal (syphilis, Lyme disease), rickettsial, viral, protozoal and Whipple bacillus infections [131]. A venous participation may occur in any type of vasculitis but is usually less important than infective arteritis.

Infection-related phlebitis is mostly caused by streptococci or staphylococci. Its nature may be exudative, suppurative, hemorrhagic, gangrenous or proliferative. Septic phlebitis is invariably followed by secondary thrombosis. The micro-organisms reach the venous wall either via the vasa vasorum or from the vessel lumen by diapedesis through the endothelial lining into intima and media. The histopathologic spectrum ranges from a necrotizing panphlebitis with predominantly polymorphonuclear infiltrate to a proliferative sclerosing phlebitis with focal or diffuse mononuclear cell infiltrate. Septic phlebitis is a very serious condition. It occurs commonly associated with intravenous drug abuse but may also be induced iatrogenically after prolonged therapeutic infusions and venous catheterization. Embolism of septic material from an infected vein may result in septic lung infarction and general pyemia.

In tuberculosis, small veins are often affected. They show the features of a granulomatous thrombophlebitis with or without characteristic tubercles intramurally or in the perivascular tissue. In leprosy, tuberculoid changes may be observed in thrombosed veins.

In rickettsial infections, mainly postcapillary venules may show endothelial swelling with perivascular and intramural infiltrates of lymphocytes, macrophages and occasional polymorphonuclear leukocytes, followed by thrombosis. In viral infections, venous participation is rare. A peculiar type of phlebitis may occur in cat-scratch disease characterized by intramural microabscesses without giant cells.

13.4.2 MIGRATING PHLEBITIS (PHLEBITIS MIGRANS SIVE SALTANS) AND MONDOR'S DISEASE

The term 'migrating phlebitis' refers to a segmental and episodic inflammation of small and middle-sized non-varicose veins, involving mostly superficial, but occasionally also visceral veins or deep veins of the extremities. The inflammation is of a focal nature, migrating along the vein or skipping to other veins. Although self-limiting and capable of resolving spontaneously, relapses are frequent occurring at irregular intervals over several years. The histopathology of early stages is characterized by a predominantly lymphocytic infiltrate around the vasa vasorum and, later, a diffuse lymphoplasmacytic infiltrate may appear within the entire vessel wall. The media may be edematous, but usually does not show fibrinoid necrosis. The intima shows fibrocellular proliferation. The internal elastic lamella is focally disrupted but the endothelial lining may remain intact for a certain period. As soon as the endothelium is damaged, secondary thrombosis develops. The hypercellular thrombus may contain 'microabscesses' of polymorphonuclear leukocytes undergoing karyorrhexis, intermingled with multinucleated giant cells of the Langhans type. These pseudogranulomas are characteristically situated at the periphery of the thrombus.

The etiology of the disease is unknown; an immune-mediated response has often been suggested. The majority of cases are primary (idiopathic migrating phlebitis). Other cases may be due to exogenous sensitizing factors. Secondary migrating phlebitis may accompany Buerger's disease. Between 35 to 70% of all cases of Buerger's disease are believed to be accompanied by relapsing bouts of migrating phlebitis [132–137], often as an early symptom preceding the clinical manifestations of arterial occlusive disease. Thrombosis but not phlebitis may be associated with but cannot predict the presence of an underlying malignancy [99,133].

(a) Mondor's disease (phlebitis chronica obliterans filiformis)

This is a special type of migrating phlebitis with prominent fibrosis of the affected vein, transforming it into a fibrous cord. The lesion has a predilection for the lateral thoracic wall area. The disease is benign and self-limiting. The cause is unknown; among the possible etiologic factors considered are mechanical irritations, local infections and dysfunction of the mammary gland. The histopathology of early stages of the disease shows the characteristics of a primary inflammatory process of the venous wall, as in migrating phlebitis, rather than an ordinary thrombosis.

13.4.3 SARCOIDOSIS (BOECK'S DISEASE)

Vascular involvement in sarcoidosis appears as typical sarcoid granulomas around and in the vessel walls. Both arteries and veins, large or small, may be affected. Sarcoidosis may involve virtually any organ and both aggregates of granulomas and granulomatous vasculitis may be seen [138]. Cerebral and hepatic veins are occasionally affected. The inflammation is typically granulomatous with non-caseating sarcoid granulomas in and around the vessel wall, or it may appear as non-specific chronic inflammation with mononuclear cell infiltrates throughout the vessel wall.

13.4.4 IMMUNE MEDIATED PHLEBITIS

Some types of phlebitis probably are the result of an immune-mediated response. A variety of different immune mechanisms (recognition of vascular structures as an antigen, direct deposition of antigen in vessels, deposition of immune complexes in vessels, delayed hypersensitivity, etc.) may be involved [138]. The inflammation may be exudative or granulomatous. An initial invasion of polymorphonuclear leukocytes is short-lived, followed by a mononuclear cell infiltrate within all wall layers. Fibrinoid necrosis of various degree may be observed. The elastic internal membrane is at first preserved but later it becomes focally destroyed. Intimal swelling and proliferation is common. As long as the endothelial layer is preserved, the occurrence of a secondary thrombosis is prevented.

Participation of veins in systemic vasculitides is not uncommon, but usually of minor importance. Systemic lupus erythematosus is frequently accompanied by venous disease with subsequent thrombosis. In hypocomplementary vasculitis, the involvement of venules is frequently encountered [139]. In Behçet's disease, inflammatory venous changes predominate over arterial involvement. In hypersensitivity angiitis, venules and small veins are commonly affected. Involvement of veins and venules by thromboangiitis is a hallmark of Buerger's disease.

Any size and localization of veins may sometimes be involved in systemic vasculitides, but small veins and venules are most commonly affected. The histologic features of inflammation are usually non-specific, with diffuse or focal infiltrates of mononuclear cells. Development of secondary thrombosis is common.

13.4.5 SECONDARY REACTIVE INFLAMMATION OF THE VEINS

A secondary inflammation of the venous wall during thrombus organization is common. Capillary sprouts with slight to moderate pericapillary mononuclear infiltrates occur within the media and adventitia and invade the thrombus through the intima. As soon as the thrombus is organized, these cellular infiltrates disappear without leaving much residuum. A certain amount of vessel wall fibrosis is not uncommon. Secondary inflammation is also observed after intravenous application of endothelium-damaging substances or as a reaction to certain toxins such as snake venom. These reactions are often non-specific histologically.

13.4.6 MISCELLANEOUS CASES

A few isolated cases of granulomatous phlebitis involving the extremity or visceral veins without simultaneous involvement of arteries and without any apparent cause, have also been reported [138,140–142]. They are extremely rare. The lesion is characterized by peri- and intravenous granulomas consisting of epithelioid and giant cells of the Langhans type, with or without necrotizing panphlebitis, and followed by thrombotic occlusion of the affected vessel. It is uncertain whether these cases actually represent a distinct new disease entity.

13.5 Malformations of the lymphatic vessels (Figures 13.30–13.35)

13.5.1 LYMPHANGIOMA

(a) **Simple lymphangioma**

Simple lymphangiomas are congenital malformations that appear soon after birth. The lesions are found in the skin and mucous membranes. They are usually small

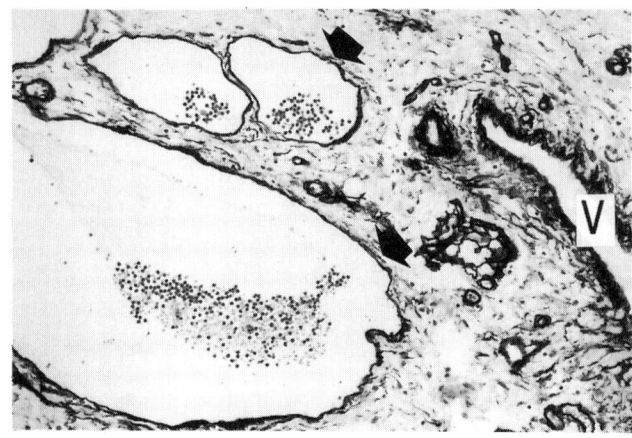

Figure 13.30 Lymphangioma. Dilated lymphatic vessels with very thin basement membranes (arrows) in comparison to the veins (V). (Type IV collagen marker (C4 Dakopatts).)

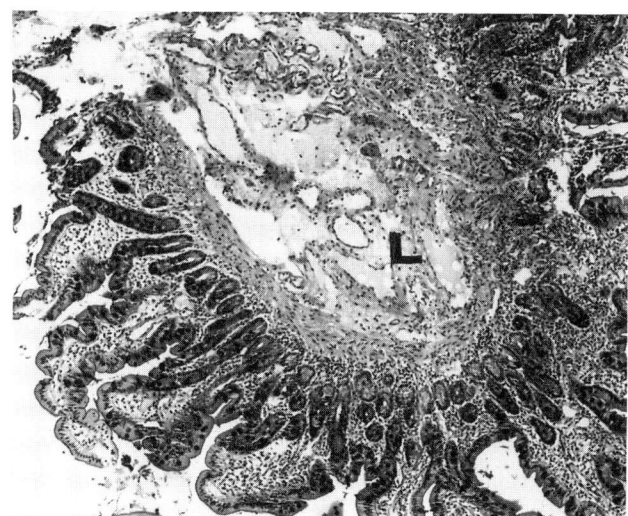

Figure 13.31 Lymphangiectases (L) in the bowel resulting in a chronic loss of protein. (H&E.)

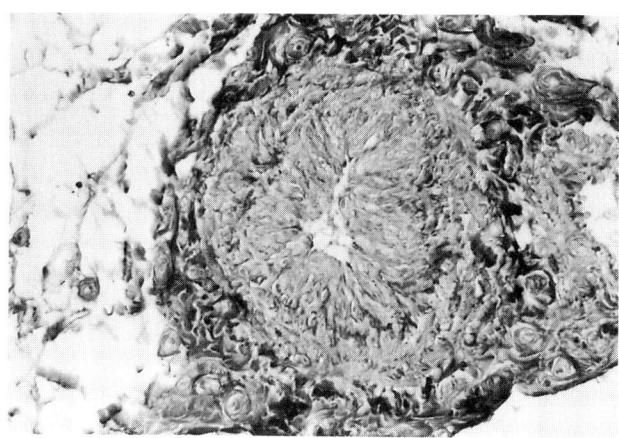

Figure 13.32 Lymphatic prefascial collector of the lower extremity with intimal sclerosis. (Van Gieson stain.)

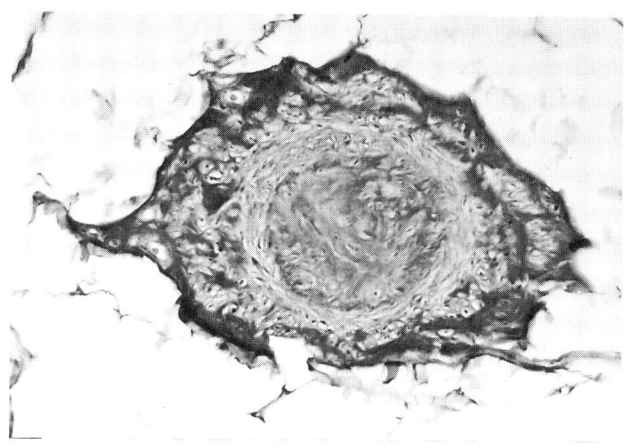

Figure 13.33 Obliterated superficial lymph collector in lymphedema. (Van Gieson stain.)

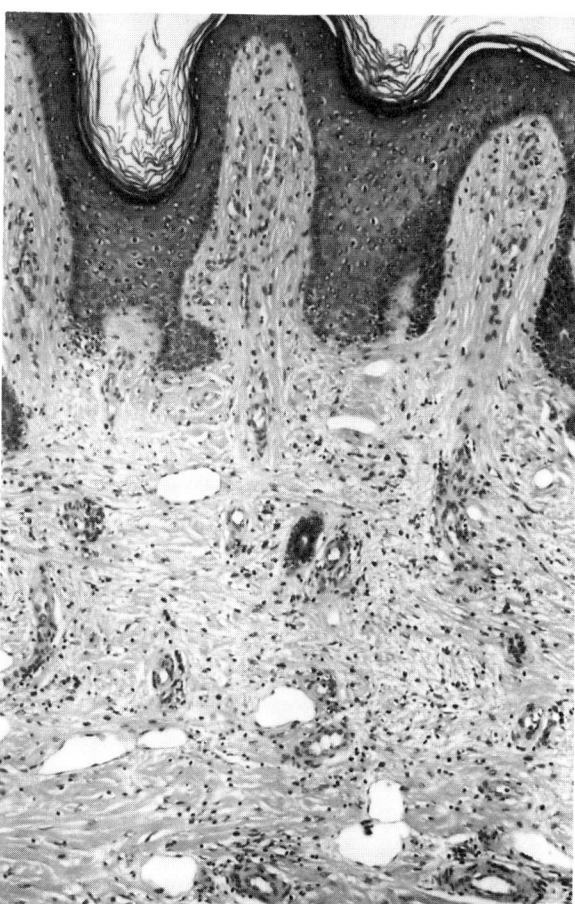

Figure 13.34 Chronic lymphedema of the leg with recurrent erysipelas. Dilated lymph capillaries and dermatitis in cutaneous and subcutaneous tissue. (H&E.)

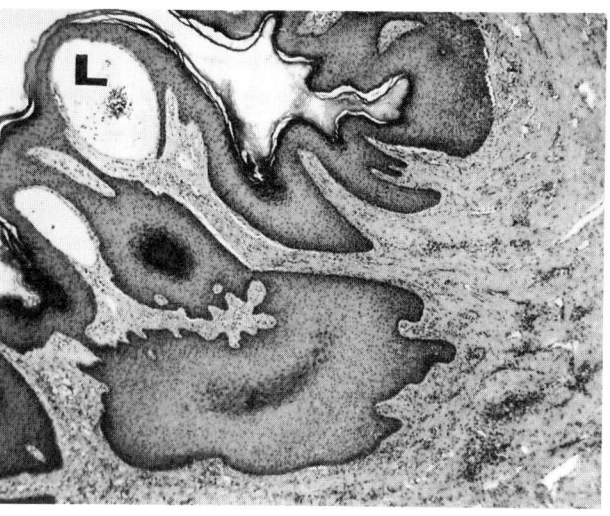

Figure 13.35 Lymphedema of the scrotum in primary lymphedema. Dilated subepidermal lymphatic vessels (L), formation of several lymph fistulae. (H&E.)

and circumscribed and contain clear fluid with few lymphocytes within dilated lymph vessels. Simple lymphangiomas may expand slowly over time from accumulation of fluid.

(b) Cavernous lymphangioma

Cavernous lymphangiomas are also congenital lesions, with a preferential distribution in the upper extremities, the axillary or scapular areas, the head and neck region including oropharynx, groin, buttock and thigh. They may be combined with malformations of the blood vessels (hemangiolymphangioma) and may contain other mesodermal derivatives such as lymph follicles, adipose and fibrous connective tissue, smooth muscle and even cartilage. Histologically, they are characterized by dilated lymphatics filled with lymph or occasionally a mixture of blood and lymph fluid. The caverns are lined by a thin endothelial layer with fibrous septa inside the lumen. The lymphangioma may reach a considerable size, and focal accumulations of lymphocytes may form lymphoid follicles around the cavernous vessels.

(c) Cystic hygroma

This is a fairly common congenital 'tumor' of the neck, rarely occurring in the axilla, groin, the retroperitoneum, thoracic wall and sacral region. It consists of an encapsulated, multilocular large mass containing serous fluid or lymph and lymphocytes. The cystic spaces are lined by a thin layer of cells with the ultrastructural characteristics of lymphatic endothelium.

13.5.2 LYMPHANGIECTASES

Generalized dilation of lymph capillaries of irregular size and shape may occur as a congenital malformation or be combined with congenital hypoplasia of the prefascial lymph collectors of the lower extremity as a cause of primary lymphedema of the leg. They may also develop as sequelae of chronic lymph stasis and cause secondary lymphedema.

Lymphangiectases may affect the extremities, sometimes linked with chromosomal abnormalities (such as Turner's syndrome, Noonan's syndrome) or occur as a symptom complex of disseminated lymphangiomatosis with other organ involvement, such as osseous lymphangiomatosis (Gorham's disease or phantom bone or disappearing bone syndrome) [143]. Other types may involve visceral organs with subsequent hydro- or chylothorax, chylopericardium, intestinal chylorrhea, chyluria and chylometrorrhea [143,145]. The brain may also be affected (lymphostatic encephalopathy) [143].

The histopathology of lymphangiectases is non-specific. Irregular cystic dilation of lymphatic vessels with normal endothelial lining, separated by fibrous collagenous septa, are the usual findings [145]. The endothelium bears the ultrastructural characteristics of a lymphatic endothelium (flat endothelial cells with short, oblique intercellular spaces, rudimentary or absent basement membrane and attachment fibers to the surrounding collagen tissue). The alterations may be combined with various other malformations of the lymphatics.

13.5.3 GORHAM'S DISEASE

This peculiar type of lymphangiomatosis consists of ectatic capillaries with flat endothelial cells lying between fibrous septa. The lumina may contain erythrocytes or merely lymph. The involvement of bones is responsible for a considerable osteolysis. Entire parts of the skeleton may disappear completely. The malformation probably derives from primitive mesenchymal cells with later differentiation into blood capillaries as well as into lymphatic capillaries. It occurs in subjects of 15–70 years with a slight predominance of males (1.7:1) [143]. The condition is usually self-limiting. However, tumor-like dissemination with involvement of entire extremities, although without evidence of malignancy has been observed [144].

13.5.4 CONGENITAL HYPOPLASIA OF PREFASCIAL LYMPH COLLECTORS

This condition is responsible for the development of primary (idiopathic) lymphedema. The distinction of congenital (Nonne–Milroy) and acquired (Meige) familial lymphedema is arbitrary and of no clinical importance. Of all primary lymphedemas, 40% are hereditary with autosomal dominance [146]. The onset of clinical manifestation varies from birth to later in life with the peak incidence just before 20 years of age. In a majority of cases, both lower extremities are affected and, in many, the edema remains unilateral in spite of the malformation.

The lymphedema may remain mild, with possible aggravation by pregnancies, infections, trauma and surgery, or it may show early progression into severe elephantiasis. Lesions with a late manifestation have a better prognosis than those with early onset and early involvement of the entire extremity [143]. Erysipelas is rarely the cause but more usually a complication of lymphedema. Lymphatic stasis is a prerequisite for the development of erysipelas, and 86–88% of the patients are women [146,147]. In milder cases of lymphedema, two pregnancies are usually well tolerated, but after further pregnancies, a serious aggravation of the edema has to be expected. The upper extremities are seldom affected, unless in combination with a systemic angiodysplasia. Lymphangiography and intracutaneous dye-injection reveal in practically all the cases various degrees of hypoplasia of the ventromedial and/or dorsolateral bundle of the prefascial lymph collections of the lower extremity, occasionally combined with hyperplasia and ectasia ('varicosis') of singular collectors [148]. When the lymph collectors are occluded, dilated and tortuous lymphatic collaterals may develop. They form irregular networks in the cutaneous and subcutaneous tissue with subsequent 'dermal reflux' of lymph.

13.5.5 SECONDARY LYMPHEDEMA

Some lymphedemas are acquired. The common causes are inflammatory diseases of lymphatics and lymph nodes from infections; tumor compression of lymph nodes and lymphatics; traumatic or iatrogenic destruction of lymph nodes and lymphatics as in postmastectomy lymphedema.

13.5.6 MORPHOLOGIC CHARACTERISTICS OF PRIMARY AND SECONDARY LYMPHEDEMA

Lymph capillaries in normal and lymphedematous tissue can be identified by their typical ultrastructural features of flat endothelial cells with short, obliquely running intercellular spaces, discontinuous basement membrane and anchoring filaments radiating obliquely from the vessel into the surrounding tissue. A combination of dilated lymph capillaries with partly dilated interendothelial spaces with an intra- and pericapillary edema is indicative of lymphedema; there are no distinguishing ultrastructural findings of primary and secondary lymphedema. The lymphatic incompetency may be demonstrated by functional assessment rather than by morphological methods [149].

Peripheral lymph collectors may be distinguished from veins by their localization, structure, and contents. The ventromedial prefascial bundle runs from the dorsum pedis to the medial side of the lower leg and along the great saphenous vein to the groin. It contains two to seven collectors each with a diameter of 0.2–0.5 mm. The lymphatics lie either directly above the fascia or halfway between the fascia and dermis. The dorsolateral prefascial bundle consists distally of three to four collectors merging to become a single channel that runs alongside the short saphenous vein to the popliteal groove. The deep collectors accompany the three leg arteries and the femoropopliteal artery before finally reaching the inguinal lymph nodes. They lie between the artery and vein or lateral to the artery. In contrast to venous drainage, the lymphatic flow runs from the deep into the superficial lymphatic system and from there into the inguinal lymph nodes. For this reason, lymphangiography does not demonstrate the deep lymphatics.

The structure of the lymph collectors consists of smooth muscle bundles that run longitudinally within intima and adventitia, but appear interwoven and spiral in the media. Collagen fibers are practically all restricted to the adventitia. The elastic fibers are thin and surround the muscle fibers without formation of a distinct internal elastic membrane. The lymphatic valves consist of fibrocollagenous structures covered by endothelium. They are numerous with spacings varying between 1 and 20 mm [150]. Ultrastructurally, they are represented by thin collagen flaps, frequently with endothelial nuclei arranged at the flap periphery and forming peculiar nodules. The contents of lymphatic collectors include a basophilic homogeneous fluid and numerous lymphocytes.

Histologically, the lymphatic collectors in primary and secondary lymphedema show numerous occlusions with or without recanalization, fibrosis of intima, media and adventitia, and occasional intramural lymphocytic infiltrates [151]. The main alterations are found in the superficial lymph collectors but occasionally also deep collectors may be similarly affected. These alterations are non-specific; the inflammatory lesions, when present, are probably due to secondary infections. Dilated lymphatics (lymph varicosities) with normal or distended valves, and hyperplastic lymphatics with smooth muscle hypertrophy may also be found.

13.5.7 COMBINED MALFORMATIONS WITH LYMPHANGIOMAS OR LYMPHEDEMA

Cavernous lymphangiomas, ectasia of lymph capillaries and lymphatic cysts, as well as various combinations of aplasia, dysplasia and hyperplasia of lymph collectors may be observed in systemic vascular malformations. They may give rise to the development of lymphatic fistulas through the skin. Lymphatic fistulas may also occur in primary and secondary lymphedema of various etiologic types. They are frequently associated with papillary hyperkeratosis of skin. Other typical alterations are a thickened epidermis and cutaneous tissue with chronic inflammation. The subcutaneous tissue appears thickened, with edema or fibrosis according to the stage of the lymphedema. There may also be atrophy of the skin appendages and occasionally loose or dense lymphocytic infiltrates in corium and subcutis. In secondary lymphedema the alterations of lymph capillaries, lymphatic collectors and skin are identical to those in primary lymphedema.

13.6 Degenerative disorders of lymphatic vessels

13.6.1 PRIMARY LYMPHANGIOSCLEROSIS

Degenerative, age-dependent alterations of superficial lymph collectors are common; they are found in 35–40% of men and women over the age of 40. This practically equal incidence in both genders is in contrast to the primary lymphedema where women predominate by a ratio of 14:1 [146]. The majority of alterations are slight and restricted to individual lymphatics as segmental, focal alterations. The lesions usually consist of intimal and/or medial fibrosis, ectasia of lymphatics and occasionally fibrotic occlusions. Inflammatory infiltrates are usually absent. A relation between age groups and severity could not be established [152]. The deep lymphatic collectors and also the thoracic duct are practically always normal even in persons of advanced age. This suggests that the deep lymphatic vessels are less prone to degeneration than the superficial lymphatics. This observation corresponds to that in the venous system.

Even in normal superficial lymph collectors, variations of the functional state are commonly observed. Both narrow lumina of sickle- or star-shaped vessels and thin walled wide-open lumina may be found. This emphasizes the importance of the active drainage function of the lymph collectors.

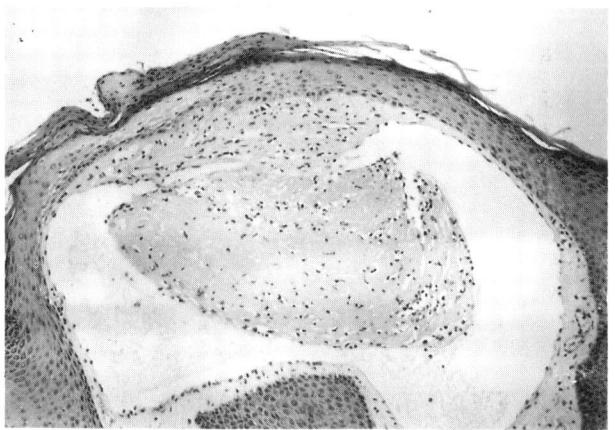

Figure 13.36 Lymph coagulum in dilated subepidermal lymphatic capillary (chronic lymphedema with lymph fistulae). (H&E.)

13.6.2 LYMPHATIC VARICES

'Varicose' lymphatics may be observed in primary lymphedema of the legs due to congenital malformations and occasionally as a sequel of a post-thrombotic chronic venous insufficiency. As a disease entity, neither condition is of great importance, but secondary lymphatic ectasia may complicate a post-thrombotic syndrome and add lymph stasis to the already existing venous congestion. The lesions appear as small saccular chain-like arranged ectasias of one or several superficial lymph collectors.

13.7 Circulatory disorders of the lymphatic vessels

13.7.1 LYMPHATIC VESSEL THROMBOSIS
[Figures 13.36, 13.37]

Lymphatic fluid contains all the coagulation factors in a lower amount (about 50–60%) than those present in the blood. The likelihood of a spontaneous coagulation is therefore much smaller and the fibrinolytic mechanisms are probably more effective than those occurring in the blood vessels [153]. Coagulation may be observed in lymphatic cysts and other lymphatic malformations. Obliteration of lymph collectors by fibrin-rich coagulum may also occur in lymphangiitis of any cause. Lymph coagulum consists entirely of fibrin with the inclusion of some lymphocytes. Organization and recanalization of the lymph coagulum take place in the same way as do thrombi in blood vessels.

Thrombosis of lymphatic vessels often accompanies arterial and venous diseases. In arterial occlusions due to peripheral arterial occlusive disease, occlusions of

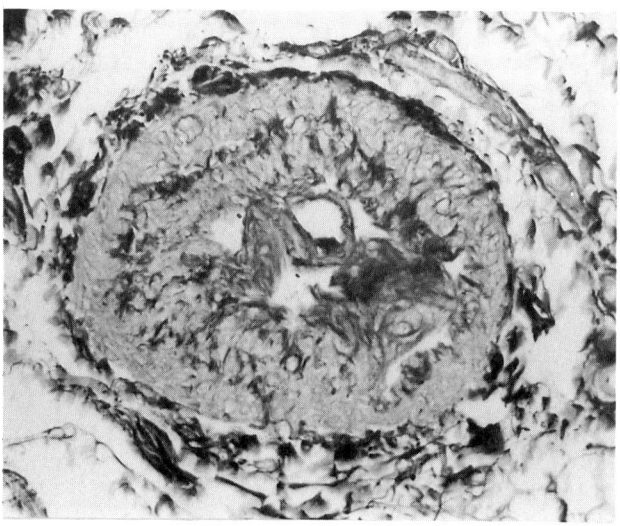

Figure 13.37 Thrombotic occlusion of a lymph collector with organization and recanalization into several small channels. (Van Gieson stain.)

deep lymphatic collectors may occur simultaneously. The question of participation of lymphatics in deep vein thrombosis has not been completely resolved. Investigations by radioisotopes have demonstrated involvement of subfascial lymph collectors in post-thrombotic states [154] as well as injury to the prefascial lymph collectors in the presence of trophic skin lesions [155]. By indirect lymphangiography it was shown that the prefascial collectors (normal diameter 0.45–0.8 mm) may appear irregularly dilated (0.6–1.1 mm) and tortuous; even calcifying lymphangiosclerosis has been observed [155]. Such changes may be responsible for the development of a secondary chronic lymphedema which frequently accompanies severe degrees of post-thrombotic syndromes.

13.8 Inflammatory diseases of lymphatic vessels

The lymphatic system has a great regenerative potential. Under normal circumstances it survives the inflammatory response as a consequence of its function as a pathway and filter for high molecular weight proteins and micro-organisms. However, certain kinds of infection are virulent enough to cause injury that cannot be overcome. The structural damage ensued leads to lymph stasis and subsequently to the formation of a protein-rich tissue exudate which in itself is a nutrient culture medium for bacteria, thus perpetuating the infection. A vicious cycle results and gives rise to permanent lymphedema.

Lymphangiitis may be due to a variety of infectious agents such as staphylococci, streptococci, coliform bacteria, pseudomonas and anaerobes [156]. A number of conditions favor the development of such infections, e.g. primary and secondary lymphedema, the post-thrombotic syndrome as well as peripheral arterial occlusive disease especially in association with diabetes mellitus. The ischemic tissue favors the development of infections. In the advanced stage of peripheral arterial occlusive disease, inflammatory alterations of deep and superficial lymph collectors have been observed [151, 157]. The post-thrombotic syndrome creates chronic venous insufficiency with trophic skin lesions and subsequent fibrous scar formation in the subcutaneous tissue which in turn causes damage to the lymphatic capillary network.

13.8.1 ERYSIPELAS

Erysipelas is a special type of streptococcus infection involving skin and subcutaneous tissue with a predilection for the lymphatic vessels. Previously it was believed that erysipelas might be responsible for the formation of a chronic lymphedema. However, recent investigations have shown that it is usually superimposed on an existing but clinically inapparent lymphedema [146,157].

The histopathology of non-specific lymphangiitis is independent of its etiology. An initial polymorphonuclear leukocyte-predominant infiltrate is soon replaced by a mononuclear cell infiltrate. Fibrinoid necrosis of the lymphatics may occur. The destruction of the endothelial layer, intima proliferation and formation of lymph thrombi are followed by a fibrous occlusion of the lumen with limited tendency to recanalization. Even if the occlusion is recanalized, the permanent loss of the lymphatic valves and the segmental fibrosis of the wall will seriously impede the normal drainage function of the vessel.

13.8.2 LYMPHANGIITIS DUE TO FILARIASIS

There is still controversy as to whether the filariasis infection represents a primary lymphangiitis or whether the inflammatory reaction is a secondary phenomenon. Some authors consider it to be a 'lymphangiosis' more than a true lymphangiitis [145]. However, more recent studies [158] showed the primary lesions to consist of eosinophilic abscesses, epithelioid and giant cell granulomas and inflammatory lesions in lymphatic and blood vessels. The dilated lymphatics have thickened walls and valves with thrombus formation, lymphangiitis and fibrosis of the perilymphatic tissues. This is believed to be indicative of injury to valves and vessel walls from lymphatic-dwelling live parasites, and the host immune reactivity [158]. Keratosis, papillomatosis, acanthosis and collagen deposition are subsequent skin alterations.

Filariasis is a parasitic infection by *Brugia malayi* or *Wucheria bancrofti*. The adult nematodes selectively attack peripheral lymphatics damaging the endothelial lining in lymphatics and lymph nodes. The filarial offspring (microfilariae) circulate throughout the vascular system triggering regional and systemic immune and inflammatory responses [158]. The disease results in a severe chronic lymphedema of the lower extremities. Apart from elephantiasis, chyluria from rupture of proximally obliterated lymphatics into the bladder, lymphangiectases, lymphorrhagia, purulent lymphangitides and thrombolymphangitides also have been reported [155].

Other parasitic diseases in which lymph–vascular participation and symptoms of lymph stasis or reflux of lymph have been observed are bilharziosis (chyluria), schistosomiasis, ascariasis, taeniasis, echinococcosis, leishmaniosis and trypanosomiasis (Chagas' disease) [145].

13.8.3 LYMPHANGIOSIS DUE TO INANIMATE IRRITANTS

This condition has been described in silicosis, after enamel inhalation, aluminum silicate, contrast media, radioactive material and vinyl chloride application [145]. The lesions are non-specific and consist of swelling and desquamation of the endothelial lining, panlymphangiitis with infiltration of mononuclear cells, fibrin precipitation in the lumen, thrombus formation with subsequent organization resulting in permanent obliteration of affected lymphatic vessels.

13.9 Neoplasias of the lymphatic vessels
[Figures 13.38–13.42]

Neoplasms of the lymphatic vessels are extremely rare. The majority of the so-called lymph vessel tumors are actually malformations without an abnormal growth

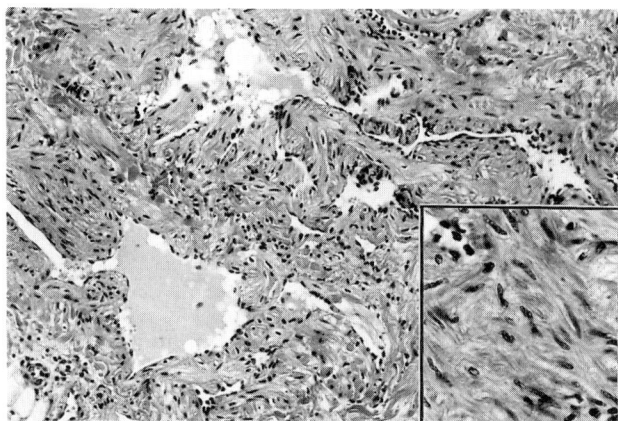

Figure 13.38 Lymphangioleiomyomatosis with proliferating smooth musculature in and around lymphatic vessels. No indications of malignancy. Inset shows higher magnification. (H&E.)

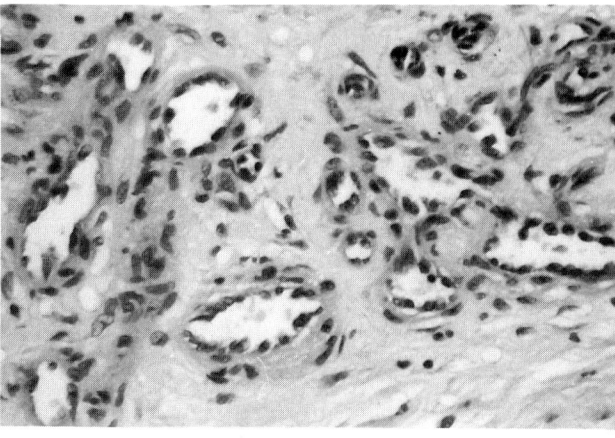

Figure 13.40 Stewart–Treves' syndrome with proliferating capillary endothelial cells. The atypical extravascular endothelial cells invade the surrounding stromal connective tissue. Kaposi's sarcoma-like type with spindle-shaped tumor cells. (H&E.)

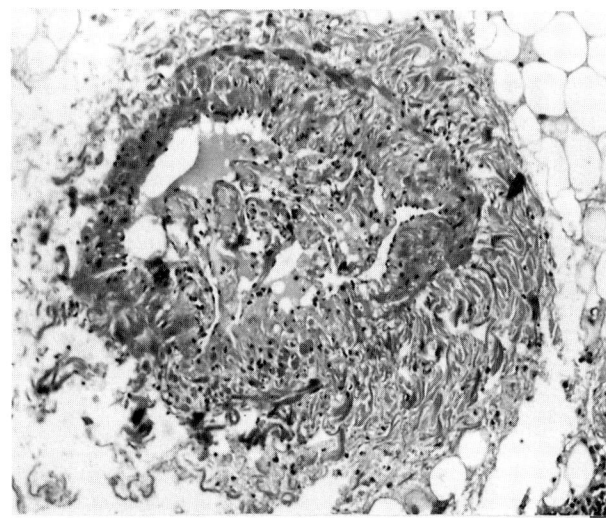

Figure 13.39 Lymphangioleiomyomatosis. Proliferation of smooth musculature into the lumen of a lymphatic collector. (H&E.)

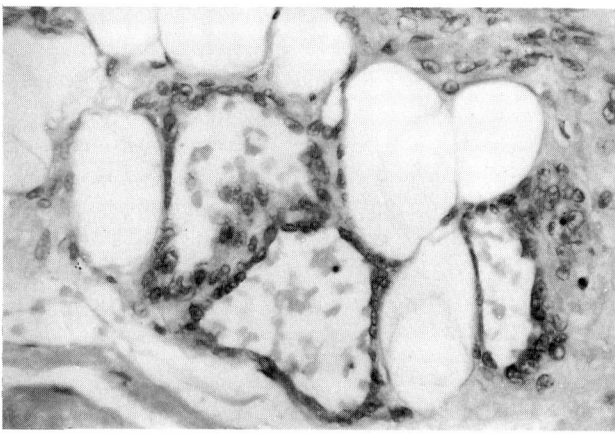

Figure 13.41 Stewart–Treves' syndrome with proliferating intralymphatic endothelial cells invading the lumen of the capillary. Hemangioendothelioma-like type with round to oval tumor cell nuclei. (H&E.)

tendency. The increase in size of lymphangiomas and lymphatic cysts represents merely a progressive dilation due to the accumulation of lymph.

13.9.1 BENIGN AND LOW-GRADE MALIGNANT LYMPHATIC VESSEL TUMORS

(a) Lymphangiopericytoma and lymphangioendothelioma

A tumor in the retroperitoneal region consisting of sharply defined cords of cells resembling pericytes covered by endothelium and surrounded by a coarse lymphatic plexus has been described and considered a lymphangiopericytoma [159]. There are also individual cases of lymphangioendotheliomas [160–162], which resemble a lymphangioma with endothelial cell proliferation forming papillary projections into the lumina or solid cell masses.

It is doubtful whether these entities represent a neoplasia derived from lymphatic endothelium. More probable is that these tumors, analogous to their hemangiomatous counterparts, derive from primitive mesenchymal cells with later differentiation into lymphatic spaces. This would correspond to similar observations in other vascular tumors such as Stewart–Treves' angiosarcoma and Kaposi's sarcoma. Both of these tumors may develop vascular spaces which resemble lymph

13.9.2 MALIGNANT TUMORS OF LYMPHATIC VESSELS

Spontaneously occurring lymphangiosarcomas probably do not exist. The term 'lymphangiosarcoma' has been applied to those tumors arising in the extremity with chronic lymphedema and presumed to originate from the endothelium of obstructed lymphatic vessels. However, the similarities between angiosarcoma and lymphangiosarcoma, as evident from ultrastructural and immunohistochemical studies, suggest that these tumors represent a common histopathologic entity and are of vascular endothelial orgin [164]. According to Enzinger and Weiss [165], it is not possible to deny the existence of a specific sarcoma of lymphatic endothelium, but there seem to be few reliable criteria to make such a distinction on histological grounds.

(a) Sarcoma of Stewart and Treves

This malignant tumor was first described by Stewart and Treves in 1948 [166]. The majority of cases are associated with chronic lymphedema following mastectomy for breast carcinoma, but only 0.45% of all women surviving 5 years following mastectomy develop this tumor [167]. Most patients are women in their seventh decade who have undergone mastectomy 4–27 years earlier. In congenital (idiopathic) lymphedema, the tumor may also occur, but these patients are younger (fourth to fifth decade) and the lymphedema is of longer duration (19–20 years in the average).

Clinically, one or more dark red or purple macules occur in the skin of the lymphedematous upper or lower extremity. As the lesions enlarge and spread, they may ulcerate. Metastases occur early and are mostly localized in the lungs. Post-mastectomy lymphangiosarcomas are usually fatal within weeks or months. The mean survival time is only 19 months for post-mastectomy sarcomas and 34 months for angiosarcomas associated with congenital chronic lymphedema [165].

It is virtually impossible to distinguish the lymphangiosarcoma and other types of angiosarcoma on histological grounds. All angiosarcomas are composed of capillaries with obviously malignant endothelial cells that infiltrate soft tissues and skin. The tumor cells may be small and poorly differentiated with scanty, ill-defined cytoplasm or large, pleomorphic and spindle-shaped or round with abundant cytoplasm. The nuclei in both cases are atypical and hyperchromatic with prominent nucleoli and increased mitotic activity.

Various forms of vascular structures may occur in angiosarcomas: caverns with flat but atypical endothelium or irregular spaces with proliferating endothelial cells forming pseudopapillae. The vascular spaces may

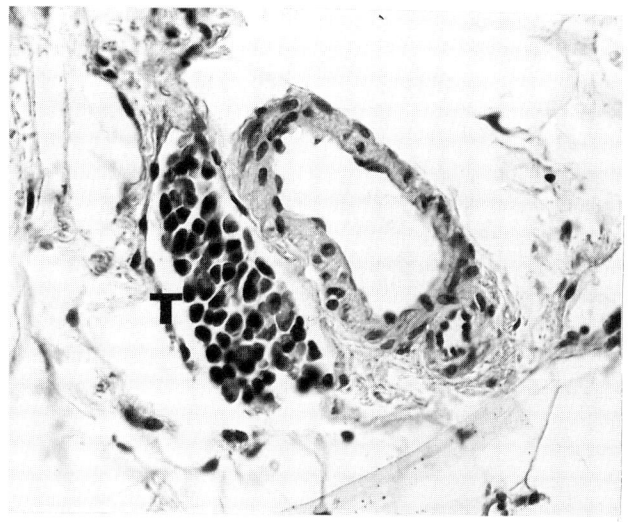

Figure 13.42 Lymphangiomatosis carcinomatosa. Tumor cells (T) in a lymph capillary accompanying a blood vessel. (H&E.)

vessels. Mesenchymal cells have a great variation of differentiation possibilities encompassing all mesenchymal cell types. In a malignant fibrous histiocytoma, for example, one may encounter endothelial cells, fibroblasts, smooth and striated muscle cells and histiocytes, all in the same tumor.

(b) Lymphangioleiomyomatosis (LAM)

This disorder is believed to start from the pelvic or retroperitoneal lymphatics, consisting of proliferation of the smooth musculature within lymphatic vessels and lymph nodes with centripetal progression into the thoracic duct, finally involving also the lymphatics within the pulmonary parenchyma. LAM occurs more frequently in women than in men. Clinical symptoms include chylascites, chylothorax and right heart failure from pulmonary hypertension. A localized type involving only lymph nodes and lymph vessels, or isolated to the lungs only, should be distinguished from the generalized variety. There is a strong association between pulmonary LAM and the tuberous sclerosis complex.

Histologically, the smooth muscle cell bundles are hypertrophied and aligned in oblique and interwoven cords. The media appears expanded and irregular and the lymphatic lumina are narrowed or obliterated. The smooth muscle cells may have enlarged and pleomorphic nuclei but atypical mitotic figures are absent. Metastases have never been observed. Concurrent proliferation of the smooth muscles in both the lymphatic and blood vessels also have been described [163].

be surrounded by cords of spindle-shaped atypical cells. This feature which is typical in Kaposi's sarcoma, may render impossible the distinction between Stewart-Treves' and Kaposi's sarcoma. If there are cavernous spaces, they may be filled with erythrocytes or by clear lymph-like fluid. The lesions surrounding the obviously malignant alterations may consist of dilated lymphatic capillaries lined by plump endothelial cells with hyperchromatic nuclei (lymphangiomatosis). These structures are believed to represent premalignant changes [165].

Ultrastructurally, the endothelial cells still express typical features such as micropinocytic vesicles, lateral desmosome-like attachments and paranuclear filaments, basement membranes, Weibel–Palade bodies and pericytes, but the nuclei are enlarged, irregularly shaped and contain prominent nucleoli. Other tumor cells resemble primitive mesenchymal cells with abundant rough-surfaced endoplasmatic reticulum, glycogen, few intercellular attachments, no Weibel–Palade bodies and no luminal differentiation between the solid cell groups.

Immunohistochemical examinations show positivity for vimentin. In well differentiated tumor cells, the reaction to factor VIII related antigen may be positive. In the more primitive cell types, immunohistochemical markers may fail to allow any differentiation [168].

In our own limited experience, the survival rate of patients with tumors resembling Kaposi's sarcoma was longer (up to 8 years) than of those with features resembling an ordinary angiosarcoma (under 1 year).

(b) Expression of lymphatic vessels in Kaposi's sarcoma

Kaposi's sarcoma is closely associated with human immunodeficiency virus infection. There is still contradictory evidence whether the tumor is derived from vascular or from lymphatic endothelium. Although the actual tumor tissue bears little resemblance to lymph–vascular structures, similar alterations of lymphatic tissue as seen in Stewart–Treves' sarcoma may be found adjacent to Kaposi's sarcoma. Immunohistochemical investigations are inconclusive. There are variations of immunoreactivity at different stages of the disease, with the early patch stage having the immunohistochemical profile of a lymphatic tumor [165].

In all probability, Stewart–Treves' sarcoma as well as Kaposi's sarcoma and ordinary angiosarcoma are closely related and derived from primitive mesenchymal cells with the capability to differentiate into either vascular or lymphatic channels. The suggestion that bone marrow-derived dermal dendrocytes might be the cells of origin of the spindle-shaped population, which characterizes Kaposi's sarcoma [169], has been refuted [170].

References

1. Todorov, A.B. (1985) Genetische Aspekte bei angeborenen Gefässfehlern, in *Angeborene Gefässfehler*, (eds S. Belov, D.A. Loose and E. Müller), Einhorn Presse Verlag, Reinbek, BRD, pp. 290–309.
2. Koch, G. (1956) Zur Klinik, Symptomatologie, Pathogenese und Erbpathologie des Klippel–Trenaunay–Weberschen Syndroms. *Actae Genet. Med. Gem.*, 5, 326–68.
3. Wellens, W. (1961) Triade de Klippel et Trenaunay. A propos de 23 cas. *Phlébologie*, 14, 21–35.
4. Schnyder, U.W. and Keller, R. (1954) Zur Klinik und Histologie der Angiome. *Arch. Dermat. Syph. (Basel)*, 198, 333–42.
5. Happle, R. (1987) Lethal genes surviving by mosaicism: a possible explanation for sporadic birth defects involving the skin. *J. Am. Acad. Dermatol.*, 16, 899–906.
6. Kontras, S.B. (1974) The Klippel–Trenaunay–Weber syndrome, in *Malformation Syndromes; Birth Defects*, (ed. D. Bergsma), Original articles series, vol. 10 (7), Grune-Stratton, New York, pp. 177–88.
7. Lindenauer, S.M. (1965) The Klippel–Trenaunay syndrome: varicosity, hypertrophy and hemangioma with no arteriovenous fistula. *Ann. Surg.*, 162, 303–14.
8. Alvoet, G.E.J., Jorens, P.G. and Roelen, L.M. (1991) Aspects génétiques dans le syndrome de Klippel–Trenaunay. *Phlébologie*, 44, 809–14.
9. Keret, D., Kam, I., Ben Arieh, Y. and Hashimonai, M. (1990) Scrotal cavernous haemangioma with a familiar history of cutaneous angiomata. *J. Roy. Soc. Med.*, 83, 402–3.
10. Boder, E. and Sedgwick, R.P. (1958) Ataxia-teleangiectasia. *Pediatrics*, 21, 526–54.
11. Rickenbacher, J. (1966) Zur Entwicklung der Venen der unteren Extremität. *Zentbl. Phlebol.*, 5, 6–14.
12. Allenby, P.A., Boesel, C.P. and Marsh, W.L. (1990) Diffuse angiomatosis of the extremities presenting as a sarcoma. *Arch. Pathol. Lab. Med.*, 114, 987–90.
13. Servelle, M. (1953) Agenesie d'une des veines principales du membre inférieur. *Coeur Med. Interne.*, 4, 53–63.
14. Malan, E. and Puglionisi, A. (1964) Congenital angiodysplasias of the extremities. *J. Cardiovasc. Surg.*, 5, 87–130; (1965) 6, 255–345.
15. May, R. and Nissl, R. (1970) Beitrag zur Klassifizierung der 'gemischten kongenitalen Angiodysplasien'. *Fortschr. Geb. Röntgenstr. Nuklearmed.*, 113, 170–89.
16. Pratesi, F. (1972) Classification of angiopathic disease of the limbs. *Folia Angiol.*, 20, 193–215.
17. Vollmar, J.P. (1976) *Arteriovenöse Fisteln, Dilatierende Arteriopathien*, (eds J.F. Vollmar and F.P. Nobbe), Thieme, Stuttgart, pp. 38–49.
18. Schobinger, R. (1977) *Periphere Angiodysplasien*, Huber; Bern, Stuttgart, Wien.
19. Malan, E. (1974) *Vascular Malformations (Angiodysplasias)*, Carlo Erba Foundation, Milan.
20. Belov, St, Loose, D.A. and Weber, J. (1989) *Vascular Malformations*, Einhorn Presse Verlag, Reinbek, Periodica Angiologica, pp. 16–29.
21. Papendiek, C.B. (1988) *Angiodysplasias in Pediatrics*, Editorial Medica Panamericana, Buenos Aires.
22. Kromhout, J.G. (1991) Vascular malformations of the extremities. Thesis, University of Amsterdam.
23. Mulliken, J.B., Glowacki, J. (1982) Haemangiomas and vascular malformations in infants and children: a classification based on endothelial characteristics. *Plast. Reconstr. Surg.*, 69, 412–22.
24. Leu, H.J. (1990) Pathomorphology of vascular malformations. Analysis of 310 cases. *Inter. Angiol.*, 9, 147–54.
25. Kappert, A. (1985) *Lehrbuch und Atlas der Angiologie*. 11. Aufl., Huber, Bern, Stuttgart, Wien, p. 306.
26. Neville, R.F., Franco, Ch.D., Anderson, R.J. et al. (1990) Popliteal artery agensis – a new anatomic variant. *J. Vasc. Surg.*, 12, 573–80.
27. Vollmar, J., Voss, E. (1979) Vena marginalis lateralis persistens – die vergessene Vene der Angiologen. *Vasa*, 8, 192–202.
28. Fischer, R. (1988) Simulation einer Parva-Stammvarikose durch eine massive Varikose der Venae nervi suralis. *Vasa*, 17, 283–7.
29. Kubik, St and Manestar, M. (1991) Gefässanatomie des Beckens, in *Das Becken*, (ed. U. Brunner), Huber, Bern, Göttingen, Toronto, pp. 12–63.
30. Leu, H.J. (1990) A rare case of angiodysplasia: penetration of inguinal lymph nodes by large superficial leg veins. *Virchows Arch. A Pathol. Anat.*, 417, 185–6.
31. Luke, J.C. (1941) The diagnosis of chronic enlargement of the leg. With a description of a new syndrome. *Surg. Gynec. Obstet.*, 73, 472–80.
32. Lodin, A. and Lindvall, N. (1958/59) Congenital absence of venous valves as a cause of leg ulcers. *Acta Chir. Scand.*, 116, 256–61.
33. Lodin, A. (1961) Congenital absence of valves in the deep veins of the leg. *Acta Derm. Venereol (Stockholm)*, 41 (suppl. 45).
34. Leu, H.J. (1974) Familial congenital absence of valves in the deep leg veins. *Humangenetik*, 22, 347–9.
35. Zamboni, P., Cossu, A., Carpanese, L. et al. (1990) The so-called primary venous aneurysms. *Phlebology*, 5, 45–50.
36. Bockenheimer, P. (1907) Ueber die genuine diffuse Phlebectasie der oberen

Extremität. *Festschrift für G.E. von Rindfleisch*, Leipzig.
37. Vogt, H.D., Altmann-Canestri, E. and Sanchez, C. (1991) La flebectasia genuina difusa del miembro superior. *Rev. Panam. Flebol. Linfol.*, 1, 35–6.
38. Moseley, J.E. and Starobin, S.G. (1964) Cystic angiomatosis of bone. *Am. J. Roentg. Rad. Therap. Nucl. Med.*, 41, 1114–20.
39. Rappaport, I. and Shiffman, M.A. (1963) Multiple phlebectasias involving jejunum, oral cavity and scrotum. *J. Am. Med. Ass.*, 185, 437–40.
40. Seckler, S.G., Rubin, H. and Rabinowitz, J.G. (1964) Systemic angiomatosis. *Am. J. Med.*, 37, 976–86.
41. Mandybur, Th.I. and Nazek, M. (1990) Cerebral arteriovenous malformations. *Arch. Pathol. Lab. Med.*, 114, 970–3.
42. Albertini, A. von (1955) *Histologische Geschwulstdiagnostik*. Thieme, Stuttgart.
43. Leu, H.J. (1989) Pathoanatomy of congenital vascular malformations, in *Vascular Malformations*, (eds St Belov, D.A. Loose and J. Weber), Einhorn Presse Verlag, Reinbek, BRD, pp. 37–45.
44. Leu, H.J. (1980) Ultrastrukturelle Veränderungen bei venöser Angiodysplasie vom Typ Klippel–Trenaunay. *Vasa*, 9, 147–51.
45. Lie, J.T. (1988) Pathology of angiodysplasia in Klippel–Trenaunay syndrome. *Pathol. Res. Pract.*, 183, 747–55.
46. Leu, H.J., Vogt, M. and Pfrunder, H. (1979) Morphological alterations of non-varicose and varicose veins. *Basic Res. Cardiol.*, 74, 435–44.
47. Leu, H.J., Vogt, M., Pfrunder, H. and Odermatt, B.F. (1991) Phlebosclerosis: disorder or disease? *Vasa*, 20, 230–6.
48. Thurner, J. and May, R. (1967) Probleme der Phlebopathie mit besonderer Berücksichtigung der Phlebosklerose. *Zentbl. Phlebol.*, 6, 404–82.
49. Leu, H.J., Rüttner, J.R. and Schneider, J. (1971) Zur Frage der Beziehungen zwischen Arteriosklerose und Phlebosklerose der Beingefässe. *Schweiz. Med. Wschr.*, 101, 1323–6.
50. Grüntzig, A. and Albrecht, H.J. (1972) Knochenmetaplasie des subkutanen Gewebes bei chronisch-venöser Insuffizienz. *Vasa*, 1, 52–61.
51. Lippmann, H.J. (1957) Subcutaneous ossification in chronic venous insufficiency. *Angiology*, 8, 378–96.
52. Leu, H.J. and Brunner, U. (1992) Verkalkende und verknöchernde Phlebosklerose. *Vasa*, 21, 11–14.
53. May, R. (1974) Die Problematik des Beckenvenensporns. *Vasa*, 3, 28–33.
54. Gullmo, Å. (1964) Periphere Venen, in *Handbuch der medizinischen Radiologie*, Bd.X/3, Springer, Berlin, p. 473.
55. Gjöres, J.E. (1965) The incidence of venous thrombosis and its sequelae in certain districts of Sweden. *Acta Chir. Scand. (Stockholm)*, suppl. 206, p. 65.
56. Widmer, L.K., Stähelin, H.B., Nissen, C. and DaSilva, A. (1981) *Venen-Arterien-Krankheiten, koronare Herzkrankheit bei Berufstätigen*. Huber, Bern, Stuttgart, Wien, p. 57.
57. Rose, S.S. and Ahmend, A. (1986) Some thoughts on the aetiology of varicose veins. *J. Cardiovasc. Surg.*, 27, 534–43.
58. Thulesius, O., Ugaily-Thulesius, L., Gjöres, J.E. and Neglen, P. (1988) The varicose saphenous vein. Functional and ultrastructural studies with special reference to smooth muscle. *Phlebology*, 3, 89–95.
59. Vogt, M. (1978) Altersabhängige morphologische Veränderungen der Vena saphena magna. *Vasa*, 7, 54–60.
60. Leu, H.J. (1978) Morphologische Veränderungen an den oberflächlichen und tiefen Venen der unteren Extremität im höheren Alter, in *Phlebologie, Lymphologie und Proktologie in verschiedenen Lebensaltern*, (ed. K. Salfeld), Schattauer, Stuttgart, pp. 31–7.
61. Rose, S.S. (1992) The aetiology of varicose veins. *Phlebology*, 6, 215–17.
62. Myers, Th.T. (1962) Diseases of the veins, in *Peripheral Vascular Diseases*, (eds E.V. Allen, N.W. Barker and E.A. Hines Jr), W.B. Saunders, Philadelphia and London, pp. 636–58.
63. Cooper Jr, A.F. Hobart, D.J. and Provenza, V. (1978) Analysis of the number and position of the valves in normal and varicose saphenous veins. *Vasc. Surg.*, 12, 308–14.
64. Kulwin, M.H. and Hines Jr, E.A. (1950) Blood vessels of the skin in chronic venous insufficiency. *Arch. Dermat. Syphil.*, 62, 293–304.
65. Basmajian, J.V. (1952) The distribution of valves in the femoral, external iliac and common iliac veins and their relation to varicose veins. *Surg. Gynec. Obstet.*, 95, 537–42.
66. Acsady, Gy., Lenguel, L. and Solti, F. (1990) Histochemical examination of the structural changes in varicose veins. *Phlebol. Proktol.*, 19, 200–4.
67. Haustein, U.F. and Herrmann, K. (1990) Lysosomale Enzyme und N-Prokollagenpeptid Typ III bei chronischer Veneninsuffizienz. *Phlebol. Proktol.*, 19, 124–6.
68. Niebes, P. (1976) *Biochemical Studies of Varicosis*. *Int. Symposium on Venous Diseases*, Nyon, Oct. 26–28, Huber, Bern, Stuttgart, Wien.
69. Lechner, W. (1982) Vergleichende elektronenoptische Untersuchungen an der Venenwand bei verschiedenen Formen und Schweregraden der primären Varikose. *Phlebol. Proktol.*, 11, 125–31.
70. Lechner, W. and Lanz, U. (1990) Veränderungen des Endothels bei haemodynamischer Fehlbelastung-Ultrastrukturelle Untersuchungsbefunde variköser Venen. *Phlebol. Proktol.*, 19, 187–90.
71. Staubesand, J. (1978) Matrixvesikel und Mediadysplasie, ein neues Konzept zur formalen Genese der Varikose. *Phlebol. Proktol.*, 7, 109–40.
72. Leu, H.J. (1980) Zur Ultrastruktur des Endothels in varikösen Venen. *Phlebol. Proktol.*, 9, 153–61.
73. Thulesius, O., Gjöres, J.E., Eriksson, D. and Berlin, E. (1984) Mechanische und biochemische Voraussetzungen der chronisch-venösen Insuffizienz. *Vasa*, 13, 195–200.
74. Vogler, E. (1953) Vasographischer Beitrag zur Aetiologie und Genese des Ulcus cruris. *Fortschr. Geb. Roentgenstr.*, 79, 79–94.
75. Haeger, K. (1967) Atraumatic arteriovenous anastomoses in the leg and foot. *Zentbl. Phlebol.*, 6492–508.
76. Hehne, H.J., Locher, J.Th., Waibel, P. and Friedrich, R. (1974) Zur Bedeutung arteriovenöser Anastomosen bei der primären Varikosis und der chronisch-venösen Insuffizienz. *Vasa*, 3, 396–8.
77. Lindemayr, W., Lofferer, O., Mostbeck, A. and Partsch, H. (1972) Arteriovenous shunts in primary varicosis? A critical essay. *Vasc. Surg.*, 6, 9–13.
78. Lofferer, O., Mostbeck, A. and Partsch, H. (1969) Arteriovenöse Kurzschlüsse der Extremitäten. Nuklearmedizinische Untersuchungen mit besonderer Berücksichtigung des postthrombotischen Unterschenkelgeschwürs. *Zentbl. Phlebol.*, 8, 2–22.
79. Gottlob, R.M.E. (1990) Morphology of valves in health and disease. *Vth European – American Symposium on Venous Disease*, Vienna, Nov. 7–10 (abstract n. 2A1).
80. Jagtman, B.A. (1983) Clinical investigation of skin elasticity. Thesis Nijmegen, The Netherlands.
81. Leu, H.J. (1991) Morphology of chronic venous insufficiency – light and electron microscopic examinations. *Vasa*, 20, 330–42.
82. Graham, J.H., Marques, A.S., Johnson, W.C. and Gray, H.R. (1972) Stasis dermatitis, in *Dermal Pathology*, (eds J.H. Graham, W.C. Johnson and B. Helwig), Harper and Row, Hagerstone, Maryland, pp. 333–60.
83. Hammersen, F. (1977) Bau und Funktion der Blutkapillaren, in *Handbuch der allgemeinen Pathologie III/7, Mikrozirkulation* (ed. H. Meessen). Springer, Berlin, Heidelberg, New York, p. 135.
84. Coleridge Smith, P.D., Thomas, P., Scurr, J.H. and Dormandy, J.A. (1988) Causes of venous ulceration: a new hypothesis. *Brit. Med. J.*, 296, 1726–7.
85. Burnand, K.G., Whimster, I., Naidoo, A. and Browse, N.L. (1982) Pericapillary fibrin in the ulcerbearing skin of the leg: the cause of lipodermatosclerosis and venous ulceration. *Brit. Med. J.*, 285, 1071–2.
86. Noordhoek, H. (1991) Stasis dermatitis and ulceration. *Phlebology*, 6 (suppl. 1), pp. 16–17.
87. Moyses, C., Cederholm-Williams, S.A. and Michel, C.C. (1987) Haemoconcentration and accumulation of white cells in the feet during venous stasis. *Int. J. Microcirc. Clin. Expl*, 5, 311–20.
88. Thomas, P.R.S., Nash, G.B. and Dormandy, J.A. (1988) White cell accumulation in dependent legs of patients with venous hypertension: a possible mechanism for trophic changes in the skin. *Brit. Med. J.*, 296, 1693–5.
89. Doerr, W. (1976) *Organpathologie*, Bd. I, Thieme, Stuttgart, p. 12.
90. Mentha, C. (1963) La Dégénérescence mucoide des veines. *Presse Méd.*, 71, 2205–6.
91. Largadièr, J. and Leu, H.J. (1984) Sogenannte zystische Adventitiadegeneration der Arteria poplitea mit Stielverbindung zum Kniegelenk. *Vasa*, 13, 267–71.
92. Leu, H.J., Largiadèr, J. and Odermatt, B. (1984) Pathogenesis of so-called cystic adventitial degeneration of peripheral blood vessels. *Virchows Archiv. A Pathol. Anat.*, 404, 289–300.
93. Lie, J.T., Jensen, P.L. and Smith, R.E. (1991) Adventitial cystic disease of the lesser saphenous vein. *Arch. Pathol. Lab. Med.*, 115, 946–8.
94. Havig, Oe. (1974) Pathogenese der tiefen Venenthrombose – eine postmortale Studie. *Vasa*, 3, 135–7.
95. Widmer, L.K., Zemp, E., Widmer, M.-Th. et al. (1985) Late results in deep vein thrombosis of the lower extremity. *Vasa*, 14, 265–8.
96. Sandritter, W. and Beneke, G. (1969) Thrombose, in *Lehrbuch der speziellen Pathologie*, Bd. I. (Erg. Bd.), (ed. E. Kaufmann), de Gruyter, Berlin, p. 464.
97. Jorns, U. (1972) Die Häufigkeit und die möglichen Einflussfaktoren der massiven Lungenembolie. Thesis, Frankfurt.
98. Feigl, W. and Schwarz, N. (1977) Häufigkeit von Beinvenenthrombosen und Lungenembolie im Obduktionsgut, in *Akute tiefe Becken- und Beinvenenthrombosen*, (ed. H. Ehringer), Huber, Bern, Stuttgart, Wien, p. 27.
99. Wegmann, D. (1981) Paraneoplastische Thrombose. Eine mortalitätsstatistische Untersuchung. *Vasa*, 10, 111–18.
100. Leu, H.J., Feigl, W. and Susani, M. (1987) Angiogenesis from mononuclear cells in thrombi. *Virchows Archiv. A Pathol. Anat.*, 411, 5–14.
101. Feigl, W., Susani, M. and Ulrich, W. (1985) Organization of experimental thrombosis by blood cells. *Virchows Archiv. A Pathol. Anat.*, 406, 133–48.
102. Tsapogas, M.J., Stirling, G.M. and Girolami, M.B. (1967) Study on the organization of experimental thrombi. *Angiology*, 18, 825–32.
103. Stirling, G.A. and Tsapogas, M.J. (1969) In vitro culture of artificial thrombi. *Angiology*, 20, 44–51.
104. Doerr, W. and Kayser, K. (1977) Koronarthrombose und Herzinfarkt, in *Der Herzinfarkt*, (ed. G. Schettgler), Schattauer, Stuttgart, p. 111.
105. Hofmann, W., Rommel, T., Schaupp, T. et al. (1980) Transformations-

vorgänge in der Frühphase der Entstehung des arteriellen Thrombus. *Virchows Archiv. A Pathol. Anat.*, **385**, 151–68.
106. Irniger, W. (1963) Histologische Altersbestimmung von Thromben und Emboli. *Virchows Archiv. A Pathol. Anat.*, **363**, 220–37.
107. Leu, H.J. (1973) Histologische Altersbestimmung von arteriellen und venösen Thromben und Emboli. *Vasa*, **2**, 265–74.
108. Bär, T., Güldner, F.H. and Wolff, J.R. (1984) 'Seamless' endothelial cells of blood capillaries. *Cell Tissue Res.*, **235**, 99–106.
109. Folkman, J. and Haudenschild, C. (1980) Angiogenesis in vitro. *Nature*, **288**, 551–6.
110. Feder, J., Masara, J.C. and Olander, J.V. (1983) The formation of capillary-like tubes by calf aortic endothelial cells grown in vitro. *J. Cell Physiol.*, **115**, 1–6.
111. Leu, H.J., Feigl, W., Susani, M. and Odermatt, B. (1988) Differentiation of mononuclear blood cells into macrophages, fibroblasts and endothelial cells in thrombus organization. *Expl Cell Biol.*, **56**, 201–10.
112. Bessis, M. (1973) *Living Blood Cells and their Ultrastructure*, Springer, Berlin, Heidelberg, New York.
113. Leu, A.J. and Leu, H.J. (1989) Spezielle Probleme bei der histologischen Altersbestimmung von Thromben und Emboli. *Pathologe*, **10**, 87–92.
114. Sachs, H. (1955) Meteorhologische Einflüsse bei den Venenthrombosen, in *Die thromboembolischen Erkrankungen und ihre Behandlung*, (eds Th. Nägeli and P. Matis), Schattauer, Stuttgart, p. 17.
115. Rappert, E. and Zandanell, P. (1958) Pathologische Veränderungen am Gefässystem bei Thrombosen. *Acta III Internationalis Angiologorum Congressus*, (ed. M. Comel), San Remo, p. 546.
116. Dodd, H. and Cockett, F.B. (1956) *The Pathology and Surgery of the Veins of the Lower Limb*. Livingstone, Edinburgh.
117. Wagenvoort, C.A. and Wagenvoort, N. (1970) Primary pulmonary hypertension. *Circulation*, **42**, 1163–84.
118. Kappert, A. (1974) Phlegmasia coerulea dolens. *Vasa*, **3**, 467–70.
119. Rohrer, M.J., Cardulo, P.A., Pappos, A.M. *et al.* (1990) Axillary artery compression and thrombosis in throwing athletes. *J. Vasc. Surg.*, **11** 761–8.
120. Baker, W.F. (1989) Clinical aspects of disseminated intravascular coagulation: a clinician's point of view. *Sem. Thromb. Hemostasis*, **15**, 1–57.
121. Masson, P. (1923) Hémangioendothéliome végétant intravasculaire. *Bull. Sci. Anat. (Paris)*, **93**, 517–32.
122. Leu, H.J. (1983) Intravaskuläre papilläre endotheliale Hyperplasie. *Pathologe*, **4**, 92–6.
123. Monreal, M., Lafoz, E., Casals, A. *et al.* (1991) Occult cancer in patients with deep venous thrombosis: a systematic approach. *Cancer*, **67**, 541–5.
124. Monreal, M., Casals, A., Boix, J. *et al.* (1993) Occult cancer in patients with acute pulmonary embolism: a prospective study. *Chest*, **103**, 816–19.
125. Brunner, U. (1988) Tiefe Venenthrombose. Vergleich des Schrifttums über verschiedene Langzeitstudien in gefässchirurgischer Sicht. *Vasa*, **17**, 247–58.
126. Feuerstein, W. (1984) Zur Pathogenese des postthrombotischen Beingeschwürs. *Phlebol. Proktol.*, **13**, 21–3.
127. Salzmann, P. (1985) Gibt es eine Korrelation zwischen dem postthrombotischen Syndrom und dem Ausmass der Veränderungen des tiefen Venensystems? *Phlebol. Proktol.*, **14**, 34–7.
128. Zimmerman, B. (1985) Thromboselokalisation und klinisches Bild des postthrombotischen Syndroms. *Phlebol. Proktol.*, **14**, 38–40.
129. Aburahma, A.F., Lucente, F.C. and Doland, J.P. (1990) Paradoxical embolism: an underestimated entity. *J. Cardiovasc. Surg.*, **31**, 685–92.
130. Diebold, J. and Löhrs, U. (1991) Venous thrombosis and pulmonary embolism (a study of 5039 autopsies). *Pathol. Res. Pract.*, **187**, 260–6.
131. Lie, J.T. (1991) Infection-related vasculitides, in *Systemic Vasculitides*, (eds A. Churg and J. Churg), Igaku-Shoin, New York, Tokyo, pp. 243–56.
132. Lie, J.T. (1987) Thromboangitis obliterans (Buerger's disease) revisited. *Pathol. Ann.*, **23** (part 2), 257–91.
133. Bollinger, A. and Leu, H.J. (1974) Thrombophlebitis saltans. *Dtsch Med. Wschr.*, **99**, 1433–6.
134. Horsch, A.K. (1988), in *Thrombangiitis obliterans – Morbus Winiwarter–Buerger*, (ed. H. Heidrich), Thieme, Stuttgart, pp. 45–7.
135. Prenner, K. (1988) Klinik der Endagiitis obliterans, in *Thrombangiitis obliterans – Morbus Winiwarter–Buerger*, (ed. H. Heidrich), Thieme, Stuttgart, pp. 49–53.
136. Pirnat, L. and Simic, Lj. (1988), in *Thrombagiitis obliterans – Morbus Winiwarter–Buerger*, (ed. H. Heidrich), Thieme, Stuttgart, pp. 47–8.
137. Shionoya, S. (1990) *Buerger's disease*, Univ. of Nagoya Press, Nagoya, Japan.
138. Churg, A. and Churg, J. (1991) *Systemic Vasculitides*, Igaku-Shoin, New York, Tokyo.
139. Grishman, E. and Spiera, H. (1991) Vasculitis in connective tissue diseases, including hypocomplementemic vasculitis, in *Systemic Vasculitides*, (A. Churg and J. Churg), Igaku-Shoin, New York, Tokyo, pp. 273–392.
140. Chakravarti, A. and Chakravarti, G. (1955) Case of giant cell polyphlebitis. *Brit. Med. J.*, **I**, 253, 255.
141. O'Donnell, M. and Kennedy, J.D. (1955) Case of primary granulomatous phlebitis. *Irish Med. J.*, 129–31.
142. Leu, H.J., Brinninger, G., Pernegger, Ch. and Odermatt, B. (1993) Primary granulomatous giant cell polyphlebitis of visceral veins. *Virchows Archiv. A Pathol. Anat.*, **423**, 519–21.
143. Heinisch, H.-M. (1983) Pediatric lymphangiology, in *Lymphangiology*, (eds M. Földi and J.R. Casley-Smith), Schattauer, Stuttgart, pp. 777–810.
144. Leu, H.J. and Brunner, U. (1981) Osteolysierende Hämangiomatose nach Trauma. *Dtsch Med. Wschr.*, **106**, 1424–8.
145. Huth, F. (1983) General pathology of the lymphvascular system, in *Lymphangiology*, (eds M. Földi and J.R. Casley-Smith), Schattauer, Stuttgart, pp. 215–300.
146. Knüsel, J. (1987) Verlauf und Prognose bei primärem Lymphödem der Beine. Eine Untersuchung an 200 Patienten. Thesis, Zürich, Switzerland.
147. Brunner, U. (1985) Hat das Manifestationsalter des primären Lymphödems hormonelle Ursachen? Referat Jahrestagung der Dtsch Ges. Angiologie, Berlin. Demeter, Gräfelfing, BRD.
148. Brunner, U. (1969) *Das Lymphödem der unteren Extremitäten*, Huber, Bern.
149. Leu, H.J. (1985) Patho-anatomical findings in the initial lymphatics, in *The Initial Lymphatics*, (eds A. Bollinger, H. Partsch and J.H.N. Wolfe), Thieme, Stuttgart, pp. 84–91.
150. Van Limborgh, J. (1966) Mikroskopische Anatomie der Lymphgefässwand, in *Morphologie und Histochemie der Gefässwand*, II. Teil, (eds M. Comel and L. Laszt), Karger, Basel, New York, p. 305.
151. Leu, H.J. (1981) Zur Pathologie der Lymphkollektoren bei primären und sekundären Lymphödemen und bei lymphologisch gesunden Verstorbenen. *Angio*, **3**, 281–6.
152. Leu, H.J. (1978) Morphologische Veränderungen an den oberflächlichen und tiefen Lymphkollektoren der unteren Extremitäten im höheren Alter, in *Phlebologie, Lymphologie und Proktologie in verschiedenen Lebensaltern. Ergebnisse der Angiologie*, Bd. 18, Schattgauer, Stuttgart, pp. 117–23.
153. Lanz, R. (1963) Ueber das Lymphödem. *Zentbl. Phlebol.*, **2**, 248–62.
154. Lofferer, O., Mostbeck, A. and Partsch, H. (1972) Nuklearmedizinische Diagnostik von Lymphabfluss-Störungen der unteren Extremitäten. *Vasa*, **1**, 94–102.
155. Tiedjen, K.U., Schultz-Ehrenburg, U. and Knorz, S. (1992) Lymphabflusstörungen bei chronischer Veneninsuffizienz. *Phlebologie*, **21**, 63–71.
156. Brunner, U., Geroulanos, St. and Leu, H.J. (1988) Infektlymphologie und Zugangslymphologie-zwei neue Begriffe in der peripheren Gefässchirurgie. *Vasa*, **17**, 275–82.
157. Brunner, U., Sonderegger, A., Fleischlin, C. and Lanz, M. (1984) Epidemiologie und Klinik des primären Lymphödems anhand von 500 Fällen, in *Die initiale Lymphstrombahn*, (eds A. Bollinger and H. Partsch), Thieme, Stuttgart.
158. Case, T., Leis, B., Witte, M. *et al.* (1991) Vascular abnormalities in experimental and human lymphatic filariasis. *Lymphology*, **24**, 174–83.
159. Enterline, H.T. and Roberts, B. (1955) Lymphangiopericytoma. *Cancer*, **8**, 582–8.
160. Hamoudi, A.B., Vassy, L.E. and Morse, T.S. (1975) Multiple lymphangioendothelioma of the spleen in a 14-year-old girl. *Arch. Pathol.*, **99**, 605–6.
161. Nather, K. (1921) Ueber ein malignes Lymphoendotheliom der Haut des Fusses. *Virchows Archiv.*, **231**, 540–56.
162. Calnan, J. and Cowdell, R.H. (1958/59) Lymphangioendothelioma of the anterior abdominal wall. *Brit. J. Surg.*, **46**, 375–8.
163. Luz, A. and Hedinger, Chr. (1973) Lymphangioleiomyomatose. *Schweiz. Med. Wschr.*, **103**, 1833–41.
164. Nash, A.D. (1989) *Soft Tissue Sarcomas*, Raven Press, New York, p. 96.
165. Enzinger, F.M. and Weiss, Sh. (1988) *Soft Tissue Tumors*, 2nd ed, Mosby, St. Louis, Washington, Toronto, p. 545.
166. Stewart, F.W. and Treves, N. (1948) Lymphangiosarcoma in postmastectomy lymphedema. *Cancer*, **1**, 64–81.
167. Shirger, A. (1962) Postoperative lymphedema: etiologic and diagnostic factors. *Med. Clins N. Am.*, **46**, 1045–50.
168. Leu, H.J. and Odermatt, B. (1989) Neue immunhistochemische Untersuchungen beim Stewart–Treves–Syndrom. *Lymphologica 89*, Medikon Verlag, München, BRD, pp. 90–1.
169. Nickoloff, B. and Griffiths, C. (1989) Factor XIIIa-expressing dermal dendrocytes in AIDS-associated cutaneous Kaposi's sarcoma. *Science*, **243**, 1736–7.
170. Kanitakis, J. and Roca-Miralles, M. (1992) Factor XIIIa-expressing dermal dendrocytes in Kaposi's sarcoma. *Virchows Archiv. A Pathol. Anat.*, **420**, 227–31.

14 ABNORMAL ARTERIOVENOUS COMMUNICATIONS AND FISTULAE

William E. Stehbens

Holman used the term 'abnormal arteriovenous communications' for those pathological lesions often termed arteriovenous malformations, aneurysms or fistulae [1]. Malformation implies maldevelopment of the blood vessels *ab initio* and further that the aetiology has been established, but it has not. The term aneurysm is not really appropriate for the essential lesion is not an aneurysm, although aneurysmal dilatations are prone to occur secondarily in the arteries and veins associated with an arteriovenous (A–V) shunt. In some instances an aortic aneurysm may produce a shunt by rupturing into the inferior vena cava. Many lesions are due to trauma or some other pathological lesion. Side-to-side communications between an artery and vein are appropriately termed fistulae without any aetiological implication. These lesions will therefore not be referred to as A–V malformations but as A–V communications with the reservation that unless otherwise indicated they are pathological rather than physiological communications.

William Hunter [2] is said to have provided the first clear description of such a communication in 1757. These lesions were frequently the result of penetrating injuries, often complicating blood-letting at the cubital fossa. It was not until Holman [1] commenced his investigations early this century that their truly pernicious character was revealed. Though relatively neglected in the past, this interesting lesion is of profound importance as a haemodynamic model for the study of vascular pathology.

A–V fistula is used in reference to A–V shunts between an artery and a neighbouring vein such as between the femoral artery and vein or the cavernous segment of the internal carotid artery and the cavernous venous sinus. These lesions are frequently traumatic in origin and often the result of perforating injuries. Their pathology in humans has not yet been carefully studied so that the best source of knowledge of such lesions is provided by experimental A–V shunts.

When an artery is anastomosed side-to-side surgically to a vein, arterial blood flows preferentially into the low pressure vein. The fistula thus formed is associated with a bruit on auscultation and a palpable thrill which imparts an uncomfortable tingling sensation to the tip of the palpating finger. The vein vibrates visibly and within a few weeks the shunt becomes more pronounced with dilatation of the proximal segment of the anastomosed artery.

The internal elastic lamina develops transversely orientated tears (Figure 14.1) proximal to the fistula within two to five days [3,4]. These become more numerous and involve the artery increasingly and further proximally with interconnecting longitudinal tears leading to extensive fragmentation of the internal elastic lamina, remnants of which appear to be functionally ineffective (Figure 14.2). The tears also involve deeper laminae (Figure 14.3) and eventually occur on the distal side of the shunt. The endothelium overlying these elastic tears may be disrupted with thrombus over the denuded surface initially. Endothelial cells undergo intense replication within the boundaries of the tears (Figure 14.4) and resume a relatively normal morphology after several weeks.

The afferent artery progresses to profound thinning of the media with patchy loss and destruction of elastic tissue and muscle (Figure 14.5) [5–7]. The wall is dilated and flaccid, sometimes with pronounced tortuosity. Some enlargement of the distal artery may ensue and aneurysmal dilatation of the proximal artery is frequent (Figure 14.6). Intimal proliferation occurs particularly close to the fistula where it is superimposed on a variable degree of medial atrophy and in the long term proximal arteries develop overt atherosclerosis (Figure 14.7). Pre-existing intimal proliferation at sites of branching proximal to a fistula thickens, extends and progresses rapidly to overt atherosclerosis independently of the diet [7]. The finding of microfractures ultra-

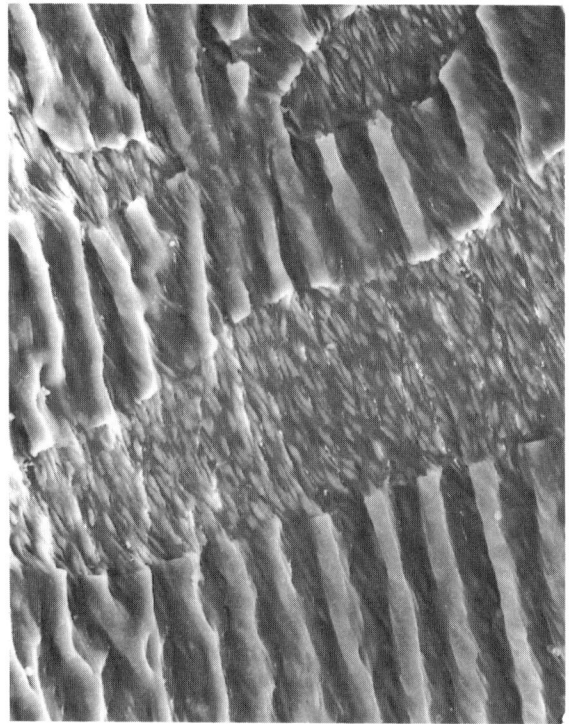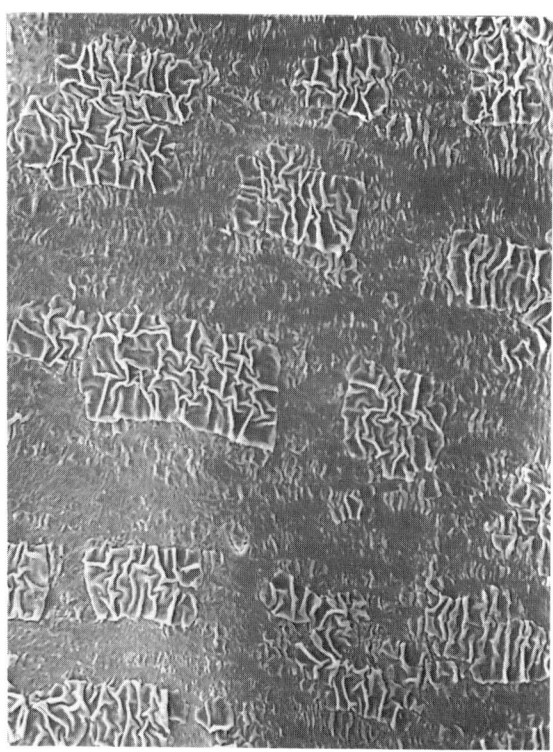

Figure 14.1 Scanning electron micrograph of transversely orientated tears of the internal elastic lamina of the common carotid artery proximal to an arteriovenous fistula in a rabbit. Note the high endothelial cell density in the floor of the tears which have sharp margins.

Figure 14.2 Scanning electron micrograph of severely fragmented internal elastic lamina with longitudinal tears interconnecting the transversely orientated tears. The residual elastic islands no longer display longitudinal corrugations and are probably of reduced functional effectiveness. Flow is from below upwards.

structurally in the internal elastic lamina adjacent to the sharp-edged tears (Figure 14.8) is consistent with mechanical or engineering failure of the elastic membrane.

The anastomosed vein becomes rapidly and irregularly dilated, its diameter increasing by four or five times and there is often narrowing to some extent opposite the shunt where the wall is more fibrotic (Figure 14.6). The dilatation extends proximally and distally and in the rabbit the eye on the homolateral side becomes exophthalmic, sometimes severely so. The inner surface of the vein adjacent to the fistula is very irregular displaying a whorling pattern of ridges and depressions which constitute the jet lesion. The endothelial cells in the jet lesion also have an irregular pattern with numerous multinucleated giant cells [8]. Beyond the jet lesion the venous wall becomes thickened initially with a loose musculoelastic intimal thickening and some enlargement (hypertrophy) of the medial muscle bundles. The intima progressively thickens by fibromusculoelastic proliferation. Ultimately it becomes fibrotic with fragmentation and loss of elastic tissue in the intima and media and

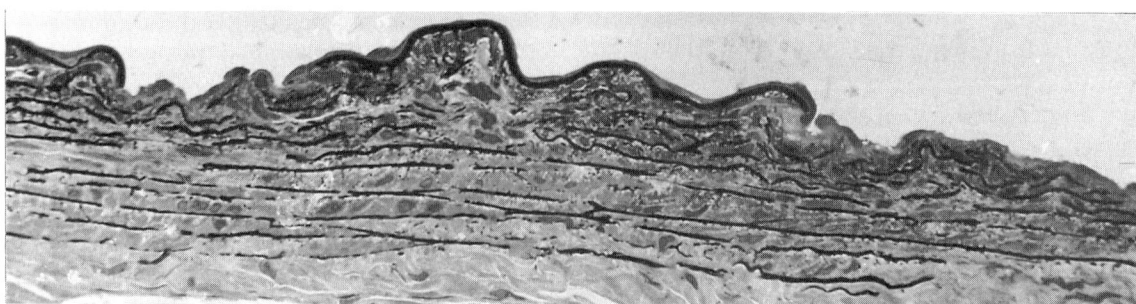

Figure 14.3 Longitudinal section of the common carotid artery proximal to an experimental arteriovenous fistula (rabbit) demonstrating fragmentation of the internal elastic lamina and underlying medial elastic laminae. Note medial thinning beneath the tears of the internal elastic lamina. (Toluidine blue.)

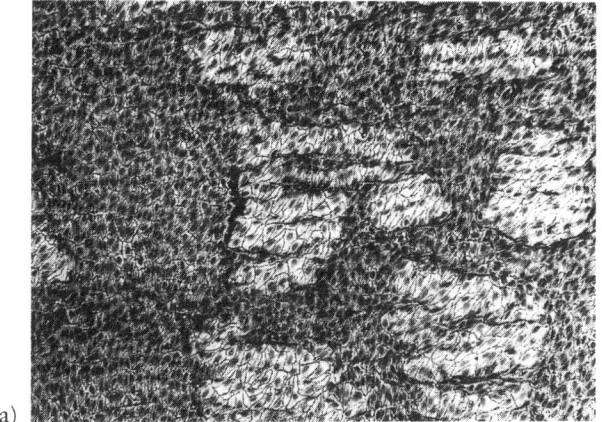

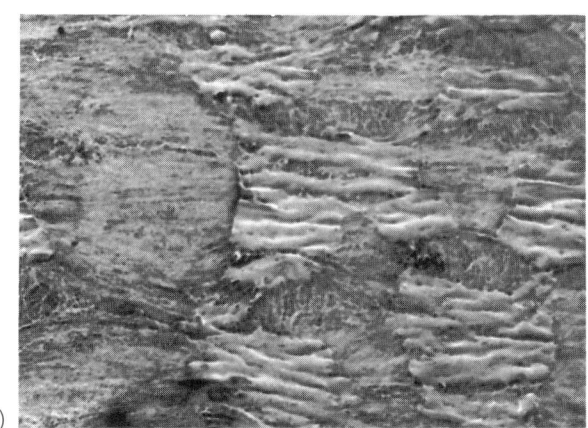

Figure 14.4 (a) *En face* preparation of endothelium of common carotid artery proximal to an arteriovenous fistula demonstrating intense endothelial replication within the flow of the tears of the internal elastic lamina. (Haematoxylin and silver nitrate.) (Reproduced with permission from Jones, Martin and Stehbens [169].) (b) A scanning electron micrograph of the underlying intima after endothelial denudation. Note the good correlation of the endothelial multiplication with the elastic tears.

often some calcification [5,6]. This intimal proliferation accumulates lipid (Figure 14.9), develops spontaneous intimal tears with limited mural dissection and mural thrombosis (Figure 14.10) [5]. Ultrastructurally the changes in the muscle, basement membranes, matrix vesicles, collagen fibril degeneration and accumulation of lipid are similar to those in experimental aneurysms and human atherosclerosis [9–11]. The thickening of the venous wall is not arterialization but is indicative of the progressive development of venous atherosclerosis although its earlier manifestations are identical to those of human phlebosclerosis.

In femoral A–V fistulae the changes are similar to those of a carotid–jugular fistula, but more rapidly progressive [7]. Tortuosity is frequent and characteristically the lower abdominal aorta bends to the left and the right common and external iliac arterial stem bends to the right with right-sided femoral fistulae. The tears in the internal elastic laminae of the muscular femoral artery appear within two days but the atrophy of the wall is much more pronounced. There can be complete loss of muscle and elastic tissue and the wall is unrecognizable as arterial. The intimal proliferation at arterial branching sites in the iliofemoral arteries and on the posterior wall of the abdominal aorta thickens, extends distally along the main stem of the arteries and progresses to overt fibrofatty atherosclerosis [7]. The changes have been regarded as the atrophic and proliferative changes of atherosclerosis respectively.

Small arteries in the neighbourhood of experimental shunts often have the histological appearance of diffuse hyperplastic sclerosis or arteriosclerosis of small peripheral arteries [12].

14.1 Haemodynamics of arteriovenous fistulae

In an acute fistula, the pressure differential is such that blood flows through the fistula as a jet into the larger diameter vein under low pressure initiating profoundly turbulent flow and is then returned to the heart for recirculation. Initially the enlargement of the afferent artery may be physiological vasodilatation. However, within days degenerative changes develop concomitantly

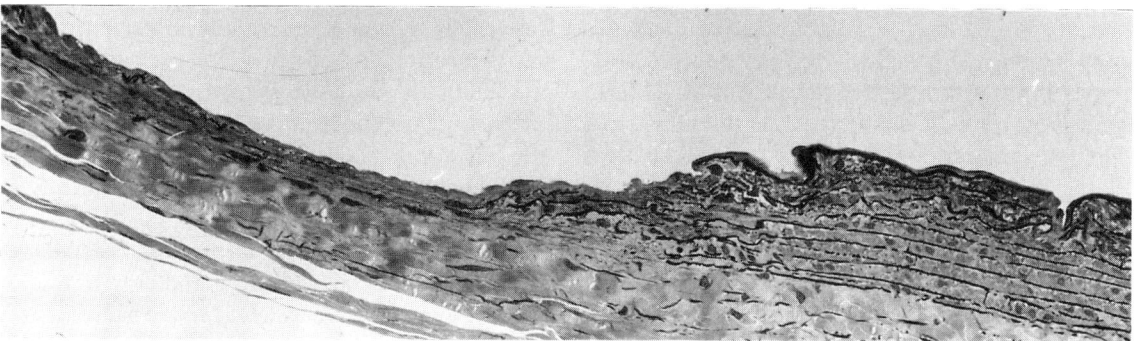

Figure 14.5 Gross atrophy of segment of the wall of the common carotid artery proximal to an arteriovenous fistula. Note almost complete loss of muscle and elastic tissue in the floor of the tear. (Toluidine blue.)

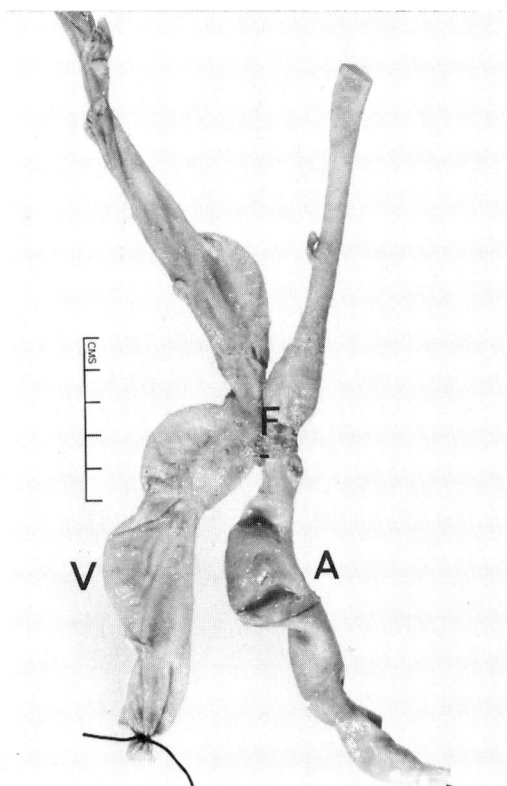

Figure 14.6 Sheep carotid–jugular arteriovenous fistula demonstrating aneurysmal dilatation of the proximal common carotid artery (A) and irregular aneurysmal dilatation of the anastomosed vein (V) both proximally and distally to the fistula at F.

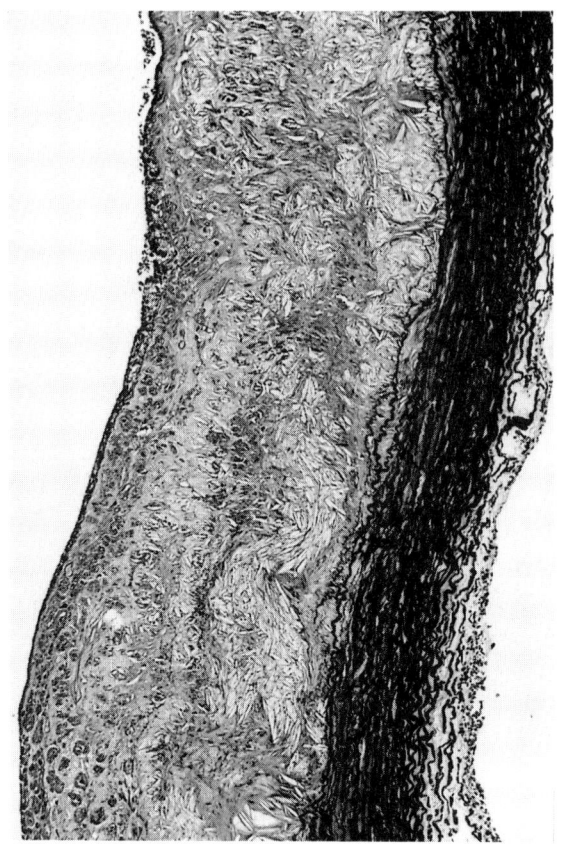

Figure 14.7 Aorta displaying overt atherosclerosis in a rabbit on a stock diet with a chronic femoral arteriovenous fistula. Note the fibromuscular proliferation over the atheromatous material deep in the intima. The lumen is to the left. (Verhoeff's elastic stain and eosin.)

with continued enlargement which progressively increases the size of the parasitic circulation.

Upon establishment of such a fistula a continuous thrill and murmur develop with systolic intensification at the site of the fistula and jet flow from the artery to the vein. The vibratory activity associated with turbulent flow is maximal over the vein adjacent to the fistula and palpable over the artery and vein proximally and distally. It is readily transmitted through the overlying tissues to the skin. The random frequencies are typical of turbulent flow and the spectral density becomes attenuated beyond 35 cps [12,13]. Small finite contributions may occur at higher frequencies but as yet have not been demonstrated. On opening the fistula the mean arterial blood pressure falls due to the low resistance through the shunt. A compensatory increase in pulse rate through a reciprocal action of the vagus and sympathetic nerves [1] together with increased venous return results in an increased cardiac output. Less blood circulates through the rest of the body with a compensatory vasoconstriction tending to offset the fall in blood pressure [14,15]. Ultimately the blood volume is increased such that the volume capacity of the aneurysmal venous segment of the parasitic circulation may be considerable.

In chronic fistulae, the systolic pressure remains at presurgical levels but the diastolic pressure falls with an increase in pulse pressure, sometimes simulating a Corrigan's or water-hammer pulse. The central venous pressure, though inconstant, is not grossly elevated [16–18].

The magnitude of the shunt depends on the calibre of the vessels anastomosed and the size of the fistula. Since the vessels enlarge substantially, the shunt increases in size. Thus unless the fistula is very small, there is little restriction to the flow. With time there is usually an increasing flow through the fistula and flow through the afferent artery may increase by a factor of at least 12 [14]. Diastolic flow in the fistulous artery is usually maintained at a level of 80–90% of the maximum systolic flow and in femoral fistulae the flow may be increased by 15 times or more and even doubled in the contralateral femoral artery [19]. The velocity in the fistulous artery has been up to 4.5 times that in the control side [19].

In the distal artery, mean and pulse pressures are

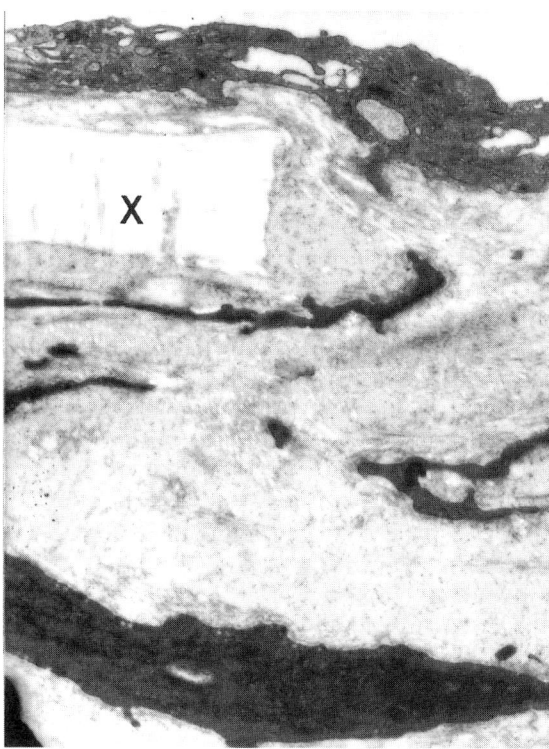

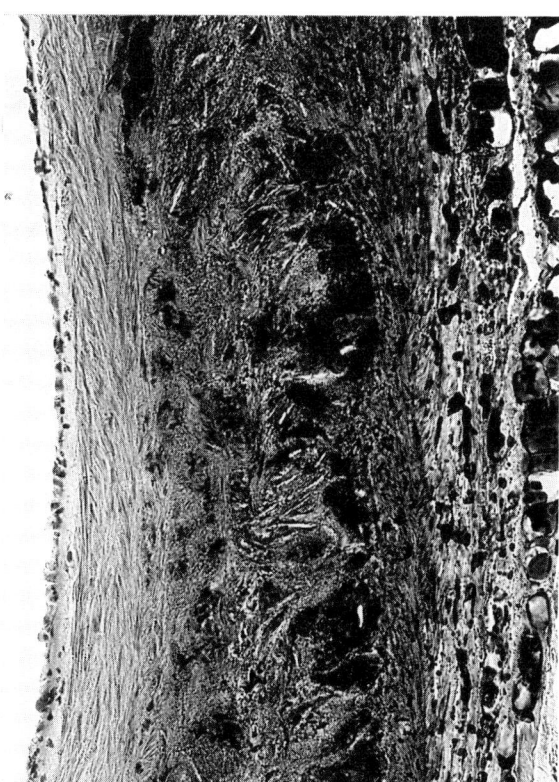

Figure 14.8 Microfracture (X) in the internal elastic lamina adjacent to an abrupt tear in the common carotid artery. Note the increased cytoplasmic density of smooth muscle cells (compared to that of endothelial cells) in the vicinity of the disrupted internal elastic lamina as if they are degenerating. This may account for the loss of muscle that is so apparent in Figure 14.5. (Courtesy of Mr G.T. Jones.)

Figure 14.9 Overt atherosclerosis in femoral vein close to a femoral arteriovenous fistula in a rabbit on a stock diet. Note the large amount of lipid and cholesterol clefts in the thickened intima. Lumen is to the left. (Haematoxylin and fat stain.)

usually lower than in the proximal artery. The flow becomes reversed, resulting in relative ischaemia distally and a need for collateral circulation to compensate, though some of this collateral flow ultimately contributes blood to the fistula.

In the proximal vein the pressure, which can vary from 0 to 15 mmHg, may be negative immediately proximal to the fistula due to a Venturi phenomenon capable of sucking air into the vein if damaged during surgery [17]. Pressures in the distal vein may be considerably elevated with flow directed towards the heart with a small fistula, and towards the periphery if the fistula and shunt are large. Valves readily become incompetent following dilatation and progressive phlebosclerosis leaving behind residual crescentic ridges to mark their previous positions. There is enlargement of the contralateral and other veins resulting in alternative collateral drainage of distal tissues and also of blood from the fistula. Pressure in the distal vein falls with time as the peripheral collaterals increase. However, there is continued venous congestion and stagnation distally.

There is always a considerable growth of both arterial and venous collaterals in the neighbourhood of a fistula and they enlarge with time. The afferent vessels continue

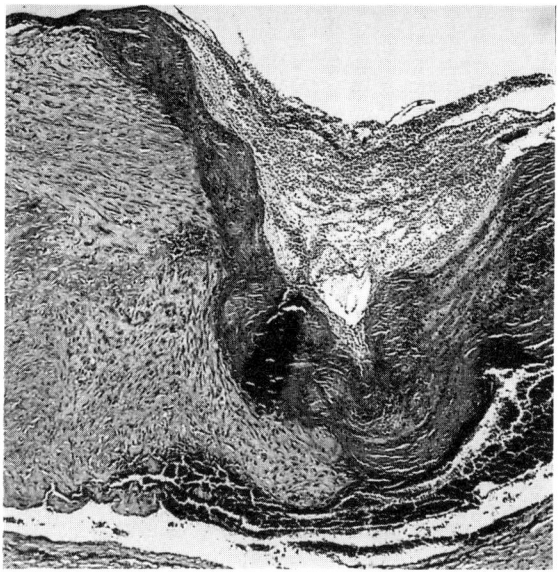

Figure 14.10 Full thickness tear of the intima of the anastomosed vein of an arteriovenous fistula in a sheep. Note the thrombus attached to the margin of the tear and floor of the ulcer so formed with dissection under the margin. (Verhoeff's elastic stain and eosin.)

to yield, thereby increasing the flow and arterial collaterals continue to enlarge providing more blood for the low pressure venous system. Even a major artery such as the contralateral common carotid artery is involved in providing blood for distal tissues and for the fistula as well and any vessel involved in the parasitic circulation can show degenerative changes. The femoral A–V fistula has demonstrated in effect that the grossly augmented flow and its attendant haemodynamic stresses result in augmentation of both atrophic and proliferative changes of atherosclerosis irrespective of the diet and serum cholesterol levels [5,7]. When a shunt involves much smaller vessels and functions for a longer period of time, there is little doubt that the vascular changes seen in A–V fistulae and aneurysms in man would eventually be reproduced. Such an experiment in a primate model, the chimpanzee preferably, would elucidate the natural history of cerebral A–V anomalies or aneurysms and differentiate those changes that are acquired from those that are developmental or due to some other pathology.

14.2 Traumatic arteriovenous fistulae and communications

Traumatic A–V communications usually arise as the result of a perforating injury of many and various sorts, including stab wounds, bullets, shrapnel, hair transplants, blood letting and less commonly, blunt and at times mild injuries. Iatrogenic injuries such as trochar or needle biopsy wounds may also be responsible. All that is needed to initiate the communication is an injury to an adjoining artery and vein and practically all major systemic arteries have been affected. It would also seem that the presence of an inherited connective tissue disorder, by increasing vascular fragility, enhances the propensity for traumatic A–V communications.

The communication may be direct or an intervening false aneurysm may form and be localized by the organization about clotted extravasated blood. The flow of arterial blood directly into the vein would be the path of least resistance and the subclinical communication becomes established at the time of trauma. Alternatively a false sac once formed may rupture secondarily into the damaged vein. In the carotid cavernous fistula, the carotid artery, possibly more susceptible to injury, is torn at the time of skull fracture and bleeding is then directly into the cavernous venous sinus so creating the fistula. These fistulae and those fashioned surgically would be expected to behave in much the same manner as experimental A–V fistulae. Current evidence is that the effects of these communications are not species-specific.

It has been demonstrated angiographically that small temporary A–V anastomoses are not uncommon in the meningeal and pial vessels of the brain following trauma. Most of these shunts close spontaneously, probably by thrombotic occlusion of the artery, vein or both. Even in experimental femoral fistulae in the rabbit, either limb of the femoral artery or the femoral vein may thrombose within a few days postoperatively. In some, the shunt may continue to function for weeks and then becomes silent due to thrombosis of one or other vessel but this does not preclude enlargement of the shunt in time unless the communication is completely occluded by thrombosis. It is not surprising that in some traumatic A–V shunts of even smaller vessels especially when contused, spontaneous occlusion results, whereas a fistula involving the larger common carotid artery and jugular vein rarely even thromboses. Occlusion of the afferent artery does not occlude the shunt. The distal artery or even a small collateral branch may remain patent and in time will enlarge the shunt. This occurs both experimentally [7] and clinically following surgical attempts to occlude feeding or afferent arteries. For this reason the modern day concept that cerebral A–V aneurysms, anomalies or malformations are possibly not always congenital but in at least some instances traumatic in aetiology has gained credence.

Traumatic A–V fistulae or communications no doubt existed in gladiatorial days, occurred through the blood-letting of the Middle Ages and are a hazard of hair transplantation, renal biopsies and carotid or vertebral angiography. Once established and recognized, surgical intervention (sometimes repeated) closes the shunt. If left alone, the veins dilate and become grossly enlarged, tortuous and varicose and the arteries will behave as in experimental models [5,7].

Many authors have been aware of degenerative changes in both the arteries and veins [1,20–22]. Callander [20] noted calcification which may occur opposite the fistula, presumably in the jet lesion.

The proximal arteries undergo dilatation, thinning, tortuosity and eventually aneurysmal dilatation. Reid [23,24] reported arterial dilatation from a traumatic femoral A–V fistula back to the heart. In chronic untreated femoral A–V fistulae, the aorta and the homolateral iliofemoral arteries proximal to a fistula develop aneurysms and severe atherosclerosis [1,21,22,25,26]. There is diminished arterial pulsation in the limb distal to the shunt [20]. Also observed in a number of subjects was that some years after surgical closure of the shunt, aneurysms developed on the feeding vessels. It has been emphasized [1,22] that closure of the shunt did not lead to regression of these degenerative changes, but that they continued to progress, suggesting that the haemodynamic stress is cumulative and that continued usage eventually causes aneurysmal dilatation. Fragility of the afferent artery has also been noted [25].

Solberg *et al.* [27] reported medial hypertrophy early in the afferent artery close to a femoral fistula. There is an increase in calibre very early after opening the fistula and there may well be proliferation and/or hypertrophy

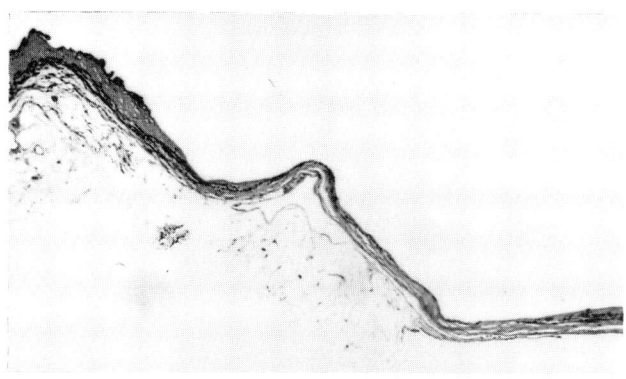

Figure 14.11 Gross atrophy of a segment of a femoral artery proximal to an arteriovenous fistula. Note the complete loss of muscle and elastic tissue in the atrophic segment. (Verhoeff's elastic stain and eosin.)

of smooth muscle cells but atrophy of the wall is the predominant change in chronic fistulae with atherosclerosis at branching sites and close to the fistula [7].

The anastomosed veins do not become arterialized nor do the arteries become vein-like. The veins develop thrombi which can give rise to emboli. Atherosclerosis can be expected to develop in the anastomosed veins as occurs in rabbits and sheep [5,7]. Haemorrhage can occur indicating that due to weakening of the vessel wall either the arteries or the veins have ruptured. Severe haemorrhage is probably more likely from an arterial source especially in view of the extreme atrophic lesions that develop (Figure 14.11). A pulsatile jet of blood has been observed in epistaxis in a sheep with a carotid–jugular fistula.

The possibility of self-cure by thrombosis must be regarded as a theoretical eventuality in moderate to large fistulae. Probably most small pial shunts and some of the larger traumatic shunts may undergo thrombosis within a few days of the injury. Established shunts may fluctuate due to thrombotic episodes but complete self cure must be rare. Recurrence of an A–V communication of the scalp has been reported in a pregnant woman 18 years after excision [28].

14.2.1 COMPLICATIONS

(a) Haemorrhage

Ectasia, tortuosity and aneurysmal dilatation are inherent features of the progression of A–V communications and haemorrhage will therefore be a major complication. This is well recognized in the cerebral lesions and thrombosis may result in haemostasis but not necessarily cure. Haemorrhage is also seen in small lesions extracranially and is often the presenting manifestation of the lesion. In view of the propensity for severe atrophy of the afferent arteries, severe bleeding is most likely to be arterial in origin.

(b) Vulnerability

Enlarged and tortuous vessels will be more vulnerable to injury and bleeding from such vessels may be fatal. Connective tissue defects aggravate the fragility of the vessels in the shunt that is responsible for both the haemorrhage and aneurysmal dilatation.

(c) Infection

Infection may complicate traumatic A–V communications which may then act as a source of septic emboli [29,30]. Such infection does not appear to complicate cerebral lesions and since extracranial shunts are not common, infected lesions are rare. The infection apparently commences in the vein and may secondarily involve the cardiac valves. Direct primary infection of the vessels may occur with traumatic lesions.

(d) Cardiac complications

The cardiac output can be grossly increased by the parasitic circulation which can constitute 50% or more of the total output. The blood volume is also increased. Exercise increases the cardiac output and increases the shunt, the result being that the total cardiac workload can be enhanced four-fold [31]. It is therefore not surprising that the heart may undergo left ventricular hypertrophy and dilatation and cardiac failure may follow [32]. This is more likely with large shunts and those that are proximal and particularly in infancy as illustrated in a 2-day-old girl with a shunt from the left subclavian artery to the left innominate vein [33]. The child had cardiomegaly, weak pulses, cyanosis, a palpable thrill and murmur. Shunts associated with 'aneurysms' of the vein of Galen are also frequently large enough to overload the heart and affected infants may be considered to have congenital heart failure. Likewise some shunts can precipitate congestive cardiac failure as when an aortic aneurysm ruptures into the inferior vena cava or when there is a diffuse shunt of unknown aetiology involving a hindquarter.

The effect of the augmented workload not only on the heart and blood vessels has been recognized but what happens to the valves is uncertain. In cardiac failure mitral incompetence is to be expected but whether a chronic shunt is responsible for aortic valve disease or incompetence [22] is unknown and awaits investigation.

Small spontaneous tears occur in the cardiac valves causing small strips of valve cusp (Lambl's excrescences) to project from the surface. Thrombosis, healing and endothelialization occur. These filiform excrescences appear to be a 'wear and tear' phenomenon and their formation could well be accentuated by the greatly augmented cardiac workload associated with an A–V shunt. Circulating bacteria become attached to such thrombi especially if already adherent to a platelet and thus initiate bacterial infection and endocarditis. Such could explain the predisposition for bacterial endocarditis. Lillehei *et al.* [34] reported the development of bacterial endocarditis within one month in a series of dogs with experimental shunts. Some animals had vegetations at the site of the fistula. This knowledge has been utilized in producing experimental endocarditis by giving an intravenous injection of a small dose of bacteria to dogs with A–V shunts. The shunts had to be large as small shunts had little effect. A similar technique has been utilized in rats. Animals with a fistula did not clear the bacteria from the blood as readily as control animals [35].

A number of cases of bacterial infection at the site of traumatic A–V fistulae has occurred in humans but after a protracted time period suggesting the infection was a secondary event. Some of these subjects subsequently developed bacterial endocarditis [29]. During long experience with A–V fistulae in experimental animals, no spontaneous endocarditis was encountered in sheep or rabbits. Instances in humans are very rare but the possibility of such vulnerability should be kept in mind.

(e) Haematological complications

Intravascular mechanically induced haemolysis and visceral siderosis are associated with chronic cardiac valvular disease in the absence of a prosthesis [36–38] and have been attributed to turbulent blood flow, shearing stresses and collisions. Intravascular erythrocyte fragmentation, poikilocytosis and evidence of haemolysis (microangiopathic haemolytic anaemia) in association with an A–V fistula disappeared following closure of the shunt. The severity of the haemolysis [39,40] has not been investigated but no doubt it will be accentuated in patients with an inherited propensity to haemolysis. If erythrocytes can be affected in this manner, it is possible that platelets may likewise be vulnerable and their lifespan reduced. This is analogous to the microangiopathic haemolytic anaemia associated with hypertension, mitral valvular stenosis, marathon running and sports.

With giant or multiple haemangiomas in small children, thrombocytopenia [41] in A–V communications [42] has been observed. The platelets are believed to be sequestered and removal of the haemangioma, thought to be associated with an A–V shunt, reverses the condition. The thrombocytopenia may be analogous to the haemolytic anaemia rather than sequestration. The bleeding tendency may be partly due to this coagulopathy.

(f) Collateral circulation

The increased blood flow to the fistula does not mean increased circulation through tissues distal to the shunt. On the contrary, distal tissues are congested but relatively anoxic because arterial collaterals will preferentially supply the fistula and venous collaterals will preferentially drain the shunt.

The development of collateral circulation in A–V shunts can be quite extreme and involves both arteries and veins. The degree of involvement of neighbouring vascular beds is well seen in cerebral lesions. This appears to be simply progressive, becoming more extensive as surgical closure or ablation of the shunt is delayed.

The stimulus to the development of the collateral circulation is not chemical stimulation from the distal tissues but hydrodynamic [17].

The gross vascularity and congeries of vessels in cerebral A–V shunts may well be acquired but their extensive involvement and replacement of brain parenchyma in association with atypical structure of arteries and veins may all be acquired changes secondary to a shunt. Most authors do not realize how very rapid and extensive the degenerative and architectural changes can be. The long-term natural history of these shunts in experimental primates requires investigation.

14.3 Left-to-right arterial shunts (systemic artery–pulmonary artery shunt)

Theoretically anastomosis of a systemic artery with a pulmonary artery (a left-to-right shunt) would not lead to the development of as great a shunt and flow rate as in A–V fistulae. Nevertheless, the afferent artery would become much enlarged and tortuous in time and atrophic lesions and atherosclerosis would develop at an accelerated rate. However, structural changes in these vessels have not been studied in detail. In 1959, Bosher *et al.* [43] reviewed 12 such cases, in nine of which the systemic artery originated from the aorta often joining the pulmonary artery after a circuitous course. Two others came from intercostal arteries. The remaining case involved the pericardiophrenic artery. It would seem that pleural adhesions can often become the site of such anastomoses. In the more recent case of an anastomotic shunt from an internal thoracic (mammary) artery to a pulmonary artery following closed chest cardiac massage, the small vessels at the shunt were said to have increased medial elastic tissue. The arteries were allegedly intermediate between a systemic and a pulmonary artery [44]. Another example of this between the left internal thoracic (mammary) artery and vessels of the left upper pulmonary lobe [45] was caused by pulmonary and pleural tuberculosis. These communications involving the internal thoracic artery are seldom sufficiently severe to produce symptoms in the adult but given time some will.

This is analogous to a patent ductus arteriosus except that the shunt in the latter is more common, usually of larger proportions, and often associated with a pulmonary artery aneurysm and at times of the ductus arteriosus itself.

An analogous situation occurs when the left coronary artery takes origin from the pulmonary trunk. Anastomoses, however small, form between the two coronary arteries. After birth, when the blood pressure differential develops between the two arteries, blood from the right coronary artery progressively becomes diverted to the left coronary artery and thence to the pulmonary trunk. Mostly the right coronary artery provides inadequate blood to the myocardium which becomes ischaemic and congestive cardiac failure follows within two years (85%). In some individuals, the right coronary though grossly dilated and tortuous, temporarily provides sufficient blood for the myocardium. In a series of patients who survived until the sixth and seventh decades, there was at times extreme dilatation of both coronary arteries but no suggestion was made of atherosclerosis [46]. Patients eventually develop angina and die of congestive cardiac failure by about 30 to 40 years of age. Ischaemia of the papillary muscles can lead to mitral valve incompetence and this aggravates the cardiac status. The flow through the left coronary artery is retrograde being in effect a vascular steal. Flow in the right coronary artery acts as the afferent artery of an A–V shunt and severe atherosclerosis develops in the right coronary, whereas the left exhibits minimal changes. The severity of the atherosclerosis must be associated with the higher pressure and augmented flow in the right coronary artery and if indeed lipid plays a role in its aetiology, it must be indeed minimal [47].

When the right coronary artery arises from the pulmonary trunk, the left coronary artery copes with the load better and such subjects may survive for a normal lifespan. The right coronary artery then acts more in the capacity of a vein [48].

When both coronary arteries arise from the pulmonary trunk, the condition is rapidly fatal. When a third coronary artery arises from the pulmonary artery, the end result depends on the size and extent of anastomosis with the two main coronary vessels. Hudson [48] described an example in a 74-year-old male known to have a systolic and diastolic murmur. The left coronary artery was enlarged and thickened. The right was grossly ectatic together with its main branches and pursued a very serpiginous route to the cardiac apex, where anastomoses occurred with a large aberrant tortuous vessel originating from the posterior sinus of Valsalva of the pulmonary trunk.

The histological features of such interarterial anastomoses require study. In all likelihood changes similar to those feeding an A–V shunt [3–7] will be exhibited but the effect of retrograde flow through an artery would also be of interest.

14.4 Congenital arteriovenous communications of the extremities

14.4.1 KLIPPEL–TRENAUNAY SYNDROME

Large congenital A–V communications may at times involve an entire extremity or part thereof. Alternatively, almost half one side of the body may be affected in combination with patchy port-wine staining of a portion of the skin of the affected part and sometimes haemangiomatous nodules together with varicose veins, and hypertrophy of the limb or affected part (Figure 14.12). These manifestations constitute the Klippel–Trenaunay syndrome [49]. It has been assumed that in the primitive capillary plexus some of the many vessels connecting the arterial to the venous end of the capillary bed persist to become sizeable channels for the A–V shunt to bypass the capillary plexus. Multiple abnormal interconnections of this nature are believed to contribute to a massive A–V shunt of blood. Associated with this unusual lesion may be gross enlargement of bones or the entire limb

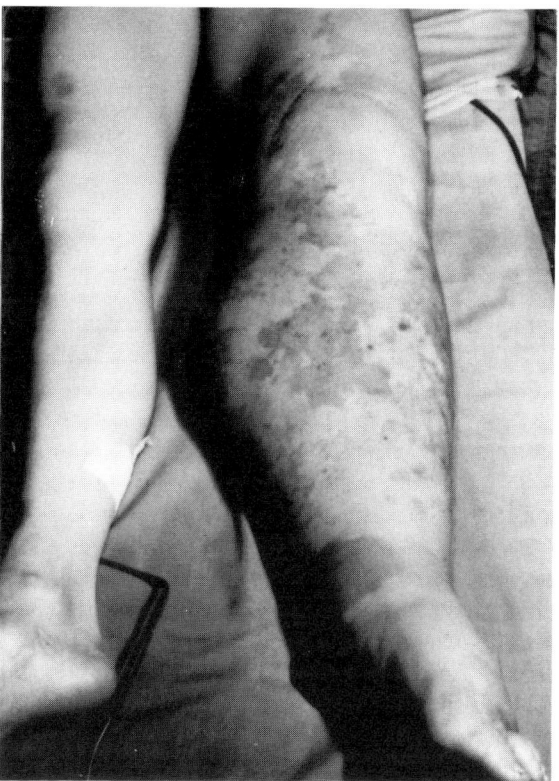

Figure 14.12 Gross enlargement of the left lower limb with blotchy port-wine discoloration of the skin in an 11-year-old girl prior to hindquarter amputation because of a diffuse arteriovenous shunt, congestive cardiac failure and increasing difficulty in managing the affected limb.

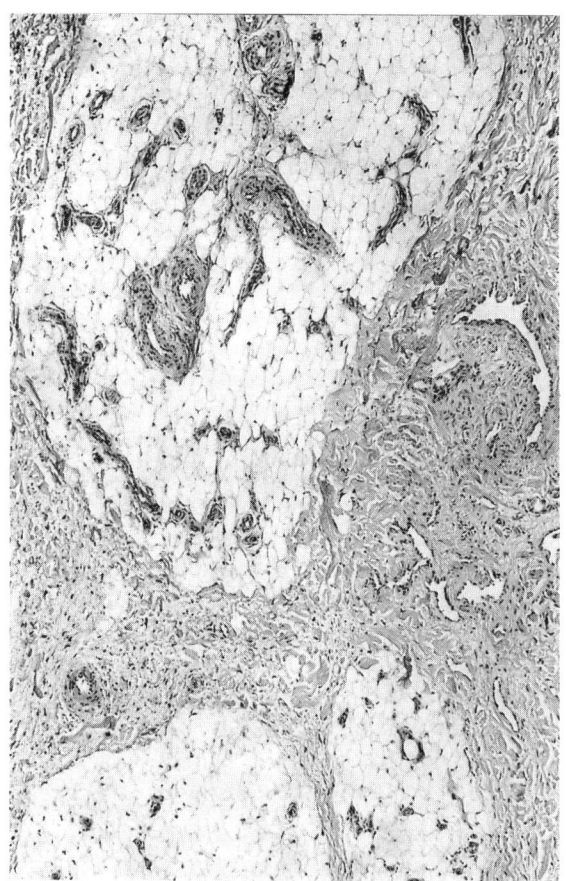

Figure 14.13 Numerous thick-walled vessels in adipose tissue but not in the broad fibrous tissue that divided the subcutaneous adipose tissue into lobules. Tissue obtained from subject with Klippel–Trenaunay syndrome (Figure 14.12). Increased vascularity was widespread throughout the limb but the thickened walls were confined to the adipose tissue. (Haematoxylin and eosin.)

and sometimes half the face. Thickening, congestion and oedema of the soft tissues with some induration, red or purplish patches of the skin and possibly even cardiac failure due to the very high cardiac output are other features encountered. A lower limb may be so enlarged that a child may have difficulty in carrying it around such that a hindlimb amputation is required. Some lesions can occur in the upper limb or on the trunk and be quite localized. Their aetiology and pathogenesis are poorly understood and the anastomoses cannot be localized.

In the case of a boy with such a large heavy arm, it had to be carried elevated in a sling and strapped to the chest. If the arm was permitted to hang down, so much blood pooled in the limb that the patient fainted [1]. In another case (an 11-year-old girl) small thick-walled vessels penetrated the soft tissues of the lower limb and homolateral buttock as if effecting some diffuse angiomatous infiltration or plexus (Figure 14.13) as Holman called it. Unfortunately, a shunt could not be localized to any particular site and a bruit and thrill were absent. The artery and vein were grossly enlarged. A hindquarter amputation was performed to relieve the congestive cardiac failure and the physical disability due to the size and weight of the limb. Increased skin temperature and varicose veins are common features and occasionally trophic changes with ulceration and recurrent haemarthrosis contribute to the grotesque appearance [1,50].

In another case a 28-year-old woman had enlargement of the entire right side of the body, including the face and a portion of the left leg and buttock. She had had bilateral painful varicose veins since early infancy [51]. The enlargement, especially of the lower limb caused pelvic tilting and scoliosis [49].

Gross ectasia of the artery and vein are usually present. Associated features that may be apparent include thrombocytopenia, hypofibrinogenaemia, syndactylism and polydactylism of all four limbs, congenital dislocation of the hip, gigantism of one or both feet, bilateral cryptorchidism and right inferior pulmonary vein varicosity. The part is usually warm and there may or may not be a palpable thrill and audible murmur. Lymphangiectasia [52] and reported 'hypoplasia' of the lymphatics [51] have been reported and there may be an absence of deep veins. Enlargement of the heart and some contractures about the joints of the affected limbs may occur [1].

Some of the features such as hemihypertrophy including bones and soft tissues of the face or of a limb are also seen in the Sturge–Weber syndrome suggesting an overlap as Furukawa and colleagues claim [53].

Therapeutic A–V shunts were once performed for congenitally short limbs but the results were poor and the limb exhibited coarse and uncontrolled growth with thickening of the limb but it was found that the type of enlargement was akin to gigantism and not the physiological growth optimistically sought. Many of the physical manifestations described above in a 'congenital' lesion are reproduced by therapeutic shunts for small limbs rather than due to a developmental anomaly. The blotchy staining of the skin is difficult to explain but it too may be a consequence of the shunt rather than a concomitant or independent feature of the syndrome and only very chronic experimental A–V fistulae are likely to clarify this relationship.

14.4.2 STURGE–WEBER SYNDROME

This syndrome has many synonyms and its true nature is obscure. It is usually considered to be unilateral and to consist of:

- an angiomatous naevus or port-wine stain at birth with a distribution corresponding to one or more areas supplied by the divisions of the trigeminal nerve;

- homolateral angiomatosis of the homolateral cerebral meninges with progressive calcification in the underlying cerebral cortex.

Others have different criteria. Poser and Taveras [54] classified the syndrome into three types:

1. Type 1 constitutes the typical Sturge–Weber syndrome (encephalotrigeminal encephalomalacia) with a port-wine naevus and at least two other features such as focal or general convulsions, hemiparesis, hemiatrophy or hemihypertrophy, mental retardation, or congenital glaucoma.
2. Type 2 is an incomplete form with skin manifestations absent, but with the other classical cerebral meningeal angiomatosis and cortical calcification.
3. Type 3 includes atypical cases with some type of vascular anomaly (not trigeminal angiomatosis) in association with other features of the syndrome. In one instance there was a raised facial haemangioma and in another a network of grossly enlarged cutaneous and subcutaneous veins. Another had cutaneous hyperpigmentation and some have café au lait spots on the trunk.

The syndrome occurs mostly in Caucasians with a preponderance in males. The haemangiomatous naevus, present at birth, is a port-wine cutaneous stain which may be blue at times with abnormal responses to stimuli. The stain may be raised above the surface as if the skin was rough and hypertrophied, though soft on palpation. The distribution involves the face and though often thought to correspond to the metameres, the anatomical boundaries are by no means accurate. Involvement of the forehead and upper eyelid is the significant distribution (Figure 14.14), there being no cerebral angiomatosis or gyriform calcification in association with angiomatosis of other regions of the face [55]. In one case closely resembling the syndrome the cutaneous lesions had a distinct A–V shunt with a strong pulsation and bruit. It is likely that the cerebral and cutaneous lesions have direct continuity. There may be variable haemangiomatous involvement of viscera, the skin including much of the trunk on one side and also mucous membranes of the mouth and pharynx. There may be thickening of facial features and even the bones in association with the haemangiomatous involvement producing considerable asymmetry. The calvarium and the skull capacity on the affected side and the contralateral limbs are reduced in size especially in the presence of long-standing hemiparesis or hemiplegia.

On surgical exploration there is increased vascularity of the scalp, thickening, sponginess and redness of the calvarium with a tendency to bleed, augmented vascularity (angiomatosis) of the dura mater, prominent diploic vessels, often with arachnoidal adhesions, and leptomeningeal angiomatosis (Figure 14.15) over the

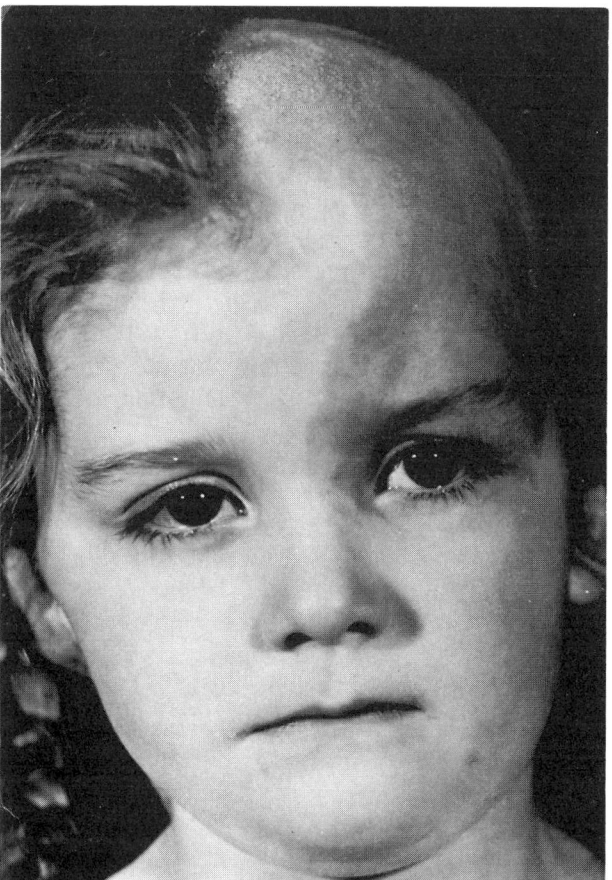

Figure 14.14 A young girl with the Sturge–Weber syndrome. The port-wine stain of the skin involves the scalp, forehead and left eye. (Reproduced with permission from Craig [170].)

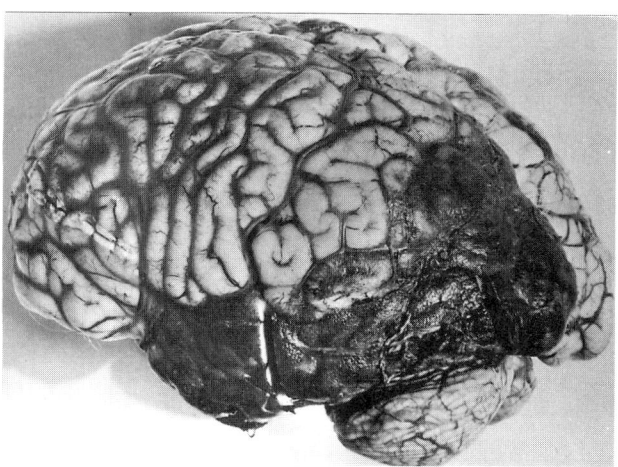

Figure 14.15 Brain exhibiting leptomeningeal angiomatosis of the temporal and occipital regions from the child with Sturge–Weber syndrome. (Reproduced with permission from Craig [170].)

parietal and occipital regions possibly extending further anteriorly but rarely ever is the cerebellum involved. The lesions are usually fairly well demarcated and there is also increased cortical vascularity, although there is cerebral hemiatrophy or atrophy of the area affected. Both cerebral hemispheres may be involved but usually it is only unilateral. The leptomeninges may be thickened and there is a layer of small tortuous veins imparting a purplish colour to the affected cortex. The vessels are of a relatively similar calibre except for larger drainage channels. The meningeal lesion occasionally has a distinct A–V shunt and it is quite apparent that there are many similarities to A–V communications involving larger vessels.

Histologically, the leptomeninges exhibit a considerable increase in the number of vessels (accentuated by their tortuosity) which are a few layers thick, sometimes filling the subarachnoid space together with some fibrosis. The pial arteries exhibit considerable intimal thickening with narrowing and mural calcification even in a 3-month-old infant. Abnormally large vessels rarely penetrate the cortex although there may be some increase in vascularity and the underlying second and third layers of the cortex exhibit extensive calcification. Initially there is granular encrustation of small cortical blood vessels, and this extends to form vascular sheaths with some involvement of intervening parenchyma. Degeneration and loss of neurones with gliosis and increased calcification ensue. There is also vascular calcification of larger vessels in the underlying white matter. The calcium deposits consist mainly of calcium phosphates and carbonates with a variable staining reaction for iron. Obliteration of small cortical vessels is frequent and there may be thrombosis of larger vessels including the middle cerebral artery.

Radiologically the typical findings, apart from the asymmetry of the skull and enlarged diploic channels, are the sinuous double-contoured tramline calcifications of the cerebral cortex (occasionally bilateral and not pathognomonic of the Sturge–Weber syndrome), cerebral atrophy with widening of the subarachnoid space and enlargement of the homolateral ventricle.

There is variation in the radiographic features [54]. Some cases are typical of an A–V communication with large arteries and veins, some associated with thrombosis of a major branch or smaller vessels supplying the area with a zone of avascularity and others have large veins coursing through the brain sometimes with dural sinus thrombosis but no conglomeration of abnormal vessels. Another group has abnormal arteries and veins or actual haemangiomas supplied by the external or internal carotid artery and there is a final group with miscellaneous findings such as a subdural haematoma and cerebral atrophy. Although believed to be characteristic of the syndrome, the venous angioma is present in only 24% of reported cases. The calcification is not always present but can appear within 15 months.

The syndrome is extremely rare and appears to be heterogeneous and until more detail is available about a number of cases it will be difficult to classify. There appears to be an A–V communication in many and with occlusion or severe narrowing of arterial channels the communication is apparently low grade.

The subjects have acute cerebral episodes suggestive of haemorrhage or ischaemia, convulsions, progressive mental retardation and hemiparesis with most dying in status epilepticus before middle age. Flow through the affected zone is rapid early in life and bleeds severely if damaged but is considerably retarded in later years.

Argument regarding its nature has included the hamartoma or dysgenesis concept and Weber [56] believed it was due to some accidental injury *in utero* but at present these views are conjectural. Light may be shed on this and related diseases when experimental A–V shunts involving different calibre vessels can be conducted to determine the natural history of such vascular abnormalities.

14.5 Vascular anomalies of the central nervous system

There is controversy over the classification of these anomalies, using the term anomaly to indicate an abnormality rather than a developmental aberration. Sako and Varco [22] express well the commonly held view that these lesions result from 'abnormal maturation in one or more of the embryologic stages in the development of the vasculature. The lesions can thus range from capillary to macroscopic sizes and vary in appearance, number, extent and behaviour'. The names of these lesions are varied and the classification used here includes telangiectases, cavernous haemangiomas, venous angiomas and A–V communications as used previously. Telangiectases and cavernous haemangiomas are often regarded as benign tumours and though this aspect will not be debated, their association with A–V shunts is pertinent to this chapter.

14.5.1 TELANGIECTASES

These are characteristically small solitary lesions usually less than 3 cm in diameter and found incidentally in middle-aged adults at autopsy. Probably they are often overlooked. They generally occur in the pons but otherwise in the cerebrum, involving the cortex or white matter and less often the cerebellum. They are usually multiple and are seen as a zone of pinkish or reddish discolouration which on closer inspection is due to red stippling occasioned by the increased density of small blood vessels or as a cluster of petechial haemorrhages

VASCULAR ANOMALIES OF THE CENTRAL NERVOUS SYSTEM   529

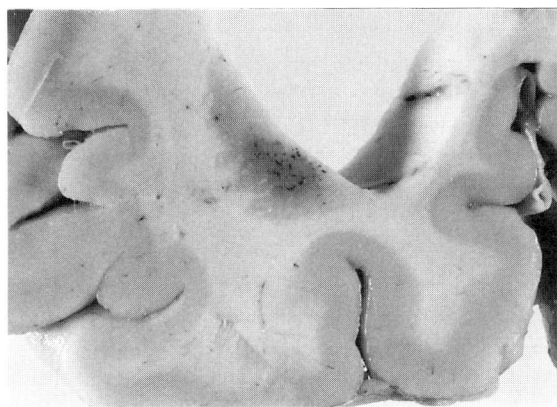

Figure 14.16 Early telangiectasis in the caudate nucleus appearing as a cluster of dark pinpoint dots. (Reproduced with permission from Stehbens [61].)

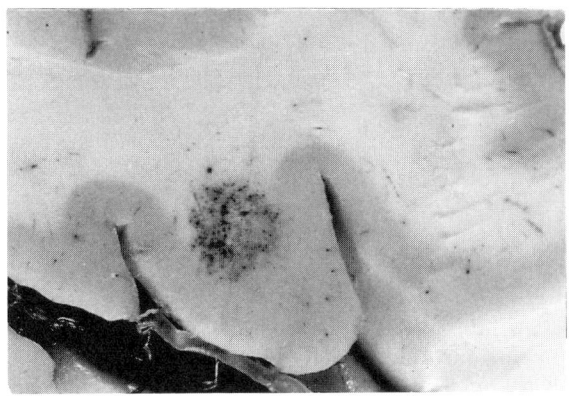

Figure 14.17 Cerebral telangiectasis at junction of white and grey matter. The vessels are large and more concentrated than in Figure 14.16. (Reproduced with permission from Stehbens [61].)

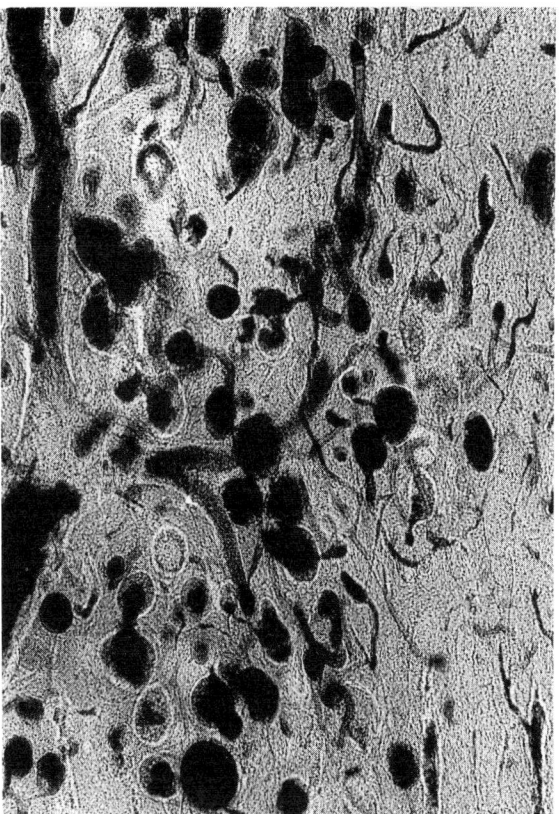

Figure 14.18 Thick paraffin section of a telangiectasis demonstrating numerous aneurysmal dilatations of small vessels and large drainage channels. (Fuchsin stain.)

(Figures 14.16, 14.17). Histologically they consist of multiple thin-walled capillary vessels that are larger than normal and possess multiple small saccular or fusiform aneurysmal dilatations (Figure 14.18) demonstrated to advantage by cutting thick sections and staining with fuchsin. Blackwood [57] considered the vessels were not more numerous and that venous channels were not enlarged but this does not always seem to be the case. Veins in some are enlarged and tortuous. There is rarely evidence of haemorrhage and some involve much of the white matter of a gyrus, extending medially as if along the venous drainage pathway. Some larger lesions consist of a massive infiltration with small blood vessels (Figure 14.19) and enlarged drainage channels which replace a considerable amount of parenchyma. There may be some calcification and gliosis of intervening parenchyma. These diffuse lesions do not conform to telangectasia or cavernous haemangioma. In some lesions the vessels are larger than capillaries. Their apparent progressive nature, the large calibre of the vessels and big drainage channels suggest there is an A–V shunt present (Figure 14.20).

In a report by Lim and Wallace [58] multiple telangiectases appeared two days after the normal delivery of a male neonate. Bleeding from the gut occurred five days later and both haematemesis and melaena over the next three weeks with progressive anaemia. Telangiectases increased in size and number on the skin and mucous membranes began to fade at age four. Multiple small pulmonary A–V shunts that had developed were held responsible for clubbing, cyanosis, dyspnoea and recurrent chest infections. The visible lesions progressively regressed leaving scars although clubbing and cyanosis persisted and no further evidence of cardiac or respiratory disorder was found. This was considered to be an instance of self-healing telangiectases [58]. It is difficult to explain this phenomenon.

14.5.2 CAVERNOUS HAEMANGIOMA

These lesions can also be found incidentally at autopsy in middle-aged adults and are no doubt more common

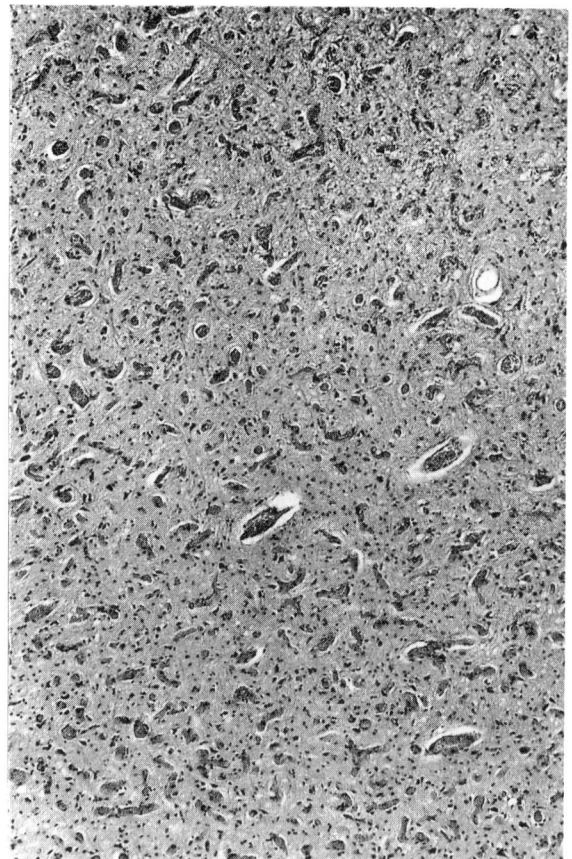

Figure 14.19 Massive diffuse vascular proliferation in brain tissue with no evidence of aneurysmal dilatation. The lesion has been classified as haemangioma. (Reproduced with permission from Stehbens [61].)

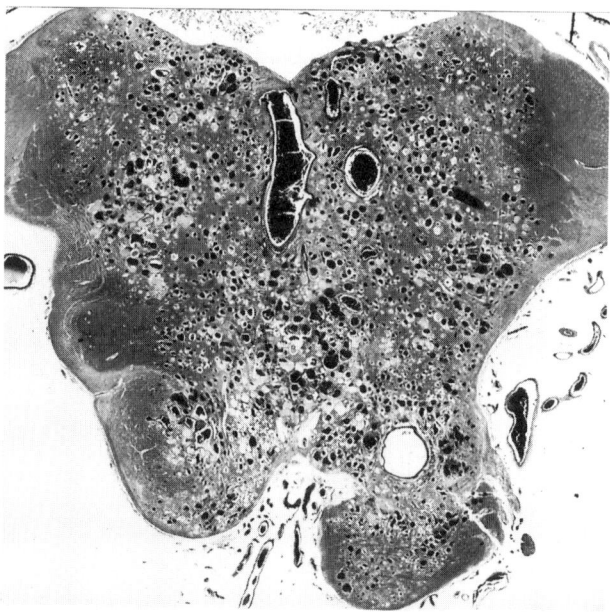

Figure 14.20 Extensive telangiectasia of the upper medulla. Abnormal vessels replace a considerable amount of parenchyma. Note the very large veins within the medulla. Most vessels are larger than capillaries. (Reproduced with permission from Farrell and Forno [171].)

than previously believed. In some instances there may be a familial form [59,60]. Whether the disorder is an inherited haemangioma or an inherited predisposition cannot be determined until more information is available regarding the aetiology and pathogenesis. They are dark red or black in cross-section and usually well circumscribed varying in size up to 3 or 4 cm in diameter. Though mostly less than 2 cm, they can be larger and even lobulated. The vessels in the main bulk of the lesion are irregularly enlarged, closely packed, vascular channels lined by endothelium with intervening hyaline trabeculae (Figures 14.21–14.23). Some may have gliosed brain tissue between channels (Figure 14.22) but it is conceivable that parenchyma can be destroyed progressively by enlarging vascular channels. It is also conceivable that these lesions may have intermediate stages [61] between the lesions depicted in Figure 14.21 and those with this appearance in Figure 14.24. The presence of an A–V shunt could account for the enlargement of blood vessels together with the haemorrhage and thromboses that are so frequent in the cavernous types (Figure 14.23). It is uncertain what part of these lesions is haemangiomatous and what is due to an A–V shunt.

Most cavernous haemangiomas show evidence of previous haemorrhage in magnetic resonance images with the haemorrhage usually localized and non-fatal. Prospectively the presenting symptoms are seizure, focal neurological deficit and headache and the annualized bleeding rate has been estimated as 0.7%. The risk of haemorrhage is greater in females than in males [62].

Some cavernous haemangiomas of the face or orbit or of the brain itself can enlarge forming tumour-like masses associated with a substantial A–V shunt with a bruit. Enlarged tortuous blood vessels participate in the shunt and are a problem in treatment as they tend to enlarge further and inadequate removal can be associated with recurrence and extension. They may erode the cranial vault, causing fatal bleeding and can involve intracranial and extracranial vessels in the arteriovenous shunt [61].

14.6 Arteriovenous communications and fistulae of the brain

These lesions are regarded as malformations or hamartomatous lesions in which there is an A–V shunt of variable degree. A–V communications are the most common vascular anomaly of the central nervous system and are probably more frequent than elsewhere in the body. Responsible for about 6% of subarachnoid haemorrhages clinically [63], they are somewhat more

ARTERIOVENOUS COMMUNICATIONS AND FISTULAE OF THE BRAIN 531

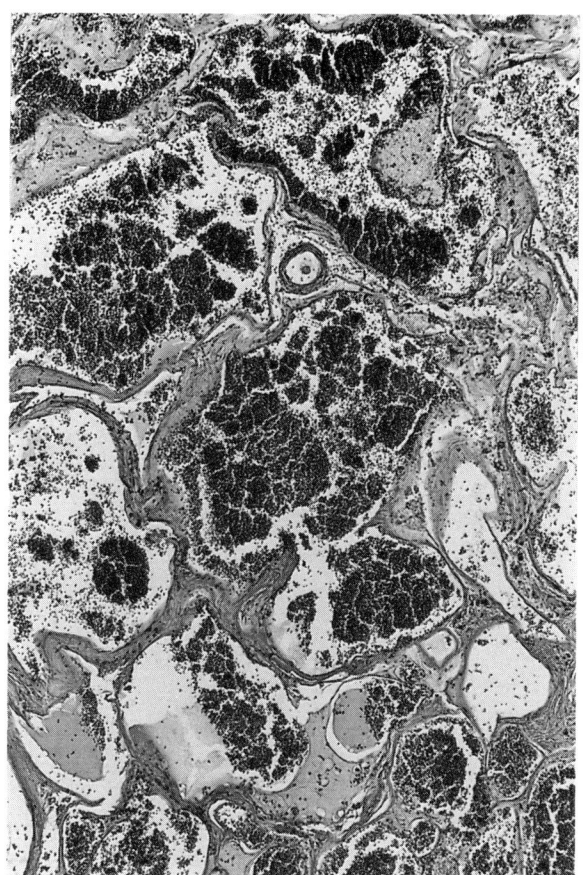

Figure 14.21 Cavernous haemangioma consisting of closely packed irregular cavernous cavities with intervening fibrous tissue. (Haematoxylin and eosin.) (Reproduced with permission from Stehbens [61].)

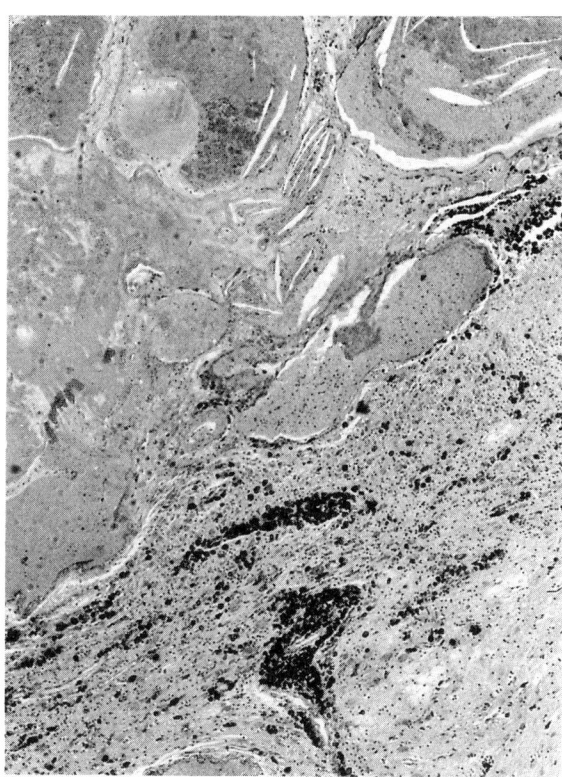

Figure 14.23 Thrombosed blood channels containing cholesterol clefts near edge of cavernous haemangioma. Large aggregates of siderophages in adjoining brain indicative of previous haemorrhage assist in identification by magnetic resonance imaging. (Haematoxylin and eosin.)

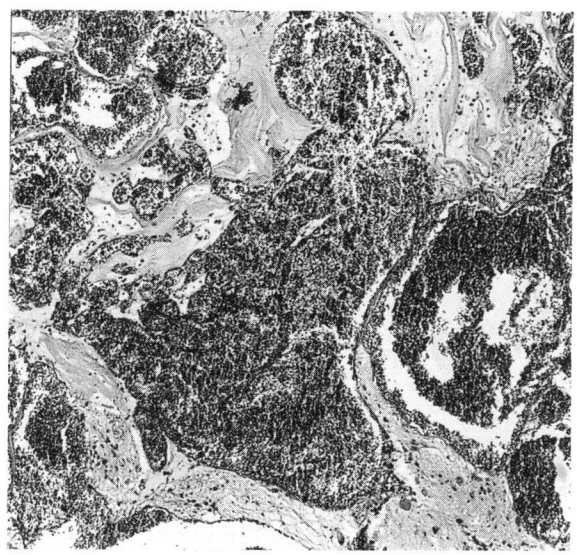

Figure 14.22 Gliosed brain between cavernous blood channels near edge of a cavernous haemangioma. (Haematoxylin and eosin.)

common in males than females. About 60–70% of such patients present clinically before the age of 40 years. There is a wide age scatter mainly in the second to sixth decades, whereas berry aneurysms tend to occur mostly after 40 years. These patients frequently suffer focal or general convulsions before the diagnosis is made and some present with a subarachnoid haemorrhage. Multiple cerebral A–V shunts are said to occur in 4–9% of cases [64].

There have also been a few reports of familial incidence of abnormal cerebral A–V communications and the observations have been alleged to support the concept that the lesions represent the persistence of the embryonic vascular pattern [65]. Anecdotal reports such as this are of doubtful significance and more convincing evidence is needed.

Supratentorial lesions are more frequent (93%) than subtentorial lesions (7%) which involve the vermis of the cerebellum particularly [66]. The middle cerebral artery is the most frequent site and also has the most extensive lesions. The middle cerebral and internal carotid arteries are the major feeders of these intracranial lesions. About 8% are mid-line and the remainder are distributed fairly equally on either side.

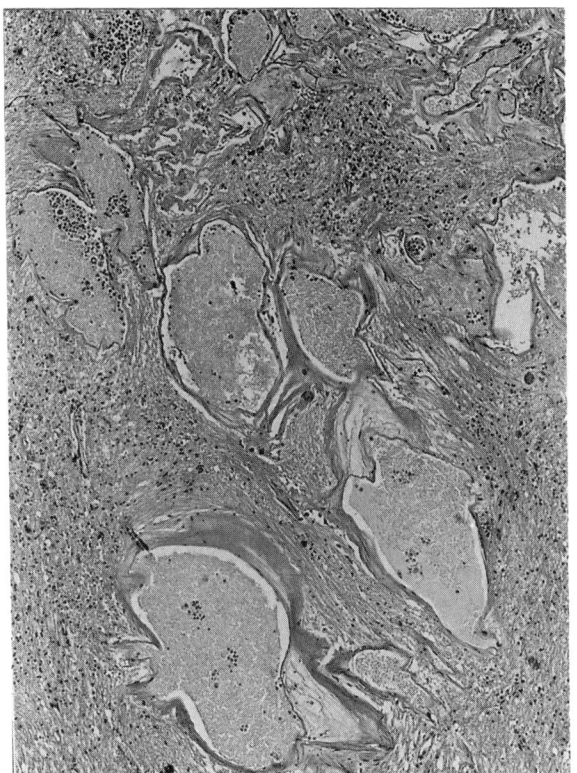

Figure 14.24 Haemangioma with large channels and hyaline fibrous walls of irregular thickness. Note intervening gliosed brain tissue between channels. (Haematoxylin and eosin.)

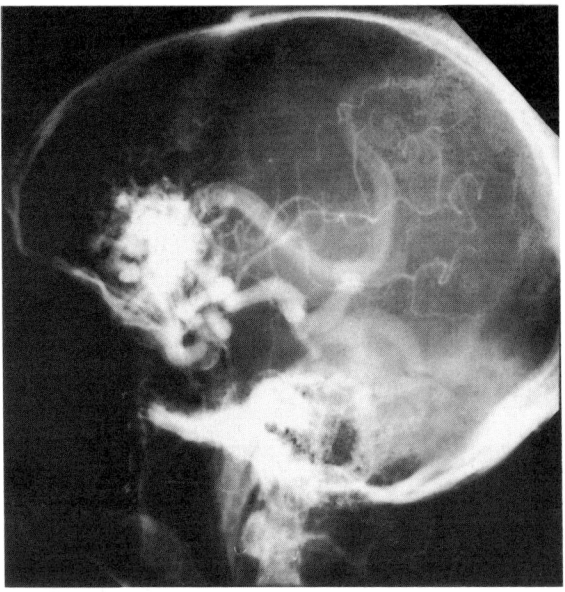

Figure 14.25 Angiogram of arteriovenous communication demonstrating large drainage channels. (Courtesy of Dr V. Balakrishnan.)

By virtue of the unique structure of the cerebral vessels with their remarkably thin walls, it is likely that they may be even more vulnerable to the degenerative changes than the femoral vessels in the rabbit, in which case histological atypia would be more pronounced than in extracranial blood vessels.

14.6.1 PATHOLOGY

There may be vascular naevi or increased vascularity of the scalp on inspection of the head and enlarged diploic channels should be sought in the calvarium. Dural vessels (both meningeal and venous sinuses) can exhibit unusual enlargement and some big channels may appear to be aberrant or alternatively primitive channels may persist, all of which may be bilateral. The subdural space can be bridged by multiple channels. Enlarged foramina in the skull may be present because of the increased calibre of vessels involved in the lesion.

A–V communications are more impressive at craniotomy than at autopsy when the overlying meninges may be shrivelled and fibrotic possibly with siderotic pigmentation indicative of past haemorrhage. There may be recent subdural, subarachnoid or intracerebral haemorrhage. There will be a variable collection of ectatic tortuous vessels over the surface of the brain and in sulci with much enlarged drainage channels. The feeding vessels and components of the circle of Willis will be ectatic and tortuous, making the circle of Willis asymmetrical, but more than one major vessel can participate in the shunt depending on its size and duration. Most of the cerebral arteries, even from the opposite side, may feed very large lesions and the head may nod rhythmically with each pulse. Pressure perfusion displays the vessels best and characteristically numerous, unusually large vessels penetrate the brain parenchyma and are associated with a disturbed vascular pattern. Some may be aneurysmally enlarged and intervening parenchyma may be softened, haemorrhagic, siderotic or gliotic.

Venous channels may be grossly enlarged (Figure 14.25) for varying distances to the extent of being aneurysmal, especially the great cerebral vein of Galen (Figure 14.26) and less often involved are the straight sinus and the superior longitudinal sagittal sinus [67,68] even at some distance from the shunt. In coronal section, the A–V communications usually present a triangular lesion, extending from the base at the meninges to an apex at or close to the ventricles in the line of the transcerebral veins. The honeycombing of the brain parenchyma with unusually large vessels is easily seen on the cut surface. The cerebral hemisphere is frequently atrophied in part due to damage to the parenchyma and possibly to post-mortem collapse of the participating vessels, some of which may be calcified. Basal arteries can exhibit pronounced atherosclerosis and in other places the walls may be thin and atrophic. Aneurysms should be sought especially on afferent and neighbouring arteries.

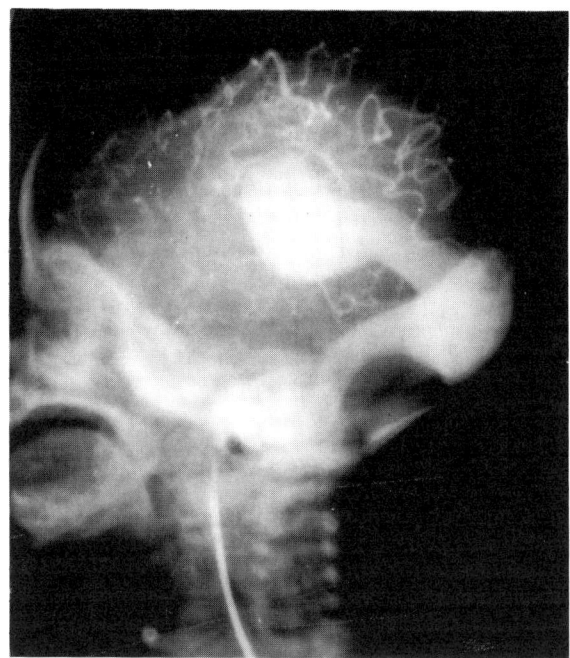

Figure 14.26 Cerebral angiogram showing aneurysm of the vein of Galen, dilated straight sinus, torcular and transverse sinus. There were also tortuous leptomeningeal vessels. (Reproduced with permission from Stehbens et al. [74].)

plexuses are involved as only part of a more extensive communication encompassing thalamus, hypothalamus and basal ganglia.

Suggested grading systems for clinical appraisal of operable risk have been suggested [70,71] and there is a need for pathological correlation with clinical grading.

14.6.2 ARTERIOVENOUS COMMUNICATIONS OF THE MID-BRAIN

Wyburn-Mason [72] reviewed A–V communications involving the mid-brain. Some subjects also had angiomatous involvement of the retina and cutaneous vascular naevi of the face and neck. In some instances the dilated and tortuous vessels extended posteriorly from the retina to involve the optic disc, nerve, chiasma and tract, thus reaching the dorsum of the mid-brain posteriorly, chiefly on one side to involve the quadrigeminal bodies, the brachia conjunctiva and red nucleus. Some extensions involve the pulvinar, hypothalamus, cerebellum, choroid plexus of the lateral ventricles and the pons. Enlarged afferent vessels, not often from the basilar and vertebral arteries, have been found and their size is commensurate with the size and duration of the shunt. Enlarged efferent vessels are numerous and involvement of the cavernous sinus accounts for the bilateral pulsating exophthalmos. The enlargement of venous sinuses, skull markings and diploic vascular channels can be observed radiologically. There is considerable destruction and degeneration of brain tissue, retina and optic pathways. The venous component may be prominent, which led some authors to interpret the lesion as a venous anomaly. The loud bruit over the side of the head and neck is inconsistent with this view.

In 27 cases of retinal A–V communications or similar lesions, 81% were associated with an intracranial A–V communication which could have involved the mid-brain. On the other hand 70% of 20 cases of known A–V communication in the mid-brain also had a retinal vascular anomaly [72]. These associations suggest that they constitute a distinct entity or syndrome which is difficult to explain on the basis of trauma, unless it occurred in embryonic life. They have been found in association with mental retardation.

14.6.3 ANEURYSMS OF THE VEIN OF GALEN

Aneurysmal dilatations of the great cerebral vein of Galen have occurred in association with a cerebral A–V communication. Some present clinically in neonates and infants. It has been suggested that some represent a congenital varix [73] but this is unlikely and in any developmental anomaly there must be reasons for such dilatation which should be sought. There may be direct anastomosis with neighbouring arteries (posterior cerebral, posterior communicating, superior cerebellar,

Dandy [69] was of the opinion that the mass of small vessels or so-called angioma in which the A–V shunt occurred is deep within brain substance. This has not been confirmed nor is it likely to be true. However, dissection and demonstration of true relationships will be a difficult exercise. The bruit and thrill are more likely to be associated with larger cortical vessels than in an angiomatous plexus.

Small A–V aneurysms, which may be multiple, are usually fed predominantly from one major cerebral artery only. By means of the distal leptomeningeal anastomoses, other major arteries, two or possibly even three, may become progressively involved. As the shunt enlarges, so do efferent drainage channels. Thrombotic episodes in the veins can lead to temporary reduction in the shunt until other collateral arteries compensate and in this way the bruit and thrill may fluctuate in intensity with time. Even extracranial vessels can participate in the shunt. Veins enlarge more so than arteries and in some lesions the tortuosity and aneurysmal enlargement of veins and sinuses can overshadow the arterial changes. The additional venous drainage may be reflected in the orbit by proptosis and in the retina by venous tortuosity and engorgement with well oxygenated blood.

A–V communications occasionally involve the choroid plexus and can be responsible for a primary intraventricular haemorrhage or even hydrocephalus. They may be bilateral but most often the choroid basilar, anterior cerebral and the anterior choroidal arteries or their branches). It is also possible that the A–V communication may drain into the great cerebral vein of Galen. Multiple openings into the aneurysmal vein of Galen have been noted but unless histology is performed on these vessels and the communications are identified as arterial, they could represent the preexisting venous tributaries carrying (arterial) oxygenated blood.

The aneurysmal vein may be half the width of the skull and irregular in shape. The straight sinus may also be irregularly dilated with the dural covering at their junction causing a constriction at that site [68]. Other veins may also be abnormally dilated and with large shunts retrograde flow is a feature in some veins and even in the superior longitudinal sagittal sinus. Some diffuse meningeal angiectasia over a cerebral hemisphere has also been observed together with gross dilatation of the straight sinus, torcular and transverse sinus (Figure 14.26) [74]. Veins of the scalp are frequently affected. Thrombosis of veins or a sinus or of the dilated afferent arteries involved in the shunt may occur and can cause massive haemorrhagic infarction of the drainage area. Spontaneous thrombotic occlusion of the dilated vein of Galen has been reported with symptoms related to hydrocephalus [75].

The dilated vein of Galen compresses the mid-brain and the aqueduct of Sylvius with resultant hydrocephalus. Haemorrhage may occur from a thin-walled dilated artery or vein into the ventricles or subarachnoid space.

Patients have been divided into three grades of severity [61].

1. The first group is born suffering from cardiac and respiratory distress due to the magnitude of the shunt such that the infants may be thought to be suffering from congenital heart disease. There are other manifestations of the disorder present but the cardiac status is the dominant feature.
2. In the second group, the infants may present from birth to nine months with hydrocephalus, convulsions, a cranial bruit, distended scalp veins and possibly haemorrhage.
3. The third group presents much later in life (average of 13 years) complaining of headache, fatigue, vertigo, hemiparesis and possibly subarachnoid haemorrhage. Radiological calcification may be present in the walls of old aneurysmal dilatations. Other sinuses and veins may undergo enormous dilatations simulating an aneurysm of the vein of Galen in association with an A–V communication near to or remote from the mid-line drainage system.

A large localized dilatation of another vein or even of a sinus producing a space-occupying mass together with a large shunt can simulate this phenomenon. Such a case was reported involving the inferior sagittal sinus [76].

These lesions are mostly considered to be congenital malformations but several patients have a history of severe head injury [77]. Some have haemangiomas of the face, lung or brain and so the congenital concept has been perpetuated but as such cases are also more likely to be reported, it is not known whether the associations are statistically significant or simply anecdotal experiences.

14.6.4 ARTERIOVENOUS COMMUNICATIONS OF THE POSTERIOR FOSSA

Large lesions in the posterior fossa are infrequent constituting only about 10% of large communications. Small subtentorial 'cryptic' A–V lesions are considerably more frequent. Mostly they involve the cerebellum. Others involve the mesencephalon, pons or medulla or all combined [78]. Their effects on the arteries and veins are similar although they have not been studied histologically in detail. The occasional lesion may be associated with multiple communications but histological confirmation of such topography is necessary.

14.6.5 SMALL OR CRYPTIC ARTERIOVENOUS COMMUNICATIONS

Although most primary intracerebral haemorrhages occur in subjects over 40 years of age, intracerebral haemorrhage happens from time to time in younger subjects without demonstrable cause even in the absence of chronic hypertension. Such haemorrhage has been attributed predominantly to small haemangiomas and cryptic A–V communications [79,80] and Potter [81] considered smaller lesions were more prone to haemorrhage than the larger lesions. The lesions are often recognized by the cluster of dilated and tortuous vessels on the cortical surface overlying the haematoma but sometimes they are buried in the depths of a sulcus. Most occur in young subjects, often in the first and second decades, and without painstaking examination of the brain they are often overlooked at autopsy. The haemorrhage may be primarily subarachnoid or intraventricular with relatively little intracerebral haemorrhage. Small occult or cryptic lesions can also be associated with an aneurysm on the afferent artery [82].

In a 45-year-old imbecile terminal haemorrhage with plaques and amyloid deposits in cerebral arterioles was attributed to multiple small arteriovenous communications, the three main features being regarded as a syndrome [83].

14.6.6 HAEMODYNAMICS

The haemodynamics of these lesions varies from time to time and the site of the actual communication would be rarely accessible because of the augmented vascularity and tortuous collateral vessels [84]. Nornes and Grip [40] estimated the flow in single afferent arteries ranged from 3 to 550 ml/min (average 180 ml/min). They further estimated the total shunt flow varied from 150 to 900 ml/min (average 490 ml/min). Pressure recordings from afferent vessels ranged from 40 to 77 mmHg (average 56 mmHg), which were well below the systemic blood pressure. However, the authors gave no indication of the pulse pressure though the water-hammer effect on the afferent arteries is of the utmost importance and may be primarily responsible for the atrophic lesions.

The incidence of bruits in abnormal communications of the brain has varied from 22 to 48% [81]. It would appear that a vein or some other vessel in the communication may partially or completely thrombose with diminution in the shunt. The bruit and thrill may then disappear but the shunt may continue to function silently. With further enlargement of vessels, the shunt may enlarge instigating reappearance of the bruit. In a series of 110 cases a bruit was found in 67% of subjects in whom the initial symptom was headache, in 50% of those with epilepsy and in only 12% of those with haemorrhage [85]. The main determining factor was size, the larger the lesion the more likely was a bruit heard. Small lesions were particularly likely to bleed and less likely to have a bruit.

Radiological findings in abnormal cerebral A–V communications include bone changes consistent with enlarged arteries, veins or sinuses, evidence of raised intracranial pressure, calcification in the vessels or in surrounding parenchyma, rapid filling of veins angiographically, a short arterial phase, bone thickening over the lesion, skull asymmetry, cerebral atrophy and evidence of haemorrhage and siderosis on magnetic resonance imaging.

14.6.7 HISTOLOGY

Histologically these abnormal A–V communications consist of many enlarged vessels of variable calibre, often in the subarachnoid space and otherwise in the parenchyma. The gross ectasia even of small vessels and their extreme tortuosity result in an apparent increased density of large vessels in a given area, imparting the impression that the vessels have not developed in a normal fashion. This view is supported by the irregular thickness and diversity of degenerative changes and mural architecture of the walls of these vessels (Figure 14.27), whether arteries or veins, all of which can be reproduced in experimental lesions. Intervening tissues will be compressed and subjected to similar vibrations to those that have damaged the blood vessel walls, resulting in cerebral atrophy and gliosis (Figure 14.28).

Many vessels possess walls of irregular fibromuscular tissue often with little residual elastic tissue and some

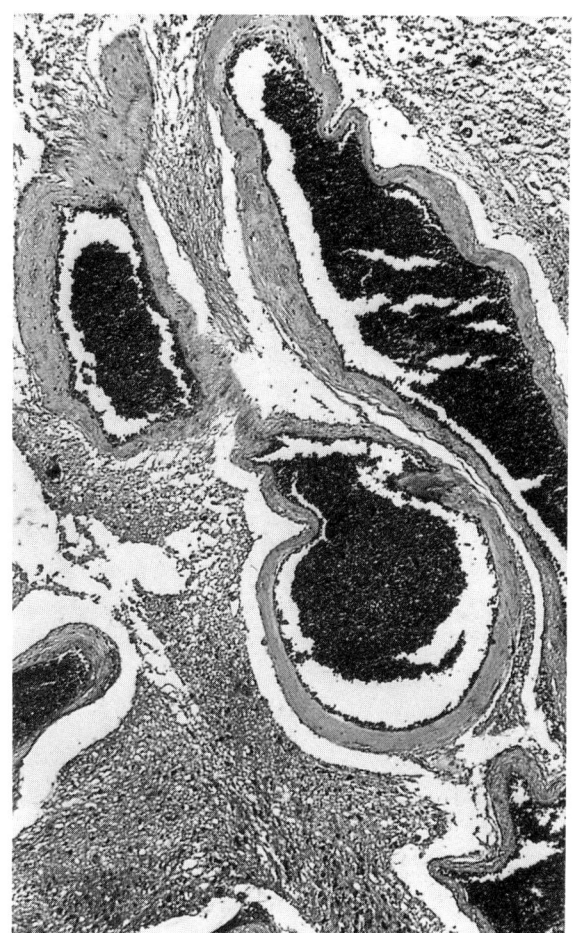

Figure 14.27 Cerebral arteriovenous communication exhibiting multiple large vessels within the parenchyma, atypical mural architecture and unusual shaped contours. (Haematoxylin and eosin.)

resemble intimal proliferation as occurs at arterial forks with destruction of the thin media. Atrophic lesions in arteries produce vessels such that their original structure and function cannot be determined. When these vessels collapse, as is seen at biopsy or autopsy, the contour of the vessels is remarkably irregular. Polypoid projections of the media into the lumen have been demonstrated by serial sections to be artifacts [86]. Some vessels are obviously dilated thin-walled veins, others possess walls identical to those of aneurysms and contain a variable amount of muscle and no elastica. Some walls will be quite hyalinized and relatively acellular. Calcification can be variable (Figure 14.29) but is usually not pronounced and evidence of thrombosis with organization is common. There may be fibrin infiltration of the wall or evidence of old or recent haemorrhage in the intervening gliotic brain tissue which exhibits demyelination and minimal calcification. Small quantities of amyloid occur in both intracranial and extracranial A–V lesions but this is not a prominent feature. Perivascular fibrosis

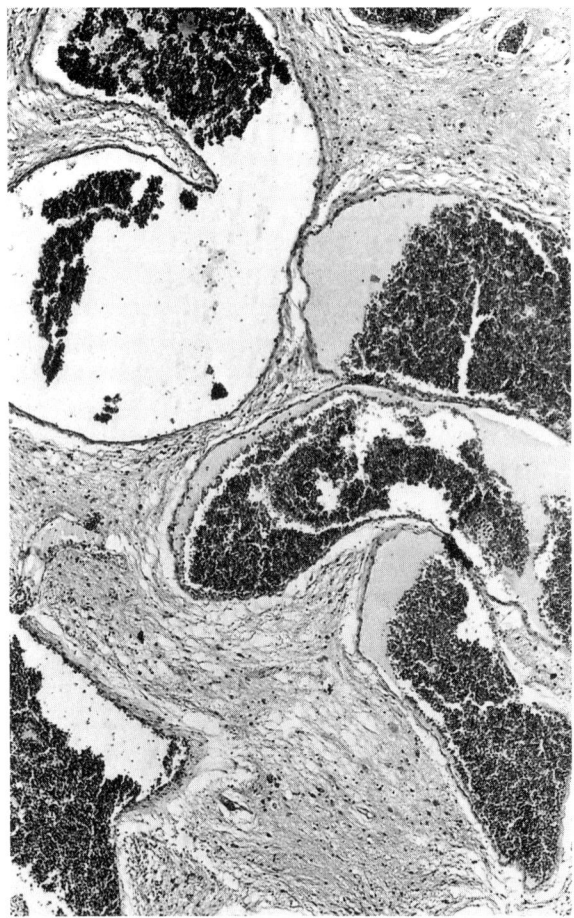

Figure 14.28 Large thin-walled vessels, probably drainage channels of a cerebral arteriovenous communication. Note degenerative changes and siderophages in the intervening brain tissue. (Haematoxylin and eosin.)

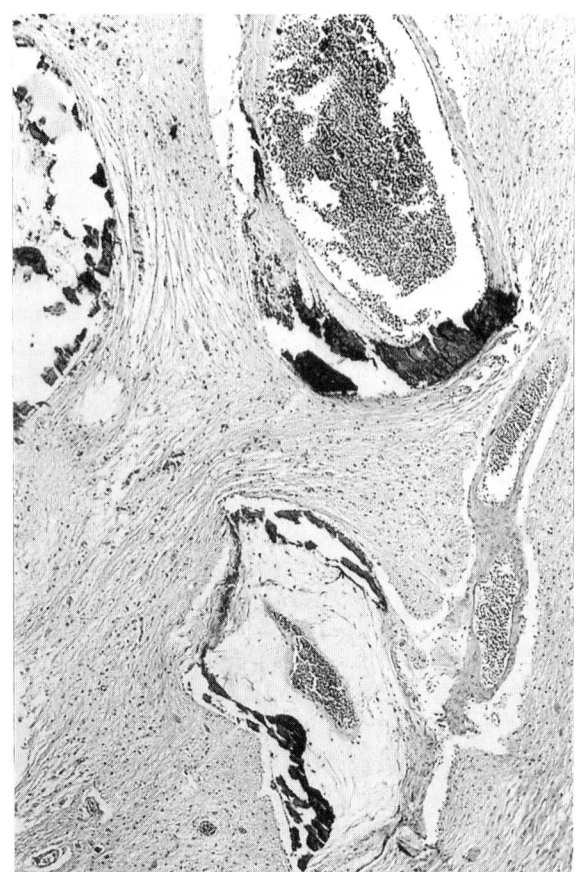

Figure 14.29 Cerebral arteriovenous communication with mural calcification of the atypical vessels. (Haematoxylin and eosin.)

may occur especially over the meningeal surface and multiple small thin-walled vessels may be numerous, as in a telangiectasia. In the adjoining parenchyma there may be increased congestion and prominence of capillaries.

Thrombotic episodes in stressed vessels will alter the rate of progression and the clinical status until collateral channels assume the role of major channels. However, most vessels are small and frankly atherosclerotic changes such as lipophages and cholesterol clefts are seldom seen. Fat stains reveal lipid in the walls of some vessels.

In 72 surgical specimens of cerebral A–V communications, sclerosis of the vessels was universal and histiocytes with clear but non-foamy cytoplasm were deep to intimal thickenings. As is usual no fat stains were performed though lipid and cholesterol were thought to be present [87]. Amyloid material may be demonstrable in thickened hyaline walls [73]. Ossification is rare.

Vessels from such communications exhibit ultrastructural changes similar to those observed in experimental A–V fistulae and atherosclerotic intima [9,88,89].

14.6.8 COMPLICATIONS

Apart from the progressive destruction of brain parenchyma, haemorrhage is the most frequent complication but these lesions do not bleed as readily as berry aneurysms. The peak incidence of subarachnoid haemorrhage stemming from them is from 10 to 30 years of age. Some 88% of those presenting with haemorrhage have no history of convulsions and only 18% of those with convulsions subsequently have a haemorrhage [90].

Haemorrhage can be the first clinical manifestation of an A–V communication. It can be subarachnoid, intracerebral or intraventricular. Often the haemorrhage is deeply placed in the cerebral hemisphere, which suggests that it may be venous bleeding but any aneurysmal dilatation within such congeries of tortuous vessels can bleed as might an aneurysm (usually berry in type) on any afferent artery. Smaller lesions have a greater tendency to bleed than larger lesions. Tönnis *et al.* [91] alleged that haemorrhage was less frequent from the lesions in cerebral and precentral regions which were more prone to be associated with convulsions. The subarachnoid haemorrhage will be most severe over the lateral aspect of the cerebral hemispheres. More than 50% of patients suffered some neurological deficit as the result of their first bleed. This equates roughly with the incidence of a significant haematoma since these lesions are not usually associated with infarcts or arterial spasm. Hemiplegia or hemiparesis of sudden or gradual onset occurs in almost half the subjects with cerebral A–V communications [61].

It has been suggested recently that increased resistance to venous drainage might predispose to haemorrhage and this could increase the pressure within the shunt, thus aggravating the mechanical effect of the vibrations but this might also reduce the magnitude of the shunt. A high rate of haemorrhage has been observed in patients with a single or impaired venous drainage or deep venous drainage alone [92,93]. Small lesions less than 2 cm in diameter usually have a single drainage vein and thus also a high rate of haemorrhage which diminish as the lesion grows and acquires more drainage veins [92].

Subdural haemorrhage is uncommon but the lesions can bleed directly into the subdural space and can be extensive, contributing to the swift demise of the patient. It can also produce a chronic haematoma [85].

Bleeding is precipitated by coughing, straining or some exertion in approximately 30% of instances, suggesting that the associated elevation of blood pressure contributes to the initiation of the haemorrhage [63]. Trauma does not appear to be a significant factor. Pregnancy has been associated with haemorrhage in a few cases but there is no statistical evidence to support a causal relationship. Massive haemorrhage can be associated with secondary pontine haemorrhage, intraocular haemorrhage and papilloedema.

(a) Progression of the lesion

Most intracranial A–V communications are slowly and relentlessly progressive. Small traumatic pial communications may spontaneously thrombose as does the occasional experimental femoral fistula in rabbits. It is rare for established fistulae to undergo spontaneous cure by thrombotic occlusion of the shunt but they have been reported [94]. Shumacker and Wayson [95] found that five of 245 intracranial communications appeared to have undergone spontaneous thrombotic occlusion and presumably self-cure. With non-fatal haemorrhage, thrombosis occurs in the bleeding vessel and the possibility is that a vital afferent artery may occlude, an infrequent event according to the evidence.

Many of the prolonged histories of these lesions indicate that following surgery, with or without an audible bruit, the lesions may remain clinically dormant as if in remission for some years before reappearance of the bruit following insidious enlargement of the shunt. In a follow-up of unruptured communications [96] the risk of death from haemorrhage was 29% while 23% of survivors had significant long-term morbidity. The mean risk of haemorrhage was 2.2% per annum. The size of the lesion was of little use as an indicator in determining which lesions would bleed. Saccular aneurysms were found in 19.3% of subjects. Exacerbations of symptoms, and sometimes fatal haemorrhage can be anticipated in the majority of lesions, including epilepsy (26–32%), periodic migrainous headache (15–24%), progressive hemiparesis (7–12%), headache (6%) and other sensory disturbances.

There is amply evidence that these communications progressively enlarge, attracting additional collaterals whether intracranial or extracranial to feed the parasitic circulation. Some enlarging intracerebral lesions develop collateral circulation via the middle meningeal artery which shows enlarged skull markings [97]. Likewise A–V communications of the face and scalp, whether traumatic or associated with a congenital angioma, are prone to enlarge incorporating ipsilateral and contralateral extracranial collaterals. They recur following inadequate surgical extirpation and ultimately recruit collateral flow from the intracranial circulation [98]. This is particularly likely with ophthalmic, ethmoidal and meningeal vessels from the internal carotid artery but the vertebral arteries too may be involved. Whilst some may become quiescent and be labelled self-cured, most, when followed, do not appear to reach an equilibrium. Such an event is dependent on thrombotic occlusion of crucial vessels and appears to occur by chance. The aggressive behaviour of many of these lesions is not due to neoplasia or simple growth of mesodermal nests of vasoformative tissues but to the unfavourable haemodynamics.

It is unlikely that new arteriovenous shunts form *de novo* although such an event could follow surgical interference or rupture of an atrophic walled afferent vessel into a dilated venous channel.

Surgical extirpation of the main lesion is followed by a significant reduction in size of the afferent and efferent vessels which resume a normal angiographic appearance in most instances [91,99].

(b) Associated intracranial saccular aneurysms

These aneurysms may or may not be of the berry type and their presence depends on the atrophic changes in afferent vessels due to the augmented haemodynamic stresses [7,61]. They may be multiple and though alleged at times not to be on afferent arteries to the shunt, this view is probably consequent upon poor evaluation of the arteries feeding the fistula [61]. Aneurysms have been found in up to 19.3% of intracranial A–V communications [96] and usually in subjects older than those with a shunt alone. Bleeding may occur from either the aneurysm or vessels of the shunt. There has been argument about whether the two lesions are related but the profound atrophy of the femoral artery and flattening and indentation of the apex of the forks proximal to experimental femoral A–V fistulae occur experimentally [7] leaving little doubt that the aneurysm is secondary to the haemodynamic effects caused by the shunt. The thinner walls of the cerebral arteries make aneurysm formation even more likely than with femoral vessels. This thesis, also supported by the development of aneurysms on the supply arteries to vascular meningiomas associated with an A–V shunt, is being increasingly acknowledged and the aneurysms are attributed to the high flow in the afferent arteries [100] and develop along the largest feeding vessel of an enlarging shunt [101]. There is certainly no reason for assuming the association of these two vascular lesions is an example of associated congenital abnormalities. Unfortunately no concerted investigation examining the cerebral vasculature histologically in detail in subjects with chronic A–V fistulae or communications has been undertaken. An aneurysm of the internal carotid artery in its cervical course has been reported in a subject with a mid-line cerebral A–V lesion [102].

In recent years aneurysms on the afferent cerebral arteries to A–V communications have been observed angiographically to regress and to almost disappear [103–105] following surgical resection or embolization of the communication. This has been considered as evidence that high flow participated in the aetiology and pathogenesis of the aneurysms but pressure changes in the afferent artery particularly the water-hammer effect must also participate. This partial regression is a remarkable observation and requires clinical and pathological follow-up. Regression is inconsistent with the development of aneurysms on afferent arteries subsequent to extirpation of an A–V fistula. Reduction in stress may allow some healing and possibly thrombosis but histological study is essential for proper interpretation. In one case [105] the aneurysms on the major artery feeding the fistula regressed. Retrograde thrombosis extended to the aneurysm which presumably underwent thrombotic occlusion. However, knowledge of the pathological changes in the afferent artery and of the natural history of aneurysms in general, especially aneurysms proximal to extracranial A–V aneurysms, suggests caution in dealing with these aneurysms that have allegedly regressed. Longer term follow-up may well reveal that they may enlarge once more. Furthermore, extirpation of the shunt does not preclude progression of the vascular changes even though less rapidly, nor the future development of aneurysms and other degenerative changes in the afferent vessels. Whatever the outcome the answer is of both academic and clinical importance.

(c) **Anatomical variation in vasculature**

Anatomical variation of the cerebral vasculature (particularly veins) has frequently been attributed to a basic developmental fault in angiogenesis. However, such variations are probably secondary phenomena attributable to the A–V shunt, which has led to gross enlargement of vessels otherwise insignificant in size. Some arterial variations such as the persistence of a trigeminal artery have been reported [61]. The association could be fortuitous or due to enlargement of a smaller vessel usually overlooked.

(d) **Cardiovascular effects**

Experimental A–V fistulae cause gross irregular enlargement and tortuosity of the anastomosed vein. Veins at a distance can enlarge sufficiently to produce exophthalmos as occurs in humans. The contralateral veins together with intercommunicating channels may also enlarge. The larger the shunt, the larger and more rapidly will these vascular changes be and in humans where the lesions are present for 15 to 20 years before becoming clinically apparent, the progressive dilatation, tortuosity and fragility of collateral vessels could well account for the troublesome vascularity encountered by surgeons. In cerebral A–V communications, in which blood vessels have thin walls, the acceleration of their already rapid blood flow and the Corrigan's pulse may greatly accelerate progression of the lesions. Reduction in haemodynamic stress should permit improved repair with increased intimal proliferation and mural thickening but the fatigue-like changes in the mural connective tissues are in all likelihood cumulative as in vibrating-tool disease. This fact could explain why aneurysmal dilatation may develop on the afferent arteries even years after extirpation of the shunt. The haemodynamic stresses will also have contributed substantially to the augmentation of atherosclerotic changes in afferent arteries [7] and this effect must be taken into account in any assessment of whether these shunts are therapeutic or not. The distal blood flow to the tissues is dependent on collateral arterial and venous circulation for both supply and drainage and it has been estimated that blood supply distally may be reduced by as much as 50% or more [31]. Congestion, stasis and oedema may be prominent. Development of the collateral circulation is to be expected in view of the poor peripheral circulation and the successful competition for collateral blood flow by the A–V shunt accounts for the distal trophic changes seen in peripheral extracranial A–V fistulae. Surgery on cerebral A–V communications results in improved vascular filling on angiography. Preoperatively there is a reduced cerebral metabolic rate [61].

A–V shunts, when small, may exert little effect on the heart but when sizeable, cause a chronic increase in cardiac output in man and experimental animals, and increased pulse rate and size. The heart may be both hypertrophied and dilated. Eventually, cardiac failure develops especially in children. It may mask the underlying cause with the shunt and rate of progression being the principal governing factors.

It has been recorded that cerebral blood flow may be increased by a factor of almost four and the size of the cerebral shunt has been estimated to be as high as 1830 cc/min [106]. The augmented cardiac workload over years cannot be assumed to be without effect on the heart and coronary arteries and sometimes must contribute to the onset of congestive cardiac failure even in adults.

Surgery on the cerebral A–V communication results in a diminution of the cerebral blood flow and size of the shunt although reduction is not always complete. It is also associated with increased peripheral resistance and A–V oxygen difference. There may be reduced ipsilateral retinal pressure. Cardiac size is reduced but the extent of the persistence of ill-effects on the heart, cardiac valves, coronary arteries, and blood vessels following extirpation of the shunt remains to be determined and the effects are likely to be cumulative.

(e) **Intellectual impairment**

Definite intellectual impairment has been observed in up to 50% of subjects with cerebral A–V shunts. There is loss of parenchymal function in the vicinity of the lesion and diminished cerebral metabolic rate, cerebral ischaemia and circulatory stagnation may all contribute to cerebral atrophy. Mental impairment can be coincidental but in a 1-year-old infant there was progressive psychomotor regression, decreased spontaneity and neurological deterioration associated with cerebral atrophy [107] indicative of the serious consequences of the shunt.

(f) **Pressure effects**

As with cerebral aneurysms, there may occasionally be pressure effects on a nerve or even on the calvarium by an aneurysmal vessel. Sometimes a cranial defect results but mostly the pressure effects are generalized especially in the presence of hydrocephalus, very great aneurysmal dilatation of a venous sinus or massive haemorrhage. Secondary pontine haemorrhage is also a possibility.

(g) **Prognosis**

These lesions are pernicious and threaten the life of the individual depending on the duration, size of the shunt and location of the primary site. The natural history of these lesions teaches the lesson that their complete extirpation should be carried out as early as possible and that angiography cannot reveal the small collaterals that can carry on the shunt after occlusion of a major afferent artery. Basically those that commence with a headache have a better prognosis with approximately 50% living for 30 years. With modern surgical practice, neurological impairment is usually remarkably mild.

The rate of major rebleeding varies from 2 to 4.0% per annum and the mortality is 1% per annum. The mean interval between the initial presentation and subsequent haemorrhage is 7.7 years.

14.7 Aetiology of arteriovenous communications

Some of these lesions of the brain and scalp are accepted as being traumatic in origin and most extracranial lesions are indeed traumatic. Most intracranial A–V shunts are assumed to be developmental anomalies and are referred to as malformations.

On considering angiogenesis in embryology and even in postnatal life, it is a wonder that direct communications between arteries and veins do not persist frequently into adult life. Other factors or events must inhibit or prevent such an occurrence. Labelling a lesion as congenital indicates its existence at birth and does not indicate its aetiology: to label a lesion as a malformation or dysgenesis suggests that the lesion has strayed from its normal developmental pathway and that the aetiology is established. Frequently both labels are conjectural and euphemisms for idiopathic or unknown etiology.

Naturally occurring physiological A–V anastomoses varying in calibre from 20 to 160 μm can be demonstrated in the pial circulation but have a wide distribution in mammals and occur in most peripheral tissues and internal organs. They have the capacity to bypass the capillary bed and to shunt arterial blood directly to the venous circulation. Rowbotham and Little [108] suggested that these could be of importance in the development of cerebral A–V communications. This must be considered a possibility, not so much in the large vessel fistulae but in the small lesions. Small cherry angiomas and the telangiectases for example have been attributed to abnormalities of the vessels or the capillary loops but the striking feature of spider naevi, cherry angiomata (Campbell de Morgan spots) and inherited haemorrhagic telangiectases is the bright red colour indicative of highly oxygenated arterial blood. Whether there are some factors which induce these physiological A–V communications to become pathological or to enlarge is unknown. This concept is supported by the readiness with which these arteriovenous anastomoses can be produced by surgical implantation of a piece of skin in sheep and the formation of small pathological lesions in pulmonary scars.

In larger telangiectases such as those in the brain, the possibility that thoroughfare channels or precapillary A–V anastomoses [109] which are normal components of the microcirculation, may on occasion enlarge relentlessly and cause small A–V shunts that in turn progressively enlarge has to be considered. That they exist under normal conditions is important and indicates that there are factors which under physiological conditions are under control although it is conceivable that they may malfunction and give rise to pathological shunts. There is need for thorough examination of the microcirculatory topography of early lesions.

Haemangiomas of the central nervous system, whether capillary or cavernous, are mostly classified as hamartomas in the belief that they are due to perverse development of embryonic vessels that either undergo angiomatous proliferation *in utero* or remain dormant for years before proliferating. There is no convincing evidence that they are hamartomatous. Campbell de Morgan (cherry red) spots of the skin are assumed to be angiomatoid malformations, yet their bright red colour suggests an arteriovenous shunt. Indeed if a small vessel shunt is to develop, this is the type of lesion that might be expected. It would account for their colour and the progressive enlargement of the vessels. Likewise in somewhat larger vessels, an A–V shunt might account for the capillary telangiectasia and even cavernous haemangiomas. Whether these are due to some local lesion or derived from the pre-existing physiological A–V communication is conjectural. Willis [110] regarded all non-malignant vascular lesions as hamartomas, reserving the term tumour for metastasizing lesions. However, the concept of an A–V shunt explains much of the behaviour of these lesions. Telangiectases, varices and cavernous haemangiomas may be only variants and stages in the natural history of an arteriovenous shunt.

Potter [81] believed that an A–V fistula was the basic pathological fault underlying these lesions and that the development of the congeries of tortuous and dilated vessels, whether predominantly arterial, venous or vessels of smaller calibre, was secondary. The co-existence of telangiectases and haemangiomas with florid A–V communications indicates possibly a similar underlying cause. Morever there is remarkable similarity of appearance and behaviour in the 'congenital' and traumatic A–V communications. The frequency of head injuries in infancy and childhood provides ample opportunity for small traumatic pial arteriovenous shunts to develop, most of which will thrombose. The occasional persistent lesion after 10–15 or more years might present clinically as a significant A–V communication. In a few instances trauma *in utero* may be responsible. Whilst this is an attractive and plausible theory, it is the association with apparently remote cutaneous angiomas, telangiectases, inherited haemorrhagic telangiectases or the diffuse shunt involving a whole limb (Figure 14.12) that is difficult to explain in our present state of knowledge. The histological appearance of blood vessels in A–V communications with atypical and unexplained architecture can no longer be regarded as support of a developmental anomaly since a femoral A–V shunt can so alter the vascular architecture as to make it unrecognizable.

The occurrence of multiple lesions especially in association with port-wine stains of the skin and a familial occurrence [65] with or without hereditary haemorrhagic telangiectasia support a developmental disorder but are not definite proof. The propensity for these A–V communications (at times multiple) in subjects with inherited connective tissue disorders manifesting acquired connective tissue fragility only emphasizes the importance of trauma in their aetiology. It is incongruous that most extracranial lesions are traumatic and most intracranial lesions are considered to be hamartomatous.

The role of pregnancy in the production of palmar erythema, spider naevi, telangiectasis and venous clusters in legs of parous women is recognized without assuming a developmental disorder but similar lesions in the central nervous system are regarded as such. While it is at present unwise to be dogmatic regarding the aetiology of these lesions, it can be said that some are acquired and due to trauma and that many of the manifestations of these lesions, irrespective of aetiology, are haemodynamically determined.

14.8 Carotid cavernous fistula

The unusual anatomical relationship of the cavernous segment of the internal carotid artery to the cavernous sinus means that trauma or leakage of an aneurysm of that segment could result in an A–V fistula. This is a rare entity, constituting about 6% of all intracranial A–V communications. Occasionally bilateral, it causes a distressing bruit and horrible facial disfigurement.

The traumatic group contains more males than females and is caused by a fracture through the base of the skull involving the sphenoid bone with an age incidence peaking in the third decade. The trauma is at times relatively trivial but can also be due to a perforating injury. It has been produced at carotid endarterectomy by passing a Fogarty catheter up the thrombosed internal carotid artery [112]. The tear in the artery varies in size up to 10 mm and in some instances the artery is completely severed. The margins of the fistula are smooth. It occurs particularly at the junction of the fixed petrous segment and the relatively free cavernous segment. In view of the degenerative changes that occur on the greater curvature of bends, it is possible that this may predispose to a tear due to trauma as might a pre-existing aneurysm. Such lesions also occur in type IV Ehlers–Danlos syndrome spontaneously [113].

The spontaneous or aneurysm group is predominantly female with a more even age distribution. Some occur in infants and children without a history of a head injury leading to the suggestion that they may be congenital but all active infants suffer head injuries.

A similar fistula has been reported between the internal carotid artery and the basilar venous plexus associated with a basal skull fracture involving the clivus [114]. It must be stressed that pulsating exophthalmos may be due to tumour in the orbit, and also carotid–jugular fistulae. Mild spontaneous A–V shunts develop between meningeal branches of the internal or external carotid arteries and dural veins in the vicinity of the cavernous sinus in middle-aged women and simulate carotid cavernous fistulae but frequently resolve spontaneously.

The fistula initiates an incessant bruit and causes gross congestion in the venous tributaries and communications with the cavernous sinus with oedema of the eyelids, face and forehead, subconjunctival haemorrhages and exophthalmos of one or both eyes, sudden diplopia and impaired vision [1]. Exophthalmos becomes pronounced, at times preventing closure of the eyelids and is often eccentric and bilateral. Its appearance may be delayed until a false aneurysmal sac bursts and may be accentuated by thrombosis within the cavernous sinus or ophthalmic veins. Pulsation of the eyeballs and engorged veins over the forehead or in the neck is common and the cardinal sign of this fistula has been pulsating exophthalmos but pulsation is not invariable.

The bruit is usually present with systolic intensification and frequently associated with a palpable thrill. Headache, intense chemosis, conjunctival congestion and possibly ulceration, extraocular palsies, optic atrophy and papilloedema are also frequent. Cardiac impairment is infrequent because it usually occurs in adults and surgery is generally instituted early. Spontaneous fistulae have been linked with pregnancy. Walker and Allègre [115] estimated that 25–30% of afflicted women develop these fistulae in the later half of pregnancy. Spontaneous rupture may have been through fusiform aneurysms.

If the fistula is of long duration, the ipsilateral internal carotid artery will enlarge and become thin walled as atrophic changes develop [5–7] and in this regard tearing of the internal carotid artery following attempted clipping [116] suggests undue fragility. Other arteries contributing to the shunt are numerous as are the venous drainage channels. The cavernous sinus enlarges and the wall thickens. The contralateral sinus becomes secondarily involved via communicating channels [61] with the microscopic changes similar to those observed in chronic experimental A–V fistulae.

Some subjects with traumatic rupture of the internal carotid artery probably die of associated injuries and escape detection. Very mild cases may also escape detection being essentially subclinical.

Death may follow trauma after an interval following haemorrhage into the sphenoid sinus and pharynx. Severe epistaxis may occur from venous haemorrhage independently of or in association with the trauma. Fatal intracranial haemorrhage from rupture of the cavernous sinus is probably a major hazard obviated by early therapy. Bleeding from enlarged communicating veins may be subdural or subarachnoid and secondary infection of the eye and orbit in chronic fistulae can be a problem. Spontaneous cure occurs sporadically due to thrombosis of the cavernous sinus or of the fistula [117]. In chronic lesions cerebral ischaemia and vascular stenosis and congestion may account for intellectual impairment and neurological deficit including hemiplegia.

Carotid ligation as a therapeutic measure by altering haemodynamics has been blamed for early or delayed cerebral haemorrhage [118].

14.9 Associated intracranial and extracranial arteriovenous communications

The majority of cranial arteriovenous communications involves cerebral vessels alone but with progressive enlargement they recruit blood from the dural vessels and ultimately there is obvious involvement of branches from the external carotid artery. A traumatic fistula between a meningeal artery and a diploic vein may close spontaneously [119]. However, progression of the shunt can then involve the external carotid and internal carotid with drainage mostly into the intracranial sinuses. A large dural shunt associated with considerable enlargement of most of the dural sinuses in a 48-year-old man was found at autopsy to have had an old thrombosis of the superior longitudinal sagittal sinus and grossly enlarged venous channels throughout the brain together with some parenchymal necrosis [120]. These channels may represent gross venous collaterals distal to the fistula and sinus obstruction and support the need for early extirpation of the shunts.

Occasionally intracranial lesions are found in association with extracranial communications of similar nature. The possibility of two lesions being initiated by the same trauma one in the scalp and one in underlying brain tissue has to be considered. Some may be manifestations of a single communication and be supplied by intracranial and extracranial vessels. Others have no definite relationship and without an obvious cause, a developmental anomaly is usually invoked.

The extracranial circulation may involve the intracranial circulation in three ways:

1. Venous drainage from extracranial A–V shunts could drain via emissary, diploic or orbital veins into dural sinuses which are involved secondarily [121]. A blood cyst or a haemangioma of the pericranium with vascular communications to intradural sinuses has

been called a sinus pericranii but this is obsolete terminology.
2. Branches of the external carotid artery (whether intracranial or extracranial) may form A–V communications with dural sinuses or meningeal veins and by progressive enlargement and erosion of the skull around participating channels, ectatic tortuous vessels are found intracranially and extracranially often with palpable bone defects. Reversal of the pulsatile flow may give the impression of multiple arteries entering directly into the lateral or sigmoid sinuses. Secondary enlargement of veins over the brain follows in chronic cases. Small anastomoses between pial and meningeal vessels may become considerably enlarged and accentuated following surgical interference or thrombosis of some crucial vessels of supply or drainage.
3. Branches of the external carotid artery may provide increasing blood supply to intracranial A–V communications via usually small insignificant anastomoses with the internal carotid or vertebrobasilar systems. There are instances of primary supply coming from the external carotid artery and most commonly this participation is via the middle meningeal artery.

14.10 Extracranial arteriovenous communications and fistulae

Trauma to the head is common but A–V communications of the head and neck are infrequent. Some may be confined to the scalp, such as that following hair transplantation for alopecia [122] but the progressive enlargement and recruitment of neighbouring arterial and venous channels including intracerebral vessels reveal the pernicious and malignant nature of these lesions which are so disfiguring and disconcerting to the victim. It would seem that if the shunt is of sufficient duration and size, involvement of intracranial vessels is inevitable. Surgical extirpation of only some feeding vessels may augment involvement of the intracranial circulation.

Cavernous haemangiomas of the scalp, forehead or orbital region are often associated with an A–V shunt of considerable proportions and involve dural and meningeal vessels. However, the feeding arteries are usually not grossly enlarged and tortuous suggesting that the shunt is not as great as in those with a more direct shunt between large arteries and veins.

14.11 Carotid–jugular fistulae

This is a rare disorder due primarily to trauma. Congenital cases have been recorded in young subjects [123] but the absence of recognized injury is not proof of a congenital aetiology. This fistula is commonly used for experimental purposes and has also been introduced as a therapeutic measure. Proven to be of no value in ameliorating mental retardation, it is a hazardous procedure, many of the subjects developing subarachnoid, intracerebral and intraventricular haemorrhage. Enlarged tortuous veins have been found at the base of the brain together with degenerative changes in the involved vessels and intravascular thrombi [124].

It has been used to counteract compression of the ipsilateral optic nerve by

- an intracranial saccular aneurysm of the internal carotid artery immediately after its emergence from the cavernous sinus;
- an aneurysm of the anterior communicating artery;
- an ectatic tortuous ophthalmic artery.

Improvement of ocular symptoms was reported and one subject died from the carotid aneurysm [125].

14.12 Vertebral arteriovenous fistulae

Most of these rare lesions have been attributed to trauma and a few have been assumed to be congenital. Penetrating injuries are by far the commonest cause though some may appear to have a spontaneous onset even from sudden alteration in head position. Vertebral angiography has been responsible for some iatrogenic fistulae. The bruit and disturbing headaches are distressing and retrograde flow has been observed in the basilar artery. Such a vascular steal can cause a cerebral deficit and gross enlargement of spinal vessels.

14.13 Arteriovenous communications of the spinal cord

Blood vessels of the spinal cord are smaller than those of the brain. The cord is less liable to injury and is infrequently examined at autopsy. It is therefore not surprising that A–V communications of the cord are rarer than those of the brain.

Telangiectases are rare in the cord but can be a cause of haematomyelia and subarachnoid haemorrhage with blood tracking up and down the cord for a variable distance. They can also cause backache, radicular pain, paraesthesia and progressive paraparesis without haemorrhage. More commonly there are cavernous haemangiomas which are believed to be more advanced stages of telangiectasia [126]. These mostly occur within the cord and usually in the posterior columns. They tend to expand within the cord and bleed leading to siderotic deposits and neurological cord disturbances. As with similar lesions elsewhere, they may be multiple within the brain and cord with an occasional cutaneous haemangioma.

Extradural spinal haemangiomas are very unusual and may produce the picture of spinal extradural haemorrhage. They can extend into the extradural fat and vertebrae and are commonly associated with cutaneous haemangiomas of the skin but rarely of the cord [126].

The commonest of these lesions in the cord are the 'venous angioma' and the A–V communications. The 'venous angioma' is allegedly more prevalent and the large ectatic or aneurysmal veins may be pulsatile and contain well oxygenated blood [127,128], suggesting that they are in reality A–V communications although with relatively small arterial supply channels insufficient to produce an audible bruit.

These spinal A–V communications are not as common as spinal cord tumours and occur between the second to the seventh decades on admission to hospital with a peak in the fifth decade but there is a pronounced shift to the left for the age at onset of symptoms.

These lesions have an extramedullary component consisting of dilated tortuous vessels around varying lengths of the cord, often causing deep impressions and possibly obstructing the spinal canal. Some vessels may develop saccular aneurysms which cause pressure symptoms. These lesions have been classified into three major morphological types [129].

1. *Single-coiled vessel* Generally in adults, it consists of only one or two afferent arteries feeding an exceedingly long tortuous venous vessel over the dorsal surface of the cord. It has a slow flow rate and is regarded as a venous angioma.
2. *Glomus type* Usually found in adults, this consists of a small localized plexus of small coiled vessels most often fed by a single afferent artery. The flow rate is slow.
3. *Juvenile type* This is the typical fast-flowing A–V communication usually found in children and young adults. It is said to have multiple feeders supplying an extensive voluminous lesion often filling the canal.

The second major component of these lesions is an associated intramedullary proliferation of small vessels simulating telangiectasis which is at times very extensive involving the grey matter particularly. Thus the cord lesions differ from the cerebral lesions in having only small vessels within the parenchyma and large vessels in the subarachnoid space. The meninges may be quite fibrotic with sideritic staining from previous haemorrhage. There may be calcification of some vessels and the surrounding bone may be eroded with enlargement of the canal. It suggests that A–V shunts may produce large vessel changes and ultimately also involve the microcirculation. The canal may be blocked by the presence of tortuous worm-like filling defects on myelography and the full extent of the lesion is usually not outlined. The vessels of the medullary venous system may be visibly pulsatile and by selective angiography only one feeder is present. Some may have involvement of the vertebrae. Mostly the lesions are in the thoracic region with the others being cervical or in the lower part of the canal.

Recently a series of patients was reported with cranial and sacral dural A–V fistulae, the nidus being at some distance from the cord with a lack of normal radicular draining veins. There was extensive involvement of the medullary venous system and spinal cord ischaemia [130]. The remote location of the shunt is significant and indicates that cases classified as venous anomalies could still have an A–V shunt.

Histologically, the lesions are similar to the cerebral A–V communications, the vessels having a propensity for thrombosis. Calcification is infrequent and the small intramedullary vessels have thick hyaline walls. The cord itself exhibits considerable gliosis with a variable degree of destruction of the cord architecture and neurons.

Spinal A–V communications have a sinister reputation because of their usually progressive nature, some 19% of subjects developing severe disability of gait within six months of onset of symptoms and 50% of subjects becoming chairbound within three years [131]. These lesions slowly but progressively destroy the cord, with the initial symptoms often being backache and radicular pain with weakness of the lower limbs followed by rapid progression to paraplegia due to complete destruction of the cord. These lesions are the single most frequent cause of spinal subarachnoid haemorrhage which is often recurrent and rarely fatal or the cause of haematomyelia.

Trauma seems to be related to the onset of bleeding in some cases and again exacerbation of symptoms from haemangiomas and A–V communications has been correlated with pregnancy [127,132].

Myelomalacia is the serious and irreversible complication and more common than in cranial lesions. Occlusive thrombosis may occur in bleeding vessels but surgical dissection of these vessels from the pial surface of the cord can be performed with relative impunity and vasospasm is infrequent. Cord compression has been incriminated but a spinal steal phenomenon may be responsible [61]. Physical exertion has been known to precipitate a flaccid paraparesis [133] sometimes with minimal sensory disturbance [134]. Transverse myelitis may occur with these lesions and the syndrome of Foix–Alajouanine (subacute necrotic myelopathy) has been attributed to a diffuse vascular cord lesion leading to paraplegia. Scoliosis probably due to muscle weakness, occasionally complicates these lesions and its onset in the first decade may be the first symptom [77].

14.13.1 FOIX–ALAJOUANINE SYNDROME

Subacute degenerative changes in the spinal cord, referred to as progressive necrosis of the spinal cord are characterized by amyotrophic paraplegia progressing from early spasticity to flaccid paraplegia with loss of tendon reflexes, sphincter control and later on, sensation. The lumbosacral segments of the cord are particularly prone to involvement with early necrosis of neurones and thickening, hyalinization and narrowing of intraspinal vessels without inflammatory changes together with pial vasculature consistent with an A–V communication [126]. The meninges may be greatly thickened and haematomyelia may result. The nature of this lesion has been a source of controversy but it is generally regarded as a manifestation of a spinal A–V communication associated with spinal cord ischaemia.

Cutaneous port-wine stains occasionally occur with spinal cord A–V communications which are usually located in the lower thoracic and lumbar segments when the cutaneous lesions are segmental. This cutaneous involvement is not always metameric but can involve underlying muscles of the corresponding metameres [132]. These cutaneous and spinal lesions are difficult to explain on an acquired basis but if continuous with the spinal lesion, they may be merely extensions of a lesion initiated *in utero*.

These lesions are usually too small to be associated with a bruit and the shunt is too small to cause cardiac embarrassment. Spinal cord A–V communications have also been associated with cerebral, retinal, vertebral, pulmonary, hepatic, renal and A–V shunts [126]. Such lesions are generally regarded as developmental as are their cerebral counterparts though this theory persists only for want of a better hypothesis. Trauma may account for some but a final decision awaits further information on their initiation, pathogenesis and natural history. The inception in some victims seems late for the appearance of developmental lesions and the young age of other instances does not preclude the possibility of some causative lesion or trauma being responsible *in utero*. The possibility of multiple lesions would be enhanced by vascular fragility associated with connective tissue disorders.

14.14 Extradural, vertebral and calvarial lesions

Haemangiomas and A–V communications or combinations of the two can occur primarily outside the dura in the skull, spinal column and adjacent tissue and depending on their size and the associated shunt, involvement of intradural structures can readily result. More detailed knowledge is required of the aetiology and early pathogenesis of haemangiomas, many of which could be acquired [61].

14.15 Ataxia telangiectasia (Louis–Bar syndrome)

Ataxia telangiectasia is an obscure disorder resulting from an autosomal recessive gene defect associated with impaired T and B lymphocyte function. The infant appears normal until about two years of age, when progressive cerebellar ataxia sets in and oculocutaneous telangiectases consisting of a faint hair-like network develop on the bulbar conjunctiva, the butterfly area of the face, ears, antecubital fossa and the neck. Considerable degenerative changes occur in the central nervous system (particularly degeneration of the Purkinje cells in the cerebellum). Immunodeficiency develops with depression of cell-mediated immunity and low levels of IgE, IgA and IgG, recurrent infections of the respiratory tract, a propensity for reticuloendothelial malignancy and carcinoma of the breast, absence or atrophy of the thymus, gonadal and endocrine abnormalities and eventually mental deterioration.

Ectasia of the veins and capillaries has been noted in the internal capsule and in the white matter of the frontal lobes as well as abnormal dilatation of subependymal veins, pial arteries and veins in cerebral sulci [61,135].

Multiple foci of telangiectasia have been noted and found diffusely in the brain in one case, with many of the vessels thickened, hyalinized and at times calcified [136]. Fresh haemorrhage or siderophages are frequent about the ectasias. There are also microabscesses, granulomas and microglial nodules and areas of demyelination in the brain.

Whilst the vascular changes in this syndrome appear to be relatively mild, and are possibly secondary to other pathological lesions or some progeric changes in the skin, the importance of this syndrome historically was said to lie in its alleged relationship to the Sturge–Weber syndrome and von Hippel–Lindau disease. Now this does not appear to be correct.

14.16 Pulmonary arteriovenous communications

These A–V shunts between pulmonary arteries and veins mostly affect adults. They vary from telangiectasia to a massive A–V shunt even with cyanosis and may be multiple [43]. They usually do not have much effect on the heart. However, by shunting poorly oxygenated blood through an enlarging parasitic circulation, some cause cyanosis, clubbing, polycythaemia and possibly osteoarthropathy, the increase in blood volume being due to the polycythaemia and elevated haematocrit with normal plasma volume. In systemic shunts there is an increase both in red cell volume and plasma with a normal haematocrit [48]. The pulmonary shunt can amount to 80% of the cardiac output.

These can occur at all ages from neonates to the elderly, with cyanosis usually present from an early age if not at birth. A massive congenital fistula in the newborn may be mistaken for cyanotic heart disease [137]. Most have a murmur over the lungs and a high percentage is associated with cutaneous angiomata.

A few cases have been reported in subjects with obstructive pulmonary disease and moderate pulmonary hypertension [138] but the disease with the greatest predisposition is hereditary haemorrhagic telangiectasia or Osler–Weber–Rendu disease or syndrome. This is an hereditary disease (autosomal dominant pattern) manifested by multiple telangiectases of the skin and mucous membranes with a tendency for troublesome bleeding. All are symptomatic by 40 years of age and 62% by 16 years. The commonest sites for lesions are the palms and nailbeds (71%), the lips and tongue (66%) and the face (20%). The lesions become more numerous with age and recurrent epistaxes is the commonest initial symptom [139]. Their bright red colour may signify the presence of an A–V shunt but these subjects also have a remarkable propensity for large A–V communications especially of the lung, the brain and the gastrointestinal tract [140]. The incidence of pulmonary shunts could approximate 25% of patients with this syndrome, which has been found in 36% of cases with a single pulmonary lesion and 57% in those with two pulmonary communications [43]. Such unexplained associations are used to support the developmental or hamartomatous concept of the A–V communications. Associations have also been recorded with multiple spider telangiectases and nodular haemangiomas of the face, neck, lips and mucous membranes.

One 52-year-old victim of this disease had a left parieto-occipital A–V communication and a berry aneurysm at the origin of the left posterior communicating artery from the left internal carotid artery. The aneurysm had bled and was probably secondary to the shunt [141]. Aggravation of this disorder has been reported during pregnancy and oestrogen therapy [142].

About half the cases have a detectable bruit and the pulmonary lesions vary considerably in size and severity of the shunt. Single lesions are more common in the lower lobes and multiple lesions occur in about one third of cases [48]. These lesions like those elsewhere may bleed into the pleural cavity or produce haemoptysis.

There seems to be no evidence that communications develop from the bronchial arteries to the pulmonary veins but presumably, if they exist, they would be substantially smaller and may be overlooked.

14.17 Coronary arteriovenous fistula

A significant communication of a coronary artery, most frequently the right, may communicate with a cardiac chamber (usually the right) or a cardiac vein. The consequence of such an event is that a pressure differential exists between the systemic circulation and the low-pressure pulmonary circulation. The artery will be grossly ectatic, tortuous and may have aneurysms. Histological changes in the coronary artery have been generally regarded as atherosclerotic and the experimental femoral A–V fistula in rabbits supports this view [7].

The venous channels exhibit phlebosclerosis. This could be overlooked and under these circumstances the true nature of a tortuous ectatic and perhaps aneurysmal coronary artery could remain undetected. A continuous murmur, if present, assists with the diagnosis.

In a 58-year-old male with angina but no heart murmur, the three main coronary arteries were found ectatic and tortuous. Two were calcified and each artery communicated with a maze of small vessels. With the presence of three communications the lesions were considered to be congenital despite the age [143].

14.18 Splanchnic arteriovenous fistulae

Significant A–V communications in the splanchnic circulation are rare and a congenital, neoplastic or inflammatory aetiology has been invoked from time to time. Trauma would be infrequent although small injuries or lesions could be responsible for some very small lesions referred to as mucosal angiectases seen in the alimentary tract [144]. However, of these an occasional lesion could develop into a significant shunt. Small A–V communications of the bowel and stomach have been incriminated in some cases of gastrointestinal bleeding of obscure origin and are often detected only by arteriography [145]. They would usually be missed at autopsy.

There has been an increase in renal A–V fistulae following the introduction of percutaneous needle biopsy. The lack of a corresponding increase in hepato-portal A–V communications which are associated with ascites, portal hypertension and hepatic congestion, is no doubt due to the much lesser importance of arterial blood supply to the liver via the hepatic artery.

A–V communications of the kidneys are mostly traumatic and due to blunt, penetrating or iatrogenic injuries including stab and bullet wounds. Iatrogenic trauma associated with needle biopsy of the kidney has been linked with an increased incidence of false aneurysms and A–V shunts which can immediately make their presence felt by haematuria and local symptoms. These may resolve spontaneously but some, failing to thrombose, persist and eventually lead to severe haemorrhage and an A–V shunt of significant proportions. Such traumatic fistulae can be bilateral [146,147]. When a fistula appears to develop *de novo* in an otherwise healthy person for no apparent reason, it is easy to invoke a congenital hypothesis. However, any trauma in the past may be long forgotten and it should be remembered that in the central nervous system or elsewhere the natural history of acquired and 'congenital' lesions is the same. Other causes invoked include an intrarenal arterial aneurysm and inflammatory lesions eroding a vessel [148]. A–V shunts may also occur in association with renal cell carcinoma.

The spleen seems to be particularly prone to blunt or non-penetrating injuries but even so A–V shunts from such trauma are rare. Splenic fistulae may be expected to follow trauma more often than eventuates but the haemorrhage from blunt splenic injuries is often so profuse as to require splenectomy which may obviate a higher incidence of splenic traumatic aneurysms and A–V communications.

Fistulae between the systemic and the portal vein are quite infrequent but have occurred following perforating injuries or rupture of an aneurysm of the hepatic or splenic artery into the hepatic vein. Occasionally they may be due to surgical trauma. Portal hypertension may be present and their size and proximity to the heart can cause cardiac embarrassment. Postoperative fistulae may develop as the result of use of mass ligatures around vascular pedicles or as a consequence of transfixion sutures [149].

14.19 Therapeutic arteriovenous shunts

During this century therapeutic A–V fistulae have been fashioned in the vain hope of improving blood flow in subjects with limb ischaemia, myocardial ischaemia, mental retardation, congenitally shortened limbs or the ill-effects of poliomyelitis [1]. Carotid–jugular fistulae were unsatisfactory, many subjects developing pulsating exophthalmos with retinopathy, congestive cardiac failure, aneurysmal dilatation of the internal jugular vein, facial asymmetry and subarachnoid haemorrhage. The overall manifestations of these therapeutic A–V fistulae are similar to those in experimental animals and to those alleged to be congenital. These therapeutic experiments aimed at improving the blood flow distally were performed without its being known that the shunts cause chronic congestion, oedema and distal ischaemia.

14.19.1 ARTERIOVENOUS SHUNTS FOR HAEMODIALYSIS

Surgically fashioned subcutaneous A–V communications in the arm or leg were introduced to replace short-term external prosthetic shunts and to improve patency rates for subjects requiring chronic haemodialysis for renal failure. The techniques used vary and many have been subjected to this surgical technique. Some communications spontaneously thrombose early but others persist for long periods of time. The veins enlarge and are engorged, ectatic and tortuous. Small aneurysms may arise and the walls thicken due to phlebosclerosis and develop severe atherosclerosis at an accelerated rate [150]. Angiographically the lumen becomes grossly irregular and severely narrowed, eventually becoming stenosed or occluded by thrombus. These shunts are small when compared with the much larger experimental carotid–jugular fistulae and give an indication of the importance of haemodynamic stress in atherogenesis. Such veins, if left intact like those elsewhere, would have shown minimal atherosclerosis for the remaining years of life, indicating a lack of importance or relevance of dietary strictures in atherosclerosis.

In an experimental study of A–V shunts for therapeutic use, the graft geometry was found to be important in reducing flow disturbances and thereby the degree of intimal-medial thickening in arteriovenous loop grafts. The thickening was found to correlate quantitatively with perivascular tissue vibratory activity [151].

14.20 Arteriovenous communications and tumours

The progressive, rapid growth and high metabolic activity of many tumours necessitate a rich blood supply and extensive drainage. There is consequently proliferation of new blood vessels and humoral angiogenic agents have been isolated from some tumours. Angiographically the presence of a tumour is likely to interrupt the normal vascular topography of the part. At times the vascular proliferation may be so prominent that participation in the neoplastic proliferation has been suggested as a possibility. However, before such an assumption is made, caution is essential.

Vascularity, including the rapid filling of veins some of which may contain red blood with high oxygen saturation is a major feature of some cerebral neoplasms. There may also be a high density of thin-walled sinusoidal veins about the tumour and the presence of an A–V shunt is apparent. Such shunts are known to occur in association with glioblastoma multiforme, vascular meningiomas, haemangioblastoma, papilloma of the choroid plexus and at times metastatic carcinoma [152]. The more vascular the tumour, the more likely there is to be an associated shunt. The A–V communication is so often such a prominent feature of haemangioblastoma that the lesion may be mistaken for an A–V communication. A bruit has been detected in subjects with haemangioblastoma and vascular meningiomas but there is no information on the frequency of such bruits.

A–V shunts are not restricted to intracranial tumours and have been associated for instance with renal cell carcinoma [153]. They are more frequently recognized with intracranial neoplasms because cerebral angiography is in more common use than selective extracranial angiography.

The vascular changes of an A–V shunt occur in association with both the cystic and the solid type of haemangioblastoma and thus are also features of von Hippel–Lindau's disease [61]. The enlarged tortuous vessels radiate from the mural nodule on the inner surface of the cyst. Histologically, the appearance of the vessels is consistent with an A–V shunt, the blood vessels being of irregular thickness and displaying peculiar angular collapsed walls. They have also been considered to be angiomatous and have intravascular thrombi with evidence of haemorrhage which may be profuse. Retinal haemangioblastomas can be mistaken for A–V communications [154] and a similar A–V lesion has been found in association with retinoblastoma [155]. Neither the cardiac output nor the cerebral blood flow in association with these tumours has been measured but a haemangiopericytoma which is similar to the haemangioblastoma had an A–V shunt about the tumour in the thigh, with a bruit. The cardiac output was 9.5 l/min preoperatively and 5.9 l/min postoperatively [156]. Similar vascular changes may occur with the angioblastic meningioma.

Spinal haemangioblastomas are small and the associated shunt may readily be mistaken for an A–V communication. Pial varicosities are likely to be prominent over the tumour mass.

The possibility is that the high degree of vascularity with its propensity to form an A–V shunt may be a feature of all intracranial tumours including metastatic deposits but with variation in degree. The shunts may develop even in a cortical scar [108,157]. The veins about these tumours can change from red to blue and back again suggesting that the flow in the shunt is variable. Such observations reveal the close relationship of trauma to the aetiology of A–V communications both intracranially and extracranially.

The blood supply to meningiomas may come from vessels normally supplying the scalp, skull, meninges and brain. The vascularity with large blood vessels and augmented vascular markings have long been recognized as features of a meningioma. These tumours may have a bruit and be associated with an increased cardiac output.

Berry aneurysms have been reported on arteries feeding some of these intracranial tumours, particularly meningiomas. It is likely the shunt has contributed to the development of the aneurysms. A wide spectrum of flow rates has been demonstrated even in the same tumour with some red veins suggestive of an A–V shunt probably producing a cerebral steal. With cerebral aneurysms being so common, the association between a tumour and berry aneurysm may be fortuitous but in the presence of an A–V shunt and with the aneurysm located on the afferent artery, the association is likely to be the result of the shunt. A highly vascular meningioma in the middle cranial fossa with a cranial bruit may be mistaken for a carotid cavernous fistula.

The blood supply to one primary melanoma of the brain was associated with an enlarged afferent artery and a very vascular tumour similar in appearances to a meningioma [158]. It is possible that small A–V shunts in association with melanoma in the central nervous system may explain the propensity for haemorrhage not seen in association with extracranial melanomata. Large dilated vessels may be found about cerebral metastases from other tumours [61].

A–V communications may be associated with renal cell carcinoma. Patients may present with congestive heart failure and an abdominal bruit is common, the diagnosis being made unexpectedly at surgery or by angiography.

A small A–V communication (called mucosal ectasia) has been found in association with an ileal leiomyoma [159] and several instances of colonic carcinoma. Such lesions were found in association with other colonic lesions and are a source of lower intestinal bleeding. They may appear independently of other lesions [160] seeming to be acquired and possibly deriving from even relatively minor injuries or subclinical infections.

14.21 Venous varicosities

Varicosity of veins is the state in which veins become elongated, tortuous and dilated in an irregular manner [12]. Varicose veins are usually relatively well localized and communicate with veins of normal calibre. In portal venous hypertension, where portal veins anastomose with systemic veins at the lower end of the oesophagus and at the anorectal junction, the veins constitute a collateral circulation from a high to a low pressure system and thus develop ectasia, elongation and tortuosity. These oesophageal varicosities and anorectal haemorrhoids (piles) are particularly prone to rupture, haemorrhage and thrombosis. The varicosities are aneurysmal and the similarity of such changes to those in anastomosed veins of A–V shunts is more than coincidental. It does not follow that there is a shunt involved but only that flow factors are important in their aetiology and pathogenesis.

Occlusion of the inferior or superior vena cava, irrespective of the cause, is followed by gross varicosities of collateral venous channels suggesting that increase in venous pressure contributes to such formation. This is seen also in anal haemorrhoids where it is thought that in pregnancy the fetus impedes flow from the pelvis. Impaired venous return from the pampiniform plexus results in a variocoele for the same reason. Gross venous enlargement appears to cause incompetence of venous valves and venous backflow results.

Thrombosis of deep veins in the lower limb causes varicose veins of the leg with secondary enlargement of collateral vessels and the mural fatigue hypothesis provides the most logical explanation for the cause of the ectasia, tortuosity, varicosities and loss of tensile strength which at certain stages can also be responsible for mural rupture. It is pertinent that abnormally shaped collagen fibrils have been found in the walls of varicose veins, such changes being associated with loss of tensile strength in inherited connective tissue disorders, experimental aneurysms, A–V fistulae and atherosclerosis.

Weakness of the wall is unlikely to be inherited, although the tendency to varicose veins may be inherited as it is in type IV Ehlers–Danlos syndrome. There is no scientific evidence that the venous valves are developmentally at fault or that their topographical distribution is responsible. There is obvious need to investigate the biochemistry and the physicochemical characteristics of vascular connective tissues with similar investigative enthusiasm and resources as have been expended on lipids in atherogenesis.

Varicose veins in various sites occur with venous obstruction and flow-induced changes in collateral flow augmented by the increased pressure which may be up to 200 mmHg in the ankle during the Valsalva manoeuvre. In the lower limb however many observations have been made suggesting that in at least some patients there is an A–V shunt involved.

Veins in the lower limb are initially slightly dilated with thickened walls due to muscle hypertrophy and intimal proliferation, and not varicose, being manifestations of phlebosclerosis. Ectasia, elongation and tortuosity then arise and with these changes, mural thinning, sacculation and fibrosis of the walls become apparent. Veins beyond the valves are swollen and may even pulsate. In the early stages of varicosities there is an unusually high oxygen saturation and oxygen partial pressure in the blood. Bright red blood may issue from an injured vein suggesting the possibility of an associated A–V shunt [161–163]. Long-standing varicosities must contain a substantial volume of blood which is venous. The degree of ectasia and varicosity will augment stasis, increase mural tension and enhance the development of phlebosclerosis. A number of authors believe that an A–V fistula underlies the development of varicose veins [161,164,165] and also explains the augmented vascularity in the adventitia and perivenous tissues in addition to the pulsation, arterial blood and phlebectasia. Gius [165] found confirmatory evidence of this thesis in 13 of 14 patients with varicose veins in the leg. On careful dissection Schalin was able to find several red vessels entering the varicose veins [164]. The possibility is that there may be a traumatic A–V shunt in the calf and that enlarged red venous tributaries draining into varicose veins may be mistaken for arterial channels. Under such circumstances where several arteries allegedly enter a large venous channel, the histological examination of such vessels is essential. In the case of type IV Ehlers–Danlos syndrome trauma to the calf may readily produce an A–V communication because of the fragility of the vessels.

The tortuosity of varicose veins has been likened to the meandering course of rivers and streams [166] and is flow-induced. The mechanism of producing these meanders differs from that of vascular tortuosity but the forces and stresses are no doubt similar and once established secondary degenerative changes will ensue, thus increasing the dilatation etc. Nylander [166] demonstrated angiographically that most of the veins have a spiral course and tortuosity, often a feature of hyperkinetic flow, is also a feature of atherosclerosis and its equivalent in small arteries.

The fatigue hypothesis most readily explains the ectasia, tortuosity, varicosities and thrombosis that are so frequent. It also explains the occasional rupture of a varix through the skin leading to severe blood loss and the vibratory activity associated with a shunt could help explain not only the fragility of the wall of the varix but the loss of tensile strength of the overlying stretched skin.

The aetiology of varicose ulceration is controversial but it is likely to be due to trophic changes associated with stasis, ischaemia and anoxia which can be explained on the basis of an A–V shunt. Trauma and infection are no doubt secondary factors that assist in perpetuation of the varicose ulceration. The concept of the involvement of an A–V shunt is becoming increasingly popular. Frank aneurysmal dilatations (up to 2.5 cm in diameter) may develop on the saphenous vein [165] and have been attributed to an associated arteriovenous shunt. The histological features of varicose veins are essentially those of phlebosclerosis progressing to severe sclerotic changes and loss of elastic tissue and muscle. Lipid is seldom sought but can be found, though usually it is mostly diffuse and extracellular. Cholesterol clefts and 'atheromata' do not occur though it is conceivable they could occur in very chronic and extreme varicosities. Calcification is infrequent. There is currently no evidence to suggest that oesophageal varices, haemorrhoids or varicocoele are associated with A–V communications. However, in the few subjects with oesophageal varices and no portal hypertension, a shunt should be considered a possibility.

14.22 Venous aneurysms and angiomas

Venous aneurysm is a term applied to a relatively localized dilatation of a vein or venous sinus of aneurysmal proportions. The giant aneurysm of the vein of Galen is probably the most widely known lesion of this type and is recognized as being associated with an A–V shunt thought to be due to a developmental anomaly. Similar aneurysmal dilatations have been described involving the saphenous vein and these too have been associated with an A–V shunt [165].

Aneurysmal dilatations of the superior vena cava, external jugular vein and others have been reported. Histologically they will exhibit moderate to severe phlebosclerosis and whilst congenital developmental errors may be invoked, it is more likely that with much

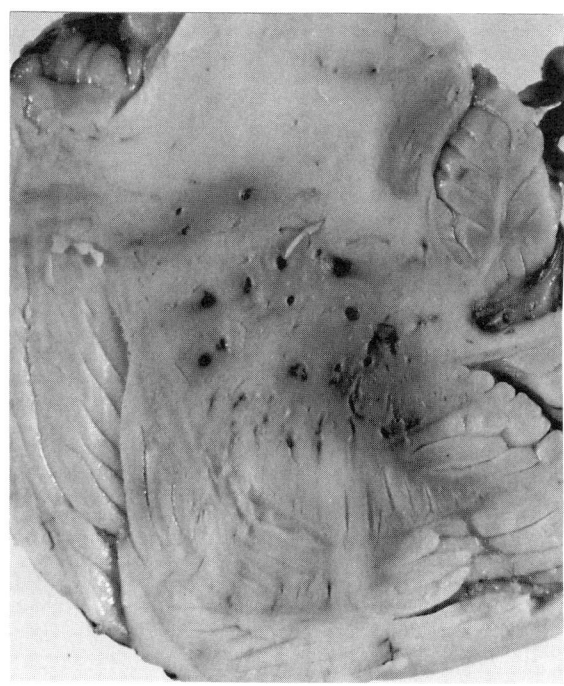

Figure 14.30 Several large veins consisting of a venous angioma in the cerebellum. (Reproduced with permission from Stehbens [61].)

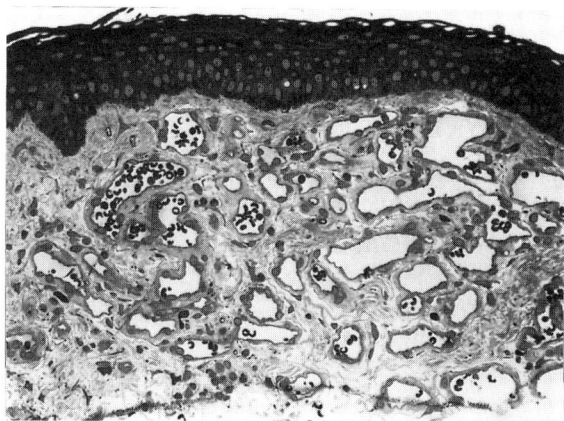

Figure 14.31 Cherry red angioma of the skin consisting of a concentration of thin walled sinusoidal vessels. (Toluidine blue.)

more detailed study an underlying, possibly cryptic A–V communication will be found responsible possibly at some distance. Some may be labelled as a venous aneurysm because of the spectacular dilatation of a vein even in the presence of an A–V shunt. It is not generally appreciated that angiography may not reveal the site of the communication.

Sometimes a long length of vein or several widely dilated veins within close proximity of each other such as in the brain (Figure 14.30) may be observed and are often referred to as a venous angioma. Some may exhibit tortuosity and their precise nature has been debated but they are usually attributed to a developmental error. It is difficult to conceive of one or a group of veins undergoing the degree of phlebectasia involved without there being appropriate internal pressure and augmented blood flow through the veins responsible for the dilatation or there being some reason for weakness and yielding of the walls. It is, therefore, more likely that an A–V shunt was involved in their development, possibly with thrombosis of one artery or vein resulting in closure of the shunt or its reduction to such a low level of activity that it is to all intents and purposes quiescent. The evidence from other lesions would suggest that regression of the phlebectasia would be minimal.

The origin of haemangiomas continues to be controversial and the possibility of at least some being neoplastic is difficult to refute. That some are associated with an A–V shunt does not mean all are due to a shunt but when thin-walled vessels continue to expand, exert pressure on surrounding tissues and bleed, an associated shunt seems likely. It is inconceivable that endothelial cells would by proliferation produce the large sinusoidal or aneurysmal vascular channels seen in some cerebral lesions without sufficient stresses to induce connective tissue weakness of the wall and an A–V communication acquired or present *ab initio* provides a plausible explanation. The development of telangiectatic vessels in the vicinity of the shunts supports this concept.

Small cherry red angiomatous spots (Campbell de Morgan spots) up to 5 mm in size, usually either flat, elevated or sometimes slightly pedunculated, occur mostly on the trunk and increase progressively in number with age. Most middle-aged and elderly people are affected (Figure 14.31). The lesions do not blanche with pressure and have been attributed to dilatation of capillary loops or of venules but their bright red colour suggests arterial blood and for this reason they may represent small A–V shunts. Ultrastructurally they are lined particularly by fenestrated endothelium [167]. They have been reported to have occurred in epidemic form and their number increased as the ambient temperature rose [168]. No infectious agent was discovered and no satisfactory explanation was forthcoming. Some older lesions become brown possibly due to thrombosis and the accumulation of haemosiderin in organization. Thus they may resolve in this way.

14.23 Significance of arteriovenous shunts

The role of physiological arteriovenous shunts is little appreciated and there is need for further information on their physiology and pathology which would be an enthralling but difficult field of study. The pathological A–V shunt, though much neglected is also one of the most fascinating fields in pathology and clinical practice.

A possible role in the pathogenesis of many cutaneous vascular lesions requires careful appraisal. The A–V shunt is likely to become a pre-eminent, valuable experimental model for the study of the effect of haemodynamics on the vessel wall and in atherogenesis. In clinical practice, the pathological arteriovenous shunt is a most pernicious lesion deserving of the utmost respect and its use in therapeutics should be considered only as a last resort, knowledge of the natural history and the pathological consequences being essential.

References

1. Holman, E. (1968) *Abnormal Arteriovenous Communications*, C.C. Thomas, Springfield.
2. Stehbens, W.E. (1958) History of aneurysms. *Med. Hist.*, 11, 274–80.
3. Greenhill, N.S. and Stehbens, W.E. (1985) Haemodynamically-induced intimal tears in experimental U-shaped arterial loops as seen by scanning electron microscopy. *Br. J. Expl. Pathol.*, 66, 577–84.
4. Greenhill, N.S. and Stehbens, W.E. (1987) Scanning electron microscopic investigation of the afferent arteries of experimental femoral arteriovenous fistulae in rabbits. *Pathology*, 19, 22–7.
5. Stehbens, W.E. (1974) Haemodynamic production of lipid deposition, intimal tears, mural dissection and thrombosis in the blood vessel wall. *Proc. Roy. Soc. London Series B*, 185, 357–73.
6. Stehbens, W.E. (1973) Experimental arteriovenous fistulae in normal and cholesterol-fed rabbits. *Pathology*, 5, 311–24.
7. Stehbens, W.E. (1992) Experimental induction of atherosclerosis associated with femoral arteriovenous fistulae in rabbits on a stock diet. *Atherosclerosis*, 95, 127–35.
8. Fallon, J.T. and Stehbens, W.E. (1972) Venous endothelium of experimental arteriovenous fistulae in rabbits. *Circ. Res.*, 31, 546–56.
9. Stehbens, W.E. (1974) The ultrastructure of the anastomosed vein of experimental arteriovenous fistulae in sheep. *Am. J. Pathol.*, 76, 377–400.
10. Stehbens, W.E. and Martin, B.J. (1993) Ultrastructural alterations of collagen fibrils in blood vessel walls. *Connect. Tissue Res.*, 29, 319–31.
11. Martin, B.J., Leppien, B. and Stehbens, W.E. (1993) Changes in collagen fibril morphology in experimental aneurysms and arteriovenous fistulae in sheep. *Int. J. Expl. Pathol.*, 74, 267–74.
12. Stehbens, W.E. (1979) *Hemodynamics and the Blood Vessel Wall*, C.C. Thomas, Springfield.
13. Simkins, T.E. and Stehbens, W.E. (1974) Vibrations recorded from the adventitial surface of experimental aneurysms and arteriovenous fistulas. *Vasc. Surg.*, 8, 153–65.
14. Schenk, W.G., Bahn, R.A., Cordell, A.R. *et al.* (1957) The regional hemodynamics of experimental acute arteriovenous fistulas. *Surg. Gynec. Obstet.*, 105, 733–40.
15. Ingebrigtsen, R. and Wehn, P.S. (1960) Local blood pressure and direction of flow in experimental arterio-venous fistula. *Acta Chir. Scand.*, 120, 142–50.
16. Holman, E. and Kolls, A.C. (1924) Experimental studies in arteriovenous fistulas. II. Pulse and blood pressure variations. *Arch. Surg.*, 9, 837–55.
17. Holman, E. and Taylor, G. (1952) Problems in the dynamics of blood flow. II. Pressure relations at site of an arteriovenous fistula. *Angiology*, 3, 415–30.
18. Schenk, W.G., Martin, J.W., Leslie, M.B. *et al.* (1960) The regional hemodynamics of chronic experimental arteriovenous fistulas. *Surg. Gynec. Obstet.*, 110, 44–50.
19. Ingebrigtsen, R., Krog, S. and Leraand, S. (1962) Velocity and flow of blood in the femoral artery proximal to an experimental arterio-venous fistula. *Acta Chir. Scand.*, 124, 45–53.
20. Callander, C.L. (1920) Study of arteriovenous fistula with an analysis of 447 cases. *Ann. Surg.*, 71, 428–59.
21. Eisenbrey, A.B. (1913) Arteriovenous aneurysm of the superficial femoral vessels. *J. Am. Med. Ass.*, 61, 2155–7.
22. Sako, Y. and Varco, R.L. (1970) Arteriovenous fistula: results of management of congenital and acquired forms, blood flow measurements, and observations on proximal arterial degeneration. *Surgery*, 67, 40–61.
23. Reid, M.R. (1925) Abnormal arteriovenous communications, acquired and congenital. *Arch. Surg.*, 11, 25–42.
24. Reid, M.R. (1925) Studies on abnormal arteriovenous communications, acquired and congenital. 1. Report of a series of cases. *Arch. Surg.*, 10, 601–38.
25. Lindenauer, S.M., Thompson, N.W., Kraft, R.O. *et al.* (1969) Late complications of traumatic arteriovenous fistulas. *Surg. Gynec. Obstet.*, 129, 525–32.
26. Shumacker, H.B. (1970) Aneurysm development and degenerative changes in dilated artery proximal to arteriovenous fistula. *Surg. Gynec. Obstet.*, 130, 636–40.
27. Solberg, L.A., Harkness, R.D. and Ingebrigtsen, R. (1970) Hypertrophy of the median coat of the artery in experimental arterio-venous fistula. *Acta Chir. Scand.*, 136, 575–8.
28. Wilkinson, H.A. (1971) Recurrence of vascular malformation of the scalp 18 years following excision. *J. Neurosurg.*, 34, 435–7.
29. Parmley, L.F., Orbison, J.A., Hughes, C.W. *et al.* (1954) Acquired arteriovenous fistulas complicated by endarteritis, and endocarditis lenta due to *Streptococcus faecalis*. *New Engl. J. Med.*, 250, 305–9.
30. Schmitt, H.J. and Grinnan, G.L.B. (1968) An infrequent complication of arteriovenous fistula. *Arch. Surg.*, 96, 829–31.
31. Sumner, D.S. (1969) Physiology and pathological anatomy, in *Collateral Circulation in Clinical Surgery*, (ed. D.E. Strandness), Saunders, Philadelphia, pp. 40–77.
32. Gupta, T.C. and Wiggers, C.J. (1951) Basic hemodynamic changes produced by aortic coarctation of different degrees. *Circulation*, 8, 17–31.
33. Walker, W.J., Mullins, C.E. and Knovick, G.C. (1964) Cyanosis, cardiomegaly and weak pulses. *Circulation*, 29, 777–81.
34. Lillehei, C.W., Bobb, J.R.R. and Visscher, M.B. (1950) The occurrence of endocarditis with valvular deformities in dogs with arteriovenous fistulas. *Ann. Surg.*, 132, 577–90.
35. Lee, S.H., Fisher, B., Fisher, E.R. *et al.* (1962) Arteriovenous fistula and bacterial endocarditis. *Surgery*, 52, 463–7.
36. Miller, D.S., Mengel, C.E., Kremer, W.B. *et al.* (1966) Intravascular hemolysis in a patient with valvular heart disease. *Ann. Int. Med.*, 65, 210–15.
37. Westring, D.W. (1966) Aortic valve disease and hemolytic anemia. *Ann. Int. Med.*, 65, 203–9.
38. Ziperovich, S. and Paley, H.W. (1966) Severe mechanical hemolytic anemia due to valvular heart disease without prosthesis. *Ann. Int. Med.*, 65, 342–6.
39. Chamberlain, J.K., O'Brien, J.F., Christ, L.M. *et al.* (1974) Intravascular hemolysis with traumatic arteriovenous fistula. *N.Y. State J. Med.*, 74, 686–8.
40. Derrick, J.R. (1970) Discussion. *Surgery*, 67, 59.
41. Katz, H.P. and Askin, J. (1968) Multiple hemangiomata with thrombopenia. *Am. J. Dis. Child*, 115, 351–5.
42. Rhodes, G.R., Cox, C.B. and Silver, D. (1973) Arteriovenous fistula and false aneurysm as the cause of consumption coagulopathy. *Surgery*, 73, 535–40.
43. Bosher, L.H., Blake, D.A. and Byrd, B.R. (1959) An analysis of the pathologic anatomy of pulmonary arteriovenous aneurysms with particular reference to the applicability of local excision. *Surgery*, 45, 91–104.
44. Stannard, M.W., Delany, D.J. and Murray, G.F. (1976) Systemic artery: pulmonary artery fistula after closed chest cardiac massage. *Br. Med. J.*, 1, 1190.
45. Cohen, E.M., Loew, D.E. and Messer, J.W. (1975) Internal mammary arteriovenous malformation with communication to the pulmonary vessels. *Am. J. Cardiol.*, 35, 103–6.
46. Purut, C.M. and Sabiston, D.C. (1991) Origin of the left coronary artery from the pulmonary artery in older adults. *J. Thor. Cardiovasc. Surg.*, 102, 566–70.
47. Burch, G.E. and De Pasquale, N.P. (1964) The anomalous left coronary artery. An experiment of nature. *Am. J. Med.*, 37, 159–61.
48. Hudson, R.E.B. (1965) *Cardiovascular Pathology*, vol. 1, Edward Arnold, London.
49. Lindenauer, S.M. (1971) Congenital arteriovenous fistula and the Klippel–Trénaunay syndrome. *Ann. Surg.*, 174, 248–63.
50. Robertson, D. (1957) Congenital arteriovenous fistulae of the extremities. *Postgrad. Med. J.*, 33, 7–13.
51. Bryer, J.V. and Grant, W. (1975) Klippel–Trénaunay syndrome. A case report and review of the literature. *S. Afr. Med. J.*, 49, 793–4.
52. Förster, C. and Kazner, E. (1973) Spinales Angiom mit Querschnittslähmung bei Klippel–Trénaunay-Syndrom. *Neuropädiatrie*, 4, 180–6.
53. Furukawa, T., Igata, A., Toyokura, Y. *et al.* (1970) Sturge–Weber and Klippel–Trénaunay syndrome with nevus of Ota and Ito. *Arch. Derm.*, 102, 640–5.
54. Poser, C.N. and Taveras, J.M. (1957) Cerebral angiography in encephalotrigeminal angiomatosis. *Radiology*, 68, 327–36.
55. Alexander, G.L. and Norman, R.M. (1960) *The Sturge–Weber Syndrome*. John Wright and Sons, Bristol.
56. Weber, F.P. (1947) *Rare Diseases and Some Debatable Subjects*, 2nd edn, Staples Press, London.
57. Blackwood, W. (1941) Two cases of benign cerebral telangiectasis. *J. Pathol. Bacteriol.*, 52, 209–11.
58. Lim, C.C. and Wallace, H.J. (1967) Multiple self-healing telangiectases with cyanosis. *Proc. Roy. Soc. Med.*, 60, 499.
59. Rigamonti, D., Hadley, M.N., Drayer, B.P. *et al.* (1988) Cerebral cavernous malformations. *New Engl. J. Med.*, 319, 343–7.
60. Clark, J.V. (1970) Familial occurrence of cavernous angiomata of the brain. *J. Neurol. Neurosurg. Psychiat.*, 33, 871–6.

61. Stehbens, W.E. (1972) *Pathology of the Cerebral Blood Vessels*, C.V. Mosby, St Louis.
62. Robinson, J.R., Awad, I.A. and Little, J.R. (1991) Natural history of the cavernous angioma. *J. Neurosurg.*, 75, 709–14.
63. Locksley, H.B. (1966) Report on the Cooperative Study of Intracranial Aneurysmns and Subarachnoid Hemorrhage, Section 5, Part 1. Natural history of subarachnoid hemorrhage, intracranial aneurysms, and arteriovenous malformations. *J. Neurosurg.*, 25, 219–39.
64. Mizutani, T., Tanaka, H. and Aruga, T. (1992) Multiple arteriovenous malformations located in the cerebellum, posterior fossa, spinal cord, dura, and scalp with associated port-wine stain and supratentorial venous anomaly. *Neurosurgery*, 31, 137–41.
65. Snead, O.C., Acker, J.D. and Morawetz, R. (1979) Familial arteriovenous malformation. *Ann. Neurol.*, 5, 585–7.
66. Houser, O.W., Baker, H.L., Svien, H.J. *et al.* (1973) Arteriovenous malformations of the parenchyma of the brain. *Radiology*, 109, 83–90.
67. Gomez, M.R., Whitten, C.F., Nolke, A. *et al.* (1963) Aneurysmal malformation of the great vein of Galen causing heart failure in early infancy. *Pediatrics*, 31, 400–11.
68. Hirano, A. and Terry, R.D. (1958) Aneurysm of the vein of Galen. *J. Neuropathol. Expl Neurol.*, 17, 424–9.
69. Dandy, W.E. (1928) Arteriovenous aneurysm of the brain. *Arch. Surg.*, 17, 190–243.
70. Shi, Y.-Q. and Chen, X.-C. (1986) A proposed scheme for grading intracranial arteriovenous malformations. *J. Neurosurg.*, 65, 484–9.
71. Spetzler, R.F. and Martin, N.A. (1986) A proposed grading system for arteriovenous malformations. *J. Neurosurg.*, 65, 476–83.
72. Wyburn-Mason, R. (1943) Arteriovenous aneurysm of the mid-brain and retina, facial naevi, and mental changes. *Brain*, 66, 163–203.
73. McCormick, W.F. (1966) The pathology of vascular ('arteriovenous') malformations. *J. Neurosurg.*, 24, 807–16.
74. Stehbens, W.E., Sahgal, K.K., Nelson, L. *et al.* (1973) Aneurysm of the vein of Galen and diffuse meningeal angiectasia. *Arch. Pathol.*, 95, 333–5.
75. Weir, B.K.A., Allen, P.B.R. and Miller, J.D.R. (1968) Excision of thrombosed vein of Galen aneurysm in an infant. *J. Neurosurg.*, 29, 619–22.
76. Seljeskog, E.L., Rogers, H.M. and French, L.A. (1968) Arteriovenous malformation involving the inferior sagittal sinus in an infant. *J. Neurosurg.*, 29, 623–8.
77. Boldrey, E. and Miller, E.R. (1949) Arteriovenous fistula (aneurysm) of the great vein of Galen and the circle of Willis. *Arch. Neurol. Psychiat.*, 62, 778–83.
78. McCormick, W.F., Hardman, J.M. and Boulter, T.R. (1968) Vascular malformations ('angiomas') of the brain, with special reference to those occurring in the posterior fossa. *J. Neurosurg.*, 28, 241–51.
79. Hawkins, C.F. and Rewell, R.F. (1946) Unheralded fatal haemorrhage in haemangiomata of the brain. *Guy's Hosp. Rep.*, 95, 88–91.
80. Noran, H.H. (1945) Intracranial vascular tumors and malformations. *Arch. Pathol.*, 39, 393–416.
81. Potter, J.M. (1955) Angiomatous malformations of the brain: their nature and prognosis. *Ann. Roy. Coll. Surg. Engl.*, 16, 227–43.
82. Deruty, R., Pelison-Guyotat, I., Mottolese, C. *et al.* (1992) Ruptured occult arteriovenous malformations associated with an unruptured intracranial aneurysm: report of three cases. *Neurosurgery*, 30, 603–7.
83. Neumann, M.A. (1960) Combined amyloid vascular changes and argyrophilic plaques in the central nervous system. *J. Neuropathol. Expl Neurol.*, 19, 370–82.
84. Nornes, H. and Grip, A. (1980) Hemodynamic aspects of cerebral arteriovenous malformations. *J. Neurosurg.*, 53, 456–64.
85. Paterson, J.M. and McKissock, W. (1956) A clinical survey of intracranial angiomas with special reference to their mode of progression and surgical treatment: a report of 110 cases. *Brain*, 79, 233–66.
86. Mandybur, T.I. and Nazek, M. (1990) Cerebral arteriovenous malformations. *Arch. Pathol. Lab. Med.*, 114, 970–3.
87. Paillas, J.E., Berard, M., Sedan, R. *et al.* (1968) The relative importance of atheroma in the clinical course of arteriovenous angioma of the brain, in *Cerebral Circulation*, vol. 30, (ed. W. Luyendijk), *Prog. Brain Res.*, pp. 419–25.
88. Stehbens, W.E. (1975) Ultrastructure of aneurysms. *Arch. Neurol.*, 32, 798–807.
89. Stehbens, W.E. (1975) Cerebral atherosclerosis. *Arch. Pathol.*, 99, 582–91.
90. Perret, G. and Nishioka, H. (1966) Arteriovenous malformations: an analysis of 545 cases of cranio-cerebral arteriovenous malformations and fistulae reported to the Cooperative Study. *J. Neurosurg.*, 25, 467–90.
91. Tönnis, W., Schiefer, W. and Walter, W. (1958) Signs and symptoms of supratentorial arteriovenous aneurysms. *J. Neurosurg.*, 15, 471–80.
92. Albert, P., Salgado, H., Polaina, M. *et al.* (1990) A study of the venous drainage of 150 cerebral arteriovenous malformations as related to haemorrhagic risks and size of the lesion. *Acta Neurochir. (Wien)*, 103, 30–40.
93. Miyasaka, K., Wolpert, S.M. and Prager, R.J. (1982) The association of cerebral aneurysms, infundibula and intracranial arteriovenous malformations. *Stroke*, 13, 196–203.
94. Santosh, C., Teasdale, E. and Molyneux, A. (1991) Spontaneous closure of an intracranial middle cerebral arteriovenous fistula. *Neuroradiology*, 33, 65–6.
95. Shumacher, H.B. and Wayson, E.E. (1950) Spontaneous cure of aneurysms and arteriovenous fistulas, with some notes on intravenous thrombosis. *Am. J. Surg.*, 79, 532–44.
96. Brown, R.D., Wiebers, D.O., Forbes, G. *et al.* (1988) The natural history of unruptured intracranial arteriovenous malformations. *J. Neurosurg.*, 68, 352–7.
97. Porter, A.J. and Bull, J. (1969) Some aspects of the natural history of cerebral arteriovenous malformation. *Br. J. Radiol.*, 42, 667–75.
98. Hurtwitz, D.J. and Kerber, C.W. (1981) Hemodynamic considerations in the treatment of arteriovenous malformations of the face and scalp. *Plastic Reconstruct. Surg.*, 67, 421–32.
99. Norlén, G. (1949) Arteriovenous aneurysms of the brain: report of ten cases of total removal of the lesion. *J. Neurosurg.*, 6, 475–94.
100. Mintz, A. and Cosgrove, G.R. (1990) Multiple peripheral aneurysms of the posterior inferior cerebellar artery associated with a cerebellar arteriovenous malformation: case report. *Neurosurgery*, 26, 533–7.
101. Azzam, C.J. (1987) Growth of multiple peripheral high flow aneurysms of the posterior inferior cerebellar artery associated with a cerebellar arteriovenous malformation. *Neurosurgery*, 21, 934–9.
102. Singer, A. (1975) Cerebral angioma and aneurysm of the cervical internal carotid artery. *Angiology*, 26, 717–22.
103. Hayashi, S., Arimoto, T., Itakura, T. *et al.* (1981) The association of intracranial aneurysms and arteriovenous malformation of the brain. *J. Neurosurg.*, 55, 971–5.
104. Shenkin, H.A., Jenkins, F. and Kim, K. (1971) Arteriovenous anomaly of the brain associated with cerebral aneurysm. *J. Neurosurg.*, 34, 225–8.
105. Kondziolka, D., Nixon, B.J., Lasjaunias, P. *et al.* (1988) Cerebral arteriovenous malformations with associated arterial aneurysms: hemodynamic and therapeutic considerations. *Canad. J. Neurol. Sci.*, 15, 130–4.
106. Shenkin, H.A., Spitz, E.B., Grant, F.C. *et al.* (1948) Physiologic studies of arteriovenous anomalies of the brain. *J. Neurosurg.*, 5, 165–72.
107. Aoki, N., Sakai, T. and Oikawa, A. (1991) Intracranial arteriovenous fistula manifesting as progressive neurological deterioration in an infant: case report. *Neurosurgery*, 52, 619–23.
108. Rowbotham, G.F. and Little, E. (1965) A new concept of the circulation and the circulation of the brain. *Br. J. Surg.*, 52, 539–42.
109. Hasegawa, T., Ravens, J.R. and Toole, J.F. (1967) Precapillary arteriovenous anastomoses: 'thorough-fare channels' in the brain. *Arch. Neurol.*, 16, 217–24.
110. Willis, R.A. (1967) *Pathology of Tumours*, 4th edn, Appleton-Century-Crofts, New York.
111. Mizutani, T., Tanaka, H. and Aruga, T. (1992) Multiple arteriovenous malformations located in the cerebellum, posterior fossa, spinal cord, dura, and scalp with associated port-wine stain and supratentorial venous anomaly. *Neurosurgery*, 31, 137–41.
112. Barker, W.F., Stern, W.E., Krayenbuhl, H. *et al.* (1968) Carotid endarterectomy complicated by carotid cavernous sinus fistula. *Ann. Surg.*, 167, 568–72.
113. Fox, R., Pope, F.M., Narcissi, P. *et al.* (1988) Spontaneous carotid cavernous fistula in Ehlers Danlos syndrome. *J. Neurol. Neurosurg. Psychiat.*, 51, 984–8.
114. Graf, C.J. (1970) Carotid-basilar venous plexus fistula. *J. Neurosurg.*, 33, 191–7.
115. Walker, A.E. and Allègre, G.E. (1956) Carotid-cavernous fistulas. *Surgery*, 39, 411–22.
116. Dandy, W.E. and Follis, R.H. (1941) On the pathology of carotid-cavernous aneurysms (pulsating exophthalmos). *Am. J. Ophthalmol.*, 24, 365–85.
117. Voigt, K., Sauer, M. and Dichgans, J. (1971) Spontaneous occlusion of a bilateral carotico cavernous fistula studied by serial angiography. *Neuroradiology*, 2, 207–11.
118. Shaw, C. and Foltz, E.L. (1968) Traumatic dissecting aneurysm of middle cerebral artery and carotid-cavernous fistula with massive intracerebral hemorrhage. *J. Neurosurg.*, 28, 475–9.
119. Ishii, R., Ueki, K. and Ito, J. (1976) Traumatic fistula between a lacerated middle meningeal artery and a diploic vein. *J. Neurosurg.*, 44, 241–4.
120. Hinokuma, K., Ohama, E., Ikuta, F. *et al.* (1990) Dural arteriovenous malformation with abnormal parenchymal vessels: an autopsy study. *Acta Neuropathol.*, 80, 656–9.
121. Robinson, J.L. and Sedzimir, C.B. (1970) External carotid transverse sinus fistula. Case report. *J. Neurosurg.*, 33, 718–20.
122. Sonder, D.E. and Bercaw, B.L. (1970) Arteriovenous fistula secondary to hair transplantation. *New Engl. J. Med.*, 283, 473–4.
123. Tekkok, I.H., Akkurt C., Suzer, T. *et al.* (1992) Congenital external carotid-jugular fistula: report of two cases and a review of the literature. *Neurosurgery*, 30, 272–6.
124. Tarlov, I.M. and Grayzel, D. (1952) Brain hemorrhage after carotid-jugular anastomosis. *Ann. Surg.*, 136, 250–60.
125. Bleasel, K. and Frew, J. (1969) Vascular compression of the optic nerves relieved by anastomosis of carotid artery to jugular vein. *J. Neurol.*

Neurosurg. Psychiat., **32**, 268–72.
126. Wyburn-Mason, R. (1944) *The Vascular Abnormalities and Tumours of the Spinal Cord and its Membranes*, C.V. Mosby, St Louis.
127. Newman, M.J.D. (1958) Spinal angioma with symptoms in pregnancy. *J. Neurol. Neurosurg. Psychiat.*, **21**, 38–41.
128. Haberland, K. (1950) Über ein spinales Angioma racemosum venosum. *Arch. Psychiat.*, **184**, 417–25.
129. Ommaya, A.K., Di Chiro, G. and Doppman, J. (1969) Ligation of arterial supply in the treatment of spinal cord arteriovenous malformations. *J. Neurosurg.*, **3**, 679–92.
130. Partington, M.D., Rüfenacht, D.A., Marsh, W.R. *et al.* (1992) Cranial and sacral dural arteriovenous fistulas as a cause of myelopathy. *J. Neurosurg.*, **76**, 615–22.
131. Logue, V. (1979) Angiomas of the spinal cord: review of the pathogenesis, clinical features, and results of surgery. *J. Neurol. Neurosurg. Psychiat.*, **42**, 1–11.
132. Fine, R.D. (1961) Angioma racemosum venosum of spinal cord with segmentally related angiomatous lesions of skin and forearm. *J. Neurosurg.*, **18**, 546–50.
133. Antoni, N. (1962) Spinal vascular malformations (angiomas) and myelomalacia. *Neurology*, **12**, 795–804.
134. Taylor, J.R. and van Allen, M.W. (1969) Vascular malformation of the cord with transient ischemic attacks. *J. Neurosurg.*, **31**, 576–8.
135. Terplan, K.L. and Krauss, R.F. (1969) Histopathologic brain changes in association with ataxia-telangiectasia. *Neurology*, **19**, 446–54.
136. Agamanolis, D.P. and Greenstein, J.I. (1979) Ataxia-telangiectasia. Report of a case with Lewy bodies and vascular abnormalities within cerebral tissue. *J. Neuropathol. Expl. Neurol.*, **38**, 475–89.
137. Hall, R.J., Nelson, W.P., Blake, H.A. *et al.* (1963) Massive pulmonary arteriovenous fistula in the newborn. *Circulation*, **31**, 762–7.
138. Balchum, O.J., Jung, R.C., Turner, A.F. *et al.* (1967) Pulmonary artery to vein shunts in obstructive pulmonary disease. *Am. J. Med.*, **43**, 178–85.
139. Porteus, M.E.M., Burn, J. and Proctor, S.J. (1992) Hereditary haemorrhagic telangiectasia: a clinical analysis. *J. Med. Genet.*, **29**, 527–30.
140. Hodgson, C.H., Burchell, H.B., Good, A. *et al.* (1959) Hereditary hemorrhagic telangiectasia and pulmonary arteriovenous fistula. *New Engl. J. Med.*, **261**, 625–6.
141. Eto, R.T., Harley, J.D., Chikos, P.M. *et al.* (1974) Subarachnoid hemorrhage in hereditary hemorrhagic telangiectasia. *Neuroradiology*, **8**, 127–30.
142. Rowley, P.T., Kurnick, J. and Cheville, R. (1970) Hereditary haemorrhagic telangiectasia: aggravation by oral contraceptives. *Lancet*, **1**, 474–5.
143. Reddy, K., Gupta, M. and Hamby, R.I. (1974) Multiple coronary arteriosystemic fistulas. *Am. J. Cardiol.*, **33**, 304–6.
144. Sprayregen, S. and Boley, S.J. (1978) Vascular ectasias of the right colon. *J. Am. Med. Ass.*, **239**, 962–4.
145. Crichlow, R.W., Mosenthal, W.T., Spiegel, P.K. *et al.* (1975) Arteriovenous malformations of the bowel. An obvious cause of bleeding. *Am. J. Surg.*, **129**, 440–8.
146. Halpern, M. (1969) Spontaneous closure of traumatic renal arteriovenous fistulas. *Am. J. Roentgen.*, **107**, 730–6.
147. Savastano, S., Feltrin, G.P., Miotto, D. *et al.* (1990) Renal aneurysm and arteriovenous fistula. Management and transcatheter embolization. *Acta Radiol.*, **31**, 73–6.
148. Itzchak, Y. and Deutsch, V. (1974) Congenital renal arterio-venous fistula. *Angiology*, **25**, 441–3.
149. Karobkin, M., Kantor, I., Pollard, J.J. *et al.* (1973) Arteriovenous fistula between systemic and portal circulations following partial gastrectomy. *Radiology*, **109**, 311–14.
150. Stehbens, W.E. and Karmody, A.M. (1975) Venous atherosclerosis associated with arteriovenous fistulas for hemodialysis. *Arch. Surg.*, **110**, 176–80.
151. Fillinger, M.F., Reinitz, E.R., Schwartz, R.A. *et al.* (1990) Graft geometry and venous intimal-medial hypoplasia in arteriovenous loop grafts. *J. Vasc. Surg.*, **11**, 556–66.
152. Dechaume, J.P., Bochu, M., Michel, D. *et al.* (1970) Pathological tumour circulation – a study of 50 cases by retrograde branchial vertebral angiography. *Neuroradiology*, **1**, 151–4.
153. Rodgers, M.V., Moss, A.J., Hoffman, M. *et al.* (1975) Arteriovenous fistulas secondary to renal cell carcinoma. *Circulation*, **52**, 345–50.
154. Sachs, M., Rancurel, G., Escourolle, R. *et al.* (1968) Maladie de von Hippel-Lindau. Hémangioblastomes médullaires simulant une malformation artério-veineuse. *Neuro-Chir.*, Paris, **15**, 575–82.
155. Bedford, M.A. and Macfaul, P.A. (1969) Retinal vascular changes in untreated retinoblastoma. *Br. J. Ophthal.*, **53**, 382–7.
156. Gensler, S., Caplan, L.H. and Laufman, H. (1966) Giant benign hemangiopericytoma functioning as an arteriovenous shunt. *J. Am. Med. Ass.*, **198**, 85–8.
157. Feindel, W. and Perot, P. (1965) Red cerebral veins. A report on arteriovenous shunts in tumors and cerebral scars. *J. Neurosurg.*, **22**, 315–25.
158. Bergdahl, L., Boquist, L., Liliequist, B. *et al.* (1972) Primary malignant melanoma of the cerebral nervous system. *Acta Neurochir.*, **26**, 139–49.
159. Fowler, D.L., Fortin, D., Wood, W.G. *et al.* (1979) Intestinal vascular malformations. *Surgery*, **86**, 377–85.
160. Stewart, W.B., Gethright, J.B. and Ray, J.E. (1979) Vascular ecstasias of the colon. *Surg. Gynec. Obstet.*, **148**, 670–4.
161. King, E.S.J. (1950) The genesis of varicose veins. *Aust. N.Z. J. Surg.*, **20**, 126–33.
162. Piulachs, P. and Vidal-Barraquer, F. (1953) Pathogenic study of varicose veins. *Angiology*, **4**, 59–100.
163. Baron, H.C. and Cassaro, S. (1986) The role of arteriovenous shunts in the pathogenesis of varicose veins. *J. Vasc. Surg.*, **4**, 124–8.
164. Schalin, L. (1980) Arteriovenous communication to varicose veins in the lower extremities studied by dynamic angiography. *Acta Chir. Scand.*, **146**, 397–406.
165. Gius, J.A. (1960) Arteriovenous anastomoses and varicose veins. *Arch. Surg.*, **81**, 299–310.
166. Nylander, G. (1969) Meanders of the great saphenous vein. *Angiology*, **20**, 587–91.
167. Stehbens, W.E. and Ludatscher, R.M. (1968) Fine structure of senile angiomas of human skin. *Angiology*, **19**, 581–92.
168. Seville, R.H., Rao, P.S., Hutchinson, D.N. *et al.* (1970) Outbreak of Campbell da Morgan spots. *Br. Med. J.*, **1**, 408–9.
169. Jones, G.T., Martin, B.J. and Stehbens, W.E. (1992) Endothelium and elastic tears in the afferent arteries of experimental arteriovenous fistulae in rabbits. *Int. J. Expl. Pathol.*, **73**, 405–16.
170. Craig, J.M. (1949) Encephalo-trigeminal angiomatosis (Sturge–Weber syndrome). *J. Neuropathol. Expl. Neurol.*, **8**, 305–18.
171. Farrell, D.F. and Forno, L.S. (1970) Symptomatic capillary telangiectasis of the brainstem without haemorrhage. *Neurology*, **20**, 341–6.

15 SYSTEMIC HYPERTENSION AND RELATED VASCULAR DISEASES
Section A: Pathophysiology Vascular Causes and Clinical Manifestations and Complications of Hypertension

Thomas F. Lüscher, Georg Noll and René R. Wenzel

15.1 Pathophysiology of hypertension

The initiating factor causing hypertension is still unknown. In chronic hypertension, elevated blood pressure is maintained by an increase in total peripheral vascular resistance, while cardiac output remains normal under most conditions (Figure 15.1) [1–3]. This observation stresses the importance of factors regulating vascular tone in the pathogenesis of high blood pressure [1,2]. However, both in man and in animal models of essential hypertension, no single derangements so far have been identified. In hypertension, the function of one or more controlling systems regulating peripheral vascular resistance is impaired. At the time the disease is detected in patients, the initiating factors may be obscured by functional and structural adaptations secondary to hypertension. Consequently, in chronic hypertension changes of vascular responsiveness may not only reflect primary dysfunction, but also secondary changes due to persistent high blood pressure.

The controlling systems governing total peripheral vascular resistance include:

1. the autonomic nervous system, which innervates the smooth muscle cells of the blood vessel wall [4,5];
2. the kidney, which adjusts salt and water excretion and produces pressor and depressor hormones [6];
3. the adrenal gland which secretes the hormones regulating water and salt metabolism and vascular tone [6,7];
4. the blood vessel wall itself, which contributes to its own responsiveness by morphological adaptation, changes in sensitivity and density of receptors of its smooth muscle and by modulatory effects of endothelium-derived vasoactive substances [1,2].

15.1.1 SYMPATHETIC NERVOUS SYSTEM

Sympathetic outflow to the resistance vessels is of utmost importance for the determination of the level of peripheral vascular resistance [1,5,7–11]. In hypertension, the sympathetic outflow to the periphery is inappropriately high only in pre-stages or early stages of hypertension, but normal in established hypertension as assessed by microneurography (Figure 15.2) [12]. In hypertensives, however, the increase of sympathetic nerve activity after stimulation with hypoxia is markedly more pronounced than in normotensive subjects [13]. A special form of hypertension in which there is an increased activity of the sympathetic nervous system is most striking in cyclosporin A-induced hypertension [14]. Furthermore, insulin which appears to play an important role in the pathogenesis of some forms of essential hypertension associated with obesity and diabetes as well as metabolic disorders, has been

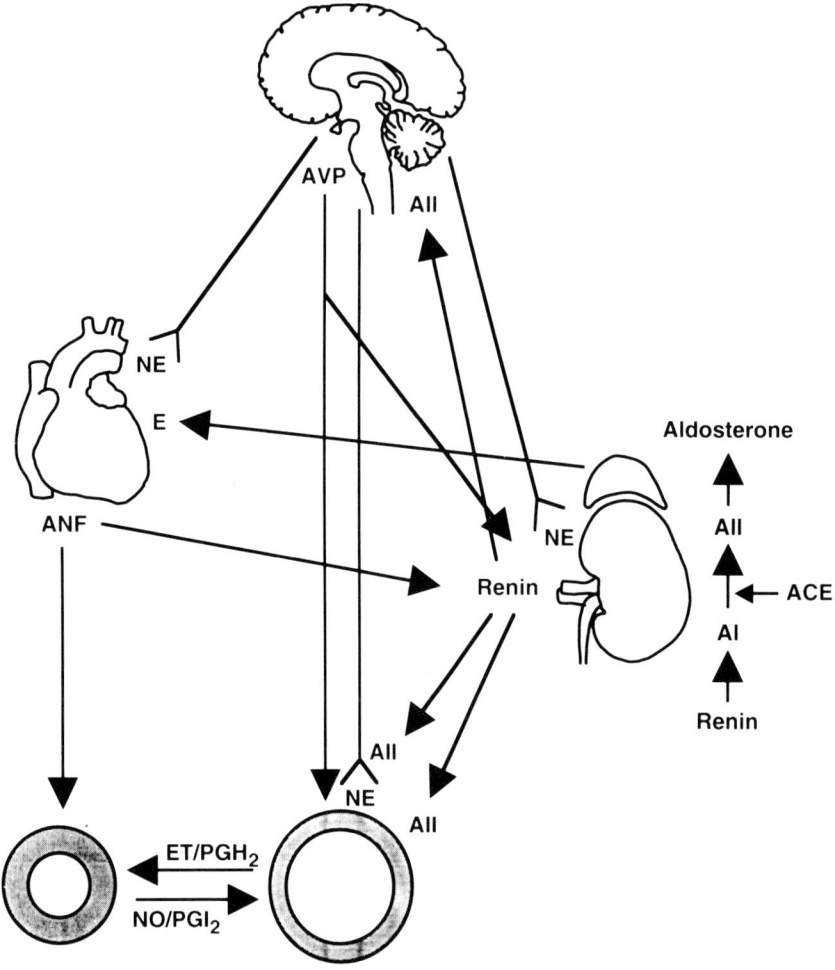

Figure 15.1 Pathophysiology of hypertension. Blood pressure is regulated by cardiac output as well as peripheral vascular resistance. Peripheral vascular resistance is determined by the lumen (radius) of resistance arteries which are regulated by numerous circulating and local factors. A = angiotensin; ACE = angiotensin converting enzyme; ANF = atrial natriuretic peptide; AVP = arginine vasopressin; E = epinephrine, ET = endothelin; NE = norepinephrine.

shown to increase peripheral sympathetic nerve activity [15]. The presence of a functioning sympathetic nervous system appears to be required for the development of hypertension. In young spontaneously hypertensive rats, the rise in blood pressure is closely related to an increase in sympathetic nerve activity [4].

The sympathetic outflow to the peripheral blood vessel originates in neurons located in the lateral parts of the reticular formation of the brain stem, i.e. the vasomotor center [1]. The activity of the center is governed by the solitary nucleus tract, which relays information from arterial and cardiopulmonary mechanoreceptors (baroreceptors and other afferents; [1]). The axons from neurons of the vasomotor center form the bulbous spinal tract and descend into the intermedial lateral column to the pre-ganglionic neurons of the spinal cord, located in the anterolateral column. The neurons of the bulbospinal tract consist of both excitatory and inhibitory neurons, which innervate the pre-ganglionic sympathetic neurons. The outflow to the periphery is determined by the interplay between these pressor and depressor neurons. Cholinergic pre-ganglionic neurons interconnect with the adrenergic post-ganglionic neurons in the sympathetic ganglia, while the post-ganglionic adrenergic neurons finally innervate the heart and the peripheral blood vessels [8,10]. All mature blood vessels are innervated by post-ganglionic sympathetic nerves. However, the density of innervation varies. In most arteries the nerves are restricted to the adventitiae–medial border, while in veins they usually penetrate into the media. Both in animals and man, the density of adrenergic innervation of the blood vessels decreases progressively with age, while the sympathetic activity of neurons as measured with microneurography increases with age [5,9,11].

The most important neurotransmitter mediating the effects of the sympathetic neurons in the blood vessel wall is noradrenaline, but adenosine triphosphate and

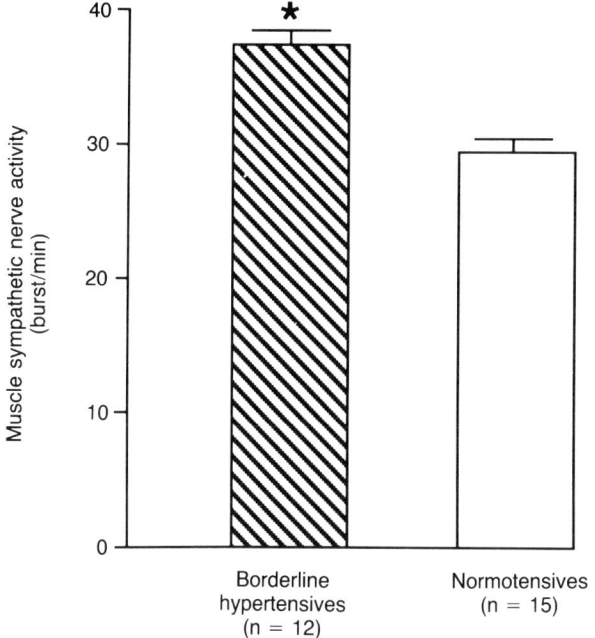

Figure 15.2 Muscle sympathetic activity as assessed by microneurography in patients with borderline hypertension as well as in normotensive subjects: Sympathetic nerve activity is higher in pre-stages of hypertension compared to normotensives (*$P < 0.01$). (Redrawn with permission from Anderson et al. [12].)

neuropeptide-Y also can contribute under certain conditions (Figure 15.3) [1]. Adrenergic neurotransmitters are released after the occurrence of an action potential and this release is facilitated by epinephrine and angiotensin II, but inhibited by norepinephrine itself (via prejunctional alpha-2 adrenergic receptors), acetylcholine, serotonin (5-hydroxytryptamine), histamine, purines and prostanoids. The released norepinephrine interacts with post-junctional alpha-1 and alpha-2 adrenergic receptors. As a rule, facilitatory mechanisms enhancing neurotransmitter release are enhanced in hypertension, while inhibitory stimuli are blunted [1,16–21].

15.1.2 RECEPTORS

The contractile response to stimulation of post-junctional receptors by adrenergic agonists is increased in several vascular beds of hypertensive animals and in humans with essential hypertension [22–26]. In chronic stages of the disease process, however, it is difficult to dissociate between hypersensitivity of the adrenoceptors and structural changes of the blood vessel wall, i.e. remodeling and hypertrophy [27,28]. The hypertensive blood vessel wall exhibits different degrees of hyperreactivity to agonists such as 5-hydroxytryptamine, angiotensin II and norepinephrine [1,22]. Most hypertensive blood vessels or vascular beds are hypersensitive to norepinephrine in some instances, even before the onset of hypertension [29–34]. This suggests that altered vascular reactivity to adrenergic stimuli may at least contribute to experimental hypertension. This hypersensitivity can be related to an enhanced alpha-1-adrenergic vasoconstriction, but also to an increased sensitivity to alpha-2-adrenergic activation.

In addition to norepinephrine, responses to other vasoconstrictors such as serotonin are also profoundly altered in hypertension [22,35]. Indeed, an increased vasoconstrictor response to serotonin is the hallmark of most forms of hypertension but may also occur with aging. In addition, the vasodilator responses to serotonin, which are mediated by the activation of the endothelium (via 5-HT$_1$-serotonergic receptors) and the release of nitric oxide, may be altered in hypertension. In the spontaneously hypertensive rat, enhanced release of endothelium-derived contracting factors in response to serotonin is responsible for altered endothelium-dependent responses to the monoamine [36]. In addition to its direct effect, the potentiating effect of serotonin on vasopressor responses to other hormones such as norepinephrine, angiotensin II and others is also increased in the hypertensive blood vessel wall [35,37,38].

15.1.3 INTRACELLULAR SIGNAL TRANSDUCTION MECHANISMS

For the increase in vascular tone characteristic of established hypertension, intracellular calcium levels are crucial mediators [39]. Intercellular calcium levels can be increased by receptor-operated activation of phospholipase C with concomitant formation of inositol trisphosphate [IP$_3$] and stimulation of protein kinase C. IP$_3$ releases calcium from intracellular stores [40–42]. On the other hand, intracellular calcium can be increased by influx of extracellular calcium, mainly through voltage-operated calcium channels.

As a rule, in most forms of experimental hypertension, activation of phospholipase C pathway and formation of its products is more pronounced [40–42]. Intracellular calcium levels also are increased in vascular smooth muscle cells obtained from hypertensive animals compared to normotensive controls [43]. Similarly, in patients with essential hypertension intracellular calcium levels in platelets are increased, but normalized during antihypertensive therapy, regardless of the agent used [44].

15.1.4 VASCULAR STRUCTURAL CHANGES

As demonstrated by Folkow, minimal peripheral vascular resistance is decreased in established experimental and human hypertension suggesting structural

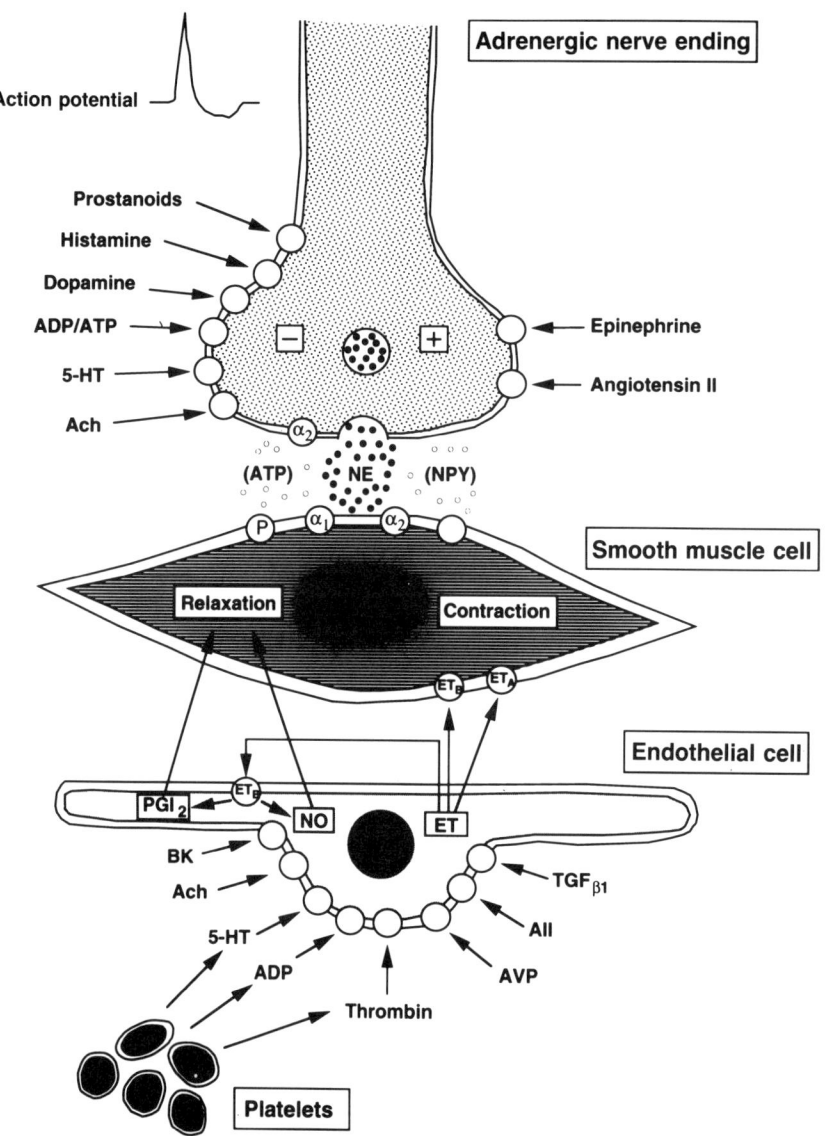

Figure 15.3 Sympathetic neurotransmission. Sympathetic nerve endings release primarily norepinephrine, but also adenosine triphosphate (ATP) and neuropeptide Y (NPY) to activate post-synaptic receptors on vascular smooth muscle. The release of these neurotransmitters is regulated primarily by inhibiting factors (left) as well as facilitatory mechanisms (right). ACh = acetylcholine; ADP = adenosine diphosphate; AII = angiotensin II; AVP = arginine vasopressin; BK = bradykinin; ET = endothelin-1; 5HT = 5-hydroxytryptamine (serotonin); NO = nitric oxide; TGF$_{\beta1}$ = transforming growth factor beta-1; PGI$_2$ = prostacyclin.

vascular changes at the resistance artery level in this disease process [27,28]. Indeed, isolated arteries obtained from experimental hypertensive animals as well as from hypertensive subjects exhibit an increased media–lumen ratio. Although originally it was hypothesized that these structural changes might be mainly related to hypertrophy and/or hypertension of vascular smooth muscle cells, more recent data strongly suggest that vascular remodelling, i.e. rearrangement of the same number of cells with comparable cellular volume, is much more important [29,45]. These structural changes may be particularly important at later stages of the hypertensive process and contribute to the maintenance of increased peripheral vascular resistance.

15.1.5 RENIN-ANGIOTENSIN SYSTEM

The renin-angiotensin system is thought to play an important role in the development and/or maintenance of high blood pressure (Figure 15.4) [45,46]. Angiotensin II is a potent vasoconstrictor hormone which also contributes to structural changes of the blood vessel wall through its proliferative and migratory properties in smooth muscle cells. Aldosterone has

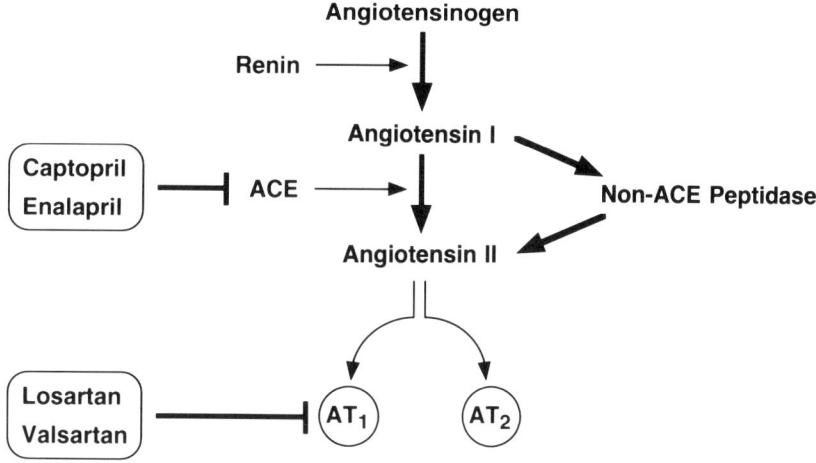

Figure 15.4 The renin-angiotensin system. Renin is the enzyme which transforms angiotensinogen (formed in the liver) into angiotensin I. Angiotensin I is further processed by the angiotensin-converting enzyme (ACE) into angiotensin II which is biologically active. In addition to ACE, non-ACE peptidases also are able to contribute to angiotensin II formation. Angiotensin II at the receptor level activates AT_1-receptors which mediate vasoconstriction, migration and proliferation of vascular smooth muscle and also AT_2-receptors, the function of which is unknown. The formation of angiotensin II is inhibited by ACE inhibitors such as captopril or enalapril. Losartan and valsartan are specific AT_1 receptor antagonists and therefore inhibit angiotensin II-induced vasoconstriction.

important renal effects, i.e. sodium and water retention. The paradigm of a form of high blood pressure in which this system is primarily involved is renovascular hypertension, particularly two-kidney/one-clip hypertension as well as ren-2 transgenic rats [47,48]. Renin is an enzyme which transforms angiotensinogen into angiotensin I which then is further processed to angiotensin II, the biologically active hormone (Figure 15.4) [45]. In addition to angiotensin converting enzymes (ACE), non-ACE peptidases are also able to transform angiotensin I into angiotensin II. This may explain why under certain conditions, even in the presence of an ACE-inhibitor, angiotensin II formation occurs [49].

At the receptor level angiotensin II primarily activates AT_1-receptors. In addition, AT_2-receptors have been delineated although their functional role is uncertain. Indeed, all known vascular effects of angiotensin II such as vasoconstriction, migration and proliferation have been shown to be mediated through AT_1-receptors [50]. The renin-angiotensin system is crucially involved in the development of hypertension. In addition to the circulating renin-angiotensin system, the vascular wall renin-angiotensin system has come much more into focus recently [46]. Indeed, the conversion of angiotensin I into angiotensin II occurs in the blood vessel wall as ACE is located in the endothelial cell membrane. In addition, several components of the renin-angiotensin system have been demonstrated in the vessel wall. The local vascular renin-angiotensin system is thought to play an important role in the local regulation of vascular tone in hypertension and also in the development of structural changes, i.e. remodeling and hypertrophy occurring during the hypertensive process.

Furthermore, the renin-angiotensin system can interact with the sympathetic nervous system both centrally as well as in peripheral neurons (Figure 15.1) [1]. Angiotensin II increases sympathetic outflow to the periphery through central mechanisms, whereas in peripheral neurons the release of neurotransmitters, in particular norepinephrine, is facilitated by the peptide. The central effect of angiotensin II could also explain the increased sympathetic nerve activity in patients with renovascular hypertension.

15.1.6 ENDOTHELIAL CONTROL OF VASCULAR TONE

More recently it has been recognized that the endothelium plays a crucial role in the regulation of local vascular tone by the release of relaxing and contracting factors (Figure 15.3) [2]. Nitric oxide formed from L-arginine via the activity of a constitutive form of nitric oxide synthase [51–53] as well as prostacyclin which is formed from arachidonic acid by the enzyme cyclo-oxygenase [55] are important relaxing factors. In addition, an endothelium-derived hyperpolarizing factor has been proposed and relaxations resistant to cyclo-oxygenase and nitric oxide inhibitors have been demonstrated in several vascular beds, in particular in the coronary circulation [55,56]. In addition, the endothelium is a source of contracting factors such as the 21-aminoacid peptide endothelin-1, cyclo-oxygenase-derived substances such as prostaglandin H_2 and thromboxane A_2 [2,57]. In addition to regulating vascular tone, these substances may also profoundly interfere with the function of circulating platelets, in

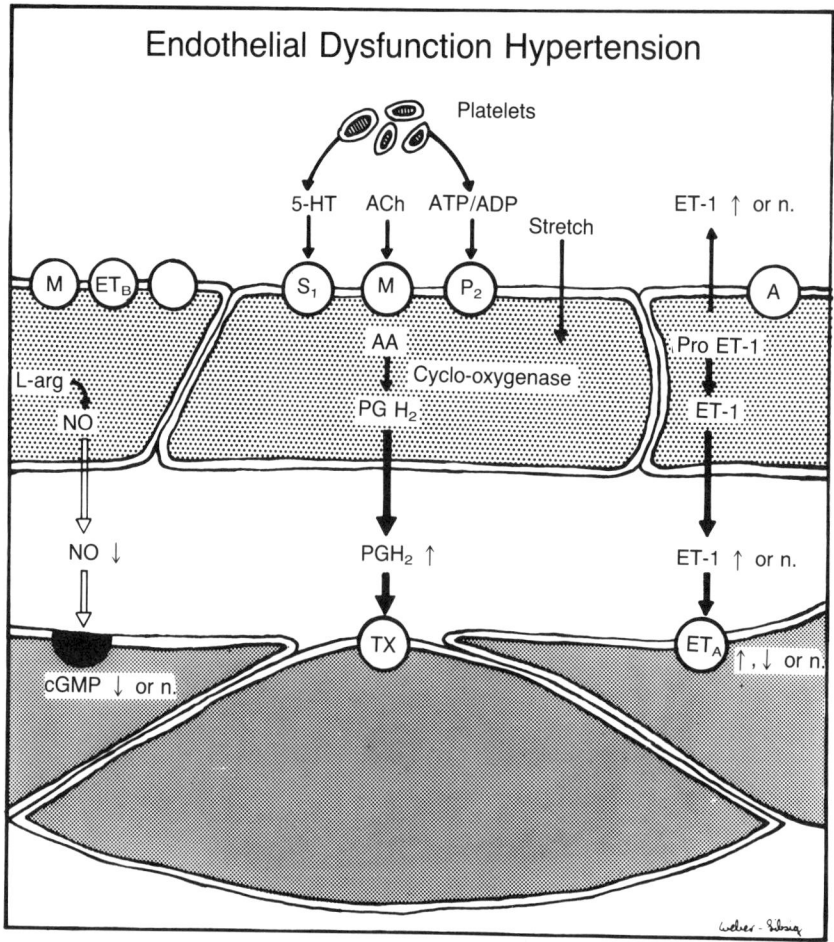

Figure 15.5 Endothelial functional changes in hypertension. The endothelium commonly becomes dysfunctional as the hypertensive process progresses. This function may involve the L-arginine (L-arg) nitric oxide (NO) pathway, with a constrictor prostaglandin such as prostaglandin H_2 (PGH_2) and/or the production and response to endothelin-1 (ET1). Open circles = receptors; AA = arachidonic acid; ACh = acetylcholine; ATP/ADP = adenosine trisphosphate/diphosphate; cGMP = cyclic 3′,5′ guanosine monophosphate; ET_A = ET_A-receptor; ET_B = ET_B-receptors; 5HT = 5-hydroxytryptamine (serotonin); M = muscarinic, P2 = P2-purinergic receptor; pro-ET1 = big endothelin or pro-endothelin; S1 = 5-HT1-serotonergic receptors; TX = thromboxane receptor; n = normal; A = angiotensin II receptor. (Reproduced with permission from Lüscher et al. [64].)

particular nitric oxide and prostacyclin which inhibit adhesion and aggregation of these cells and monocytes [58,59]. Furthermore, they also inhibit migration and proliferation of vascular smooth muscle (in particular nitric oxide and prostacyclin; [60,61]). Endothelin has no significant direct effects on platelets, although it may inhibit the cells through its capacity to stimulate endothelial prostacyclin production. On the other hand, endothelin appears to be a stimulator of vascular smooth muscle cell migration and proliferation [63].

In hypertension a number of derangements of endothelial cell function have been described which in large part appear to be secondary to the hypertensive process (Figure 15.5) [1,64]. In particular, the basal formation of nitric oxide appears to be reduced [65,66], while receptor-stimulated activation of the L-arginine nitric oxide pathway appears to be blunted as well [67–80]. Indeed, endothelium-dependent relaxations or vasodilation respectively, are reduced in experimental models of hypertension as well as in the forearm circulation and the coronary circulation of most hypertensive patients (Table 15.1). The mechanism responsible for impaired endothelium-dependent relaxations in hypertension differ depending on the vascular bed studied and the experimental model of hypertension used (Figure 15.5) [64]. In the spontaneously hypertensive rat, an enhanced formation of endothelium-derived contracting factors, most likely prostaglandin H_2 is an important determinant, while in other forms of hypertension, the L-arginine nitric oxide pathway may be inhibited and/or the responsiveness of vascular smooth muscle to nitric oxide reduced. These changes in endothelial function may not only contribute to the increased peripheral vascular resistance, but also to structural changes in

Table 15.1 Effects of intra-arterial infusion of acetylcholine on forearm coronary blood flow in patients with hypertension as compared to normotensive controls in various studies published in the literature

References	Normotensives (n)	Hypertensives (n)	Results
Forearm Circulation			
67	8	8	Impaired in HT
68	18	18	Impaired in HT
70	15	15	Impaired in HT
71	10	11	Impaired in HT
69	12	14	Impaired in HT
73	14	12	Impaired in HT
74	15	21	Impaired in HT
75	12	12	Impaired in HT
76	18	24	Normal in HT
Coronary Circulation			
77	18	12	Reduced in microcirculation in hyperlipidemia and less so in HT
78	15	14	Reduced in HT
79	9	10	Reduced in HT with LVH

HT = hypertension; LVH = left ventricular hypertrophy.

Table 15.2 Studies reporting circulating endothelin levels in systemic and pulmonary hypertension

Control (pg/ml)	Hypertension (pg/ml)	P	Reference
1.4 ± 0.1*	1.4 ± 0.1*	NS	81
1.6 ± 0.1†	1.7 ± 0.1†	NS	81
5.1 ± 0.5‡	5.7 ± 0.5‡	NS	82
44.7 ± 3.5	42.3 ± 4.9	NS	83
0.24 ± 0.02‡	0.23 ± 0.01§	NS	84
1.4 ± 0.5	2.3 ± 1.1	0.025	85
0.5 ± 0.2	1.1 ± 0.7	0.05	86
18.5 ± 0.9	30.2 ± 1.4	0.01	87
18.5 ± 0.9	30.1 ± 1.4	0.01	88

Data are expressed as mean ± SEM. * At the age of 20–34 years, male; † at the age of 35–39 years, male; ‡ data expressed as picomoles per liter in this reference; § severe uncontrolled hypertension.

large conduit arteries (where the complications of hypertension occur, particularly in the coronary circulation), but also in the resistance circulation.

The production of endothelin in hypertension generally appears to be normal as judged from the circulating levels of endothelin (Table 15.2) [64,81–88]. Indeed, circulating levels of endothelin as measured in patients and in animal models of hypertension are normal except in the presence of vascular disease such as atherosclerosis and/or renal failure. However, since most endothelin is released abluminally rather than luminally [89], circulating levels may not reflect the local vascular production of endothelin. Indeed, in deoxycorticosteroid (DOCA) hypertension, an increased local vascular production of endothelin has been suggested in spite of normal circulating levels of endothelin [90,91]. Similarly, in the spontaneously hypertensive rat, endothelin receptor antagonists do lower blood pressure in spite of the normal circulating levels of the peptide [92,93]. These contradictory results can be explained by the capacity of endothelin to potentiate other vasoconstrictor responses at very low concentrations [94]. Hence, an increased endothelin production which may not lead to increased circulating levels of the peptide, may still contribute significantly to an increase in vascular tone and possibly structure.

15.1.7 ROLE OF THE KIDNEY IN BLOOD PRESSURE REGULATION

The kidney plays a particularly important role in the long-term regulation of blood pressure [6,95]. A key component in this context is the renal-body fluid feedback due to pressure-natriuresis mechanisms, which stabilize arterial blood pressure as long as renal excretory capacity is not impaired. However, abnormalities of renal function that impair the excretory capacity require increased arterial pressure to restore renal body fluid to normal so that intake and output of salt and water remains balanced [6]. If the pressure-natriuresis mechanism is inhibited (e.g. by servocontrolling renal arterial pressure at the normal level in experimental hypertension) sodium and water excretion remain below the intake and therefore this results in severe increases in body-fluid volumes and cardiovascular collapse. Thus, a central hypothesis put forward by Guyton and co-workers [96] suggests that essential hypertension may be a compensatory response for an inability of the kidney to excrete the required amounts of sodium and water at a normal arterial pressure. A common feature of all renal disease causing hypertension is a decrease in the ratio of glomerular filtration rate to tubular absorbtion. This may come about due to primary reductions in glomerular filtration rate (e.g. due to increased preglomerular resistance as it occurs in Goldblatt hypertension or a decreased filtration co-efficient K_f as it occurs in glomerular nephritis). The primary increase of tubular reabsorption due to excessive formation of antinatriuretic hormones may also be involved.

In spite of this extensive experimental work, the renal abnormalities responsible for essential hypertension remain elusive. This may be due to the insiduous onset of human hypertension as well as compensatory changes that mask many of the initial mechanisms within the kidney leading to hypertension.

15.2 Vascular causes of secondary hypertension

Various forms of vascular disease can induce hypertension [48]. Most commonly, atherosclerotic disease of one or both renal arteries or fibromuscular dysplasia of these blood vessels is associated with renovascular hypertension. Furthermore, coarctation of the aorta can lead to high blood pressure.

15.2.1 ATHEROSCLEROTIC RENOVASCULAR DISEASE

Atherosclerotic and fibromuscular dysplasia are the most common causes of renovascular disease [96]. The two conditions are of similar frequency among younger patients, but atherosclerotic disease predominates in older patients [96–98]. Atherosclerotic lesions of the renal circulation are common in men over 50 years of age. Typically, the patients are overweight, smoke and have other risk factors for cardiovascular disease. A considerable number of these patients exhibit atherosclerotic vascular lesions in other parts of the circulation such as the coronary, carotid and peripheral vascular bed. Renal function is also more likely to be impaired in patients with atherosclerotic renovascular disease.

Particularly in the group of patients with atherosclerotic renovascular disease, it is often difficult to decide whether the renal artery lesions are a cause or a consequence of pre-existing essential hypertension [48]. Indeed, the duration of hypertension is longer and the incidence of a positive family history for high blood pressure is higher in these patients than in those with other forms of renovascular disease.

Atherosclerotic lesions have a different anatomical distribution in the renal circulation to that in other forms of renovascular lesions, as they primarily affect the proximal part of the main renal artery (Figure 15.6) [48]. The lesions are more frequently eccentric than concentric and have a more irregular appearance than fibromuscular renovascular lesions and they can be associated with superimposed thrombosis, dissection, embolism and aneurysms in the renal artery. Larger atherosclerotic plaques of the aortic wall near the orifice of the renal artery can also impair renal blood flow and cause renovascular hypertension. Abdominal aortic aneurysms often are associated with unilateral or bilateral renal artery stenosis.

Renal atheroembolism is often an unsuspected cause of renal failure and renovascular hypertension in the elderly. Renal atheroembolism occurs particularly in the setting of diffuse and severe atherosclerotic disease of the abdominal aorta. While spontaneous embolization takes place, surgical manipulation of the aorta or diagnostic angiographic procedures have been increasingly recognized as the most important precipitating cause of symptomatic or occult renal atheroembolism.

Atherosclerosis is most commonly a progressive disease, either due to further growth of existing lesions, superimposed thrombi with vascular occlusion and/or the development of new lesions in previously unaffected

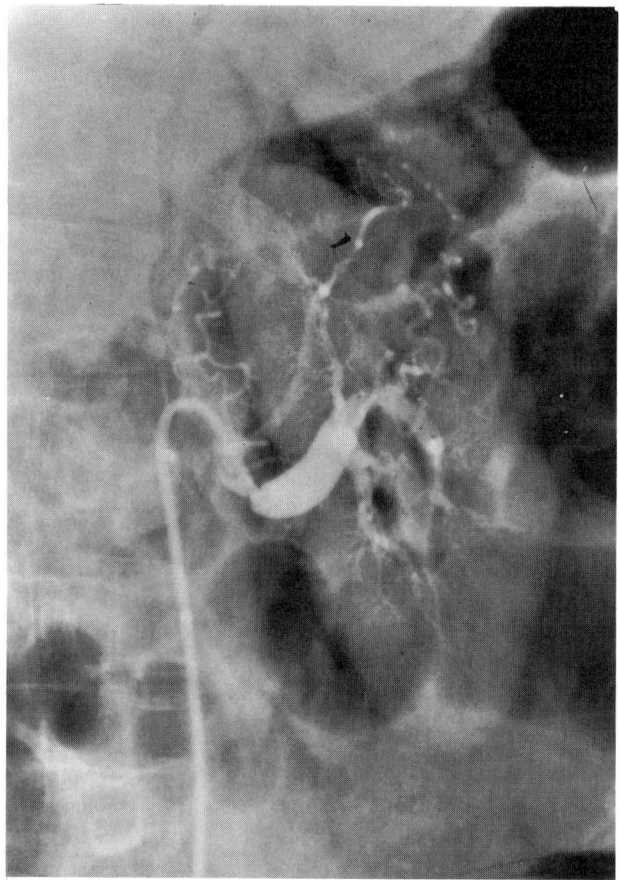

Figure 15.6 Angiographic presentation of an atherosclerotic stenosis of the left renal artery. Note the proximal subtotal stenosis.

segments. The exact cause of atherosclerosis remains unknown [99,100]. Most modern concepts of atherosclerosis focus on local morphological and/or functional changes of the vascular endothelium as a primary step in the disease process. The response-to-injury hypothesis of atherogenesis proposed that injury to the endothelium can initiate the atherosclerotic process. Indeed, removal of the endothelium by means of a balloon catheter is a very reliable stimulus to induce the development of an atherosclerotic plaque. Repetitive microinjuries of the endothelium at sites of high shear stress may explain why atherosclerotic lesions primarily involve branching sites of the arterial circulation.

Functional changes of the endothelium and the interaction of platelets and monocytes with the vessel wall are important steps in the development of the atherosclerotic process [99,100]. Growth factors and inhibitors are synthesized and released from endothelial cells, macrophages, vascular smooth muscle cells and platelets. Important growth inhibitors produced by the endothelium are heparin and heparan sulfate as well as endothelium-derived nitric oxide which modulates vascular proliferation via a cyclic GMP-dependent mechanism. Under certain experimental conditions, endothelial cells can also produce growth factors such as platelet-derived growth factor. Although endothelin may facilitate growth under certain conditions [64], it appears to be a much weaker growth factor than platelet-derived growth factor. Platelets, on the other hand, are an important source of substances evoking proliferation and migration of vascular smooth muscle cells such as platelet-derived growth factor, epidermal growth factor and transforming growth factor-β. Increased interactions between platelets and blood vessel walls, as occur after endothelial injury and in states of endothelial dysfunction such as hypertension, hyperlipidemia, smoking and atherosclerosis, may contribute significantly to the development of the atherosclerotic plaque [100].

In diet-induced atherosclerosis of non-human primates, monocytes adhere to the endothelial layer shortly after initiating a high-cholesterol diet [99]. In human atherosclerotic blood vessels, a marked polymorphism with small, normal-sized and giant endothelial cells and, as a consequence, a decreased number of cells per square millimeter has been noted. The attached monocytes are particularly prominent in junctional areas and between endothelial cells, from where they may migrate into the subendothelial space, accumulate fat and become foam cells. The foam cells from the fatty streaks are early lesions in the atherosclerotic process. Smooth muscle cells migrating from the media into the intima may also accumulate fat and take part in the formation of these lesions. Fatty streaks may be converted into fibrous plaques. While macrophages are the predominant cell of fatty streaks, the fibrous cap of the more advanced lesions primarily contains smooth muscle cells. In both lesions, the endothelial cell layer, although markedly separated from the media by the grossly expanded subendothelial layer, remains morphologically intact. Only in very late stages of the disease process does the endothelial layer begin to separate, particularly at branching sites, and the subendothelial space may be exposed to the circulating blood with consequent platelet adherence. At sites where platelets adhere and aggregate, vasoactive substances such as thromboxane A_2, serotonin and adenosine nucleotide are released, as well as platelet-derived growth factor. This further promotes smooth muscle cell proliferation and vasospasm and eventually occlusion at the site of an atherosclerotic lesion.

15.2.2 ARTERIAL FIBROMUSCULAR DYSPLASIA

Fibromuscular dysplasia [FMD] is a non-atherosclerotic and non-inflammatory vascular disease that primarily involves medium-sized and small arteries, most commonly the renal (Figure 15.7) and carotid arteries [96].

FMD is diagnosed in about 4% of potential kidney

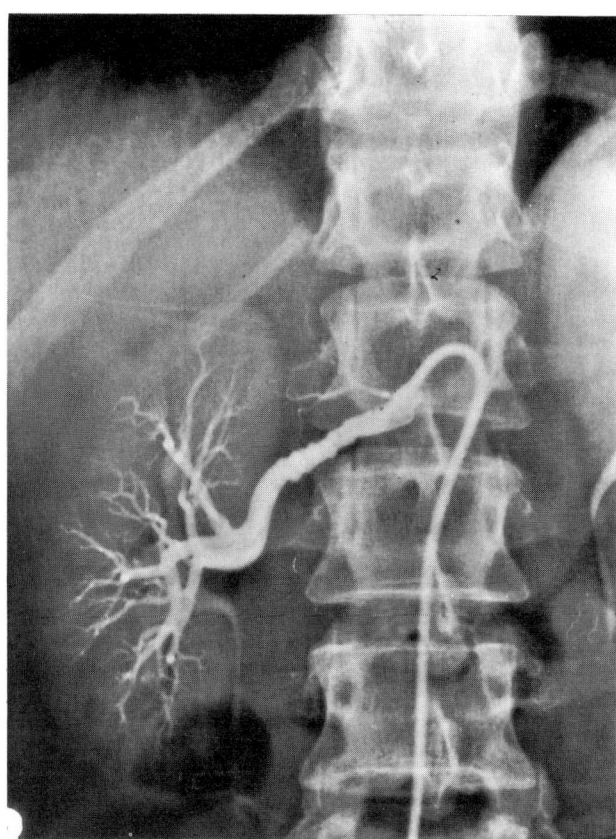

Figure 15.7 Fibromuscular dysplasia of the right renal artery. Note the involvement of the middle portion of the right renal artery with typical 'string of beads' stenosis. This angiographic presentation commonly can be classified histologically as medial fibromuscular dysplasia.

donors at angiography [103]. In an autopsy study the incidence was about 1% [104]. Similarly FMD was found in 1% or less of patients undergoing carotid angiography [96]. In the hypertensive population, renovascular FMD is the underlying cause in about 2–5%. In patients with renovascular hypertension, FMD is the underlying arterial lesion in 20–50%.

The majority of patients with FMD have renovascular disease (Figure 15.8), whereas in about in one-third, the cerebral circulation is involved [96]. Multivessel involvement is common, particularly in patients with bilateral FMD lesions. Less frequent manifestations of FMD involve the mesenteric, subclavian and iliac arteries.

The pathologic classification of FMD was introduced by Harrison and McCormack in 1971 [105]. The classification is based on the site of involvement within the arterial wall, i.e. intima, media or adventitia (Figure 15.8). Thus, three main forms of FMD have been delineated: intimal fibroplasia, medial fibromuscular dysplasia and periarterial fibroplasia. Lesions involving the medial layer of the blood vessel wall have been further subclassified into medial fibroplasia, perimedial

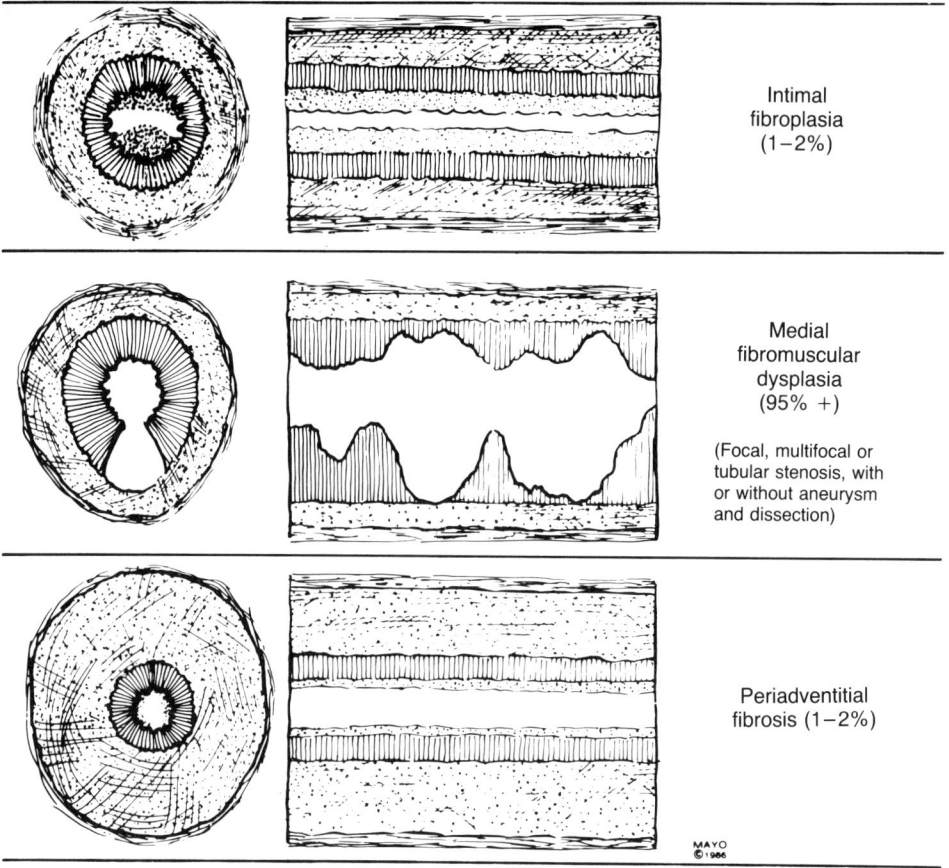

Figure 15.8 Histological classification of fibromuscular dysplasia. (Reproduced with permission from Lüscher et al. [96].)

fibroplasia, and medial hyperplasia. Medial dissection, which originally was considered a fourth subtype of medial fibromuscular dysplasia, is a complication of FMD rather than a separate or distinct disorder (Figure 15.8). This classification of FMD has the advantage of showing an excellent correlation between the angiographic appearance and the pathologic findings.

Medial fibromuscular dysplasia and in particular its subtype, **medial fibroplasia**, are the most common forms of FMD, accounting for 70–95% of all fibromuscular lesions (Figure 15.8). Angiographically, medial fibroplasia appears as the classical 'string of beads' stenosis (Figure 15.7). The 'beads' exceed the diameter of the proximal unaffected part of the artery. Thickened fibromuscular ridges alternating with areas of thinning and widening of the arterial wall are the pathologic basis of the radiologic aspects. In the renal artery the distal two-thirds (often extending into the branch arteries) are typically involved.

In **perimedial fibroplasia** the 'beads' are usually less numerous and are smaller in diameter than those in the proximal unaffected part of the artery (Figure 15.8). In histologic examinations, perimedial fibroplasia exhibits marked fibroplasia of the outer half of the media, and the external elastic membrane often is effaced. This fibroplasia is almost exclusively seen in young women with right-sided renal artery stenosis, marked collateral circulation and hypertension.

Medial hyperplasia is characterized by focal concentric stenosis that is caused by excessive medial smooth muscle proliferation without associated fibrosis (Figure 15.8). The stenosis is usually smooth, severe and sometimes tubular in shape. As in other forms of FMD, medial hyperplasia typically involves the middle or distal part of the affected artery (Figure 15.8). This is an unusual type of FMD, probably accounting for less than 5% of fibroplastic stenoses.

Intimal hyperplasia is angiographically indistinguishable from medial hyperplasia. Histologically, however, it is characterized by a circumferential or eccentric accumulation of fibrous tissue in the intima (Figure 15.8). The internal elastic lamina can always be identified. In contrast to features of atherosclerosis, no inflammatory changes and no lipid accumulation occur. The lesion is rare and accounts for only 1–5% of all fibromuscular arterial lesions. In young patients, long tubular stenoses are common, while smooth focal stenoses predominate in elderly patients.

Periarterial fibroplasia is the rarest form of FMD. Here, fibroplasia with collagen encompasses the adventitia and extends into the surrounding tissue.

Progression of FMD has been documented on repeated angiograms as well as through the course of clinical symptoms, although it occurs slower than with atherosclerotic renovascular disease [106,107]. Progression was more common in older patients with focal or tubular stenoses than in those with medial fibroplasia, but it did not lead to total occlusion. Rarely, spontaneous reversal of FMD with reversal of hypertension may occur. In patients with renovascular hypertension the natural history of FMD is influenced by superimposed arteriosclerotic changes, particularly in smokers, who make up a large percentage of patients with renovascular FMD.

The cause of FMD remains unknown, but humoral, mechanical and genetic factors as well as smoking and ischemia of the blood vessel wall have been suspected [96]. FMD is much more frequent in females than in males. Although nephroptosis is frequently associated with FMD of the right renal artery, an increased renal mobility is not associated with a higher risk for FMD. In line with this clinical finding, experimental studies revealed only minor histologic changes in response to stretching of the renal artery. The importance of genetic factors in the pathogenesis of FMD is supported by a high incidence in some families and in Caucasians. The inheritance pattern appears to be consistent with an autosomal dominant trait, with variable penetrance [108]. Renovascular hypertension is much less frequent in adult blacks than in Caucasians and, if present, usually can be attributed to atherosclerotic lesions. Furthermore, the HLA-DRW6 antigen is associated with an increased risk for FMD. Experimental occlusion of arterial vasa vasorum causes distinct vascular changes. In the media the amount of extracellular connective tissue increases and myofibroblasts appear [96]. Thus, a decreased blood supply to the vascular wall due to functional or morphologic obstruction of the vasa vasorum might lead to proliferative responses. Smoking is strongly associated with FMD in a dose-dependent manner. The way in which smoking is related to the pathogenesis of the disease process, however, remains uncertain. Finally, FMD has been considered to be the end stage of some form of vasculitis or an immunologic process. Vascular changes ascribed to the rubella syndrome show similarities with FMD [96]. The clinical presentation of FMD depends on the arteries involved, the degree of vascular obstruction, and the presence or absence of a collateral circulation. Thus, patients may be asymptomatic or may have signs and symptoms of occlusive vascular disease. As compared with patients with renal arteriosclerosis, patients with renovascular FMD are younger, typically female and have a shorter duration of hypertension [96]. In some series, a family history of hypertension is less common in FMD, while others report a high incidence of hypertension, stroke or other cardiovascular disease in relatives of these patients. Impaired kidney function is rare in renovascular FMD, even in the presence of bilateral disease.

Renal arterial aneurysms can cause hypertension as a result of concomitant stenosis, dissection, compression of arteries or renal tissue or peripheral emboli [102]. The rupture of FMD aneurysms occurs very rarely, even in the presence of hypertension. The rupture of fibromuscular aneurysms into a renal vein, however, may cause renal arteriovenous fistulas. Dissection of the renal artery in patients with FMD seems to occur much less frequently than in the cerebrovascular circulation. Renal infarction is a potential complication of renovascular FMD, particularly in the presence of a dissection or large aneurysm. The emboli may cause abdominal or flank pain and hypertension in some patients. Selective renal venous renin samplings in the branches of the renal vein may be useful to collect in order to detect local renin oversecretion in hypertensive patients with renal embolization.

The treatment of renovascular disease with either surgery, percutaneous transluminal renal angioplasty (PTRA) or antihypertensive drugs may be indicated to normalize blood pressure or to preserve renal function [108–112]. In contrast to patients with atherosclerotic renovascular disease, drugs are rarely used as a first-line measure in the treatment of FMD. PTRA is the treatment of choice for renovascular FMD. About one-half to two-thirds of the patients are cured after the intervention. The results of both surgery and PTRA are best in patients with unilateral FMD, poorer in those with bilateral FMD and poorest in those with systemic FMD.

15.2.3 RENOVASCULAR VASCULITIS AND OTHER VASCULAR DISEASES

Besides arteriosclerosis, the differential diagnosis of FMD includes inflammatory vascular diseases such as Takayasu's arteritis and vascular lesions of neurofibromatosis [96]. True idiopathic intimal hyperplasia is very rare and structurally indistinguishable from atherosclerotic intimal fibrosis. On an angiogram, intimal and medial hyperplasia can be distinguished from atherosclerotic plaques by their anatomic location. Atherosclerotic stenoses usually occur within 1 cm of the orifice of the main renal or internal carotid artery, are often eccentric and are associated with atherosclerotic changes in the abdominal aorta. FMD almost always involves the middle or distal parts of the renal or carotid artery; the focal stenoses are concentric and typically have a smooth appearance. Classic 'string of beads' stenoses are easily recognized and consistent with FMD (Figure 15.7).

Takayasu's arteritis almost always involves the aorta

564 PATHOPHYSIOLOGY, CAUSES AND CLINICAL ASPECTS OF HYPERTENSION

and its major branch arteries at or near their origin and in its active stage usually is accompanied by laboratory evidence of inflammation [113]. Ehlers–Danlos syndrome sometimes leads to aneurysms of major arteries similar to those seen in patients with FMD. Patients with the syndrome have characteristic clinical signs such as joint laxity and increased skin elasticity [114]. In neurofibromatosis, stenoses at the orifices of the renal, celiac and superior mesenteric arteries can occur, as can narrowing of the abdominal aorta, although this happens less frequently. The proximal site of arterial involvement along with stigmata of neurofibromatosis of the skin and bones usually is diagnostic in patients with this disorder. Congenital abdominal coarctation also may be associated with proximal renal artery stenosis.

15.3 Clinical manifestations and complications of hypertension

Major cardiovascular risk factors [115–117] are:

- Age
- Hypertension
- Dyslipidemia (hypercholesteremia, low HDL, LDLs, hyperglycemia, increased Lp-levels)
- Diabetes mellitus (both type I and type II)
- Smoking
- Coagulation disorders
- Platelet disorders
- Genetic factors.

Table 15.3 Compications of hypertension

Disease	Complications
Coronary artery disease	Angina pectoris
	Myocardial infarction
	Sudden death
	Congestive heart failure
Cerebrovascular disease	Transient ischemic attack
	Amaurosis fugax
	Ischemic stroke
	Hemorrhagic stroke
Peripheral vascular disease	Intermittent claudication
	Gangrene (amputation)
Aortic vascular disease	Aortic aneurysm
	Aortic dissection
	Leriche syndrome
Renal vascular changes	Renovascular hypertension
	Renal failure

All of these are associated with an increased risk of coronary artery disease, sudden death, stroke, peripheral vascular occlusive disease and renal failure.

In contrast to most other attempts to reduce cardiovascular risk factors, hypertension has been shown to be treatable with currently available drugs and the reduction in blood pressure is clearly associated with a decreased frequency of complications of the hypertensive process such as stroke, congestive heart failure,

Before

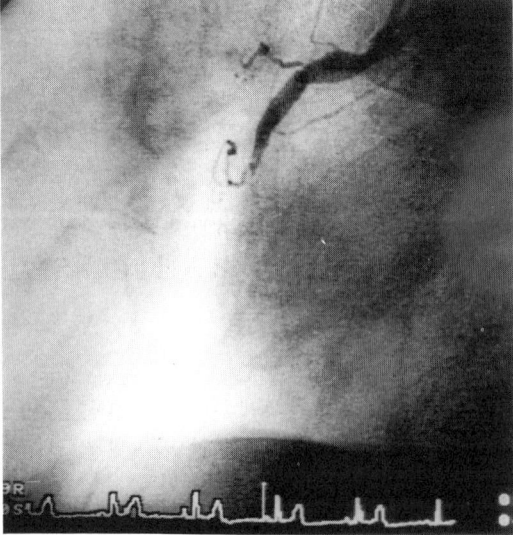

After

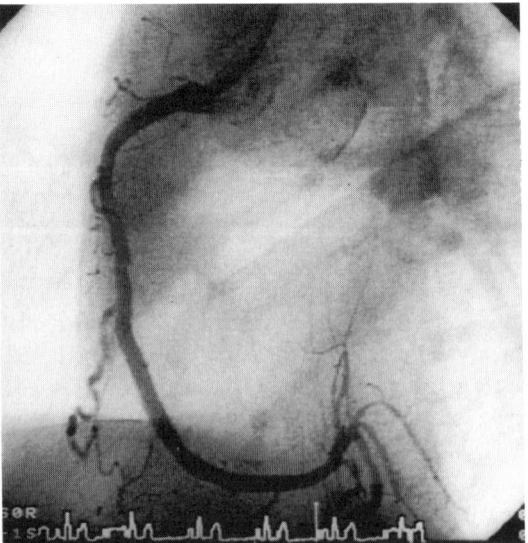

Figure 15.9 Angiographic presentation of acute myocardial infarction with occlusion of the proximal right coronary artery. After percutaneous transluminal angioplasty (PTCA) the entire previously occluded vessel becomes visible.

Figure 15.10 Dissection of the abdominal aorta. In the magnetic resonance image, dissection of the descending aorta becomes visible with the true and false lumen. At the top of the false lumen a thrombus is visible. The false and true lumina are separated by an intimal flap. The brighter parts of the dissection channel indicate low flow (a) (sagittal view). In the transverse view (b), the aortic arch becomes visible with the true lumen in the center surrounded by the false channel which is filled by a thrombus. (By courtesy of Peter Buser.)

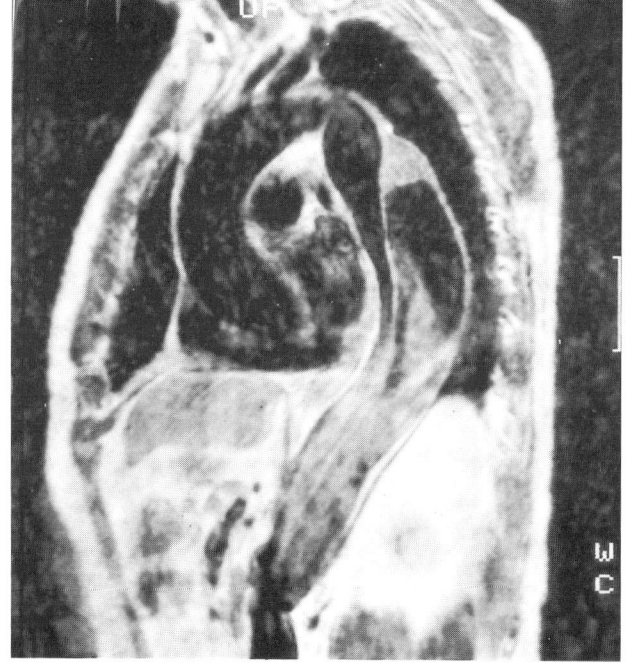

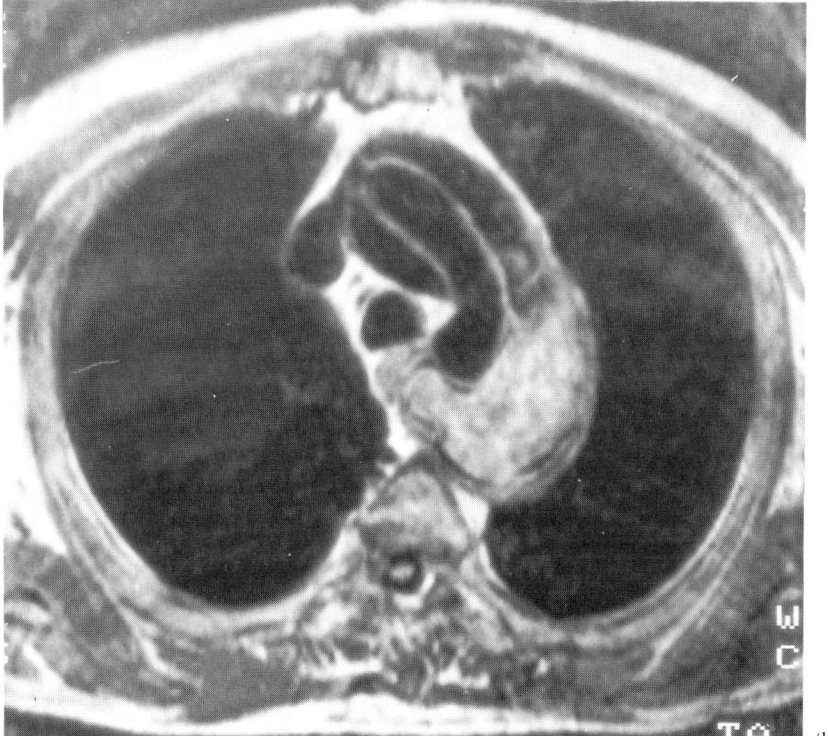

renal failure and most likely also coronary artery disease (although this effect of antihypertensive therapy is less striking) [118–120].

The clinical manifestations of the complications of hypertension include most manifestations of coronary artery disease such as angina pectoris, myocardial infarction (Figure 15.9) and sudden death, aneurysms of the aorta, atherothrombotic obstruction of the abdominal aorta and its branches, cerebrovascular accidents as well as renal failure (Table 15.3) [117].

About half of the deaths from coronary artery disease are sudden, most commonly due to ventricular fibrillation [121–130]. About a third of these patients who die suddenly have a history of hypertension and about another third have increased heart weight, suggesting a history of high blood pressure. Angina pectoris is

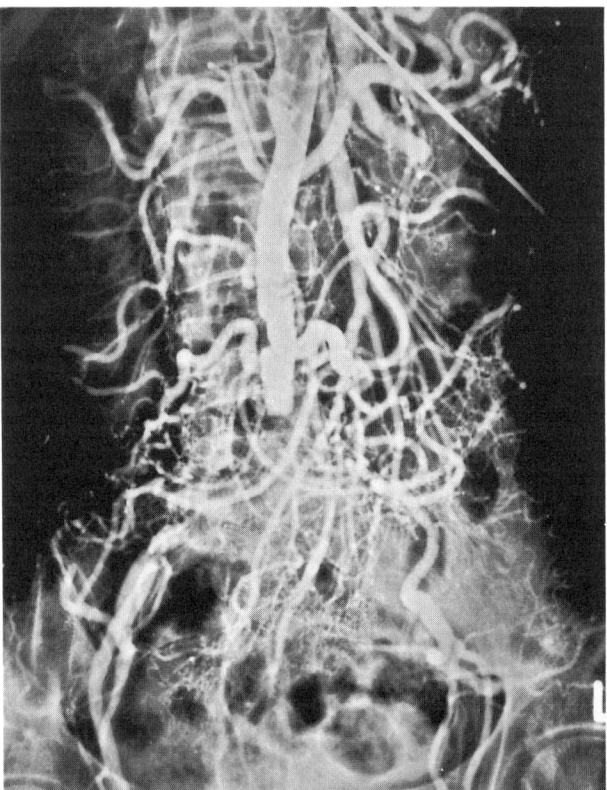

Figure 15.11 Angiographic presentation of an occlusion of the abdominal aorta just above the bifurcation leading to the clinical syndrome described by Leriche. Due to the occlusion of the main aorta just above the bifurcation a huge number of collaterals develop and filling of the iliac arteries through these collaterals is visible.

also more frequently found in hypertensive than in normotensive subjects and this association increases continuously as blood pressure rises. Indeed, hypertension is present in about half of the patients with angina pectoris and probably even more so in women. Similarly, a substantial number of patients with fatal acute transmural myocardial infarction have a history of hypertension or cardiomegaly at necropsy. Hypertension not only increases the risk of having an acute myocardial infarction, but also impairs prognosis after this event [131–134].

Abdominal aortic aneurysms most commonly occur in aortic vascular segments with atherosclerosis and/or dissection (Figure 15.10) [135–140]. These events are far more frequent in hypertensive than in normotensive patients. Indeed, hypertension together with Marfan's syndrome and pregnancy are the most common predisposing factors for aortic dissection [141–153]. The higher the blood pressure the more likely aortic dissection is to occur in hypertensive patients.

Atherothrombotic obstruction of the abdominal aorta and its branches is also a typical vascular disease associated with hypertension. Indeed, the syndrome of thrombotic obliteration of the aortic bifurcation as described by Leriche in 1940 [154–157] is known to be associated with hypertension (Figure 15.11). Similarly, atherosclerotic obstruction of the leg arteries leading to intermittent claudication is more commonly seen in hypertensive than in normotensive patients.

One of the strongest associations of hypertension with cardiovascular disease is that of cerebrovascular accidents and high blood pressure [115–117,158,159]. Indeed, after age, hypertension is the most common and potent predictor of atherothrombotic cerebrovascular infarction as well as hemorrhagic stroke. In patients with asymptomatic hypertension, the risk of a cerebrovascular accident is about four times higher than in normotensive subjects [160]. On the other hand, half to three-quarters of the patients with cerebrovascular disease are hypertensive. As in the case of acute myocardial infarction, the presence of hypertension increases the mortality rate of acute cerebrovascular accidents [116,161]. Also, recurrent cerebrovascular ischemia is much more common in hypertensives than in normotensive patients. On the other hand, treatment of hypertension has been shown to diminish the frequency of cerebrovascular events, most strikingly hemorrhagic strokes [118–120].

In certain patients rather than major strokes, lacunar strokes and infarcts, usually multiple small and cystic infarcts of the basal ganglia or pons resulting from occlusion of penetrating branches chiefly from the middle and posterior cerebral artery or basilar arteries occur [162,164]. Usually these events are associated with only minor or no neurologic deficit [165].

The Charcot–Bouchard aneurysms are aneurysms of very small cerebral arteries, most commonly perforating arteries of less than 1 mm in diameter, especially in basal ganglia and subcortical regions. These changes are found in almost half of hypertensive patients at necropsy but rarely in normotensive patients matched for age and sex [165]. Rupture of such aneurysms may be responsible for hemorrhage in hypertensive patients [164–167]. In addition to hypertension, age also appears to increase the formation of these aneurysms and the risk of cerebrovascular bleeding.

Renal disease can be both cause and effect of hypertension (see 15.2.1) [48]. Indeed, all forms of renovascular and renoparenchymatous disease are associated with hypertension. On the other hand, hypertension, particularly untreated, is known to impair renal function. Hence, in an individual patient, it is often difficult to determine whether renal disease is the cause or consequence of hypertension [6,48]. Classically, in nephrosclerosis the kidneys are involved uniformly leading to the classical 'granular' surface at necropsy and marked changes of the arterial tree in particular arterioles with narrowing of the lumen. These vascular changes are associated with severe parenchymal damage with infarction of the glomeruli, tubular degeneration and cellular infiltration of the interstitium. These morphological changes on the other hand lead to marked functional changes of the kidney as well as the secretion of vasoactive substances, in particular renin and other factors further enhancing blood pressure and in turn renal damage [45].

References

1. Vanhoutte, P.M. and Lüscher, T.F. (1986) Peripheral mechanisms in cardiovascular regulation: transmitters, receptors and the endothelium, in *Handbook of Hypertension*, vol. 8, (eds A. Zanchetti and R.C. Tarazzi), Elsevier, Amsterdam, New York, Oxford, pp. 96–123.
2. Lüscher, T.F. and Vanhoutte, P.M. (1990) *The Endothelium Modulator of Cardiovascular Function*, CRC Press, Boca Raton, Fla./USA, pp. 1–25.
3. Lund-Johansen, P. (1980) Haemodynamics in essential hypertension. *Clin. Sci.*, 59 (suppl.), 343s.
4. Judy, W.V., Watanabe, A.M., Henry, D.P. *et al.* (1976) Sympathetic nerve activity: role in regulation of blood pressure in spontaneously hypertensive rat. *Circ. Res.*, 38 (suppl. 2), II-21.
5. Wallin, B.G., Sunlof, G., Eriksson, B.-M. *et al.* (1981) Plasma noradrenaline correlates to sympathetic muscle nerve activity in normotensive man. *Acta Physiol. Scand.*, 11, 9.
6. Hall, J.E. and Guyton, A.C. (1991) The kidney and regualtion of blood pressure, in *Renovascular and Renal Parenchymatous Hypertension*, (eds T.F. Lüscher and N.M. Kaplan), Springer-Verlag, Berlin, Heidelberg, New York, London, Paris, Tokyo, Hong Kong, Barcelona, Budapest, p. 3.
7. Goldstein, D.S. and Lake, C.R. (1984) Plasma norepinephrine and epinephrine levels in essential hypertension. *Fed. Proc.*, 43, 57.
8. Frewin, D.B., Hume, W.R., Waterson, J.G. and Whelan, R.F. (1971) The histochemical localisation of sympathetic nerve endings in human gingival blood vessels. *Aust. J. Expl Biol. Med. Sci.*, 49, 573.
9. Waterson, J.G., Frewin, D.B. and Soltys, J.S. (1974) Age-related differences in catecholamine fluorescence of human vascular tissue. *Blood Vessels*, 11, 79.
10. Gerke, D.C., Frewin, D.B. and Soltys, J.S. (1975) Adrenergic innervation of human mesenteric blood vessels. *Aust. J. Expl Biol. Med. Sci.*, 53, 241.
11. Berkowitz, B.A. and Kohler, C. (1980) Vascular catecholamines and aging, in *Vascular Neuroeffector Mechanisms*, (eds J.A. Bevan, R.A. Maxwell, T. Godfraind and P.M. Vanhoutte), Raven Press, New York, p. 335.
12. Anderson, E.A., Sinkey, C.A., Lawton, W.J. and Mark, A.L. (1989) Elevated sympathetic nerve activity in borderline hypertensive humans. Evidence from direct intraneural recordings. *Hypertension*, 14, 177–83.
13. Somers, V.K., Mark, A.L. and Abboud, F.M. (1988) Potentiation of sympathetic nerve responses to hypoxia in borderline hypertensive subjects. *Hypertension*, 11, 608–12.
14. Scherrer, U., Vissing, S.F., Morgan, B.J. *et al.* (1990) Cyclosporine-induced sympathetic activation and hypertension after heart transplantation. *New Engl. J. Med.*, 323, 693–9.
15. Anderson, E.A., Hoffman, R.P., Balon, T.W. *et al.* (1991) Hyperinsulinemia produces both sympathetic neural activation and vasodilation in normal humans. *J. Clin. Invest.*, 87, 2246–52.
16. Collis, M.G., De Mey, C. and Vanhoutte, P.M. (1979) Enhanced release of noradrenaline in the kidney of the young spontaneously hypertensive rat. *Clin. Sci.*, 57, 233S.
17. Yamori, Y. (1977) Pathogenesis of spontaneous hypertension as a model for essential hypertension. *Jpn Circ. J.*, 41, 259.
18. Zimmermann, B.G., Rolewiez, T.F., Dunham, E.W. and Gisslen, J.L. (1969) Transmitter release and vascular responses in skin and muscle of hypertensive dogs. *Am. J. Physiol.*, 217, 798.
19. Ester, M., Julius, S., Zweifler, A. *et al.* (1977) Mild high-renin essential hypertension: neurogenic human hypertension? *New Engl. J. Med.*, 296, 405.
20. Franco-Morselli, R., Elghorzi, J.L., Joly, E. *et al.* (1977) Increased plasma adrenaline concentrations in benign essential hypertension. *Br. Med. J.*, 2, 1251.
21. Kubo, T. and Su, C. (1983) Effects of serotonin and some other neurohumoral agents on adrenergic neurotransmission in spontaneously hypertensive rat vasculature. *Clin. Expl Hypertens. Theory/Practice*, A5, 1501.
22. Collis, M.G. and Vanhoutte, P.M. (1977) Vascular reactivity of isolated perfused kidneys from male and female spontaneously hypertensive rats. *Circ. Res.*, 41, 759.
23. Bevan, J.A., Bevan, R.D., Chang, P.C. *et al.* (1975) Analysis of changes in reactivity of rabbit arteries and veins two weeks after induction of hypertension by coarctation of the abdominal aorta. *Circ. Res.*, 37, 183.
24. Whall, C.W., Myers, M.M. and Halpern, W. (1980) Norepinephrine sensitivity, tension development and neuronal uptake in resistance arteries from spontaneously hypertensive and normotensive rats. *Blood Vessels*, 17, 1.
25. Webb, R.C. and Vanhoutte, P.M. (1979) Sensitivity to norepinephrine in isolated tail arteries from spontaneously hypertensive rats. *Clin. Sci.*, 57, 31S.
26. Baum, T. and Shropshire, T. (1967) Vasoconstriction induced by sympathetic stimulation during development of hypertension. *Am. J. Physiol.*, 212, 1020.
27. Mulvany, M.J. (1993) Control of vascular structure. *Am. J. Med.*, 94 (suppl. 4A), 205–38.
28. Folkow, B. (1956) Physiological aspects of primary hypertension. *Physiol. Rev.*, 62, 347.
29. McQueen, E.G. (1956) Vascular reactivity in experimental renal and renoprival hypertension. *Clin. Sci.*, 15, 523.
30. Bereck, K.H., Stocker, M. and Gross, F. (1980) Changes in renal vascular reactivity at various stages of deoxycorticosterone hypertension in rats. *Circ. Res.*, 46, 619.
31. Bereck, K.H. and Bohr, D.F. (1977) Structural and functional changes in vascular resistance and reactivity in the deoxycorticosterone acetate (DOCA)-hypertensive pig. *Circ. Res.*, 40 (suppl. I), I–146.
32. Lais, L.T. and Brody, M.J. (1978) Vasoconstrictor hyperresponsiveness: an early pathogenic mechanism in the spontaneously hypertensive rat. *Eur. J. Pharmacol.*, 47, 177.
33. Amann, F.W., Bolli, P., Kiowski, W. and Bühler, F.R. (1981) Enhanced alpha-adrenoceptor mediated vasoconstriction in essential hypertension. *Hypertension*, 3 (suppl. I), I-119.
34. Pettinger, W.A., Sanchez, A., Saavedra, J. *et al.* (1982) Altered renal alpha$_2$-adrenergic receptor regulation in genetically hypertensive rats. *Hypertension*, 4 (suppl. II), II-188.
35. Lüscher, T.F. and Vanhoutte, P.M. (1986) Endothelin-dependent responses to platelets and serotonin in the aorta of the spontaneously hypertensive rat. *Hypertension*, 8 (suppl. II), 55–60.
36. Luscher, T.F., Bühler, F.R. and Vanhoutte, P.M. (1988) Serotonin and the cardiovascular system, in *Neurocardiology*, (eds H.E. Kulbertus and G. Franck), Futura Publishing, New York.
37. Tabuchi, Y., Nakamaru, M., Rakugi, H. *et al.* (1989) Endothelin enhances adrenergic vasoconstriction in perfused rat mesenteric arteries. *Biochem. Biophys. Res. Commun.*, 159, 1304.
38. Yang, Z., Richard, V., von Segesser, L. *et al.* (1990) Threshold concentrations of endothelin-1 potentiate contractions to norepinephrine and serotonin in human arteries: a new mechansim of vasospasm? *Circulation*, 82, 188.
39. Resink, T.J. and Bühler, F.R. (1989) Dysfunctions of calcium extrusion in hypertension, in *Blood Cells and Arteries in Hypertension and Atherosclerosis*, (eds P. Meyer and P. Marche), *Atherosclerosis Reviews*, vol. 19, Raven Press, New York, pp. 157–69.
40. Resink, T.J., Grigorian, G.Y., Moldabaeva, A.K. *et al.* (1987a) Histamine-induced phosphoinositide metabolism in cultured human umbilical vein endothelial cells. Association with thromboxane and prostacyclin release. *Biochem. Biophys. Res. Commun.*, 44, 438–46.
41. Resink, T.J., Scott-Burden, T., Jones, C.R. *et al.* (1987b) Increased proliferation rate and phosphoinositide turnover in cultured smooth muscle cells from spontaneously hypertensive rats. *J. Hypertension*, 5 (suppl. 5), S145–8.
42. Resink, T.J., Scott-Burden, T. and Bühler, F.R. (1988) Endothelin stimulates phospholipase C in cultured vascular smooth muscle cells. *Biochem. Biophys. Res. Commun.*, 157, 1360–8.
43. Sugiyama, T., Yoshizumi, M., Takaku, F. and Yazaki, Y. (1990) Abnormal calcium handing in vascular smooth muscle cells of spontaneously hypertensive rats. *Hypertension*, 17, 603–11.
44. Erne, P., Bolli, P., Bürgisser, E. and Bühler, F.R. (1984) Correlation of platelet calcium with blood pressure. Effect of antihypertensive therapy. *New Engl. J. Med.*, 310, 1084–8.
45. Sealey, J.E. and Laragh, J.H. (1990) The renin angiotensin aldosterone system for normal regulation of blood pressure and sodium and potassium homeostasis, in *Hypertension, Pathophysiology, Diagnosis, and Management*, (eds L.H. Laragh and B.M. Brenner), Raven Press, New York, p. 1287.
46. Dzau, V.J. (1986) Significance of the vascular renin-angiotensin pathway. *Hypertension*, 8, 553.
47. Lüscher, T.F., Jäger, K., Müller, F.B. and Bühler, F.R. (1990) Renovascular hypertension: update on diagnosis and treatment, in *Handbook of Hypertension, The Management of Hypertension*. vol. 13, (eds F.R. Bühler and J.H. Laragh), Elsevier, Amsterdam, p. 90.
48. Lüscher, T.F., Lie, J.T. and Sheps, S.G. (1992) Pathology and pathogenesis of renovascular hypertension, in *Renovascular and Renal Parenchymatous Hypertension*, (eds T.F. Lüscher and N.M. Kaplan), Springer, Berlin.
49. Yang, Z., Arnet, U., von Segesser, L. *et al.* (1993) Different effects of angiotensin-converting enzyme inhibition in human arteries and veins. *J. Cardiovasc. Pharmacol.*, 22 (suppl. 5), 517.
50. Timmermans, P.M.B.W.M., Benfield, P., Chiu, A.T. *et al.* (1992) Angiotensin II receptors and functional correlates. *Am. J. Hypertension*, 5, 221.

51. Palmer, R.M.J., Ferrige, A.G. and Moncada, S. (1987) Nitric oxide release accounts for the biological activity of endothelium-derived relaxing factor. *Nature*, 327, 524.
52. Palmer, R.M.J., Ashton, D.S. and Moncada, S. (1968) Vascular endothelial cells synthesize nitric oxide from L-arginine. *Nature*, 333, 664–6.
53. Bredt, D.S., Hwang, P.M., Glatt, C.E. *et al.* (1991) Cloned and expressed nitric oxide synthase structurally resembles cytochrome P-450 reductase. *Nature*, 351, 714.
54. Moncada, S. and Vane, J.R. (1987) Pharmacology and endogenous roles of prostaglandin endoperoxides, thromboxane A2 and prostacyclin. *Pharmacol. Rev.*, 30, 293.
55. Vanhoutte, P.M. (1987) The end of the quest. *Nature*, 327, 459.
56. Richard, V., Tanner, F.C., Tschudi, M. and Lüscher, T.F. (1990) Different activation of L-arginine pathway by bradykinin, serotonin, and clonidine in coronary arteries. *Am. J. Physiol.*, 259, H1433.
57. Yanagisawa, M., Kurihara, H., Kimura, S. *et al.* (1988) A novel potent vasoconstrictor peptide produced by vascular endothelial cells. *Nature*, 332, 411.
58. Radomski, M.W., Palmer, R.M.J. and Moncada, S. (1990) An L-arginine/nitric oxide pathway present in human platelets regulates aggregation. *Proc. Natl. Acad. Sci. USA*, 87, 5193.
59. Radomski, M.W., Palmer, R.M.J. and Moncada, S. (1987) Endogenous nitric oxide inhibits human platelet adhesion to vascular endothelium. *Lancet*, ii, 1057.
60. Garg, U.C. and Hassid, A. (1989) Nitric oxide-generating vasodilators and 8-bromo-cyclic guanoside monophosphate inhibit mitogenesis and proliferation of cultured rat vascular smooth muscle cells. *J. Clin. Invest.*, 83, 1774–7.
61. Dubey, R.K., Ganten, D. and Lüscher, T.F. (1993) Enhanced migration of smooth muscle cells from Ren-2 transgenic rats in response to angiotensin II: inhibition by nitric oxide (abstract). *Hypertension*, 22, 412.
62. Warner, T.D., Mitchell, J.A., de Nucci, G. and Vane, J.R. (1989) Endothelin-1 and endothelin-3 release EDRF from isolated perfused arterial vessels of the rat and rabbit. *J. Cardiovasc. Pharmacol.*, 13 (suppl. 5), 85–88.
63. Dubin, D., Pratt, R.E., Cooke, J.P. and Dzau, V.J. (1989) Endothelin, a potent vasoconstrictor, is a vascular smooth muscle mitogen. *J. Vasc. Med. Biol.*, 1, 13.
64. Lüscher, T.F., Boulanger, C.M., Dohi, Y. and Yang, Z. (1992) Endothelium-derived contracting factors (brief review). *Hypertension*, 19, 117–30.
65. Dohi, Y. and Lüscher, T.F. (1991) Endothelin-1 in hypertensive resistance arteries: intraluminal and extraluminal dysfunction. *Hypertension*, 18, 543.
66. Calver, A., Collier, J., Moncada, S. and Vallance, P. (1992) Effect of local intra-arterial N^G-monomethyl-L-arginine in patients with hypertension: the nitric oxide dilator mechanism appears abnormal. *J. Hypertension*, 10, 1025.
67. Linder, L., Kiowski, W., Bühler, F.R. and Lüscher, T.F. (1990) Indirect evidence for release of endothelium-derived relaxing factor in human forearm circulation in vivo: blunted response in essential hypertension. *Circulation*, 81, 1762.
68. Panza, J.A., Quyyumi, A.A., Brush Jr, J.E. and Epstein, S.E. (1990) Abnormal vascular endothelium-dependent vascular relaxation in patients with essential hypertension. *N. Engl. J. Med.*, 323, 22.
69. Panza, J.A., Casino, P.R., Badar, D.M. and Quyyumi, A.A. (1993) Effect of increased availability of endothelium-derived nitric oxide precursor on endothelium-dependent vascular relaxation in normals and in patients with essential hypertension. *Circulation*, 87, 1475.
70. Panza, J.A., Quyyumi, A.A., Callahan, T.S. and Epstein, S.E. (1993) Effect of antihypertensive treatment on endothelium-dependent vascular relaxation in patients with essential hypertension. *J. Am. Coll. Cardiol.*, 21, 1145–51.
71. Panza, J.A., Casino, P.R., Badar, D.M. and Quyyumi, A.A. (1993) Effect of increased availability of endothelium-derived nitric oxide precursor on endothelium-dependent vascular relaxation in normal subjects and in patients with essential hypertension [see comments]. *Circulation*, 87, 1475–81.
72. Lüscher, T.F. and Haefeli, W.E. (1993) The L-arginine pathway in the clinical arena: tool or remedy? (editorial comment). *Circulation*, 87, 1746–8.
73. Hirooka, Y., Imaizumi, T., Masaki, H. *et al.* (1992) Captopril improves impaired endothelium-dependent vasodilation in hypertensive patients. *Hypertension*, 20, 175–80.
74. Creager, M.A., Roddy, M.A., Coleman, S.M. and Dzau, V.J. (1992) The effect of ACE inhibition on endothelium-dependent vasodilation in hypertension. *J. Vasc. Res.*, 29, 97.
75. Taddei, S., Virdis, A., Mattei, P. and Salvetti, A. (1994) Vasodilation to acetylcholine in primary and secondary forms of human hypertension. *Hypertension* (in press).
76. Cockcroft, J.R., Chowiencyk, P.J., Benjamin, N. and Ritter, J.M. (1994) Preserved endothelium-dependent vasodilation with essential hypertension. *N. Engl. J. Med.*, 330, 1036.
77. Zeiher, A.M., Drexler, H., Saurbier, B. and Just, H. (1993) Endothelium-mediated coronary blood flow modulation in humans. Effects of age, atherosclerosis, hypercholesterolemia, and hypertension. *J. Clin. Invest.*, 92, 652–62.
78. Treasure, C.B., Manoukian, S.V., Klein, J.L. *et al.* (1992) Epicardial coronary artery responses to acetylcholine are impaired in hypertensive patients. *Circ. Res.*, 71, 776–81.
79. Treasure, C.B., Klein, J.L., Vita, J.A. *et al.* (1993) Hypertension and left ventricular hypertrophy are associated with impaired endothelium-mediated relaxation in human coronary resistance vessels. *Circulation*, 87, 86–93.
80. Lüscher, T.F., Tanner, F.C., Tschudi, M.R. and Noll, G. (1993) Endothelial dysfunction in coronary artery disease. *Ann. Rev. Med.*, 44, 395–418.
81. Miyauchi, T., Yanagisawa, M., Suzuki, N. *et al.* (1989) Venous plasma concentrations of endothelin in normal and hypertensive subjects (abstract). *Circulation*, 80 (suppl. II), II-2280.
82. Davenport, A.P., Ashby, M.J., Easton, P. *et al.* (1990) A sensitive radioimmunoassay measuring endothelin-like immunoreactivity in human plasma: comparison of levels in patients with essential hypertension and normotensive control subjects. *Clin. Sci.*, 78, 261–4.
83. Schrader, J., Tebbe, U., Borries, M. *et al.* (1990) Plasma Endothelin bei Normalpersonen und Patienten mit nephrologisch-rheumatologischen und kardiovaskulären Erkrankungen. *Klin. Wchschr.*, 68, 774–9.
84. Schiffrin, E.L. and Thibault, G. (1991) Plasma endothelin in human essential hypertension. *Am. J. Hypertens.*, 4, 303–8.
85. Shihiri, M., Hirata, Y., Ando, K. *et al.* (1990) Plasma endothelin levels in hypertension and chronic renal failure. *Hypertension*, 15, 493–6.
86. Kohno, M., Yasunari, K., Murakawa, K. *et al.* (1990) Plasma immunoreactive endothelin in essential hypertension. *Am. J. Med.*, 88, 614–18.
87. Saito, Y., Nakao, K., Mukoyama, M. *et al.* (1990) Application of monoclonal antibodies for endothelin to hypertensive research. *Hypertension*, 15, 734–8.
88. Saito, Y., Nakao, K., Mukoyama, M. and Imura, H. (1990) Increased plasma endothelin level in patients with essential hypertension. *New Engl. J. Med.*, 322, 205.
89. Wagner, O., Christ, G., Wojta, J. *et al.* (1992) Polar secretion of endothelin-1 by cultured endothelial cells. *J. Biomed. Chem.*, 267, 16066.
90. Larivière, R., Thibault, G. and Schiffrin, E.L. (1993) Increased endothelin-1 content in blood vessels of deoxycorticosterone acetate-salt hypertensive rats but not in spontaneously hypertensive rats. *Hypertension*, 21, 294–300.
91. Deng, L.Y. and Schiffrin, E.L. (1992) Effects of endothelin on resistance arteries of DOCA-salt hypertensive rats. *Am. J. Physiol.*, 262, H1782–7.
92. Nguyen, P.V., Parent, A., Deng, L.Y. *et al.* (1992) Endothelin vascular receptors and responses in deoxycorticosterone acetate-salt hypertensive rats. *Hypertension*, 19 (suppl. II), II-98–104.
93. Nishikibe, M., Tsuchida, S., Okada, M. *et al.* (1993) Antihypertensive effect of a newly synthesized endothelin antagonist, BQ-123, in a genetic hypertensive model. *Life Sci.*, 52, 717–24.
94. Yang, Z., Richard, V., von Segesser, L. *et al.* (1990) Threshold concentrations of endothelin potentiate contraction to norepinephrine. *Circulation*, 82, 188.
95. Guyton, A.C. (1991) Blood pressure control – special role of the kidneys and body fluids. *Science*, 252, 1813–16.
96. Lüscher, T.F., Lie, J.T., Stanson, A.W. *et al.* (1987) Arterial fibromuscular dysplasia. *Mayo Clin. Proc.*, 62, 931–52.
97. Meany, T.F., Dustan, H.P. and McCormack, L.J. (1968) Natural history of renal arterial disease. *Radiology*, 91, 881–7.
98. Pohl, M.A. and Novick, A.C. (1985) Natural history of atherosclerotic and fibrous renal artery disease: clinical implications. *Am. J. Kidney Dis.*, 5, A120–30.
99. Ross, R. (1986) The pathogenesis of atherosclerosis – an update. *New Engl J. Med.*, 314, 488–500.
100. Lüscher, T.F., Espinosa, E., Dubey, R.K. and Yang, Z. (1993) Vascular biology of human coronary artery and bypass graft disease. *Curr. Opinion Cardiol.*, 8, 963–74.
101. Lüscher, T.F., Vetter, H., Studer, A. *et al.* (1980) Extrarenaler Gefässbefall bei fibromuskulär bedingter renovaskulärer Hypertonie. *Klin. Wschr.*, 58, 493–500.
102. Lüscher, T.F., Vetter, H., Pouliadis, G. *et al.* (1991) Rare forms of renal hypertension. *Klin. Wschr.*, 59, 35–45.
103. Cragg, A.H., Smith, T.P., Thompson, B.H. *et al.* (1989) Incidental fibromuscular dysplasia in potential renal donors: long-term clinical follow-up. *Radiology*, 172, 145–7.
104. Heffelfinger, M.J., Holley, K.E. and Harrison, E.G. (1970) Arterial fibromuscular dysplasia studied at autopsy (abstract). *Am. J. Clin. Pathol.*, 54, 274.
105. Harrison, E.G. and McCormack, L.J. (1971) Pathologic classification of renal arterial disease in renovascular hypertension. *Mayo Clin. Proc.*, 46, 161–7.
106. Felts, J.H., Whitley, N.O. and Johnston, F.R. (1979) Progression of medial fibroplasia of the renal artery and the development of renovascular hyper-

tension. *Nephron*, **24**, 89–90.
107. Sheps, S.G., Kincaid, O.W. and Hunt, J.C. (1972) Serial renal function and angiographic observations in idiopathic fibrous and fibromuscular stenoses of the renal arteries. *Am. J. Cardiol.*, **30**, 55–60.
108. Rushton, A.R. (1980) The genetics of fibromuscular dysplasia. *Arch. Intern. Med.*, **140**, 233–6.
109. Foster, J.H., Maxwell, M.H. Franklin, S.S. et al. (1975) Renovascular occlusive disease: results of operative treatment. *J. Am. Med. Ass.*, **231**, 1043–8.
110. Gruentzig, A., Kuhlmann, U., Vetter, W. et al. (1978) Treatment of renovascular hypertension with percutaneous transluminal dilatation of a renal artery stenosis. *Lancet*, **i**, 801–2.
111. Lüscher, T.F., Keller, H.M., Imhof, H.G. et al. (1986) Fibromuscular hyperplasia: extension of the disease and therapeutic outcome. *Nephron*, **44** (suppl. 1), 109–14.
112. Sos, T.A., Pickering, T.G., Sniderman, K. et al. (1983) Percutaneous transluminal renal angioplasty in renovascular hypertension due to atheroma or fibromuscular dysplasia. *New Engl. J. Med.*, **309**, 274–9.
113. Sheps, S.G. and McDuffie, F.C. (1980) Vasculitis, in *Peripheral Vascular disease*, (eds J.L. Inergens, J.A. Spittell and J.F. Fairbairn), W.B. Saunders, Philadelphia-London-Toronto, pp. 493–554.
114. Lüscher, T.F., Essandoh, L.K., Lie, J.T. et al. (1987) Renovascular hypertension: a rare cardiovascular manifestation of the Ehlers–Danlos syndrome. *Mayo Clin. Proc.*, **62**, 223–9.
115. Kannel, W.B. and Stokes III, J. (1985) The epidemiology of coronary artery disease, in *Diagnosis and Therapy of Coronary Artery Disease*, (ed. P.F. Cohn), Martinus Nijhoff Publishing, Boston, Dordrecht, Lancaster, p. 63.
116. Kannel, W.B., Gordon, T. and Schwartz, M.J. (1971) Systolic versus diastolic blood pressure and risk of coronary heart disease. The Framingham study. *Am. J. Cardiol.*, **27**, 335.
117. Roberts, W.C. (1980) The hypertensive diseases, in *Topics in Hypertension*, (ed. J.H. Laragh), Yorke Medical Books, New York, 368–88.
118. Veterans Administration Cooperative Study Group on Antihypertensive Agents (1967) Effects of treatment on morbidity in hypertension. Results in patients with diastolic blood pressures averaging 115 through 129 mmHg. *J. Am. Med. Ass.*, **202**, 1028.
119. Veterans Administration Cooperative Study Group on Antihypertensive Agents (1970) Effects of treatment on morbidity in hypertension. II. Results in patients with diastolic blood pressure, averaging 90 through 114 mmHg. *J. Am. Med. Ass.* **213**, 1143.
120. MacMahon, S., Peto, R., Cutler, J. et al. (1990) Blood pressure, stroke, and coronary heart disease. Part 1, Prolonged differences in blood pressure: prospective observational studies corrected for the regression dilution bias. *Lancet*, **335**, 765–74.
121. Moritz, A.R. and Zamcheck, N. (1946) Sudden and unexpected deaths in young soldiers: diseases responsible for such deaths during World War II. *Arch. Pathol.*, **42**, 459.
122. Spain, D.M., Bradess, V.A. and Mohr, C. (1960) Coronary atherosclerosis as a cause of unexpected and unexplained death. *J. Am. Med. Ass.*, **174**, 384.
123. Kuller, I. (1966) Sudden and unexpected non-traumatic deaths in adults: a review of epidemiological and clinical studies. *J. Chronic Dis.*, **19**, 1165.
124. Kuller, I., Lilienfeld, A. and Fisher, R. (1966) Epidemiological study of sudden and unexpected deaths due to arteriosclerotic heart disease. *Circulation*, **34**, 1056.
125. Kuller, I., Lilienfeld, A. and Fisher, R. (1967) An epidemiological study of sudden and unexpected deaths in adults. *Medicine*, **46**, 341.
126. Shapiro, S., Weinblatt, F., Frank, C.W. et al. (1969) Incidence of coronary heart disease in a population insured for medical care (HIP): myocardial infarction, angina pectoris, and possible myocardial infarction. *Am. J. Public Health*, **59** (suppl. II), 1.
127. Fulton, M., Julian, D.G. and Oliver, M.F. (1969) Sudden death and myocardial infarction. *Circulation* **39**, **40** (suppl. IV), 182.
128. Chang, B.N., Perlman, L.V., Fulton, M. et al. (1970) Predisposing factors in sudden cardiac deaths in Tecumseh, Michigan. *Circulation*, **41**, 31.
129. Gordon, T. and Kannel, W.B. (1971) Premature mortality from coronary heart disease. The Framingham study. *J. Am. Med. Ass.*, **215**, 1617.
130. Kuller, L.H., Cooper, M., Perper, J. et al. (1973) Myocardial infarction and sudden death in an urban community. *Bull. N.Y. Acad. Med.*, **49**, 532.
131. Roberts, W.C. and Buja, L.M. (1972) The frequency and significance of coronary arterial thrombi and other observations in fatal acute myocardial infarction. A study of 107 necropsy patients. *Am J. Med.*, **52**, 425.
132. Eppinger, E.G. and Levine, S.A. (1984) Angina pectoris. Some clinical considerations, with special reference to prognosis. *Arch. Intern. Med.*, **53**, 120.
133. Block Jr, W.J., Crumpacher, E. and Dry, T.J. (1952) Prognosis of angina pectoris, observations in 6,882 cases. *J. Am. Med. Ass.*, **150**, 259.
134. Seim, S. (1950) Angina pectoris: a prognostic study. *Acta Med. Scand.*, **166**, 255.
135. Estes Jr, J.E. (1950) Abdominal aortic aneurysm: a study of one hundred and two cases. *Circulation*, **2**, 258.
136. Crane, C. (1955) Arteriosclerotic aneurysm of the abdominal aorta. Some pathological and clinical correlations. *New Engl. J. Med.*, **253**, 954.
137. Wheelock, F. and Shaw, R.S. (1956) Aneurysm of the abdominal aorta and iliac arteries. *New Engl. J. Med.*, **255**, 72.
138. Brindley, P. and Stembridge, V.A. (1956) Aneurysms of the aorta. A clinicopathologic study of 369 necropsy cases. *Am. J. Pathol.*, **32**, 67.
139. Sommerville, R.L., Allen, E.V. and Edwards, J.E. (1959) Bland and infected arteriosclerotic abdominal aortic aneurysms: a clinicopathologic study. *Medicine*, **38**, 207.
140. Halpert, B. and Willms, R.K. (1962) Aneurysms of the aorta. An analysis of 249 necropsies. *Arch. Pathol.*, **74**, 1653.
141. Maccallum, W.G. (1909) Dissecting aneurysm. *Bull. Johns Hopkins Hosp.*, **20**, 9.
142. Tyson, M.D. (1931) Dissecting aneurysms. *Am. J. Pathol.*, **7**, 581.
143. Shennan, T. (1934) *Dissecting Aneurysms*. Medical Research Council, Special Report Series, No. 193, His Majesty's Stationery Office, London.
144. Weiss, S. (1935) The clinical course of spontaneous dissecting aneurysm of the aorta. *Med. Clin. N. Amer.*, **18**, 177.
145. McGeachy, T.E. and Paullin, J.E. (1937) Dissecting aneurysm of the aorta. *J. Am. Med. Ass.*, **108**, 1690.
146. Glendy, R.E., Castleman, B. and White, P.D. (1937) Dissecting aneurysm of aorta: clinical and anatomic analysis of 19 cases (13 acute) with notes on differential diagnosis. *Am. Heart J.*, **13**, 129.
147. David, P., McPeak, E.M., Vivas-Salas, E. et al. (1947) Dissecting aneurysm of the aorta: a review of 17 autopsied cases of acute dissecting aneurysm of the aorta encountered at the Massachusetts General Hospital from 1937 to 1946 inclusive, eight of which were correctly diagnosed ante mortem. *Ann. Intern. Med.*, **27**, 405.
148. Levinson, D.C., Edmeades, D.T. and Griffith, C.C. (1950) Dissecting aneurysm of the aorta. Its clinical, electrocardiographic and laboratory features. Report of fifty-eight autopsied cases. *Circulation*, **1**, 360.
149. Gore, I. and Seiwert, V.J. (1952) Dissecting aneurysm of the aorta. Pathologic aspects: an analysis of eighty-five fatal cases. *Arch. Pathol.*, **53**, 121.
150. Gore, I. (1955) Pathogenesis of dissecting aneurysm of the aorta. *Arch. Pathol.*, **53**, 142.
151. Burchell, H.B. (1955) Aortic dissection (dissecting hematoma; dissecting aneurysm of the aorta). *Circulation*, **12**, 1068.
152. Halpert, B. and Brown, C.A. (1955) Dissecting aneurysms of the aorta. Study of 12 cases. *Arch. Pathol.*, **60**, 378.
153. Hirst Jr, A.E., Jones Jr, V.J. and Kime Jr, S.W. (1958) Dissecting aneurysm of aorta: a review of 505 cases. *Medicine*, **37**, 217.
154. Leriche, R. (1940) De la resection du carrefour aortoviliaque avec double sympathectomie lobaire pour thrombose arteritique de l'aorte: le syndrome de l'obliteration terminoaortique par arterite. *Presse Med.*, **48**, 601.
155. Gross, H. and Philips, B. (1940) Complete occlusion of the abdominal aorta: a review of seven cases. *Am. J. Med. Sci.*, **200**, 203.
156. Lueth, H.C. (1940) Thrombosis of the abdominal aorta: a report of four cases showing the variability of symptoms. *Ann. Intern. Med.*, **13**, 1167.
157. Leriche, R. and Morel, A. (1948) The syndrome of thrombotic obliteration of the aortic bifurcation. *Ann. Surg.*, **127**, 193.
158. Hicks, S. and Warren, S. (1951) Infarction of the brain without thrombosis. An analysis of one-hundred cases with autopsy. *Arch. Pathol.*, **52**, 403.
159. Low-Beer, T. and Phear, D. (1961) Cerebral infarction and hypertension. *Lancet*, **1**, 103.
160. Kannel, W.B., Wolf, P.A., Verter, J. et al. (1970) Epidemiologic assessment of the role of blood pressure in stroke. The Framingham study. *J. Am. Med. Ass.*, **214**, 301.
161. David, N.J. and Heyman, A. (1960) Factors influencing the prognosis of cerebral thrombosis and infarction due to atherosclerosis. *J. Chronic Dis.*, **11**, 394.
162. Fisher, C.M. (1965) Lacunes: small deep cerebral infarcts. *Neurology*, **15**, 774.
163. Fisher, C.M. (1972) Cerebral miliary aneurysms in hypertension. *Am. J. Pathol.*, **66**, 313.
164. Fisher, C.M. (1969) The arterial lesions underlying lacunes. *Acta Neuropathol.*, **12**, 1.
165. Fisher, C.M. (1967) The lacunar stroke. The dysarthria-clumsy hand syndrome. *Neurology*, **17**, 614.
166. Cole, F.M. and Yates, F.O. (1967) The occurrence and significance of intracerebral micro-aneurysms. *J. Pathol. Bact.*, **93**, 393.
167. Stehbens, W.E. (1972) *Pathology of the Cerebral Blood Vessels*, C.V. Mosby Co. St Louis, p. 284.

15 Section B: Pathologic Aspects of Hypertension

Jacob Churg and Marvin H. Goldstein

15.4 Reactive changes in blood vessels

Hypertension, i.e. increase of intravascular pressure occurs in all segments of circulation, including capillaries and veins, but unless otherwise specified, it commonly refers to the arterial pressure. In addition to arterial hypertension, hypertension in the portal vein will be considered in this section.

Arterial hypertension is usually divided into 'primary' or 'essential', and 'secondary' accompanying other diseases, e.g. those of the kidney, adrenal gland, etc. Both types of hypertension occur in two forms: 'benign' where the rise of blood pressure is moderate and usually chronic and 'malignant' characterized by rapidly progressive and severe elevation of pressure with acute damage to the blood vessels and frequently renal failure.

The origin and nature of essential hypertension is uncertain and subject to much speculation. Perhaps it represents, by analogy with diabetes mellitus, an inappropriate relic inherited from our primitive ancestors. Quite likely in hunting societies, periods of feast when large amounts of meat were consumed and stored as body fat, alternated with famine, when survival depended upon fat reserves. This led to the development of efficient lipid metabolism at the expense of carbohydrate metabolism. Civilization has stabilized the food supply mainly by providing more carbohydrates and thus increasing the incidence of diabetes in individuals predisposed by heredity. Similarly, a rapid but temporary rise of blood pressure might have been an important and favorable element of the 'fight or flight' response, shunting more blood to the vital organs, e.g. the heart. In civilized societies such inherited response may become a burden, because sudden fright is much less common than moderate but persistent stress which would not allow the blood vessels to relax.

This section will be devoted to the changes in arteries and arterioles related to hypertension and will concentrate on the more recent information. Data from the earlier literature can be found in the 1980 review by Lie [1]. It should be remembered that similar, but milder and less frequent alterations occur in older people with normal blood pressure and that progressive intimal thickening is a common manifestation of aging.

Arterial changes vary with the severity of hypertension, the size and location of the arteries and perhaps also with individual predisposition, due to genetic or environmental factors. Severity of hypertension is expressed in the rapidity of its onset (acute vs chronic), the level of blood pressure (diastolic being more important than systolic) and its duration. It affects large conduit arteries (aorta, its branches, large muscular arteries) in a manner different from the medium-sized muscular arteries, and the latter, from small arteries and arterioles (so-called resistance vessels). The vessels of some organs are especially susceptible, e.g. those of the kidney.

Genetic and environmental factors affecting the blood pressure have been discussed in Section A of this chapter. There is also some experimental evidence that vascular smooth muscle cells in animals prone to hypertension (spontaneously hypertensive rat) differ from those of a non-hypertensive strain, being more able to proliferate and to show a stronger response to contractile stimuli [2,3].

It may be easier to follow the development of changes in the vascular walls by examining patients who have chronic 'benign' hypertension, supplemented by data from experimental animals. In benign essential hypertension the cardiac output is normal but the peripheral resistance is increased. The site of resistance is located in the small arteries and arterioles with an internal diameter of less than 200 µm and especially those under 100 µm [4]. The first morphologic change is narrowing of the vascular lumen and thickening of its wall, or more specifically, of its medial layer. Initially this is due to the contraction of smooth muscle cells and can be relieved by appropriate relaxants. Contraction may not be equally distributed among the resistance vessels and some may be narrowed to the point of closure. This rarefaction of the vascular bed may contribute in some degree to the increase of peripheral resistance, at least in

Vascular Pathology. Edited by W.E. Stehbens and J.T. Lie. Published in 1995 by Chapman & Hall, London. ISBN 0 412 48640 7

experimental animals (spontaneously hypertensive rat) [5].

Contraction of the smooth muscle cells has been ascribed to a variety of causes: stretching of the wall by the increased intravascular pressure and increased sympathetic tone, the earlier mentioned increased responsiveness of their muscle cells and perhaps, at least in humans a defect of vasodilating mechanisms [6–8]. It has been noted that smooth muscle cells in other locations, e.g. gastrointestinal tract, also become more responsive [9]. In all of these situations, stretching of the smooth muscle may be the first or primary event [10]. There is a recent proposal that hypertension and its vascular effects are due to an imbalance between the endothelium-derived relaxing and contracting factors [11]. Another suggestion, increased amounts of vasoconstrictive substances in the circulation, has never been substantiated [10], except for the increased production of renin and angiotensin in malignant hypertension.

In a relatively short time, perhaps only a few weeks of persistent contraction, structural changes supervene, beginning with hypertrophy and hyperplasia of the smooth muscle cells [12,13]. Hyperplasia appears to be an earlier event [14] and is predominantly seen in small vessels, while hypertrophy affects mainly the large vessels [12] (Figure 15.12). Hyperplasia probably also accounts for the smooth muscle cells that migrate from the media into the intima. In experimental animals these changes are preceded by increased incorporation of tritiated thymidine and increased DNA in the nuclei [2]. This increase reflects multiplication of nuclei in hyperplasia, and nuclear enlargement and polyploidy in hypertrophy [14]. The stimuli that promote hyperplasia and hypertrophy are essentially the same as those that cause contraction: tension or stretching of smooth muscle cells by the increased intravascular pressure [15], perhaps abetted by such factors as increased sympathetic activity [16–18], activity of growth factors [19] and possibly overproduction of endothelin [20].

The thickened media narrows the vascular lumen and prevents its full expansion during the diastolic phase. As mentioned earlier it had been suggested that in the small resistance vessels of experimental animals the luminal narrowing may be caused not by hypertrophy or hyperplasia of the media but by its remodelling with rearrangement of cells [12]. Such vessels respond only incompletely to relaxing agents.

If hypertension persists, the next step is deposition in the media and the intima of connective tissue elements, such as glycosaminoglycans of the ground substance, elastic fibers and collagen [15,21]. This connective tissue is laid down mainly by smooth muscle cells [22], perhaps with contribution of the fibroblasts normally present in the media and intima, the endothelial cells and the blood cells (monocytes) that penetrate the stressed endothelium and acquire fibroblastic pro-

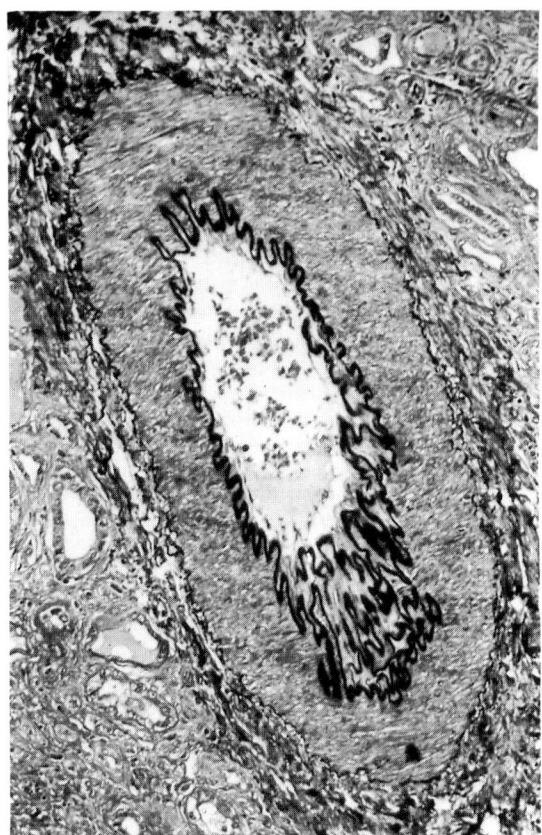

Figure 15.12 Benign hypertension. Early stage of benign nephrosclerosis: hypertrophy of smooth muscle cells in the arterial media. (Verhoeff-Van Gieson stain.)

perties. In turn the extracellular matrices influence the behavior and the function of the cells [23]. Deposition of connective tissue is promoted by androgens and inhibited by estrogens [24]. This is in keeping with generally more severe hypertension in males. It is believed that vascular sclerosis does not initiate hypertension (except when it occurs, under certain conditions in the kidney) but undoubtedly it can perpetuate and even aggravate the elevation of blood pressure.

In the large conduit vessels (aorta, its major branches and large muscular arteries), intimal atherosclerosis and its sequelae are markedly promoted by hypertension. The same holds true of the so-called cystic medianecrosis, i.e. degeneration and fibrous replacement of the smooth muscle cells and consequent fragmentation of the elastic lamellae. The cause of medianecrosis is not known, although there is some experimental evidence linking it to the deprivation of renal function and to sodium overload [25–27]. Medianecrosis has been also produced by substances that cause excessive contraction or are toxic to the smooth muscle [26]. Hypertension may cause a tear in the insufficiently supported intima of the aorta followed by penetration of blood into the media and by large stretches of dissection in the vascular

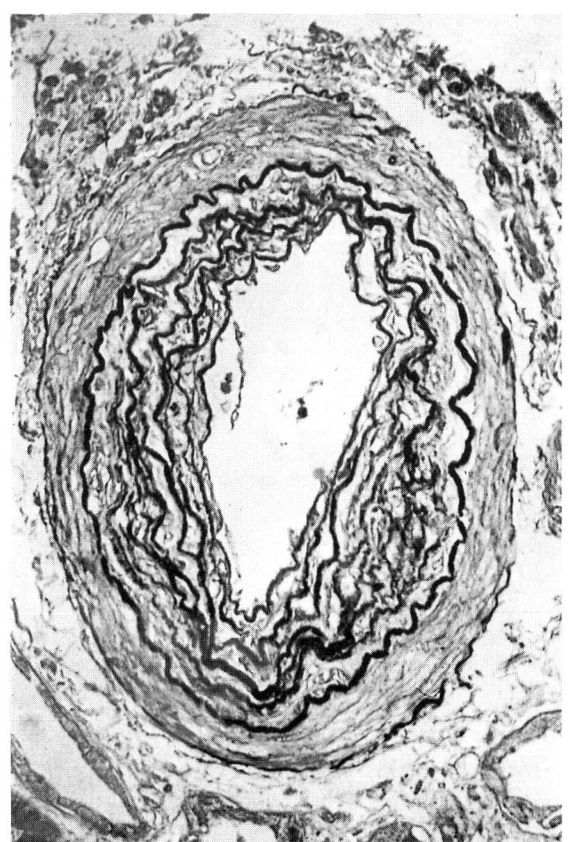

Figure 15.13 Benign hypertension. Fibroelastic thickening of arterial intima. Multiple new layers of elastic tissue internal to the original internal elastic lamina. The medial layer is preserved. (Crystal violet stain.)

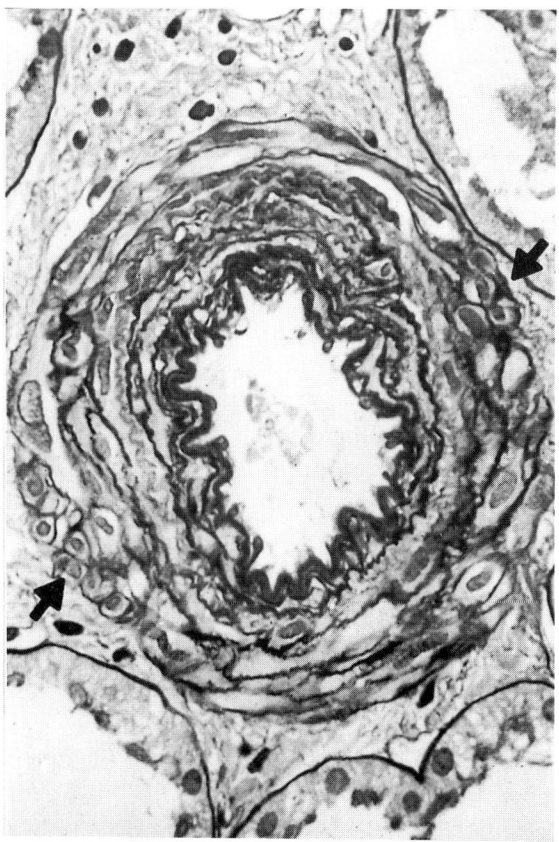

Figure 15.14 Benign hypertension. Small artery showing extensive replacement of the media by fibrous tissue. Only small clusters of smooth muscle cells are visible in the outer media (arrows). The subendothelial basal lamina is thickened. (PAS stain.)

wall. A more gradual effect of hypertension superimposed upon the medial degeneration is the development of arterial aneurysms.

Intimal thickening in the medium-sized and small arteries is greatly enhanced by so-called elastic reduplication, i.e. formation of new, secondary, replicated layers of the internal elastic lamina (Figure 15.13). The important consequence of intimal sclerosis is the gradual compression of the media with atrophy of the smooth muscle cells, often accompanied by fibrosis (Figure 15.14). In the larger muscular arteries, e.g. those of the extremities, cystic medianecrosis similar to that in the aorta, is a frequent occurrence. It seldom leads to arterial dissection, but usually ends in medial calcification (Monckeberg sclerosis), which further decreases the elasticity of the wall, although it does not result in luminal stenosis.

Changes in the small arteries and arterioles (less than 200 μm in diameter) differ somewhat from those in the larger vessels. In hypertension, more of the increased intravascular pressure is transmitted to these vessels because their parent arteries have become less elastic and less able to absorb or dampen the pressure. In the early stages of hypertension medial contraction undoubtedly occurs. In man it is followed by hyperplasia in the arteries and arterioles and perhaps also by rearrangement of smooth muscle cells in the media of smaller vessels believed to occur in experimental animals. Intimal collagenization is also observed, but the most characteristic although non-specific lesion is infiltration of the vessel wall, i.e. the intima and the media by hyalin (Figure 15.15). Hyalin is a homogeneous 'glassy' substance which stains strongly with eosin and with periodic acid-Schiff's reagent (PAS). It contains blood proteins as demonstrated by the presence of immunoglobulins (especially IgM) and complement (C3 and its derivatives), some fibrin or fibrinogen as well as a certain amount of lipid and complex carbohydrates. The lipid may impart a very finely vacuolated appearance to the hyalin. The proteins are apparently denatured, or firmly anchored, forming insoluble deposits. It has been suggested that complement, specifically IC3b, becomes attached to the hyaluronic acid of the ground substance [28]. Hyalin also contains layers of basement membrane, perhaps newly formed, or more likely representing the

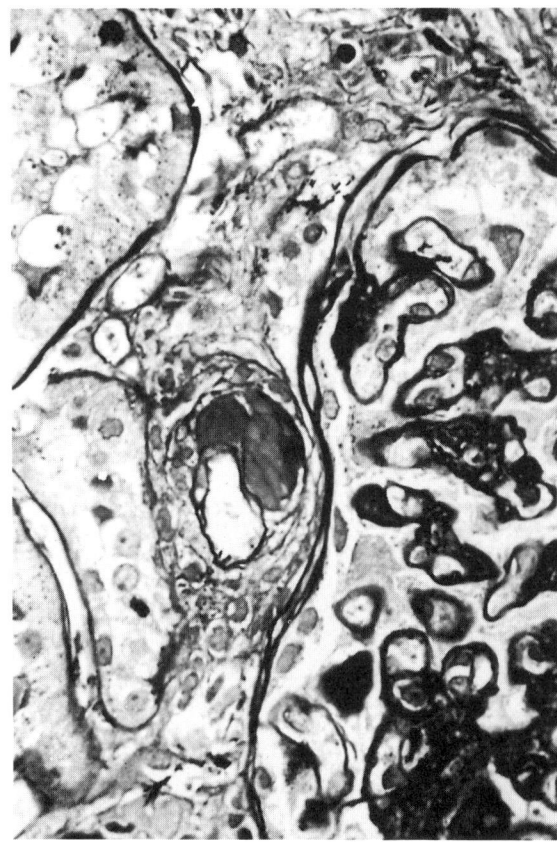

Figure 15.15 Benign hypertension. Juxtaglomerular arteriole with a thick wall and a dark deposit of hyalin, extending from the intima into the media. (PAS stain.)

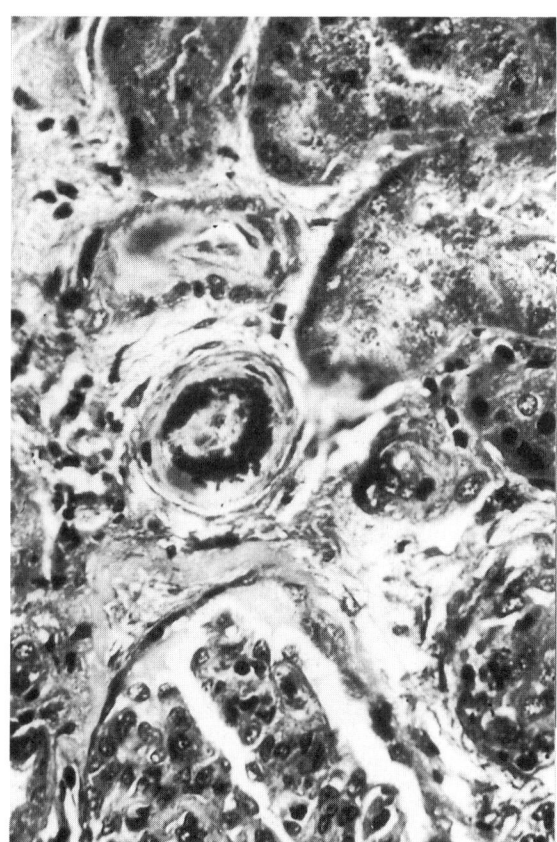

Figure 15.16 Malignant hypertension. Fibrinoid necrosis in a renal arteriole. (Courtesy Dr Steen Olsen.) (Trichrome stain.)

remnants of the basal laminae that surround muscle cells of the media. Possibly some of the protein is derived from the cytoplasm of these cells.

Hyaline infiltration occurs mainly in vessels that normally lack or have only an attenuated internal elastic lamina. This deficiency, apparently exaggerates the stretching effect of the intravascular pressure, damaging the endothelial cells, or widening the interendothelial spaces, and driving blood plasma into the wall. Hyalin first appears as small subendothelial patches which invade the media and spread circumferentially, narrowing the lumen.

Hyalinization of arterioles also occurs in non-hypertensive older individuals. It is seen to a striking degree in diabetes mellitus, perhaps because of increased permeability of the endothelium and of the underlying basement membranes.

Very high (usually over 180/120 mmHg) and rapidly developing hypertension ('malignant' hypertension) leads to a different set of changes in the resistance vessels. Contracting of the smooth muscle layer which is thinner and weaker than that in the larger arteries, is insufficient to contain the intravascular pressure. The lumen dilates, usually in a segmental fashion, alternating with contraction ('string-of-sausages' effect). In the dilated segments the endothelium is acutely stretched and damaged [29] with increased permeability of the vascular wall, extravasation of blood plasma and red cells and often, thrombosis. This can be clearly seen in the ocular fundi, where rapid rise of blood pressure induces microvascular aneurysms, focal hemorrhages, edema of the retina and ischemic necrosis ('cotton-wool spots'). Malignant hypertension also affects the intracranial circulation and may lead to rupture of cerebral aneurysms and those of the circle of Willis [30].

Dilated arterial segments predispose to platelet activation with release of platelet-derived growth factor and thromboxane. These substances stimulate intermittent constriction of the vessel as well as proliferation of smooth muscle cells and their migration into the intima [29].

The characteristic change of malignant hypertension is fibrinoid necrosis of the arterioles (Figure 15.16) and very small arteries, most often seen in the kidney and the brain, but also in the periadrenal and peripancreatic tissue, intestine, gallbladder and, less often, elsewhere in the body. Fibrinoid necrosis affects the vessels of the same caliber as hyalin deposition of 'benign' hypertension. There is also similarity of microscopic appearance,

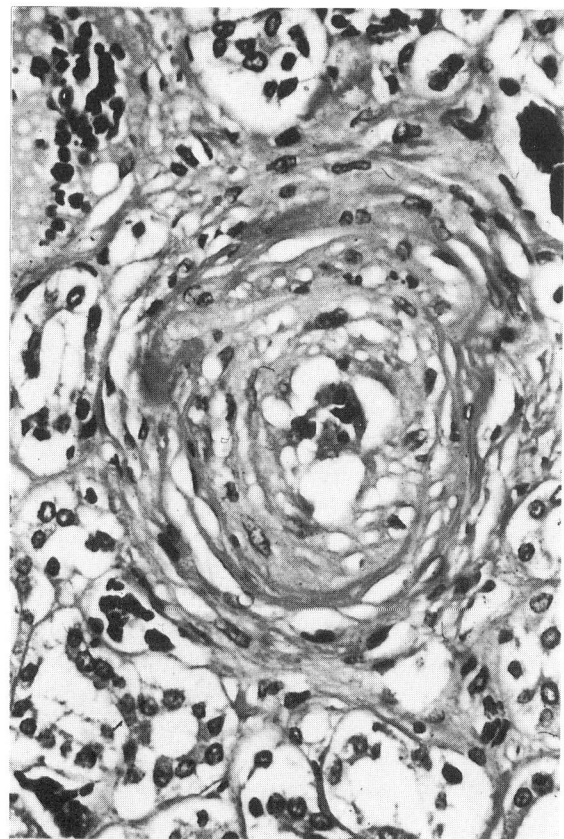

Figure 15.17 Malignant hypertension. 'Mucoid' thickening of the arterial intima with narrowing of the lumen. (H&E stain.)

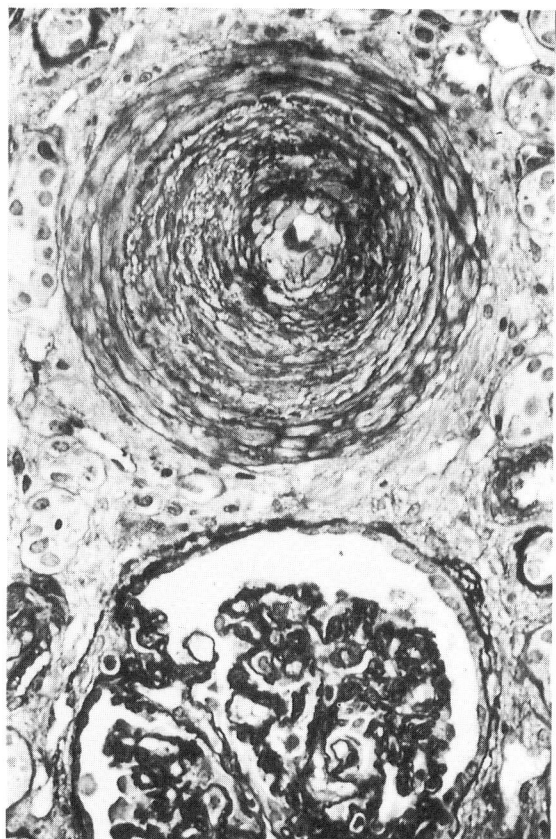

Figure 15.18 Malignant hypertension. Striking 'onion peel' thickening of the arterial intima with marked narrowing of the lumen. A nearby glomerulus shows ischemic changes with collapse of the tuft and wrinkling of capillary walls. (PAS stain.)

although fibrinoid is non-homogeneous and does not have sharply defined outlines (Figure 15.16). Similarly, fibrinoid consists of plasma proteins, but with considerable participation of fibrin or fibrinogen and their derivatives, of necrotic smooth muscle cells and occasionally of red blood cells. Inflammatory exudate, mainly polymorphonuclear leukocytes, is uncommon in man, but is a regular feature of fibrinoid necrosis in some animal species, e.g. rat [31]. When blood pressure is lowered by appropriate therapy, fibrinoid necrosis regresses and is often replaced by connective tissue, or by plexiform 'angioblastic nodules' composed of loose connective tissue, endothelial cells and fibrin [32] with partial restoration of blood flow.

In contrast to arterioles, arteries respond to malignant hypertension by marked thickening of the intima and severe narrowing of the lumen (Figure 15.17), caused by deposition of nearly acellular 'mucoid' ground substance, mostly glycoproteins. The source of this substance has not been established; it is unlikely that it is manufactured by the relatively few intimal cells, particularly when malignant hypertension is 'primary', i.e. not preceded by a phase of 'benign' hypertension. Perhaps it is produced by the smooth muscle cells of the media, or, to some extent, by transudation from the blood stream. In time, the number of cells increases and other elements of connective tissue appear. The cells and the accompanying matrix are often arranged in concentric layers ('onion-peel') (Figure 15.18), perhaps indicating episodes of dilatation and contraction. 'Onion-peel' thickening also occurs in the more severe cases of benign hypertension.

In contrast to fibrinoid necrosis, mucoid thickening often persists, despite the lowering of blood pressure, and becomes organized with permanent narrowing of the lumen. Furthermore, malignant hypertension may be accompanied by thrombotic microangiopathy which causes severe damage to the arteries and arterioles (Figure 15.19). Mucoid thickening and microangiopathy also occur as primary lesions leading to hypertension, especially in hemolytic-uremic syndrome and in scleroderma. In these cases severe narrowing of vascular lumina in the kidney may be followed by malignant hypertension of the 'primary' type, in contrast to the 'secondary' type which develops after a period of benign hypertension of whatever origin. To repeat, malignant

576 PATHOLOGY OF HYPERTENSION

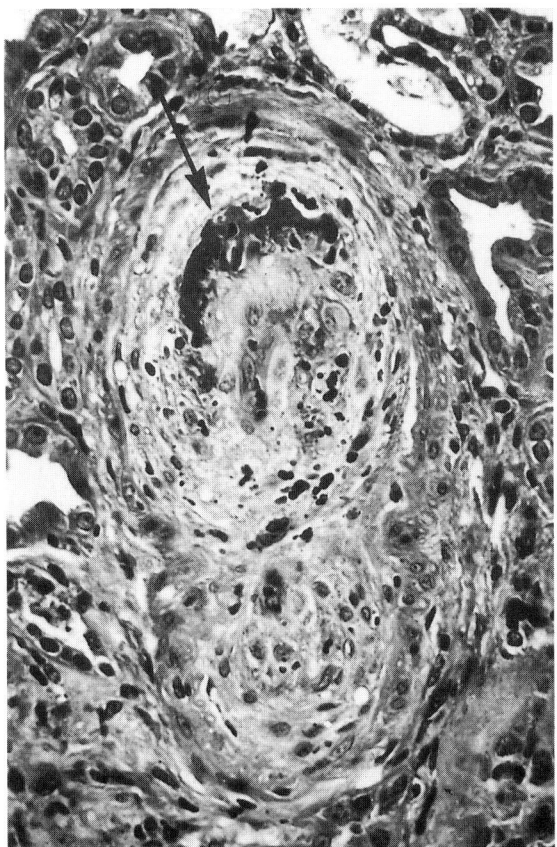

Figure 15.19 Malignant hypertension. Thrombotic microangiopathy affecting the artery. Severe intimal swelling almost completely occludes the lumen. In addition to the scattered intimal or myointimal cells, intima contains a few inflammatory cells and red blood cells many of which are fragmented. A thin dark semicircle represents fibrin deposit (arrow). (H&E stain.)

hypertension may induce hemolytic-uremic syndrome, or may be caused by it. Once established, severe narrowing of the renal vessels predisposes to a 'vicious circle' where progressively higher blood pressure leads to further constriction of the vascular lumina and in turn to further elevation of blood pressure.

15.5 Complications of hypertension

15.5.1 KIDNEY

Hypertension damages the kidney by two different mechanisms. In the first, chronic ischemia caused by advanced vascular sclerosis induces glomerular collapse and tubular atrophy, ending in parenchymal fibrosis and scarring. The second mechanism involves transmission of the elevated blood pressure into the glomerular capillaries, where it causes hyperperfusion and damages the capillary walls, followed by thrombosis, necrosis and often crescent formation. The first mechanism operates mainly in benign hypertension, and the second, in malignant hypertension, but there are undoubtedly cases of overlap where both mechanisms are present simultaneously or sequentially. It should be also remembered that the kidney can initiate hypertension, usually of the malignant type, and that benign nephrosclerosis can probably maintain and even aggravate the pre-existing hypertension. As is well known, 'clipping' of one main renal artery in an experimental animal (dog) causes hypertension, which eventually leads to arterial sclerosis in the opposite 'unprotected' kidney and to permanent hypertension that cannot be abolished by unclipping or removal of the clipped kidney.

Benign hypertension of whatever origin leads to sclerotic changes, described earlier, in the renal arteries and arterioles which reduce the blood flow to the affected segment of the kidney. Most often these changes infringe in a scattered fashion upon the minority of the vessels and produce small areas of chronic ischemia and scarring, while most of the parenchyma remains normal or nearly normal. Ischemia develops at a different pace in different individuals, generally more rapidly in those with higher blood pressure. Furthermore, vascular sclerosis and parenchymal scarring occur even with normal blood pressure, but usually only in a mild degree.

If vascular disease is sufficiently severe and widespread, considerable parenchymal atrophy ensues (Figure 15.20) and renal function deteriorates, occasionally ending in renal failure. Such outcome is seen in less than 5% of patients with benign hypertension. However, because of the frequency of hypertension in the general population, the total number of patients who develop renal failure is considerable. Statistically, some 25% of end-stage renal disease has been ascribed to hypertensive nephropathy [33].

Arteriosclerosis sometimes occurs in chronic glomerular diseases, such as IgA nephropathy (Berger's disease) or focal segmental sclerosis, before the onset of hypertension. These sclerotic changes are usually mild and do not cause significant narrowing of the lumen [34]. The mechanism is not clear; perhaps it is similar to the process that damages the glomeruli. When hypertension eventually develops, parenchymal damage may progress rapidly.

(a) Parenchymal renal changes

Hypertension usually causes contraction of the afferent arterioles which protects the glomerular capillaries from excessive intravascular pressure. In experimental animals (spontaneously hypertensive rat) this protection is further augmented by maintaining or even increasing the inner diameter of the efferent arterioles [35]. However in the DOCA-salt model, where hypertension develops rapidly, these compensating mechanisms are

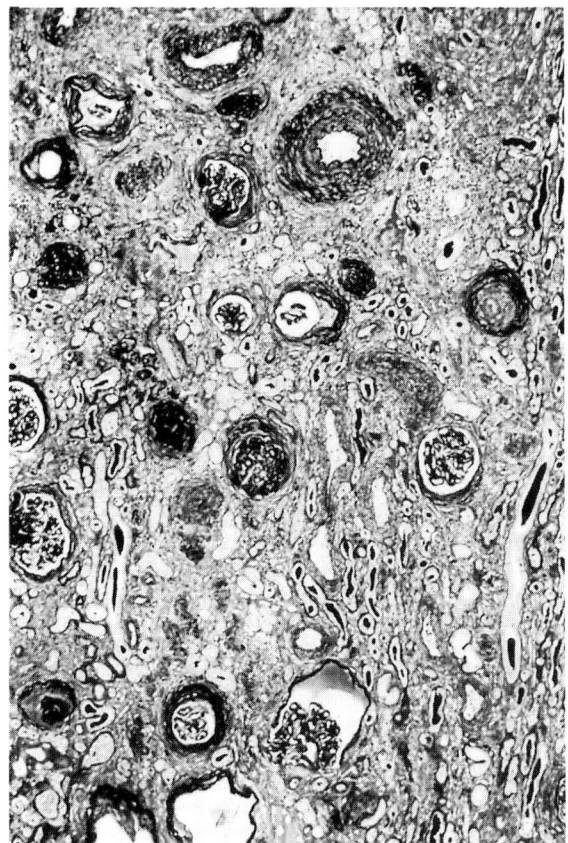

Figure 15.20 Benign hypertension. Advanced nephrosclerosis. Variable thickening and narrowing of small arteries, collapse and sclerosis of glomeruli, extensive atrophy of tubules. (PAS stain.)

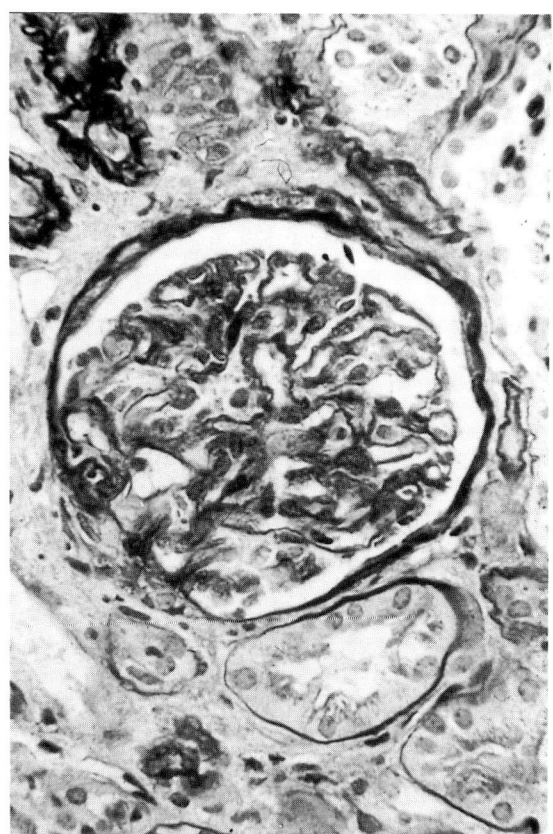

Figure 15.21 Benign hypertension. Early ischemic changes in the glomerulus manifested by partial collapse of capillaries and wrinkling of the walls. (PAS stain.)

insufficient to prevent severe arteriolosclerosis and glomerular damage [36]. Possibly a direct injury to the smooth muscle cells [27] limits the effectiveness of arteriolar contraction.

In benign hypertension in man, the main consequence of arteriolosclerosis is diminished blood flow through the glomerulus. This leads to decrease in the size of the capillary lumina, and thickening and wrinkling of their walls (Figure 15.21), followed by complete capillary collapse and loss of glomerular function. This ischemic glomerulosclerosis differs from that seen in chronic glomerulonephritis, where progressive deposition of matrix and collagen in the mesangial areas causes secondary compression of the capillaries. Although in the ischemic glomeruli, the mesangium appears to be enlarged, this is only relative to the decreased luminal cross section, and not a true mesangial expansion. The ischemic changes of hypertensive glomerulopathy are best demonstrated in thin (less than 3 μm) histologic sections.

Collapse of the capillary tuft is often accompanied by thickening of the Bowman's capsule, due to widening and splitting of its basement membrane and to formation of a layer of collagen on its inner aspect. Similar changes also occur in the healing stage of crescentic glomerulonephritis. However, these are usually limited and segmental in extent, with the capillary collapse clearly related to the overlying fibrous crescent. Although large crescents may compress the entire tuft, their eccentric origin and nature can usually be noted in at least some glomeruli. Furthermore even the fibrous crescents often contain a few cells.

Tubular and interstitial changes follow sclerosis of arterioles and glomeruli (Figure 15.20). The tubules atrophy and become smaller. They are lined by flattened cells which have lost many of their organelles. Tubular basement membranes are thickened and split. The space between the contracted tubules is filled by proliferating connective tissue and often by collections of lymphocytes together with a few histiocytes. Polymorphonuclear leukocytes and plasma cells, indicators of true inflammation, are seldom seen. The end result is a small cortical scar and focal atrophy in the medulla. Scarring produces limited shallow depressions on the surface of the kidney interspersed with areas of normal tissue. The eventual outcome is a pale and firm contracted kidney with a thin cortex and a surface resem-

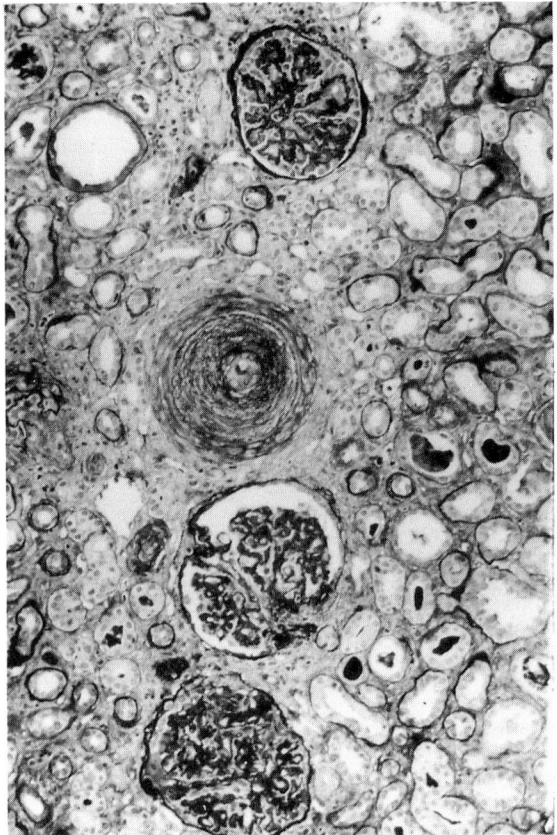
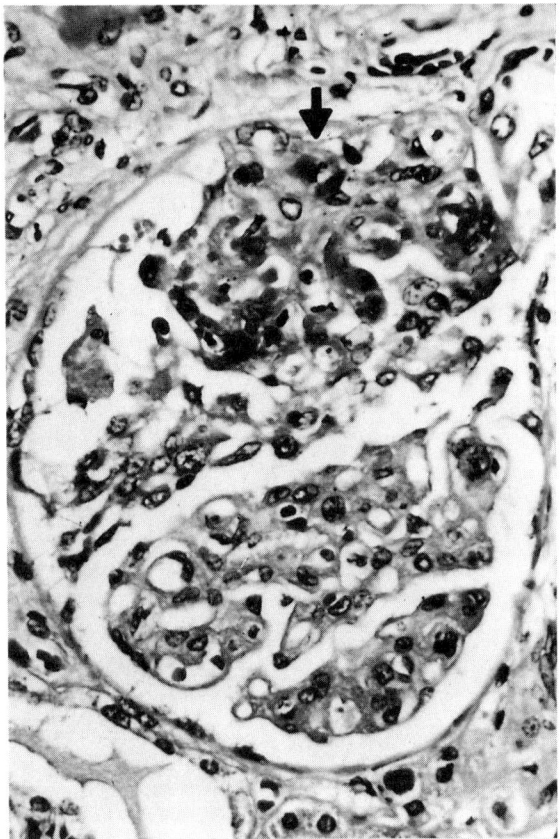

Figure 15.22 Malignant hypertension with severe malignant nephrosclerosis. There is 'onion peel' thickening of the arterial intima and ischemic collapse of the glomerular capillaries. The tubules are fairly well preserved, indicating recent onset of hypertension. (PAS stain.)

Figure 15.23 Glomerulus in malignant hypertension. There are several capillary thrombi in the lobule indicated by the arrow. (H&E stain.)

bling grained leather, which tends to adhere to the renal capsule.

The renal changes in malignant hypertension, so-called malignant nephrosclerosis (Figure 15.22) are seen in their pure form when the process is 'primary', arising in a previously normotensive patient, or when it is superimposed on benign 'essential' hypertension of short duration. The vascular damage in the kidney is usually more pronounced than elsewhere in the body, and it often affects most of the parenchyma leading to acute renal failure [37].

As mentioned earlier, the glomerular changes are mainly due to transmission of high intravascular pressure into the capillaries of the tuft. Basically these changes are similar to those in the arterioles, including segmental necrosis and thrombosis (Figure 15.23), modest cellular proliferation in the mesangium, adhesions to the Bowman capsule and sometimes crescent formation. Crescents may suggest the diagnosis of extracapillary rapidly progressing glomerulonephritis with renal failure, but in that situation the crescents are large and numerous and the vessels lack the changes of malignant hypertension.

Advancing arteriolar narrowing may add ischemic changes manifested by capillary wrinkling and collapse (Figures 15.18, 15.22). Hyperplasia and hypergranularity of the juxtaglomerular apparatus is probably the basis for the high levels of renin and angiotensin in the blood.

In cases where malignant hypertension is secondary to the narrowing of small arteries by hemolytic–uremic syndrome, the glomeruli may show characteristic changes consisting of widening of subendothelial spaces in the capillaries, mesangiolysis and fragmented red blood cells [38].

The renal parenchyma supplied by the severely narrowed or obstructed vessels often becomes infarcted. The necrotic cortical foci may be recognized on the surface of the kidney and they may also extend down to the medulla. Punctate parenchymal hemorrhages are often numerous; they represent small collections of blood in the urinary spaces of the badly damaged glomeruli or in their corresponding tubules.

In malignant hypertension superimposed upon a long-standing benign hypertension, or upon parenchymal renal disease, there will be an appropriate mixture of morphologic changes.

As mentioned earlier, the dividing line between the malignant and the benign hypertension is not sharp since blood pressure levels in the hypertensive population form a continuum. In a group of borderline cases called by Fahr [39] 'decompensated benign nephrosclerosis', glomerular damage due to high intravascular pressure may be more prominent than changes in the arterioles and may end in considerable glomerular sclerosis [40]. The juxtamedullary glomeruli are predominantly involved and parenchymal scars are often based in that region, with the apex directed toward the capsule [40]. Possibly sclerosis of arterioles caused by long-standing and severe 'benign' hypertension facilitates the transmission of pressure into the glomeruli.

Effective treatment of malignant hypertension by drugs of the vasodilator type, especially the angiotensin-converting enzyme (ACE) inhibitors, assisted where necessary by temporary dialysis, has reduced 1-year mortality from 80% to less than 20% and 5-year survival to over 50%. As mentioned earlier, the fibrinoid necrotic lesions in the arterioles and small arteries recede, with at least partial improvement of blood flow and of renal function. However, a long term follow-up of patients treated continuously for up to 4 years, showed that many eventually develop renal failure [41]. At autopsy, improvement in the small vessels was counterbalanced by residual thickening of the wall and sometimes by occlusion of the lumen by fibrous tissue and old thrombi in the interlobular and arcuate arteries. Even more striking were similar changes in the large arteries, the size of hilar and interlobar, although in untreated patients dying early in renal failure, these vessels appeared to be normal. No obvious explanation is available. Perhaps there were minor submicroscopic changes which progressed over a sufficiently long period of time, and perhaps very early and effective treatment may prevent them. In any event the treated patients developed appreciable diffuse atrophy and fibrosis of the parenchyma and also focal scars with sclerosed glomeruli which could often be traced to an old thrombosis in an interlobular artery [41].

15.5.2 HEART

Hypertensive cardiomyopathy is directly related and is roughly proportional to the degree of hypertension, but not to its duration [42]. It is the major cause of hypertension related deaths, accounting for some 35–45% of cases [43]. Its main anatomical manifestation is left ventricular hypertrophy of the concentric type, with a small chamber and thick wall. The enlarged heart usually weighs over 500 g but seldom exceeds 800 g. Muscular hypertrophy is occasionally accompanied by endocardial thickening and fibrosis. With the onset of congestive heart failure, the left ventricle eventually becomes dilated and pulmonary hypertension may develop, followed by hypertrophy and then dilatation of the right ventricle.

Microscopically, individual muscle fibers are at first enlarged, but later undergo degenerative changes and replacement by fibrous tissue. Hypertension of the malignant type may lead to myocyte necrosis [44]. Coronary atherosclerosis and the resulting coronary heart disease is markedly aggravated by hypertension with higher degrees of atherosclerosis and more severe myocardial ischemia, both chronic accompanied by myocardial fibrosis, and acute due to occlusion of coronary arteries. Myocardial fibrosis increases the incidence and severity of congestive heart failure, while myocardial infarction accounts for a considerable number of deaths in hypertensive patients.

15.5.3 BRAIN

Hypertensive encephalopathy is usually the result of malignant hypertension, but sometimes occurs with only moderately elevated pressure, e.g. in eclampsia and, especially in children, with glomerulonephritis, particularly in those treated with corticosteroids. It is manifested by severe headaches, nausea, vomiting, confusion and visual disturbances, progressing to seizures, stupor and coma. The symptoms can be usually reversed by lowering the blood pressure with appropriate medications. On pathologic examination the brain may appear normal, but sometimes there is evidence of edema with a cerebellar pressure cone. Microscopically, in some cases widespread vascular disease is seen especially fibrinoid necrosis and also thrombosis of small arteries and arterioles, with multiple minute hemorrhages and infarcts.

Hypertension often leads to **cerebral hemorrhage**. There are two forms of intracranial bleeding that are related to hypertension. Subarachnoidal hemorrhage usually originates in an aneurysm of the circle of Willis, saccular or 'berry' aneurysms, which are due to developmental defects of smooth muscle and elastic tissue in the arterial media, especially at the bifurcations. Some of these defects are associated with connective tissue disorders: Ehlers–Danlos syndrome, polycystic kidney disease, etc. There is progressive weakening of the vascular wall with time, due to hemodynamic stress of normal pulsating blood flow. Hypertension contributes to but does not initiate these berry aneurysms. Small aneurysms are common in the general population and remain asymptomatic. If they attain a larger size (over 0.5–1 cm in diameter) they may produce symptoms and may rupture, especially with a sudden rise of blood pressure of any cause, e.g. emotional stress or physical effort [45]. Berry aneurysms can be treated surgically.

The second important form of intracranial hemorrhage is most often due to rupture of an aneurysm of a small parenchymal cerebral artery (Charcot–Bouchard aneurysms); these aneurysms are much more common in hypertensive then in non-hypertensive populations [46]. Effects of intracerebral bleeding, especially of a large size, are more serious than those of subarachnoidal bleeding, and surgical approach to the treatment of cerebral aneurysms is more difficult.

As with other organs, atherosclerosis of the arteries supplying the brain, beginning with the carotids, is aggravated by hypertension. Atherosclerosis greatly predominates over hemorrhage as the cause of 'strokes'. Severe narrowing or occlusion of arteries leads to ischemic infarcts in the brain, but ischemia may also be due to atheromatous emboli or to emboli arising from the arterial thrombi.

15.6 Complications of therapy of hypertension

15.6.1 MESENTERIC VASCULAR NECROSIS AFTER SURGICAL CORRECTION OF AORTIC COARCTATION

Mesenteric arteritis is a syndrome of hypertension and arterial or arteriolar fibrinoid necrosis that occurs in about 10% of patients after surgical repair of aortic coarctation [47,48]. The vessels involved are those below the coarctation. The symptoms usually appear on the third postoperative day and consist of elevation of pressure above the preoperative level, fever, leukocytosis, abdominal pain, vomiting and gastrointestinal bleeding. If left untreated, bowel gangrene, perforation and peritonitis may follow.

Pathologic examination discloses fibrinoid necrosis and almost always neutrophilic inflammation [49,50] in the arteries of mesentery, abdominal viscera, gastrointestinal tract, as well as in the intercostal and diaphragmatic arteries and branches of abdominal aorta. Aneurysms and thrombosis are frequent. Appropriate antihypertensive therapy lowers the blood pressure, prevents serious complications and initiates the healing process.

The syndrome is most likely due to sudden exposure of the thin-walled previously 'protected' arteries, below the coarctation, to high pulsating pressure, causing vascular spasm and hypertension, followed by necrosis and inflammation. An experimental counterpart of this process has been produced by Byrom and Dodson [51], using repeated forceful injection of bland liquid (Ringer's solution) into the arterial system of a rat and thus severely raising the blood pressure. This was followed by necrosis of the arterial media usually accompanied by inflammation.

15.6.2 COMPLICATIONS IN THE USE OF PHARMACOLOGIC AGENTS IN THE TREATMENT OF HIGH BLOOD PRESSURE

There are many different drugs available for treating hypertension, all of which may produce adverse effects [52]. Unfortunately, the frequency of side-effects makes it difficult for some patients to continue their long-term use. While monotherapy is preferable, it is often necessary to use a second or even a third drug to control blood pressure effectively, further increasing the likelihood that the patient will experience untoward reactions. The main groups of drugs used to lower blood pressure are indicated in Table 15.4. A brief discussion of the usefulness and complications associated with each of these groups follows.

Table 15.4 Antihypertensive agents and their adverse effects

Class	Adverse effect
Diuretics	
Thiazides	Sudden death (arrhythmia or other causes); hypokalemia (except with K^+-sparing diuretics); glucose intolerance; elevated lipids, uric acid and calcium; sexual dysfunction
Loop diuretics	
Potassium-sparing diuretics	
Beta-adrenergic receptor blockers	
Non-selective (propranolol)	Bronchospasm; aggravated congestive heart failure and peripheral vascular disease; decreased mental acuity; bradycardia and heart block
Selective (atenolol, metoprolol)	
Alpha-adrenergic receptor blockers	
Prazosin	Orthostatic hypotension; headache; edema
Terazosin	
Calcium-channel blockers	
Verapamil, Dilitiazem, Dihydropyridines (nifedipine, isradipine, etc.)	Constipation; headache; edema; tachycardia
Angiotensin-converting enzyme inhibitors	
Captopril	Hyperkalemia; cough; rash; angioneurotic edema; decreased renal function, neutropenia
Enalapril	
Lisinopril	
Central-acting alpha agonists	
Clonidine	Fatigue; drowsiness; orthostatic hypotension; rebound hypertension
Guanabenz, Guanfacine	
Methyldopa	Liver damage; hemolytic anemia
Vasodilators	
Hydralazine	Headache; fluid retention; nasal congestion, lupus-like syndrome
Minoxidil	Hypertrichosis; pleural and pericardial effusion

(a) Diuretics

Diuretics are effective antihypertensive agents, especially in patients with congestive heart failure, stroke and renal failure [53]. They are generally inexpensive and well-tolerated. Thiazide diuretics have been used for the longest period of time, and therefore, data are more complete with these agents [53]. Complications associated with their use include the following: hypokalemia, which may induce cardiac arrhythmias; an increased incidence of sudden death (possibly related to arrhythmias), but also noted in diabetics and patients with known coronary artery disease; alterations in the lipid profile (increased total cholesterol, LDL cholesterol and triglycerides), glucose intolerance, elevations of serum uric acid and serum calcium, decrease in serum magnesium; hyponatremia and metabolic alkalosis [54–57]. Loop diuretics may induce similar metabolic changes but are more effective in patients with marked congestive heart failure and renal insufficiency [58]. The potassium-sparing diuretics are efficacious as secondary agents and in limiting hypokalemia, but must be used with close monitoring in patients with diabetes mellitus, renal insufficiency and when used in conjunction with ACE inhibitors and beta-adrenergic blocking agents [59].

(b) Beta-adrenergic receptor blocking agents

This group of drugs is favored in hypertensive patients with coronary artery disease and prior myocardial infarction, in younger patients and those with evidence of sympathetic hyperactivity, i.e. rapid pulse and wide pulse pressure [60]. They may be safely combined with most other antihypertensive agents [61]. The antihypertensive action of the beta-blockers is due primarily to their negative inotropic and chronotropic properties and they must be used with caution in combination with drugs with similar effects (i.e. some calcium channel blockers and in patients with congestive heart failure, cardiac conduction abnormalities and bradycardia) [62]. Other adverse effects include bronchospasm, peripheral vascular constriction and decrease in mental acuity, rendering them less useful in patients with chronic obstructive pulmonary disease, peripheral vascular disease and neurologic disease [63].

(c) Alpha-adrenergic receptor blocking agents

The mechanism of action of these drugs is primarily by inhibiting norepinephrine-induced vasoconstriction of vascular smooth muscle [64]. They may be used in combination with all the major classes of antihypertensive agents (especially with beta-blockers) [65]. There is minimal alteration in heart rate, cardiac output and renal blood flow, and they do not cause undesirable lipid abnormalities, central nervous system depression, fatigue or sexual dysfunction. The major side effects are orthostatic hypotension, headache and fluid retention [65,66].

(d) Calcium-channel blockers

These agents decrease peripheral vascular resistance by blocking calcium influx into vascular smooth muscle cells and thereby inhibiting contraction [67]. They are useful in the majority of hypertensive patients and, like diuretics, are particularly efficacious in elderly and black patients [68]. They are generally free of adverse metabolic effects, but because of their negative inotropic effects must be used with caution in patients with poor left ventricular function [69]. Other side effects include constipation (especially verapamil), flushing, tachycardia and edema (especially the dihydropyridine derivatives, such as nifedipine) [70].

(e) Angiotensin-converting enzyme (ACE) inhibitors

This group of drugs inhibits the production of the potent vasoconstrictor angiotensin II, leading to reduction of peripheral vascular resistance as well as renal sodium and water reabsorption [71]. They are the agents of choice in patients with congestive heart failure, diabetic nephropathy and renovascular hypertension [72]. Acute renal failure may be induced in patients with renal artery stenosis with a solitary kidney and in patients with bilateral renal artery stenosis. Other adverse effects include hyperkalemia, angioedema, cough, rash and taste disturbances [72,73].

(f) Central-acting alpha-agonists

These agents stimulate adrenoceptors in the brain stem and hypothalamus, thereby inhibiting sympathetic outflow from the central nervous system, decreasing peripheral vascular resistance, heart rate and blood pressure [74]. They have no significant effects on glucose regulation, serum lipid levels or renal function [75]. Their usefulness is limited by the high incidence of side effects, primarily drowsiness, fatigue, orthostatic hypotension and altered mental acuity. Abrupt discontinuation of these drugs may lead to a rebound hypertension that may reach very high levels [75].

(g) Vasodilators

By directly dilating arterial smooth muscle, these drugs reduce peripheral vascular resistance [76]. The fall in blood pressure is associated with a reflex-mediated increase in heart rate, stroke volume and cardiac output [77]. Tachycardia, fluid retention, headache, palpitations and nasal congestion are common side effects [54].

They are often used in combination with diuretics and beta-blockers to minimize the fluid retention and increase in heart rate, and as adjunctive therapy in patients with severe refractory hypertension [77,78].

15.7 Portal hypertension

The term portal hypertension refers to increased blood pressure in the portal vein and its tributaries, exceeding as a rule 30 cm H_2O. Most often hypertension is caused by increased resistance to the outflow of blood, usually located in the liver, but in some cases it is due to increased inflow, mainly generated by an enlarged spleen [79].

The ensuing changes in the portal vein can be described in relatively simple terms: phlebosclerosis, i.e. thickening and fibrosis of the wall, and luminal thrombosis, either primary or superimposed upon the damaged wall. If the thrombus becomes recanalized, it gives rise to so-called cavernous transformation of the portal vein [80]. Clinical manifestations are either those of diseases causing portal hypertension, or those due to sequelae of hypertension, particularly its effect on the collateral circulation. In the following pages both anatomical and clinical abnormalities will be briefly reviewed.

A very large spleen due to a hematologic disorder can cause portal hypertension by dint of high blood flow, and even an enlarged spleen secondary to liver cirrhosis can contribute to some degree. Large spleen can also produce symptoms of hypersplenism, including leukopenia, thrombocytopenia and anemia. Another mechanism of high blood flow is a vascular fistula between the hepatic artery and portal vein, caused by trauma (e.g. liver biopsy), or of congenital origin [81].

More frequently portal hypertension is due to increased resistance to the blood flow [82]. This resistance may be located in the portal vein before its entry into the liver, in the circulatory system of the liver or in the hepatic veins. Prehepatic obstruction may be caused by pressure or infiltration by a tumor; by thrombosis of the portal or splenic vein due to infection, secondary to pyelophlebitis or gangrenous appendicitis; or intra-abdominal thrombosis due to a hypercoagulable state, such as polycythemia vera or pregnancy. Thrombosis is generally more common in children. In some cases the cause of portal hypertension is unknown (idiopathic), although there are suggestions that environmental factors (e.g. toxins) play a role in its development.

Most instances of portal hypertension are caused by intrahepatic disease [83]. Obstruction to the blood flow may be presinusoidal, sinusoidal or post-sinusoidal, each associated with somewhat different changes in the liver parenchyma and with different etiologies. However there may be some overlap between these three types or locations, depending upon the nature and extent of the pathologic process.

Presinusoidal obstruction occurs with abnormalities in the portal areas [82], including those caused by toxins (organic arsenicals, vinyl chloride, copper); schistosomiasis; sarcoidosis; leukemic infiltrates; metastatic carcinomatosis; congenital cystic hepatic fibrosis. Space-occupying infiltrates, inflammation, fibrosis and direct damage, singly or in combination, lead to the occlusion of small portal veins. Thus in schistosomiasis, parasitic ova are trapped in the venules and cause granulomatous inflammation, followed by fibrosis, which may extend into the sinusoids. In presinusoidal obstruction, liver parenchyma is at first little affected and liver function tests are normal or near normal, but eventually parenchymal atrophy and liver failure develops in some patients.

Sinusoidal obstruction is usually secondary to parenchymal disease and often occurs together with pre- and post-sinusoidal obstruction. In essence, cirrhosis causes severe alteration, distortion and narrowing of the vascular channels. In acute alcoholic hepatitis, destruction of hepatocytes is most prominent near the terminal hepatic venules and the venules themselves undergo sclerosis and obliteration. These changes may regress, at least in part, with abstinence from alcohol. In chronic active hepatitis and in biliary cirrhosis, obstruction is at first most prominent in the portal areas, but later tends to spread to the sinusoids.

Intrahepatic postsinusoidal obstruction is typically seen in veno-occlusive disease (VOD) [84], due mainly to subintimal fibrosis in the small hepatic veins, progressing to occlusion. Etiology varies. In some countries ingestion of pyrrolizidine alkaloids (constituents of so-called 'bush tea') is responsible, and the damage can be reversed in most patients (usually children) by abstention. In the developed countries VOD may follow cancer chemotherapy, arsphenamines, and probably also cytotoxic agents used for immunosuppression after bone marrow and kidney transplants. VOD is a serious illness, with ascites, jaundice, hepatomegaly, abdominal pain and considerable mortality in the transplanted patients.

Extrahepatic postsinusoidal obstruction is seen in Budd–Chiari syndrome, due to thrombosis of hepatic veins often extending into the inferior vena cava [84]. It occurs after abdominal trauma, in myeloproliferative disorders, intra-abdominal carcinoma, pregnancy or with oral contraceptives. The main symptoms include ascites, enlargement of the liver and spleen and abdominal pain, predominately in the liver area. The course may be acute, subacute or chronic and mortality is high, up to 50% in 2 years. Liver biopsy shows severe centrilobular congestion and necrosis, or more often atrophy of hepatocytes. Eventually, fibrosis of the affected zones and cirrhosis may develop.

Sequelae of the portal hypertension depend to a degree upon the level of obstruction. Generally, presinusoidal obstruction has less effect on the structure and function of hepatocytes than post-sinusoidal obstruction, while sinusoidal obstruction is more often the result than the cause of liver damage. Some of the sequelae, such as abnormal liver function tests, ascites, enlargement of the spleen and hypersplenism have already been mentioned. The most serious effect of portal hypertension is the stress placed on the collateral connections between the portal system and the veins of systemic circulation. Dilatation of the collaterals and formation of varices in the mucosa of lower esophagus and gastric fundus predisposes to rupture and exsanguinating hemorrhages [84]. A similar process also occurs in other locations, e.g. the anus, but with less danger of hemorrhage. An unusual complication of portal hypertension, with or without cirrhosis, is the development of pulmonary hypertension usually associated with plexogenic arteriopathy [85,86].

References

1. Lie, J.T. (1980) The structure of the normal vascular system and its reactive changes, in *Peripheral Vascular Diseases*, (eds J.L. Juergens, J.A. Spittel Jr and J.F. Fairbairn II), Allen-Barker-Hines, W.B. Saunders, Philadelphia, pp. 51–81.
2. Hadreva, V., Tremblay, J. and Hamet, P. (1989) Abnormalities of growth characteristics of aortic smooth muscle cells in spontaneously hypertensive rats. *Hypertension*, 13, 589–97.
3. Bolzon, B.J. and Cheung, D.W. (1989) Isolation and characterization of single vascular muscle cells from spontaneously hypertensive rats. *Hypertension*, 14, 137–44.
4. Benditt, E.P. and Schwartz, S.M. (1988) Blood vessels, in *Pathology*, (eds E. Rubin and J.L. Farber), J.B. Lippincott Co., Philadelphia, pp. 477–81.
5. Henrich, H., Hertel, R. and Assmann, R. (1970) Structural differences in the mesentery microcirculation between normotensive and spontaneously hypertensive rats. *Pflügers Arch.*, 375, 153–9.
6. Mendlowitz, M. and Naftchi, N. (1958) Work of digital vasoconstriction produced by infused norepinephrine in primary hypertension. *J. Appl. Physiol.*, 13, 247–51.
7. Winquist, R.J., Bunting, P.B., Baskin, E.P. and Wallace, A.A. (1984) Decreased endothelium dependent relaxation in New Zealand Genetic Hypertensive Rats. *J. Hypertens.*, 2, 541–5.
8. Itah, H., Pratt, R.E. and Dzan, V.J. Atrial natriuretic peptide inhibits hypertrophy of vascular smooth muscle cells. *J. Clin. Invest.*, 86, 1690–7.
9. Sakai, Y., Kwan, C.Y. and Daniel, E.E. (1984) Contractile responses of vasa deferentia from rats with genetic and experimental hypertension. *J. Hypertens.*, 2, 631–8.
10. Rorive, G.L., Carlier, P.G. and Foidart, G.M. (1986) The structural responses of the vascular wall in experimental hypertension, in *Handbook of Hypertension*, vol. 7, (eds A. Zanchetti and R.C. Farazzi), Elsevier, Amsterdam, pp. 431–52.
11. Luscher, T.F. (1990) Imbalance of endothelium-derived relaxing and contracting factors: a new concept of hypertension. *Am. J. Hypertens.*, 3, 317–30.
12. Heagerty, A.M., Bund, S.J. and Izzard A.S. (1991) Long-term structural changes in human hypertensive vessels. *Basic Res. Cardiol.*, 86 (suppl. 1), 19–23.
13. Owens, G.K. (1989) Control of hypertrophic versus hyperplastic growth of vascular smooth muscle cells. *Am. J. Physiol.*, 257, H1755–65.
14. Owens, G.K. and Schwartz, S.M. (1982) Alterations in the vascular smooth muscle mass in the spontaneously hypertensive rat: role of cellular hypertrophy, hyperploidy and hyperplasia. *Circ. Res.*, 51, 280–9.
15. Wolinsky, H. (1970) Response of rat aortic media to hypertension: morphological and chemical studies. *Circ. Res.*, 26, 507–22.
16. Nakada, T. and Lovenberg, W. (1978) Lysine incorporation in vessels of spontaneously hypertensive rats: effect of adrenergic drugs. *Eur. J. Pharmacol.*, 48, 87–96.
17. Head, R.J. (1989) Hypernoradrenergic innervation: its relationship to functional and hyperplastic changes in the vasculature of the spontaneously hypertensive rat. *Blood Vessels*, 26, 1–20.
18. Albert, V. and Campbell, G.R. (1990) Relationship between the sympathetic nervous system and vascular smooth muscle: a morphometric study of adult and juvenile spontaneously hypertensive rat/Wistar-Kyoto rat caudal artery. *Heart Vessels*, 5, 129–39.
19. Scott-Burden, T., Resink, T.J. and Buhler, F.R. (1989) Enhanced growth and growth factor responsiveness of vascular smooth muscle cells from hypertensive rats. *J. Cardiovasc. Pharmacol.*, 14 (suppl. 6), S16–21.
20. Mortensen, L.H., Pawloski, C.M., Kanagy, N.L. and Fink, D.G. (1990) Chronic hypertension produced by infusion of endothelin. *Hypertension*, 15, 729–33.
21. Hollander, W., Kramsch, D.M., Famelant, M. and Madoff, I.M. (1968) Arterial wall metabolism in experimental hypertension of coarction of the aorta of short duration. *J. Clin. Invest.*, 47, 1221–9.
22. Foidart, J.M., Savolainen, E.R., Carlier, P. et al. (1985) Effect of pregnancy and hypertension on biosynthesis of collagen and proteoglycans by normotensive or hypertensive rat aortas. *Clin. Expl Hypertens.*, B4, 183–206.
23. Kleinman, H.K., Klebe, R.J. and Martin, G.R. (1981) The role of collagenous matrices in the addition and growth of cells. *J. Cell Biol.*, 88, 473–85.
24. Sirek, O.V., Sirek, A. and Fikar, K. (1977) The effect of sex hormones on glycosaminoglycan content of aorta and coronary arteries. *Atherosclerosis*, 27, 227–33.
25. Braun-Menendez, E. and von Euler, U.S. (1947) Hypertension after bilateral nephrectomy in the rat. *Nature*, 160, 905.
26. Churg, J. (1963) Renal and renoprival vascular disease in the rat. *Arch. Pathol.*, 75, 547–57.
27. Salgado, E.D. (1970) Medial aortic lesions with metacorticoid hypertension. *Am. J. Pathol.*, 58, 305–27.
28. Gamble, C.N. (1986) The pathogenesis of hyaline arteriolosclerosis. *Am. J. Pathol.*, 122, 410–20.
29. Kincaid-Smith, P. (1980) Malignant hypertension: mechanisms and management. *Pharmacol. Ther.*, 9, 245–69.
30. Kannel, W.B., Wolf, P.A., Verter, J. and McNamara, P.M. (1970) Epidemiologic assessment of the role of blood pressure in stroke: the Framingham study. *J. Am Med. Ass.*, 214, 301–10.
31. Zeek, P.M., Smith, C.C. and Weeter, J.C. (1948) Studies on periarteritis nodosa III. The differentiation between the vascular lesions of periarteritis nodosa and of hypersensitivity. *Am. J. Pathol.*, 24, 889–917.
32. Hughson, M.D., Harley, R.A. and Hennigar, G.R. (1982) Cellular arteriolar nodules: their presence in heart, pancreas and kidneys of patients with malignant nephrosclerosis. *Arch. Pathol. Lab. Med.*, 106, 71–74.
33. US Renal Data System (USRDS) (1990) Annual Report. The National Institutes of Health, National Institute of Diabetes, Digestive and Kidney Diseases. Bethesda, MD.
34. Baldwin, D.S. and Neugarten, J. (1985) Treatment of hypertension in renal disease. *Am. J. Kidney Dis.*, 5, A57–70.
35. Kimura, K., Nanba, S., Tojo, A. et al. (1989) Variations in arterioles in spontaneously hypertensive rats. Morphometric analysis of afferent and efferent arterioles. *Virchows Arch. A Pathol. Anat.*, 415, 565–9.
36. Tojo, A., Kimura, K., Nanba, S. et al. (1990) Variations in renal arteriolar diameter in deoxy-corticosterone acetate-salt hypertensive rats. A microvascular cast study. *Virchows Arch. A Pathol. Anat.*, 417, 389–93.
37. Goldstein, M.H., Wright, J.L. and Churg, J. (1991) Vasculitis and hypertension, in *Systemic Vasculitides*, (eds A. Churg and J. Churg), Igaku-Shoin, New York, pp. 359–72.
38. Linton, A.L., Gavras, H., Gleadle, R.I. et al. (1969) Micro-angiopathic hemolytic anemia and the pathogenesis of malignant hypertension. *Lancet*, I, 1277–82.
39. Fahr, T. (1934) Pathologische Anatomic des Morbus Brightii, in *Handbuch der speziellen pathologischen Anatomie und Histologie*, vol. VI/2, (eds F. Henke and O. Lubarsch), Springer Verlag, Berlin.
40. Bohle, A. and Rutscheck, M. (1982) The compensated and decompensated form of benign nephrosclerosis. *Pathol. Res. Pract.*, 174, 357–67.
41. McCormack, L.F., Beland, J.E., Schneckloth, R.E. and Corcoran, A.C. (1958) Effect of antihypertensive treatment on the evolution of renal lesions in malignant nephrosclerosis. *Am. J. Pathol.*, 34, 1011–21.
42. Stein, B.R. and Barnes, A.R. (1948) Severity and duration of hypertension in relation to amount of cardiac hypertrophy. *Am. J. Med. Sci.*, 216, 661–4.
43. Smith, D.E., Odel, H.M. and Kernohan, J.W. (1950) Causes of death in hypertension. *Am. J. Med.*, 9, 516–29.
44. Koepsell, J.E., Kuzma, J.F. and Murphy, F.D. (1950) Hypertensive cardiovascular disease (acute) (malignant hypertension) clinical and pathologic study of 39 cases. *Arch. Int. Med.*, 85, 432–58.
45. Chason, J.L. and Hindman, W.M. (1958) Berry aneurysms of the circle of Willis. *Neurology*, 8, 41–44.
46. Cole, F.M. and Yates, F. (1967) Intracerebral microaneurysms and small cerebral lesions. *Brain*, 90, 759–68.
47. Benson, W.R. and Sealy, W.C. (1956) Arterial necrosis following resection of coarctation of the aorta. *Lab. Invest.*, 5, 359–76.
48. Ho, E.C. and Moss, A.J. (1972) The syndrome of 'mesenteric arteritis' following surgical repair of aortic coarctations. *Pediatrics*, 49, 40–45.
49. Lober, P.H. and Lillehei, C.W. (1954) Necrotizing panarteritis following repair of coarctation of aorta. *Surgery*, 35, 950–6.
50. Hurt, R.L. and Hanbury, W.J. (1957) Intestinal vascular lesions simulating

poly-arteritis nodosa after resection of coarctation of the aorta. *Thorax*, **12**, 258–63.
51. Byrom, F.B. and Dodson, L.F. (1949) The causation of acute arterial necrosis in hypertensive disease. *J. Pathol. Bacteriol.*, **60**, 357–68.
52. Struthers, A.D. and Dollery, C.T. (1988) Antihypertensive drugs: pharmokinetics, pharmacodynamics, metabolism, side effects & drug interactions, in *Handbook of Hypertension*, vol. 11, (eds W.H. Birkenhager and J.L. Reid), Elsevier, New York, pp. 1–40.
53. Collins, R., Peto, R., Macmahon, S. *et al.* (1990) Blood pressure, stroke and coronary heart disease. Part 2. Short term reductions in blood pressure: overview of randomised drug trials in their epidemiological context. *Lancet*, **336**, 827–38.
54. Medical Research Council Working Party (1985) MRC trial of treatment of mild hypertension: principal results. *Br. Med. J.*, **291**, 97–104.
55. Multiple Risk Factor Intervention Research Group (1985) Baseline rest electrocardiographic abnormalities, antihypertensive treatment and mortality in the Multiple Risk Factor Intervention Trial. *Am. J. Cardiol.*, **56**, 1–15.
56. Ames, R.P. (1987) The influence of non-beta-blocking drugs on the lipid profile: are diuretics outclassed as initial therapy for hypertension? *Am. Heart J.*, **116**, 1790–6.
57. Maclean, D. and Tudhope, G.R. (1983) Modern diuretic treatment. *Br. Med. J.*, **286**, 1419–22.
58. The Joint National Committee on Detection, Evaluation and Treatment of High Blood Pressure (1980) The 1980 Report of the Joint National Committee on Detection, Evaluation, and Treatment of High Blood Pressure. *Arch. Intern. Med.*, **140**, 1280–5.
59. Greenblatt, D.J. and Koch-Weser, J. (1973) Adverse reactions to spironolactone. *J. Am. Med. Ass.*, **225**, 40.
60. Dollery, C.T. (1988) Beta-adrenoceptor blockage. Past, present, and future. *J. Cardiovasc. Pharmacol.*, **11** (suppl. 2), S1–S4.
61. Veterans Administration Cooperative Study Group on Antihypertensive Agents (1983) Efficacy of nadolol alone and combined with bendroflumethiazide and hydralazine for systemic hypertension. *Am. J. Cardiol.*, **52**, 1230–7.
62. McMahon, F.G. (1990) Beta-blocking drugs and their hybrids, in *Management of Essential Hypertension: The Once-A-Day Era*, 3rd edn, (ed. F. Gilbert McMahon), Futura Publishing Inc., Mount Kisco N.Y., pp. 225–93.
63. Beumer, H.M. (1974) Adverse effects of beta-adrenergic receptor blocking drugs on respiratory function. *Drug*, 7, 130.
64. Graham, R.M., Oates, H.F., Stoker, L.M. *et al.* (1977) Alpha blocking action of the antihypertensive agent, prazosin. *J. Pharmacol. Expl Ther.*, **201**, 747–52.
65. Blaufox, M.D., Ross, L., Koshy, K. *et al.* (1981) Physiologic effects of prazosin HCl: consequences of diuretic combination therapy. *Nephron*, **29**, 85–89.
66. Lowenstein, J. and Neusy, A.J. (1981) The biochemical effects of antihypertensive agents and the impact on atherosclerosis. *J. Cardiovasc. Pharmacol.*, **3** (suppl. 3), 256–60.
67. Fleckenstein, A., Fleckenstein-Grun, F., Frey, M. *et al.* (1989) Calcium antagonism and ACE inhibition: two outstandingly effective means of interference with cardiovascular calcium overload, high blood pressure and arteriosclerosis in spontaneously hypertensive rats. *Am. J. Hypertens.*, **2**, 194–204.
68. Dahlof, B., Eggertsen, R. and Hannson, L. (1989) Calcium antagonists combined with beta-blockers or ACE inhibitors in the treatment of hypertension. *J. Cardiovasc. Pharmacol.*, **12** (suppl. 6), S104–8.
69. Lehtonen, A., Gordin, A. and Salo, H. (1987) Comparisons of sustained release verapamil and hydrochlorathiazide in hypertension effect on blood pressure and metabolic variables. *Int. J. Clin. Pharmacol. Ther. Toxicol.*, **35**, 301–5.
70. McMahon, F.G. (1990) Calcium channel blockers (CCBs), in *Managment of Essential Hypertension: The Once-A-Day Era*, 3rd edn, (ed. F. Gilbert McMahon), Futura Publishing Inc, Mount Kisco N.Y., pp. 117–75.
71. Dzau, V.J. (1987) Vascular angiotensin pathways: a new therapeutic target. *J. Cardiovasc. Pharmacol.*, **10** (suppl. 7), S9–S16.
72. The CONSENSUS Trial Study Group (1987) Effects of enalapril on mortality in severe congestive heart failure: results of the Cooperative North Scandinavian Enalapril Survival Study (CONSENSUS). *New Engl J. Med.*, **316**, 1429–35.
73. Canzanello, V.J., Madaio, M.F. and Madias, E. (1987) Enalapril in the management of hypertension associated with renal artery stenosis. *J. Clin. Pharmacol.*, **27**, 32–40.
74. Lowenstein, J. (1980) Clonidine. *Ann. Intern. Med.*, **92**, 74–77.
75. Houston, M.C. (1982) Clonidine hydrochloride. *South. Med. J.*, **75**, 713–21.
76. Eggersten, R. and Hansson, L. (1985) Vasodilators in hypertension – a review with special emphasis on the combined use of vasodilators and beta-adrenoceptor blockers. *Int. J. Clin. Pharmcol. Ther. Toxicol.*, **23**, 411–23.
77. Ramcay, L.E., Parnell, L. and Waller, P.C. (1987) Comparison of nifedipine, prazosin and hydralazine added to the treatment of hypertensive patients uncontrolled by thiazide diuretic plus beta-blocker. *Postgrad. Med. J.*, **63**, 99–103.
78. Moulds, R.F.W. (1985) Clinical pharmacology of vasodilator drugs. *Med. J. Aust.*, **142**, 398–401.
79. Boyer, T.D. (1990) Portal hypertension and bleeding esophageal varices, in *Hepatology*, 2nd edn, (eds D. Zakim and T.D. Boyer), W.B. Saunders, Philadelphia, p. 574.
80. Gibson, J.B. and Richards, R.L. (1955) Cavernous transformation of the portal vein. *J. Path. Bact.*, **70**, 81–96.
81. Waes, L.V., Demeulanaere, L., Damme, W. *et al.* (1979) Hepaticoportal fistula and portal hypertension. *Dig. Dis. Sci.*, **24**, 565–9.
82. Boyer, T.D. (1990) Portal hypertension and bleeding esophageal varices, in *Hepatology*, 2nd edn, (eds D. Zakim and T.D. Boyer), W.B. Saunders, Philadelphia, pp. 586–7.
83. Craig, J.R. (1990) Liver, in *Anderson's Pathology*, 9th edn, (ed. J.M. Kissane), CV Mosley, St Louis, pp. 1248, 1249.
84. Bras, G. and Brandt, K.H. (1987) Vascular disorders, in *Pathology of the Liver*, (eds R.N.M. McSween, P.P. Anthony and P.J. Scheuer), Churchill Livingstone, Edinburgh, pp. 482–502.
85. Edwards, B.S., Weir, E.K., Edwards, W.D. *et al.* (1987) Coexistent pulmonary and portal hypertension: morphologic and clinical features. *J. Am. Coll. Cardiol.*, **10**, 1233–8.
86. McDonnell, P.J., Toye, P.A. and Hutchins, G.M. (1983) Primary pulmonary hypertension and cirrhosis: are they related? *Am. Rev. Respir. Dis.*, **127**, 437–41.

16 PULMONARY HYPERTENSION AND RELATED VASCULAR DISEASES

William D. Edwards

16.1 General features

16.1.1 DEFINITION

Pulmonary hypertension is defined clinically as pulmonary arterial pressure consistently in excess of 30/15 mmHg, or a mean pressure greater than 25 mmHg. It results from vasoconstrictive or obstructive lesions within the pulmonary vessels and thereby represents a hemodynamic consequence rather than a specific disease state.

16.1.2 PREVALENCE

In a recent population study, the incidence of pulmonary hypertension, though low in women, was 13% for men older than 34 years and 28% for those older than 64 years [1]. Most patients had *secondary* forms of pulmonary hypertension that were due to underlying ischemic or valvular heart disease or chronic pulmonary disease and, therefore, were potentially reversible. By comparison, although *primary* pulmonary hypertension has been the focus of many recent studies, it is a relatively rare disorder that affects women more frequently than men and is often progressive and irreversible.

16.1.3 CLASSIFICATION

Because pulmonary hypertension has numerous causes, several classifications have been proposed that emphasize certain distinguishing features. Categories include the duration of illness (acute, subacute or chronic), origin of lesions (primary or secondary), location of lesions (precapillary or postcapillary), microscopic patterns (plexogenic, thromboembolic, and others), and etiologic groupings (postcapillary obstruction, chronic hypoxia, pulmonary vascular disease, and left-to-right shunts) [2].

In practice, diagnostic terms generally incorporate several of these features (e.g. chronic thromboembolic pulmonary hypertension, or primary plexogenic pulmonary hypertension). In this chapter, **chronic secondary** pulmonary hypertension is classified according to the site of obstruction (precapillary or postcapillary) and is further categorized by microscopic patterns and underlying causes. Separate sections are devoted to the **acute and subacute** forms and to the **primary** forms of pulmonary hypertension.

16.1.4 PATHOPHYSIOLOGY

Recent observations in the field of vascular biology have provided new insights and interpretations regarding the pathophysiology of pulmonary hypertension. Studies dealing with the endothelium have targeted the importance of shear forces, surface charge, endothelial injury and endothelial-derived vasoactive substances. The role of vascular smooth muscle cells, including myointimal cells, cannot be overemphasized, and much basic research has been directed towards understanding their proliferation, migration and response to various angiogenic and growth factors. Finally, the importance of thrombosis in certain forms of pulmonary hypertension has led to a renewed interest in platelet function and altered coagulation, including diminished thrombolytic activity in the pulmonary vasculature of patients with pulmonary hypertension. Although a more detailed discussion of these topics is beyond the scope of this chapter, several recent reviews are available [3–5].

16.2 Normal pulmonary vasculature

16.2.1 GENERAL FEATURES

A review of the normal pulmonary vasculature is provided to facilitate recognition of the hypertensive patterns. The pulmonary circulation represents a low-pressure and low-resistance vascular bed and its struc-

Table 16.1 Comparison of pulmonary and systemic circulations

Feature	Pulmonary Range	(mean)	Systemic Range	(mean)
Arterial pressure (mmHg)	22/10	(13)	120/80	(90)
Capillary pressure (mmHg)	6–9	(7)	10–30	(17)
Venous pressure (mmHg)	1–4	(2)	0–10	(6)
Arterial M/D ratio (%)	3–7	(5)	15–25	(20)
Venous M/D ratio (%)	2–5	(3)	3–6	(4)
Vascular resistance (U·m^2)	1–4	(3)	10–25	(15)
Blood flow (l/min)	4–6	(5)	4–6	(5)

M/D ratio = ratio of medial thickness to external diameter of vessel.

Table 16.2 Diameters of histologic types of pulmonary arteries

Histologic type	Diameter (μm)	Adjacent airways
Elastic	>1000 (1 mm)	Lobar, segmental, and subsegmental bronchi
Musculoelastic	500–1500	Subsegmental bronchi
Muscular	50–1000	Subsegmental bronchi and terminal bronchioles
Arteriole	15–150	Respiratory bronchioles, alveolar ducts and alveolar walls (acinar level)

ture reflects these hemodynamic features. Thus, it is characterized by pulmonary arteries and veins that are normally thin-walled and differ appreciably from vessels in the systemic circulation (Table 16.1). Synonyms for the pulmonary vascular bed include the central circulation and the lesser circulation.

16.2.2 PULMONARY ARTERIES

In humans, pulmonary arteries accompany their respective airways. From the level of the pulmonary valve to the small (1 mm) subsegmental bronchi, these vessels are elastic in structure. They function as conduits that readily distend during increased pulmonary blood flow. If elastic arteries become obstructed, pulmonary hypertension may result.

The pulmonary trunk and ascending aorta share a common adventitia, reflecting their origin from division of the truncus arteriosus. Normally, the diameters of the two great arteries are similar. However, beyond six months of age, the wall thickness of the pulmonary trunk is only about half that of the ascending aorta and elastic fibers are less plentiful and more fragmented than in the aorta.

Pulmonary arteries become muscular at the level of subsegmental bronchi, and they maintain this structure until they enter the pulmonary acinus, at the level of the respiratory bronchiole (Table 16.2). In normal lungs, the presence of medial smooth muscle beyond this level is age-related. Elastic and muscular arteries have diameters that are similar to their accompanying airways, although some muscular pulmonary arteries are smaller (Figure 16.1).

The primary role of muscular pulmonary arteries is to control pulmonary vascular resistance. In humans, there is appreciable individual variability in the arterial response to oxygen and other vasoactive substances. Subjects with hyper-reactive pulmonary vascular beds may be particularly prone to develop certain forms of pulmonary hypertension.

Pulmonary arterioles travel either beside respiratory bronchioles and alveolar ducts or within alveolar walls and, thereby, represent intra-acinar structures. In adults, as they taper, the arterioles gradually lose their medial smooth muscle and internal elastic membrane. Because they contribute little to vascular resistance in the normal lung, the clinical term arteriolar resistance is anatomically misleading.

16.2.3 PULMONARY MICROCIRCULATION

Pulmonary capillaries form an extensive network within the alveolar walls, primarily for the purpose of gas exchange. At rest, most capillary beds in the lung are only partially open. With exercise, however, the beds open further to accomodate an increased blood flow, without an appreciable increase in pulmonary vascular resistance. Extensive loss of the intra-acinar microcirculation may prevent this response and contribute to the development of pulmonary hypertension [6]. It is recognized that the capillary network also serves a metabolic function, including the primary site of activity for angiotensin-converting enzyme.

16.2.4 PULMONARY VEINS

Small venules travel within alveolar walls and are similar to pulmonary arterioles in both location and structure, whereas larger venules occupy the periphery of the acinus. Pulmonary veins travel in the interlobular septa and have an indistinct external elastic membrane (Figure 16.2). Thus, in contrast to venules, they differ from pulmonary arteries in both location and structure. The pulmonary veins function as distensible conduits for blood flow, and their obstruction may lead to the development of pulmonary hypertension.

16.2.5 PULMONARY LYMPHATICS

Lymphatic channels are located in the interlobular septa and along the pleural surface. They are distinguished

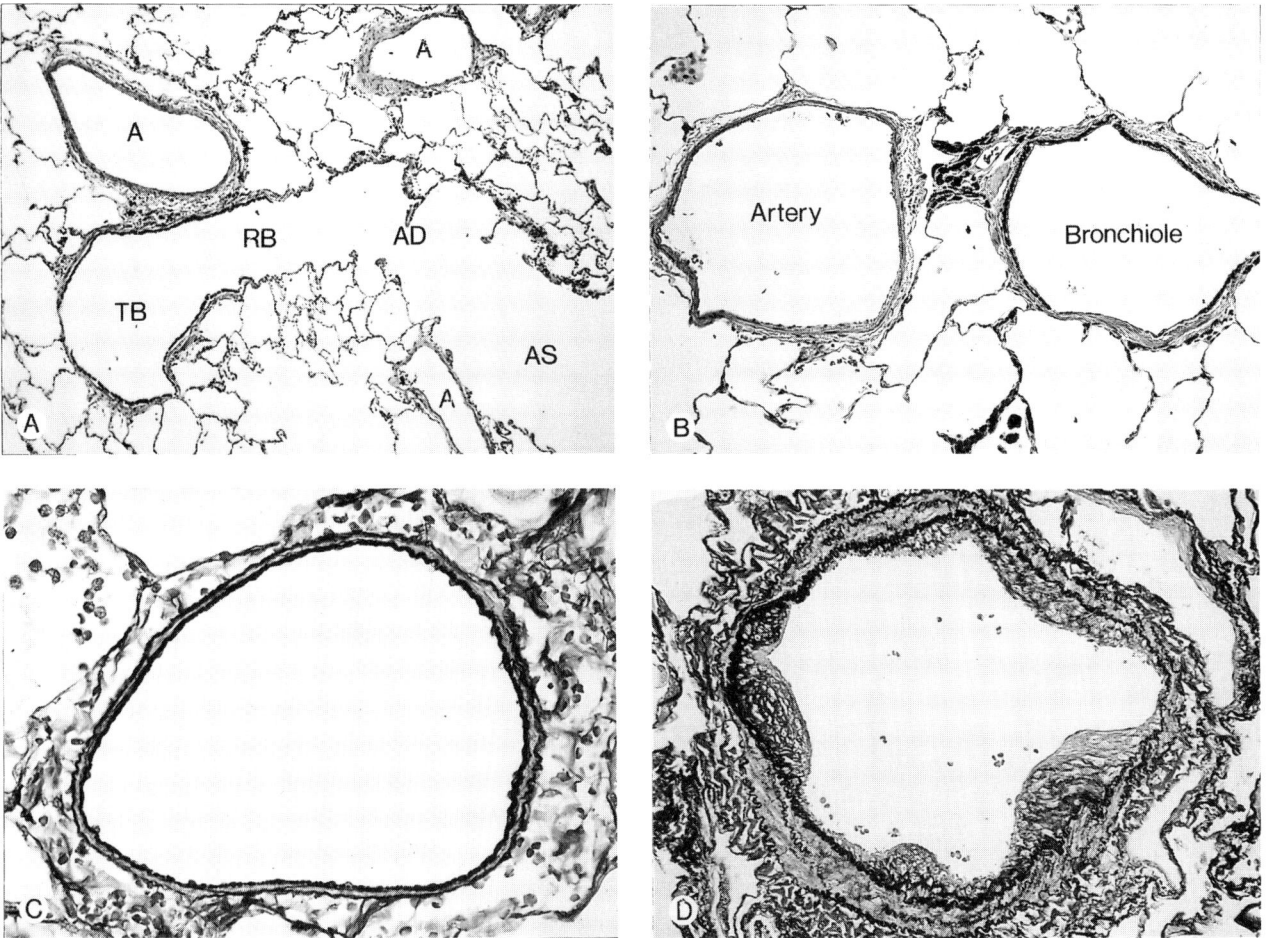

Figure 16.1 Normal muscular pulmonary arteries, shown in cross-section. (A) Small artery (A) travelling with adjacent distal airways. AD = alveolar duct; AS = alveolar sac; RB = respiratory bronchiole; TB = terminal bronchiole. (B) Similar diameters of small artery and adjacent bronchiole. (C) Artery with normally thin media. (D) Age-related fibrous intimal pads and mild increase in medial thickness. ((A, B) Hematoxylin–eosin; (C, D) elastic-van Gieson.)

from veins by the presence of valves and by the absence of luminal red blood cells. Their primary role is to maintain dry alveoli by draining excess interstitial fluid from the lungs.

16.2.6 BRONCHIAL CIRCULATION

In general, bronchial arteries arise from the descending thoracic aorta at the level of the carina, although small branches may originate from the coronary arteries. Bronchial veins normally drain either into the left atrium or into the azygos or hemiazygos veins. The bronchial circulation functions to nourish the tracheobronchial tree and the pulmonary vasculature (through the vasa vasora). Arterial bronchopulmonary anastomoses occur in the lung less frequently than do their venous counterparts. Pulmonary and bronchial arteriovenous anastomoses are rare in the normal lung.

16.2.7 AGE-RELATED CHANGES

During fetal life, the combined effects of a patent ductus arteriosus, the relative hypoxia of fetal blood and the collapsed state of the lungs contribute to the development of a high-pressure and high-resistance pulmonary vascular bed. This physiologic form of transient pulmonary hypertension is manifested morphologically by medial hypertrophy of muscular and elastic pulmonary arteries and by right ventricular hypertrophy.

At birth, profound hemodynamic changes take place that rapidly transform the pulmonary vascular bed into a low-pressure and low-resistance circulation. Pulmonary vasoconstriction abates as the ductus arteriosus closes, the arterial oxygen saturation increases and the lungs expand. Complete regression of medial hypertrophy in the pulmonary arteries generally occurs by the age of six months, as does regression of right ventricular hypertrophy.

During childhood and adolescence, remodeling of the

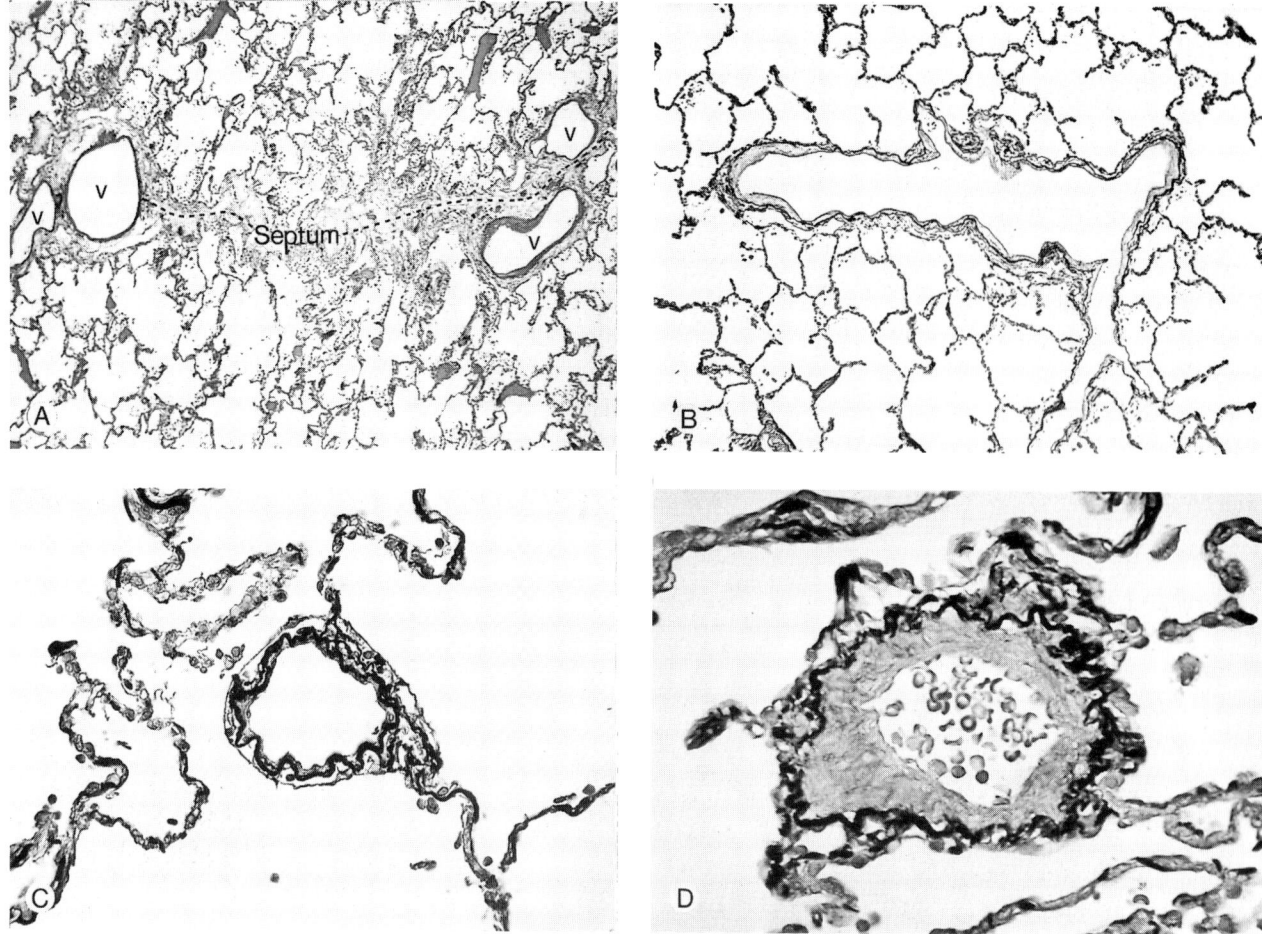

Figure 16.2 Normal small pulmonary veins. (A) Veins (V) travelling in interlobular septum (dotted line). (B) Small vein in pulmonary acinus. (C) Venule within alveolar wall. (D) Age-related fibrous intimal thickening. (Elastic-van Gieson.) ((D) Reproduced from Edwards with permission [2].)

pulmonary vasculature occurs, such that smooth muscle progressively extends into the small intra-acinar pulmonary arteries [6,7]. Age-related loss of medial muscle in the very small (<100 μm) arteries has also been reported at this time [8]. During young adult life and middle age, the structure of the pulmonary vascular bed remains relatively stable.

In the elderly, however, the pulmonary trunk becomes mildly dilated and a few shallow atheromas may be observed in the elastic pulmonary arteries. Moreover, mild medial thickening and shallow eccentric intimal fibrosis commonly involve the muscular pulmonary arteries (Figure 16.3). With age, capillaries also become slightly thicker and veins often develop intimal hyalinization with mild luminal narrowing.

16.3 Acute and subacute pulmonary hypertension

16.3.1 PERSISTENT PULMONARY HYPERTENSION OF THE NEWBORN

In some full-term infants and some premature infants with hyaline membrane disease, the transition from a fetal to an extrauterine pulmonary circulation fails to occur and pulmonary hypertension persists after birth. This may represent a primary (idiopathic) disorder or can result from hypoxemia and acidosis, due to intrauterine or perinatal asphyxia, meconium aspiration, pneumonia, thromboembolism, sepsis, shock or pulmonary hypoplasia. Right-to-left shunts exist at the levels of the foramen ovale and patent ductus arteriosus. Although respiratory symptoms usually develop within the first few postnatal days and resolve within two weeks, in some patients the process is fatal or becomes chronic.

In fatal cases, the pulmonary vasculature exhibits

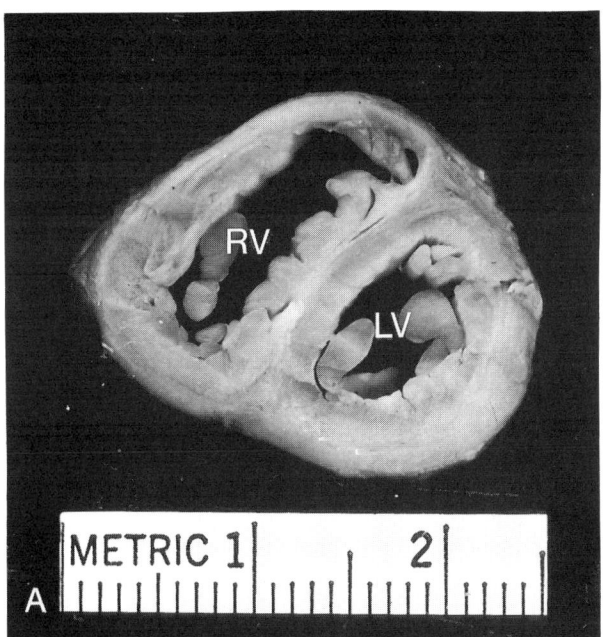
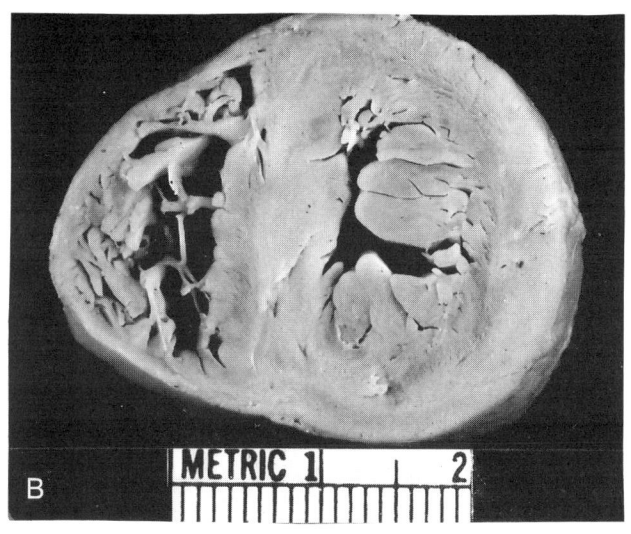
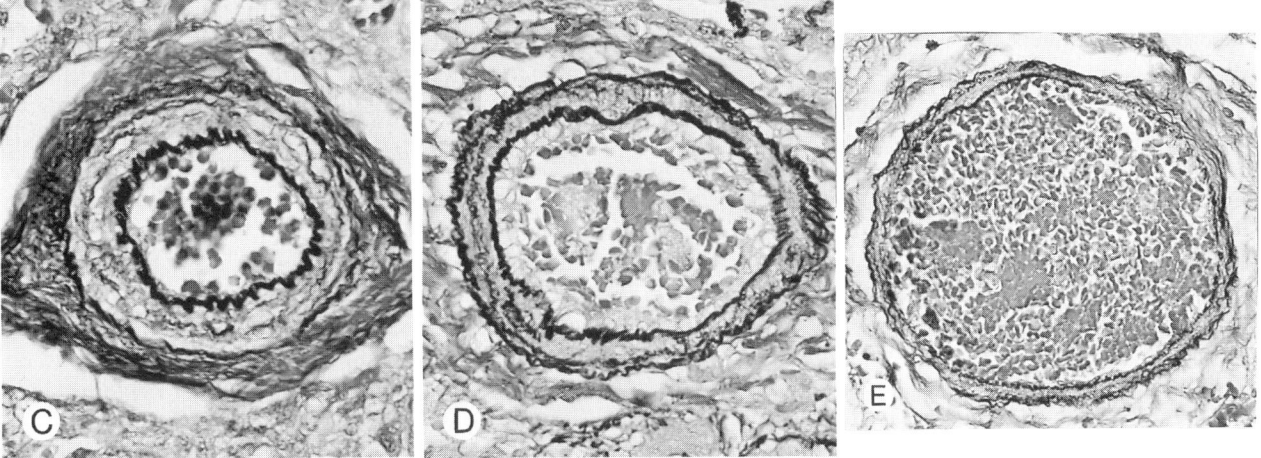

Figure 16.3 Cardiopulmonary changes at birth. (A, B) Postnatal decrease in right ventricular (RV) wall thickness compared to left ventricular (LV) wall. Compare fetal heart (A) with heart from 3-month-old infant (B). (C–E) Postnatal decrease in medial thickness of muscular pulmonary arteries. Compare artery at birth (C) with those at age 5 months (D) and 7 months (E). ((C–E) Elastic-van Gieson.) ((A) Reproduced with permission from Edwards [2].)

not only the normal degree of medial hypertrophy in muscular pulmonary arteries that is expected in a neonate but also abnormal extension of smooth muscle within small arteries and arterioles. Platelet-fibrin thrombi are frequently observed, and adventitial fibrosis is prominent in some cases. Moreover, recent studies have documented an increased number of periarterial nerves with vasoconstrictor activity, as well as a perinatal imbalance in the production of leukotrienes, prostacyclins, and other humoral factors [9,10]. Thus, persistence of the fetal cardiopulmonary circulation appears to involve both prenatal and postnatal factors.

16.3.2 ACUTE PULMONARY THROMBOEMBOLISM

Depending on their size, extent and rate of recurrence, pulmonary thromboemboli may be asymptomatic or may result in pulmonary infarction, pulmonary hypertension or sudden death. During an acute episode, some patients without previous thromboembolic events develop acute pulmonary hypertension. In this setting, pulmonary arterial pressure rarely exceeds 40 mmHg, unless there is pre-existing cardiopulmonary disease [11]. Acute thromboembolic pulmonary hypertension appears to be related not only to arterial obstruction but also to hypoxemic pulmonary vasoconstriction and to the release of vasoactive substances such as serotonin.

With time, most non-fatal pulmonary thromboemboli either lyse or organize and recanalize. Consequently, pulmonary arterial pressure usually returns toward normal. It is doubtful that chronic pulmonary hypertension ever develops after only a single episode of pulmonary thromboembolism. Thus, if the hypertension persists or progresses after an acute event, then the pulmonary arteries will generally also harbor old thrombotic lesions indicative of previous embolic events. It is recognized that non-thrombotic emboli (such as fat, air, amniotic fluid and neoplasms) may also produce acute pulmonary hypertension.

16.3.3 ACUTE LUNG INJURY

Acute lung injury, in the setting of either acute alveolar damage or sepsis, may be associated with the development of acute pulmonary hypertension. The mechanisms are poorly understood and appear to vary among patients. Some investigators have implicated hypercapnia, while others have emphasized the role of platelet-fibrin thrombi, thrombi rich in leukocytes, vasoconstriction due to neural stimulation or humoral factors and other obstructive lesions [12,13]. The morphologic features of chronic pulmonary hypertension are not observed.

16.3.4 ACUTE LEFT HEART FAILURE

Left ventricular failure with secondary pulmonary venous hypertension can occur abruptly in patients with acute myocardial infarction, myocarditis or acute aortic or mitral regurgitation. Grossly, the lungs are congested, heavy and wet, and pleural effusions may be present. Microscopically, the lungs exhibit diffuse acute congestion and interstitial and alveolar edema. The pulmonary vasculature shows no evidence of medial hypertrophy or other chronic hypertensive lesions, unless preexistent heart failure or ventricular hypertrophy also pertains.

16.3.5 NEOPLASTIC EMBOLIC PULMONARY HYPERTENSION

Among subjects with neoplastic involvement of the lungs, there exists a group in whom pulmonary arterial obstruction by tumor emboli represents the most prominent microscopic feature. Clinically, such cases are characterized by subacute pulmonary hypertension that tends to be severe and rapidly progressive. Death generally occurs one to three months after the development of respiratory symptoms and is usually attributable to right ventricular failure or massive neoplastic embolization. Microscopically, there is widespread pulmonary arterial obstruction by neoplastic emboli, with or without admixed thrombus. Medial hypertrophy of the muscular arteries is either absent or only mild, due to the short duration of the disease.

The five most common primary sites, accounting for more than 80% of the cases, include carcinomas of the breast, lung, stomach, prostate and cervix [14]. Overall, 98% are malignant tumors and most are high grade, although three patients with right atrial myxomas have been reported. Patients in whom a clinical diagnosis of malignancy antedates the development of pulmonary symptoms typically have primary carcinomas of the breast, lung, prostate, cervix or colon. In contrast, patients with pulmonary symptoms before a diagnosis of malignancy is made tend to have primary carcinomas of the stomach, kidneys, liver or pancreas.

16.4 Chronic pulmonary hypertension

16.4.1 GENERAL FEATURES

More commonly, pulmonary hypertension is chronic in nature, rather than acute or subacute, and develops over the course of years. In this regard, it is important to emphasize that obstructive vascular lesions form progressively not only after symptoms appear but also during the preclinical phase of the disease. In individual cases, the duration of the asymptomatic stage is usually speculative but is thought to range from months to years.

Microscopically, various patterns of pulmonary vascular lesions allow the classification of pulmonary hypertension into several distinct histopathologic forms. Despite these differences, however, all forms of chronic pulmonary hypertension also share certain pulmonary and cardiac features in common [15]:

- Pulmonary vascular features
  - Dilatation and atheromas of elastic arteries
  - Medial hypertrophy of elastic and muscular arteries
  - Intimal proliferation in muscular arteries
  - Muscularization of arterioles
- Cardiac features
  - Hypertrophy and dilatation of right ventricle
  - Straightening of ventricular septum
  - Regurgitation of pulmonary and tricuspid valves
  - Dilatation of right atrium and venae cavae
- Other features
  - Compression of bronchi (obstructive pneumonias)
  - Compression of left recurrent laryngeal nerve (hoarseness)
  - Distension of jugular veins
  - Congestion of liver and spleen.

16.4.2 PULMONARY VASCULAR FEATURES

The mediastinal and intrapulmonary elastic arteries are characteristically dilated, a feature that is readily detected radiographically. Medial hypertrophy is also present, but its extent may be masked by dilatation (Figure 16.4). Microscopically, the media is thickened and frequently exhibits focal degeneration (cystic medial necrosis). Chronically elevated pressure in the pulmonary arteries, like that in the systemic circulation, is often associated with the development of atherosclerosis. However, pulmonary intimal lesions differ substantially from systemic atheromas. Plaques tend to be shallow, non-obstructive and limited to the elastic arteries. Microscopically, pulmonary atheromas consist of smooth muscle cells and foam cells but rarely exhibit degenerating thrombus, cholesterol clefts, iron pigment or calcification.

Medial hypertrophy of muscular pulmonary arteries is thought to represent the morphologic counterpart of chronic vasoconstriction. It is a constant finding in all types of chronic pulmonary hypertension, although the severity of medial hypertrophy often varies from vessel to vessel (Figure 16.5). It tends to be most marked in the venous and plexogenic forms of pulmonary hypertension and least severe in the embolic and hypoxic forms. Muscularization of arterioles is another commonly observed feature, but its presence correlates better with increased pulmonary blood flow that with pressure [6].

Proliferative intimal lesions of the muscular pulmonary arteries generally accompany most forms of chronic pulmonary hypertension. They are composed of smooth muscle cells and myofibroblasts, considered to be of medial origin, and an extracellular matrix that is rich in collagen, elastin and glycoaminoglycans (Figure 16.6). Such lesions tend to be eccentric rather than concentric and are thought to represent the aftermath of an arterial response to injury or the organization of shallow *in situ* mural thrombus.

Regardless of the severity of these medial and intimal lesions, however, they are each considered to be potentially reversible if the cause of pulmonary hypertension can be removed (for example, repair or replacement of a stenotic mitral valve or patch closure of a ventricular septal defect) [16]. Although pulmonary vascular pressure and resistance generally fall dramatically following such operative procedures, their return to normal values may take months to years, as attenuation and remodeling of the pulmonary vasculature takes place.

16.4.3 CARDIAC FEATURES

Right ventricular hypertrophy, like medial hypertrophy, is a constant feature of chronic pulmonary hypertension and is referred to clinically as cor pulmonale (Figure 16.7). With time, right ventricular dilatation occurs and causes obliteration of the retrosternal space, which may be detected radiographically in the lateral view. Dilatation also results in straightening of the ventricular septum, such that both ventricles attain a D-shape in cross-section. In severe cases, the right ventricle achieves a circular shape, with a crescentric left ventricular chamber. These changes in ventricular shape, coupled with hypoxemia, partly explain the **left ventricular dysfunction** that is commonly observed in patients with chronic pulmonary hypertension.

Microscopically, right ventricular myocytes exhibit hypertrophy, with increased cell diameters and enlarged hyperchromatic nuclei. In dilated hearts, attenuation (stretching) of myocytes produces cells with near-normal diameters and thereby masks the severity of hypertrophy. Interstitial fibrosis is also commonly observed, particularly in the subendocardium, and represents a pericellular or patchy process. Myocyte hypertrophy and interstitial fibrosis form the morphologic substrate for decreased right ventricular compliance. Occasionally, mild focal lymphocytic myocarditis affects the right ventricle, particularly in cases of sudden death.

With time, chronic dilatation of the pulmonary trunk and its valvular annulus may lead to the development of pulmonary incompetence. Similarly, dilatation of the right ventricle and tricuspid annulus often results in tricuspid regurgitation. Chronic insufficiency eventually leads to mild valvular thickening, without calcification. Right atrial dilatation may be quite striking and, in

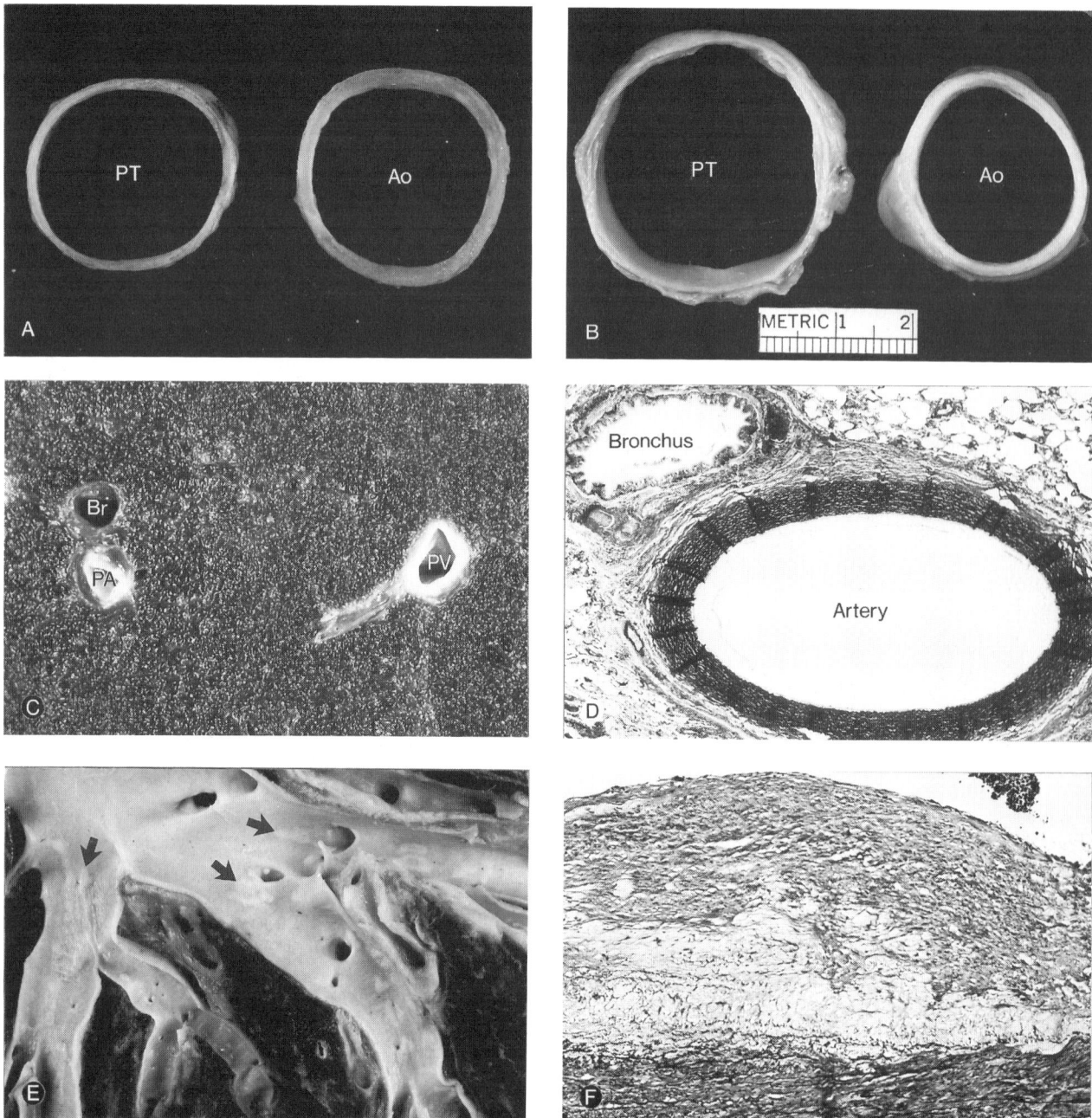

Figure 16.4 Elastic pulmonary arteries in chronic pulmonary hypertension. (A, B) Similar diameters of pulmonary trunk (PT) and ascending aorta (Ao) in normal state (A), compared to dilated pulmonary trunk in chronic pulmonary hypertension (B). (C, D) Similar diameters of elastic pulmonary artery (PA) and adjacent bronchus (Br) in normal lung (C), compared to dilated pulmonary artery in chronic pulmonary hypertension (D). PV = pulmonary vein. (E, F) Gross and microscopic appearances, respectively, of intimal atheromas (arrows). ((D, F) Elastic-van Gieson.) ((D, E) Reproduced from Edwards with permission [2].)

some cases, is associated with aneurysmal leftward bowing of the valve of the fossa ovalis. If the foramen ovale is patent, an appreciable right-to-left shunt can develop, and an avenue is available for paradoxical embolization. In addition, elevated right atrial pressure may be associated with dilatation of the coronary sinus and decreased coronary perfusion pressure.

16.4.4 OTHER FEATURES

Dilated pulmonary arteries can cause significant distortion of adjacent structures. Compression of the left main and right intermediate bronchi leads to recurrent obstructive pneumonias in some patients, particularly children with compliant bronchi [17]. In the setting of

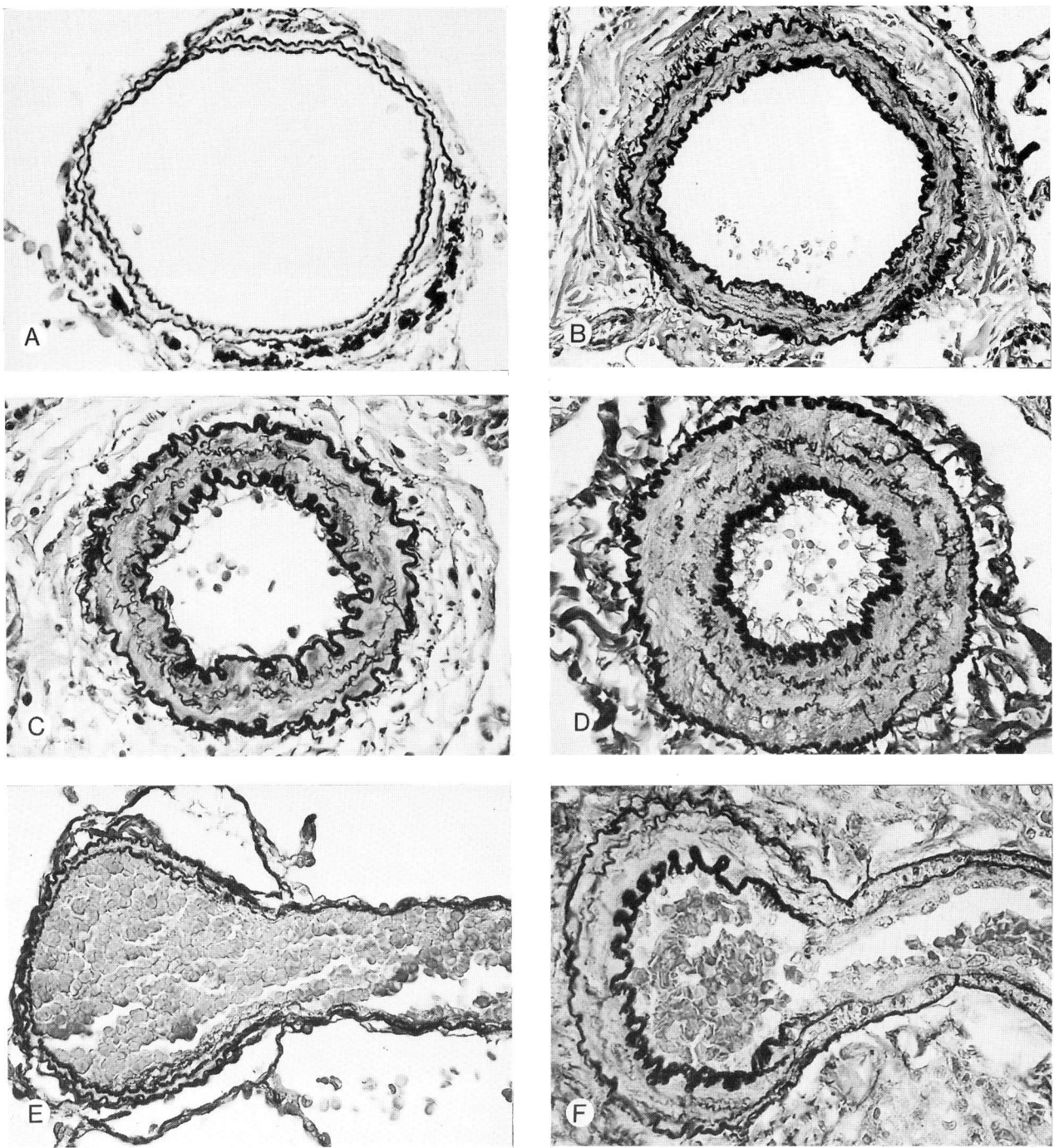

Figure 16.5 Media of muscular pulmonary arteries in chronic pulmonary hypertension. (A–D) Varying extents of medial hypertrophy. Normal artery (A) compared to mild (B), moderate (C), and severe (D) degrees of hypertrophy. (E, F) Muscularization of arteriole. Normal small artery and arteriolar branch (E) compared to vessel of similar size, showing medial hypertrophy and muscularized arteriole (F). (Elastic-van Gieson.) ((E, F) reproduced with permission from Edwards [2].)

mitral stenosis with chronic pulmonary venous hypertension, entrapment of the left bronchus between the distended left atrium, below, and the dilated left pulmonary artery, above, results in a hemodynamic vise that not only elevates the bronchus but also compresses it. Finally, rightward displacement of the aortic arch by a dilated pulmonary artery can cause compression of the left recurrent laryngeal nerve, between the aorta and trachea, and thereby produce hoarseness.

Dilatation of the venae cavae and their tributaries is associated with jugular venous distension and congestive hepatosplenomegaly. With time, steatosis and

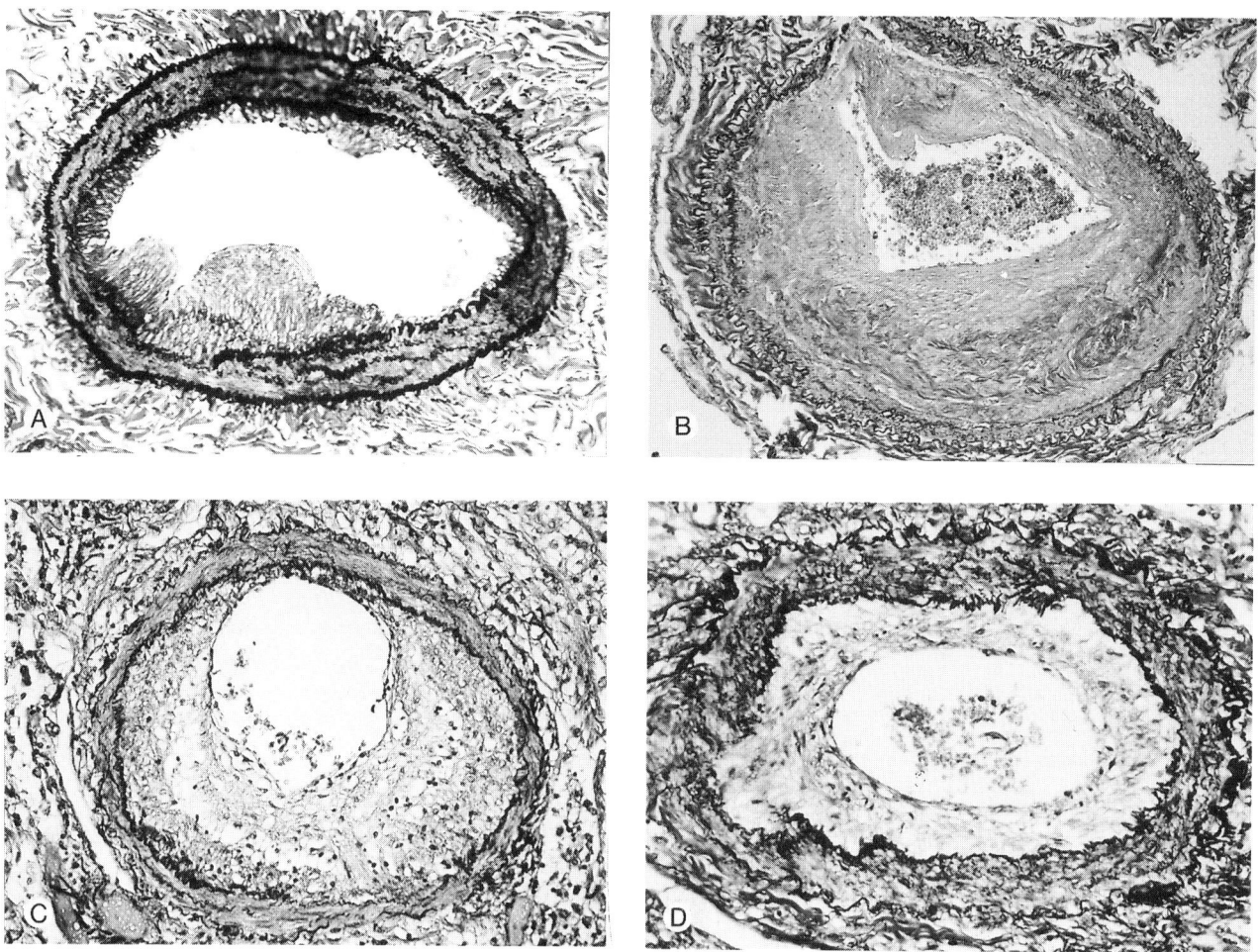

Figure 16.6 Intima of muscular pulmonary arteries in chronic pulmonary hypertension. (A) Shallow eccentric intimal pads. (B) Dense eccentric intimal fibrosis. (C) Eccentric intimal proliferation. (D) Concentric nonlaminar intimal proliferation. (Elastic-van Gieson.) (A, C, D) Reproduced with permission from Edwards [2], (B) from Bjornsson and Edwards [97].)

atrophy of centrilobular hepatocytes occur and may be accompanied by varying degrees of fibrosis and by abnormalities in liver function. These changes do not represent cirrhosis and regenerative nodules do not develop. Terminally, acute hemorrhagic centrilobular necrosis (shock liver) may occur.

16.4.5 COEXISTENT FORMS

In general, the major site of pulmonary vascular obstruction is either precapillary or postcapillary (Figure 16.8). Within these two broad categories, certain causes of pulmonary hypertension are associated with relatively specific types of microscopic lesions. These three interrelated features – location, etiology, and histopathology – provide the basis for a classification of pulmonary hypertension that is currently most favored among pathologists. Precapillary forms of chronic pulmonary hypertension include plexogenic, embolic, hypoxic and dietary-related arteriopathies, as well as cases associated with pulmonary fibrosis. The postcapillary forms, in contrast, are represented by pulmonary capillary hemangiomatosis, veno-occlusive disease and venous hypertension.

Occasionally, two or more forms of pulmonary vascular disease may coexist and each contribute to the hypertensive state. For example, an individual with chronic heart failure and chronic bronchitis might exhibit lesions of both the venous and hypoxic forms of pulmonary hypertension. Similarly, a patient with mitral stenosis and pulmonary venous hypertension could, because of limited activity and sluggish blood flow, develop venous thrombosis and thromboembolic pulmonary hypertension. In elderly patients with atrial septal defects, pulmonary hypertension may be attributable more to coexistent ischemic or valvular heart disease than to the congenital anomaly. Clinically, recognition of coexistent forms may be important for accurately accessing their potential reversibility.

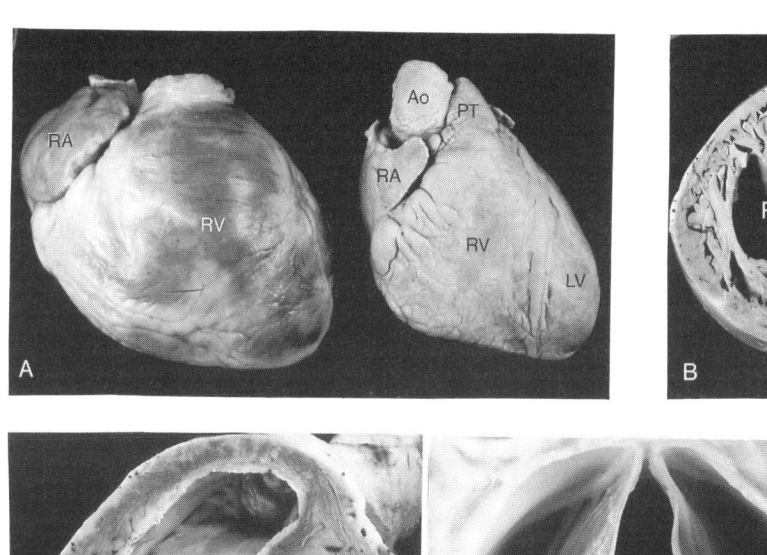
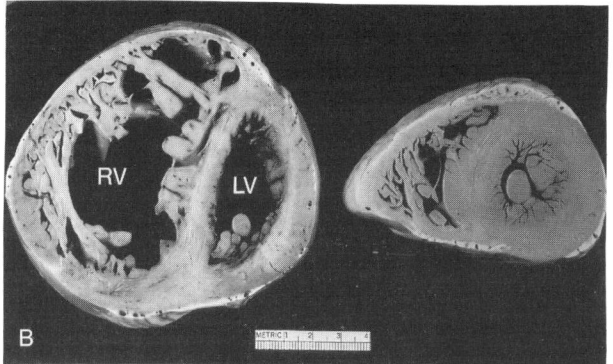
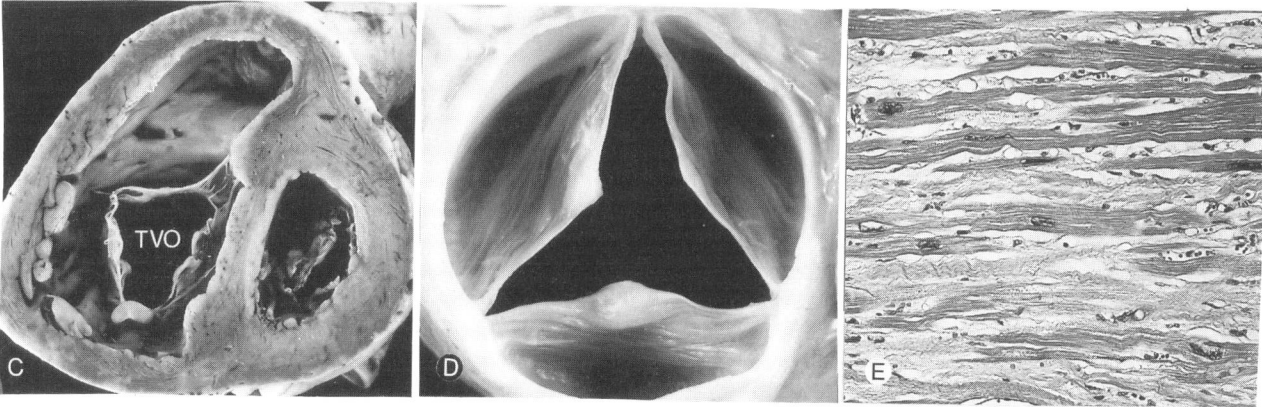

Figure 16.7 Cardac manifestations of chronic pulmonary hypertension. (A) Right ventricular (RV) and right atrial (RA) dilatation, with normal heart at right for comparison. Ao aorta; LV = left ventricle; PT = pulmonary trunk. (B) Right ventricular hypertrophy, dilatation and straightening of ventricular septum, with normal heart at right for comparison. (C, D) Valvular regurgitation, due to annular dilatation, involving tricuspid (C) and pulmonary (D) valves. TVO = tricuspid valve orifice. (E) Hypertrophied right ventricular myocytes, with interstitial fibrosis. ((E) Hematoxylin-eosin.) ((A, C) reproduced with permission from Edwards[2].)

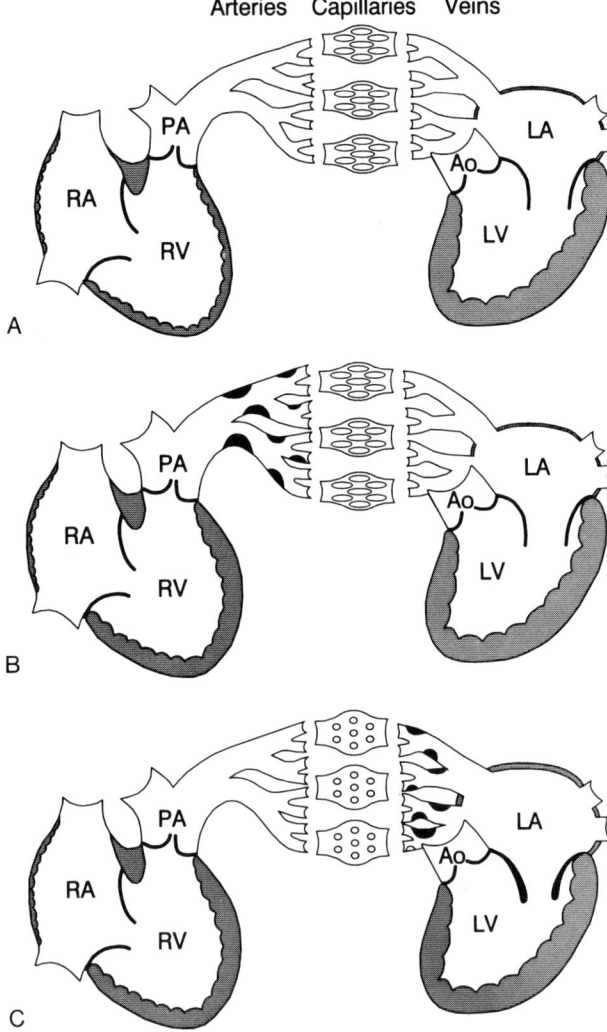

Figure 16.8 Pulmonary vascular bed. (A) Normal pulmonary vasculature and right heart, for comparison. (B) Precapillary forms of pulmonary hypertension, with obstructive lesions in pulmonary arteries and secondary right ventricular hypertrophy. (C) Postcapillary forms of pulmonary hypertension, with obstructive lesions (such as mitral stenosis, shown here) distal to capillaries. Ao = ascending aorta; LA = left atrium; LV = left ventricle; RA = right atrium; RV = right ventricle. (Redrawn with permission from Edwards [15].)

16.5 Chronic precapillary pulmonary hypertension

16.5.1 PLEXOGENIC PULMONARY HYPERTENSION

(a) General features

Plexogenic disease occurs as either a primary (idiopathic) or a secondary disorder. Disorders associated include:

- Primary pulmonary hypertension
- Secondary pulmonary hypertension
- Congenital cardiac left-to-right shunts
- Portal hypertension (cirrhosis or portacaval shunts)
- Autoimmune connective tissue diseases
- Human immunodeficiency virus (HIV-1)
- Pulmonary schistosomiasis (intra-arterial ova)
- Aminorex fumarate (appetite suppressant)
- Denatured rapeseed oil (toxic oil syndrome).

It represents a histopathologic form of pulmonary hypertension that is characterized by a constellation of lesions affecting the muscular arteries. In addition to non-specific medial hypertrophy and muscularization of arterioles, the arteries also exhibit concentric intimal proliferation, concentric laminar intimal fibrosis, fibrinoid degeneration, necrotizing arteritis, dilatation lesions and plexiform lesions. The relative proportion of these lesions varies from case to case and even within the lung. Thus, if lung biopsy specimens are too small, sampling error can result in an inaccurate assessment of the severity of pulmonary vascular disease.

In addition to the aforementioned lesions, the muscular arteries may also harbor eccentric intimal fibrosis and fresh or organized thrombi, particularly near sites of high-grade obstruction. Although the microcirculation and veins are relatively uninvolved, focal clusters of alveolar siderophages (iron-laden macrophages) are occasionally encountered. Interestingly, hyperplasia of bronchiolar endocrine cells has also been reported in patients with pulmonary hypertension and appears to be most prevalent in plexogenic arteriopathy [18]. Because of the variety of arterial lesions observed in this disorder, some investigators consider the term 'plexogenic' to be too restrictive or potentially misleading. Regardless of terminology, however, this is the only disorder, other than neoplastic embolic disease, that commonly results in systemic or suprasystemic pressure in the pulmonary circulation (i.e. systolic pressure greater than 120 mmHg).

(b) Microscopic features

Medial hypertrophy is variable in severity and appears to represent the morphologic counterpart of chronic vasoconstriction. Interestingly, the presence of appreciable hypertrophy is thought to delay the development of the more ominous intimal fibroproliferative lesions and, thereby, to impart an element of protection to the pulmonary arteries [19]. A substantial loss of distal arteries and arterioles, as evidenced by a decreased numerical density of arteries relative to alveoli, has also been reported [6,7]. However, this is a controversial topic in which not all investigators are in agreement [8,20].

Intimal proliferative lesions tend to be concentric rather than eccentric (Figure 16.9). Initially, the smooth muscle cells and myofibroblasts migrate from the media

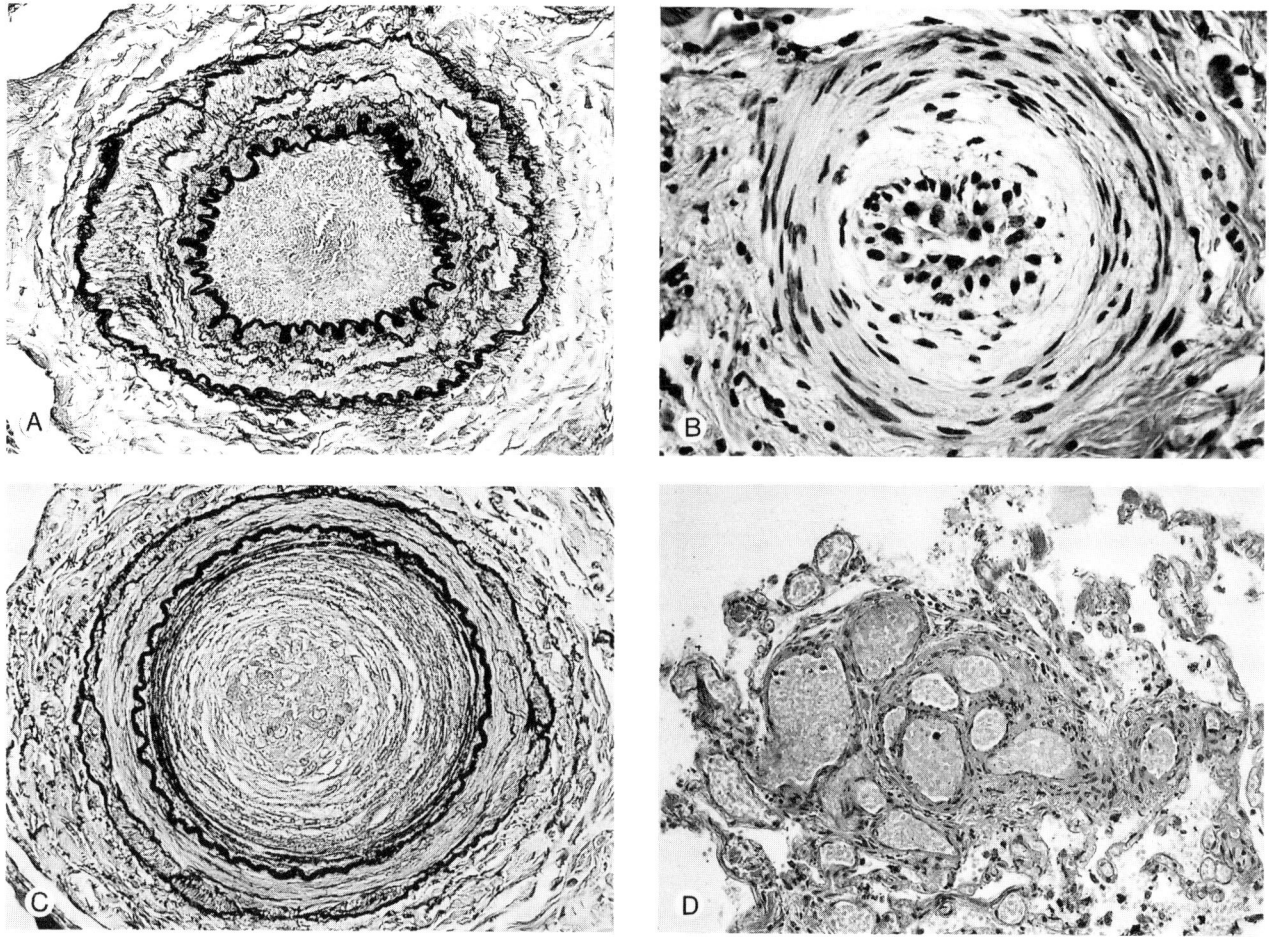

Figure 16.9 Plexogenic pulmonary hypertension, involving muscular arteries. (A) Medial hypertrophy (grade 1). (B) Concentric intimal proliferation (grade 2). (C) Concentric laminar intimal fibrosis (grade 3). (D) Dilatation lesion (grade 5). (E) Fibrinoid degeneration (arrow) (grade 6). (F) Necrotizing arteritis (arrow) (grade 6). (G, H) Plexiform lesions (grade 4), shown in longitudinal section (G) and cross-section (H). ((A, C, F, H) Elastic-van Gieson; (B, D, E, G) Hematoxylin-eosin.) (Reproduced with permission from Edwards [2] (B, E, G, H) and from Bjornsson and Edwards [97] (D).)

and grow in a radial pattern, with their nuclei arranged like spokes about the narrowed lumen [21]. As the intimal cells become more numerous, they begin to align circumferentially, like medial cells. With time, the extracellular matrix produced by intimal cells changes from glycosaminoglycans to collagen and elastin. The resulting concentric laminar intimal fibroelastosis produces an onion-skin or target-like appearance. Such lesions are generally observed in small muscular pulmonary arteries and often form prominent sphincter-like mounds just proximal to the origins of smaller branches.

Dilatation, or angiomatoid, lesions are characterized by clusters of dilated and tortuous arterial channels that develop as post-stenotic lesions or in association with medial degeneration. Fibrinoid degeneration and necrotizing arteritis are destructive medial lesions that probably represent the aftermath of severe prolonged vasospasm. Focal medial damage results in the formation of microaneurysms, which are considered to be the precursors of plexiform lesions.

Plexiform lesions typically involve small muscular pulmonary arteries near their origins from larger parent vessels. They are characterized by focal medial disruption and aneurysmal dilatation, within which forms a complex proliferative tuft of intimal cells and capillary channels (hence, the older designation as glomeruloid lesions). The proliferative tissue is composed of smooth muscle cells, myofibroblasts and fibrillary cells that resemble vasoformative reserve cells [22]. Within the complex labyrinth of capillary channels, platelets and fibrin frequently adhere and may be phagocytosed by the fibrillary cells. Distally, multiple thin-walled and dilated arterial vessels are commonly observed.

In some cases, distinction between plexiform lesions and organizing thrombi may be difficult. However, in contrast to plexiform lesions, thrombi tend to involve arteries of various sizes and are rarely associated with

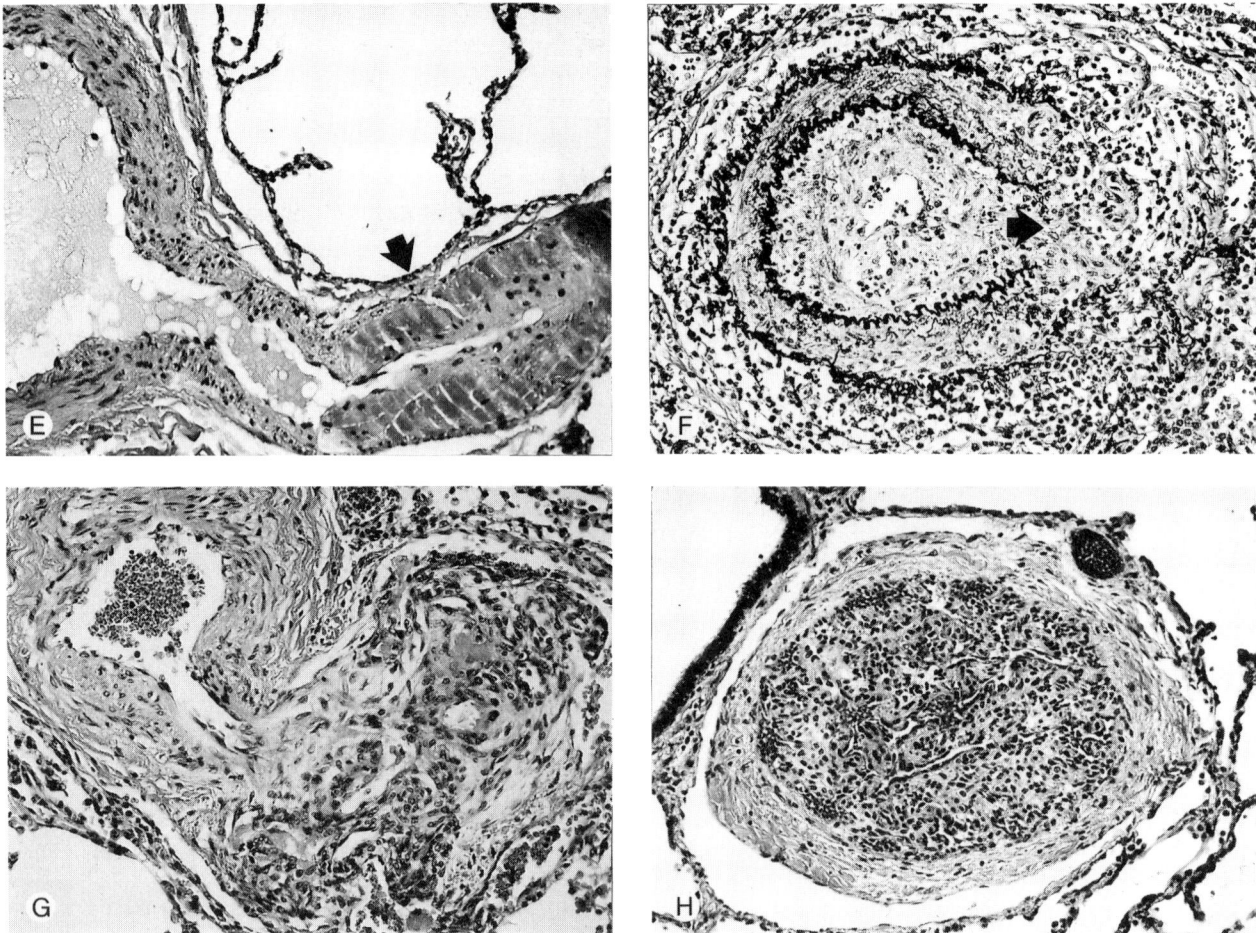

Figure 16.9 Continued

medial disruption, microaneurysms or the presence of concentric laminar intimal fibrosis. Furthermore, organizing thrombi are usually less cellular than plexiform lesions and have fewer but larger recanalization channels. In this regard, it is important to note that older plexiform lesions may become hypocellular and fibrotic.

(c) Congenital cardiac left-to-right shunts

Among patients with unoperated congenital cardiac shunts and unobstructed pulmonary blood flow, there is a tendency to develop progressive hypertensive pulmonary vascular disease. Eventually, the extent of high-grade obstructive lesions in the muscular pulmonary arteries is sufficient to render the pulmonary hypertension irreversible. At this stage, the underlying congenital heart disease becomes inoperable. Thus, the rationale for early operative intervention is to prevent the development of irreversible pulmonary vascular disease.

The types of lesions encountered and their order of appearance were first described over 35 years ago by Heath and Edwards [23]. This classification has since been modified by Wagenvoort [24] and by Rabinovitch and colleagues [25]. It is important to emphasize that use of the modified Heath–Edwards classification (Table 16.3) should be restricted *only* to patients with

Table 16.3 Modified Heath–Edwards classification

Grade	Lesion	Reversible
1A	Muscularization of arterioles	Yes
1B	Medial hypertrophy	Yes
1C	Loss of intra-acinar arteries	Yes*
2	Concentic intimal proliferation	Yes
3	Concentric laminar intimal fibrosis	Borderline†
5	Dilatation lesions	Borderline†
6	Fibrinoid degeneration	No
6	Necrotizing arteritis	No
4	Plexiform lesions	No

* Although arterial loss is irreversible, the percentage of involved vessels is usually small, such that the entire pulmonary vascular bed still exhibits potentially reversible disease. † If grade 3 or 5 lesions are mild in extent, the overall pulmonary vascular disease is generally reversible. If moderate, the disease may regress, remain unchanged or progress. If severe, however, the pulmonary vascular disease tends to be irreversible and progressive.

congenital cardiac left-to-left shunts and should *not* be applied to other forms of pulmonary hypertension. Various studies have shown that grade 1 and grade 2 lesions are potentially reversible, whereas grades 3 and 5 are borderline, with unpredictable behavior. Grades 4 and 6 represent the morphologic hallmarks of irreversible disease [26–28]. The extent to which small peripheral arteries are lost tends to increase with the higher grades [8].

There is no universal agreement concerning the grading of individual cases. For some authors, the grade applied to the whole case simply represents the highest grade lesion observed in the available lung tissue. Others advocate the use of a semiquantitative descriptive diagnosis, owing to the complexity of the various lesions [29,30]. These recommendations apply primarily to older children and adults, in whom the higher grade lesions are expected. For infants and young children, however, intimal proliferation (grade 2) is often the most severe lesion encountered. In this setting, use of the modified Heath–Edwards classification is limited because the presence of potentially reversible disease does not always correlate with operability [31]. Some infants exhibit severe pulmonary hypertension in the immediate postoperative period, presumably on a vasospastic basis, and some cases are fatal.

In the setting of congenital heart disease, the severity of pulmonary vascular disease is related not only to the patient's age but also to the underlying congenital anomaly and to individual differences in pulmonary vascular reactivity. Among subjects with an isolated atrial septal defect, the likelihood of ever developing **irreversible plexogenic pulmonary hypertension** is less than 10% [32]. Microscopically, all patients exhibit medial hypertrophy of muscular pulmonary arteries, muscularization of arterioles and dilatation of the entire pulmonary vascular bed [33,34]. Loss of intra-acinar arteries is variable. In adults, vascular dilatation is often accompanied by organized thrombi, medial fibroelastosis, mild intimal and adventitial fibrosis in the muscular arteries and by mild medial hypertrophy and intimal fibrosis in the veins [35]. It is important to emphasize that, in elderly patients with atrial septal defects, pulmonary venous hypertension due to coexistent left ventricular hypertrophy may contribute to the hypertensive state.

In contrast to interatrial communications, individuals with large unoperated ventricular septal defects are at high risk for the development of irreversible plexogenic disease. Virtually all patients who do not die of heart failure or infective endocarditis will eventually succumb to the ravages of pulmonary hypertension, usually in the third or fourth decade. Microscopically, medial hypertrophy of muscular arteries and muscularization of arterioles represent the dominant lesions during the first year of life. Between six months and one year of age, intimal hyperplasia begins to develop in the pre-acinar arteries, and the size and number of intra-acinar arteries begin to diminish [24,36–38]. Progressive intimal obstruction causes increased pulmonary vascular resistance and decreased medial hypertrophy distally. Concentric laminar intimal fibrosis and irreversible high-grade lesions usually do not develop before two years of age, but exceptions have been reported [39]. Although the sequence of vascular changes is predictable, the rate and extent of development are not and are probably determined primarily by individual differences in pulmonary vascular reactivity. Herein lies the rationale for closure of large ventricular septal defects before the age of two and perhaps during the first year of life.

Historically, in 1950, Civin and Edwards [40] observed that an adult patient with a ventricular septal defect *and* subpulmonary stenosis did not develop obstructive pulmonary vascular disease, in contrast to patients without infundibular stenosis. With this background, in 1952, Muller and Dammann [41] reported the first case of surgical narrowing of the pulmonary trunk, to prevent the development of severe and irreversible pulmonary hypertension until closure of the ventricular septal defect could be safely performed when the child was older. Since that time, regression of pulmonary vascular lesions after banding procedures has been well documented in lung biopsy specimens [16]. Although pulmonary artery banding is still being performed under certain circumstances, primary repair of the underlying anomaly at an early age is favored in most cases today.

Transposition of the great arteries warrants special mention because severe pulmonary vascular disease can develop even in the absence of a ventricular septal defect or patent ductus arteriosus. Pulmonary hypertension also tends to progress more rapidly than for isolated ventricular septal defects. Thus, transposition is the most common underlying anomaly among infants with irreversible pulmonary hypertension in the first year of life [39]. For older patients, irreversible disease develops in 8% with an intact septum and in 40% with a ventricular septal defect. The propensity for high-grade lesions to form at an early age may be related to the fact that subjects with transposition generally show less medial hypertrophy than those with isolated ventricular septal defects [19]. Between two and seven months of age, intimal proliferation is first observed in the preacinar arteries and intimal fibrosis commences thereafter. However, the arterial density decreases only after plexiform lesions develop [42]. Organized microthrombi are also commonly identified and appear to contribute to the progression of pulmonary hypertension.

Among patients with atrioventricular septal defects, those with Down's syndrome develop obstructive pulmonary vascular disease at an appreciably earlier age than individuals without this syndrome [43]. The ability of muscular pulmonary arteries to develop medial hypertrophy appears to be impaired in subjects with Down's syndrome [44]. As a result, intimal hyperplasia represents the primary vascular response to elevated pulmonary artery pressure, and it often becomes prominent during the first year of life. These changes are similar to those described for transposition of the great arteries, but they are generally less severe. Rarely, however, the development of irreversible disease, with plexiform lesions, occurs by the age of one year. Subjects with Down's syndrome may also exhibit upper airway obstruction (due to nasal hypoplasia and enlarged tonsils, adenoids and tongue), laryngomalacia, obstructive sleep apnea, inadequate clearance of secretions, recurrent pneumonias and alveolar hypoplasia, resulting in chronic hypoxia that contributes to the severity of pulmonary hypertension [45].

Plexogenic pulmonary hypertension has also been described in detail for other forms of congenital heart disease associated with shunts, including truncus arteriosus and double inlet left ventricle [46,47]. During the first year of life, observed arterial lesions include medial hypertrophy, muscularization of arterioles and intimal proliferation. Higher grade lesions generally occur in a time frame similar to that described for isolated ventricular septal defects.

(d) **Pulmonary and portal hypertension**

The coexistence of pulmonary and portal hypertension, although rare, appears to represent more than just a coincidental association. In almost all cases, the clinical diagnosis of portal hypertension either precedes or is made concurrently with that of pulmonary hypertension [48]. Hepatic cirrhosis is the most common cause of portal hypertension in this group, and many patients have undergone surgical creation of a shunt between their portal and systemic venous circulations. These observations suggest that the underlying liver disease contributes to the development of pulmonary hypertension, not *vice versa*. Currently, it is thought that dietary substances with pulmonary vasoactive properties, that normally would have been metabolized by the liver, gain access to the pulmonary circulation and induce vasoconstriction, thrombosis or intimal proliferation. It is also possible that the diseased liver produces vasoactive substances.

Microscopically, the pulmonary arteries are involved by medial hypertrophy and by intimal proliferation and fibrosis. In some patients, fibrosis and old thrombotic lesions are the major causes of luminal obstruction. Most cases, however, represent the plexogenic form of pulmonary hypertension [49]. It is of interest that platelet thrombi are frequently identified in the small arteries (and even within plexiform lesions) in fatal cases and that ante-mortem studies often demonstrate abnormalities in platelet function in these patients.

(e) **Other causes of plexogenic disease**

Plexogenic pulmonary hypertension is also known to occur in other settings (see p. 596). Pulmonary schistosomiasis has been implicated in the development of severe pulmonary hypertension and microscopic studies reveal arterial ova associated with plexiform lesions and other vascular abnormalities. It has also been reported following the use of the appetite suppressant aminorex fumarate or ingestion of denatured rapeseed oil (toxic oil syndrome), and these two topics are discussed in section 16.5 dealing with dietary-related pulmonary hypertension. Plexogenic disease can affect patients with autoimmune connective tissue disorders, as discussed in section 16.5.4 on pulmonary fibrosis. Finally, it has been reported among subjects infected with the human immunodeficiency virus (HIV-1). Currently, the virus is thought to promote the release of mediators, rather than to directly infect the pulmonary vascular endothelium [50,51].

(f) **Primary plexogenic pulmonary hypertension**

The plexogenic form of pulmonary hypertension is considered primary (idiopathic) if no cause can be established clinically. By the time the disease is diagnosed, the entire constellation of arterial lesions is usually well established, including high-grade irreversible obstructions. Consequently, even though the microscopic features are virtually identical to those described for congenital cardiac left-to-right shunts, the modified Heath–Edwards classification does not appear to be useful prognostically. The topic of primary pulmonary hypertension is covered in section 16.7.

16.5.2 EMBOLIC PULMONARY HYPERTENSION

(a) **General features**

Embolic obstruction of the pulmonary arteries, if extensive, causes elevated pulmonary vascular resistance and the development of pulmonary hypertension. The vast majority of cases are related to recurrent pulmonary thromboembolism, although non-thrombotic emboli can also produce the hypertensive state. Embolic material may obstruct the large mediastinal or lobar pulmonary arteries or, more commonly, the segmental and more peripheral elastic arteries, as well as the muscular arteries.

(b) **Chronic recurrent thromboembolism**

Thromboembolic disease generally occurs in adults and affects women more frequently than men [52]. Most emboli originate from venous thrombi in the legs or pelvis. Perhaps recurrent showers of small thromboemboli from periuterine veins, associated with the menstrual cycle, account in part for the propensity of this disease to affect young and middle-aged women. Rarely, emboli arise from thrombi elsewhere in the circulation, including the right atrium and the surfaces of indwelling catheters, such as ventriculoatrial shunts for hydrocephalus.

In general, the clinical course is characterized by classic episodes of recurrent pulmonary embolism, with acute dyspnea and chest pain, with or without pulmonary infarction. In some cases, however, the disease progresses without obvious embolic events. In this setting, thought to be the result of recurrent showers of small emboli, even ventilation-perfusion scans often fail to suggest an embolic process, and primary (idiopathic) pulmonary hypertension may be diagnosed clinically [53]. When only the small muscular pulmonary arteries are involved, even at autopsy it may be impossible to distinguish thromboembolic disease from primary thrombosis.

If untreated, patients with recurrent thromboembolic disease generally succumb within two to five years after clinical diagnosis. The most common causes of death are right heart failure and sudden death. Occasionally, paradoxical systemic embolization occurs across a patent foramen ovale and is associated with acute cerebral ischemic events [54].

Large emboli in the mediastinal or lobar pulmonary arteries commonly undergo necrosis and mummification, often with focal calcification, but with little organization and fibrosis. Although they can cause severe luminal obstruction, some are amenable to surgical extraction [55]. In classic cases of recurrent thromboembolic disease, the intrapulmonary elastic arteries characteristically show fibrous webs or bands, representing thromboemboli that have undergone partial lysis and subsequent organization.

Microscopically, the intrapulmonary elastic and muscular arteries harbor thromboemboli that generally vary in age. Old chronic lesions usually predominate and include luminal fibrous webs, recanalized channels and occlusive fibrous plugs, as well as focal eccentric fibrous intimal pads (Figure 16.10). Recent emboli include fresh and organizing thrombi and organizing lesions often have a loose myxoid appearance. Iron is commonly observed in large organized thromboemboli but is usually absent in smaller lesions. Only rarely are the muscular arteries the site of concentric laminar intimal fibrosis or medial defects suggestive of healed arteritis. Plexiform and dilatation lesions are not encountered.

Medial hypertrophy of the muscular arteries occurs in response to elevated pulmonary vascular resistance and tends to be less severe in thromboembolic disease than in the other forms of pulmonary hypertension. This indicates that the major cause of pulmonary hypertension in the setting of recurrent embolization is mechanical obstruction rather than vasoconstriction. Distal to sites of obstruction, the medial thickness of muscular arteries and arterioles is generally normal; the microcirculation and pulmonary veins are uninvolved.

(c) **Non-thrombotic embolic disease**

Rarely, non-thrombotic emboli occur in sufficient quantity to produce pulmonary hypertension. Emboli composed of fat, gas or amniotic fluid can result in fatal acute pulmonary hypertension and right ventricular failure. Moreover, in the setting of head trauma or birth trauma, embolization of brain tissue to the lungs may cause sudden death [56,57]. Neoplastic pulmonary emboli were discussed earlier as a potential cause of subacute disease that is rapidly progressive and may produce systemic levels of pulmonary artery pressure [14].

Chronic pulmonary hypertension due to embolization of non-thrombotic material most commonly occurs with helminthic infestations and intravenous drug abuse (Figure 16.11). In endemic regions, schistosomiasis is frequently associated with pulmonary hypertension. Schistosome ova impact in small muscular pulmonary arteries and incite an arteritis with secondary thrombosis, fibrosis and plexiform lesions [58]. Only rarely do other infestations, such as echinococcosis or filariasis, cause pulmonary hypertension. In the setting of chronic intravenous drug abuse, insoluble microcrystals (such as talc, starch or cellulose) accumulate in the muscular pulmonary arteries and frequently produce vascular injury and secondary thrombosis [59].

Certain conditions can mimic embolic pulmonary hypertension. Primary sarcomas of the pulmonary artery, although rare, often form intraluminal masses that resemble thromboemboli angiographically. Extrinsic compression of the mediastinal pulmonary arteries and veins may occur in patients with mediastinal fibrosis or its variant, chronic idiopathic pulmonary hilar fibrosis, and thereby also mimic embolic disease.

16.5.3 HYPOXIC PULMONARY HYPERTENSION

Chronic alveolar hypoxia is one of the most potent pulmonary vasoconstrictors known in humans. It has numerous potential causes, the most common of which is chronic bronchitis. Other causes include:

- Residence at high altitude
- Chronic upper airway obstruction
  - Congenital webs
  - Enlarged soft tissues (sleep apnea)

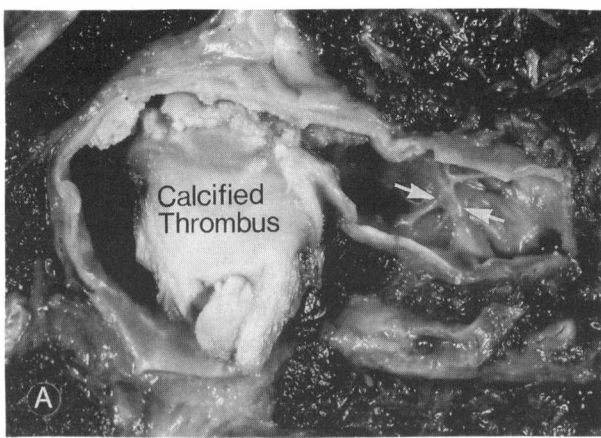
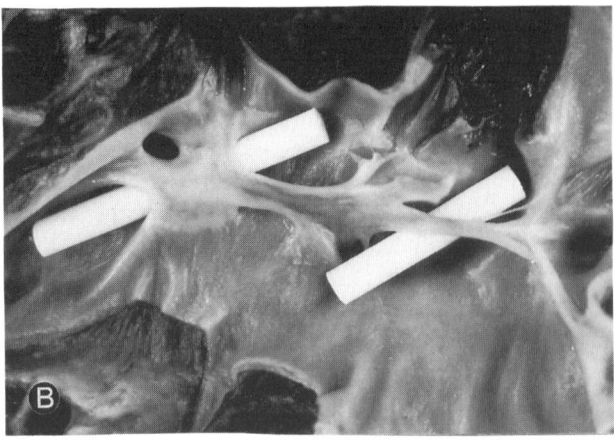
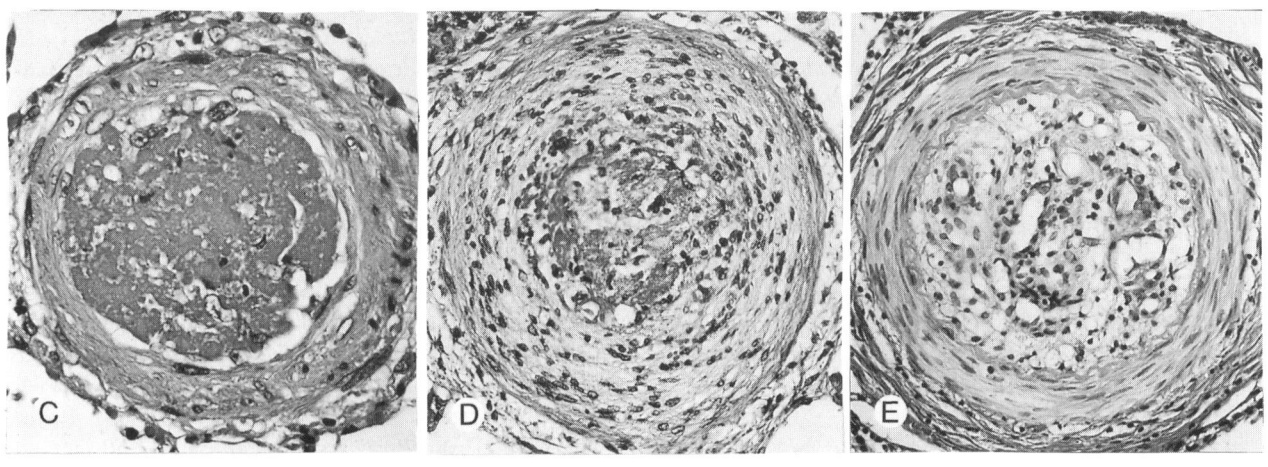
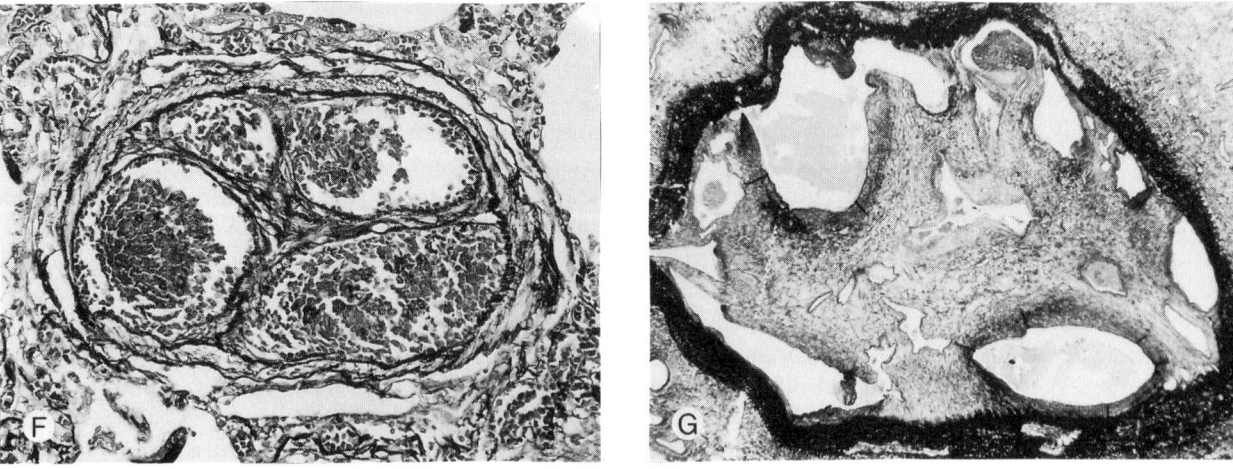

Figure 16.10 Thromboembolic pulmonary hypertension. (A, B) Gross appearances. (A) Necrotic and calcified embolus in lobar artery, and fibrous web (arrows) in segmental branch. (B) Fibrotic luminal webs (white probes) in segmental artery. (C–G) Microscopic appearances. (C) Fresh thromboembolus. (D) Organizing thrombus. (E) Early organization and recanalization (compare with plexiform lesion). (F, G) Old organized and recanalized thromboemboli, involving small muscular (F) and large elastic (G) arteries. ((C, D, E) Hematoxylin-eosin; (F, G) Elastic-van Gieson.) ((A, E, and F) Reproduced with permission from Edwards [2].)

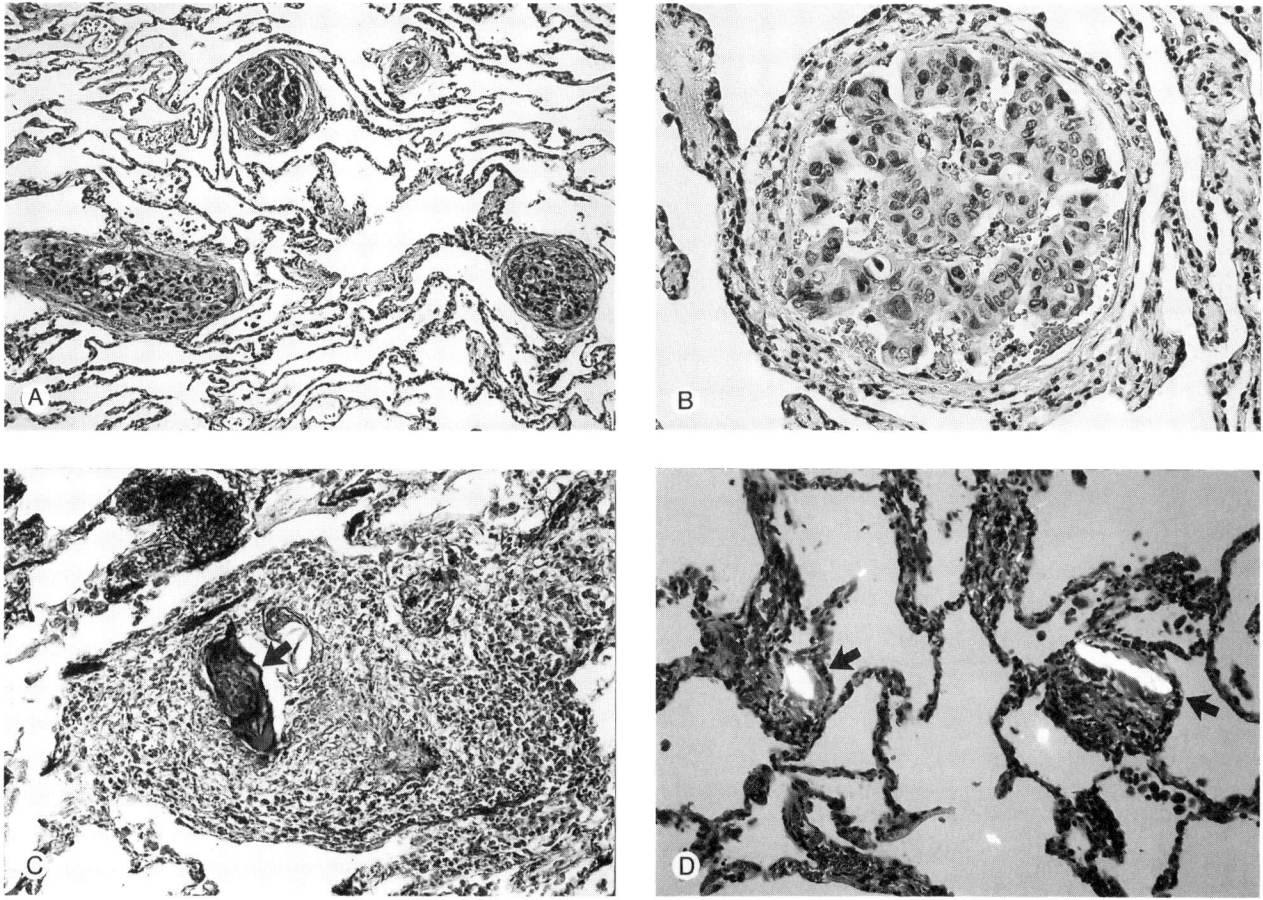

Figure 16.11 Non-thrombotic embolic pulmonary hypertension. (A, B) Neoplastic emboli. Low-power view (A) showing widespread arterial obstruction, and high-power view (B) demonstrating neoplastic nature of embolus. (C) Schistosome egg (arrow), with secondary pulmonary arteritis and intimal proliferation. (D) Arterial obstruction due to foreign-body response to talc emboli (arrows: polarized light) in chronic intravenous drug abuse. (Hematoxylin-eosin.) (Reproduced with permission from Shields and Edwards [14] (A, B) and from Edwards [2] (C).)

- Enlarged tonsils
- Enlarged tongue (Down's syndrome)
- Impaired thoracic excursion
  - Extreme obesity (Pickwickian syndrome)
  - Kyphoscoliosis
  - Thoracic ankylosing spondylitis
  - Diffuse pleural fibrosis
  - Progressive muscular dystrophy
  - Chronic poliomyelitis
- Pulmonary parenchymal diseases
  - Pulmonary emphysema
  - Chronic bronchitis
  - Asthmatic bronchitis
  - Cystic fibrosis
  - Bronchiectasis.

In most cases, polycythemia and acidosis develop in addition to the hypoxia and also contribute to the hypertensive state [60,61]. It is unclear whether the observed arterial lesions are induced by hypoxia *per se* or by secondary vasoconstriction. Subjects with Down's syndrome often exhibit several causes of chronic hypoxia, as discussed previously [44].

The most prevalent microscopic findings are medial hypertrophy of muscular pulmonary arteries and muscularization of arterioles (Figure 16.12) [62,63]. Longitudinal muscle bundles commonly involve the arterial intima, media, adventitia and the venous media, and eccentric intimal fibrosis is frequently identified. However, concentric laminar intimal fibrosis, pulmonary arteritis, dilatation lesions, and plexiform lesions are not encountered.

In destructive pulmonary parenchymal disorders such as emphysema, focal loss of capillary beds may be substantial. Bronchial arteries and veins are generally dilated and tortuous, and arterial bronchopulmonary anastomoses are prevalent, particularly in patients with bronchiectasis. Although the pulmonary vascular lesions due to chronic alveolar hypoxia are potentially reversible, the underlying cause of hypoxia often is not.

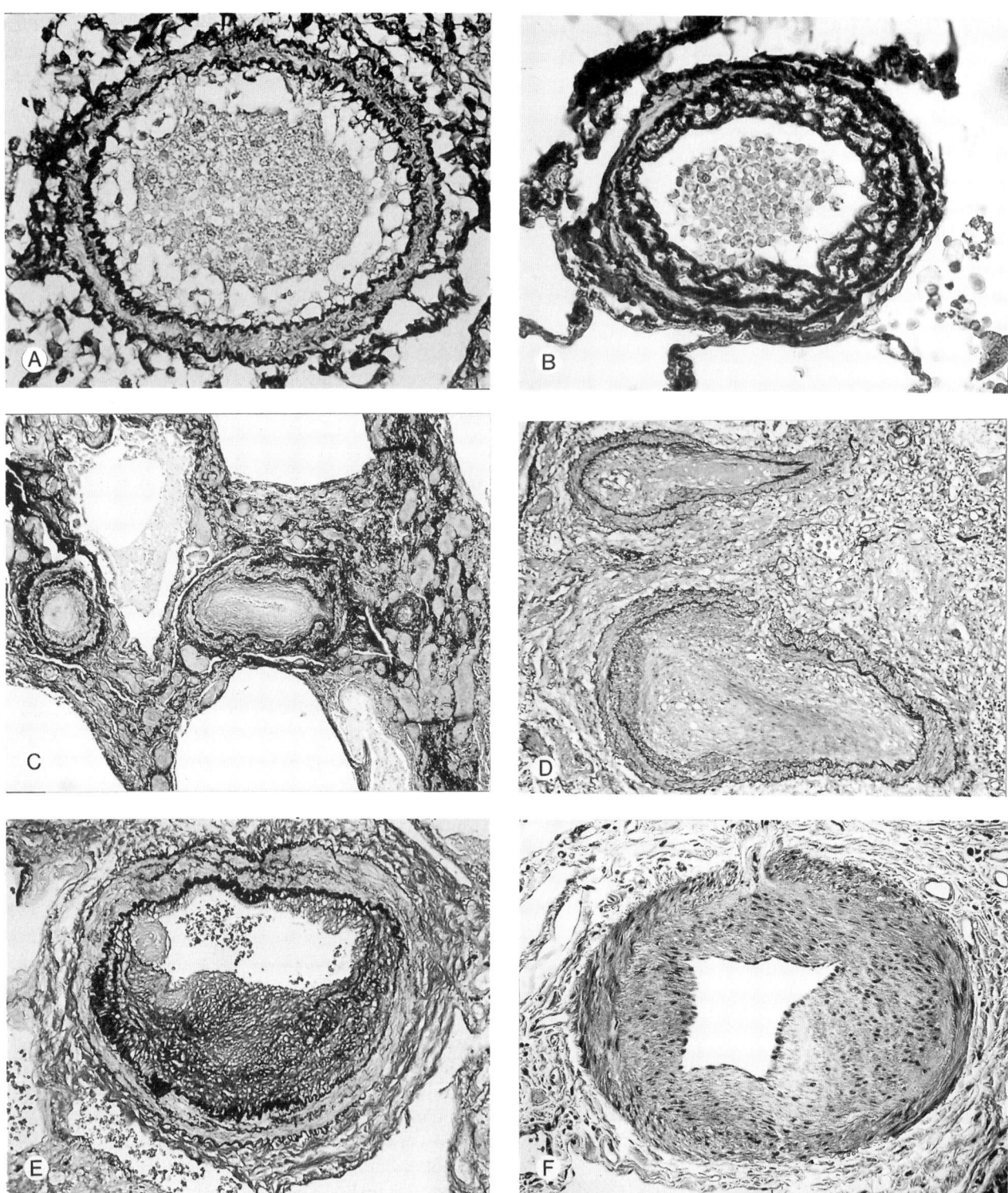

Figure 16.12 Pulmonary hypertension in chronic hypoxia and pulmonary fibrosis. (A, B) Hypoxic pulmonary hypertension, with muscular pulmonary arteries involved by medial hypertrophy (A) and longitudinal bundles of intimal smooth muscle cells (B). (C–F) Pulmonary hypertension in scleroderma with pulmonary fibrosis, showing muscular pulmonary arteries with intimal fibrosis in area of interstitial fibrosis (C), intimal fibrous plugs (D), eccentric intimal fibroelastosis (E) and concentric non-laminar intimal proliferation (F). (A–E) Elastic-van Gieson; (F) hematoxylin-eosin. ((B) Reproduced with permission from Edwards [2].)

16.5.4 PULMONARY HYPERTENSION WITH PULMONARY FIBROSIS

Patients with various chronic fibrosing disorders of the lung may develop pulmonary hypertension:

- Pulmonary interstitial fibrosis
- Pneumoconioses
- Sarcoidosis
- Autoimmune diseases
  - Scleroderma (progressive systemic sclerosis)
  - Systemic lupus erythematosus
  - Mixed connective tissue disease
  - Dermatomyositis
  - Rheumatoid arthritis.

In most cases, the vascular lesions are considered to be a result of parenchymal fibrosis and chronic alveolar hypoxia [64]. In addition, *in situ* thrombosis frequently occurs, due to stasis or vascular injury. Among patients with autoimmune connective tissue disease, particularly those with scleroderma or the CREST syndrome, it is intriguing that severe pulmonary hypertension can develop even in the absence of pulmonary fibrosis.

Microscopically, the most severely obstructive lesions are generally limited to the small pulmonary arteries, microcirculation and pulmonary veins (Figure 16.12). Medial hypertrophy and eccentric intimal fibrosis are commonly observed in both arteries and veins [65]. Other frequently encountered lesions include organized and recanalized thrombi and occlusive fibrous plugs [66]. Capillary beds are usually obliterated in areas of parenchymal fibrosis, and the aforementioned arterial and venous lesions are also most prevalent in fibrotic regions. Bronchial vessels and arterial bronchopulmonary anastomoses are dilated and may be quite prominent. Rarely, the histopathologic lesions are characteristic for plexogenic pulmonary hypertension or pulmonary veno-occlusive disease [67–70].

16.5.5 DIETARY-RELATED PULMONARY HYPERTENSION

Ingested substances, or their metabolites, may adversely affect the pulmonary circulation and induce vasoconstrictive or obstructive lesions that result in the development of pulmonary hypertension. However, because there is considerable variability in pulmonary vascular reactivity, substances that produce pulmonary hypertension in some individuals may not necessarily do so in others or in experimental animals. Thus, the results observed in animal models of pulmonary hypertension are not always applicable to humans. For example, the pyrrolizidine alkaloids, such as monocrotaline and fulvine, cause pulmonary hypertension in several animal species but not in humans [71,72]. Moreover, Jamaican bush tea, which contains pyrrolizidine alkaloids, produces hepatic veno-occlusive disease, cirrhosis and portal hypertension in humans, but it does not cause pulmonary hypertension.

Between 1967 and 1972, use of the appetite suppressant aminorex fumarate in Switzerland, West Germany and Austria was associated with an epidemic of pulmonary hypertension. In fatal cases, microscopic examination of the lungs revealed plexogenic disease in most subjects, although thrombotic lesions were prominent in some [72,73]. It is of interest that aminorex fumarate does not produce pulmonary hypertension in experimental animals.

In Spain during 1981 and 1982, the illegal use of denatured rapeseed oil as a cooking substitute for olive oil resulted in the toxic oil syndrome. Among some patients with the syndrome, particularly women, pulmonary hypertension developed as a late manifestation and was fatal in a substantial number. Microscopically, the muscular pulmonary arteries showed medial hypertrophy with focal degeneration or destruction, luminal thrombi of varying ages, eccentric intimal proliferation that was often highly obstructive, focal plexiform lesions and adventitial cuffing by lymphocytes and plasma cells [74,75]. Arterioles were muscularized, and pulmonary veins exhibited eccentric intimal proliferation and fibrosis.

Other substances have also been implicated. Recently, a case of pulmonary veno-occlusive disease was associated with the use of oral contraceptives [76].

16.6 Chronic postcapillary pulmonary hypertension

16.6.1 PULMONARY CAPILLARY HEMANGIOMATOSIS

This very rare disorder was first described in 1978 [77]. It affects adolescents and adults and may be familial. Pulmonary hypertension develops in most patients and is often considered primary (idiopathic) clinically. In contrast to other histopathologic forms of primary pulmonary hypertension that most commonly affect women, this entity shows no gender predilection. Death is usually attributable to respiratory insufficiency or right heart failure. It is unclear whether pulmonary capillary hemangiomatosis represents a neoplastic, hamartomatous or angiogenic disorder.

By low-power microscopy, patchy areas of apparent pulmonary congestion or fibrosis are observed. At higher magnification, however, the patches are characterized by a proliferation of capillary-size channels within the pulmonary parenchyma (Figure 16.13). Although this vasoformative tissue primarily invades the walls of alveoli and veins, it may also infiltrate the walls of arteries and airways, as well as the pleura and

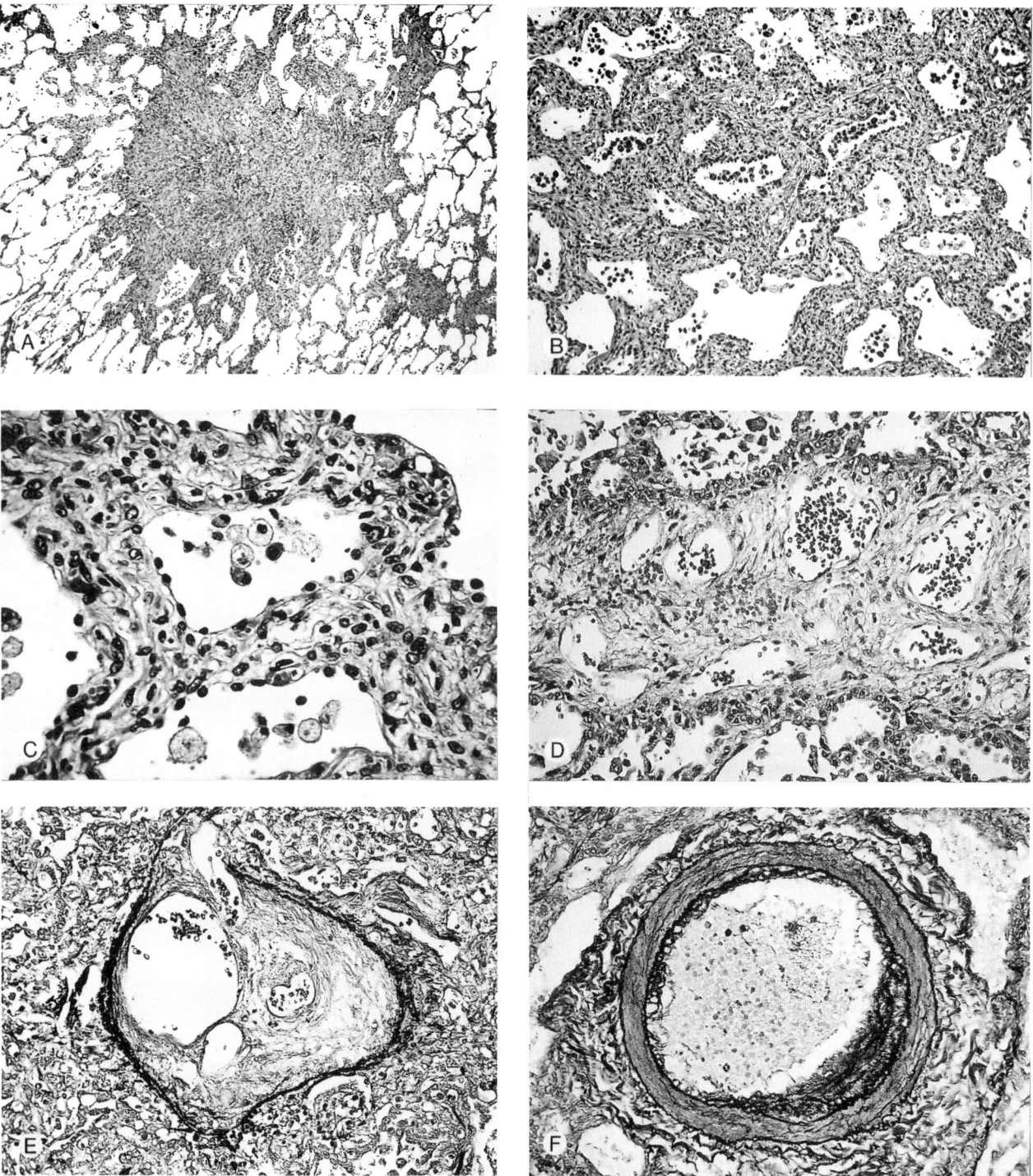

Figure 16.13 Pulmonary capillary hemangiomatosis. (A) Low-power view, showing focal nodular distribution. (B) Medium-power view, with thickened alveolar walls. (C, D) High-power views, showing capillary proliferation in alveolar walls (C) and interlobular septum (D). (E) Organized and recanalized thrombus in small pulmonary vein. (F) Medial hypertrophy and eccentric intimal fibrosis of muscular pulmonary artery. ((A–D) Hematoxylin-eosin; (E, F) elastic-van Gieson.)

interlobular septa [78–81]. Projection of vascular channels along both sides of affected alveolar walls is a characteristic feature. Luminal extension and obstruction are most prominent in veins but may also involve airways.

16.6.2 PULMONARY VENO-OCCLUSIVE DISEASE

This rare disorder primarily affects children, adolescents and young adults, although occurrences in infants and older adults have been described. Some cases are familial, and some are associated with hypertrophic cardiomyopathy [82]. There appears to be no gender predilection. Like most forms of pulmonary hypertension, the disease is characterized by progressive dyspnea. Although some cases are clinically thought to represent primary plexogenic disease, pulmonary congestion and interstitial edema are commonly observed radiographically and suggest postcapillary obstruction. Death usually occurs within two to three years after diagnosis of the hypertensive state and may be sudden or related to right ventricular failure. Rarely, the disease has a more rapid subacute course [83].

The microscopic hallmark of pulmonary veno-occlusive disease is the presence of organized and recanalized thrombi within pulmonary venules and veins (Figure 16.14) [84]. Eccentric intimal fibrosis also commonly effects these vessels and is considered to represent organized mural thrombus. Only rarely, however, is fresh thrombus observed. Veins are also involved by medial hypertrophy and by so-called arterialization (i.e. the acquisition of a distinct external elastic lamina). Occasionally, active pulmonary phlebitis is identified and may be granulomatous. In this regard, it is important to note that sarcoidosis may simulate pulmonary veno-occlusive disease [85].

As pressure becomes elevated in the pulmonary vascular bed proximal to the venous obstructions, numerous secondary microcirculatory and arterial lesions develop, including capillary congestion, interstitial and pleural edema, dilatation of interstitial and pleural lymphatics and alveolar clusters of siderophages (hemosiderin-laden macrophages). In addition to medial hypertrophy, seen in all forms of chronic pulmonary hypertension, the small muscular arteries may exhibit eccentric intimal fibrosis and organized thrombus, similar to the lesions described within pulmonary veins [86]. Not observed, however, are concentric laminar intimal fibrosis, pulmonary arteritis, dilatation lesions or plexiform lesions.

16.6.3 PULMONARY VENOUS HYPERTENSION

Overall, the most common cause of pulmonary hypertension is obstruction distal to the pulmonary veins. The causes of obstruction are numerous and include left ventricular hypertrophy or dysfunction, mitral or aortic valve disease, and others:

- Pulmonary veins
  - Fibrosing mediastinitis
  - Mediastinal neoplasm
  - Congenital pulmonary vein stenosis
  - Anomalous pulmonary venous connection
- Left atrium
  - Cardiac myxoma
  - Ball valve thrombus
  - Cor triatriatum
- Mitral valve
  - Mitral stenosis
  - Mitral regurgitation
- Left ventricle
  - Chronic heart failure
  - Constrictive pericarditis
  - Restrictive cardiomyopathy
  - Hypertrophic cardiomyopathy
  - Congenital subaortic stenosis
- Aortic valve
  - Aortic stenosis
  - Aortic regurgitation
- Thoracic aorta
  - Supravalvular aortic stenosis
  - Coarctation of aorta.

Chronic pulmonary venous hypertension is associated with engorgement of the entire pulmonary vascular bed, which may interfere with pulmonary function [87]. Secondary medial and intimal lesions develop, all of which are potentially reversible if the cause of obstruction is relieved, but their regression may take months to years [88,89].

Microscopically, the pulmonary veins and venules are involved by dilatation, medial hypertrophy, arterialization (with acquisition of a distinct external elastic lamina) and focal eccentric intimal fibrosis (Figure 16.15) [90]. Microcirculatory lesions are prominent and include capillary congestion and dilatation, septal and pleural edema, dilatation of interstitial and pleural lymphatics, focal alveolar edema, hemorrhages and clusters of siderophages [91]. This constellation of findings serves to distinguish the postcapillary forms of pulmonary hypertension from precapillary forms. Edema and fibrosis of interlobular septa are responsible for the Kerley B lines seen radiographically. In contrast to veno-occlusive disease, organized and recanalized venous thrombi are not a feature of pulmonary venous hypertension.

As a result of increased blood flow through bronchopulmonary venous anastomoses, the bronchial veins appear congested and dilated [92]. Arterioles are muscularized and muscular pulmonary arteries are commonly involved by prominent medial hypertrophy, as well as by appreciable intimal and adventitial fibrosis [93]. The intimal lesions are thought to represent organized *in situ* thrombi, due to stasis. Rarely, pulmonary arteritis occurs [94]. However, regardless of the severity or duration of pulmonary venous hypertension, there is no development of concentric laminar intimal fibrosis, dilatation lesions or plexiform lesions.

16.7 Primary pulmonary hypertension

16.7.1 GENERAL FEATURES

Among patients with pulmonary hypertension, there exists a group in whom no underlying cardiopulmonary

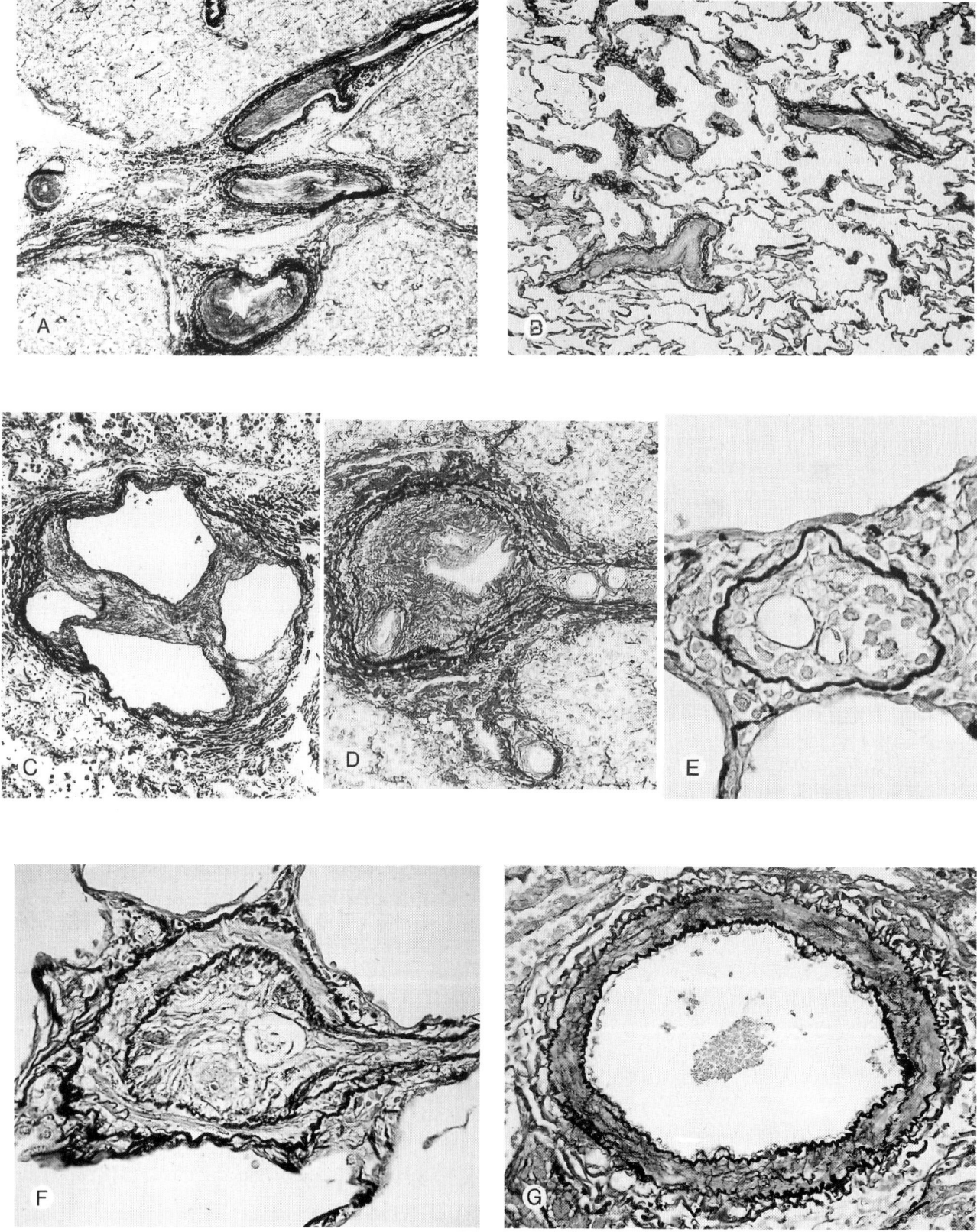

Figure 16.14 Pulmonary veno-occlusive disease. (A, B) Low-power views, showing obstructive intimal fibrosis of pulmonary veins in interlobular septum (A) and pulmonary interstitium (B). (C–E) Organized and recanalized thrombi, involving small veins (C, D) and venule (E). (F, G) Arterial lesions, showing organized thrombus (F) and medial hypertrophy (G). (See Figure 16.15 for other lesions encountered with pulmonary veno-occlusive disease.) (Elastic-van Gieson.)

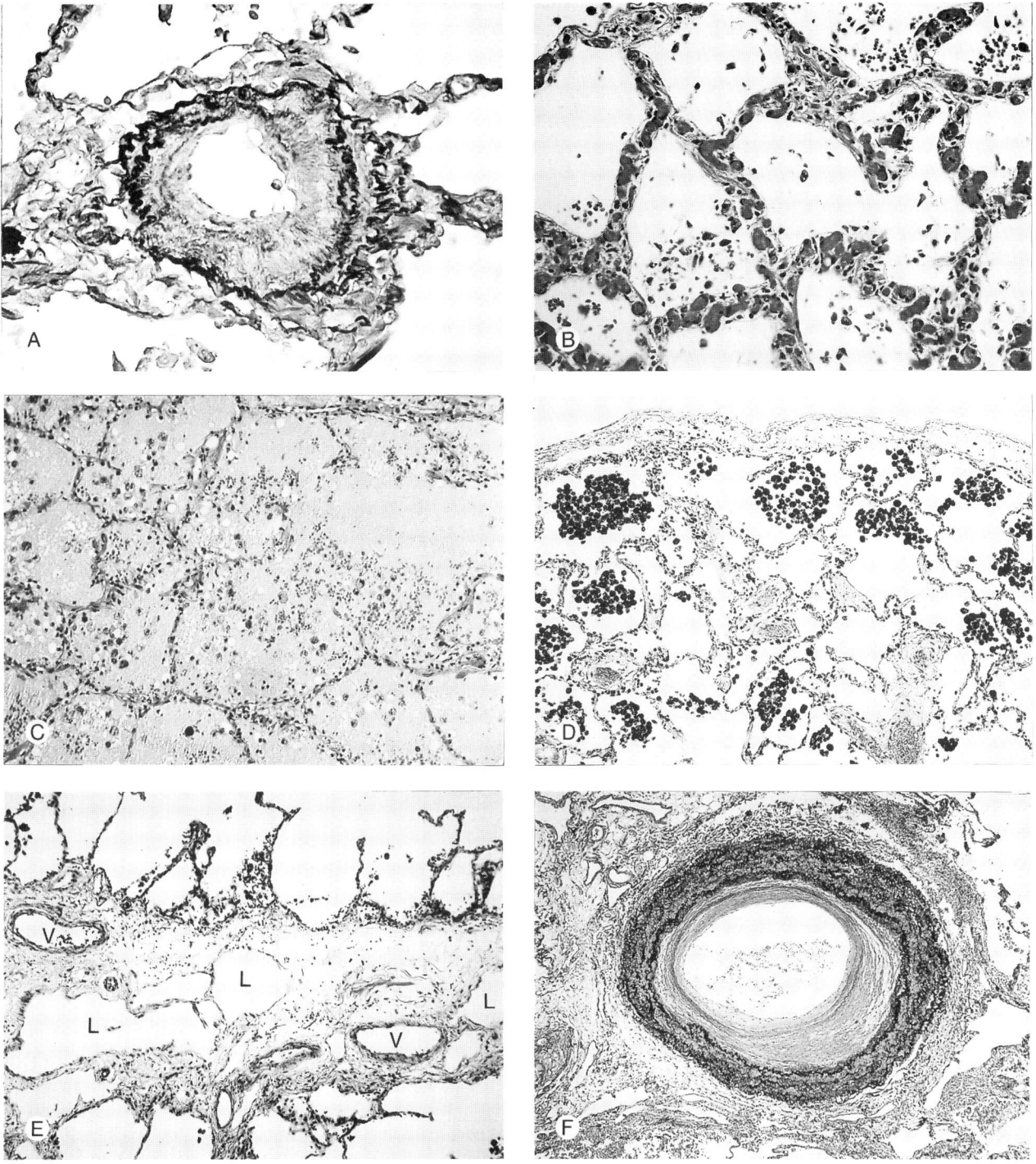

Figure 16.15 Chronic pulmonary venous hypertension. (A) Pulmonary vein, showing arterialization and eccentric intimal fibrosis. (B) Engorgement of microcirculation. (C) Hemorrhagic pulmonary edema. (D) Alveolar clusters of siderophages. (E) Dilatation of septal lymphatics (L), and edema of interlobular septum, V = pulmonary vein. (F) Secondary medial hypertrophy and eccentric intimal fibrosis of pulmonary artery. ((A, F) Elastic-van Gieson; (B–E) hematoxylin-eosin.) ((C–E) Reproduced with permission from Edwards [2].)

disorder can be identified to explain the hypertensive state clinically. Such patients are considered to have primary (idiopathic) pulmonary hypertension. Although this disorder represents a single entity clinically, several different patterns have been identified microscopically. The plexogenic and thrombotic forms of pulmonary hypertension are the two most commonly observed patterns (Table 16.4) [94a–99].

Table 16.4 Features of primary pulmonary hypertension in five clinicopathologic studies

Year of study	Cases (n)	Age in years (mean (range))	Gender ratio (F:M (n))	Histopathologic type (n (%))			
				Plexogenic	Thrombotic	PVOD	Other
1970 [99]	156	28 (1–76)	2.1 (105:51)	110 (71)	31 (20)	5 (3)	10 (6)
1980 [98]	40	34 (2–63)	1.0 (20:20)	14 (35)	12 (30)	2 (5)	12 (30)
1985 [97]	80	35 (2–71)	1.7 (50:30)	22 (28)	45 (56)	5 (6)	8 (10)
1989 [96]	58	34 (6–66)	1.5 (35:23)	25 (43)	19 (33)	7 (12)	7 (12)
1991 [95]	101	33 (2–66)	0.9 (49:52)	56 (56)	13 (13)	25 (25)	7 (7)
Total	435	32 (1–76)	1.5 (259:176)	228 (52)	120 (28)	44 (10)	44 (10)

PVOD = pulmonary veno-occlusive disease.

Table 16.5 Features of primary pulmonary hypertension in five clinical studies

Year of study	Cases (n)	Age in years (mean (range))	Gender ratio (F:M (n))	Symptoms to diagnosis (yr)	Diagnosis to death (yr)	Symptoms to death (yr)
1984 [107]	120	34 (3–64)	2.6 (87:33)	–	5*	–
1986 [106]	34	30 (1–45)	3.3 (26:8)	3	4	7
1987 [105]	87	33 (14–69)	3.6 (68:19)	–	3	–
1987 [104]	90	30 (13–48)	2.6 (65:25)	2	3.5	5.5
1987 [103]	187	36 (1–81)	1.7 (118:69)	2	–	–
Total	518	34 (1–81)	2.4 (364:154)	2–3	3–5	5.5–7

* Within five years, 79% were dead, but 21% survived longer.

Some investigators consider these patterns to be distinct and, therefore, indicative of several possible basic defects in the pulmonary vasculature. Others, however, interpret the numerous microscopic patterns to be more consistent with individual variability in response to a single basic defect. Different investigators have proposed that the basic lesion is most likely vasoconstriction, endothelial injury, intimal proliferation or arteriolar loss [100,101]. However, because pulmonary tissue from biopsy or autopsy is usually available only late in the course of the disease, the vascular lesions are generally advanced and highly obstructive. Consequently, the primary lesion in most cases is probably masked, altered or destroyed, such that its identification becomes more a matter of speculation than observation. Our current understanding of the pathobiology of primary pulmonary hypertension is insufficient to determine with certainty either the nature or number of basic defects.

Primary pulmonary hypertension occurs in women twice as frequently as in men and tends to affect young and middle-aged adults. Familial cases have also been reported [102]. The time interval between diagnosis and death is generally three to five years (Table 16.5) [103–107]. Survival rates at one, three and five years are approximately 65%, 50% and 35%, respectively [108]. Thus, it is important to emphasize that nearly one-third of patients are still alive five years after diagnosis. Subjects with thrombotic disease tend to have a longer survival than those with plexogenic or other forms [97]. Rarely, primary pulmonary hypertension regresses spontaneously [106,109].

Clinically, the mean pulmonary arterial pressure is usually about 60 mmHg, although systemic levels have been reported [95,103–105]. Survival, however, depends more on the integrity of right ventricular function than on pulmonary arterial pressure, and right heart failure is the most common cause of death. Sudden death claims about 25% of the patients, occurs twice as often with plexogenic disease as in the other histopathologic forms, and is prevalent among patients with severe hypoxemia. Occasionally, sudden death represents the initial manifestation of primary pulmonary hypertension and is investigated as a forensic case [110].

It is also recognized that certain secondary forms of pulmonary hypertension can mimic primary disease and should be included in the differential diagnosis. These include recurrent thromboembolism, chronic alveolar hypoxia, pulmonary fibrosis, mediastinal fibrosis, veno-occlusive disease and capillary hemangiomatosis. Schistosomiasis, sarcoidosis, neoplasms and amyloidosis may also present clinically like primary pulmonary hypertension [14,99,111]. In some patients, the distinction between primary and secondary disease can only be resolved by microscopic evaluation of lung tissue, either at open lung biopsy or autopsy.

16.7.2 NOMENCLATURE

In 1973, a meeting of the World Health Organization (WHO) was convened to discuss primary pulmonary hypertension; three histopathologic forms were recognized:

1. plexogenic pulmonary arteriopathy;
2. recurrent pulmonary thromboembolism;
3. pulmonary veno-occlusive disease [112].

Since that time, concepts have changed and additional microscopic patterns have been described, such that the original classification warrants modification.

According to the WHO report, plexogenic disease included not only cases with plexiform lesions but also those with only medial hypertrophy or concentric laminar intimal fibrosis. This is based on the assumption that the primary form progresses in a manner similar to that observed with congenital cardiac left-to-right shunts. However, because this developmental sequence has not been demonstrated in patients with primary pulmonary hypertension, it seems premature to diagnose plexogenic disease in cases that lack plexiform lesions [97].

The embolic nature of recurrent pulmonary thromboembolism is also being questioned. Because *in situ* thrombosis is likely in some cases, the designation of this category as thrombotic disease is probably more accurate. Additionally, in the absence of fresh thrombus or luminal fibrous webs, the interpretation of eccentric intimal fibrosis and luminal fibrous plugs as thrombotic in origin seems speculative and fibrotic disease may be a better term.

It is generally agreed that when plexiform lesions coexist with thrombotic or fibrotic lesions, plexogenic disease is considered the primary disorder and the other processes represent secondary features. Expanding this concept, some investigators have perceived plexogenic disease as the only true form of primary pulmonary hypertension [113]. However, because thrombotic and fibrotic lesions may be idiopathic processes, the removal of thrombotic or veno-occlusive disease from the group of disorders known collectively as primary pulmonary hypertension seems unwarranted at the present time.

For these reasons, a more descriptive system of nomenclature is recommended (Table 16.6). Until a better understanding of the disease is achieved, a classification system based on the unchanging microscopic features seems preferable to one based on potentially changing perceptions about the underlying pathogenesis.

16.7.3 HISTOPATHOLOGIC PATTERNS

Plexogenic disease represents the most prevalent microscopic form of primary pulmonary hypertension and accounts for about 50% of the cases. Microscopic findings include medial hypertrophy of muscular pulmonary arteries, muscularization of arterioles, intimal proliferation, concentric laminar intimal fibrosis, dilatation lesions, fibrinoid degeneration, necrotizing arteritis and plexiform lesions (Figure 16.16). Although the relative proportion of the different abnormalities varies from case to case, all are characterized by unequivocal plexiform lesions. Concentric laminar intimal fibrosis tends to be more prominent in adults than in children [114]. Organized thrombi are also commonly observed as secondary lesions [115]. In some cases, fresh platelet-fibrin thrombi are plentiful, particularly within plexiform lesions.

Taken collectively, the thrombotic and fibrotic patterns account for about 30% of all cases of primary pulmonary hypertension and have a somewhat better prognosis than the plexogenic or veno-occlusive forms [96,97]. Although there is no clinical evidence of thrombotic obstruction within the mediastinal, lobar or segmental pulmonary arteries, the muscular and small elastic arteries exhibit organized and recanalized thrombi microscopically (Figure 16.17). Eccentric fibrosis and luminal fibrous plugs are also characteristic and may represent the only obstructive lesions encountered (Figure 16.18). The high-grade lesions of plexogenic disease are not observed.

Table 16.6 Histopathologic forms of primary pulmonary hypertension

Descriptive diagnosis	WHO classification
Primary pulmonary hypertension	
Plexogenic type	Plexogenic pulmonary arteriopathy
Thrombotic type	Recurrent pulmonary thromboembolism
Fibrotic type (concentric or occlusive)	Recurrent pulmonary thromboembolism
Fibrotic type (concentric laminar)	Plexogenic pulmonary arteriopathy
Arteritis type	Plexogenic pulmonary arteriopathy
Medial hypertrophy type	Plexogenic pulmonary arteriopathy
Medial defect type	Not designated
Misaligned vessel type	Not designated
Pulmonary veno-occlusive disease	Pulmonary veno-occlusive disease
Pulmonary capillary hemangiomatosis	Not designated

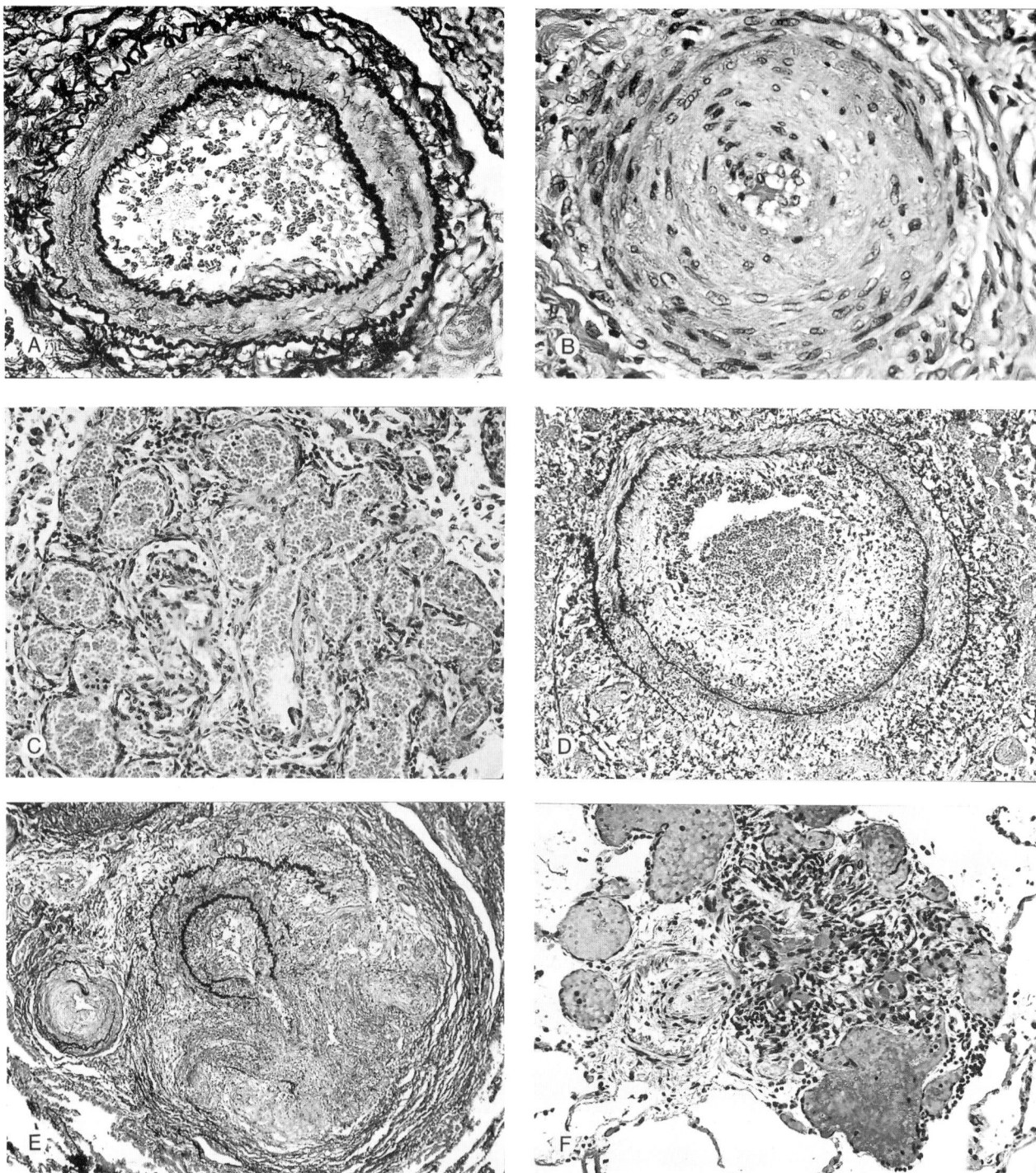

Figure 16.16 Primary pulmonary hypertension, plexogenic type, involving muscular pulmonary arteries. (A) Medial hypertrophy. (B) Concentric laminar intimal proliferation. (C) Dilatation lesion. (D) Pulmonary arteritis. (E, F) Plexiform lesions. ((A, D, E) Elastic-van Gieson; (B, C, F) hematoxylin-eosin.) ((C, E) Reproduced with permission from Edwards [2].)

Idiopathic non-granulomatous pulmonary arteritis represents a very rare disorder that affects elastic and muscular vessels in children and young adults [97,116]. Although it is characterized by focal arterial destruction and secondary thrombosis, it appears to differ from the plexogenic and thrombotic forms of primary pulmonary hypertension (Figure 16.19). Giant cell pulmonary arteritis has also been described as a cause of pulmonary hypertension.

Cases without plexiform lesions, but which primarily exhibit the other microscopic features of plexogenic pulmonary hypertension, are best categorized according

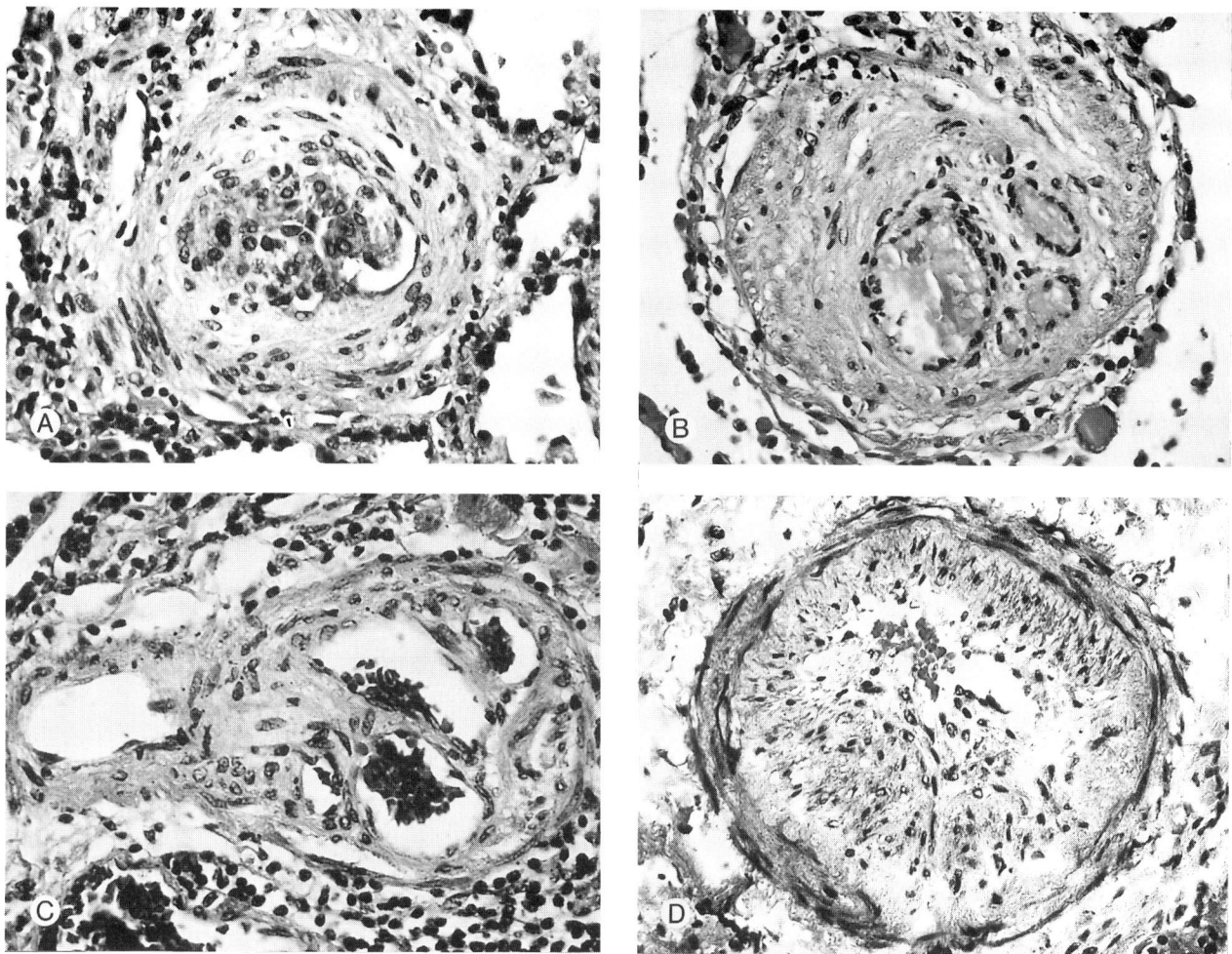

Figure 16.17 Primary pulmonary hypertension, thrombotic type, involving small muscular pulmonary arteries. (A) Organizing thrombus. (B, C) Old organized and recanalized thrombi. (D) Eccentric intimal fibrosis. (Hematoxylin-eosin.)

to the most severe lesions identified. In some patients, medial hypertrophy is the only observed lesion and, rarely, its extent is surprisingly mild (Figure 16.19) [96,97]. In other cases, medial hypertrophy is accompanied by concentric laminar intimal fibrosis, with or without arteritis [117].

Pulmonary veno-occlusive disease represents an idiopathic disorder that accounts for about 10% of the cases of primary pulmonary hypertension. If pulmonary congestion and edema are not particularly prominent, the postcapillary nature of the disease may be inapparent clinically and can resemble the arterial forms of hypertensive pulmonary vascular disease. Microscopically, however, fibrosis and organized thrombi within pulmonary veins are widespread.

The remaining 10% of cases include such rare disorders as pulmonary capillary hemangiomatosis. Recently, two new forms of pulmonary hypertension that appear to be congenital in nature have been described: medial defects in pulmonary arteries, associated with intimal proliferation and fibrosis and misaligned pulmonary vessels [118,119].

16.7.4 RATIONALE FOR THERAPY

Medial hypertrophy is present in virtually all forms of primary pulmonary hypertension and is thought to represent the morphologic counterpart of chronic vasoconstriction [21]. Intimal proliferation of smooth muscle cells and myofibroblasts is another prevalent feature of primary pulmonary hypertension. Migration of these cells from the media and their expansion in the intima are related to the release of various mediators, including platelet-derived growth factor from smooth muscle cells [100,101]. Thrombosis also plays a prominent role in most forms of primary pulmonary hypertension, either as a primary or secondary phenomenon.

These observations provide the rationale for clinical therapy with pulmonary vasodilators, platelet inhibitors

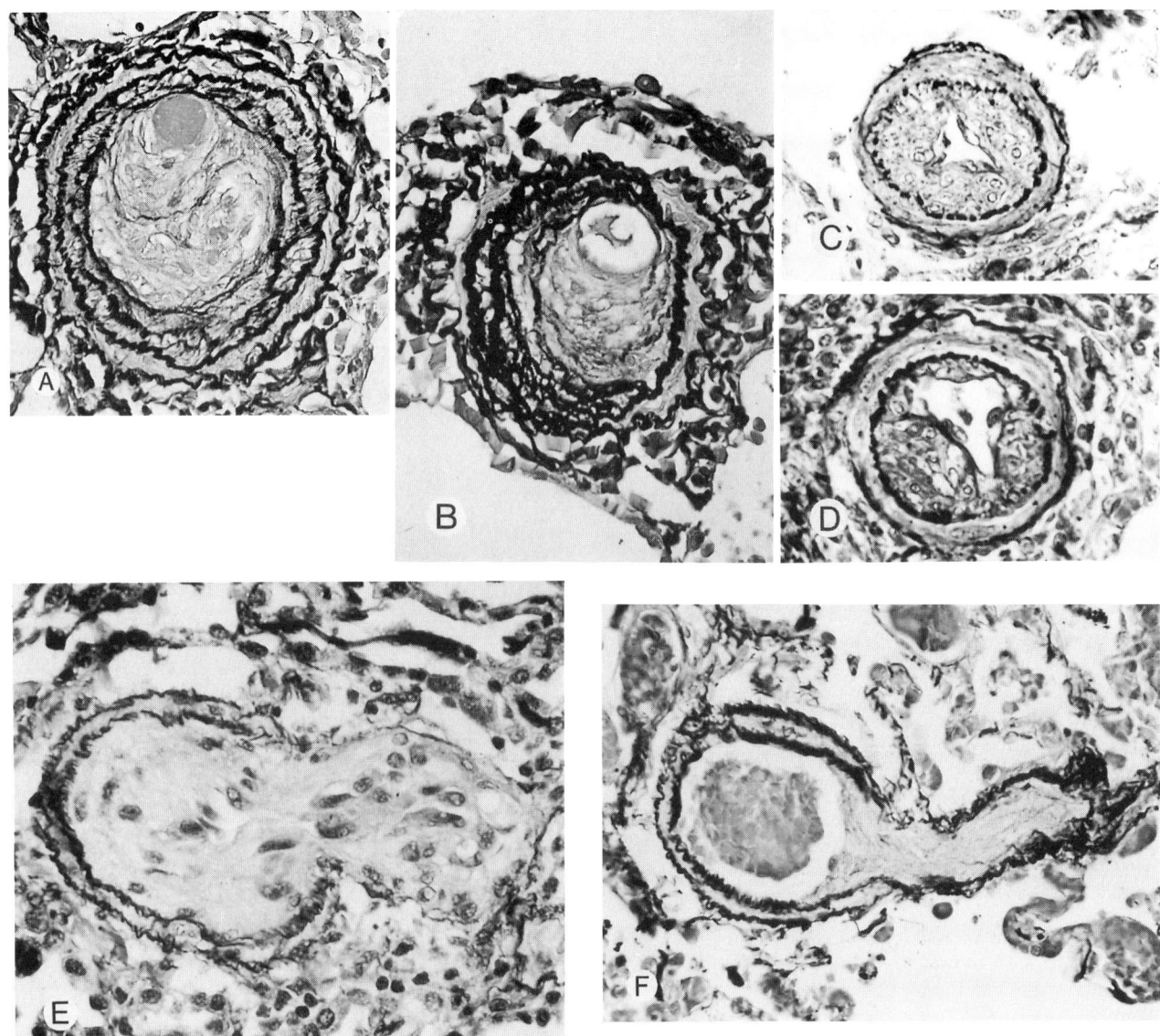

Figure 16.18 Primary pulmonary hypertension, fibrotic type, involving small muscular pulmonary arteries. (A, B) Eccentric intimal fibrosis. (C, D) Proliferative intimal pads. (E) Obstructive intimal proliferation involving small artery and arteriolar branch. (F) Fibrous plug in pulmonary arteriole. (Elastic-van Gieson.) ((C–F) Reproduced with permission from Edwards [2].)

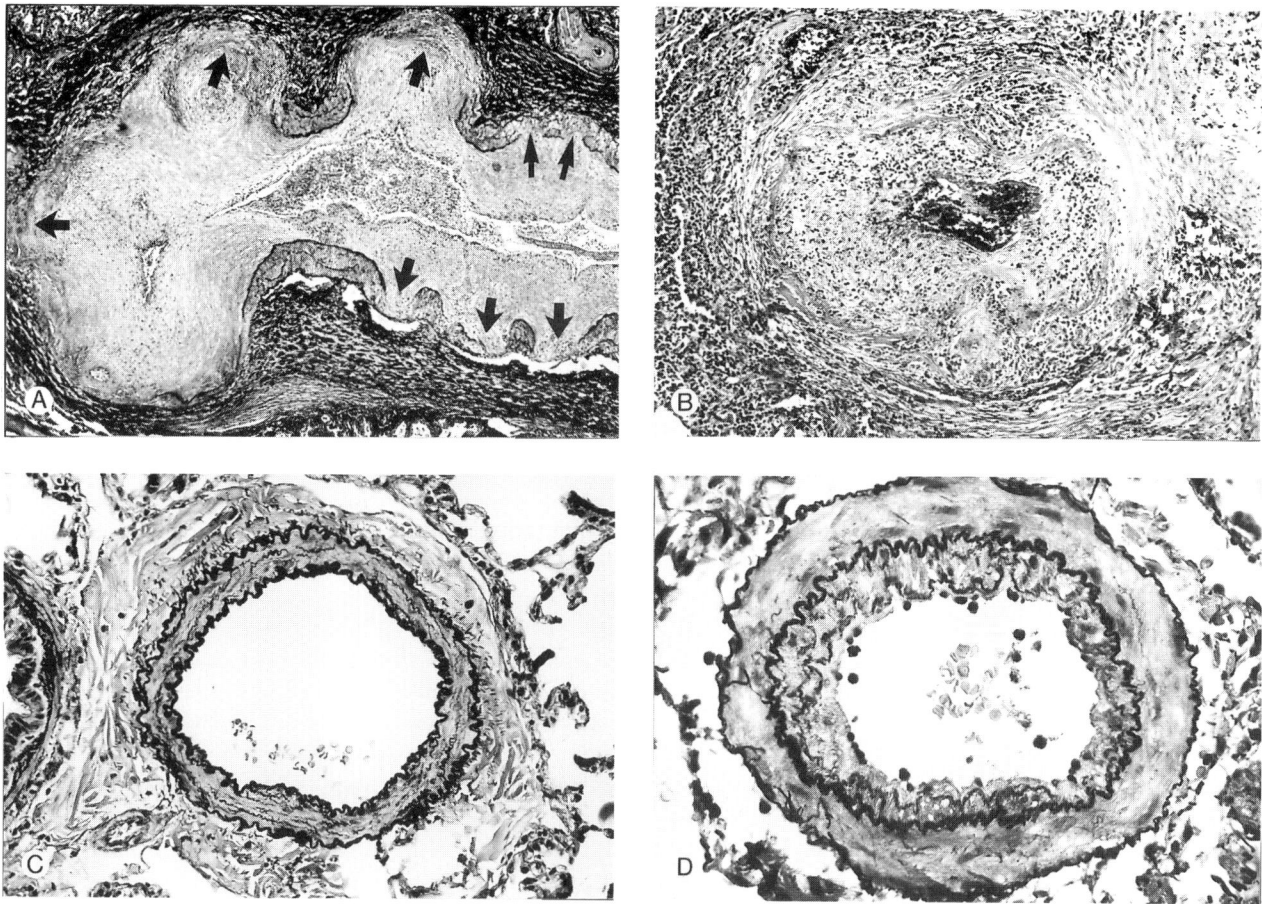

Figure 16.19 Primary pulmonary hypertension, other types, involving muscular pulmonary arteries. (A, B) Pulmonary arteritis in 11-year-old girl, with numerous medial disruptions (arrows) and secondary intimal proliferation (A) and inflammatory infiltrate (B). (C, D) Isolated medial hypertrophy in 8-year-old boy (C) and 68-year-old woman (D). Mild intimal thickening is considered age-related (D). ((A, C, D) Elastic-van Gieson; (B) hematoxylin-eosin.) ((A) Reproduced with permission from Edwards [2].)

and anticoagulants. For vasodilators, however, limited effectiveness in the pulmonary circulation and adverse reactions in the systemic circulation have appreciably restricted their usefulness. The success of antiplatelet and anticoagulation therapy has also been sporadic. Currently, the use of high-dose calcium channel blockers and the continuous intravenous infusion of prostacyclin are being investigated and appear efficacious [120].

The relatively high rate of unsuccessful medical treatment probably reflects the advanced and presumably irreversible nature of the obstructive pulmonary vascular lesions that already exist at the time of initial clinical diagnosis. Although the duration of the asymptomatic stage of primary pulmonary hypertension is unknown, at least two to three years usually elapse between the onset of symptoms and diagnosis. Better therapeutic results may depend in part on earlier detection of the hypertensive state. Presently, if medical treatment fails, lung transplantation is an option for selected patients [121–123].

16.8 Open lung biopsy

16.8.1 GENERAL FEATURES

Open lung biopsy may be useful in the evaluation of patients with primary pulmonary hypertension or underlying congenital heart disease. In addition, biopsy specimens from patients with dyspnea and pulmonary parenchymal disease may also show appreciable pulmonary vascular lesions. To minimize the likelihood of sampling error, specimens should be at least 2 cm in greatest dimension and should not be limited to the immediate subpleural region. If the vascular disease is not uniform in distribution, then biopsies of both lungs or of the upper and lower lobes may be indicated. Whether vascular changes in lingular biopsies are representative of the remainder of the lung, however, is controversial [124,125].

Fixation of the lung biopsy tissue in a distended state is recommended and is best achieved by transbronchial or transalveolar injection of formalin under low manual pressure from a syringe with a 27-gauge needle [126]. After fixation, the specimen should be sectioned in multiple parallel planes such that the arteries and their adjacent airways are cut in cross-section. Slides should be prepared from at least three levels in the paraffin block and stained with hematoxylin–eosin and elastic-van Gieson. Iron and trichrome stains are considered optional.

For the proper interpretation of biopsy tissues, pathologists must have access to certain clinical information. This includes the patient's age, gender, history of cardiopulmonary and systemic disorders, pulmonary artery and wedge pressures, results of ventilation–perfusion scans, if performed, and the lobe from which the biopsy specimen was taken. For patients with congenital heart disease, it is important to know not only the nature of the underlying anomalies but also the previous cardiac operations and the planned future operations.

16.8.2 PRIMARY PULMONARY HYPERTENSION

Among patients with clinically unexplained pulmonary hypertension, open lung biopsy is useful in selected cases to exclude secondary forms of the disease and to define the microscopic pattern of disease [98]. Currently, however, therapy is not different for the various subtypes, and the results of therapeutic regimens have not been evaluated based on the morphologic patterns. In addition, when lung transplantation is planned, some surgeons consider postbiopsy pleural adhesions to be a contraindication [127].

If an open lung biopsy is performed, it is important to emphasize that unequivocal plexiform lesions should be identified before rendering a diagnosis of plexogenic pulmonary hypertension [96]. An elastic-van Gieson stain is particularly helpful for distinguishing plexiform lesions from organizing thrombus. Plexiform lesions affect small muscular pulmonary arteries at sites of previous arteritis and microaneurysm formation, whereas organizing thrombi involve arteries of varying sizes and generally show no evidence of previous arteritis or aneurysmal dilatation. Other microscopic patterns of primary pulmonary vascular disease were discussed earlier (Table 16.6). Use of the modified Heath–Edwards classification is **not** appropriate for primary pulmonary hypertension.

16.8.3 CONGENITAL HEART DISEASE

Numerous studies have substantiated the usefulness of open lung biopsy for evaluating operability in the setting of congenital heart disease [16,25–28,31,33,36–38,42,46,47,128]. For infants and young children, the most prominent pulmonary arterial lesions are medial hypertrophy, muscularization of arterioles, focal intimal proiferation and, in some, loss of peripheral vessels. At this age, vascular reactivity changes as lung maturation occurs, and postnatal persistence of pulmonary hypertension tends to be associated with a labile vascular system. As a result, the presence of reversible lesions does not always correspond to a successful postoperative outcome [42,128]. After surgical repair of the congenital malformation, some patients exhibit severe episodic or continuous pulmonary hypertension, presumably on the basis of vasospasm or persistent vasoconstriction, respectively.

Use of the modified Heath–Edwards classification is recommended for older children and adults with congenital heart disease. Medial hypertrophy and intimal proliferation are considered reversible processes (Table 16.3). In patients with intimal fibrosis or dilatation lesions, the pulmonary vascular disease is borderline, and it may regress, remain unchanged or progress, in an unpredictable manner, postoperatively. Fibrinoid degeneration, necrotizing arteritis and plexiform lesions represent the histopathologic hallmarks of irreversible pulmonary vascular disease. Absence of medial hypertrophy in a patient with high pulmonary resistance suggests that the obstruction, usually due to intimal fibrosis, is present in pre-acinar arteries that were not included in the biopsy specimen [37,42].

For patients with congenital cardiac left-to-right shunts, the lesions of plexogenic pulmonary hypertension should be designated both qualitatively and semiquantitatively. However, for those with left-sided cardiac obstructions or heart failure, the features of chronic pulmonary venous hypertension may also be observed, and the modified Heath–Edwards classification is **not** applicable to this form of pulmonary hypertension.

In the setting of only a single functional ventricle (as in tricuspid atresia or double inlet left ventricle), a Fontan atriopulmonary anastomosis may be performed. Because right atrial blood flows directly into the pulmonary arteries, there is no ventricular pumping chamber for the pulmonary circulation. Postoperatively, pulmonary blood flow is maintained primarily by the respiratory bellows action of the thorax and, to a lesser extent, by right atrial contractions. As a result, even only moderate degrees of medial hypertrophy or intimal fibrosis may be associated with pulmonary vascular resistances high enough to hinder adequate pulmonary blood flow. The presence of medial hypertrophy is more detrimental in patients with double-inlet left ventricle than in those with tricuspid atresia [129]. With sluggish blood flow, mural thrombi can develop in the right atrium and provide a source for recurrent pulmonary thromboembolism.

16.8.4 UNEXPLAINED CHRONIC DYSPNEA

Among patients with unexplained chronic dyspnea in whom pulmonary parenchymal disease is considered a possible cause, an open lung biopsy may be performed. In most, an interstitial or airway disorder is identified that explains the dyspnea. In areas of fibrosis, some may also harbor obstructive pulmonary vascular lesions, as discussed in the sections on hypoxic pulmonary hypertension (16.5.3) and on pulmonary hypertension with pulmonary fibrosis (16.5.4). There may be a clinical history of underlying autoimmune connective tissue disease, as well.

For other patients, however, pulmonary parenchymal disease is minimal or absent, and obstructive pulmonary vascular lesions represent the major abnormality. In this setting, the most commonly observed microscopic patterns are recurrent thromboembolism, the thrombotic and fibrotic forms of primary pulmonary hypertension, pulmonary veno-occlusive disease and chronic pulmonary venous hypertension. Evidence of heart failure, left-sided valvular disease, or other postcapillary obstructions should be sought if venous hypertension is identified. Similarly, if the features of thrombotic, fibrotic and venous hypertension coexist, a source of extrinsic vascular compression, such as mediastinal fibrosis or neoplasm, should be considered [130,131].

16.9 Related vascular disorders

16.9.1 PULMONARY VASCULITIS

Inflammation of pulmonary blood vessels may represent an isolated disorder of the lungs or part of systemic vasculitis, and it can occur with other inflammatory systemic disorders, particularly the autoimmune connective tissue diseases [117,132]. Pulmonary vasculitis is also commonly associated with granulomatous disease of the lungs or alveolar hemorrhage [133–138]. This topic is discussed in detail in Chapter 17.

Pulmonary arteritis, as a fibrinoid or necrotizing process, also occurs in the setting of pulmonary hypertension. In plexogenic disease, it is thought to result in the formation of microaneurysms that are considered to be precursors of plexiform lesions. Thus, pulmonary arteritis is not only a feature of primary pulmonary hypertension but also that associated with congenital cardiac left-to-right shunts, portal hypertension, autoimmune connective tissue diseases, human immunodeficiency virus (HIV-1), pulmonary schistosomiasis, aminorex fumarate and the toxic oil syndrome. Rarely, giant cell arteritis affects the pulmonary vasculature, either as an isolated disorder or in association with giant cell aortitis [139,140].

Pulmonary phlebitis has been observed in patients with veno-occlusive disease and tends to be a granulomatous process. In this regard, sarcoidosis has been reported to mimic pulmonary veno-occlusive disease [85].

16.9.2 PULMONARY ARTERY ANEURYSMS AND DISSECTIONS

Most pulmonary artery aneurysms are associated with one or more of the following conditions:

- congenital heart disease
- pulmonary hypertension
- weakened vessels.

This is usually as a result of cystic medial necrosis, vasculitis, or infection [141–143]. The most commonly observed forms of congenital heart disease are patent ductus arteriosus and atrial septal defect. When pulmonary hypertension pertains, it usually represents primary or secondary plexogenic disease, and the aneurysm almost always affects the mediastinal pulmonary arteries, rather than the intrapulmonary vessels. Grossly, pulmonary artery aneurysms are saccular and may harbor intimal tears and partial dissections [142]. They characteristically exhibit prominent cystic medial necrosis microscopically.

Dissection and fatal rupture of the mediastinal pulmonary arteries may also complicate chronic pulmonary hypertension, especially in patients with a patent ductus arteriosus [144–146]. Intimal tears are irregular, often multiple, and usually confined to the pulmonary trunk and its bifurcation (Figure 16.20). Thus, the fate of an intimal tear is similar to that in the aorta. The tear may remain uncomplicated, can stretch and form a so-called partial dissection, may be associated with development of an intramedial dissection, or can progress to become a through-and-through rupture. Microscopically, cystic medial necrosis is the rule.

16.9.3 PULMONARY VASCULAR NEOPLASMS

Metastatic involvement of the pulmonary vasculature has been associated with the development of subacute pulmonary hypertension or massive fatal neoplastic emboli, as discussed previously [14]. Primary tumors of the mediastinal pulmonary arteries may also produce or mimic pulmonary hypertension. Approximately 75% represent undifferentiated sarcomas, myogenous tumors (leiomyosarcomas and rhabdomyosarcomas), or fibrocytic tumors (fibrosarcomas and fibromyxosarcomas) [147–149]. The remainder include chondrosarcomas, osteosarcomas, angiosarcomas, mesenchymomas and malignant fibrous histiocytomas [150]. Angiographically, they tend to form luminal masses that may resemble large pulmonary emboli.

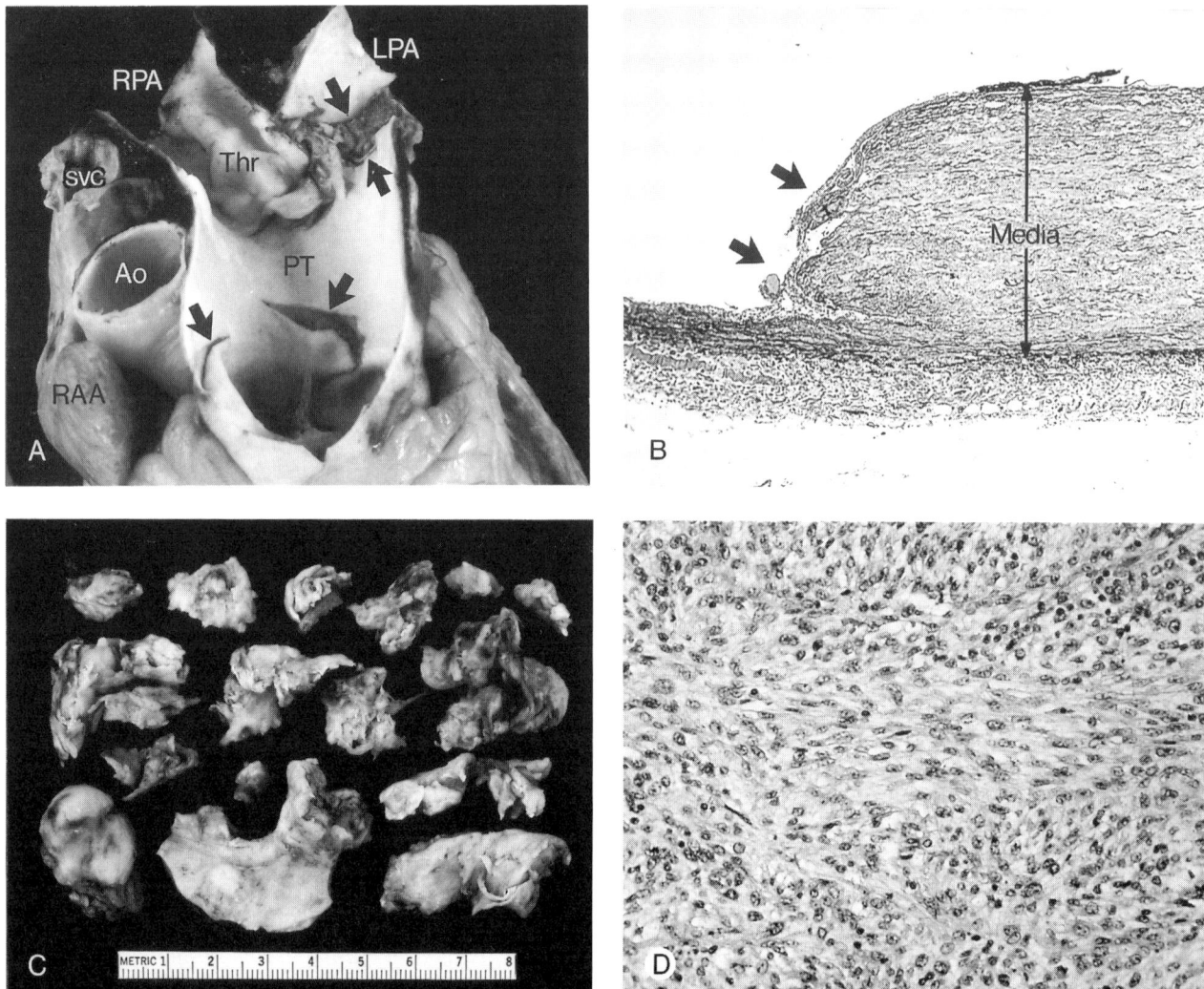

Figure 16.20 Related pulmonary vascular disorders. (A, B) Fatal rupture of pulmonary artery, involving multiple sites (arrows), in patient with chronic thromboembolic pulmonary hypertension. Ao = ascending aorta; LPA = left pulmonary artery; PT = pulmonary trunk; RAA = right atrial appendage; RPA = right pulmonary artery; SVC = superior vena cava; Thr = old organized thromboembolus. (C, D) Surgically resected leiomyosarcoma of pulmonary trunk, resembling chronic thromboembolic pulmonary hypertension angiographically. ((B) Elastic-van Gieson; (D) hematoxylin-eosin.)

Some are amenable to surgical resection (Figure 16.20). This topic is discussed in detail in Chapter 21.

References

1. Rich, S., Chomka, E., Hasara, L. et al. (1989) The prevalence of pulmonary hypertension in the United States: adult population estimates obtained from measurements of chest roentgenograms from the NHANES II survey. Chest, 96, 236–41.
2. Edwards, W.D. (1989) Pathology of pulmonary hypertension. Cardiovasc. Clin., 18, 321–59.
3. Rich, S. and Brundage, B.H. (1989) Pulmonary hypertension: a cellular basis for understanding the pathophysiology and treatment. J. Am. Coll. Cardiol., 14, 545–50.
4. Newman, J.H. and Ross, J.C. (1989) Primary pulmonary hypertension: a look at the future. J. Am. Coll. Cardiol., 14, 551–5.
5. Rabinovitch, M. (1991) Investigational approaches to pulmonary hypertension. Toxicol. Pathol., 19, 458–69.
6. Meyrick, B. and Reid, L. (1983) Pulmonary hypertension: anatomic and physiologic correlates. Clin. Chest. Med., 4, 199–217.
7. Haworth, S.G. and Hislop, A.A. (1983) Pulmonary vascular development: normal values of peripheral vascular structure. Am. J. Cardiol., 52, 578–83.
8. Takahashi, T., Wagenvoort, N. and Wagenvoort, C.A. (1983) The density of muscularized pulmonary arteries in normal lungs: a morphometric study. Arch. Pathol. Lab. Med., 107, 19–22.
9. Raine, J., Hislop, A.A., Redington, A.N. et al. (1991) Fatal persistent pulmonary hypertension presenting late in the neonatal period. Arch. Dis. Child., 66, 398–402.
10. Patterson, K., Kapur, S.P. and Chandra, R.S. (1988). Persistent pulmonary hypertension of the newborn: pulmonary pathologic aspects. Perspect. Pediatr. Pathol., 12, 139–54.
11. Rosenow III, E.C., Osmundson, P.J. and Brown, M.L. (1981) Pulmonary embolism. Mayo. Clin. Proc., 56, 161–78.
12. Spapen, H. and Vincken, W. (1991) Pulmonary arterial hypertension in sepsis and the adult respiratory distress syndrome. Acta Clin. Belg., 47, 30–41.
13. Tomashefski Jr, J.F., Davies, P., Boggis, C. et al. (1983) The pulmonary vascular lesions of the adult respiratory distress syndrome. Am. J. Pathol., 112, 112–26.
14. Shields, D.J. and Edwards, W.D. (1992) Pulmonary hypertension attributable to neoplastic emboli: an autopsy study of 20 cases and a review of literature. Cardiovasc. Pathol., 1, 279–87.
15. Edwards, J.E. (1974) Pathology of chronic pulmonary hypertension. Pathol. Ann., 9, 1–25.

16. Wagenvoort, C.A., Wagenvoort, N. and Draulans-Noë, Y. (1984). Reversibility of plexogenic pulmonary arteriopathy following banding of the pulmonary artery. *J. Thorac. Cardiovasc. Surg.*, 87, 876–86.
17. Dailey, M.E., O'Laughlin, M.P., and Smith, R.J. (1990) Airway compression secondary to left atrial enlargement and increased pulmonary artery pressure. *Int. J. Pediatr. Otorhinolaryngol.*, 19, 33–44.
18. Gosney, J., Heath, D., Smith, P. *et al.* (1989) Pulmonary endocrine cells in pulmonary arterial disease. *Arch. Pathol. Lab. Med.*, 113, 378–80.
19. Yamaki, S. and Wagenvoort, C.A. (1981) Plexogenic pulmonary arteriopathy: significance of medial thickness with respect to advanced pulmonary vascular lesions. *Am. J. Pathol.*, 105, 70–5.
20. Mooi, W. and Wagenvoort, C.A. (1983) Decreased numbers of pulmonary blood vessels: reality or artifact? *J. Pathol.*, 141, 441–7.
21. Caslin, A.W., Heath, D., Madden, B. *et al.* (1990) The histopathology of 36 cases of plexogenic pulmonary arteriopathy. *Histopathology*, 16, 9–19.
22. Heath, D., Smith, P. and Gosney, J. (1988) Ultrastructure of early plexogenic pulmonary arteriopathy. *Histopathology*, 12, 41–52.
23. Heath, D. and Edwards, J.E. (1958) The pathology of hypertensive pulmonary vascular disease: a description of six grades of structural changes in the pulmonary arteries with special reference to congenital cardiac septal defects. *Circulation*, 18, 533–47.
24. Wagenvoort, C.A. (1973) Hypertensive pulmonary vascular disease complicating congenital heart disease: a review. *Cardiovasc. Clin.*, 5, 43–60.
25. Rabinovitch, M., Haworth, S.G., Vance, Z. *et al.* (1980) Early pulmonary vascular changes in congenital heart disease studied in biopsy tissue. *Hum. Pathol.*, 11, 499–509.
26. Yamaki, S., Mohri, H., Haneda, K. *et al.* (1989) Indications for surgery based on lung biopsy in cases of ventricular septal defect and/or patent ductus arteriosus with severe pulmonary hypertension. *Chest*, 96, 31–39.
27. Braunlin, E.A., Moller, J.H., Patton, C. *et al.* (1986) Predictive value of lung biopsy in ventricular septal defect: long-term follow-up. *J. Am. Coll. Cardiol.*, 8, 1113–18.
28. Wagenvoort, C.A. (1985) Open lung biopsies in congenital heart disease for evaluation of pulmonary vascular disease: Predictive value with regard to corrective operability. *Histopathology*, 9, 417–36.
29. Wagenvoort, C.A. (1981) Grading of pulmonary vascular lesions: a reappraisal. *Histopathology*, 5, 595–8.
30. Haworth, S.G. (1987) Understanding pulmonary vascular disease in young children (editorial). *Int. J. Cardiol.*, 15, 101–3.
31. Bush, A., Busst, C.M., Haworth, S.G. *et al.* (1988) Correlations of lung morphology, pulmonary vascular resistance and outcome in children with congenital heart disease. *Br. Heart J.*, 59, 480–5.
32. Steele, P.M., Fuster, V., Cohen, M. *et al.* (1987) Isolated atrial septal defect with pulmonary vascular obstructive disease: long-term follow-up and prediction of outcome after surgical correction. *Circulation*, 76, 1037–42.
33. Yamaki, S., Horiuchi, T., Miura, M. *et al.* (1987) Secundum atrial septal defect with severe pulmonary hypertension: open lung biopsy diagnosis of operative indication. *Chest*, 91, 33–38.
34. Haworth, S.G. (1983) Pulmonary vascular disease in secundum atrial septal defect in childhood. *Am. J. Cardiol.*, 51, 265–72.
35. Schamroth, C.L., Sareli, P., Pocock, W.A. *et al.* (1987) Pulmonary arterial thrombosis in secundum atrial septal defect. *Am. J. Cardiol.*, 60, 1152–6.
36. Hall, S.M. and Haworth, S.G. (1992). Onset and evolution of pulmonary vascular disease in young children: abnormal postnatal remodelling studied in lung biopsies. *J. Pathol.*, 166, 183–93.
37. Haworth, S.G. (1987) Pulmonary vascular disease in ventricular septal defect: structural and functional correlations in lung biopsies from 85 patients, with outcome of intracardiac repair. *J. Pathol.*, 152, 157–68.
38. Fried, R., Falkovsky, G., Newburger J. *et al.* (1986). Pulmonary arterial changes in patients with ventricular septal defects and severe pulmonary hypertension. *Pediatr. Cardiol.*, 7, 147–54.
39. Alt, B. and Shikes, R.H. (1983) Pulmonary hypertension in congenital heart disease: irreversible vascular changes in young infants. *Pediatr. Pathol.*, 1, 423–34.
40. Civin, W.H. and Edwards, J.E. (1950) Pathology of the pulmonary vascular tree: I. A comparison of the intrapulmonary arteries in Eisenmenger complex and in stenosis of ostium infundibuli associated with biventricular origin of the aorta. *Circulation*, 2, 545–52.
41. Muller Jr, W.H. and Dammann, J.F. Fr (1952) The treatment of certain congenital malformations of the heart by the creation of pulmonic stenosis to reduce pulmonary hypertension and excessive pulmonary blood flow. *Surg. Gynecol. Obstet.*, 95, 213–9.
42. Haworth, S.G., Radley-Smith, R. and Yacoub, M. (1987) Lung biopsy findings in transposition of the great arteries with ventricular septal defect potentially reversible pulmonary vascular disease is not always synonymous with operablility. *J. Am. Coll. Cardiol.*, 9, 327–33.
43. Clapp, S., Perry, B.L., Farooki, Z.Q. *et al.* (1990) Down's syndrome, complete atrioventricular canal, and pulmonary vascular obstructive disease. *J. Thorac. Cardiovasc. Surg.*, 100, 115–21.
44. Yamaki, S., Horiuchi, T. and Sekino, Y. (1983) Quantitative analysis of pulmonary vascular disease in simple cardiac anomalies with the Down syndrome. *Am. J. Cardiol.*, 51, 1502–6.
45. Spicer, R.L. (1984) Cardiovascular disease in Down syndrome. *Pediatr. Clin. N. Am.*, 31, 1331–43.
46. Juaneda, E. and Haworth, S.G. (1984) Pulmonary vascular disease in children with truncus arteriosus. *Am. J. Cardiol.*, 54, 1314–20.
47. Juaneda, E. and Haworth, S.G. (1985) Double inlet ventricle: lung biopsy findings and implications for management. *Br. Heart J.*, 53, 515–19.
48. Robalino, B.D. and Moodie, D.S. (1991) Association between primary pulmonary hypertension and portal hypertension: analysis of its pathophysiology and clinical, laboratory and hemodynamic manifestations. *J. Am. Coll. Cardiol.*, 17, 492–8.
49. Edwards, B.S., Weir, E.K., Edwards, W.D. *et al.* (1987) Coexistent pulmonary and portal hypertension: morphologic and clinical features. *J. Am. Coll. Cardiol.*, 10, 1233–8.
50. Polos, P.G., Wolfe, D., Harley, R.A. *et al.* (1992) Pulmonary hypertension and human immunodeficiency virus infection: two reports and a review of the literature. *Chest*, 101, 474–8.
51. Mette, S.A., Palevsky, H.I., Pietra, G.G. *et al.* (1992) Primary pulmonary hypertension in association with human immunodeficiency virus infection: a possible viral etiology for some forms of hypertensive pulmonary arteriopathy. *Am. Rev. Respir. Dis.*, 145, 1196–200.
52. Palevsky, H.I. (1989) Pulmonary hypertension and thromboembolic disease in women. *Cardiovasc. Clin.*, 19, 267–83.
53. Rich, S., Pietra, G.G., Kieras, K. *et al.* (1986) Primary pulmonary hypertension: radiographic and scintigraphic patterns of histologic subtypes. *Ann. Intern. Med.*, 105, 499–502.
54. Lang, I., Steurer, G., Weissel, M. and Burghuber, O.C. (1988) Recurrent paradoxical embolism complicating severe thromboembolic pulmonary hypertension. *Eur. Heart J.*, 9, 678–81.
55. Moser, K.M., Auger, W.R., Fedullo, P.F. and Jamieson, S.W. (1992) Chronic thromboembolic pulmonary hypertension: clinical picture and surgical treatment. *Eur. Respir. J.*, 5, 334–42.
56. Torry, J.M. (1987) Massive brain tissue and fat pulmonary embolism following severe head injury. *Med. Sci. Law*, 27, 128–31.
57. Hauck, A.J., Bambara, J.F. and Edwards, W.D. (1990) Embolism of brain tissue to the lung in a neonate: report of a case and review of the literature. *Arch. Pathol. Lab. Med.*, 114, 217–18.
58. Chaves, E. (1966). The pathology of the arterial pulmonary vasculature in Manson's schistosomiasis. *Dis. Chest*, 50, 72–7.
59. Tomashefski Jr, J.F. and Hirsch, C.S. (1980) The pulmonary vascular lesions of intravenous drug abuse. *Hum. Pathol.*, 11, 133–45.
60. Archer, S.L., McMurtry, I.F. and Weir, E.K. (1989) Mechanisms of acute hypoxic and hyperoxic changes in pulmonary vascular reactivity. *Lung Biol. Health Dis.*, 38, 241–90.
61. Reid, L.M. (1986) Structure and function in pulmonary hypertension: new perceptions. *Chest*, 89, 279–88.
62. Wright, J.L., Petty, T. and Thurlbeck, W.M. (1992) Analysis of the structure of the muscular pulmonary arteries in patients with pulmonary hypertension and COPD: National Institutes of Health nocturnal oxygen therapy trial. *Lung*, 170, 109–214.
63. Heath, D., Williams, D., Rios-Dalenz, J. *et al.* (1990) Small pulmonary arterial vessels of Aymara Indians from the Bolivian Andes. *Histopathology*, 16, 565–71.
64. Morgan, J., Griffiths, J., du Bois, R. and Evans, T. (1991) Hypoxic pulmonary vasoconstriction in systemic sclerosis and primary pulmonary hypertension. *Chest*, 99, 551–6.
65. Pronk, L.C. and Swaak, A.J. (1991) Pulmonary hypertension in connective tissue disease: report of three cases and review of the literature. *Rheumatol. Int.*, 11, 83–86.
66. Yousem, S.A. (1990) The pulmonary pathologic manifestations of the CREST syndrome. *Hum. Pathol.*, 21, 467–74.
67. Sato, T., Matsubara, O., Tanaka, Y. and Kasuga, T. (1993) Association of Sjögren's syndrome with pulmonary hypertension: Report of two cases and review of the literature. *Hum. Pathol.*, 24, 199–205.
68. Morassut, P.A., Walley, V.M. and Smith, C.D. (1992) Pulmonary veno-occlusive disease and the CREST syndrome. *Can. J. Cardiol.*, 8, 1055–8.
69. Roncoroni, A.J., Alvarez, C. and Molinas, F. (1992) Plexogenic arteriopathy associated with pulmonary vasculitis in systemic lupus erythematosus. *Respiration*, 59, 52–56.
70. Sharma, S., Vaccharajani, A. and Mandke J. (1990) Severe pulmonary hypertension in rheumatoid arthritis. *Int. J. Cardiol.*, 26, 220–2.
71. Meyrick, B.O. and Reid, L.M. (1982) Crotalaria-induced pulmonary hypertension: Uptake of ^{3}H-thymidine by the cells of the pulmonary circulation and alveolar walls. *Am. J. Pathol.*, 106, 84–94.
72. Heath, D. and Kay, J.M. (1978) Diet, drugs, and pulmonary hypertension. *Prog. Cardiol.*, 7, 125–40.
73. Kay, J.M., Smith, P. and Heath, D. (1971) Aminorex and the pulmonary circulation. *Thorax*, 26, 262–70.
74. Gómez-Sánchez, M.A., Saenz de la Calzada, C., Gomez-Pajuelo, C. *et al.* (1990) Clinical and pathologic manifestations of pulmonary vascular disease in the toxic oil syndrome. *J. Am. Coll. Cardiol.*, 18, 1539–45.
75. Gómez-Sánchez, M.A., Mestre de Juan, M.J., Gómez-Pajuelo, C. *et al.* (1989) Pulmonary hypertension due to toxic oil syndrome: a clinico-

pathologic study. *Chest*, **95**, 325–31.
76. Townend, J.N., Roberts, D.H., Jones, E.L. and Davies, M.K. (1992) Fatal pulmonary venoocclusive disease after use of oral contraceptives. *Am. Heart J.*, **124**, 1643–14.
77. Wagenvoort, C.A., Beetstra, A. and Spijker, J. (1978) Capillary haemangiomatosis of the lungs. *Histopathology*, **2**, 401–6.
78. Wagenaar, S.S., Mulder, J.J.S., Wagenvoort, C.A. and van den Bosch, JMM. (1989) Pulmonary capillary haemangiomatosis diagnosed during life. *Histopathology*, **14**, 212–4.
79. Langleben, D., Heneghan, J.M., Batten, A.P. *et al.* (1988) Familial pulmonary capillary hemangiomatosis resulting in primary pulmonary hypertension. *Am. Intern. Med.*, **109**, 106–9.
80. Tron, V., Magee, F., Wright, J.L. *et al.* (1986) Pulmonary capillary hemangiomatosis. *Hum. Pathol.*, **17**, 1144–50.
81. Heath, D. and Reid, R. (1985) Invasive pulmonary haemangiomatosis. *Br. J. Dis. Chest*, **79**, 284–94.
82. Chetty, R., Rose, A.G., Commerford, P.J. and Taylor, D.A. (1992) Pulmonary veno-occlusive disease associated with hypertrophic cardiomyopathy. *Cardiovasc. Pathol.*, **1**, 289–93.
83. Nawaz, S., Dobersen, M.J., Blount Jr, S.G. *et al.* (1990) Florid pulmonary veno-occlusive disease. *Chest*, **98**, 1037–9.
84. Kay, J.M., de Sa, D.J. and Mancer, J.F.K. (1983) Ultrastructure of lung in pulmonary veno-occlusive disease. *Hum. Pathol.*, **14**, 451–6.
85. Hoffstein, V., Ranganathan, N. and Mullen, J.B.M. (1986) Sarcoidosis simulating pulmonary veno-occlusive disease. *Am. Rev. Respir. Dis.*, **134**, 809–11.
86. Wagenvoort, C.A., Wagenvoort, N. and Takahashi, T. (1985) Pulmonary veno-occlusive disease: involvement of pulmonary arteries and review of the literature. *Hum. Pathol.*, **16**, 1033–41.
87. Hosenpud, J.D., Stibolt, T.A., Atwal, K. and Shelley, D. (1990) Abnormal pulmonary function specifically related to congestive heart failure: comparison of patients before and after cardiac transplantation. *Am. J. Med.*, **88**, 493–6.
88. Levine, M.J., Weinstein, J.S., Diver, D.J. *et al.* (1989) Progressive improvement in pulmonary vascular resistance after percutaneous mitral valvuloplasty. *Circulation*, **79**, 1061–7.
89. Camara, M.L., Aris, A., Padro, J.M. and Caralps, J.M. (1988) Long-term results of mitral valve surgery in patients with severe pulmonary hypertension. *Ann. Thorac. Surg.*, **45**, 133–6.
90. Randhawa, R.S., Chopra, P. and Tandon, H.D. (1983) Autopsy study of pulmonary vascular changes in patients with rheumatic mitral stenosis. *Indian J. Med. Res.*, **78**, 681–8.
91. Haworth, S.J., Hall, S.M. and Patel, M. (1988) Peripheral pulmonary vascular and airway abnormalities in adolescents with rheumatic mitral stenosis. *Int. J. Cardiol.*, **18**, 405–16.
92. Ohmichi, M., Tagaki, S., Nomura, N. *et al.* (1988) Endobronchial changes in chronic pulmonary venous hypertension. *Chest*, **94**, 1127–32.
93. Wagenvoort, C.A. and Wagenvoort, N. (1982) Smooth muscle content of pulmonary arterial media in pulmonary venous hypertension compared with other forms of pulmonary hypertension. *Chest*, **81**, 581–5.
94. Cornell, W.B., Rosenkranz, E., Moodie, D.S. and Ratliff, N.B. (1991). Pulmonary hypertension with necrotizing arteritis secondary to congenital mitral stenosis. *Pediatr. Cardiol.*, **12**, 184–5.
94a. Rubin, L.J. (1993) Primary pulmonary hypertension (ACCP consensus statement). *Chest*, **104**, 230–50.
95. Burke, A.P., Farb, A. and Virmani, R. (1991) The pathology of primary pulmonary hypertension. *Mod. Pathol.*, **4**, 269–82.
96. Pietra, G.G., Edwards, W.D., Kay, J.M. *et al.* (1989) Histopathology of primary pulmonary hypertension: a qualitative and quantitative study of pulmonary blood vessels from 58 patients in the National Heart, Lung, and Blood Institute, primary pulmonary hypertension registry. *Circulation*, **80**, 1198–206.
97. Bjornsson, J. and Edwards, W.D. (1985) Primary pulmonary hypertension: a histopathologic study of 80 cases. *Mayo Clin. Proc.*, **60**, 16–25.
98. Wagenvoort, C.A. (1980) Lung biopsy specimens in the evaluation of pulmonary vascular disease. *Chest*, **77**, 614–25.
99. Wagenvoort, C.A. and Wagenvoort, N. (1970) Primary pulmonary hypertension: a pathologic study of the lung vessels in 156 clinically diagnosed cases. *Circulation*, **42**, 1163–84.
100. Heath, D., Smith, P., Gosney, J. *et al.* (1987) The pathology of the early and late stages of primary pulmonary hypertension. *Br. Heart J.*, **58**, 204–13.
101. Haworth, S.G. (1983) Primary pulmonary hypertension. *Br. Heart J.*, **49**, 517–21.
102. Loyd, J.E., Atkinson, J.B., Pietra, G.G. *et al.* (1988) Heterogeneity of pathologic lesions in familial primary pulmonary hypertension. *Am. Rev. Respir. Dis.*, **138**, 952–7.
103. Rich, S., Dantzker, D.R., Ayres, S.M. *et al.* (1987) Primary pulmonary hypertension: a national prospective study. *Ann. Intern. Med.*, **107**, 216–23.
104. Glanville, A.R., Burke, C.M., Theodore, J. and Rovin, E.D. (1987). Primary pulmonary hypertension: length of survival in patients referred for heart-lung transplantation. *Chest*, **91**, 675–81.
105. Kanemoto, N. (1987) Natural history of pulmonary hemodynamics in primary pulmonary hypertension. *Am. Heart J.*, **114**, 407–13.
106. Rozkovec, A., Montanes, P. and Oakley, C.M. (1986) Factors that influence the outcome of primary pulmonary hypertension. *Br. Heart J.*, **55**, 449–58.
107. Fuster, V., Steele, P.M., Edwards, W.D. *et al.* (1984) Primary pulmonary hypertension: natural history and the importance of thrombosis. *Circulation*, **70**, 580–7.
108. D'Allonzo, G.E., Barst, R.J., Ayres, S.M. *et al.* (1991) Survival in patients with primary pulmonary hypertension: results from a national prospective registry. *Ann. Intern. Med.*, **115**, 343–9.
109. Fujii, A., Rabinovitch, M. and Matthews, E.C. (1981) A case of spontaneous resolution of idiopathic pulmonary hypertension. *Br. Heart J.*, **46**, 574–7.
110. Ackermann, D.M. and Edwards, W.D. (1987) Sudden death as the initial manifestation of primary pulmonary hypertension: report of four cases. *Am. J. Forensic Med.*, **8**, 97–102.
111. Veinot, J.P., Edwards, W.D. and Kyle, R.A. (1993) Pulmonary vascular amyloid causing pulmonary hypertension: report of a case and review of literature. *Cardiovasc. Pathol.*, **2**, 231–5.
112. Hatano, S. and Strasser, T. (1975) *Primary Pulmonary Hypertension: Report on a WHO Meeting*, Geneva, October 15–17, 1973. WHO, Geneva, pp. 9–45.
113. Anderson, E.G., Simon, G. and Reid, L. (1973) Primary and thromboembolic pulmonary hypertension: a quantitative pathological study. *J. Pathol.*, **110**, 273–93.
114. Yamaki, S. and Wagenvoort, C.A. (1985) Comparison of primary plexogenic arteriopathy in adults and children: a morphometric study in 40 patients. *Br. Heart J.*, **54**, 428–34.
115. Wagenvoort, C.A. and Mulder, P.G. (1993) Thrombotic lesions in primary plexogenic arteriopathy: similar pathogenesis or complication? *Chest*, **103**, 844–9.
116. Clausen, K.P. and Geer, J.C. (1969) Hypertensive pulmonary arteritis. *Am. J. Dis. Child.*, **118**, 718–24.
117. Juaneda, E., Watson, H. and Haworth, S.G. (1985) An unusual case of rapidly progressive primary pulmonary hypertension in childhood. *Int. J. Cardiol.*, **7**, 306–9.
118. Wagenvoort, C.A. (1986) Medial defects of lung vessels: a new cause of pulmonary hypertension. *Hum. Pathol.*, **17**, 722–6.
119. Wagenvoort, C.A. (1986) Misalignment of lung vessels: a syndrome causing persistent neonatal pulmonary hypertension. *Hum. Pathol.*, **17**, 727–30.
120. Palevsky, H.I. and Fishman, A.P. (1991) The management of primary pulmonary hypertension. *J. Am. Med. Ass.*, **265**, 1014–20.
121. Starnes, V.A., Stinson, E.B., Oyer, P.E., *et al.* (1991) Single lung transplantation: A new therapeutic option for patients with pulmonary hypertension. *Transplant. Proc.*, **23**, 1209–10.
122. Maurer, J.R., Winton, T.L., Patterson, G.A. and Williams, T.R. (1991) Single-lung transplantation for pulmonary vascular disease. *Transplant. Proc.*, **23**, 1211–12.
123. Levine, S.M., Gibbons, W.J., Bryan, C.L. *et al.* (1990) Single lung transplantation for primary pulmonary hypertension. *Chest*, **98**, 1107–15.
124. Gianoulis, M. and Wright, J.L. (1990) An autopsy study of the structure of the small vessels in biopsies from the lingula and upper and lower lobes: implications for vascular assessment. *Mod. Pathol.*, **3**, 567–9.
125. Newman, S.L., Michel, R.P. and Wang, N.-S. (1985) Lingular lung biopsy: is it representative? *Am. Rev. Respir. Dis.*, **132**, 1084–6.
126. Churg, A. (1983) An inflation procedure for open lung biopsies. *Am. J. Surg. Pathol.*, **7**, 69–71.
127. Nicod, P. and Moser, K.M. (1989) Primary pulmonary hypertension: the risk and benefit of lung biopsy. *Circulation*, **80**, 1486–8.
128. Wilson, N.J., Seear, M.D., Taylor, G.P. *et al.* (1990) The clinical value and risks of lung biopsy in children with congenital heart disease. *J. Thoracic Cardiovasc. Surg.*, **99**, 460–8.
129. Geggel, R.L., Mayer Jr, J.E., Fried, R. *et al.* (1990) Role of lung biopsy in patients undergoing a modified Fontan procedure. *J. Thorac. Cardiovasc. Surg.*, **99**, 451–9.
130. Espinosa, R.E., Edwards, W.D., Rosenow III, E.C. and Schaff, H.V. (1993) Idiopathic pulmonary hilar fibrosis: an unusual cause of pulmonary hypertension. *Mayo Clin. Proc.*, **68**, 778–82.
131. Berry, D.F., Buccigrossi, D., Peabody, J. *et al.* (1986) Pulmonary vascular occlusion and fibrosing mediastinitis. *Chest*, **89**, 296–301.
132. Okubo, S., Kunieda, T., Ando, M. *et al.* (1988) Idiopathic isolated pulmonary arteritis with chronic cor pulmonale. *Chest*, **94**, 665–6.
133. Lie, J.T. (1989) Classification of pulmonary angiitis and granulomatosis: histopathologic perspectives. *Sem. Respir. Med.*, **10**, 111–21.
134. Churg, A. (1983) Pulmonary angiitis and granulomatosis revisited. *Hum. Pathol.*, **14**, 868–83.
135. Fulmer, J.D. and Kaltreider, H.B. (1982) The pulmonary vasculitides. *Chest*, **82**, 615–24.
136. Takemura, T., Matsui, Y., Saiki, S. and Mikami, R. (1992) Pulmonary vascular involvement in sarcoidosis: a report of 40 autopsy cases. *Hum. Pathol.*, **23**, 1216–23.

137. Myers, J.L. and Katzenstein, A.A. (1986) Microangiitis in lupus-induced pulmonary hemorrhage. *Am. J. Clin. Pathol.*, **85**, 552–6.
138. Mark, E.J. and Ramirez, J.F. (1985) Pulmonary capillaritis and hemorrhage in patients with systemic vasculitis. *Arch. Pathol. Lab. Med.*, **109**, 413–18.
139. Ladanyi, M. and Fraser, R.S. (1987) Pulmonary involvement in giant cell arteritis. *Arch. Pathol. Lab. Med.*, **111**, 1178–80.
140. Wagenaar, S.S., van den Bosch, J.M.M., Westermann, C.J.J. *et al.* (1986) Isolated granulomatous giant cell vasculitis of the pulmonary elastic arteries. *Arch. Pathol. Lab. Med.*, **110**, 962–4.
141. Bartter, T., Irwin, R.S. and Nash, G. (1988) Aneurysms of the pulmonary arteries. *Chest*, **94**, 1065–75.
142. Butto, F., Lucas Jr, R.V. and Edwards, J.E. (1987) Pulmonary arterial aneurysm: a pathologic study of five cases. *Chest*, **91**, 137–41.
143. Nienaber, C.A., Spielmann, R.P., Montz, R. *et al.* (1986) Development of pulmonary aneurysm in primary pulmonary hypertension: a case report. *Angiology*, **37**, 319–24.
144. Coard, K.C.M. and Martin, M.P. (1992) Ruptured saccular pulmonary artery aneurysm associated with persistent ductus arteriosus. *Arch. Pathol. Lab. Med.*, **116**, 159–61.
145. Walley, V.M., Virmani, R., and Silver, M.D. (1990) Pulmonary arterial dissections and ruptures: to be considered in patients with pulmonary arterial hypertension presenting with cardiogenic shock or sudden death. *Pathology*, **22**, 1–4.
146. Yamamoto, M.E., Jones, J.W. and McManus, B.M. (1988) Fatal dissection of the pulmonary trunk: an obscure consequence of chronic pulmonary hypertension. *Am. J. Cardiovasc. Pathol.*, **1**, 353–9.
147. McGlennen, R.C., Manivel, J.C., Stanley, S.J. *et al.* (1989). Pulmonary artery trunk sarcoma: a clinicopathologic, ultrastructural, and immunohistochemical study of four cases. *Mod. Pathol.*, **2**, 486–94.
148. Nonomura, A., Kurumaya, H., Kono, N. *et al.* (1988) Primary pulmonary artery sarcoma: report of two autopsy cases studied by immunohistochemistry and electron microscopy, and review of 110 cases reported in the literature. *Acta Pathol. Jap.*, **38**, 883–96.
149. Baker, P.B. and Goodwin, R.A. (1985) Pulmonary artery sarcomas: a review and report of a case. *Arch. Pathol. Lab. Med.*, **109**, 35–39.
150. Glock, Y., Binon, J.P., Rocchichioli, J.P. *et al.* (1989) Primary malignant fibrous histiocytoma of the right ventricle and main pulmonary trunk with a review of the literature. *Texas Heart Inst. J.*, **16**, 296–304.

17 SYSTEMIC, PULMONARY, AND CEREBRAL VASCULITIS

J.T. Lie

17.1 Definition

Vasculitis has a deceptively simple morphologic definition but a seemingly endless variety of clinical manifestations. Vasculitis can be defined as inflammation of the blood vessels that is often accompanied by vessel necrosis and occlusive changes. Vasculitis may arise *de novo* as a primary disorder of blood vessels (e.g. polyarteritis nodosa) or it may occur secondarily to a diverse group of systemic diseases (e.g. seropositive rheumatoid arthritis.) Vasculitis may be generalized or localized; it may be clinically silent or it may have a multitude of symptoms and serious consequences. The distribution of vasculitic lesions may be systemic or predominantly pulmonary or isolated to the central nervous system [1–9]. A definitive diagnosis of vasculitis depends on the correct interpretation of histologic changes because virtually none of the vasculitic syndromes have pathognomonic clinical and laboratory findings.

17.2 Etiology and pathogenesis

With the exception of vasculitis associated with infectious diseases [10,11] the cause and pathogenesis of all other systemic and isolated vasculitides are either unknown or incompletely understood. The prevailing theory is that most vasculitic syndromes are produced by immune complex-mediated or cell-mediated immunopathogenetic mechanisms [12–19]. However, the probable antigen of vasculitis in man has been identified in very few instances, notably in some patients with hepatitis Bs antigenemia [20,21]. Furthermore, a variety of clinical features of vasculitis and variation in the size of vessel involvement have been identified with hepatitis Bs antigen. Hepatitis Bs antigen may be associated with small-vessel vasculitis limited to skin [22] or kidney [23], with cryoglobulinemia [24] or with polyarteritis nodosa involving multiple organs and various-sized blood vessels [25].

Evidence for immune complex-mediated disease is derived from detection of circulating immune complexes using a variety of techniques: from demonstrations of their presence as cryoglobulins, from the development of hypocomplementemia and from the demonstration of immune reactants in tissue by direct immunofluorescence [14–18]. Not only do multiple factors determine whether immune complexes wll be deposited, but the subsequent pathogenesis of tissue injury triggered by their deposition depends on several mediators including complements, neutrophil infiltration and possibly the coagulation and kallikrein–kinin system [17,19]. The occasional finding of immune complex deposits in small blood vessels without the usual histologic features of vasculitis would indicate that secondary pathogenetic mechanisms must be involved to produce vascular inflammation [18]. The classification of vasculitis using immunological techniques has also proved ineffectual. Paronetto [12] demonstrated that immunofluorescent localization of immunoglobulins and complements in tissue was frequent in polyarteritis but it was also frequent in hypersensitivity angiitis and granulomatous angiitis.

Antineutrophil cytoplasmic antibodies (ANCA), classified as either cytoplasmic (c-ANCA) or perinuclear (p-ANCA) in the fluorescent staining pattern, have been recently recognized as an important serologic marker for the diagnosis and monitoring of disease activity of systemic vasculitis. However, ANCA may also be detected in many non-vasculitic conditions. Detection of these autoantibodies has been most useful in distinguishing Wegener's granulomatosis from other forms of systemic vasculitis, but it has not replaced or lessened the need for the biopsy diagnosis of vasculitis, including Wegener's granulomatosis [5,26–30].

17.3 Clinicopathological classification

To date, there is still no standardized or universally accepted classification of vasculitis. A definitive classification of vasculitis has been hampered not only by insufficient knowledge of the etiology and pathogenesis of vasculitis, but also by the considerable clinical and

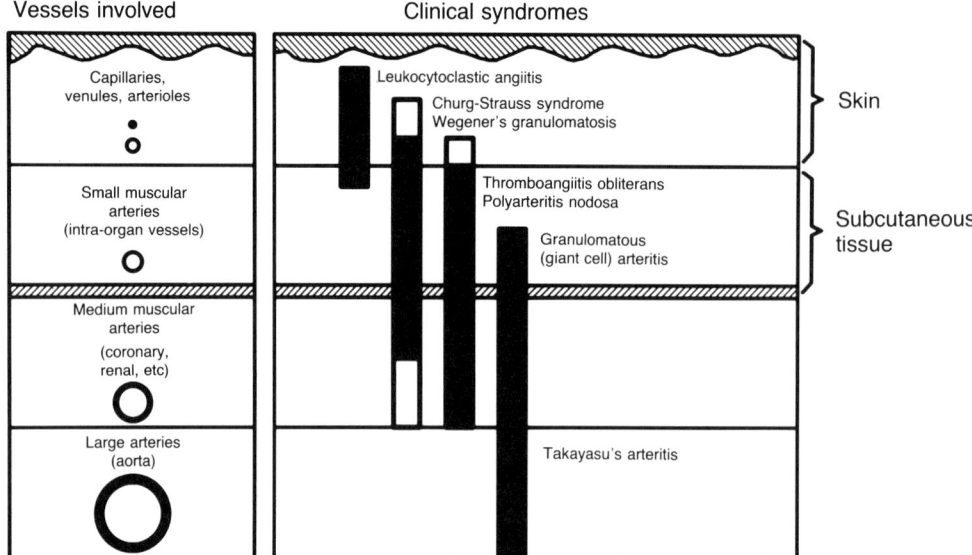

Figure 17.1 Overlapping nature of the level and size of blood vessels involved in major types of vasculitis. (Redrawn from Gilliam and Smiley [52], with permission.)

pathological overlap between many of the vasculitic syndromes [15,18,31].

As the prototype of systemic necrotizing vasculitis, **periarteritis nodosa** was first described in 1866 by Adolf Küssmaul, the clinician, and Rudolf Maier, the pathologist [32]. Ferrari [33] introduced the alternative name **polyarteritis,** pointing out that the arterial inflammation was more often transmural than merely in the outer wall. Involvement of pulmonary arteries in polyarteritis was subsequently described by Mönckeberg [34], in 1905, and by Ophöls [35] in 1923, as were necrotizing lesions of veins. Periarteritis (or polyarteritis) nodosa then became the designation for almost any necrotizing vasculitis in which the etiology could not be established.

It was not until the early 1950s that a serious attempt was made to classify vasculitides; by then, several additional types of vasculitis other than polyarteritis nodosa became known: Takayasu arteritis or 'pulseless disease' [36–38], thromboangiitis obliterans or Buerger's disease [39,40], temporal arteritis [41–43], allergic granulomatosis and angiitis (or Churg–Strauss syndrome) [39,40], and Wegener's granulomatosis [46,47]. Zeek [48,49] in 1952, was the first to recognize hypersensitivity vasculitis as a distinct entity quite separate from polyarteritis nodosa. Zeek proposed the generic term **necrotizing angiitis** to designate the vascular lesions, both arterial and venous, the fully developed stage of which consisted of fibrinoid necrosis and inflammatory reaction involving all three coats of the vessel walls. Zeek's classification [48,49] encompassed five types of necrotizing angiitis: hypersensitivity angiitis; allergic granulomatous angiitis; rheumatic arteritis; periarteritis nodosa and temporal arteritis. A notable omission in this scheme was Wegener's granulomatosis, which was first described by German pathologists in the 1930s, but did not appear in the English-language literature until 1954 [46,47].

In addition to differences in clinical and pathological features, the caliber and types of blood vessels involved were important criteria in utilizing Zeek's classification of vasculitis [48,49]. However, a strict and complete separation of different types of vasculitis according to the size of vessel involvement is not feasible (Figure 17.1), and the vasculitis syndromes with overlapping clinical and pathological features remain a constant source of nosologic confusion [31]. Despite its limitation, Zeek's classification of vasculitis is practical and has served as the blueprint for later investigators to formulate alternative schemes of classification, of which there have been many [1–10,13,15,18,50–59], but as yet none is ideal [57,58].

A practical classification of primary and secondary vasculitis, incorporating the predominant type and size of vessel involvement is shown in Table 17.1. This classification offers the clinician guidelines for when to suspect and what to expect in the histologic diagnosis of vasculitis. A new category of vasculitis look-alikes may be added to accommodate clinicopathologic entities that are not true vasculitis but may mimic vasculitis either in their clinical presentations, angiographic appearances, histopathologic findings or a combination thereof [7,8].

Classification aids diagnostic procedures and facilitates the appropriate course of action in the management of vasculitis. Early and correct diagnosis of vasculitis becomes vital not only for instituting immunosuppressive treatment of more aggressive forms

Table 17.1 A practical classification of vasculitis

- Primary vasculitis
  - Affecting large, medium and small-sized blood vessels
    - Takayasu arteritis
    - Giant cell (temporal) arteritis
    - Primary angiitis of the central nervous system
  - Affecting predominantly medium and small-sized blood vessels
    - Polyarteritis nodosa
    - Churg–Strauss syndrome
    - Wegener's granulomatosis
  - Affecting predominantly small-sized blood vessels
    - Microscopic polyangiitis
    - Schönlein–Henoch syndrome
    - Leukocytoclastic vasculitis
  - Miscellaneous conditions
    - Buerger's disease
    - Behçet's disease
    - Kawasaki disease
- Secondary vasculitis
  - Infection-related vasculitis (bacterial, fungal, ickettsial, viral)
  - Vasculitis secondary to connective tissue disease
  - Drug hypersensitivity-related vasculitis
  - Vasculitis secondary to mixed essential cryoglobulinemia
  - Malignancy-related vasculitis
  - Hypocomplementemic urticarial vasculitis
  - Organ transplant vasculitis
  - Pseudovasculitic syndromes (myxoma, endocarditis, Sneddon syndrome).

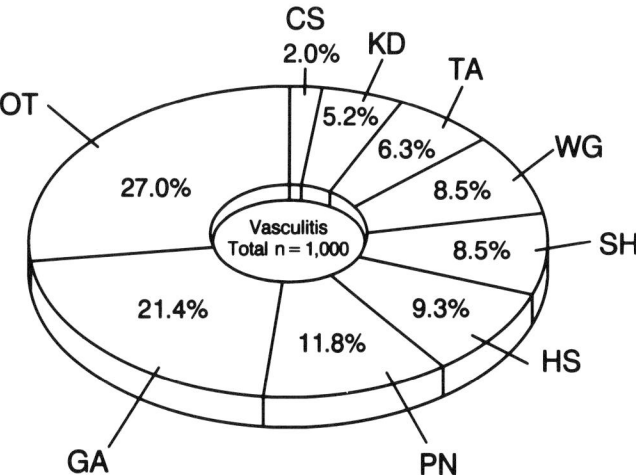

Figure 17.2 Frequency distribution of eight selected categories of vasculitis in the American College of Rheumatology Classification Criteria study of a selected series of 1000 cases. CS = Churg–Strauss syndrome; TA = Takayasu arteritis; HS = hypersensitivity angiitis; WG = Wegener's granulomatosis; SH = Schönlein–Henoch purpura; PN = polyarteritis nodosa; GA = giant cell (temporal) arteritis; OT = other type-unspecified systemic vasculitis.

of vasculitis to prevent irreversible tissue damage, but also for withholding cytotoxic agents when their use is unwarranted. The discussion to follow will focus on only the major types of systemic, pulmonary and cerebral angiitis. Data from the American College of Rheumatology-sponsored 12-year study on the classification criteria of vasculitis provide an indication of the relative frequency of eight selected categories of vasculitic syndromes, excluding cerebral angiitis, in the hospital referral practice patient population (Figure 17.2).

17.4 Giant cell arteritides

There are three groups of clinicopathologic entities in which giant cell arteritis characterizes the pathologic lesions of the affected blood vessels ranging in size from the aorta at one end to arterioles and venules at the other end of the spectrum. These entities are Takayasu arteritis, the arteritis of some rheumatic diseases and temporal arteritis.

17.4.1 TAKAYASU ARTERITIS

Takayasu arteritis (aortic arch syndrome, pulseless disease, primary or non-specific arteritis) is an inflammatory vascular disease of unknown etiology, affecting usually the aorta and its brachiocephalic branches and, less commonly, pulmonary arteries, visceral arteries, coronary arteries and arteries of the upper and lower extremities [36–38,60–63]. The disease has a worldwide distribution and affects all age groups, but is decidedly more common in the Orient and occurs typically in young women aged between 15 and 45 years. In the USA, the estimated incidence rate of 2.6 cases per million persons per year for Takayasu arteritis is almost identical to that of Wegener's granulomatosis, similar to that of polyarteritis nodosa and about one tenth that of temporal arteritis [63].

The early description of the disease emphasized its aortic arch manifestations, but it is now well known that the entire aorta and its major branches may be involved, producing coarctation, occlusion or aneurysmal dilatation [36–38,60–63]. The clinical manifestations of Takayasu arteritis may be separated into the acute and subacute stage with features of a systemic illness predominating, and a chronic phase or end-stage disease in which the sequelae of vascular occlusion such as hypertension, pulse deficit and/or limb claudication in a young adult become evident. The early-phase symptoms are therefore non-specific and include fever, anemia, malaise, arthralgia, myalgia or diffuse pain, skin rashes, headache and an elevated erythrocyte sedimentation rate (ESR). The incidence of these symptoms has been reported to vary from 14 to 63% [60–63] and a correct clinical diagnosis of Takayasu's arteritis at this early phase of the disease was made in less than 10% of patients according to a recent US study [63].

The correct diagnosis is usually initiated by a high index of clinical suspicion and requires a total arteriography to ascertain the pattern and distribution of arterial lesions [61]. There are no specific laboratory tests for Takayasu arteritis. Various immunologic abnormalities in patients with Takayasu arteritis have been reported. Circulating immune complexes have been detected in up to 50% of patients, but they do not appear to correlate with the disease activity, nor can they be implicated as a causative factor [64,65].

During the early phase of Takayasu arteritis, corticosteroids may play a role in reducing or controlling the disease activity [66]. Reconstructive or bypass surgery may be necessary in selected cases, but is usually postponed until the disease is in a 'burn-out' phase with a normal ESR [62,67,68]. When surgery is performed at the active phase of Takayasu arteritis, full-thickness biopsies of the aortic wall should be attempted to obtain a conclusive histologic diagnosis of the disease [63,66–68].

Hypotheses for the etiology of Takayasu arteritis include an autoimmune disease and genetically related disorder [60,64,65,69–73]. Rare instances of familial cases and siblings with Takayasu arteritis also have been reported [68]. Patients with Takayasu arteritis have a statistically higher frequency of the haplotype BW52, DR2, and DR4 antigens compared with healthy Japanese and North American subjects [70–72]. Of interest, both DR2 and DR4 are associated with several autoimmune diseases, including rheumatoid arthritis and giant cell arteritis [64]; Takayasu arteritis has been reported to occur in patients with rheumatoid arthritis, ankylosing spondylitis, Reiter's syndrome, temporal arteritis, polymyalgia rheumatica, scleroderma, thyrotoxicosis and inflammatory bowel disease [60].

Anatomically, Takayasu arteritis has been classified into four types [38], based on the location and extent of the vascular involvement (Figure 17.3). Type I represents the classic pulseless-disease type with involvement of the aortic arch and its brachiocephalic vessels and type IA is the aneurysmal ascending aorta variant that often presents as aortic insufficiency clinically; type II designates involvement of the thoracoabdominal aorta, sparing the aortic arch; type III denotes the combination of type I and type II; and type IV refers to pulmonary artery involvement, which may or may not be associated with involvement of the aorta and systemic arteries. The diagnosis of type IV is usually based on angiographic findings only.

Pathologically, the characteristic long segmental tapering and often irregular arterial narrowing is caused by the undulated intimal proliferation and fibrotic contraction of the media and adventitia. These changes, together with the coexisting age-related atherosclerosis (if present in an older person) and mural thrombosis, account for the typical stenosis, coarctation and post-

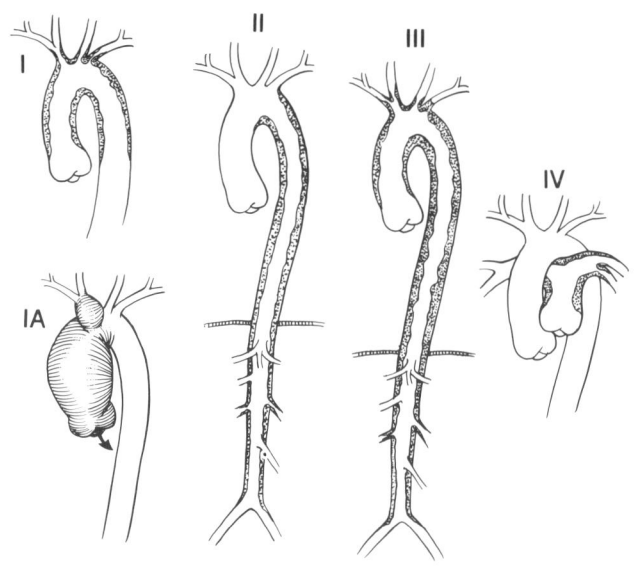

Figure 17.3 Topographical classification of Takayasu arteritis: type I, involvement of the aortic arch; type IA, aneurysmal ascending aorta; type II, involvement of the thoracoabdominal aorta; type III, combination of types I and II; type IV, involvement of the pulmonary arteries.

stenotic dilatations that can be visualized on angiograms [61]. Aneurysm formation and arterial dissection are the less commonly known complications of Takayasu arteritis, and aortic insufficiency may occur in 10–20% of the patients due to aortic root dilatation [38].

Takayasu arteritis is usually suspected clinically and/or angiographically, taking into consideration the patient's age and gender and the anatomic distribution of vascular lesions. The diagnosis should be confirmed whenever possible by examination of biopsy or autopsy specimens, bearing in mind that the disease has distinctive patterns of histopathologic changes at different stages of its chronologic development [38,60–63]. In the early or active phase, as seen in surgical biopsies (Figure 17.4), the disease is characterized by a granulomatous arteritis with patchy destruction of the medial musculoelastic lamellae. The cellular infiltrate is predominantly lymphoplasmacytic and most prominent in the media. Both Langhans and foreign-body type giant cells may be present in variable numbers, as may the eosinophils, but the latter tend to be scarce in most cases. There is usually some adventitial and intimal fibrosis following the panarteritis inflammatory process. A band of infarct-like necrosis of the media may be observed occasionally [74,75]. Within this morphologic spectrum of basically a granulomatous lymphoplasmacytic arteritis, the severity of medial disruption and fibrosis and the segmental nature of arteritis vary greatly between cases, as does the intensity of the inflammatory cell infiltrate and the number of giant cells present.

In the chronic phase or end-stage of the disease,

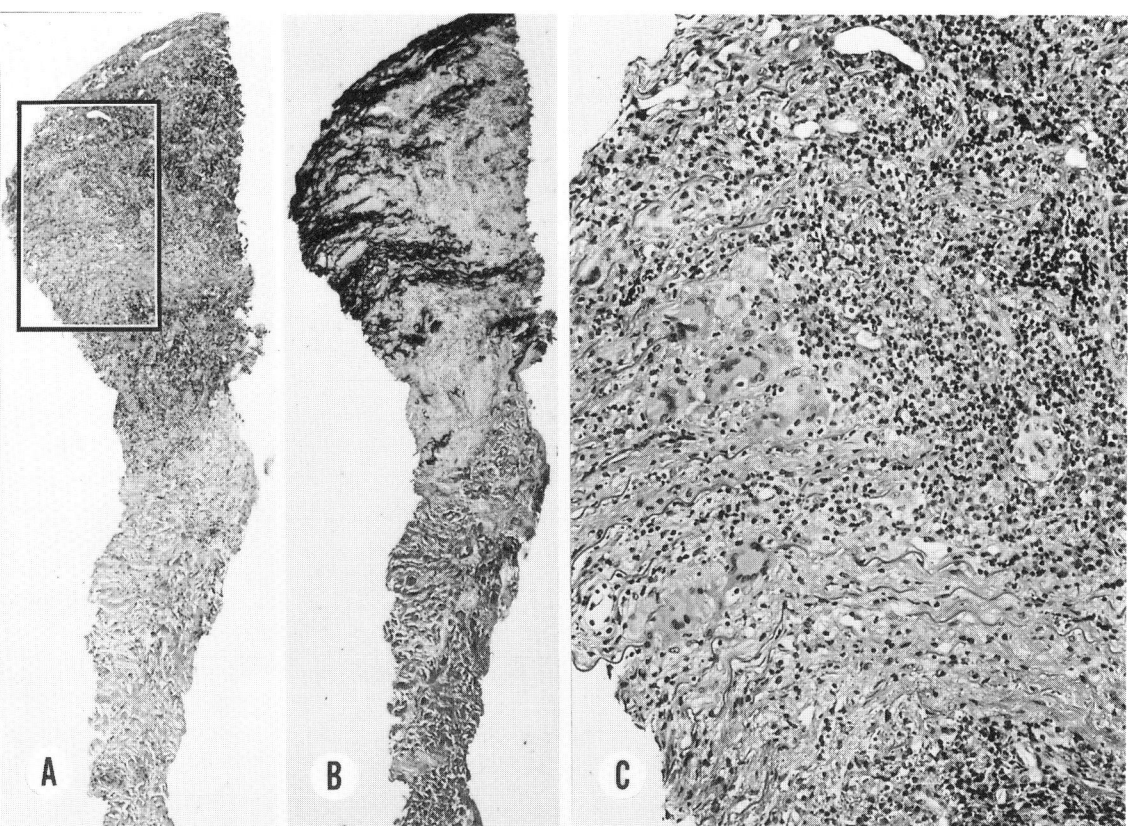

Figure 17.4 Histopathology of active phase of Takayasu arteritis, as seen in this surgical biopsy of the aorta. Matching H&E (A) and elastic stain (B) sections, showing granulomatous aortitis with disruption of medial elastic lamellae. (C) is close-up view of the framed area in (A) showing a cluster of giant cells in the predominantly lymphoplasmacytic infiltrate. (A and B ×40; C ×160)

transmural sclerosis with scanty or no inflammatory cell infiltrate becomes the histologic hallmark of Takayasu arteritis (Figure 17.5). The degree of intimal and adventitial fibrosis is proportional to the duration and severity of the arteritis. Secondary thrombosis occurs not infrequently and it poses an additional threat to complete occlusion of the affected artery. It is in the burnt-out stage of the disease that a Takayasu arteritis may escape recognition, and is likely to be mistaken as arteriosclerosis by pathologists who examine the scarred fibrotic artery as a surgical biopsy or autopsy specimen.

Takayasu arteritis, as described, has been given a variety of other names in reports by different authors to emphasize certain aspects of its protean clinical manifestations, and also in reports originating from different geographic regions describing the same pathologic entity. The proliferation of synonyms for Takayasu arteritis (Table 17.2) is a major source of nosologic confusion and creates difficulties for comparing the disease's prevalence and treatment results in different communities or geographic regions.

The large vessel arteritis of rheumatic diseases (most commonly associated with rheumatoid arthritis, ankylosing spondylitis and systemic lupus erythromatosus) is also a granulomatous arteritis and, histopathologically, may be indistinguishable from Takayasu arteritis or extracranial giant cell (temporal) arteritis [38,63,74–76]. In contrast, the medium-sized and small vessel vasculitis of rheumatoid arthritis and of systemic lupus erythromatosus resembles the polyarteritis type necrotizing angiitis [77–81].

17.4.2 TEMPORAL ARTERITIS AND POLYMYALGIA RHEUMATICA

In the Western hemisphere, giant cell arteritis occurs most commonly in two maladies of the elderly; it is *sine qua non* of temporal arteritis and it may be found in 25–35% of patients with polymyalgia rheumatica [82–87]. Temporal arteritis and polymyalgia rheumatica are closely related clinical syndromes; both occur almost exclusively in persons over 50 years of age and, in both, women are affected about two to three times as commonly as men. An increase in the reported incidence of temporal arteritis and polymyalgia rheumatica over the past three decades probably reflects a greater awareness of these syndromes [83–86]. There are geographical differences in the incidence of temporal arteritis world-

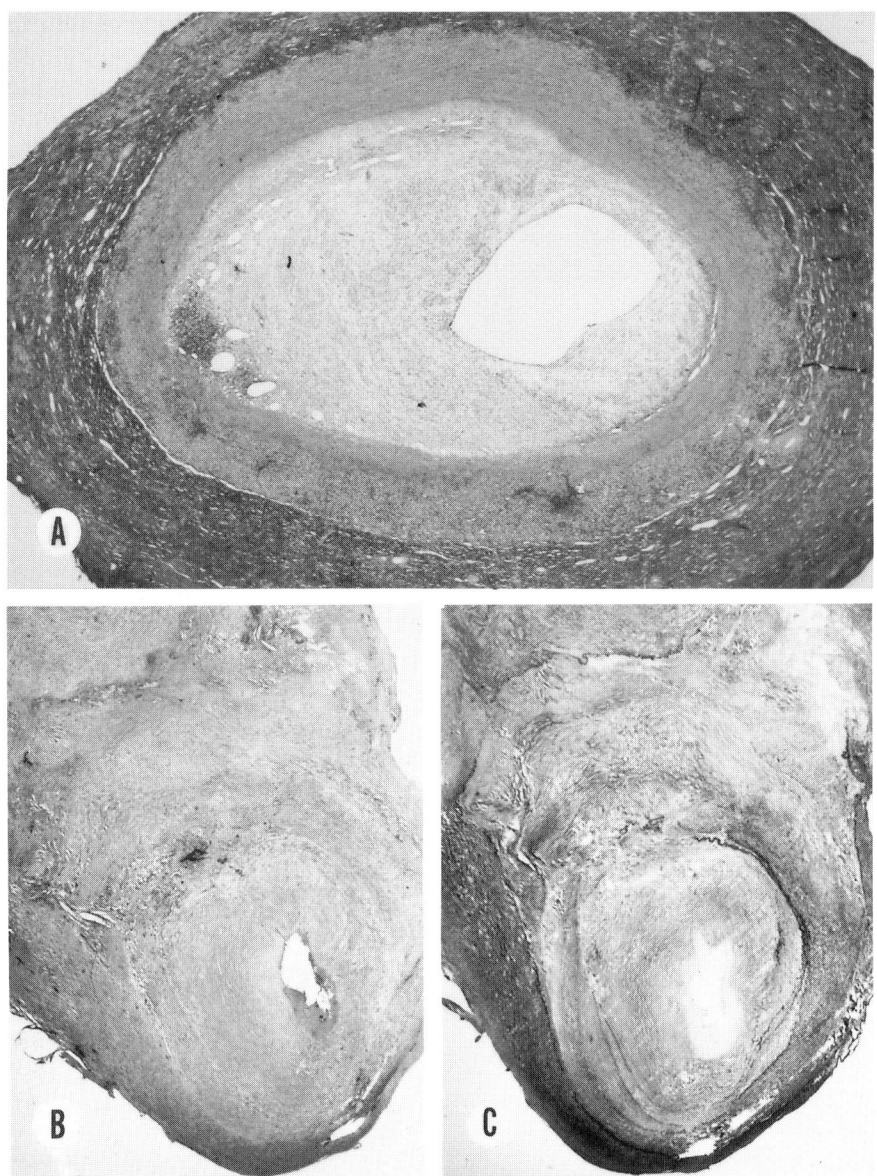

Figure 17.5 Histopathology of evolving chronic phase of Takayasu arteritis. (A) Early chronic phase intimal and adventitial fibrosis with scanty residual inflammatory infiltrate; (B and C) matching H&E and elastic stain sections, respectively, of late chronic phase occlusive transmural fibrosis without inflammatory infiltrate, indistinguishable from arteriosclerosis. (A, B, and C ×16.)

wide and within the United States [87]. Where the disease is prevalent, temporal arteritis may be found in about 1 in 750 persons 50 years of age or older, with a reported annual incidence of approximately 1 in 10 000 in population studies [82,85]; polymyalgia rheumatica occurs in about 1 in 250 persons 50 years of age or older [83,84]. An old autopsy study in Sweden [88] suggested that the true incidence of temporal arteritis and polymyalgia rheumatica might be higher; histologic evidence of giant cell arteritis was present in 1.7% of 889 unselected autopsies.

Although temporal arteritis and polymyalgia rheumatica are clinically related syndromes, they usually occur independently and the cause of either is unknown. Diagnosis of both conditions is based on recognition of the characteristic history and clinical findings, with an almost invariably elevated ESR in the range of 40–160 mm/h (Westergren). About 40–50% of patients with temporal arteritis have symptoms of polymyalgia rheumatica, but only 25–35% of patients with polymyalgia rheumatica have biopsy-proven temporal arteritis [82–84]. In contrast to Takayasu's arteritis, both temporal arteritis and polymyalgia rheumatica occur much more commonly among the Caucasians and they are rare in Asian, African-American, Native American, and Hispanic patients [87]. Among African-

Table 17.2 Selected synonyms for Takayasu arteritis

- Sclerosing aortitis (Beneke, 1925)
- Reverse coarctation (Griffin, 1939)
- Aortic arch syndrome (Frövig, 1946)
- Pulseless disease (Shimizu and Sano, 1951)
- Takayasu's disease (Caccamise and Whitman, 1952)
- Obliterative arteritis (Learmonth, 1952)
- Young female arteritis (Ross and McKusick, 1953)
- Martorell syndrome (Martorell and Fabre, 1954)
- Takayasu syndrome (DeBes et al., 1955)
- Primary arteritis (Barker and Edwards, 1955)
- Non-specific arteritis (Kalmansohn and Kalmansohn, 1957)
- Obliterative brachiocephalic arteritis (Gibbons and King, 1957)
- Idiopathic aortitis (Issacson, 1964)
- Stenosing aortitis (Sen et al., 1962)
- Atypical coarctation (Inada et al., 1962)
- Takayasu arteritis (Judge et al., 1962)
- Middle aortic syndrome (Sen et al., 1963)
- Takayasu's arteriopathy (Strachan, 1964)
- Truncoarteritis productiva obliterans (Nasu and Mamiya, 1966)
- Occlusive thromboarteriopathy (Maekawa and Ishikawa, 1966)
- Acquired aortoarteritis (Domingo et al., 1967)
- Aortitis syndrome (Committee Report, 1968)
- Idiopathic medial aortoarteripathy (Marquis et al., 1968)
- Non-specific aortoarteritis (Sen et al., 1973)

Americans, only 34 biopsy-proven cases of temporal arteritis have been described between 1950 and 1990, though there may have been some undiagnosed or unreported cases [89,90].

In patients with **temporal arteritis**, the illness may begin abruptly or insidiously with headache, jaw claudication or visual disturbances as the major presenting complaint. Non-specific constitutional symptoms such as malaise, fatigue, weight loss, fever and anemia are common [84,91] and may mislead the unsuspected clinician to undertake a lengthy, expensive and futile search for a more sinister or unusual disease [92]. Partial or complete unilateral or bilateral blindness occurs in 10–20% of patients; once the visual loss is fixed, it usually becomes permanent [91].

Polymyalgia rheumatica is a clinical syndrome characterized by pain and stiffness in shoulders and pelvic girdles without muscle atrophy or weakness, often accompanied by non-specific constitutional symptoms as in temporal arteritis and a moderately elevated ESR, followed by a quick and dramatic response to treatment with low to moderate doses of corticosteroids. Diagnosis is usually not made until symptoms have been present for at least a month; about 25–35% of patients may have a biopsy-proven temporal arteritis [84].

A temporal artery biopsy is recommended in all patients suspected to have giant cell arteritis [93,94]. When the artery is clearly abnormal by inspection and palpation, a shorter segment (2 cm) biopsy may be sufficient to establish the diagnosis. If the artery is not obviously abnormal, a minimum 4 cm segment is needed and multiple cross-sections of the artery should be examined for evidence of arteritis [93,95]. If the first temporal artery biopsy is negative for arteritis, the opposite side should be biopsied. In 15–20% of cases, histologic evidence of temporal arteritis is obtained only after the second examination of a bilateral biopsy [93].

Extracranial systemic-vessel giant cell arteritis occurs in 10–15% of patients with temporal arteritis and polymyalgia rheumatic [96]. It may manifest as the aortic arch syndrome in the elderly, or cause limb claudication and ischemia [97–100]. More dramatically, it can be an unsuspected cause of lethal aortic dissection or ruptured aortic aneurysm [96,101]. Involvement of the coronary arteries with fatal myocardial infarction has also been reported [102–105]. Small-vessel (arterioles and venules) granulomatous angiitis (Figure 17.6) occurs in two uncommon syndromes: disseminated visceral giant cell angiitis and primary (granulomatous) angiitis of the central nervous system; both are relatively new clinical entities and each has a high mortality rate according to the case studies reported in the literature [106,107].

(a) Histopathology of temporal arteritis

The histopathology of temporal arteritis has been described in varying details by many investigators in the past 50 years, but confusion on this subject lingers because the classic granulomatous (giant cell) arteritis is seen in less than 50% of positive temporal artery biopsies from symptomatic patients [4,108–115]. The clinical significance of the known morphologic variants of temporal arteritis remains uncertain since both the granulomatous and non-granulomatous variants may be observed in the same biopsy. The number of giant cells, the intensity and the predominant focus of inflammatory cell infiltrate are also highly variable. There is no evidence that the duration of symptoms, elevation of ESR or any other clinical and laboratory finding in a patient can be consistently correlated with a particular histopathologic pattern of temporal arteritis [111–115].

The identification of active inflammatory changes in the vessel wall, but not the presence of giant cells, is usually considered obligatory for a histologic diagnosis of arteritis. *Three major histologic variants of temporal arteritis have been described: the classic giant cell or granulomatous arteritis* (Figures 17.7 and 17.8) *and the atypical or non-granulomatous arteritis*, characterized by intimal proliferation with focal and scanty inflammatory cell infiltrate predominantly in the adventitia (Figure 17.9). Healed temporal arteritis is characterized by intimal fibrosis and medial scarring with the tell-tale

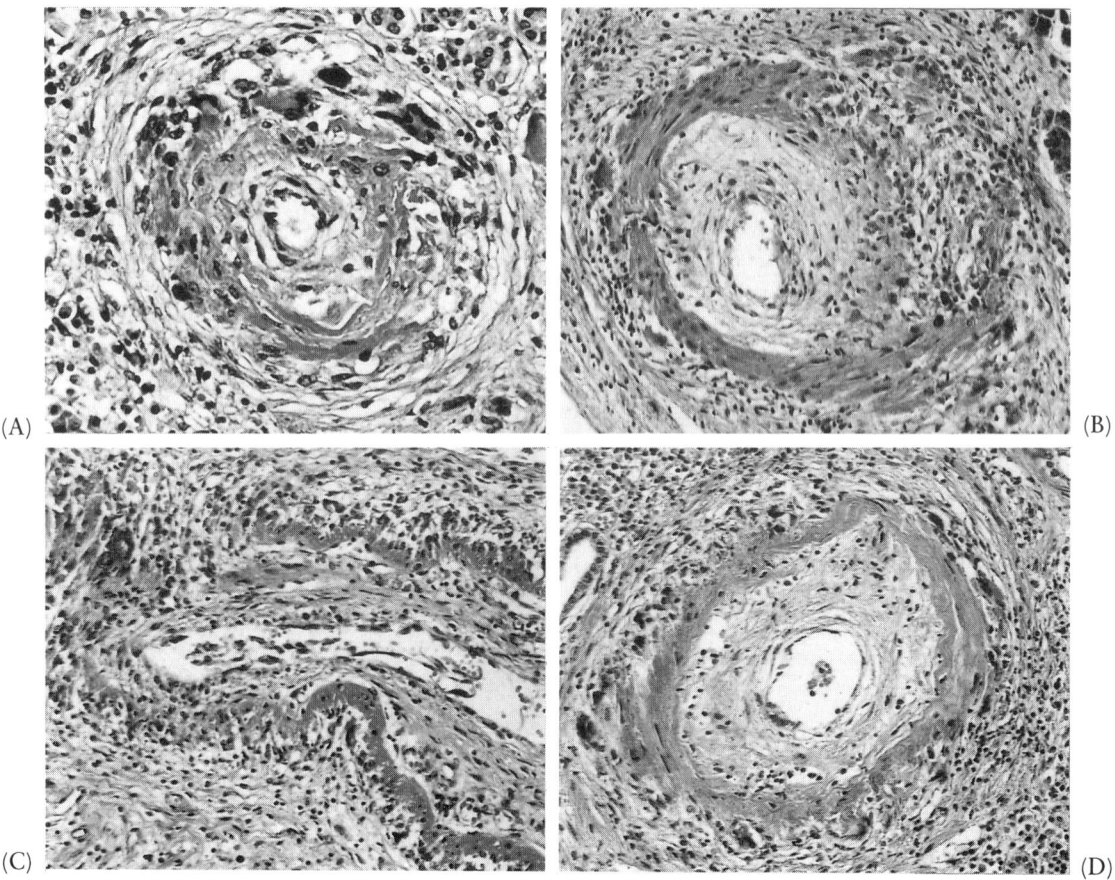

Figure 17.6 Small-vessel (arterioles and venules) granulomatous angiitis of pancreas (A), liver (B), spleen (C) and kidney (D) in disseminated giant cell angiitis. (H&E × 160.)

disorderly and segmental disruption of the internal elastic lamina, indicative of the asymmetry of previous transmural arterial inflammation (Figure 17.10). Fragmentation and fraying of the internal elastic lamina *per se* is such a constant feature of aging change of all arteries, the temporal artery included [108], that it alone is not diagnostic of active or healed arteritis. Inappropriate emphasis on this non-specific histologic finding (disruption of the internal elastic lamina) as a diagnostic feature of arteritis is a common pitfall in the interpretation of the temporal artery biopsy.

Fibrous intimal proliferation is a regular feature of all histologic variants of temporal arteritis and, more than thrombosis, the cause of vascular stenosis and occlusion (Figures 17.7 and 17.9). The intimal proliferation characteristically consists of loosely arranged stellate and spindle-shaped smooth muscle cells in a myxoid stroma (Figure 17.11). The classic temporal arteritis is distinctly granulomatous in character; the inflammatory process may be focal and confined to the media or it may be transmural and circumferential in distribution. The cellular infiltrate is invariably mixed, but usually lymphomononuclear with prominent plasma cells, histiocytes and, infrequently, eosinophils. The multi-nucleated giant cells, which may be Langhans or foreign-body type, are usually found in the intima–media junction, at close proximity to the fragmented external elastic lamina. The number of giant cells present in temporal arteritis is highly variable, and they occur focally and irregularly in the affected artery. Not infrequently, a solitary giant cell may be found outside the media and is detected only by chance after the examination of multiple serial sections (Figure 17.12). Giant cells are seen in less than 50% of all positive temporal artery biopsies. Their presence is not required for the diagnosis of temporal arteritis.

17.5 Polyarteritis group of systemic vasculitis

The polyarteritis group of systemic vasculitis comprises, in addition to the classic polyarteritis nodosa (PAN), microscopic polyarteritis, infantile polyarteritis (or the vasculitis of Kawasaki disease), hypersensitivity angiitis as defined by Zeek [7,48,49] and Churg–Strauss syndrome [2,6,44,45]. Churg–Strauss syndrome will be discussed later in section 17.6.

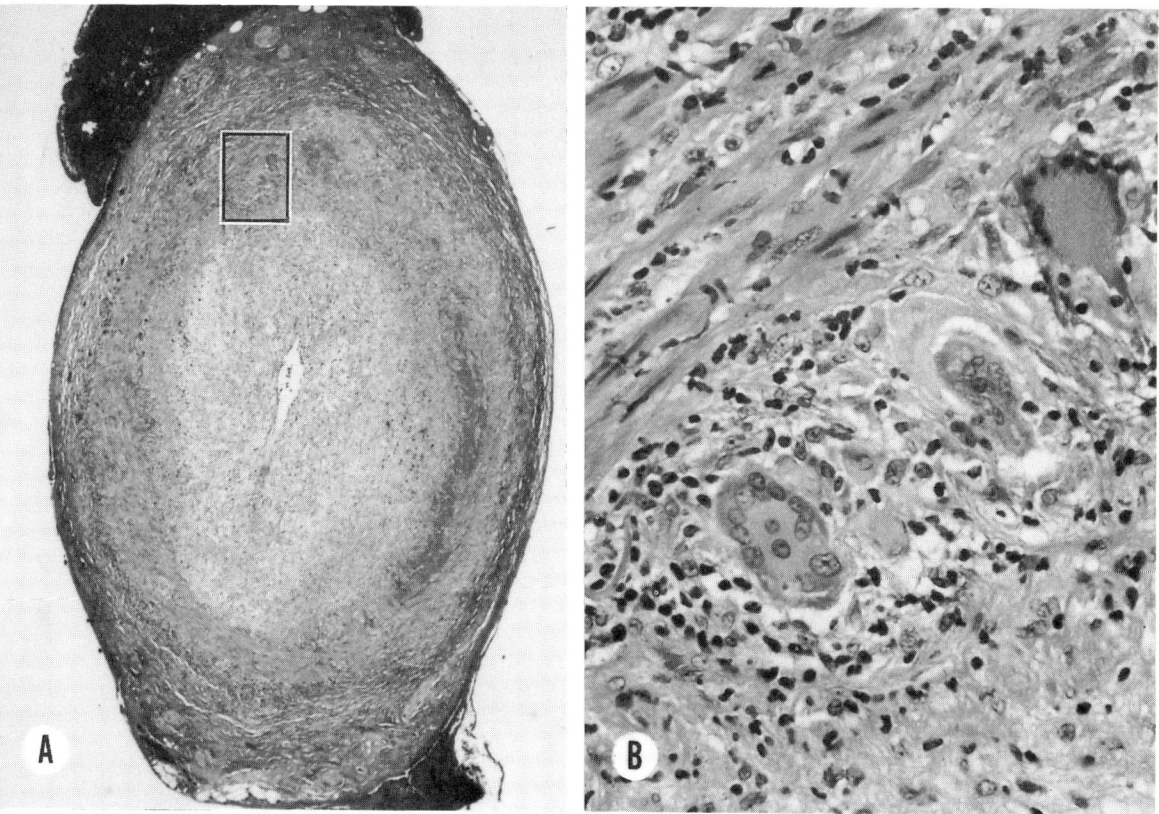

Figure 17.7 A typical giant cell temporal arteritis. (A) shows occlusive intimal fibrosis with diffuse granulomatous inflammation of the media. (B) is close-up view of the framed area in (A) showing both the Langhans and foreign-body type giant cells. (A ×40; B ×400.)

17.5.1 CLASSIC POLYARTERITIS NODOSA

Although classic PAN can occur at any age, the mean age of onset of disease is 40–50 years and men are affected twice as often as women. The clinical manifestations of classic polyarteritis nodosa (PAN) are highly variable [7,15,20,116–118]. PAN is a chronic systemic disease with a propensity for exacerbations and remissions, and if untreated, an alarmingly high mortality. The clinical presentation of PAN is often quite non-specific, with fever, weight loss, malaise, myalgia, arthralgia and headache as common complaints. Hypertension is frequently observed. Evidence of organ or tissue ischemia may be prominent and includes skin rashes, purpura or ulcerations, livedo reticularis, abdominal pain, peripheral neuropathy and renal insufficiency. Renal involvement and mononeuritis multiplex are seen in up to 70% of adult cases; the heart and gastrointestinal organs are involved in 30–40%, and the lungs only rarely [7].

There are no diagnostic laboratory tests for PAN: non-specific abnormal tests may include an elevated ESR, leukocytosis, anemia, proteinuria, hematuria, abnormal urinary sediments and positive HBsAg serology in 10–30% depending on the case selection. The diagnosis is usually suggested by a combination of the pertinent clinical features and characteristic angiographic findings, and confirmed with positive biopsy findings where possible. Biopsies of symptomatic sites, preferably at the height of the disease activity and prior to drug treatment, usually have the greatest diagnostic yield. The results of blind biopsies and biopsies done late in the course of the disease are inconclusive and less helpful. Biopsies of the muscle, nerve, kidney, rectum and other viscera are preferable to skin biopsy which, even when positive, is less diagnostic and not indicative of systemic involvement. Abnormal visceral (renal, celiac and mesenteric) angiography, particularly with microaneurysms, may be observed in up to 50% of classic PAN. However, such angiographic finding is not specific for PAN, and may be seen in a diverse group of other vasculitic and non-vasculitic conditions [116].

Pathologically, PAN is a necrotizing vasculitis of medium-sized and small arteries; the veins and venules are involved only occasionally [7,119]. The vascular lesions are characteristically focal and segmental, in different stages of development, and have a predilection for branching points of vessels. While any given indi-

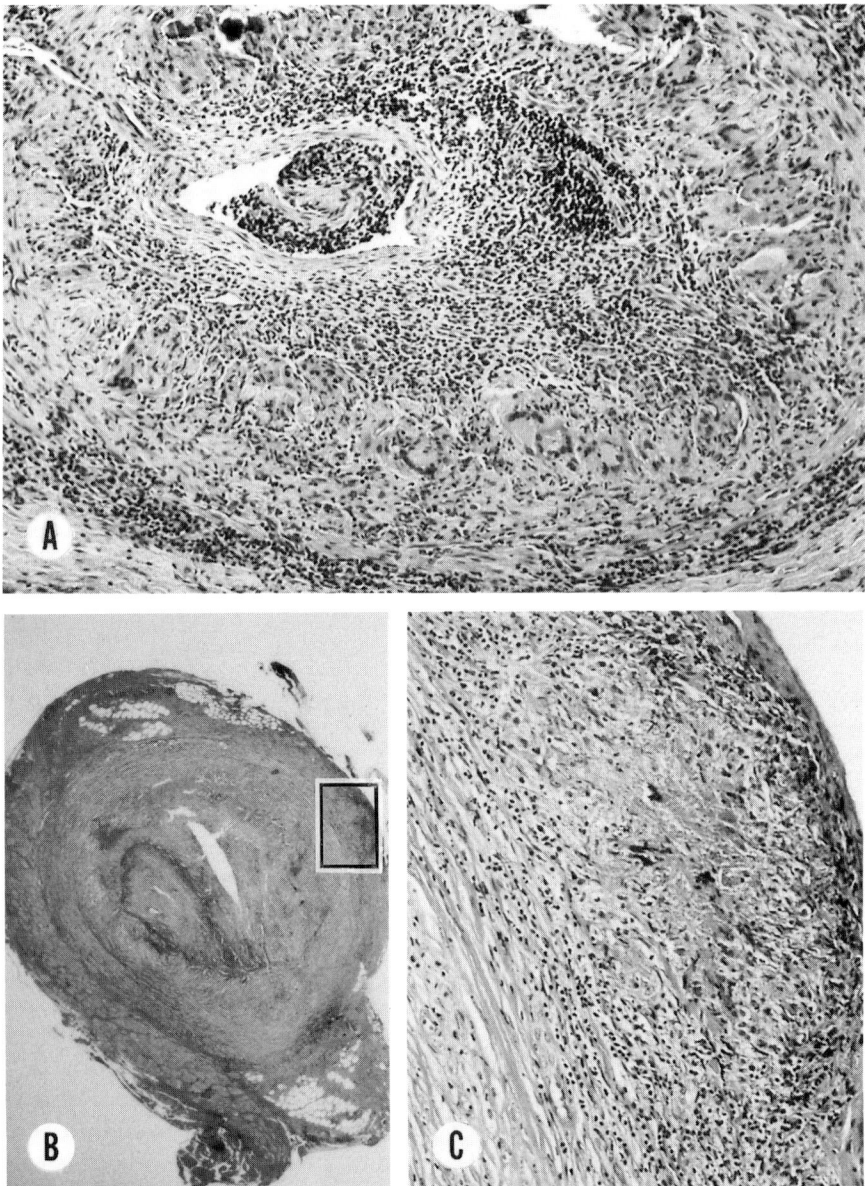

Figure 17.8 Variants of granulomatous temporal arteritis. (A) An intense transmural lymphocytic infiltrate admixed with giant cells. (B) Scanty or no giant cells but there is a necrobiotic granuloma in the adventitia (framed area). (C) Close-up view of the adventitial granuloma in (B). (A and C × 160; B ×16.)

vidual arterial lesion may not be diagnostic, the coexistence of acute, healing and healed lesions intermingled with seemingly normal uninvolved arterial segments are uniquely unmistakable histopathologic hallmarks of PAN (Figure 17.13).

The destructive vasculitis with fibrinoid necrosis (Figure 17.13) represents an early or active lesion and may be observed in both medium-sized (up to 5 or 6 mm in diameter) and small (down to 50 μm in diameter) arteries and arterioles. The damaged vessel wall appears to be replaced by a flame-like amorphous eosinophilic material, tinctorially resembling fibrin (hence the term 'fibrinoid necrosis'). An intense mixed-cell inflammatory infiltrate almost invariably accompanies fibrinoid necrosis, as may thrombosis. Granulomatous vasculitis with or without giant cells (Figure 17.14) may also be seen in PAN, but only rarely. However, fibrinoid necrosis alone is not specific for PAN; it occurs with regularity, for instance, in small blood vessels of patients with malignant hypertension.

Fibrous intimal proliferation and segmental or diffuse scarring of the media with destruction or loss of the underlying elastic lamellae signify the healing and healed lesions of PAN (Figures 17.15 and 17.16). The residual inflammatory infiltrate in healing lesions is almost exclusively lymphocytic (Figure 17.15) and

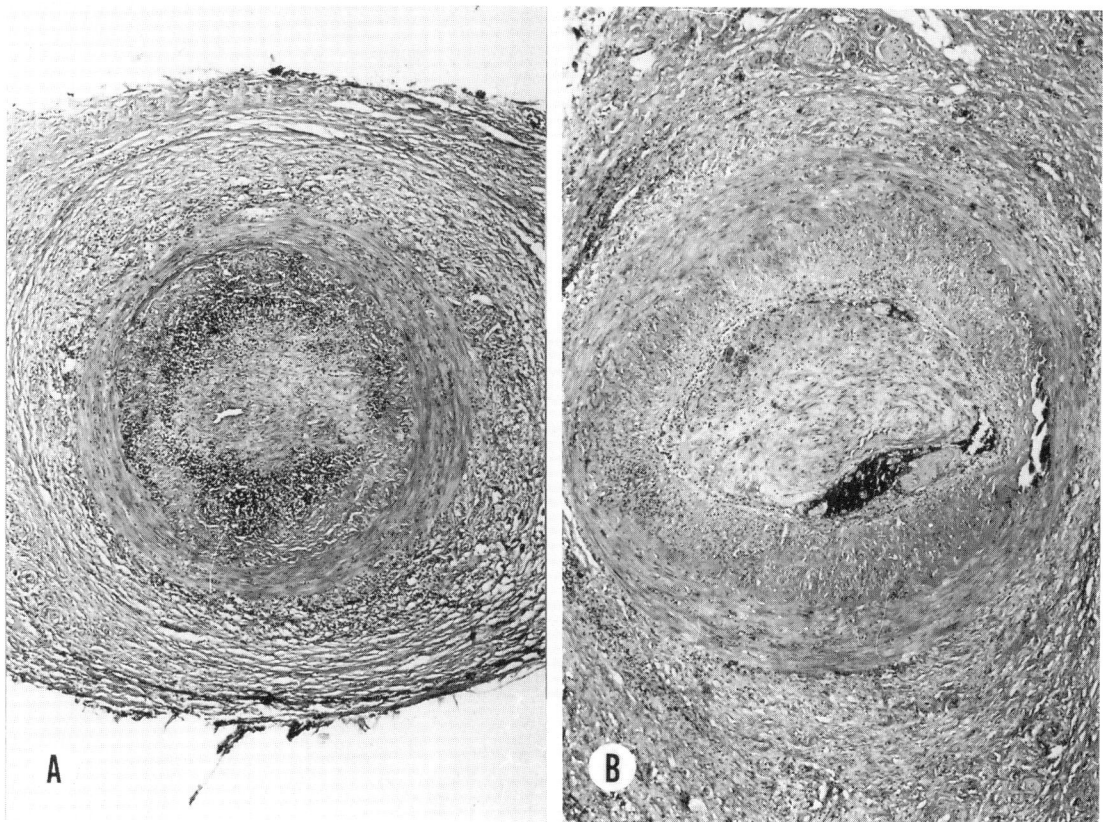

Figure 17.9 Atypical, nongranulomatous temporal arteritis. (A) Intimal and adventitial lymphocytic infiltrate. (B) Adventitial cell infiltrate only. Neither has giant cells. (A and B ×40.)

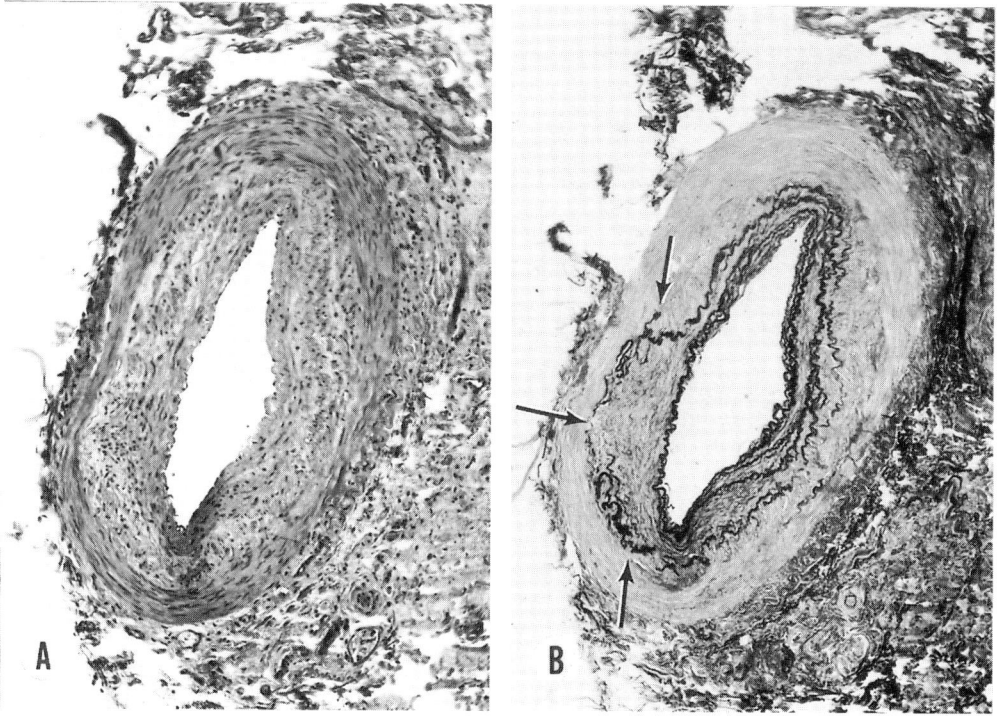

Figure 17.10 Healed temporal arteritis: (A) H&E section shows asymmetric fibrous scarring of the media. (B) Elastic stain section shows eccentric disruption of the internal elastic lamina (arrows). (A and B ×64.)

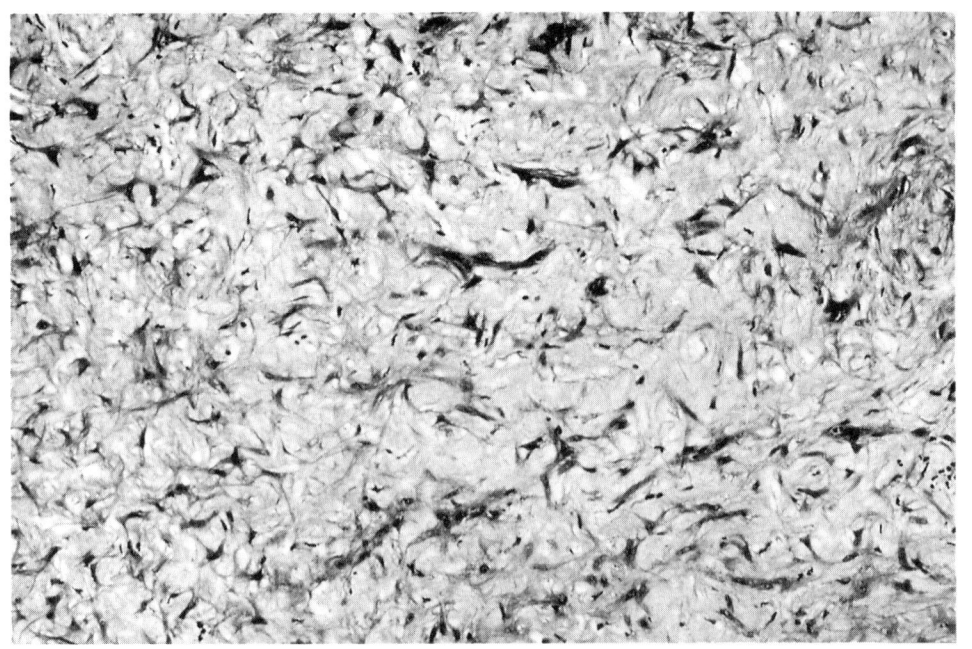

Figure 17.11 Stellate and spindle cell proliferation in a loose myxoid stroma of intimal fibrosis in temporal arteritis. (H&E ×240.)

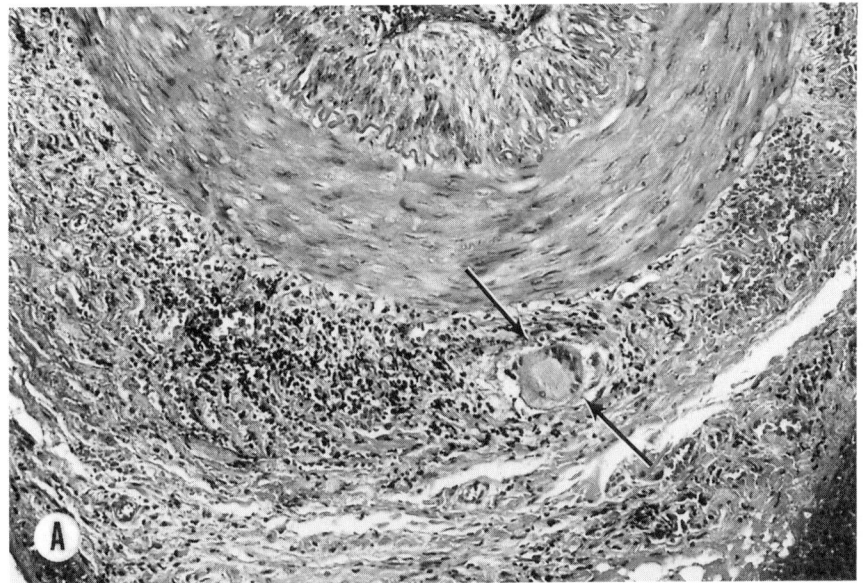

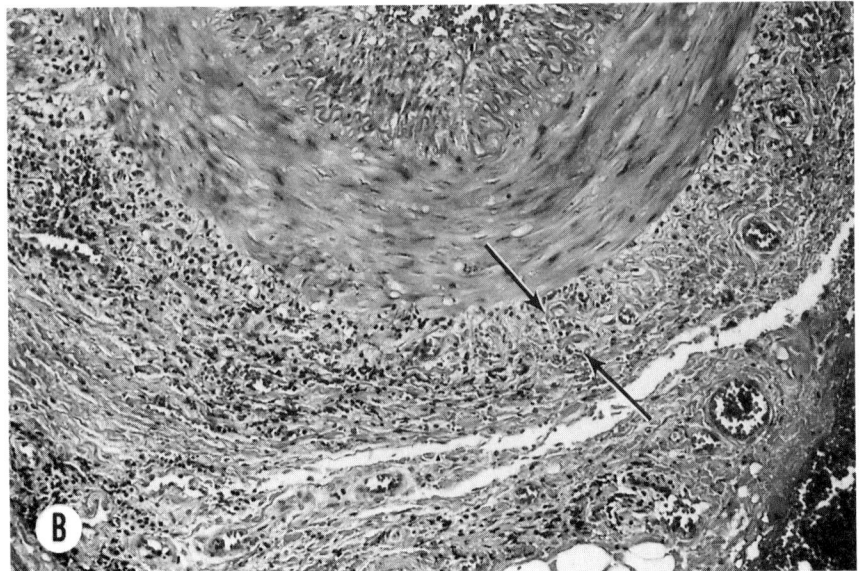

Figure 17.12 The vagary of finding or not finding giant cells in biopsies of temporal arteritis. (A and B) Serial sections of the same biopsy tissue block, 50 μm apart; a giant cell is present in section (A) and absent in the corresponding area of section (B) (arrows). (A and B ×160.)

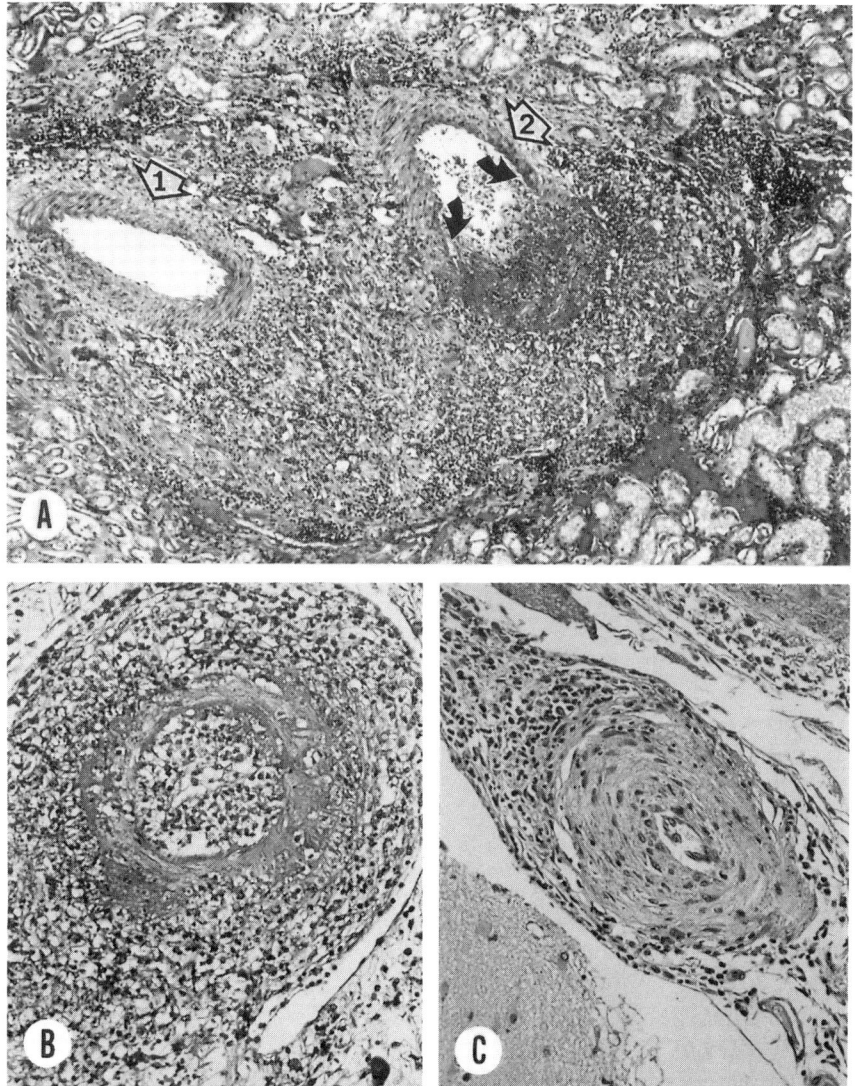

Figure 17.13 Variegated lesions in different arteries occurring simultaneously in a typical case of classic polyarteritis nodosa. (A) Two different segments of the same interlobar artery of the kidney: segment 1 appears normal while segment 2 shows a focal necrosis with microaneurysm (arrows). (B) Typical necrotizing vasculitis with fibrinoid necrosis. (C) Proliferative endarteritis typical of healing stage of vascular lesion in polyarteritis. (H&E A ×64, B and C ×160.)

becomes progressively more scarce in end-stage lesions (Figure 17.16).

It is commonly believed that the lungs are not involved in PAN [120], but this is certainly incorrect (Figure 17.17). PAN with pulmonary involvement is a clinically distinct subgroup of systemic vasculitis. Two separate series of cases from the Mayo Clinic [121,122] reported 28 and 32% of patients who had PAN with involvement of the lungs. Rose and Spencer [123], in their classic study of 111 autopsy cases of PAN, also recognized 32 cases (29%) with pulmonary involvement.

17.5.2 MICROSCOPIC POLYARTERITIS

A distinction between microscopic polyarteritis and classic polyarteritis nodosa is justified since the distribution of vascular lesions, clinical manifestations and the complications differ in these two conditions [124]. In 1948, Davson et al. [125] linked the presence of primary systemic vasculitis with segmental necrotizing glomerulonephritis in a subgroup of patients, suggesting that such patients had a 'microscopic form' of polyarteritis which was distinct from the classic PAN described by Kussmaul and Maier [32]. Later, Wainwright and Davson [126] provided a morphological basis for this concept by suggesting that the glomerular lesions were themselves a manifestation of vasculitis since the glomerulus can be regarded as differentiated micro-vasculature. In microscopic polyarteritis, blood vessels of calibers larger than the arterioles are seldom, if even, involved (Figure 17.18).

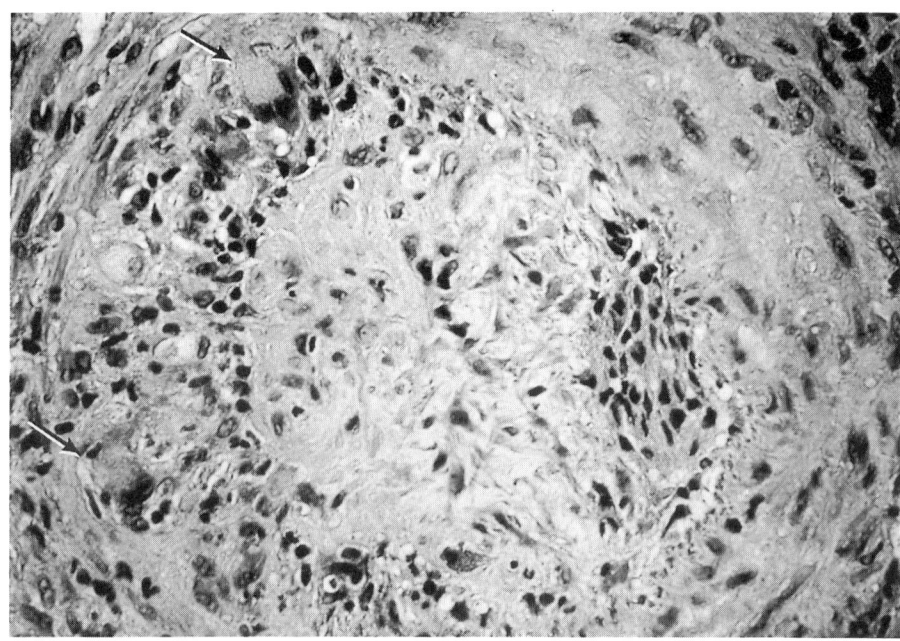

Figure 17.14 A granulomatous variant of acute phase lesion of polyarteritis nodosa with giant cells (arrows). (H&E ×400.)

17.5.3 INFANTILE POLYARTERITIS AND KAWASAKI DISEASE

Although polyarteritis has been reported to occur in a newborn under one month of age [127], it is generally uncommon in infants and children. Only 26 cases of polyarteritis in infancy were reported through 1973 and less than 150 cases in older children were reported in the literature through 1976 [128,129]. Infantile polyarteritis shows a special predilection for cardiac involvement as coronary vasculitis and multiple arterial aneurysms (Figures 17.19 and 17.20), with infrequent involvement of the skeletal muscle, kidneys and other viscera, whereas the childhood form is similar to adult PAN in the distribution of organ involvement [128,130]. Most investigators [128–132] have concluded that infantile polyarteritis is indistinguishable clinically and pathologically from fatal cases of Kawasaki disease, also known as the acute febrile mucocutaneous lymph node syndrome [132].

17.5.4 HYPERSENSITIVITY ANGIITIS (CUTANEOUS AND SMALL-VESSEL ANGIITIS)

Necrotizing angiitis involving small blood vessels has many synonyms and is commonly associated with a large and heterogeneous group of clinical syndromes. Zeek [48,49] had originally used the term 'hypersensitivity angiitis' to describe disseminated necrotizing vasculitis of arterioles and venules, both systemic and pulmonary and considered it to be distinguishable from polyarteritis nodosa. Clinically, the vascular lesions are seen most commonly in the skin, where they usually appear as purpura or urticaria. The term hypersensitivity angiitis has been used by others [15,121] to refer to conditions in which skin involvement dominates and visceral involvement is absent or occurs only rarely. Other investigators prefer such synonyms as 'allergic vasculitis' [133] and 'leukocytoclastic vasculitis' [134].

Because they are easily accessible for biopsy, cutaneous lesions of hypersensitivity vasculitis have been studied more extensively than those in other sites, and much of our understanding of small vessel vasculitis is based on cutaneous vasculitis. Current belief is that the

lating immune complexes in vessel walls that activate the complement cascade [16,54,134]. Joints, muscles, peripheral nerves, kidneys and the gastrointestinal tract are the more common sites of systemic involvement. Clinically, significant involvement of the lungs, heart and the central nervous system occurs less frequently and is seen mainly in patients with hypersensitivity angiitis and essential mixed cryoglobulinemic vasculitis [25]. Polymorphonuclear leukocytes then migrate to the area and release lysosomal enzymes that damage blood vessels and lead to diapedesis of erythrocytes, fibrin deposition and local tissue necrosis.

It has been suggested that cutaneous necrotizing vasculitis can be divided into neutrophilic (Figure 17.21) and lymphocytic (Figure 17.22) vasculitis. The former frequently is associated with hypocomplementemia, whereas the latter is not [135,136]. However, they may simply be different evolutional stages of the same

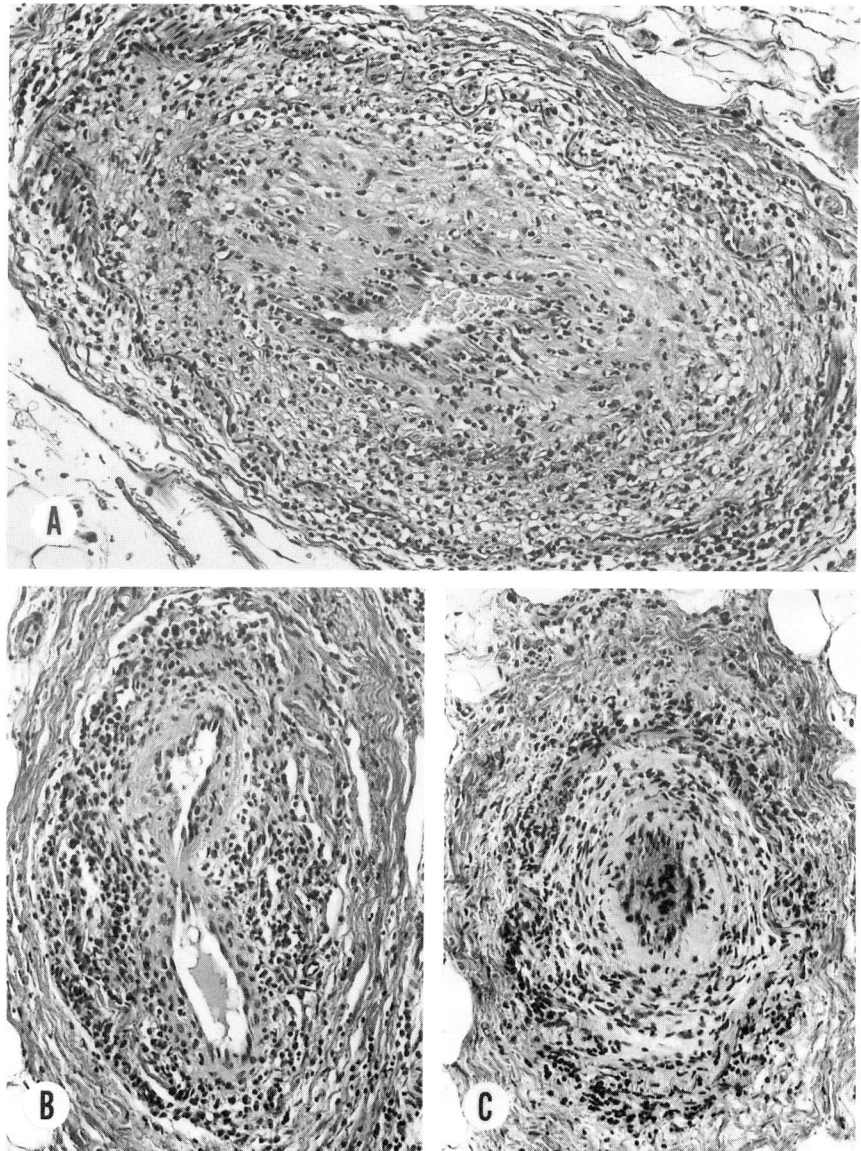

Figure 17.15 Healing lesions of polyarteritis nodosa (A, B and C) appearing in different segment of the surgically resected ischemic bowel. (H&E ×160.)

disease process and hypocomplementemia cannot serve as an independent diagnostic feature. Indeed, sequential biopsies in cutaneous leukocytoclastic vasculitis have shown that the inflammatory cell infiltrate changes progressively from a neutrophilic predominant to a lymphocytic predominant type over a five-day period [137].

Hypersensitivity angiitis (Figure 17.22) may be seen as the primary clinicopathological process in serum sickness, Schönlein–Henoch syndrome, drug hypersensitivity reaction and essential mixed cryoglobulinemia. The identical type of vasculitis can also be seen in association with a variety of systemic disorders, immune-mediated diseases and selected type of malignancies (Table 17.1). The diagnostic approach is similar to that recommended for polyarteritis nodosa. The management plan for hypersensitivity angiitis should include identification and removal of an offending agent, treatment of the underlying disease and a judicious use of immunosuppressive therapy.

17.6 Pulmonary angiitis and granulomatosis

'Pulmonary angiitis' means, literally, inflammation of blood vessels in the lungs, irrespective of the cause. 'Pulmonary granulomatosis' refers to inflammatory changes in the lung parenchyma characterized by clustered infiltrates rich in lymphocytes, plasma cells, epithelioid cells or histiocytes, with or without the

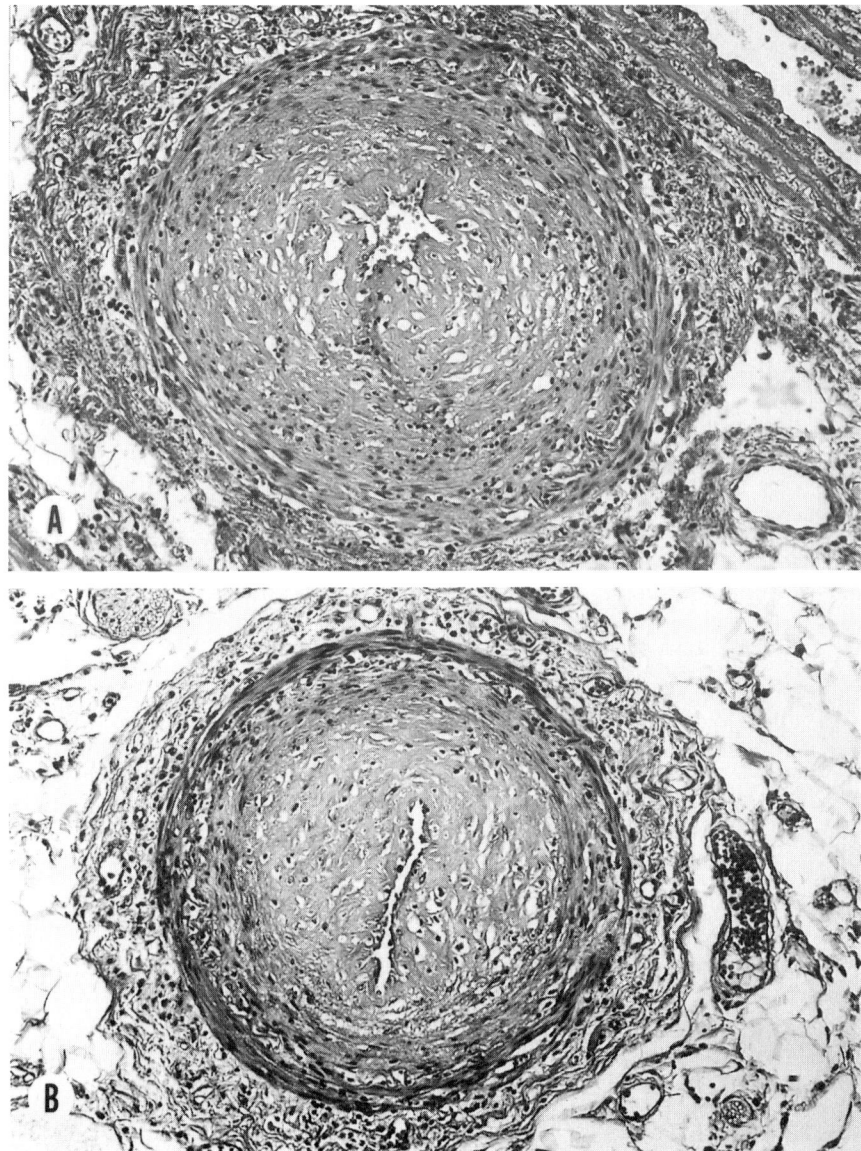

Figure 17.16 Healed lesions of polyarteritis nodosa (A and B) appearing in different segments of the surgically resected ischemic bowel from the same patient as shown in Figure 17.15. (H&E ×160.)

presence of multinucleate giant cells and with or without tissue necrosis. The term 'pulmonary angiitis and granulomatosis' is used when inflammation of blood vessels coexists with granulomatous inflammation of the lung parenchyma. Should fibrinoid necrosis of blood vessels or the surrounding tissue, or both, become a dominant feature, the descriptive terms 'necrotizing angiitis' and 'necrotizing granulomatosis' may apply. The preponderance of eosinophilic granulocyte in the inflammatory infiltrate may be an additional distinguishing histopathologic feature of pulmonary angiitis and granulomatosis, such as in Churg–Strauss syndrome [1,2,6,45].

17.6.1 CLASSIFICATION OF PULMONARY ANGIITIS AND GRANULOMATOSIS

Current classifications of pulmonary angiitis and granulomatosis [1,6] are at best arbitrary, but necessary, for a rational approach to the diagnosis and treatment of these disorders. A practical scheme of classification, incorporating both the clinical and pathologic characteristics of pulmonary vasculitides, seems most useful in offering the clinician guidelines for when to suspect and what to expect in the histologic diagnosis of vasculitis (Table 17.3).

In 1973, Liebow [138] first described five varieties of

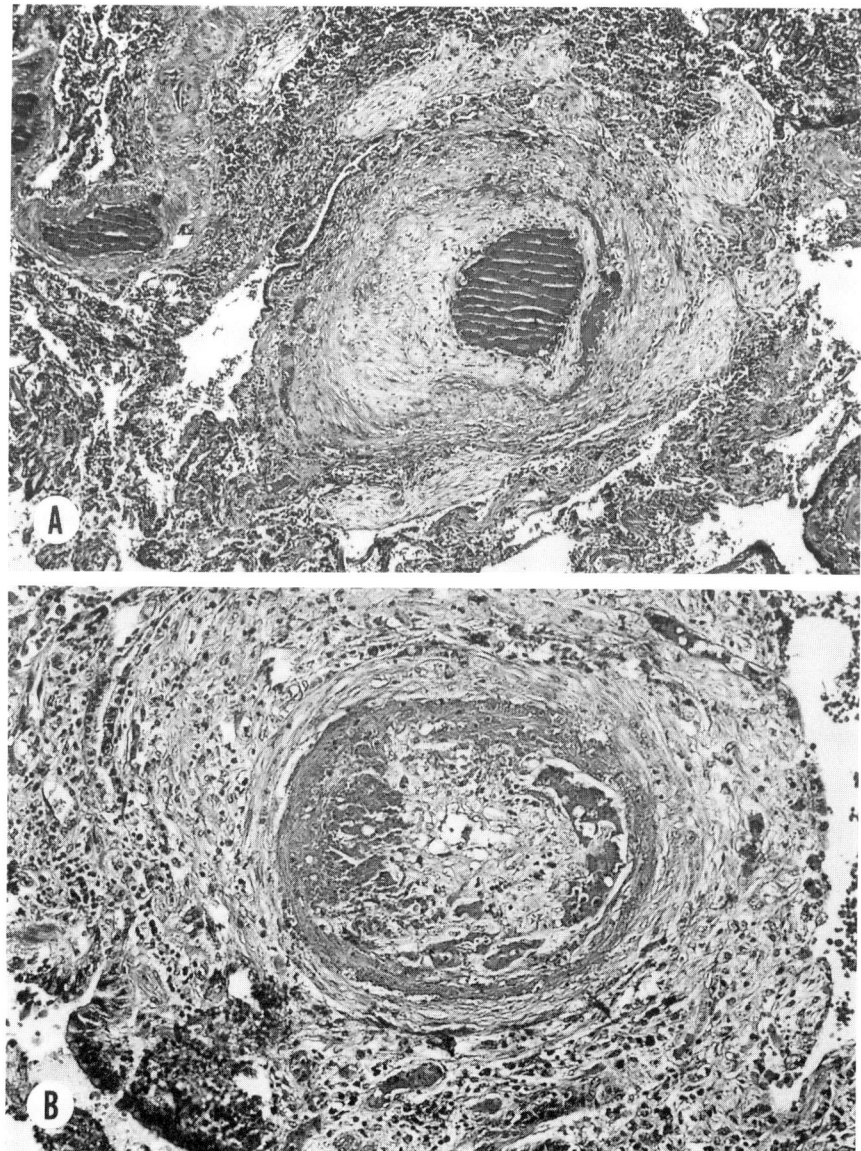

Figure 17.17 Lung involvement in polyarteritis nodosa: necrotizing vasculitis of a small pulmonary artery (A) and bronchial artery (B). (H&E A ×64, B ×160.)

some similarities in the histologic characteristics and natural history of these disorders. They were:

- classic Wegener's granulomatosis
- limited angiitis and granulomatosis of the Wegener's type
- lymphomatoid granulomatosis
- necrotizing sarcoid angiitis and granulomatosis
- bronchocentric granulomatosis.

This group of heterogeneous disorders was unified by tissue necrosis accompanied by a granulomatous inflammatory reaction and angiitis that is nearly always present in pulmonary vessels and sometimes in systemic vessels as well. In Liebow's view, any implication that these conditions are necessarily 'variants' of the same disease is unwarranted, since the cause and pathogenesis are both unknown. On this premise, the reason is unclear for the non-inclusion of allergic granulomatosis and angiitis (Churg–Strauss syndrome) in Liebow's classification [138].

17.6.2 WEGENER'S GRANULOMATOSIS

What is now known as Wegener's granulomatosis was probably first described by Klinger [139] several years before Wegener's reports in the 1930s [140,141]. Classic Wegener's granulomatosis is characterized by the triad of aseptic granulomatous necrosis of the upper and lower respiratory tract, necrotizing angiitis and focal glomerulonephritis [142–144]. Wegener's granulo-

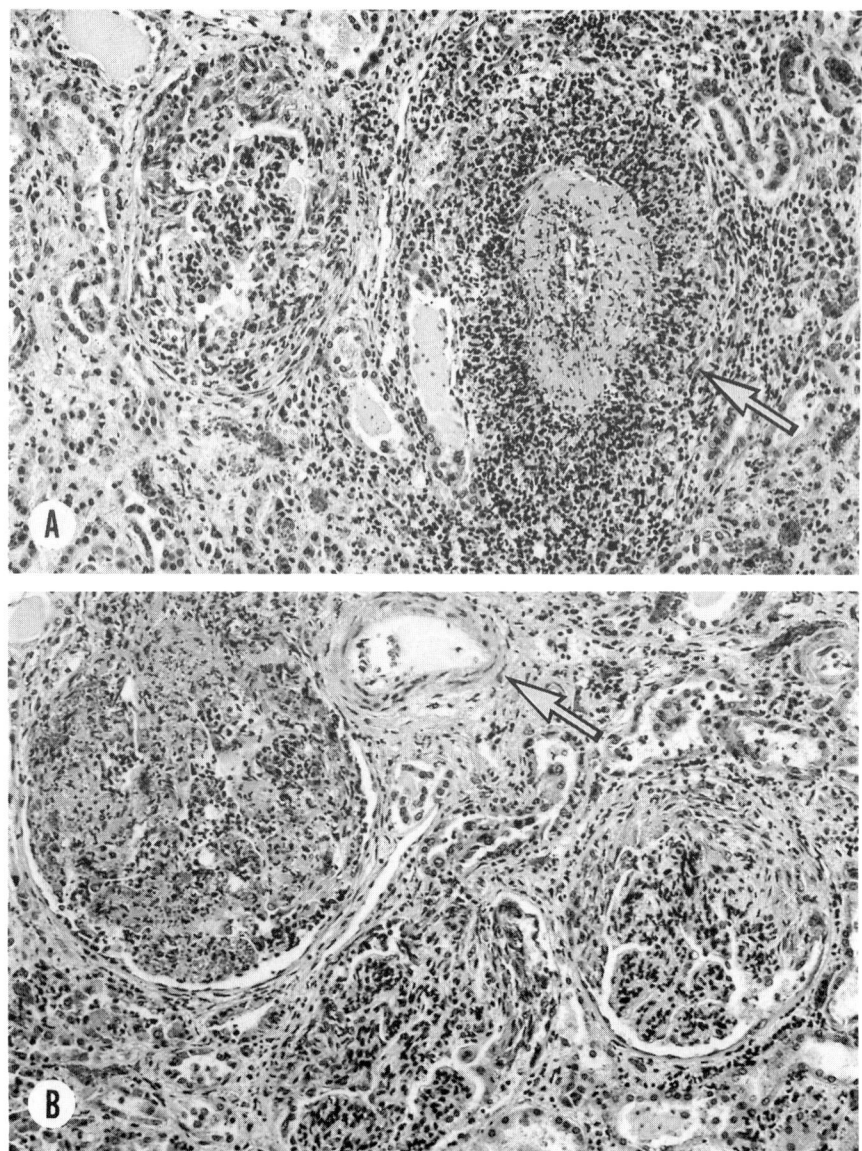

Figure 17.18 (A) Arterial lesion (arrow) in microscopic polyarteritis. (B) Necrotizing glomerulitis in microscopic polyarteritis with a normal arteriole (arrow) from a different part of the same kidney as in (A) (H&E ×160.)

matosis has the potential to involve almost any organ system of the body [145]. The disease is somewhat more common in men, with a peak incidence in the fifth decade. Untreated patients die within about five months of the onset of symptoms, usually of renal failure, unless treated aggressively with cytotoxic agents [144,145].

The concept of the so-called limited forms of Wegener's granulomatosis [146] has been modified in recent years, since these cases probably represent early, occult or protracted stages of the disease that may later expand or transform into the classic disseminated forms [147].

The typical lung lesions of Wegener's granulomatosis are necrotizing granulomatosis combined with vasculitis (Figure 17.23). The granulomas may be discrete or confluent, forming an irregular geographic pattern of necrosis (Figure 17.24). The central zone of necrosis is surrounded by a dense cluster of lymphocytes, plasma cells and palisading histiocytes. Eosinophils may be present but are generally not prominent. The number of giant cells that can be identified is highly variable and they may be found remote from areas of granulomatous necrosis (Figure 17.25). The vascular lesions are essentially a necrotizing angiitis, and not necessarily a granulomatous angiitis, affecting some small and large blood vessels and sparing others. Thus, granulomatous tissue necrosis is a constant histopathologic feature, but not the necrotizing angiitis, in a given biopsy of the lung and the upper respiratory tract (nasal mucosa and sinuses) in Wegener's granulomatosis.

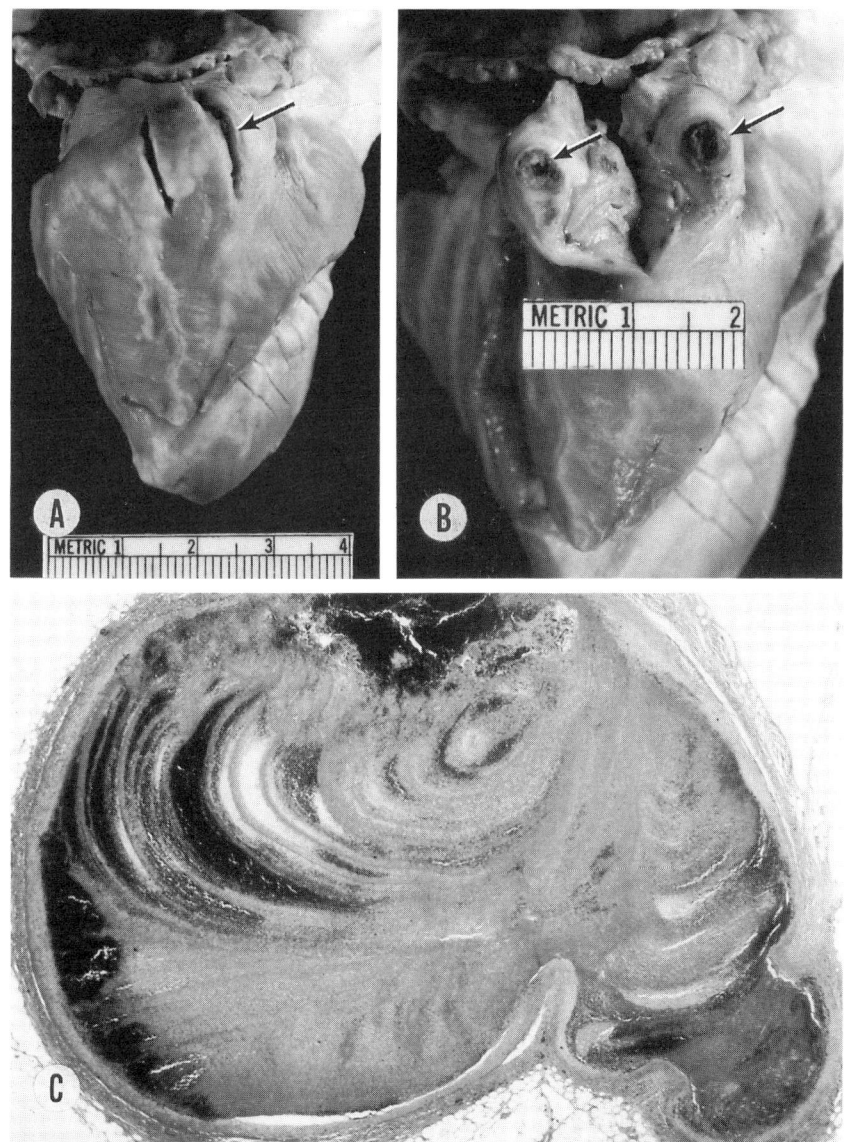

Figure 17.19 Coronary arterial lesions in Kawasaki disease. (A and B) Aneurysmal right coronary artery with occlusive thrombosis (arrows). (C) Photomicrograph of the aneurysmal coronary artery. (H&E ×16.)

17.6.3 CHURG–STRAUSS SYNDROME

Also known as allergic granulomatosis and angiitis [2,44,45,148], Churg–Strauss syndrome is a relatively uncommon systemic disease with clinical and pathologic features that overlap both polyarteritis nodosa and Wegener's granulomatosis. The syndrome is characterized by pulmonary and systemic necrotizing angiitis, extravascular granulomas and eosinophilia, occurring almost exclusively in patients with asthma or an allergic history [2,148]. Churg–Strauss syndrome is probably more common than the number of reported cases in the literature would indicate [2], and many were previously described as variants of polyarteritis nodosa with pulmonary involvement [123]. Lanham and associates [148] suggest that Churg–Strauss syndrome has often gone undiagnosed, not only because of the narrow focus on fulfilling the histopathologic criteria, but also because different disease entities that form components of the syndrome are recognized individually but remain unintegrated. The fact that Lanham and colleagues [148] were able to identify 154 cases of Churg–Strauss syndrome in the English literature surveyed up to June 1982 would support their contention.

The pulmonary lesions of Churg–Strauss syndrome may resemble chronic eosinophilic pneumonia with granulomatous necrosis and vasculitis. The necrotizing angiitis, with prominent eosinophilic infiltrate, charac-

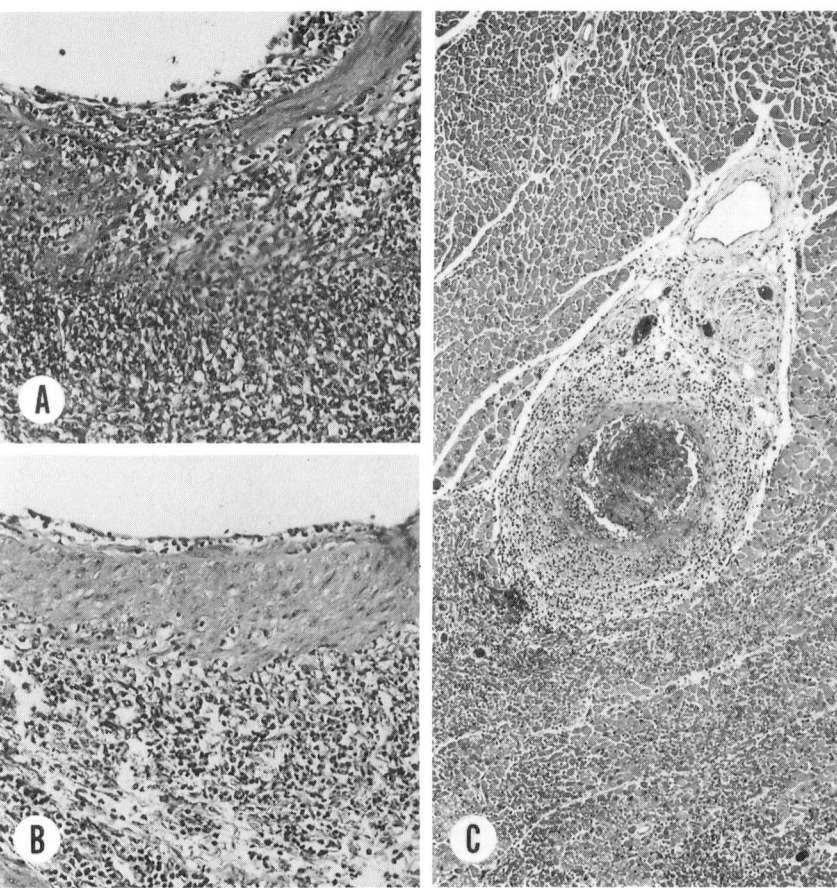

Figure 17.20 Coronary arterial lesions in Kawasaki disease. (A and B) Typical variegated appearance of necrotizing vasculitis affecting the epicardial coronary artery. (C) Necrotizing vasculitis of an intramural branch of the coronary artery. (H&E A&B ×160, C ×64.)

Table 17.3 Classification of pulmonary angiitis and granulomatosis

- Vasculitis of known cause and confined to the lungs
  - Infective vasculitis (bacterial, fungal, parasitic, viral)
  - Reactive vasculitis to embolic material (cotton, gauze, talc)
  - Primary pulmonary hypertension (plexogenic arteriopathy)
  - Secondary pulmonary hypertension (recurrent thromboembolism)
  - Pulmonary veno-occlusive disease
  - Pulmonary hypertension associated with cirrhosis or anorectic drug
- Vasculitis of unknown cause with lung as primary target organ (pulmonary angiitis and granulomatosis)
  - Wegener's granulomatosis (classic and limited forms)
  - Allergic angiitis and granulomatosis (Churg–Strauss syndrome)
  - Necrotizing sarcoid granulomatosis
  - Bronchocentric granulomatosis
- Systemic vasculitis that may involve the lungs
  - Polyarteritis nodosa
  - Rheumatoid arthritis
  - Systemic lupus erythematosus
  - Scleroderma (systemic sclerosis)
  - Dermatopolymyositis
  - Mixed connective tissue disease
  - Hypersensitivity vasculitis
  - Behçet syndrome/Hughes–Stovin syndrome
  - Takayasu arteritis
  - Disseminated and isolated giant cell angiitis

teristically involves both the arteries and veins (Figure 17.26) in distinction to polyarteritis, and the angiitis may affect the systemic and pulmonary blood vessels with equal frequencies. Bronchioles elsewhere in the lung generally show changes of chronic asthma and may also have extravascular eosinophilic granulomas (Figure 17.27). Pulmonary and/or systemic eosinophilic granulomas are a histopathologic hallmark of Churg–Strauss syndrome [45]; the cutaneous extravascular necrotizing granuloma, however, lacks diagnostic specificity and may be found in a diverse variety of systemic diseases [149].

17.6.4 NECROTIZING SARCOID GRANULOMATOSIS

Necrotizing sarcoid granulomatosis superficially resembles Wegener's granulomatosis [150–153]. Some patients are asymptomatic, whereas others present with non-specific symptoms of malaise, fever, cough and pleuritic pain. About one fourth of patients have abnormal chest radiographs, but cavitation does not occur and hilar lymph node enlargement is uncommon. In contrast to a slight male predominance in Wegener's granulomatosis, necrotizing sarcoid granulomatosis is four times more common in females. The age range is wide and the disease sometimes occurs in children or teenagers [6].

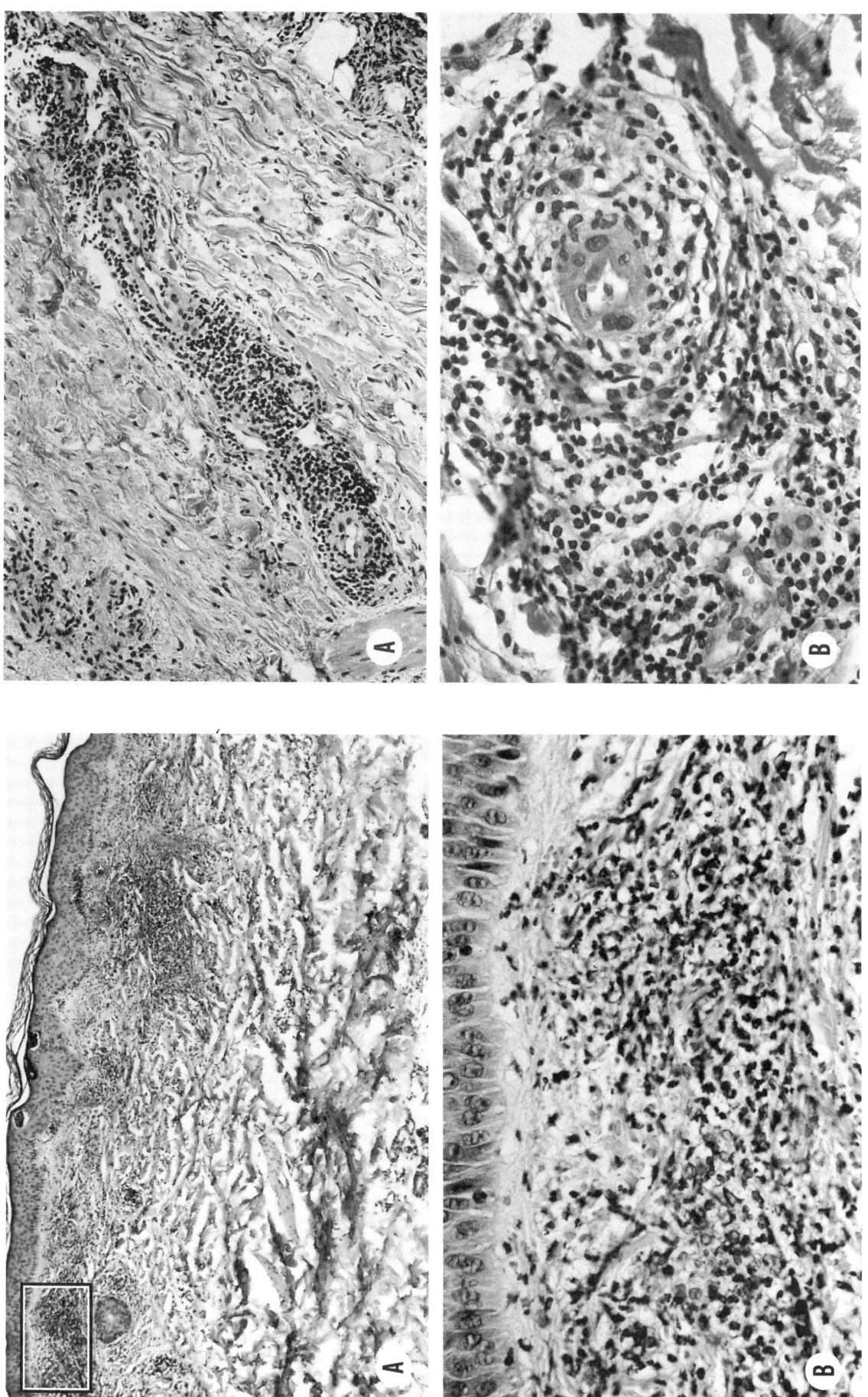

Figure 17.21 (A) Typical leukocytoclastic vasculitis of dermal arterioles and venules; the boxed area is shown at higher magnification in (B). (H&E A ×64, B ×400.)

Figure 17.22 Drug hypersensitivity vasculitis (A) is morphologically indistinguishable from the non-specific lymphocytic vasculitis (B), as seen in a variety of malignant diseases and retroperitoneal fibrosis. (H&E A ×160, B ×400.)

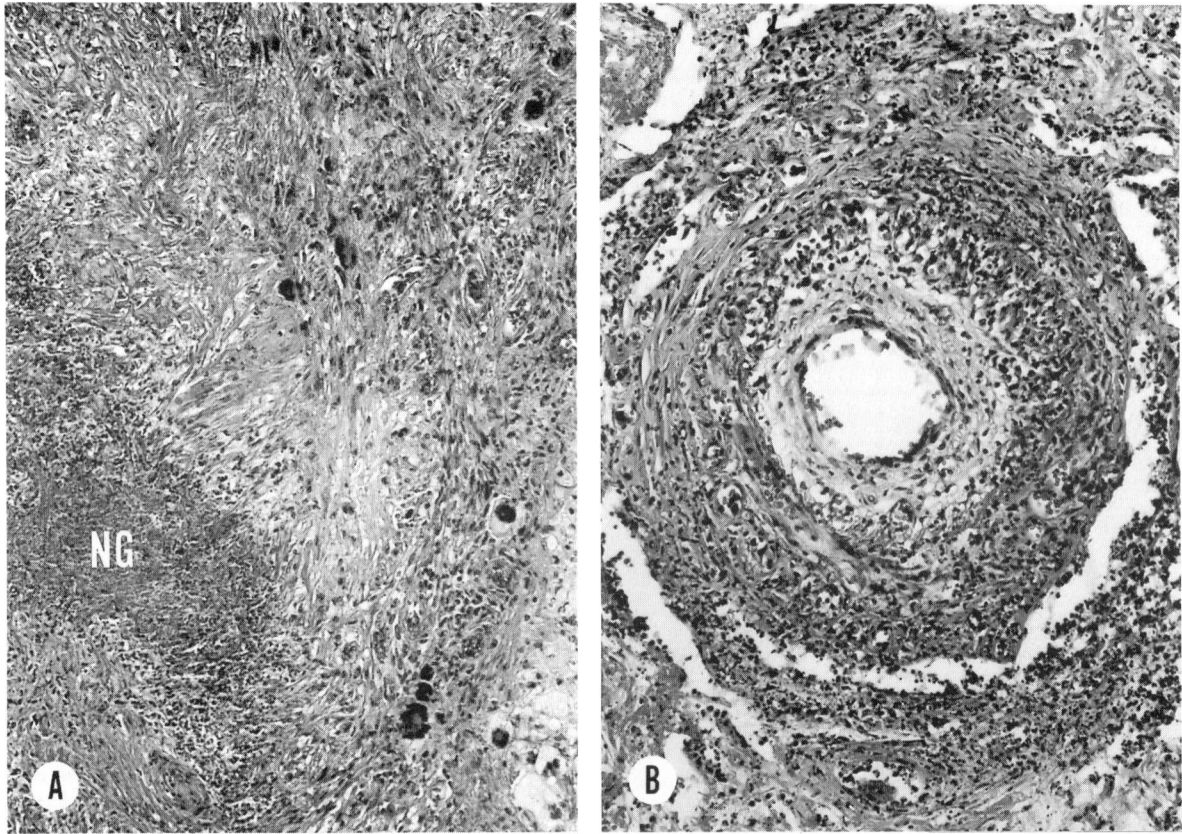

Figure 17.23 Typical pulmonary lesions of Wegener's granulomatosis. (A) Necrotizing granuloma (NG) surrounded by several giant cells. (B) Necrotizing vasculitis of a small artery. (H&E ×160.) (Reproduced with permission from Lie [6].)

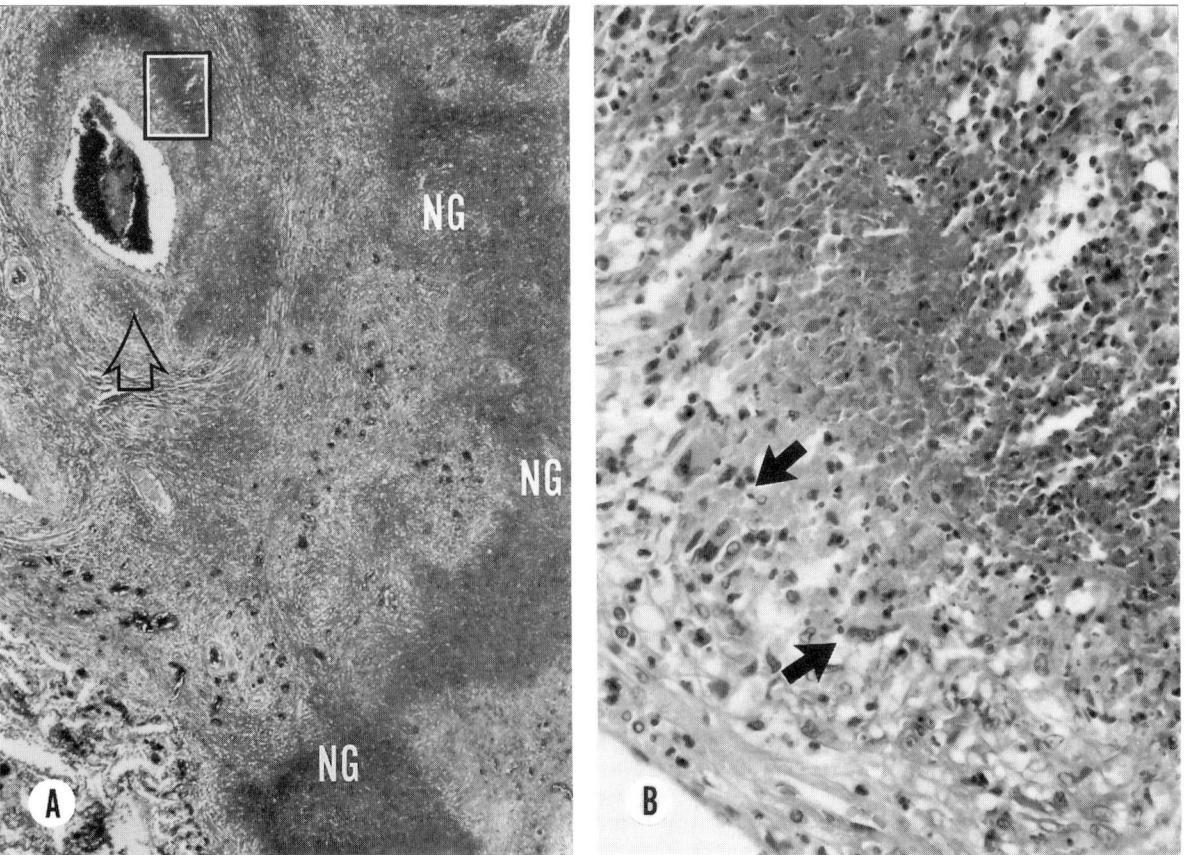

Figure 17.24 (A) Wegener's granulomatosis with necrotizing vasculitis of a medium-sized artery (arrow) in an area of the lung with a geographic pattern of confluent necrotizing granulomas (NG). (B) Close-up of the boxed area in (A) showing giant cells in the arterial wall. (H&E A ×40, B ×400.) (Reproduced with permission from Lie [6].)

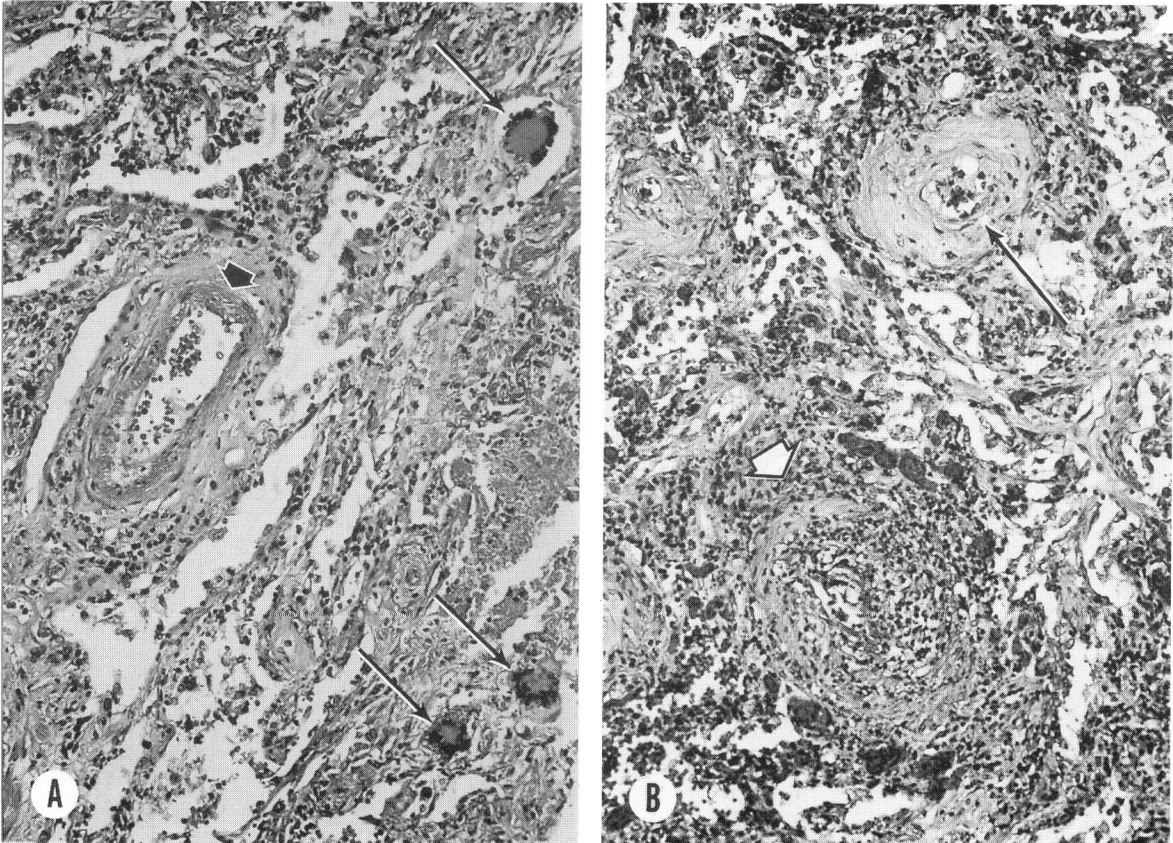

Figure 17.25 Variations of the histopathologic changes of the lung in Wegener's granulomatosis. (A) Absence of vasculitis (short arrow) and isolated giant cells (long arrows) without granulomatous necrosis of the lung. (B) Two small arteries of the lung, side by side, one with necrotizing vasculitis (short arrow) and one without (long arrow). (H&E ×160.) (Reproduced with permission from Lie [6].)

The distinctive morphologic feature is the presence of numerous sarcoid-like granulomas, which are not seen in any other form of pulmonary angiitis and granulomatosis. The vasculitis in necrotizing sarcoid granulomatosis affects both the arteries and veins, but seldom appears as 'destructive' as in other forms of necrotizing angiitis (Figure 17.28). Its histologic appearance varies from compression or infiltration of the vessel wall by non-caseating granulomas and multinucleated giant cells to non-specific transmural infiltration by lymphocytes and plasma cells. Systemic vasculitis is not a feature of necrotizing sarcoid granulomatosis [152,153].

The validity of necrotizing sarcoid granulomatosis as an independent entity separate from pulmonary sarcoidosis is questionable. In two separate surveys of the diagnosis of pulmonary sarcoidosis by open lung biopsy, Carrington and associates [150] and Rosen and co-workers [151] reported the prevalence of granulomatous angiitis to be 42 and 69%, respectively. The prognostic significance of pulmonary sarcoidosis with necrotizing granulomas is unclear.

17.7 Cerebral vasculitis

The central nervous system may be the seat of a wide variety of vasculitides, all but one of which are associated with a known underlying disease.

Because in most patients cerebral vasculitides are diagnosed clinically without a biopsy confirmation, one should be aware of a host of non-vasculitic conditions that may simulate vasculitis clinically or angiographically (Table 17.4).

17.7.1 PRIMARY (GRANULOMATOUS) ANGIITIS OF THE CENTRAL NERVOUS SYSTEM

Primary (granulomatous) angiitis of the central nervous system (PANS) was probably first described in 1922, by Harbitz, among the 'unknown forms of arteritis' [154]. This condition later became known as 'non-infectious granulomatous angiitis involving the central nervous system' [155], 'granulomatous angiitis of the nervous system' [156], or 'isolated angiitis of the central nervous

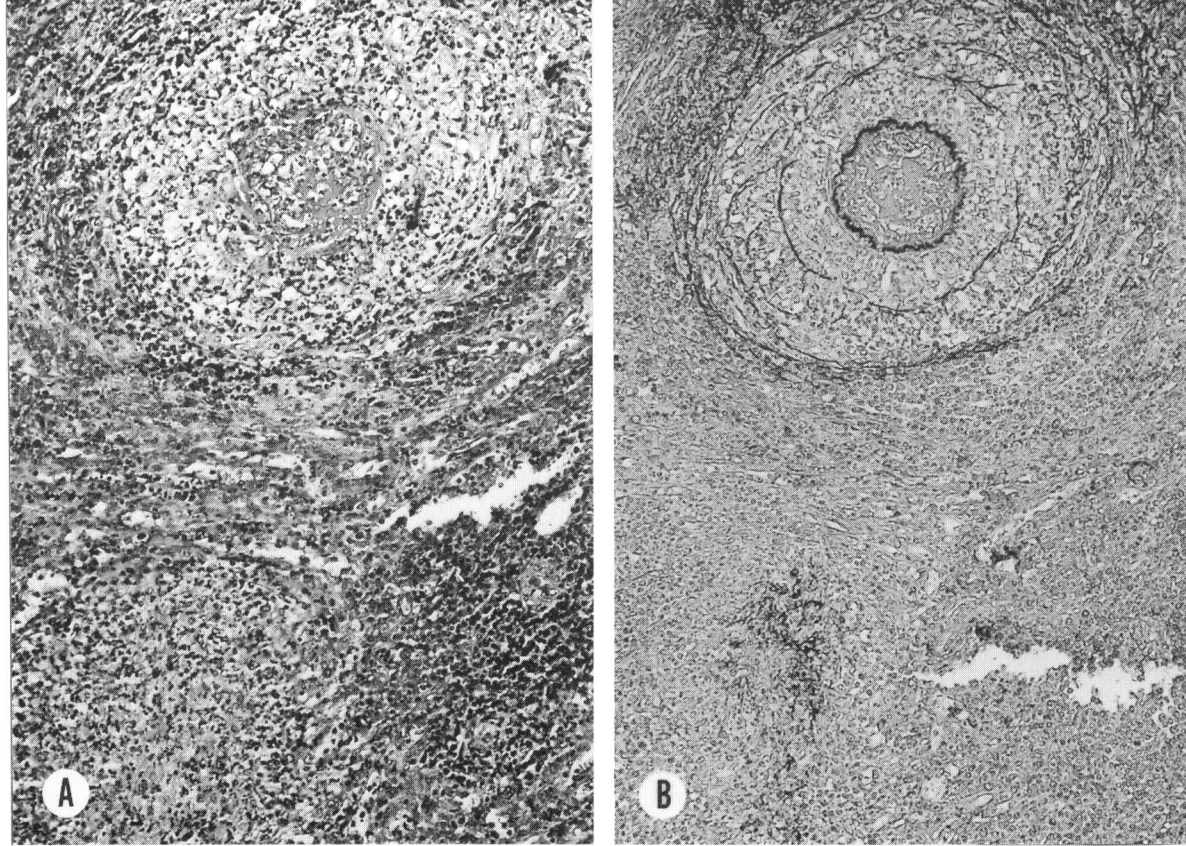

Figure 17.26 (A) Necrotizing vasculitis of a small pulmonary vein in Churg–Strauss syndrome with prominent eosinophils in the cellular infiltrate. (B) A matching section stained with elastic van Gieson to illustrate that the small blood vessel is a vein, not an artery. ((A) H&E; (B) elastic stain. ×160.) (Reproduced with permission from Lie [6].)

Table 17.4 Angiitis of the central nervous system

- Primary cerebral angiitis
  - Granulomatous angiitis of the nervous system
- Secondary cerebral angiitis
  - Infective angiitis (bacterial, fungal, protozoal, rickettsial, viral)
  - Systemic diseases
    - Giant cell arteritis (temporal arteritis, Takayasu arteritis)
    - Polyarteritis nodosa
    - Wegener's granulomatosis
    - Churg–Strauss syndrome
    - Hypersensitivity angiitis
    - Systemic lupus erythematosus or other connective tissue disease
    - Behçet syndrome
    - Cogan syndrome
    - Necrotizing sarcoid granulomatosis and sarcoid angiitis
    - Inflammatory bowel disease
  - Drug-induced or drug-related
    - Allopurinol
    - Amphetamines
    - Cocaine
    - Ephedrine
    - Heroin
  - Malignancy related
    - Hodgkin's lymphoma
    - Non-Hodgkin's lymphoma
    - Lymphomatoid granulomatosis
    - Leukemia
    - Metastatic small cell lung cancer
- Vasculitis simulators
  - Fibromuscular dysplasia
  - Moyamoya disease
  - Antiphospholipid syndrome
  - Vasospasm or acute arterial hypertension
  - Thrombotic thrombocytopenic purpura
  - Cardiac myxoma embolism
  - Sickle cell anemia
  - Radiation vasculopathy
  - Acute meningoencephalitis
  - Malignant angioendotheliomatosis

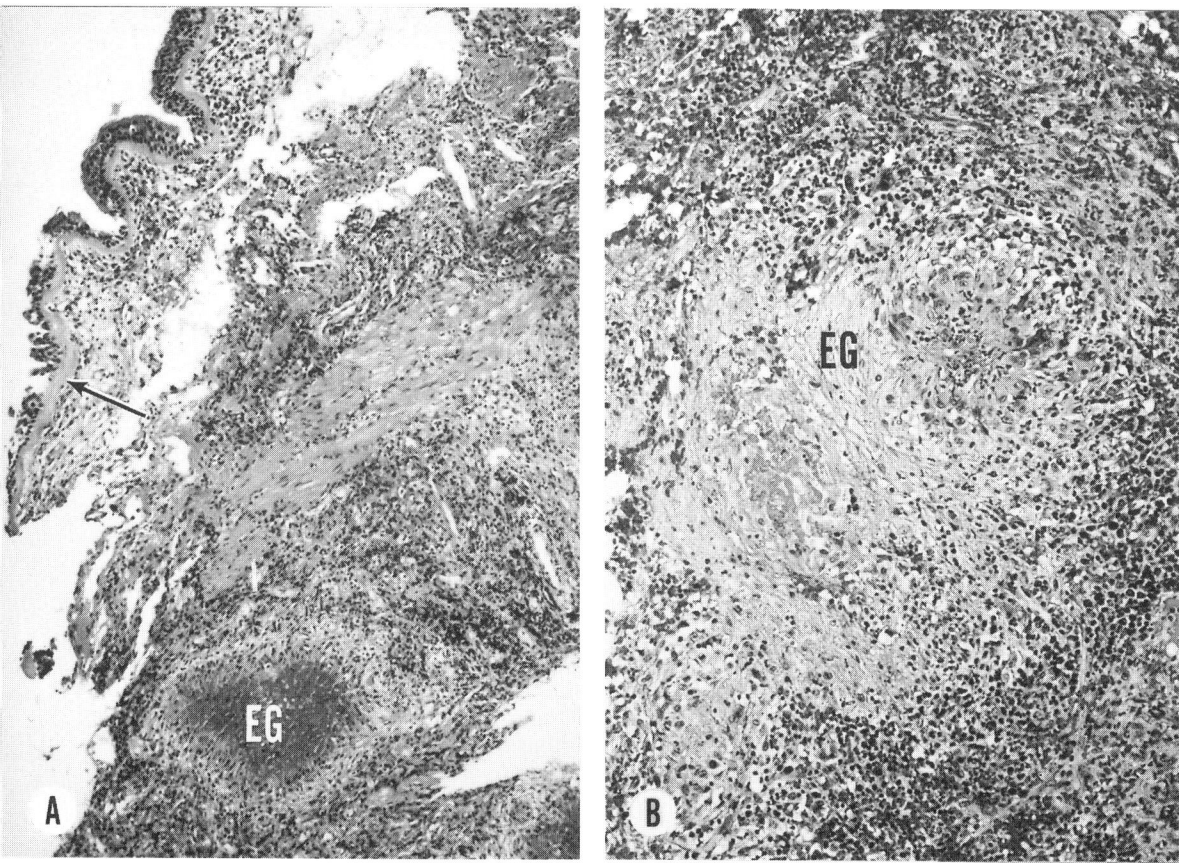

Figure 17.27 Churg–Strauss syndrome. (A) Bronchial biopsy showing the thick basement membrane (arrow) of an asthmatic and submucosal extravascular eosinophilic granuloma (EG). (B) Extravascular eosinophilic granulomas (EG) of the spleen. (H&E A ×64, B ×160.) (Reproduced with permission from Lie [6].)

system' [157]. Identical lesions have also been reported in the literature as 'giant-cell arteritis involving small meningeal and intracerebral vessels' [158]. Although PANS is usually restricted to the central nervous system, autopsies in some of the previously reported cases have shown a variable degree of involvement of extracranial arteries, including pulmonary and abdominal visceral angiitis. Thus, the designation of 'isolated angiitis' of the central nervous system is inappropriate.

PANS is uncommon and probably little more than 120 cases have been reported in the English language literature to date [9,159–163]. The disease occurs in patients of all ages (mean age 44 years and range 3 to 75 years) with a 5:3 or 4:3 slight male preponderance [162]. Although the definitive diagnosis of PANS requires biopsy-proven documentation, most of the cases reported were diagnosed clinically and angiographically or only at autopsy [160,162]. Biopsy, on the other hand, may not always be conclusive because of the focal nature of the distribution of PANS and the inherent sampling problem for small biopsies. Such is the dilemma that applies to the diagnosis of virtually all other systemic and isolated vasculitides [7].

PANS is a distinct nosologic entity with well charac-terized clinical, angiographic and histopathologic diagnostic features (Table 17.5).

In about two thirds of the reported cases, the presenting clinical features include headache, confusion, altered mental status and progressive intellectual deterioration. Diplopia, blurred vision, nystagmus, pupillary

Table 17.5 Diagnostic features of primary granulomatous angiitis of the nervous system

Clinical
Unexplained acute progressive encephalopathy without evidence of extracranial or systemic vasculitis; sometimes associated with history of herpes zoster infection, Hodgkin's lymphoma or illicit drug use; mean age 44 (range 3–75) years with 4:3 male preponderance.

Angiographic
Multifocal segmental irregularity, stenosis and dilatation of small and medium-sized intracranial arteries; alterations in blood flow or associated mass; rarely normal angiograms.

Histopathologic
Focal, segmental, necrotizing or granulomatous angiitis of leptomeningeal and parenchymal small blood vessels, commonly with skipped lesions, and coexistence of acute, healing and healed lesions.

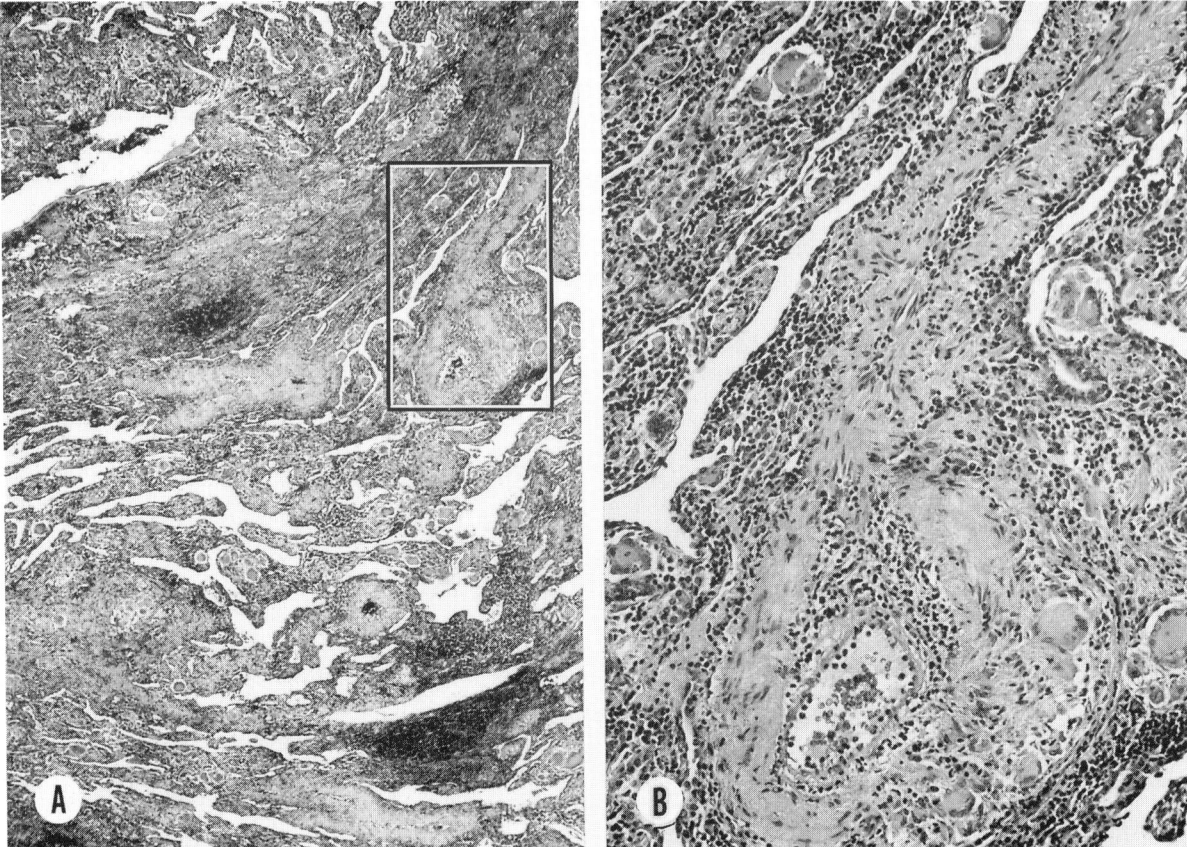

Figure 17.28 (A) Characteristic pulmonary histopathologic features of necrotizing sarcoid granulomatosis. (B) Close-up view of the boxed area in (A) showing granulomatous vasculitis with numerous giant cells. (H&E A ×40, B ×160.) (Reproduced with permission from Lie [6].)

abnormalities and dysarthria are indications of possible cranial nerve involvement. Hemiparesis and focal cerebral manifestations are not uncommon, whereas extrapyramidal signs and brain-stem strokes occur infrequently. Involvement of the spinal cord is also rare [9].

Angiographic findings in cerebral vasculitis are not entirely specific though they are quite characteristic [164,165]. Stenosis of the affected arteries may be focal or diffuse, partial or complete, circumferential or eccentric and smooth or irregular. Dilatation of the blood vessels tends to be discrete and aneurysmal. Changes in blood flow may be accelerated or diminished. Distribution of arterial alterations may be localized or widespread, usually affecting the smaller leptomeningeal and intraparenchymal blood vessels.

Although angiography may correctly suggest the presence of a cerebral vasculitis, it is incapable of revealing the histologic type of vasculitis, which only a positive biopsy can provide. Acute blood pressure elevation can mimic the angiographic appearance of cerebral vasculitis [166]. Unusual distribution of PANS involving the larger anterior and posterior cerebral arteries as well as both carotid siphons has also been reported [167]. In addition to its diagnostic usefulness, angiography is the only means currently available to monitor disease activity and the outcome of drug treatment in cerebral vasculitis.

Pathologically, PANS affects the small and medium-sized arteries and only rarely the veins and venules of the nervous system and meninges. It is characterized by a segmental, necrotizing or granulomatous vasculitis, often accompanied by thrombosis. Skipped lesions are common. The inflammatory infiltrate is predominantly lymphocytic with a smaller number of neutrophils, eosinophils, histocytes and plasma cells (Figure 17.29). Both Langhans and foreign body-type giant cells may be present and in variable numbers (Figure 17.30). Intimal fibrosis signifies the results of healing. Morphologically acute, healing and healed lesions frequently coexist in different segments of the same artery or adjacent arteries (Figure 17.31), reminiscent of polyarteritis nodosa [7].

17.7.2 SECONDARY ANGIITIS OF THE CENTRAL NERVOUS SYSTEM

Secondary angiitis of the central nervous system may be associated with infections, systemic vasculitis, rheumat-

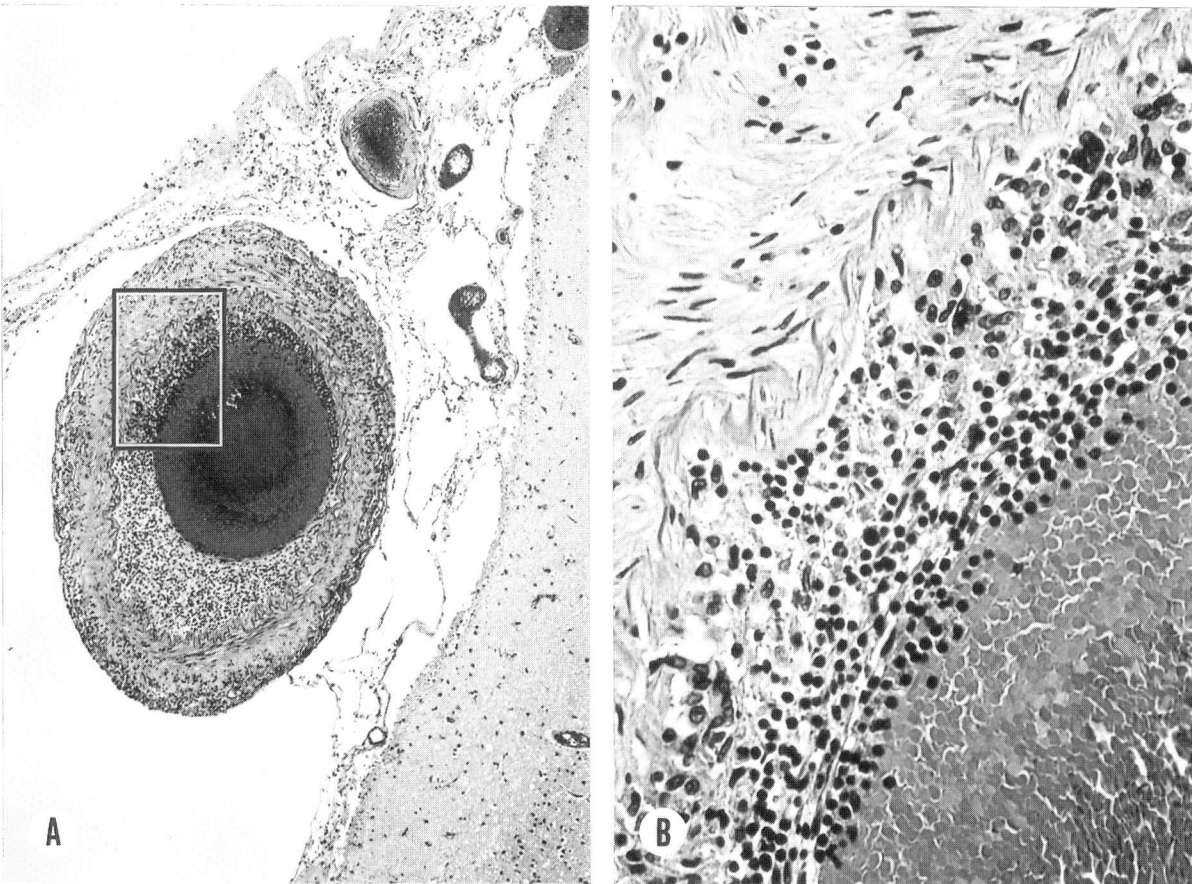

Figure 17.29 (A) Necrotizing angiitis of a leptomeningeal artery. (B) Close-up view of the boxed area in (A) to show the intense lymphoplasmacytic infiltrate without giant cells. (H&E A × 64, B ×400.)

ologic disorders, drug hypersensitivity, illicit drug abuse and malignancy (see Table 17.4). Only selected examples of secondary angiitis of the central nervous system are briefly reviewed here.

(a) Giant cell arteritis

The giant cell arteritis group comprises temporal arteritis and Takayasu arteritis, two distinct syndromes that have in common, histologically, a granulomatous inflammation of small, medium-sized and large arteries [4]. Although neurologic dysfunction and peripheral neuropathy are not uncommon in both temporal arteritis [168] and Takayasu arteritis [169], angiitis of the intracerebral and peripheral nerve blood vessels is distinctly rare.

(b) Polyarteritis nodosa and Churg–Strauss syndrome

Neurologic abnormalities occur in 25% to 50% of patients with polyarteritis nodosa, more commonly in the form of peripheral neuropathy. The onset of central nervous system disease tends to occur later in the course of polyarteritis nodosa than peripheral neuropathies [170]. Neurological abnormalities of Churg–Strauss syndrome, including vasculitis, are similar in their frequency and pattern of involvement to those in polyarteritis nodosa.

(c) Wegener's granulomatosis

Based on clinical and pathologic criteria, the frequency of central nervous system involvement in Wegener's granulomatosis varies from 22 [171] to 54% [172]. Necrotizing granulomatosis or focal vasculitis occurs independently more often than in combination. Cyclophosphamide therapy has reduced the incidence of neurologic complications of Wegener's granulomatosis, but treatment failure still occurs [173].

(d) Hypersensitivity angiitis

The incidence of neurologic complications in hypersensitivity angiitis is unknown. As is exemplified by the classic serum sickness or Schönlein–Henoch purpura [174], the central nervous system abnormalities include

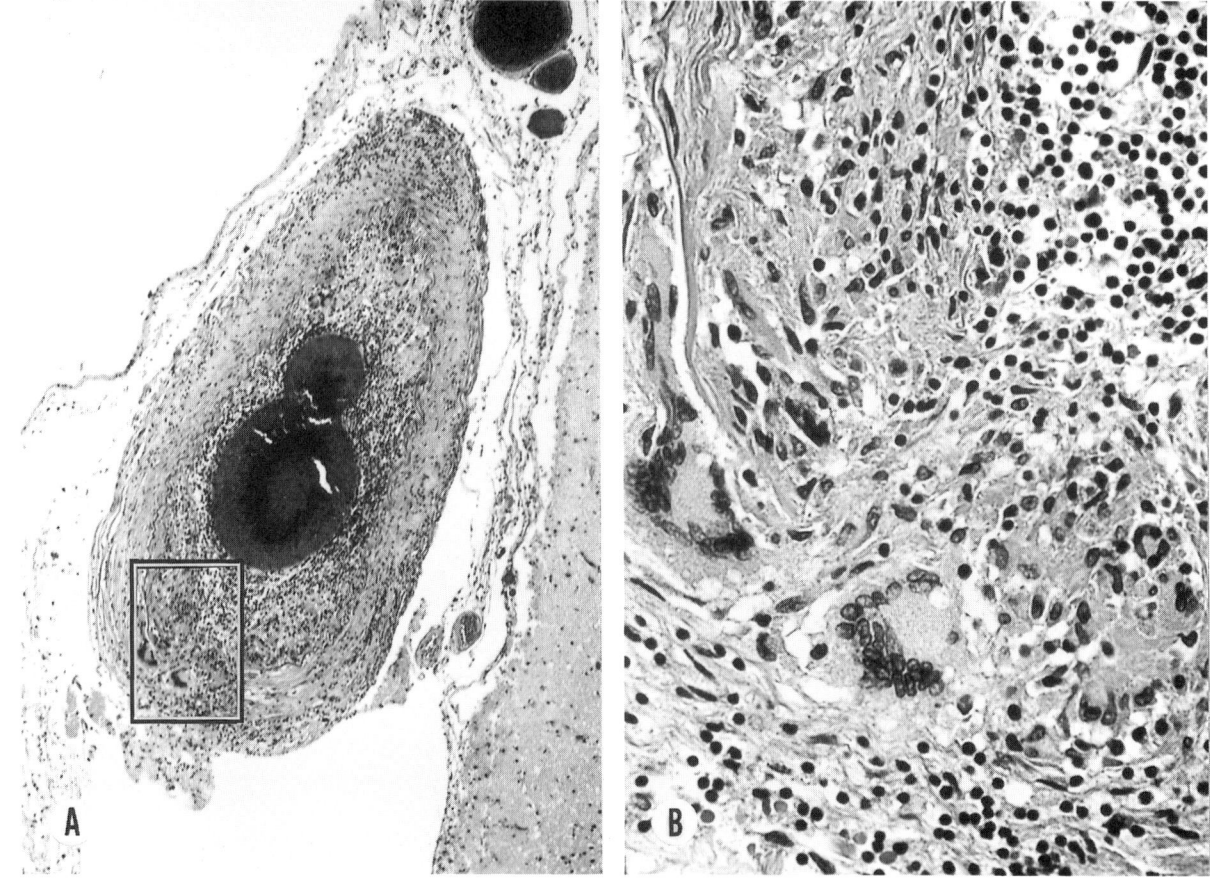

Figure 17.30 (A) Granulomatous angiitis of a leptomeningeal artery. (B) Close-up view of the boxed area in (A) to show a collection of the Langhans-type giant cells. (H&E A ×64, B ×400.)

encephalopathy, seizures, coma and peripheral neuropathies. Cerebral vasculitis is uncommon, but peripheral nerve necrotizing vasculitis frequently accompanies cutaneous vasculitis or visceral hypersensitivity angiitis.

(e) Rheumatic connective tissue disease

Central nervous system disease may be part of the clinical presentation of systemic lupus erythematosus in 25–75% of cases, of which about 30% are noninflammatory thrombotic vasculopathy of systemic lupus erythematosus and only 12.5% true vasculitis [175].

Central nervous system disease is uncommon in progressive systemic sclerosis; it has been reported to occur in 4% of 442 consecutive cases of progressive systemic sclerosis in one series [176], none of which could be attributed to vasculitis. Among the three cases of progressive systemic sclerosis presumed to have angiitis of the central nervous system, two had angiograms compatible with cerebral angiitis without biopsy confirmation [177,178], and the third was found to have only a right thalamic hemorrhage at post-mortem examination [179].

While vasculitis-related peripheral neuropathy is common in rheumatoid arthritis, angiitis of the central nervous system is exceedingly rare. A survey of the literature up to 1987 shows that there are only 12 reported cases of rheumatoid cerebral vasculitis [180]. These 12 cases had documented rheumatoid arthritis 1 to 30 years prior to the clinical onset of neurologic complications. Equally uncommon is systemic necrotizing vasculitis involving cerebral blood vessels in rheumatic heart disease, dermatopolymyositis, primary Sjögren's syndrome [181] and relapsing polychondritis [182].

(f) Behçet's syndrome

Bechçet's syndrome is a systemic disease with vasculitis as the common basis of its protean clinical manifestations. Behçet's syndrome may be a relatively benign disease, but the presence of neurologic involvement worsens the prognosis. About 30% of patients with Behçet's syndrome may have neurologic abnormalities

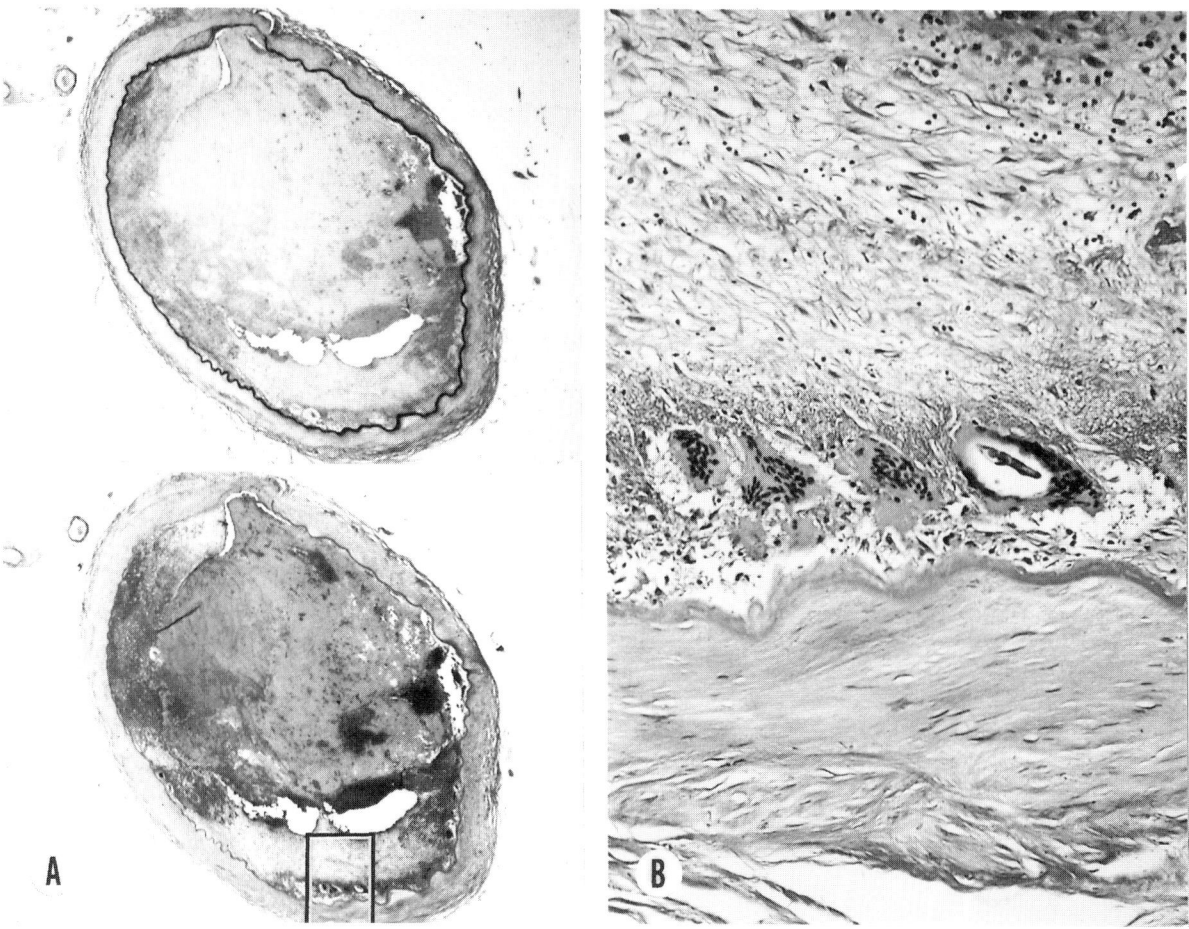

Figure 17.31 (A) Elastic stain and H&E stain of a healing granulomatous angiitis of the posterior cerebral artery from the same brain as that shown in Figures 17.29 and 17.30. (B) Close-up view of the boxed area in (A) to show intimal fibrosis and the foreign-body type giant cells. (A ×16, B ×160.)

that include meningoencephalitis, corticospinal tract involvement, cerebral ataxia, pseudotumor, pseudobulbar palsy, paraplegia, sensory disturbances and seizures [183,184].

The central nervous system pathologic findings in Behçet's syndrome include venous thrombosis, meningeal inflammation, perivascular cell loss and demyelination and a non-specific small-vessel lymphocytic vasculitis (Figure 17.32). Angiographically, resolution of cerebral vasculitis can be demonstrated after the successful treatment of Behçet's syndrome with combined cytotoxic agents and corticosteroids [185].

(g) Cogan syndrome

Cogan syndrome is an uncommon disease characterized by non-syphilitic interstitial keratitis associated with vestibuloauditory dysfunction, usually in young adults and with an equal sex distribution. At least 130 cases have been reported in the literature up to 1990 [186]. The prevalence of systemic vasculitis has been estimated to range from 15 to 72% [187]. Small-vessel vasculitides in Cogan syndrome are histopathologically indistinguishable from the polyarteritis nodosa-type necrotizing vasculitis and aortitis is the most common form of large-vessel vasculitis; involvement of intracerebral blood vessel is rare.

(h) Cerebral vasculitis associated with drug use and drug abuse

Systemic necrotizing angiitis associated with drug abuse was first reported in 1970 [188,189]. This was soon followed by a description of 19 patients with cerebral vasculitis associated with drug abuse, most of whom used intravenous methamphetamines, who had tissue-proven cerebral vasculitis or small-vessel occlusive disease on cerebral angiograms [190]. Since then, cerebral vasculitis has been reported in patients who are polydrug abusers and those who use heroin, ephedrine or cocaine exclusively [191].

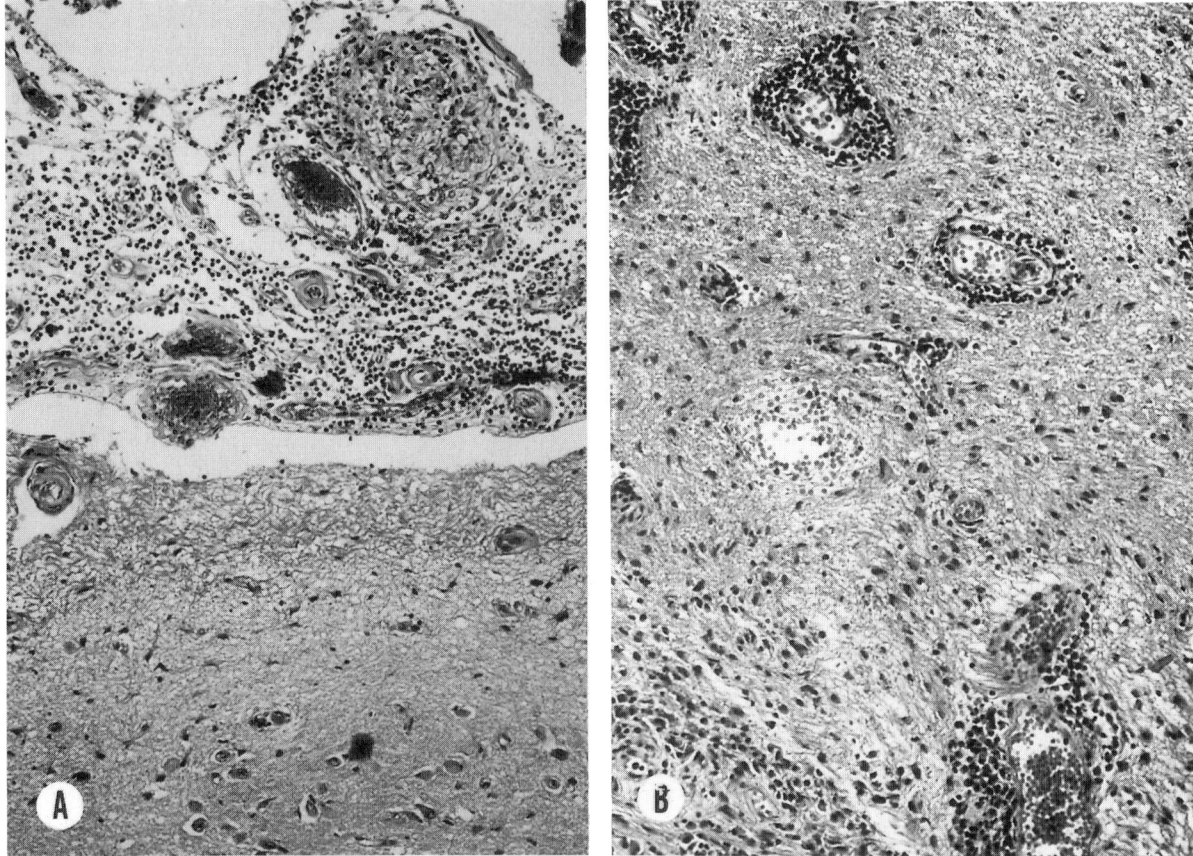

Figure 17.32 Small vessel vasculitis of the brain in Behçet's syndrome. (A) A necrotizing vasculitis of the leptomeningeal blood vessels. (B) Lymphocytic vasculitis of small intracerebral blood vessels. (H&E A and B ×160.)

17.7.3 CNS ANGIITIS MIMICKERS

The central nervous system may be involved in a variety of systemic diseases and some of these cases have clinical or angiographic features that mimic cerebral vasculitis.

Lymphomatoid granulomatosis (LMG) is not a vasculitis, but a peripheral T-cell lymphoma with angioinvasive and angiodestructive features that mimic vasculitis. Central nervous system dysfunction and peripheral neuropathy may occur in 15–20% of LMG patients. There has been a report of one patient in whom clinical evidence of LMG was confined to the central nervous system [192].

Moyamoya disease is a peculiar clinical entity associated with transient ischemic attacks, stroke or intracerebral hemorrhage in young adults, being most prevalent in Japan where it was first described. The name 'moyamoya disease' is coined (after a Japanese expression for something hazy, just like 'a puff of cigarette smoke drifting in the air') for the wispy appearance of collaterals demonstrated by cerebral angiography [193]. Histopathologic changes in the brain in autopsy cases do not suggest vasculitis; these changes have been commonly described as thickening of the affected vessels with hyperplasia of the intima, disorganization of the internal elastic lamina and medial fibrosis [194].

Fibromuscular dysplasia may mimic extracranial vasculitis angiographically, but it rarely affects the intracerebral arteries.

Antiphospholipid syndromes are diseases associated with the presence of autoantibodies in the blood against the negatively charged phospholipids, principally lupus anticoagulant and anticardiolipin antibodies. Antiphospholipid syndromes may be primary (not associated with a known underlying disease) or secondary (associated with systemic lupus erythematosus, lupus-like disease or another connective tissue disease). The syndromes have a wide spectrum of clinical manifestations, including recurrent arterial and venous thrombosis, recurrent fetal loss, thrombocytopenia, hemolytic anemia, livedo reticularis, verrucous endocarditis, transient ischemic attacks and strokes [195]. Coagulopathy rather than vasculitis appears to be the pathologic basis of occlusive vascular disease in antiphospholipid syndromes [196,197].

Cardiac myxoma embolism may occur in systemic or cerebral circulation, and neurologic abnormalities are

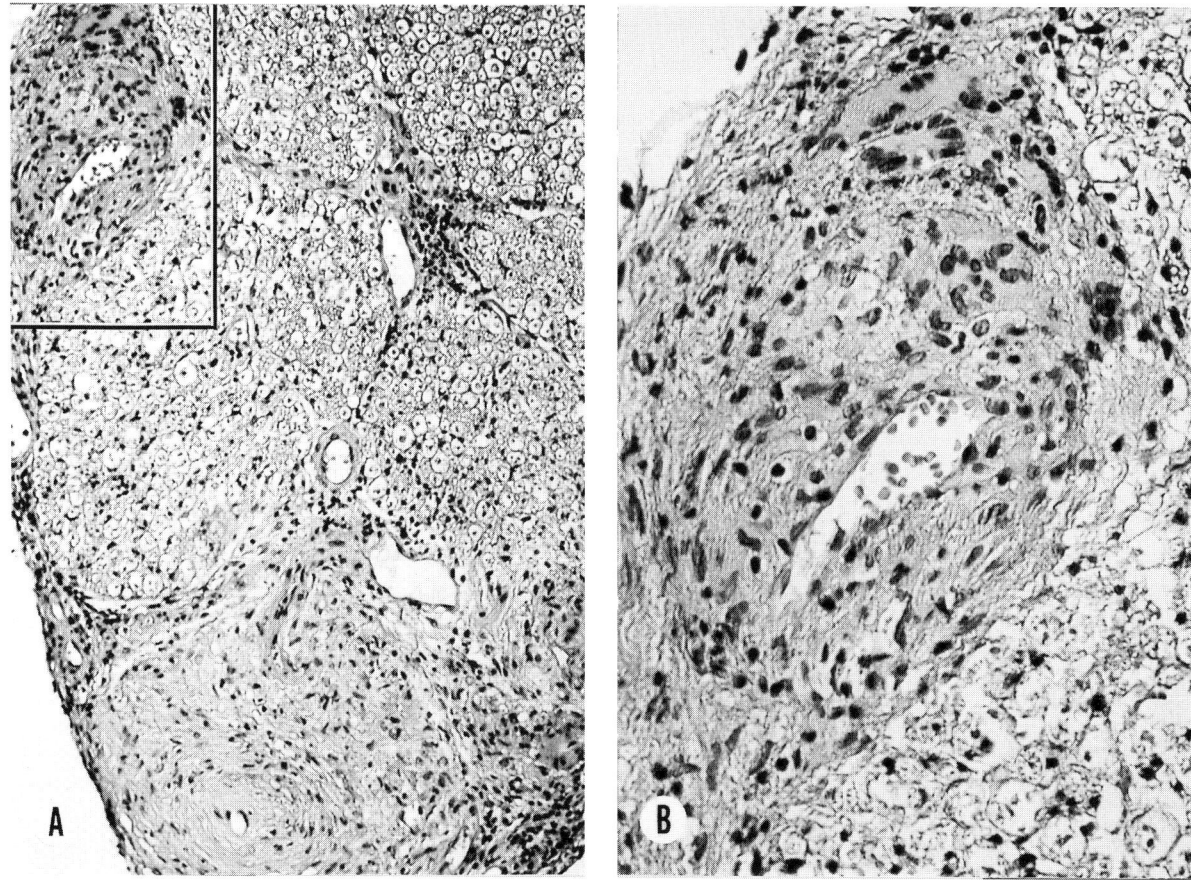

Figure 17.33 (A) Granulomatous angiitis of the spinal cord artery in Hodgkin's disease. (B) Close-up view of the boxed area in (A) to show the Langhans-type giant cells of the granulomatous angiitis. (H&E A× 160, B ×400.)

the presenting manifestation in about one third of patients with cardia myxomas [198,199]. Cerebral angiography often reveals microaneurysms that mimic vasculitis, which may progress or regress after surgery for the removal of cardic myxomas, as may the neurologic deficits.

Rarely, **PANS** may be a reverse mimicker, simulating lymphoma or Hodgkin's disease of the central nervous system or spinal cord (Figure 17.33) [220].

17.7.4 CONCLUSIONS

There are many causes of cerebral angiitis, and many non-vasculitic conditions may simulate cerebral angiitis. PANS, though relatively uncommon, is clinically the most important type of cerebral angiitis because of the overall unfavorable prognosis. Cerebral angiitis is usually suspected clinically and by suggestive angiographic findings, but a definitive diagnosis still requires histologic documentation of the presence of a true vasculitis. A positive biopsy is diagnostic for the disease in question, but a single negative biopsy does not necessarily exclude primary or secondary cerebral vasculitis because of the focal nature of the lesions and the unavoidable sampling errors associated with small biopsies.

References

1. Lie, J.T. (1977) Nosology of pulmonary vasculitides. *Mayo Clin. Proc.*, **52**, 520–2.
2. Lie, J.T. (1986) The classification of vasculitis and a reappraisal of allergic granulomatosis and angiitis (Churg–Strauss syndrome). *Mt Sinai J. Med.*, **53**, 429–39.
3. Lie, J.T. (1987) Coronary vasculitis: a review in the current scheme of classification of vasculitis. *Arch. Pathol. Lab. Med.*, **111**, 224–33.
4. Lie, J.T. (1987) The classification and diagnosis of vasculitis in large and medium-sized blood vessels. *Pathol. Annu.*, **22**(1), 125–62.
5. Lie, J.T. (1988) Classification and immunodiagnosis of vasculitis: a new solution or promises unfulfilled? *J. Rheumatol.*, **15**, 728–32.
6. Lie, J.T. (1989) Classification of pulmonary angiitis and granulomatosis: histopathologic perspectives. *Sem. Respir. Med.*, **10**, 111–21.
7. Lie, J.T. (1989) Systemic and isolated vasculitis: a rational approach to classification and pathologic diagnosis. *Pathol. Annu.*, **24**(1), 25–114.
8. Lie, J.T. (1992) Vasculitis, 1815 to 1991: classification and diagnostic specificity. (The 1991 Dunlop–Dottridge Lecture.) *J. Rheumatol.*, **19**, 83–9.
9. Lie, J.T. (1992) Primary (granulomatous) angiitis of the central nervous system: a clinicopathologic analysis of 15 new cases and review of the literature. *Hum. Pathol.*, **23**, 164–71.
10. Lie, J.T. (1991) Infection-related vasculitis, in *Systemic Vasculitides*, (eds A. Churg and J. Churg), Igaku Shoin, New York, pp. 243–56.
11. Manion, W.C. (1963) Infectious angiitis, in *The Peripheral Blood Vessels*,

(eds J.L. Orbison and D.E. Smith), Williams & Wilkins, Baltimore, pp. 221–31.
12. Paronetto, F. (1976) Systemic nonsupportive necrotizing angiitis, in *Textbook of Immunopathology*, (eds P.A. Miescher and H.J. Muller-Eberhard), Grune & Stratton, New York, pp. 1012–24.
13. Christian, C.L. and Sergent, J.S. (1976) Vasculitis syndromes: clinical and experimental models. *Am. J. Med.*, 61, 385–92.
14. Conn, D.L., McDuffie, F.C., Holley, K.E. and Schroeter, A.L. (1976) Immunologic mechanisms in systemic vasculitis. *Mayo Clin. Proc.*, 51, 511–18.
15. Fauci, A.S., Hayne, B.F. and Katz, P. (1978) The spectrum of vasculitis: clinical, pathogenic, immunologic, and therapeutic considerations. *Ann. Intern. Med.*, 89, 660–76.
16. Soter, N.A. and Austen, K.F. (1980) Pathogenetic mechanisms in necrotizing vasculitides. *Clin. Rheum. Dis.*, 6, 233–53.
17. Nydegger, M.E. and Lampert, P.H. (1980) The role of immune complexes in the pathogenesis of necrotizing vasculitides. *Clin. Rheum. Dis.*, 6, 255–78.
18. McCluskey, R.T. and Fienberg, R. (1983) Vasculitis in primary vasculitides, granulomatoses, and connective tissue diseases. *Hum. Pathol.*, 14, 305–15.
19. Savage, C.O.S. and Ng, Y.C. (1986) The etiology and pathogenesis of major systemic vasculitides. *Postgrad. Med. J.*, 62, 627–36.
20. Sergent, J.S., Lockshin, M.D., Christian, C.L. and Gocke, D.J. (1976) Vasculitis with hepatitis B antigenemia: long-term observations in nine patients. *Medicine (Baltimore)*, 55, 1–18.
21. Sergent, J.S. (1980) Vasculitis associated with viral infections. *Clin. Rheum. Dis.*, 6, 339–50.
22. Gianotti, F. (1973) Papular acrodermatitis of childhood: an Australia antigen disease. *Arch. Dis. Child.*, 48, 794–9.
23. Kohler, P.F., Cronin, R.E., Hammon, W.S.S. et al. (1974) Chronic membranous glomerulonephritis caused by hepatitis B antigen-antibody immune complexes. *Ann. Intern. Med.*, 81, 448–51.
24. Levo, Y., Gorevic, P.D., Kassab, H.J. et al. (1977) Association between hepatitis B virus and essential mixed cryoglobulinemia. *New Engl. J. Med.*, 296, 1501–4.
25. Gorevic, P.D., Kassab, H.J., Levo, Y. et al. (1980) Mixed cryoglobulinemia: clinical aspects and long-term follow-up of 40 patients. *Am. J. Med.*, 69, 287–308.
26. Savage, C.O. and Lockwood, C.M. (1990) Antineutrophil antibodies in vasculitis. *Adv. Nephrol.*, 19, 225–36.
27. Cohen Tervaert, J.W., Goldschmeding, R., Elema, J.D. et al. (1990) Association of autoantibodies to myeloperoxidase with different forms of vasculitis. *Arthritis Rheum.*, 33, 1264–72.
28. Roberts, D.E. (1992) Antineutrophil cytoplasmic autoantibodies. *Clin. Lab. Med.*, 12, 85–98.
29. Kallenberg, C.G.M., Mulder, A.H.L. and Cohen Tervaert, J.W. (1992) Antineutrophil cytoplasmic antibodies: a still-growing class of autoantibodies in inflammatory disorders. *Am. J. Med.*, 93, 675–82.
30. Fienberg, R., Mark, E.J., Goodman, M. et al. (1993) Correlation of antineutrophils cytoplasmic antibodies with the extrarenal histopathology of Wegener's (pathergic) granulomatosis and related forms of vasculitis. *Hum. Pathol.*, 24, 160–8.
31. Leavitt, R.Y. and Fauci, A.S. (1986) Polyangiitis overlap syndrome: classification and prospective clinical experience. *Am. J. Med.*, 81, 79–85.
32. Kussmaul, A. and Maier, R. (1866) Ueber eine bisher nicht beschrievene eigenthümliche Arterienerkrankung (Periarteritis nodosa), die mit Morbus Brightü und rapid fortschreitender allgemeiner Muskellähmung einhergeht. *Dtsch. Arch. Klin. Med.*, 1, 484–518.
33. Ferrari, E. (1903) Ueber Polyarteritis acuta nodosa (sogenannte Periarteritis nodosa) und ihre Beziehungen zur Polymyositis and Polyneuritis acts. *Beitr. Path. Anat.*, 34, 350–86.
34. Mönckeberg, J.G. (1905) Ueber Periarteritis nodosa. *Beitr path. Anat.*, 38, 101–34.
35. Ophüls, W. (1923) Periarteritis acuta nodosa. *Arch. Intern. Med.*, 32, 870–98.
36. Shimigu, K. and Sano, K. (1951) Pulseless disease. *J. Neuropath. Expl. Neurol.*, 1, 37–47.
37. Judge, R.D., Currier, R.D., Gracie, W.A. and Figley, M.M. (1962) Takayasu's arteritis and the aortic arch syndrome. *Am. J. Med.*, 32, 379–92.
38. Lie, J.T. (1991) Takayasu arteritis, in *Systemic Vasculitides*, (eds A. Churg and J. Churg), Igaku Shoin, New York, pp. 159–79.
39. Buerger, L. (1908) Thromboangiitis obliterans: a study of the vascular lesions leading to presenile gangrene. *Am. J. Med. Sci.*, 136, 567–80.
40. Lie, J.T. (1988) Thromboangiitis obliterans (Buerger's disease) revisited. *Pathol. Annu.*, 23(2), 257–91.
41. Hutchinson, J. (1890) Diseases of the arteries. On a peculiar form of thrombotic arteritis of the aged which is sometimes productive of gangrene. *Arch. Surg. (London)*, 1, 323–9.
42. Horton, B.T., Magath, T.B. and Brown, G.E. (1934) Arteritis of the temporal vessels. *Arch. Intern. Med.*, 53, 400–10.
43. Huston, K.A., Hunder, G.G., Lie, J.T. et al. (1978) Temporal arteritis: a 25-year epidemiological, clinical and pathological study. *Ann. Intern. Med.*, 88, 162–7.
44. Churg, J. and Strauss, L. (1951) Allergic granulomatosis, allergic angiitis, and periarteritis nodosa. *Am. J. Pathol.*, 27, 277–94.
45. Churg, J. (1963) Allergic granulomatosis and granulomatous vasculitis syndromes. *Ann. Allergy*, 21, 619–28.
46. Fahey, J., Leonard, E., Churg, J. and Godman, G. (1954) Wegener's granulomatosis. *Am. J. Med.*, 17, 168–79.
47. Godman, G. and Churg, J. (1954) Wegener's granulomatosis: pathology and review of the literature. *Arch. Pathol. Lab. Med.*, 58, 533–53.
48. Zeek, P.M. (1952) Periarteritis nodosa: a critical review. *Am. J. Clin. Pathol.*, 22, 777–90.
49. Zeek, P.M. (1953) Periarteritis and other forms of necrotizing angiitis. *New Engl. J. Med.*, 248, 764–72.
50. Copeman, P.W.M. and Ryan, T.J. (1970) The problems of classification of cutaneous angiitis with reference to histopathology and pathogenesis. *Br. J. Dermatol.*, 82 (suppl. 5), 3–14.
51. deShazo, R.D. (1975) The spectrum of systemic vasculitis: a classification to aid diagnosis. *Postgrad. Med.*, 58, 78–82.
52. Gilliam, J.N. and Smiley, J.D. (1976) Cutaneous necrotizing vasculitis and related disorders. *Ann. Allergy*, 37, 328–39.
53. Alarcón-Segovia, D. and Brown Jr, A.L. (1964) Classification and etiologic aspects of necrotizing angiitides. *Mayo Clin. Proc.*, 39, 205–22.
54. Alarcón-Segovia, D. (1977) The necrotizing vasculitides: a new pathogenetic classification. *Med. Clin. N. Am.*, 61, 241–60.
55. Alarcón-Segovia, D. (1980) Classification of the necrotizing vasculitides in man. *Clin. Rheum. Dis.*, 6, 223–31.
56. Churg, J. and Churg, A. (1989) Idiopathic and secondary vasculitis: a review. *Mod. Pathol.*, 2, 144–60.
57. Lie, J.T. (1994) Nomenclature and classification of vasculitis: plus ça change, plus c'est la même chose. *Arthritis. Rheum.*, 37, 181–6.
58. Jeanette, J.C., Falk, R.J., Andrassy, K. et al. (1994) Nomenclature of systemic vasculitides: the proposal of an international consensus conference. *Arthritis Rheum.*, 37, 187–92.
59. American College of Rheumatology (1990) Classification Criteria for vasculitis. *Arthritis Rheum.*, 33, 1065–144.
60. Hachiya, J. (1970) Current concepts of Takayasu's arteritis. *Semin. Roentgenol.*, 5, 245–59.
61. Lande, A. and Berkmen, Y.M. (1976) Aortitis: pathologic, clinical, and angiographic review. *Radiol. Clin. N. Am.*, 14, 219–40.
62. Lupi-Herrera, E., Sánchez-Torres, G., Marcushamer, J. et al. (1977) Takayasu's arteritis: clinical study of 107 cases. *Am. Heart J.*, 93, 94–103.
63. Hall, S., Barr, W., Lie, J.T. et al. (1985) Takayasu's arteritis: a study of 32 North American patients. *Medicine (Baltimore)*, 64, 89–99.
64. Numano, F., Maezawa, H., Sawada, S. et al. (1981) Circulating immune complexes in Takayasu disease: lack of evidence for a causative role. *Arch. Intern. Med.*, 141, 162–3.
65. Alcocer-Varela, J., Reyes-Lopez, P.A., Sanchez-Torres, G. and Alarcon-Sagovia D. (1989) Immunologic studies in patients with Takayasu's arteritis. *Clin. Expl. Rheumatol.*, 7, 345–50.
66. Shelhamer, J.H., Volkman, D.J., Parrillo, J.E. et al. (1985) Takayasu's arteritis and its therapy. *Ann. Intern. Med.*, 103, 121–6.
67. Duncan, J.M. and Cooley, D.A. (1986) Surgical considerations in aortitis, in *Aortitis: Clinical, Pathologic, and Radiographic Aspects*, (eds A. Lande, Y.M. Berkman and H.A. McAllister), Raven Press, New York, pp. 243–72.
68. Scott, D., Awang, H., Sulieman, B., Wang, F. et al. (1986) Surgical repair of visceral artery occlusions in Takayasu's disease. *J. Vasc. Surg.*, 3, 904–10.
69. Meda, H., Saito, Y., Yamaguchi, H. et al. (1967) Immunological studies of aortitis syndrome. *Jap. Heart J.*, 8, 4–18.
70. Moriuchi, J., Wakisaka, A., Aizawa, M. et al. (1982) HLA-linked susceptibility gene of Takayasu's disease. *Hum. Immunol.*, 4, 87–91.
71. Isohisa, I., Numano, F., Maezawa, H. and Sasazuki, T. (1982) Hereditary factors in Takayasu's disease. *Angiology*, 33, 98–104.
72. Volkman, D.J., Mann, D.L. and Fauci, A.S. (1982) Association between Takayasu's arteritis and a B-cell alloantigen in North Americans. *New Engl. J. Med.*, 306, 464–5.
73. Kodama, Y., Kida, O., Morotomi, Y. and Tanaka, K. (1986) Male siblings with Takayasu's arteritis suggest genetic etiology. *Heart and Vessels*, 2, 51–4.
74. Zvaifler, N.J. and Weintraub, A.M. (1963) Aortitis and aortic insufficiency in chronic rheumatic disorders: a reappraisal. *Arthritis Rheum.*, 6, 241–5.
75. Heggtveit, H.A., Henningar, G.R. and Morrione, T.G. (1963) Panaortitis. *Am. J. Pathol.*, 42, 151–72.
76. Reimer, K.A., Rodgers, R.F. and Oyasu, R. (1976) Rheumatoid arthritis with rheumatoid heart disease and granulomatous aortitis. *J. Am. Med. Ass.*, 235, 2510–12.
77. Pagel, W. (1951) Polyarteritis nodosa and the 'rheumatic' diseases. *J. Clin. Path.*, 4, 137–57.
78. Cruickshank, B. (1954) The arteritis of rheumatoid arthritis. *Ann. Rheum. Dis.*, 13, 136–46.

79. Schmid, F.R., Cooper, N.S., Ziff, M. and McEwwn, C. (1961) Arteritis in rheumatoid arthritis. *Am. J. Med.*, **30**, 56–83.
80. Scott, D.G.I., Bacon, P.A. and Tribe, C.R. (1981) Systemic rheumatoid vasculitis: a clinical and laboratory study of 50 cases. *Medicine (Baltimore)*, **60**, 288–97.
81. Ansari, A., Larson, P.H. and Bates, H.D. (1985) Cardiovascular manifestations of systemic lupus erythematosus: current perspective. *Prog. Cardiovasc. Dis.*, **27**, 421–34.
82. Huston, K.A., Hunder, G.G., Lie, J.T. et al. (1978) Temporal arteritis: a 25-year epidemiologic, clinical and pathologic study. *Ann. Intern. Med.*, **88**, 162–7.
83. Chuang, T.Y., Hunder, G.G., Ilstrup, D.M. and Kurland, L.T. (1982) Polymyalgia rheumatica: a 10-year epidemiologic and clinical study. *Ann. Intern. Med.*, **97**, 672–80.
84. Hunder, G.G. and Michet, C.J. (1986) Giant cell arteritis and polymyalgia rheumatica. *Clin. Rheum. Dis.*, **11**, 471–83.
85. Machado, E.B.V., Michet, C.J., Ballard, D.J. et al. (1988) Trends in incidence and clinical presentation of temporal arteritis in Olmsted County, Minnesota, 1950–1985. *Arthritis Rheum.*, **31**, 745–9.
86. Bengtsson, B.A. and Malmvall, B.E. (1981) The epidemiology of giant cell arteritis including temporal arteritis and polymyalgia rheumtica. *Arthritis Rheum.*, **24**, 899–904.
87. Healey, L.A. (1993) On the epidemiology of polymyalgia rheumatica and temporal arteritis. *J. Rheumatol.*, **20**, 1639–40.
88. Ostberg, G. (1973) On arteritis: with special reference to polymyalgia arteritica. *Acta Pathol. Microbiol. Immunol. Scand.*, **237**, 1–59.
89. Love, D.C., Rapkin, J., Lesser, G.R. et al. (1980) Temporal arteritis in blacks. *Ann. Intern. Med.*, **105**, 387–9.
90. Lie, J.T. (1992) Giant cell temporal arteritis in a Laotian Chinese. *J. Rheumatol.*, **19**, 1651–2.
91. Calamia, K.T. and Hunder, G.G. (1980) Clinical manifestations of giant cell (temporal) arteritis. *Clin. Rheum. Dis.*, **6**, 389–403.
92. Case Records of the Massachusetts General Hospital (1986) Case 35. *New Engl. J. Med.*, **315**, 631–9.
93. Hall, S., Lie, J.T., Kurland, L.T. et al. (1983) The therapeutic impact of temporal artery biopsy. *Lancet*, **2**, 1217–20.
94. Hall, S. and Hunder, G.G. (1984) Is temporal artery biopsy prudent? *Mayo Clin. Proc.*, **59**, 793–6.
95. Klein, R.G., Campbell, R.J., Hunder, G.G. and Carnery, J.A. (1976) Skip lesions in temporal arteritis. *Mayo Clin. Proc.*, **51**, 504–10.
96. Klein, R.G., Hunder, G.G., Stanson, A.W. and Sheps, S.G. (1975) Large vessel involvement in giant cell (temporal) arteritis. *Ann. Intern. Med.*, **83**, 806–12.
97. Rivers, S.P., Baur, G.M., Inahara, T. and Porter, J.M. (1982) Arm ischemia secondary to giant cell arteritis. *Am. J. Surg.*, **143**, 554–8.
98. Perruquet, J.L., Davis, D.E. and Harrington, T.M. (1986) Aortic arch arteritis in the elderly: an important manifestation of giant cell arteritis. *Arch. Intern. Med.*, **146**, 289–91.
99. Fiore, W., Penn, T.E., Quill, T. et al. (1986) Giant cell arteritis in a 20-year-old black man: a cause of intermittent calf claudication. *J. Vasc. Surg.*, **4**, 192–5.
100. Green, G.M., Lain, D., Sherwin, R.M. et al. (1986) Giant cell arteritis of the legs: clinical isolation of severe disease with gangrene and amputations. *Am. J. Med.*, **81**, 727–33.
101. Harris, M. (1968) Dissecting aneurysm of the aorta due to giant cell arteritis. *Br. Heart J.*, **30**, 840–4.
102. Morrison, A.N. and Abitbol, M. (1955) Granulomatous arteritis with myocardial infarction: a case report with autopsy findings. *Ann. Intern. Med.*, **42**, 691–700.
103. Martin, J.F., Kittas, C. and Triger, D.R. (1980) Giant cell arteritis of coronary arteries causing myocardial infarction. *Br. Heart J.*, **43**, 487–9.
104. Säve-Söderbergh, J., Malmvall, B.E., Andersson, R. and Bengtsson, B.A. (1985) Giant cell arteritis as a cause of death: report of nine cases. *J. Am. Med. Ass.*, **255**, 493–6.
105. Lie, J.T., Failoni, D.D. and Davis Jr, D.C. (1986) Temporal arteritis with giant cell aortitis, coronary arteritis, and myocardial infarction. *Arch. Pathol. Lab. Med.*, **110**, 857–60.
106. Lie, J.T. (1978) Disseminated visceral giant cell arteritis: histopathologic description and differentiation from other granulomatous vasculitides. *Am. J. Clin. Pathol.*, **69**, 299–305.
107. Lie, J.T. (1992) Primary granulomatous angiitis of the central nervous system: a clinicopathologic analysis of 15 new cases and review of the literature. *Hum. Pathol.*, **23**, 164–71.
108. Lie, J.T. Brown Jr, A.L. and Carter, E.T. (1970) Spectrum of aging changes in temporal arteries: its significance in interpretation of biopsy of temporal artery. *Arch. Pathol.*, **90**, 278–85.
109. Gilmour, J.R. (1941) Giant cell arteritis. *J. Pathol. Bacteriol.*, **53**, 263–77.
110. Harrison, C.V. (1948) Giant cell or temporal arteritis: a review. *J. Clin. Pathol.*, **1**, 197–211.
111. Mambo, N.C. (1979) Temporal (granulomatous) arteritis: a histopathological study of 32 cases. *Histopathology*, **3**, 209–21.
112. Allsop, C.J. and Gallagher, P.J. (1981) Temporal artery biopsy in giant cell arteritis: a reappraisal. *Am. J. Surg. Pathol.*, **5**, 317–23.
113. McDonnell, P.J., Moore, G.W., Miller, N.R. et al. (1986) Temporal arteritis: a clinicopathologic study. *Ophthalmology*, **93**, 518–30.
114. Lie, J.T. (1990) Diagnostic histopathology of major systemic and pulmonary vasculitic syndromes. *Rheum. Dis. Clin. N. Am.*, **16**, 269–92.
115. Lie, J.T. (1990) American College of Rheumatology: illustrated histopathologic classification criteria for selected vasculitis syndromes. *Arthritis Rheum.*, **33**, 1074–87.
116. Travers, R.L., Allison, D.J., Brettle, R.P. and Hughes, G.R.V. (1979) Polyarteritis nodosa: a clinical and angiographic analysis of 17 cases. *Sem. Arthritis Rheum.*, **8**, 184–99.
117. Cohen, R.D., Conn, D.L. and Ilstrup, D.M. (1980) Clinical features, prognosis and response to treatment in polyarteritis. *Mayo Clin. Proc.*, **55**, 146–55.
118. Scott, D.G.I., Bacon, P.A., Elliott, P.J. et al. (1982) Systemic vasculitis in a district general hospital 1972–1980: clinical and laboratory features, classification and prognosis of 80 cases. *Q. J. Med.*, **51**, 292–311.
119. Arkin, A. (1930) A clinical and pathological study of periarteritis nodosa: a report of five cases, one histologically healed. *Am. J. Pathol.*, **6**, 401–26.
120. Cupps, T.R. and Fauci, A.S. (1981) *The Vasculitides*, W.B. Saunders, Philadelphia.
121. Symposium on periarteritis nodosa (1949) *Mayo Clin. Proc.*, **24**, 17–43.
122. Moskowitz, R.W., Baggenstoss, A.H. and Slocumb, C.H. (1963) Histopathologic classification of periarteritis nodosa: a study of 56 cases confirmed at autopsy. *Mayo Clin. Proc.*, **38**, 345–57.
123. Rose, G.A. and Spenser, H. (1957) Polyarteritis nodosa. *Q. J. Med.*, **26**, 43–81.
124. Savage, C.O.S., Winearles, C.G., Evans, D.J. et al. (1985) Microscopic polyarteritis: presentation, pathology and prognosis. *Q. J. Med.*, **56**, 467–83.
125. Davson, J., Ball, J. and Platt, R. (1948) The kidney in polyarteritis nodosa. *Q. J. Med.*, **17**, 175–202.
126. Wainwright, J. and Davson, J. (1950) The renal appearances in microscopic form of polyarteritis nodosa. *J. Pathol. Bacteriol.*, **62**, 189–96.
127. Wilmer, H.A. (1945) Two cases of periarteritis nodosa occurring in the first month of life. *Bull. Johns Hopkins Hosp.*, **77**, 275–86.
128. Ettlinger, R.E., Nelson, A.M., Burke, E.C. and Lie, J.T. (1979) Polyarteritis nodosa in childhood: a clinical pathologic study. *Arthritis Rheum.*, **22**, 820–5.
129. Reimold, E.W., Weinberg, A.G., Fink, C.W. and Battles, N.D. (1976) Polyarteritis in children. *Am. J. Dis. Child.*, **130**, 534–41.
130. Tanaka, N., Sekimoto, K. and Naoe, S. (1976) Kawasaki disease: relationship with infantile periarteritis nodosa. *Arch. Pathol. Lab. Med.*, **100**, 81–86.
131. Landing, B.H. and Larson, E.J. (1977) Are infantile periarteritis nodosa with coronary artery involvement and fatal mucocutaneous lymph node syndrome the same? Comparison of 20 patients from North America with patients from Hawaii and Japan. *Pediatrics*, **59**, 651–62.
132. Yanagihala, R. and Todd, J.K. (1980) Acute febrile mucocutaneous lymph node syndrome. *Am. J. Dis. Child.*, **134**, 603–14.
133. McCombs, R.P. (1965) Systemic allergic vasculitis. *J. Am. Med. Ass.*, **194**, 1059–64.
134. Sams Jr, W.J., Thorne, E.R., Small, P. et al. (1976) Leukocytoclastic vasculitis. *Arch. Dermatol.*, **112**, 219–26.
135. Soter, N.A., Mihm Jr, M.C., Gigli, I. et al. (1976) Two distinct cellular patterns in cutaneous necrotizing vasculitis. *J. Invest. Dermatol.*, **66**, 344–50.
136. Massa, M.C. and Su, W.P.D. (1984) Lymphocytic vasculitis: is it a specific clinicopathologic entity? *J. Cutan. Pathol.*, **11**, 132–9.
137. Zax, R.H., Hodge, S.J. and Callen, J.P. (1990) Cutaneous leukocytoclastic vasculitis: Serial histopathologic evaluation demonstrates the dynamic nature of the infiltrate. *Arch. Dermatol.*, **126**, 69–72.
138. Liebow, A.A. (1973) The J Burns Ambersons Lecture: pulmonary angiitis and granulomatosis. *Am. Rev. Respir. Dis.*, **108**, 1–18.
139. Klinger, H. (1931) Grenzformen der Periarteritis nodosa. *Frankfurt Z. Pathol.*, **42**, 455–80.
140. Wegener, F. (1936) Über generalisierte, septische Gefässerkrankugen. *Verh. dt. Pathol. Ges.*, **29**, 202–10.
141. Wegener, F. (1939) Über eine eigenartige rhinogene Granulomatose mit besonderer Beteiligung des Arteriensystems und der Nieren. *Beitr. Pathol. Anat.*, **102**, 36–68.
142. Fahey, J., Leonard, E., Churg, J. and Godman, G. (1954) Wegener's granulomatosis. *Am. J. Med.*, **17**, 168–79.
143. Godman, G. and Churg, J. (1954) Wegener's granulomatosis: pathology and review of the literature. *Arch. Pathol. Lab. Med.*, **58**, 533–53.
144. Walton, E.W. (1958) Giant cell granuloma of the respiratory tract (Wegener's granulomatosis). *Br. Med. J.*, **2**, 265–70.
145. Hoffman, G.S., Kerr, G.S., Leavitt, R.Y. et al. (1992) Wegener's granulomatosis: a prospective analysis of 158 patients. *Ann. Intern. Med.*, **116**, 488–98.
146. Carrington, C.B. and Liebow, A.A. (1966) Limited forms of angiitis and granulomatosis of Wegener's type. *Am. J. Med.*, **41**, 497–527.
147. Fienberg, R. (1981) The protracted superficial phenomenon in pathergic (Wegener's) granulomatosis. *Hum. Pathol.*, **12**, 458–67.

148. Lanham, J.G., Elkon, K.B., Pusey, C.D. et al. (1984) Systemic vasculitis with asthma and eosinophilia: a clinical approach to the Churg–Strauss syndrome. Medicine (Baltimore), 63, 65–81.
149. Finan, M.C. and Winkelmann, R.K. (1983) The cutaneous extravascular necrotizing granuloma (Churg–Strauss granuloma) and systemic disease: a review of 27 cases. Medicine (Baltimore), 62, 142–58.
150. Carrington, C.B., Gaensler, E.A., Mikus, J.P. et al. (1976) Structure and function in sarcoidosis. Ann. N.Y. Acad. Sci., 278, 265–82.
151. Rosen, Y., Moon, S., Huang, C.T. et al. (1977) Granulomatous pulmonary angiitis in sarcoidosis. Arch. Pathol. Lab. Med., 101, 170–4.
152. Churg, A., Carrington, C.B. and Gupta, R. (1979) Necrotizing sarcoid granulomatosis. Chest, 76, 406–13.
153. Koss, M.N., Hochholzer, L., Feigin, D.S. et al. (1980) Necrotizing sarcoid-like granulomatosis: clinical, pathologic, and immunopathologic findings. Hum. Pathol., 11 (suppl. 1), 510–519.
154. Harbitz, F. (1922) Unknown forms of arteritis with special reference to their relation to syphilitic arteritis and periarteritis nodosa. Am. J. Med., 163, 250–72.
155. Newman, W., Wolf, A. (1952) Non-infectious granulomatous angiitis involving the central nervous system. Trans. Am. Neurol. Assoc., 77, 114–17.
156. Budzilovich, G.N., Feigin, I. and Siegel, H. (1963) Granulomatous angiitis of the nervous system. Arch. Pathol. Lab. Med., 76, 250–6.
157. Cupps, T.R., Morre, P.M. and Fauci, A.S. (1983) Isolated angiitis of the central nervous system. Am. J. Med., 74, 97–106.
158. McCormick, H.M. and Neuberger, K.T. (1958) Giant-cell arteritis involving small meningeal and intracerebral vessels. J. Neuropathol. Expl. Neurol., 17, 471–8.
159. Burger, P.C., Burch, J.G. and Vogel, F.S. (1977) Granulomatous angiitis. Stroke, 8, 29–35.
160. Calabrese, L.H. and Mallek, J.A. (1988) Primary angiitis of the central nervous system: report of 8 new cases, review of the literature, and proposal for diagnostic criteria. Medicine, 67, 20–39.
161. Moore, P.M. (1989) Diagnosis and management of isolated angiitis of the central nervous system. Neurology, 39, 167–73.
162. Calabrese, L.H., Furlan, A.J., Gregg, L.A. and Ropes, T.J. (1992) Primary angiitis of the central nervous system: diagnostic criteria and clinical approach. Cleve. Clin. J. Med., 59, 293–306.
163. Sabharwal, U.K., Keogh, L.H., Weisman, M.H. and Zvaifler, N.J. (1982) Granulomatous angiitis of the nervous system: case report and review of the literature. Arthritis Rheum., 25, 342–5.
164. Ferris, E.J. and Levine, J. (1973) Cerebral arteritis: classification. Radiology, 109, 327–41.
165. Sole-Llenas, J., Mercader, J.M. and Mirosa, F. (1978) Cerebral arteritis. Angiology, 29, 713–18.
166. Garner, B.F., Burns, P., Bunning, R.D. and Laureno, R. (1990) Acute blood pressure elevation can mimic arteriographic appearance of cerebral vasculitis. J. Rheumatol., 17, 93–7.
167. Husein, A.M.A. and Haq, N. (1990) Cerebral arteritis with unusual distribution. Clin. Radiol., 41, 353–4.
168. Caselli, R.J., Hunder, G.G. and Whisnant, J.P. (1988) Neurologic disease in biopsy-proven giant cell (temporal) arteritis. Neurology, 38, 352–9.
169. Currier, R.D., DeJong, R.N. and Bole, G.G. (1954) Pulseless disease: central nervous system manifestations. Neurology, 4, 818–30.
170. Moore, P.M. and Fauci, A.S. (1981) Neurologic manifestations of systemic vasculitis: a retrospective and prospective study of the clinical copathologic features and responses to therapy in 25 patients. Am. J. Med., 71, 517–24.
171. Fauci, A.S., Haynes, B.F., Katz, P. and Wolff, S.M. (1983) Wegener's granulomatosis: prospective clinical and therapeutic experience with 85 patients for 21 years. Ann. Intern. Med., 98, 76–85.
172. Drachmann, D.A. (1963) Neurological complications of Wegener's granulomatosis. Arch. Neurol., 8, 145–55.
173. Kroneman III, O.C. and Pevzner, M. (1986) Failure of cyclophosphamide to prevent cerebritis in Wegener's granulomatosis. Am. J. Med., 80, 526–7.
174. Lewis, I.C. and Philpott, M.G. (1956) Neurological complications in the Schönlein-Henoch syndrome. Arch. Dis. Child., 31, 369–71.
175. Johnson, R.T. and Richardson, E.P. (1968) The neurological manifestations of systemic lupus erythematosus: a clinical pathological study of 24 cases and review of the literature. Medicine, 47, 337–69.
176. Farrell, D.A. and Medsger Jr, T.A. (1982) Trigeminal neuropathy in progressive systemic sclerosis. Am. J. Med., 73, 57–2.
177. Lee, J.L. and Haynes, J.M. (1967) Carotid arteritis and cerebral infarction due to scleroderma. Neurology, 17, 18–22.
178. Estey, E., Liebermann, A., Pinto, R. et al. (1979) Cerebral arteritis in scleroderma. Stroke, 5, 595–7.
179. Wise, T.N. and Ginzler, E.M. (1975) Scleroderma cerebritis, an unusual manifestation of progressive systemic sclerosis. Dis. Nerv. System, 36, 60–2.
180. Sigal, L.H. (1987) The neurologic presentation of vasculitis and rheumatologic syndromes: a review. Medicine, 66, 157–80.
181. Andonopoulos, A.P., Lagos, G., Drosos, A.A. and Moutsopoulos, H.M. (1990) The spectrum of neurological involvement in Sjögren's syndrome. Br. J. Rheumatol., 29, 21–23.
182. Stewart, S.S., Ashizawa, T., Dudley Jr, A.W. et al. (1988) Cerebral vasculitis in relapsing polychondritis. Neurology, 38, 150–2.
183. Chajek, T. and Fainaru, M. (1975) Behçet's disease: report of 41 cases and a review of the literature. Medicine, 54, 179–96.
184. Shimizu, T., Ehrlich, G.E., Inaba, G. and Hayashi, K. (1979) Behçet's disease (Behçet's syndrome). Sem. Arthritis Rheum., 8, 223–60.
185. Zelenski, J.D., Capraro, J.A., Holden, D. and Calabrese, L.H. (1989) Central nervous system vasculitis in Behçet's syndrome: angiographic improvement after therapy with cytotoxic agents. Arthritis Rheum., 32, 217–20.
186. Bielory, I., Conti, J. and Frohman, L. (1990) Cogan's syndrome. J Allergy Clin. Immunol., 85, 808–15.
187. Vollertsen, R.S., McDonald, T.J., Younge, B.R. et al. (1986) Cogan's syndrome: 18 cases and a review of the literature. Mayo Clin. Proc., 61, 344–61.
188. Gocke, D.J., Hsu, K., Morgan, C. et al. (1970) Association between polyarteritis and Australia antigen. Lancet, ii, 1149–53.
189. Citron, B.P., Halperin, M. and McCarbon, M. (1970) Necrotizing angiitis associated with drug abuse. New Engl. J. Med., 283, 1003–11.
190. Rumbauch, C.L., Bergeron, R.T., Fang, H.C.H. and McCormack, R. (1971) Cerebral angiographic changes in the drug abuse patient. Radiology, 101, 335–44.
191. Kaye, B.R. and Fainstat, M. (1987) Cerebral vasculitis associated with cocaine abuse. J. Am. Med. Ass., 258, 2104–6.
192. Kokmen, E., Billman Jr, K. and Abell, M.R. (1977) Lymphomatoid granulomatosis clinically confined to the CNS. Arch. Neurol., 34, 782–4.
193. Suzuki, J. and Takaku, A. (1969) Cerebrovascular 'Moyamoya' disease. Arch. Neurol., 20, 288–99.
194. Yamashita, M., Oka, K. and Tanaka, K. (1983) Histopathology of the brain vascular network in Moyamoya disease. Stroke, 14, 50–8.
195. Love, P.E. and Santoro, S.A. (1990) Antiphospholipid antibodies: anti-cardiolipin and the lupus anticoagulant in systemic lupus erythematosus (SLE) and in non-SLE disorders. Ann. Intern. Med., 112, 682–98.
196. Lie, J.T. (1989) Vasculopathy in the antiphospholipid syndromes. J. Rheumatol., 16, 713–15.
197. Lie, J.T. (1994) Vasculitis in the antiphospholipid syndrome: culprit or consort? J. Rheumatol., 21, 397–9.
198. Wold, L.E. and Lie, J.T. (1980) Cardiac myxomas: a clinicopathologic profile. Am. J. Pathol., 101, 219–39.
199. Roeltgen, D.P., Weimer, G.R. and Patterson, L.F. (1981) Delayed neurologic complications of left atrial myxoma. Neurology, 31, 8–13.
200. Inwards, D.J., Piepgras, D.G., Lie, J.T. et al. (1991) Granulomatous angiitis of the spinal cord associated with Hodgkin's disease. Cancer, 68, 1318–22.

18 BUERGER'S DISEASE (THROMBOANGIITIS OBLITERANS)

Shigehiko Shionoya, Hans Jörg Leu and J.T. Lie

Thromboangiitis obliterans (TAO), commonly known by the eponym Buerger's disease or the von Winiwarter–Buerger disease, is a non-atherosclerotic, segmental and usually recurrent inflammatory occlusive vascular disease of unknown etiology. The disease occurs predominantly in young male tobacco users with onset of clinical signs and symptoms commonly before the age of 40–50 years. It involves principally the medium-sized and small arteries and veins of the lower and upper limbs. It affects the visceral, pulmonary and cerebral blood vessels only rarely, and the disease is not known to occur in the aorta.

Thromboangiitis obliterans is an uncommon but not rare disease. The disease has a worldwide distribution, being more prevalent in the Orient, southeast Asia, India, Middle East and Eastern Europe. Imprecise and ill-conceived clinical and pathologic criteria are largely responsible for the widespread and continued uncertainty and confusion in the diagnosis and management of Buerger's disease. As has been pointed out by Papa and Adar [1], because of the wide variation in the selection of diagnostic criteria and documentation of TAO, many clinical and laboratory investigations in the past were carried out on poorly defined patient populations, casting serious doubt on the validity of the conclusions. Familiarity with the nosologic evolution and the unique clinico-angiographic features of TAO is essential for the avoidance of over- or under-diagnosis of the disease, and a prerequisite for mastering the correct interpretation of the histopathology at different stages of the disease [2,3].

18.1 Historical perspective

The earliest detailed description of TAO was provided by a little known young apprentice surgeon to Theodor Billroth, Felix von Winiwarter (1852–1931), in 1879 in Vienna [4,5]. By coincidence, that happened to be the year and place of birth of the American surgeon, Leo Buerger (1879–1943) who gave the first English-language account of the same disease 40 years later, when he was working at the Mount Sinai Hospital in New York City.

In 1877, at Billroth's request, Winiwarter dissected and studied in detail the amputated right leg of a 57-year-old man who had 'spontaneous gangrene' of the right foot. In a 25-page-long case report, with hand-drawn microscopic illustrations, Winiwarter painstakingly described the pathologic findings. He considered the nature of occlusive vascular lesions in the leg not as thrombosis or arteriosclerosis but as primarily an inflammatory disease with fibrosis involving both the arteries and veins, and he named the lesions 'endarteritis obliterans and endophlebitis', breaking the then tradition of calling every occlusive vascular disease that results in a gangrene 'arteriosclerosis' [6].

At the Meeting of the Association of American Physicians, Washington, DC, in May 1908, Leo Buerger [7] read a paper entitled 'Thromboangiitis obliterans: a study of the vascular lesions leading to presenile spontaneous gangrene', on the basis of detailed pathological studies of the blood vessels dissected from 11 amputated limbs. In this first of a series of articles on TAO, Buerger summarized the clinical characteristics of the disease as follows:

1. onset between 20–40 years;
2. attack of ischemic rest pain in the foot, calf or toes, and particularly of a sense of numbness or coldness whenever the weather is unfavorable;
3. one or both feet are markedly blanched, almost cadaveric in appearance, cold to the touch, and when the foot becomes warm, some color gradually returns;
4. absent ankle pulses;
5. rheumatic pain in the leg;

6. recurrent intermittent claudication;
7. trophic disturbances after months or years: erythromelalgia, a bright red blush of the toes and the foot in the pendent position, a blister, hemorrhagic bleb or ulcer near the tip of the toe, usually on the big toe, under the nail, and severe pain;
8. cyanotic discoloration and gangrene.

Buerger emphasized the extensive thrombotic obliteration of the arteries and veins except the largest and the smallest ones, and the importance of the disease's frequent association with migrating thrombophlebitis of superficial veins of the arms and legs. Thromboses of different histologic ages were found. Miliary foci of polymorphonuclear leukocyte collections ('microabscesses'), with a central area of fibrin deposition and one or more phagocytic giant cells made their intraluminal presence near the periphery in the thrombus. They were observed much more commonly in the affected veins than in the arteries [2,7].

Although Buerger placed more emphasis on thrombosis than on changes in the vessel wall at first, he finally made a non-committal statement that an acute inflammatory process of the blood vessel might be an initial manifestation of the pathologic process of the disease, **thromboangiitis obliterans**. The which-came-first, thrombosis-or-angiitis, question remains unresolved, but the evidence favors angiitis as the initiating process of Buerger's disease [2].

Buerger concluded as follows: 'Taking the true nature of the lesion into consideration, I would suggest that the names 'endarteritis obliterans' and 'arteriosclerotic gangrene' be discarded in this connection, and that we adopt the term 'obliterating thromboangiitis' of the lower extremities when we wish to speak of the disease under discussion.' Buerger's detailed observation and description about the clinical and pathohistological features of the disease was so clear and complete that the malady became known as 'Buerger's disease'. The crucial statement 'of the disease under discussion' was soon forgotten by many, however, and there was a time that all cases of lower-limb gangrene, occurring at any age, came to be diagnosed as 'thromboangiitis obliterans' [8].

After the Second World War, skepticism about this ill-defined disease entity resurfaced. In 1960, Wessler and his associates [9] claimed that the disease described by Buerger was indistinguishable from arteriosclerosis, systemic embolization or idiopathic peripheral arterial thrombosis, on the basis of 84 patients, from 1928 through 1956 in their series, with onset of arterial insufficiency before the age of 45 years. This assertion prompted an editorial [10] in the *Lancet*, entitled 'Does Buerger's disease exist?' and numerous other rebuttals [2] which argued strongly in favor of the recognition of Buerger's disease as a distinct clinicopathologic entity.

Although Buerger in his first paper [7] had already pointed out the inevitable coexistence of arteriosclerotic lesions in older patients with thromboangiitis obliterans, opponents of Buerger's disease as a distinct entity attributed the cause of the occlusive process solely to arteriosclerosis, even when the large-vessel proximal arteriosclerotic lesions are absent [1,8–10]. Currently, controversy regarding the existence of TAO has abated, and there is irrefutable proof of the occurrence of this peculiar form of occlusive disease afflicting the peripheral arteries and veins of susceptible young smokers, irrespective of their gender. As the specificity of the disease is derived from its clinical characteristics, the eponym 'Buerger's disease' is more appropriate than 'thromboangiitis obliterans', which tends to be more rigidly identified with the often unavailable or impractical histopathologic criteria.

18.2 Etiology and pathogenesis

The cause of Buerger's disease is not completely understood and a number of etiologic factors have been suggested, such as cold injury, tobacco allergy or hypersensitivity, infection (syphilis, typhus, streptococcus, dermatomycoses, rickettsia and viruses), autoimmunity, metabolic abnormalities and hypercoagulable state, but none of these hypotheses has been proven or can be substantiated.

Various hypotheses suggesting an autoimmune mechanism in the pathogenesis of Buerger's disease have been examined recently. Evidence for this included an increase in complement factor C4, anti-elastin [11] and anti-collagen antibody, cellular sensitivity to human type I or III collagen [12], and circulating immune complexes in patients with the disease: both organ-specific autoantibodies (IgM, IgG, IgA) and C3 component have been observed in the diseased blood vessels [13,14]. However, whether these findings are primary or secondary phenomenon with respect to the vascular lesions of Buerger's disease is uncertain and the significance of these immunologic mechanisms remains to be elucidated.

While the cause of Buerger's disease remains unresolved, tobacco use is very closely related with the initiation, exacerbations and remissions of the disease [2]. The vasoconstricting effect of tobacco on the peripheral vessels was demonstrated in man by Bruce *et al.* [15], as early as in 1909, using the volume changes in the hand and arm. In 1933, Harkavy [16] studied skin reaction following intracutaneous injection with 0.01 ml of tobacco extract in 87 patients with Buerger's disease, 36 with coronary disease and 262 controls: positive skin reactions were found in 87%, 36% and 16%, respectively. From this observation, Harkavy [16] concluded that tobacco hypersensitivity might play an important role in the pathogenesis of Buerger's disease.

Astrup [17] observed that the oxygen dissociation curve of a patient with Buerger's disease showed a shift to the left at low tension; that is to say, increased affinity of hemoglobin for oxygen: this is almost entirely due to a raised carboxy-hemoglobin level. Mukaiyama et al. [18] proposed that smoking might induce a prethrombotic state of hypercoagulability and reduced fibrinolytic activity, often occurring in blood vessels with damaged endothelium.

Is there a genetic predisposition factor to the development of Buerger's disease from smoking? Ohtawa et al. [19], in 1974, first noted an increase in the incidence of HLA-A9, BW10 and a Japanese specific antigen J-1-1 together with an absence of HLA-A12 in Japanese patients with Buerger's disease. Subsequent HLA-typing studies were reported by McLoughlin et al. [20] and more Japanese investigators [21], and they also found a high frequency of BW22.2, J-1-1, A9 or B5 and a low frequency of B12, but the results are more variable in the other antigens. Although some disagreement remains, most investigators agree there may be a gene in human chromosomes that determines susceptibility to the disease, linked to the presence or absence of certain HLA-antigens which may vary in different ethnic populations.

It remains uncertain whether non-smokers can develop Buerger's disease; the difficulty might be the lack of objective evidence for true non-smokers. The hazard of environmental tobacco smoke and passive smoking has recently attracted mounting attention [22]. Much work is being undertaken to identify sensitive markers with which to measure tobacco smoke exposure in non-smokers. The detection and measurement of nicotine and cotinine in the body fluid have received the most attention, with cotinine becoming increasingly accepted as a short-term marker in epidemiologic studies because of its relatively long half-time (20 hours, as compared with 2 hours for nicotine), lack of susceptibility to fluctuations during exposure to smoking, and the non-invasive method of collecting urine and saliva specimens [22,23].

There is a strong correlation, including a dose-response relation, between urinary cotinine levels and self-reported exposure to tobacco smoke. Matsushita et al. [23] recommended that those with urinary cotinine levels above 50 ng/mg creatinine be considered as **active smokers**; those with levels between 10 and 50 ng/mg creatinine as **passive smokers**; and those with levels below 10 ng/mg creatinine as **non-smokers** or without significant exposure to tobacco smoke. The measurement of urinary cotinine levels in patients with Buerger's disease confirmed that the patient's self-reporting smoking habit is quite unreliable. Passive smoking reduced platelet sensitivity to the antiaggregation effects of prostaglandins, this effect being more marked in non-smokers than in smokers [24]. Furthermore, passive exposure to tobacco smoke enhanced platelet aggregate formation and increased the number of damaged, anuclear, endothelial cells in the blood [25].

These epidemiological and clinical studies show that passive smoking can and does occur at home, in the workplace and the community, and heighten our attention to the health hazards of involuntary smoking. Based on the evidence of both the endothelial cell injury and platelet activation induced by exposure to tobacco smoke, even passive smoking may conceivably predispose thrombus formation in the blood vessels.

However, it is still uncertain whether true 'passive smokers' could develop Buerger's disease. Only a multicenter epidemiologic and clinical study that is based on the long-term evaluation of health effects of involuntary exposure to tobacco smoke may provide objective evidence to support the hypothesis that passive smoking could influence the occurrence of Buerger's disease and the aggravation of the disease process.

Although other factors may have an etiologic role in Buerger's disease, it is indisputable that smoking holds the key to the solution. If the health hazards of involuntary smoking could be explicated, it would remove a major objection to considering tobacco as the most important if not the sole cause of Buerger's disease.

18.3 Epidemiology

Although Buerger's disease has a worldwide distribution, it is more prevalent in the Middle, Near and Far East regions than in the North America and Western Europe.

18.3.1 USA AND EUROPE

The reported number of new patients with Buerger's disease in the USA and Europe has decreased mainly through the adoption of stricter diagnostic criteria. Before the late 1960s, over-diagnosis of Buerger's disease occurred even at the Mount Sinai Hospital, where Buerger began his work on TAO: of the 205 cases diagnosed as Buerger's disease at the Hospital from 1933 through 1963, only 33 were later considered to be compatible with the correct diagnosis; the diagnosis was questionable in 28 cases, and incorrect in 144 cases [26].

At the Mayo Clinic, over a 40-year period (1947–86), the annual patient registration has increased from 166 232 in 1947 to 221 000 in 1986 but the prevalence rate of patients with the diagnosis of Buerger's disease has steadily declined from 104 per 100 000 patient registrations in 1947 to 12.6 per 100 000 patient registrations in 1986 [2,3,27].

At the International Symposium on Buerger's disease in Bad Gastein, Austria in 1986, Cachovan [28] reported the following prevalence rate of Buerger's disease in patients with peripheral arterial occlusive disease in

Europe and other countries: 1–3% in Switzerland, 0.5–5% in West Germany, 1.2–5.6% in France, 4% in Belgium, 0.5% in Italy, 0.25% in the United Kingdom, 3.3% in Poland, 6.7% in East Germany, 11.5% in Czechoslovakia, 39% in Yugoslavia, 80% in Israel (Ashkenazim), 45–63% in India and 16–66% in Korea and Japan. These rates were calculated from selected series of patients treated at specialized institutions rather than from the general population as a whole.

18.3.2 ASIA

In Asia, a much higher proportion of patients with limb ischemia has been attributed to Buerger's disease than that in the USA and Europe. In 1980, Nigam et al. [29] in Delhi reported that Buerger's disease accounted for 63%, arteriosclerosis obliterans for 15% and miscellaneous causes for 22% out of 169 cases of limb ischemia during a 3-year period. At the Christian Medical College Hospital in Vellore, South India [30] in 1989, 186 (53%) of 352 patients with peripheral vascular disease were diagnosed as Buerger's disease and the remaining 166 (47%) as arteriosclerosis obliterans.

In 1931, reviewing the data of 50 cases of the disease in Korea, Ludlow [31] reported that the ratio of the number of patients with Buerger's disease to all inpatients was 1:400 and to the male inpatients only it was 1:250. In 1961, McKusick and Harris [32] reported 28 cases of Buerger's disease reviewed at the Presbyterian Medical Center in Chonju, Korea. All patients were male and smokers; 23 of the 28 patients were farmers or farm laborers, and all 23 were of the lowest socioeconomic status.

In 1973, Hill and colleagues [33] described an analysis of 106 patients with Buerger's disease in Java, Indonesia: all the patients were cigarette smokers and only one was a woman. In general, the patients were from the lower socioeconomic sector of the community and there were no patients who could be judged middle-class even by Indonesian standards. They concluded that the environmental factors of significance in this disease as it occurred in Java appeared to be tobacco, cold injury and a past history of mycotic infection.

In 1931, Noble [34] described 15 cases (14 men and 1 woman) of Buerger's disease in Bangkok, Thailand. The majority of them had an outdoor job; all but one were heavy smokers and the one exception was a woman who habitually chewed betel nut. In China, Whyte [35], a missionary surgeon in Swatow, reported the clinical features of two patients with Buerger's disease in 1917. Although it is well-known that the disease occurs widely throughout Asia, to date, no nationwide epidemiologic study has been carried out in all these countries.

In 1976, the Buerger's Disease Research Committee of the Ministry of Health and Welfare of Japan [21] analyzed 3034 patients (2930 men and 104 women) with the disease from all over Japan and estimated its incidence to be about 5 per 100 000 population. In 1986, the Epidemiology of Intractable Disease Research Committee of the Ministry of Health and Welfare of Japan [36] estimated that there were 8858 patients with the disease who were treated at various medical institutions in Japan; they found also that there were about 5 per 100 000 population and that there was no significantly greater prevalence among manual laborers. The number of new patients with Buerger's disease in Japan seems to be decreasing slightly, but the number of the patients under the care of a physician remains almost unchanged due to recurrences. At the senior author's institution in Japan, the current ratio of new patients with Buerger's disease to new patients with arteriosclerosis obliterans is about 1:3 (Shionoya, unpublished data).

18.3.3 BUERGER'S DISEASE IN WOMEN

Buerger's disease was uncommon in women; the reported incidence was 1–2% in most published series of cases before 1970. Several recently published series showed a much higher prevalence of women with the disease: Lie's report [27] showed that 12 (11%) of 109 cases of the disease from 1981 to 1985 in Rochester, Minnesota, were female; there were 5 (19%) of 26 in the 1987 Oregon study [37], 48 (14%) of 355 from 1975 to 1984 in Yugoslavia [38], 12 (22.6%) of 53 patients in a Swiss study [39] and 26 (23%) of 112 from 1970 to 1987 in another study from the USA [40]. It is unclear whether the greater number of smokers among young women in recent years is solely responsible for the increased prevalence of Buerger's disease in women, or the reported incidence varied with the diagnostic criteria adopted. The prevalence of Buerger's disease in Japanese women remains relatively low compared to the increased number of female smokers.

18.4 Clinical and angiographic characteristics

18.4.1 CLINICAL PRESENTATION

In Buerger's disease, the vaso-occlusive lesions seem to begin in the peripheral blood vessels and extend proximally. The disease may progress insidiously until the occlusive lesions involve the forearm or crural arteries, and the early clinical manifestations are multifarious, including coldness, paresthesia, skin color changes, rest pain and intermittent claudication. Therefore, Fontaine's stepwise classification, which is useful for the clinical staging of arterial insufficiency due to arteriosclerosis obliterans, is not useful in gauging the severity of ischemia in Buerger's disease. Gangrene or ulceration does not always follow claudication and may even precede it [41].

Characteristically, the fingers or toes are cold and damp to the touch. The patient often complains of paresthesia of the finger or foot after manual labor or walking, respectively. The skin color changes are characteristic of the disease; the affected fingers and toes are purplish red, particularly with pendency. Differences in the delay of the return of skin color or in the degree of reactive hyperemia reflect regional differences in the severity of ischemia.

Although foot claudication is the usual symptom associated with ischemia due to infrapopliteal arterial occlusion, calf claudication may be experienced if the disease progresses to the suprapopliteal segment. Gangrene and ulceration may occur spontaneously, but in the majority of cases, such trophic lesions follow various forms of trauma, including iatrogenic injury. Necrotic lesions develop most commonly on the tip of a digit, particularly the big toe. As a result of secondary infection, such lesions spread proximally and are associated with intractable pain. Rest pain is characteristically localized to the digits or immediately adjacent areas and often precedes gangrene or ulceration. Recurrent superficial thrombophlebitis develops frequently on the arm, lower leg or foot. Redness of the skin over the affected vein and tenderness usually disappears in two to three weeks, leaving a black-brown pigmentation.

18.4.2 CLINICAL CORRELATION

From 1977 through 1988, 255 new patients with Buerger's disease were treated at the senior author's institution [41], comprising 249 men (98%) and 6 women (2%). The age at onset of symptoms ranged from 19 to 49 years (average 35.8 ± 7.7 years). The major presenting symptoms were paresthesia, coldness or cyanosis in 94 patients (36.9%), gangrene or ulcer in 47 (18.4%), foot claudication in 38 (14.9%), calf claudication in 42 (16.5%), rest pain in 26 (10.2%) and thrombophlebitis in 8 (3.1%). From the onset of symptoms to the end of follow-up necrotic lesions occurred in 184 (72.2%) of the 255 patients, phlebitis migrans in 109 (42.7%) and involvement of the upper extremity in 230 (90.2%).

Two limbs were affected in 17% of the 255 patients, three in 43% and all four in 40%; 83% of all the cases had involvement of three or four limbs and none had single limb involvement. The accompanying veins of the main crural arteries were often involved, but no disturbance of venous return was clinically detectable [41].

18.4.3 ARTERIOGRAPHIC FINDINGS

Angiographically, multiple segmental occlusions of distal extremity arteries are characteristic of Buerger's disease, with each occlusion being either tapered or abrupt. The arterial lumen proximal to the occlusion is usually smooth. A corrugated or accordion-like appearance is sometimes seen, mostly in the femoral or crural arteries, which may represent an associated arterial spasm. There is usually an extensive network of collateral vessels around each occlusion so that arterial circulation in the extremity is maintained by collaterals in spite of occlusion of almost all the main feeder arteries; these collateral vessels have a 'corkscrew' or 'rootlike' appearance (Figures 18.1 and 18.2). The arteriographic appearance of the upper extremity involvement is the same as that in the lower extremity [41]. Unlike arteriosclerosis obliterans, neither calcification of the vessel wall nor a moth-eaten defect of the arterial silhouette is seen in TAO (Table 18.1).

18.4.4 CLINICAL DIAGNOSIS

Our clinical diagnostic criteria for Buerger's disease are:

- smoking history
- onset before the age of 40 years
- infrapopliteal arterial occlusive lesions
- either upper limb involvement or migrating phlebitis
- absence of atherosclerotic risk factors other than smoking.

A tentative clinical diagnosis of Buerger's disease can be made when all five requirements are met; arteriographic findings serve as supporting evidence [41]. Table 18.2 summarizes the clinical distinctions between Buerger's disease and arteriosclerosis obliterans.

According to Papa and Adar [1], in addition to the three basic observations emphasized by Buerger – young age, male gender, tobacco use – one needs to consider three other essential features for the clinical diagnosis of TAO:

- upper extremity involvement (UEI)
- superficial thrombophlebitis (STP)
- vasospastic phenomenon (VSP).

At least two of these three additional features (UEI, STP, VSP) are required for a 'definite' diagnosis of TAO, and one or none for 'probable' or 'suspected' category, respectively. Thus, the criteria for diagnosis of 'definite' cases of Buerger's disease proposed by Papa and Adar [1] are virtually the same as those proposed by Shionoya [41].

18.5 Pathology

Buerger's disease is fundamentally an inflammatory thrombosis that affects both arteries and veins, and the histopathology of the involved blood vessels varies according to the chronologic age of the disease at which the tissue sample is obtained for examination.

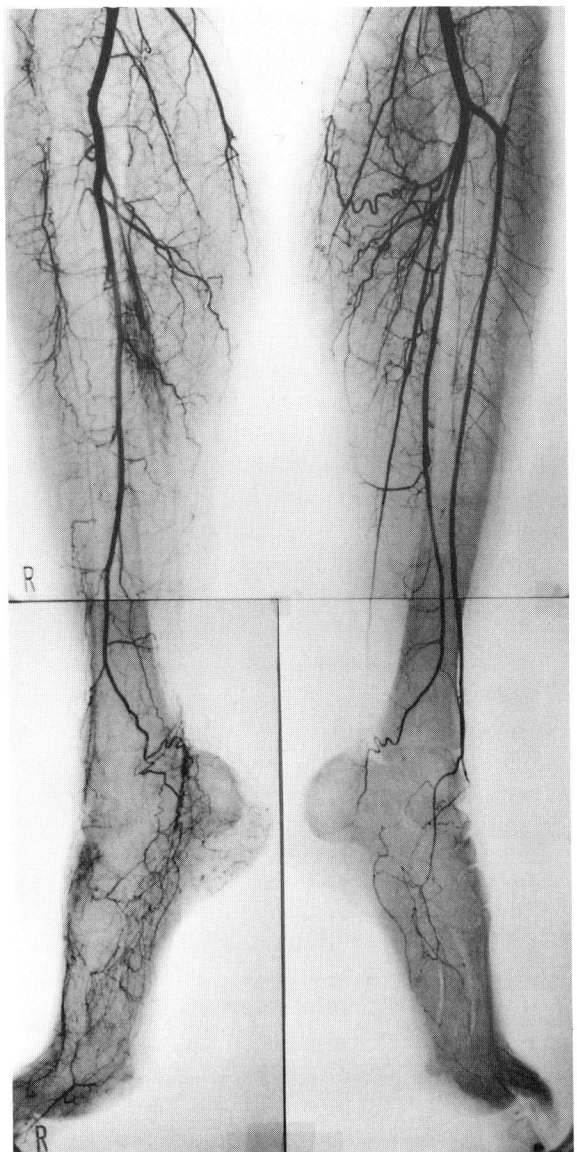

Figure 18.1 Bilateral femoral arteriogram of a 31-year-old man with Buerger's disease. In addition to multiple arterial occlusions in the feet and toes, the anterior and posterior tibial arteries are occluded in the right leg; the anterior tibial artery is abruptly occluded and the posterior tibial artery shows a tapering occlusion, respectively, at the left ankle.

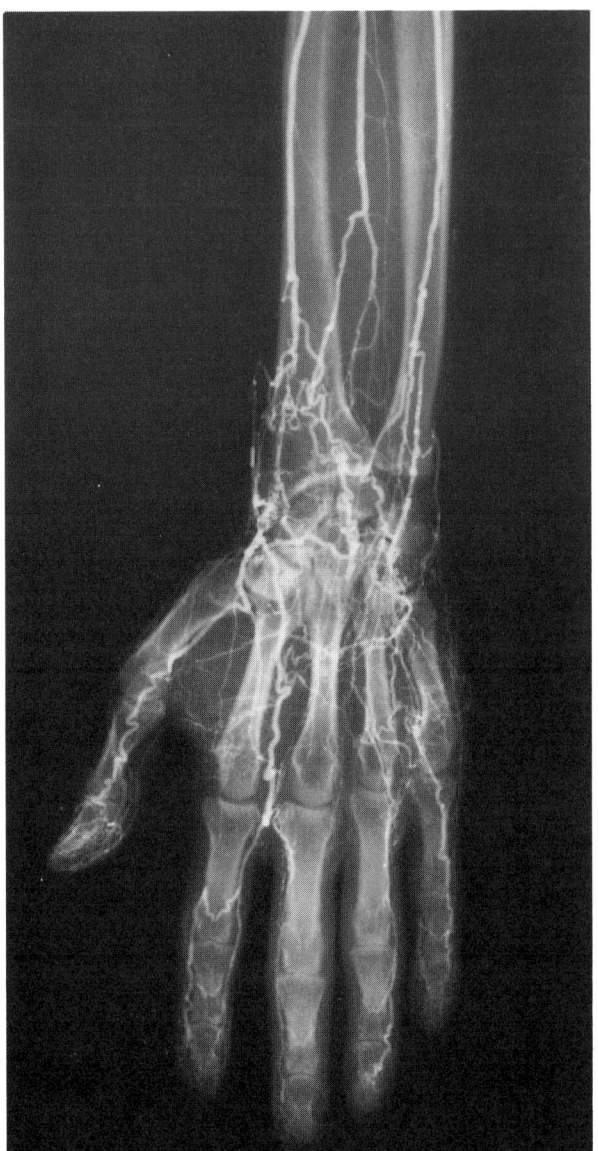

Figure 18.2 Right brachial arteriogram of a 46-year-old man with Buerger's disease. Despite multiple occlusions of the arteries of the forearm, hand and fingers, the affected upper extremity remains asymptomatic.

The histopathology is most likely to be diagnostic at the acute phase of the disease. It evolves to changes being consistent with or suggestive of the disease in the appropriate clinical setting at the immediate stage or subacute phase and becomes virtually indeterminate at end-stage or chronic phase, when all that remains is organized thrombus and fibrosis of the blood vessels [2,7,32,39, 42–44].

Dible [42], almost 30 years ago, had acknowledged that the pathological diagnosis of Buerger's disease was by no means always secure: 'there is so much variation from case to case, depending upon the stage of the disease and the characteristic capriciousness of the lesions, that it is difficult to give a succinct account of the histology . . .'. Nevertheless, Dible [42] believed that the histologic distinction between Buerger's disease and arteriosclerosis obliterans was so clear-cut that a differentiation could be made with a high degree of accuracy by simply examining tissue sections containing digital arteries and veins, the small blood vessels that are not normally affected by arteriosclerosis in individuals under the age of 40.

Table 18.1 Angiographic distinctions between thromboangiitis obliterans and arteriosclerosis obliterans*

Angiographic feature	Thromboangiitis obliterans	Arteriosclerosis obliterans
General appearance of blood vessels	Small and tapering	Large and tortuous
Flow of dye	Arterial fade out with or without early venous filling	Delayed filling of distal arteries
Size and location of vessels involved	Small and medium-sized, distal vessels often involved	Any size but large proximal vessels most often involved
Extent of occlusion	Segmental and often multifocal	Diffuse and segmental
Appearance of artery proximal to site of occlusion	Smooth outline and of even caliber	Irregular caliber and lumen of vessel
Extremity involved	Often both lower and upper, and digits	Lower extremities predominantly
Appearance of collateral circulation	Tree root or spider legs configuration around point of abrupt occlusion	Not specific

* Reproduced with permission from Lie [2].

Table 18.2 Clinical distinctions between thromboangiitis obliterans and arteriosclerosis obliterans*

Clinical feature	Thromboangiitis obliterans (%) (n = 234)	Arteriosclerosis obliterans (%) (n = 317)
Average age (range) at onset of disease in years	29 years (17–44)	59 years (33–79)
Male patients in army personnel	100	99
Male patients in civilian practice	96	45
Use of tobacco	100	44
Diabetes mellitus	0	30
Migratory thrombophlebitis	34	0
Raynaud's phenomenon	24	4
Involvement of aorta and visceral arteries	Rare	Common
Involvement of upper extremities	50	17
Intermittent claudication as initial symptom	66	90
Ischemic peripheral neuritis	5	30
Ulcers and gangrene in smokers	72	6
Ulcers and gangrene in non-smokers	2	22
Amputation of fingers and toes	18	2
Below-knee amputation	12	3
Above-knee amputation	8	4
10-year survival rate	94	66

* Reproduced with permission from Lie [2].

18.5.1 ACUTE PHASE LESIONS

The early, or active, phase lesion is characterized by acute inflammation involving all coats of the vessel wall, in association with occlusive thrombosis. Around the periphery of the thrombus, there are frequently what appear to be collections of polymorphonuclear leukocytes with karyorrhexis, the so-called 'microabscesses', in which one or more multinucleated giant cells may be present. This histologic finding is most characteristic of, but may not be specific for, Buerger's disease [45]. This striking inflammatory thrombotic lesion occurs with greater regularity in veins than in arteries (Figure 18.3) and is infrequently seen when organization of the thrombus is well under way.

Whether the vascular lesions of Buerger's disease are primarily thrombotic or primarily inflammatory has never been satisfactorily settled and probably never will. In either event, the intense inflammatory infiltration and cellular proliferation seen in the acute stage lesions is peculiar and distinctive (Figure 18.3). If, by chance, the acute and often tender nodular subcutaneous phlebitic lesion is biopsied at an early stage, one may indeed observe in different segments of the same affected vein several coexisting lesions. These are acute phlebitis without thrombosis (Figure 18.4), acute phlebitis with

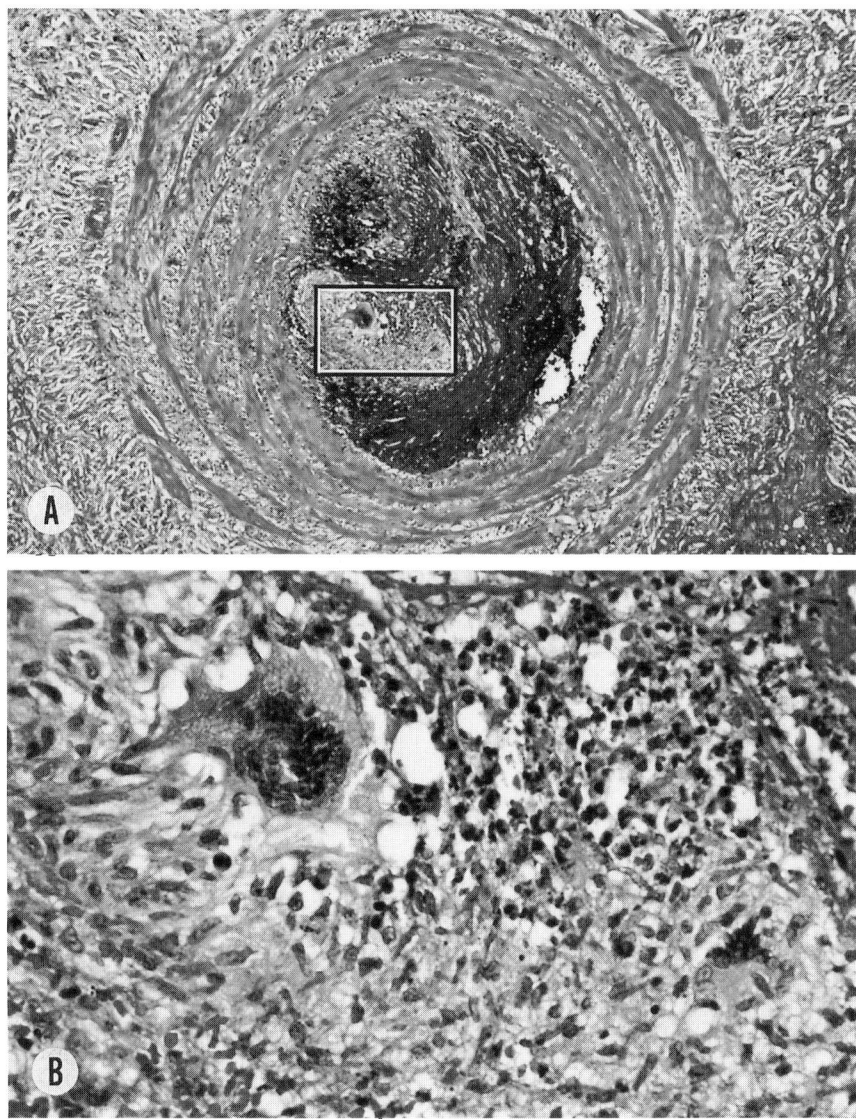

Figure 18.3 (A) Typical acute phase histologic lesion of Buerger's disease in a vein with intense thromboangiitis. (B) Close-up view of the boxed area in (A) showing microabscesses in the thrombus and 2 multinucleaed giant cells. (H&E A ×64, B ×400.) (Reproduced with permission from Lie [2].)

thrombosis (Figure 18.5) and acute phlebitis with thrombus containing microabscesses and giant cells (Figure 18.6). Rarely, giant cells are present in granulomatous inflammation of the organizing thrombus without microabscesses (Figure 18.7).

Wessler [9] has seriously questioned the specificity of the acute vascular lesions in thromboangiitis obliterans, and he was also critical of the veracity of the photomicrographs of acute vascular lesions in several of Buerger's articles on the subject [2]. Wessler [9] concluded that '... although Buerger may indeed have seen an acute arterial lesion, he did not at any time present documentary proof of its existence'. Although less frequently observed, the acute phase lesions undoubtedly occur in arteries (Figure 18.8), sometimes as late as when the thrombus is undergoing organization (Figure 18.9).

18.5.2 INTERMEDIATE PHASE AND END-STAGE LESIONS

The intermediate, or subacute, phase signifies progressive organization of the occlusive thrombus in the arteries and veins, which is usually accompanied by a prominent inflammatory cell infiltrate within the thrombus and less so in the vessel wall (Figure 18.10). The chronic phase or end-stage is characterized by completed organization of the occlusive thrombus with extensive recanalization, prominent vascularization of the media and adventitial and perivascular fibrosis

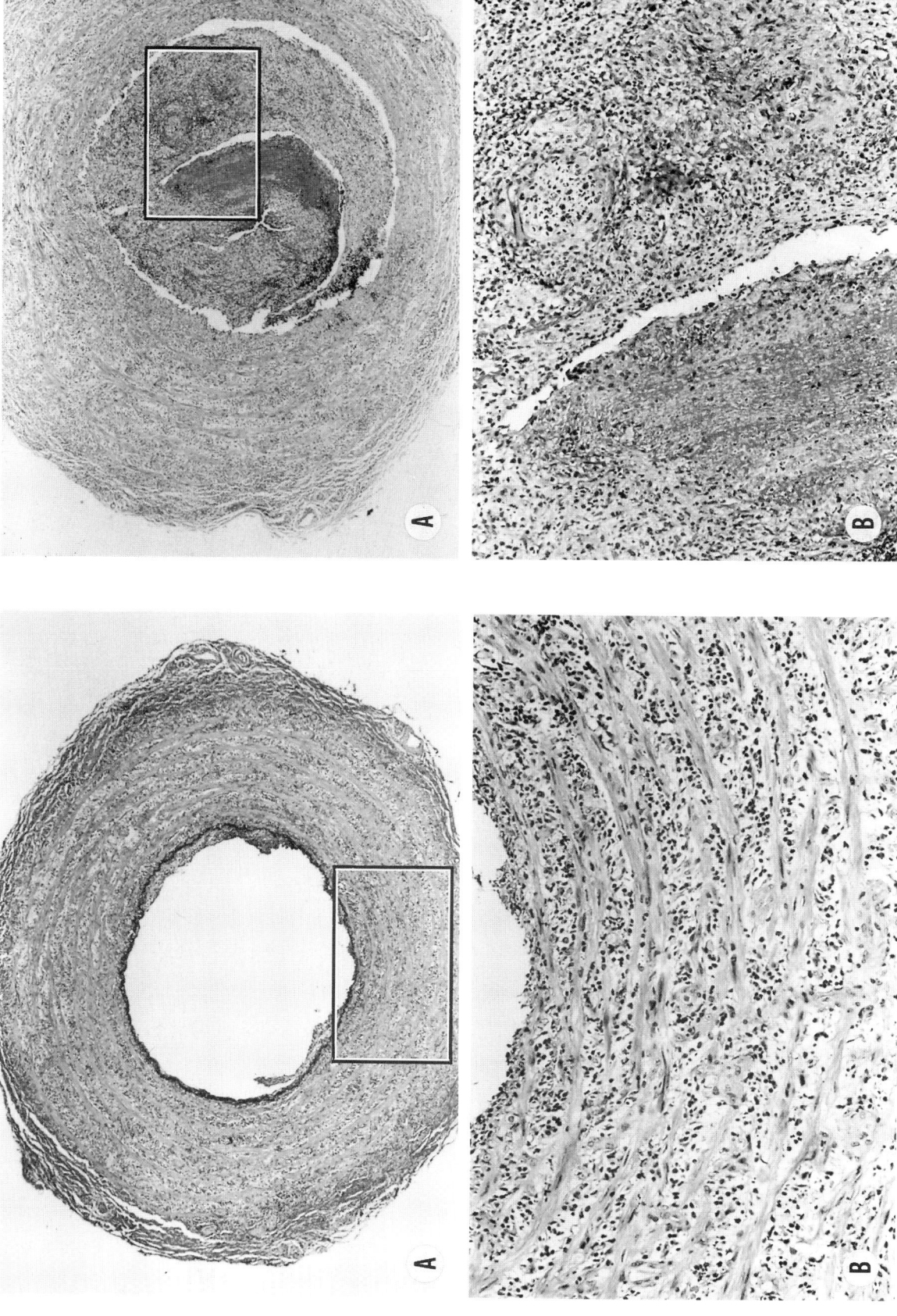

Figure 18.4 (A) Acute phlebitis without thrombus. (B) Close-up view of the boxed area in (A) showing the intense mixed-cell inflammatory infiltrate throughout the vessel wall. (H&E A ×40, B ×160.) (Reproduced with permission from Lie [2].)

Figure 18.5 (A) Acute phlebitis with thrombosis. (B) Close-up view of the boxed area in (A) showing a granulomatous inflammatory focus and microabscesses within the occlusive thrombus but no giant cells. (H&E A ×40, B ×160.) (Reproduced with permission from Lie [2].)

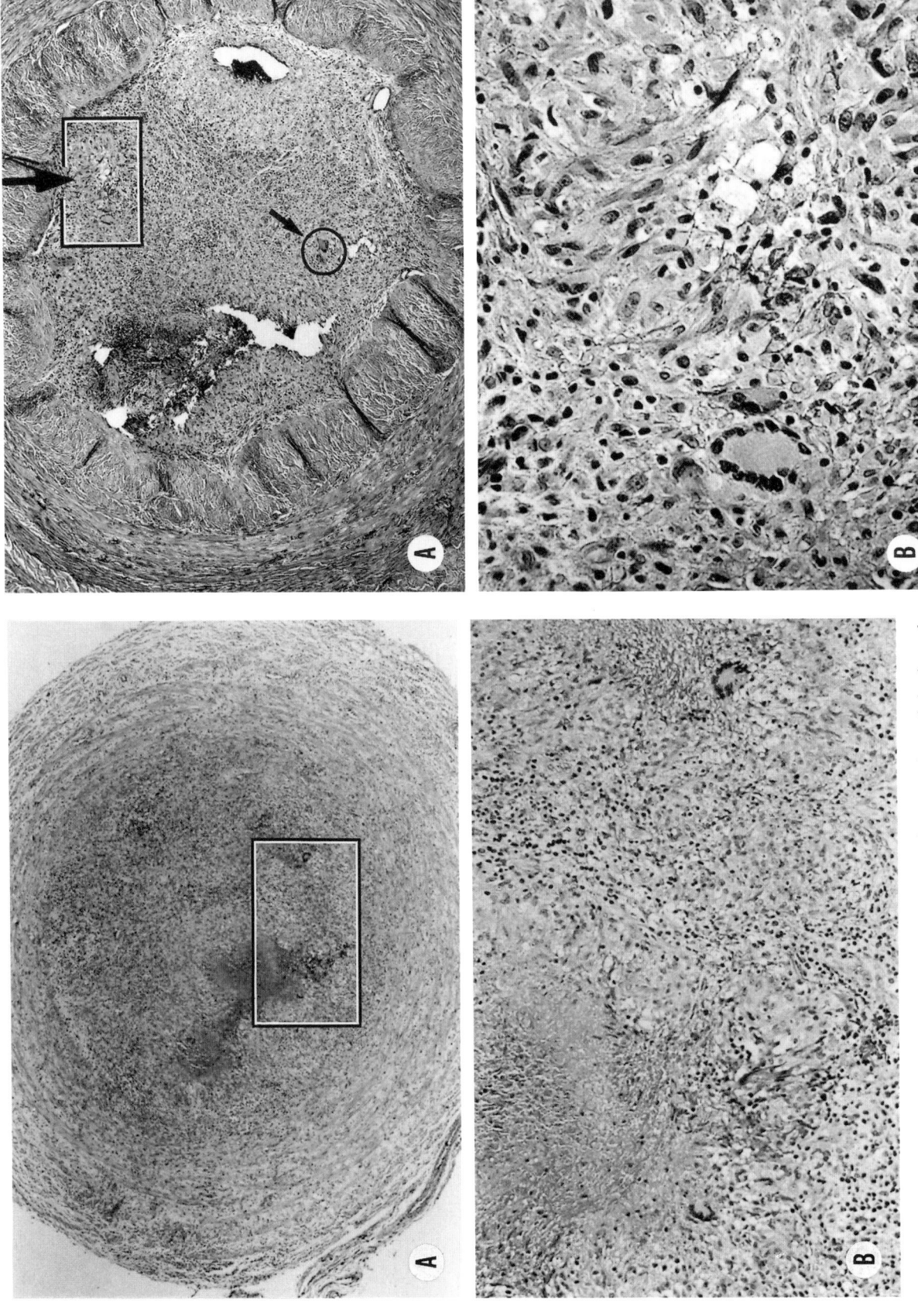

Figure 18.6 (A) Acute phlebitis with thrombosis. (B) Close-up view of the boxed area in (A) showing granulomatous foci, microabscesses and giant cells within the occlusive thrombus. (H&E A × 40, B × 160.) (Reproduced with permission from Lie [2].)

Figure 18.7 (A) Thrombophlebitis in Buerger's disease with intraluminal granulomatous inflammation of the occlusive thrombus containing multinucleated giant cells in areas outlined by the rectangle and circle. (B) Close-up view of the

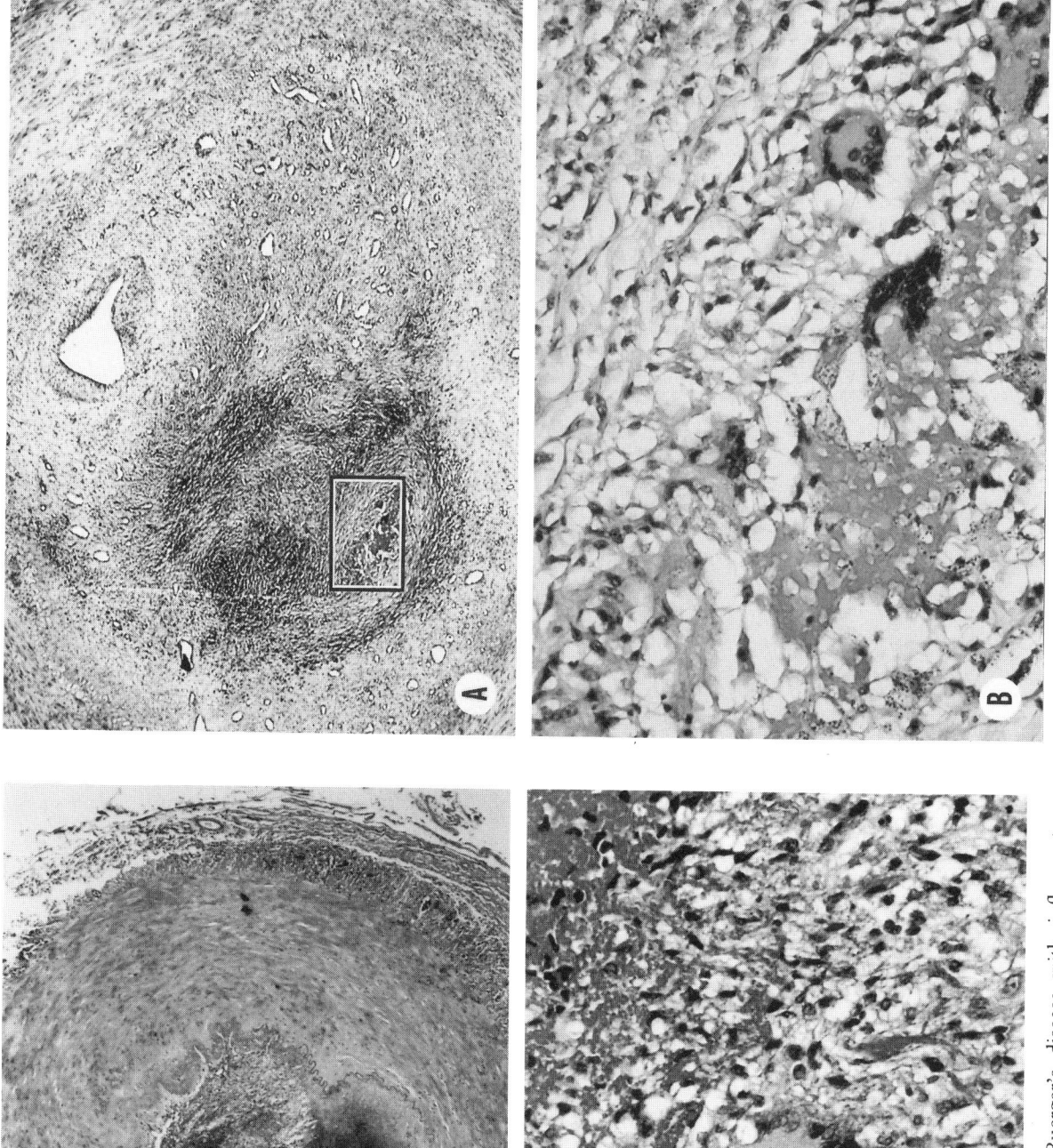

Figure 18.8 (A) Acute arterial lesion in Buerger's disease with inflammatory thrombosis and microabscess within the thrombus. (B) Close-up view of the boxed area in (A) showing a giant cell in microabscess within the thrombus. (H&E A ×40, B ×400.) (Reproduced with permission from Lie [2].)

Figure 18.9 (A) Femoral artery in Buerger's disease with an organizing thrombus has a rarely seen microabscess (boxed area). (B) Close-up view of the boxed area in (A) to show several giant cells in the microabscess of an organizing thrombus. (H&E A ×64, B ×400.)

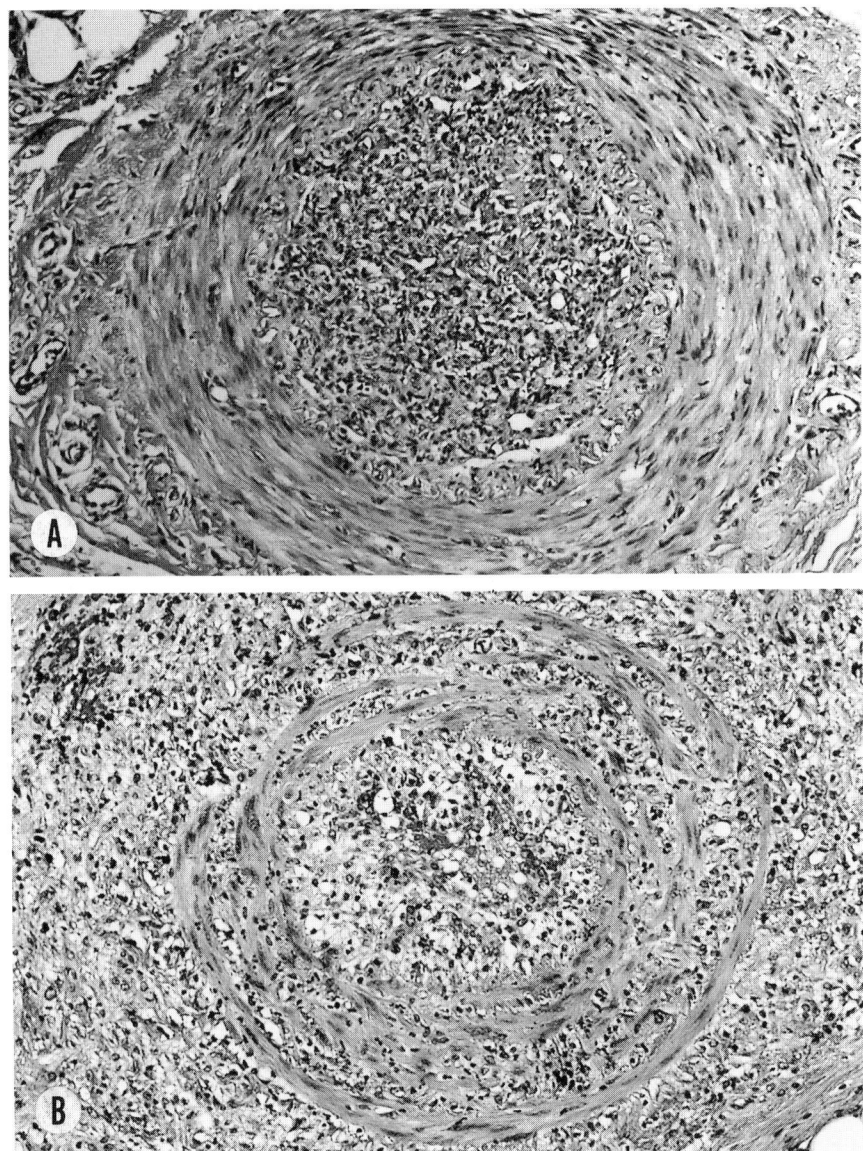

Figure 18.10 (A) Digital artery and (B) digital vein of intermediate stage lesion in Buerger's disease; both show early organization of an occlusive thrombus with prominent inflammatory cell infiltrate. (H&E. A and B ×64.) (Reproduced with permission from Lie [2].)

(Figure 18.11). In all three stages, the normal architecture of the vessel wall subjacent to the occlusive thrombus and including the internal elastic lamina remains essentially intact (Figures 18.10, 18.11, and 18.12). These findings distinguish thromboangiitis obliterans from arteriosclerosis and from other systemic vasculitides in which there is usually more striking disruption of the internal elastic lamina and the media, disproportional to those attributable to aging change.

Buerger's disease is segmental in distribution; 'skip' areas of normal vessels between diseased ones are common, and the intensity of the periadventitial reaction may be quite variable in different segments of the same vessel. Bland arterial and venous thrombosis with little or no cellular reaction often intermingle with inflammatory thrombosis in the vascular bed (Figure 18.13).

18.5.3 OTHER DIAGNOSTIC FEATURES

Histological diagnosis of Buerger's disease is usually inconclusive or tentative at best when only the amputated specimens or occluded arteries and veins are examined. The intermediate and chronic stage lesions have far fewer characteristic features and are seldom diagnostic. The intermediate lesions coincide with the early phase of organization of the occlusive thrombi in arteries and veins of all sizes (Figures 18.10, 18.12, 18.14, 18.15, and 18.16). This process is characteristic

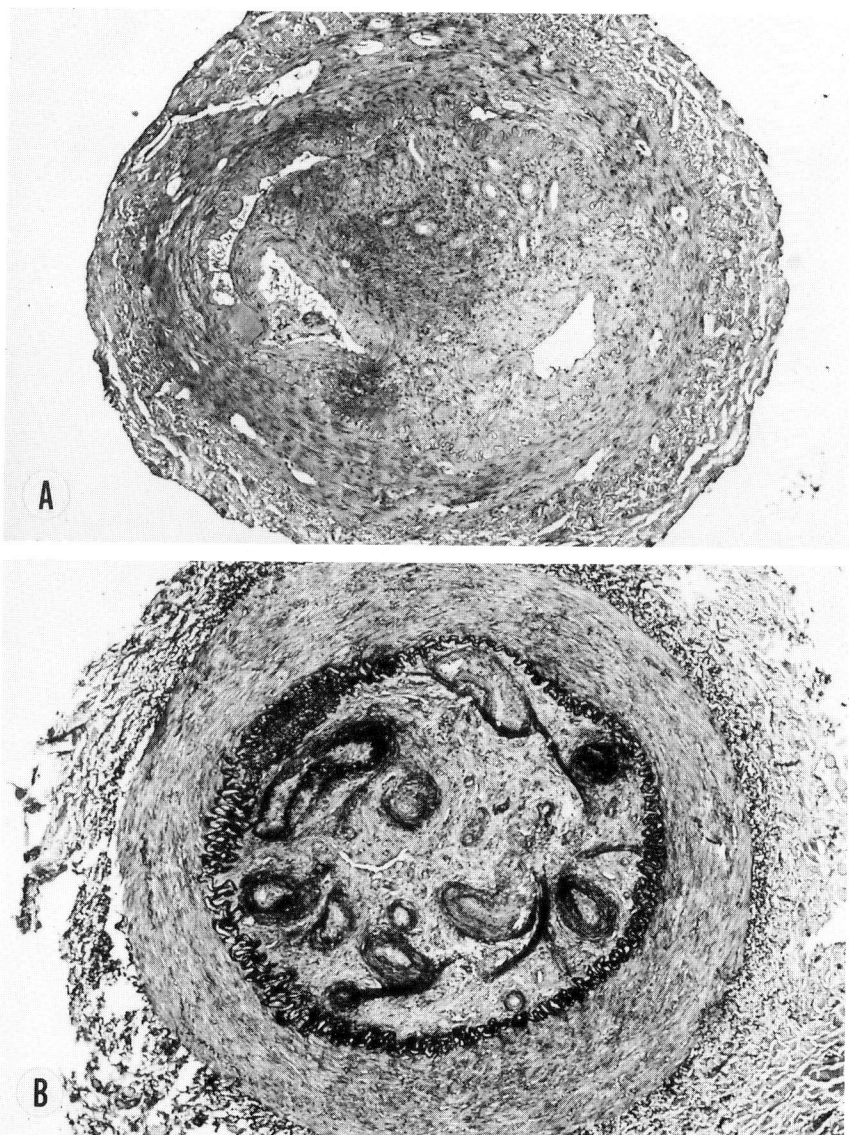

Figure 18.11 Chronic stage lesion of Buerger's disease in a radial artery. Note extensive recanalization of the organized thrombus with prominent vascularization of the media, intact internal elastic lamina and some residual lymphomononuclear cell infiltrate. (A: H&E ×64; B: elastic-van Gieson stain.) (Reproduced with permission from Lie [2].)

if not unique to Buerger's disease, because of the marked cellular proliferation and inflammatory infiltrate (Figure 18.10) which are rarely seen in the organization of the ordinary, bland arterial and venous thrombi. Lymphohistiocytic cells and, to a much lesser extent, granulocytic leukocytes, contribute to the inflammatory infiltrates. Eosinophils may be present but seldom in excessive numbers. The elastic laminae usually remain essentially intact. These changes are frequently observed in small digital blood vessels which are not normally affected by arteriosclerosis or atherosclerosis.

The end-stage chronic lesions are understandably the least distinctive of the three morphologic stages of Buerger's disease. The lesions are characterized by occluded arteries and veins with organized and recanalized thrombi accompanied by fibrosis and neovascularization of the vessel walls (Figure 18.11). As such, they represent the end products of vascular injury and occlusive thrombosis. The degree of perivascular fibrosis and lymphoid infiltration observed in the organized thrombi and vessel walls varies throughout the obliterated vascular segments. Focal residual inflammatory reaction of the organized thrombus may still be sufficiently characteristic to suggest Buerger's disease (Figure 18.17). Overall, these features are consistent with a disease process in which focal or segmental vasculitis, combined with thrombosis and endarteritic changes, effect a variable pattern of vascular obliteration that is quite distinct from arteriosclerosis with bland thrombosis. One hardly needs to be reminded that

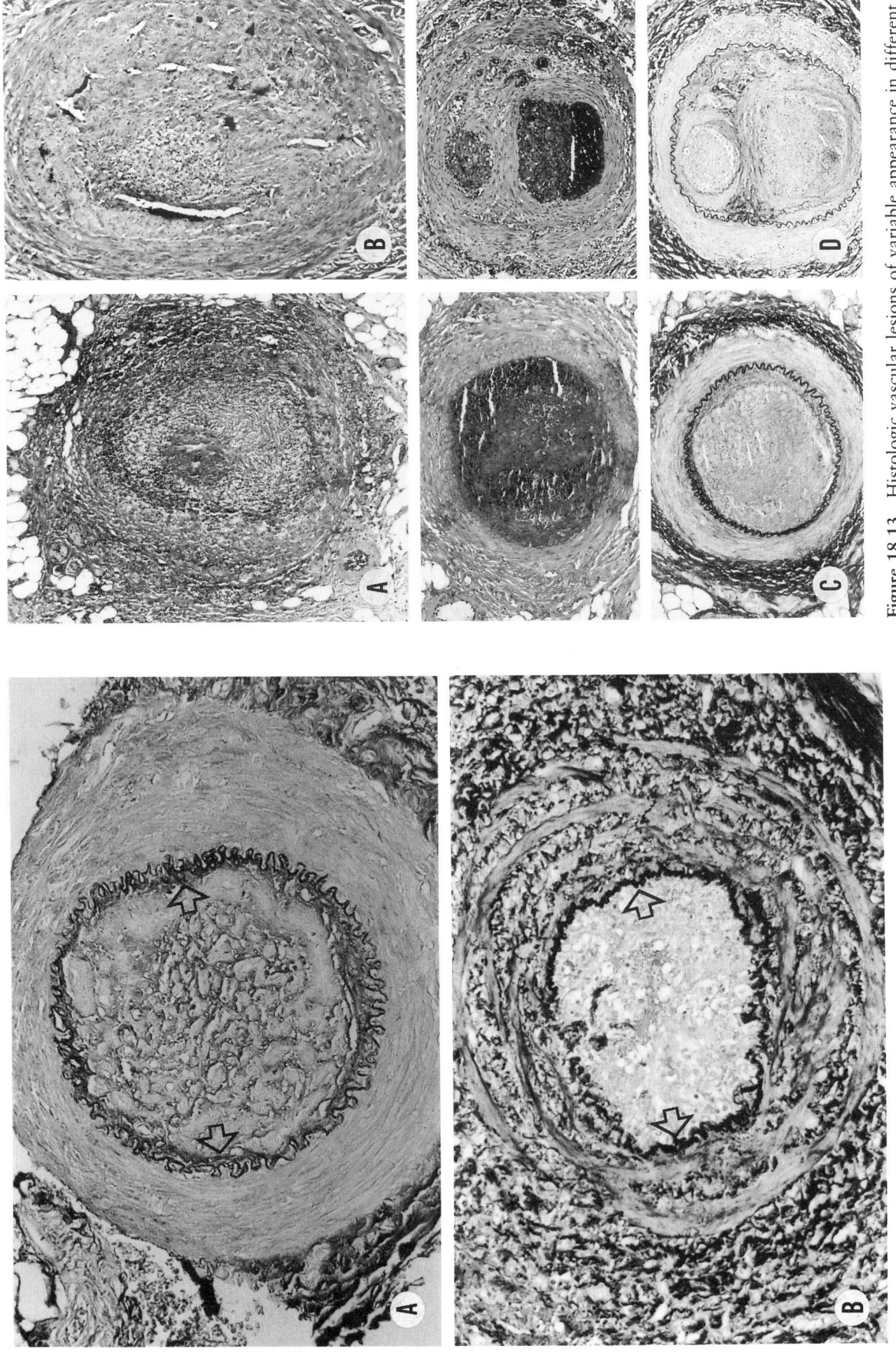

Figure 18.13 Histologic vascular lesions of variable appearance in different blood vessels of the same amputation specimen. (A) Acute lesion in a vein with intensely cellular thromboangiitis. (B) Intermediate lesion in a vein with an organizing inflammatory thrombus. (C and D) Rather plain-looking bland arterial thrombosis with hematoxylin-eosin sections above and elastic stain sections below (A–D ×64.) (Reproduced with permission from Lie [2].)

Figure 18.12 (A) Digital artery and (B) digital vein of intermediate stage lesion in Buerger's disease, corresponding to those shown in Figure 18.10, showing essentially normal architecture of the vessel wall subjacent to the occlusive thrombus. (Elastic-van Gieson stain: A and B × 64.) (Reproduced with permission from Lie [2].)

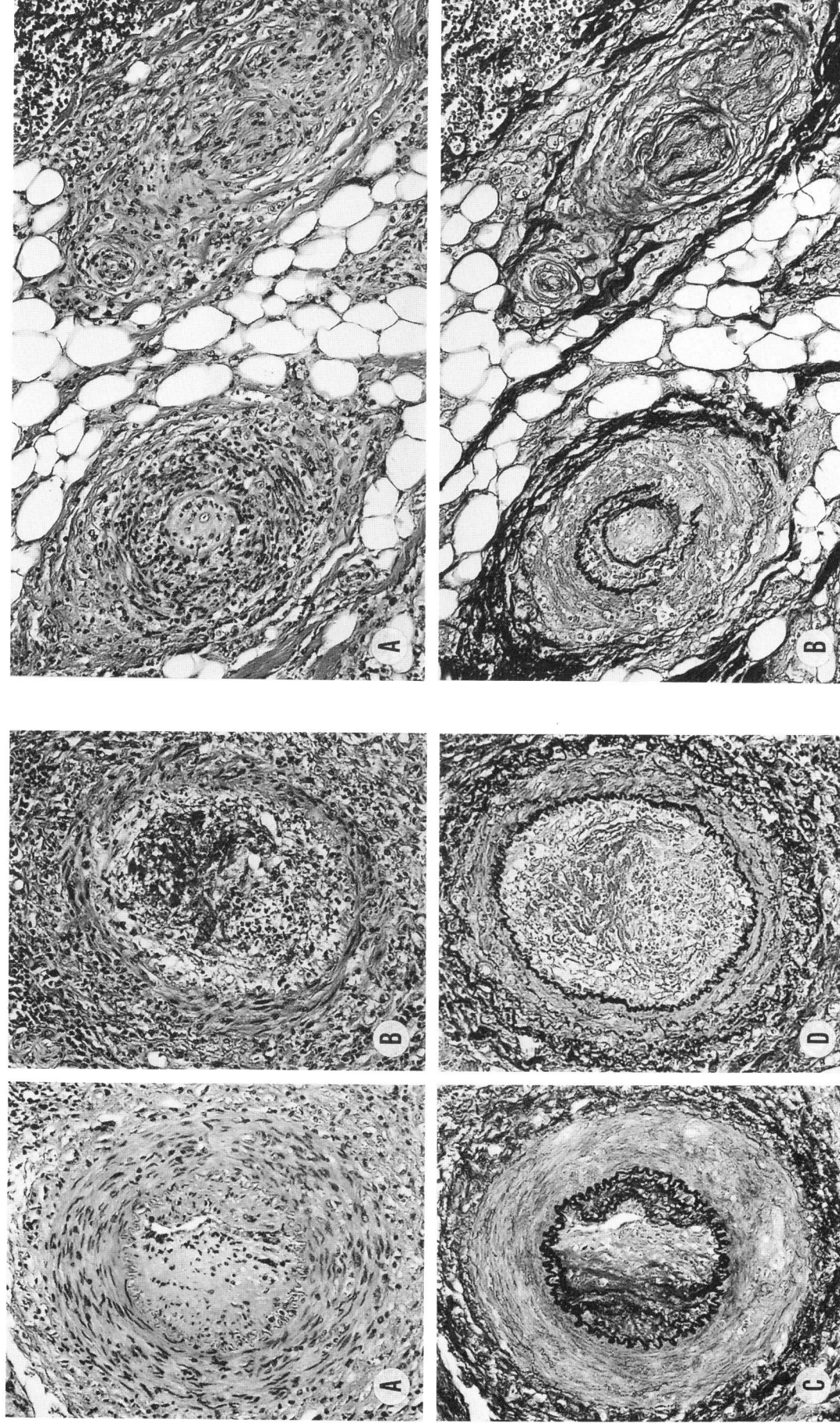

Figure 18.14 Intermediate lesions of digital artery (A and C) and digital vein (B and D) with organizing thrombi and residual inflammatory reaction (A, B: H&E; C, D: elastic stain × 160.) (Reproduced with permission from Lie [2].)

Figure 18.15 Corresponding H&E (A) and elastic stain (B) sections of a small artery (left) and vein (right) with intermediate stage lesions of Buerger's disease. Without an elastic stain the distinction between the artery and vein may not be so readily apparent. (A, B H&E; C, D: elastic stain × 160.) (Reproduced with permission from Lie [2].)

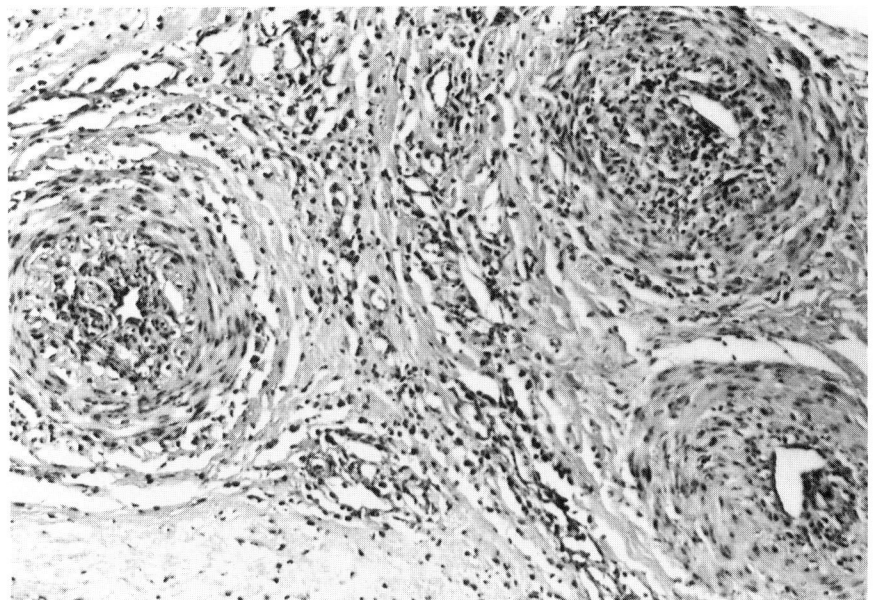

Figure 18.16 The small-vessel lesions in Buerger's disease with resolving angiitis and early occlusive intimal proliferation. Vessels of this caliber usually escape damage in atherosclerosis. (H&E ×160.) (Reproduced with permission from Lie [2].)

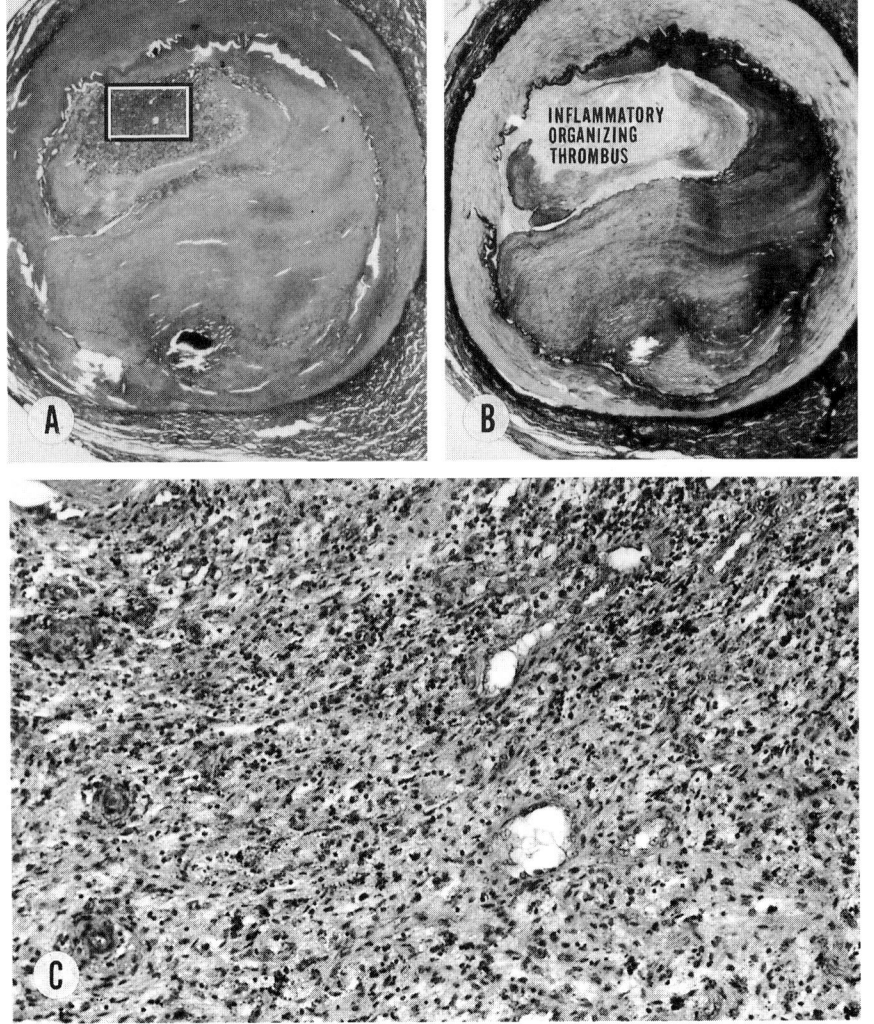

Figure 18.17 (A) H&E and (B) elastic stain sections of a chronic lesion in Buerger's disease. (C) Close-up view of the boxed area in (A) showing the residual predominantly lymphocytic infiltrate in the thrombus. (A and B ×16; C ×160.) (Reproduced with permission from Lie [2].)

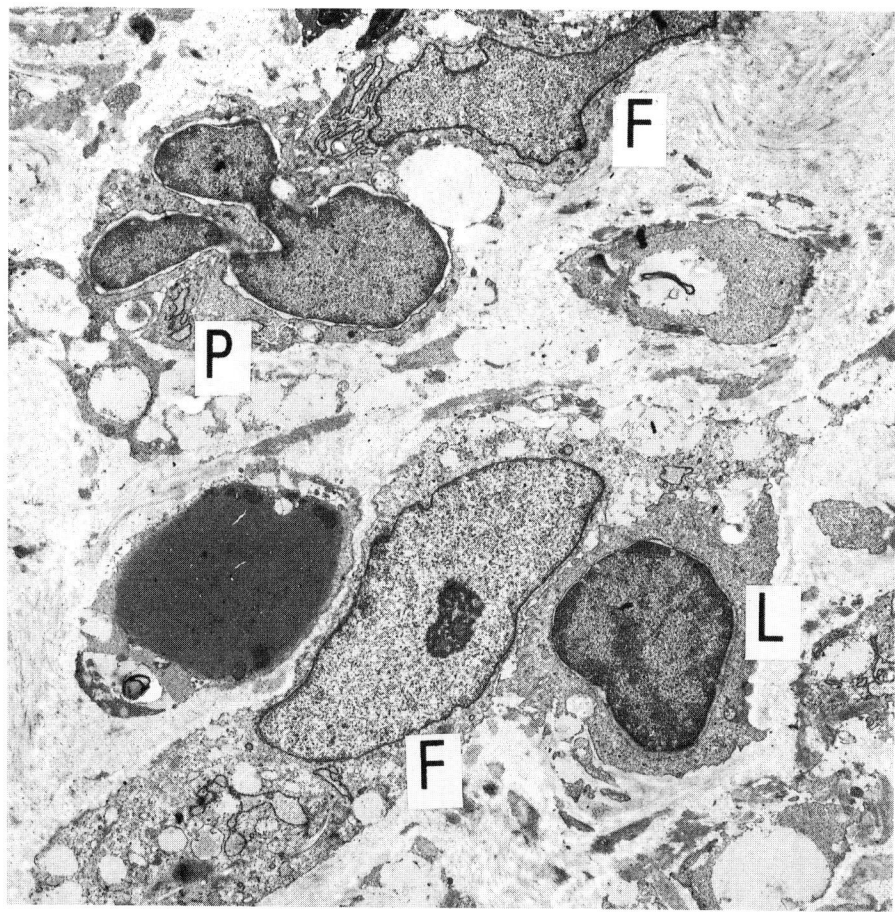

Figure 18.18 Ultrastructure of the arterial wall in Buerger's disease with a mixed inflammatory infiltrate: polymorphonuclear leukocytes (P), lymphocytes (L) and fibroblasts (F). (Phosphate-buffered glutaraldehyde × 5300.)

in some patients, especially those over the age of 40, both Buerger's disease and arteriosclerosis may coexist, thus creating further diagnostic uncertainty and controversy. Buerger's disease does not confer an immunity to atherosclerosis or arteriosclerosis that is aging related.

18.5.4 IMMUNOHISTOCHEMISTRY

To date, there have been very few published studies focusing on the cytoskeleton and immunohistochemistry of the cellular elements in Buerger's disease.

Soon after the thrombus has occluded the vessel lumen, spindle cells begin to appear in the periphery of the thrombus. They originate in the media and pass through fenestrations along the internal elastic lamella into the intima and from there into the thrombus. These cells express vimentin and alpha-1-actin (monoclonal marker for smooth muscle actin) and are derived from smooth muscle cells of the media. Capillaries also appear in the marginal zones of the thrombus. The endothelial cells express factor VIII-related antigen and *Ulex europaeus* agglutinin [46].

In later stages of thrombus organization, the spindle cells in the thrombus lose their positive staining for alpha-1-actin along with their differentiation into fibroblasts. The demonstration of the internal elastic lamella by collagen type IV markers (Dakopatts C4) confirms that the lamella is intact and that the smooth media muscle cells migrate inward through existing fenestrations to enter the intima. The newly-formed capillaries within the thrombus are surrounded by a thin basement membrane mainly composed of type IV collagen produced by the endothelial cells.

In summary, the process of thrombus organization in TAO is essentially identical to that in ordinary thrombosis but with an added inflammatory component. The invasion of organizing smooth muscle cells from the media of the blood vessel appears more intensified resulting in a hypercellular thrombus with rapid organization. Prominent inflammatory cell infiltrate in thrombus organization is a hallmark of Buerger's disease. Initial preservation of the internal elastic lamina is another distinguishing feature from arteriosclerosis/atherosclerosis and necrotizing vasculitis.

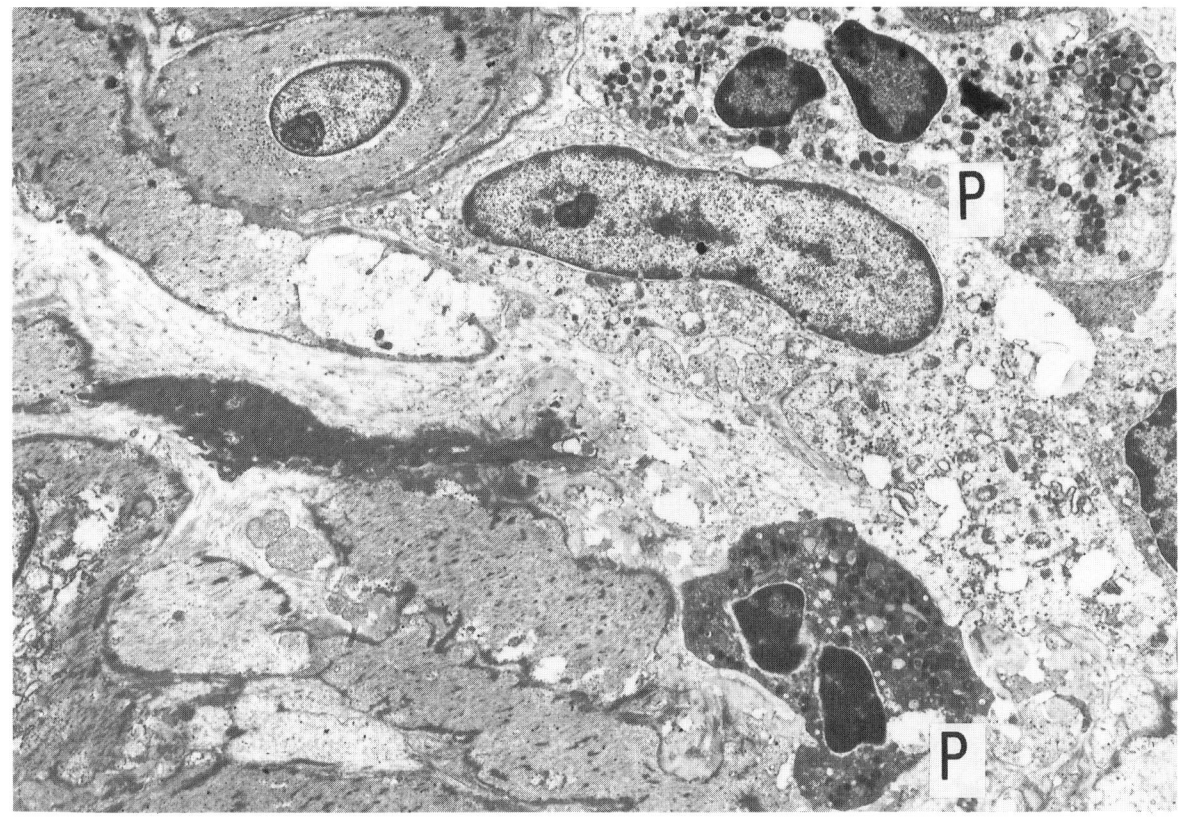

Figure 18.19 Ultrastructure of migrating phlebitis in Buerger's disease with polymorphonuclear leukocyte (P) predominating infiltrate. (Phosphate-buffered glutaraldehyde × 5300.)

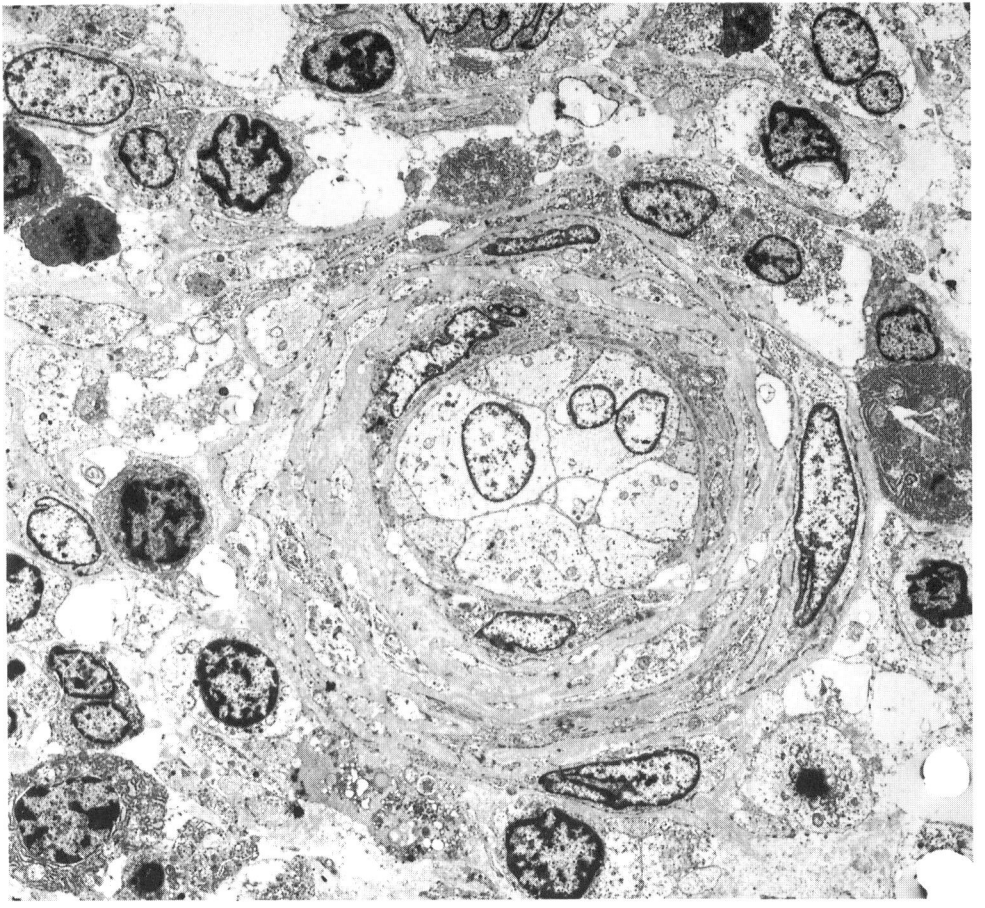

Figure 18.20 Occluded vasa vasorum in the arterial wall of Buerger's disease, surrounded by a mixed chronic inflammatory infiltrate mainly of lymphocytes and plasma cells. (Phosphate-buffered glutaraldehyde × 2600.)

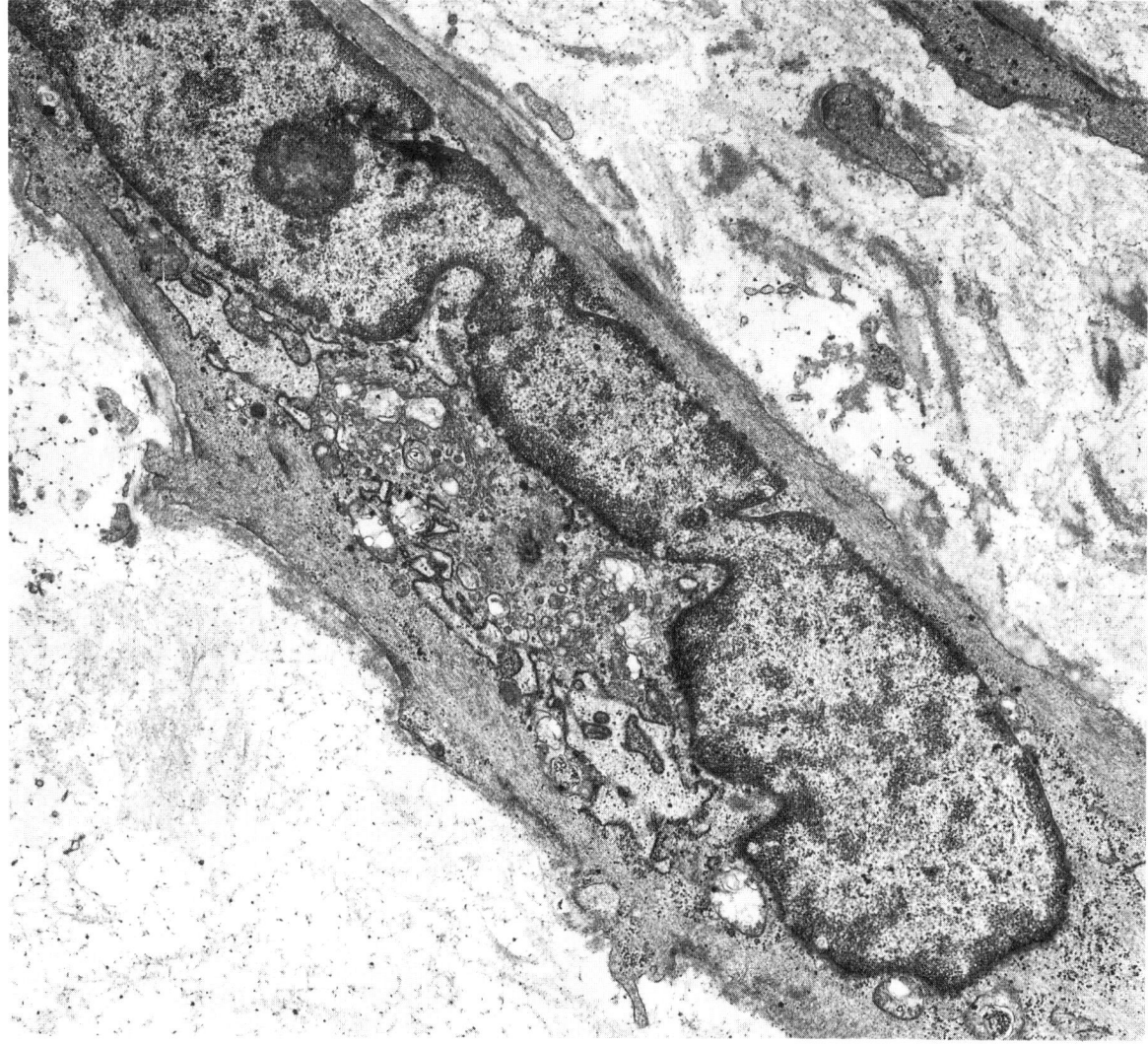

Figure 18.21 Ultrastructure of the arterial wall in Buerger's disease showing an activated myocyte with abundant endoplasmatic reticulum. (Phosphate-buffered glutaraldehyde ×11900.)

18.5.5 ELECTRON MICROSCOPY

The acute phase vascular lesions of TAO are most characteristic but they are seldom biopsied and even more rarely studied by electron microscopy. The ultrastructural changes are non-specific and have no diagnostic value (Figure 18.18) [44]. The tunica media of the affected arteries and veins show necrotic foci with infiltration of lymphocytes, macrophages and occasional polymorphonuclear leukocytes (Figures 18.19 and 18.20). Capillary sprouting may also be observed while some of the vasa vasora are occluded (Figure 18.19). Many smooth muscle cells show ultrastructural features of activation with the cytoplasm containing an increased number and dilated endoplasmatic reticulum (Figure 18.21). In the intima, similar inflammatory cell infiltrates are present and, occasionally, eosinophils and epithelioid cells may also be observed.

18.6 Buerger's disease of blood vessels in unusual locations

Buerger's disease, as already noted, is almost exclusively a disease of the blood vessels in the lower and upper limbs. There have been only occasional reports, usually without adequate histologic proof, of involvement of large elastic arteries such as the aorta, the pulmonary artery and iliac arteries. Although Buerger [47] had described that vascular obliteration could affect blood vessels other than those of the limbs, the involvement of the cerebral arteries, coronary arteries, renal arteries and mesenteric arteries has been documented in only a handful of patients, almost all as single case reports [2,48,49]. The most spectacular case of Buerger's disease with combined peripheral and visceral involvement was that of an 18-year-old male cigarette smoker who, in a span of 15 years, underwent bilateral lumbar and dorsal

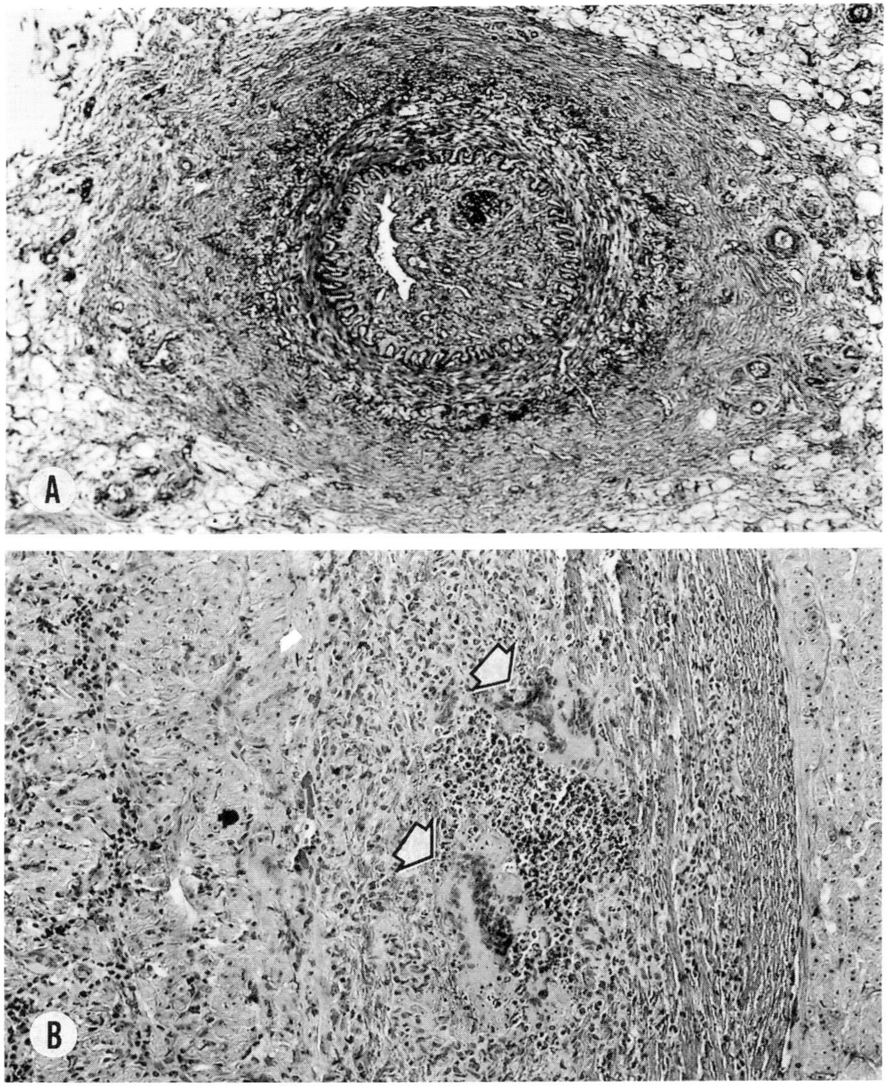

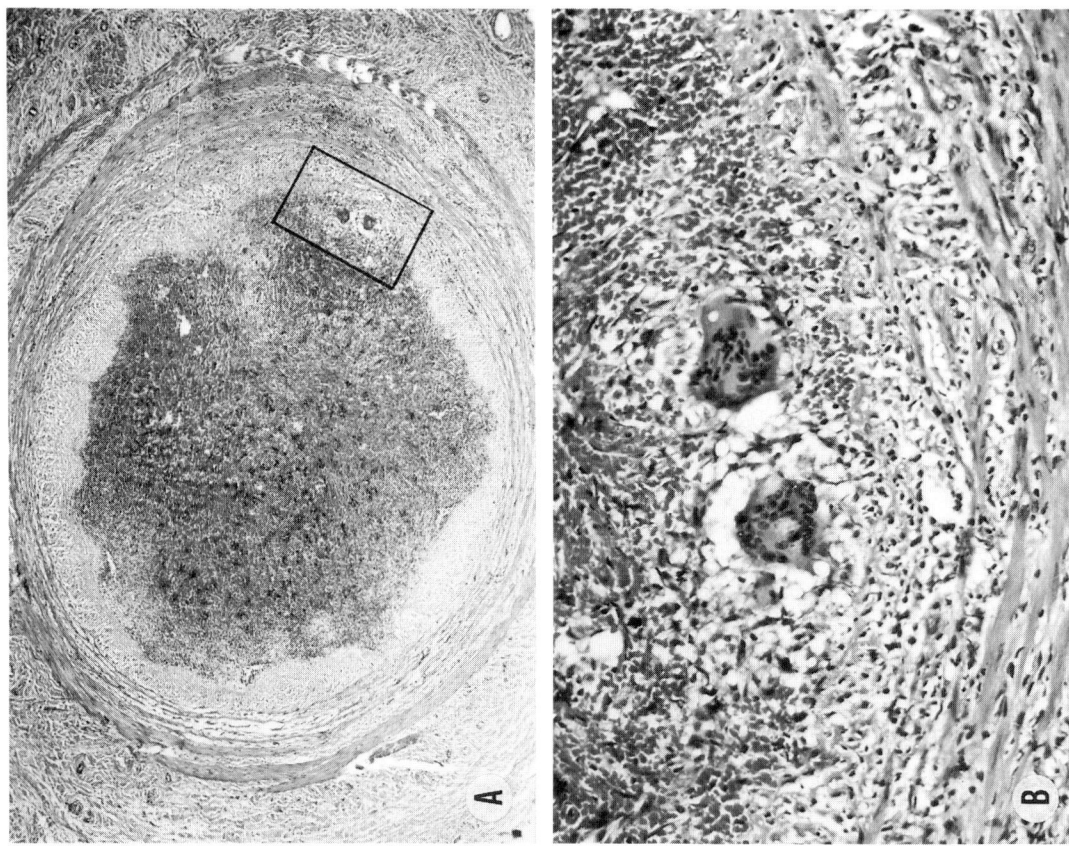

Figure 18.22 Vascular lesions of artery (A) and vein (B) in visceral and coronary thromboangiitis obliterans, histologically identical to those of the limbs, including microabscesses and giant cells (arrows) within the thrombus. (A ×64, B ×160.) (Reproduced with permission from Lie [2].)

Figure 18.23 (A) Coronary artery bypass saphenous vein graft with thromboangiitis obliterans. (B) Close-up view of the boxed area in (A) showing microabscess with giant cells within the acute occlusive thrombus. (H&E A ×64, B ×400.) (Reproduced with permission from Lie [2].)

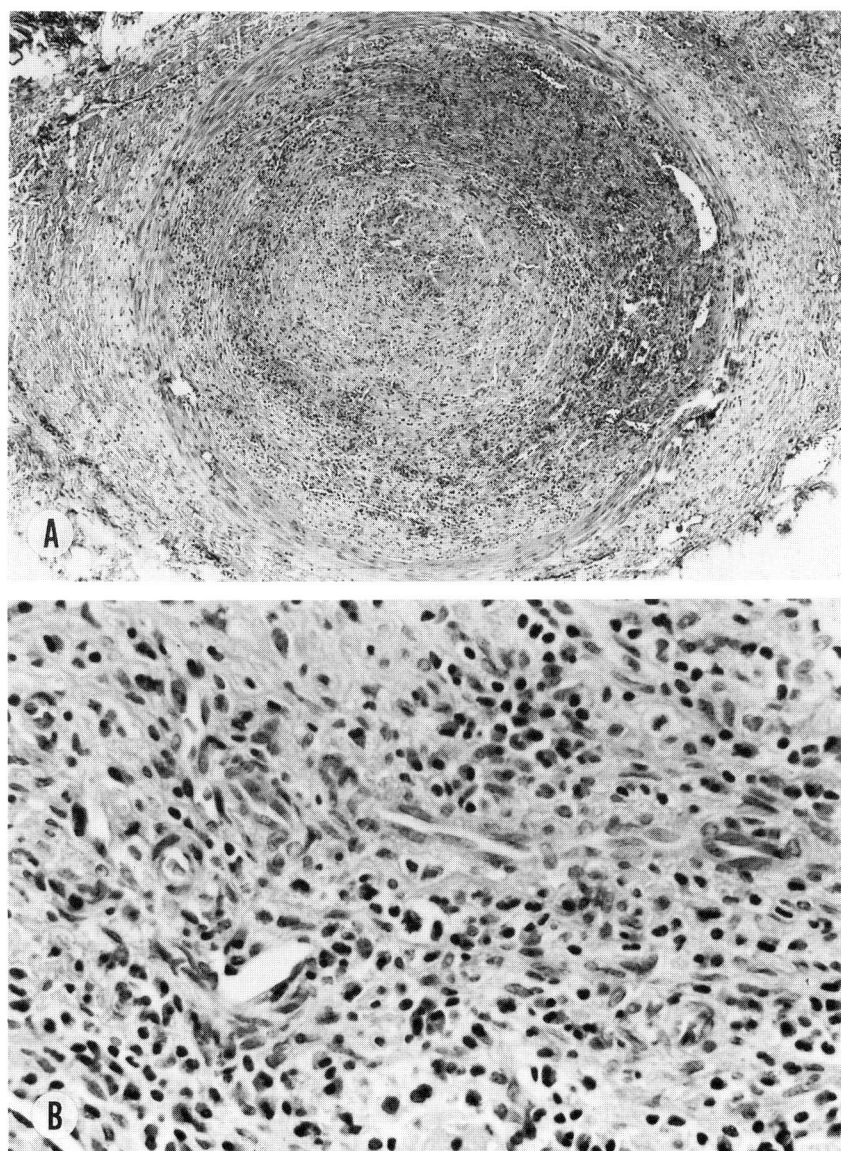

Figure 18.24 (A) Acute thromboangiitis of the temporal artery with intense inflammatory cell infiltrate. (B) Close-up view of the inflammatory infiltrate with prominent eosinophils. (H&E A ×64, B ×400.) (Reproduced with permission from Lie [2].)

sympathectomies, two bowel resections and 13 amputations, including bilateral above-elbow and above-knee amputations, before he succumbed at age 33 to another episode of bowel infarction from recurrent Buerger's disease of the mesenteric arteries and veins [50].

The histopathology of visceral thromboangiitis obliterans is identical to that observed in blood vessels of the limbs with involvement of both arteries and veins (Figure 18.22). Verging on being true pathological curiosities are a unique case of Buerger's disease in a saphenous vein arterial graft (Figure 18.23) [51] and the unusual examples of Buerger's disease in the temporal arteries of young smokers, with or without peripheral ischemia requiring amputations (Figure 18.24) [52].

Also not widely known is the occurrence of Buerger's disease in testicular and spermatic arteries and veins, as was originally described by Buerger [47] and in patients who are either ex-smokers or tobacco-chewers [53,54].

18.7 Conclusion

Buerger's disease (thromboangiitis obliterans) is a specific clinicopathological entity quite distinct from arteriosclerosis. The cause of thromboangiitis obliterans is unknown, but it is principally a disease of young male smokers. The disease is more prevalent in certain geographic areas than in others, and there is also a definite ethnic predisposition. At present, validation for the diagnosis of Buerger's disease is initiated clinically on the concordant gender, age and smoking habit of the patient, plus a constellation of characteristic signs and symptoms, radiological support with the unique features of the arteriography, and pathological confirmation where possible by the specificity of the acute phase lesions. A set of strict and well defined clinical diagnostic criteria is essential for any study of Buerger's disease to ensure the homogeneity of the selected patient population for valid comparisons.

References

1. Papa, M.Z. and Adar, R. (1992) A critical look at thromboangiitis obliterans (Buerger's disease). *Persp. Vasc. Surg.*, 5, 1–21.
2. Lie, J.T. (1988) Thromboangiitis obliterans (Buerger's disease) revisited, *Pathol. Annu.*, 23(2), 257–91.
3. Lie, J.T. (1989) The rise and fall and resurgence of thromboangiitis obliterans (Buerger's disease). *Acta. Pathol. Jap.*, 39, 153–8.
4. Lie, J.T., Mann, R.J. and Ludwig, J. (1979) The brothers von Winiwarter, Alexander (1848–1917) and Felix (1852–1931), and thromboangiitis obliterans. *Mayo Clin. Proc.*, 54, 802–7.
5. Winiwarter, F. (1879) Über eine eigenthümliche Form von Endarteriitis und Endophlebitis mit Gangrän des Fusses. *Arch. Klin. Chir.*, 23, 202–26.
6. Zoege-Manteuffel, W. (1891) Über angiosclerotische Gangrän. *Arch. Klin. Chir.*, 42, 569–74.
7. Buerger, L. (1908) Thrombo-angiitis obliterans: a study of the vascular lesions leading to presenile spontaneous gangrene. *Am. J. Med. Sci.*, 136, 567–80.
8. Eastcott, H.H.G. (1992) *Arterial Surgery*, 3rd edn, Churchill Livingstone, Edinburgh, pp. 153–73.
9. Wessler, S., Ming, S.C., Gurewich, V. et al. (1960) A critical evaluation of thromboangiitis obliterans. The case against Buerger's disease. *New Engl. J. Med.*, 262, 1149–62.
10. Editorial. (1960) Does Buerger's disease exist? *Lancet*, 2, 969–70.
11. Bollinger, A., Hollman, B., Schneider, E. et al. (1979) Thromboangiitis obliterans: Diagnose und Therapie im Licht neuer immunologischer Befunde. *Schweiz. Med. Wschr.*, 109, 537–43.
12. Adar, R., Papa, M.Z., Halpern, Z. et al. (1983) Cellular sensitivity to collagen in thromboangiitis obliterans. *New Engl. J. Med.*, 308, 1113–16.
13. Gulati, S.M., Madhra, K., Thusoo, T.K. et al. (1982) Autoantibodies in thromboangiitis obliterans. *Angiology*, 33, 642–50.
14. Roncon, A., Delgado, L., Correia, P. et al. (1989) Circulating immune complexes in Buerger's disease. *J. Cardiovasc. Surg.*, 30, 821–5.
15. Bruce, J.W., Miller, J.R. and Hooker, D.R. (1909) The effect of smoking upon blood pressure and upon the volume of the hand. *Am. J. Physiol.*, 24, 104–16.
16. Harkavy, J. (1933) Tobacco sensitiveness in thromboangiitis obliterans, migrating phlebitis and coronary artery disease. *Bull. N.Y. Acad. Med.*, 9, 318–28.
17. Astrup, P. (1964) An abnormality in the oxygen-dissociation curve of blood from patients with Buerger's disease and patients with non-specific myocarditis. *Lancet*, 2, 1152–4.
18. Mukaiyama, H., Matsumoto, T., Shionoya, S. et al. (1988) Effects of cigarette smoking on platelet MAO activity, coagulation-fibrinolysis, plasma levels of prostaglandins, catecholamines and serotonin, and circulating endothelial cell counts. *J. Jap. Coll. Angiol.*, 28, 331–8.
19. Ohtawa, T., Juji, T., Kawano, N. et al. (1974) HL-A antigen in thromboangiitis obliterans. *J. Am. Med. Ass.*, 230, 1128.
20. McLoughlin, G.A., Helsby, C.R., Evans, C.C. et al. (1976) Association of HLA-A9 and HLA-B5 with Buerger's disease. *Br. Med. J.*, 2, 1165–6.
21. *Annual Report of the Buerger's Disease Research Committee of the Ministry of Health and Welfare of Japan* (1976), (ed. K. Ishikawa), Tokyo, pp. 3–15, 86–97.
22. Fielding, J.E. and Phenow, K.J. (1988) Health effects of involuntary smoking. *New Engl. J. Med.*, 319, 1452–60.
23. Matsushita, M., Matsumoto, T., Shionoya, S. et al. (1991) Urinary cotinine measurement in patients with Buerger's disease – Effects of active and passive smoking on the disease process. *J. Vasc. Surg.*, 14, 53–8.
24. Sinzinger, H. and Kefalides, A. (1982) Passive smoking severely decreases platelet sensitivity to antiaggregatory prostaglandins. *Lancet*, 2, 392–3.
25. Davis, J.W., Shelton, L., Watanabe, I.S. et al. (1989) Passive smoking affects endothelium and platelets. *Arch. Intern. Med.*, 149, 386–9.
26. Herman, B.E. (1975) Buerger's syndrome. *Angiology*, 26, 713–16.
27. Lie, J.T. (1987) Thromboangiitis obliterans (Buerger's disease) in women. *Medicine*, 64, 65–72.
28. Cachovan, M. (1988) Epidemiologie und geographisches Verteilungsmuster der Thromboangiitis obliterans, in *Thromboangiitis obliterans Morbus Winiwarter–Buerger*, (ed. H. Heidrich), Georg Thieme, Stuttgart, New York, pp. 31–6.
29. Nigam, R., Narayanan, P.S., Sharma, S.R. et al. (1980) Thromboangiitis obliterans and arteriosclerosis obliterans as cause of limb ischemia in Delhi. *Ind. J. Surg.*, 42, 9–15.
30. Booshanam, V.M. (1989) Role of sympathectomy in Buerger's disease. Read at the 7th Congress of the Asian Surgical Association in Penang (personal communication).
31. Ludlow, A.I. (1931) Thromboangiitis: a review and report of the disease in Koreans. *China Med. J.*, 45, 487–514.
32. McKusick, V.A. and Harris, W.S. (1961) The Buerger syndrome in the Orient. *Bull. Johns Hopkins Hosp.*, 109, 241–91.
33. Hill, G.L., Moeliono, J., Tumewu, F. et al. (1973) The Buerger syndrome in Java: a description of the clinical syndrome and some aspects of its aetiology. *Br. J. Surg.*, 60, 606–13.
34. Noble, T.P. (1931) Thromboangiitis obliterans in Siam. *Lancet*, 220, 288–91.
35. Whyte, G.D. (1917) Thromboangiitis obliterans. *China Med. J.*, 31, 371–8.
36. Nishikimi, N., Shionoya, S., Mizuno, S. et al. (1987) Result of national epidemiological study of Buerger's disease. *J. Jap. Coll. Angiol.*, 27, 1125–30.
37. Mills, J.L., Taylor, L.M. and Porter, J.K. (1987) Buerger's disease in the modern era. *Am. J. Surg.*, 154, 123–54.
38. Pirnat, L., Simic, L.J. (1988) Epidemiologie und geographisches Verteilungsmuster der Endangiitis obliterans, in *Thromboangiitis obliterans Morbus Winiwarter–Buerger*, (ed. H. Heidrich), Georg Thieme, Stuttgart, New York, pp. 36–8.
39. Leu, H.J. (1985) Thrombangiitis obliterans Buerger. Pathologisch-anatomische Analyse von 53 Fällen. *Schweiz. Med. Wschr.*, 115, 1080–6.
40. Olin, J.W., Young, J.R., Graor, R.A. et al. (1990) The changing clinical spectrum of thromboangiitis obliterans (Buerger's disease). *Circulation*, 82 (suppl. IV), 3–8.
41. Shionoya, S. (1990) *Buerger's Disease. Pathology, Diagnosis and Treatment*, The University of Nagoya Press, Nagoya, pp. 261.
42. Dible, J.H. (1966) *The Pathology of the Limb Ischaemia*, Oliver & Boyd, Edinburgh, pp. 79–96.
43. Williams, G. (1969) Recent view on Buerger's disease. *J. Clin. Pathol.*, 22, 573–8.
44. Leu, H.J. (1975) Early inflammatory changes in thromboangiitis obliterans. *Path. Microbiol.*, 43, 151–6.
45. Leu, H.J. and Bollinger, A. (1978) Phlebitis saltans sive migrans, *Vasa*, 7, 440–2.
46. Leu, H.J. and Odermatt, B.F. (1989) Immunhistochemische Differenzierung proliferierender Intima- und Thromboszellen in Arterien und Venen bei Thromboangiitis Obliterans, in *Symposium d. Dtsch. Ges. f. Angiologie*, Frankfurt, June 23–24.
47. Buerger, L. (1924) *The Circulatory Disturbance of the Extremities: Including Gangrene, Vasomotor and Trophic Disorders*, W.B. Saunders, Philadelphia.
48. Deitch, E.A. and Sikkema, W.W. (1981) Intestinal manifestation of Buerger's disease. *Am. Surg.*, 47, 326–8.
49. Rosen, N., Sommer, I. and Knobel, B. (1985) Intestinal Buerger's disease. *Arch. Pathol. Lab. Med.*, 109, 962–3.
50. Cebezas-Moya, R. and Dragstedt III, L.R. (1970) An extreme example of Buerger's disease. *Arch. Surg.*, 101, 632–4.
51. Lie, J.T. (1987) Thromboangiitis obliterans (Buerger's disease) in a saphenous vein arterial graft. *Hum. Pathol.*, 18, 402–4.
52. Lie, J.T. and Michet Jr, C.J. (1988) Thromboangiitis obliterans with eosinophilia (Buerger's disease) of the temporal arteries. *Hum. Pathol.*, 19, 598–602.
53. Lie, J.T. (1987) Thromboangiitis obliterans (Buerger's disease) in an elderly man after cessation of cigarette smoking – a case report. *Angiology*, 38, 864–7.
54. Lie, J.T. (1988) Thromboangiitis obliterans (Buerger's disease) and smokeless tobacco. *Arthritis Rheum.*, 31, 812–13.

19 NON-ATHEROSCLEROTIC AND NON-VASCULITIC DISEASES OF CORONARY ARTERIES

Renu Virmani, Andrew Farb and Allen P. Burke

The most frequent cause of death in the western world today is atherosclerosis, especially when it involves the coronary arteries [1]. In order of frequency, atherosclerosis affects abdominal aorta, the coronary arteries, peripheral arteries and the cerebral arteries; however, its prime target for morbidity and mortality are the heart and brain [2–5]. Although 90% of all ischemic syndromes are caused by atherosclerosis, it is still useful to recognize a large number of non-atherosclerotic and non-vasculitic conditions, i.e. congenital and acquired diseases that may affect the vascular system:

- Metabolic and intimal proliferative diseases
  - Mucopolysaccharidosis
  - Hyperoxaluria
  - Homocystinuria
  - Fabry's disease
  - Pseudoxanthoma elasticum
  - Amyloidosis
  - Idiopathic arterial calcification of infancy
  - Thrombosis and intimal hyperplasia with contraceptive steroids or in the peripartum period
- Vascular malformations
  - Anomalous origin
  - Arteriovenous malformations
  - Hereditary hemorrhagic telangiectasia (Osler–Weber–Rendu disease)
  - Fibromuscular dysplasia
- Aneurysms
  - Congenital
    - Berry aneurysm
    - Sinus of Valsalva aneurysm
    - Fibromuscular dysplasia
    - Coronary aneurysm
  - Traumatic
    - True
    - False
    - Dissecting
  - Dissecting
    - Spontaneous
    - Secondary to hypertension
    - Marfan's syndrome
- Embolic diseases
  - Spontaneous
    - Infectious emboli (infective endocarditis)
    - Non-infectious (left atrium, marantic endocarditis, left ventricle, atheroemboli, disseminated intravascular coagulation, paradoxical, tumor, normal tissue, parasitic, fat and calcium)
  - Induced
    - Iatrogenic (atheromatous, calcium, silicon, teflon, plastic gelfoam, valve prosthesis, catheters, sutures, needles, air, vegetable fibers and talc)
    - Traumatic (air, fat, bone marrow and bullets)
- Trauma, penetrating and non-penetrating
  - Lacerations
  - Thrombosis
  - Dissection
  - Radiation, electrical and thermal trauma.

In this chapter, these non-atherosclerotic, non-vasculitic pathologic conditions will be described with special emphasis on disorders involving the coronary artery/myocardial vascular bed which are associated with the most frequent clinical manifestations:

- Coronary artery spasm
  - Prinzmetal's angina

- Cocaine-induced spasm
- Industrial nitroglycerin withdrawal
- Small vessel disease (Syndrome X)
- Myocardial oxygen supply–demand imbalance
  - Myocardial hypertrophy (aortic stenosis, aortic regurgitation, hypertrophic cardiomyopathy)
  - Prolonged hypotension
  - Carbon monoxide poisoning
  - Thyrotoxicosis
  - Pheochromocytoma
  - Massive injection of isoproterenol or epinephrine
- Coronary artery mural thickening secondary to metabolic and intimal proliferation disease
  - Mucopolysaccharidosis (Hurler's disease)
  - Pseudoxanthoma elasticum
  - Amyloidosis
  - Idiopathic arterial calcification of infancy
  - Fabry's disease
  - Thrombosis and intimal hyperplasia with contraceptive steroids
- Coronary artery anomalies
  - Coronary arteriovenous malformation
  - Coronary–cameral fistula
  - Anomalous origin of left coronary artery from pulmonary artery
  - Anomalous origin of coronary artery from aorta (left-from-right sinus of Valsalva or right-from-left sinus of Valsalva)
- Coronary embolism secondary to cardiomyopathies, mitral stenosis, left ventricular aneurysms, iatrogenic, marantic or infective endocarditis, from prosthetic valves, papillary fibroelastoma of aortic valve, myxoma
- Coronary thrombosis from thrombocythemia or coronary spasm with minimal atherosclerosis
- Coronary ostial occlusion
  - From catheters (especially after balloon angioplasty)
  - Intimal proliferation due to flow trauma
  - With aortic Starr–Edward's valve
  - With congenital aortic supravalvular stenosis
- Arterial dissections with coronary luminal compression
  - Aortic dissection with proximal extension
  - Isolated coronary artery dissection (spontaneous, iatrogenic from guide catheters, etc.)
  - Compression of coronary artery from sinus of Valsalva, aneurysm or tumor compression
- Traumatic injuries
  - Penetrating (puncture, laceration, complete transection, partial transection, aneurysm, arteriovenous fistula and dissection)
  - Non-penetrating injury (external compression or blast effect) (intimal contusion, intimal flap, intimal injury and thrombosis).

19.1 Pathophysiology of coronary circulation

The coronary vascular bed, consisting of the major left and right epicardial coronary arteries and intramyocardial coronary arteries, provides essential oxygen and metabolic needs of the myocardium. Normal myocardial function is dependent upon the balance between myocardial oxygen supply and demand. Myocardial oxygen supply is determined by coronary blood flow and oxygen carrying capacity, whereas oxygen demand is dependent upon heart rate, myocardial contractility and systolic wall tension. Coronary blood flow is influenced by the driving pressure across the coronary vascular bed and the resistance of the small vessels within the myocardium. The epicardial arteries are the conductance vessels which, under normal conditions, offer very little resistance to flow. As these vessels become intramyocardial, they give rise to small penetrating branches which arise approximately at right angles and are responsible for the large drop in intravascular pressure. These vessels have been designated as 'resistance vessels' and morphologically are the coronary arterioles (Figure 19.1). The arterioles control myocardial blood flow and therefore serve a regulatory function [6]. The normal myocardium is an extremely vascular organ, rich in capillaries (approximately 4000 capillaries/mm^2); however, capillaries are not uniformly patent.

The blood flow to the heart is determined by the aortic pressure and the resistance offered by the intramyocardial vessels. Coronary pressure is slightly below aortic pressure because of the Venturi effect. The coronary circulation is unique in that the resistance to blood flow is influenced by the phasic contraction (systole) and relaxation (diastole) of the myocardium. Because the intramyocardial vessels are compressed during systole, two-thirds of coronary blood flow occurs during diastole. There is an increased susceptibility of the subendocardium to ischemia compared to the subepicardium because of a greater reduction in systolic flow due to extravascular compressive forces. Under physiologic conditions, the ratio of endocardial to epicardial flow throughout the cardiac cycle is approximately 1.25:1 as a result of increased dilatation of the subendocardial vasculature which compensates for the increased wall stress and oxygen consumption in the subendocardium [7]. The vasodilatory reserve of the subendocardium is much less than in the subepicardium because of greater wall stress, greater resistance to flow and higher metabolic needs; these account for the ST-segment depression seen with decreased endocardial blood flow [8,9].

While epicardial coronary artery stenosis can reduce myocardial blood flow, the intramyocardial vascular bed has the capacity to reduce resistance to approxi-

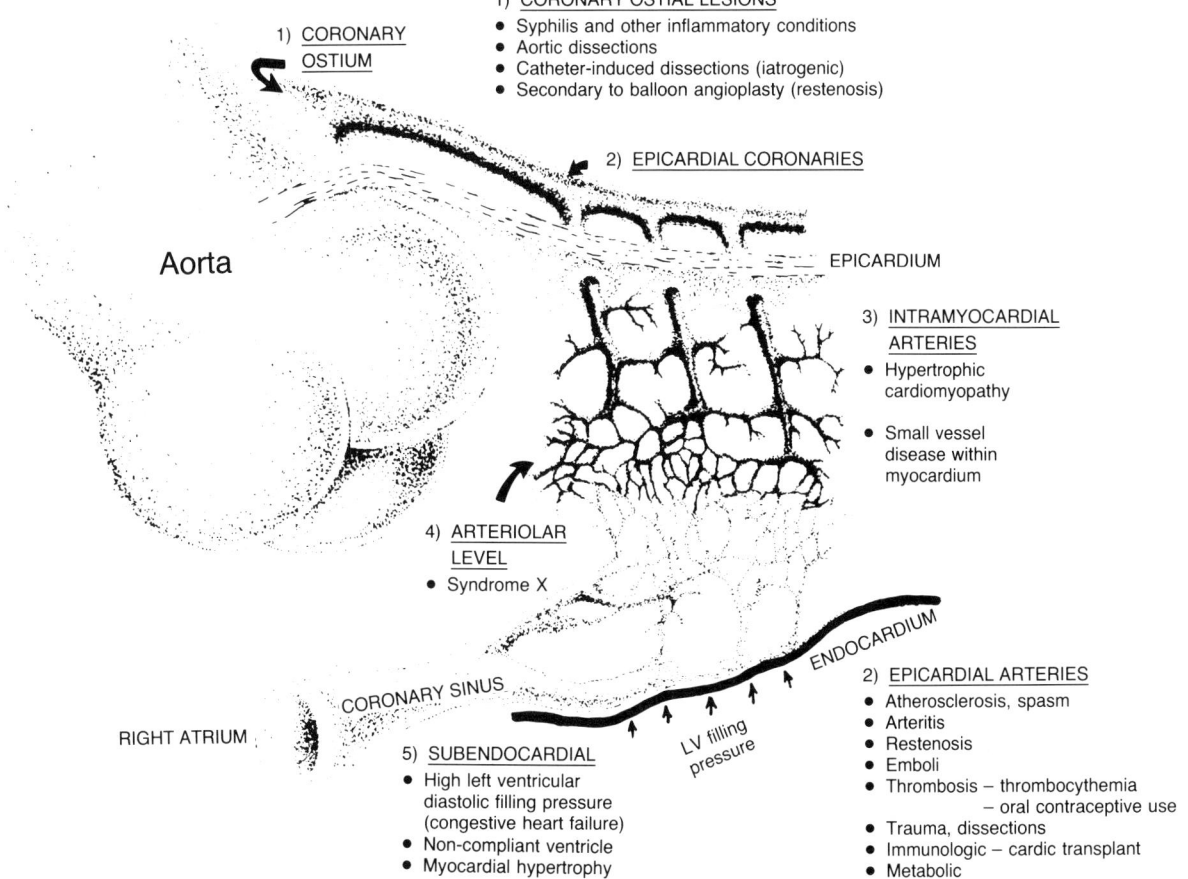

Figure 19.1 Pathologic conditions other than atherosclerosis that may affect the coronary arteries at various levels: coronary ostium, epicardial coronaries, intramural arteries, arteriolar level and at the subendocardium. (Redrawn with permission from Cheitlin [76].)

mately 15–20% of basal levels [10,11]. A greater than 80% cross-sectional luminal narrowing of an epicardial coronary artery is necessary to overcome the vasodilatory reserve of the intramyocardial coronary resistance vessels for ischemia to become manifest at basal conditions. With exercise, a 60% coronary narrowing begins to limit the ability of coronary blood flow to meet the metabolic demand [12].

Coronary blood flow is markedly affected by changes in vascular tone. These changes may be mediated by neural, metabolic, hormonal or chemical factors, as well as by local vasodilator and vasoconstrictor substances released by endothelium. The coronary arteries are richly innervated by the sympathetic and parasympathetic nervous system [13]. Alpha-adrenergic stimulation causes vasoconstriction via release of norepinephrine, and beta-adrenergic stimulation leads to vasodilatation of large and small coronary arteries [13–15]. Parasympathetic stimulation dilates small coronary arteries [16]. Adenosine, a metabolite of adenine nucleotides, is a powerful vasodilator [17] and is considered to be an important mediator of vasodilatation in response to reduced coronary flow. Considerable evidence exists linking imbalance in the oxygen supply-to-demand ratio with increased adenosine formation [18,19].

The endothelium has recently been appreciated to be an active paracrine organ producing potent vasoactive, anticoagulant, procoagulant and fibrinolytic substances [20]. In the human heart, there are approximately 10^{12} endothelial cells occupying an area greater than $1000\,m^2$ [10]. Therefore, significant abnormalities in the structure and function of endothelial cells in vascular diseases may greatly influence the vascular tone. Endothelium-derived relaxing factor (EDRF), described by Furchgott in 1983, is a powerful vasodilator of most blood vessels [21]. EDRF has now been characterized as nitric oxide and is derived from amino acid L-arginine [22,23]. Several important mediators of EDRF release have been categorized: acetylcholine, thrombin, bradykinin, thromboxane A_2, histamine and aggregating platelets [24,25]. Release of endogenous EDRF in the basal state maintains resting arterial tone [26]. In the presence of endothelial injury, many substances that cause vasodilatation with intact endothelium cause vasoconstriction and a consequent fall in myocardial blood flow [27]. This has been well documented in coronary angiographic studies in patients with atherosclerosis. Further, it has been shown that both hypertension and hypercholesterolemia impair release of EDRF [28]. Patients more than 30 years in age with angiographically normal arteries undergoing diagnostic catheterization may display a vasoconstrictor response to intracoronary acetylcholine, suggesting the presence of dysfunctional endothelium in association with mild atherosclerosis [29].

Platelets release powerful vasoconstrictors like thromboxane A_2 which may cause endothelial injury and a decrease in production of the vasodilator prostacycline leading to a further increase in vascular tone. Platelet activation can occur in both non-atherosclerotic and non-obstructed atherosclerotic coronary arteries in which the endothelium has been damaged. The response to thrombus formation is vasoconstriction, platelet aggregation and further reduction in myocardial blood flow [27]. The release of the endothelium-derived peptide, endothelin, causes a prolonged, potent vasoconstriction of coronary arteries and, therefore, may also be an important modulator of coronary tone.

19.2 Disease categories and their consequences

A complete description of all non-atherosclerotic, non-vasculitic disease processes that affect the vascular system is beyond the scope of this chapter. Rather, a short discussion of the important entities, differential diagnosis and pathogenesis will be presented.

19.2.1 VARIANT ANGINA PECTORIS (PRINZMETAL'S ANGINA)

In 1959, Prinzmetal and colleagues described an unusual syndrome of chest pain at rest, unrelated to previous exertion or emotional stress, associated with electrocardiographic ST-segment elevation [30]. It has now been confirmed that variant angina is due to vasospasm. Vasospasm most often occurs at a site of adjacent atherosclerotic plaque. The vasospasm is characterized by a transient, sudden marked reduction in the lumen of the epicardial coronary artery which occurs in the absence of increase in myocardial oxygen demand (i.e. unrelated to an increase in heart rate or blood pressure). It has been shown that these atherosclerotic segments are hypercontractile, possibly due to endothelial dysfunction, in response to a variety of agents, including acetylcholine, leukotrienes, serotonin and other circulating vasoconstrictors [31,32]. At the site of vasoconstriction, there is fibrin deposition. Further fibrinopeptide A, a breakdown product of fibrinogen, is elevated in the plasma indicating ongoing thrombotic activity [33]. There is a circadian variation (with peak frequency early morning and low frequency in the afternoon), and heparin suppresses both the circadian variation and fibrinopeptide A release in variant angina but not in stable angina [34]. Additionally, an increase in the number of adventitial mast cells of vasospastic arteries, in the absence of severe coronary atherosclerosis, has been demonstrated [35]. Several studies have suggested that magnesium ions may play a role in variant angina. Magnesium sulphate has been shown to alleviate or prevent cold-pressor-induced chest pain in patients with variant angina [36].

19.2.2 DRUG ABUSE

Cocaine abusers may have myocardial ischemic syndromes secondary to coronary thrombosis in the presence or absence of underlying coronary artery atherosclerosis (Figure 19.2) [37]. The underlying mechanisms are poorly understood. Cocaine inhibits the re-uptake of norepinephrine by the sympathetic nerve terminals, thereby potentiating the effects of endogenous catecholamines [38]. Like those with variant angina, subjects with cocaine-associated coronary thrombosis have a greater number of adventitial mast cells with and without underlying severe atherosclerosis compared to subjects with non-cocaine-induced coronary thrombosis or cocaine overdose [37]. These findings suggest that adventitial mast cells may play an important role in the pathogenesis of atherosclerosis, vasospasm, thrombosis and myocardial ischemia in long-term cocaine abusers.

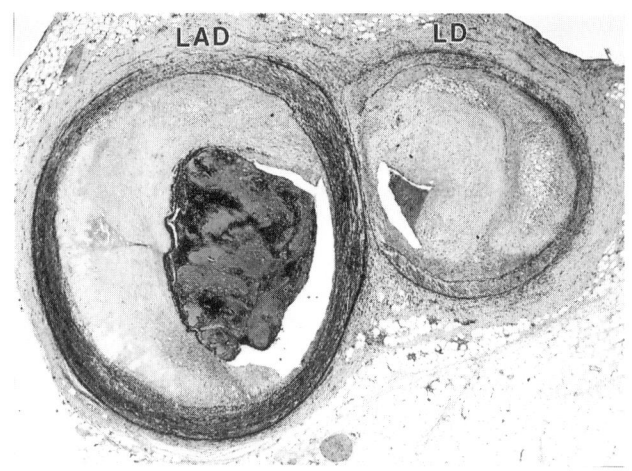

Figure 19.2 A 36-year-old black male with history of recent intranasal abuse of cocaine presented with chest pain. At autopsy, normal heart weight and thrombotic occlusion of left anterior descending (LAD) and left diagonal (LD) arteries were seen with underlying atherosclerotic luminal narrowing of 60% and 95% in cross-sectional area, respectively.

19.2.3 INDUSTRIAL NITROGLYCERIN WITHDRAWAL

Since the First World War, it has been recognized that ammunition workers are exposed to substantial levels of aerosolized nitrates which can be absorbed via the lungs and skin. Workers may demonstrate an acute illness manifested by headache, hypotension, palpitations and gastrointestinal disturbance. Over time, tolerance to these effects usually develops. However, withdrawal from chronic nitroglycerin exposure may result in angina unrelated to exertion or emotion. Acute myocardial infarction and spontaneous coronary spasm have been documented during a period of withdrawal [39,40].

19.2.4 CHEST PAIN WITH A NORMAL CORONARY ARTERIOGRAM (SYNDROME X)

The syndrome of angina or angina-like chest pain with angiographically normal coronary arteries in the absence of large vessel spasm is often referred to as Syndrome X [41]. These patients typically constitute as many as 10–20% of patients undergoing coronary arteriography because of chest pain suspicious of angina [42]. Ergonovine challenge fails to illicit vasospasm, and there is impairment of the ability to reduce coronary resistance and increase coronary blood flow in response to atrial pacing [43]. The inability to increase coronary blood flow with exercise may be associated with wall motion abnormalities and perfusion defects on thallium tomography [44]. Of the patients with atypical chest pain and normal coronary arteries, a substantial number have a positive exercise test [45]. Some may exhibit lactate production and ST-segment depression during exercise [46]. The prognosis is excellent: there is 96% survival at 7 years in patients with at least 50% ejection fraction [47]. The etiology of Syndrome X is unknown. Maseri and colleagues have proposed that there is focal pre-arteriolar constriction as a result of impaired EDRF flow-mediated vasodilatation [48].

19.2.5 MYOCARDIAL OXYGEN SUPPLY–DEMAND IMBALANCE

(a) Increased oxygen demand

Myocardial oxygen supply–demand imbalance most commonly arises from any condition that causes excessive pressure or volume overload resulting in increased wall stress of the involved ventricle. Myocardial hypertrophy is a compensatory process that results in normalization of wall stress [49,50]. However, myocardial hypertrophy may be associated with a decrease in coronary vasodilatory reserve and capillary density may be altered within the myocardium [51]. Not all stimuli of cardiac hypertrophy lead to adverse changes in the coronary vasculature [50]. Many factors may influence the adaptation of the coronary vasculature to cardiac hypertrophy, and these include the stimulus that provokes the hypertrophy (pressure and/or volume overload), the age of the patient, stabilization of the hypertrophy and normalization of wall stress, duration of hypertrophy and ventricle involved [52–57]. Myocardial oxygen consumption is elevated in the setting of a hypertrophied left ventricle, increased systolic pressure and prolongation of ventricular ejection [58]. Increased pressure on intramural coronary arteries may exceed the coronary perfusion pressure thereby decreasing coronary blood flow [59,60]. The left-ventricular end-diastolic pressure is also elevated which lowers the aortic left-ventricular gradient in diastole, resulting in decreased myocardial perfusion, subendocardial ischemia and angina [59–61]. Increased myocardial lactate production can also be demonstrated with exercise or with isoproterenol infusion in patients without epicardial coronary narrowing [62].

The conditions giving rise to marked left-ventricular hypertrophy include aortic stenosis and/or regurgitation, hypertrophic cardiomyopathy and chronic uncontrolled systemic hypertension. Aortic stenosis may be at the valvular, supravalvular and subvalvular levels. In hypertrophic cardiomyopathy, myocardial ischemia is common and multifactorial [62,63]. Possible etiologies include impaired vasodilatory reserve secondary to thickening and narrowing of intramyocardial coronary arteries and increased oxygen demand, especially in patients with outflow gradients [64]. Similarly, approximately 25–50% of patients with left-ventricular hypertrophy from dilated cardiomyopathy or congestive heart failure can develop chest pain. The chest pain may be due to simultaneous occurrence of coronary atherosclerosis or reduction in the vasodilatory reserve of the coronary microvasculature [65–67]. In all of these conditions, there is increased myocardial oxygen demand due to high left-ventricular systolic pressure and increased left-ventricular mass.

Thyrotoxicosis results in increase in total body oxygen demand, as well as myocardial oxygen consumption (MVO_2). The usual cardiovascular manifestations include palpitations, dyspnea, tachycardia and systolic hypertension; congestive heart failure, angina pectoris and myocardial infarction have also been reported [68–71]. In most cases, the clinical appearance of heart failure and myocardial ischemia associated with thyrotoxicosis signifies underlying myocardial or coronary vascular disease. Some cases are primarily due to severe hyperthyroidism with increased myocardial oxygen demand in otherwise structurally normal heart [71]. Experimental and clinical studies provide evidence that thyrotoxicosis can precipitate myocardial ischemia and/or congestive heart failure: congestive heart failure can be produced in animals by administering thyroxine;

children with thyrotoxicosis develop congestive heart failure without underlying cardiac disease, and angina and myocardial infarction have been reported in patients with normal coronary arteries [69–72].

Finally, while the major cardiovascular manifestation of pheochromocytoma is hypertension, myocardial ischemia, myocarditis, catecholamine cardiomyopathy and even myocardial infarction have been reported [71,73–77].

(b) **Reduced oxygen supply**

Hypotension of any etiology which persists will cause a marked decrease in myocardial blood flow. This results in an increase in sympathetic tone and increased catecholamine release which further increases the metabolic demand and worsens myocardial supply–demand imbalance. When the oxygen delivery is insufficient to maintain normal aerobic metabolism, circumferential subendocardial ischemia and infarction may occur [78–80].

In carbon monoxide poisoning there is higher affinity of carbon monoxide for hemoglobin than for oxygen leading to reduced oxygen delivery to the tissues. The central nervous system findings usually dominate the clinical presentation but fatal cardiac abnormalities may occur from either myocardial hypoxia or a direct toxic effect of the gas on myocardial mitochondria [81–83]. Additionally, carbon monoxide, through its influence on platelets and permeability of vessel wall, may precipitate coronary spasm and thrombosis [84].

19.2.6 CORONARY ARTERY MURAL THICKENING SECONDARY TO METABOLIC AND INTIMAL PROLIFERATIVE DISEASES

Metabolic diseases that can lead to severe luminal narrowing include mucopolysaccharidosis, pseudoxanthoma elasticum, amyloidosis, idiopathic infantile arterial calcification, Fabry's disease and intimal hyperplasia with contraceptive steroid use.

Mucopolysaccharidosis is characterized by deficiencies of lysosomal enzymes involved in the degradation of acid mucopolysaccharides [86]. Hurler's syndrome, a type of mucopolysaccharidosis Type I, is the cause of the most severe coronary narrowing seen in children and is due to the accumulation in the intima of vacuolated smooth muscle cells (gargoyle cells) filled with acid mucopolysaccharide [87–90]. The arterial narrowing is circumferential (Figure 19.3). Patients usually die during the first or second decade of life. Clinical and electrocardiographic evidence of ischemia is rare. Other involved arteries include the aorta and pulmonary artery [86].

Pseudoxanthoma elasticum is a genetically heterogenous disorder of unknown cause [91]. Histologically, it is a disorder of elastic tissue which shows fragmentation and calcification [92]. The skin (yellowish papules), the eye (retinal angioid streaks), gastrointestinal (hemorrhage) and the cardiovascular systems are most severely affected. Coronary artery disease is characterized by elastic fiber thickening and calcification with superimposed atherosclerosis and luminal narrowing (Figure

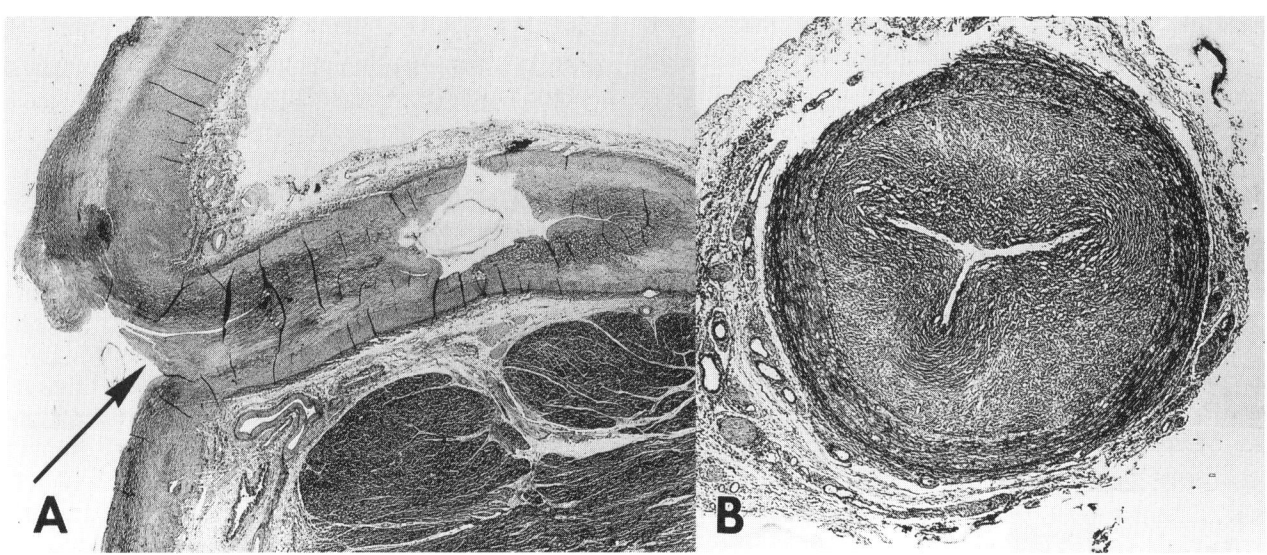

Figure 19.3 (A) Section through the left main coronary artery at the ostium (arrow) of a patient with Hurler's disease. Notice intimal hyperplasia obliterating the lumen. (B) Cross-section of left anterior descending coronary artery showing intimal hyperplasia secondary to mucopolysaccharide infiltration of smooth muscle cells as well as increase in collagen deposition. (Reproduced with permission from Cheitlin [77].)

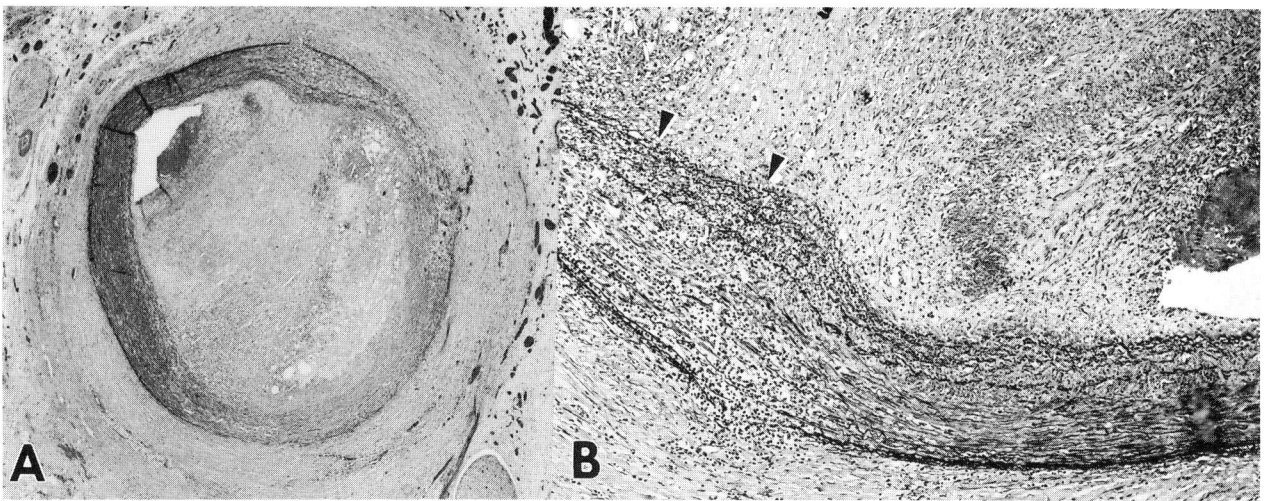

Figure 19.4 Microscopic section of the left anterior descending epicardial coronary artery from 23-year-old woman with pseudoxanthoma elasticum. (A) Note marked intimal proliferation and premature atherosclerosis almost obliterating the lumen and a superimposed thrombus. (B) The internal elastic lamina (arrowheads) is fragmented and partially destroyed. (Movat stain.) (Reproduced with permission from Cheitlin [76].)

19.4) [91–94]. The radial and ulnar arteries may be involved resulting in absence of pulses [91].

Amyloidosis is characterized by the extracellular deposition of fibrillar proteins within a β-pleated sheet formation which involves different pathogenic mechanisms associated with a variety of underlying etiologies [95]. Characteristically, amyloid deposits cause compression of adjacent cells and tissues causing atrophy and mechanical rigidity. Deposits occur in the intramyocardial muscular arteries and arterioles involving all layers of the vessel and can lead to vascular compromise of the lumen and a reduction in blood supply [94–97] (Figure 19.5). Amyloid deposits have been described in vessels of most organs, the aorta, epicardial coronary arteries, veins and capillaries [98].

Idiopathic infantile arterial calcification (juvenile arterial sclerosis, occlusive infantile arteriopathy) is a rare and fatal disease of muscular arteries of unknown etiology characterized by fragmentation and diffuse calcification of the internal elastic lamina accompanied by intimal proliferation with severe luminal narrowing (Figure 19.6) [99–103]. The frequency of involvement of arteries is as follows: coronary 90%; renal, pancreatic and splenic 50%; aorta, thyroidal and thymic arteries 36%; carotid and extremities 29% [99]. Death usually occurs at a mean age of 6 months, mostly from cardiac involvement.

Fabry's disease is caused by a deficiency of α-galactosidase A (ceramide trihexosidase) and is inherited as an X-linked recessive [104]. The diagnosis is usually not made until adulthood by which time organ damage has already occurred [105–108]. There is deposition of ceramide trihexosidase in lysosomes in endothelial cells, smooth muscle cells and pericytes

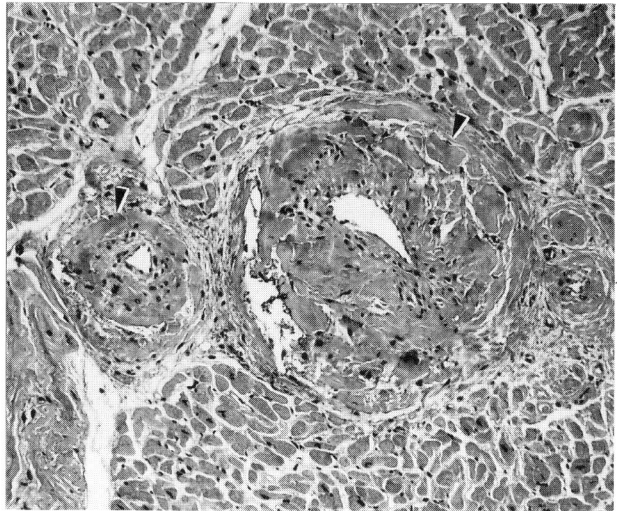

Figure 19.5 Microscopic section showing markedly thickened intramural coronary arteries (arrowheads) in a 41-year-old man who died suddenly during induction of anesthesia. Thickening is secondary to infiltration of the wall with a hyaline substance which had apple-green birefringence with Congo red stain characteristic of amyloid protein. (H&E.) (Reproduced with permission from Cheitlin [76].)

of the vascular system, especially within the coronary arteries (Figure 19.7), renal glomerular and tubular cells, cardiac myocytes, myocardial conduction fibers and cardiac valvular fibroblasts [108]. Under light microscopy, the deposits of ceramide trihexosidase appear as vacuoles; they are sudanophilic and PAS positive and strongly birefringent [107]. By electron microscopy, the deposits are intralysosomal irregular aggregates of concentric or parallel lamellae of alter-

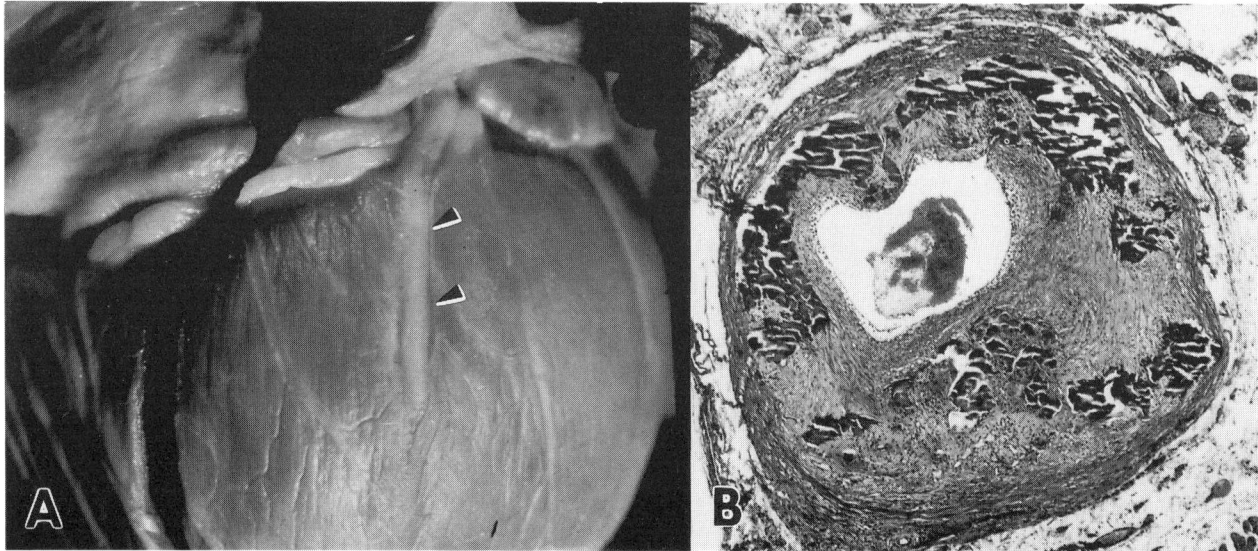

Figure 19.6 (A) External surface of the heart of an infant with juvenile intimal sclerosis (JIS). Notice enlarged, prominent and thickened obtuse marginal coronary artery (arrowheads). (B) Left anterior descending coronary artery from a patient with JIS; note marked calcification (black areas) at the level of internal elastic lamina and within the intima with marked narrowing of the lumen by fibrointimal proliferation characteristic of juvenile intimal sclerosis. (H&E.)

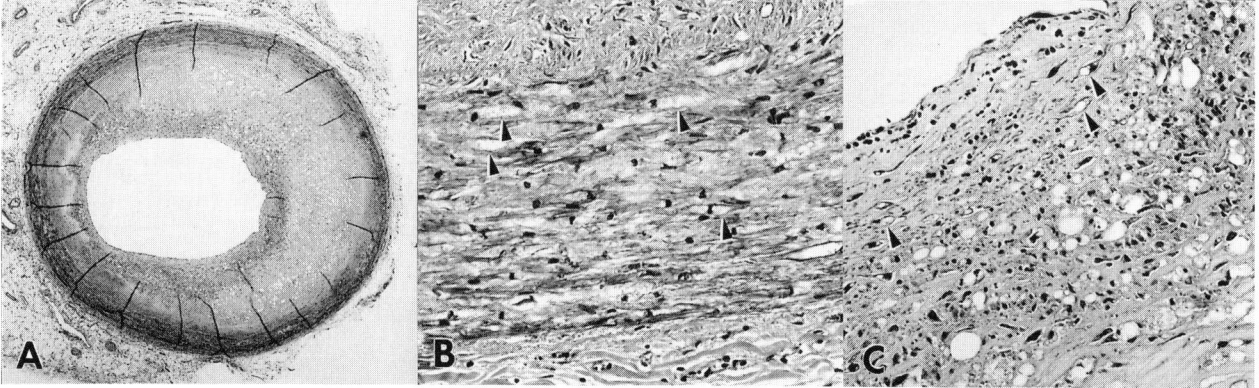

Figure 19.7 (A) Photomicrographs of a histologic section of the left anterior descending coronary artery from a 64-year-old man with Fabry's disease with 70% cross-sectional area luminal narrowing. (B) High power of the media showing vacuolization of smooth muscle cells (arrowheads). C. Vacolated smooth muscle cells are also present in the intima (arrowheads). (H&E.)

nating light and dark bands spaced 4–5.5 nm apart [107]. Clinical manifestations include angiokeratomas, congestive heart failure (cardiomyopathy, dilated or hypertrophic), angina, dysrrhythmias and hypertension [105].

Thrombosis and **intimal hyperplasia** has been linked to oral contraceptive steroid use (Figure 19.8). Oral contraceptives increase the risk of overt and subclinical thromboembolic injury and/or thrombosis [109]. The estrogen component of the oral contraceptive decreases antithrombin III activity, and this effect is exacerbated in women with an impaired fibrinolytic response to intravascular clot formation. Oral contraceptive use is associated with an increased risk of myocardial infarction, and thrombotic and hemorrhagic stroke. The risk of untoward effects is further augmented by other cardiovascular risk factors especially smoking, hypertension and hypercholesterolemia. The incidence of myocardial infarction among non-smoking women aged 30–39 years and 40–44 years on oral contraceptives is similar in both groups averaging 3 to 4 per 100 000 per year. However, when one combines smoking and oral contraceptive use, the incidence of myocardial infarction increases to 185 per 100 000 per year [111–112]. The increased risk of coronary thrombosis may occur through a variety of mechanisms. Oral contraceptives accelerate platelet aggregation and increase platelet prothrombin-converting (factor III) activity [109]. Oral

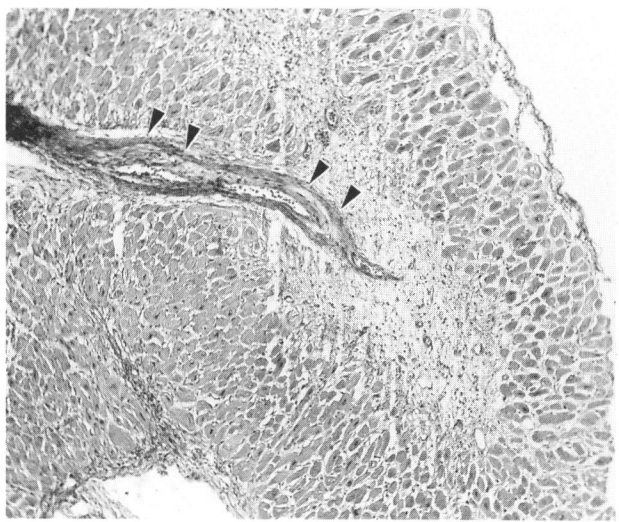

Figure 19.8 Microscopic section of the myocardium from an 18-year-old postpartum woman, showing an intramural coronary artery cut longitudinally (arrowheads) with intimal hyperplasia. Surroundng this vessel there is evidence of myocyte drop out and collapse with early fibrosis consistent with myocardial ischemic injury. (Movat stain.) (Reproduced with permission from Cheitlin [77].)

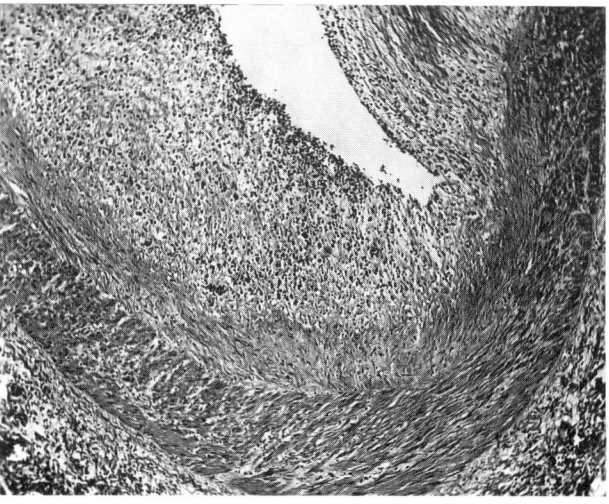

Figure 19.9 Microscopic cross-section of an epicardial coronary artery from a patient who died with myocardial infarction. Note intimal thickening with round-cell inflammatory infiltrate, especially in the intima, consistent with a non-specific coronary arteritis. (H&E.) (Reproduced with permission from Cheitlin [77].)

contraceptives also increase blood pressure and decrease glucose tolerance [112–113]. The increased thrombotic risk is attributable to both the estrogen and progestogen components of oral contraceptives. However, since the 1970s the use of 'very low dose' oral contraceptives has resulted in a decrease in the overall risk of cardiovascular disease.

Most of the collagen vascular diseases cause specific vasculitic pathologic changes in the vessel wall, especially polyarteritis nodosa and rheumatoid arthritis; however, there is evidence that non-specific arteritis, possibly of viral etiology can cause luminal narrowing and myocardial ischemia (Figure 19.9). Similarly, accelerated coronary artery disease is a major cause of morbidity and mortality among cardiac transplant recipients [117]. At Stanford University, 23% of deaths in patients who live more than 1 year after transplantation are due to coronary artery disease [117]. There is accelerated intimal proliferation in epicardial arteries consisting of smooth muscle cells, collagen, foam cells and inflammatory cells causing concentric luminal narrowing (Figure 19.10). It has been postulated that transplant atherosclerosis occurs as a consequence of repeated immunologic damage [118–120].

19.2.7 CORONARY ARTERY ANOMALIES

Coronary artery anomalies are found in approximately 1% of all patients undergoing angiography and in approximately 0.3% of patients undergoing autopsy [114–116]. Five major classifications of coronary artery anomalies have been used:

1. anomalous origin or one or more coronary arteries from pulmonary trunk;
2. anomalous origin of one or more coronary arteries from aorta;
3. single coronary artery ostium;
4. hypoplastic coronary arteries;
5. coronary artery fistula.

When angina or myocardial infarction is seen in a young individual, the presence of congenital coronary artery anomaly should be considered.

When the left main coronary artery arises from the pulmonary trunk, there is decreased perfusion of the left ventricle in the postnatal period as the pulmonary artery pressure falls. Poor myocardial blood flow results in poor cardiac output, an elevation in left atrial pressure and pulmonary hypertension. During this period coronary collateral circulation may develop between the right and left coronary arteries [99]. The extent of the collateral circulation will determine the severity of myocardial ischemic injury. Typically myocardial infarction involves the anterolateral papillary muscle and is associated with subsequent endocardial fibroelastosis [121]. Most patients suffer myocardial infarction and congestive heart failure within one to two months of birth, with death occurring within the first two years of life.

Anomalous origin of coronary arteries from the aorta was previously considered to be of no functional significance. However, Cheitlin and colleagues in 1974 reported the occurrence of sudden death and myocardial

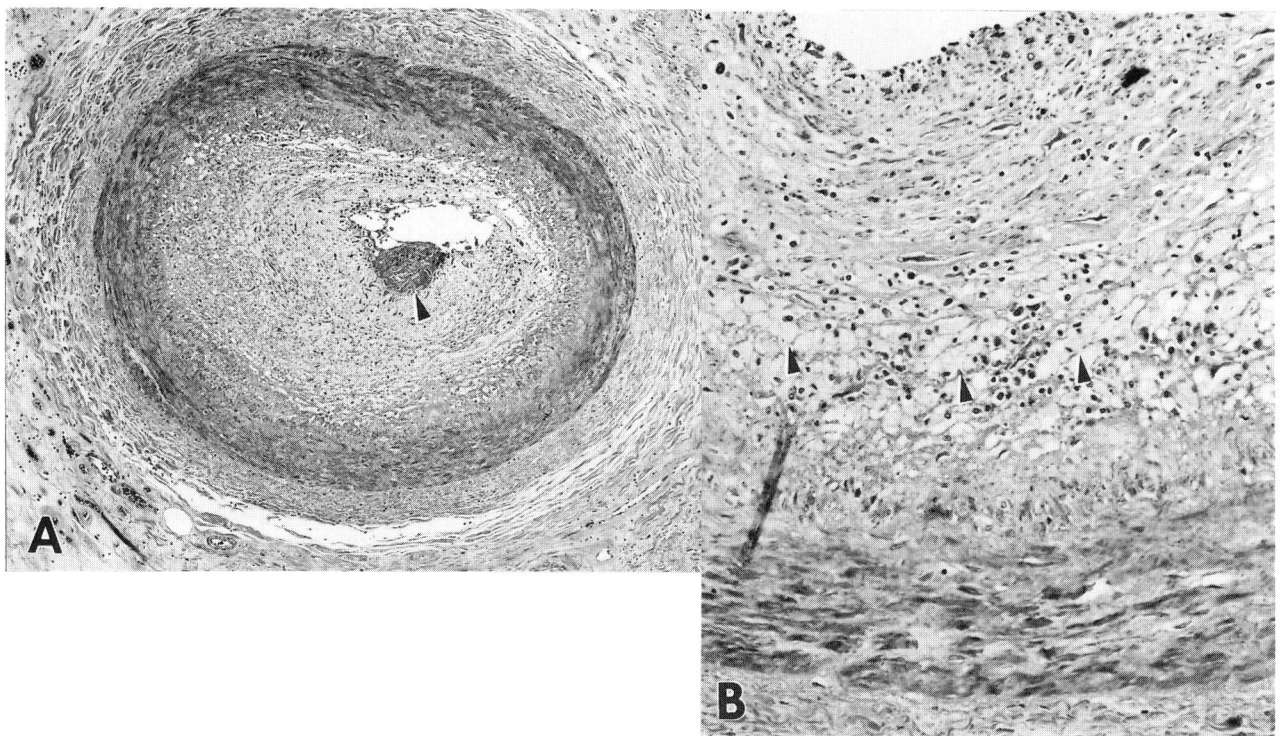

Figure 19.10 (A) Epicardial coronary artery from a 19-year-old man who died suddenly 2 years after cardiac transplant. There is marked luminal compromise by fibrointimal proliferation and superimposed thrombosis (arrowhead). (B) High power view of the wall of epicardial artery showing foam cells (arrowheads) and chronic lymphocytic infiltration. (H&E.) (Reproduced from Virmani *et al.* [155].)

ischemia in patients with origin of left coronary artery from the right sinus of Valsalva (Figure 19.11) [122]. Sudden death typically occurs in individuals in the second decade of life usually during exercise (57%). It has also been reported in individuals with the right coronary artery arising from the left coronary but the incidence is much less (25%) than when the left arises from the right sinus [123]. Other coronary anomalies – left circumflex or left anterior descending and right coronary arteries from the right aortic sinus, left main or right coronary artery from posterior aortic sinus, single coronary ostium, hypoplastic coronary arteries, and coronary artery fistula (Figure 19.12) – are rare causes of death in comparison with left main or right coronary artery arising from the opposite sinus [123].

Myocardial bridging of the left anterior descending coronary artery is a common variant of the normal course of coronary arteries and is seen in 30% of autopsy cases and 1% of coronary angiograms [124]. Recently Morales and colleagues [125] have shown that the depth of the myocardial muscle bridge (tunnelled coronary artery) is associated with myocardial fibrosis. The length and depth of the tunnel may determine whether patients are symptomatic or asymptomatic. Cases of sudden death associated with a tunnelled left anterior descending have been reported (Figure 19.13) [126].

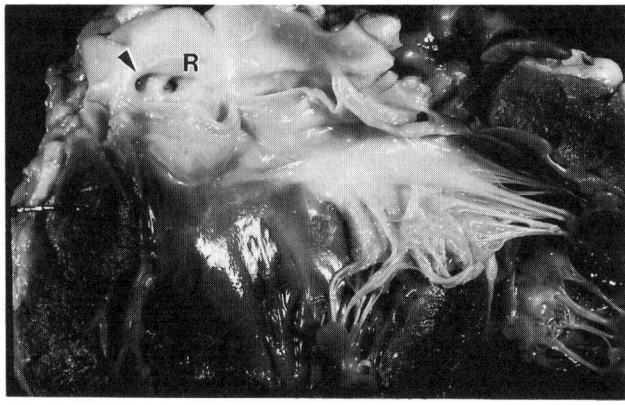

Figure 19.11 Heart of a 14-year-old boy who died suddenly while playing soccer. The only abnormality was the right (R) and left coronary arteries (arrowhead) which arose from the right sinus of Valsalva. The left coursed between the aorta and the pulmonary trunk before dividing into left anterior descending and left circumflex coronary arteries.

19.2.8 ARTERIOVENOUS MALFORMATIONS

Arteriovenous malformations (AVMs) are abnormal communications between arteries and veins without an intervening capillary bed. Both congenital and acquired AVM are described; the acquired are usually traumatic in origin, while the congenital are present at birth but become apparent soon after birth or occasionally are asymptomatic until adulthood [127]. AVMs may be present anywhere in the body. Approximately 50% are located in the head and neck and other locations include central nervous system, extremities, lung, heart, liver and kidney. Because blood flows preferentially from artery to vein, where the resistance is lower than the surrounding systemic capillary bed, the cardiac output and blood volume may increase as compensatory mechanisms. AVMs may be small or large and the pulmonary AVMs are often associated with Osler–Weber–Rendu disease. In large AVMs of the lung, cyanosis may be present at birth or develop in childhood. If not resected surgically, complications are frequent and significant [127].

19.2.9 FIBROMUSCULAR DYSPLASIA

Fibromuscular dysplasia is a term used to describe a group of structural abnormalities of one or more layers of medium size and large arteries that result in luminal narrowing by fibromuscular tissue with or without associated aneurysms and dissections of the media. The disease is considered a congenital malformation of the arterial structure. It most often affects young Caucasian women and most commonly involves the renal and carotid arteries [128]. There are three main histologic types: intimal fibroplasia, medial fibromuscular dysplasia and periadventitial fibroplasia. The most common is **medial fibromuscular dysplasia** which accounts for 70–95% of all fibromuscular dysplasia (Figure 19.14A). Angiographically, fibromuscular dysplasia appears as a 'string of beads' with stenosis alternating with aneurysms due to fibrous and smooth muscle cell ridges alternating with marked thinning of the vascular wall which is replaced by fibrous tissue. Medial fibromuscular dysplasia affects the distal two-thirds of the renal artery, the carotid, mesenteric, hepatic, iliac and coronary arteries [129].

Intimal fibroplasia comprises 1–5% of all cases and occurs in all age groups, but is most frequent in women of childbearing age. Angiographically, a corkscrew or irregular, long tubular luminal stenosis is seen. Histologically, there is circumferential intimal proliferation by fibrous tissue and smooth muscle cells in the absence of lipid deposition or inflammation (Figure 19.14B). Renal arteries are most often affected but carotid, vertebral and splanchnic arteries may also be involved [129].

Adventitial fibroplasia is extremely rare and consists of dense collagenous replacement of the loose fibrous tissue of the arterial adventitia which extends into the surrounding adipose tissue.

19.2.10 CORONARY EMBOLISM

Coronary thrombosis with underlying severe atherosclerosis (>75% cross-sectional area luminal nar-

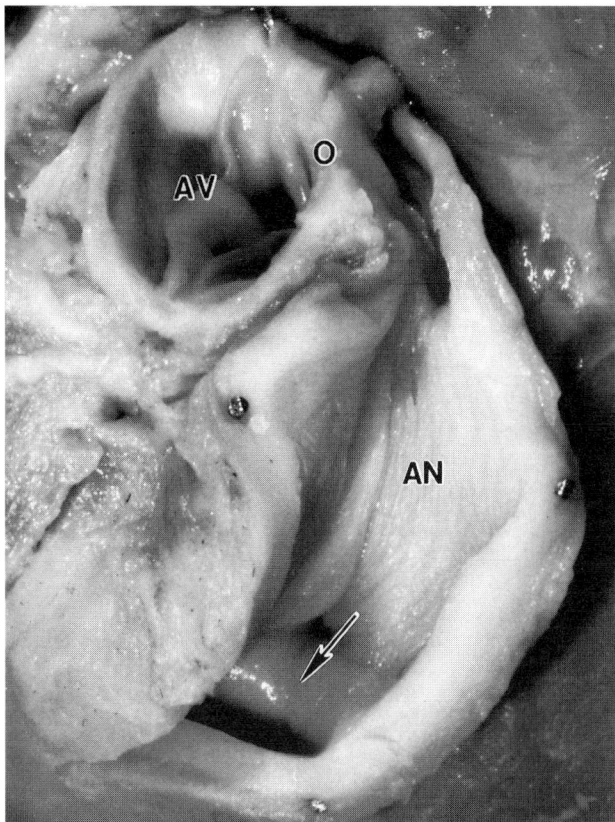

Figure 19.12 Coronary artery fistula from left coronary artery to the right ventricle (arrow) in a 12-day-old infant. The coronary artery wall is aneurysmally dilated and thickened. AN = aneurysm; AV = aortic valve; O = ostium of the left coronary artery. (Reproduced with permission from Robinowitz et al. [156].)

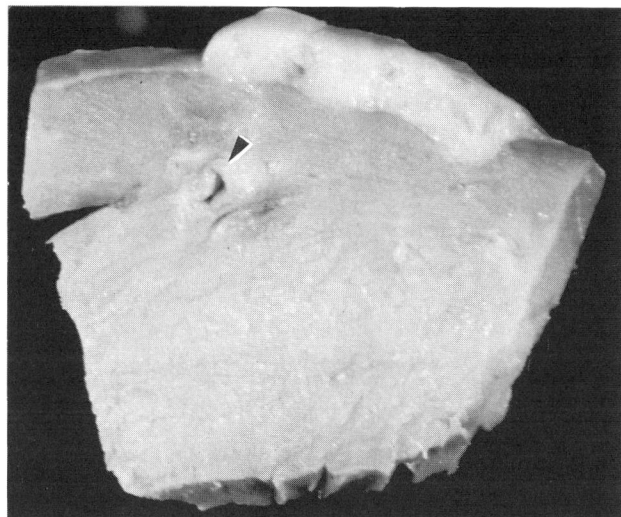

Figure 19.13 Myocardial muscle bridge. Section of myocardium of left ventricular anterior wall showing the left anterior descending coronary artery (arrowhead) in cross-section buried 0.4 cm under the epicardium. (Reproduced with permission from Cheitlin [76].)

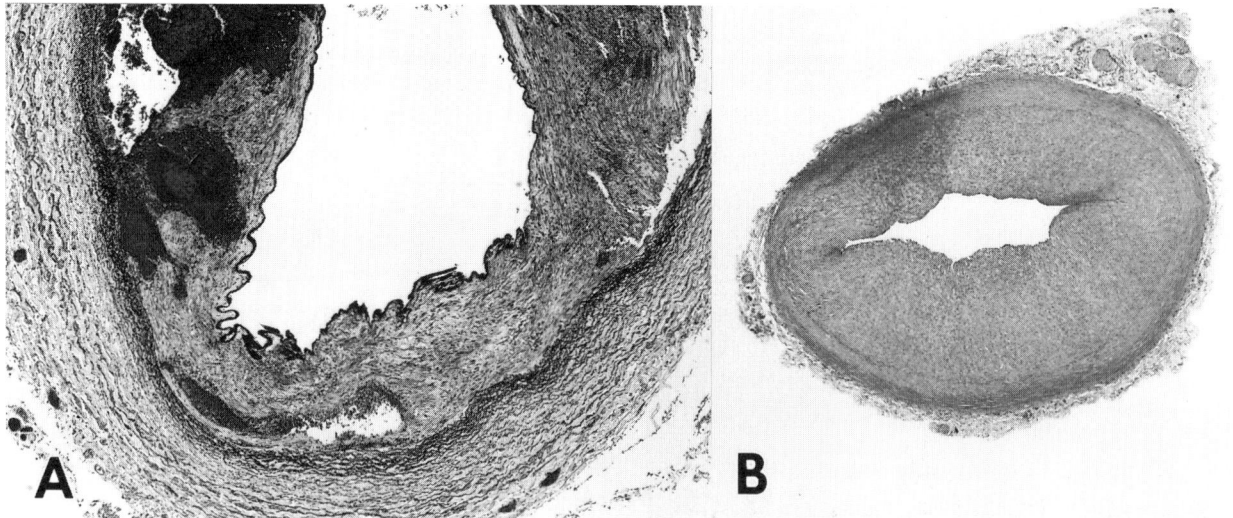

Figure 19.14 (A) Histologic section of the renal artery from a 50-year-old woman showing medial fibromuscular dysplasia and associated dissection of the media. (Movat.) (B) Histologic section of renal artery showing severe luminal narrowing by intimal fibroplasia consisting of smooth muscle cells and collagen. Note normal media and adventitia. (H&E.)

rowing) as a cause of acute myocardial infarction is seen in 90% of patients and is related to the underlying atherosclerotic plaque morphology, i.e. hemorrhage into a plaque and plaque rupture with superimposed thrombus. Coronary embolism as a cause of coronary occlusion in the absence of underlying atherosclerosis is rare. Previously, it was exclusively associated with infective endocarditis; however, with newer interventions, including invasive techniques, the incidence has increased, and other etiologies are now recognized. The natural causes of emboli include: infective (Figure 19.15A and B) and non-infective endocarditis; emboli from mural thrombi (associated with atrial fibrillation, myocardial infarction or cardiomyopathies); tumor emboli which may originate in the heart from myxomas (Figure 19.16) or from primary malignancies of the lungs, kidneys, colon, etc.; and fat emboli, especially marrow emboli in patients with fractures or after resuscitation [130]. Rarely, myocardial tissue may embolize from myocardial infarction with cardiac rupture.

With the advent of cardiac surgery, the incidence of systemic air embolism has increased. Calcium emboli which almost always originate from the aortic and mitral valves, may occur during valvular surgery or after valvular balloon dilatation [131]. Other unusual emboli include silicone from an oxygen pump, teflon, suture material, talc and cholesterol. Fragments of atherosclerotic material (atheroemboli) may be dislodged from the aorta during catheterization or surgery. Similarly, atherosclerotic material may embolize into distal coronary arteries in patients undergoing percutaneous coronary artery or saphenous vein graft angioplasty with the incidence being higher in vein grafts (Figure 19.17) [132].

19.2.11 CORONARY THROMBOSIS

While most thrombotic events in the heart occur secondary to coronary atherosclerosis, damage to the arterial wall and endothelium can occur from iatrogenic causes (catheters, trauma) or vasospasm. Vasospasm has been documented to occur in areas of mild coronary atherosclerosis with superimposed thrombosis. As noted previously, coronary thrombosis has been shown to occur after cocaine use, in women on oral contraceptives (especially in combination with smoking) and in normal or mildly atherosclerotic arteries [31,109,133,134]. Diffuse multiorgan thrombosis, as well as thrombosis within the intramyocardial small coronary arteries, can occur with disseminated intravascular coagulation (DIC). Histologically, DIC appears as fibrin-platelet thrombi or hyaline thrombi [135]. Other disorders of coagulation which may cause similar widespread thrombosis include thrombotic thrombocytopenic purpura, thrombocytosis and deficiencies of antithrombin III, protein C or protein S [136,137]. Defective fibrinolysis secondary to the 'lupus anticoagulant' or due to the presence of anticardiolipin antibodies also increases the risk of thrombosis [138].

19.2.12 CORONARY OSTIAL OCCLUSION

Coronary ostial occlusion prior to the advent of balloon angioplasty was traditionally seen in syphilitic aortitis and Takayasu's disease (Figure 19.18) [83,139,140].

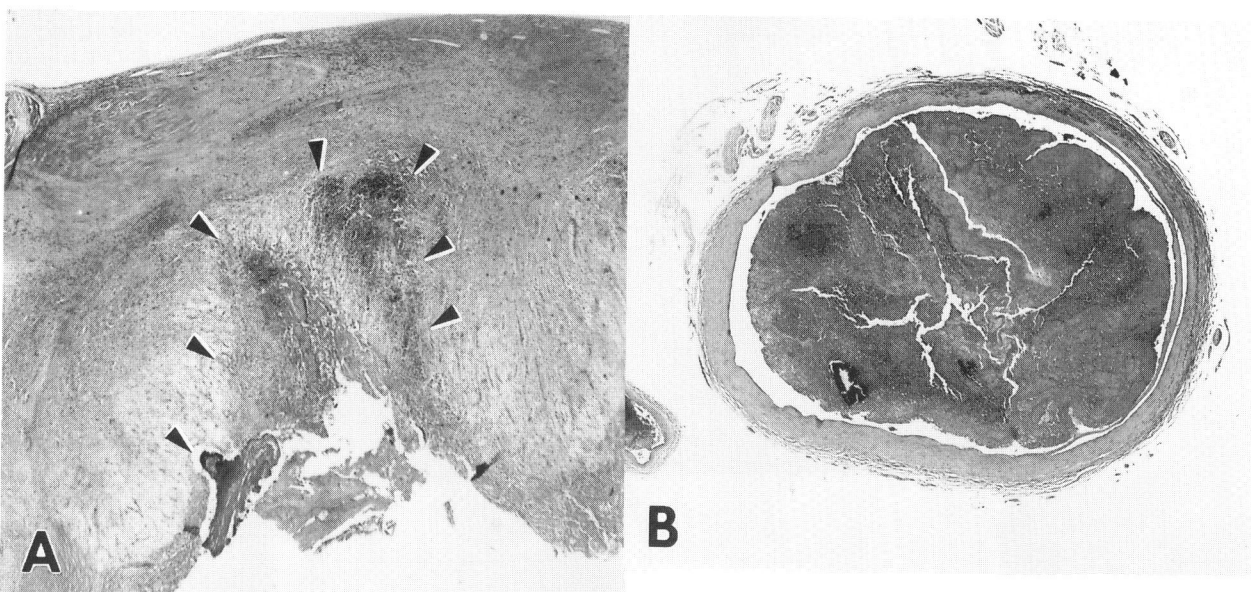

Figure 19.15 Microscopic section of the mitral valve (A) with chronic rheumatic valvulitis and superimposed infective endocarditis (arrowheads) with embolization to the left coronary artery (B) from a patient who developed sudden onset of chest pain and ECG changes of myocardial infarction. The embolus is seen totally occluding an underlying normal coronary artery. (H&E.) (Reproduced with permission from Cheitlin [76].)

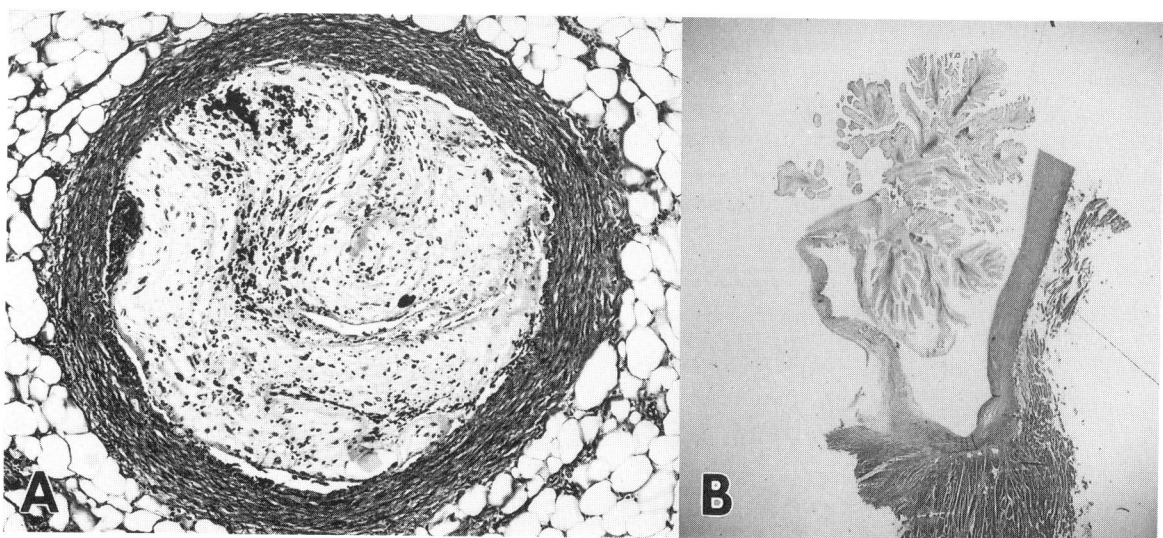

Figure 19.16 (A) Small left epicardial coronary artery containing an embolus from a left atrial myoxoma in a patient who died suddenly. (B) Longitudinal section of the aortic valve with a papillary fibroelastoma arising from the edge of the leaflet that extended to the coronary ostia. (H&E.) (Reproduced with permission from Cheitlin [76].)

Since the advent of balloon angioplasty it is not unusual to observe intimal smooth muscle cell proliferation in the ostium of left main or right coronary arteries after angioplasty (Figure 19.19) [141]. Turbulence caused by abnormal flow around centrally obstructing prosthetic valve such as the Starr–Edward valve may also lead to intimal proliferation around the coronary ostia, and this may occur as early as one month after valve implantation [142]. In supravalvular aortic stenosis, the membrane attachment may extend to the coronary ostium and cause stenosis [143].

19.2.13 ARTERIAL DISSECTIONS WITH CORONARY LUMINAL COMPRESSION

Aortic dissection, which involves the ascending aorta (type I and II), may extend proximally to involve the coronary ostia. Ostial compression occurs in 8% of

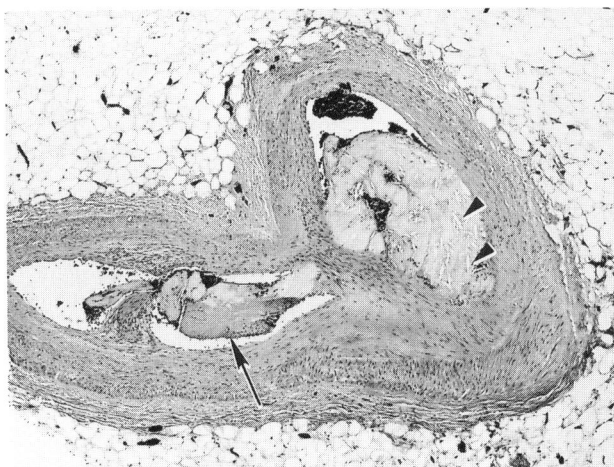

Figure 19.17 Atheroembolus in a distal small epicardial coronary artery; the lumen shows presence of pultaceous debris, cholesterol clefts (arrowheads) and thrombus (arrow). (H&E.)

these cases [144]. Most often, both the left main and right coronary arteries are dissected concomitantly. Less commonly, isolated dissection of the right coronary artery is present and isolated left main dissection is rare [145]. Clinically, isolated dissection of the right coronary artery causes inferior wall infarction, whereas involvement of the left main coronary artery causes sudden death. Spontaneous coronary artery dissections occur most frequently in women (80%) with the dissection plane between the inner two-thirds and outer one-third

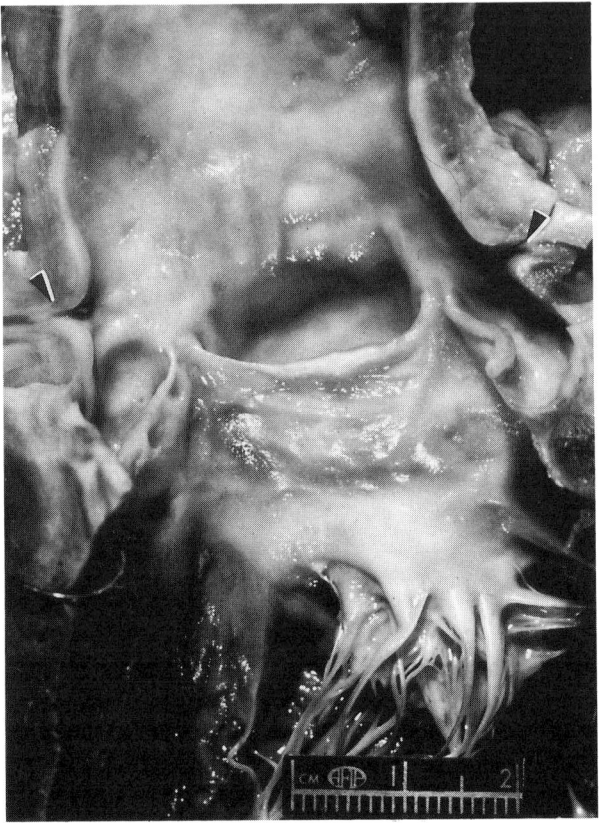

Figure 19.18 Left ventricular outflow tract, aortic valve and ascending aorta showing marked narrowing of both coronary artery ostia (arrowheads) with marked thickening of the ascending aorta in a 51-year-old white female with Takayasu's aortitis.

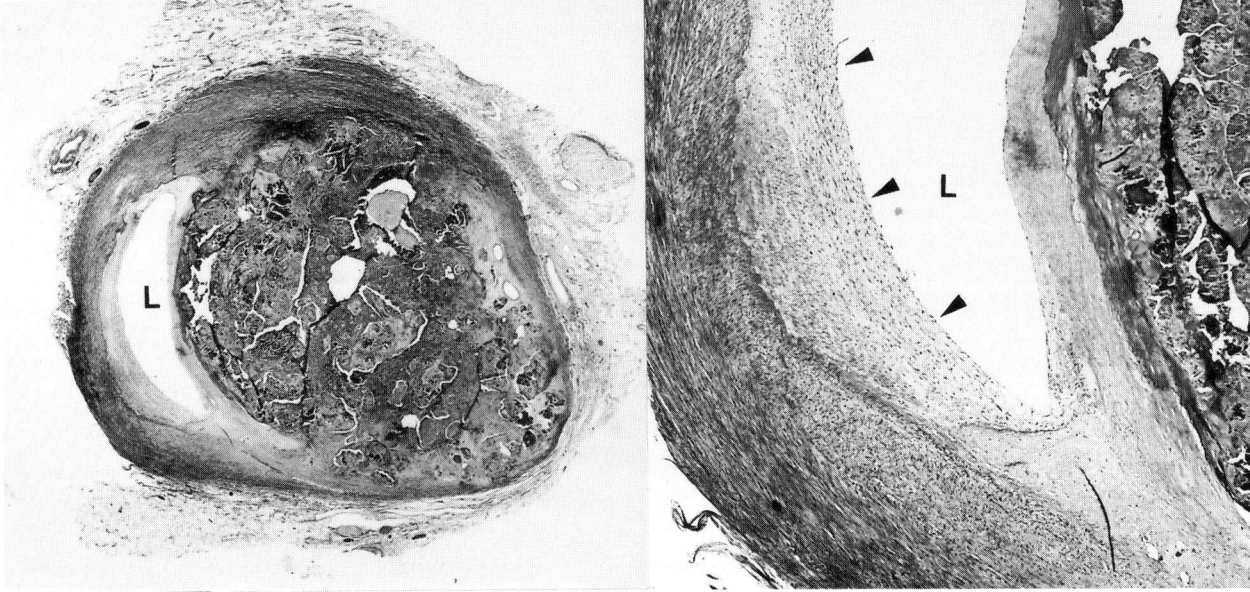

Figure 19.19 An 81-year-old man who underwent coronary balloon angioplasty of right coronary ostium 3 months prior to death showing marked calcification and severe luminal (L) narrowing with fibrointimal proliferation (arrowheads) causing restenosis. (Movat.)

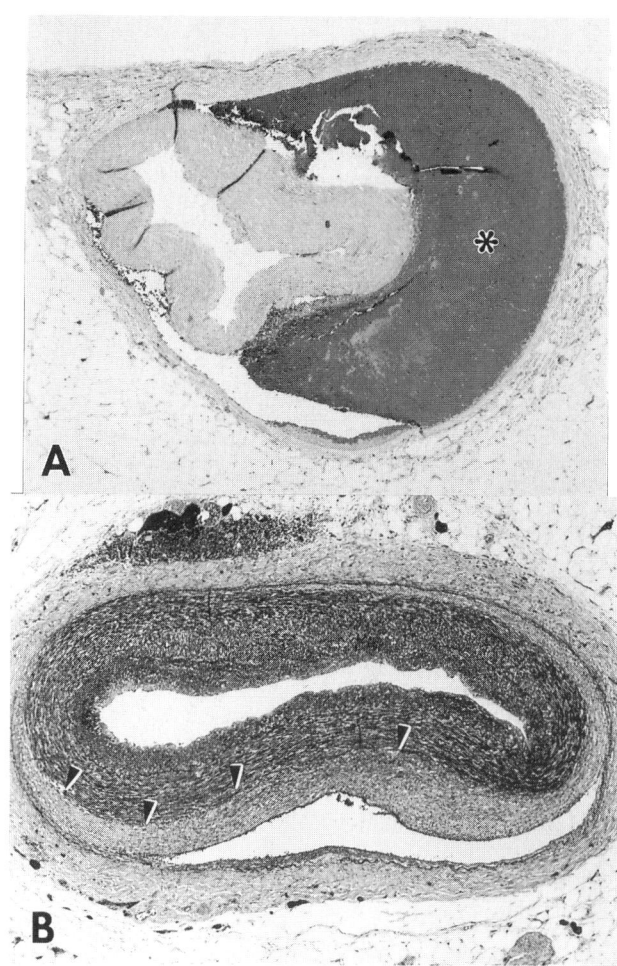

Figure 19.20 (A) A 39-year-old white female with sudden death at autopsy had acute dissection of the left anterior descending coronary artery (*) which resulted in acute myocardial infarction of the anterior wall of the left ventricle. (B) She also had a healed dissection (arrowheads) of the right coronary artery with a healed transmural posterior wall infarction of the left ventricle. (Movat stain.) (Reproduced with permission from Virmani and Forman [157].)

of the arterial wall (Figure 19.20). All patients present with sudden onset of chest pain and most have electrocardiograhic evidence of infarction [145]. Catheter-induced coronary artery dissections (Figure 19.21A and B), although well described, are extremely rare, with the reported incidence between 0.03 and 0.3% [83]. There have been rare instances of coronary compression from sinus of Valsalva aneurysms which have caused myocardial ischemia and infarction [146]. Rare examples of coronary artery tumor infiltration have also resulted in myocardial infarction [147].

19.2.14 TRAUMATIC INJURIES

Coronary artery injury may occur from many types of trauma. Injuries leading to blunt trauma are motor vehicle accidents, blows to the chest (steering wheel or crushing injuries), kicks from animals, etc. Penetrating injuries can occur from knife wounds, gunshot or shrapnel. Blunt injuries occur principally as a result of high-speed motor vehicle collisions that lead to rapid deceleration. One in every five patients with blunt trauma to the chest has some degree of cardiac injury [148] consisting of coronary artery injury, myocardial contusion or rupture, disruption of a valve or pericardial laceration. Coronary artery occlusion usually involves the left anterior descending coronary artery and may lead to intimal tear, spasm, thrombosis, dissections and pseudoaneurysms [149]. However, the ECG changes of myocardial infarction that are seen after blunt trauma usually are the consequence of myocardial contusion as coronary lacerations and thrombosis are rare [150].

In penetrating injuries, especially gunshot wounds, the width of the track around the missile path is proportional to the square of the velocity and the mass of the missile [151]. Therefore, the coronary artery can be lacerated and thrombosed simply by being in the area of the path of the missile. While the incidence of coronary injury is low (3.1–4.4% of all penetrating heart wounds), the mortality is extremely high [152]. As might be expected, the left anterior descending coronary artery is most commonly involved, and the surgical treatment is suture ligation of the cut vessel with coronary bypass grafting.

As mentioned above, the most rapidly increasing type of trauma to coronary arteries is occurring in the era of coronary angioplasty and other newer non-surgical coronary interventions. Coronary artery dissections occur most often during coronary angioplasty with the incidence of major ischemic complications varying from 2–9% in patients with multivessel disease [153]. The most frequent reason for the acute closure during angioplasty is coronary dissection and flaps (Figure 19.22A) or thrombotic occlusion which require use of other devices or emergency bypass surgery (performed in 1% to 4% of patients undergoing angioplasty) [154]. Late closure (restenosis), one to three months after angioplasty, is secondary to fibrointimal proliferation (Figure 19.22B and C).

19.3 Summary

This review is by no means exhaustive but provides a framework for classifying non-atherosclerotic disease of blood vessels with emphasis on the disorders of the coronary circulation which are associated with the greatest morbidity and mortality. Overall, when a young patient with low atherosclerotic risk factor profile presents with an ischemic cardiac syndrome, these unusual causes of myocardial ischemia and infarction should be considered in the differential diagnosis.

694 CORONARY NON-ATHEROSCLEROTIC AND NON-VASCULITIC DISEASES

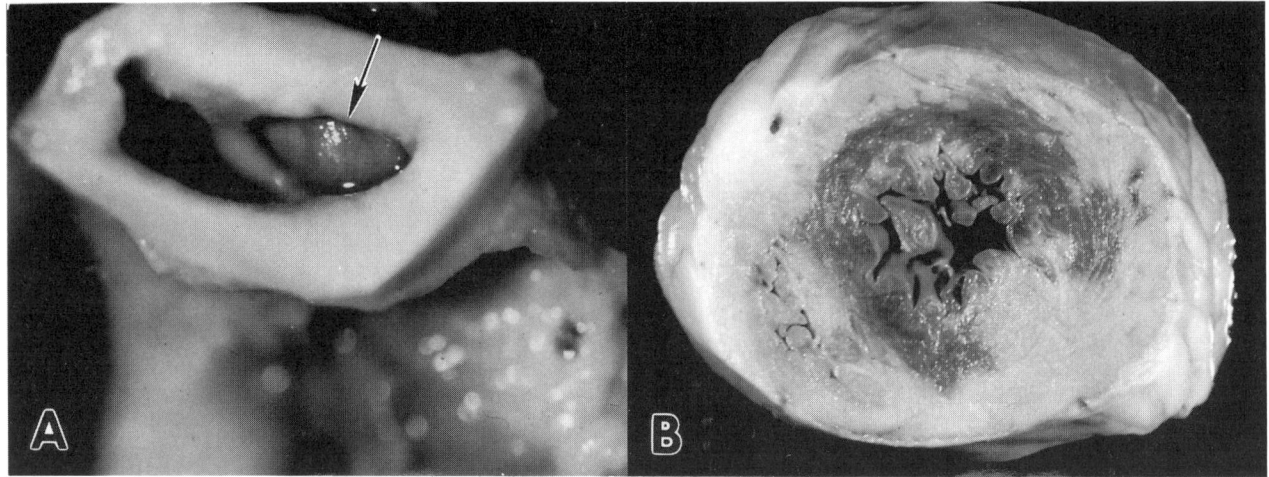

Figure 19.21 (A) Left main coronary ostium showing acute dissection (arrow) from a patient who died 24 hours after coronary catheterization. (B) Bread-loaf slice of the apical half of left ventricle showing subendocardial hemorrhagic infarct.

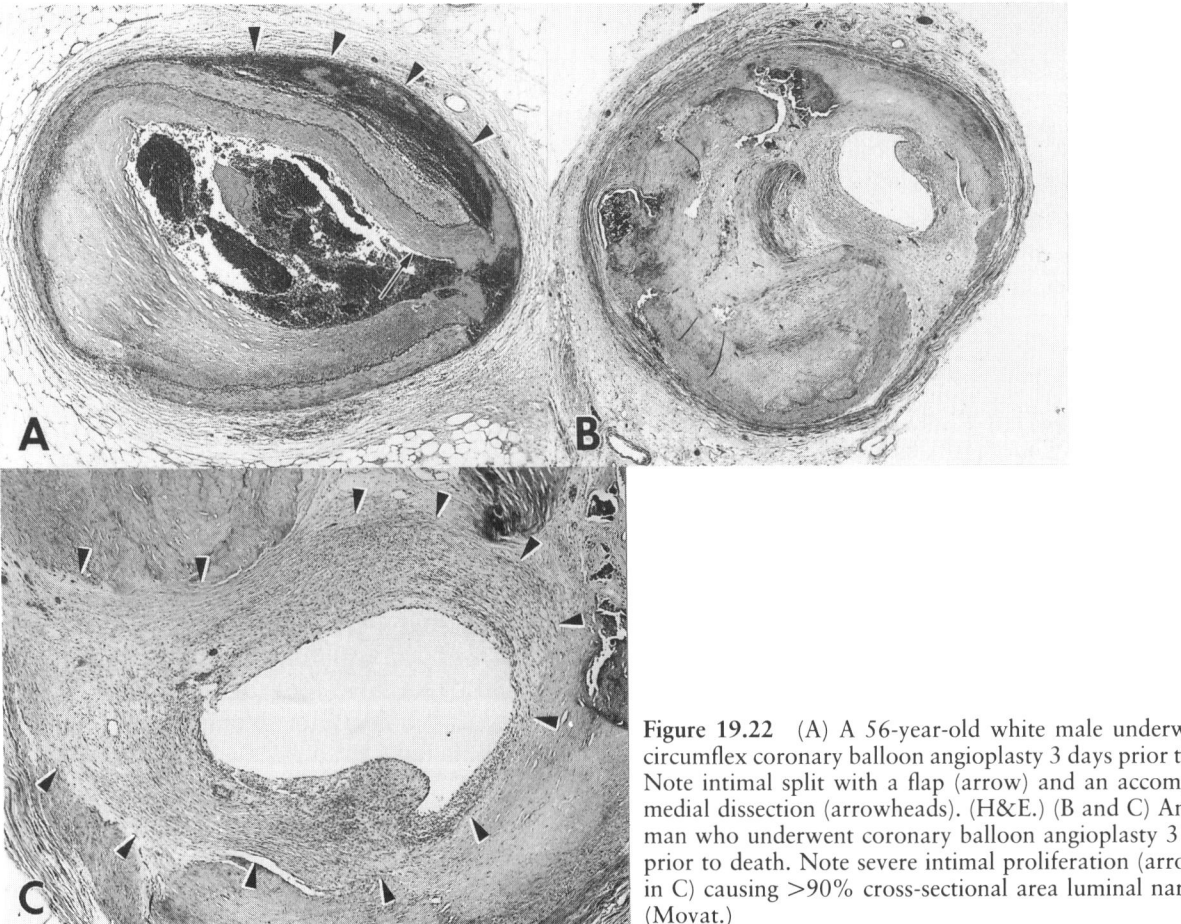

Figure 19.22 (A) A 56-year-old white male underwent left circumflex coronary balloon angioplasty 3 days prior to death. Note intimal split with a flap (arrow) and an accompanying medial dissection (arrowheads). (H&E.) (B and C) An elderly man who underwent coronary balloon angioplasty 3 months prior to death. Note severe intimal proliferation (arrowheads in C) causing >90% cross-sectional area luminal narrowing. (Movat.)

References

1. Report of the Working Group on Atherosclerosis of the National Heart, Lung, and Blood Institute (1981) vol. 2, DHEW Publication No. (NIH) 82-2035, Washington, DC, US Government Printing Office.
2. Glagov, S. (1972) Hemodynamic risk factors: Mechanical stress, mural architecture, medial nutrition and vulnerability of arteries to atherosclerosis, in *The Pathogenesis of Atherosclerosis*, (eds R.W. Wissler and J.C. Geer), Williams and Wilkins, Baltimore, pp. 164–87.
3. Strong, J.P. and McGill Jr, H.C. (1962) The natural history of coronary atherosclerosis. *Am. J. Pathol.*, **40**, 37–49.
4. Pells, S. and Fayerweather, W.E. (1985) Trends in the incidence of myocardial infarction and in associated mortality and morbidity. *New Engl. J. Med.*, **312**, 1005–11.
5. McGill Jr, H.C. et al. (1963) Natural history of human atherosclerosis, in *Atherosclerosis and Its Origin*, (eds M. Sandler and G.H. Bourne), Academic Press, New York, pp. 42–65.

6. Provenza, D.V. and Scherlis, S. (1959) Coronary circulation in dog's heart: demonstration of muscle sphincter in capillaries. *Circ. Res.*, **7**, 318–34.
7. Klocke, F.J. (1976) Coronary blood flow in man. *Prog. Cardiovasc. Dis.*, **19**, 117–66.
8. Sabbah, H.N. and Stein, P.D. (1982) Effect of acute regional ischemia on pressure in the subepicardium and subendocardium. *Am. J. Physiol.*, **242**, H240–4.
9. Brazier, J., Cooper, N. and Buckberg, G. (1974) The adequacy of subendocardial oxygen delivery: the interaction of determinants of flow, arterial oxygen content and myocardial oxygen need. *Circulation*, **49**, 968–77.
10. Braunwald, E. and Sobel, B.E. (1992) Coronary blood flow and myocardial ischemia, in *Heart Disease: A Textbook of Cardiovascular Medicine*, (ed. E. Braunwald), W.B. Saunders Company, Philadelphia, pp. 1161–99.
11. Marcus, M.L. (1983) Metabolic regulation of coronary blood flow, in *The Coronary Circulation in Health and Disease*, (ed. M.L. Marcus), McGraw-Hill, New York, pp. 1085–126.
12. Gould, K.L., Lipscomb, K. and Hamilton, G.W. (1974) Physiologic basis for assessing critical coronary stenosis, instantaneous flow response and regional distribution during coronary hyperemia as measure of coronary flow reserve. *Am. J. Cardiol.*, **33**, 87–94.
13. Young, M.A. and Vatner, S.F. (1986) Regulation of large coronary arteries. *Circ. Res.*, **59**, 579–96.
14. Woodman, O.L. and Vatner, S.F. (1987) Coronary vasoconstriction mediated by alpha 1 and alpha 2 adrenoceptors in the conscious dog. *Am. J. Physiol.*, **253**, H388–93.
15. Vatner, D.E., Knight, D.R., Homcy, C.J. et al. (1986) Subtypes of beta-adrenergic receptor in bovine coronary arteries. *Circ. Res.*, **59**, 463–73.
16. Higgins, C.B., Vatner, S.F. and Braunwald, E. (1973) Parasympathetic control of the heart. *Pharmacol. Rev.*, **25**, 119–28.
17. Rubio, R. and Berne, R.M. (1969) Release of adenosine by the normal myocardium and its relationship to the regulation of coronary resistance. *Circ. Res.*, **25**, 407–15.
18. Sparks Jr, H.V. and Bardenheuer, H. (1986) Regulation of adenosine formation by the heart. *Circ. Res.*, **58**, 193–201.
19. Bardenheuer, H. and Schrader, J. (1986) Supply-to-demand ratio for oxygen determines formation of adenosine by the heart. *Am. J. Physiol.*, **250**, H173–80.
20. Henderson, A.H. (1991) Endothelium in control. *Br. Heart J.* **65**, 116–25.
21. Furchgott, R.F. (1983) Role of endothelium in responses of vascular smooth muscle. *Circ. Res.*, **55**, 557–72.
22. Palmer, R.M.J., Ferrige, A.G. and Moncada, S. (1987) Nitric oxide release accounts for the biological activity of endothelium-derived relaxing factor. *Nature*, **327**, 524–6.
23. Palmer, R.M.J., Ashton, D.S. and Moncada, S. (1988) Vascular endothelial cells synthesize nitric oxide from L-arginine. *Nature*, **333**, 664–6.
24. Yasue, H., Horio, Y., Nakamura, N. et al. (1986) Induction of coronary spasm by acetylcholine in patients with variant angina: possible role of parasympathetic nervous system in the pathogenesis of coronary artery spasm. *Circulation*, **74**, 955–63.
25. Dinerman, J.L. and Mehta, J.L. (1990) Endothelial, platelet, and leukocyte interactions in ischemic heart disease: insights into potential mechanisms and their clinical relevance. *J. Am. Coll. Cardiol.*, **16**, 207–22.
26. Schini, V.B. (1991) Nitric oxide and vascular reactivity. *Coronary Artery Dis.*, **2**, 293–314.
27. Vanhoutte, P.M. and Shimokawa, H. (1989) Endothelium-derived relaxing factor and coronary vasospasm. *Circulation*, **80**, 1–9.
28. Andrews, H.E., Bruckdorfer, K.R., Dunn, R.C. and Jacobs, M. (1987) Low-density lipoproteins inhibit endothelium-dependent relaxation in rabbit aorta. *Nature* **327**, 237–9.
29. Yasue, H., Matsuyama, K., Matsuyama, K. et al. (1990) Responses of angiographically normal human coronary arteries to intracoronary injection of acetylcholine by age and segment. Possible role of early coronary atherosclerosis. *Circulation*, **81**, 482–90.
30. Prinzmetal, M., Kennamer, R., Merliss, R. et al. (1959) Angina pectoris, I: a variant form of angina pectoris. Preliminary report. *Am. J. Med.*, **27**, 375–88.
31. Ganz, P. and Alexander, R.W. (1985) New insights into the cellular mechanisms of vasospasm. *Am. J. Cardiol.*, **56**, 11E–15E.
32. McFadden, E.P., Clarke, J.G., Davies, G.J. et al. (1991) Effect of intracoronary serotonin on coronary vessels in patients with stable angina and patients with variant angina. *New Engl. J. Med.*, **324**, 648–54.
33. Irie, T., Imaizumi, T., Matuguchi, T. et al. (1989) Increased fibrinopeptide A during anginal attack in patients with variant angina. *J. Am. Coll. Cardiol.*, **14**, 589–94.
34. Ogawa, H., Yasue, H., Oshima, S. et al. (1989) Circadian variation of plasma fibrinopeptide A level in patients with variant angina. *Circulation*, **80**, 1617–26.
35. Forman, M.B., Oates, J.A., Robertson, D. et al. (1985) Increased adventitial mast cells in a patient with coronary spasm. *New Engl. J. Med.*, **313**, 1138–41.
36. Cohen, L. and Kitzes, R. (1986) Prompt termination and/or prevention of cold-pressor-stimulus-induced vasoconstriction of different vascular beds by magnesium sulphate in patients with Prinzmetal's angina. *Magnesium*, **5**, 144–9.
37. Kolodgie, F.D., Virmani, R., Cornhill, J.F. et al. (1991) Increase in atherosclerosis and adventitial mast cells in cocaine abusers: an alternative mechanism of cocaine-associated coronary vasospasm and thrombosis. *J. Am. Coll. Cardiol.*, **17**, 1553–60.
38. Richie, J.M. and Cohen, J. (1980) Local anesthetics, in *The Pharmacologic Basis of Therapeutics*, (eds L.S. Goodman and A. Gilman), Macmillan, New York, pp. 307–8.
39. Lange, R.L., Reid, M.S., Tresch, D.D. et al. (1972) Nonatheromatous ischemic heart disease following withdrawal from chronic industrial nitroglycerine exposure. *Circulation*, **46**, 666–78.
40. Przybojewski, J.Z. and Heyns, M.H. (1983) Acute coronary vasospasm secondary to industrial nitroglycerin withdrawal. *S. Afr. Med. J.*, **63**, 158–65.
41. Hutchison, S.J., Poole-Wilson, P.A. and Henderson, A.H. (1988) Angina with normal coronary arteries. A review. *Q. J. Med.*, **72**, 677–88.
42. Rutherford, J.D. and Braunwald, E. (1992) Chronic ischemic heart disease, in *Heart Disease. A Textbook of Cardiovascular Medicine*, (ed. E. Braunwald), W.B. Saunders Company, Philadelphia, pp. 1292–364.
43. Cannon III, R.O., Schenke, W.H., Quyyumi, A., et al. (1991) Comparison of exercise testing with studies of coronary flow reserve in patients with microvascular angina. *Circulation*, **83** (suppl. III), 77–88.
44. Cannon, R.O., Bonow, R.O., Bacharach, S.L. et al. (1985) Left ventricular dysfunction in patients with angina pectoris, normal epicardial coronary arteries and abnormal vasodilatory reserve. *Circulation*, **71**, 218–26.
45. Geltman, E.M., Henes, C.G., Senneff, M.J. et al. (1990) Increased myocardial perfusion at rest and diminished perfusion reserve in patients with angina and angiographically normal arteries. *J. Am. Coll. Cardiol.*, **16**, 586–96.
46. Berland, J., Cribier, A., Cazor, J.L. et al. (1984) Angina pectoris with angiographic normal coronary arteries: a clinical, hemodynamic, and metabolic study. *Clin. Cardiol.*, **7**, 485–92.
47. Kemp, H.G., Kronmal, R.A., Vlietstra, R.E. and Frye, R.L. (1986) Seven-year survival of patients with normal or near normal coronary arteriograms. A CASS Registry study. *J. Am. Coll. Cardiol.*, **7**, 479–83.
48. Maseri, A., Crea, F., Kaski, J.C. and Crake, T. (1991) Mechanism of angina pectoris in Syndrome X. *J. Am. Coll. Cardiol.*, **17**, 499–506.
49. Meerson, F.Z. (1969) The myocardium in hypertension, hypertrophy, and heart failure. *Circ. Res.*, **25** (suppl. II), 1–163.
50. Dellsperger, K.C. and Marcus, M.L. (1989) Influence of cardiac hypertrophy on the functional capacity of the coronary circulation, in *Nonatherosclerotic Ischemic Heart Disease*, (eds R. Virmani and M.B. Forman), Raven Press, New York, pp. 107–23.
51. Mueller, T.M., Marcus, M.L., Kerber, R.E. et al. (1978) Coronary blood flow in experimental canine left ventricular hypertrophy. *Circ. Res.*, **42**, 543–9.
52. Gascho, J.A., Mueller, T.M., Eastham, C. and Marcus, M.L. (1982) Effect of volume-overload hypertrophy on the coronary circulation in awake dog. *Cardiovasc. Res.*, **16**, 288–92.
53. Marcus, M.L., Mueler, T.M., Gascho, J.A. and Kerber, R.E. (1979) Effect of cardiac hypertrophy secondary to hypertension on coronary circulation. *Am. J. Cardiol.*, **44**, 1023–8.
54. Malike, A.B., Ahe, T., O'Kane, H. and Geha, A.S. (1973) Cardiac function, coronary flow and oxygen consumption in stable left ventricular hypertrophy. *Am. J. Physiol.*, **225**, 186–91.
55. Tarazi, R.C. (1985) The heart in hypertension. *N. Engl. J. Med.*, **312**, 308–9.
56. Wangler, R.D., Peters, K.G., Marcus, M.L. and Tomanek, R.J. (1982) Effect of duration of arterial hypertension and cardiac hypertrophy on coronary vasodilator reserve. *Circ. Res.*, **51**, 10–18.
57. Marcus, M.L., Doty, D.B., Hiratzka, L.F. et al. (1982) Decreased coronary reserve. *New Engl. J. Med.*, **307**, 1362–6.
58. Smucker, M.L., Tedesco, C.L. and Manning, S.B. (1988) Demonstration of an imbalance between coronary perfusion and excessive load as a mechanism of ischemia during stress in patients with aortic stenosis. *Circulation*, **78**, 573–82.
59. Vinten-Johansen, J. and Weiss, H.R. (1980) Oxygen consumption in subepicardial and subendocardial regions of the canine left ventricle – the effect of experimental acute valvular aortic stenosis. *Circ. Res.*, **46**, 139–45.
60. Matsuo, S., Tsuruta, M., Hayano, M. et al. (1988) Phasic coronary blood flow velocity determined by doppler flow meter catheter in aortic stenosis and aortic regurgitation. *Am. J. Cardiol.*, **62**, 917–22.
61. Marcus, M.L., Dot, D.B., Hiratzka, L.F. et al. (1982) Decreased coronary reserve. A mechanism for angina pectoris in patients with aortic stenosis and normal coronary arteries. *New Engl. J. Med.*, **307**, 1362–6.
62. Braunwald, E. (1992) Valvular heart disease, in *Heart Disease. A Textbook of Cardiovascular Medicine*, (ed. E. Braunwald), W.B. Saunders Company, Philadelphia, pp. 1007–77.
63. Cannon, R.O., Schenke, W.H., Maron, B.J. et al. (1987) Differences in coronary flow and myocardial metabolism at rest and during pacing between patients with obstructive and patients with nonobstructive hyper-

trophic cardiomyopathy. *J. Am. Coll. Cardiol.*, **10**, 53–62.
64. Tamaka, M., Fujiwara, H., Onodera, T. *et al.* (1987) Quantatative analysis of narrowing of intramyocardial small arteries in normal hearts, hypertensive hearts, and hearts with hypertrophic cardiomyopathy. *Circulation*, **75**, 1130–9.
65. Cannon, R.O., Cunnion, R.E., Parrillo, J.E. *et al.* (1987) Dynamic limitation of coronary vasodilatory reserve in patients with dilated cardiomyopathy and chest pain. *J. Am. Coll. Cardiol.*, **10**, 1190–200.
66. Treasure, C.B., Vita, J.A., Cox, D.A. *et al.* (1990) Endothelium dependent dilatation of the coronary microvasculature is impaired in dilated cardiomyopathy. *Circulation*, **81**, 772–9.
67. Opherk, D., Mall, G., Zebe, H. *et al.* (1984) Reduction of coronary reserve. A mechanism for angina pectoris in patients with arterial hypertension and normal coronary arteries. *Circulation*, **69**, 1–7.
68. Skelton, C.L. (1982) The heart and hyperthyroidism. *N. Engl. J. Med.*, **307**, 1206–8.
69. Kotler, M.N., Michaelides, K.M., Bouchard, R.J. and Warbasse, J.R. (1973) Myocardial infarction associated with thyrotoxicosis. *Arch. Intern. Med.*, **132**, 723–8.
70. Featherstone, H.J. and Stewart, D.K. (1983) Angina in thyrotoxicosis. Thyroid-related coronary artery spasm. *Arch. Intern. Med.*, **143**, 554–5.
71. Williams, G.H. and Braunwald, E. (1992) Endocrine and nutritional disorders and heart disease, in *Heart Disease: A Textbook of Cardiovascular Medicine*, (ed. E. Braunwald), W.B. Saunders Company, Philadelphia, pp. 1827–55.
72. Cavallo, A., Joseph, C.J. and Casta, A. (1984) Cardiac complications in juvenile hyperthyroidism. *Am. J. Dis. Child.*, **138**, 479–82.
73. McManus, B.M., Fleury, T.A. and Roberts, W.C. (1981) Fatal catecholamine crisis in pheochromocytoma: curable form of cardiac arrest. *Am. Heart J.*, **102**, 930–2.
74. Sardesai, S.H., Mourant, A.J., Sivathandon, Y. *et al.* (1990) Phaeochromocytoma and catecholamine-induced cardiomyopathy presenting as heart failure. *Br. Heart J.*, **63**, 234–7.
75. Haas, G.J., Tzagournis, M. and Boudoulas, H. (1988) Pheochromocytoma. Catecholamine-mediated electrocardiographic changes mimicking ischemia. *Am. Heart J.*, **116**, 1363–5.
76. Cheitlin, M.D. and Virmani, R. (1989) Myocardial infarction in the absence of coronary atherosclerotic disease, in *Nonatherosclerotic Ischemic Heart Disease*, (eds R. Virmani and M.B. Forman), Raven Press, New York, pp. 1–30.
77. Cheitlin, M.D., McAllister, H.A. and deCastro, C.M. (1975) Myocardial infarction without atherosclerosis. *J. Am. Med. Ass.*, **231**, 951–9.
78. Hackel, D.B., Ratliff, N.B. and Mikat, E. (1974) The heart in shock. *Circ. Res.*, **35**, 805–11.
79. Greenhout, J.H. and Reichenbach, D.D. (1969) Cardiac injury and subarachnoid hemorrhage. *J. Neurosurg.*, **30**, 521–36.
80. Jones, C.E., Smith, E.E., DuPont, E. and Williams, R.D. (1978) Demonstration of nonperfused myocardium in late hemorrhagic shock. *Circ. Shock*, **5**, 97–104.
81. Grace, T.W. and Platt, F.W. (1981) Subacute carbon monoxide poisoning. Another great imitator. *J. Am. Med. Ass.*, **246**, 1698–700.
82. Penney, D.G. (1988) A review: hemodynamic response to carbon monoxide. *Environ. Hlth Perspec.*, **77**, 121–30.
83. Marius-Nunez, A.L. (1990) Myocardial infarction with normal coronary arteries after acute exposure to carbon monoxide. *Chest*, **97**, 491–4.
84. Ebisuno, S., Yasuno, M., Yamada, Y. *et al.* (1986) Myocardial infarction after acute carbon monoxide poisoning: case report. *Angiology*, **37**, 621–4.
85. Ferry, D.R., Henry, R.L. and Kern, M.J. (1986) Epinephrine-induced myocardial infarction in a patient with angiographically normal arteries. *Am. Heart J.*, **111**, 1193–5.
86. Pierpont, M.E.M. and Moller, J.H. (1989) Cardiac manifestations of systemic disease, in *Moss' Heart Disease in Infants, Children, and Adolescents*, 4th edn, (eds F.H. Adams, G.C. Emmanouilides and T.A. Riemenschneider), Williams & Wilkins, Baltimore, pp. 778–801.
87. McKusick, V.A., Neufeld, E.F. and Kelly, T.E. (1978) The mucopolysaccharide storage diseases, in *The Metabolic Basis of Inherited Disease*, (eds J.B. Stanbury, J.B. Wyngaarden and D.S. Frederickson), 4th edn, McGraw-Hill, New York, pp. 1282–310.
88. Ferrans, V.J. (1991) Metabolic and familial disease, in *Cardiovascular Pathology*, 2nd edn, (ed. M.D. Silver), Churchill Livingstone, New York, pp. 1073–149.
89. Brosius, F.C. and Roberts, W.C. (1981) Coronary artery disease in the Hurler syndrome. Qualitative and quantitative analysis of the extent of coronary narrowing at necropsy in six children. *Am. J. Cardiol.*, **47**, 649–53.
90. Krovetz, L.J., Lorincz, A.E. and Schiebler, G.L. (1965) Cardiovascular manifestations of the Hurler syndrome: hemodynamic and angiographic observations in 15 patients. *Circulation*, **31**, 132–41.
91. Goodman, R.M., Smith, E.W., Paton, D. *et al.* (1963) Pseudoxanthoma elasticum: a clinical and histopathological study. *Medicine*, **42**, 297–334.
92. Mendelsohn, G., Bulkley, B.H. and Hutchins, G.M. (1978) Cardiovascular manifestations of pseudoxanthoma elasticum. *Arch. Pathol. Lab. Med.*, **102**, 298–302.
93. Schachner, L. and Young, D. (1974) Pseudoxanthoma elasticum with severe cardiovascular disease in a child. *Am. J. Dis. Child.*, **127**, 571–5.
94. Dardir, M., Ferrans, V.J. and Robert, W.C. (1989) Coronary artery disease in familial and metabolic disorders, in *Nonatherosclerotic Ischemic Heart Disease*, (eds R. Virmani and M.B. Forman), Raven Press, New York, pp. 185–235.
95. Gertz, M.A. and Kyle, R.A. (1989) Primary systemic amyloidosis – a diagnostic primer. *Mayo Clin. Proc.*, **64**, 1505–19.
96. Smith, T.J., Kyle, R.A. and Lie, J.T. (1984) Clinical significance of histopathologic patterns of cardiac amyloidosis. *Mayo Clin. Proc.*, **59**, 547–55.
97. Olson, L.J., Gertz, M.A., Edwards, W.D. *et al.* (1987) Senile cardiac amyloidosis with myocardial dysfunction. Diagnosis by endomyocardial biopsy and immunohistochemistry. *New Engl. J. Med.*, **317**, 738–42.
98. Buja, L.M., Khoi, N.B. and Roberts, W.C. (1970) Clinically significant cardiac amyloidosis. Clinicopathologic findings in 15 patients. *Am. J. Cardiol.*, **26**, 394–405.
99. Takahashi, M. and Lurie, P.R. (1989) Abnormalities and diseases of the coronary vessels, in *Moss' Heart Disease in Infants, Children, and Adolescents*, 4th edn, (eds F.H. Adams, G.C. Emmanouilides and T.A. Riemenschneider), Williams & Wilkins, Baltimore, pp. 627–47.
100. Anderson, K.A., Burbach, J.A., Fenton, L.J. *et al.* (1985) Idiopathic arterial calcification of infancy in newborn siblings with unusual light and electron microscopic manifestations. *Arch. Pathol. Lab. Med.*, **109**, 838–42.
101. Moran, J.J. (1975) Idiopathic arterial calcification of infancy: a clinicopathologic study. *Pathol. Annu.*, **10**, 393–417.
102. Stolte, M. and Jurowich, B. (1975) Arteriopathia calcificans infantum. *Basic Res. Cardiol.*, **70**, 307–25.
103. Witzleben, C.L. (1970) Idiopathic infantile arterial calcification – a misnomer? *Am. J. Cardiol.*, **26**, 305–9.
104. Desnick, R.J. and Sweeley, C.C. (1983) Fabry's disease: Alpha-galactosidase A deficiency, in *The Metabolic Basis of Inherited Disease*, 5th edn, (eds J.B. Stanbury, J.B. Wyngaarden and D.S. Fredrickson), McGraw-Hill, New York, pp. 906–35.
105. Pyeritz, R.E. (1992) Genetics and cardiovascular disease, in *Heart Disease. A Textbook of Cariovascular Medicine*, 4th edn, (ed. E. Braunwald), W.B. Saunders Company, Philadelphia, pp. 1622–55.
106. Morgan, S.H. and Crawford, M, d'A. (1988) Anderson–Fabry disease. A commonly missed diagnosis. *Br. Med. J.*, **297**, 872–3.
107. Ferrans, V.J., Hibbs, R.G. and Burda, C.D. (1969) The heart in Fabry's disease. A histochemical and electron microscopic study. *Am. J. Cardiol.*, **24**, 95–110.
108. Colucci, W.S., Lorell, B.H., Scohen, F.J. *et al.* (1982) Hypertrophic cardiomyopathy due to Fabry's disease. *New Engl. J. Med.*, **307**, 926–8.
109. Stadel, B.V. (1981) Oral contraceptives and cardiovascular disease. *New Engl. J. Med.*, **305**, 612–18; 672–8.
110. Mann, J.I., Vessey, M.P., Thorgood, M. and Doll, R. (1975) Myocardial infarction in young women with special reference to oral contraceptives practice. *Br. Med. J.*, **2**, 241–5.
111. Mann, J.I. and Inman, W.W. (1975) Oral contraceptives and death from myocardial infarction. *Br. Med. J.*, **2**, 241–5.
112. Merians, D.R., Haskell, W.L., Vranizan, K.M. *et al.* (1985) Relationship of exercise, oral contraceptive use, and body fat to concentration of plasma lipids and lipoprotein cholesterol in young women. *Am. J. Med.*, **78**, 913–19.
113. Webber, L.S., Hunter, S.M., Baugh, J.G. *et al.* (1982) The interaction of cigarette smoking, oral contraceptive use and cardiovascular risk factor variables in children: the Bogalusa Heart Study. *Am. J. Publ. Health.*, **72**, 266–74.
114. Baltaxe, H.A., Wixson, D. (1977) The incidence of congenital anomalies of the coronary arteries in the adult population. *Radiology*, **122**, 47–52.
115. Hobbs, R.E., Millit, H.D., Raghaven, P.V. *et al.* (1981) Congenital coronary anomalies: Clinical and therapeutic complications. *Cardiovasc. Clin.*, **12**, 43–58.
116. Alexander, R.W. and Griffith, G.C. (1956) Anomalies of the coronary arteries and their clinical significance. *Circulation*, **14**, 800–5.
117. Gao, S.Z., Schroeder, J.S., Hunt, S. and Stinson, E.B. (1988) Retransplantation for severe accelerated coronary vascular disease in heart transplant recipients. *Am. J. Cardiol.*, **52**, 867–81.
118. Billingham, M.E. (1987) Cardiac transplant atherosclerosis. *Transplant. Proc.*, **19** (suppl. 5), 19–25.
119. Gao, S.Z., Alderman, E.L., Schroeder, J.S. *et al.* (1990) Progressive coronary luminal narrowing after cardiac transplantation. *Circulation*, **82** (suppl. IV), IV269–75.
120. Johnson, D.E., Alderman, E.L., Schroeder, J.S. *et al.* (1991) Transplant coronary artery disease: histopathologic correlations with angiographic morphology. *J. Am. Coll. Cardiol.* **17**, 449–57.
121. Askenazi, J. and Nadas, A.S. (1975) Anomalous left coronary artery originating from the pulmonary artery. Report in 15 cases. *Circulation*, **51**, 976–87.

122. Cheitlin, M.D., DeCastro, C.M. and McAllister, H.A. (1974) Sudden death as a complication of anomalous left coronary origin from the anterior sinus of Valsalva. *Circulation*, **50**, 780–7.
123. Taylor, A.J., Rogan, K.M. and Virmani, R. (1992) Sudden cardiac death with congenital coronary artery anomalies. *J. Am. Coll. Cardiol.*, **20**, 640–7.
124. Morales, A.R., Romanelli, R. and Boucek, R.J. (1980) The mural left anterior descending coronary artery, strenuous exercise, and sudden death. *Circulation*, **82**, 230–7.
125. Morales, A.R., Romanelli, R., Tate, L.G. *et al.* (1993) Intramural left anterior descending coronary artery. Significance of the depth of the muscle tunnels. *Hum. Pathol.*, **24**, 693–701.
126. Virmani, R., Farb, A. and Burke, A.P. (1993) Ischemia from myocardial bridging: fact or fancy? *Hum. Pathol.*, **24**, 687–8.
127. Virmani, R., Darcy, T. and Robinowitz, M. (1992) Congenital malformatons of the vasculature, in *Vascular Medicine*, (eds J. Loscalzo, M.A. Creager and V.J. Dzau), Little, Brown and Company, New York, pp. 1115–44.
128. Harrison Jr, E.G. and McCormack, L.J. (1971) Pathological classification of renal arterial disease in renovascular hypertension. *Mayo Clin. Proc.*, **46**, 161–7.
129. Luscher, T.F., Lie, J.T., Stanson, A.W. *et al.* (1987) Arterial fibromuscular dysplasia. *Mayo Clinic Proc.*, **62**, 931–52.
130. Atkinson, J.B., Forman, M.B. and Virmani, R. (1989) Emboli and thrombi in coronary arteries, in *Nonatherosclerotic Ischemic Heart Disease*, (eds R. Virmani and M.B. Forman), Raven Press, New York, pp. 355–85.
131. Roberts, W.C. (1978) Coronary embolism: a review of causes, consequences, and diagnostic considerations. *Cardiovasc. Med.*, **3**, 699–710.
132. Saber, R.S., Edwards, W.B., Holmes Jr, D.R. *et al.* (1988) Balloon angioplasty of saphenous vein bypass grafts: a histopathologic study of six grafts from five patients, with emphasis on restenosis and embolic complications. *J. Am. Coll. Cardiol.*, **12**, 1501–9.
133. Kolodgie, F.D., Virmani, R., Cornhill, J.F. *et al.* (1991) Increase in atherosclerosis and adventitial mast cells in cocaine abusers: an alternative mechanism of cocaine-associated coronary vasospasm and thrombosis. *J. Am. Coll. Cardiol.*, **17**, 1553–60.
134. McKenna, W.J., Chew, C.Y.C. and Oakley, C.M. (1980) Myocardial infarction with normal coronary angiogram. Possible mechanism of smoking risk in coronary artery disease. *Br. Heart J.*, **43**, 493–8.
135. Ridolfi, R.L., Hutchins, G.M. and Bell, W.R. (1979) The heart and cardiac conduction system in thrombotic thrombocytopenic purpura. *Ann. Intern. Med.*, **91**, 357–63.
136. Schafer, A.I. (1985) The hypercoagulable states. *Ann. Intern. Med.*, **102**, 814–28.
137. Virmani, R., Poposky, M.A. and Roberts, W.C. (1979) Thrombocytosis, coronary thrombosis, and acute myocardial infarction. *Am. J. Med.*, **67**, 498–506.
138. Love, P.E. and Santoro, S.A. (1990) Antiphospholipid antibodies: anticardiolipin and lupus anticoagulant in systemic lupus erythematosis (SLE) and in non-SLE disorders. *Ann. Int. Med.*, **112**, 682–98.
139. Virmani, R. and McAllister Jr, H.A. (1986) Pathology of the aorta and major arteries, in *Aortitis: Clinical, Pathologic and Radiographic Aspects*, (eds A. Lande, Y.M. Berkmen and H.A. McAllister), Raven Press, New York, pp. 7–53.
140. Virmani, R., Lande, A. and McAllister Jr, H.A. (1986) Pathological aspects of Takayasu's arteritis, in *Aortitis: Clinical, Pathologic, and Radiographic Aspects*, (eds A. Lande, Y.M. Bermen and H.A. McAllister), Raven Press, New York, pp. 55–79.
141. Waller, B.F., Pinkerton, C.A. and Foster, L.N. (1987) Morphologic evidence of accelerated left main coronary artery stenosis: a late complication of percutaneous transluminal balloon angioplasty of the proximal left anterior descending coronary artery. *J. Am. Coll. Cardiol.*, **9**, 1019–23.
142. Yates, J.D., Kirch, M.M., Sodeman, T.M. *et al.* (1974) Coronary ostial stenosis. A complication of aortic valve replacement. *Circulation*, **49**, 530–4.
143. Gibson, R., Nihill, M.R., Mullins, C.E. *et al.* (1981) Congenital coronary artery obstruction associated with aortic valve anomalies in children. Report of two cases. *Circulation*, **64**, 857–61.
144. Hirst, A.E., Johns, V.J. and Kime, S.W. (1958) Dissecting aneurysm of the aorta. A review of 505 cases. *Medicine*, **37**, 217–79.
145. Robinowitz, M., Virmani, R. and McAllister, H.A. (1982) Spontaneous coronary artery dissection and eosinophilic inflammation. A cause and effect relationship. *Am. J. Med.*, **72**, 923–7.
116. Brandt, J., Jogi, P. and Lührs, C. (1985) Sinus of Valsalva aneurysm obstructing coronary arterial flow. Case report and collective review of the literature. *Eur. Heart J.*, **6**, 1069–73.
147. Miyazaki, T., Toshida, T., Mori, H. *et al.* (1985) Intractable heart failure, conduction disturbances and myocardial infarction by massive myocardial invasion of malignant lymphoma. *J. Am. Coll. Cardiol.*, **3**, 937–41.
148. Gay, W. (1982) Blunt trauma to the heart and great vessels. *Surgery*, **91**, 507–9.
149. Lascault, G., Komajda, M., Drobinski, G. and Grosgogeat, Y. (1986) Left coronary artery aneurysm and anteroseptal acute myocardial infarction following blunt chest trauma. *Eur. Heart J.*, **7**, 538–40.
150. Arto, M.J., Cokins, S.G. and Jonas, E. (1984) Acute anterior wall myocardial infarction secondary to blunt chest trauma. *Angiology*, **35**, 802–4.
151. Amato, J.J. and Rich, N.M. (1972) Temporary cavity effects in blood vessel injury by high velocity missiles. *J. Cardiovasc. Surg.*, **13**, 147–55.
152. Merrill, W.H. (1989) Coronary artery injuries secondary to trauma, in *Nonatherosclerotic Ischemic Heart Disease*, (eds R. Virmani and M.B. Forman), Raven Press, New York, pp. 387–96.
153. Ellis, S.G., Vandormael, M.G., Cowley, M.J. *et al.* and the Multivessel Angioplasty Prognosis Study Group (1990) Coronary morphologic and clinical determinants of procedural outcome with angioplasty for multivessel coronary disease. Implications for patient selection. *Circulation*, **82**, 1193–202.
154. DiSciasco, G., Cowley, M.J., Vetrovec, G.W. *et al.* (1988) Triple vessel coronary angioplasty: acute outcome and long-term results. *J. Am. Coll. Cardiol.*, **12**, 42–8.
155. Virmani, R., Robinowitz, M. and Daruy, T.P. (1991) Coronary vasculitis, in *Cardiovascular Pathology*, (eds R. Virmani, J.B. Atkinson and J.J. Fenoglio), W.B. Saunders, Philadelphia, p. 177.
156. Robinowitz, M., Forman, M.B. and Virmani, R. (1989) Nonatherosclerotic coronary aneurysms, in *Nonatherosclerotic Ischemic Heart Disease*, (eds R. Virmani and M.B. Forman), Raven Press, New York, p. 279.
157. Virmani, R. and Forman, M.B. (1989) Coronary artery dissections, in *Nonatherosclerotic Ischaemic Heart Disease*, (eds R. Virmani and M.B. Forman), Raven Press, New York, pp. 334–5.

20 DIAGNOSTIC ANGIOGRAPHY, IMAGING AND INTERVENTION

Anthony W. Stanson

The various methods of imaging blood vessels produce pictures that represent some of the gross morphologic characteristics of normal and pathologic vessels. These images do not replace the microscopic diagnosis, but they often substitute for an *in vivo* gross pathologic diagnosis. There are a few diseases, however, in which such imaging can accurately predict the microscopic diagnosis. The greatest benefit of imaging studies is that they provide helpful information in planning patient treatment. The focus of this chapter is discussion of those diseases that have characteristic vascular imaging findings that lead to a diagnosis. Therefore, of the many vascular diseases, only a few will be presented here.

20.1 Imaging modalities

The traditional imaging modality for vascular disease is **angiography**. This represents the most invasive and expensive modality, but also the one that offers the most specific information on the peripheral and visceral arteries. **Ultrasonography** is the simplest and least expensive imaging modality and serves many important functions such as detection of abdominal aortic aneurysms, carotid artery stenosis, deep venous thrombus of the extremities, renal transplant failure, pulsatile hematoma following arterial punctures, hepatic and portal vein thrombosis and surveillance of vascular grafts in the extremities. Between the opposite levels of complexity and expense of angiography and ultrasound, are **magnetic resonance imaging** and **computed tomography**. Each imaging modality has a unique and complementary role in diagnosing vascular disease, and while it is not always possible to predict which modality would best image any particular vascular disease problem, certain situations are more suited to one or the other.

Before examining the specific characteristics and diagnostic capabilities of these modalities, one should consider what morphologic feature can be detected by each: the vessel lumen, the wall and the surrounding tissue. Vessel lumens are best evaluated by angiography.

The appearance of the lumen can be an important indicator of specific disease. An angiogram allows appreciation of subtle variations of caliber. When a stenosis is encountered, pressure measurements can be taken and, when appropriate, a balloon catheter can be applied to dilate the lesion. If an occlusion is discovered, its specific appearance can provide evidence of an acute or chronic occlusion and possibly indicate etiology. The angiogram also provides a global view of an arterial bed; small vessels can be seen, at a diameter of less than a millimeter. Having such a range of vessel sizes on a film provides valuable information in diagnosing vascular disease. Other imaging modalities cannot display such a range.

What the angiogram does not do is to provide a view of the vessel wall. Even mural thrombus is often not appreciated. The other three imaging modalities show the vessel wall with differing degrees of specificity, although their ability to display small vessels is limited. At times, it is important to have both the lumen of the vessel and its wall characteristics displayed to evaluate a disease process [1,2]. In addition to morphologic characteristics, ultrasonography (US), magnetic resonance imaging (MRI) and angiographic cine filming can provide information regarding flow and velocity, which is not feasible with computed tomography (CT). However, fast CT, with electron beam technology, can provide information of blood flow and organ perfusion.

20.2 Morphology

There are a limited number of pathologic responses that a vessel can display on any particular imaging modality. The lumen can be narrow, large, irregular or occluded. The wall can be thick, calcified or interrupted. Major vascular anomalies also can be identified, such as at the aortic arch including coarctations [3] (Figure 20.1). Specific alterations of the lumen and wall, as well as their distribution in the vascular bed, allow most diagnoses to be made. There are many overlapping imaging features among diseases often making specific

Vascular Pathology. Edited by W.E. Stehbens and J.T. Lie. Published in 1995 by Chapman & Hall, London. ISBN 0 412 48640 7

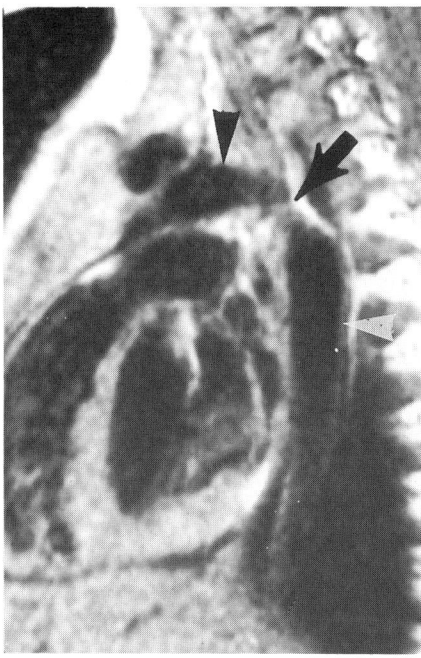

Figure 20.1 MR scan taken in sagittal projection. Coarctation of the thoracic aorta (arrow). With this scan sequence the vascular structures are black. A segment of the aortic arch (black arrowhead) and the descending thoracic aorta (white arrowhead) are identified.

order. Consideration of the disease process is particularly important when considering lower quality filming systems such as digital subtraction angiography and cine filming. These systems are in widespread use and are not capable of providing diagnostic images in certain diseases.

20.3 Arterial diseases

20.3.1 ARTERIOSCLEROSIS

Arteriosclerosis is the most common disease encountered in the course of imaging blood vessels. The spectrum of findings is very broad, from slight irregularity of vessel lumen to extreme shagginess (Figures 20.2, 20.3). The distribution varies throughout the arterial bed depending upon the underlying etiologic factors as well as the age of the patient. Angiography offers the best imaging modality overall for making the diagnosis and evaluating its distribution within the vascular bed. There are, however, features of other imaging systems which also make them valuable. Ultrasound is excellent to detect stenoses at the carotid artery bifurcation and of the larger arteries of the extremities, and computed tomography is ex-

diagnoses difficult. However, usually a specific pathologic diagnosis can be made if enough imaging is provided. This is possible by having a great understanding of the imaging patterns of disease, not unlike those principles underlying the practice of pathology.

Before addressing imaging findings of arterial disease, some description of normal vessels and characteristics of angiographic systems are in order. Arteries have walls that are smooth and parallel. There follows a branch and a reduction in caliber. There should be no zones of expansion or tapering. If either of these findings exist, there is an underlying disease condition, even if only spasm is the etiology. Attention to such details in interpretation can be the difference between making or missing an early diagnosis. It is therefore intrinsic to this interpretive process that film quality be the highest possible in terms of spatial and contrast resolution. Spatial resolution refers to the ability of the film system to resolve the smallest distance between a pair of lines, while contrast resolution refers to the ability of the film system to distinguish the smallest difference of radiographic density between two tissues, that is, detectable shades of gray. Obviously, if the structure being studied is large, such as the aorta or a main primary artery, then it is not so critical that the imaging system be of such high quality, but if the disease process is affecting the digital arteries or the distal arteries of the abdominal viscera, then the film quality must be of the highest

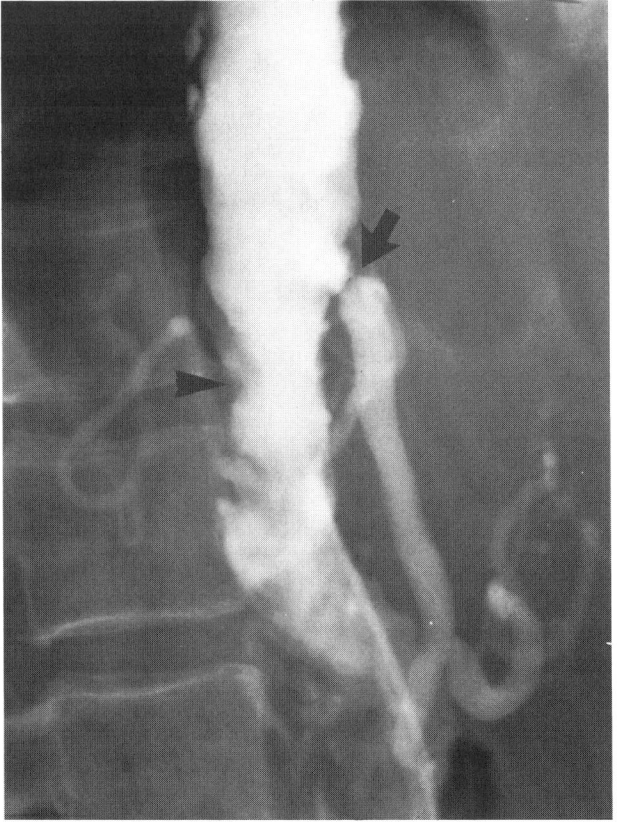

Figure 20.2 Lateral view of the abdominal aorta shows stenosis of the superior mesenteric artery (arrow). The celiac artery is not seen because of occlusion. Note the large plaques on the posterior wall of the aorta (arrowhead).

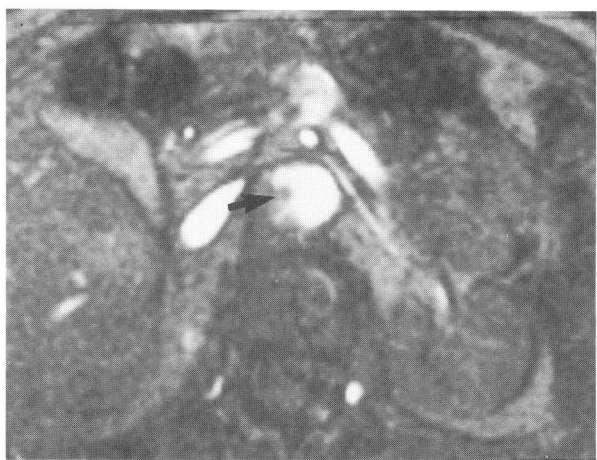

Figure 20.3 MRI cross-section through the abdomen above the renal arteries. The irregularity of the right side of the aorta from 6 o'clock to 10 o'clock (arrow) is probably atheromatous disease but could be old thrombus.

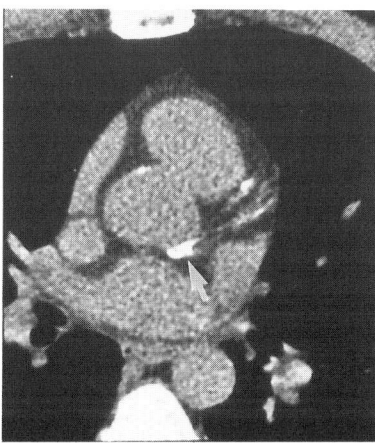

Figure 20.4 Fast-CT scan taken without contrast material through the upper heart in a patient with advanced coronary artery disease. Note the dense atheromatous calcification at the origin of the main left coronary artery (arrow). There are also calcific plaques in the left anterior descending and its diagonal branch.

cellent to identify atheromatous calcification in arteries to a limit of about 2 mm in diameter (Figure 20.4).

The angiographic findings of atheromatous disease are of two categories; those that are specific to the arterial lumen and those that consider the distribution of disease in the vascular bed. The appearance of atheromatous disease varies greatly throughout the course of the disease process. Early, and in a young patient, the lesion will appear as a smooth plaque on the wall of the artery either as an eccentric plaque or as a focal stenosis that is somewhat concentric and tapered. There may be only a few lesions scattered at the origins of primary and secondary branches, such as the sub-

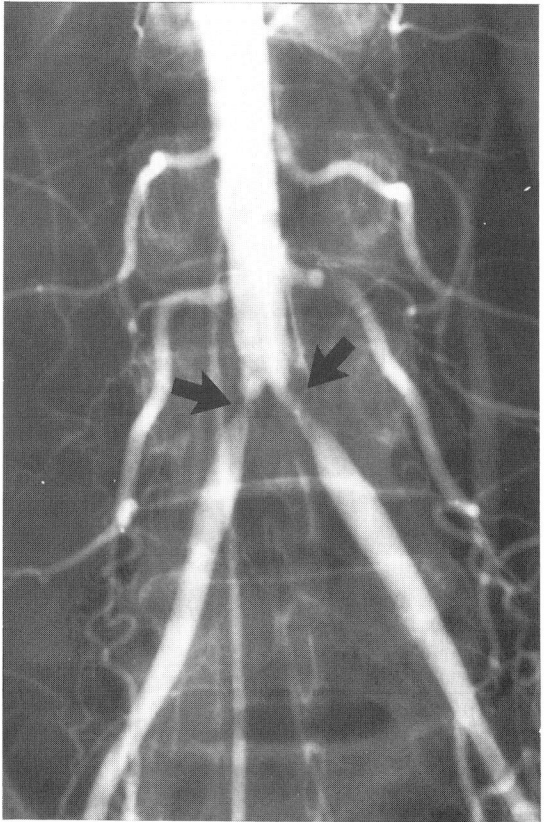

Figure 20.5 Abdominal aortogram. Bilateral iliac artery stenosis (arrows) of atheromatous disease from cigarette smoking in this 50-year-old patient. Note the mild irregularity of the wall of the lower aorta. Distal to the iliac stenoses, the arteries are normal.

clavian, internal carotid and renal arteries. Such patients usually have a history of cigarette smoking and are susceptible to so-called premature atherosclerosis. The main morphologic feature of such lesions in young patients is smooth borders. If only the primary aortic branches are affected and these smooth lesions produce a tapered stenosis, it is possible to confuse the diagnosis with Takayasu's arteritis, but with adequate experience and with angiograms of both the thoracic and abdominal aortic segments, rarely should this mistake be made. Areas of minimal vascular abnormality and their distribution can be clues to the correct diagnosis.

Another common site of early atherosclerotic lesion in the patient who smokes, is at the lower abdominal aorta and the proximal common iliac arteries (Figure 20.5). In contrast to the smooth appearance of early lesions involving the primary and secondary branches, aortoiliac lesions often have irregular borders. The disease involvement, when first found, is usually very focal or extends for only a few centimeters from the aortic bifurcation. The onset of symptoms, the most common being claudication, can occur as early as the beginning of the fourth decade of life. In such young patients,

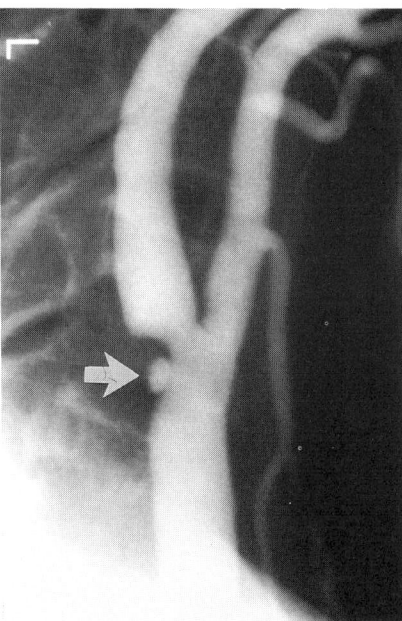

Figure 20.6 Carotid arteriogram at the bifurcation shows an atheromatous plaque with an ulcer (arrow).

the distal arteries, from the external iliac segments throughout the femoral, popliteal and tibial distribution, are almost always normal by angiography. The predilection for cigarette smoking to produce isolated and extensive atheromatous lesions at the aortoiliac site is so unique that finding it on an angiogram in a patient, who is under 60 years of age, confidently predicts that smoking is the etiology. This is an example of an angiographic appearance and distribution of a disease process allowing not only the diagnosis to be made but the etiology also to be assigned. Many such examples exist in diagnostic vascular imaging.

For most patients, the atheromatous disease related to cigarette smoking seems to begin at the aortoiliac site and spread cephalad and caudad over the course of many years until the sites of involvement are widespread. The other group of patients, who first have symptoms from lesions at origins of primary and secondary aortic branches, as mentioned above, also will have some degree of atheromatous disease at the aortoiliac site.

A different distribution of atheromatous lesions is found in elderly patients who do not have a smoking history. The lesion sites are predominantly in the arteries of the lower extremities. The appearance of the lesions and their pattern of distribution are somewhat similar to that found in diabetic patients; stenoses and occlusions are present in the tibial arteries and in the distal superficial femoral and popliteal arterial segments. There is either relative or complete sparing of the aortoiliac segment in many of these patients. However, they often have advanced disease in the internal iliac arteries and in the deep femoral branches. These two arterial beds are usually unaffected in the young smoking population unless Buerger's disease is present. It is of interest to note that the arteries of the upper extremities, except the proximal subclavian sites, are often uninvolved by advanced atheromatous disease in both the smoking population and in elderly patients who do not smoke, while those same arteries are so often severely affected in the insulin-dependent diabetic population.

In all of these atherosclerotic patients, the angiographic appearance of the lesions has a wide variation and the lesions are not necessarily bilateral. In the same patient, with advanced disease, there may be shelf-like

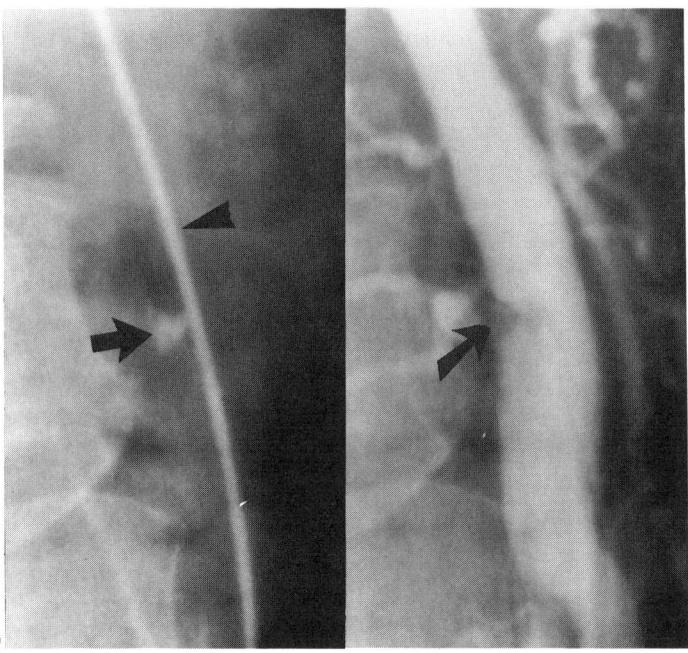

Figure 20.7 (a) Lateral view of the low abdominal aorta shows a calcific density (arrow) just posterior to the intraaortic catheter (arrowhead). This is an atheromatous plaque projecting as a sessile polyp into the aorta. (b) The aorta has been injected with contrast material and the calcific atheromatous sessile polyp is seen as a filling defect (arrow). Note that in the presence of contrast material within the aortic lumen it is not possible to detect the calcific nature of the plaque.

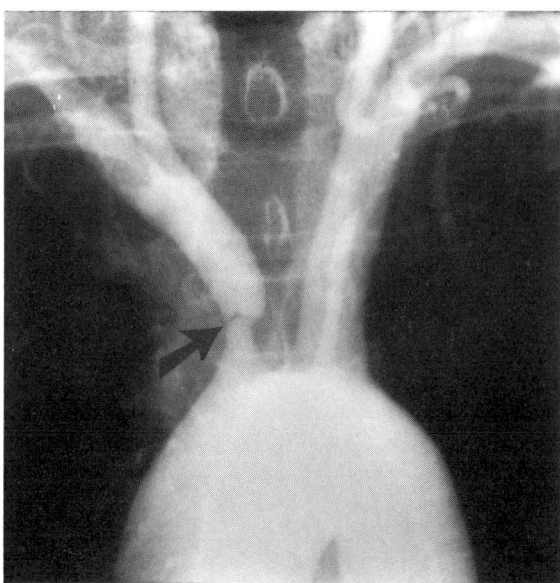

Figure 20.8 Thoracic aortogram in anteroposterior view shows stenosis of the innominate artery with a shelf-like lesion (arrow). This is an atheromatous lesion. This patient has almost no evidence of disease elsewhere.

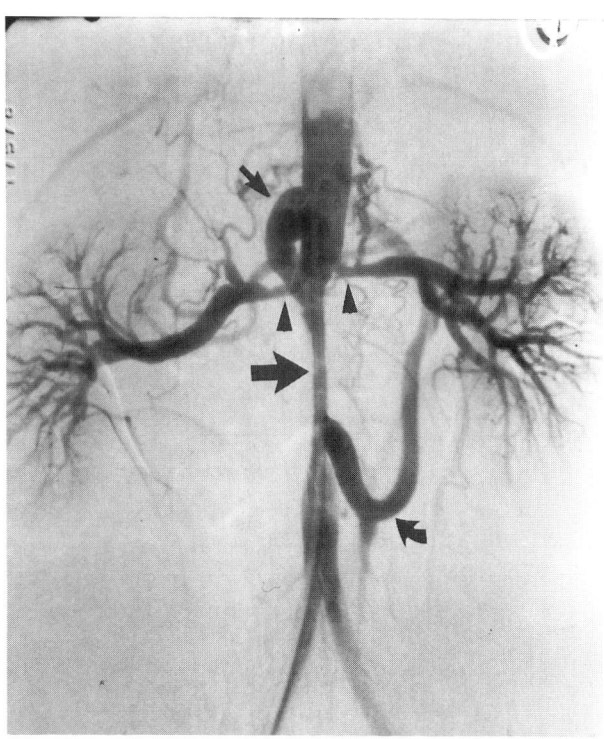

Figure 20.9 Abdominal aortogram. Takayasu's disease with segmental stenosis of the infrarenal aorta (horizontal arrow). The renal arteries (arrowheads) are stenotic proximally. The inferior mesenteric artery (curved arrow) is enlarged and supplies collateral filling of the celiac artery which is occluded at its origin. Note that the proximal superior mesenteric artery is aneurysmal (top arrow).

plaques, sessile plaques, ulcers, focal asymmetric or symmetric stenoses, long segmental stenoses, irregular luminal borders without stenosis and occlusions [4,5,6] (Figures 20.6, 20.7, 20.8). This multifaceted appearance is characteristic of atheromatous disease. Occasionally, it may mimic other vascular disease such Buerger's disease, temporal arteritis or Takayasu's disease. It is important to be familiar with differences in the appearance and distribution of lesions in each disease condition and for each patient age group.

20.3.2 VASCULITIS

Vasculitis is a complex collection of diseases that have variable effects upon blood vessels of differing sizes and distribution depending on the etiology of vasculitis. Many involve arteries that are too small to identify angiographically. A few of them affect larger arteries in certain patterns and distributions which allows angiographic diagnosis. The angiogram shows bilateral involvement that is not necessarily uniformly symmetric. The constellation of angiographic findings allows differentiation of the type of vasculitis in many cases.

(a) Takayasu's and temporal arteritis

Both Takayasu's and temporal arteritis can present with similiar angiographic findings, i.e. bilateral stenotic changes of the subclavian, axillary and proximal brachial arteries and rarely of the femoral, popliteal and proximal tibial arteries [5,7–9]. The major distinguishing feature is involvement of the aorta and its primary branches found in Takayasu's disease. Also, from a clinical standpoint, Takayasu's disease occurs in patients under 40 years of age and temporal arteritis occurs in patients over 50 years of age. These simple guidelines apply in at least 95% of the cases. If the age of the patient is not known and the radiologist must make a diagnosis from the angiograms alone, then complete assessment must be made of each arterial bed. The more areas covered by the angiogram, the more accurate will be the diagnosis.

Because of the overlap of the arterial involvement of Takayasu's and temporal arteritis, details that distinguish these two diseases must be sought. Takayasu's disease has certain angiographic characteristics that are unique. The aorta and its primary branches are virtually always affected. The aortic findings are irregularity of the lumen, narrowing of the lumen, thickening of the wall and aneurysmal changes. The distribution of these findings are predominately: the ascending segment, the descending area just beyond the arch, above the diaphragmatic hiatus and the zone through the abdominal viscera (Figure 20.9). Of course, in some cases the entire aorta is abnormal. Occasionally, calcification of the aortic wall occurs, probably as a manifestation of the healing phase. This may be found in young patients

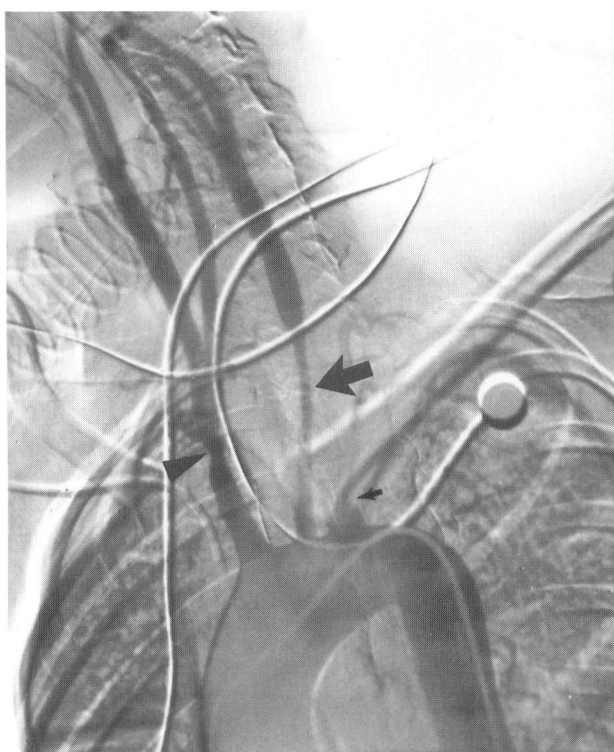

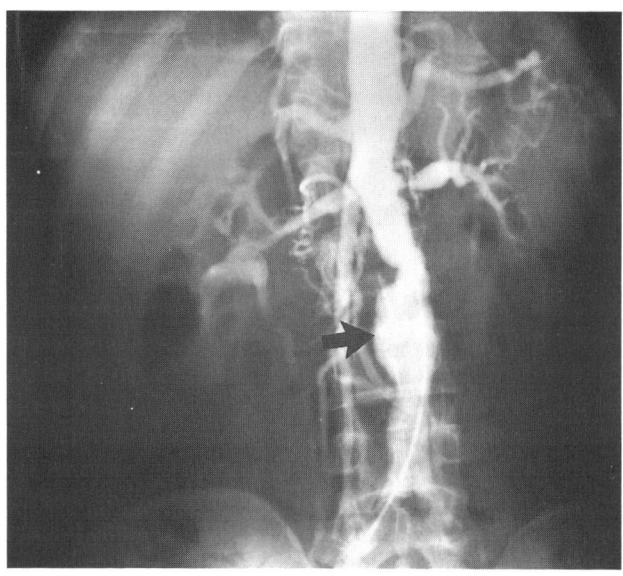

Figure 20.11 Abdominal aortogram in a teenage boy with Takayasu's disease. There is marked irregularity of the infrarenal aorta with one area of moderate narrowing and aneurysm formation below it (arrow). There is also high grade stenosis in the proximal left main renal artery.

Figure 20.10 Aortic arch injection in the left anterior oblique view shows abnormalities of the brachiocephalic arteries compatible with Takayasu's disease. The left subclavian is occluded in a flame-shaped point (small arrow). The proximal left common carotid (large arrow) has diffuse tubular narrowing. The distal innominate artery (arrowhead) has focal narrowing. The right subclavian artery is occluded.

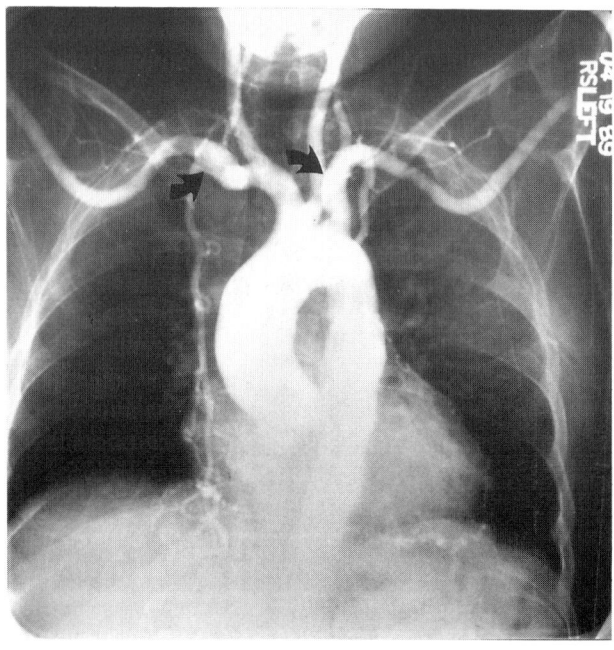

Figure 20.12 Thoracic aortogram in a young woman with Takayasu's disease. Note the diffuse irregularity of the lumen with slight ectasia involving the thoracic aorta. There is also ectasia of the proximal subclavian arteries (arrows).

in whom there would be no differential diagnosis of atherosclerosis. Such a finding gives confidence to the diagnosis of Takayasu's disease.

Sometimes the entire aorta appears normal. It is then that the angiographic appearance of the primary branches becomes especially important [8]. Considering how young this population is, any abnormalities of the aortic branches should raise speculation of Takayasu's disease (Figure 20.10). In the absence of cigarette smoking, almost no other disease affects this distribution of arteries. The same imaging findings that are found in the aorta are to be searched for in the primary branches, namely: irregularity, stenosis and aneurysm, with the addition of occlusions which are preceded by concentric tapering. Involvement can also be found in secondary and tertiary branches. About one-third of Takayasu's patients have aneurysmal changes, the aorta being more often affected than the branches (Figures 20.11, 20.12). The abdominal visceral arteries are often involved by proximal stenotic lesions, the superior mesenteric and renal arteries more often than the celiac and inferior mesenteric arteries. Renal artery stenosis is a major cause of hypertension in these patients. However, aortic stenosis may also be severe enough to cause hypertension.

The stenotic lesions of Takayasu's disease, and also of temporal arteritis, are smooth and tapered in most instances. The tapering can be very long and involves

ARTERIAL DISEASES 705

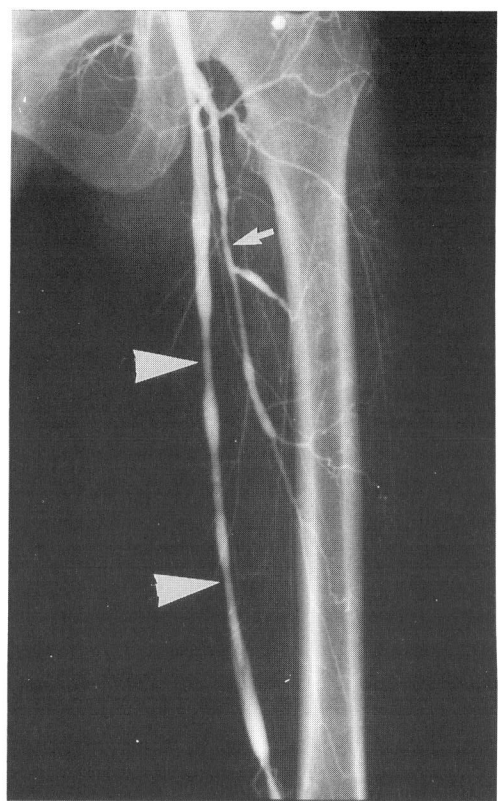

Figure 20.13 Femoral arteriogram of a young woman with Takayasu's disease. There are multiple areas of smooth stenoses (arrowheads) alternating with normal zones in the course of the superficial femoral artery. Similar disease is present in the deep femoral artery (arrow).

both ends of the stenotic segment. Furthermore, the tapered lesions are relatively concentric as they become stenotic (Figure 20.13). These are important characteristics because many cases of atherosclerosis demonstrate tapered stenoses, but usually only the proximal end of the stenosis is tapered. The distal end is usually more rounded or squared (Figure 20.14). Also, if the distal end is found to be somewhat tapered, it is rarely concentric.

Narrowing of arteries by arteritis may be very slight and subtle, perhaps representing only a 5 or 10% reduction of the lumen. This is easily overlooked, but may be the only sign of arteritis. The previously mentioned point about arterial walls being parallel until a branch divides is an important observation in detecting arteritis. In the acute phase of Takayasu's disease, the walls of the vessels may be thickened (Figure 20.15). The one place where this can be seen by angiography is the aorta where the wall is outlined by the air in the lung: the right side of the ascending segment and the left side of the descending segment. Otherwise, arterial wall thickness cannot be assessed by angiography. However, computed tomography, ultrasound and magnetic resonance images can display vessel wall thickness.

Temporal arteritis (giant cell arteritis) can be detected in about 10–20% of the patients with the disease by angiography of the brachiocephalic arteries and rarely of the femoral arteries [9]. The usual method of diagnosis is from a temporal artery biopsy, but for those few patients who manifest large artery involvement, angio-

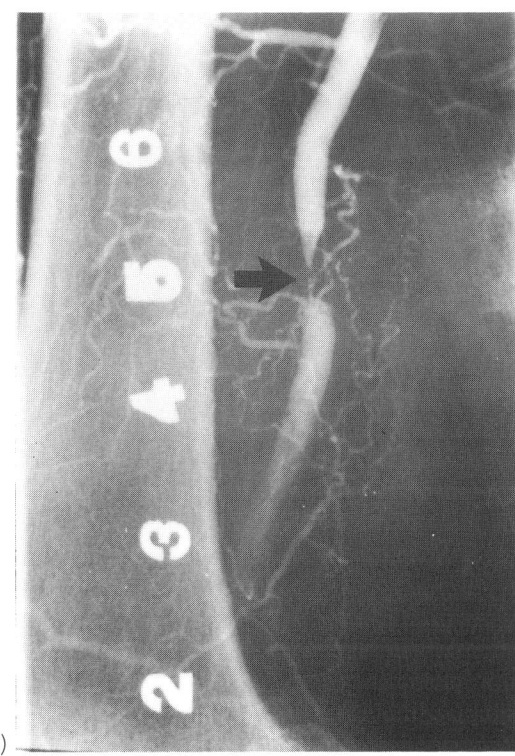 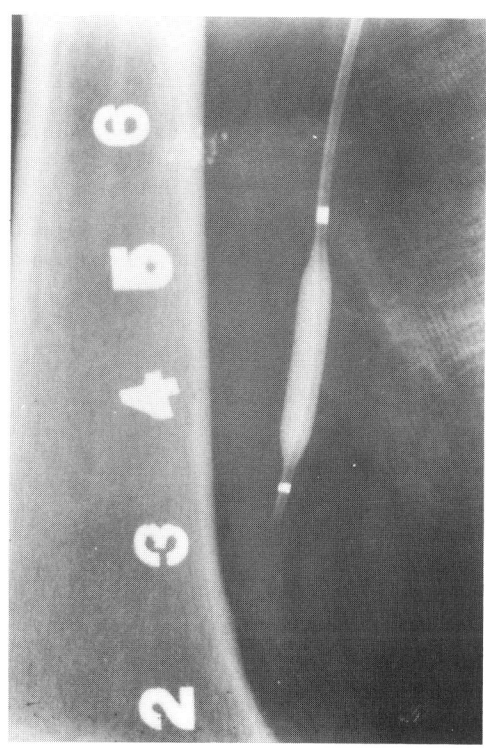

(a) (b)

Figure 20.14a,b

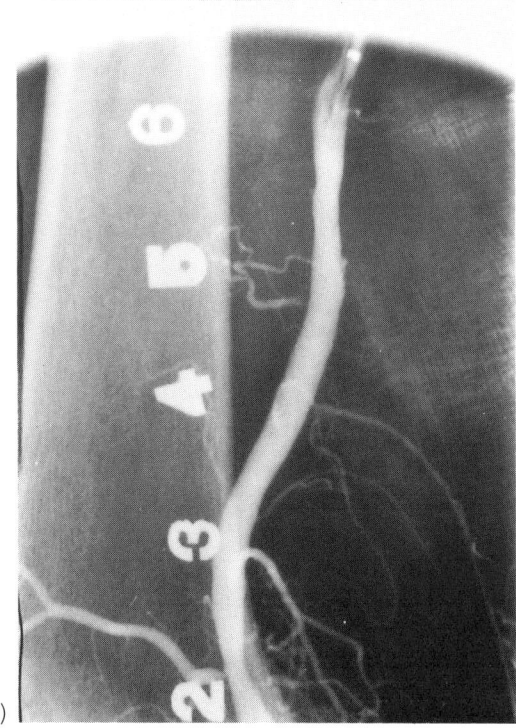

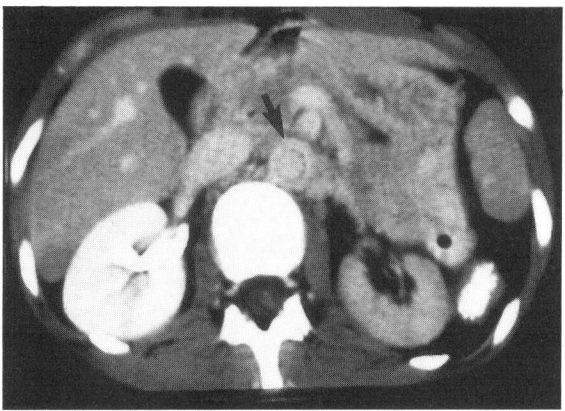

Figure 20.15 CT scan through the renal level. Acute phase of Takayasu's arteritis shows a high density ring (arrow) around the aorta. This disappeared after a few weeks of steroid therapy.

Figure 20.14 (a) Femoral angiogram shows a high grade atheromatous stenosis (arrow) at the femoral–popliteal junction. Note the proximal tapering of the lesion while the distal segment has a flat border. This is a typical atheromatous lesion in a young patient or a lesion early in the course of the disease process. (b) A balloon catheter has been placed across the stenosis and inflated. (c) After the balloon catheter dilatation there is considerable improvement in the caliber of the artery.

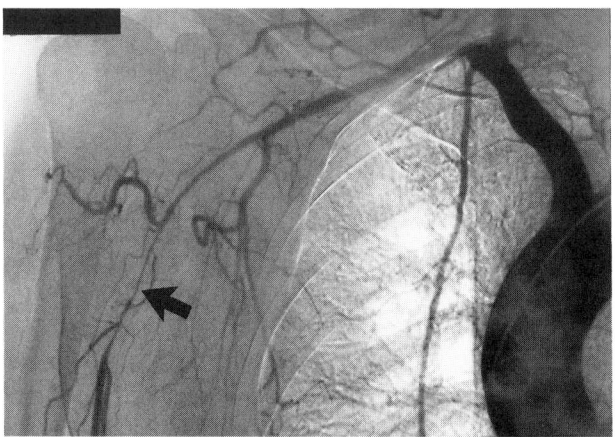

Figure 20.16 Arch aortogram with filming over the right shoulder. Temporal arteritis. The segmental stenosis of the axillary and brachial artery junction (arrow) has the typical appearance of either temporal arteritis or Takayasu's arteritis, but in this patient who is 60 years of age the diagnosis is the former.

graphy can make the specific diagnosis (Figure 20.16). The angiographic changes in the brachiocephalic arteries are those of stenoses, occlusions and rarely small fusiform aneurysms. The subclavian and axillary artery segments are the most commonly affected and often there is extension into the proximal brachial artery. In contrast to Takayasu's disease, the common carotid arteries are not affected, nor are the innominate and proximal left subclavian arterial segments. Furthermore, no other primary branch of the aorta is affected. The aorta is rarely affected, unlike the high frequency of involvement in Takayasu's disease. Lesions of the aorta in temporal arteritis are focal false aneurysms or dissections, and while they often lead to death, they are not often documented by any imaging.

In a few patients with temporal arteritis, leg claudication is the predominant symptom. The femoral angiogram shows a somewhat similar pattern of arterial involvement as that seen in the brachiocephalic arteries. The stenotic arterial segments are often long and show alternating zones of involvement. The prominent feature is concentric tapering of the arteries at the stenotic junctions. The involvement can extend into the proximal tibial arteries (Figure 20.17). The branches of the deep femoral arteries are a particularly good place to find evidence of temporal arteritis. This arterial bed is resistant to disease in many patients with atherosclerosis except for the proximal 1 or 2 cm. Whenever diffuse stenotic disease is found here, something unusual should be considered in the diagnosis, such as vasculitis or ergot toxicity. However, patients with advanced diabetic arteriopathy or elderly patients with advanced arteriosclerosis often have severe occlusive disease of the deep femoral branches, but the lumen of the vessels show coarse irregularity rather than the smooth walls of long segments of stenosis and concentric tapering as is found with temporal arteritis (and Takayasu's arteritis).

The angiographic findings of both temporal arteritis

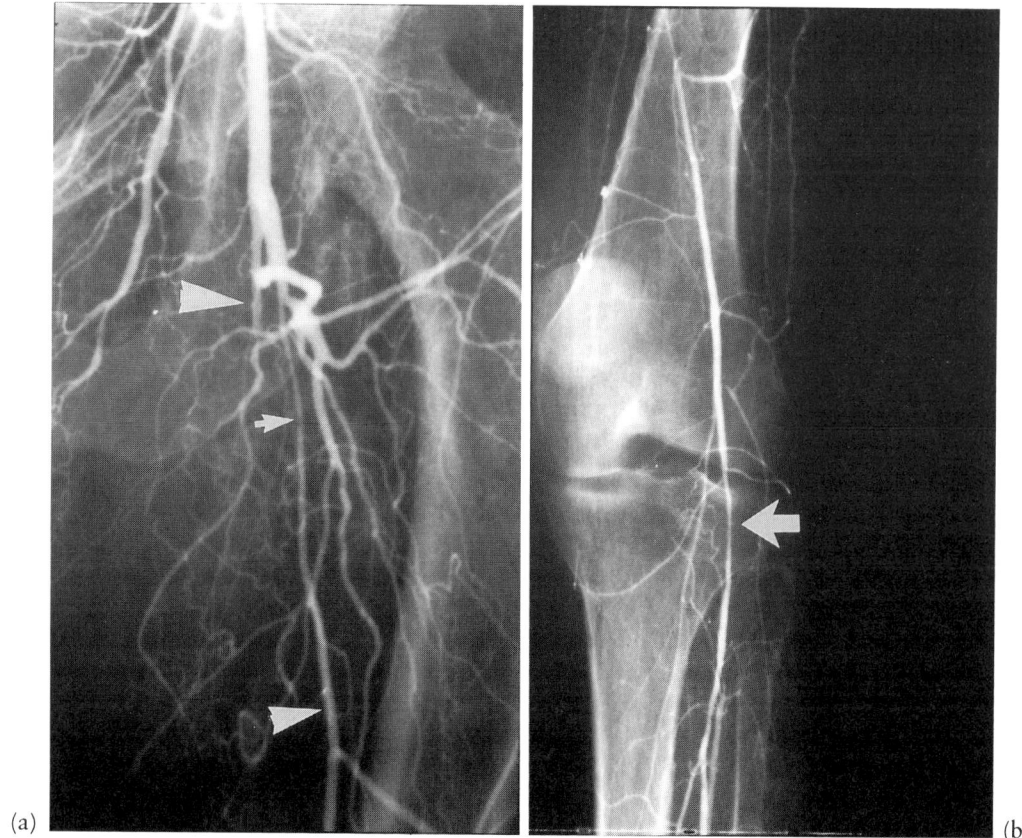

Figure 20.17 Temporal arteritis in a 65-year-old patient. (a) Femoral angiogram over the proximal thigh shows a long area of smooth narrowing in the deep femoral artery (arrow). Note the caliber of the artery returns to normal distally (lower arrowhead). There is also occlusion of the superficial femoral artery (top arrowhead) which has diffuse narrowing in its proximal segment. (b) In the popliteal segment there is diffuse narrowing at and below the knee joint level (arrow). There is also slight narrowing of the posteriotibial trunk. At the proximal popliteal segment there is diffuse narrowing. These skip areas of smooth stenoses are typical for temporal arteritis.

and Takayasu's disease are usually so classic in appearance and distribution that the diagnosis would be virtually certain by an experienced angiographer. This is true for at least three-quarters of the cases encountered. It would seem to be unnecessary to seek a biopsy for proof in such cases. Indeed, many patients with Takayasu's disease are diagnosed by angiography and placed on a course of steroid therapy without submitting to a biopsy. Of course, there is no suitable superficial arterial source for a biopsy in Takayasu's disease as there is in temporal arteritis, namely, the superficial temporal artery. Therefore, if faith is placed in the angiographic interpretation, two factors should be considered: the experience of the angiographer and the angiographic evidence of the disease. To a certain extent, these are related and inseparable.

Two important diseases must be differentiated from Takayasu's disease and one from temporal arteritis. For the stenotic form of Takayasu's disease, early atherosclerosis must be excluded. For the aneurysmal form, an elastic tissue disease such as Ehlers–Danlos syndrome and Marfan syndrome must be excluded. Usually, this is possible. In the case of temporal arteritis, atherosclerosis may be a major point of differential contention. This disease is prevalent in the elderly population. The overlap of simultaneously occurring diseases is frequent and needs to be differentiated. The experience of the angiographer is indeed pivotal and, when a confident diagnosis can be made, it will be supported by the biopsy or by the outcome of the treatment.

(b) Buerger's disease

Buerger's disease is another vascular disease that often has unique angiographic findings. These patients have an extraordinary sensitivity to cigarette smoke which causes obliteration of distal arteries of the extremities. The disease moves proximally over several years. The occlusive pattern has some characteristics that distinguish it from arteriosclerosis [5,10]. The distal small branches are stenotic and occluded before similar changes progress proximally. There are skip areas of arterial involvement in the hands and feet. The terminal segments of normal arteries often show tapered ends

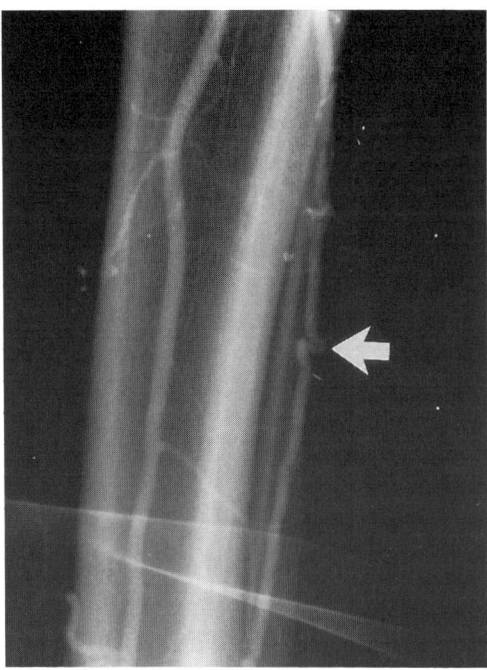

Figure 20.18 Tibial arteriogram in Buerger's disease manifesting as marked irregular tortuousity (arrow) of the anterior tibial artery. This is a so-called corkscrew appearance which in this location is specific for this disease.

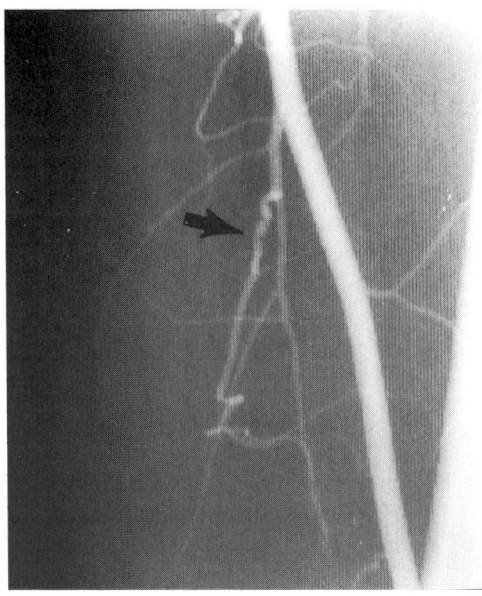

Figure 20.19 Femoral angiogram in Buerger's disease. The irregularity of this branch (arrow) of the superficial femoral artery is direct evidence of Buerger's disease.

similar to other types of vasculitis. A paucity of collateral arteries is in contrast with the extensive number that so frequently accompanies arteriosclerosis. One unique type of collateral pathway found is the persistence of the vasa vasorum of the occluded tibial arteries. They become enlarged and tortuous and are commonly seen in Buerger's disease and rarely seen in occlusions of atherosclerosis. Another characteristic angiographic finding is at the ends of occluded main arteries of the lower leg and forearm. An irregular tapering of the main artery is found several millimeters beyond the last adjacent branch. This is in contrast to the chronic occlusions of atheromatous disease which have a rounded, convex end, which is immediately distal to an adjacent patent branch that serves as a collateral for distal refilling. The above arterial findings contribute to the overall appearance of Buerger's disease but are not entirely diagnostic. However, there is a more specific arterial abnormality which is only occasionally identified; an intraluminal irregularity involving a short segment near the proximal limit of the involved major artery (Figure 20.18). It is also found in branches of the deep femoral artery and in the small branches of the distal superficial femoral artery and is frequently encountered (Figure 20.19). The appearance is that of an irregular stenosis that sometimes has a corkscrew path similar to the angiographic appearance of some forms of medial fibroplasia. This is a unique finding which in some cases provides the only direct evidence of Buerger's disease when otherwise the distal occlusive arterial pattern is non-specific. This is another example where the appearance of disease of the deep femoral arterial branches provides a window of opportunity to make a definitive diagnosis. In difficult diagnostic cases, having an angiogram that includes the deep femoral artery can make the difference between a diagnosis and a mystery.

It is important to distinguish this intra-arterial corkscrew appearance of Buerger's disease, from highly tortuous regional collateral arteries that can be found around zones of occlusion in atherosclerosis and from the similar appearance of the highly tortuous vasa vasorum in occlusions of thromboangiitis obliterans. A prominent and tortuous vasa vasorum is not as specific for Buerger's disease as is the intraluminal corkscrew appearance.

There are two additional angiographic findings that warrant attention in Buerger's disease: ectasia of regional arteries and spasm. The ectasia is most often identified in the popliteal artery but also can be found in the hand arteries. Spasm is usually encountered only in arteries of the hands and feet. Angiograms taken before and after an intra-arterial injection of a vasodilator drug can demonstrate this.

The main differential diagnostic considerations for Buerger's disease are arteriosclerosis and embolic disease. Because Buerger's disease has its onset in young patients and because it starts in distal arteries, atheromatous disease is usually not difficult to rule out, except in insulin-dependent diabetic patients. Occasionally, an elderly patient is encountered who had developed Buerger's disease when younger and had avoided cigarette smoking for the ensuing years, but carries permanent occlusive arterial disease. The characteristic angiographic findings of Buerger's disease no longer would be evident. This is probably true for many types of vasculitis that heal with the result that the angiogram looks similar to arteriosclerosis. The other problematic differential is previous embolic disease that has a residual of partial recanalization. This may result in a non-specific angiographic appearance which can be difficult to distinguish unless the more specific, direct angiographic findings of Buerger's disease are present.

(c) Polyarteritis nodosa

Polyarteritis nodosa (PAN) is another vasculitis that has unique angiographic findings that permit a somewhat specific diagnosis. Actually, such angiographic findings support a diagnosis of a necrotizing vasculitis of which PAN is the most frequently encountered in patients coming to angiography. Rarely, other types of vasculitis, such as rheumatoid and Churg–Strauss syndrome, may present at angiography with similar changes to PAN. The main arterial beds to be studied for PAN are the abdominal viscera, which include the kidneys, the gut, the liver and the spleen [10,11]. Occasionally, arteries of the extremities are affected. The angiographic findings are stenoses, occlusions and aneurysms. Aneurysms are the hallmark of a necrotizing vasculitis (Figures 20.20, 20.21). They are present in less than half of the PAN patients coming to angiography. Polyarteritis manifests itself in the terminal arteries of the viscera and extends proximally to arteries of a diameter of 3–4 mm. The aneurysms are found more often in the mid- to upper size range of these vessels and the stenoses and occlusions are found distally. Excellent film quality is required to detect the early arterial abnormalities of PAN. It is important that the diagnostic angiogram include injections of each of the abdominal visceral arteries, at least until one of them reveals aneurysms. Often, only one of the vascular beds will show the disease.

The differential diagnosis of PAN depends upon what angiographic abnormality is found, occlusions or aneurysms and, to some extent, in which arterial bed the abnormalities are found. If only occlusions or stenoses are present in the terminal arteries, they have no specific angiographic characteristic. If this involves the mesenteric arteries, it is a non-specific finding and is to be interpreted only in the context of the clinical history. If found in the renal arteries, the differential diagnosis includes many renal diseases. If multiple aneurysms are found, then the confidence for diagnosing PAN is high, although other types of necrotizing vasculitis are non-excluded. Another possible disease condition to consider would be disseminated mycotic aneurysms. Rarely, patients with fibromuscular dysplasia may have scattered

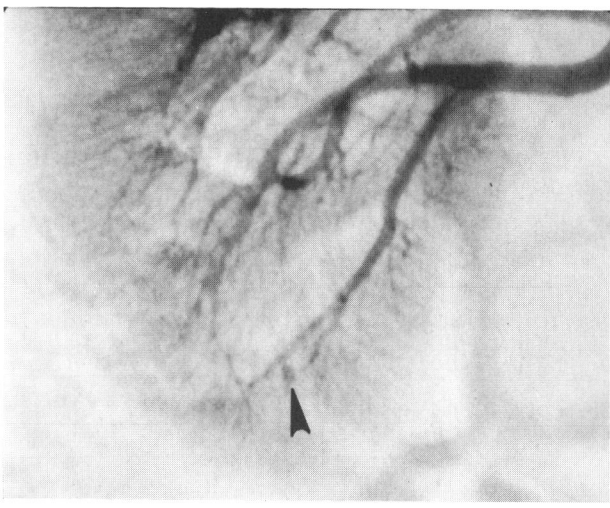

Figure 20.20 Right renal arteriogram in a patient with polyarteritis nodosa shows a microaneurysm in the lower pole at the level of an arcuate artery (arrowhead).

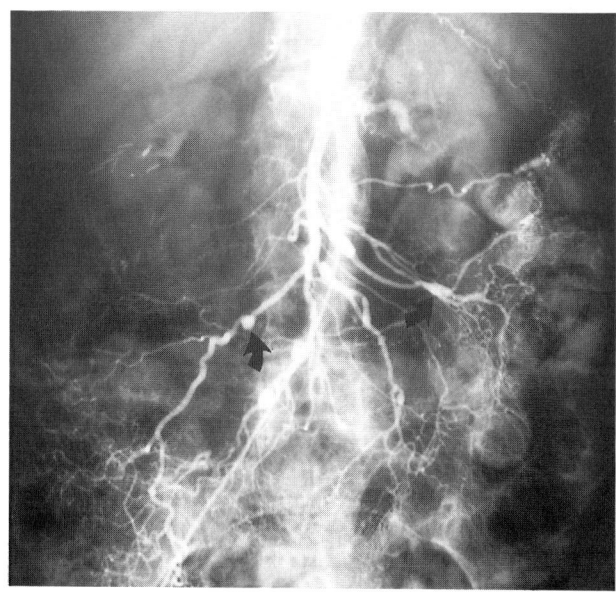

Figure 20.21 Superior mesenteric angiogram shows scattered areas of vascular ectasia and irregularity (arrows). This appearance is compatible with necrotizing vasculitis. This patient has polyarteritis nodosum.

aneurysms in the visceral arteries, but usually it is limited to larger branches than are found in PAN. Finally, patients in cardiogenic shock or presenting with diffuse spasm of the mesenteric arteries from other causes, may have an angiographic pattern that mimics stenoses or multiple aneurysms because of alternating degrees of spasm.

(d) Miscellaneous vasculitis

Vasculitis associated with connective tissue diseases, such as rheumatoid, as well as other types of rare vasculitis, do not have a specific angiographic appearance. Those patients with connective tissue disease who come to angiography most often have symptoms of hand ischemia and a non-specific vascular occlusive disease is evident. Sometimes characteristic findings of vasculitis are present, i.e. alternating zones of stenosis with occlusions.

20.3.3 ANEURYSM

Aneurysms of the major arteries are well suited to be studied by CT scanning, MRI and ultrasound (US), while the value of angiography is to provide preoperative identification of adjacent major branches or to evaluate for distal embolization. The advantage of CT, MRI and US is that they detect the outer wall of the aneurysm, while the angiogram only identifies the patent lumen which may be much smaller than the outer wall diameter in the presence of mural thrombus [1,2,12,13]. CT scanning provides more specific information about the characteristics of an aneurysm than does ultrasound, such as rupture, infection, inflammatory tissue, false aneurysms and complications of vascular grafts.

The most common aneurysm is found at the infrarenal aorta. Ultrasound is usually the only imaging modality required because size and extent can be determined. However, for those patients with diffuse aneurysmal disease (arteriomegaly), CT or angiography are more suitable to evaluate the iliac arteries and the thoracic aorta. These patients have a high incidence of femoral and popliteal aneurysms for which angiography provides the best global view for surgical planning, especially below the knee [14]. Patients with Ehlers–Danlos syndrome also may have aneurysms in multiple locations including the aorta, the visceral arteries, and in the peripheral arteries. Patients with Marfan syndrome often have an aneurysm of the ascending aorta (Figure 20.22). In both of these syndromes, dissections are commonly associated [4,15].

(a) Aneurysm complications

Complications of aneurysms are best evaluated by CT scanning which overall provides the most specific imaging information. Rupture of an aortic aneurysm is detected on CT scan sections by hemorrhage causing obliteration of the surrounding fat-tissue planes (Figure 20.33). The resulting hematoma in the retroperitoneum is displayed as a high CT density compared to the surrounding structures. Therefore, it is not necessary to use i.v. contrast material to identify a ruptured aneurysm of the aorta and iliac arteries. If i.v. contrast material is

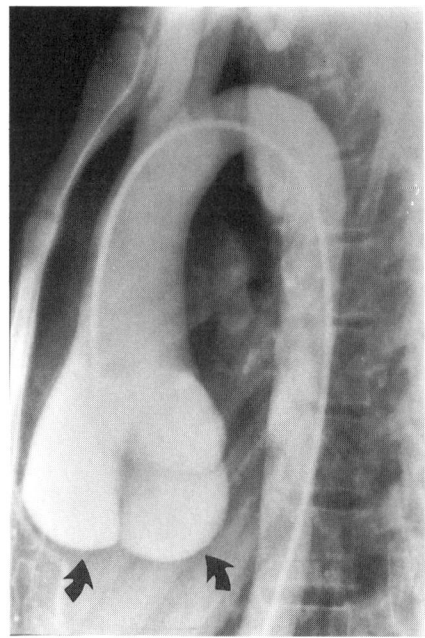

Figure 20.22 Thoracic aortogram in lateral view shows aneurysmal dilatation of the sinuses of Valsalva (arrows) and the proximal ascending thoracic aorta. This patient has Marfan syndrome.

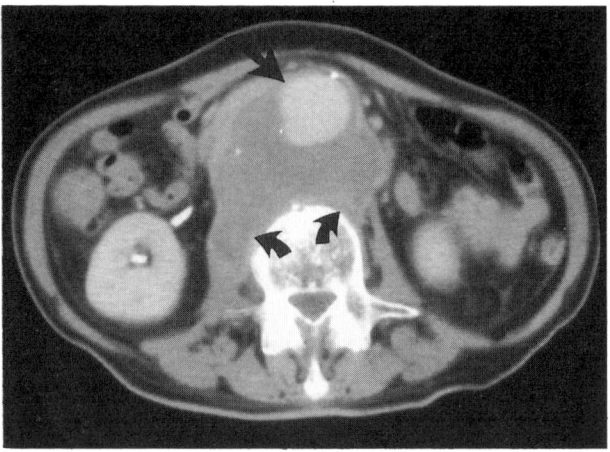

Figure 20.23 CT scan through the abdominal aorta below the renal artery level. There is a large aneurysm with a contained rupture and a relatively small lumen (arrow). There is obliteration by the aneurysm of the normally expected fat tissue planes adjacent to the spine (curved arrows).

used, it may be possible to define the site of the rupture if the contrast material is extravasated beyond the walls of the aneurysm. The use of CT scanning is helpful to confirm the presence of a rupture. Clinically, this may be difficult to establish because other conditions can mimic the pain of a symptomatic aneurysm, such as periaortic adenopathy, periaortitis and hemorrhage within the psoas or rectus muscle. Ultrasonography does not provide enough specific imaging information of the

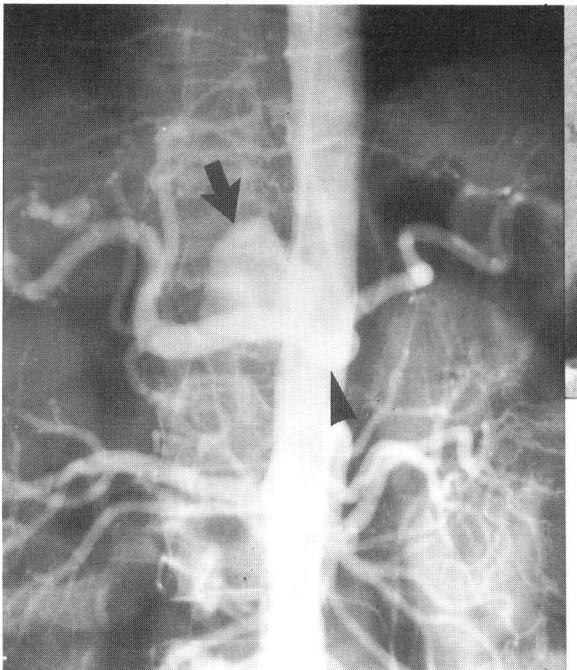
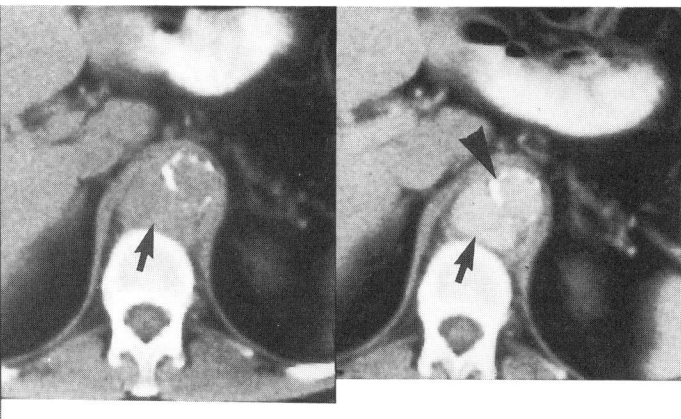

Figure 20.24 (a) Abdominal aortogram shows a false aneurysm (arrow) arising from the right side of the aorta just above the level of the celiac artery (arrowhead). (b) CT scan taken through the level of the false aneurysm (arrow) which is seen posteriorly on this non-contrast scan. (c) CT scan taken through the same level with i.v. contrast material shows opacification of the false aneurysm (arrow). The abdominal aorta (arrowhead) is densely calcified throughout most of its circumference.

retroperitoneum to be helpful, although it can prove the existence of an aneurysm of the aorta and in most cases also of the common iliac arteries. MRI provides diagnostic information similar to the findings of the CT scan.

(b) Mycotic aneurysm

Mycotic aneurysm of the aorta almost always has irregular borders and may show some evidence of destruction of the wall. The CT image is not diagnostic for infection but it is suggestive, especially if the location of the aneurysm is in an unusual site when compared to the much more frequent arteriosclerotic ones. The surrounding tissue of an infected aneurysm may show a low density fluid collection, indicating abscess. Mycotic aneurysms also may show obliteration of the surrounding soft tissue fat as the wall becomes destroyed and the lumen expands and is contained only by reactive, inflammatory tissue. This also represents one of the CT scan findings of a false aneurysm irrespective of etiology.

(c) False aneurysm

False aneurysm detection by an imaging modality depends upon the morphologic characteristics of the vascular pathology. If sufficient calcification of the intima is present, evidence for a false aneurysm may be detected by CT scanning. The ability of CT to detect calcification in arterial walls makes it valuable in displaying pathologic conditions and in diagnosing vascular disease. More than any other imaging technique, including plain films, CT images show calcification. In patients with arterioscleroses, the location of the most prominent calcification of the aorta and the primary branches is in the intima. Thus, the inner border demarcates the lumen. Extension of a portion of an aneurysm lumen beyond the confines of the intimal calcification indicates a false aneurysm (Figure 20.24). This is an important observation in the interpretation of vascular disease and adds specificity to the diagnosis. In the aorta, false aneurysms are found in various sizes from tiny and asymptomatic to huge and ruptured. Most of the small ones are related to ulceration of atheromatous plaques. Other etiologies include; infection, arteritis, contained rupture and trauma. Most traumatic aortic aneurysms, of those patients who survive to have a CT scan or aortogram, occur at the region of the ligamentum arteriosum and are secondary to a deceleration injury to the chest. Both CT and aortography have important roles in the diagnosis. The diagnosis is made by identifying a disruption of the inner wall of the aorta which sometimes involves the entire circumference and at other times presents as a small focal intimal disruption that is barely discernible. At times an old traumatic aneurysm is detected by CT scanning incidental to another indication for the examination. The location of the lesion and its irregular contour usually suggest the nature of the aneurysm.

(d) Inflammatory aneurysm

Inflammatory aneurysm of the aorta, also called periaortitis, has a unique CT appearance. In the region of the infrarenal abdominal aorta, a rind of hypervas-

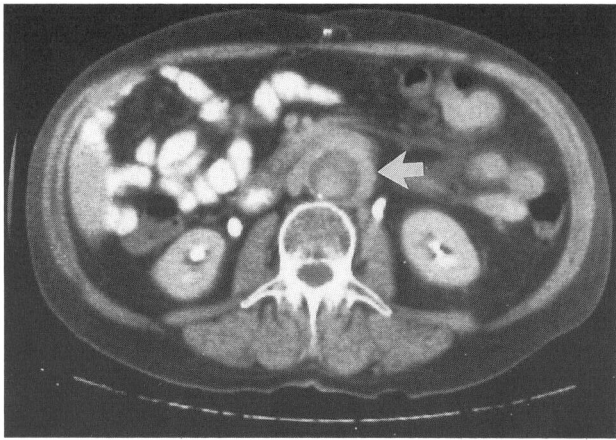

Figure 20.25 CT scan obtained with i.v. contrast material and through the infrarenal portion of the aorta. There is a small aneurysm with a thick rind of enhancing tissue (arrow) indicating periaortitis.

cular tissue is adherent to the anterior wall of the aorta. Hypervascularity is described as enhancement of the CT density following i.v. contrast material. The lesion extends to the sides of the aorta as a thinner layer than at the anterior portion (Figure 20.25). The posterior wall of the aorta is spared. The length of involvement is variable, sometimes extending to the iliac arteries. The ureters may become entrapped, which can be seen on the CT scan, and sometimes produce hydronephrosis. Periaortitis is a specific type of retroperitoneal fibrosis, one that has a characteristic CT scan appearance. The ultrasound image is also somewhat specific for this entity. The wall thickening is displayed as a hypoechoic zone anterior to the aortic lumen. However, the specificity is not as great as with CT images. Also, if the rind is thin, US may not detect the abnormality. Rarely this idiopathic inflammatory process originates in the thoracic aorta and may extend to the abdominal region in some cases. In the thoracic variety, the rind of inflammatory tissue surrounds the aortic wall rather than being just on the anterior and lateral walls. If the disease process is limited to the infrarenal segment of the aorta, almost no other disease condition has a similar appearance [16]. However, in some cases the abnormal tissue has an irregular, nodular appearance. In such cases the differential diagnosis would include adenopathy. Above the level of the renal arteries, if the inflammatory tissue encircles the aorta, then the differential diagnosis would include the acute phase of Takayasu's disease.

(e) Visceral artery aneurysm

Aneurysms of the abdominal visceral arteries occur from a variety of etiologies such as several types of necrotizing vasculitis, fibromuscular dysplasia, idiopathic dissection, arteriosclerosis, infection and Ehlers–Danlos syndrome. Angiography is an ideal modality to identify and assess their extent and character. However, CT scanning offers important information in some cases. Arteriosclerotic aneurysms usually have calcified borders which are easily detected by CT. Without the calcification, i.v. contrast material sometimes allows CT scan detection although an aneurysm would need a minimum diameter of nearly one centimeter to be visible (Figure 20.26). There are times when an unsuspected visceral artery aneurysm ruptures and a CT scan identifies the hematoma which would not have been appreciated at angiography. Together these two imaging procedures provide the best approach in complicated cases. Indeed, once a ruptured aneurysm is identified, it may be feasible to embolize it to stop the hemorrhage. This is especially true in the retroperitoneal location where surgical approach is limited.

(f) Peripheral aneurysms

In the peripheral vascular beds, similar etiologic types of aneurysms occur as those found in the viscera. Angiography is the most useful diagnostic modality, although MRI and US also have important roles in detection and surveillance. The most common type of aneurysm in the periphery is that which is related to arteriomegaly. They are almost always limited to the thigh and the popliteal area, the upper extremity rarely being involved (Figure 20.27). These aneurysms are diffuse, involving long segments. The walls are often markedly scalloped because of laminated mural thrombus. These tend to embolize and the angiogram is particularly useful for studying the length of the extremity and for providing a surgical map. Traumatic aneurysms of the extremities are usually evaluated satisfactorily by US, although some may require angiography, especially if they are deep or if the condition of the overlying tissue does not allow placement of the ultrasound probe.

20.3.4 DISSECTION

Aortic dissection is detected by all imaging modalities. The important findings are two lumens (one is false) and an intimal flap between them (Figure 20.28). In the thoracic area, transesophageal ultrasound offers superior images to transthoracic ones. MRI shows aortic dissections in any plane, which can facilitate visualization of the extent of the dissection. CT images can be obtained before and after the intravenous administration of contrast material. The scans taken before i.v. contrast material can identify the position of atheromatous calcification of the intima which, if displaced away from the wall, indicates some type of dissection is present. Also, adjacent hemorrhage can be detected. Use of contrast material allows complete anatomic display of the extent of the dissection [17]. If the CT scans are obtained

ARTERIAL DISEASES 713

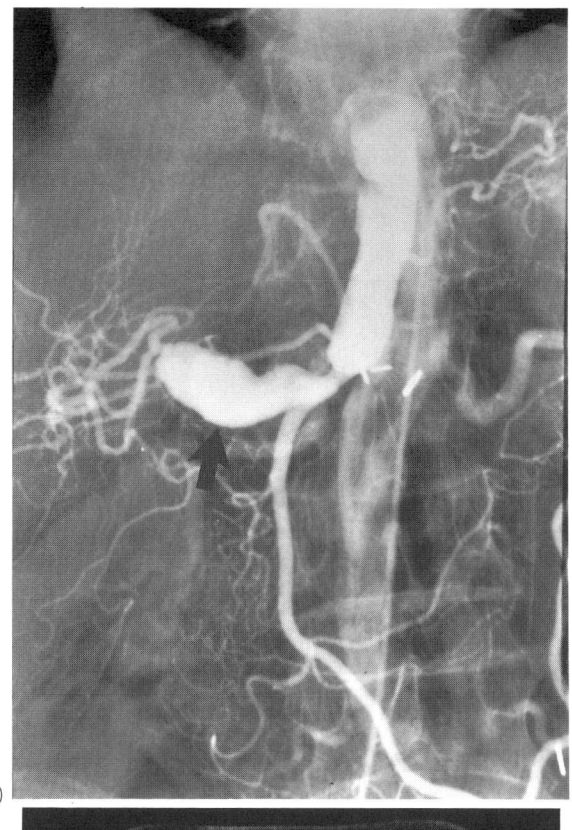

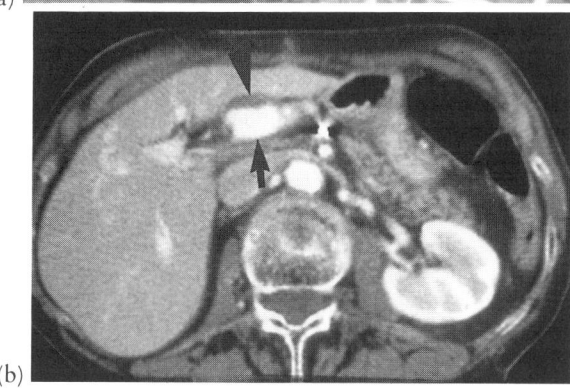

Figure 20.26 (a) Celiac angiogram. Iatrogenic dissection of the common hepatic artery (arrow). The aneurysm formation is secondary to the expansion of the dissection. (b) CT scan through the liver. The use of i.v. contrast material shows the dissecting aneurysm of the common hepatic artery (arrow). The thin zone of lucency anterior to the contrast within the lumen is thrombus (arrowhead).

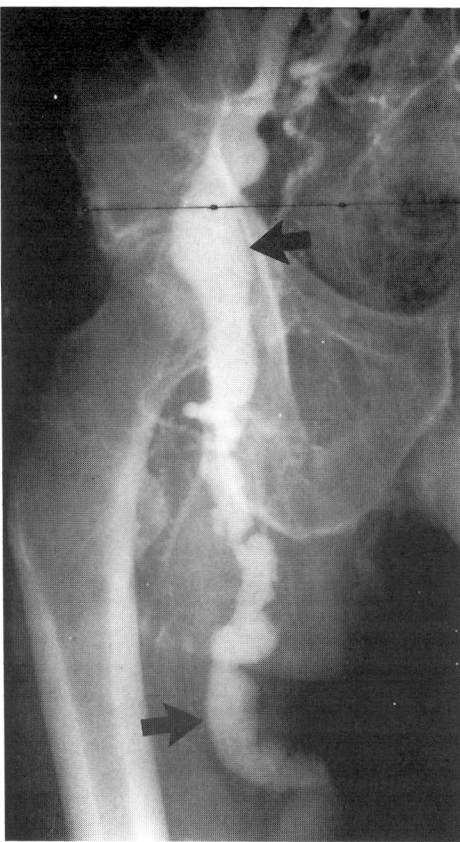

Figure 20.27 Femoral arteriogram showing the diffuse irregular ectatic appearance of arteriomegaly of the common femoral (top arrow) and superficial femoral (bottom arrow) artery segments. The deep femoral artery is occluded.

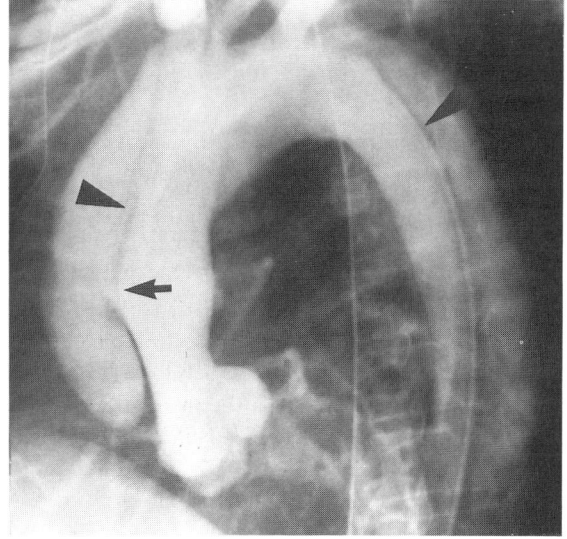

Figure 20.28 Thoracic aortogram in left anterior oblique position shows diffuse dissection with an entry site above the valve level (arrow). The intimal flap is identified in the ascending and descending segments (arrowheads).

at consecutive thin sections, the relationship of the primary branches and the dissection lumens can be identified. It is not often that the entry and re-entry sites are identified by CT scanning. These sites can be located accurately during angiography using an intra-aortic catheter and digital subtraction angiography technique. Angiography also displays the primary branches and their relationship to the true and false lumens.

Chronic dissections have a variable natural history, which can be followed by CT scanning. In some cases,

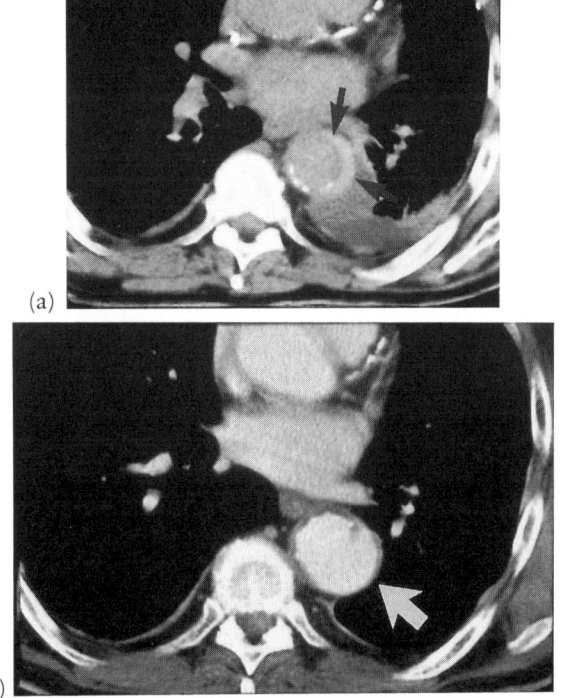

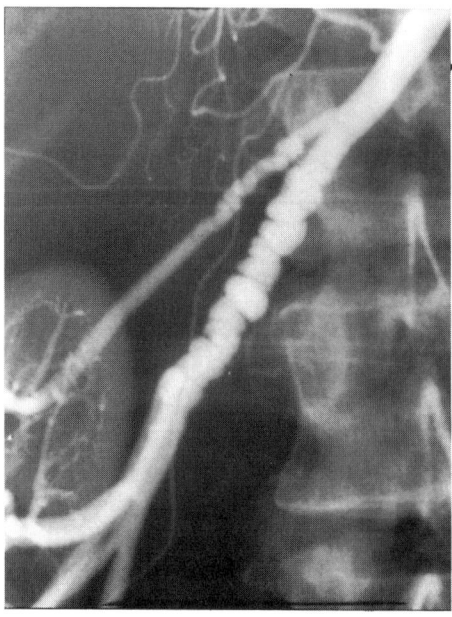

Figure 20.29 (a) CT scan of the descending thoracic aorta shows a high density crescent (arrows) along the left wall of the aorta. This is an intramural hematoma from a penetrating atheromatous ulcer. (b) CT scan obtained five weeks later at this same level shows expansion of the aorta (arrow) and resorption of the hematoma.

Figure 20.30 Right renal arteriogram shows fibromuscular dysplasia of the string-of-beads type of medial fibroplasia.

the false lumen persists; in others, some degree of thrombosis occurs. The dissection may extend more proximally or distally. There may be a generalized expansion of the caliber over the course of months to years. One particular finding that is interesting to observe is calcification of the inner wall of the false lumen which can occur as early as two years after the initial event.

20.3.5 AORTIC ULCER WITH HEMATOMA

There is a variant of dissection which presents as an intramural hematoma in the acute setting instead of an intimal flap and a false lumen. Therefore, the imaging characteristics are entirely different from the better known classic form of dissection and the etiology is different: penetration of an atheromatous ulcer [18]. In this condition, the CT scans taken before i.v. contrast material show a crescent-shaped high CT density within the wall of the aorta [19] (Figure 20.29(a)). The hematoma extends for a variable distance cephalad and caudad from the atheromatous ulcer. Resorption of the hematoma occurs within a few weeks and often leaves its mark as an eccentric expansion of the aorta centered at the site of the original ulcer [20] (Figure 20.29(b)).

These ulcers are found almost always at the middle and distal thirds of the descending thoracic aorta. MRI shows parallel findings to those of the CT scan. However, MRI is so sensitive to produce a high signal intensity from hematoma, that even mural thrombus can have a crescent-shaped appearance. Furthermore, intimal calcification does not have a signal by MRI; therefore, one would not be able to distinguish intramural from mural thrombus.

20.3.6 FIBROMUSCULAR DYSPLASIA

After arteriosclerosis and related aneurysmal disease, fibromuscular disease (FMD) is the most common arterial abnormality encountered. In most patients, it is limited to the renal arteries and is an incidental finding. The classic angiographic appearance is that of a string of beads. The involved arterial segment has a course, serrated lumen with variable degrees of stenoses. This appearance is the most common and is found in the renal arteries at the middle and distal portions [6,21] (Figure 20.30). It may also be seen in the proximal external iliac arteries and in the proximal internal carotid arteries. Angiography is the imaging modality best able to display FMD. This string-of-beads type of FMD manifests itself in variations of length, numbers of beads, aneurysmal size of the beads, separation between the beads and degree of stenosis. Between the tightly packed beads are webs of thin tissue which may cause diaphragm-like stenoses, which in turn may lead to hypertension in patients with renal artery involvement. It is not feasible to search for stenotic webs because many oblique angiographic views would need to be taken to see them in profile. This lesion lends itself to a high success rate of treatment with balloon catheter dilatation.

The string-of-beads pattern of FMD belongs to a subgroup of other variations of medial FMD which includes perimedial fibroplasia and medial hyperplasia. They have a variety of angiographic appearances which are not as easily distinguished by angiography as at pathologic examination. Perimedial fibroplasia in some instances looks like the string-of-beads pattern of medial fibroplasia except the beads are less numerous and are smaller in diameter than the main artery. In other cases, this type of medial FMD has an appearance of irregular or smooth stenosis that is indistinguishable from medial hyperplasia or intimal fibroplasia. Intimal fibroplasia is not classified within the subgroup of medial type FMD. Sometimes this intimal type of FMD presents as a single, focal stenosis, anywhere along the length of usually a renal artery, which is a relatively specific finding but which can have the angiographic appearance of a variant of perimedial fibroplasia. The adventitial type of FMD often has a non-specific angiographic appearance of a long segment of smooth narrowing of the renal artery. It may also present as a smooth, segmental stenosis with elongated shoulders.

The differential diagnosis of FMD varies according to the subtype. The string of beads type of FMD, if mild, needs to be distinguished from a variety of appearances of spasm either from catheter tip stimulation or from a shock wave of the contrast material injection. This latter finding has the appearance of perfect harmonic wave form with a constant internodal distance. Such perfect symmetry is not found in disease conditions. Catheter tip-induced spasm has an irregular appearance that can simulate the appearance of an atheromatous lesion, perimedial fibroplasia or intimal hyperplasia. The clue is its relationship to the end of the catheter and its absence on the preliminary aortic injection.

Three other appearances of FMD are identified at angiography: dissection, aneurysm and occlusion. These are rarely encountered and are most often found in the internal carotid arteries, the renal arteries and, very rarely, in the celiac and superior mesenteric arteries.

Idiopathic dissection may extend into the primary and secondary branches and frequently leads to branch occlusions and subsequent segmental infarction. Rarely, the same patient may develop spontaneous dissection in two or three vascular beds though not usually synchronously (Figure 20.31). In most patients dissection occurs in only one vascular bed [5]. When dissection is recognized from the angiogram, an intimal flap needs to be seen to be certain of the diagnosis. However, the projection of the artery may not allow detection of the intimal flap, and its presence may be only suggested because of a persistent collection of contrast material

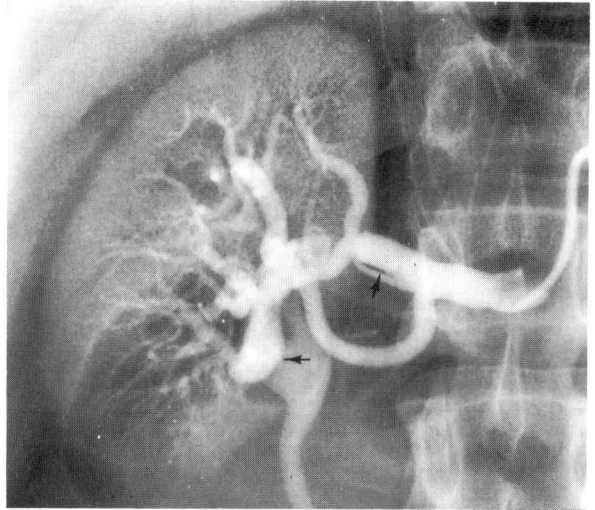

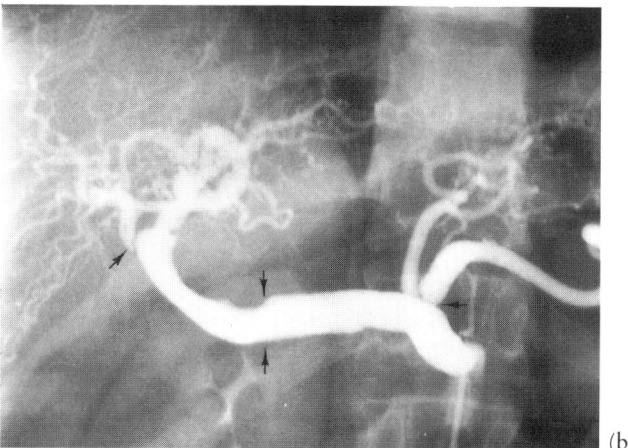

Figure 20.31 (a) Right renal arteriogram shows idiopathic dissection of the renal artery with a small intimal flap at the distal main segment (upper arrow). The aneurysm of the lower segmental artery (lower arrow) is also an indication of a dissection with contrast in the false lumen. The intimal flap is not identified here in this projection. (b) The same patient as Figure 20.31(a). The celiac artery injection shows additional evidence of dissection (arrows). Also, there is diffuse ectasia of the common hepatic artery which is compatible with fibromuscular dysplasia in view of the overall findings in the celiac, superior mesenteric and renal arteries.

within a segment of the artery producing an appearance of a fusiform aneurysm. The collection of contrast material is trapped by an intimal flap oriented in a plane not detected by the angiogram. Often the disease is recognized indirectly because of the irregular appearance of the lumen indicative of subintimal fluid (hemorrhage) collection. This will produce an eccentric, segmental stenosis. Weeks later, the angiogram often shows partial or complete resolution of the subintimal fluid, and the angiogram returns to a normal or near normal appearance. In some cases, the initial angiogram shows occlusion. Also, non-occlusive thrombus can develop in the artery adjacent to a dissection. This may result in embolization.

Aneurysms in the proximal distribution of the celiac and superior mesenteric arteries are another manifestation of FMD. The angiographic appearance is not specific for the diagnosis, but FMD should be considered in the differential diagnosis. Aneurysms in this location are indeed rarely encountered and may be either an isolated finding of FMD or associated with dissection.

Finally, in some cases of vascular involvement of FMD, the angiographic findings are occlusions or stenoses of the origins of the superior mesenteric or celiac artery in the presence of renal artery FMD. The angiographic findings are not specific, but in the absence of atherosclerosis, and without evidence of a vasculitis, then FMD is the most likely diagnosis.

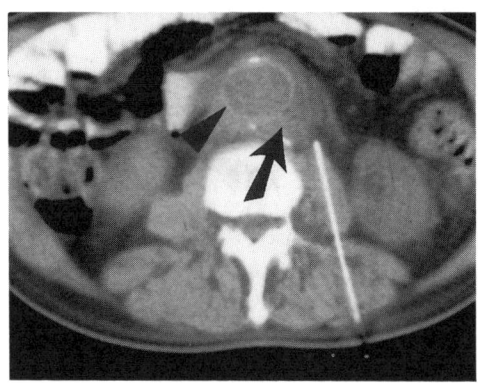

Figure 20.32 CT scan taken through the infrarenal portion of the abdomen without i.v. contrast material. An aortic synthetic graft (arrowhead) is surrounded by a perigraft fluid collection (arrow). A needle has been placed through the left side of the back to aspirate this fluid to prove that it is infected.

20.3.7 VASCULAR GRAFTS

Vascular grafts within the abdomen are often best studied by CT scanning [23]. In the extremities, US is the diagnostic examination of choice, because of its noninvasive nature and low cost. In the normally healed state, the graft bed contains the graft, which should be round and should opacify with i.v. contrast material. The anastomoses should be of the same caliber as the graft or only slightly larger. Following aneurysm repair there usually is perigraft fluid that lasts for several weeks or months. This slowly resorbs in almost every case. Complications of vascular grafts include infection, anastomotic aneurysm, aneurysm of the synthetic graft material and graft occlusion. CT findings of graft infection are perigraft air and fluid. Perigraft air within one month of surgery can be normal, but if present after that time, infection is present. Perigraft fluid that increases in quantity over time is almost always a sign of infection (Figure 20.32). An isotope study is the diagnostic procedure of choice for infection, but sometimes postoperative hematoma can cause confusion in the interpretation. Rarely, an anastomotic aneurysm can cause hematoma to develop in a perigraft location, giving a misleading appearance of infection. Aneurysms that develop at the ends of grafts are either of the adjacent native aorta (or artery) or are a breakdown of the anastomosis. CT scanning displays these processes very well. Many synthetic grafts are visible as a thin dense circle by the CT scan cross-section. Being able to establish the site of the graft contributes to a more accurate assessment of the pathologic process.

20.3.8 MISCELLANEOUS VASCULAR DISEASES

(a) **Arteriovenous malformations**

Arteriovenous malformations (AVMs) are a large assortment of lesions that have a wide variation in appearance by angiography. Any organ is susceptible to involvement and in patients with certain syndromes, such as Rendu–Osler–Weber, multiple organs may be affected. Angiography and MRI are equally important imaging modalities in the evaluation and diagnosis of AVMs. In the classic lesion, the angiogram shows a large disordered network of dilated arteries which then leads to a dense parenchymal vascular phase and, in many cases, the next phase is rapid opacification of the draining veins [5,6] (Figure 20.33). At times, pronounced venous shunting is a major finding. Also, the draining veins may be irregularly dilated.

Some AVMs are predominantly venous and are poorly identified from an arterial injection. This is found in Klippel–Trenaunay syndrome and in deep muscular venous malformations (Figure 20.34). These lesions are comprised of a complex network of dilated venous structures which may require direct puncture for the venogram to reveal the anatomy. In these cases, MRI is especially valuable to identify the lesion, its depth of involvement and precise location within an organ or extremity (Figure 20.35). For treatment planning, either by surgery or catheter embolization, this is valuable information.

The differential diagnosis of AVMs includes neoplasms and hemangiomas. In the extremities, certain soft tissue sarcomas may simulate an AVM by their angiographic appearance of dilated arteries and venous shunting. The major distinguishing feature is the clinical history; an AVM is congenital.

Angiodysplasia of the intestinal tract is a lesion with specific angiographic findings and which may have the appearance of an arteriovenous fistula [24]. The lesion itself may be acquired, but the propensity to develop it may be congenital. These lesions are most often identified in the ascending colon but sometimes are found in the small bowel. Angiography is the only

ARTERIAL DISEASES 717

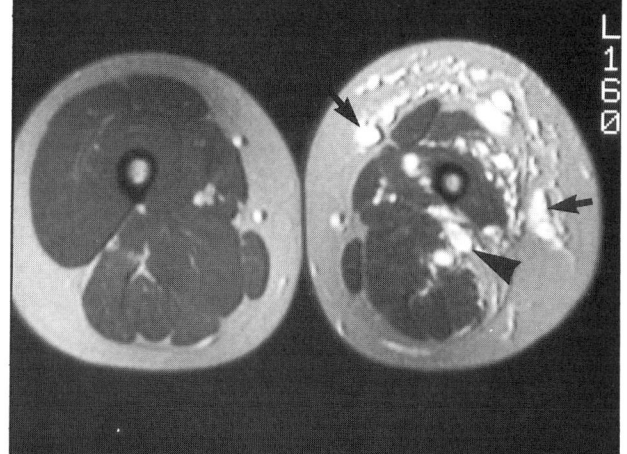

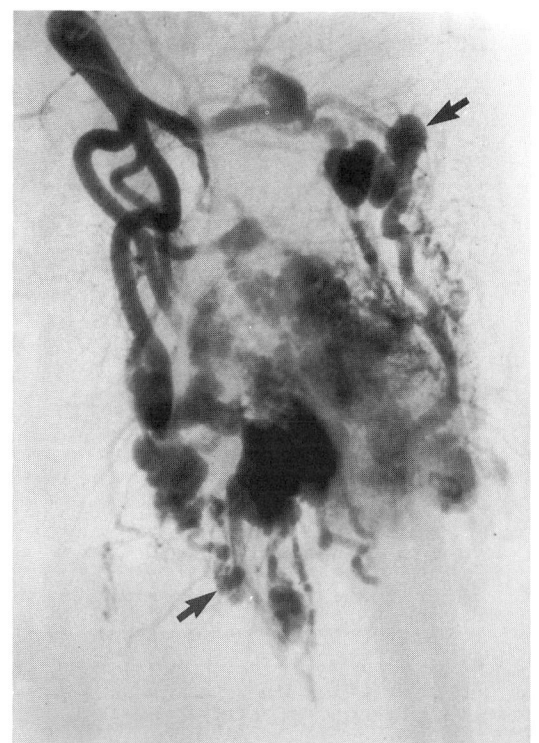

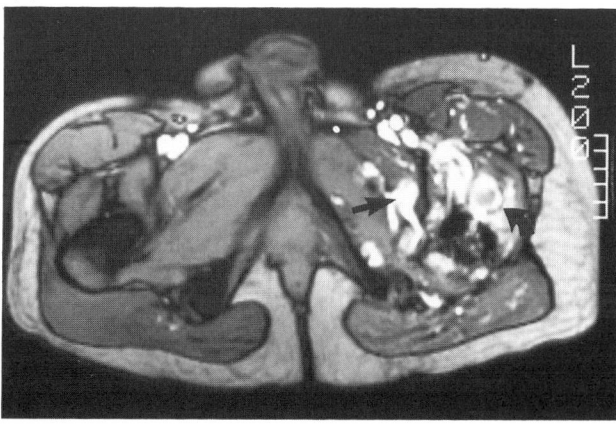

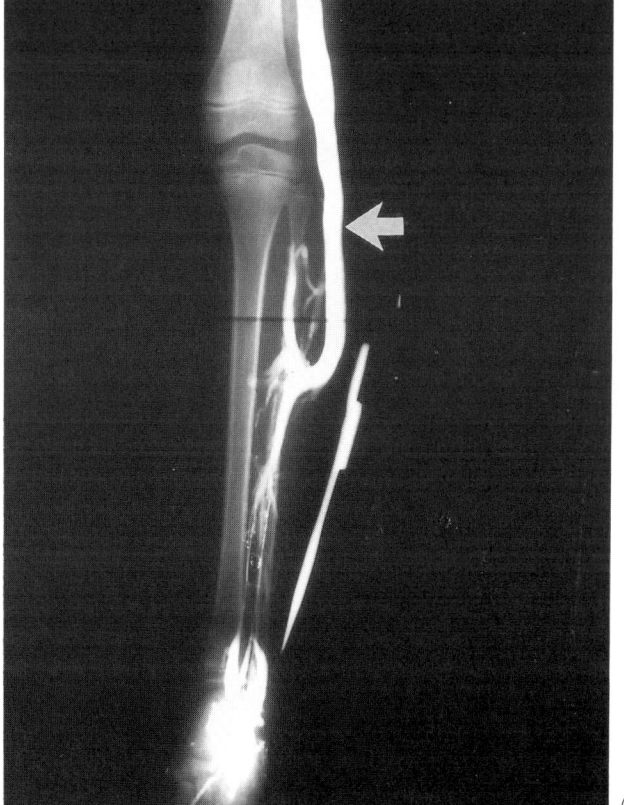

Figure 20.33 (a) Subtraction angiogram over the left hip with injection of the inferior gluteal artery shows a complex arterioverous malformation (AVM) with multiple aneurysms (arrows) and diffuse hypervascular stain. The venous phase is not yet apparent. (b) MRI scan through the hips. The AVM is manifested around the left hip as a high density (arrows) collection of vessels in and around the regional muscles.

Figure 20.34 (a) MRI scan through the mid-thighs shows a diffuse venous malformation manifested by the high density white areas (arrows) in the subcutaneous fat anteriorly and laterally. There is also a prominent embryologic sciatic vein (arrowhead). This is the typical appearance of Klippel–Trenaunay syndrome. (b) Left leg venogram of the same patient showing an anomalous lateral vein (arrow) of the upper calf and thigh. This appearance is compatible with Klippel–Trenaunay syndrome.

imaging modality that can detect them. Gastrointestinal bleeding is the sign that leads to the angiogram. At angiography, multiple foci of various sizes (millimeters) manifested by hypervascularity are identified in the bowel wall (Figure 20.36). The draining vein appears early and persists longer than the adjacent normal veins. These lesions range widely in size and extent. Active bleeding is rarely identified.

(b) **Cystic adventitial disease and arterial entrapment**

The popliteal artery is the most frequent site of involvement by cystic adventitial disease [25]. The angiogram shows an intramural filling defect of the wall of the

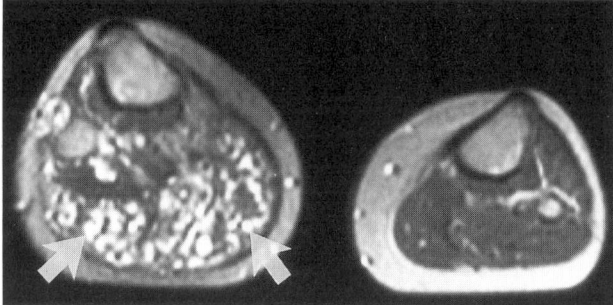

Figure 20.35 MRI scan through the mid-calf region shows an abnormally large right leg in a patient with Klippel–Trenaunay syndrome. There is diffuse permeation of the gastrocnemius muscles by an extensive network of veins (arrows).

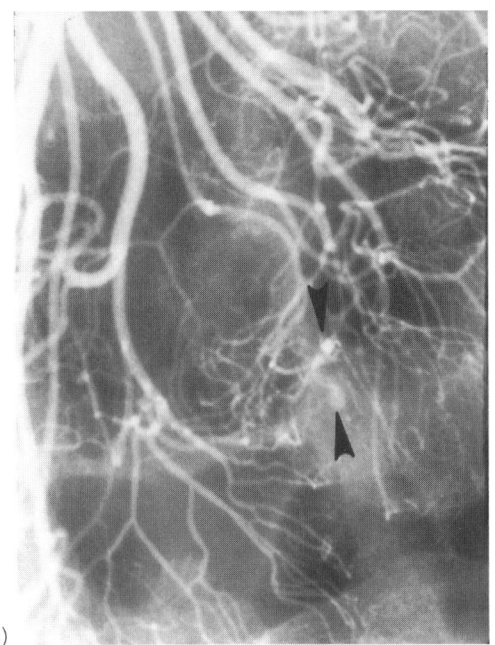

(a)

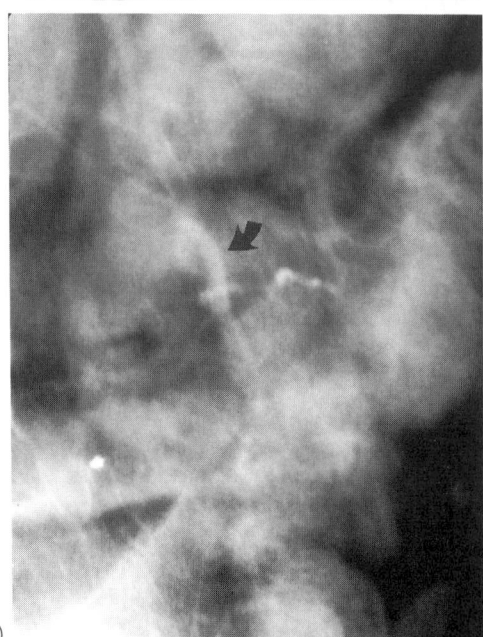

(b)

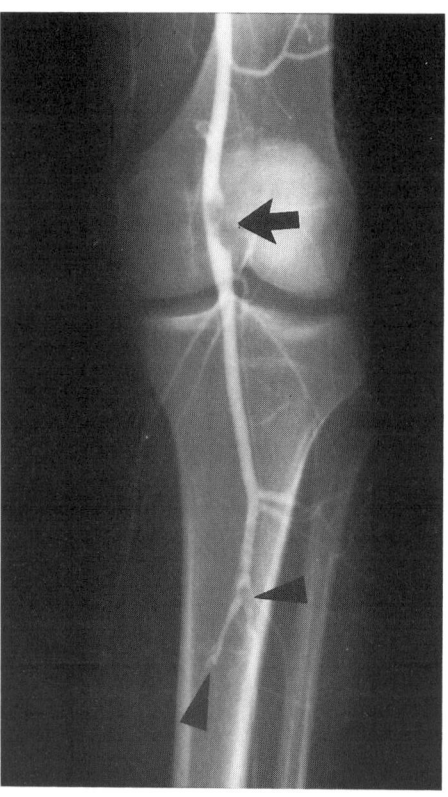

Figure 20.37 Popliteal arteriogram shows a filling defect resulting in stenosis of the mid-popliteal artery (arrow). This has resulted in distal embolization into the tibial arteries (arrowheads). In a young patient this lesion is either thrombus secondary to injury from popliteal artery entrapment, which is the diagnosis in this young boy, or the lesion could represent cystic adventitial disease except in this entity the distal embolization would not be compatible.

artery near the level of the knee joint space [10]. The degree of stenosis is variable. This lesion can be similar in appearance to entrapment of the popliteal artery by the gastrocnemius muscle. Therefore, a specific diagnosis is difficult to make at angiography. Examination by CT scanning or US may be helpful in identifying the thick wall of the artery found with cystic disease. Popliteal entrapment can cause a filling defect of the lumen because of intimal hyperplasia and thrombus secondary to trauma by the abnormal position of usually the medial head of the gastrocnemius muscle (Figure 20.37). Angiographic distinction can be difficult between the two diseases, but the maneuver of plantar flexion during the angiogram will cause an increase in the degree of stenosis of the popliteal artery if the etiology is entrap-

Figure 20.36 (a) Superior mesenteric angiogram over the mid-small bowel region shows two focal areas of dilated vessels (arrowheads). (b) Late phase of the angiogram shows early venous drainage (arrow) at the vicinity of the dilated vessels. This combination of findings is compatible with angiodysplasia responsible for gastrointestinal blood loss.

ment. In the resting state, there is often medial deviation of the popliteal artery above the level of the joint space.

(c) Ergot toxicity

Arterial changes of ergot toxicity are manifested by spasm. The angiographic pattern is multiple, focal stenoses or long, segmental ones [5] (Figure 20.38). They are usually found in the arteries of the lower extremities, although many arterial beds can be affected. The arterial caliber returns to normal in a few days after drug withdrawal. The onset seems to be related to an overdosage of the suppository form of ergot medication. Angiography is the best modality to make the diagnosis. Arterial spasm is found bilaterally but is often not symmetric in appearance. At times, the angiographic findings are far more pronounced in one leg compared to the other. The differential diagnosis includes spasm from any cause, such as cardiogenic shock or toxicity from other vasospastic drugs. Vasculitis also needs to be considered in the differential diagnosis.

There is one form of ergot toxicity that causes permanent arterial stenosis. The drug form is methysergide maleate. It induces a type of retroperitoneal fibrosis which encases the aorta and iliac arteries which can lead to occlusion. Peripheral arteries are rarely affected.

(d) Hemangioma

Hemangiomas are studied either by angiography or MRI. In the extremities, capillary hemangiomas and some cavernous hemangiomas may not be detected by angiography but will be detected by MRI as masses. Similar to the imaging of AVMs, MRI accurately displays the location of hemangiomas. However, the vascular component of a capillary hemangioma does not have a specific MRI appearance. However, cavernous hemangiomas have a structure which has a relatively specific MRI appearance of high signal intensity as found within the liver. The angiogram shows cloud-like collections of contrast material that begin at the periphery of the lesion in the mid-arterial phase and last for the 30 s of filming while gradually becoming larger by filling in towards the center (Figure 20.39). The CT scan appearance shows patches of contrast staining beginning at the periphery of the lesion and extending inward over the next few minutes. US imaging shows a hyperechoic lesion of fairly characteristic appearance but which is only suggestive and not specific for the diagnosis and must be distinguished from certain types of metastases. MRI of high signal intensity also cannot always be differentiated from neoplasm.

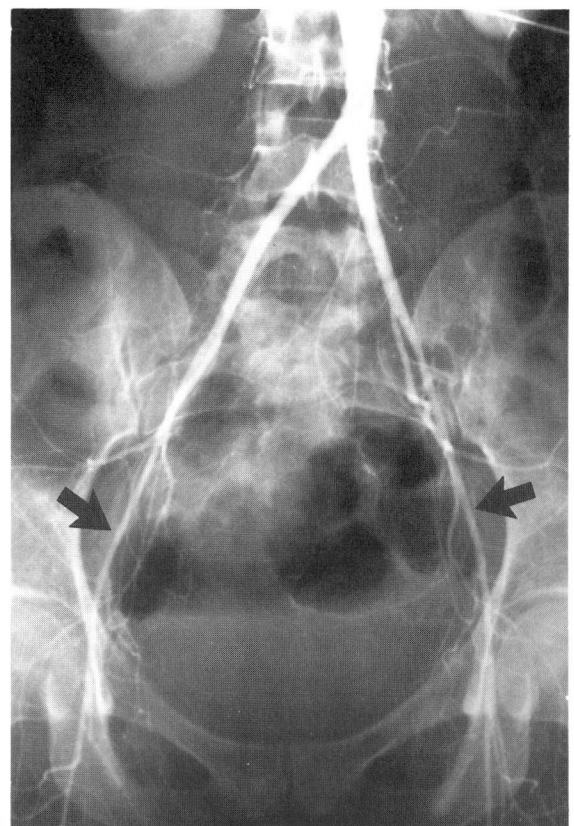
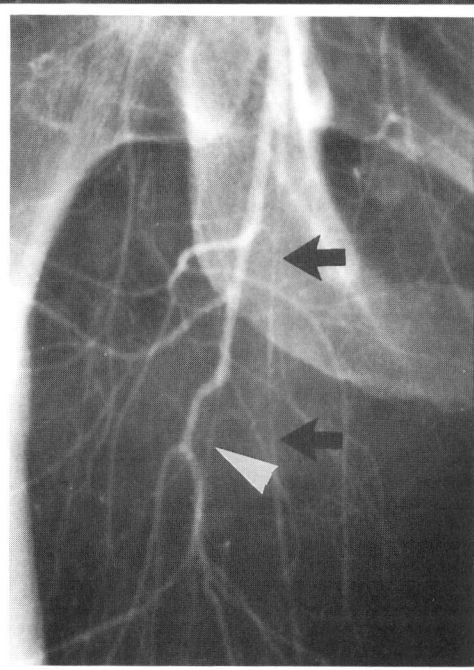

Figure 20.38 (a) Abdominal aortogram shows diffuse narrowing of the external iliac artery segments (arrows); the branches of the internal iliac arteries are also stenotic. This is compatible with ergot toxicity. (b) Close-up view of the upper thigh shows diffuse narrowing of the superficial femoral artery (arrows) and of a segment of the deep femoral artery (arrowhead).

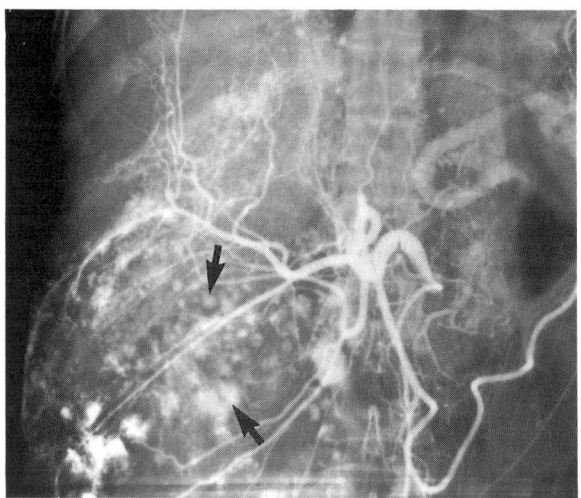

Figure 20.39 Hepatic angiogram shows diffuse patchy parenchymal staining in the liver (arrows) compatible with cavernous hemangioma.

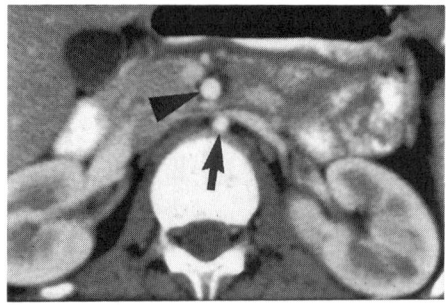

Figure 20.40 CT scan through the renal level in a patient with neurofibromatosis. The aorta (arrow) is very stenotic and has a diameter less than the superior mesenteric artery anteriorly (arrowhead).

(e) Neurofibromatosis

Vascular abnormalities related to neurofibromatosis are centered about the abdominal aorta and the visceral artery origins (Figure 20.40). The most typical finding is alteration of the caliber of the aorta; it may be diffusely ectatic or narrowed or both. It is common for the adjacent visceral arteries to be stenotic or even occluded at the origins. Angiography is the best imaging modality to evaluate this, although sagittal and coronal scanning by MRI could display the abnormality in more advanced cases. The angiogram will provide the highest resolution images which may prove important to differentiate this condition from two other conditions which can look similar: congenital coarctation and Takayasu's disease (Figure 20.41). However, it may not be possible to make this determination. It especially can be difficult to distinguish coarctation from neurofibromatosis [26]. Specific features to look for are ectasia of the aorta and the visceral arteries proximally, which are not found with coarctation, except for post-stenotic dilatation. If the aortic abnormality is that of ectasia, neurofibromatosis is difficult to distinguish from the aneurysmal form of Takayasu's disease. Takayasu's disease usually involves other vascular beds which distinguishes it from the other two conditions.

(f) Radiation fibrosis

This vascular disease results in obliteration of the arteries in the field of the radiation treatment. It begins to be evident a few years after the treatments and leads to slowly progressive arterial occlusion [27]. Angiography is the most specific imaging modality. The arterial abnormalities are usually long segments of stenoses but

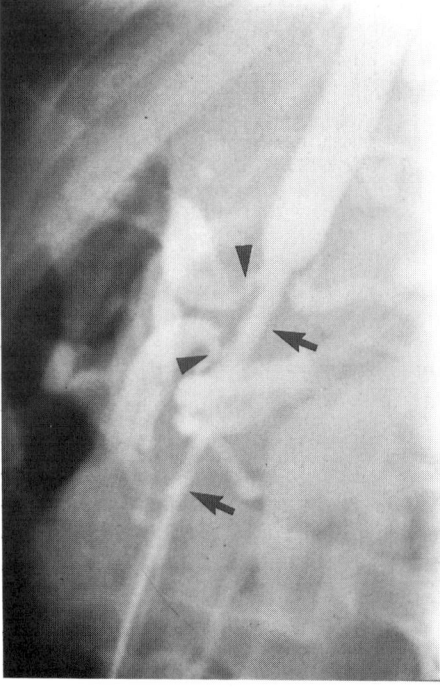

Figure 20.41 Abdominal aortogram in lateral view shows diffuse narrowing of the aorta (arrows). There is also proximal stenosis of the celiac artery (upper arrowhead) and of the superior mesenteric artery (lower arrowhead). This is a congenital coarctation of the abominal aorta.

can be mixed with multiple, focal stenoses. Such angiographic findings are not specific by themselves, but the history of radiation therapy and the correlation of the site of the disease process to the field of treatment allow interpretation of the vascular occlusive disease.

20.4 Arterial intervention

The emergence of angiographic interventional procedures in the past 15 years has led to the development of a complex array of therapeutic procedures that may

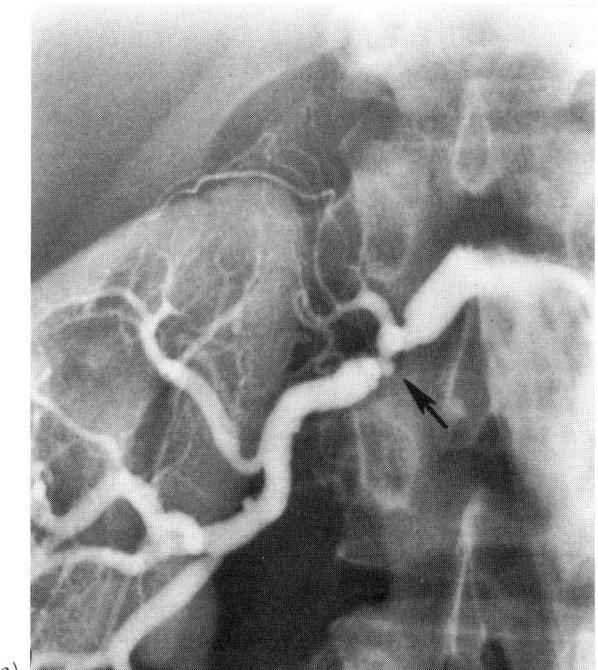 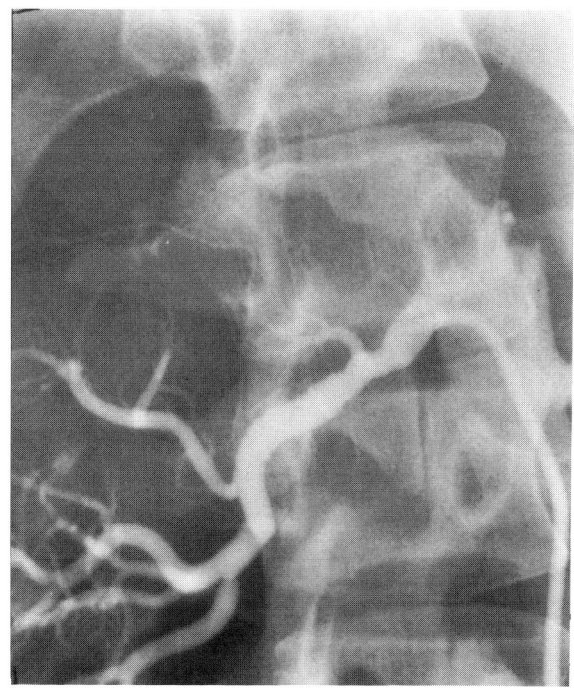

Figure 20.42 (a) Renal arteriogram (right side) showing fibromuscular dysplasia, medial group, probably perimedial type. The middle and distal portion of the main artery and the proximal portions of three primary branches are involved with irregularity of the lumen and high grade stenosis (arrow) at the middle third. (b) Angiogram performed after balloon catheter dilatation shows a residual stenosis of about 20%.

accompany diagnostic imaging. At the leading edge of this process is the placement of stented vascular grafts through angiographic catheters [28].

The first interventional procedure that made a significant impact was percutaneous transluminal angioplasty (PTA) with the use of an inflatable balloon catheter (see Figure 20.14). This remains the most frequently performed interventional procedure. It is used to dilate stenotic arteries (and veins). There is a large range of balloon sizes from small ones for renal and coronary artery branches up to large ones for the pulmonary artery and the aorta. The object is to dilate the diseased vessel up to the expected normal diameter or to the level of the adjacent patent lumen. In most cases, the innate elasticity of the vessel is overcome and the lumen remains patent. Predicting the outcome of the procedure depends mostly upon the disease being treated and the morphology of the stenosis. A single, focal, atheromatous stenosis in a common iliac artery has a 90% chance to stay patent within a 2-year period if the patient does not smoke. In the lower popliteal artery, this probability drops to about 50%. The mechanism of action is thought to be stretching of the arterial wall until there is loss of compliance by destroying the elasticity of the arterial wall components. This includes denervation of the vasa vasorum and necrosis of some cellular components of the diseased wall. For those lesions that recur, the mechanism is not completely understood. Sometimes there appears to be recoil of the elastic properties of the vessel wall. At other times, there is abundant intimal proliferation. Stenotic lesions of renal FMD treated by PTA have a relatively high success rate if the lesion is of the medial type and has focal and not segmental stenoses and if no dissection is present (Figure 20.42). In contrast, stenotic lesions caused by arteritis, in the acute phase, respond poorly and have a high recurrence rate. Likewise, those lesions secondary to intimal hyperplasia following arterial surgery have a poor response to PTA.

In an attempt to offer better therapy for complex types of atheromatous lesions and stenosis caused by intimal hyperplasia, a variety of ablation devices have been employed. These include cutting atherectomy devices, grinding devices and a variety of laser catheters. In certain specific morphologic lesions, some of these devices have proved to be beneficial but overall the rate of recurrence of the lesions remains similar to that of PTA.

Immediately following PTA of an atheromatous lesion, there is frequently identified an intimal dissection at the site of the previous stenotic lesion. Such intimal cracks seem to be part of the mechanism of a successful dilatation (Figure 20.43). In effect, it represents a partial endarterectomy and releases that portion of the arterial wall from the constricting effect of the circumferential atheromatous lesion. At times, such dissections are large

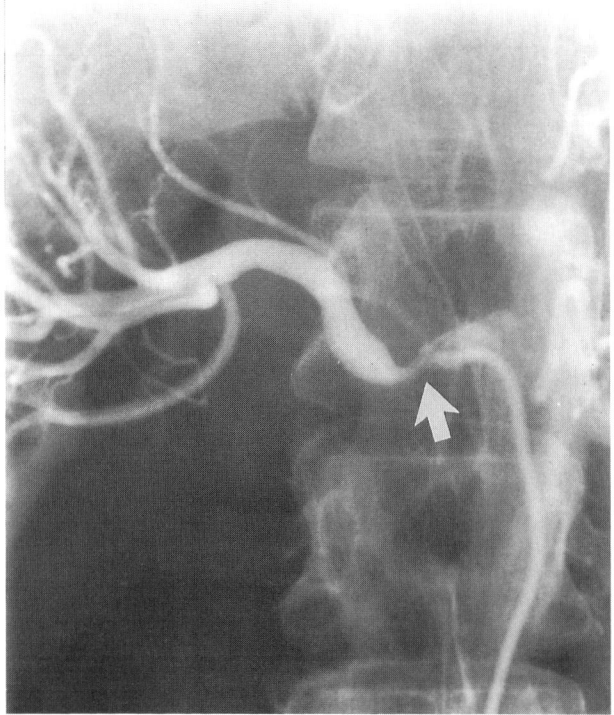 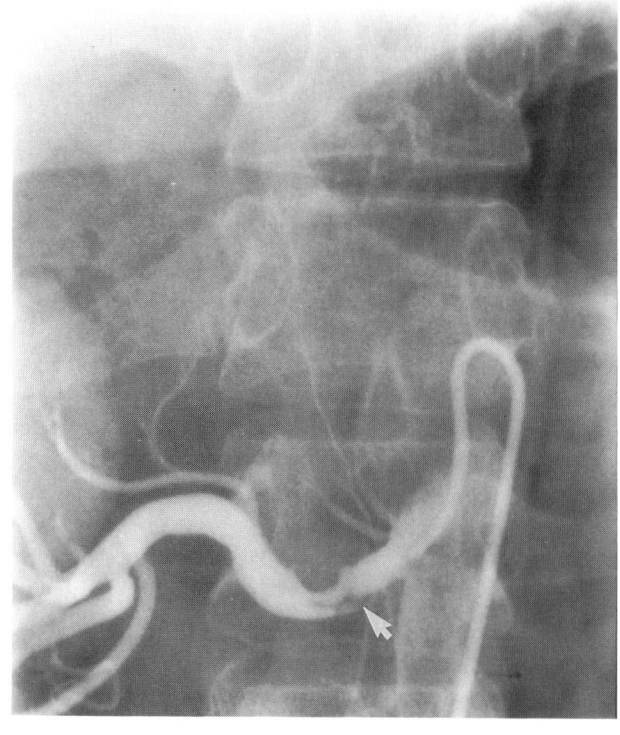

Figure 20.43 (a) Right renal arteriogram shows a high grade proximal stenosis (arrow) from atheromatous disease. (b) Shows the result after balloon catheter dilatation. There is an intimal crack (arrow) but the lumen remains stenotic.

and lead to a secondary occlusion of the artery and, in rare cases, the dissection of the atheromatous plaque is completely circumferential and the entire plaque becomes dislodged and embolizes. Another complication of PTA is embolization of atheromatous debris. This is estimated to occur in as many as 3% of procedures but it is rarely of clinical significance. Aneurysm formation or rupture of the dilated artery is a rare complication of PTA. Making careful measurements of the artery to be dilated and matching this with the balloon diameter are important considerations. Also, in the older patient, it is important not to overdilate a lesion. In a younger patient, such overdilatation, by 1 or 2 mm, is commonly performed in an attempt to overcome the elasticity of the tissues. In cases of FMD, the main concern of a complication is perforation through one of the aneurysmal 'beads'. With the string-of-beads type lesion, the wall of these focal aneurysm-like areas is thin and subjected to perforation by the guidewire during placement of the balloon catheter (Figure 20.44).

Intra-arterial stent placement by catheters is a technology that is designed to enhance the success rate of balloon catheter dilatation. Early results indicate slightly better patency rates over simple PTA. However, it is too early yet to determine when and where this expensive technology is best applied. The newest innovations of intravascular stents are those that support graft fabric. These are placed into stenotic arteries and through the

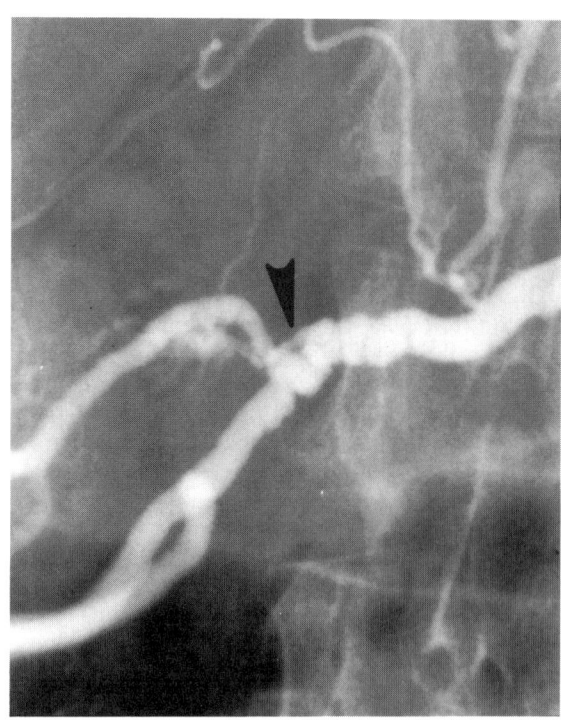

Figure 20.44 Right renal arteriogram shows a complication of balloon catheter dilatation of the underlying fibromuscular dysplasia. There is a perforation (arrowhead) with local extravasation of contrast material resulting from catheter and guidewire injury of the thin wall of this dysplastic lesion.

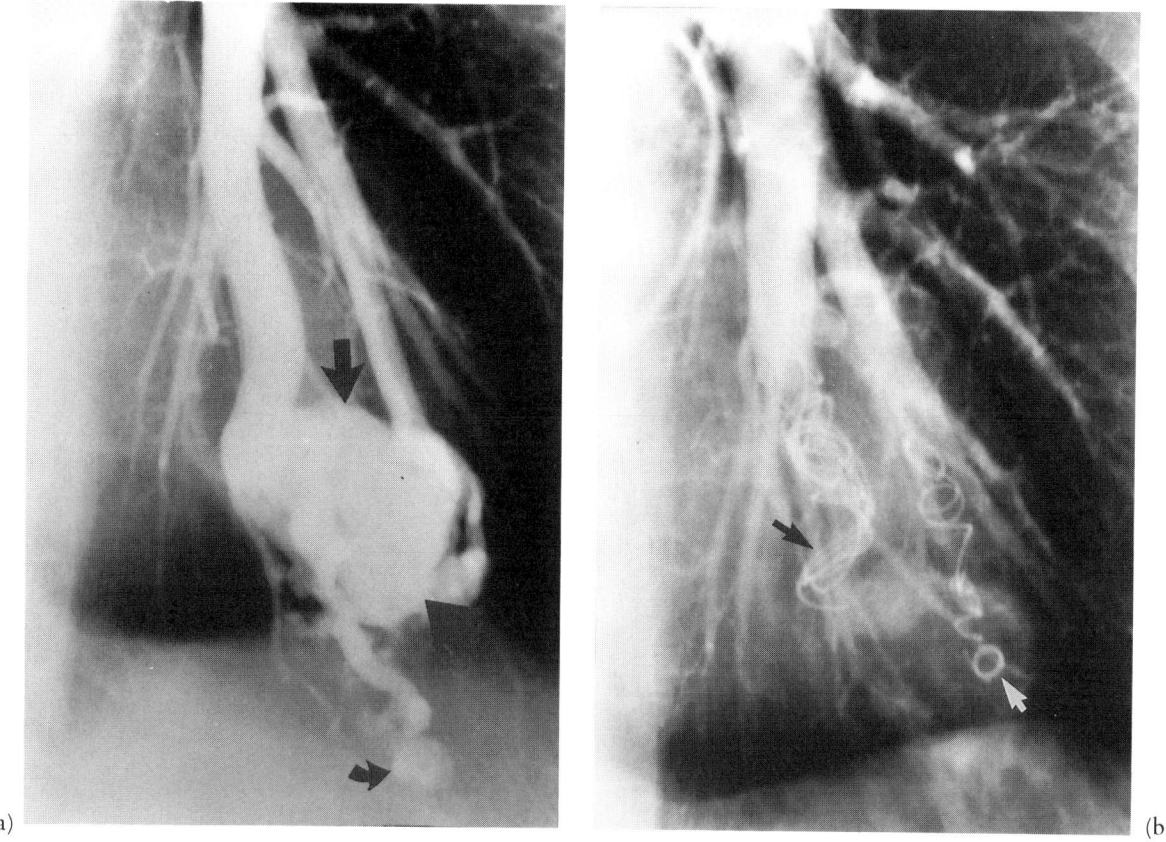

Figure 20.45 (a) Pulmonary angiogram showing complex arteriovenous fistula (arrows) of the left lower lobe artery with multiple feeding arteries. This is an early arterial phase and the venous return is not seen yet. (b) Postembolization, the pulmonary angiogram shows occlusion of the arteries that were supplying the arteriovenous fistula. Multiple Gianturco coils (arrows) were used.

path of aneurysm, as in the treatment of an aortic aneurysm or dissection. This intervention is too new for data to predict its success.

A large segment of interventional procedures pertains to therapeutic embolization of lesions. This includes a large variety of clinical situations including traumatic bleeding, neoplasms, hemangiomas and arteriovenous malformations. Embolic material includes metallic coils of various configurations, gelatin particles, synthetic sponge particles, silk sutures, detachable balloons and ethanol (Figure 20.45). Some of these procedures stand alone in their therapeutic effort, others augment the surgical approach, and yet others offer palliation.

For thrombotic and embolic disease, the main interventional procedure involves thrombolytic therapy delivered by selective catheter placement and subsequent prolonged infusion of a thrombolytic agent. This is an effective method of dissolving thrombus if it is not organized. Usually, another interventional procedure, such as PTA or stent placement, accompanies lytic therapy because an underlying lesion is often encountered. Distal embolization frequently accompanies the long process of lytic therapy and it is important to continue the infusion of the lytic agent to manage this embolic debris.

20.5 Venous diseases

20.5.1 IMAGING

The most frequently encountered venous disease is thromboembolism. All imaging modalities play a role in making the diagnosis. Venography is the traditional imaging study and is definitive in most areas of the body. However, at times, US is the modality of choice by being non-invasive and inexpensive to use, especially for deep venous thrombosis (DVT) of the extremities. This is true in the legs from the popliteal to common femoral venous segments, and in the arm from the brachial to the subclavian venous segments. Below the knee, however, US is not able to adequately evaluate all five sets of main deep veins. Contrast venography is an excellent diagnostic modality in this area. Diagnostic capacity of US is good for studying the jugular, hepatic, portal and splenic veins, as well as the inferior vena cava. MRI is capable of displaying venous thrombosis

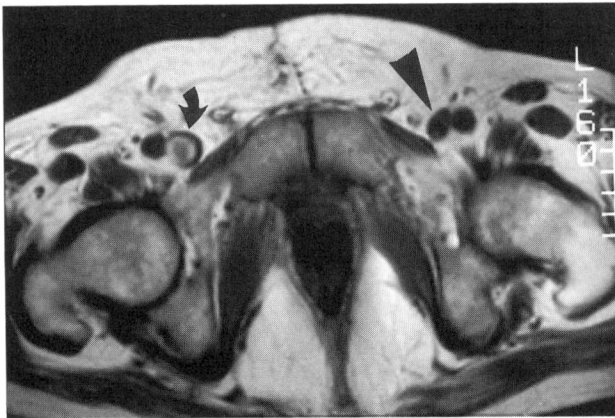

Figure 20.46 MRI of the pelvis at the inguinal region. Thrombosis of the right femoral vein (arrow) is shown as a higher signal intensity than the adjacent right femoral artery. Also, note that the diameter of the right vein is larger than the left one (arrowhead). This is a sign of acute thrombus.

anywhere in the body (Figure 20.46). Fresh thrombus will appear as an absent flow void (a static structure) within the vein lumen in addition to presenting evidence of surrounding edema. However, in the veins of the lower leg, MRI images are not as clearly depicted as are venogram images. This can lead to uncertainty in determining the status of the thrombotic process. In comparison the contrast venogram produces anatomic images of superior quality that are very familiar to all clinicians and, therefore, give confidence of interpretation to the untutored observer. Also venographic images allow estimation of the age of the thrombus. In cases of recanalized thrombus, the residual intraluminal fibrotic tissue would be difficult to appreciate with any other imaging study.

20.5.2 THROMBUS

When thrombus is fresh, contrast material from a venogram surrounds the thrombus producing a pair of tracks along the wall as seen tangentially [5,6] (Figure 20.47). Another imaging feature of acute thrombus is found in expansion of the vein caliber. The accretion process of progressive thrombosis results in radial expansion as well as central propagation. The diagnostic feature by US in this acute thrombolic setting, is an expanded vein which cannot be compressed when moderate pressure is applied. There continues to be lack of compressibility in the subacute thrombotic state before recanalization occurs. It may be difficult to detect a small retracted thrombus by US or by MRI. In certain clinical settings it is important to establish the relative age of thrombus for therapeutic planning purposes. The venogram is the most specific examination for this purpose.

After 3–5 days, thrombus develops adhesion to the

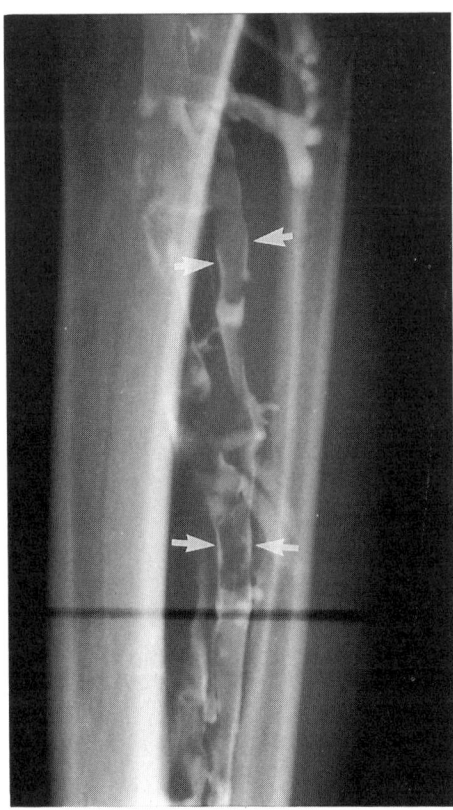

Figure 20.47 Acute deep venous thrombosis of the left leg. The venogram shows the outline of the fresh thrombus as a pair of tracks (arrows).

vein walls, thus precluding the peripheral passage of contrast material. At this phase the vein is occluded and in such a state one cannot make further interpretation about the vein or the thrombus. In some cases, eventual recanalization occurs whereby multiple paths are created in the core of the occluding thrombus. This may appear as multiple string-like filling defects (Figure 20.48). In the extreme case, there is complete recanalization. This results in a smooth lumen narrower than the original (Figure 20.49). The walls become permanently plastered with organized thrombus and the valves are lost. In those cases in which the thrombus does not adhere to the walls, retraction of the thrombus presents as a serpentine filling defect with a relatively thick peripheral zone of contrast material compared to the very thin peripheral line of contrast material in the acute state. Eventually this retracting thrombus disappears and the residual veins appear normal because the valves are not incorporated into the walls as adherent fibrous tissue.

The appearance of thrombus, acute, subacute and chronic, in leg veins, applies to all other vascular beds. Usually venography is used to study most of the venous system. But CT, US and MRI have important roles especially in the abdomen and CT and MRI are important imaging modalities in the chest. However,

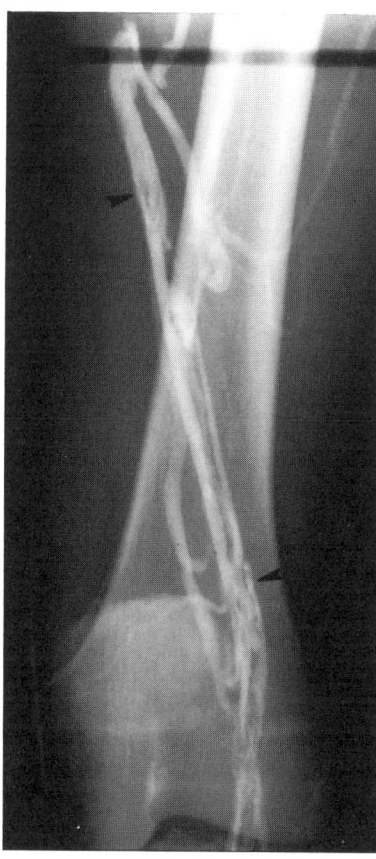

Figure 20.48 Venogram of the left distal thigh and popliteal area shows old deep vein thrombosis with partial recanalization (arrowheads). The dark linear stripes within the lumen are areas of old thrombus that have not yet recanalized.

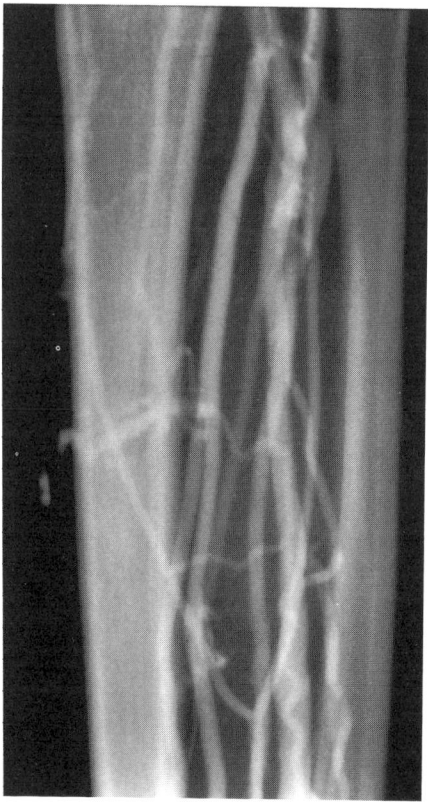

Figure 20.49 Venogram of the left lower leg shows smooth walled veins without valves. This is the appearance of complete recanalization of old deep vein thrombosis.

they will not be as accurate at determining the age of thrombus as venography.

20.5.3 PULMONARY EMBOLUS

The target organ of venous thrombotic disease is the lung. Pulmonary emboli have similar angiographic appearances as thrombotic disease has in the legs or elsewhere [5,6] (Figure 20.50), but in the central pulmonary arteries, old emboli present as a laminated plaque on the wall or as foci of stenoses (Figure 20.51). Angiography is usually the only modality used to make the direct diagnosis of pulmonary embolism at all branch levels. However, fast CT is excellent in detecting acute or chronic emboli in the main and lobar arteries, and transesophageal echo is good for detecting proximal emboli.

The differential diagnosis of pulmonary emboli includes: Takayasu's disease, pulmonary leiomyosarcoma, primary pulmonary artery hypertension and fibrosing mediastinitis. In Takayasu's disease there may be multiple pulmonary artery stenoses and sometimes aneurysms. The involvement is usually at the central arterial level and mimics chronic pulmonary emboli. Leiomyosarcoma of the pulmonary artery presents as an intraluminal filling defect that by most modalities would be indistinguishable from embolus. However, it is theoretically possible that MRI would depict such a mass as a tumor and not as an embolus. Some patients with primary pulmonary artery hypertension have pruning of the terminal pulmonary arteries that mimics the appearance of chronic peripheral small emboli. Finally, patients with fibrosing mediastinitis can develop pulmonary artery stenoses at multiple sites in the central and hilar regions. Also bronchogenic carcinoma can cause pulmonary artery stenosis which would be unifocal. Pulmonary angiography cannot be used to distinguish etiologies of such pulmonary artery stenoses. However, fast-CT scanning would be an ideal imaging modality to evaluate the mediastinum; fibrosing mediastinitis and neoplasm are readily displayed.

20.5.4 BUDD–CHIARI SYNDROME

Budd–Chiari syndrome has various venographic manifestations: occlusive disease involving the intrahepatic inferior vena cava (IVC) or the hepatic veins and their branches. All imaging modalities can detect occlusive

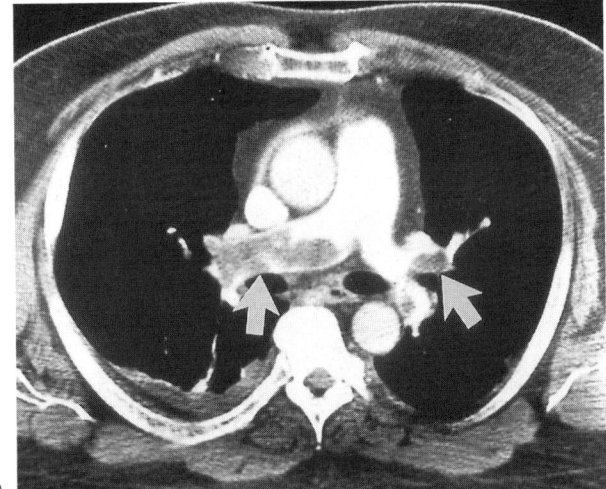

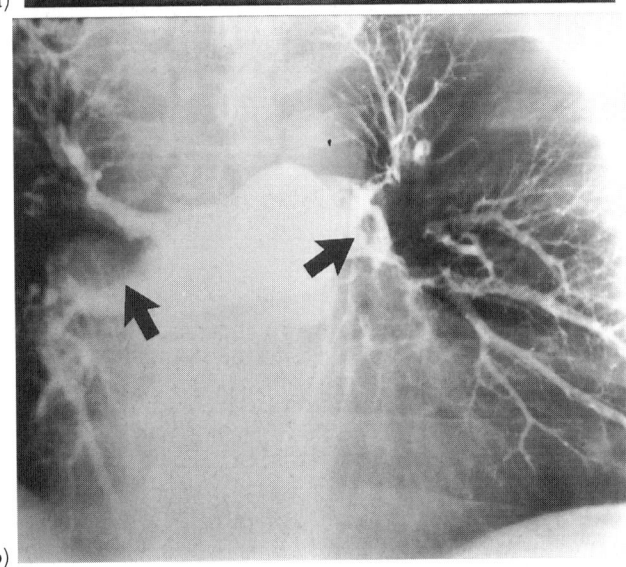

(a)

(b)

Figure 20.50 (a) Fast-CT scan through the pulmonary arteries showing large bilateral pulmonary emboli (arrows). (b) Pulmonary angiogram of the same patient as in Figure 20.50(a) shows the large, bilateral pulmonary emboli (arrows). In both the CT and the angiogram, the intraluminal filling defects indicate acute emboli.

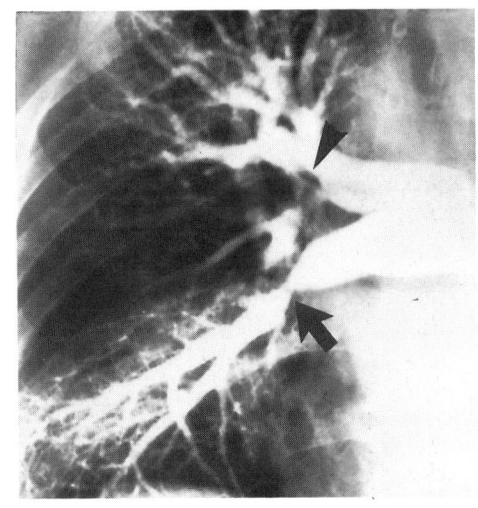

Figure 20.51 Right pulmonary artery angiogram shows stenosis of the lower lobe artery (arrow) and slight narrowing of the upper lobe artery (arrowhead) compatible with old pulmonary embolism. These stenotic sites by themselves are not specific for old pulmonary embolism. Takayasu's disease could produce this appearance as could fibrosing mediastinitis. A fast-CT scan would provide specific diagnostic information.

thrombus within the intrahepatic IVC and the main hepatic veins, but if only stenosis is present, then angiography is the best imaging modality. It also offers the opportunity to measure pressures across the stenotic lesions and to apply balloon catheter dilatation to eliminate the pressure differences which may relieve the symptoms (Figure 20.52). Urokinase treatment is also effective in eliminating fresh thrombus, and this also can be most effectively delivered at the time of angiography. Some patients with Budd-Chiari syndrome have occlusive disease of the small, intrahepatic vein branches which has a unique and specific angiographic appearance when an injection is performed with the catheter wedged into the patent portion of an hepatic vein. The appearance is that of a 'spider web' network of small collaterals within the parenchyma [4,6] (Figure 20.53). This is also the angiographic appearance of veno-occlusive disease.

20.6 Venous intervention

Interventional procedures upon veins include lytic therapy, balloon catheter dilatation, vena cava filter and stent placement [28]. None of these is as successful in the venous beds as they are in the peripheral arteries, presumably because of the lower flow status in veins which seems to promote eventual thrombolic response upon vein walls at the treatment site. However, lytic therapy for pulmonary embolism is very effective to dissolve emboli. In this location it is easy for the lytic agent to bathe the emboli continuously as the pulmonary arteries are in a convenient downstream position relative to venous flow. In other venous beds there is opportunity for the lytic agent to bypass the thrombosed area in lieu of a low resistance patent pathway. Indeed in the hepatic, renal or portal venous sites it is difficult to apply a lytic agent directly from an upstream site which would be the most effective for lysis.

One interventional vascular procedure is unique to the venous system: vena cava filter placement for thromboembolic disease. Several designs of filters are available. The objective is to trap emboli at the level of the inferior vena cava (sometimes also at the superior vena cava level). These devices are placed from a venous

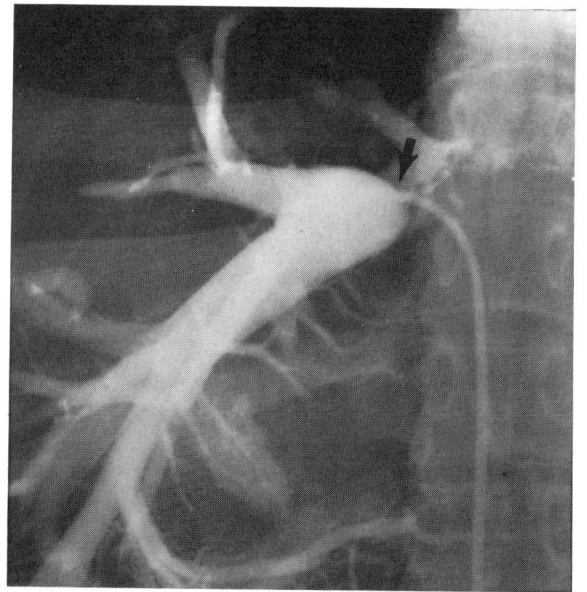

(a)

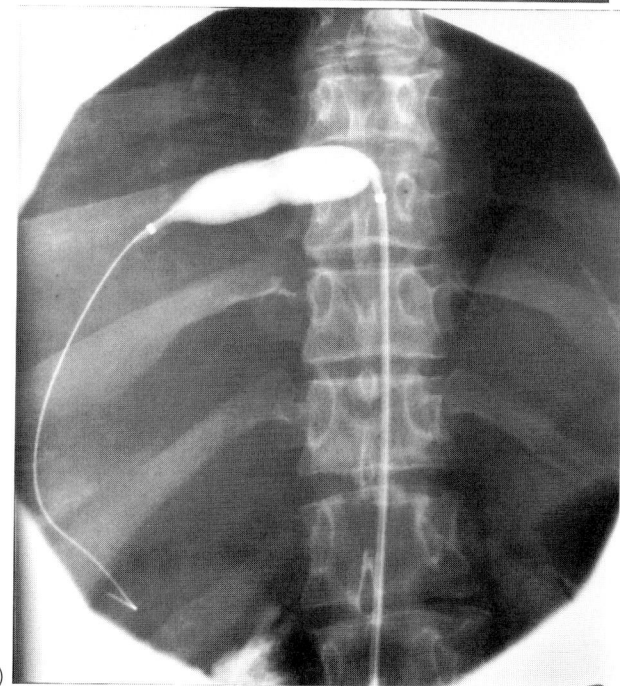

(b)

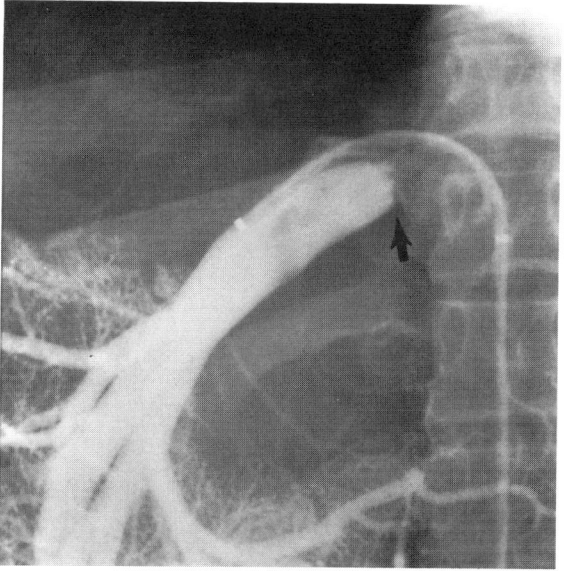

(c)

Figure 20.52 (a) Selective injection of the right hepatic vein in a patient with Budd–Chiari syndrome shows high-grade stenosis (arrow) at the orifice. (b) Balloon catheter dilatation of the stenotic orifice of the right hepatic vein. (c) Follow-up hepatic venogram shows improvement in the diameter of the hepatic vein orifice (arrow).

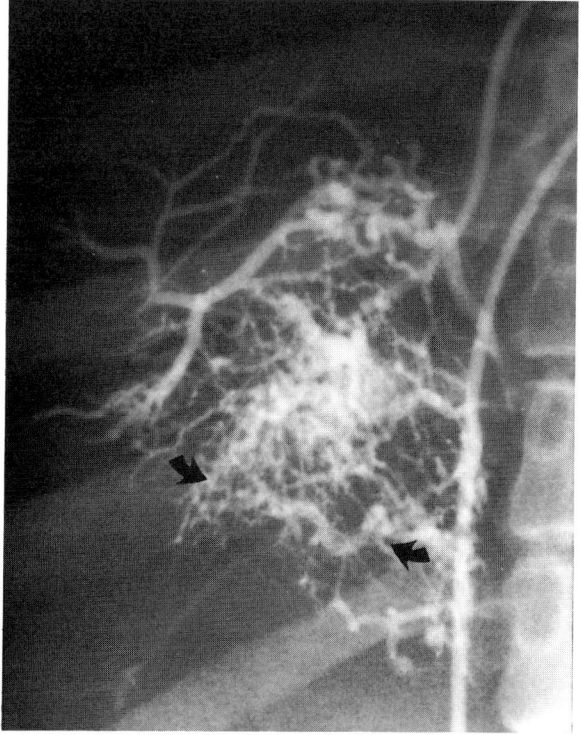

Figure 20.53 Wedged hepatic venogram in a patient with Budd–Chiari syndrome where the majority of the hepatic veins have become obliterated by thrombosis. There is a diffuse spider web-like network (arrows) indicating intrahepatic venous collaterals.

catheterization entry point and can be delivered at a relatively accurate location within the vena cava. They are considered to be more than 95% effective in trapping emboli. Complications related to these devices are: migration of the device, perforation of an anchoring leg through the vena cava and thrombotic occlusion of the vena cava. Migration and perforation are rarely encountered with recent improvements in designs. Thrombosis of the vena cava, secondary to filter placement, ranges between 5 and 20% and may actually be related to clot trapping efficiency rather than to local mechanical influences of the device.

References

1. Machida, K. and Tasala, A. (1980) CT patterns of mural thrombus in aortic aneurysms. *J. Comput. Assist. Tomogr.*, **4**, 840.
2. Torres, W.E., Maurer, D.E., Steinberg, H.V. *et al.* (1988) CT of aortic aneurysms: the distinction between mural and thrombus calcification. *Am. J. Roentgenol.*, **150**, 1317–19.
3. Predey, T.A., McDonald, V., Demos, T.C. and Moncada, R. (1989) CT of congenital anomalies of the aortic arch. *Semin. Roentg.*, **24**, 96–111.
4. Kadir, S. (1986) *Diagnostic Angiography*, W.B. Saunders, Philadelphia.
5. Neiman, H.L. and Yao, J.S.T. (1985) *Angiography of Vascular Disease*, Churchill Livingstone, Edinburgh.
6. Abrams, H.L. (1983) *Abrams Angiography*, 3rd edn, Little, Brown and Company, Boston.
7. Yamato, M., Lecky, J.W., Hiramatsu, K. and Kohda, E. (1986) Arteritis: radiographic and angiographic findings in 59 patients. *Radiology*, **161**, 329.
8. Hall, S., Barr, W., Lie, J.T. *et al.* (1985) Takayasu arteritis: a study of 32 North American patients. *Medicine*, **64**, 89–99.
9. Klein, R.G., Hunder, G.G. and Stanson, A.W. (1975) Large-artery involvement in giant cell (temportal) arteritis (GCA). *Ann. Intern. Med.*, **83**, 806.
10. Young, J.R., Graor, R.A., Oliv, J.W. and Bartholomew, J.R. (1991) *Peripheral Vascular Disease*, Mosby Year Books, St Louis.
11. Conn, D.L. (1990) *Vasculitis Syndromes, Rheumatic Disease of Clinics of North America*, vol. 16:2, W.B. Saunders Co., Philadelphia.
12. Vowden, P., Wilkinson, D., Ausobsky, J.R. and Kester, R.C. (1989) A comparison of three imaging techniques in the assessment of an abdominal aortic aneurysm. *J. Cardiovasc. Surg.*, **30**, 891–6.
13. Pavone, P., Di Cesare, E., Di Renzi, P. *et al.* (1990) Abdominal aortic aneurysm evaluation: comparison of US, CT, MRI, and angiography. *Mag. Reson. Imag.*, **8**, 199–204.
14. Hollier, L.H., Stanson, A.W., Gloviczki, P. *et al.* (1983) Arteriomegaly: classification and morbid implications of diffuse aneurysmal disease. *Surgery*, **93**, 700–8.
15. McKusick, V.A. (1972) *Heritable Disorders of Connective Tissue*, 4th edn, C.V. Mosby Company, St Louis.
16. Pennell, R.C., Hollier, L.H., Lie, J.T. *et al.* (1985) Inflammatory abdominal aortic aneurysms: a thirty-year review. *J. Vasc. Surg.*, **2**, 859–69.
17. Bis, K.G. and Farah, M. (1993) Precise evaluation crucial in aortic dissection. *Diag. Imag.*, **15**, 88–97.
18. Stanson, A.W., Kazmier, F.J., Hollier, L.H. *et al.* (1986) Penetrating atherosclerotic ulcers of the thoracic aorta: natural history and clinicopathologic correlations. *Ann. Vasc. Surg.*, **1**, 15–23.
19. Welch, T.J., Stanson, A.W., Sheedy, P.F. *et al.* (1990) Radiographic evaluation of penetrating aortic atherosclerotic ulcer. *Radiographics*, **10**, 675–85.
20. Hussain, S., Glover, J.L., Bree, R. and Bendick, P.J. (1989) Penetrating atherosclerotic ulcers of the thoracic aorta. *J. Vasc. Surg.*, **9**, 710–17.
21. Kincaid, O.W., Davis, G.D., Hallermann, F.J. and Hunt, J.C. (1968) Fibromuscular dysplasia of the renal arteries: arteriographic features, classification, and observations on natural history of the disease. *Am. J. Roentg.*, **104**, 271–82.
22. Edwards, B.S., Stanson, A.W., Holley, K.E. and Sheps, S.G. (1982) Isolated renal artery dissection: presentation, evaluation, management, and pathology. *Mayo Clin. Proc.*, **57**, 564–71.
23. Brown, O.W., Stanson, A.W., Pairolero, P.C. and Hollier, L.H. (1982) Computerized tomography following abdominal aortic surgery. *Surgery*, **91**, 716–22.
24. Boley, S.J., Sprayregen, S., Sammartano, R.J. *et al.* (1977) The pathophysiologic basis for the angiographic signs of vascular ectasias of the colon. *Radiology*, **125**, 615–21.
25. Flanigan, D.P. *et al.* (1979) Summary of cases of adventitial cystic disease of the popliteal artery. *Ann. Surg.*, **189**, 165.
26. Lewis III, V.D., Meranze, S.G., McLean, G.K. *et al.* (1988) The midaortic syndrome: diagnosis and treatment. *Radiology*, **167**, 111–13.
27. Butler, M.J., Lane, R.H.S. and Webster, J.H.H. (1980) Irradiation injury to large arteries. *Br. J. Surg.*, **67**, 341.
28. Castaneda-Zuniga, W.R. and Tadavarthy, S.M. (1992) *Interventional Radiology*, 2nd edn, Williams and Wilkins, Baltimore.

21 NEOPLASMS OF LARGE ARTERIES AND VEINS, AND TUMOR ANGIOGENESIS

A.P. Burke and R. Virmani

Neoplasms that arise in large blood vessels can be classified by location in the intima, medial wall or adventitia; by the histologic features, or by the type of vessel involved. For purposes of this review, tumors will be classified by the vessel of origin. There is usually no doubt that a neoplasm originates from a vessel if it is grossly present within the lumen and is attached to the intimal surface. Some neoplasms of vessels have a minor intraluminal component and are attached to the medial wall. In order to diagnose a tumor of vessel origin, a segment of attached vessel must be removed during the surgical procedure, the parenchyma of another organ must not be involved by the tumor and the operative report must indicate that in the opinion of the surgeon the tumor arose within the vessel.

Soft tissue neoplasms that arise in small vessels obscure their origins when they exceed 1 or 2 cm in diameter. The following discussion will concentrate on tumors that occur in elastic or muscular arteries and large veins.

21.1 Tumors of arteries

21.1.1 SARCOMAS OF THE AORTA

(a) Incidence

The majority of primary tumors of arteries involve the aorta or pulmonary artery. Primary tumors of the aorta are exceptionally rare. The majority are sarcomas, of which there are approximately 50 cases reported in the medical literature [1–12].

(b) Classification

We support a classification of aortic sarcomas proposed by Haber and Truong [7]. In this classification, the term 'intimal sarcoma' refers to aortic sarcomas that are luminal or predominantly luminal. The term 'intimal' does not designate a histologic type but rather indicates the putative site of origin [7]. The normal aortic intima is composed of endothelial cells, fibroblasts and smooth muscle cells. It is not surprising that aortic sarcomas can consist of cells of any one or a combination of these types and may have a variety of histologic appearances.

Those aortic tumors that are attached to the aortic media and grow into the adventitia and periaortic soft tissue, with little luminal growth, are classified by their histologic subtype similar to other sarcomas of soft tissue. These non-intimal aortic sarcomas are less common than the intimal variety.

(c) Gross features

By definition, intimal sarcomas are either entirely intraluminal, in which case they grossly resemble thrombi, or are predominantly luminal with focal extension into the wall or adventitia. Occasionally, intimal sarcomas can cause thinning and aneurysmal dilatation of the aortic wall. When they occur in the abdominal aorta, they can be mistaken by the surgeon for an atherosclerotic aneurysm.

Unlike sarcomas of the venae cavae, aortic sarcomas rarely appear to arise in the wall of the great vessel. Those rare examples that have little luminal component and are predominantly mural are histologically more likely to be differentiated leio- or angiosarcomas.

Most aortic sarcomas occur in the abdominal aorta between the celiac artery and the iliac bifurcation; approximately 30% occur in the descending thoracic aorta. There have been several reported cases of aortic sarcomas arising at the site of a synthetic aortic graft anastomosis [1,12]. It is not unusual for the initial diagnosis to be made on the basis of embolectomy material, grossly considered by the surgeon to be a thrombus.

(d) Histologic features

Intimal aortic sarcomas are usually poorly differentiated sarcomas of fibroblastic or myofibroblastic differentiation. They are composed of mitotically active spindle cells with varying degrees of atypia, necrosis and pleomorphism. The luminal surface is often composed of dense fibrous tissue with a layering of spindle cells which are only minimally atypical (Figure 21.1). There may be an epithelioid appearance to tumor cells (Figure 21.2) and a mixture of pleomorphic fibro- and histiocytic cells resembling malignant fibrous histiocytoma (Figure 21.3). Some intimal aortic sarcomas have, for this reason, been classified as malignant fibrous histiocytomas [11]. The intimal surface of the aorta adjacent to gross tumor may demonstrate a lining of atypical cells that has been termed 'dysplasia'. These cells occasionally demonstrate endothelial differentiation, which has been cited as evidence of endothelial derivation of the tumor. However, there are few intimal sarcomas that are easily classified as angiosarcomas (Figure 21.4). Most poorly differentiated intimal sarcomas do not have immunohistochemical features of endothelial cells, but are more similar to tumors of myofibroblastic origin (Figures 21.5, 21.6).

Leiomyosarcomas, with characteristic fascicular

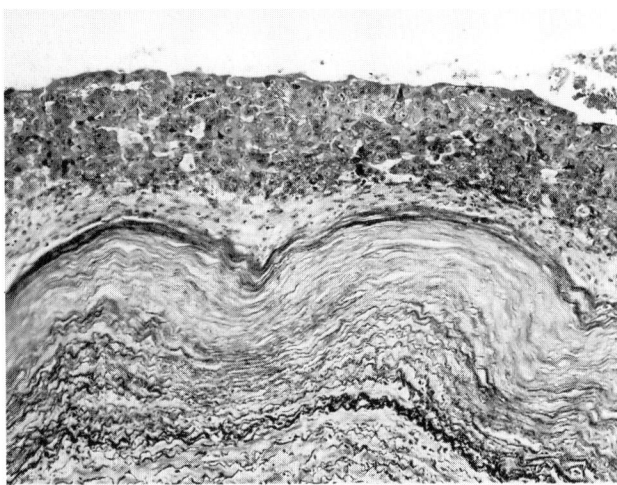

Figure 21.2 Sarcoma of the aorta. At the margin of the tumor there is layering of sarcoma directly over the intima, which in this case shows mild fibrointimal thickening. There can be an epithelioid appearance to sarcoma cells. This tumor was taken from a 63-year-old woman with Leriche's syndrome. (Movat pentachrome stain.) (Reproduced with permission from Burke and Virmani [51].)

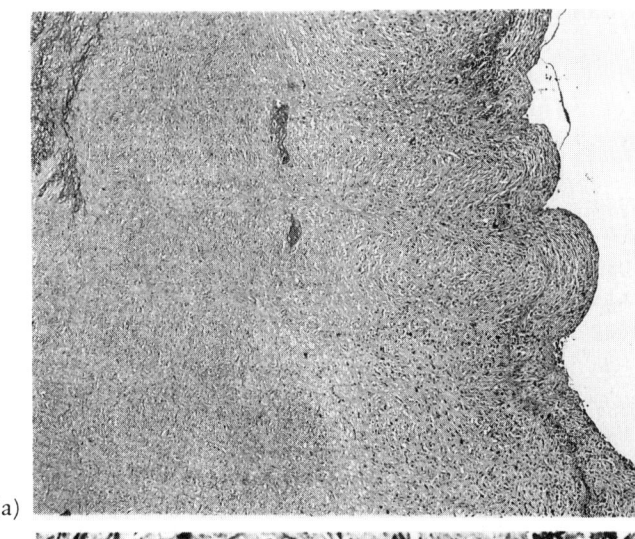

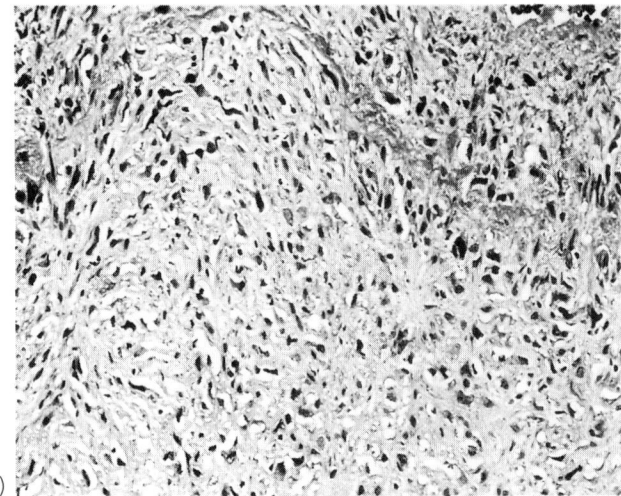

Figure 21.1 (a) Sarcoma of the aorta. Layering of atypical spindled cells over an inner fibrous area is typical of intimal aortic sarcomas. This tumor was resected from a 75-year-old man who had lower extremity claudication. The tumor was located in the thoracoabdominal aorta. (H&E.) (b) A higher magnification of the interface between the sarcoma and the fibrous layer. (H&E.)

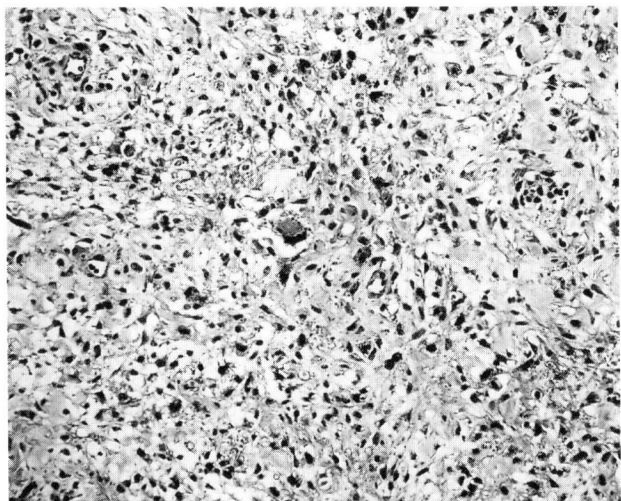

Figure 21.3 Sarcoma of the aorta. In this example tumor cells are pleomorphic, resembling malignant fibrous histiocytoma. (H&E.)

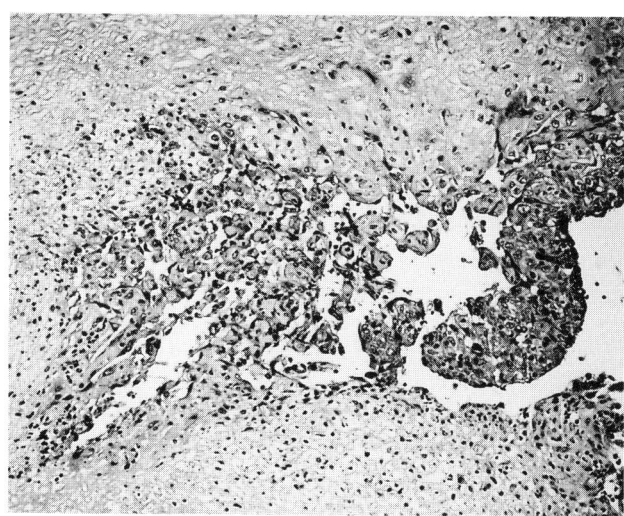

Figure 21.4 Sarcoma of the aorta. Occasionally, aortic intimal sarcomas have areas of angiosarcoma. This tumor was located in the abdominal aorta of a 58-year-old man who experienced leg pain while jogging. An abdominal aneurysm, that was clinically suspected to be atherosclerotic, was removed. (H&E.)

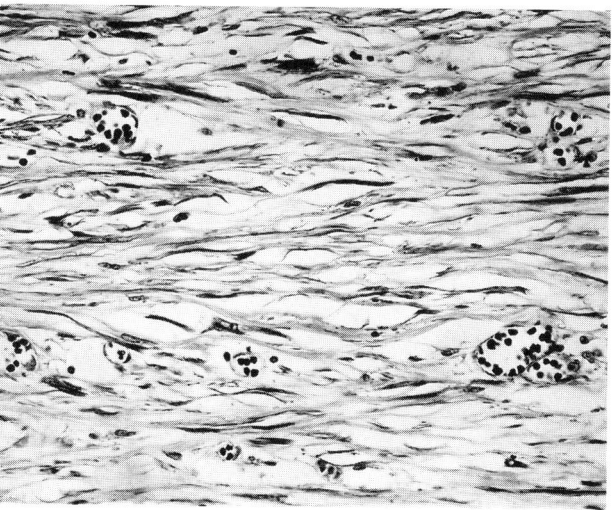

Figure 21.5 Sarcoma of the aorta. Spindled areas can have a deceptively bland appearance; thorough sampling of luminal aortic tumors is important to diagnose sarcoma. (H&E.)

growth, intracytoplasmic glycogen and ultrastructural characteristics of smooth muscle cells are extremely rare as are luminal (intimal) aortic sarcomas.

Sarcomas of the aorta that have only a minor luminal component are, in contrast to intimal sarcomas, generally better differentiated. The few examples that we have encountered are leiomyosarcomas, similar to sarcomas of the venae cavae, or angiosarcomas.

(e) Clinical features

Most patients with sarcomas of the aorta are middle aged; in a recent series the mean age was 62 years [1] (Table 21.1). In the largest series of reported cases, there was no sex predilection [1,2]. Because most tumors are intraluminal, the most common symptoms are related to embolic phenomena. Claudication and absent pulses, usually of the lower extremities, are common complaints of patients with aortic sarcoma. Other symptoms include back pain, abdominal pain because of mesenteric artery occlusion, shock from rupture of aneurysm formed by the tumor and symptoms related to malignant hypertension [6]. Treatment consists of surgical removal of the affected aortic segment with repair by synthetic graft. Occasionally, the surgical diagnosis is atherosclerotic aneurysm and the diagnosis of malignancy is made first at histologic examination of a repaired aortic aneurysm.

The prognosis of intimal sarcomas of the aorta is generally poor, because of a high incidence of metastases. The most common sites of metastases are skeleton, peritoneum, liver and mesenteric lymph nodes. There

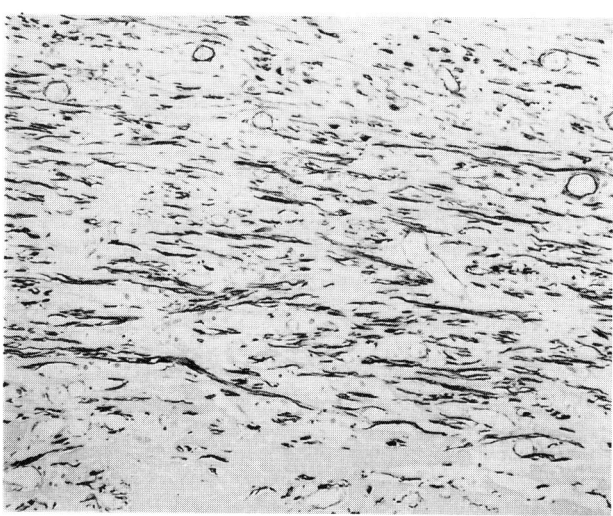

Figure 21.6 Sarcoma of the aorta. Immunoperoxidase preparation with antismooth muscle actin (same tumor as in Figure 21.5), demonstrating spindled cells positive. Most intimal aortic sarcomas are consistent with myofibroblastic derivation. (Avidin-biotin complex.) (Reproduced with permission from Burke and Virmani [51].)

are notable exceptions, however, of patients who live for years without symptoms after surgery.

21.1.2 NON-SARCOMATOUS AORTIC NEOPLASMS

Benign tumors of the aorta are exceedingly rare. We have seen a few examples of benign fibrous histiocytomas and inflammatory pseudotumors of the aortas in young adults and children. These tumors are attached to the aortic adventitia, are cured by resection and usually occur in the proximal aorta.

Table 21.1 Sarcomas of the great vessels: clinicopathologic features*

Data	Great vessels		
	Aorta	Pulmonary artery	Inferior vena cava
Number	12	18	17
Mean age of patient (years)	64	44	51
Male:female ratio	6:6	13:5	4:13
Site (number of tumors)	thoracic (4)	right (12)	upper† (6)
	abdominal (8)	left (4)	lower (8)
		both (2)	both (3)
Relation to vessel (number of tumors)			
luminal	10	17	2
mural	2	1	15
Histology (number of tumors)			
undifferentiated	10	14	1
angiosarcoma	1	1	0
leiomyosarcoma	1	1	16
osteo/chondrosarcoma	0	5	0

* Adapted from Burke et al. [1]. † Bulk of tumor at level of hepatic veins and above.

The soft tissue adjacent to the aortic adventitia contains dispersed paraganglia that function similarly to the carotid body. These paraganglia are located predominantly near the ligamentum arteriosus and at the inferior mesenteric artery (organ of Zuckerkandl). Occasionally, normal or hyperplastic paraganglia can cause confusion to the surgical pathologist who is not familiar with the presence of paraganglial tissues near the aorta. Neoplasms of these paraganglia occur which are several times rarer than paragangliomas of the carotid body, and are likewise found near the ligamentum arteriosus, at which site they are usually termed aortopulmonary or aortic paragangliomas, and at the site of the organ of Zuckerkandl in the retroperitoneum [13–15]. In the latter site, a segment of aorta is usually removed with removal of the tumor. Both benign and malignant paragangliomas adjacent to the aorta have been described [13–15]. Although not primary neoplasms of the aorta, paragangliomas should be considered in the differential diagnosis of tumor involving the aortic wall. The histologic, immunohistochemical and ultrastructural features of aortic paragangliomas are identical to other paragangliomas.

21.1.3 NEOPLASMS OF THE PULMONARY ARTERY

(a) Incidence

Approximately 100 primary sarcomas of the pulmonary artery have been reported [1,2,16–25].

(b) Classification

Neoplasms of the pulmonary arteries are virtually limited to sarcomas. It is simplest to classify sarcomas of the pulmonary artery similarly to sarcomas of the aorta. There are several similarities between pulmonary sarcomas and aortic sarcomas: most pulmonary artery sarcomas are predominantly luminal, present as thromboemboli and not easily classified by histologically appearance. Those pulmonary artery sarcomas that are intraluminal are best classified as intimal sarcomas; these have a wide variety of histologic appearance. Those very rare tumors that arise from the wall of the pulmonary artery are classified by their histologic subtype. These tumors are very difficult to distinguish from sarcomas of lung parenchyma.

(c) Gross features

Grossly, the typical sarcoma of the pulmonary artery resembles a mucoid clot (Figures 21.7, 21.8). It often extends distally along the lumen of the pulmonary arterial branches and occasionally infiltrates into pulmonary parenchyma. The pulmonary trunk is usually involved, and for unknown reasons, extension along the right pulmonary artery is more common than along the left.

(d) Histologic features

Microscopically, sarcomas of the pulmonary artery resemble those of the aorta. However, the range of histologic appearances is more varied; mucoid, osteosarcomatous and chondrosarcomatous areas are more common (Figure 21.9). Malignant cell layering over dense collagen is present less often than in aortic sarcomas. Because of the histologic variety, sarcomas of the pulmonary arteries, in contrast to aortic sarcomas, have been given a large variety of histologic diagnoses.

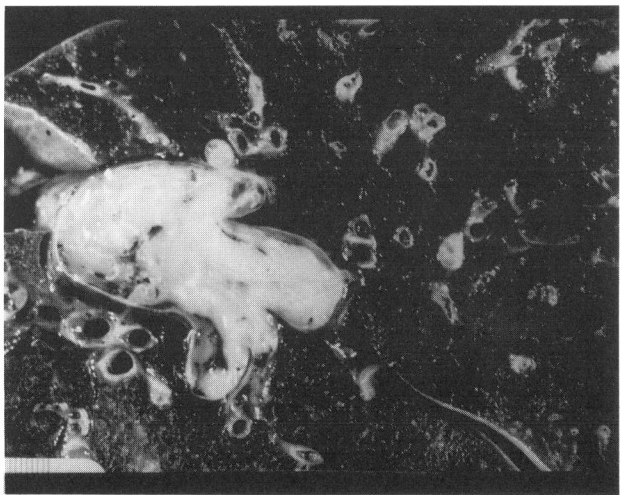

Figure 21.7 Sarcoma of pulmonary artery. Typically, there is filling of pulmonary arteries with mucoid tumor resembling clot. This patient died after several months treatment for presumed embolic pulmonary hypertension. A tissue diagnosis was not made during life.

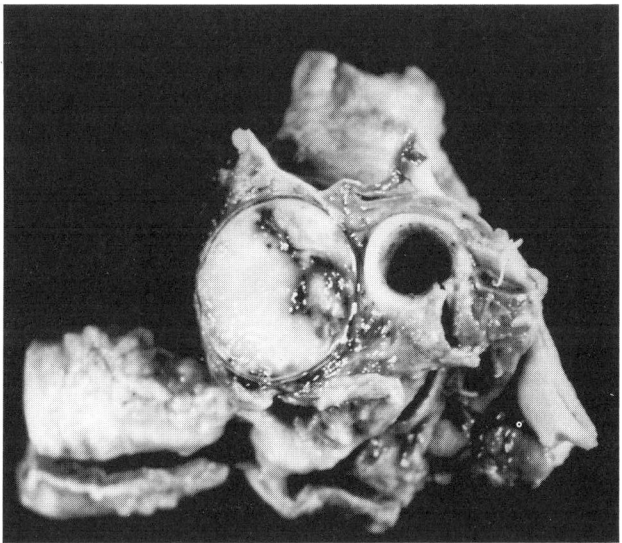

Figure 21.8 Sarcoma of pulmonary artery. In this example from a different patient, note the distended pulmonary artery without extension beyond the vessel wall.

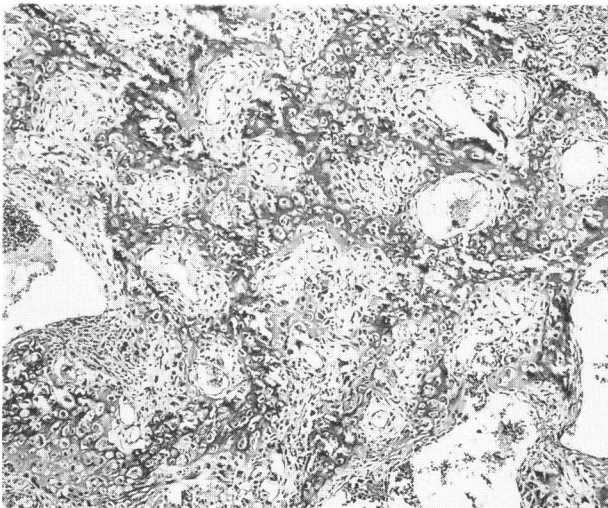

Figure 21.9 Sarcoma of pulmonary artery. Osteosarcoma is found more frequently in intimal pulmonary artery sarcomas than intimal aortic sarcomas. This tumor was removed by endarterectomy from a 41-year-old man with multiple pulmonary emboli refractory to medical therapy. Subsequently he developed metastases to the lungs and skeleton (not shown). (H&E.) (Reproduced with permission from Burke and Virmani [51].)

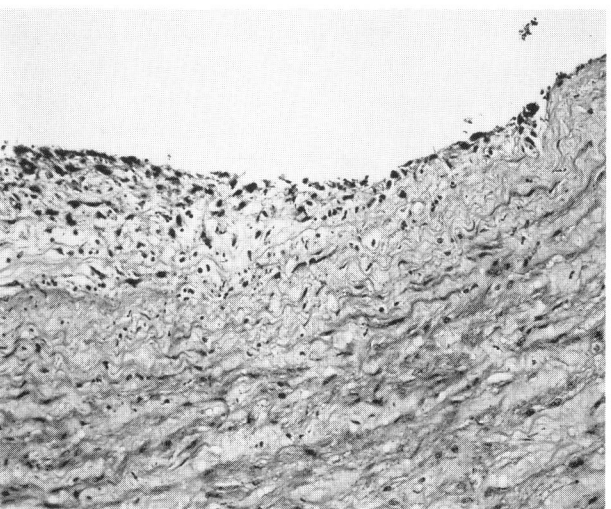

Figure 21.10 Sarcoma of the pulmonary artery. The margin of this tumor demonstrates the transition of the tumor with the surrounding intima, which is lined by atypical cells. These cells have been cited as evidence for endothelial dysplasia. This tumor was diagnosed at the autopsy of a 69-year-old woman who died of pulmonary embolism. (H&E.)

There have been reports of luminal leiomyosarcomas, rhabdomyosarcomas, angiosarcomas and malignant fibrous histiocytomas [2,25]. Not all of these reports provided ultrastructural or immunohistochemical documentation of specific differentiation. Similar to intimal sarcomas of the aorta, the intima at the margins of the tumor is often lined by atypical cells suggestive of endothelial derivation (Figure 21.10). Also similar to aortic sarcomas, however, endothelial differentiation in the tumor is difficult to demonstrate.

Because most sarcomas of the pulmonary arteries involve the pulmonary trunk, it has been hypothesized that they arise from primitive cells of the bulbus cordi [21]. Reports of immunohistochemistry are few [1,21,24], and generally demonstrate positivity for vimentin, smooth muscle and muscle-specific actin.

These staining patterns are not specific and are compatible with myofibroblastic origin.

(e) Clinical features

Because pulmonary artery sarcomas are very rare, and because they cause symptoms similar to recurrent pulmonary emboli, the diagnosis is virtually never considered early in the patient's disease. There is usually a prolonged course of anticoagulants [17,18,21] for the presumed clinical diagnosis of pulmonary emboli. The histologic diagnosis is made usually only at autopsy, although the diagnosis is occasionally made at endarterectomy. Patients with pulmonary artery sarcoma can sometimes die suddenly without previous symptoms [17].

Most reviews of pulmonary artery sarcomas have shown no sex predilection, with the exception of two large series that have shown a predominance of male patients [1,2] (Table 21.1). Although sarcomas of the pulmonary artery only rarely occur in children [16], the mean age at presentation is younger than that of aortic or caval sarcomas [1].

Sarcomas of the pulmonary artery are less likely to metastasize to distant sites than are their counterparts in the aorta. However, metastases to the kidney, brain, lymph nodes and skin have been reported [1]. A clinical course of over two years without metastases or treatment is common [1,19,20], but survival at five years is rare. Patients in whom curative resection has been attempted have a longer disease-free course than those without curative surgery. There is no good evidence at this time that chemo- or radiation therapy benefits patients with sarcomas of the pulmonary artery.

21.1.4 NEOPLASMS OF MUSCULAR ARTERIES

Muscular arteries can rarely give rise to neoplasms; most of these have been reported as leiomyosarcomas [26].

21.2 Neoplasms of veins

21.2.1 SARCOMAS

(a) Classification

Most sarcomas of veins occur in the inferior vena cava, arise in the vessel wall and are typical leiomyosarcomas on histologic evaluation [1,2,27,28]. Rarely, sarcomas of the inferior vena cava are confined to the lumen (Figure 21.11) and could be classified as intimal. Leiomyosarcomas of the superior vena cava, femoral vein, popliteal vein and pulmonary veins are quite rare [1,29–32].

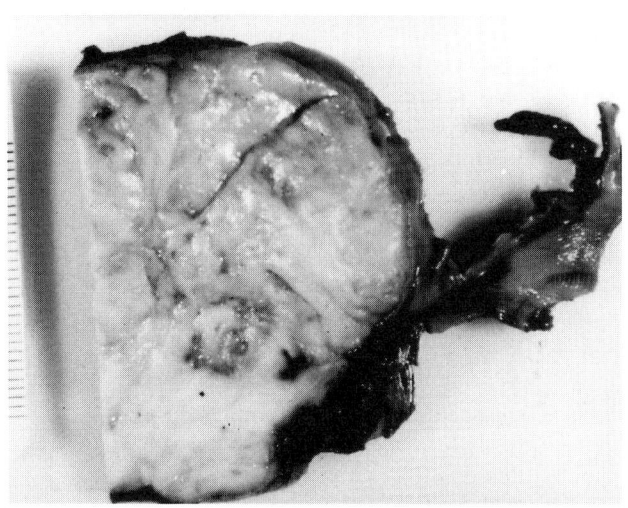

Figure 21.11 Sarcoma of inferior vena cava. This tumor was entirely luminal. Most sarcomas of the inferior vena cava are attached to the wall and extend into surrounding soft tissue. This tumor was removed from a 55-year-old woman with an obstruction in her inferior vena cava below the kidney.

(b) Incidence

The incidence of sarcomas of the venae cavae, based on reports in the literature, is approximately two to three times greater than that of sarcomas of great arteries. The true incidence is probably higher, because origin in the inferior vena cava can be difficult to prove. These lesions are typically larger than sarcomas of arteries and often remain asymptomatic for a long period because luminal growth can be minimal. Many retroperitoneal leiomyosarcomas may have originated in the inferior vena cava but have obscured their site of origin after reaching a large size.

(c) Gross features

Grossly, leiomyosarcomas of the inferior vena cava are firmly attached to the wall of the vessel and form discrete masses that extend into the retroperitoneum. Rarely, they fill the lumen without significant spread into the vessel wall. The location of the sarcoma in the inferior vena cava can affect the clinical presentation (see below).

(d) Microscopic features

Histologically, most sarcomas of the inferior vena cava are typical of leiomyosarcomas. There is a fascicular growth pattern of fuchsinophilic spindle cells that contain glycogen, often have perinuclear vacuoles and possess blunt-ended nuclei. Characteristically, there are areas of growth in which the fascicles lie at right angles to one another (Figure 21.12). Slightly over one half

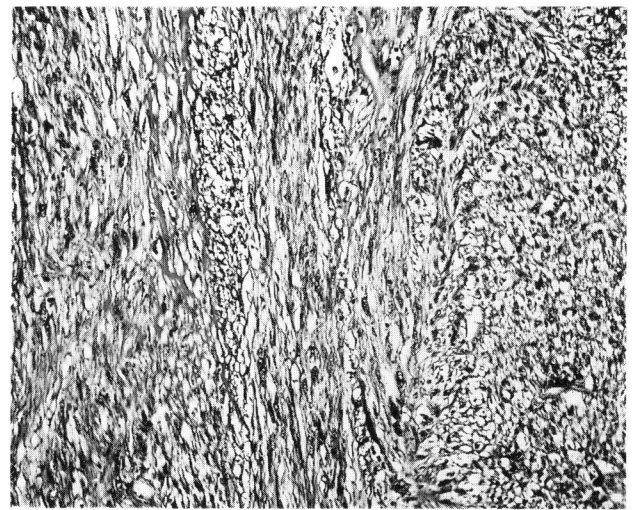

Figure 21.12 Leiomyosarcoma of the inferior vena cava. A histologic section from the tumor shown in Figure 21.10. The fascicles of leiomyosarcoma often lie at right angles to one another. (H&E.)

will demonstrate intracytoplasmic desmin with the use of immunohistochemical techniques. Desmin is more specific for leiomyosarcoma than are antibodies to actin, which is prevalent in many types of soft tissue proliferations.

Luminal sarcomas of the inferior vena cava are exceptionally rare. Grossly and microscopically, these tumors resemble intimal sarcomas of great arteries. Unusual venous sarcomas that have been reported include angiosarcomas of the superior vena cava, synovial sarcomas of the superior vena cava and leiomyosarcomas of the pulmonary, femoral and iliac veins [1].

(e) Clinical features

The majority of leiomyosarcomas of the inferior vena cava arise in women and the average age at presentation is approximately 60 years [1] (Table 21.1). The presenting symptom depends on the tumor location: those at the level of the liver present with Budd–Chiari syndrome and have the worst prognosis; those in the middle portion of the inferior vena cava present with pain, and distal lesions have the best long-term outcome and present typically with IVC syndrome [27,28]. Other modes of presentation include recurring pulmonary emboli and metastatic disease; rarely, sarcomas of the inferior vena cava can be incidental findings. Survival is longer in patients with sarcomas of the inferior vena cava than in patients with sarcomas of the aorta and pulmonary arteries, with an average of about three years. Metastases can occur in a variety of sites, including the lungs, kidneys, pleura, chest wall, liver and bones [1].

21.2.2 LEIOMYOMAS

Small, incidental leiomyomas of peripheral veins are quite common (Figures 21.13, 21.14), and usually present as masses that can be painful. Leiomyomas of the inferior vena cava are much rarer (Figure 21.15) and are generally luminal [33], in contrast to leiomyosarcomas of the venae cavae, most of which are attached to the vessel wall. The majority of leiomyomas that occur within the lumen of the inferior vena cava are extensions of uterine leiomyomas and represent so-called intravenous leiomyomatosis [34]. Less often they arise from the lining of the vena cava itself, or are extensions of leiomyomas which originate in the hepatic, femoral or more distal veins [35].

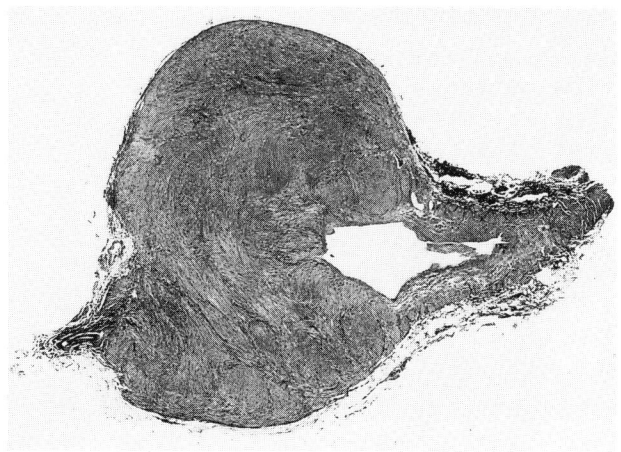

Figure 21.13 Leiomyoma of popliteal vein. This lesion presented as a tender nodule over the right calf of a 21-year-old woman. (H&E.)

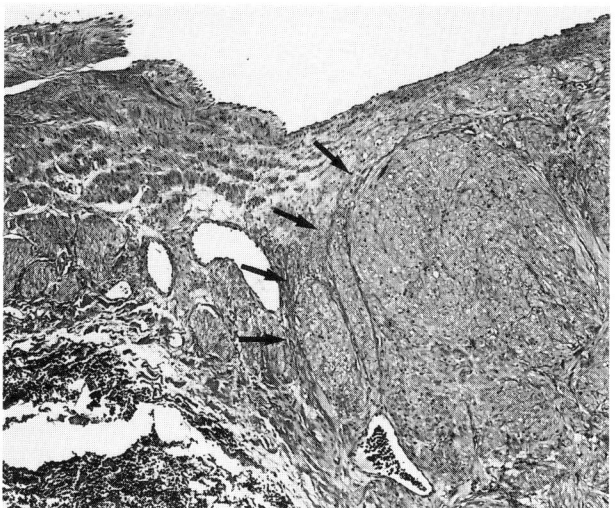

Figure 21.14 Higher power magnification of Figure 21.11 demonstrates the junction between leiomyoma and wall of vein. (H&E.)

736 ARTERIAL AND VENOUS NEOPLASMS

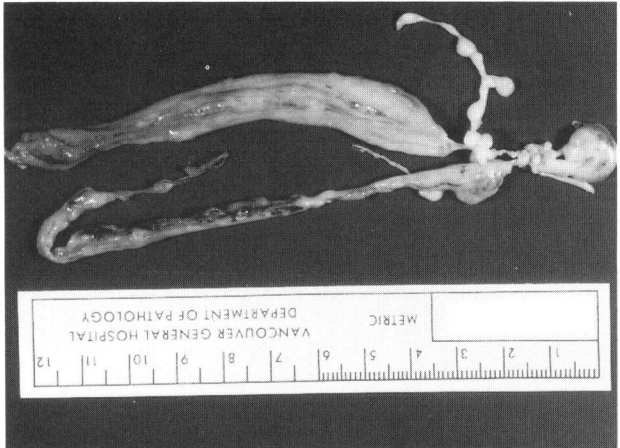

Figure 21.15 Leiomyoma of inferior vena cava. Luminal leiomyomas can fill the inferior vena cava, as primary neoplasms or extension from pelvic leiomyomas (intravenous leiomyomatosis). (Figure courtesy of Dr John English, Vancouver General Hospital, British Columbia.)

21.3 Tumor angiogenesis

21.3.1 DEFINITION

Angiogenesis, which strictly denotes new vessel formation, occurs not only as an integral part of tumor growth and metastasis, but also plays a central role in inflammation, organ development and reproduction [36].

21.3.2 CELLULAR AND HUMORAL COMPONENTS OF ANGIOGENESIS

The cellular components of the tumor angiogenic process include endothelial cells of capillaries, tumor cells, macrophages and mast cells. The protein signals that modulate blood vessel growth are the focus of great interest and have largely been discovered only in the past decade. The first endothelial cell growth factor to be purified was later identified as basic fibroblast growth factor. Since that time, other growth factors that stimulate endothelial cell growth *in vitro* have been identified. These include acidic fibroblast growth factor, vascular endothelial growth factor (vascular permeability factor), platelet-derived endothelial cell growth factor and transforming growth factor-alpha. Only the endothelial cell growth factors are specific for endothelial cells; fibroblast growth factor and platelet-derived growth factor are pleiotrophic and are mitogenic for a wide variety of cell types.

Several studies have demonstrated an effect *in vitro* of a variety of peptides on endothelial differentiation, a variety of peptides on endothelial differentiation, division and DNA synthesis. However, the interaction *in vivo* of these various substances with regard to tumor growth is poorly understood. *In situ* hybridization and immunohistochemistry are well established techniques

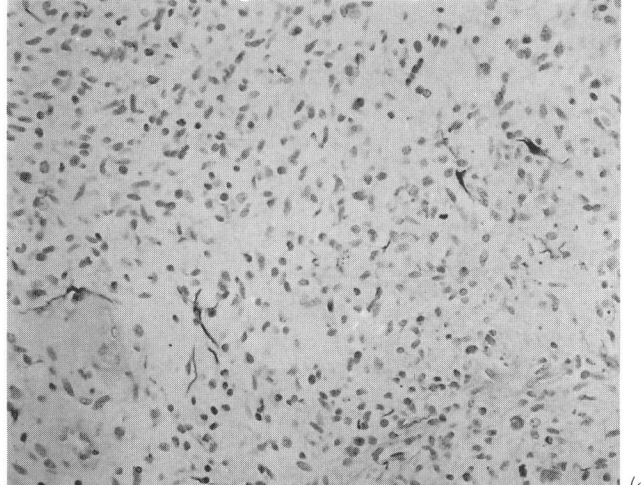

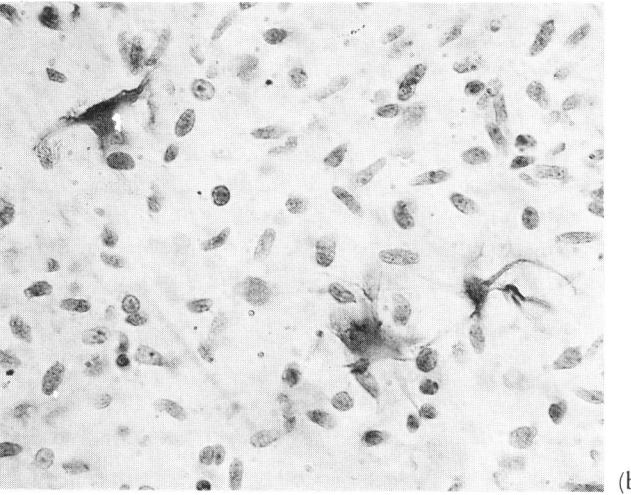

Figure 21.16 (a) High-grade astrocytoma. Immunoperoxidase preparation demonstrating positivity for transforming growth factor-beta within astrocytic tumor cells; note long positive cell processes. (b) Higher power magnification of (a). (Avidin-biotin complex.)

that localize proteins and messenger RNA in tissue sections and thereby determine those cells in a tumor milieu that are expressing growth factors. A limitation of these techniques is their relatively low sensitivity, which restricts their usefulness in identifying peptides that are present in very small concentration. Nevertheless, several reports have demonstrated the expression of angiogenic growth factors within tissue samples of high grade astrocytomas [37,38]. These malignancies are well known to possess large numbers of proliferating vessels. Transforming growth factor-alpha mRNA and acidic fibroblast growth factor mRNA have been identified by *in situ* hybridization within malignant astrocytes, as well as the corresponding proteins by immunohistochemistry (Figure 21.16). Basic fibroblast growth factor has also been demonstrated within proliferating blood vessels in glioblastoma multiforme. In our laboratory we have demonstrated both acidic and basic fibroblast growth factor as well as transforming growth factor-alpha within malignant astrocytes and blood vessels of high grade astrocytomas. Filtrates of human glioblastoma cell lines contain soluble factors that induce transformational alterations in endothelial cell cultures; these factors have yet to be characterized [39].

21.3.3 PHYSIOLOGY OF ANGIOGENESIS

The biology of the action of angiogenic growth factors on endothelial cell proliferation and tumor growth is poorly understood. Constituents of the extracellular matrix, such as heparin, heparan sulfate and related polysaccharides appear to affect the activity of acidic fibroblast growth factor and basic fibroblast growth factor. The mechanism of this action appears to involve modification of cell surface receptors, conformational changes in the protein to allow receptor binding, protection for degradation by proteases and acid, and facilitation of diffusion of growth factors. The degradation of the extracellular matrix by the endothelial cell may contribute to the angiogenic process. Binding of basic fibroblast growth factor to heparan sulfate may result in the sequestration and inactivity of basic fibroblast growth factor, which is reversed by the secretion of heparanases [40]. Inhibitors of metalloproteinases, proteolytic enzymes that break down connective tissue matrices, may concomitantly inhibit the angiogenic process [41].

The relationship between tumor cell expression of angiogenic growth factors and invasive and metastatic potential is not clear. Tumor suppressor genes and angiogenic inhibitors such as thrombospondin may participate in a complex interactive balance that, when disturbed, results in excessive vascular growth [42]. Transforming growth factor-beta and tumor necrosis factor-alpha, although they are angiogenic inhibitors *in vitro*, may actually contribute to the growth of tumor blood vessels by attracting monocytes which possess angiogenic activity, as well as mast cells, which are loaded with heparin granules.

21.3.4 CLINICAL CORRELATES OF TUMOR ANGIOGENESIS

The degree of angiogenesis can be estimated by a quantitation of microvessels within a section of tumor that is the most highly vascularized. There is evidence that the degree of angiogenesis in breast cancer correlates with the presence of axillary and distant metastases [43], as well as survival in early stage patients [44]. Currently, estimation of the degree of angiogenesis in other types of malignancy is being correlated with the presence of metastasis and prognosis [45].

The measurement of certain angiogenic factors, especially basic fibroblast growth factor, in body fluids may provide prognostic data and estimation of tumor burden or recurrence in patients with malignancies [46]. Basic fibroblast growth factor determinations in serum, cerebrospinal fluid and urine have been performed in a number of patients with solid malignancies, and there is evidence that basic fibroblast growth factor levels in urine correlate with the presence of transitional cell carcinoma of the bladder.

A major area of research is the development of factors that inhibit angiogenesis [47]. These factors have the potential for tumor suppression and use as chemotherapeutic agents. *In vitro*, alpha-interferon is mildly angioinhibitory. It has been used successfully in the treatment of infantile hemangiomas [48] and Kaposi's sarcoma [49]. Medroxyprogesterone (tamoxifen), an antihormonal agent widely used for the treatment of breast cancer, may have angioinhibitory functions [50]. It remains to be seen what role more powerful and specific angioinhibitory substances will play in the chemotherapeutics of malignancies in the coming decade [47].

References

1. Burke, A.P. and Virmani, R. (1993) Sarcomas of the great vessels. *Cancer*, **69**, 387–95.
2. Fenoglio Jr, J.J. and Virmani, R. (1988) Primary malignant tumors of the great vessels, in *Pathology of the Heart and Great Vessels*, vol. 12, (ed. B. Waller), Churchill Livingstone, New York, pp. 429–38.
3. Josen, A.S. and Khine, M. (1989) Primary malignant tumor of the aorta. *J. Vasc. Surg.*, **9**, 493–8.
4. Pruszczynski, M., Coronel, C.M., Naudin ten Cate, L. *et al.* (1988) Immunohistochemical and ultrastructural studies of a primary aortic intimal sarcoma. *Pathology*, **20**, 173–8.
5. Becquemin, J.P., Lebbe, C., Saada, F. and Avril, M.F. (1988) Sarcoma of the aorta: report of a case and review of the literature. *Ann. Vasc. Surg.*, **2**, 225–30.
6. Nishikawa, H., Miyakoshi, S., Nishimura, S. *et al.* (1989) A case of aortic intimal sarcoma manifested with acutely occurring hypertension and aortic occlusion. *Heart Vessels*, **5**, 54–8.
7. Haber, L.M. and Truong, L. (1988) Immunohistochemical demonstration of the endothelial nature of aortic intimal sarcoma. *Am. J. Surg. Pathol.*, **12**, 798–802.
8. Fitzmaurice, R.J. and McClure, J. (1990) Aortic intimal sarcoma; an unusual case with pulmonary vasculature involvement. *Histopathology*, **15**, 457–62.
9. Herzberg, A.J. and Pizzo, S.V. (1988) Primary undifferentiated sarcoma of the thoracic aorta. *Histopathology*, **13**, 571–4.
10. Wright, E.P., Glick, A.D., Virmani, R. and Page, D.L. (1985) Aortic intimal sarcoma with embolic metastases. *Am. J. Surg. Pathol.*, **9**, 890–7.
11. Tejada, E., Becker, G.J. and Waller, B.F. (1991) Malignant myxoid emboli as the presenting feature of primary sarcoma of the aorta (myxoid malignant fibrous histiocytoma): a case report and review of the literature. *Clin. Cardiol.*, **14**, 425–30.
12. Weinberg, D.S. and Maini, B.S. (1980) Primary sarcoma of the aorta associated with a vascular prosthesis: a case report. *Cancer*, **15**, 398–401.
13. Faure, G., Carpentier, E., Berthet, E. *et al.* (1980) [Paraganglioma of the organs of Zuckerkandl. A case report (author's transl)]. *J. Urol. (Paris)*, **86**, 671–4.
14. Lack, E.E., Stillinger, R.A., Colvin, D.B. *et al.* (1979) Aortic-pulmonary paraganglioma: report of a case with ultrastructural study and review of the literature. *Cancer*, **43**, 269–78.
15. Duff, C., van Segesser, L., Schmid, E.R. *et al.* (1989) [Surgery of retroperitoneal pheochromocytoma]. *Helv. Chir. Acta*, **56**, 151–3.
16. Farooki, Z.Q., Chang, C.H., Jackson, W.L. *et al.* (1988) Primary pulmonary artery sarcoma in two children. *Pediatr. Cardiol.*, **9**, 243–51.
17. Varriale, P. and Chryssos, B. (1991) Pulmonary artery sarcoma: another cause of sudden death. *Clin. Cardiol.*, **14**, 160–4.

18. Promisloff, R.A., Segal, S.L., Lenchner, G.S. et al. (1988) Sarcoma of the pulmonary artery. *Chest*, **93**, 207–8.
19. Fer, M.F., Greco, F.A., Haile, K.L. et al. (1981) Unusual survival after pulmonary artery sarcoma. *South. Med. J.*, **74**, 624–6.
20. Klinke, W.P., Gelfand, E.T. and Baron, L. (1985) Primary sarcoma of the pulmonary trunk: successful surgical intervention and prolonged survival. *Clin. Cardiol.*, **8**, 437–40.
21. McGlennen, R.C., Manivel, J.C., Stanley, S.J. et al. (1989) Pulmonary artery trunk sarcoma: a clinicopathological, ultrastructural, and immunohistochemical study of four cases. *Mod. Pathol.*, **2**, 486–94.
22. Baker, P.B. and Goodwin, R.A. (1985) Pulmonary artery sarcomas. Review and report of a case. *Arch. Pathol. Lab. Med.*, **109**, 35–39.
23. Kruger, I., Borowski, A., Horst, M. et al. (1990) Symptoms, diagnosis and therapy of primary sarcomas of the pulmonary artery. *Thorac. Cardiovasc. Surg.*, **38**, 91–95.
24. Nonomura, A., Kurumaya, H., Kono, J. et al. (1988) Primary pulmonary artery sarcoma. Report of two autopsy cases studied by immunohistochemistry and electron microscopy, and review of 110 cases reported in the literature. *Acta Path. Jap.*, **38**, 883–96.
25. Van Damme, H., Vaneerdeweg, W. and Schoofs, E. (1987) Malignant fibrous histiocytoma of the pulmonary artery. *Ann. Surg.*, **205**, 203–7.
26. Leeson, M.C., Malaei, M. and Makley, J.T. (1990) Leiomyosarcoma of the popliteal artery. A report of two cases. *Clin. Orthop.*, **253**, 225–30.
27. Griffin, A.S. and Sterchi, J.M. (1987) Primary leiomyosarcoma of the inferior vena cava: a case report and review of the literature. *J. Surg. Oncol.*, **34**, 53–60.
28. Bruyninckx, C.M. and Derksen, O.S. (1986) Leiomyosarcoma of the inferior vena cava. Case report and review of the literature. *J. Vasc. Surg.*, **3**, 652–6.
29. Leu, H.J. and Makek, M. (1986) Intramural venous leiomyosarcomas. *Cancer*, **57**, 1395–400.
30. Taheri, S.A. and Conner, G.W. (1983) Leiomyosarcoma of iliac veins. *Surgery*, **94**, 516–20.
31. Basu, S.K., Scott, T.D., Wilmshurts, C.C. et al. (1988) Leiomyosarcomata of the popliteal vessels: rare primary tumours. *Eur. J. Vasc. Surg.*, **2**, 423–5.
32. Fischer, M.G., Gelb, A.M., Nussbaum, M. et al. (1982) Primary smooth muscle tumors of venous origin. *Ann. Surg.*, **21**, 238–40.
33. Payan, M.J., Xerri, L., Choux, R. et al. (1989) Giant leiomyoma of the inferior vena cava. *Ann. Pathol.*, **9**, 44–46.
34. Norris, H.J. and Parmley, T. (1975) Mesenchymal tumors of the uterus. V. Intravenous leiomyomatosis. A clinical and pathologic study of 14 cases. *Cancer*, **36**, 2164–78.
35. Dunlap, H.J. and Udjus, K. (1990) Atypical leiomyoma arising in an hepatic vein with extension into the inferior vena cava and right atrium. Report of a case in a child. *Pediat. Radiol.*, **20**, 202–3.
36. Folkman, J. and Shing, Y. (1992) Angiogenesis. *J. Biol. Chem.*, **267**, 10931–4.
37. Maxwell, M., Nabler, S.P., Wolfe, H.J. et al. (1991) Expression of angiogenic growth factor genes in primary human astrocytomas may contribute to their growth and progression. *Cancer Res.*, **51**, 1345–51.
38. Stefanik, D.F., Rizkalla, L.R., Soi, A. et al. (1991) Acidic and basic fibroblast growth factors are present in glioblastoma multiforme. *Cancer Res.*, **51**, 5760–5.
39. Silbergeld, D.J., Ali-Osman, F. and Winn, H.R. (1991) Induction of transformational changes in normal endothelial cells by cultured human astrocytoma cells. *J. Neurosurg.*, **75**, 604–12.
40. Vladavsky, I., Korner, G., Ishai-Michaeli, R. et al. (1990) Extracellular matrix-resident growth factors and enzymes: possible involvement in tumor metastasis and angiogenesis. *Cancer Metastasis Rev.*, **9**, 203–26.
41. Moses, M.A. and Langer, R. (1991) A metalloproteinase inhibitor as an inhibitor of neovascularization. *J. Cell. Biochem.*, **47**, 230–5.
42. Good, D.J., Polverini, P.J., Rastinejad, F. et al. (1990) A tumor suppressor-dependent inhibitor of angiogenesis is immunologically and functionally indistinguishable from a fragment of thrombospondin. *Proc. Natl Acad. Sci. USA*, **87**, 6624–78.
43. Weidner, N., Semple, J.P., Welch, W.R. and Folkman, J. (1991) Tumor angiogenesis and metastasis – correlation in invasive breast carcinoma. *N. Engl. J. Med.*, **324**, 1–8.
44. Weidner, N., Folkman, J., Pozza, F. et al. (1992) Tumor angiogenesis: a new significant and independent prognostic indicator in early-stage breast carcinoma. *J. Natl Cancer Inst.*, **84**, 1875–87.
45. Weidner, N., Carroll, P.R., Flax, J. et al. (1993) Tumor angiogenesis correlates with metastasis in invasive prostate carcinoma. *Am. J. Pathol.*, **143**, 401–9.
46. Fujimoto, K., Ichimori, Y., Kakizoe, T. et al. (1991) Increased serum levels of basic fibroblast growth factor in patients with renal cell carcinoma. *Biochem. Biophys. Res. Commun.*, **180**, 386–92.
47. Folkman, J. and Ingber, D. (1992) Inhibition of angiogenesis. *Semin. Cancer Biol.*, **3**, 89–96.
48. White, C.W., Sondheimer H.M., Crouch E.C. et al. (1989) Treatment of pulmonary hemangiomatosis with recombinant interferon alpha 2a. *New Engl. J. Med.*, **320**, 1197–200.
49. Mitsayasu, R.T. (1991) Interferon alpha in the treatment of AIDS-related Kaposi's sarcoma. *Br. J. Haematol.*, **79** (suppl. 1), 69–73.
50. Billington, D.C. (1991) Angiogenesis and its inhibition: potential new therapies in oncology and non-neoplastic diseases. *Drug Des. Discov.*, **8**, 3–35.
51. Burke, A.P. and Virmani, R. (1993) Sarcomas of the great vessels. *Cancer*, **71**, 1761–73.

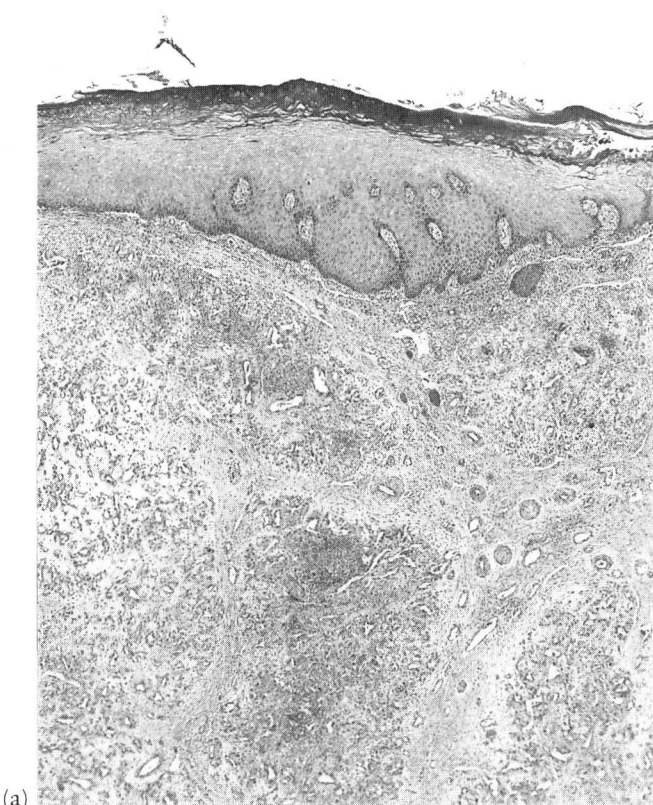

Figure 22.1 Bacillary angiomatosis: (a) Lobules of well-formed capillaries reminiscent of pyogenic granuloma. (b) Lobules punctuated by foci with leukocytoclastic debris, neutrophils, and flocculent or granular material. (c) Warthin–Starry stain (pH 4.0) demonstrating curved organisms appearing singly and in small clusters. (Oil.)

In fact, some reports, in the earlier literature, of 'disseminated pyogenic granuloma', may actually be examples of BA [3,14]. However, in contrast to pyogenic granuloma, BA contains vessels lined by plumper, more atypical appearing endothelial cells and, most importantly, it exhibits acute inflammatory foci, even in the absence of surface ulceration.

Kaposi's sarcoma enters into the differential diagnosis of BA since both processes have a predilection for immunosuppressed, especially HIV-positive, individuals and both are frequently characterized by the presence of multiple cutaneous lesions. However, Kaposi's sarcoma lacks a well formed, lobulated vascular pattern with plump, protruding endothelium as is seen in bacillary angiomatosis and, instead, is often dominated by spindle cells with slit-like vascular channels. It also differs by featuring a lymphoplasmacytic, rather than polymorphonuclear, inflammatory reaction. Periodic acid-Schiff-positive, diastase-resistant hyaline globules, especially when present in a clustered, grape-like arrangement, are a well recognized feature of the plaque and nodular stages of Kaposi's sarcoma which further aid in its distinction.

BA should be at the forefront of the differential diagnosis when evaluating vascular proliferations arising in immunocompromised patients, especially if leukocytoclastic debris or acute inflammation is present. This disease, if left untreated, can prove fatal [3].

22.1.2 VERRUGA PERUANA (CARRION'S DISEASE, OROYA FEVER)

In the course of the construction of a railway between Lima and La Oroya, Peru, at least 7000 individuals are

22 TUMORS AND TUMEFACTIONS OF PERIPHERAL VESSELS*

Elizabeth A. Montgomery and John F. Fetsch

22.1 Reactive lesions of peripheral vessels

This group includes vascular proliferations which result from infectious processes, immunologic disturbances or host response to a variety of other etiologies, including trauma. Angiolymphoid hyperplasia with eosinophilia (epithelioid hemangioma) is included in this section, in part, to highlight its contrasting features with Kimura's disease, with which it has been confused in the past and, in part, as a reflection of our belief that some examples have features consistent with a reactive tumefaction. This view is controversial, however, and we acknowledge the fact that some lesions are sufficiently exuberant as to suggest a true, albeit benign, neoplasm. Both benign and so-called malignant angioendotheliomatosis are included in this section, primarily to clarify confusion which arose prior to the advent of immunohistochemical staining. Whereas the former appears to be a reactive vascular proliferation caused by protean immunological disturbances, the latter has now been shown to represent an angiotropic form of lymphoma. Pyogenic granuloma has not been included in this section as the current trend has been to regard it as a benign neoplasm, lobular capillary hemangioma, a view which is also open to debate.

22.1.1 BACILLARY ANGIOMATOSIS

Bacillary (epithelioid) angiomatosis (BA) is a pseudo-neoplastic vascular proliferation, first described in HIV-infected individuals [1]. The disease has a predilection for, but is not restricted to, immunocompromised patients [2,3]. A newly recognized fastidious Gram-negative, Warthin–Starry-positive, rickettsia-like microorganism, *Rochalimaea henselae* [4,5,6], appears to be the predominant pathogen, although other closely related agents, including *Afipia felis* [7,8] and *Rochalimaea quintana* [9], have also been implicated. These organisms are susceptible to antibiotics, including erythromycin, rifampin and doxycycline, which often must be administered for a 4–6-week course to avoid relapse. Although cutaneous lesions are the most frequently recognized manifestation of this disease, a systemic infection typically ensues in the immunosuppressed host with reported sites of involvement including the lymph nodes [10], bone marrow, spleen, liver, soft tissue [11,12], conjunctivae and mucosal surfaces [3]. In immunocompetent individuals, lesions are believed to remain localized to the inoculation site [13].

The lesions of BA typically contain a lobulated proliferation of capillary-sized vessels which are often well formed (Figure 22.1(a)). The endothelium lining the vessels may be plump with an 'activated' or mildly atypical appearance. Aggregates of neutrophils, leukocytoclastic debris and granular flocculent material are present both within the vascular lobules and the adjacent soft tissue (Figure 22.9(b)). The infectious agent is harbored within these foci and appears, with the aid of the Warthin–Starry stain (pH 4.0), as clumps of small curved rods approximately 0.5–1.0 µm in length (Figure 22.1(c)).

The differential diagnosis of BA revolves primarily around three entities: pyogenic granuloma, Kaposi's sarcoma and Carrion's disease. A detailed discussion of the latter is presented in the following section and so it will not be reiterated here, other than to note that it is rarely seen outside of its endemic areas in South America.

Dermal examples of BA bear a superficial resemblance to pyogenic granuloma (lobular capillary hemangioma).

---

* The opinions or assertions contained herein are the private views of the authors and are not to be construed as official or reflecting the views of the Departments of the Army, Navy, Air Force or Defense.

Vascular Pathology. Edited by W.E. Stehbens and J.T. Lie. Published in 1995 by Chapman & Hall, London. ISBN 0 412 48640 7

said to have died from a severe febrile illness which came to be known by Peruvian doctors as Oroya fever [15]. The condition is also referred to as Carrion's disease, after Daniel A. Carrion, a medical student, who established the relationship between the febrile condition and cutaneous lesions, designated 'verruga peruana nodules', which may subsequently develop. He accomplished this by inoculating himself with blood from a cutaneous lesion of an affected individual and thereafter developed a febrile episode consistent with Oroya fever which lead to his death. In endemic areas, the term *la verruga* is used to encompass both manifestations of this biphasic disease [15].

The etiologic agent is *Bartonella bacilliformis*, a hemotropic, mobile, pleomorphic, Gram-negative bacteria which has been shown to elaborate an angiogenesis factor *in vitro* [16,17]. On the basis of both the former feature and the organism's phylogenetic similarities to the *Rochalimaea* and *Afipia* genera [18] described earlier, some observers have drawn parallels between this disease process and bacillary angiomatosis [9,10]. Carrion's disease is transmitted by *Lutzomyia (Phlebotomus) verrucarum*, a nocturnal sandfly. Humans are the only known reservoir.

After an incubation period of approximately three weeks, individuals without prior tolerance develop a fever and an acute, severe, hemolytic anemia, the result of virtually 100% parasitization of circulating erythrocytes by the micro-organism. Infiltration of the reticuloendothelial system ensues with resultant hepatosplenomegaly and lymphadenopathy. In the pre-antibiotic era, the mortality at this stage was approximately 40%; the current figure is around 8%. A tissue phase which signals improvement in the patient's condition, appears approximately two months after the hematic phase and is characterized by the development of verruga peruana nodules which primarily involve the face and extremities. In endemic areas, where more than 60% of asymptomatic individuals have antibodies to *B. bacilliformis*, infections may follow an abbreviated course, and, in fact, healthy individuals harboring the organism have been identified. This latter group may serve as the natural reservoir for the infection [15].

The lesions of Carrion's disease can be subclassified histologically as miliary, when small and confined to the papillary dermis, nodular, when small to medium-sized and present in the reticular dermis or subcutis, or mular, when large and involving both skin and subcutaneous tissue [19]. All contain vasoformative elements, commonly admixed with inflammatory cells, and typically arranged in a multinodular or lobulated pattern (Figure 22.2). Superficial examples may be polypoid and, when accompanied by well formed vessels with patent lumina, may be suggestive of a pyogenic granuloma or bacillary angiomatosis. Lesions which arise in less distensible tissues may exhibit more solid 'angioblastic' growth

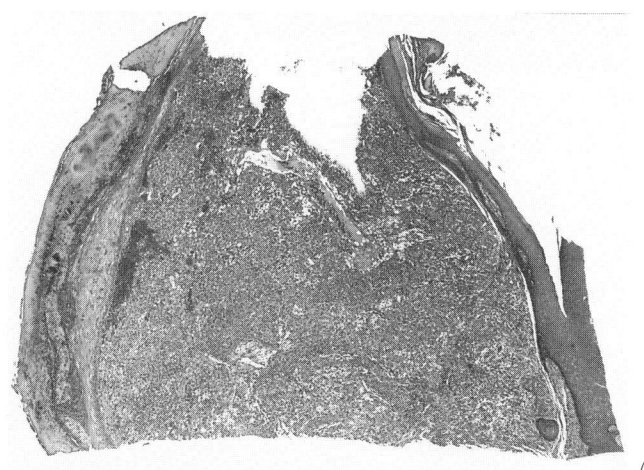

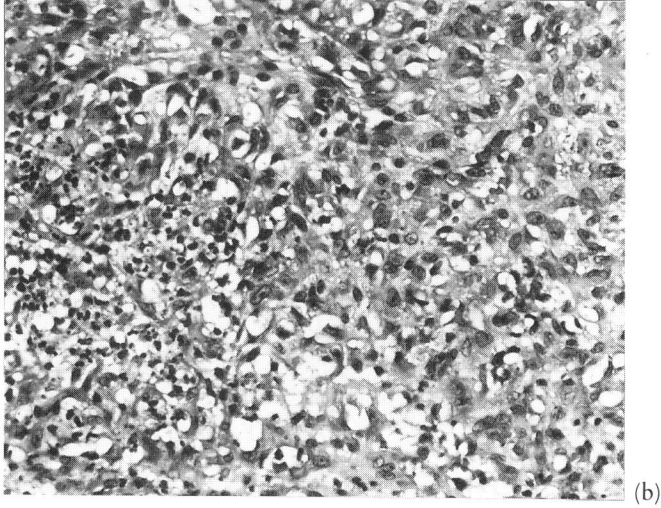

Figure 22.2 (a) Verruga peruana lesion. Scanning power shows demonstrates an exuberant, vaguely lobulated vascular proliferation with crusted overlying skin. (b) Endothelial cells with varying degrees of atypia are associated with neutrophils; Rocha–Lima inclusions may be fleeting. (Courtesy of Dr J. Arias-Stella Jr)

suggestive of a neoplastic process [20]. All examples are unified by the presence of plump atypical endothelial (verruga) cells. Depending on the stage of the lesions, lymphocytes and plasma cells or polymorphonuclear leukocytes with microabscess formation may be the predominant inflammatory constituents. Fibrin deposition, cellular necrosis, and fibrosclerosis may also be evident. Superficial lesions generally resolve over a period of 4–6 weeks whereas deeper nodules may persist for up to 4 months. The identification of Rocha–Lima inclusions, which may be fleeting, assists in confirming the diagnosis. These granular structures are best seen when tissues are fixed in buffered neutral formalin, embedded in glycol methacrylate and stained with Giemsa [20]. They also stain lightly, though less convincingly, with the Warthin–Starry and PAS/D stains.

When inclusions are not found, the diagnosis rests on clinicopathologic correlation.

22.1.3 PAPILLARY ENDOTHELIAL HYPERPLASIA

This benign reactive process which represents an unusually exuberant form of organizing vascular thrombus, was first described in 1923 by Pierre Masson as 'vegetant intravascular hemangioendothelioma' [21], a designation which reflected his belief that it was instead neoplastic. Others [23] have referred to lesions of this type as 'intravascular angiomatosis'.

Papillary endothelial hyperplasia (PEH) may occur at any age and involve virtually any vessel, including those of neoplastic processes and vascular malformations [164]. However, in its 'pure' form, it typically presents as a solitary, superficial, firm, bluish or erythematous mass, involving the fingers, head and neck or anorectal regions. Commonly, physical examination reveals limited mobility of the process about its longitudinal axis. Astute gross examination by the surgeon or the pathologist may reveal confinement of the process to the lumen of a dilated vessel, usually a vein.

The initial report by Masson eloquently describes the proliferation of endothelial cells within vessels (hemorrhoidal) forming papillary fronds associated with thrombus (Figure 22.3(a)). The fronds contain a core of fibrin or hyalinized collagen, depending upon the stage of the lesion, and are lined by a single layer of endothelial cells which may be plump or swollen but lack significant atypia and mitotic activity [21–28] (Figure 22.3(b)–(d)). Occasionally, due to the plane of sectioning or an actual event, the fronds appear to be 'free-floating' within the vessel lumen. Extravascular extension may occasionally be seen, although it is usually not extensive. However, large, predominantly extravascular examples arising in hematomas have also been reported [28]. The following features help differentiate PEH from angiosarcoma, a tumor with which it has occasionally been confused:

1. the frequent confinement of the process to a vascular lumen;
2. a lack of cellular pleomorphism;
3. the typical arrangement of the endothelium in a monolayer;
4. a low mitotic rate;
5. a paucity of cellular necrosis.

22.1.4 INTRAVASCULAR FASCIITIS

Nodular fasciitis is a well characterized reactive pseudosarcomatous myofibroblastic proliferation which usually arises in the superficial fascia, subcutis or muscle. In these locations, it generally evolves into a relatively well circumscribed mass which stabilizes at a size of less than 3 cm after a period of initial rapid growth. Similar proliferations may also develop in other sites such as the periosteum (parosteal fasciitis) and within blood vessels (intravascular fasciitis) [29]. Recurrence following simple local excision is uncommon, regardless of the location.

Intravascular fasciitis can be seen at any age and has no gender predilection. However, it occurs most frequency in children and young adults, where it favors the upper extremities and head and neck region [29–31]. Although the number of reported cases is relatively small, there is a suggestion that lesions of this type may, on average, evolve somewhat more slowly than their subcutaneous or fascial counterparts. Gross examination reveals one or more masses with either a circumscribed or somewhat infiltrative appearance. Close scrutiny sometimes reveals the intimate association with one or more vessels, usually veins.

Intravascular fasciitis shares many histologic features with nodular fasciitis, the key distinction being the former's association with vasculature (Figure 22.4(a)). A solitary round or oval mass, a serpentine growth or a multinodular or plexiform proliferation (Figure 22.4(b)) may be noted, depending on the extent of the process and the number and type of vessels involved. The intima, media and adventitia of the vessel wall, as well as the juxtaposed soft tissue, are often involved by the loose 'feathery' proliferation of myofibroblastic cells. Extravasated erythrocytes and scattered lymphocytes are usually present. Osteoclast-like giant cells, cystic degeneration and keloid-like collagen are additional features which may be noted and seem to imply intralesional maturation. Ganglion-like myofibroblasts, a characteristic feature of proliferative fasciitis and proliferative myositis, are typically absent. Mitoses may be numerous and this feature, in conjunction with focal cellularity or a history of rapid growth, may lead to an incorrect diagnosis of sarcoma. However, if appropriate attention is given to the bland nuclear morphology, the relatively small size of the proliferation and its general circumscription, as well as the occasional presence of features which suggest intralesional maturation, a correct diagnosis can almost always be rendered.

In contrast to vascular smooth muscle tumors, intravascular fasciitis is less likely to exhibit a discrete fascicular growth pattern. Also, smooth muscle cells are usually somewhat larger than myofibroblasts due to more abundant eosinophilic cytoplasm and they more frequently feature blunt-ended nuclei and juxtanuclear vacuoles. Finally, longitudinal cytoplasmic striations, as demonstrated with Masson's trichrome stain, are a characteristic feature of smooth muscle but are infrequently seen and less well developed in myofibroblasts.

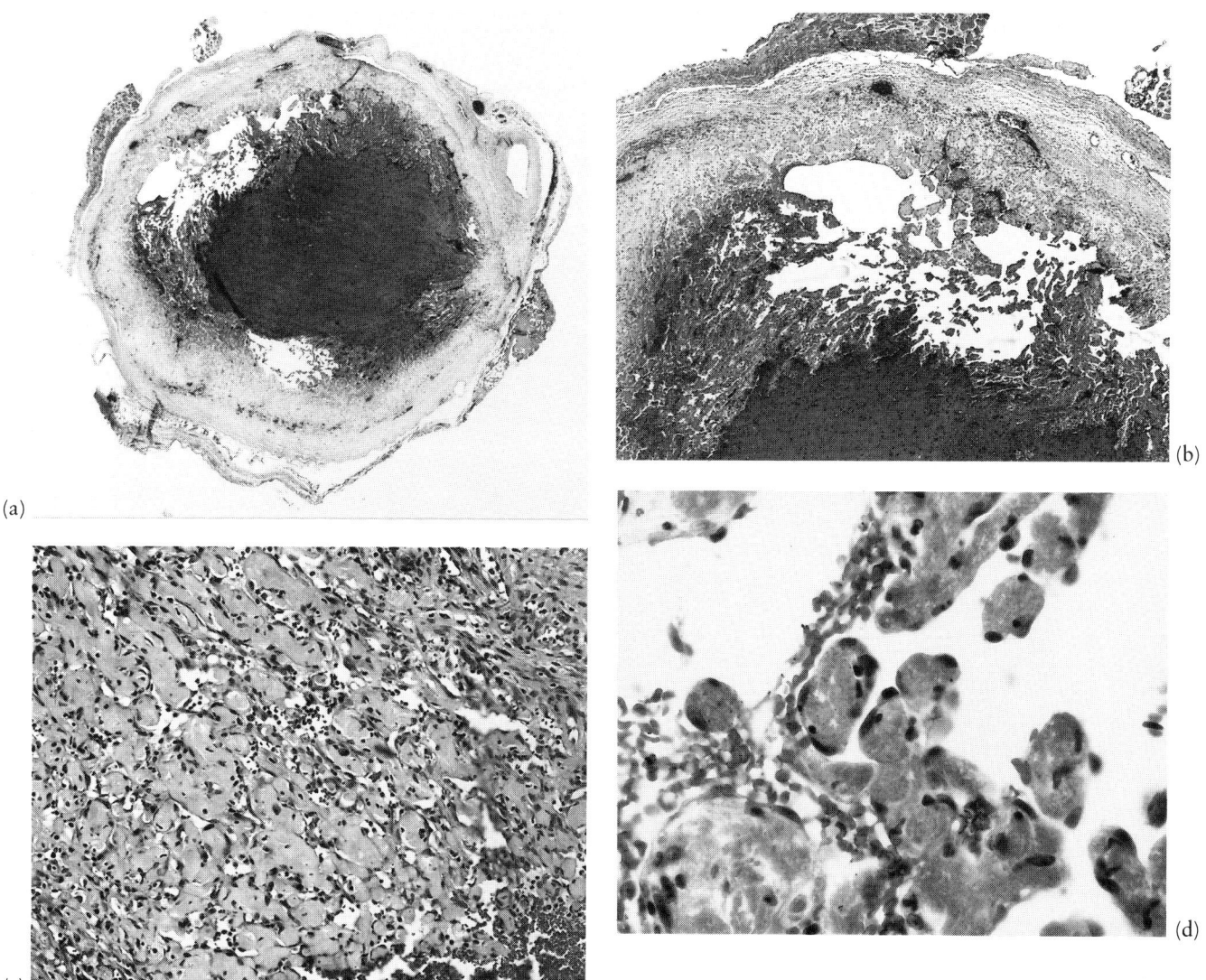

Figure 22.3 Papillary endothelial hyperplasia. (a) Cross-section of a vessel containing thrombus with a papillary endothelial proliferation. (b) Higher power view of (a). (c) Exuberant lesions may appear similar to angiosarcoma but in contrast tend to feature a monolayer of endothelial cells, a lack of mitoses and the absence of pleomorphism. (d) Higher power shows acellular fibrin cores 'coated' by plump amitotic endothelial cells.

22.1.5 ANGIOENDOTHELIOMATOSIS

This term, introduced some thirty years ago by Pfleger and Tappeiner [32], has been used to describe intravascular proliferations which are frequently associated with systemic manifestations [33]. Both benign and malignant clinical courses have been recognized but the morphologic distinction between these subgroups was not fully appreciated until the advent of immunohistochemistry [34]. It is now clear the most fatal examples previously referred to as 'malignant angioendotheliomatosis' are actually intravascular lymphomas of B-cell or, much less frequently, T-cell phenotype.

The majority of patients with intravascular lymphoma exhibit involvement of the skin subcutis and/or central nervous system [35–41]. Superficial lesions in the form of nodules or plaques primarily involve the trunk and extremities. Telangiectasia, hemorrhage and ulceration may be present in these areas. The most frequent central nervous system manifestation is progressive dementia although other findings can include decreased visual acuity, blindness, speech disturbances including aphasia, lethargy, headaches and progressive paralysis. The temporary nature of some neurologic manifestations is suggestive of transient ischemic attacks. Approximately one-third of patients exhibit serologic anomalies (i.e. rheumatoid factor, antinuclear antibodies) which postdate the onset of disease. Extravascular large cell lymphoma involving the lymph nodes, spleen, gastrointestinal tract, or other sites [34,36,37,41] may be de-

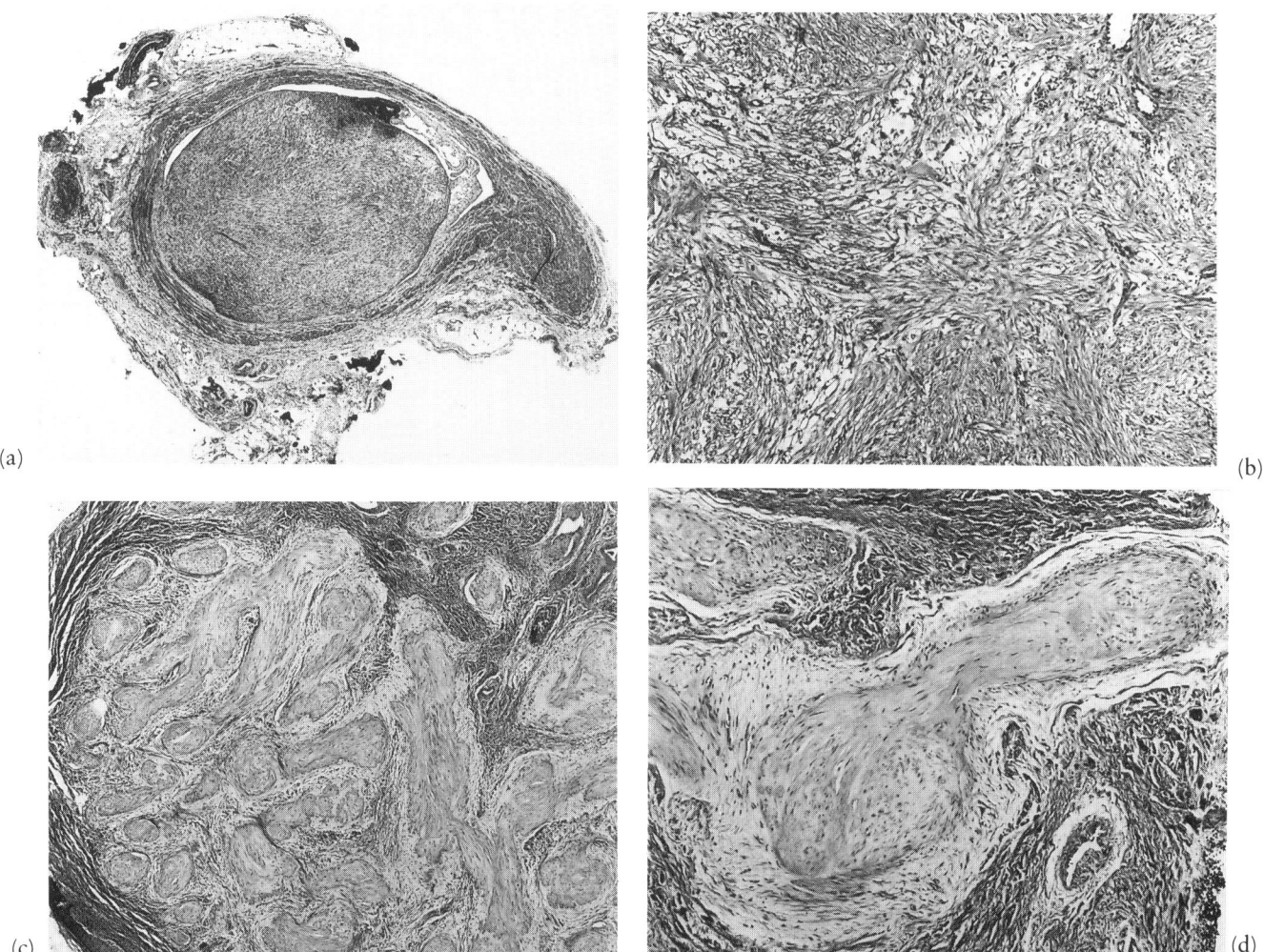

Figure 22.4 Intravascular fasciitis. (a) Spindle cell proliferation confined to the intravascular space. (b) The higher power appearance is identical to nodular fasciitis, consisting of cytologically bland myofibroblasts arranged in a loose storiform pattern. (c) Intravascular myofibroblastic proliferation of the corpus cavernosum of the penis with features suggestive of a late stage of intravascular fasciitis. Note the plexiform configuration. (d) The intravascular nature of the process is readily apparent at higher magnification; note the smooth muscle layer of the vessel wall.

monstrable in 25% or more of cases. However, the bone marrow is typically uninvolved.

On histologic examination, intravascular lymphomatosis features vessels of normal or dilated caliber with an intraluminal collection of large atypical cells exhibiting high nuclear to cytoplasmic ratios, nuclear hyperchromasia and nucleolar prominence (Figure 22.5(a)). These cells may be few in number or they may be present to such an extent as to occlude the vascular lumen. When cellular crowding is present, it can produce a false impression of cohesiveness and lead to an erroneous diagnosis of carcinoma. Occasionally, the tumor cells are enmeshed within fibrin thrombi. The malignant infiltrate sometimes spills over into the surrounding tissues and regional necrosis may be present. The neoplastic cells are typically immunoreactive with anti-leukocyte common antigen, as well as B- or, rarely, T-cell subset markers.

Benign (reactive) angioendotheliomatosis encompasses an uncommon group of cutaneous lesions characterized by activated immune status [34,42–46], either as a result of an ongoing infection (i.e. bacterial endocarditis, tuberculosis) or an allergic/hypersensitivity reaction. The anatomic distribution and apparently the clinical appearance of these lesions overlaps somewhat with the findings in intravascular lymphomatosis. However, patients with benign angioendotheliomatosis do not exhibit profound neurologic manifestations and typically improve spontaneously or following treatment (i.e. antibiotics, steroids) directed at the underlying cause of the immunologic derangement.

Benign angioendotheliomatosis features a proliferation of endothelial cells with a somewhat cohesive appearance, exhibiting relatively bland vesicular nuclei with small, distinct nucleoli. The presence of abundant amphophilic cytoplasm results in a relatively normal

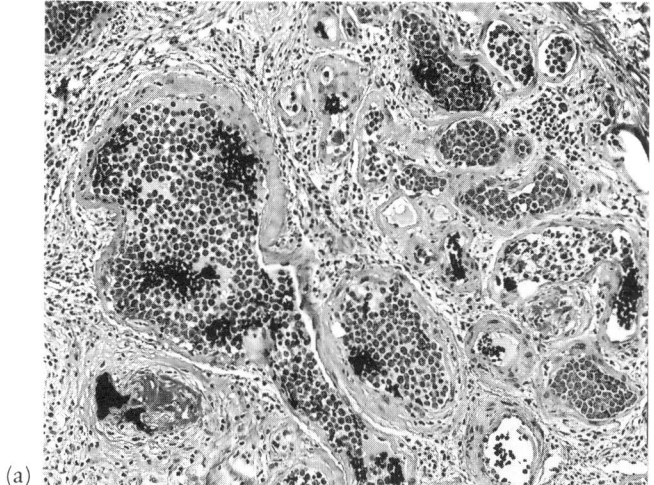
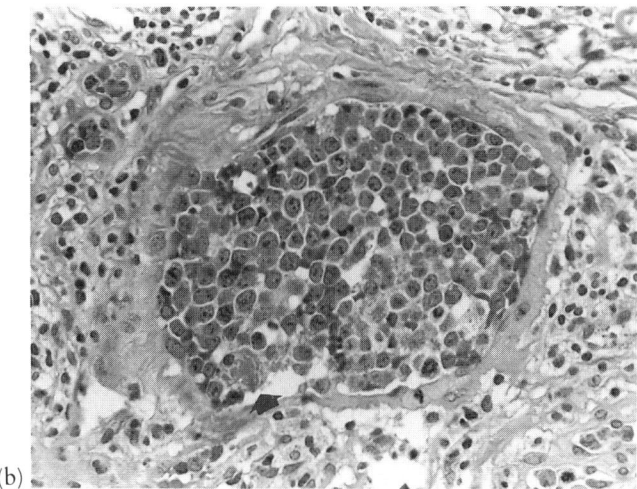
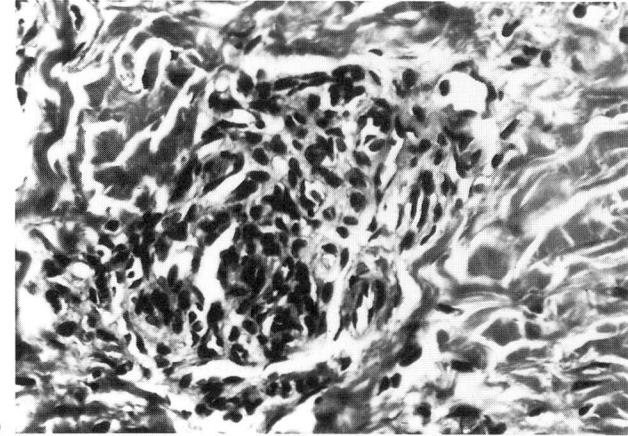

Figure 22.5 (a) Intravascular lymphomatosis ('malignant angioendotheliomatosis'). Cytologically malignant cells filling the vascular spaces, imparting a false impression of cohesiveness. These cells stained strongly with antileukocyte common antigen and L26, a B-cell marker. (b) A higher power view of an occluded vascular space. Note the fibrin deposition (arrow). (c) Reactive angioendotheliomatosis, consisting of a proliferation of endothelial cells and supporting elements lacking cytologic atypia. (Courtesy of Dr M. Wick.)

nuclear to cytoplasm ratio (Figure 22.5(b)). Subtotal vascular occlusion, fibrin thrombi and recanalized vessels with a 'glomeruloid' architecture may be present. The surrounding soft tissue is often edematous with a mild perivascular inflammatory infiltrate consisting primarily of mature lymphocytes. The proliferating endothelial cells are typically immunoreactive with antifactor VIII related antigen. However, a word of caution is warranted. A variety of cells, including those of intravascular lymphoma, may adsorb FVIIIrAg when exposed to plasma, therefore a panel approach to immunohistochemical studies is essential in order to minimize interpretation errors.

22.1.6 KIMURA'S DIASEASE

The condition which is now widely known as Kimura's disease [47] was actually first described in 1937 by Kimm and Szeto [48], as 'eosinophilic hyperplastic lymphogranuloma' in the *Proceedings of the Chinese Medical Society*. Over the years, a number of descriptive designations have been used for this disorder and include eosinophilic lymphofolliculoid granuloma, eosinophilic lymphoid granuloma of soft tissues, eosinophilic lymphofolliculopathy, eosinophilic granuloma of soft tissue and eosinophilic lymphofolliculosis of the skin. Although confusion with angiolymphoid hyperplasia with eosinophilia (epithelioid hemangioma) exists in the literature, these disorders are currently viewed as two separate and distinct entities [49–52].

Kimura's disease appears almost exclusively in the Orient, where it presents as a mass lesion, sometimes of impressive magnitude, primarily in the head and neck region. Other reported sites of involvement include the groin, upper limb, axilla and chest wall [47,52]. The masses may be multifocal or bilateral. Regional lymphadenopathy and peripheral blood eosinophilia are commonly noted. An elevation in the serum IgE may also be present. Renal disease, usually a nephrotic syndrome, has infrequently been observed but it appears to occur with greater frequency in this group than in the general population [53–55].

The pathogenesis of this peculiar disorder remains obscure although it is speculated to be the result of an aberrant immunologic response to an as yet undetermined antigenic stimulus [67].

The condition is characterized, histologically, by a poorly marginated fibroinflammatory mass (Figure 22.6(a)) predominantly involving the subcutaneous tissue but also occasionally extending into the dermis, underlying musculature or adjacent structures such as the salivary glands. Although the microscopic features vary somewhat with the duration of the lesion, all stages feature fibrosis (Figure 22.6(b)), a reactive vascular proliferation and an inflammatory infiltrate dominated by eosinophils and lymphocytes. Earlier examples typi-

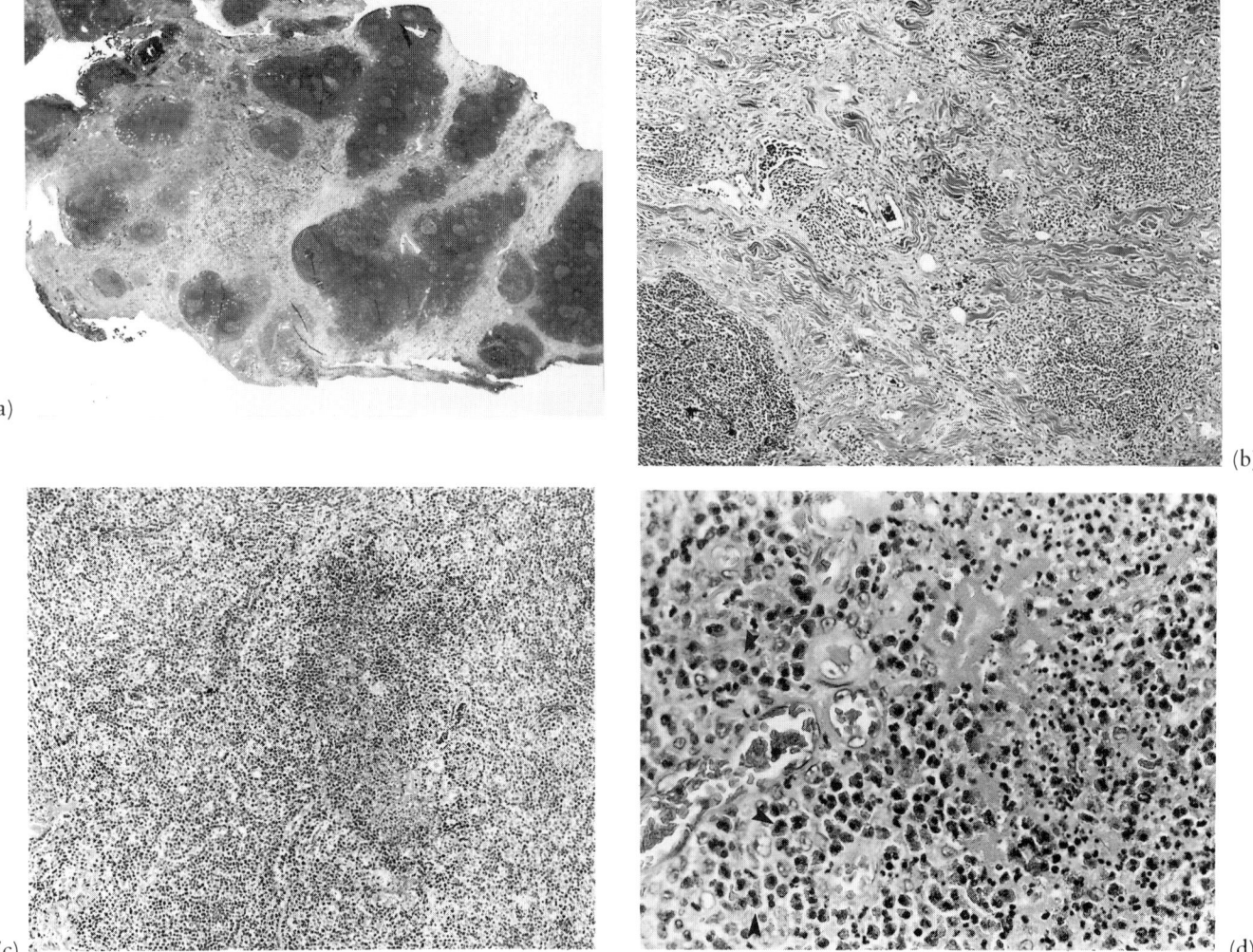

Figure 22.6 Kimura's disease. (a) Fibrosis and lymphoid follicle formation are the salient features at scanning power. (b) Note the relatively inconspicuous appearance of the vessels. (c) Eosinophilic micro-abscesses are a frequent and helpful feature. (d) Bilobated eosinophils within a microabscess.

cally exhibit a more pronounced inflammatory reaction while later stages are more fibrotic. Lymphoid follicles are a universal finding and are generally distributed through the process. Eosinophilic microabscesses are also sometimes present. The constellation of features seen in regional lymph nodes associated with Kimura's disease is well documented in the literature and will not be reiterated here [56,57].

In contrast to angiolymphoid hyperplasia with eosinophilia (epithelioid hemangioma), the vessels in Kimura's disease are typically well canalized, lack epithelioid morphology, and, for the most part, tend to be a relatively minor or inconspicuous component of the process. Whereas the differential diagnosis for angiolymphoid hyperplasia with eosinophilia revolves primarily around vascular neoplasia, one is more likely to consider fibroinflammatory conditions when viewing an example of Kimura's disease.

22.1.7 ANGIOLYMPHOID HYPERPLASIA WITH EOSINOPHILIA (EPITHELIOID HEMANGIOMA)

In 1969, Wells and Whimster published a group of nine lesions under the descriptive designation 'angiolymphoid hyperplasia with eosinophilia' (ALHE) [58]. All of the lesions arose in the head and neck region and were predominantly located in the subcutaneous tissues. A review of these cases casts some doubt as to whether a single clinicopathologic entity is represented. Urabe and colleagues [51] consider four of the nine cases to be more accurately classified as Kimura's disease, a disorder which is now viewed as a separate and distinct entity [Table 22.1].

The year following Wells and Whimster's article, Kandil [59] suggested the concept of ALHE should be broadened to include dermal lesions previously classified as 'atypical pyogenic granuloma(s)' by Peterson and

Table 22.1 Clinicopathologic features of subcutaneous angiolymphoid hyperplasia with eosinophilia (epithelioid hemangioma) versus Kimura's disease

Data	Kimura's disease	ALHE
Geographic distribution	Asia	Worldwide
Duration	Months to years	Months to years
Peak decade (age)	Third	Third
Sex	M > F	M = F
Bilaterality	Yes	No
Size	Average = 3–6 cm	Average = 1 cm
Peripheral blood	Increased serum IgE and blood eosinophilia	Normal serum IgE rarely increased eosinophils
Recurrences	20–30%	20–35%
Associated nephrotic syndrome	Yes, occasionally	Very rare
Histologic features	Fibrosis, extensive lymphoid follicle formation, eosinophilic microabscesses	Vasocentric process with minimal fibrosis, lymphoid follicles restricted to periphery, eosinophils prominent without abscess formation
	Poor margination	Well marginated
	Inconspicuous vascular proliferation, endothelial cells lack epithelioid morphology	Prominent vascular proliferation abundant epithelioid endothelial cells

colleagues [60] and 'inflammatory angiomatous nodules' by Wilson-Jones and Bleehen [61]. This view has generally been accepted although certain morphologic differences exist between the dermal and subcutaneous forms of the disease.

In 1979, Rosai and colleagues introduced the term 'histiocytoid hemangioma' [62] as a descriptive designation to encompass a group of lesions unified by histiocytoid (epithelioid) morphology. It is now recognized that at least three clinicopathologic entities were included under this rubric: angiolymphoid hyperplasia with eosinophilia, epithelioid hemangioendothelioma and the so-called 'benign endocardial angioreticuloma'. The latter actually represents a mesothelial process [63]. Thus, although important from a conceptual viewpoint, 'histiocytoid hemangioma' seems to have little utility as a diagnostic term since it does not correlate with a specific clinical profile nor does it imply a prognosis. As a result, we do not utilize this term as a pathologic diagnosis.

Epithelioid hemangioma is a designation previously proposed by Weiss [64] to encompass the benign vascular lesions included in the histiocytoid hemangioma spectrum [65–67], thus delineating them from epithelioid hemangioendothelioma, a low grade malignant neoplasm which has proven metastatic potential. Vascular lesions which have or may exhibit epithelioid endothelium include:

- angiolymphoid hyperplasia with eosinophilia (epithelioid hemangioma)
- epithelioid hemangioendothelioma
- spindle cell hemangioendothelioma
- angiosarcoma (especially epithelioid variant)
- Dabska tumor (malignant endovascular papillary angioendothelioma)
- verruga peruana/Carrion's disease
- bacillary angiomatosis
- papillary endothelial hyperplasia (more often 'plump' than epithelioid)
- hemangioma/lymphangioma (occasional minor component).

Hence, epithelioid hemangioma and angiolymphoid hyperplasia with eosinophilia have been used synonymously. From a teleologic perspective, which of these two designations is preferred might reflect whether a given lesion is viewed as a reactive tumefaction or a true neoplasm.

Both Kimura's disease and ALHE have a predilection for the skin and subcutaneous tissue of the head and neck region. Both disorders may also be multifocal and associated with regional adenopathy and peripheral blood eosinophilia [68]. Therefore, from a clinical perspective, it is not surprising that confusion between these processes exists in the literature. However, while adenopathy and peripheral eosinophilia may be seen in both, they are less frequent in ALHE. The latter also typically presents as a smaller mass which is almost invariably unilateral [51]. Furthermore, ALHE does not exhibit a geographic or racial preference whereas Kimura's disease occurs almost exclusively in the Orient.

Despite the clinical similarities, the histology of ALHE (Figure 22.7) [58–74] is distinctly different from Kimura's disease. Subcutaneous examples of ALHE are characterized by a prominent proliferation of capillary-

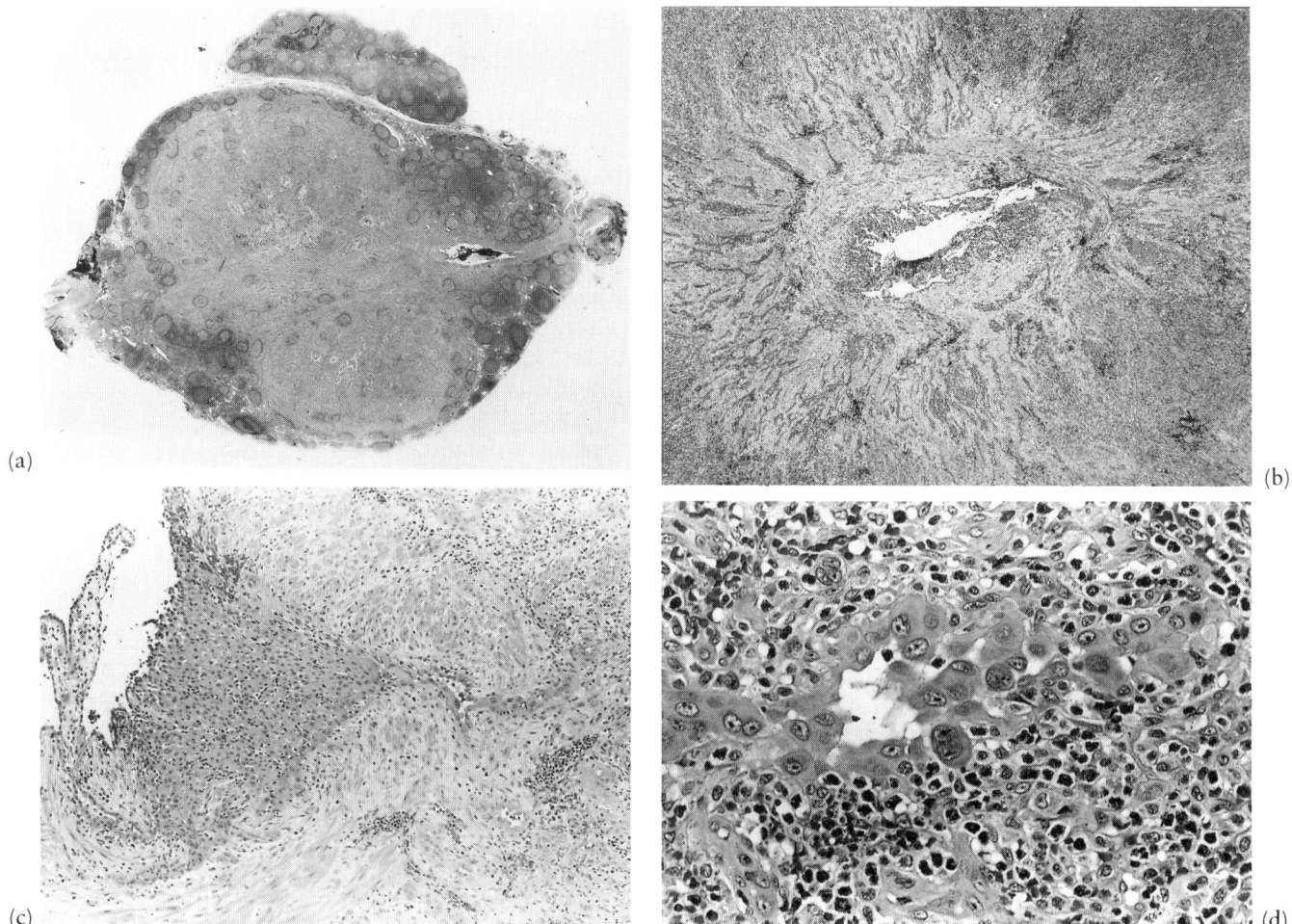

Figure 22.7 Angiolymphoid hyperplasia with eosinophilia (epithelioid hemangioma) (compare with Figure 22.6). (a) The process is symmetrically distributed about a medium-sized vessel which, on close inspection, proved to be an artery (case 1). Subcutaneous examples are well circumscribed and frequently surrounded by lymphoid follicles. (b) The small vessels with prominent endothelial cells radiate from a larger central vessel (case 2). Note the intraluminal endothelial proliferation with features of papillary endothelial hyperplasia. (c) A solid intraluminal epithelioid endothelial proliferation with extension through a vessel wall, possibly at a branch point (case 3). (d) A capillary channel with early canalization. lined by epithelioid endothelium. The background contains mixed inflammatory elements with many eosinophils. Although mild 'atypia' is evident, note the absence of features commonly associated with malignancy (e.g. sharp angulation of nuclear membrane, clumping of chromatin along the nuclear membrane).

sized vessels which, although well formed, often have an 'immature', uncanalized appearance. Many of these vessels are lined by plump epithelioid (histiocytoid) endothelial cells. Mild cytologic atypia may be noted but generally the nuclei have small nucleoli, an abundance of euchromatin and little heterochromatin clumping along the nuclear membranes (Figure 22.7(d)). Lobulation and folds in the nucleus may occasionally be observed. The vascular proliferation is frequently centered about, and emanates radially from, a medium-sized artery or vein which shows histologic evidence of damage [74] (Figure 22.7(b),(c)). The process is commonly well marginated and bordered peripherally by lymphoid follicles (Figure 22.7(d)). An inflammatory milieu rich in eosinophils and lymphocytes is almost invariably present (Figure 22.7(d)). Eosinophilic microabscesses, an occasional finding in Kimura's disease, are not a feature of ALHE. Fibrosclerosis is minimal or absent.

Dermal examples of ALHE [69] also contain a proliferation of small vessels, lined by epithelioid endothelium, and an inflammatory infiltrate rich in lymphocytes and eosinophils. However, in this location, the vascular proliferation is somewhat less well marginated. It more frequently has a mature, canalized appearance and is not generally associated with a medium-sized artery or vein. Lymphoid follicles are also a less commonly observed in this superficial location.

Features which suggest that at least some examples of ALHE are reactive in nature include:

1. a predilection for superficial sites with minimal soft tissue padding;
2. a historical account or trauma in some instances;
3. the localized, relatively marginated and symmetrical arrangement of the capillary proliferation about a medium-sized vessel, in many subcutaneous examples;
4. evidence of damage to involved larger vessels (e.g. fibrointimal proliferation, discontinuity of the elastic lamina, mural disruption);
5. the identification of features consistent with intralesional maturation (i.e. a transition from 'immature' small vessels without patent lumina to vessels with well defined lumina, sometimes without epithelioid endothelium);
6. a pronounced inflammatory reaction.

Local recurrence has been noted in up to one third of patients [69]. Whether this is the result of a persisting underlying vascular anomaly (i.e. arteriovenous shunt) or an indication of inherent neoplastic potential is unresolved. Occasional patients have been reported to have lesions in several sites. However, this seems more logically attributed to multicentricity rather than evidence of metastases since there are no reported deaths due to this process [67,69,70]. (One case reported by Reed and Terezakis [70] may have given rise to a regional lymph node metastasis but this is a unique occurrence. The patient was followed for 5 years and there was no evidence of recurrent disease.) Optimal management is considered to be complete local excision.

22.2 Benign vascular tumors

22.2 GENERAL FEATURES OF BENIGN VASCULAR TUMORS

In general, the following morphologic features in a vascular tumor support a benign diagnosis [75]:

- zonated or lobular growth;
- bland morphology with minimal mitotic activity;
- arrangement of the endothelium in a monolayer;
- presence of a 'mature' vascular pattern with appropriate supporting elements or evidence of intralesional maturation.

However, as is commonly the case in surgical pathology, no single feature can be relied upon with absolute certainty. For example, angiosarcomas may contain deceptively bland foci closely reminiscent of hemangioma, and pediatric vascular tumors (infantile or juvenile hemangiomas) are often cellular with an immature appearance and prominent mitotic activity. These examples illustrate the necessity of thorough tumor sampling for accurate classification and the importance of clinical data as malignant vascular tumors are uncommon in children.

Hemangiomas of all types often contain additional supporting elements which include pericytes, smooth muscle and interstitial fibroblast-like cells. These components are frequently more pronounced in pediatric tumors and can be highlighted with special histochemical stains (e.g. reticulin, Movat, pentachrome), as well as by immunohistochemical techniques.

In this section, we have included a brief discussion of macular stains, as they apply to the differential diagnosis of capillary hemangioma, but refer the reader to other sources for a comprehensive review of telangectasias and the various dysmorphic syndromes which have benign vascular proliferations as a component [76].

22.2.1 PYOGENIC GRANULOMA (LOBULAR CAPILLARY HEMANGIOMA)

The term pyogenic granuloma is an etiologic and pathologic misnomer which has been retained over time. Poncet and Dor [81] are credited with the first report in 1897. They believed the lesions to be examples of botryomycosis and that the process was analagous to 'champignons de castration' (castration fungus) seen in horses. Hartzell [82], who is credited with popularizing the term 'pyogenic granuloma' in 1904, also considered the lesions infectious and attributed them to *Staphylococcus*. An infectious etiology has now, however, largely been disproved and current observers favor either an exaggerated vascular hyperplasia with granulation tissue-like features or a lobular variant of capillary hemangioma [83,84].

The lesions may involve mucosal, cutaneous, subcutaneous or even intravascular sites. Affected individuals under the age of 18 years are predominantly males, whereas women vastly outnumber men between the ages of 19 and 40 years. In adults older than 40 years, pyogenic granuloma affects the sexes equally [85]. A history of trauma is reported in approximately one third of cases [86,87]. Local recurrence develops in up to 16% of cases treated by simple excision. In Kerr's series [87] of 289 cases, the most common sites of involvement, in decreasing order of frequency were the gingiva, fingers, lips, face and tongue. Tumors of the oral and nasal mucosa show a marked predilection for women in their reproductive years [86,88]. However, no sex predilection has been identified for other anatomic sites.

Approximately 1% of pregnant women are said to develop pyogenic granulomas involving the oral mucosa [87], especially in the interdental regions of the gingiva. These examples, which are also referred to as granuloma gravidarum, epulis or gingival tumor of pregnancy, typically have an onset in the first trimester. Regression, although not always complete, often occurs in the postpartum period. Similar lesions may develop with oral contraceptive use. This association suggests a hormonally sensitive process although receptor analysis by immunohistochemical staining has thus far proven negative [89].

Pyogenic granulomas are usually solitary, although on rare occasion, multiple lesions may develop. Disseminated lesions have been reported to occur spontaneously in otherwise healthy individuals [97,99,100], as well as in patients with underlying malignancies [102]. An account of multiple asynchronous lesions within the distribution of a port-wine stain is also recorded [101]. Finally, multiple pyogenic granulomata with a 'satellite' distribution may arise following trauma to [95,96,98], or the surgical manipulation of [90–94, 96] a previously isolated lesion. This latter phenomena seems to occur most frequently in teenage and young adult males with truncal tumors, particularly in the scapular region. Awareness of this infrequent occurrence may help alleviate undue alarm and overly aggressive intervention.

Superficial pyogenic granulomata, involving the mucous membranes or skin, may be sessile, polypoid or pedunculated. They frequently have a rapid onset but stabilize at a maximum size of several millimeters to a few centimeters after several weeks or months. The lesions range in color from bluish purple to bright red. Their epithelial surface may be attenuated or ulcerated.

On histological examination, pyogenic granuloma is characterized by a relatively well marginated proliferation of small capillary-sized vessels arranged in a multilobular pattern (Figure 22.8). Larger feeder vessels may be seen in association with the vascular lobules. The process is set in a fibromyxoid stroma which, in the absence of surface ulceration, is inflammatory cell poor. Both endothelial and stromal elements may exhibit brisk mitotic activity. Polypoid or pedunculated lesions commonly possess a collarette of hyperplastic epithelium. Examples which are more deep-seated tend to exhibit less stromal edema and vascular dilatation than their superficial counterparts.

An intravascular form of pyogenic granuloma [105, 106] has also been described. These lesions have a predilection for small to medium-sized venous channels of the neck and upper extremities. The mean and median ages at presentation are in the third decade of life. Most cases seem to develop over a period of 2–8 weeks. On gross examination, the lesions frequently have light coloration, a firm consistency and exhibit a polypoid intraluminal architecture. Apart from an intravascular location, their histology is typical of pyogenic granuloma.

The differential diagnosis of pyogenic granuloma includes vascular tumefactions which result from treatable infections (e.g. bacillary angiomatosis, Carrion's disease). Bacillary angiomatosis (BA) warrants special attention since it occurs worldwide (whereas Carrion's

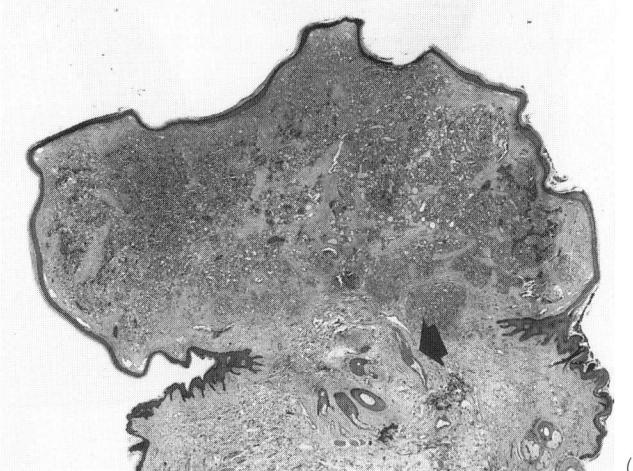

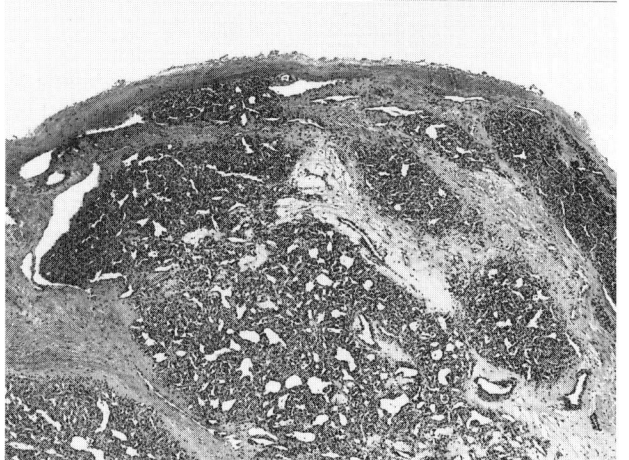

Figure 22.8 (a) and (b) Pyogenic granuloma (lobular capillary hemangioma) with a pedunculated appearance. Note the lobules of well formed vessels separated by loose fibromyxoid stroma. Many of the capillary channels have an 'open' appearance. A 'feeder vessel' is apparent in this example.

disease, for practical purposes, is restricted to endemic regions in South America) and since its 'low power' appearance can bear a particularly close resemblance to pyogenic granuloma. In fact, some debilitated patients, previously interpreted as having a disseminated form of pyogenic granuloma, may have actually had BA [3,14]. Both processes feature a lobulated capillary proliferation set in a fibromyxoid stroma. However, BA differs from pyogenic granuloma by containing scattered foci of necrosis with flocculent material, neutrophils and leukocytoclastic debris. These foci are typically present even in the absence of surface ulceration and harbor short, curved, Warthin–Starry-positive bacilli. When multifocal pyogenic granuloma-like lesions are encountered in the setting of debilitation or immunosuppression, bacillary angiomatosis warrants strong consideration as it can occasionally prove fatal if untreated.

Pyogenic granuloma must be also be distinguished

from malignant vascular tumors such as angiosarcoma and the nodular stage of Kaposi's sarcoma. Angiosarcoma differs from pyogenic granuloma by exhibiting more infiltrative growth with interanastomosing vascular channels lined by plump, atypical endothelial cells. Necrosis and atypical mitoses are also commonly present.

A single nodular lesion of Kaposi's sarcoma can bear a close clinical resemblance to pyogenic granuloma. However, Kaposi's disease, in contrast to pyogenic granuloma, is frequently a multifocal process associated with immunosuppression (e.g. AIDS, transplant recipients) and has an increased incidence in certain ethnic groups. From a histologic perspective, the nodular lesions of Kaposi's sarcoma do not feature a well-formed lobular capillary proliferation but are instead dominated by spindle cells with slit-like vascular spaces. Intracytoplasmic, periodic acid-Schiff-positive/diastase-resistant, eosinophilic hyaline globules and a peripheral plasma-cell response are additional features characteristically present at this stage of Kaposi's sarcoma but which are not typically seen in pyogenic granuloma.

Finally, multifocal lesions with a clinical appearance similar to pyogenic granuloma have been reported in patients treated with isotrentinoin (Accutane) for severe cystic acne [103,104]. These, however, have a histologic appearance more in keeping with granulation tissue. Spontaneous resolution usually follows cessation of isotrentinoin therapy.

22.2.2 CAPILLARY HEMANGIOMA

Capillary hemangiomas are common and, in fact, are the most frequent tumor of infancy, seen in about 10% of term and 20% of preterm babies [108,109]. They may, on rare occasion, be associated with right-sided aortic arch coarctation, sternal clefting, mid-line abdominal raphe, and sacral and genitourinary tract defects [145]. There is a distinct female preponderance with a female to male ratio up to 3:1 [110], although lower figures have been reported [77,116]. In the pediatric population, capillary hemangiomas are typically cellular and have been referred to as infantile hemangioendothelioma [111], juvenile hemangioma, strawberry nevus [110,113] and, perhaps most appropriately, cellular capillary hemangioma [112,115] (Figure 22.9).

These lesions most frequently involve the skin or subcutis of the head and neck region, although a wide variety of other sites may also be involved. Rarely, they may grow to sufficient size to damage adjacent structures and even less frequently, they may have life-threatening or fatal consequences. The vast capillary surface area associated with large examples can cause platelet trapping, thrombocytopenia and a coagulopathy. This phenomenon was first described in 1943 by Kasabach and Merritt [117]. They reported a male infant with a large congenital capillary hemangioma of the thigh which progressed to involve most of the torso by 3 months of age and led to a consumptive coagulopathy. The lesion was treated with irradiation and in the ensuing 21 months regressed, leaving residual scarring and atrophy. The syndrome, which bears their names, is now known to occur with a variety of large vascular lesions of diverse histologic type and biologic potential [118–123,272–277,572].

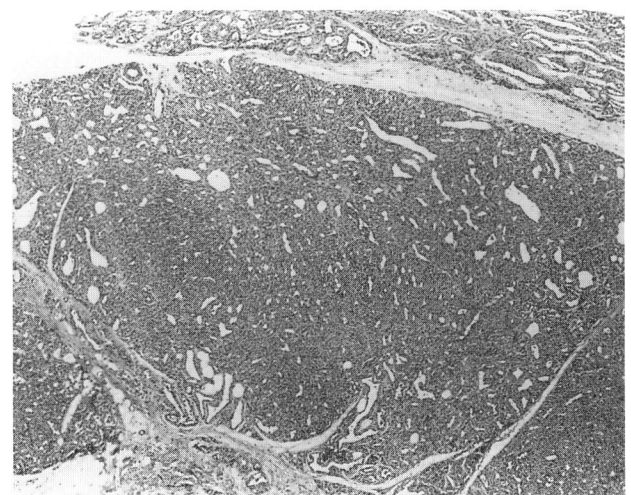
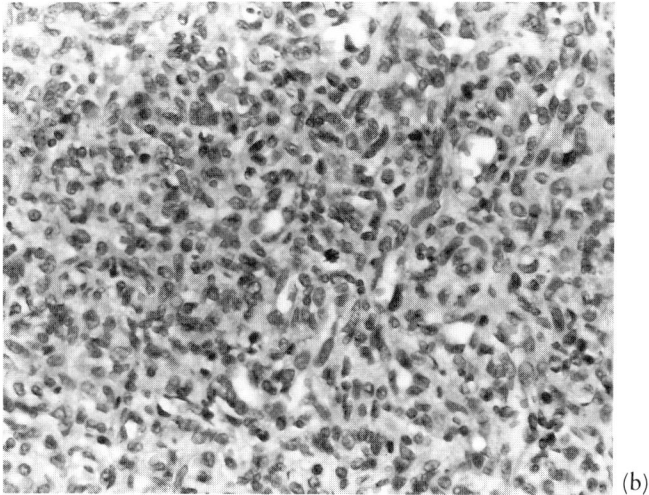

Figure 22.9 Cellular capillary hemangioma ('infantile hemangioendothelioma'). (a) Note the marginated and somewhat lobular appearance of the small vessel proliferation (b) While cellular, immature and mitotically active, the architectural features of the lesion and young age of the patient support a benign process. (Courtesy of Dr E. Lack.)

Capillary hemangiomas typically have a clinical course characterized by proliferation in the first few months of life, followed by regression and, in many instances, virtually complete involution. Lister [113] and others [110,114] have demonstrated that approximately half of untreated patients with superficial lesions are left with unblemished skin by 5 years of life and from 70 to 90% of patients are 'cured' by 7 years of age. These results do not appear to be influenced by gender, duration of the proliferative phase, size or site of the lesions [110]. Thus, treatment is usually a matter of 'benign neglect'. The rare examples with life-threatening or severely disfiguring consequences due to massive size or strategic location have, in recent years, been managed, with varying degrees of success, by selective embolization and laser resection, corticosteroid therapy and, more recently, interferon alpha-2A [126–130].

During the proliferative phase, capillary hemangiomas are characterized histologically by an exuberance of endothelial cells, pericytes and fibroblast-like cells [115, 124,125]. The endothelial cell nuclei can have prominent nucleoli and mitotic activity may be pronounced. Many of the vessels may lack apparent lumina, although tubular or cord-like angiogenic growth can be highlighted with a reticulin stain. On low power examination, the lesions often have a marginated or circumscribed appearance and the proliferating vessels are typically arranged in a lobular pattern. Maturation is often first noted at the periphery of these lobules and is characterized by the presence of flattened, or less active appearing endothelium lining vessels with patent lumina. Over time, a greater percentage of the capillaries assume this morphology. The vascular lobules also become more accentuated due to an ingrowth of fibrous and adipose connective tissue.

Superficial capillary hemangioma (strawberry nevus or hemangioma) needs to be differentiated from vascular stains. The term nevus flammeus has been used to encompass a wide variety of congenital macular stains, including both small, transient lesions and the larger, persistent, port-wine stains. The former group includes birthmarks fatuously known as a 'salmon patch' (nevus simplex), 'stork bite', or an 'angel's kiss'. Common sites of involvement include the glabella, eyelids and the nape of the neck [76,133,134]. In the latter location they are also referred to as nevus flammeus nuchae, erythema nuchae and Unna's nevus [76]. These macular stains are very common, occurring in a third or more of newborn infants [131–133]. Those located in the center of the face commonly disappear by 1 year of life, whereas nape lesions fade more slowly and often incompletely with faint vestiges persisting into adulthood. Port-wine stains (nevus venosus), on the other hand, occur far less frequently. They consist of larger macules with irregular borders which tend to enlarge in proportion to the growth of the child and generally do not fade [135,136]. They are typically flat in infancy and childhood but may become elevated and nodular later in life.

Lateral facial port-wine stains occurring in the distribution of the trigeminal nerve with abrupt termination at the midline are a component of the Sturge–Weber (leptomeningeal nevus flammeus or encephalotrigeminal angiomatosis) syndrome. Port-wine stains are also associated with the Klippel–Trenaunay (osteohypertrophic nevus flammeus) and Parkes Weber syndromes.

Unlike capillary hemangiomas, congenital macular stains are not characterized by endothelial proliferation [125]. In fact, when biopsied early in life, they typically reveal minimal or no apparent histologic abnormality [107,136]. Persistent, laterally located lesions of the port-wine stain type, however, eventually develop pronounced capillary ectasia [107,135,137] which may be attributable to impaired neural modulation of the vessels [136]. Macular stains are thus more accurately regarded as telangiectasias than true hemangiomas.

22.2.3 CAVERNOUS HEMANGIOMA

Cavernous hemangiomas are common vascular tumors in both children and adults [77,78]. They accounted for almost 70% percent of 1363 vascular tumors from 1056 patients reviewed by Watson and McCarthy [138]. There appears to be a predilection for the upper half of the body. Roughly equal numbers of males and females are affected. Unlike capillary hemangiomas, cavernous hemangiomas do not frequently regress [125]. Examples occurring in deep soft tissue and organs (liver [138], bone [139], intestines [140], lung [141]) are well-known. Rarely, large deep seated examples may be associated with the Kasabach–Merritt consumptive coagulopathy syndrome.

Cutaneous cavernous hemangiomas are soft, elevated, dark blue or purplish masses which compress easily and blanch with pressure. Deep-seated examples may be inapparent clinically and, on occasion, are incidental radiologic findings during the evaluation of unrelated disorders. The histology is characterized by either a lobulated or poorly marginated collection of engorged

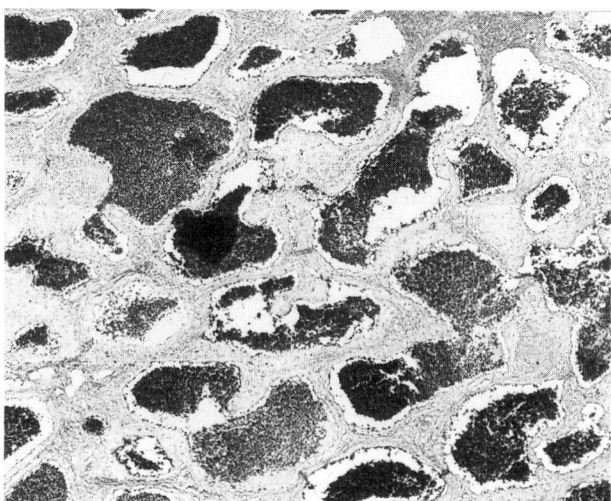

Figure 22.10 Cavernous hemangioma showing ectatic engorged vessels.

thin-walled vascular channels lined by flattened endothelium (Figure 22.10). Supporting elements (pericytes, smooth muscle cells and fibroblastic cells) are often less pronounced than in capillary hemangiomas. Sometimes, especially in the superficial portion of cutaneous tumors, a coexisting small vessel component may be evident. Recently Calonje and Fletcher [142], have described 'sinusoidal hemangioma', a variant which occurs in adults and consists of clustered markedly dilated interconnecting (sinusoidal) vascular spaces.

Cavernous hemangiomas have been listed as a component of a number of dysmorphic and genetic syndromes [144,145,149] including blue-rubber bleb nevus [164–168], Maffucci's [150–163], Klippel–Trenaunay [146,148] and Parkes Weber [147] syndromes. However, critical review of the vascular lesions described and/or illustrated in these reports reveals a heterogeneous group which includes macular stains, arteriovenous hemangiomas or malformations, capillary and cavernous hemangiomas, and spindle cell hemangioendotheliomas. Moreover, since vascular lesions are common in infancy and childhood, it has been argued that some of the associations which have been described in dysmorphic syndromes may not be statistically relevant [145]. A comprehensive review of these syndromes is beyond the scope of this chapter and is available elsewhere [76], but Maffucci's syndrome and the blue-rubber bleb nevus syndrome merit further comment.

Maffucci is credited with the first description of the syndrome of dyschondroplasia and hemangiomata. It is a congenital but non-hereditary syndrome with no sex predilection [150–163] heralded by the appearance of multiple vascular lesions shortly after birth or prior to puberty. The osseous pathology appears later when skeletal growth is rapid, in the form of extensive enchondromatosis which may eventually give rise to chondrosarcomas in approximately 15% of patients [156]. While the vascular lesions in some reports seem to represent cavernous hemangiomas [154,155,158], many appear to be examples of spindle cell hemangioendothelioma, a tumor of uncertain biologic potential [159–163] discussed elsewhere in this chapter.

Blue-rubber bleb nevus syndrome was so named by Bean in 1958 but Gascoyen (1860) has been credited with the first report [164]. Affected patients present with multiple small dome-shaped vascular lesions involving the skin and internal organs [164–168]. Profound iron deficiency, as first highlighted by Berlyne [165], is common and attributable to numerous lesions lining the gastrointestinal tract, especially the small bowel. There is some evidence that this syndrome can be transmitted in an autosomal dominant fashion [164,165].

Biopsied cutaneous lesions demonstrate relatively well demarcated congeries of dilated thin-walled vessels, situated in the upper and mid-reticular dermis and lined by attenuated endothelium. The overlying skin is flattened and hyperkeratotic. Gastrointestinal tract lesions have similar vessels, which may be located in any layer of the bowel wall, but frequently protrude into the mucosa [165,168] where they are prone to ulceration. The presence of prominent strands of organized smooth muscle and wisps of elastic lamina in some vessel walls has been cited as evidence that these lesions are actually multiple vascular malformations of venous type rather than cavernous hemangiomas [164]. Not surprisingly, papillary endothelial hyperplasia has been observed within these anomalous vessels [166].

22.2.4 SUPERFICIAL ARTERIOVENOUS TUMOR/HEMANGIOMA

A group of acquired cutaneous arteriovenous hemangiomas with a predilection for the perioral region and the extremities of adults was described by Girard and co-workers in 1974 [169]. Similar lesions were subsequently reported as 'acral arteriovenous tumors' by Carapeto and colleagues [170] and Connelly and Winkelmann [171]. Clinically, they are small (less than 1 cm) red or purple papules with little tendency for spontaneous regression. Some examples may resemble basal cell carcinoma or a nevus. Local excision is usually curative.

On microscopic examination, the tumors consist of relatively well circumscribed masses of thick- and thin-walled vessels, located primarily in the dermis of the skin or submucosa of the lip. Many of the vessels have a 'transitional' appearance between arteries and veins and in some cases, a direct communication between the latter may be noted [169]. The endothelial cells may be plump but are not cytologically atypical.

22.2.5 DEEP ANGIOMATOUS LESIONS

Benign deep vascular lesions represent a disease spectrum with considerable clinicopathologic overlap. All share the capacity to be infiltrative and therefore may be difficult to cure with local surgical excision. Acknowledging these points and given evidence which suggests that the predominant vessel pattern and anatomic location seem to have little influence on the recurrence rate, it has been recently proposed that the intramuscular tumors be grouped under the generic designation of 'angioma' [179]. We can find little fault with this approach, especially if one attempts to include, for future reference and study, a description of the vessel types in the body of the pathology report. However, lesions which conform to the definition of angiomatosis, as used elsewhere in this section, warrant separate distinction since they appear to exhibit a higher recurrence rate than tumors confined to one soft tissue site. Extensive arteriovenous malformations may also

(a) Arteriovenous malformations

Lesions which have arteriovenous anastomoses may be either acquired or congenital. The former are usually solitary and traumatic in origin [172,173]. Congenital arteriovenous connections are often multiple, involving a significant portion of an extremity or the head and neck region [146–148,174–177]. This latter group appears to have a female predilection [148,176]. Arteriovenous malformations which have a prominent superficial component, associated with substantial shunting, present as pulsating collections of tortuous vessels and are sometimes referred to as cirsoid aneurysms, racemose aneurysms, aneurysms by anastomosis or pulsating angiomas [172,173]. Examples which contain large dilated vessels have been designated arteriovenous aneurysms.

The age at which patients come to medical attention is typically related to the conspicuousness of a surface component [176]. The most common presenting complaint is swelling of the extremity, followed by cosmetic disfigurement and visible pulsations. Pain is less common. Superficial varicosities, increased warmth, and thrills or bruits are often present over the affected site. Systemic hemodynamic effects, such as cardiac enlargement, high-output cardiac failure and Branham's sign (bradycardia elicited by digital pressure on the afferent arterial supply), are identified only rarely in congenital arteriovenous malformations [148,176]. Traumatic fistulas, however, are somewhat more likely to be associated with these findings. This difference has been attributed to more extensive, tortuous and narrower arteriovenous communications in congenital examples which allow the peripheral resistance to be maintained [176].

In 1900, Klippel and Trenaunay summarized a group of patients with the following triad: a lower extremity port wine stain, varicose veins and skeletal and soft tissue hypertrophy of the affected site with lengthening of the limb [146,148]. Seven years later, Parkes Weber [147] described a similar group of cases but included two individuals who also had extensive arteriovenous malformations. Patients with all four of the above features are now regarded as having the Parkes Weber or Klippel–Trenaunay–Weber syndrome.

The diagnosis of arteriovenous malformation is frequently made with greater accuracy on the basis of clinical and radiographic findings than by histologic examination. Arteriography [178] is imperative not only to confirm the presence of arteriovenous anastomoses but also to identify cases where superficial varicosities are attributable to deep venous obstruction or the congenital absence of deep veins rather than an arteriovenous malformation; excision of superficial veins in the latter cases is contraindicated [148]. Further, arteriography is needed to assess the feasibility of surgery since arteriovenous malformations often have several feeding vessels and there is a tendency for recurrence via collateral circulation if incompletely excised.

The histology of arteriovenous malformations may vary considerably from one area to the next and foci identical to capillary or cavernous hemangiomas may be present. The identification of direct arteriovenous anastomoses may require extensive tissue sampling. When these are not seen, the presence of juxtaposed medium-sized or larger arteries and veins and the identification of arterialized veins, characterized by prominent fibrointimal hyperplasia and medial muscular hypertrophy aid this diagnosis [176].

(b) Intramuscular hemangiomas

Intramuscular hemangiomas/angiomas are relatively uncommon, accounting for 0.8–4.4% of all vascular tumors in two large series [138,179]. There does not appear to be a distinct gender predilection [179–182]. The majority of cases are identified in the first three decades of life. Beham and Fletcher recently studied 74 intramuscular angiomatous lesions and found that 12% were evident at birth and 69% manifested by the age of 20 years [179]. In Allen and Enzinger's study of 89 cases, published in 1972 [181], the peak incidence was in the third decade.

The lower extremity, in particular the quadriceps femoris, is the most frequent site affected. However, any muscle may be involved and a substantial number of cases have been reported in the upper extremity (especially the forearm), the chest and the head and neck region. Many examples are less than 5 cm in maximum dimension at the time of diagnosis, although tumors over 20 cm in size have been recorded [181]. Soft tissue swelling and pain are the most frequent sign and symptom, respectively.

The recurrence rates in recent series range from a low of 18% [181] to a high of 61% [179]. This wide discrepancy may be attributable to a shorter follow-up period in the former study. Recurrent disease is directly attributable to incomplete excision.

The gross appearance varies widely, depending on the type and size of vessels which predominate and the extent to which supporting elements such as adipose and fibrous connective tissue are represented. Tumors composed predominantly of small capillary-sized vessels (Figure 22.11) tend to be poorly marginated and vary in color from whitish tan to reddish brown. This group is the least likely to be correctly interpreted as a vascular tumor by the surgeon [181]. Tumors dominated by a large vessel pattern (e.g. cavernous spaces, dilated veins) are much more likely to be recognized grossly as vascular

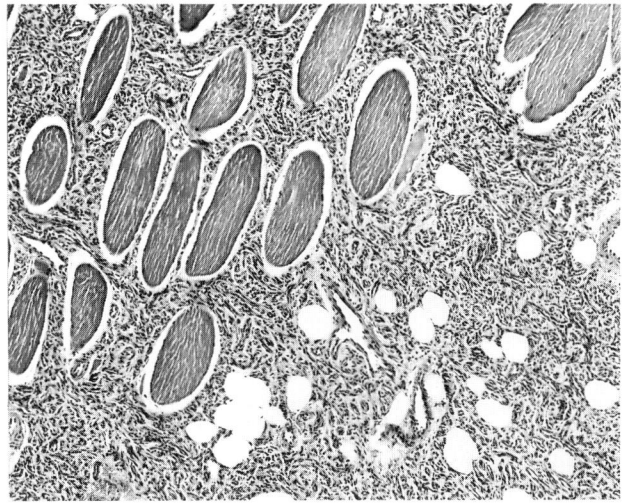

Figure 22.11 Intramuscular hemangioma. This example contains numerous well formed capillaries admixed with a small amount of adipose tissue. When the latter component is prominent, the lesion may be mistaken for an intramuscular lipoma.

anomalies. When intramuscular hemangiomas are accompanied by abundant adipose tissue, an incorrect diagnosis of lipoma or liposarcoma may be entertained both clinically and histologically. Lesions with this appearance have, in the past, been referred to as 'infiltrating angiolipomas' [183–186]. Occasionally foci of ossification may be seen [179,181]; this seems to occur most frequently in lesions with a complex vascular pattern, containing an arteriovenous component [179].

In the past, most authors have categorized benign intramuscular vascular tumors according to vessel size or type [181,182]. However, it has been recently proposed that all of these lesions, including capillary, cavernous, arteriovenous, lymphangiomatous and complex malformation types be regarded as intramuscular 'angiomas' [179]. This reasoning is based on the fact that most examples have mixed features, despite a frequently dominant vessel pattern and that a lack of correlation between the predominant vessel type and the clinical outcome has been noted. Although this approach has validity, it is worth remembering that there is some correlation between vessel pattern and anatomic site. For example, intramuscular capillary hemangiomas and lymphangiomas favor the upper half of the body.

The differential diagnosis of intramuscular hemangioma/angioma includes angiomatosis, angiosarcoma and lipoma/liposarcoma. Angiomatosis is primarily a clinical diagnosis, based on extent of the process.

Angiosarcoma may be entertained when dealing with a cellular small vessel variant of intramuscular hemangioma. However, the latter lacks an interanastomosing sinusoidal pattern, nuclear pleomorphism and atypical mitotic activity. When considering this differential, one should be aware of the rarity of primary angiosarcomas of skeletal muscle. The youthful age of many patients with intramuscular hemangioma also militates against a diagnosis of angiosarcoma.

As mentioned earlier, intramuscular hemangiomas with abundant fat can be confused with lipogenic neoplasms. However, the latter rarely contain large, dilated or 'gaping' vasculature and their small vessel pattern lacks the exuberance of that seen in hemangiomas. The absence of lipoblasts is a key feature which differentiates intramuscular hemangioma with fatty overgrowth from liposarcoma.

(c) Venous hemangiomas

Venous hemangiomas are rare tumors which often involve deep structures. Adults are reported to be affected more frequently than children. Sites which may be involved include the skeletal muscle [182,188,189], bones [139,190], mediastinum [191], joint spaces [192], mucosa-lined hollow organs [193] and the spinal cord [194]. Due to sluggish blood flow and thrombosis of feeding vessels, these lesions are often not visualized by arteriography [187a]. As a result, venography, including direct injection, is better suited for their demonstration.

On microscopic examination one sees blood-filled, endothelial-lined channels with prominent muscular walls. These walls frequently have disorganized smooth muscle bundles and there is often a paucity of elastic tissue [64,187]. It is the thickened muscular walls which distinguish venous from cavernous hemangiomas. However, many lesions reported as venous hemangiomas contain a cavernous component and, in fact, some authors have used the terminology interchangably [195,196].

(d) Angiomatosis

Angiomatosis is a term which over the years has been applied to a variety of processes, including papillary endothelial hyperplasia [23], encephalofacial vascular malformations in Sturge–Weber syndrome [76,144,145], and extensive multifocal benign vascular proliferations in children which may be associated with a poor prognosis due to organ compromise or hemorrhage [197]. For the purposes of this discussion, angiomatosis is used as recently emphasized by Rao and Weiss [198], who defined the process as a histologically benign vascular proliferation growing contiguously in multiple tissue planes or extensively in tissues of the same type (e.g. apposed muscles). Multifocal vascular proliferations were excluded from their definition. Similar criteria were provided by Howat and Campbell in 1987 [199]. The lesions tend to be based in the deep subcutaneous tissue and muscles, but more superficial tissues or underlying bone may also be involved.

Although the true incidence of these lesions is unknown, they appear to be relatively rare. For example, in a review by Watson and McCarthy [138], of 1056 patients with benign vascular lesions, only seven individuals, briefly mentioned under the heading 'diffuse systemic hemangiomata', would seem to fulfill current definitional criteria for a diagnosis of angiomatosis.

Rao and Weiss' recent series included 31 females and 20 males. Over half of the patients were brought to medical attention prior to the age of 20 years, and of these, 11 were evaluated in the first year of life. This finding is supportive of the view that many examples arise on a congenital basis.

The most common symptoms are persistent diffuse swelling, pain and tenderness. Limb hypertrophy is present only infrequently. Vascular lesions are, in many instances, not suspected clinically since superficial discoloration is frequently absent and arteriovenous shunting is usually not apparent. The lower extremity, including the buttock, is the most frequently affected site, followed by the trunk and the upper extremity. Less commonly, the head and neck, back, pelvis and retroperitoneum may be involved.

Angiomatosis is characterized histologically by an admixture of large irregular venous segments with disorganized muscular walls, cavernous vessels and capillary channels, scattered diffusely throughout tissue planes and often associated with large amounts of adipose tissue. Arteries and lymphatic channels may also be noted but are typically not seen in direct communication with the former. Features which are said to be distinctive, though not specific, include the presence of capillary-sized vessels proliferating adjacent to, and within the walls of, the disorganized venous segments [198,199].

Angiomatosis, as defined above, is a vascular anomaly with a strong propensity for local recurrence and, based on past experience, this can be expected in the majority of patients [198,199]. Management appears to reflect a balance between complete extirpation of the lesion and obviating excessive morbidity. Malignant transformation has not been reported.

The differential diagnosis of angiomatosis revolves primarily around intramuscular hemangioma and diffuse arteriovenous malformation. The former distinction is primarily clinical, based on extent of the process. However, the histologic features described earlier, which are somewhat distinctive for angiomatosis, may assist in the differentiation. Diffuse arteriovenous malformation can have an extensive clinical appearance similar to angiomatosis but, in general, it is more likely to be associated with edema, phlebectasia, increased warmth, a bruit and other features consistent with shunting. Arteriography is an invaluable aid in the diagnosis of this process. In general, arteriovenous malformation differs histologically from angiomatosis by featuring a greater abundance of thick-walled arteries and juxtaposed 'arterialized' veins.

(e) Other benign deep angiomatous lesions

Synovial and tendinous [200–209], neural [210–216] and intraosseous hemangiomas [139,218,219] are all well documented in the literature.

Synovial hemangiomas most frequently affect the knee joint. They produce signs and symptoms which often begin during childhood, including pain, swelling and recurrent joint effusions. **Hemangiomas arising within peripheral nerves** are rare and there is no established age predilection or favored site of involvement. Signs and symptoms may include pain, hypoesthesia and muscle wasting of the innervated region. Both synovial and neural hemangiomas are often of the cavernous type.

Hemangiomas of bone most frequently affect the skull and vertebrae. They are usually first noted in adulthood and are more frequently solitary than multifocal. The majority of these lesions are asymptomatic, incidental radiographic findings. However, they may be associated with local pain, swelling and, infrequently, a pathologic fracture. The vasculature may have cavernous, capillary or, rarely, venous or arteriovenous features.

Diffuse skeletal hemangiomatosis (diffuse cystic angiomatosis) refers to extensive, multicentric angiomatous lesions of bone. This disorder is often associated with visceral and soft tissue hemangiomas [221–224].

A rare disease initially described by Gorham and Stout [217] as 'massive osteolysis', but also referred to as 'disappearing' or 'phantom bone disease', is of uncertain pathogenesis although it may be linked to some form of vascular derangement or angiomatosis. This disease, which predominantly affects individuals under the age of 40 years, is characterized by extensive osteolysis of a single bone or a contiguous group of bones [218,220]. The process eventually stabilizes but the extent of intervening destruction is unpredictable.

22.2.6 RECENTLY RECOGNIZED LESIONS

(a) Microvenular hemangioma

This recently described lesion [251] generally presents as a small solitary nodule or plaque involving the extremities of young adults. The 10 patients reported by Hunt and colleagues ranged in age from 9 to 39 years (median age 29.5 years). The clinical features are in keeping with a diagnosis of hemangioma although the acquired nature of the lesion, evidence of lesional growth and an origin within an extremity may occasionally lead one to consider the possibility of the patch stage of Kaposi's sarcoma in the differential diagnosis.

The histology of microvenular hemangioma is characterized by a permeative proliferation of small irregularly branching vessels which are well-formed but often have collapsed, somewhat inconspicuous lumina. The vessel walls are said to be thicker than those of capillary hemangiomas. The endothelium lacks cytologic atypia and inflammation is only rarely noted. Hemosiderin deposits may be present. In contrast to Kaposi's sarcoma, microvenular hemangioma lacks the promontory sign (i.e. an irregular proliferation of small vessels, adjacent to and protruding into a more ectatic vessel), a spindle cell element, apoptotic endothelium, intracytoplasmic hyaline globules and an inflammatory infiltrate rich in plasma cells.

(b) Glomeruloid hemangioma

Glomeruloid hemangioma occurs as a component of the POEMS syndrome, which was first described in 1968 by Dr Shimpo in the Japanese literature (225 as cited in 226). This syndrome, also known as Takatsuki syndrome, Crow–Fukase syndrome and plasma cell dyscrasia with polyneuropathy and endocrine disorder, is characterized by the following features:

- Polyneuropathy
- Organomegaly (hepatosplenomegaly and lymphadenopathy)
- Endocrinopathy (amenorrhea, gynecomastia, hypothyroidism, adrenal insufficiency and glucose intolerance)
- Monoclonal protein (marrow plasmacytosis, paraproteinemia)
- Skin lesions including glomeruloid and cherry angiomas, acanthosis, hyperpigmentation and hypertrichosis.

The syndrome differs from ordinary myeloma in that bone lesions tend to be sclerotic, plasma cells are frequently only mildly increased in the marrow, the paraprotein titer commonly is lower and the patients are typically younger. Enlarged lymph nodes in POEMS patients frequently show features of Castleman's disease [229].

Glomeruloid hemangiomas are commonly multifocal [226–230]. The majority of examples involved the skin of the trunk or proximal extremities where they appear as pin-sized to pea-sized papules. However, internal structures may also be affected [229]. Histologic examination reveals dilated, ectatic vessels with intraluminal capillary conglomerates, architecturally resembling renal glomeruli (Figure 22.12). The vessels are lined by flattened or slightly plump endothelium with bland nuclear features. Interposed between the capillary loops are plump 'stromal' cells with clear cytoplasm. These

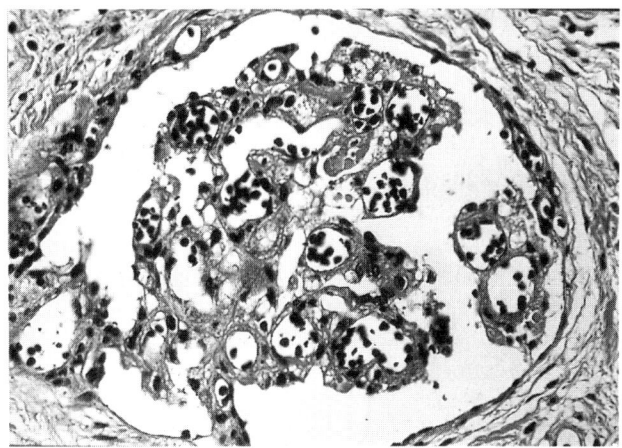

Figure 22.12 Glomeruloid hemangioma. The lobular collection of capillaries within a larger vessel is reminiscent of a renal glomerulus. (Courtesy of Dr J. Rosai.)

latter cells occasionally contain PAS-positive, diastase-resistant globules which are believed to represent phagocytized immunoglobulin.

As noted earlier, cherry hemangiomas have also been described in POEMS syndrome [228–230] and a few lesions having hybrid features with glomeruloid hemangioma have been identified. Thus, it has been suggested that, in this setting, the two hemangioma types may represent either a different stage in the evolution of a single process or a variation in the degree of the vascular response to the angiogenic stimuli [229].

The exact mechanism by which angiogenesis is induced in POEMS syndrome is not known, although both the stimulation of endothelial cells by way of immunoglobulin deposition and the secretion of angiogenic factors by activated lymphocytes are proposed factors [229]. Since this is, in all likelihood, a reactive rather than neoplastic vascular proliferation, it could be viewed as a form of reactive angioendotheliomatosis.

For those unfamiliar with the rather characteristic appearance of glomeruloid hemangioma, the presence of multiple cutaneous vascular lesions, some harboring eosinophilic globules, may raise a question of Kaposi's sarcoma. However, the former is easily distinguished by its restricted intravascular growth, well formed vascular channels and lack of a spindled component.

The presence of eruptive vascular lesions as described above should prompt a search for other stigmata of POEMS syndrome. Patients with this disorder tend to do poorly as a result of their underlying disease.

(c) Angioblastoma (acquired tufted angioma, progressive capillary hemangioma)

Nakagawa has been credited with the first description of this tumor in 1949 [231]. He described a 35-year-old housewife with small firm dark nodules of her upper left arm which had appeared at age 17 or 18 and slowly progressed. Numerous publications subsequently appeared in the Japanese literature but the tumor was largely unrecognized in Europe and North America until Wilson-Jones' brief account of 10 patients under the designation 'acquired tufted angioma' in 1976 [232]. Additional reports have since appeared in the English language [233–238] including a detailed summary of 20 cases by Wilson-Jones and Orkin [234].

Almost 60% of cases have an onset in the first year of life and over 70% are evident before the age of 10 years. The lesions are frequently painful. They typically develop insidiously, with slow growth for several years before stabilizing. Occasionally, however, more rapid growth is noted. Spontaneous regression or involution is rare. Metastases have not been reported.

The most frequent sites of involvement are the neck, upper chest and shoulders. There is considerable variability in size and appearance although commonly they are macular or plaque-like, with slight granularity or nodularity due to a superimposed papular component.

Scanning a section of the tumor at low magnification reveals tightly packed clusters of capillaries with a rounded or ovoid ('cannonball') appearance (Figure 22.13(a),(b)). The process is usually concentrated in the mid- and deep dermis, although involvement of the papillary dermis and superficial subcutis may also be evident. The intervening dermal collagen has a normal appearance with minimal, if any, inflammation. Coalescence of the capillary aggregates occasionally results in the presence of larger, more geographic, vascular expanses. The vascular tufts contain plump or spindled endothelium, pericytes and occasional smooth muscle cells, all with bland morphology. The constituents are frequently arranged in a whorled or concentric pattern such that individual capillary lumina are compressed and slit-like (Figure 13(c)). Dilated vascular channels may be evident at the periphery of the capillary aggregates. Mitotic activity is usually scant. Mast cells may be abundant in and about the tumor.

Since the morbidity associated with angioblastoma appears to be primarily cosmetic, aggressive intervention is not required. Soft X-ray therapy or surgical excision are the primary treatment modalities. Local recurrence may occur following incomplete excision.

The differential diagnosis for angioblastoma includes cellular capillary hemangioma (juvenile or benign hemangioendothelioma), pyogenic granuloma (lobular capillary hemangioma), angiosarcoma and Kaposi's sarcoma. However, with the exception of cellular capillary hemangioma, none of these considerations could be described as exhibiting a relatively extensive, yet superficially zonated, multinodular and lobular vascular proliferation with bland cytologic features and essentially normal intervening stroma with little, if any, inflammation. Cellular capillary hemangioma differs in that it generally features larger tumor lobules and frequently extends deeper. Pyogenic granuloma (lobular capillary hemangioma) is typically a more confined process, often having a polypoid appearance. The capillary channels in pyogenic granuloma also tend to be less compressed and slit-like than those seen in angioblastoma. In contrast to the relatively normal stroma which intervenes between vascular tufts in angioblastoma, the stroma of pyogenic granuloma typically has a fibromyxoid appearance.

(d) Targetoid hemosiderotic hemangioma (THH)

Recognition of this recently described benign vascular lesion is primarily of importance because its histology overlaps somewhat with Kaposi's sarcoma [239–241]. However, its clinical presentation is distinctive. It typically occurs as a solitary lesion on the trunk or extremities of young adults: Seven of the 10 patients described to date have been males. Early lesions have a central purple, violaceous or brown-black papule, bordered by an inner pale zone and a more peripherally situated ecchymotic ring. As such, these lesions resemble a target. The outer ring fades with maturation, leaving behind a small papule which can clinically resemble a fibrous histiocytoma.

The histology of targetoid hemosiderotic hemangioma varies with the duration of the lesion. Early on, it is characterized by ectatic thin-walled vascular channels situated in the superficial dermis and lined by plump, sometimes epithelioid, endothelium. Intraluminal papillary endothelial projections and fibrin thrombi may be present. Deeper vessels, located in the reticular dermis, have an angulated, irregular and slit-like appearance. They exhibit a permeative, collagen 'dissecting', growth pattern and are lined by attenuated, relatively inconspicuous endothelium. Extension into the superficial subcutis may also be noted. Hemorrhage, hemosiderin deposition, edema and a mild lymphocytic infiltrate are commonly present. In later stages, the superficial ectatic vacular channels are lost and collapsed, and anastomosing, small vessels predominate.

The histopathologic differential diagnosis of targetoid hemosiderotic hemangioma revolves primarily around Kaposi's sarcoma and acquired progessive lymphangioma (benign lymphangioendothelioma) [387–389]. From a clinical perspective, Kaposi's sarcoma differs by being a more extensive, multifocal process with a predilection for immunosuppressed patients and those of Mediterranean ancestry. Kaposi's sarcoma differs histologically by containing apoptotic endothelial cells, clusters of intracytoplasmic eosinophilic hyaline globules and a plasma cell infiltrate.

Acquired progressive lymphangioma differs clinically from targetoid hemosiderotic hemangioma in that it is generally a more extensive, slowly progressive process,

BENIGN VASCULAR TUMORS 759

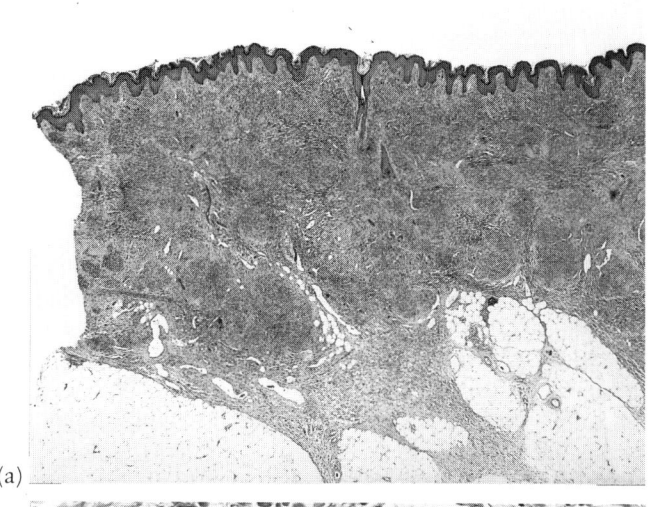
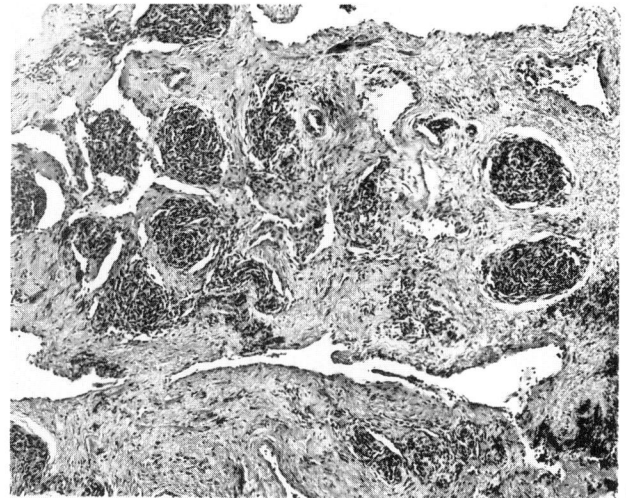
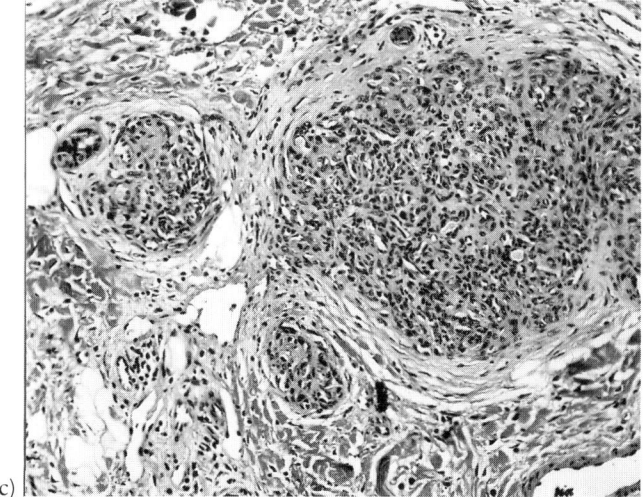

Figure 22.13 Angioblastoma of Nakagawa (acquired tufted angioma). (a) At scanning power, 'cannonball' aggregates of proliferating capillary-sized vessels, distributed throughout the dermis, are apparent. Note that the process stops rather abruptly at the dermal–subcutaneous junction. (b) At higher magnification, tight whorled capillary channels with a collapsed appearance compress larger, more ectatic, crescent-shaped vessels. (c) The presence of well formed capillaries with supporting elements (e.g. pericytes) arranged in lobules, are features in keeping with a benign interpretation.

often having the appearance of a large bruise-like macule. Histologically, both entities feature numerous anastomosing vascular channels with a 'collagen dissection' pattern. However, acquired progressive lymphangioma typically lacks hemosiderin deposition and its vascular channels are generally bloodless.

Of note, cutaneous lesions with a targetoid appearance may also be observed in erythema multiforme, erythema chronicum migrans of Lyme disease and within cherry angiomas in patients with primary amyloidosis. However, the clinical features and histology of these disease processes are substantially different from targetoid hemosiderotic hemangioma.

The histogenesis of targetoid hemosiderotic hemangioma is unknown. Currently, observers favor either a *de novo* reactive lesion or traumatization of a pre-existing hemagioma with resultant 'atypical' features.

22.2.7 OTHER LESIONS

Other benign vascular lesions worthy of mention include angiokeratoma [80,242–244], verrucous hemangioma [245] and angioma serpiginosum [80,247–250].

There are five clinical forms of **angiokeratoma**. The generalized systemic type (angiokeratoma corpus diffusum) is associated with Fabry's disease, fucosidosis and a deficiency of β-galactosidase. The lesions are characterized histologically by the presence of dilated vessels which are primarily restricted to the uppermost dermis and are bordered or enclosed by elongate rete ridges. With time, the overlying epidermis often becomes hyperkeratotic and, sometimes, papillomatous. The process is commonly regarded as a form of telangiectasia rather than true neoplasm.

Verrucous hemangioma shares many similarities with angiokeratoma, the key distinction being the added presence of an underlying hemangioma/vascular malformation within the deep dermis or subcutis. This entity is reported to have a high local recurrence rate attributable to incomplete resection of the anomalous vascular proliferation. A recently described congenital lesion, digital verrucous fibroangioma [246], may be related to verrucous hemangioma.

Angioma serpiginosum is a benign vascular ectasia with a distinct gyrate or serpiginous clinical appearance. It typically appears in females in the first two decades of life and favors the lower extremities. Although there may be periods of relative stability, this process has a tendency for slow progession.

In an attempt to be complete, we also note several newly described lesions which, although not fully characterized, have been included by others [79,80] in the discussion of vascular tumors: giant cell angioblastoma [252], multinucleated cell angiohistiocytoma [253–255] and proliferative cutaneous angiomatosis [256]. Based on available information, the latter appears to be a true vascular tumor. However, the histogenesis of the others is unclear. The interested reader is referred to the cited references.

22.3 Lesions of indeterminate biologic potential

The three lesions described below are rare and not without their controversies. Although the first six Dabska tumors were described in 1969, less than a dozen total cases have been reported to date. Spindle cell hemangioendothelioma and kaposiform infantile hemangioendothelioma were recognized more recently and experience with large numbers of patients with long-term follow-up is lacking. Consequently, the histogenesis and biologic potential or these lesions is not fully resolved. While spindle cell hemangioendothelioma was initially regarded as a borderline or low grade malignant neoplasm, authors of more recent reports have tended to favor either a benign tumor or a non-neoplastic, possibly reactive, vascular process which develops as a result of aberrant blood flow. In a similar vein, kaposiform infantile hemangioendothelioma has been interpreted by some authors as a variant of juvenile (cellular capillary) hemangioma and by others as a borderline or low grade malignancy.

22.3.1 SPINDLE CELL HEMANGIOENDOTHELIOMA

This distinctive vascular proliferation was first characterized as a clinicopathologic entity by Weiss and Enzinger in 1986 [257]. It typically presents as a superficial slow-growing painless mass involving the dermis and/or subcutis. Although the largest example thus far reported has measured 11 cm in greatest dimension [260], the vast majority are 2 cm or less in size [257,258,263]. This lesion may develop at any age, although preliminary data suggest a predilection for the third and fourth decades [257–265]. More than 50% of the cases involve the hands or feet with the remainder occurring elsewhere in the extremities or on the trunk. Multifocality is common. A small number of cases have been associated with other disease processes including Milroy's disease [257,260], Maffucci's disease [159–163,257,258], Klippel–Trenaunay syndrome [260] and an early onset of varicose veins [260].

The histology of spindle cell hemangioendothelioma (SCHE) is highly characteristic. The process is typically well marginated and is dominated by two components: cavernous vascular spaces, similar to those seen in a cavernous hemangioma, and a spindle cell proliferation vaguely reminiscent of Kaposi's sarcoma (Figure 22.14(a),(b)). The former element frequently features phleboliths. Smooth muscle may be evident at the periphery (Figure 22.14(c)) or within the lesion, in association with the cavernous spaces or the more solid spindled areas. Epithelioid endothelial cells, sometimes with intracytoplasmic lumina, are an additional feature of this process. The latter element, as well as the lack of grape-like clusters of PAS-positive, diastase-resistant hyaline globules and no known association with HIV status, aid in distinguishing this entity from Kaposi's sarcoma.

SCHE was initially regarded as a variant of low-grade angiosarcoma based on a perceived proclivity for local recurrence, an association with epithelioid hemangioendothelioma in one instance, and a single documented example which metastasized after a 40-year period punctuated by 19 local recurrences and a course of radiation therapy [257]. Several recent reports have taken the view that SCHE is a non-neoplastic, possibly reactive process [260,263,264], which arises in response to abnormal blood flow, in turn related to a pre-existing vascular malformation [260]. This view is based on the occasional presence of malformed vessels adjacent to the lesions and the belief that many examples which have been interpreted as recurrences, are in fact, new lesions developing as a result of a field-effect phenomenon [260].

Pending the accumulation of additional cases with long-term follow-up, we have tentatively chosen to include this entity in the indeterminate category. Although metastases in uncomplicated examples with typical histology have not been reported, local and regional recurrences are a problem in a high percentage of cases. In addition, we have seen a few cases with sufficient cytologic atypia to warrant some concern as to biologic potential. The documentation of angiosarcoma [247,260] and epithelioid hemangioendothelioma, or a proliferation similar to it [257,259,260], arising at the site of or in close proximity to SCHE is also difficult to dismiss. These latter findings raise the possibility that this proliferation may possess increased potential for malignant transformation. We believe management decisions for this tumor need to be individualized. Attempts at complete resection to minimize the possibility of recurrence should be tempered with a desire to preserve function. In instances of incomplete excision,

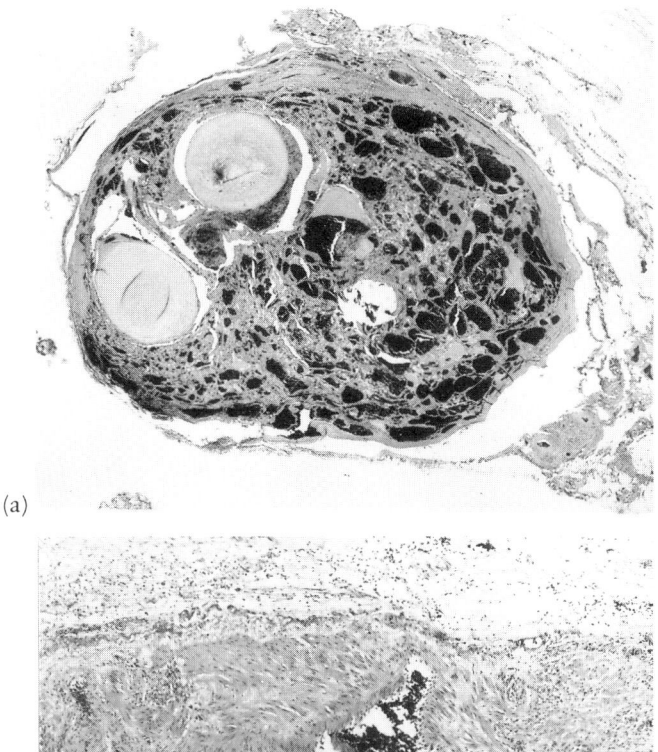
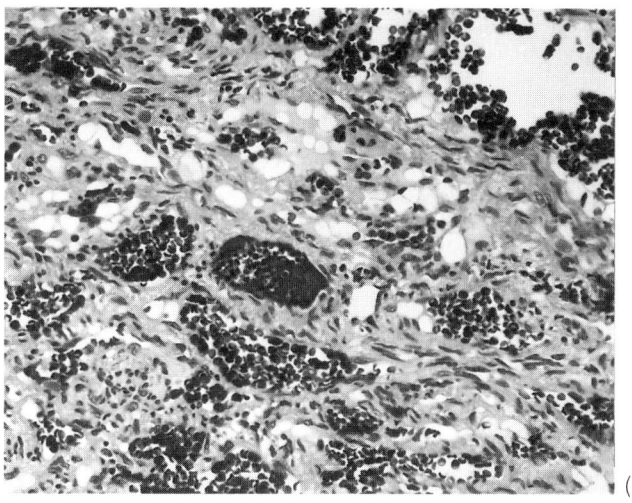
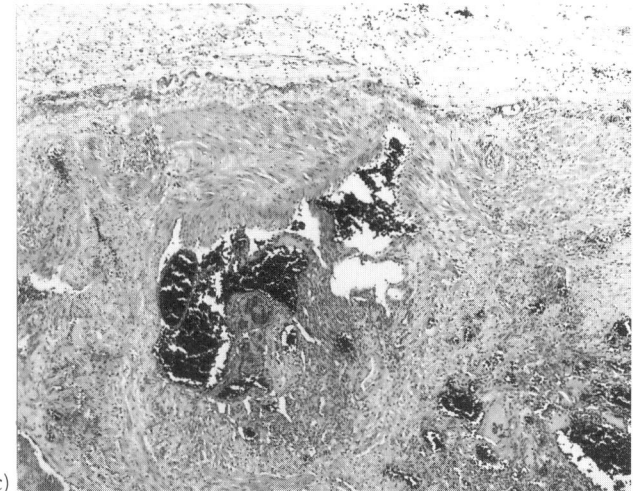

Figure 22.14 (a) Spindle cell hemangioendotheliomas are typically well marginated, as seen in this example, and have both a spindled element reminiscent of Kaposi's sarcoma and cavernous hemangioma-like vascular spaces. Phleboliths are a common feature. (b) A higher magnification demonstrating the spindled cells, cavernous spaces, and several vacuolated endothelial cells. (c) Smooth muscle is occasionally seen at the periphery or within these lesions.

follow-up is advised. Careful evaluation of surgical specimens is recommended to exclude a more ominous component with definite metastatic potential, such as is described above. Additional experience with this process has been presented in abstract form.

22.3.2 (MALIGNANT) ENDOVASCULAR PAPILLARY ANGIOENDOTHELIOMA (DABSKA TUMOR)

This exceedingly rare tumor was first recognized in 1969 by Maria Dabska [266]. With the exception of isolated case reports, little has been added to the literature since the initial description [266–270]. Although two examples are purported to have metastasized to lymph nodes [266], a point of contention with some authors [268], no patient is known to have died of this tumor. Given this limited potential for aggressive behavior, we currently favor the inclusion of this tumor in the borderline category.

Although the majority of these tumors appear to occur in infants and children, A.F.I.P. experience indicates rare examples may also be seen in adults [271]. The tumors tend to be superficial, primarily involving of the skin and subcutis, but left untreated, they possess a capacity for expansile growth with deep extension into underlying structures including muscle and bone. At this point in time, no anatomic site appears to be favored.

Histologic examination reveals a tumor composed of intercommunicating vascular channels of varying caliber, some large and irregular with a cavernous appearance, others smaller and capillary-like (Figure 22.15). The vessels contain endothelium with diverse morphology, ranging from a normal flattened appearance to plump and epithelioid to distinctly columnar. The latter endothelial variants may exhibit cytologic atypia and are sometimes arranged in papillary (primitive glomeruloid) tufts with a central avascular hyaline core (Figure 22.15(a)). This feature is the true *sine qua non* of the process. Endothelial cells lining the papillae have nuclei which are eccentrically located along the luminal aspect of the tuft, a feature which Dabska has likened to the appearance of match heads [266]

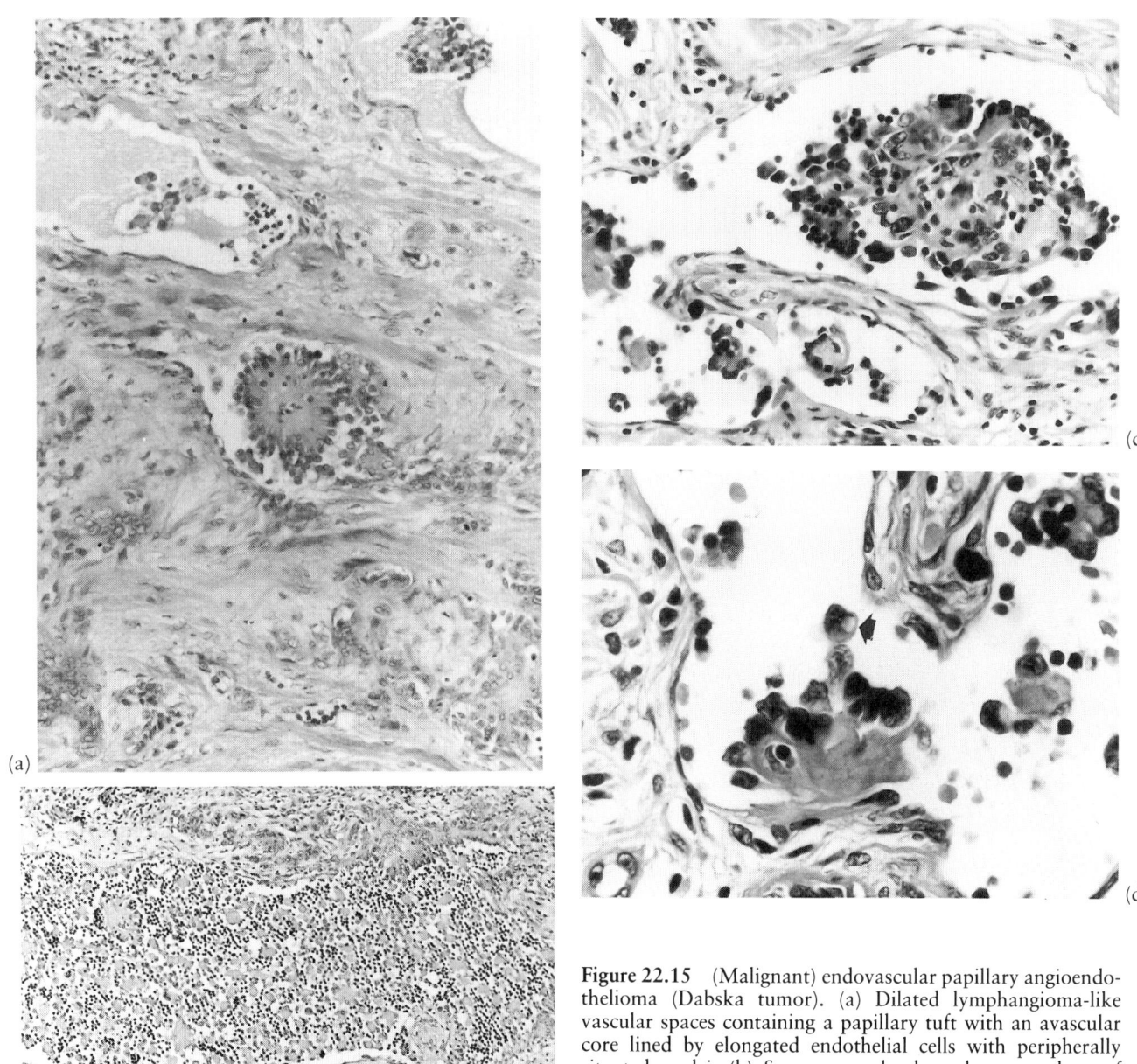

Figure 22.15 (Malignant) endovascular papillary angioendothelioma (Dabska tumor). (a) Dilated lymphangioma-like vascular spaces containing a papillary tuft with an avascular core lined by elongated endothelial cells with peripherally situated nuclei. (b) Some examples have large numbers of lymphocytes within the ectatic vascular spaces and (c) intimately associated with the endothelial tufts. (d) A high power view demonstrating tall, columnar-shaped endothelium with abluminal nuclei. One epithelioid endothelial cell (arrow) may be exhibiting 'primitive' intracytoplasmic lumen formation, a feature shared with several other vascular lesions.

(Figure 22.15(d)). Ultrastructural examination has demonstrated the hyaline core to consist of basal lamina-like material.

Intravascular lymphocytes may be prominent (Figure 22.15(b)) and are sometimes intimately associated with the endothelium (Figure 22.15(c)). The surrounding soft tissue can have a relatively normal appearance or it may be fibrotic. Occasionally lymphoid aggregates, foci of hemorrhage and degenerative elements (e.g. cholesterol clefts, siderophages) are noted.

The presence of epithelioid endothelium, sometimes with vacuolated cytoplasm consistent with early lumen formation, is a feature Dabska tumor shares with several other vasoformative processes including spindle cell hemangioendothelioma, epithelioid hemangioendothelioma and angiolymphoid hyperplasia with eosinophilia (epithelioid hemangioma).

The histogenesis of endovascular papillary angioendothelioma remains unresolved. The presence of intravascular lymphocytes intimately associated with the endothelium of some tumors has led one group to hypothesize differentiation towards 'high' endothelium of the postcapillary venules. A lymphatic derivation has also been considered, since the dilated vessels are often devoid of erythrocytes and the intervening stroma is occasionally fibrotic with lymphoid aggregates, features not unlike those seen in cutaneous lymphangioma or chronic obstructive lymphedema [268].

22.3.3 KAPOSIFORM INFANTILE HEMANGIOENDOTHELIOMA

Kaposiform infantile hemangioendothelioma (KIH) is a rare but distinctive vascular tumor which primarily affects infants and children [276,277]. The tumor generally manifests as a large retroperitoneal mass which is frequently associated with a consumptive coagulopathy (Kasabach–Merritt syndrome) and is sometimes complicated by intestinal obstruction, jaundice and hemoperitoneum [272–277]. Although the tumor has proven lethal for the majority of patients with intra-abdominal disease, due to aggressive local behavior, distant metastases have not been reported. One reported lesion of an upper extremity exhibited a growth pattern which was interpreted as being more in keeping with extensive local metastases than multifocality or contiguous extension. However, the patient is alive with no evidence of disease 6 years following amputation and radiation therapy [275,277]. Similar tumors occurring in the extremities, scalp and neck, have had a more favorable outcome [277]. An association with lymphangiomatosis has been reported [277].

A consensus approach to management of intra-abdominal examples has not been developed; treatment has ranged from supportive care to attempts at surgical resection. With varying degrees of success, prednisone, radiation and chemotherapy have also been utilized in an attempt to reduce tumor burden. Optimal management for peripherally situated examples is believed to be wide local excision [277].

The tumors are characterized histologically by infiltrative, lobular growth with intervening fibrous septa (Figure 22.16(a)). Well formed capillaries, sometimes containing fibrin thrombi, are admixed with short fascicles of spindle cells with slit-like vascular lumina (Figure 22.16(b)). The latter component results in a pattern reminiscent of Kaposi's sarcoma and serves as a distinguishing feature from other pediatric vascular tumors such as cellular capillary hemangioma (juvenile or infantile hemangioendothelioma). The lobulated growth pattern, lack of a prominent interanastomosing vascular pattern, and paucity of significant cytologic atypia aid in distinguishing this tumor from angiosarcoma.

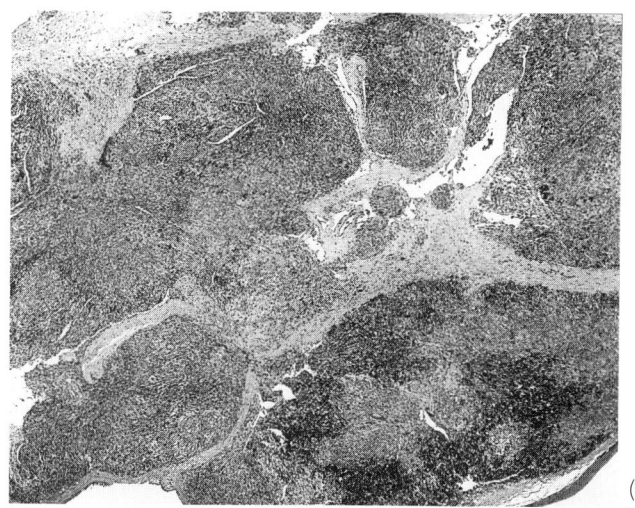
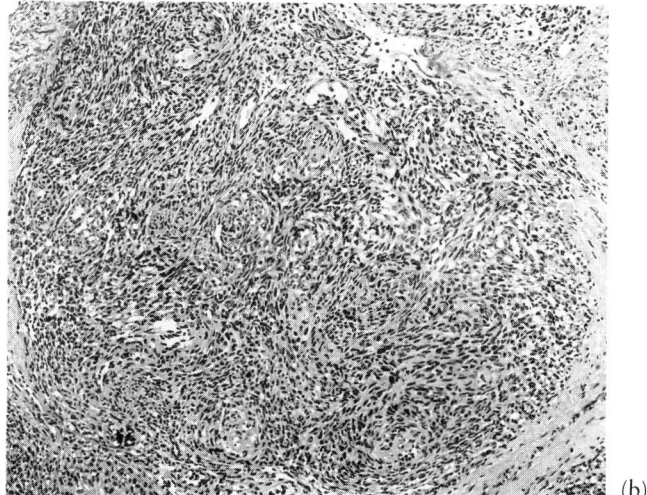

Figure 22.16 Kaposiform infantile hemangioendothelioma. (a) Note the prominent lobulated architecture. (b) At higher magnification, one sees a cellular spindle cell proliferation reminiscent of Kaposi's sarcoma. (Courtesy of Dr S.W. Weiss.)

Features which distinguish KIH from Kaposi's sarcoma include:

1. the young age of the patients;
2. the apparent lack of an association with HIV status;
3. confinement of the process to one general site or location which is usually deep-seated;
4. the lobulated architecture of the vascular proliferation;
5. a less pronounced inflammatory (lymphoplasmacytic) response;
6. the relative abundance of pericytic cells within the process, a feature common to other vascular tumors of childhood [85].

Although hyaline globules have been documented in KIH [277], their occurrence appears to be considerably less frequent than in Kaposi's sarcoma.

22.4 Malignant vascular tumors

Included in this section are epithelioid hemangioendothelioma (a tumor which is frequently regarded as low grade but is fully capable of metastases), Kaposi's sarcoma and angiosarcoma. The latter entity is also sometimes referred to as 'Kaposi's disease', reflecting the belief of some investigators that, at least in its initial stages, it may be an abnormal hyperplasia rather than a true neoplasm. We have included it here based on its capacity to be widely disseminated and the large collective number of fatal cases.

22.4.1 EPITHELIOID HEMANGIOENDOTHELIOMA

Epithelioid hemangioendothelioma (EHE) is a malignant vascular tumor which generally pursues a less aggressive course than angiosarcoma. It can occur at any age although it is rare in childhood. The predominant sites of involvement are the soft tissue, lungs, liver and bones.

Soft tissue examples [278–281,291] have been reported to occur with equal frequency in males and females. However, this data is primarily based on A.F.I.P. material and therefore may be male biased. The median age at presentation is in the fifth decade. The tumors are typically solitary and have a predilection for the extremities. Either the subcutis or deeper soft tissue sites may be involved. More than 50% of cases are associated with a medium-sized or larger vessel, usually a vein [278,279]. Involvement of the jugular, femoral and iliac veins has been documented. In the largest soft tissue series thus far reported, metastases and tumor-related deaths have occurred in 31 and 13% of patients, respectively, with a mean follow-up period of 48 months [279]. Features which may correlate with more aggressive biologic behavior in this location include: mitotic counts of greater than 1 mitosis per 10 high power fields, spindled tumor-cell morphology, the presence of necrosis, and 'significant' cytologic atypia [278,279].

Intravascular bronchioloalveolar tumor (IVBAT), sclerosing endothelial tumor, sclerosing interstitial vascular sarcoma, primary chondrosarcoma of the lung and pulmonary deciduosis is a partial list of designations previously used to describe examples of EHE of the lungs [282–285]. Approximately 80% of patients are women. The median age at presentation is 40 years. Multiple and bilateral nodules, commonly 1 cm or less in size, are typically noted at presentation. At least 65% of patients eventually succumb to disease, some as many as 15 years after diagnosis [282]. Preliminary observations suggest the following features may be associated with an adverse outcome for patients with pulmonary EHE:

- clinical symptoms at the time of diagnosis
- extensive intravascular, endobronchial, interstitial and pleural spread
- peripheral lymphadenopathy, even in the absence of documented nodal metastases
- hepatic metastases [282].

Although both the pattern and extent of disease in pulmonary EHE suggest a metastatic process, this has generally been viewed as a primary, possibly multicentric, neoplasm since past experience has indicated that an extrapulmonary primary does not become apparent clinically. Previous autopsy studies have also supported this view. However, many of these data were compiled prior to the recognition of a soft tissue disease counterpart, which favors the extremities. Imaging studies and autopsy examinations are commonly limited to the torso and, as such, some extremity tumors may have escaped detection. Therefore, we believe that all patients with EHE involving the lungs should be thoroughly evaluated for evidence of an extrapulmonary primary, with special attention being paid to the limbs. Several recent reports lend some support to this view [280,281].

Before the vascular nature of EHE was recognized, hepatic examples [286–289] were interpreted as sclerosing hepatic carcinomas, cholangiocarcinomas or calcifying mixed malignant tumors. Hepatic involvement is commonly multifocal and bilobar. Approximately two-thirds of the affected patients are women. The mean age at presentation is approximately 50 years. In the A.F.I.P. hepatic series [286], the largest thus far reported, 35% of patients died of disease with the interval to death ranging from less than 2 to approximately 10 years after diagnosis. However, given the fact that at least 80% of patients alive at last follow-up (mean 9.8 years) had untreated disease, the mortality figure for this tumor will undoubtedly prove to be substantially higher. A relationship to oral contraceptive use has been suggested although it has not been statistically confirmed [288]. As with pulmonary examples, identification of EHE in the liver should prompt a thorough clinical investigation to exclude the possibility of metastases from other potential primary sites.

Skeletal EHE [279,290] typically manifests in the second and third decades of life. The tumor predominates in males, is frequently multicentric (in over 60%) and has a predilection for the bones of the extremities, especially those of the lower limb. The mortality rate for osseous examples is not known since the number of reported cases is small and follow-up limited. However, preliminary data suggest a relatively indolent course in most instances. For reasons which are not clear, patients with multifocal bone disease seem to fare better than individuals with solitary osseous tumors [279,290].

The gross and microscopic features of EHE are similar in all sites [278–288,290–292]. The tumor nodules have a white-tan, well-margined appearance and a firm, rubbery or 'cartilaginous' consistency. Calcifications may occasionally be present. Microscopic examination reveals a tumor composed of epithelioid (histiocytoid) and, occasionally, spindle or dendritic cells, embedded singly, in cord-like arrangements, or clusters within a matrix variably described as 'myxohyaline' or 'chondromyxoid' (Figure 22.17(a)). The matrix frequently has a hyalinized or collagenized appearance centrally and a more myxoid quality peripherally. All of these features belie the vascular nature of the process. However, close scrutiny frequently reveals the presence of scattered neoplastic cells with prominent cytoplasmic vacuoles (Figure 22.17(b)). Occasionally, the vacuoles may contain intraluminal erythrocytes, a sign of 'early' or 'primitive' vasoformative differentiation. This finding, along with the sporadic presence of a well-formed neoplastic vascular component and the frequent association of the process with a pre-existing medium-sized or larger vessel (Figure 22.17(a)), should assist the pathologist in recognizing the tumor's vascular nature.

EHE generally features mild to moderate atypical cytology, although, on rare occasions, foci with significant pleomorphism may be noted. Tumors with the latter appearance can sometimes be difficult to distinguish from epithelioid angiosarcoma, a finding which suggests the possibility of a histologic (diagnostic) continuum. However, in most instances, epithelioid angiosarcoma is readily distinguished by its paucity of myxohyaline matrix and its tendency for considerably more atypism, cellularity, mitotic activity and necrosis. Interanastomosing vascular channels, which can be highlighted with a reticulin stain, are also more prevalent in angiosarcoma. Finally, the nuclei of epithelioid angiosarcoma frequently feature prominent, melanoma-like nucleoli, a finding generally absent in EHE.

The following features of EHE serve to distinguish it from angiolymphoid hyperplasia with eosinophilia (epithelioid hemangioma):

1. a growth pattern which is more infiltrative;
2. a less pronounced inflammatory response;
3. a more architecturally and cytologically primitive vascular pattern (i.e. endothelial cells present singly or in clusters or cord-like arrangements);
4. the presence of a myxohyaline matrix;
5. cytologic atypia may be more pronounced;
6. large, deep-seated, vessels are more often affected (e.g. jugular and femoral veins).

We acknowledge the existence of vascular lesions which seem to exhibit hybrid features between these two relatively distinct entities. Such lesions are uncommon and are best diagnosed descriptively with a recommendation for complete excision and close follow-up.

Additional infrequent considerations in the differential diagnosis of EHE include: epithelioid sarcoma, metastatic sclerosing carcinomas (especially signet ring adenocarcinoma) and chondrosarcoma. Epithelioid sar-

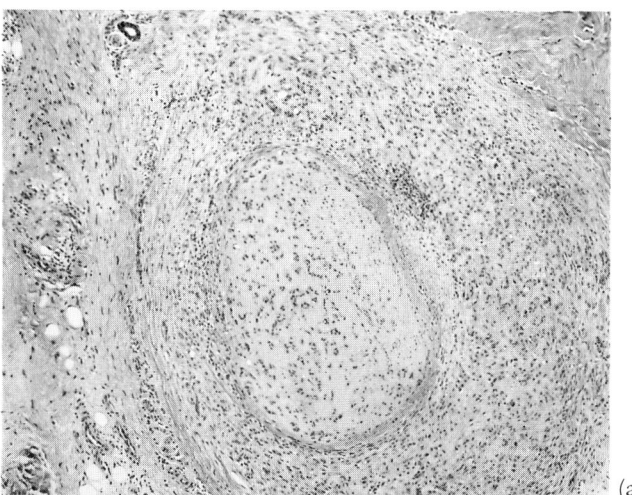
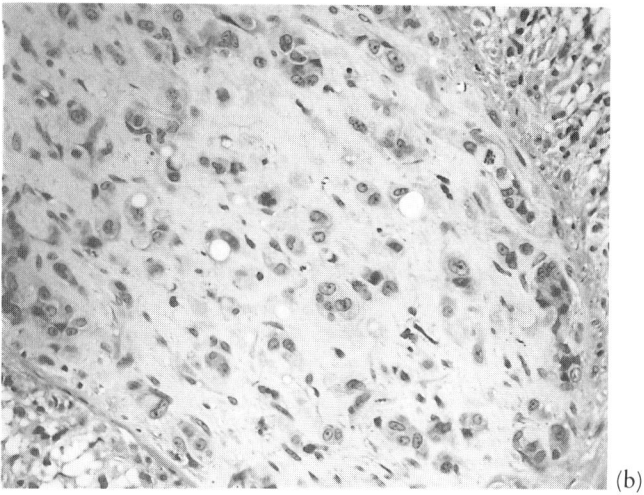

Figure 22.17 (a) Epithelioid hemangioendothelioma occluding the lumen of a medium-sized vessel, and expanding into adjacent soft tissue. (b) Note the myxohyaline matrix and the epithelioid endothelial cells. Rudimentary intracytoplasmic lumina are well demonstrated in this illustration.

coma differs from a clinical perspective by having a strong predilection for the tendons and aponeuroses. It differs histologically by featuring a rather distinctive geographic or garland-like growth pattern with central necrosis. Signet ring carcinoma differs histochemically by featuring mucicarmine positive vacuoles; the cytoplasmic vacuoles of EHE are either mucicarmine-negative, or at best, weakly positive along the luminal border. Both carcinomas and epithelioid sarcoma are typically immunoreactive with antibodies directed against keratin and epithelial membrane antigen and are non-reactive with anti-factor VIII related antigen. The opposite is generally true of EHE. However, this is not always the case. Epithelial and non-vascular mesenchymal tumors may occasionally exhibit weak reactivity with anti-factor VIII-related antigen due to antigen adsorption and EHE sometimes exhibit immunoreactivity with antikeratins, especially those antibodies directed against low molecular weight keratin polypeptides [577]. Therefore a panel approach is prudent when evaluating immunhistochemical studies in this setting.

Like chondrosarcoma, the stromal matrix of EHE is reported to contain sulfated acid mucins which can be highlighted with aldehyde fuschin at pH 1.0 [278]. However, in contrast to chondrosarcoma, the neoplastic cells of epithelioid hemangioendothelioma typically lack S100 protein expression.

Two uncommon considerations in the differential diagnosis are also worth brief mention. First, EHE exhibiting pleural or peritoneal extension can grow in an organ-encasing manner and produce a pattern reminiscent of malignant mesothelioma. Second, intraosseous EHE, especially if multifocal, can be confused histologically with myeloma since both tumors may feature coarse granular nuclear chromatin and hyaline-like eosinophilic cytoplasm. However, if appropriate attention is given to clinical parameters (e.g. in mesothelioma, historical and other clinical evidence of asbestos exposure; in myeloma, paraproteinemia), and a battery is used when ordering histochemical and/or immunohistochemical studies, the correct diagnosis can usually be made without substantial difficulty.

22.4.2 KAPOSI'S SARCOMA

(a) Background

Although Köbner is credited with the first report in 1869 [293], Moriz Kaposi's series published three years later established this tumor as a distinct clinicopathologic entity [294]. Kaposi's paper, entitled 'idiopathic multiple pigmented sarcoma of the skin' describes in detail five adult male patients, aged 40–68 years, and briefly mentions a boy aged 8–10 years. He believed the condition to be a generalized disease which proved rapidly fatal. Interest in the condition remained relatively dormant in the literature for the next 100 years until the disease began manifesting in immunosuppressed individuals, first in the setting of iatrogenic immunosuppression associated with solid organ transplantation and later as a feature of the acquired immunodeficiency syndrome (AIDS).

(b) Epidemiologic subtypes of Kaposi's sarcoma

In the 'classic' or European form of the disease, Kaposi's sarcoma (KS) typically affects male patients between the ages of 50 and 80 years. The peak incidence is in the sixth [295] or seventh [296] decade. Combining data from two large series [295,296] gives a male to female ratio of 11:1 although ratios as high as 15:1 have been observed [297]. A racial predilection is evident, with an increased incidence in men of Mediterranean descent or of Ashkenazic Jewish extraction. Isolated familial cases have been reported [298]. While some investigators have noted an association with HLA-DR5 antigen [299], this has been refuted by others [300]. The disease frequently follows an indolent course [295,301]. Patients typically survive an average of 10–15 years following their initial diagnosis and commonly die of an unrelated cause. Secondary malignancies have been reported in more than 35% of the patients [301] with approximately half of these tumors being of hematopoietic/lymphoreticular derivation (e.g. leukemia, lymphoma, multiple myeloma). In most instances, the patients are clinically well at presentation, having no anemia or abnormal leukocyte counts. Cutaneous lesions are usually first noted in the distal portion of the lower extremities and evolve in stages, consisting initially of purple patches, followed by plaques and nodules. Over time, the lesions extend proximally, gradually coalesce and may ulcerate. Some foci may regress while others progress. Upper extremity and internal involvement may develop although the latter is often clinically silent [302,303].

The African or 'endemic' form of KS [302,304–306] has its highest incidence in the north-east Zaire–northwest Ugandan region. The incidence decreases as one travels radially from this vicinity with more rapid decline in the northerly direction [302]. This disease reportedly accounts for 9% of malignancies in Ugandan males and approximately 10% of all cancers in Zaire. Two distinct age groups are affected: young to middle-aged adults and children. The median age at presentation for the adult population is in the fourth decade, and 90–97% of these individuals are males [305]. The majority have a clinically benign, nodular form of the disease although both florid and aggressive variants also occur. Affected children have a male to female ratio of 3:1 and a mean age at presentation of 3 years. They typically exhibit prominent lymph node involvement unaccompanied by cutaneous manifestions [302,307,308]. In contrast to most adult cases, the disease in children is usually fulminant and fatal within 2 or 3 years. A recent study from Rwanda suggests that, at least in recent years, many of the patients living in endemic areas with aggressive disease are also HIV seropositive, whereas those with localized cutaneous disease are seronegative [306].

A third epidemiologic subgroup at risk for KS is composed of individuals (primarily transplant patients) receiving potent, high-dose or long-term immunosuppressive therapy. The overall risk to these patients is relatively low. Kaposi's sarcoma is estimated to occur in 0.4% of renal transplant patients [309] and is said to account for 3.4% of all malignancies in the transplant population [310]. The mean interval to onset after transplantion is 16.5 months [310]. Many of these individuals are also of Jewish or Mediterranean descent. However, females comprise a higher percentage of those affected;

the male to female ratio ranges from 2:1 to 3:1 [309, 311–316]. Although KS may assume a chronic or aggressive course in these patients, regression frequently follows discontinuation of the immunosuppressive treatment. In some instances, regression evolves into a complete remission while in other cases further therapy may be required [310]. Patients receiving immunosuppressive agents as treatment for systemic lupus erythematosus [317] and various other collagen vascular and skin disorders [318,319] are also included in this category.

The 'epidemic' or AIDS-related form of KS occurs in HIV-positive individuals. The clinical definition for AIDS-KS is lymphadenopathic and/or oral, genital, gastrointestinal, pulmonary or disseminated cutaneous KS sarcoma [320]. These criteria were developed in Uganda where they have allowed distinction between 'endemic' and 'epidemic' (i.e. HIV-seropositive) KS with 91 and 95% sensitivity and specificity, respectively [320]. The presence of oral KS is particularly helpful, having a sensitivity of 73% and a predictive value of 99% for HIV seropositivity [320]. Since the pair of reports from the CDC in 1981 describing 26 homosexual men with KS in California and New York City [321,322], AIDS-KS has become the largest epidemiologic subgroup of this disease. As in classic KS, an association with the HLA-DR5 antigen has been observed in some studies [323].

The risk of developing KS for an AIDS patient is estimated to be 300 times greater than that of other immunosuppressed individuals and 20 000 times greater that of the general population [324]. In this group, KS frequently assumes an aggressive course. Due to increased awareness, the patients often present with small, subtle clinical lesions. Areas prone to KS in the adult AIDS population include: the oral cavity, especially the hard palate, the tip of the nose, behind the ears, and the trunk, penis, legs and feet. A predisposition for skin-cleavage lines has also been noted [325]. Lesions more often involve the upper half of the body than in classic KS [326]. Post-mortem studies have demonstrated a high incidence of concurrent disease in lymph nodes, the gastrointestinal tract and lungs [327,328]. Pediatric cases of AIDS-KS have a proclivity for lymphadenopathic disease [77,329], although dermatopathic cases have been reported [330].

Of interest, the various groups of AIDS patients have unexplained differences in the incidence of KS [331–333]. For example, KS is reported to occur in 21% [324] to 36% of homosexual or bisexual males with AIDS but it has been identified in only 4.3, 1.9 and 1.6% of intravenous drug abusers, transfusion recipients and hemophiliacs with AIDS, respectively [333]. Also women infected with HIV through contact with bisexual men are at greater risk of developing KS than those infected though contact with other high risk groups (e.g. intravenous drug abusers, transfusion recipients, hemophiliacs) [324,334]. Various sexual practices such as increased oral–anal contact and receptive anal intercourse may also be associated with an increased frequency of KS [324,335,336] although this is a point of contention [337–339]. These and other findings have led to the speculation that there may be sexually transmitted cofactor(s) in the pathogenesis of AIDS-KS.

Cytomegalovirus antigens (CMV-DNA and/or CMV-RNA) have been detected in KS via immunohistochemical, immunofluorescent, *in situ* hybridization, polymerase chain reaction and Southern blot hybridization techniques [341,342]. As a result, CMV is the infectious agent most commonly suspected of being a cofactor in the pathogenesis of this disease [340–343]. However, its role remains controversial [344] for the follow reasons:

1. the CMV genome does not appear to be integrated into Kaposi's sarcoma cells [343];
2. there is no consistent association between CMV infection and classical Kaposi's sarcoma [340,341];
3. CMV is so ubiquitous in the populations at risk for KS (e.g. iatrogenic immunosuppression, African 'endemic' [344] and AIDS 'epidemic' forms) that its presence may represent nothing more than a coexisting generalized infection (i.e. a 'passenger' agent).

Earlier findings suggesting associations between KS and herpes simplex [345,346], hepatitis A and hepatitis B viruses have given rise to similar conclusions. More recently, human papilloma virus (HPV) has also been implicated as a potential factor in the pathogenesis of this disease [347,348]. Finally, HIV itself may contribute to the development, growth and maintenance of KS in seropositive individuals. Through its action on infected cells (e.g. CD4+ lymphocytes, KS cells), HIV has been shown to incite the production of cytokines (e.g. Oncostatin M, tumor necrosis factor-alpha, interleukin-1) [349] and angiogenic growth factors [350–355,403]. At present, however, additional work is required to determine whether any of these agents has a direct role in initiating the disease process and, if so, how it interrelates with other potential factors including the patient's genetic profile and hormonal status.

(c) Clinical patterns of disease

Three clinical disease patterns of KS have been recognized [302]: nodular, aggressive and generalized. This format was based on early studies of patients with 'endemic' (African) disease but serves as a useful construct for evaluating all KS patients. Nodular disease is characterized by the presence of circumscribed cutaneous or subcutaneous nodules. It usually pursues an indolent course, although internal involvement, which is frequently asymptomatic, is often present at the time of

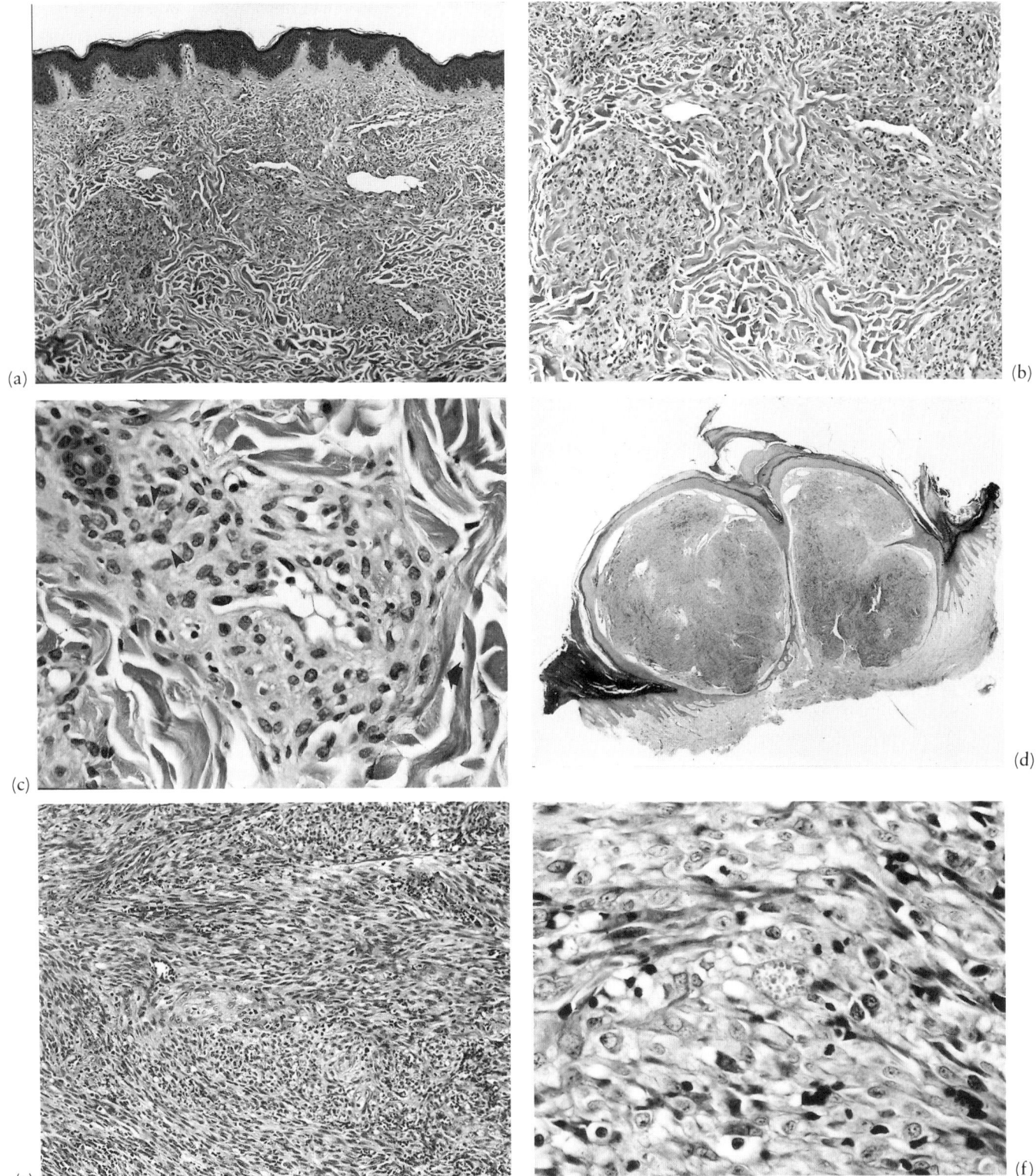

Figure 22.18 (a and b) Kaposi's sarcoma (patch-plaque stage). Note the increased cellularity around pre-existing dermal vessels and a collagen-dissecting pattern. (c) Higher magnification demonstrating the small-vessel proliferation. Rare hyaline globules (arrow head) and hemosiderin deposition (arrow) are evident. (d) Nodular Kaposi's sarcoma with a polypoid configuration and an epithelial collarette. (e) Spindle cells are arranged in sweeping fascicles with slit-like spaces containing red blood cells. (f) Hyaline-globules as they appear in an H&E-stained section.

death. The aggressive form of KS generally arises from a background of pre-existing nodular disease. It is characterized by extensive exophytic and ulcerative or deep infiltrative growth usually involving the extremities. Osseous and visceral involvement are commonly present but may be clinically silent. The generalized form of KS includes lymphadenopathic disease with or without systemic involvement. As mentioned erlier, lymphadenopathic disease with or without systemic involvement occurs primarily in children.

(e) Histogenesis

Over time, a large variety of cell types has been put forth as the progenitor for Kaposi's lesions including: blood vessel and lymphatic endothelium, pericytes, smooth muscle cells, (myo)fibroblasts, histiocytes and even Schwann cells [356]. Most observers now believe KS is a vascular or vascular-related process and as such, endothelium and vascular-derived supporting cells (i.e. pericytes) are considered to be the key elements. Recently, debate has focused on whether the endothelial cells, and thus the lesions in general, are of lymphatic or blood vessel derivation. Results of immunohistochemical and ultrastructural studies have been conflicting in this regard with some observers favoring the former [357–359], others [360,361] the latter, and still others an amalgam of both [356].

The following features have led to the speculation that KS may be an unusual hyperplasia ('Kaposi's disease') rather than a true neoplasm:

1. a tendency for multifocal development as opposed to the presence of a primary tumor with subsequent metastases;
2. a strong association with immunodeficiency and a capacity for regression with the reinstatement of normal immune function (i.e. the regression of KS with discontinuation of iatrogenic immunosuppression);
3. a pronounced predilection for the male sex, a feature which implies a hormonal influence;
4. the existence of an endemic form of the disease within certain regions of Africa [362–364].

Microspectrophotometric [364] and flow cytometric [365,366] analyses of Kaposi's lesions have produced diploid results, additional findings consistent with, although not unequivocally indicative of, a reactive process. It has been postulated [362,364] that KS begins as a reactive/reparative response to an acquired immune deficiency. At this stage, it may be reversible. However, through a 'second hit' mechanism (viral cofactor, other), lesions may acquire the capacity for autonomous growth, thus becoming truly neoplastic. For the time being, it would seem preferable to retain the 'sarcoma' designation for Kaposi's lesions since:

1. they have a tendency, in many instances, to progess despite medical management;
2. there are clinically aggressive forms of the disease which may prove rapidly fatal;
3. pleomorphic or anaplastic morphologic variants have been documented which have both morphologic and clinical resemblance to angiosarcomas [296,303, 367].

(f) Histologic patterns

There are no well defined morphologic or immunohistochemical differences between the classical, endemic, iatrogenic (immunosuppressive) and AIDS-associated forms of KS. While the histologic diagnosis of well developed nodular or plaque lesions is generally not difficult, early, patch (macular) lesions may have sufficiently subtle morphology that a definite diagnosis can not be rendered. In the latter instance, little is usually lost by adopting a conservative stance, providing supportive medical management and rebiopsying the patient at a later date when more typical lesions are present.

In the early, patch stage of KS [359,368–370], changes predominate in the upper half of the reticular dermis where one sees a proliferation of capillaries around pre-existing dermal vessels and adnexa (Figure 22.18(a)–(c)). These newly formed vessels often have a collapsed, jagged or angulated appearance but on occasion, they may be somewhat ectatic. The endothelial lining is flattened or slightly plump. Some endothelial cells may contain apoptotic nuclei, a feature of diagnostic value [359]. The protrusion of small proliferating capillary channels into the vascular lumen of a larger, pre-existing dermal vessel, the 'promontory' sign, also has diagnostic importance [325]. Bland-appearing spindle cells may be associated with the neovasculature, although at this stage they tend to be a minor component. A variable inflammatory infiltrate dominated by lymphocytes, with or without plasma cells, is frequently present. Extravasated erythrocytes, hemosiderin deposition and intracytoplasmic PAS-positive, diastase-resistant, hyaline globules may or may not be noted [370]. As the process progresses to involve the full thickness of the dermis, it becomes palpable and is clinically recognized as a plaque.

In the plaque stage, the spindled component of KS becomes more prominent. These cells are dispersed amongst the dermal collagen bundles and are also noted in and around the network of new vessels. They form slit-like spaces which frequently contain red blood cells. Plasma cells and hemosiderin deposits are also usually apparent. Eosinophilic hyaline spherules, 1–7 μm in size, are commonly present and form grape-like agglomerations which are predominantly intracellular (Figure 22.18(c)). They are believed by many investigators to represent various stages of erythrophagolysosomes

[371,372] and are a helpful, although not entirely specific, feature. Similar inclusions, though usually not as abundant, may be seen in a variety of other vascular proliferations, both benign and malignant [277,373].

Nodular Kaposi's lesions represent further development and organization beyond the plaque stage. On gross examination, cutaneous lesions have a well circumscribed, violaceous, dome-shaped or polypoid appearance. The spindle cell population often dominates, forming fascicles and sheets which may resemble well differentiated fibrosarcoma or even leiomyosarcoma (Figure 22.18(d),(e)). Extravasated erythrocytes, siderophages, hyaline globules (Figure 22.18(f)), and a peripheral lyphoplasmacytic infiltrate are typically present. Single cell necrosis is also seen.

Plemorphic or anaplastic change ('malignant transformation') has, on rare occasions, been reported in KS. Lesions with this morphology are believed capable of true metastases. In some instances, the morphology is indistinguishable from a spindled or poorly differentiated angiosarcoma. Other examples have been likened to fibrosarcoma or undifferentiated malignancies [296, 302,303,367].

A lymphangioma-like variant of classic KS has also been described [379–381]. Its clinical presentation does not appear to vary substantially from more typical cases. However, its histology differs by featuring a predominance of ectatic lymphatic-like channels which permeate the dermis. Associated inflammation is minimal but hemosiderin deposition is seen. A minor, ill defined, spindle cell component may be present, but it is not usually intermingled with the vascular clefts as in more typical Kaposi's lesions.

KS may involve lymph nodes [374–378], either as an initial, sometimes isolated, manifestation, or as a later component of disseminated disease. Like cutaneous examples, it is readily recognized when the disease is fully established but is difficult to characterize in its initial stages. Early changes include subcapsular sinus ectasia and intrasinusoidal vascular proliferation. Step sectioning may be required to identify a spindle cell component. Caution is advised when diagnosing early nodal KS, especially when clinical details are not at hand, since other intranodal vascular proliferations may exhibit some morphologic overlap (i.e. vascular transformation of sinuses/nodal angiomatosis) [391, 393]. Intranodal palisaded myofibroblastoma, a recently characterized benign myofibroblastic proliferation which occurs predominantly in the inguinal lymph nodes of adults also shares some morphologic resemblance to advanced intranodal KS [400–402].

(g) Differential diagnosis

The clinical differential of KS is quite long due to the various stages through which the disease passes. It includes (acro-)angiodermatitis, bacillary angiomatosis, pyogenic granuloma, melanoma, cutaneous lymphoma, blue nevus, dermatofibroma (fibrous histiocytoma), hemangioma, cicatrix, purpura pigmentosa chronica, postinflammatory pigmentation and a number of other conditions [382]. However, in spite of this rather lengthy list, many cases of KS, for the experienced physician, are sufficiently typical in their clinical appearance as to be essentially diagnosable without biopsy [302]. The challenge lies in recognizing early stages of the disease as well as unusually aggressive examples. An accurate diagnosis in these instances is dependent on a high index of suspicion and appropriate clinicopathological correlation. AIDS and its attendant KS epidemic have resulted in the recent delineation of several histologic mimics of this disease. In the interest of brevity, the following discussion is primarily skewed toward these newly described entities.

(Acro-)angiodermatitis [383–386], secondary to chronic venous insufficiency, occasionally bears sufficient clinical and morphologic resemblance so as to be dubbed a 'pseudo-Kaposi's sarcoma'. Such lesions have been described in association with diabetes mellitus [383,384], arteriosclerosis [383], post-traumatic venous insufficiency [383], a paralyzed limb [386] and arteriovenous shunting [384,385]. Patients typically present with plaques, scaly patches or violaceous nodules involving the distal portions of the lower extremity, especially the foot and ankle. On histologic examination, a background featuring extravasated erythrocytes, hemosiderin deposition, fibroblastic proliferation and scattered inflammatory elements is frequently noted, thus resembling the mileau of KS. However, the small vessel proliferation of the former is generally lobular and well formed, as opposed to the haphazard, collapsed appearance typically associated with early stages of KS. Attention to the clinical features and recognition of the lobular architecture of the vascular proliferation should avert misdiagnosis.

Targetoid hemosiderotic hemangioma (THH) [239–241] bears a histological resemblance to KS, but the clinical presentation is quite different. The lesions are typically solitary and in their early stages of evolution, they exhibit a rather characteristic target-like gross appearance. For a more detailed discussion of this 'entity', we refer the reader to the preceding section of the text dealing with benign vascular tumors.

Acquired progressive lymphangioma (benign lymphangioendothelioma) has been reported in both children and adults but, to our knowledge, has not been described in immunocompromised patients [387–389]. This lesion presents as a solitary macule or plaque which slowly enlarges. Cure has generally been achieved by local excision. The lesions are characterized, histologically, by interanastomosing endothelial-lined vascular clefts, with a collagen-dissecting pattern, distributed throughout the dermis. Extension into the subcutis may be noted. The endothelial cells may be plumper and more prevalent than would normally be expected in association with lymphatic channels but atypia is absent. The vascular lumina sometimes contain proteinaceous material; red blood cells are generally absent. Extravasated erythrocytes, hemosiderin deposition, endothelial cell apoptosis, hyaline globules and a plasma cell infiltrate are features of KS which serve to distinguish it from acquired progressive lymphangioma.

Bacillary angiomatosis enters into the differential diagnosis since it has both a predilection for immunosuppressed patients and is typically a multifocal or generalized process. In fact, in the AIDS population, it is not uncommon for this disease to coexist with KS [11]. Its proper distinction is important since it is the result of a treatable infection, which, if unmanaged, can prove fatal. For a detailed discussed of this entity, we refer the reader to the earlier section of this chapter dealing with reactive vascular proliferations.

Nodular Kaposi's sarcoma features a prominent spindled component which commonly contains areas with a fascicular growth pattern. As a result, **fibrosarcoma** and **leiomyosarcoma** may occasionally be considered in the differential diagnosis. All three tumors contain cells capable of reacting with immunohistochemical antibodies directed against muscle specific and smooth muscle actins [390]. Although longitudinal cytoplasmic fibrillations may also be seen in all three, they are much more prevelant and better defined in leiomyosarcoma. The latter entity differs further from the other two by featuring blunt-ended nuclei and more abundant eosinophilic cytoplasm. The plasma cell infiltrate, slit-like vascular spaces, degree of red blood cell extravasation and hyaline globules in KS set it apart from both leiomyosarcoma and fibrosarcoma. Other spindle cell tumors which might also be included in the differential diagnosis include spindle cell hemangioendothelioma [257–265] and the spindled variant of angiosarcoma [419].

Although a variety of vascular proliferations have been described as primary intranodal processes [391], **vascular transformation of sinuses** is probably the most likely to be mistaken for KS [392–394]. This entity was first described by Haferkamp in 1971 [392] and is believed to be due to complete occlusion of the efferent lymphatic channels with or without coexisting partial occlusion of the nodal veins [395,396]. A recent series of 76 patients published by Chan and co-workers [393] highlights a large morphologic spectrum for this process. They describe four major vascular patterns: cleft-like, rounded or oval, solid and plexiform. Most lesions contained more than one pattern. The vascular proliferation expands the subcapsular, intermediate and medullary sinuses of the lymph node to varying degrees. There is frequently associated fibrosclerosis and red blood cell extravasation. The intervening lymphoid parenchyma may be mildly or markedly depleted depending on the extent of the sinusoidal expansion. 'Nodal angiomatosis' [398,399] and 'plexiform vascularization of lymph nodes' [397] probably represent part of the morphologic spectrum described above. The lack of spindled fascicles, the associated fibrosis of the sinusoidal tissue and the paucity of extrasinusoidal and extracapsular extension help distinguish vascular transformation of sinuses from KS. While hyaline globules may be seen in both entities, they are more abundant in KS.

(h) Treatment of KS

Treatment of KS is, in most instances, palliative. It should also be recognized that most patients with this disease die of unrelated causes (e.g. second malignancy, AIDS-related opportunistic infections, etc.). In general, classic KS responds well to local therapies, iatrogenic KS often exhibits regression with the reduction or discontinuation of immunosuppressive therapy, and patients with the African ('endemic') form of the disease, excluding those with the lymphadenopathic variant, are said to have favorable results with systemic single or multi-agent chemotherapy. An excellent review which highlights therapeutic options for AIDS-KS been published by Tappero and colleagues [403]. Although several staging systems exist [404,405], their discussion is based on the one developed by Krown and co-workers [406]. This approach incorporates the extent of lesions, the absolute numbers of CD4+ T cells, and whether there is evidence of systemic illness:

1. a history of opportunistic infections;
2. 'B' symptoms (unexplained fever, night sweats, >10% involuntary weight loss, persistent diarrhea for >2 weeks);
3. a Karnofsky performance status <70% [407].

Using these criteria, patients are divided into low and high risk groups for aggressive disease. Low risk individuals with cosmetically disfiguring or symptomatic lesions are generally treated conservatively with local therapies (e.g. liquid nitrogen cryotherapy, intralesional vinblastine or vincristine, intralesional interferon alpha, laser therapy, surgical removal or irradiation) [408–412]. High risk patients are frequently managed with systemic therapy, often with the use of a multi-agent approach in order to minimize toxicity and unwanted side-effects.

Therapies which may show promise for the future include anti-angiogenic modulators such as recombinant platelet factor-4 [413], synthetic analogues of fumagillin [414], vitamin D3 analogues [415], synthetic heparin substitutes [416] and bacterial cell wall complexes with properties similar to those of an *Arthro-*

bacter sp. [417]. Cytokine inhibitors and cytokine receptor blockers may also prove useful [403].

22.4.3 ANGIOSARCOMA

(a) Background

In this chapter, angiosarcoma is used in a generic sense to encompass fully malignant neoplasms of endothelial derivation whether originating from lymphatics (lymphangiosarcoma) or blood vessels (hemangiosarcoma). This seems justifiable for the following reasons:

1. it can be difficult or impossible to make a definitive statement with regard to the precise origin of a malignant endothelial tumor;
2. the morphologic, immunohistochemical and ultrastructural features of tumors previously classified as lymphangiosarcoma or hemangiosarcoma overlap;
3. there appears to be little if any therapeutic or prognostic relevance to the distinction.

Angiosarcoma is a rare tumor, estimated to comprise less than 1% of all sarcomas [418]. It can develop in practically any site but there is a particularly strong predilection for the skin and subcutis. In this superficial location angiosarcoma occurs in three distinct clinical settings:

- the face and scalp of the elderly [418–425,439]
- the extremities of patients with chronic lymphedema [428,430–435,569]
- at sites previously subjected to radiation therapy [446–475].

Other key primary sites for angiosarcoma are the breast parenchyma, liver, deep soft tissue, skeleton, heart and spleen. There are reports of this tumor developing in association with foreign bodies [562–566,559,572] and defunctionalized arteriovenous fistulae in transplant recipients [567,568]. Also, an increased frequency has been reported in neurofibromatosis [556–561] where the tumor may occur either as an independent finding or in association with benign or malignant peripheral nerve sheath tumors. Finally, isolated case reports have documented angiosarcoma developing in the site of a previous a herpes zoster infection [574] and in the setting of xeroderma pigmentosum [532].

Arsenical compounds (e.g. Fowler's solution, arsenical insecticides) [509,523–525], vinyl chloride [508, 509,518] and thorium dioxide (Thorotrast) [502,509, 511,517,522] exposure have been implicated in the development of approximately 25% of angiosarcomas arising in the liver but only rarely are they cited as a potential factor in the development of extrahepatic tumors [503,504]. Anabolic steroids [511], DES [510], inhaled copper salts [526] and oral contraceptives [523] may also incite hepatic angiosarcomas, although their association remains to be confirmed.

(b) Angiosarcoma of the face and scalp

The most common location for angiosarcoma is the scalp and mid-facial region. The vast majority of affected individuals are Caucasian and in their seventh or eight decade of life. The disease is uncommon under the age of 50 years. Due to a remarkable variability in clinical appearance, superficial angiosarcomas can be misinterpreted as a bruise, hemangioma, lymphangioma, infectious process, focus of chronic edema or myxedema, scarring alopecia, malignant melanoma or even primary or metastatic carcinoma. The neoplasms may be well marginated or ill defined, solitary or multifocal and flat, elevated, nodular or cystic. Consistency varies from firm and solid to soft and fluctuant or spongy. The majority of tumors are red or bluish purple, a feature which attests to their vascular nature. However, a few edematous examples may retain normal skin coloration. Large or long-standing lesions frequently ulcerate and may become secondarily infected. Factors which may contribute to the dismal outcome of patients with this disease include:

1. delayed presentation due to a lack of symptoms or slow, insidious growth;
2. a low clinical index of suspicion resulting in a postponed biopsy diagnosis;
3. erroneous histopathologic diagnoses of biopsy specimens due to deceptively bland morphology;
4. large size and/or multifocality at the time of diagnosis,
5. underestimation of the extent of disease when instituting management.

In the largest reported series, the 5-year survival rate was 12%, with half of the patients dying within 15 months of presentation [422]. The single most important prognostic factor is tumor size [419,422]. Neoplasms smaller than 5 cm tend to recur and metastasize less frequently than larger examples [419]. Tumors with a prominent lymphoid reaction may also be associated with a better prognosis [419]. The location, clinical appearance and histologic grade of the tumor, as well as the patient's age and sex have not been shown to correlate statistically with survival. The cervical lymph nodes and lungs are the most frequent metastatic sites, followed in frequency by the liver, spleen, skeleton, kidneys and heart. The best chance for cure seems to entail radical surgical removal of the primary tumor, supplemented with wide-field electron beam radiotherapy and, in selected instances, regional lymph node clearance [425]. Adjuvant radiotherapy is usually required since these tumors typically extend well beyond their grossly apparent confines and complete resection is often not possible [419]. When surgery is not considered an option, radiotherapy also plays an important palliative role.

(c) Lymphedema-associated angiosarcoma

In 1948, Stewart and Treves [427] reported six patients, treated for breast carcinoma by radical mastectomy with or without supplemental irradiation, who developed (lymph)angiosarcoma in the ipsilateral extremity following chronic postoperative edema. This complication is said to be rare, occurring in 0.45% of postmastectomy patients surviving at least 5 years [426]. However, given the frequency of breast cancer, it is not surprising that approximately 190 additional cases had been added to the literature up to 1981 [428,430–433, 439,440,468,569]. The incidence of this complication is decreasing, given the current, more conservative surgical approach to breast carcinoma.

Chronic lymphedema is considered the predominant factor in the development of these tumors. However, the mechanism by which it induces the development of angiosarcoma is not known. Several theories, which may not be mutually exclusive, have been proposed. The oldest, put forth by Stewart and Treves, suggests the existence of a systemic carcinogen which, while circulating within the lymph, induces malignant transformation [427]. Others have suggested that the body's ongoing attempt to establish a lymphatic colateral circulation eventually goes awry, failing to respond to normal control mechanisms (so-called 'morbid lymphangiomatosis') [429,584]. More recently, it has been proposed that chronic lymphedema results in the development of an immunologically 'privileged' site which lacks normal immune surveillance and thus is more prone to malignant transformation [428].

Adjuvant radiotherapy, utilized in over 50% of reported cases, has probably contributed to the development of some of these tumors, either indirectly, by augmenting the damaging effects of surgery with the resultant promotion of lymphedema or, more directly, though the inadvertent inclusion of the affected site in the irradiation field. The latter scenario is believed uncommon.

The average interval from the onset of postmastectomy lymphedema to the appearance of angiosarcoma is approximately 9.25 years (range approximately 1 [433a and b] to 24 [427] years) [433]. Gross examination typically reveals pitting, indurated or 'pachydermatous' skin with red or bluish purple macular, papular, polypoid or fungating lesions. The tumors may be either solitary or multicentric. Sometimes, a dominant mass with multiple satellite lesions is noted.

Similar neoplasms are reported following persistent lymphedema associated with other postoperative settings [432,437], including segmental mastectomy complicated by mastitis [435]. Angiosarcoma may also develop in association with chronic congenital [432, 428,436–441], post-traumatic [432,438,440], idiopathic [432,438,440,441], postirradiation and filariasis-associated [443–445] lymphedema. Examples arising in the setting of chronic congenital and idiopathic lymphedema often have a later onset (mean 23 [438] to 26 years [433]) and the affected individuals appear to have a somewhat longer mean survival [432,433] than patients with postmastectomy lymphedema-associated tumors. Although the number of reported cases [443–445] is small, patients with filariasis-associated angiosarcoma also appear to have a longer latency period (mean 20 years) than the postmastectomy group.

Optimal management is generally considered to be early, radical and ablative surgery in the form of limb, forequarter or hindquarter amputation. Local recurrence following lesser surgical intervention is common and regarded as an ominous event. When this occurs, amputation is usually ineffective in preventing metastases and death [439].

(d) Postirradiation angiosarcoma

Postirradiation angiosarcomas have a predilection for the skin and subcutis, although they occasionally arise in more deep-seated sites (e.g. small or large bowel [448, 452], breast parenchyma [464,466], lungs [465,466], omentum [450], vagina and bladder [448]). Affected individuals can be subdivided into two groups, based on whether radiotherapy was given for a benign disorder (e.g. eczema, sinusitis [425], hemangiomas [468,470–472] or lymphangiomas [468,469]) or a malignancy. Approximately 29% of the 45 postirradiation angiosarcomas reviewed by Goette and Detlefs [447] and Edeiken and co-workers [465] occurred following treatment of a benign tumor. The majority of the remaining patients received irradiation as part of a therapeutic protocol for managing gynecologic [419,447,448–452] or breast carcinomas. The mean interval to angiosarcoma was shorter in the group treated for a malignancy, approximately 11 years (range 2.5–25 years) versus 22 years (range 4–52 years) for benign conditions. This difference could be due to the use of higher irradiation dosages in the malignant group.

We are aware of 19 reported examples of postirradiation angiosarcoma involving the breast or chest wall which developed after radiotherapy was utilized in combination with a total or segmental mastectomy, wide local excision, excisional biopsy or lumpectomy, with or without axillary sampling or dissection [419,447, 453–455,460–465]. The mean and median intervals to the diagnosis of angiosarcoma were 6.1 and 5.5 years, respectively (range 2.4–13 years). Lymphedema, localized to the treated site, was documented as a complicating factor in a few instances. As with other postirradiation angiosarcomas, the skin and subcutis were the predominant sites involved. However, a small number of individuals had additional or exclusive involvement of their remaining breast parenchyma [435,454,464].

(e) Angiosarcoma of deep soft tissue

The true incidence of angiosarcoma arising in deep soft tissue is unknown. Enzinger and Weiss have estimated that 24% of 366 angiosarcomas reviewed over a 10-year period at the Armed Forces Institute of Pathology involved this location, although this figure could be somewhat inflated due to the inadvertent inclusion of tumors extending from a more superficial site [497]. This assumption is supported by the rarity of published examples [494–497]. Deep soft tissue angiosarcomas [495–497] are said to occur throughout life, without predilection for one age group. The extremities and abdominal cavity are favored sites. In general, soft tissue angiosarcomas seem to have a propensity for high-grade histology. Epithelioid morphology is well documented in the group (Figure 22.19(a)) and may lead to an erroneous diagnosis of carcinoma or melanoma [495]. Some deep-seated examples appear to originate from medium or large-sized vessels [495,496].

(f) Angiosarcoma of the breast parenchyma

Over 200 cases of primary, non-iatrogenic angiosarcomas of the breast parenchyma have been reported in the literature [468,476–85]. These tumors have occurred in patients between the ages of 14 [485] and 85 [480] years. The mean age at presentation in a review of 87 cases by Chen and co-workers was 35 years [478]. The most common presentation is that of a painless, soft mass with bluish red or black discoloration of the overlying skin. The outcome, in general, has been poor with a mean interval to death of 22 months and a 3-year disease-free survival rate of only 14% given in Chen's review [478]. However, recent reports suggest survival rates may be substantially better for patients who have tumors with a uniformly well differentiated appearance [479,480,484]. While some authors have also suggested that tumor size [456,479] and the duration of clinical symptoms [456] may have prognostic significance, others have not found this to be the case [480,483,484].

Optimal management is generally considered to be complete surgical excision with a wide resection margin as tumors of this type typically invade well beyond their grossly apparent confines. This usually necessitates at least a simple mastectomy and may, in some cases with deeply situated neoplasms, require the removal of pectoral muscle as well [479]. Axillary lymph node removal is reserved for the rare case in which there is

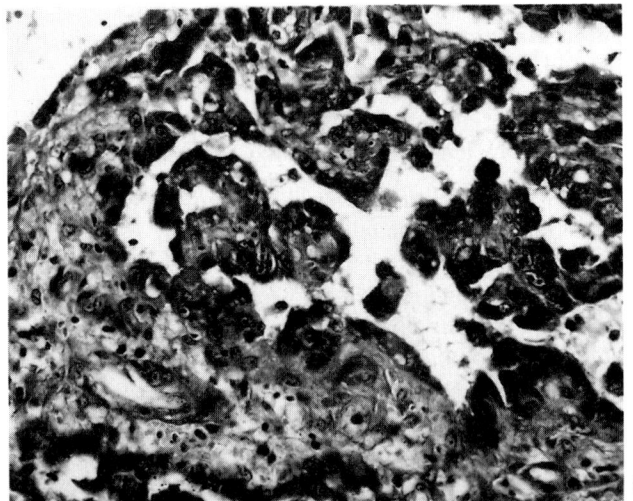

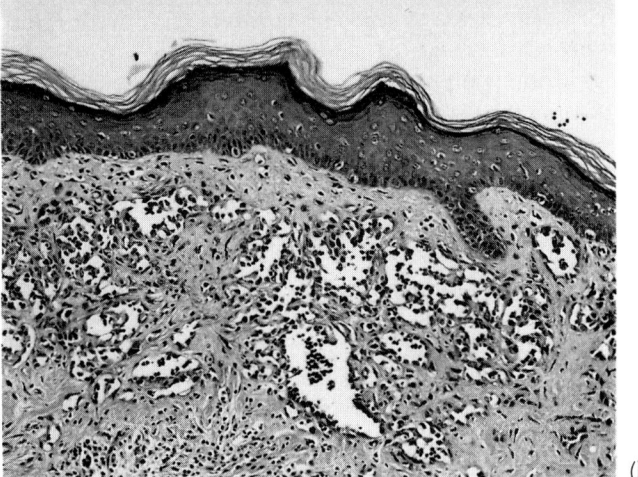

Figure 22.19 (a) Deep angiosarcoma. Note the prominent epithelioid morphology in this example. (b) Superficial angiosarcoma. Although atypia is not pronounced in this example, note the focal piled-up appearance of the endothelial cells. This lesion was multifocal, had deep extension, and contained areas with more pronounced atypia.

clinical evidence of metastatic involvement or when removal is necessary to provide an adequate resection margin. The role of adjunct therapy is not firmly established although it may have a beneficial effect in selected instances [484]. Contralateral breast involvement has been reported in up to 21% of cases [478]. This may be the result of either a separate primary or metastatic disease; the latter scenario is believed to be considerably more common. Frequent sites of metastases include the lungs, skin/subcutis, bones, liver and the central nervous system.

The differential diagnosis for primary angiosarcoma of the breast parenchyma includes a variety of hemangiomas (e.g. perilobular, venous) [488–491,493], angiomatosis [492], hemangiopericytoma [486] and lymphangioma [487]. Hemangiomas are the most common of these considerations; they tend to be small and are often incidental microscopic findings. We agree with the view of others [490] that vascular lesions of the breast should, in most instances, be removed in their entirety so that they may be thoroughly evaluated before a final diagnosis is rendered. This approach is necessary since angiosarcoma of the breast often contains areas with deceptively bland morphology.

(g) Foreign body-associated angiosarcoma

Infrequently, angiosarcoma has developed in association with foreign body material (e.g. Dacron vascular graft, shrapnel, bullet, surgical sponge, metallic orthopedic appliances). We are aware of 11 [562–566,572] published examples of this phenomenon. The tumors have manifested after a latency period of 3 to 63 years. Solid-state tumorigenesis [570,571] and foreign body–host chemical interactions [562,564,573] have been implicated as potential factors in the pathogenesis. The former is believed dependent on three variables:

- the configuration of the implant;
- a host response with development of a fibrous (pseudo)capsule;
- a latency period in which active remodeling of the intracapsular microenvironment occurs, isolated and unchecked by normal regulatory measures, resulting in the production of a malignant clone.

As with other angiosarcomas, the tumors are typically aggressive and lethal.

(h) Morphology of angiosarcoma

Angiosarcoma has a broad morphologic spectrum. At one extreme, the tumor may consist entirely of well developed hemangioma or lymphangioma-like vascular spaces (angiomatous or collagen dissection pattern) (Figure 22.19(b)), in which the only clues of malignancy are the interanastomosing and infiltrative nature of the process, the presence of mild nuclear hyperchromasia and an occasional crowding or piling up of the endothelium, sometimes forming small papillations. The opposite end of the spectrum includes both a spindle cell pattern reminiscent of fibrosarcoma or Kaposi's sarcoma and an 'undifferentiated' pattern which consists of plump epithelioid neoplastic cells with prominent nucleoli and diffuse sheet-like growth, suggestive of carcinoma or melanoma (Figure 22.19(b)). A high index of suspicion, knowledge of the clinical findings and thorough tumor sampling are essential to establish the correct diagnosis at these morphologic extremes. Since angiosarcomas frequently exhibit a diversity of patterns adequate sampling will often allow one to identify both vasoformative architecture and cytologically malignant features. Where the histologic grade has been shown to have prognostic significance, as in the breast, sampling is also critical to assure appropriate stratification of patients for consideration of adjuvant therapy [484].

When well developed vessels are not apparent, the presence of cytoplasmic vacuolization consistent with early lumen development and a red blood cell or hemosiderin-rich milieu may serve as important clues which point one in the direction of a vascular tumor. A reticulin stain can help highlight tube-like vascular growth which may be inapparent in hematoxylin and eosin stained sections.

Immunohistochemistry can prove invaluable when vasoformative architecture is minimal or absent. However, we strongly advise the use of a panel approach for the following reasons. First, the antibodies (e.g. anti-FVIIIrAg, anti-CD34 [QBEND/10, My10]) and lectin (*Ulex europaeus* agglutinin I, UEAI), most frequently utilized in the identification of endothelial cells react with different antigenic determinants and have different sensitivities and specificities [575,578,580,581,586,588]. As a result, these tests can prove complementary. For example, while anti-factor VIIIrAg has the greatest specificity for endothelium, poorly differentiated vascular tumors sometimes lack reactivity with this marker or only express it to a minor degree. These same neoplasms may continue to express CD34 antigen and bind with UEAI. Although the latter studies lack the specificity of anti-FVIIIrAg, positive results in the proper setting and, in the absence of other compelling immunohistochemical evidence to the contrary, can help confirm a histologic impression of angiosarcoma. Second, angiosarcomas, especially those with epithelioid morphology, are fully capable of reacting with antibodies directed against cytokeratin [495,553a,577,582,583,585] and B72.3 [535,553a], results commonly equated with epithelial differentiation. However, these neoplasms have been demonstrated to be negative for epithelial membrane antigen (EMA) [495,553a,577,582] and immunoreactivity for FVIIIrAg, CD34 and UEAI may be retained. Too narrow an immunoprofile in such cases could lead to an incorrect diagnosis of carcinoma and the undue dismissal of angiosarcoma from the differential diagnosis.

(i) Other

For a review of angiosarcoma arising in the liver [502, 505–526], spleen [527–531,531a], heart and great vessels [538,539,564], orbits [589], intestines [140], bones [139,218,219,498–501], central nervous system [533,537], serous membranes [555], lungs [550,551], kidneys [542,543], bladder [544], prostate [546, 554], seminal vesicles [534], female genital tract [545, 547], adrenal glands [504,536,553a] and thyroid gland [540,541,582], we refer the reader to the cited references.

Acknowledgements

The authors wish to thank Drs Javier Arias-Stella Jr, Franz Enzinger, Ernest Lack, Juan Rosai, Sharon Weiss and Mark Wick for graciously providing materials from their collections for illustrative purposes. We also thank Dr Norio Azumi for translating selected articles from the Japanese literature.

References

1. Stoler, M.H., Bonfiglio, T.A. and Steigbigel, R.T. (1983) An atypical subcutaneous infection associated with acquired immune deficiency syndrome. *Am. J. Clin. Pathol.*, 80, 714–18.
2. LeBoit, P.E., Berger, T.G., Egbert, B.M. et al. (1989) Bacillary angiomatosis. The histopathology and differential diagnosis of a pseudoneoplastic infection in patients with human immunodeficiency virus disease. *Am. J. Surg. Pathol.*, 13, 909–20.
3. Cockerell, C.J. and LeBoit, P.E. (1990) Bacillary angiomatosis: a newly characterized, pseudoneoplastic, infectious, cutaneous vascular disorder. *J. Am. Acad. Dermatol.*, 22, 501–12.
4. Relman, D.A., Loutit, J.S., Schmidt, T.M. et al. (1990) The agent of bacillary angiomatosis: an approach to the identification of uncultured pathogens. *New Engl. J. Med.*, 323, 1573–80.
5. Relman, D.A., Falkow, S., LeBoit, P.E. et al. (1991) The organism causing bacillary angiomatosis, peliosis hepatis, and fever and bacteremia in immunocompromised patients. *New Engl. J. Med.*, 324, 1514 (letter).
6. Reed, J.A., Brigati, D.J., Flynn, S.D. et al. (1992) Immunocytochemical identification of *Rochalimea henselae* in bacillary (epithelioid) angiomatosis, parenchymal bacillary peliosis, and persistent fever with bacteremia. *Am. J. Surg. Pathol.*, 16, 650–7.
7. English, C.K., Wear, D.J., Margileth, A.M. et al. (1988) Cat scratch disease: isolation and culture of the bacterial agent. *J. Am. Med. Ass.*, 259, 1347–52.
8. Brenner, D.J., Hollis, D.G., Moss, C.W. et al. (1991) Proposal of *Afipia* gen. nov., with *Afipia felis* sp. nov. (formerly the cat scratch disease bacillus), *Afipia clevelandensis* sp. nov. (formerly the Cleveland Clinic Foundation strain), *Afipia broomeae* sp. nov., and three unnamed genospecies. *J. Clin. Microbiol.*, 29, 2450–60.
9. Schwartzman, W.A. (1992) Infections due to *Rochalimaea*: the expanding clinical spectrum. *Clin. Infect. Dis.*, 15, 893–902.
10. Chan, J.K.C., Lewin, K.J., Lombard, C.M. et al. (1991) Histopathology of bacillary angiomatosis of lymph node. *Am. J. Surg. Pathol.*, 15, 430–7.
11. Steeper, T.A., Rosenstein, H., Weiser, J. et al. (1992) Bacillary epithelioid angiomatosis involving the liver, spleen, and skin in an AIDS patient with concurrent Kaposi's sarcoma. *Am. J. Clin. Pathol.*, 97, 713–18.
12. Leong, S.S., Cazen, R.A., Yu, G.S.M. et al. (1992) Abdominal visceral peliosis associated with bacillary angiomatosis: Ultrastructural evidence of endothelial destruction by bacilli. *Arch. Pathol. Lab. Med.*, 116, 866–71.
13. Cockerell, C.J., Bergstresser, P.R., Myrie-Williams, C. et al. (1990) Bacillary epithelioid angiomatosis occurring in an immunocompetent individual. *Arch. Dermatol.*, 126, 787–90.
14. Nappi, O. and Wick, M.R. (1986) Disseminated lobular capillary hemangioma (pyogenic granuloma): a clinicopathologic study of two cases. *Am. J. Dermatopathol.*, 8, 379–85.
15. Howe, C. (1943) Carrion's disease: immunologic studies. *Arch. Intern. Med.*, 72, 147–67.
16. Recavarren, S. and Lumbreras, H. (1986) Pathogenesis of the verruga in Carrion disease. *Am. J. Pathol.*, 10, 595–610.
17. Garcia, F.U., Wojta, J., Broadley, K.N. et al. (1990) *Bartonella bacilliformis* stimulates endothelial cells in vitro and is angiogenic in vivo. *Am. J. Pathol.*, 136, 1125–35.
18. O'Connor, S.P., Dorsch, M., Steigerwalt, A.G. et al. (1991) 16S rRNA sequences of *Bartonella bacilliformis* and cat scratch disease bacillus reveal phylogenetic relationships with the alpha-2 subgroup of the class *Protobacteria*. *J. Clin. Microbiol.*, 29, 2144–50.
19. Arias-Stella, J., Lieberman, P.H., Erlandson, R.A. et al. (1986) Histology, immunohistochemistry, and ultrastructure of the verruga in Carrion's disease. *Am. J. Surg. Pathol.*, 10, 595–610.
20. Arias-Stella, J., Lieberman, P.H., Garcia-Caceres, U. et al. (1987) Verruga peruana mimicking malignant neoplasms. *Am. J. Dermatopathol.*, 9, 279–91.
21. Masson, P. (1923) Hémangioendotheliome végétant intravasculaire. *Bull. Soc. Anat. Paris*, 93, 517–23.
22. Hashimoto, H., Daimaru, Y. and Enjoji, M. (1983) Intravascular papillary endothelial hyperplasia: a clinicopathologic study of 91 cases. *Am. J. Dermatopathol.*, 5, 539–46.
23. Salyer, W.R. and Salyer, D.C. (1975) Intravascular angiomatosis: development and distinction from angiosarcoma. *Cancer*, 36, 995–1101.
24. Kuo, T., Sayers, P.M. and Rosai, J. (1976) Masson's 'vegetant intravascular hemangioendothelioma': a lesion often mistaken for angiosarcoma. Study of seventeen cases located in the skin and soft tissues. *Cancer*, 38, 1227–36.
25. Clearkin, K.P. and Enzinger, F.M. (1976) Intravascular papillary endothelial hyperplasia. *Arch. Pathol. Lab. Med.*, 100, 441–4.
26. Stern, Y., Braslavsky, D., Segal, K. et al. (1991) Intravascular papillary endothelial hyperplasia in the maxillary sinus. A benign lesion that may be mistaken for angiosarcoma. *Arch. Otolaryngol. Head Neck Surg.*, 117, 1182–84.
27. Amerigo, J. and Berry, C.L. (1980) Intravascular papillary endothelial hyperplasia in the skin and subcutaneous tissue. *Virchows Archiv. A Pathol. Anat. Histopathol.*, 387, 81–90.
28. Pins, M.R., Rosenthal, D.I., Springfield, D.S. et al. (1993) Florid extravascular papillary endothelial hyperplasia (Masson's pseudoangiosarcoma) presenting as a soft-tissue sarcoma. *Arch. Pathol. Lab. Med.*, 117, 259–63.
29. Patchefsky, A.S. and Enzinger, F.M. (1981) Intravascular fasciitis. A report of 17 cases. *Am. J. Surg. Pathol.*, 5, 29–32.
30. Kahn, M.A., Weathers, D.R. and Johnson, D.M. (1987) Intravascular fasciitis: a case report on an intraoral location. *J. Oral. Pathol.*, 16, 303–6.
31. Freedman, P.D. and Lumerman, H. (1986) Intravascular fasciitis: a report of two cases and review of the literature. *Oral. Surg. Oral. Med. Oral. Pathol.*, 62, 549–54.
32. Pfleger, L. and Tappeiner, J. (1959) Zu Kenntnis der systemisierten endotheliomatose der cutanen Blutgefasse (reticuloendotheliomiose?). *Hautarzt*, 10, 359–63.
33. Person, J.R. (1977) Systemic angioendotheliomatosis: a possible disorder of a circulating angiogenic factor. *Br. J. Dermatol.*, 96, 329–31.
34. Wick, M.R. and Rocamora, A. (1988) Reactive and malignant 'angioendotheliomatosis': a discriminant pathologic study. *J. Cutan. Pathol.*, 15, 260–71.
35. Dolman, C.L., Sweeney, V.P. and Magil, A. (1979) Neoplastic angioendotheliomatosis. The case of the missed primary. *Arch. Neurol.*, 36, 5–7.
36. Ansell, J., Bhawan, J., Cohen, S. et al. (1982) Histiocytic lymphoma and angioendotheliomatosis. One disease or two? *Cancer*, 50, 1506–12.
37. Bhawan, J., Wolff, S.M., Ucci, A.O. et al. (1985) Malignant lymphoma and malignant angioendotheliomatosis: one disease. *Cancer*, 55, 570–76.
38. Wrotnowski, V., Mills, S.E. and Cooper, P.H. (1985) Malignant angioendotheliomatosis: an angiotropic lymphoma? *Am. J. Clin. Pathol.*, 83, 244–8.
39. Sheibani, K., Battifora, H., Winberg, C.D. et al. (1986) Further evidence that 'malignant angioendotheliomatosis' is an angiotropic large cell lymphoma. *New Engl. J. Med.*, 314, 943–8.
40. Bhawan, J. (1987) Angioendotheliomatosis proliferans systemisata: an angiotropic neoplasm of lymphoid origin. *Semin. Diagn. Pathol.*, 4, 18–27.
41. Ferry, J.A., Harris, N.L., Picker, L.J. et al. (1988) Intravascular lymphomatosis (malignant angioendotheliomatosis): a B-cell neoplasm expressing surface homing receptors. *Mod. Pathol.*, 1, 444–52.
42. Ruiter, D. and Mandema, E. (1964) New cutaneous syndrome in subacute bacterial endocarditis. *Arch. Intern. Med.*, 113, 175–82.
43. Scott, P.W.B., Silvers, D.N. and Helwig, E.B. (1975) Proliferating angioendotheliomatosis. *Arch. Pathol.*, 99, 323–6.
44. Pasyk, K. and Depowski, M. (1978) Proliferating systematized angioendotheliomatosis of a 5-month-old infant. *Arch. Dermatol.*, 114, 1512–5.
45. Martin, S., Pitcher, D., Tschen, J. et al. (1980) Reactive angioendotheliomatosis. *J. Am. Acad. Dermatol.*, 2, 117–23.
46. Eisert, J. (1980) Skin manifestations of subacute bacterial endocarditis mimicking Tappeiner's angioendotheliomatosis. *Cutis*, 25, 394–5.
47. Kimura, T., Yoshimura, S. and Ishikawa, E. (1948) Abnormal granuloma with proliferation of lymphoid tissue. *Nippon Byori Gakkai Kaishi*, 37, 179–80.
48. Kimm, H.T. and Szeto, C. (1937) Eosinophilic hyperplastic lymphogranuloma, comparison with Mikulicz's disease. *Proc. Chin. Med. Soc.*, 329. (Cited by Kung, I.T.M. and Chan, J.K.C. (1988), in *Am. J. Surg. Pathol.*, 12, 804 (letter) and by Allen, P.W., Ramakrishna, B. and MacCormack, L.B. (1992), in *Pathol. Annu.*, 27, 51–87.)
49. Chan, J.K.C., Hui, P.K., Ng, C.S. et al. (1989) Epithelioid hemangioma (angiolymphoid hyperplasia with eosinophilia) and Kimura's disease in Chinese. *Histopathology*, 15, 557–74.
50. Googe, P.B., Harris, N.L. and Mihm, M.C. (1987) Kimura's disease and angiolymphoid hyperplasia with eosinophils: two distinct histopathological entities. *J. Cutan. Pathol.*, 14, 263–71.
51. Urabe, A., Tsuneyoshi, M. and Enjoji, M. (1987) Epithelioid hemangioma versus Kimura's disease: a comparative clinicopathologic study. *Am. J. Surg. Pathol.*, 11, 758–66.
52. Kung, I.T.M., Gibson, J.B. and Bannatyne, P.M. (1984) Kimura's disease: a clinicopathological study of 21 cases and its distinction from

angiolymphoid hyperplasia with eosinophilia. *Pathology*, **16**, 39–44.
53. Matsumoto, K., Katayama, H. and Hatano, M. (1988) Minimal-change nephrotic syndrome associated with subcutaneous lymphoid granuloma (Kimura's disease). *Nephron*, **49**, 251–4.
54. Qunibi, W.Y., Al-Sibai, M.B. and Akhtar, M. (1988) Mesangioproliferative glomerulonephritis associated with Kimura's disease. *Clin. Nephrol.*, **30**, 111–4.
55. Yamada, A., Mitsuhashi, K., Miyakawa, Y. et al. (1982) Membranous glomerulonephritis associated with eosinophilic folliculitis of the skin (Kimura's disease): report of a case and review of the literature. *Clin. Nephrol.*, **18**, 211–15.
56. Kuo, T.-T., Shih, L.-Y. and Chan, H.-L. (1988) Kimura's disease. Involvement of regional lymph nodes and distinction from angiolymphoid hyperplasia with eosinophilia. *Am. J. Surg. Pathol.*, **12**, 843–54.
57. Hui, P.K., Chan, J.K.C., Ng, C.S. et al. (1989) Lymphadenopathy of Kimura's disease. *Am. J. Surg. Pathol.*, **13**, 177–86.
58. Wells, G.C. and Whimster, I.W. (1969) Subcutaneous angiolymphoid hyperplasia with eosinophilia. *Br. J. Dermatol.*, **81**, 1–15.
59. Kandil, E. (1970) Dermal angiolymphoid hyperplasia with eosinophilia versus pseudopyogenic granuloma. *Br. J. Dermatol.*, **83**, 405–8.
60. Peterson, W.C., Fusaro, R.M. and Goltz, R.W. (1964) Atypical pyogenic granuloma. A case of benign hemangioendotheliomatosis. *Arch. Dermatol.*, **90**, 197–201.
61. Wilson-Jones, E. and Bleehen, S.S. (1969) Inflammatory angiomatous nodules with abnormal blood vessels occurring about the ears and scalp (pseudo or atypical pyogenic granuloma). *Br. J. Dermatol.*, **81**, 804–16.
62. Rosai, J., Gold, J. and Landy, R. (1979) The histiocytoid hemangiomas: a unifying concept embracing several previously described entities of skin, soft tissue, large vessels, bone, and heart. *Hum. Pathol.*, **10**, 707–30.
63. Luthringer, D.J., Virmani, R., Weiss, S.W. et al. (1990) A distinctive cardiovascular lesion resembling histiocytoid/epithelioid hemangioma, evidence suggesting mesothelial participation. *Am. J. Surg. Pathol.*, **14**, 993–1000.
64. Enzinger, F.M. and Weiss, S.W. (1988) Benign tumors and tumorlike lesions of blood vessels, in *Soft Tissue Tumors*, 2nd edn, C.V. Mosby, Philadelphia, pp. 489–532.
65. Rosai, J. (1982) Angiolymphoid hyperplasia with eosinophilia of the skin. Its nosological position in the spectrum of histiocytoid hemangioma. *Am. J. Dermatopathol.*, **4**, 175–84.
66. Rosai, J. and Ackerman, L.R. (1974) Intravenous atypical vascular proliferation. *Arch. Dermatol.*, **109**, 714–17.
67. Allen, P.W., Ramakrishna, B. and MacCormack, L.B. (1992) The histiocytoid hemangiomas and other controversies. *Pathol. Annu.*, **27**, 51–87.
68. Tsanh, W.Y.W. and Chan, J.K.C. (1993) The family of epithelioid vascular tumors. *Histol. Histopath.*, **8**, 187–212.
69. Olsen, T.G. and Helwig, E.B. (1985) Angiolymphoid hyperplasia with eosinophilia: a clinicopathologic study of 116 patients. *J. Am. Acad. Dermatol.*, **12**, 781–96.
70. Reed, R.J. and Terezakis, N. (1972) Subcutanous angioblastic lymphoid hyperplasia with eosinophilia (Kimura's disease). *Cancer*, **29**, 489–97.
71. Angervall, L., Kindblom, L.G., Karlsson, K. et al. (1985) Atypical hemangioendothelioma of venous origin: a clinicopathologic, angiographic, immunohistochemical, and ultrastructural study of two endothelial tumors within the concept of histiocytoid hemangioma. *Am. J. Surg. Pathol.*, **9**, 504–16.
72. Castro, C. and Winkelmann, R.K. (1974) Angiolymphoid hyperplasia with eosinophilia in the skin. *Cancer*, **34**, 1696–1705.
73. Grimwood, R., Swinehart, J.M. and Aeling, J.L. (1979) Angiolymphoid hyperplasia with eosinophilia. *Arch. Dermatol.*, **115**, 205–7.
74. Fetsch, J.F. and Weiss, S.W. (1991) Observations concerning the pathogenesis of epithelioid hemangioma (angiolymphoid hyperplasia). *Mod. Pathol.*, **4**, 449–55.
75. Weiss, S.W. (1989) Vascular tumors: a deductive approach to diagnosis. *Surg. Pathol.*, **2**, 185–201.
76. Esterly, N.B. (1987) Cutaneous hemangiomas, vascular stains, and associated syndromes. *Curr. Prob. Pediatr.*, **17**, 7–69.
77. Coffin, C.M. and Dehner, L.P. (1993) Vascular tumors in children and adolescents: A clinicopathologic study of 228 tumors in 222 patients. *Pathol. Annu.*, **1**, 97–120.
78. Johnson, W.C. (1976) Pathology of cutaneous vascular tumors. *Int. J. Dermatol.*, **15**, 239–70.
79. Tsang, W.Y.W., Chan, J.K.C. and Fletcher, C.D.M. (1991) Recently characterized vascular tumors of the skin and soft tissues. *Histopathology*, **19**, 489–501.
80. Hunt, S.J. and Santa Cruz, D.J. (1992) Acquired benign-and 'borderline' vascular lesions. *Dermatol. Clin.*, **10**, 97–115.
81. Poncet, M.M. and Dor. (1897) De la botyromycose humaine. *Rev. Chir. (Paris)*, **18**, 996–7.
82. Hartzell, M.B. (1904) Granuloma pyogenicum (botryomycosis of French authors). *J. Cutan. Dis.*, **22**, 520–5.
83. Mills, S.E., Cooper, P.H. and Fechner, R.E. (1980) Lobular capillary hemangioma: the underlying lesion of pyogenic granuloma: a study of 73 cases from the oral and nasal mucus membranes. *Am. J. Surg. Pathol.*, **4**, 471–9.
84. Cooper, P.H. and Mills, S.E. (1982) Subcutaneous granuloma pyogenicum – lobular capillary hemangioma. *Arch. Dermatol.*, **118**, 30–33.
85. Michelson, H.E. (1925) Granuloma pyogenicum: a clinical and histologic review of twenty nine cases. *Arch. Dermatol.*, **12**, 495–505.
86. Leyden, J.J. and Master, G.H. (1979) Oral cavity pyogenic granuloma. *Arch. Dermatol.*, **108**, 226–8.
87. Kerr, D.A. (1951) Granuloma pyogenicum. *Oral Surg.*, **4**, 158–76.
88. McDonald, R.H. (1956) Granuloma gravidarum: pregnancy tumor of the gingiva. *Am. J. Obstet. Gynecol.*, **72**, 1132–6.
89. Nichols, G.E., Gaffey, M.J., Mills, S.E. et al. (1992) Lobular capillary hemangioma: an immunohistochemical study including steroid hormone receptor status. *Am. J. Clin. Pathol.*, **97**, 770–5.
90. Taira, J.W., Hill, T.L. and Everett, M.A. (1992) Lobular capillary hemangioma (pyogenic granuloma) with satellitosis. *J. Am. Acad. Dermatol.*, **27**, 197–300.
91. Coskey, R.J. and Mehregan, A.H. (1967) Granuloma pyogenicum with multiple satellite recurrences. *Arch. Dermatol.*, **96**, 71–73.
92. Amerigo, J., Gonzalez-Campora, R., Galera, H. et al. (1983) Recurrent pyogenic granuloma with multiple satellites: Clinicopathological and ultrastructural study. *Dermatologica*, **166**, 117–21.
93. Warner, J. and Wilson-Jones, E. (1968) Pyogenic granuloma recurring with multiple satellites: a report of 11 cases. *Br. J. Dermatol.*, **80**, 218–27.
94. Evans, C.D. and Warin, R.P. (1957) Pyogenic granuloma with local recurrences. *Br. J. Dermatol.*, **69**, 106.
95. Foldvari, F. (1935) Post-traumatic angioma. *Br. J. Dermatol.*, **47**, 463–7.
96. Zaynoun, S.T., Juljulian, H.H. and Kurban, A.K. (1974) Pyogenic granuloma with multiple satellites. *Arch. Dermatol.*, **109**, 689–91.
97. Wilson, B.B., Greer, K.E. and Cooper, P.H. (1989) Eruptive disseminated lobular capillary hemangioma (pyogenic granuloma). *J. Am. Acad. Dermatol.*, **21**, 391–4.
98. Frain-Bell, W. (1958) Multiple pyogenic granulomata. *Br. J. Dermatol.*, **70**, 428–9.
99. Juhlin, L., Sven-Olof, H., Ponten, J. et al. (1970) Disseminated granuloma pyogenicum. *Acta Derm. Venereol. (Stockh.)*, **50**, 134–6.
100. Strohal, R., Gillitzer, R., Zonzits, E. et al. (1991) Localized vs generalized pyogenic granuloma. *Arch. Dermatol.*, **127**, 856–61.
101. Swerlick, R.A. and Cooper, P.H. (1983) Pyogenic granuloma (lobular capillary hemangioma) within port-wine stains. *J. Am. Acad. Dermatol.*, **8**, 627–30.
102. Pembroke, A.C., Grice, K., Levantine, A.V. et al. (1978) Eruptive angiomata in malignant disease. *Clin. Expl Dermatol.*, **3**, 147–56.
103. Exner, J.H., Dahod, S. and Pochi, P.E. (1983) Pyogenic granuloma-like acne lesions during isotretinoin therapy. *Arch. Dermatol.*, **119**, 808–11.
104. Valentic, J.P., Barr, R.J. and Weinstein, G.D. (1983) Inflammatory neovascular nodules associated with oral isotretinoin treatment of severe acne. *Arch. Dermatol.*, **119**, 871–2.
105. Cooper, P.H., McAllister, H.A. and Helwig, E.B. (1979) Intravenous pyogenic granuloma: a study of 18 cases. *Am. J. Surg. Pathol.*, **3**, 221–8.
106. Ulbright, T.M. and Santa Cruz, D.J. (1980) Intravenous pyogenic granuloma. *Cancer*, **45**, 1646–52.
107. Lever, W.F. and Schaumberg-Lever, G. (1983) Vascular tumors, in *Histopathology of the Skin*, 6th edn, J.B. Lippincott, Philadelphia, pp. 623–651.
108. Holmdahl, K. (1955) Cutaneous hemangiomas in premature and mature infants. *Acta Paediatr. Scand.*, **44**, 370–9.
109. Amir, J., Metzker, A., Krikler, R. et al. (1986) Strawberry hemangioma in preterm infants. *Pediatr. Dermatol.*, **3**, 331–2.
110. Bowers, R.E., Graham, E.A. and Tomlinson, K.M. (1960) The natural history of the strawberry nevus. *Arch. Dermatol.*, **82**, 667–80.
111. Stout, A.P. (1943) Hemangio-endothelioma; a tumor of blood vessels featuring vascular endothelial cells. *Ann. Surg.*, **118**, 445–64.
112. Pasky, K.A., Grabb, W.C. and Cherry, G.W. (1983) Crystalloid inclusions in endothelial cells of cellular and capillary hemangiomas: a possible sign of immaturity. *Arch. Dermatol.*, **119**, 134–7.
113. Lister, W.A. (1938) The natural history of strawberry nevus. *Lancet*, **1**, 1429–34.
114. Sachatello, C.R. and McSwain, B. (1968) Regression of cutaneous capillary hemangioma. *Am. J. Surg.*, **116**, 113–4.
115. Gonzalez-Crussi, F. and Reyes-Mugica, M. (1991) Cellular hemangiomas of infancy ('hemangioendotheliomas'). Light microscopic, immunohistochemical, and ultrastructural observations. *Am. J. Surg. Pathol.*, **15**, 769–78.
116. Watson, W.L. (1939) Blood and lymph vessel tumors in children. *J. Pediatr.*, **15**, 401–7.
117. Kasabach, H.H. and Merritt, K.K. (1940) Capillary hemangioma with extensive purpura: Report of a case. *Am. J. Dis. Child.*, **59**, 1063–70.
118. Seo, W., Kishimoto, M., Minato, T. et al. (1993) Submandibular hemangioma as the initial manifestation of Kasabach-Merritt syndrome. *Int. J. Pediatr. Otolaryngol.*, **25**, 269–76.
119. Karabocuoglu, M., Balsarer, N., Aydogan, •• et al. (1992) Development of Kasabach-Merritt syndrome following needle aspiration of a

hemangioma. *Pediatr. Emerg. Care*, 8, 218–20.
120. Currie, B.G., Schell, D. and Bowring, A.C. (1991) Giant hemangioma of the arm associated with cardiac failure and the Kasabach-Merritt syndrome in a neonate. *J. Pediatr. Surg.*, 26, 734–7.
121. El-Dessouky, M., Azmy, A.F., Raine, P.A.M. et al. (1988) Kasabach-Merritt syndrome. *J. Pediatr. Surg.*, 23, 109–11.
122. Henley, J.D., Danielson, C.F.M., Rothenberger, S.S. et al. (1993) Kasabach-Merritt syndrome with profound platelet support. *Am. J. Clin. Pathol.*, 99, 628–30.
123. de Prost, Y., Teillac, D., Bodemer, C. et al. (1991) Successful treatment of Kasabach-Merritt syndrome with pentoxifylline. *J. Am. Acad. Dermatol.*, 25, 854–5.
124. Glowacki, J. and Mulliken, J.B. (1982) Mast cells in hemangiomas and vascular malformations. *Pediatrics*, 70, 48–51.
125. Mulliken, J.B. and Glowacki, J. (1982) Hemangiomas and vascular malformations in infants and children: a classification based on endothelial characteristics. *Plast. Reconstr. Surg.*, 70, 48–51.
126. Folkman, J. (1989) Successful treatment of angiogenic disease. *New Engl. J. Med.*, 320, 1211–12.
127. White, C.W., Sondhein, H.M., Crouch, E.C. et al. (1989) Treatment of pulmonary hemangiomatosis with recombinant interferon ALFA-2a. *New Engl. J. Med.*, 320, 1197–200.
128. Enjolras, O., Riche, M.C., Merland, J.J. et al. (1990) Management of alarming hemangiomas of infancy: a review of 25 cases. *Pediatrics*, 85, 491–8.
129. Apfelberg, D.B., Lane, B. and Marx, M.P. (1991) Combined (team) approach to hemangioma management: arteriography with superselective embolization plus YAG laser/sapphire tip resection. *Plast. Reconstr. Surg.*, 88, 71–82.
130. Ezekowitz, R.A., Mulliken, J.B. and Folkman, J. (1992) Interferon alfa-2a therapy for life-threatening hemangiomas of infancy. *New Engl. J. Med.*, 326, 1456–63.
131. Osburn, K., Schosser, R.H. and Everett, M.A. (1987) Congenital pigmented and vascular lesions in newborn infants. *J. Am. Acad. Dermatol.*, 16, 788–92.
132. Margileth, A.M. and Museles, M. (1965) Current concepts in diagnosis and management of congenital cutaneous hemangiomas. *Pediatrics*, 36, 410–16.
133. Pratt, A.G. (1953) Birthmarks in infants. *Arch. Derm. Syph.*, 67, 302–5.
134. Tan, K.L. (1972) Nevus flammeus of the nape, glabella, and eyelids. A clinical study of frequency, racial distribution, and association with congenital anomalies. *Clin. Pediatr.*, 11, 112–18.
135. Barsky, S.H., Rosen, S., Geer, D.E. et al. (1980) The nature and evolution of port wine stains: a computer-assisted study. *J. Invest. Dermatol.*, 74, 154–7.
136. Smoller, B.R. and Rosen, S. (1986) Port wine stains. A disease of altered neural modulation of blood vessels. *Arch. Dermatol.*, 122, 177–9.
137. Finley, J.L., Noe, J.M., Arndt, K.A. et al. (1984) Port wine stains. Morphologic variations and developmental lesions. *Arch. Dermatol.*, 120, 1453–5.
138. Watson, W.L. and McCarthy, W.P. (1940) Blood and lymph vessel tumors: 1056 cases. *Surg. Gynecol. Obstet.*, 71, 569–88.
139. Wold, L.E., Swee, R.G. and Sim, F.H. (1985) Vascular lesions of bone. *Pathol. Annu.*, 20, 101–37.
140. Gentry, R.W., Dockerty, M.B. and Clagett, O.T. (1949) Vascular malformations and vascular tumors of the gastrointestinal tract. *Int. Abstr. Surg.*, 88, 281–322.
141. Galliani, C.A., Beatty, J.F. and Grosfeld, J.L. (1992) Cavernous hemangioma of the lung in an infant. *Pediatr. Pathol.*, 12, 105–11.
142. Calonje, E. and Fletcher, C.D.M. (1991) Sinusoidal hemangioma. A distinctive benign vascular neoplasm within the group of cavernous hemangiomas. *Am. J. Surg. Pathol.*, 15, 1130–5.
143. Weiss, S.W. (1988) Pedal hemangioma (venous malformation) occurring in Turner's syndrome: an additional manifestation of the syndrome. *Hum. Pathol.*, 19, 1015–18.
144. Smith, D.W. (1982) *Recognizable Patterns of Human Malformations*, 3rd edn, W.B. Saunders, Philadelphia.
145. Burns, A.J., Kaplan, L.C. and Mulliken, J.B. (1991) Is there an association between hemangiomas and syndromes with dysmorphic features? *Pediatrics*, 88, 1257–67.
146. Klippel, M. and Trenaunay, P. (1900) Du naevus variqueux ostéo-hypertrophique. *Arch. Gén. Méd. (Paris)*, 185, 641–72.
147. Parkes Weber, F. (1907) Angioma formation in connection with hypertrophy of limbs and hemihypertrophy. *Br. J. Dermatol.*, 19, 231–5.
148. Lindenauer, S.M. (1971) Congenital arteriovenous fistula and the Klippel–Trenaunay syndrome. *Ann. Surg.*, 174, 248–63.
149. Stephen, M.J., Hall, B.D., Smith, D.W. et al. (1975) Macrocephaly in association with unusual cutaneous angiomatosis. *J. Pediatr.*, 87, 353–9.
150. Umansky, A.L. (1946) Dyschondroplasia with hemangiomata (Maffucci's syndrome). Report of a case with mild osseous manifestations. *Bull. Hosp. Joint. Dis.*, 7, 59–68.
151. Andren, J.-F., Elner, A. and Hogeman, K.-E. (1963) Maffucci's syndrome. Report of four cases. *Acta Chir. Scand.*, 126, 397–405.

152. Anderson, I.F. (1965) Maffucci's syndrome. Report of a case and review of the literature. *S. Afr. Med. J.*, 39, 1066–70.
153. Mullins, J.F. and Livingood, C.S. (1951) Maffucci's syndrome (dyschondroplasia with hemangiomas): a case with early osseous changes. *Arch. Dermatol.*, 63, 478–82.
154. Bean, W.B. (1955) Dyschondroplasia and hemangiomata (Maffucci's syndrome). *Arch. Intern. Med.*, 95, 767–78.
155. Bean, W.B. (1958) Dyschondroplasia and hemangiomata (Maffucci's syndrome) II. *Arch. Intern. Med.*, 102, 544–50.
156. Lewis, R.J. and Ketcham, A. (1973) Maffucci's syndrome: Functional and neoplastic significance. *J. Bone Joint Surg.*, 55A, 1465–79.
157. Berlin, R. (1965) Maffucci's syndrome. Dyschondroplasia with vascular hamartomas. *Acta Med. Scand.*, 177, 299–307.
158. Johnson, T.E., Nasr, A.M., Nalbandian, R.M. et al. (1990) Enchondromatosis and hemangioma (Maffucci's syndrome) with orbital involvement. *Am. J. Ophthalmol.*, 110, 153–9.
159. Kuzma, J.F. and King, J.M. (1948) Dyschondroplasia with hemangiomatosis (Maffucci's syndrome) and teratoid tumor of the ovary. *Arch. Pathol.*, 46, 74–82.
160. Howard, F.M. and Lee, R.E. (1971) The hand in Maffucci's syndrome. *Arch. Surg.*, 103, 752–6.
161. Fanburg, J.C., Meis, J.M. and Rosenberg, A.E. (1993) Maffucci's syndrome: multiple enchondromas and spindle cell hemangioendotheliomas. *Mod. Pathol.*, 6, 6A.
162. Lawson, J.P. and Scott, G. (1990) Case report 602. *Skel. Radiol.*, 19, 158–62.
163. Sakurane, H.F., Sugai, T. and Saito, T. (1967) The association of the blue rubber bleb nevus and Maffucci's syndrome. *Arch. Dermatol.*, 95, 28–36.
164. Fine, R.M., Derbes, V.J. and Clark, W.H. (1961) Blue rubber bleb nevus. *Arch. Dermatol.*, 84, 144–7.
165. Berlyn, G.M. and Berlyne, N. (1960) Anaemia due to 'blue-rubber-bleb' naevus disease. *Lancet*, 2, 1275–7.
166. Kumakiri, M., Fukaya, T. and Miura, Y. (1981) Blue rubber bleb nevus syndrome with Masson's vegetant intravascular hemangioendothelioma. *J. Cutan. Pathol.*, 8, 365–73.
167. Fretzin, D.F. and Potter, B. (1965) Blue rubber bleb nevus. *Arch. Intern. Med.*, 116, 924–9.
168. Rice, J.S. and Fischer, D.S. (1962) Blue rubber bleb nevus syndrome. *Arch. Dermatol.*, 86, 503–11.
169. Girard, C., Graham, J.H. and Johnson, W.C. (1974) Arteriovenous hemangioma (arteriovenous shunt): a clinicopathologic and histochemical study. *J. Cutan. Pathol.*, 1, 73–87.
170. Carapeto, F.J., Garcia-Perez, A. and Winkelmann, R.K. (1977) Acral arteriovenous tumor. *Acta Derm. Venereol. (Stockh.)*, 57, 155–8.
171. Connelly, M.G. and Winkelmann, R.K. (1985) Acral arteriovenous tumor: a clinicopathologic review. *Am. J. Surg. Pathol.*, 9, 15–21.
172. Reid, M.R. (1925) Studies on abnormal arteriovenous communications, acquired and congenital. I. Report of a series of cases. *Arch. Surg.*, 10, 601–38.
173. Reid, M.R. (1925) Abnormal arteriovenous communications, acquired and congenital. II. The origin and nature of arteriovenous aneurysms, cirsoid aneurysms, and simple angiomas. *Arch. Surg.*, 10, 996–1009.
174. Pemberton, J.D.J. and Saint, J.H. (1928) Congenital arteriovenous communications. *Surg. Gynecol. Obstet.*, 46, 471–83.
175. Seeger, S.J. (1938) Congenital arteriovenous anastomoses. *Surgery*, 3, 264–305.
176. Szilagyi, D.E., Elliot, J.P., DeRusso, F.J. et al. (1965) Peripheral congenital arteriovenous fistulas. *Surgery*, 57, 61–81.
177. Lawton, R.L., Tidrick, R.T. and Brintall, E.S. (1975) A clinico-pathologic study of multiple congenital arteriovenous fistulae in the lower extremity. *Angiology*, 8, 161–9.
178. Zelch, M.G. and Geisinger, M.A. (1990) Arteriography of the extremities, in *Radiology. Diagnosis – Imaging – Intervention*, vol. 2, (eds J.M. Taveras, J.T. Ferrucci and E. Buonocore), Lippincott, St Louis. pp. 1–16.
179. Beham, A. and Fletcher, C.D.M. (1991) Intramuscular angioma: a clinicopathological analysis of 74 cases. *Histopathology*, 18, 53–59.
180. Fergusson, I.L.C. (1972) Haemangiomata of skeletal muscle. *Br. J. Surg.*, 59, 634–7.
181. Allen, P.W. and Enzinger, F.M. (1972) Hemangiomas of skeletal muscle: an analysis of 89 cases. *Cancer*, 29, 8–23.
182. Shallow, T.A., Eger, S.A. and Wagner, F.B. (1944) Primary hemangiomatous tumors of skeletal muscle. *Ann. Surg.*, 119, 700–40.
183. Gonzales-Crussi, F., Enneking, W.F. and Arean, V.M. (1966) Infiltrating angiolipoma. *J. Bone Joint Surg.*, 48A, 1111–24.
184. Stimpson, N. (1971) Infiltrating angiolipomata of skeletal muscle. *Br. J. Surg.*, 58, 464–6.
185. Lin, J.J. and Lin, F. (1974) Two entities in angiolipoma. *Cancer*, 34, 720–7.
186. Austin, R.M., Mack, G.R., Townsend, C.M. et al. (1980) Infiltrating (intramuscular) lipomas and angiolipomas. *Arch. Surg.*, 115, 281–4.
187. Niechaje, I.A. and Sternby, N.H. (1983) Diagnostic accuracy and pathology of vascular tumors and tumor-like lesions. *Chir. Plastica*, 7, 153–61.
187a. Madewell, J.E. and Sweet, D.E. (1988) Tumors and tumor-like lesions in

188. Jenkins, H.P. and Delaney, L.A. (1932) Benign angiomatous tumors of skeletal muscle. *Surg. Gynecol. Obstet.*, **55**, 464–80.
189. Light, R.A. (1943) Venous hemangioma of skeletal muscle. *Ann. Surg.*, **118**, 465–8.
190. Gunge, M. and Yamamoto, H. (1987) An immunohistochemical and electron microscopic study of a central venous hemangioma of the mandible. *Arch. Otorhinolaryngol.*, **244**, 30–35.
191. Horimoto, H., Sasaki, M., Kuroda, K. et al. (1990) [A case of venous hemangioma in mediastinum.] *Kyobu Geka*, **43**, 1000–3.
192. Krner, K. and Fruensgaard, S. (1989) Synovial venous hemangioma of the knee joint. *Arch. Orthop. Trauma Surg.*, **108**, 253–4.
193. Jones, W.P., Keller, F.S., Odrezin, G.T. et al. (1987) Venous hemangioma of the gallbladder. *Gastrointest. Radiol.*, **12**, 319–21.
194. Helen, P., Mattila, J., Suonpaa, M. et al. (1986) Bleeding of a venous hemangioma inside the filum terminale. *Ann. Clin. Res.*, **18** (suppl. 47), 47–50.
195. Flores, J.T. and Apfelberg, D.B. (1983) Regarding venous or cavernous hemangioma [letter]. *J. Dermatol. Surg. Oncol.*, **9**, 424.
196. Fulton, M.N. and Sosman, M.C. (1942) Venous angiomas of skeletal muscle. Report of four cases. *J. Am. Med. Ass.*, **119**, 324–7.
197. Holden, K.R. and Alexander, F. (1970) Diffuse neonatal angiomatosis. *Paediatrics*, **46**, 411–21.
198. Rao, V.K. and Weiss, S.W. (1992) Angiomatosis of soft tissue: an analysis of the histologic features and clinical outcome in 51 cases. *Am. J. Surg. Pathol.*, **16**, 764–71.
199. Howat, A.J. and Campbell, P.E. (1987) Angiomatosis: a vascular malformation of infancy and childhood. *Pathology*, **19**, 377–82.
200. Bennett, G.E. and Cobey, M.C. (1939) Hemangioma of joints. *Arch. Surg.*, **38**: 487–500.
201. Harkins, H.N. (1937) Hemangioma of a tendon or tendon sheath. Report of a case with a study of twenty-four cases from the literature. *Arch. Surg.*, **34**, 12–22.
202. Bate, T.H. (1954) Hemangiomata of the tendon sheath. *J. Bone Joint Surg.*, **36A**, 104–9.
203. Moon, N.F. (1973) Synovial hemangioma of the knee joint. A review of previously reported cases and inclusion of two new cases. *Clin. Orthop.*, **90**, 183–90.
204. DePalma, A.F. and Mauler, G.G. (1964) Hemangioma of synovial membrane. *Clin. Orthop.*, **32**, 93–99.
205. Larsen, I.J. and Landry, R.M. (1969) Hemangioma of the synovial membrane. *J. Bone Joint Surg.*, **51A**, 1210–15.
206. Atkinson, T.J., Wolf, S., Anavi, Y. et al. (1988) Synovial hemangioma of the temporomandibular joint: Report of a case and review of the literature. *J. Oral Maxillofac. Surg.*, **46**, 804–8.
207. Aalberg, J.R. (1990) Synovial hemangioma of the knee. A case report. *Acta Orthop. Scand.*, **61**, 88–89.
208. Mehregan, D.R., Mehregan, A.H., Collier, D.U. et al. (1991) Synovial hemangioma. *J. Am. Acad. Dermatol.*, **25**, 851–2.
209. Linson, M.A. and Posner, I.P. (1979) Synovial hemangioma as a cause of recurrent knee effusions. *J. Am. Med. Ass.*, **242**, 2214–15.
210. Losli, E.J. (1952) Intrinsic hemangiomas of the peripheral nerves. *Arch. Pathol.*, **53**, 226–32.
211. Purcell, F.H. and Gurdjian, E.S. (1935) Hemangiomata of peripheral nerves. With report of a case of cavernous hemangioma of the sciatic nerve. *Am. J. Surg.*, **30**, 541–4.
212. Peled, I., Iosipovich, Z., Rousso, M. et al. (1980) Hemangioma of the median nerve. *J. Hand Surg. [Am.]*, **5**, 363–5.
213. Patel, C.B., Tsai, T.-M. and Kleinert, H.E. (1986) Hemangioma of the median surg. a report of two cases. *J. Hand Surg. [Am.]*, **11**, 76–79.
214. Maruoka, N., Yamakawa, Y. and Shimauchi, M. (1988) Cavernous hemangioma of the optic nerve. Case report. *J. Neurosurg.*, **69**, 292–4.
215. Lo, W.M.W., Brackmann, D.E. and Shelton, C. (1989) Facial nerve hemangioma. *Ann. Otol. Rhinol. Laryngol.*, **98**, 160–1.
216. Bilge, T., Kaya, A., Alatli, M. et al. (1989) Hemangioma of the peroneal nerve: Case report and review of the literature. *Neurosurgery*, **25**, 649–52.
217. Gorham, L.W. and Stout, A.P. (1955) Massive osteolysis (acute spontaneous absorption of bone, phantom bone, disappearing bone). Its relation to hemangiomatosis. *J. Bone Joint Surg. [Am.]*, 985–1004.
218. Dorfman, H.D., Steiner, G.C. and Jaffee, H.L. (1971) Vascular tumors of bone. *Hum. Pathol.*, **2**, 349–76.
219. Unni, K.K., Ivins, J.C., Beabout, J.W. et al. (1971) Hemangioma, hemangiopericytoma, and hemangioendothelioma (angiosarcoma) of bone. *Cancer*, **27**, 1403–14.
220. Fornaiser, V.L. (1970) Hemangiomatosis with massive osteolysis. *J. Bone Joint Surg.*, **52B**, 444–51.
221. Schajowicz, F., Aiello, C.L., Francone, M.V. et al. (1978) Cystic angiomatosis (hamartous haemolymphangiomatosis) of bone. A clinicopathological study of three cases. *J. Bone Joint Surg.*, **60B**, 100–6.
222. Boyle, W.J. (1972) Cystic angiomatosis of bone. *J. Bone Joint Surg.*, **54B**, 626–36.
223. Spjut, H.J. and Lindbom, A. (1962) Skeletal angiomatosis. *Acta Pathol. Microbiol. Scand.*, **55**, 49–58.
224. Reid, A.B., Reid, I.L., Johnson, G. et al. (1989) Familial diffuse cystic angiomatosis of bone. *Clin. Orthop.*, **238**, 211–8.
225. Shimpo, S., Nishitani, H., Tsunemura, T. (1968) Solitary plasmacytoma with polyneuritis and endocrine disturbance. *Nippon Rinsho*, **26**, 2444–56.
226. Ishikawa, O., Nihei, Y. and Ishikawa, H. (1987) The skin changes of POEMS syndrome. *Br. J. Dermatol.*, **117**, 523–6.
227. Zak, F.G., Solomon, A. and Fellner, M.J. (1966) Viscerocutaneous angiomatosis with dysproteinemia phagocytosis: its relation to Kaposi's sarcoma and lymphoproliferative disorders. *J. Pathol.*, **92**, 594–9.
228. Puig, L., Moreno, A., Domingo, P. et al. (1985) Cutaneous angiomas in POEMS syndrome. *J. Am. Acad. Dermatol.*, **112**, 961–4.
229. Chan, J.K.C., Fletcher, C.D.M., Hicklin, G.A. et al. (1990) Glomeruloid haemangioma. a distinctive cutaneous lesion of multicentric Castleman's disease associated with POEMS syndrome. *Am. J. Surg. Pathol.*, **14**, 1036–46.
230. Kanitakis, J., Roger, H., Soubrier, M. et al. (1988) Cutaneous angiomas in POEMS syndrome. An ultrastructural and immunohistochemical study. *Arch. Dermatol.*, **124**, 695–8.
231. Nakagawa, K. (1949) Case report of angioblastoma of the skin. *Hifuka Seibyoka Zasshi*, **59**, 92–94.
232. Wilson Jones, E. (1976) Dowling oration 1976. Malignant vascular tumors. *Clin. Expl Dermatol.*, **1**, 287–312.
233. Scott, O.L.S. and Wilson-Jones, E. (1977) Tufted haemangioma. *J. Roy. Soc. Med.*, **70**, 283.
234. Wilson Jones, E. and Orkin, M. (1989) Tufted angioma (angioblastoma). A benign progressive angioma, not to be confused with Kaposi's sarcoma or low-grade angiosarcoma. *J. Am. Acad. Dermatol.*, **20**, 214–25.
235. Alessi, E., Bertani, E. and Sala, F. (1986) Acquired tufted hemangioma. *Am. J. Dermatopathol.*, **8**, 68–75.
236. Padilla, R.S., Orkin, M. and Rosai, J. (1987) Acquired tufted angioma (progressive capillary hemangioma), a distinctive clinicopathologic entity related to lobular capillary hemangioma. *Am. J. Dermatopathol.*, **9**, 292–300.
237. Kumakiri, M., Muramoto, F., Tsukinga, I. et al. (1983) Crystalline lamellae in the endothelial cells of a type of hemangioma characterized by the proliferation of immature endothelial cells and pericytes – angioblastoma (Nakagawa). *J. Am. Acad. Dermatol.*, **8**, 68–75.
238. Hiraiwa, A., Takai, K., Fukui, Y. et al. (1990) Nonregressing lipodystrophia centrifugalis abdominalis with angioblastoma (Nakagawa). *Arch. Dermatol.*, **126**, 206–9.
239. Santa Cruz, D.J. and Aronberg, J. (1988) Targetoid hemosiderotic hemangioma. *J. Am. Acad. Dermatol.*, **19**, 550–8.
240. Rapini, R.P. and Golitz, L.E. (1990) Targetoid hemosiderotic hemangioma. *J. Cutan. Pathol.*, **17**, 233–5.
241. Vion, B. and Frenk, E. (1992) Targetoid hemosiderotic hemangioma. *Dermatology*, **184**, 300–2.
242. Imperial, R. and Helwig, E.B. (1967) Angiokeratoma: a clinicopathologic study. *Arch. Dermatol.*, **95**, 166–75.
243. Epinette, W.W., Norins, A.L., Drew, A.L. et al. (1973) Angiokeratoma corporis diffusum. *Arch. Dermatol.*, **101**, 754–7.
244. Whyte, M.P. (1978) Angiokeratoma serpiginosum. *Int. J. Dermatol.*, **17**, 793–8.
245. Imperial, R. and Helwig, E.B. (1967) Verrucous hemangioma. A clinicopathologic study of 21 cases. *Arch. Dermatol.*, **96**, 247–53.
246. Kohda, H. and Narisawa, Y. (1992) Digital verrucous fibroangioma: A new variant of verrucous hemangioma. *Acta Derm. Venereol. (Stockh.)*, **72**, 303–4.
247. Frain-Bell, W. (1957) Angioma serpiginosum. *Br. J. Dermatol.*, **69**, 2551–68.
248. Barker, L.P. and Sachs, P.M. (1965) Angioma serpiginosum. A comparative study. *Arch. Dermatol.*, **92**, 613–20.
249. Stevenson, J.R. and Lincoln, C.S. (1967) Angioma serpiginosum. *Arch. Dermatol.*, **95**, 16–22.
250. Marriott, P.J., Munr, D.D. and Ryan, T. (1975) Angioma serpiginosum – familial incidence. *Br. J. Dermatol.*, **93**, 701–6.
251. Hunt, S.J., Santa Cruz, D.J. and Barr, R.J. (1991) Microvenular hemangioma. *J. Cutan. Pathol.*, **18**, 235–40.
252. Gonzales-Crussi, F., Chou, P. and Crawford, S.E. (1991) Congenital, infiltrating giant cell angioblastoma. A new entity? *Am. J. Surg. Pathol.*, **15**, 175–83.
253. Smith, N.P. and Wilson-Jones, E. (1985) Multinucleate cell angiohistiocytoma – a new entity. *Br. J. Dermatol.*, **113** (suppl. 29), 15.
254. Smith, N.P. and Wilson-Jones, E. (1986) Multinucleate cell angiohistiocytoma: a new entity. *J. Cutan. Pathol.*, **13**, 77.
255. Smolle, J., Auboeck, L., Gogg-Retzer, I. et al. (1989) Multinucleate cell angiohistiocytoma: a clinicopathological, immunohistochemical and ultrastructural study. *Br. J. Dermatol.*, **121**, 113–21.
256. Brooks, J., Elenitas, R., Hicks, D. et al. (1993) Proliferative cutaneous angiomatosis: a cellular tumor mimicking angiosarcoma and Kaposi's

sarcoma. *Mod. Pathol.*, **6**, 5A.
257. Weiss, S.W. and Enzinger, F.M. (1986) Spindle cell hemangioendothelioma: a low grade angiosarcoma resembling a cavernous hemangioma and Kaposi's sarcoma. *Am. J. Surg. Pathol.*, **10**, 521–30.
258. Scott, G.A. and Rosai, J. (1988) Spindle cell hemangioendothelioma: report of seven additional cases of a recently described vascular neoplasm. *Am. J. Dermatopathol.*, **10**, 281–8.
259. Zoltie, N. and Roberts, P.F. (1989) Spindle cell haemangioendothelioma in association with epithelioid haemangioendothelioma. *Histopathology*, **15**, 544–6.
260. Fletcher, C.D.M., Beham, A. and Schmid, C. (1991) Spindle cell haemangioendothelioma: a clinicopathological and immunohistochemical study indicative of a non-neoplastic lesion. *Histopathology*, **18**, 291–301.
261. Steinbach, L.S., Omisky, S.H., Shpall, S. *et al.* (1991) MR imaging of spindle cell hemangioendothelioma. *J. Comput. Assist. Tomogr.*, **15**, 155–7.
262. Terashi, H., Itami, S., Kurata, S. *et al.* (1991) Spindle cell hemangioendothelioma: report of three cases. *J. Dermatol.*, **18**, 104–11.
263. Ding, J., Hashimoto, H., Imayama, S. *et al.* (1992) Spindle cell hemangioendothelioma: probably a benign vascular lesion not a low grade angiosarcoma. *Virchows Archiv. A Pathol. Anat. Histopathol.*, **420**, 77–85.
264. Imayama, S., Murakamai, Y., Hashimoto, H. *et al.* (1992) Spindle cell hemangioendothelioma exhibits the ultrastructural features of a reactive vascular proliferation rather than of angiosarcoma. *Am. J. Clin. Pathol.*, **97**, 279–87.
265. Ono, C.M., Mitsunaga, M.M. and Lockett, L.J. (1992) Intragluteal spindle cell hemangioendothelioma. An unusual presentation of a recently described vascular neoplasm. *Clin. Orthop.*, **281**, 224–8.
266. Dabska, M. (1969) Malignant endovascular papillary angioendothelioma of the skin in childhood. Clinicopathologic study of six cases. *Cancer*, **24**, 503–10.
267. Patterson, K. and Chandra, R.S. (1985) Malignant endovascular papillary angioendothelioma. Cutaneous borderline tumor. *Arch. Pathol. Lab. Med.*, **109**, 671–3.
268. Manivel, J.C., Wick, M.R., Swanson, P.E. *et al.* (1986) Endovascular papillary angioendothelioma of childhood: a vascular lesion characterized by 'high' endothelial cell differentiation. *Hum. Pathol.*, **17**, 1240–4.
269. Magnin, P.H., Schroh, R.G. and Barquin, M.A. (1987) Endovascular papillary angioendothelioma in children. *Pediatr. Dermatol.*, **4**, 332–5.
270. Morgan, J., Robinson, M.J., Rosen, L.B. *et al.* (1989) Malignant endovascular papillary angioendothelioma (Dabska tumor). A case report and review of the literature. *Am. J. Dermatopathol.*, **11**, 64–68.
271. Enzinger, F.M. and Weiss, S.W. (1988) Hemangioendothelioma: vascular tumors of intermediate malignancy, in *Soft Tissue Tumors*, 2nd edn, C.V. Mosby, Philadelphia, pp. 533–44.
272. Pearl, G.S. and Matthews, W.H. (1979) Congenital retroperitoneal hemangioendothelioma with Kasabach–Merritt syndrome. *South. Med. J.*, **72**, 239–40.
273. Weinblatt, M.E., Kahn, E. and Kochen, J.A. (1984) Hemangioendothelioma with intravascular coagulation and ischemic colitis. *Cancer*, **54**, 2300–4.
274. Niedt, G.W., Greco, M.A., Wieczorek, R. *et al.* (1989) Hemangioma with Kaposi's sarcoma-like features: report of 2 cases. *Pediatr. Pathol.*, **9**, 567–75.
275. Lai, F.M., Allen, P.W., Yuen, P.M. *et al.* (1991) Locally metastasizing vascular tumor: spindle cell, epithelioid or unclassified hemangioendothelioma. *Am. J. Clin. Pathol.*, **96**, 660–3.
276. Tsang, W.Y.W. and Chan, J.K.C. (1991) Kaposi-like infantile hemangioendothelioma: a distinctive vascular neoplasm of the retroperitoneum. *Am. J. Surg. Pathol.*, **15**, 982–9.
277. Zukerburg, L.R., Nickoloff, B.J. and Weiss, S.W. (1993) Kaposiform hemangioendothelioma of infancy and childhood. An aggressive neoplasm associated with Kasabach–Merritt syndrome and lymphangiomatosis. *Am. J. Surg. Pathol.*, **17**, 321–8.
278. Weiss, S.W. and Enzinger, F.M. (1982) Epithelioid hemangioendothelioma: a vascular tumor often mistaken for a carcinoma. *Cancer*, **50**, 970–81.
279. Weiss, S.W., Ishak, K.G., Dail, D.H. *et al.* (1986) Epithelioid hemangioendothelioma and related lesions. *Semin. Diagn. Pathol.*, **3**, 259–87.
280. Zagzag, D., Yang, G., Seidman, I. *et al.* (1993) Malignant epithelioid hemangioendothelioma arising in an intramuscular lipoma. *Cancer*, **71**, 764–8.
281. Vebeken, E., Beyls, J., Moerman, P. *et al.* (1985) Lung metastases of malignant epithelioid hemangioendothelioma mimicking a primary intravascular bronchioalveolar tumor. A histologic, ultrastructural, and immunohistochemical study. *Cancer*, **55**, 1741–6.
282. Dail, D.H., Liebow, A.A. and Gmelich, J.T. (1983) Intravascular, bronchiolar, and alveolar tumor of lung: an analysis of twenty cases of a peculiar sclerosing endothelial tumor. *Cancer*, **51**, 452–64.
283. Corrin, B., Manners, B., Millard, M. *et al.* (1979) Histogenesis of the so-called 'intravascular bronchioloalveolar tumor'. *J. Pathol.*, **128**, 163–7.
284. Azumi, N. and Churg, A. (1981) Intravascular sclerosing bronchiolo-aveolar tumor. *Am. J. Surg. Pathol.*, **5**, 587–96.
285. Weldon-Linne, C.M., Victor, T.A., Christ, M.L. *et al.* (1981) Angiogenic nature of the 'intravascular bronchioalveolar tumor' of the lung: an electron microscopic study. *Arch. Pathol. Lab. Med.*, **105**, 174–9.
286. Ishak, K.G., Sesterhenn, I.A., Goodman, Z.G. *et al.* (1984) Epithelioid hemangioendothelioma of the liver: a clinicopathologic and follow up study of 32 cases. *Hum. Pathol.*, **15**, 839–52.
287. Fukayama, M., Nehei, Z., Takizawa, T. *et al.* (1984) Malignant epthelioid hemangioendothelioma of the liver, spreading through the hepatic veins. *Virchows Arch. A Pathol. Anat. Histopathol.*, **404**, 275–87.
288. Dean, P.J., Haggitt, R.C. and O'Hara, C.J. (1985) Malignant epithelioid hemangioendothelioma of the liver in young women: relationship to oral contraceptive use. *Am. J. Surg. Pathol.*, **9**, 695–704.
289. Miller, W.J., Dodd, G.D., Federle, M.P. *et al.* (1992) Epithelioid hemangioendothelioma of the liver: imaging findings with pathologic correlation. *Am. J. Roentgenol*, **159**, 53–57.
290. Tsuneyoshi, M., Dorfman, H.D. and Bauer, T.W. (1986) Epithelioid hemangioendothelioma of bone: a clinicopathologic, ultrastructural, and immunohistochemical study. *Am. J. Surg. Pathol.*, **10**, 754–64.
291. Ellis, G.L. and Kratochvil, F.J. (1986) Epithelioid hemangioendothelioma of the head and neck: a clinicopathological report of 12 cases. *Oral Surg. Oral Med. Oral Pathol.*, **61**, 61–68.
292. Marin, I.R., Todo, S., Tzakis, A.G. *et al.* (1988) Treatment of hepatic epithelioid hemangioendothelioma with liver transplantation. *Cancer*, **62**, 2079–84.
293. Köbner, H. (1869) Zur Kenntniss der allgemeinen sarcomatose und der hautsarcome im besonderen. *Arch. Dermatol. Syph.*, **1**, 369–81.
294. Kaposi, M. (1872) Idiopathic multiple pigmented sarcoma of the skin. *Arch. Dermatol. Syph.*, **4**, 265–73. (Translated from German in *CA – A Cancer Journal for Clinicians* (1982) **32**, 342–347.)
295. Reynolds, W.A., Winkelmann, R.K. and Soule, E.H. (1965) Kaposi's sarcoma: a clinicopathologic study with particular reference to its relationship to the reticuloendothelial system. *Medicine*, **44**, 419–43.
296. Cox, F.H. and Helwig, E.B. (1959) Kaposi's sarcoma. *Cancer*, **12**, 289–98.
297. Oettle, A.G. (1962) Geographical and racial differences in the frequency of Kaposi's sarcoma as evidence of environmental or genetic causes. *Acta Un. Int. Cancr.*, **18**, 330–63.
298. Finlay, A.Y. and Marks, R. (1979) Familial Kaposi's sarcoma. *Br. J. Dermatol.*, **100**, 323–6.
299. Pollack, M.S., Safai, B., Myskowski, P.L. *et al.* (1983) Frequencies of HLA and Gm immunogenetic markers in Kaposi's sarcoma. *Tissue Antigens*, **21**, 1–8.
300. Tzfoni, E.E., Scherman, L., Battat, S. and Brautbar, H. (1993) No HLA antigen is significant in classic Kaposi's sarcoma. *J. Am. Acad. Dermatol.*, **28**, 118–19.
301. Safai, B., Mike, V., Giraldo, G. *et al.* (1980) Association of Kaposi's sarcoma with second primary malignancies: possible etiopathogenic implications. *Cancer*, **45**, 1472–9.
302. Templeton, A.C. (1981) Kaposi's sarcoma. *Pathol. Annu.*, **2**, 315–36.
303. Reed, W.B., Kamath, H.M. and Weiss, L. (1974) Kaposi sarcoma, with emphasis on internal manifestations. *Arch. Dermatol.*, **110**, 115–18.
304. Lee, F.D. (1968) A comparative study of Kaposi's sarcoma and granuloma pyogenicum in Uganda. *J. Clin. Pathol.*, **21**, 119–28.
305. Lothe, F. (1963) Kaposi's sarcoma in Uganda Africans. *Acta Pathol. Microbiol. Scand.*, (suppl. 161), 1–70.
306. Ngendahayo, P., Mets, T., Bugingo, G. *et al.* (1989) Le sarcoma de Kaposi au Rwanda: aspects clinico-pathologiques et épidémiologiques. *Bull. Cancer (Paris)*, **76**, 383–94.
307. Dutz, W. and Stout, A.P. (1960) Kaposi's sarcoma in infants and children. *Cancer*, **13**, 684–94.
308. Olweny, C.L.M., Kaddumukasa, A., Atine, I. *et al.* (1976) Childhood Kaposi's sarcoma: clinical features and therapy. *Br. J. Cancer*, **33**, 555–60.
309. Harwood, A.R., Osoba, D., Hofstader, S.L. *et al.* (1979) Kaposi's sarcoma in recipients of renal transplants. *Am. J. Med.*, **67**, 759–65.
310. Penn, I. (1983) Kaposi's sarcoma in immunosuppressed patients. *J. Clin. Lab. Immunol.*, **12**, 1–10.
311. Shmueli, D., Shapira, Z., Yussim, A. *et al.* (1989) The incidence of Kaposi's sarcoma in renal transplantation patients and its relation to immunosuppression. *Transpl. Proc.*, **21**, 3209–13.
312. Penn, I. (1979) Kaposi's sarcoma in organ transplantation recipients. *Transplantation*, **27**, 8–11.
313. Siegel, J.H., Janis, R., Alper, J.C. *et al.* (1969) Disseminated visceral Kaposi's sarcoma: appearance after human renal allograft rejection. *J. Am. Med. Ass.*, **207**, 1493–6.
314. Myers, B.D., Kessler, E., Levi, J. *et al.* (1974) Kaposi's sarcoma in kidney transplant patients. *Arch. Intern. Med.*, **110**, 602–4.
315. Qunibi, W.Y., Barri, Y., Alfurayh, O. *et al.* (1993) Kaposi's sarcoma in renal transplant recipients: a report of 26 cases from a single institution. *Transplant. Proc.*, **25**, 1402–5.
316. Straehley, C.J., Santos, J.I., Downey, D.M. *et al.* (1975) Kaposi sarcoma in a renal transplant recipient. *Arch. Pathol.*, **99**, 611–13.
317. Klein, M.B., Pereira, F.A. and Kanntor, I. (1974) Kaposi sarcoma com-

plicating systemic lupus erythematosis treated with immunosuppression. *Arch. Dermatol.*, 110, 602–4.
318. Klepp, O., Dahl, O. and Stenwig, J.T. (1978) Association of Kaposi's sarcoma and prior immunosuppressive therapy. *Cancer*, 42, 2626–30.
319. Gange, R.W. and Wilson-Jones, E. (1978) Kaposi's sarcoma and immunosuppressive therapy: an appraisal. *Clin. Expl Dermatol.*, 3, 135–46.
320. Desmond-Hellmann, S.D., Mbidde, E.K., Kizito, A. et al. (1991) The value of a clinical definition for epidemic KS in predicting HIV seropositivity in Africa. *J. Acq. Immune Defic. Synd.*, 4, 647–51.
321. Centers for Disease Control (1981) Follow-up on Kaposi's sarcoma and pneumocystis pneumonia. *MMWR Morb. Mortal. Wkly Rep.*, 30, 409–10.
322. Friedman-Kien, L., Laubenstein, L., Marmor, M. et al. (1981) Kaposi's sarcoma and pneumocystis pneumonia among homosexual men – New York City and California. *MMWR Morb. Mortal. Wkly Rep.*, 30, 305–30.
323. Friedman-Kien, E.A., Laubenstein, L.J., Rubinstein, P. et al. (1982) Disseminated Kaposi's sarcoma in homosexual men. *Ann. Intern. Med.*, 96, 693–700.
324. Beral, V., Peterman, T.A., Berkelman, R.L. and Jaffee, H.W. (1990) Kaposi's sarcoma among persons with AIDS: a sexually transmitted infection. *Lancet*, 335, 123–8.
325. Gottlieb, G.J. and Ackerman, A.B. (1982) Kaposi's sarcoma: an extensive disseminated form in young homosexual men. *Hum. Pathol.*, 13, 882–92.
326. Safai, B. (1984) Clinical features of Kaposi's sarcoma/acquired immune deficiency syndrome and its management. *Antibiot. Chemother.*, 32, 54–70.
327. Lemlich, G., Schwam, L. and Lebwohl, M. (1987) Kaposi's sarcoma and acquired immunodeficiency syndrome. Post mortem findings in twenty-four cases. *J. Am. Acad. Dermatol.*, 16, 319–25.
328. Welch, K., Finkbeiner, W., Alpers, C.E. et al. (1984) Autopsy findings in the acquired immunodeficiency syndrome. *J. Am. Med. Ass.*, 252, 1152–9.
329. Orlow, S.J., Cooper, D., Petrea, S. et al. (1993) AIDS-associated Kaposi's sarcoma in Romanian children. *J. Am. Acad. Dermatol.*, 2, 449–53.
330. Connor, E., Boccon-Gibod, L., Joshi, V. et al. (1990) Cutaneous acquired immunodeficiency syndrome-associated Kaposi's sarcoma in pediatric patients. *Arch. Dermatol.*, 126, 791–3.
331. DeJarlais, D.C., Marmor, M., Thomas, P. et al. (1984) Kaposi's sarcoma among four different AIDS risk groups [letter]. *New Engl. J. Med.*, 310, 1119.
332. Centers for Disease Control (1982) Epidemiologic aspects of the current outbreak of Kaposi's sarcoma and opportunistic infections. *New Engl. J. Med.*, 306, 248–52.
333. Haverkos, H.W. and Drotman, D.P. (1985) Prevalence of Kaposi's sarcoma among patients with AIDS [letter]. *New Engl. J. Med.*, 312, 1518.
334. Biggar, R.J., Burnett, W., Mikl, J. and Nasca, P. (1989) Cancer among New York men at risk of acquired immunodeficiency syndrome. *Int. J. Cancer*, 43, 979–85.
335. Beral, V., Bull, D., Darby, S. et al. (1992) Risk of Kaposi's sarcoma and sexual practices associated with faecal contact in homosexual or bisexual men with AIDS. *Lancet*, 339, 632–5.
336. Darrow, W.W., Peterman, T.A., Jaffee, H.W. et al. (1992) Kaposi's sarcoma and exposure to faeces [letter]. *Lancet*, 339, 685.
337. Elford, J., Tindall, B. and Sherkey, T. (1992) Kaposi's sarcoma and insertive rimming [letter]. *Lancet*, 339, 938.
338. Matondo, P. (1992) Kaposi's sarcoma and faecal-oral exposure. [letter]. *Lancet*, 339, 1490.
339. Page-Bodkin, K., Tappero, J., Samuel, M. et al. (1992) Kaposi's sarcoma and faecal-oral exposure [letter]. *Lancet*, 339, 1490.
340. Giraldo, G., Beth, E., Henle, G. et al. (1978) Antibody patterns to herpesviruses in Kaposi's sarcoma. II. Serological association of American Kaposi's sarcoma with cytomegalovirus. *Int. J. Cancer*, 22, 126–31.
341. Giraldo, G., Beth, E. and Huang, E.-S. (1980) Kaposi's sarcoma and its relationship to cytomegalovirus (CMV). III. CMV DNA and CMV early antigens in Kaposi's sarcoma. *Int. J. Cancer*, 26, 23–29.
342. Iochim, H.L., Dorsett, B., Melamed, J. et al. (1992) Cytomegalovirus, angiomatosis, and Kaposi's sarcoma: new observations on a debated relationship. *Mod. Pathol.*, 5, 169–78.
343. Drew, W.L., Conant, M.A., Miner, R.C. et al. (1982) Cytomegalovirus and Kaposi's sarcoma in young homosexual men. *Lancet*, 2, 125–7.
344. Ambinder, R.F., Newman, C., Hayward, G.S. et al. (1987) Lack of association of cytomegalovirus with endemic African Kaposi's sarcoma. *J. Infect. Dis.*, 156, 193–7.
345. Giraldo, G., Beth, E. and Haguenau, F. (1972) Herpes-type virus particles in tissue culture of Kaposi's sarcoma from different geographic regions. *J. Natl Cancer Inst.*, 49, 1509–26.
346. Giraldo, G., Beth, E., Coeur, P. et al. (1972) Kaposi's sarcoma: a new model in the search for viruses associated with human malignancies. *J. Natl Cancer Inst.*, 49, 1495–507.
347. Huang, Y.Q., Rush, M.G., Polesz, B.J. et al. (1992) HPV-16-related DNA sequences in Kaposi's sarcoma. *Lancet*, 339, 515–18.
348. Nickoloff, B.J., Huang, Y.Q., Li, J.J. and Friedman-Kien, A.E. (1992) Immunohistochemical detection of papillomavirus antigens in Kaposi's sarcoma. *Lancet*, 339, 548–9.
349. Miles, S.A., Martinez-Maza, O., Rezai, A. et al. (1992) Oncostatin M as a potent mitogen for AIDS-Kaposi's-sarcoma-derived cells. *Science*, 253, 1432–4.
350. Vogel, J., Hinrichs, S.H., Reynolds, R.K. et al. (1988) The HIV tat gene induces dermal lesions resembling Kaposi's sarcoma in transgenic mice. *Nature*, 335, 606–11.
351. Ensoli, B., Barillari, G., Salahuddin, S.Z. et al. (1990) Tat protein of HIV-1 stimulates growth of cells derived from Kaposi's sarcoma lesions of AIDS patients. *Nature*, 345, 84–86.
352. Salahuddin, S.Z., Nakamura, S., Biberfeld, P. et al. (1988) Angiogenic properties of Kaposi's sarcoma-derived cells after long-term culture in vitro. *Science*, 242, 430–3.
353. Nakamura, S., Salahuddin, S.Z., Biberfeld, P. et al. (1988) Kaposi's sarcoma cells: long-term culture with growth factor from retrovirus-infected CD4+ T cells. *Science*, 242, 426–30.
354. Ensoli, B., Nakamura, S., Salahuddin, S.Z. et al. (1989) AIDS-Kaposi's sarcoma-derived cells express cytokines with autocrine and paracrine growth factors. *Science*, 243, 223–6.
355. Bovi, P.D., Curatola, A.M., Kern, F.G. et al. (1987) An oncogene isolated by transfection of Kaposi's sarcoma DNA encodes a growth factor that is a member of the FGF family. *Cell*, 50, 729–37.
356. Ruszczak, Z., Mayer-Da Silva, A. and Orfanos, C.E. (1987) Kaposi's sarcoma in AIDS. Multicentric neoplasia in early skin lesions. *Am. J. Dermatopathol.*, 9, 388–98.
357. Hodak, E., Trattner, A., David, M., Kornbrot, N. et al. (1993) Quantitative and qualitative assessment of plasma von Willebrand factor in classic Kaposi's sarcoma. *J. Am. Acad. Dermatol.*, 28, 217–21.
358. Beckstead, J., Wood, G. and Fletcher, V. (1985) Evidence for the origin of Kaposi's sarcoma from lymphatic endothelium. *Am. J. Pathol.*, 119, 294–300.
359. McNutt, N.S., Fletcher, V. and Conant, M.A. (1983) Early lesions of Kaposi's sarcoma in homosexual men. An ultrastructural comparison with other vascular proliferations in skin. *Am. J. Pathol.*, 111, 62–77.
360. Rutgers, J.L., Wieczorek, R., Bonette, F. et al. (1986) The expression of endothelial cell surface antigens by AIDS-associated Kaposi's sarcoma. *Am. J. Pathol.*, 122, 493–9.
361. Scully, P.A., Steinman, H.K., Kennedy, C. et al. (1988) AIDS-related Kaposi's sarcoma displays differential expression of endothelial surface antigens. *Am. J. Pathol.*, 130, 244–51.
362. Costa, J. and Rabson, A.S. (1983) Generalised Kaposi's sarcoma is not a neoplasm [letter]. *Lancet*, 1, 58.
363. Brooks, J.J. (1986) Kaposi's sarcoma: A reversible hyperplasia. *Lancet*, 2, 1309–11.
364. Auerbach, H.E. and Brooks, J.J. (1989) Kaposi's sarcoma: neoplasia or hyperplasia. *Surg. Pathol.*, 2, 19–28.
365. Bisceglia, M., Bosman, C. and Quirke, P. (1992) A histologic and flow cytometric study of Kaposi's sarcoma. *Cancer*, 69, 793–8.
366. Fukunaga, M. and Silverberg, S.G. (1990) Kaposi's sarcoma in patients with acquired immune deficiency syndrome. A flow cytometric DNA analysis of 26 lesions in 21 patients. *Cancer*, 66, 758–64.
367. Smith, K.J., Skelton, H.G., James, W.D. et al. (1991) Angiosarcoma arising in Kaposi's sarcoma (pleomorphic Kaposi's sarcoma) in a patient with human immunodeficiency disease. *J. Am. Acad. Dermatol.*, 24, 790–2.
368. Schwartz, R.A., Burgess, G.H. and Hoshaw, R.A. (1980) Patch stage Kaposi's sarcoma. *J. Am. Acad. Dermatol.*, 2, 509–12.
369. Schwartz, J.L., Muhlbauer, J.E. and Steigbigel, R.T. (1984) Pre-Kaposi's sarcoma. *J. Am. Acad. Dermatol.*, 11, 377–80.
370. Chor, P.J. and Santa Cruz, D.J. (1992) Kaposi's sarcoma: a clinicopathologic review and differential diagnosis. *J. Cutan. Pathol.*, 19, 6–20.
371. Kao, G.F., Johnson, F.B. and Sulica, V. (1990) The nature of the hyaline (eosinophilic) globules and vascular slits of Kaposi's sarcoma. *Am. J. Dermatopathol.*, 12, 256–67.
372. Kostianovsky, M., Lamy, Y. and Greco, M.A. (1992) Immunohistochemical and electron microscopic profiles of cutaneous Kaposi's sarcoma and bacillary angiomatosis. *Ultrastruct. Pathol.*, 16, 629–40.
373. Fukunaga, M. and Silverberg, S. (1991) Hyaline globules in Kaposi's sarcoma: a light microscopic and immunohistochemical study. *Mod. Pathol.*, 4, 187–90.
374. Ecklund, R.E. and Valaitis, J. (1962) Kaposi's sarcoma of lymph nodes. *Arch. Pathol.*, 74, 224–9.
375. Ramos, W., Taylor, H.B., Hernandez, B.A. et al. (1976) Primary Kaposi's sarcoma of lymph nodes. *Am. J. Clin. Pathol.*, 66, 998–1003.
376. O'Connell, K.M. (1977) Kaposi's sarcoma of lymph nodes: histologic study of lesions in 16 cases in Malawi. *J. Clin. Pathol.*, 30, 696–703.
377. Amazon, K. and Rywlin, A.M. (1979) Subtle clues to diagnosis by conventional microscopy: lymph node involvement in Kaposi's sarcoma. *Am. J. Dermatopathol.*, 1, 173–6.
378. Bhana, D., Templeton, A.C., Master, S.P. and Kyalwazi, S.K. (1970) Kaposi's sarcoma of lymph nodes. *Br. J. Cancer*, 24, 464–70.
379. Gange, R.W. and Wilson-Jones, E. (1979) Lymphangioma-like Kaposi's

sarcoma: A report of three cases. *Br. J. Dermatol.*, 100, 327–334.
380. Leibowitz, M.R., Dagliotto, M., Smith, E. et al. (1980) Rapidly fatal lymphangioma-like Kaposi's sarcoma. *Histopathology*, 4, 559–66.
381. Ronchese, F. and Kern, A.B. (1957) Lymphangioma-like Kaposi's sarcoma. *Arch. Dermatol.*, 75, 418–27.
382. Blumenfeld, W., Egbert, B.M. and Sagebiel, R.W. (1985) Differential diagnosis of Kaposi's sarcoma. *Arch. Pathol. Lab. Med.*, 109, 123–7.
383. Mali, J.W.H., Kuiper, J.P. and Hamers, A.A. (1965) Acro-angiodermatitis of the foot. *Arch. Dermatol.*, 92, 515–18.
384. Bluefarb, S.M. and Adams, L.A. (1967) Arteriovenous malformation with angiodermatitis: stasis dermatitis simulating Kaposi's disease. *Arch. Dermatol.*, 96, 176–81.
385. Earhart, R.N., Aeling, J.A., Nuss, D.D. et al. (1974) Pseudo-Kaposi sarcoma. *Arch. Dermatol.*, 10, 907–10.
386. Meynadier, J., Malbos, S., Guilhou, J.-J. et al. (1980) Pseudo-angiosarcomatose de Kaposi sur membre paralytique. *Dermatologica*, 160, 190–7.
387. Watanabe, M., Kishiyama, K. and Ohkawara, A. (1983) Acquired progressive lymphangioma. *J. Am. Acad. Dermatol.*, 8, 663–7.
388. Tadaki, T., Aiba, S., Masu, S. et al. (1988) Acquired progressive lymphangioma as a flat erythematous patch on the abdominal wall of a child. *Arch. Dermatol.*, 124, 699–701.
389. Wilson Jones, E., Winkelmann, R.K., Zachary, C.B. et al. (1990) Benign lymphangioendothelioma. *J. Am. Acad. Dermatol.*, 23, 229–35.
390. Weich, H.A., Salahuddin, S.Z., Gill, P. et al. (1991) AIDS-associated Kaposi's sarcoma-derived cells in long-term culture express and synthesize smooth muscle alpha-actin. *Am. J. Pathol.*, 139, 1251–8.
391. Chan, J.K.C., Frizzera, G., Fletcher, C.D.M. et al. (1992) Primary vascular tumors of lymph nodes other than Kaposi's sarcoma. Analysis of 39 cases and delineation of two new entities. *Am. J. Pathol.*, 16, 335–50.
392. Haferkamp, O., Rosenau, W. and Lennert, K. (1971) Vascular transformation of lymph node due to venous obstruction. *Arch. Pathol.*, 92, 81–83.
393. Chan, J.K.C., Warbke, R.A. and Dorfman, R. (1991) Vascular transformation of sinuses of lymph nodes. A study of its morphologic spectrum and distinction from Kaposi's sarcoma. *Am. J. Surg. Pathol.*, 15, 732–43.
394. Ostrowski, M.L., Siddiqui, T., Barnes, R.E. et al. (1990) Vascular transformation of lymph node sinuses. A process displaying a spectrum of histologic features. *Arch. Pathol. Lab. Med.*, 114, 656–60.
395. Steinmann, G., Földi, E., Földi, M. et al. (1982) Morphologic findings in lymph nodes after occlusion of the efferent lymphatic vessels and veins. *Lab. Invest.*, 47, 43–50.
396. Davies, J.D. and Stansfeld, G. (1972) Spontaneous infarction of superficial lymph nodes. *J. Clin. Pathol.*, 25, 689–96.
397. Lucke, V.M., Davies, J.D., Wood, C.M. et al. (1987) Plexiform vascularization of lymph nodes: an unusual but distinctive lymphadenopathy in cats. *J. Comp. Pathol.*, 97, 109–19.
398. Fayemi, A.O. and Toker, C. (1975) Nodal angiomatosis. *Arch. Pathol.*, 99, 170–2.
399. Bedrosian, S.A. and Goldman, R.L. (1984) Nodal angiomatosis: relationship to vascular transformation of lymph nodes. *Arch. Pathol. Lab. Med.*, 108, 864–5.
400. Weiss, S.W., Gnepp, D.R. and Bratthauer, G.L. (1989) Palisaded myofibroblastoma. A benign mesenchymal tumor of lymph node. *Am. J. Surg. Pathol.*, 13, 341–6.
401. Suster, S. and Rosai, J. (1989) Intranodal hemorrhagic spindle cell tumor with amianthoid fibers. Report of six cases of a distinctive mesenchymal neoplasm of the inguinal region that simulated Kaposi's sarcoma. *Am. J. Surg. Pathol.*, 13, 347–57.
402. Fletcher, C.D.M. and Starling, R.W. (1990) Intranodal myofibroblastoma presenting in the submandibular region: evidence of a broader clinical and histologic spectrum. *Histopathology*, 16, 287–94.
403. Tappero, J.W., Conant, M.A., Wolfe, S.F. et al. (1993) Kaposi's sarcoma. Epidemiology, pathogenesis, histology, clinical spectrum, staging criteria and therapy. *J. Am. Acad. Dermatol.*, 28, 371–95.
404. Mitsuyasu, R.T. (1987) Clinical variants and staging of Kaposi's sarcoma. *Semin. Oncol.*, 14 (suppl. 3), 13–18.
405. Krigel, R.L., Lauberstin, L.J. and Muggia, F.M. (1983) Kaposi's sarcoma: A new staging classification. *Cancer Treat. Rep.*, 67, 531–4.
406. Krown, S.E., Metroka, C. and Wernz, J.C. (1989) Kaposi's sarcoma in the acquired immunodefiency syndrome: a proposal for uniform evaluation, response, and staging criteria. *J. Clin. Oncol.*, 7, 1201–7.
407. Karnofsky, D.A., Abelmann, W.H., Craver, L.F. and Burchenal, J.H. (1948) The use of the nitrogen mustards in the palliative treatment of carcinoma. With particular reference to bronchogenic carcinoma. *Cancer*, 1, 634–56.
408. Boudreaux, A.A., Smith, L.L., Cosby, C.D. et al. (1993) Intralesional vinblastine for cutaneous Kaposi's sarcoma associated with acquired immunodeficiency syndrome. A clinical trial to evaluate efficacy and discomfort associated with infection. *J. Am. Acad. Dermatol.*, 28, 6–65.
409. Myskowski, P.L. (1992) Intralesional interferon alpha-2b produces responses in KS. *Dermatology*, 3, 11.
410. Krown, S.E., Gold, J.M.W., Niedzwiecki, D. et al. (1990) Interferon-alpha with zidovudine: safety, tolerance, and clinical and virologic effects in patients with Kaposi's sarcoma associated with the acquired immunodeficiency syndrome (AIDS). *Ann. Intern. Med.*, 112, 812–21.
411. Groopman, J.E., Gottlieb, M.S., Goodman, J. et al. (1984) Recombinant alpha-2 interferon therapy for Kaposi's sarcoma associated with acquired immunodeficiency syndrome. *Ann. Intern. Med.*, 100, 671–6.
412. Rios, A., Mansell, P.W., Newell, G.R. et al. (1985) Treatment of acquired immunodeficiency syndrome-related Kaposi's sarcoma with lymphoblastoid interferon. *J. Clin. Oncol.*, 3, 506–12.
413. Maione, T.E., Gray, G.S., Petro, J. et al. (1990) Inhibition of angiogenesis by recombinant platelet factor-4 and related peptides. *Science*, 247, 77–79.
414. Ingber, D., Fujita, T., Kishimoto, S. et al. (1990) Synthetic analogues of fumagillin that inhibit angiogenesis and suppress tumor growth. *Nature*, 348, 555–7.
415. Oikawa, T., Hirotani, K., Ogasawara, H. et al. (1990) Inhibition of angiogenesis by vitamin D_3 analogues. *Eur. J. Pharmacol.*, 178, 247–50.
416. Folkman, J., Weisz, P.B., Joulie, M.M. et al. (1989) Control of angiogenesis with synthetic heparin substitutes. *Science*, 243, 1490–3.
417. Nakamura, S., Sakurada, S., Salahuddin, S.Z. et al. (1992) Inhibition of development of Kaposi's sarcoma-related lesions by a bacterial wall complex. *Science*, 255, 1437–40.
418. Bardwil, J.M., Mocega, E.E., Butler, J.J. and Russin, D.J. (1968) Angiosarcomas of the head and neck region. *Am. J. Surg.*, 116, 548–53.
419. Maddox, J.C. and Evans, H.L. (1981) Angiosarcoma of skin and soft tissue: a study of 44 cases. *Cancer*, 48, 1907–21.
420. Rosai, J., Sumner, H.W., Kostianovsky, M. and Perez-Mesa, C. (1976) Angiosarcoma of the skin. A clinicopathologic and fine structural study. *Hum. Pathol.*, 7, 83–109.
421. Cooper, P.H. (1987) Angiosarcomas of the skin. *Semin. Diag. Pathol.*, 4, 2–17.
422. Holden, C.A., Spittle, M.F. and Jones, E.W. (1987) Angiosarcoma of the face and scalp: prognosis and treatment. *Cancer*, 59, 1046–57.
423. Reed, R.J., Palomeque, F.E., Hairston III, M.A. and Krementz, E.T. (1966) Lymphangiosarcomas of the scalp. *Arch. Derm.*, 94, 396–402.
424. Haustein, U.-F. (1991) Angiosarcoma of the face and scalp. *Int. J. Dermatol.*, 30, 851–6.
425. Hodgkinson, D.J., Soule, E.H. and Woods, J.E. (1979) Cutaneous angiosarcoma of the head and neck. *Cancer*, 44, 1106–13.
426. Schirger, A. (1962) Postoperative lymphedema: etiologic and diagnostic factors. *Med. Clin. North. Am.*, 46, 1045–50.
427. Stewart, F.W. and Treves, N. (1948) Lymphangiosarcoma in post-mastectomy lymphedema. A report of six cases in elephantiasis chururgica. *Cancer*, 1, 64–81.
428. Schreiber, H., Barry, F.M., Russell, W.C. et al. (1979) Stewart–Treves syndrome: a lethal complication of post-mastectomy lymphedema and regional immune deficiency. *Arch. Surg.*, 114, 82–5.
429. Martorell, F. (1951) Tumorigenic lymphedema. *Angiology*, 2, 386–92.
430. McConnell, E.M. and Harris, H.R. (1966) Angiosarcoma in post-mastectomy lymphoedema. *Brit. J. Surg.*, 53, 572–6.
431. Fitzpatrick, P.J. (1969) Lymphangiosarcoma and breast cancer. *Can. J. Surg.*, 12, 172–7.
432. Woodward, A.H., Ivins, J.C. and Soule, E.H. (1972) Lymphangiosarcoma arising in chronic lymphaedematous extremities. *Cancer*, 30, 562–72.
433. Eby, C.S., Brennan, M.J. and Fine, G. (1967) Lymphangiosarcoma: a lethal complication of chronic lymphedema. Report of two cases and review of the literature. *Arch. Surg.*, 94, 223–30.
433a.Birge, R.F., Peisen, C.J., Thornton, F.E. et al. (1957) Angiosarcoma in post-mastectomy. *J. Iowa Med. Soc.*, 47, 491–5.
433b.Sternby, N.H., Gynning, I. and Hogeman, K.-E. (1961) Postmastectomy angiosarcoma. *Acta Chir. Scand.*, 121, 420–32.
434. McSwain, B., Whitehead, W. and Bennett, L. (1973) Angiosarcoma: report of three cases of postmastectomy lymphangiosarcoma and one of hemangiosarcoma. *South. Med. J.*, 66, 102–6.
435. Benda, J.A., Al-Jurf, A.S., Benson III, A.B. (1987) Angiosarcoma of the breast following segmental mastectomy complicated by lymphedema. *Am. J. Clin. Pathol.*, 87, 651–5.
436. Merrick, T.A., Erlandson, R.A. and Hajdu, S.I. (1971) Lymphangiosarcoma of a congenitally lymphedematous arm. *Arch. Pathol.*, 91, 365–71.
437. Alessi, E., Sala, F. and Berti, E. (1986) Angiosarcomas in lymphedematous limbs. *Am. J. Dermatopathol.*, 8, 371–8.
438. Mackenzie, D.H. (1971) Lymphangiosarcoma arising in chronic congenital and idiopathic lymphoedema. *J. Clin. Pathol.*, 24, 524–9.
439. Sordillo, P.P., Chapman, R., Hajdu, S.I. et al. (1981) Lymphangiosarcoma. *Cancer*, 48, 1674–9.
440. Taswell, H.F., Soule, E.H. and Coventry, M.B. (1962) Lymphangiosarcoma arising in chronic lymphedematous extremities. *J. Bone Joint Surg.*, 44A, 277–94.
441. Aird, I., Weinbren, K. and Walter, L. (1956) Angiosarcoma in a limb the seat of spontaneous lymphedema. *Brit. J. Cancer*, 10, 424–30.
442. Huey, G.R., Stehman, F.B., Roth, L.M. and Ehrlich, C.E. (1985) Lymphangiosarcoma of the edematous thigh after radiation therapy for carcinoma of the vulva. *Gynecol. Oncol.*, 20, 394–401.

443. Muller, R., Hajdu, S.I. and Brennan, M.F. (1987) Lymphangiosarcoma associated with chronic filarial lymphedema. *Cancer*, 59, 174–83.
444. Devi, K.R. and Bahuleyan, C.K. (1977) Lymphangiosarcoma of the lower extremity associated with chronic lymphedema. *Ind. J. Cancer*, 14, 176–8.
445. Sordillo, E.M., Sordillo, P.P., Hajdu, S.I. *et al.* (1981) Lymphangiosarcoma after filarial infection. *J. Dermatol. Surg. Oncol.*, 7, 235–9.
446. Paik, H.H. and Komorowski, R. (1976) Hemangiosarcoma of the abdominal wall following irradiation therapy of endometrial carcinoma. *Am. J. Clin. Pathol.*, 66, 810–14.
447. Goette, D.K. and Detlefs, R.L. (1985) Postirradiation angiosarcoma. *J. Am. Acad. Dermatol.*, 12, 922–6.
448. Chen, K.T.K., Hoffman, K.D. and Hendricks, E.J. (1979) Angiosarcoma following therapeutic irradiation. *Cancer*, 44, 2044–8.
449. Wolov, R.B., Sato, N., Azumi, N. *et al.* (1991) Intra-abdominal 'angiosarcomatosis'. Report of two cases after pelvic irradiation. *Cancer*, 67, 2275–9.
450. Westenberg, A.H., Wiggers, T., Henzen-Logmans, S.C. *et al.* (1989) Postirradiation angiosarcoma of the greater omentum. *Eur. J. Surg. Oncol.*, 15, 175–8.
451. Morgan, M.A., Moutos, D.D.M., Pippitt, A.H. *et al.* (1989) Vaginal and bladder angiosarcoma after therapeutic irradiation. *South. Med. J.*, 82, 1434–6.
452. Nanus, D.M., Kelson, D. and Clark, G.C. (1987) Radiation-induced angiosarcoma. *Cancer*, 60, 777–9.
453. Stokkel, M.P.M. and Peterse, H.L. (1992) Angiosarcoma of the breast after lumpectomy and radiation therapy for adenocarcinoma. *Cancer*, 69, 2965–8.
454. Moskaluk, C.A., Merino, M.J., Danforth, D.N. and Medeiros, L.J. (1992) Low-grade angiosarcoma of the skin of the breast: a complication of lumpectomy and radiation therapy for breast carcinoma. *Hum. Pathol.*, 23, 710–14.
455. Otis, C.N., Peschel, R., Mckhann, C. *et al.* (1986) The rapid onset of cutaneous angiosarcoma after radiotherapy for breast cancer. *Cancer*, 57, 2130–14.
456. Steingaszner, L.C., Enzinger, F.M. and Taylor, H.B. (1965) Hemangiosarcoma of the breast. *Cancer*, 18, 352–61.
457. Davies, J.D., Rees, G.J.G. and Mera, S.L. (1983) Angiosarcoma in irradiated post-mastectomy chest wall. *Histopathology*, 7, 947–56.
458. Sessions, S.C. and Smink, R.D. (1992) Cutaneous angiosarcoma of the breast after segmental mastectomy and radiation therapy. *Arch. Surg.*, 127, 1362–3.
459. Rubin, E., Maddox, W.A. and Mazur, M.T. (1990) Cutaneous angiosarcoma of the breast 7 years after lumpectomy and radiation therapy. *Radiology*, 174, 258–60.
460. Hamels, J., Blondiau, P. and Mirgaux, M. (1981) Cutaneous angiosarcoma arising in a mastectomy scar after therapeutic irradiation. *Bull. Cancer (Paris)*, 68, 353–6.
461. Shaikh, N.A., Beaconsfield, T., Walker, M. and Ghilchik, M.W. (1988) Postirradiation angiosarcoma of the breast – a case report. *Eur. J. Surg. Oncol.*, 14, 449–51.
462. Body, G., Sauvanet, E., Calais, G. *et al.* (1987) Angiosarcoma cutané du sein apres adenocarcinome mammaire opéré et irradié. *J. Gyn. Obstet. Biol. Reprod. (Paris)*, 16, 479–83.
463. Kuten, A., Sapir, D., Cohen, Y. *et al.* (1985) Postirradiation soft tissue sarcoma occurring in breast cancer patients: report of seven cases and results of combination chemotherapy. *J. Surg. Oncol.*, 28, 168–71.
464. Givens, S.S., Ellerbroek, N.A., Butler, J.J. *et al.* (1989) Angiosarcoma rising in an irradiated breast: a case report and review of the literature. *Cancer*, 64, 2214–16.
465. Edeiken, S., Russo, D.P., Knecht, J. *et al.* (1992) Angiosarcoma after tylectomy and radiation therapy for carcinoma of the breast. *Cancer*, 70, 644–7.
466. Segal, S.L., Lenchner, G.S., Cichelli, A.V. *et al.* (1988) Angiosarcoma presenting as diffuse alveolar hemorrhage. *Chest*, 94, 214–16
467. Stotter, A.T., McNeese, M.D., Ames, F.C. *et al.* (1989) Predicting the rate and extent of locoregional failure after breast conservation therapy for early breast cancer. *Cancer*, 64, 2217–25.
468. McCarthy, M.D. and Pack, G.T. (1950) Malignant blood vessel tumors. A report of 56 cases of angiosarcoma and Kaposi's sarcoma. *Surg. Gynecol. Obstet.*, 91, 465–82.
469. Girard, C., Johnson, W.C. and Graham, J.H. (1970) Cutaneous angiosarcoma. *Cancer*, 26, 868–83.
470. Bennett, R.G., Keller, J.W. and Ditty, J.F. (1978) Hemangiosarcoma subsequent to radiotherapy for a hemangioma of infancy. *J. Dermatol. Surg. Oncol.*, 4, 881–3.
471. Ward, C.M. and Buchanan, R. (1977) Haemangiosarcoma following irradiation of a haemangioma of the face (case report). *J. Maxillofac. Surg.*, 5, 164–6.
472. Amendola, B.E., Amendola, M.A., McClatchey, K.D. and Miller, C.H. (1989) Radiation-associated sarcoma: a review of 23 patients with postradiation sarcoma over a 50-year period. *Am. J. Clin. Oncol.*, 12, 411–15.
473. Cancellieri, A., Eusebi, V., Mambelli, V. *et al.* (1991) Well-differentiated angiosarcoma of the skin following radiotherapy. *Pathol. Res. Pract.*, 187, 301–6.
474. Prescott, R.J. and Mainwaring, A.R. (1990) Irradiation-induced penile angiosarcoma. *Postgrad. Med. J.*, 66, 576–9.
475. Ulbright, T.M., Clark, S.A. and Einhorn, L.H. (1985) Angiosarcoma associated with germ cell tumors. *Hum. Pathol.*, 16, 268–72.
476. Hunter, T.B., Martin, P.C., Dietzen, C.D. *et al.* (1985) Angiosarcoma of the breast. Two case reports and review of the literature. *Cancer*, 56, 2099–106.
477. Shore, J.H. (1957) Haemangiosarcoma of the breast. *J. Path. Bact.*, 74, 289–93.
478. Chen, K.T.K., Kirkgaard, D.D. and Bocian, J.J. (1980) Angiosarcoma of the breast. *Cancer*, 46, 368–71.
479. Donnell, R.M., Rosen, P.P., Lieberman, P.H. *et al.* (1981) Angiosarcoma and other vascular tumors of the breast: pathologic analysis as a guide to prognosis. *Am. J. Surg. Pathol.*, 5, 629–42.
480. Merino, M.J., Berman, M. and Carter, D. (1983) Angiosarcoma of the breast. *Am. J. Surg. Pathol.*, 7, 53–60.
481. Gulesserian, H.P. and Lawton, R.L. (1969) Angiosarcoma of the breast. *Cancer*, 24, 1021–6.
482. York, N.G. (1972) Malignant haemangioendothelioma of the breast. *Med. J. Aust.*, 2, 1361–3.
483. Rainwater, L.M., Martin, J.K., Gaffey, T.A. *et al.* (1986) Angiosarcoma of the breast. *Arch. Surg.*, 121, 669–72.
484. Rosen, P.P., Kimmel, M. and Ernsberger, D. (1988) Mammary angiosarcoma. The prognostic significance of tumor differentiation. *Cancer*, 62, 2145–51.
485. Alvarez-Fernandez, E. and Salinero-Paniagua, E. (1981) Vascular tumors of the mammary gland. A histochemical and ultrastructural study. *Virchows Arch. A Pathol. Anat. Histopathol.*, 394, 31–47.
486. Tavassoli, F.A. and Weiss, S.W. (1981) Hemangiopericytoma of the breast. *Am. J. Surg. Pathol.*, 5, 745–52.
487. Sieber, P.R. and Sharkey, F.E. (1986) Cystic hygroma of breast. *Arch. Pathol. Lab. Med.*, 110, 353–5.
488. Rosen, P.P., Jozefczyk, M.A. and Boram, L.H. (1985) Vascular tumors of the breast. IV. Venous hemangioma. *Am. J. Surg. Pathol.*, 9, 659–65.
489. Rosen, P.P. and Ridolfi, R.L. (1977) The perilobular hemangioma. *Am. J. Clin. Pathol.*, 68, 21–23.
490. Jozefczyk, M.A. and Rosen, P.P. (1985) Vascular tumors of the breast. II. Perilobular hemangiomas and hemangiomas. *Am. J. Surg. Pathol.*, 9, 491–503.
491. Lesueur, G.C., Brown, R.W. and Bhathal, P.S. (1983) Incidence of perilobular hemangioma in the female breast. *Arch. Pathol. Lab. Med.*, 107, 308–10.
492. Rosen, P.P. (1985) Vascular tumors of the breast. V. Nonparenchymal hemangiomas of mammary subcutaneous tissues. *Am. J. Surg. Pathol.*, 9, 723–9.
493. Nielsen, B. (1983) Haemangiomas of the breast. *Pathol. Res. Pract.*, 176, 253–7.
494. Conway, J.D. and Smith, M.B. (1951) Hemangio-endothelioma originating in a peripheral nerve. Report of a case. *Ann. Surg.*, 134, 138–41.
495. Fletcher, C.D.M., Beham, A., Bekir, S. *et al.* (1991) Epithelioid angiosarcoma of deep soft tissue: a distinctive tumor readily mistaken for an epithelial neoplasm. *Am. J. Surg. Pathol.*, 15, 915–24.
496. Bricklin, A.S. and Rushton, H.W. (1977) Angiosarcoma of venous origin arising in radial nerve. *Cancer*, 39, 1556–8.
497. Enzinger, F.M. and Weiss, S.W. (1988) Malignant vascular tumors, in *Soft Tissue Tumors*, 2nd edn, C.V. Mosby, Philadelphia, pp. 545–80.
498. Campanacci, M., Boriani, S. and Guinti, A. (1980) Hemangioendothelioma of bone: a study of 29 cases. *Cancer*, 46, 804–14.
499. Abdelwahab, I.F., Kenan, S., Klein, M.J. and Lewis, M.M. (1992) Case report: Angiosarcoma occurring in a bone infarct. *Clin. Radiol.*, 45, 412–14.
500. Wold, L.E., Unni, K.K., Beabout, J.W. *et al.* (1982) Hemangioendothelial sarcoma of bone. *Am. J. Surg. Pathol.*, 6, 59–70.
501. Larsson, S.E., Lorentzen, A.R., Boquist, L. *et al.* (1975) Malignant hemangioendothelioma of bone. *J. Bone Joint Surg.*, 57A, 84–89.
502. MacMahon, H.E., Murphy, A.S. and Bates, M.I. (1947) Endothelial-cell sarcoma of liver following thorotrast injections. *Am. J. Pathol.*, 23, 585–613.
503. Ghandur-Mnaymneh, L. and Gonzalez, M.S. (1981) Angiosarcoma of the penis with hepatic angiomas in a patient with low vinyl chloride exposure. *Cancer*, 47, 1318–24.
504. Livaditolu, A., Alexiou, G., Floros, D. *et al.* (1991) Epithelioid angiosarcoma of the adrenal gland associated with chronic arsenic intoxication? *Pathol. Res. Pract.*, 187, 284–9.
505. Rennke, H., Prat, G.A., Etcheverry, R.B. *et al.* (1971) Hemangioendotelioma maligno del higado y arsenicismo cronico. *Rev. Med. Chile*, 99, 664–8.
506. Selby, D.M., Stocker, J.T. and Ishak, K.G. (1992) Angiosarcoma of the liver in childhood: a clinicopathologic and follow-up study of 10 cases. *Pediatr. Pathol.*, 12, 485–98.

507. Neshiwat, L.F., Friedland, M.L., Somorr-Lesnick, B. *et al.* (1992) Hepatic angiosarcoma. *Am. J. Med.*, 93, 219–22.
508. Makk, L., Delmore, F., Creech, J.L. *et al.* (1976) Clinical and morphologic features of hepatic angiosarcoma in vinyl chloride workers. *Cancer*, 37, 149–63.
509. Popper, H., Thomas, L.B., Telles, N.C. *et al.* (1978) Development of hepatic angiosarcoma in man induced by vinyl-chloride, thorotrast and arsenic. *Am. J. Pathol.*, 92, 349–76.
510. Hoch-Ligeti, C. (1978) Angiosarcoma of the liver associated with diethylstilbestrol. *J. Am. Med. Ass.*, 240, 1510–1.
511. Falk, H., Thomas, L.B., Popper, H. and Ishak, K. (1979) Hepatic angiosarcoma associated with androgenic anabolic steroids. *Lancet*, 2, 1120–2.
512. Alrenga, D.P. (1975) Primary angiosarcoma of the liver. Review article. *Int. Surg.*, 60, 198–203.
513. Block, J.B. (1974) Angiosarcoma of the liver following vinyl chloride exposure. *J. Am. Med. Ass.*, 229, 53–54.
514. Ludwig, J. and Hoffman, H.N. (1975) Hemangiosarcoma of the liver. Spectrum of morphologic changes and clinical findings. *Mayo Clin. Proc.*, 50, 255–63.
515. Kauffman, S.L. and Stout, A.P. (1961) Malignant hemangioendothelioma in infants and children. *Cancer*, 14, 1186–96.
516. Sussman, E.B., Nydick, I. and Gray, G.F. (1974) Hemangioendothelial sarcoma of the liver and hemochromatosis. *Arch. Pathol. Lab. Med.*, 97, 39–42.
517. da Silva Horta, J. (1956) Late lesions in man caused by colloidal thorium dioxide (Thorotrast). *Arch. Pathol. Lab. Med.*, 62, 403–18.
518. Thomas, L.B., Popper, H., Berk, P.D. *et al.* (1975) Vinyl-chloride-induced liver disease. From idiopathic portal hypertension (Banti's syndrome) to angiosarcoma. *New Engl. J. Med.*, 292, 17–22.
519. Creech, J.L. and Johnson, M.N. (1974) Angiosarcoma of liver in the manufacture of polyvinyl chloride. *J. Occup. Med.*, 16, 150–1.
520. Noronha, R. and Gozalez-Crussi, F. (1984) Hepatic angiosarcoma in childhood. A case report and review of the literature. *Am. J. Surg. Pathol.*, 8, 863–71.
521. Kojiro, M., Nakashima, T., Ito, Y. *et al.* (1985) Thorium dioxide-related angiosarcoma of the liver. Pathomorphologic study of 29 autopsy cases. *Arch. Pathol. Lab. Med.*, 109, 853–7.
522. Kohiro, M., Kawano, Y., Kawasaki, H. *et al.* (1982) Thorotrast-induced hepatic angiosarcoma and combined hepatocellular and cholangiocarcinoma. *Cancer*, 49, 2161–4.
523. Falk, H., Herbert, J.T., Edmonds, L. *et al.* (1981) Review of four cases of childhood hepatic angiosarcoma – elevated environmental arsenic exposure in one case. *Cancer*, 47, 382–91.
524. Lander, J.J., Stanley, R.J., Sumner, H.W. *et al.* (1975) Angiosarcoma of the liver associated with Fowler's solution (postassium arsenate). *Gastroenterology*, 68, 1582–6.
525. Regelson, W., Kim, U., Ospina, J. *et al.* (1968) Hemangioendothelial sarcoma of liver from chronic arsenic intoxication by Fowler's solution. *Cancer*, 21, 514–22.
526. Cortez Pimentel, J. and Peixoto Menezes, A. (1977) Liver disease in vineyard sprayers. *Gastroenterology*, 72, 275–83.
527. Wolkinson, H.A., Lucas, J.C. and Foote, F.W. (1968) Primary splenic angiosarcoma. *Arch. Pathol. Lab. Med.*, 85, 213–18.
528. Autrey, J.R. and Weitzner, S. (1975) Hemangiosarcoma of the spleen with spontaneous rupture. *Cancer*, 35, 534–9.
529. Aranha, G.V., Gold, J. and Grage, T.B. (1976) Hemangiosarcoma of the spleen: report of a case and review of previously reported cases. *J. Surg. Oncol.*, 8, 481–7.
530. Chen, K.T.K., Bolles, J.C. and Gilbert, E.F. (1979) Angiosarcoma of the spleen. *Arch. Pathol. Lab. Med.*, 103, 122–4.
531. Smith, V.C., Eisenberg, B.L. and McDonald, E.C. (1985) Primary splenic angiosarcoma. Case report and literature review. *Cancer*, 55, 1625–7.
531a. Falk, S., Krishnan, J. and Meis, J.M. (1993) Primary angiosarcoma of the spleen. A clinicopathologic study of 40 cases. *Am. J. Surg. Pathol.*, 17, 959–70.
532. Leake, J., Sheehan, M.P., Rampling, D. *et al.* (1992) Angiosarcoma complicating xeroderma pigmentosum. *Histopathology*, 21, 179–81.
533. Mena, H., Ribas, J.L., Enzinger, F.M. *et al.* (1991) Primary angiosarcoma of the central nervous system. *J. Neurosurg.*, 75, 73–76.
534. Lamont, J.S., Hesketh, P.J., de las Morenas, A. *et al.* (1991) Primary angiosarcoma of the seminal vesicle. *J. Urol.*, 146, 165–7.
535. Sirgi, K.E., Wick, M.R. and Swanson, P.E. (1993) B72.3 and CD34 immunoreactivity in malignant epithelioid soft tissue tumors. Adjuncts in the recognition of endothelial neoplasms. *Am. J. Surg. Pathol.*, 17, 179–85.
536. Kareti, L.R., Katlein, S. and Blauvelt, A. (1988) Angiosarcoma of the adrenal gland. *Arch. Pathol. Lab. Med.*, 112, 1163–5.
537. Cookston, M., Cotter, G.W., Schlitt, M. *et al.* (1991) Primary angiosarcoma of the brain. *South. Med. J.*, 84, 517–20.
538. Burke, A.P. and Virmani, R. (1993) Sarcomas of the great vessels. A clinicopathologic study. *Cancer*, 71, 1761–73.
539. Janigan, D.T., Husian, A. and Robinson, N.A. (1986) Cardiac angiosarcoma. A review and a case report. *Cancer*, 57, 852–9.
540. Pfaltz, M., Hedinger, C., Saramaslani, P. *et al.* (1983) Malignant hemangioendothelioma of the thyroid and Factor VIII-related antigen. *Virchows Arch. A Pathol. Anat. Histopathol.*, 401, 177–84.
541. Ruchti, C., Gerbert, H.A. and Schaffner, T. (1984) Factor VIII-related antigen in malignant hemangioendothelioma of the thyroid: additional evidence for the endothelial origin of this tumor. *Am. J. Clin. Pathol.*, 82, 474–80.
542. Allred, C.D., Cathey, W.J. and McDivitt, R.W. (1981) Primary renal angiosarcoma: a case report. *Hum. Pathol.*, 12, 665–8.
543. Cason, J.D., Waisman, J. and Plaine, L. (1987) Angiosarcoma of kidney. *Urology*, 30, 281–3.
544. Stroup, R.M. and Chang, Y.C. (1987) Angiosarcoma of the bladder: a case report. *J. Urol.*, 137, 984–5.
545. Ongkasuwan, C., Taylor, J.E., Chik-Kwun, T. and Prempree, T. (1982) Angiosarcomas of the uterus and ovary. Clinopathologic report. *Cancer*, 49, 1469–75.
546. Smith, D.M., Manivel, C., Kapps, D. *et al.* (1986) Angiosarcoma of the prostate: report of 2 cases and review of the literature. *J. Urol.*, 135, 382–4.
547. Milne, D.S., Hinshaw, K., Malcolm, A.J. *et al.* (1990) Primary angiosarcoma of the uterus: a case report. *Histopathology*, 16, 203–5.
548. Alles, J.U. and Bosslet, K. (1988) Immunocytochemistry of angiosarcomas. A study of 19 cases with special emphasis on the applicability of endothelial cell specific markers to routinely prepared tissues. *Am. J. Clin. Pathol.*, 89, 463–71.
549. Ehrmann, R.L. and Griffiths, C.T. (1979) Malignant hemangioendothelioma of the uterus. *Gynecol. Oncol.*, 8, 376–83.
550. Case records of the Massachusetts general hospital (1954) Case 40191. *New Engl. J. Med.*, 250, 837–43.
551. Tralka, G.A. and Katz, S. (1963) Hemangioendothelioma of the lung. *Am. Rev. Respir. Dis.*, 87, 107–15.
552. Prince, C. (1942) Primary angio-endothelioma of the kidney: report of a case and brief review. *J. Urol.*, 47, 787–92.
553. Ben-Izhak, O., Auslander, L., Rabison, S. *et al.* (1992) Epithelioid angiosarcoma of the adrenal gland with cytokeratin expression: report of a case with accompanying mesenteric fibromatosis. *Cancer*, 69, 1808–12.
553a. Wenig, B.M., Abbondanzo, S.L. and Heffess, C.S. (1994) Epithelioid angiosarcoma of the adrenal glands. A clinicopathologic study of nine cases with a discussion of the implications of finding 'epithelial-specific' markers. *Am. J. Surg. Pathol.*, 18, 62–73.
554. Chan, K.W. (1990) Case report: angiosarcoma of the prostate. An immunohistochemical study of a case. *Pathology*, 22, 108–10.
555. McCaughey, W.T.E., Dardick, I. and Barr, J.R. (1983) Angiosarcoma of serous membranes. *Arch. Pathol. Lab. Med.*, 107, 304–7.
556. Brown, R.W., Tornos, C. and Evans, H.L. (1992) Angiosarcoma arising from malignant schwannoma in a patient with neurofibromatosis. *Cancer*, 70, 1141–4.
557. Chauduri, B., Ronan, S.G. and Manaligod, J.R. (1980) Angiosarcoma arising in a plexiform neurofibroma. *Cancer*, 46, 605–10.
558. Millstein, D.I., Chik-Kwun, T. and Campbell, E.W. (1981) Angiosarcoma developing in a patient with neurofibromatosis (von Recklinghausen's disease). *Cancer*, 47, 950–4.
559. Lederman, S.M., Martin, A.C., Laffey, K.T. *et al.* (1987) Hepatic neurofibromatosis, malignant schwannoma, and angiosarcoma in von Recklinghausen's disease. *Gastroenterology*, 92, 234–9.
560. Macaulay, A.A. (1978) Neurofibrosarcoma of the radial nerve in von Recklinghausen's disease with metastatic angiosarcoma. *J. Neurol. Neurosurg. Psychiatry*, 41, 474–8.
561. Riccardi, V.M., Wheeler, T.M., Pickard, L.R. and King, B. (1984) The pathophysiology of neurofibromatosis: II. Angiosarcoma as a complication. *Cancer Genet. Cytogenet.*, 12, 275–80.
562. Weiss, W.M., Riles, T.S., Gouge, T.H. and Mizrachi, H.H. (1991) Angiosarcoma at the site of a dacron vascular prosthesis: a case report and literature review. *J. Vasc. Surg.*, 14, 87–91.
563. Hayman, J. and Huygens, H. (1983) Angiosarcoma developing around a foreign body. *J. Clin. Pathol.*, 36, 515–18.
564. Fehrenbacher, J.W., Bowers, W., Strate, R. *et al.* (1981) Angiosarcoma of the aorta associated with a dacron graft. *Ann. Thorac. Surg.*, 32, 297–301.
565. Dube, V.E. and Fisher, D.E. (1972) Hemangioendothelioma of the leg following metallic fixation of the tibia. *Cancer*, 30, 1260–6.
566. Jennings, T.A., Peterson, L., Axiotis, C.A. *et al.* (1988) Angiosarcoma associated with foreign body material. A report of three cases. *Cancer*, 62, 2436–44.
567. Keane, M.M. and Carney, D.N. (1993) Angiosarcoma arising from a defunctionalized arteriovenous fistula. *J. Urol.*, 149, 364–5.
568. Byers, R.J., McMahon, R.F.T., Freemont, A.J. *et al.* (1992) Epithelioid angiosarcoma arising in an arteriovenous fistula. *Histopathology*, 21, 87–9.
569. Hermann, J.B. (1965) Lymphangiosarcoma of the chronically edematous extremities. *Surg. Gynecol. Obstet.*, 121, 1107–15.
570. Bischoff, F. and Bryson, G. (1964) Carcinogenesis through solid state surfaces. *Prog. Expl Tumor. Res.*, 5, 85–133.

571. Brand, K.G., Johnson, K.H. and Buoen, L.C. (1976) Foreign body tumorigenesis. *CRC Crit. Rev. Toxicol.*, **4**, 353–94.
572. Ben-Izhak, O., Kerner, H., Brenner, B. *et al.* (1992) Angiosarcoma of the colon developing in a capsule of a foreign body. *Am. J. Clin. Pathol.*, **97**, 416–20.
573. Oppenheimer, B.S., Oppenheimer, E.T., Stout, A.P. *et al.* (1958) The latent period in carcinogenesis by plastics in rats and its relation to the presarcomatous stage. *Cancer*, **11**, 204–13.
574. Hudson, C.P., Hanno, R. and Callen, J.P. (1984) Cutaneous angiosarcoma in a site of healed herpes zoster. *Int. J. Dermatol.*, **23**, 404–7.
575. Mackay, B., Ordonez, N.G. and Huang, W.-L. (1989) Ultrastructural and immunocytochemical observations on angiosarcomas. *Ultrastruct. Pathol.*, **13**, 97–110.
576. Marrogi, A.J., Hunt, S.J. and Santa Cruz, D.J. (1990) Cutaneous epithelioid angiosarcoma. *Am. J. Dermatopathol.*, **12**, 350–6.
577. Gray, M.H., Rosenberg, A.E., Dickersin, G.R. *et al.* (1990) Cytokeratin expression in epithelioid vascular neoplasms. *Hum. Pathol.*, **21**, 212–17.
578. Leader, M., Collins, M., Patel, J. *et al.* (1986) Staining for factor VIII related antigen and *Ulex europaeus* agglutinin (UEA-I) in 230 tumours. An assessment of their specificity for angiosarcoma and Kaposi's sarcoma. *Histopathology*, **10**, 1153–62.
579. Guarda, L.A., Ordonez, N.G., Smith, J.L. *et al.* (1984) Immunoperoxidase localization of Factor VIII in angiosarcomas. *Arch. Pathol. Lab. Med.*, **108**, 129–32.
580. Little, D., Said, J.W., Siegel, R.J. *et al.* (1986) Endothelial cell markers in vascular neoplasms: an immunohistochemical study comparing Factor VIII-related antigen, blood group specific antigens, 6-Keto-PGFl alpha, and *Ulex europaeus* I lectin. *J. Pathol.*, **149**, 89–95.
581. Sehested, M. and Hou-Jensen, K. (1981) Factor VIII-related antigen as an endothelial marker in benign and malignant diseases. *Virchows Arch. A Pathol. Anat. Histopathol.*, **391**, 217–25.
582. Eusebi, V., Carcangiu, M.L., Dina, R. *et al.* (1990) Keratin-positive epithelioid angiosarcoma of the thyroid. A report of four cases. *Am. J. Surg. Pathol.*, **14**, 737–47.
583. Maiorana, A., Fante, R., Fano, R.A. *et al.* (1991) Epithelioid angiosarcoma of the buttock. Case report with immunohistochemical study on the expression of keratin polypeptides. *Surg. Pathol.*, **4**, 325–32.
584. McConnell, E.M. and Haslem, P. (1959) Angiosarcoma in postmastectomy lymphoedema. A report of five cases and review of the literature. *Br. J. Surg.*, **46**, 322–32.
585. Ramani, P., Bradley, N.J. and Fletcher, C.D.M. (1990) QBEND/10, a new monoclonal antibody to endothelium: assessment of its diagnostic utility in paraffin sections. *Histopathology*, **17**, 237–42.
586. Traweck, S.T., Kandalaft, P.L., Mehta, P. *et al.* (1991) The human progenitor cell antigen (CD34) in vascular neoplasia. *Am. J. Clin. Pathol.*, **96**, 25–31.
587. Battifora, H. (1990) Expression of keratins by endothelial cells: Atavism or anarchy? *Ultrastruct. Pathol.*, **14**, iii–v (editorial).
588. Ordonez, N.G. and Batsakis, J.G. (1984) Comparison of *Ulex europaeus* I lectin and Factor VIII-related antigen in vascular lesions. *Arch. Pathol. Lab. Med.*, **108**, 129–32.
589. Messmer, E.P., Font, R.L., McCrary III, J.A. *et al.* (1983) Epithelioid angiosarcoma of the orbit presenting as Tolosa–Hunt syndrome. A clinicopathologic case report with review of the literature. *Ophthalmology*, **90**, 414–21.

INDEX

Page numbers appearing in **bold** refer to figures and page numbers appearing in *italic* refer to tables.

Abducent nerve, compression by vertebral artery 440
Abetalipoproteinemia (Bassen–Kornzweig syndrome) 146–7
Abnormal arteriovenous communication 517–50
Acetylcholine 555, **556**
Acid lipase deficiency 139
Acid maltase (alpha-1-glucosidase) deficiency 409
Acquired progressive lymphangioma (benign lymphangioendothelioma) 770
Acquired tufted angioma (angioblastoma; progressive capillary haemangioma) 757–758
Acral arteriovenous tumors 753
(Acro)-angiodermatitis (pseudo-Kaposi's syndrome) 770
Acromegaly 16, 399
Adaptation 16–18, 204
Adenosine diphosphate **556**, **558**
Adenosine triphosphate 447, 554, **556**, **558**
Adhesion molecules 333, 345–6
Adrenal gland, hyaline globules 454
Adrenergic neurotransmitters 555
Adventitial cystic degeneration or disease 262
Aggrecan 107
Aging (senescence) 224
Alcoholism, subdural hematoma associated 463
Aldosterone 556–7
Alkaline phosphatase 322
Alkaline phosphatase–anti-alkaline phosphatase 320
Allergic vasculitis (hypersensitivity vasculitis) 636–7, 649–50
α-/β-adrenergic receptor blocking agents 581
Alpha-1-glucosidase (acid maltase) deficiency 409
Alport's syndrome 99
Alzheimer's disease 480
Aminoacid metabolism diseases 147–50
β-aminoproprionitrile 118–19
Aminorex fumarate 605
Amyloidosis 157–60, 262, 477, 685
    AA amyloidosis 158
    AL amyloidosis 158–9
    ATTR 159
    extensive 478
    hemodialysis associated 158
    hereditary 158
    senile cardiovascular 159–60
Anal hemorrhoids 547
Anaphylatoxin C5a 334
Aneurysms 2, 353–409
    abdominal aorta 556
    acid maltase deficiency associated 409
    aortic, *see* Aortic aneurysm
    aortic sinus 33, **36**, 368
    berry, *see* Berry aneurysm
    carotid
        cavernous segment 378
        extracranial 369
    celiac artery 373–4
    cerebral arteries 254, 377
        in acromegalics 16
        in infants 409
    Charcot–Bouchard 566, 580
    colic arteries 373
    coronary arteries 372–3
    diagnostic angiography 710–12
    dissecting 354, 404–7
        cerebral arteries 405–7
        cervical arteries 404
        splanchnic arteries 404–5
    false 80, 353, **354**, 408
    femoral artery 370
    fungal (mycotic) 403
    fusiform 353–4, **358**, 378–9
    gastric arteries 373
    gastroepiploic artery 373
    hemodynamic stress in 375–6
    iatrogenic 408–9
    iliac artery 370
    infections 377
    inflammatory 338, 340, 349
    intracranial saccular 537–8
    jejunal artery 373–4
    mesenteric arteries 373–4
    miliary (microaneurysm) 254, 354, 407, 455, 474–5, 480
        hemorrhage from 468
        retinal 407
        skin capillaries 407
    murmurs induced by 7
    mycotic (septic emboli) 401–3
    neoplastic (oncotic) 403–4
    neurofibromatosis associated 409
    osteogenesis imperfecta associated 409
    pancreaticoduodenal artery 373–4
    parasitic 403
    popliteal artery 370–1
    progeria associated 409
    progressive enlargement 376
    pulmonary artery 368–9
        dissecting 369
        Rasmussen's 368
    renal artery 373
    rupture 374–7
        in pregnancy 375
    saccular 354
        unrelated to forks 379–80
    spinal arteries 400
    splanchnic arteries 371
    splenic artery 373
    subclavian artery 370
    thoracic duct 408
    3-M associated 409
    thrombosis in 376
        mural 376–7
    traumatic 80
    cerebral arteries 401
    peripheral arteries 400–61
    true 353, **354**
    umbilical artery 374
    vein of Galen 548
    venous 407–8, 548–9
        therapeutic 408
    vertebral artery 369–70
Angiitis, *see* Vasculitis
Angina pectoris 565
    variant (Prinzmetal's angina) 682
Angioblast 13–14
Angioblastoma (acquired tufted angioma; progressive capillary hemangioma) 757–8, 759
Angiocytic matrix vesicles 212–14
Angiodysplasia 489
Angioendotheliomatosis 743–5
    benign (reactive) 744–5
    malignant 743, 745
Angiogenesis 13–15, 736–7
    post-natal 15
    tumor 737
Angiography 691
Angiokeratoma 752
Angiokeratoma corporis diffusum universale (Fabry's disease) 137–8
Angiolymphoid hyperplasia with eosinophilia (epithelioid hemangioma) 746–9
Angiomalacia 245
Angioma serpiginosum 760
Angiomas 754
    acquired tufted (angioblastoma; progressive capillary hemangioma) 757, 759
Angiomatosis 755
Angioplasty effects 82
Angiosarcomas 319, 749, 755, 772–5
    breast parenchyma 774–5
    deep soft tissue 774
    face and scalp 712–13
    foreign body associated 775
    lymphedema associated 773
    morphology 775
    postirradiation 773
Angiotensin 554
    I 557
    II 555–7
Angiotensin converting enzyme 554, 557
    inhibitors 581
Ankylosing spondylitis 341
Anterior cerebral artery compression 441
Anterior inferior cerebellar artery, compression effect 440
Antibodies
    handling 319
    monoclonal, used in immunophenotyping *318*, 319
    screening 319
    storage 319
    to modified lipoproteins 331

used in vascular pathology 318–19
Anticoagulant therapy 481
Antihypertensive agents *580*
Antineutrophil cytoplasmic antibodies 623
Antioxidants 240–1
Antiphospholipid syndromes 652
Aorta
  abdominal coarctation 31–2
  aneurysm, see Aortic aneurysm
  anomalies 27–42
  arch, see Aortic arch
  ascending aorta hypoplasia 28
  ascending aorta obstruction 27–8
    hourglass type 27, **28**
    hypoplastic type 27, **28**
    membranous type 27–8
  atherosclerosis, see under Atherosclerosis
  benign tumors 731–2
  coarctation 13, 396
    aortic dissection 28, 32
    between left common carotid and left subclavian arteries 42
    infection 28, 33
    mesenteric vascular necrosis after surgical correction 580
    thoracic 31–2
  complete severance 80
  dissection
    diagnostic angiography 712–14
    with coronary luminal compression 691–2
  false aneurysm 80
  hypertension degeneration 367
  intimal tear 572–3
  leiomyosarcoma 730–1
  medial degeneration (medionecrosis) 252–3
  non-penetrating injury 80
  non-sarcomatous neoplasms 731–2
  post-stenotic dilatation 362–3
  sarcoma 729–31, **732**
Aortic aneurysm 2, 184, 338, 339, 340, 355–7
  abdominal 556
    inflammatory 362
  associated conditions 341
  atherosclerotic 357–62
  children 362
  complications 360
  death from 359–60
  dissection 363–8
    aortic valve stenosis associated 367
    associated conditions 366–7
    blunt abdominal injury causing 366
    cocaine associated 368
    rupture 365
    types 365
  elastolytic 361
  neonatal, post-umbilical artery catheterization 361–2
  post-leg amputation 361
  proteolyic activity in 361
  rupture 359, 362
  syphilitic 355–7
  tuberculous 357
  young adults 361
Aortic arch
  abnormal course and/or branching 35
    with intact arch/arches 35–42
  aneurysm 2
  arch-descending aorta junction coarctation 29–31
  cervical 42
  double 35–8

hypothetical double aortic arch of Edwards 35, **36**, **37**
  interruption 38
interruption 32–3, **34**, 35
  left-sided 38
    with right descending aorta 39
  right 39–42
    mirror image branching, without retroesophageal segment 40
    with isolation of left subclavan artery 40, **41**
    with left descending aorta 37, 40
    with retroesophageal segment 40–1
    with right descending aorta/aberrant left subclavian artery 40
  tubular hypoplasia 28–9
Aortic arch syndrome, see Takayasu arteritis
Aortic associated lymphoid tissue 344
Aortic root dilatation 367
Aortic stenosis/regurgitation 683
Aortic ulcer with hematoma, diagnostic angiography 714
Aortic valve
  bicuspid 32
  stenosis 367
Aortitis 341, 625–9
Aorto-left ventricular tunnel 34, **36**
Apo-A$_1$ 284, 285
  chemical/physical characterization in arteries 292–3
Apo-AI$_{Milano}$ 144
Apo-B 274, 277–82, 291, 299
Apo-C$_{III}$ 275
Apocrine secretion 212
Apoprotein E-deficient rat 143
Aortopulmonary septal defect 21–3
  associated conditions 23
Arachidonic acid 558
Arginine vasopressin 554, 556
Arterialization 16
Arteriectasis 254, 353, 355, 377–8
Arteries 2–9
  anatomical nomenclature of sites about forks 7
  anatomical variations 11
  angle of bifurcation 3–4
  aplasia 12
  area ratio (branching coefficient) 5–6
  calibre 2
  compression by 2–3
  cross-sectional area at fork 4–5
  hypoplasia 12
  medial defects of Forbus (medial raphes) 8–9
  murmurs induced in 6–7
  structure 2
    intima 7
    medial elastic lamellar units 7–8
Arterioles 9
  fibrinoid necrosis 574–5
Arterioliths 80
Arteriolosclerosis 175
Arteriomegaly 16, 353–4, 360
Arteriosclerosis (diffuse hyperplastic sclerosis) 175, 253–5
Arteriovenous communications (anastomoses) 9, 354, 546–7
Arteriovenous fistula 76, 250–1, 354, 517–50, 543
  acute 519
  artery pressures 520–1
  artery proximal 6, 17
  bruit 517, 520
  chronic 520

  collateral vessels 521–2, 524
  cranial dural 543
  erythrocyte life span 212
  femoral 519
  hemodynamics 519–22
  magnitude of shunt 520
  proximal vein pressure 521
  sacral dural 543
  thrill 517, 520
  traumatic 522–3
    complications 523–4
    self-cure by thrombosis 523
Arteriovenous malformations 680–1, 754
  diagnostic angiography 716–17
Arteriovenous shunts 549–50
  therapeutic 546
    for hemodialysis 546
Arteriovenous shunts with tumors 547
Arteritis
  atheroembolism-induced 426–7
  non-specific 679
  see also Vasculitis
Astrocytoma, see Glioblastoma multiforme
Ataxia telangiectasia (Louis–Bar syndrome) 489, 493, 544
Atheroembolism 415–33
  arteritis due to 426–7
  cerebral 422
    experimental 429–31
  clinical effects 416
  coronary 421–2
  cutaneous 417–19
    dermal nodules 418
  distribution 415–16
  experimental models 425
  gastrointestinal tract 422–63
    subnecrotizing ischemia 423
  impaction of platelet aggregates 417
  impaction sequences *430*
  incidence 415–16
  lower limb 417–19, 420–1
    cutaneous necrosis 418
    experimental 431–3
    gangrene 418, 420
    intermittent claudication 418
    pain 417–18
    proximal ulcerated atheroma 421
    purple toes 418
  pathogenesis 429
  platelet reaction to atheroma contents 425–6
  renal 419–20
    experimental 427–9
  surgical problem 423–5
  visceral 419
Atherogenesis 271–308
  smooth muscle cells in 211–12
  thrombogenic hypothesis 83–5, 242–7
Atheroma 175
Atherosclerosis 68, 119–21, 175–252, 329, 560
  aetiology 225–52
    epidemiological evidence 239–40
    experimental evidence 238
    pathological evidence 237–8
  angiocytic matrix vesicles 212
  aorta 177–84, **185**
    aneurysm 180, 184
    intimal proliferation 181, 183
    ulceration 179, 180
    vasa vasorum 184
  associated disorders 219–25
    aging 224
    connective tissue disorder 222

copper deficiency 223
diabetes mellitus 221
emotional stress 221
homocystinuria 222–3
hypertension 220–1
immunological 221–2
Menkes' syndrome 223
progeria 224–5
virus-induced atherosclerosis 222
vitamin C 223
Werner's syndrome 225
zinc deficiency 223
carotid arteries 194–5
 internal 12
cerebral 185–91
 electron microscopy 190–1
 microscopy 187–90
collagen changes 119–20
complications 197–202
 aneurysmal dilatation 197–8
 calcification 201
 ectasia 197–8
 hypertension 201–2, 202
 intimal tear 199–200
 ischaemia 201
 rupture 199–200
 stenosing intimal proliferation 201
 thromboembolism 200–1
 tortuosities 198–9
 ulceration 199–200
coronary 191–3, 679
diagnostic methods 700–3
 angiography 700, 701–3
 computed tomography 700
 ultrasound 700
diet effect 347
diet-induced (non-human primates) 561
drug effects 347
early lesions 196–7
 proliferative lesion 196
 tears in internal elastic lamina 196–7
endothelial cells 209
Evans blue staining 215
exercise effect 251–2
genetics 220
haemodynamic models 247–9
 carotid jugular arteriovenous
  fistulae 247
 experimental aneurysms 247
 experimental arterial forks 248
 femoral arteriovenous fistulae 248–9
 half-ring bypass graft with stenosis 248
 hypercholesterolemia/altered
  hemodynamics 249
 nephrectomy 248
 tortuosities 247
 U-bends 248
history 175–6
hypotheses
 fatigue 246–7
 imbibition 213–14
 intimal injury 180, 204, 208, 242–3
 lipid 225–37
 lipid oxidation 240–1
 mechanical/haemodynamic 244–6
  trauma 245–6
  wear and tear 245
 monoclonal 243–4
 thrombogenic 241–2
 unifying 244
inflammation associated, see Inflammation,
 atherosclerosis associated
intimal proliferation
 in infancy 203–5

in lower animals 207
 localization 205–6
limbs 202
localization 202–3
 factors localizing lesions to specific sites
  202–3
 general topography 202
lower animals 207–8
malignant tumours associated 252
mass transport phenomenon 245
oxyradical damage 240
peripheral vascular disease 195
proteoglycan changes 120
pulmonary arteries 195
regression 238–9
severity assessment 219
sex differences 219–20
single umbilical artery effect 203
small vessels 254
splanchnic arteries 193
tears in internal elastic lamina 206–7
therapeutic models 249–51
 arteriovenous fistula 250–61
 venous bypass graft 249–50
umbilical arteries 196
vascular rejection in organ transplant 252
veins 203
 of arteriovenous shunt 203
vertebral arteries 194–5
virus-induced 222
Atherosclerotic renovascular disease 560–1
Atherosis 257
Atrial natriuretic peptide **554**
Atrioventricular septal defects 599–600
Autoimmune diseases
 chronic periaortitis compared 347–8
 connective tissue 600
Avidin-biotin system 320, **321**

Bacillary angiomatosis 739–40, 771
Bacterial endocarditis, cerebral embolism
 451
Bassen–Kornzweig syndrome
 (abetalipoproteinemia) 146–7
Batten's disease 139–40
Battered baby syndrome 463
Behçet's disease 650–1
Benign lymphangioendothelioma (acquired
 progressive lymphangioma) 770
Benign vascular tumors 749–60
Berry aneurysms 354, 376, 380–94, 481,
 547
 aetiology 399–400
 associated conditions 394–9
  anatomical variation of circle of Willis
   395
  cerebral arteriovenous communications
   396
  cerebral tumors 398–9
  coarctation of aorta 396
  congenital abnormalities 396
  Ehlers–Danlos syndrome 397
  fibromuscular dysplasia/hyperplasia
   397
  fusiform dilatation of carotid artery 399
  growth hormone effect on arteries 399
  headache 399
  hypertension 395
  Marfan's syndrome 398
  moyamoya disease 398
  orbital pain 399
  phaeochromocytoma 399
  polycystic disease of kidney 396
  pseudoxanthoma elasticum 395

  sickle cell anaemia 399
  systemic lupus erythematosus 399
  tuberous sclerosis 399
 initiation/development 388–90
 pathology 381–90
  cerebellar degeneration 394
  embolism 393
  ischaemic lesions 393
  microevagination 389–90
  perianeurysmal gliosis 393
  steer-horn (funnel-shaped dilatation)
   389
  thinning areas 393
 pressure effects 393–4
 prognosis 394
 rupture 391–2
  sequelae 394
 subarachnoid haemorrhage 394
 transient ischaemic attacks 393
 ultrastructure 388
Biglycan 107
Biliary cirrhosis 235
Binswanger's disease 484–5
Blalock–Taussig procedure 444
Blood dyscrasias 481–2
Blue rubber bleb syndrome 489, 752
Blue toe syndrome 419
Boecks disease **504**, 506
Bone
 adaptation to stress 18
 fractures, stress/pathological 199, 251
 remodelling 18, 204
 stress deprivation 18
Brachial-basilar insufficiency (subclavian
 steal syndrome) 443–4
Brachiocephalic (innominate) stenosis 444
Bradykinin 556
Brain
 Ammon's horn, arterial supply reduction
  440–1
 arteriovenous communication 530–40
  aetiology 539–40
  anatomical variations 538
  cardiovasculature effects 538–9
  complications 536–9
  haemodynamics 534–5
  histology 535–6
  intellectual impairment 539
  intracranial saccular aneurysms
   associated 537
  midbrain 533
  pathology 532–3
  posterior fossa 534
  pressure effect 539
  prognosis 539
  progression of lesion 537
  small/cryptic 534
 fistulae 530–3
 occipital lobe necrosis 440
 tissue compression 440–1
 vasomotor centre 554
Brain stem
 haemorrhage 476–7
 ischaemia 455
Branham's sign 754
Bronchial artery–pulmonary vein
 anastomosis 545
Bronchus-associated lymphoid tissue 344
Bronchus suis 49
Bruits, see Murmurs
Budd–Chiari syndrome 500, 502, 582
Buerger's disease (thromboangiitis obliterans)
 505, 657–78
 arteriographic findings 637–9

arteriosclerosis distinctions 663
clinical correlation 661
clinical diagnosis 661
clinical presentation 660–1
diagnostic angiography 707–9
diagnostic features 668–73
electron microscopy 675
epidemiology 659–60
etiology 658–9
historical perspective 657–8
immunohistochemistry 673
migrating phlebitis **674**
pathogenesis 658–9
pathology 661–75, **665–72**
   acute phase 663–4, **665–7**
   end-stage 664, **669, 672**
   intermediate phase 664, **668, 670, 671**
   unusual locations 675–7
   vasa vasorum **674**
Bulbospinal tract 554

Cachetin (tumour necrosis factor) 121, 332, 345
Caisson disease 456
Calcinosis (pallidal siderosis; vascular siderosis) 483–4
Calcium channel blockers 581
Calcospherites 212
Calf muscle pump impairment 497
Campbell de Morgan spots 549
Capillaries
  bed 9
  fibrosis 258
  growth/development 14
    postnatal 15
  hemangioma 751–3
Carbon monoxide poisoning 451, 684
Cardiac left-to-right shunts, congenital 598–600
Cardiac myxoma embolus 341, 652
Cardiac transplant rejection 331
Cardiopulmonary changes at birth 589
Carotid-basilar venous plexus fistula 541
Carotid cavernous fistula 540–1
Carotid-jugular arteriovenous fistula 247, 542
Carotid ligation 541
Carotid sinus, ball thrombi in 80
Carotid syphon 2
Carotidynia 439
Carrion's disease (verruga peruana; Oroya fever) 740–2
Castleman's disease 757
Cathepsin G 110
Cavernous hemangioma 529–30, 752–3
Cavernous sinus thrombosis 457
Cell debris 212–14
Cellular immune mechanisms 331
Central-acting alpha-agonists 581
Central nervous system, vascular anomalies 528–30
  see also Brain
Cerebellum
  hemorrhage 472
  herniation 441
    tonsillar necrosis 441
  infarct 446, 449
    red 449
Cerebral amyloid angiopathy (congophilic angiopathy) 477–80
Cerebral arteries
  anatomical displacement 439–40
  atheroembolism 422
  coiling 439–40

kinking 439–40
media 8
neonatal 10, **11**
tortuosity 247, 439–40
  diffuse in children 262
Cerebral arteriovenous communications 396
Cerebral atherosclerosis 441
Cerebral circulation 10–11
Cerebral haemorrhage, serum cholesterol 438
Cerebral infarction (encephalomalacia) 444–54
  laboratory data 454
  pathology 445–54
    adrenal hyaline globules 454
    cardiovascular disease 454
    cerebral swelling 453–4
    distribution of infarcts 449–50
    large vessel embolism 453
    microscopic 447–9
    neurogenic ulceration 454
    pathogenesis of cerebral ischaemia 450–3
    secondary degeneration 454
    small vessel embolism 453
  prognosis 454
Cerebral swelling 453–4
Cerebral tumours 480–1
Cerebral vasculitis 645–53
Cerebral vein thrombosis 457–8
Cerebrospinal blood vessels 10–11
Cerebrotendinous xanthomatosis 147
Cerebrovascular disease 437–85
  cerebral vein thrombosis 457–8
  compression by 440–1
  dural sinus thrombosis 457–8
  epidemiology 438–9
  haematological disorders 456
  hypertension related 439
  lacunar softenings (état lacunaire) 454–5
  microcirculatory occlusions 456
  mortality 437–8
  murmurs 441–2
    arteriovenous fistula 441
    atherosclerotic stenosis 441
    intracranial arterial aneurysm 441–2
    tumours 442
  veins compressed 440
Cerebrovascular insufficiency 442–4
  steal syndromes 443–4
  transient ischaemic attacks 442–3
Ceroid 314, 335
Cervical rib 370
Chest injury 80–1
Chiropractic manipulation of head/neck, embolism precipitated by 453
Cholesterol 214, 428–9, 438
  crystal embolism (rabbits, dogs) 426
  granuloma 426
Cholesterol-fed animals 226–9
Cholesteryl ester-rich particles 304
  uptake 304–6
Cholesteryl ester storage disease 139
Chondrocytic matrix vesicles 212–14
Chondroitin 4-sulphate 106
Chondroitin 6-sulphate 106, 217
Choriocarcinoma 404, 468, 481
Choroid plexus
  haemorrhage 482
  papilloma 398, 482
Chronic dyspnea, unexplained 617
Chronic obstructive jaundice 235
Chronic periaortitis 336–49
  activation/proliferation markers 343–4

aortic associated lymphoid tissue 344
atherosclerosis complication 346–9
  computed tomography 346–7
autoimmune diseases compared 347–8
clinical 338–40, 346
cytokines in 344–5
dilated aorta (inflammatory aneurysm) 340–1
lymphocyte populations 343
theories 348–9
Chronic periarteritis 343
Churg–Strauss syndrome 341, 641, **646, 647**
  central nervous system 648
Circle of Willis 12, 13
  aneurysms 30, 395, 409
  infarction limitation/contribution 451
  postnatal development 16
  steal syndrome associated 444
  variations 11, 12, 395, 473
Circulatory arrest 455
Circulatory changes during maturation 15–16
Coagulation (red) thrombus 500
Coarctation of the aorta 13, 396
  abdominal 31–2
  aortic dissection 28, 32
  berry aneurysms 396
  between left common carotid and left subclavian arteries 42
  infection 28, 33
  mesenteric vascular necrosis 580
  thoracic 31–2
Cocaine abuse 451, 483, 690
Coeliac artery, see Celiac artery
Cogan syndrome 651
Collagens 89–99
  biochemical properties 111
  biosynthesis stages 91
  blood vessel wall containing 216–17
  classification of types 89–90
  Crosslinking 92–5
    copper deficiency effect 118
    lysyl oxidase 92
    non-enzymatic glycosylation 95
    other components 94–5
    reducible crosslink formation 92–4
  FACIT 96–7
  fibril dystrophic arrangement 216
  fibrillary 90–2, 95–6
    assembly 90–2
    biosynthesis 90–2
    structure 90–2
  interaction with low density lipoproteins (LDLs) 276
  type I 90, 90, 95
  type II 90
  type III 90, 95–6
    deficiency 357
  type IV 90, 98–9
  type V 90, 96
  type VI 90, 97, **98**, 99
  type VII 90
  type VIII 90, 97–8
  type IX 90, 97
  type X 90, 98
  type XI 90, 96
  type XII 90, 97
  type XIV 14, 90, 97
Collateral circulation, naturally occurring 12–13
Colonic infarction 360
Congenital anomalies of blood vessels 21–59

Congenital hypoplasia of prefascial lymph
    collectors 508–9
Congophilic angiopathy (cerebral amyloid
    angiopathy) 477–80
Connective tissue (blood vessel walls)
    89–121
  biochemical properties 111
  degradation 108–11
  proteolysis 111
  turnover 108–11
Connective tissue diseases 150–7, 222
Copper deficiency 116–19, 223, 361, 362
  animal models 116–18
  effects on:
    collagen crosslinking 118
    elastin crosslinking 118
  human genetic diseases 119
  sites of action in connective tissue
      metabolism 116
Copper metabolism disorders 163–5
  dietary deficiency 165
Coronary arteries 42–6, 671–85, **694**
  atheroembolism 421–2
    death from 421–2
  atherosclerosis 191–3, 71
  cardiac transplant recipient 687
  dissection 685
  embolism 681–2, **691**
  fistula 680, **689**
  left dominance 12, 25
  luminal compression, with arterial
      dissections 691–3
  mural thickening 684–7
  myocardial bridging of left anterior
      descending artery 688, **689**
  non-atherosclerotic/non-vasculitic diseases
      679–93, **694**
  origin variations 24, 687–8
  origin variations: aorta 42–4
    communication with vessel/cardiac
        chamber 44, **45**
    ectopic origin 42–3
    single coronary artery 43–4
    stenosis of origin 44
  origin variations: pulmonary artery 12,
      44–6, 525
    both arteries 46
    left artery 46, **47**, 525
    right artery 46
  pathophysiology of coronary circulation
      680–2
  right dominance 12
  trauma 693
Coronary arteriovenous fistula 545
Coronary heart disease (CHD) 176, 233
  copper deficiency 223
  coronary artery stenosis 233
  deaths 192
    in joggers, marathon runners 251
  epidemiology 239–40
  familial hypercholesterolaemia associated
      229
  genetic factors 220
  hypertension associated 220
  plasma cholesterol concentration 226
  ochronosis associated 237
  open lung biopsy 618
  right/left coronary artery dominance 12
  smoking effect 226
  type A personality 221
Coronary ostial occlusion 690–1
Coronary sinus 52–3
Coronary thrombosis 690
Coronary thrombolysis 482

Coronary venous bypass graft 372–3
Corrigan's pulse 356, 538
Corticosteroids 347
CREST syndrome 605
Crow–Fukase syndrome (POEMS syndrome;
    Takatsuki syndrome; plasma cell
    dyscrasia) 757
Crutches, vascular injury due to 81
Cryoglobulinemia 625
Cutaneous/small vessel angiitis
    (hypersensitivity angiitis) 636–7, 649
Cutis laxa 115, 119, 153, 357
Cyanotic heart disease, congenital,
    thromboembolic cerebral lesions
    associated 451
Cyclo-oxygenase 557
Cystic adventitial disease 717–19
Cystic hygroma 508
Cystic medionecrosis 252–3, 572
Cystinuria 115
Cytokines (interleukins) 331–3
  polymerase chain reaction 345

Dabska tumor (endovascular papillary
    angioendothelioma) 762, **762**
Decompensated benign nephrosclerosis 579
Decorin 107
Deep angiomatous lesions 753–6
Deep vein thrombosis, lower limb 547–8
Dementia 484
Deoxypyridinoline (lysyl-pyridinoline) 93,
    94
Dermatan sulphate 106
Desmosine 100, **101**
Diabetes mellitus 135–7, 221, 234–5
  animals 137
  arteriolar hyalinization 574
  cardiac dysfunction 136
  polyneuropathy 136
  polyol pathway 137
  renal vascular changes 136
  stroke associated 438
Diagnostic angiography 699–727
  aneurysms 710–12
    complications 710
    false 711
    inflammatory 711–12
    mycotic 711
    peripheral 712
    visceral artery 712
  aortic dissection 712–14
  aortic ulcer with hematoma 714
  arterial entrapment 717–19
  arterial intervention 720–3
  arteriosclerosis 700–3
  arteriovenous malformations 717–18
  Budd–Chiari syndrome 725–6, **727**
  Buerger's disease 707–9
  cystic adventitial disease 717–19
  ergot toxicity 719
  fibromuscular dysplasia 714–16
  hemangioma 719, **720**
  imaging modalities 699
  morphology 699–700
  neurofibromatosis 720
  polyarteritis 709
  pulmonary embolus 725
  radiation fibrosis 720
  vascular grafts 716
  vasculitis 703–7, 710
  venous diseases 723–7
    imaging 723–4
    intervention 726–7
    thrombus 724–5

3,3′-diaminobenzidine 321
Diffuse cystic angiomatosis (diffuse skeletal
    hemangiomatosis) 756
Diffuse hyperplastic sclerosis 175, 253–5
Diffuse phlebectasia of Bockenheimer 491
Diffuse skeletal hemangiomatosis (diffuse
    cystic angiomatosis) 756
Dihydroxylysinonorleucine 94
Disappearing bone disease (phantom bone,
    Gorham's disease) 508, 756
Disseminated intravascular coagulation
    503
Disseminated lipogranulomatosis (Farber's
    disease) 139
Diuretics 581
Down's syndrome 480, 600, 602–3
  atrioventricular septal defects 599–600
  obstructive pulmonary vascular disease
      600
Drug abuse
  cardiovascular effects 483
  cerebral vasculitis associated 651
  necrotizing angiitis 403
Ductus arteriosus
  absence 25
  double 36, 42
Duplication syndrome-9q34 153
Dural sinus thrombosis 457–8

Eclampsia 482
Ehlers–Danlos syndrome 113–15, 155–7,
    397
  aortic aneurysm 357
  aortic sinus dilatation 368
  aortic valve incompetence 368
  arterial aneurysm 564
  biochemical defects 114–15, 155
  menstruation effect 220
  phenotype classification 113–14
  vertebral artery aneurysm 369
  type IV 216, 540
    calf trauma 548
Elastase 110
Elastic membrane 276
Elastin 99–103
  biochemical properties 111
  biosynthesis 99
  blood vessel wall-contained 215
  composition 99–100
  crosslinking 100
    copper deficiency 118
  distribution 100–3
  extensibility 103
  function 100–3
Embolism 504
Encephalomalacia, see Cerebral infarction
Endarterectomy 200
Endarteritis obliterans 257
Endothelial control of vascular tone 557–9
Endothelialitis 331
Endothelin 554, 558, 559
Endothelin-1 **556**, 557
Endothelium 209–10
  cell identification 319
Endothelium-derived relaxant factor 210
Endovascular papillary angioendothelioma
    (Dabska tumor) 762, **762**
Entactin (nidogen) **102**, 104, 217
Enzyme-linked immunosorbent assay
    (ELISA) 345
Epidermal growth factor 417
Epinephrine 554
Epithelioid hemangioendothelioma 764–6
Epithelioid hemangioma (angiolymphoid

hyperplasia with eosinophilia) 746–9
Epulis (granuloma gravidarum; gingival tumor of pregnancy) 749
Erdheim's cystic medial necrosis 366
Ergot toxicity 719
Erysipelas 511
Erythrocytes (red cells) 70, 456
　degeneration 211
　life-span shortening 212
　plasma membrane fragments 212
　sludging 70, 451, 456
E-selectin 333, 345–6
Essential cryoglobulinemia 625
Evans blue 215
Exercise 251–2
Exophthalmos, pulsating 541
External carotid artery steal (internal-external carotid steal) 444
Extracranial arteriocommunications, fistulae 542
Extradural haematoma, cerebral 460–2
　causes 460
　mortality 462
　pathology 461–2
Extradural haematoma, spinal 462
Extrahepatic postsinusoidal obstruction 582

Fabry's disease (angiokeratoma corporis diffusum universale) 137–8, 236, 685–6
Familial apo-AI deficiency 144
Familial apolipoprotein B-100 deficiency 234
Familial apoprotein cII deficiency 141
Familial CIII deficiency 144
Familial dysbetalipoproteinemia (hyperlipoproteinemia III) 142–3
Familial hyperalphalipoproteinemia 144
Familial hypercholesterolemia 141–2, 229–34
　animal model 142
　atherosclerosis compared 231–2
Familial hyperlipoproteinemia, type III 234
Familial hypertriglyceridemia (hyperlipoproteinemia type IV) 143–4
Familial hypoalphalipoproteinemia 144
Familial lecithin-cholesterol acyltransferase (LCAT) deficiency 144–5
Familial lipid metabolic disorders 234–5
Familial lipoprotein lipase deficiency 140–1
Familial Mediterranean fever 158
Farber's disease (disseminated lipogranulomatosis) 139
Fasciitis, intravascular 742, **744**
Fat 313
　dietary 70
　embolism 456
Fatigue hypothesis 246–7
Fatty acids 70
Fetal circulation 2
Fibrillin **102**, 104–5
Fibrinoid necrosis 630–7
Fibroglycan 107
Fibromodulin 107
Fibromuscular dysplasia, arterial 371, 397, 561–3, 689, **690**
　adventitial 689
　central nervous system 652
　diagnostic angiography 714–16
　medial hyperplasia 562
　periarterial hyperplasia 563
Fibromusculointimal proliferation 210–11

Fibronectin **102**, 104, 217
Filariasis 511
Fish-eye disease 144–5
Fluorescein isothiocyanate 321
Foam cell necrosis 329–30
Foix–Alajouanine syndrome 543–4
Fontan atriopulmonary anastomosis 417
Foreign body giant cell 218
Fragile X syndrome (Martin–Bell syndrome) 157
Free fatty acids 427
Fucosidosis 133
Fulvine 605

Galactosemic dogs 137
Galactosyl-hydroxylysine 91
Gaucher's disease (glucosyl ceramide lipidosis) 138–9
Gelatinases A/B *109*, 110
Giant cell aortitis 341
Giant cell (temporal) arteritis 319, 625–30, **634**
　atypical, non-granulomatosis 629, 633
　biopsy 629
　central nervous system 648
　diagnostic angiography 703–7
　granulomatous **632**
　healed 630, **633**
　histopathology 629–30
Gingival tumour of pregnancy (epulis; granuloma gravidarum) 749
Glioblastoma multiforme (astrocytoma types III/IV) 398
　haemorrhage into/about 468, 480
Glucosyl-galactosyl-hydroxylysine 91
Glycogen storage diseases 129
Glycoproteins 103–5
　sub-unit structure **102**
Glycosaminoglycans 272, 275–6
Glucosyl ceramide lipidosis (Gaucher's disease) 138–8
Glypican 107
Gold particles 322
Goodpasture's syndrome 99
Gorham's disease (phantom bone; disappearing bone disease) 508, 756
Granuloma gravidarum (epulis; gingival tumour of pregnancy) 749
Granulomatosis
　lymphomatoid 347, 652
　necrotizing sarcoid 642
　pulmonary angiitis and 637–45
Granulomatous angiitis 649, **650**
Great vein of Galen 441, 457, 458, 548
Gut-associated lymphoid tissue 344

Haemangioblastoma 398
Haemangiolymphangioma 491–2
Haemangioma 719, **720**, 749
　calvarial lesions, extradural/vertebral 544
　capillary 751–2
　cavernous 529–30
　giant 524
　glomeruloid 757
　intramuscular 747–8
　intraosseous 756
　microvenular 756
　multiple 524
　origin 549
　peripheral nerves 756
　progressive capillary (angioblastoma; acquired tufted angioma) 757, **759**
　synovial 756
　targetoid hemosiderotic 758–9, 770

　tendinous 756
　venous 491
　verrucous 752
Haemangioreticulum of Albertini 491
Haemoglobinopathies 161–2
Haemolytic uraemic syndrome 576
Haemorrhoids 13
Haemostasis, thrombosis associated 64–5
Hashimoto's thyroiditis 344
Head injury
　dissecting aneurysm following 453
　false aneurysm following 453
　internal carotid artery thrombosis 453
Head traction effect 81
Heart
　anastomotic channels 78
　congenital disease, open lung biopsy 616
　physical training effect 251
Heath–Edwards classification, modified 599, 616
Heat stroke 482
Hemodynamic hypothesis 246–7
Hemodynamic stress 375–6, 519–22
Heparan sulphate 106
Heparin 106
Hepatitis B antigen 623
Hepatolenticular degeneration (Wilson's disease) 115, 164
Hereditary haemorrhagic telangiectasia (Osler–Weber–Rendu disease) 372, 545
Herpes viruses 331
High density lipoproteins (HDLs) 234, 240, 271
　accumulation in arteries 284–5
　deficiency with planar xanthomas 144
Hippel–Lindau syndrome 489, 493, 546–7
Histidino-hydroxylysinonorleucine 93
Histidino-hydroxymerodesmosine 94
Histochemistry 313–15
　lectin 314–15
　lipid 313–14
　methods 313–15
　　elastic-van Gieson staining 313
　　haematoxylin and eosin 313
　　Nile blue sulphate 314
　　oil-red-O-method 314
　　periodic acid–Schiff 314
Homocystinuria 149, 222–3, 236
Hodgkin's disease 653
Horner's syndrome 39
Human immune mechanisms 331
Human immunodeficiency virus-1 600
Hurler's syndrome (mucopolysaccharidosis II) 129, 130, 131–2, 236–7, 684
Hurler–Scheie syndrome 129
Hutchinson–Gilford syndrome (childhood progeria) 162–3, 224–5,
Hyalin 573–4
Hyaline arteriolosclerosis 255–6, 573–4
Hyaluronic acid 106
Hydroxylase enzyme 91
Hydroxylysine aldehyde (hydroxyallysine) 93
(hydroxy)lysino-5-oxo-norleucine 93
Hydroxylysin-norleucine 93
Hydroxylysin-pyridinoline (pyridinoline) 93, 94
4-hydroxyproline 91
3-hydroxypyridinium crosslinks 93
5-hydroxytryptamine (serotonin) 555, **556**, **558**
Hypercholesterolemia 85, 214, 249, 259–60
Hyperlipidemia 70, 438

Hyperlipoproteinemias 140–4
  III (familial dysbetalipoproteinemia) 142–6
  IV (familial hypertriglyceridemia) 143–4
Hyperoxalurias (oxalosis) 134–5
Hypersensitivity angiitis (cutaneous/small vessel angiitis; allergic vasculitis; leukocytoclastic vasculitis) 636–7, 646
Hypertension, deoxycorticosteroid 559
Hypertension, neoplastic emboli pulmonary 590
Hypertension, portal, see Portal hypertension
Hypertension, systemic 212, 220–1, 553–83
  benign 571, **572**, 573
  cerebral aneurysm associated 395
  cerebral infarction associated 451
  chronic uncontrolled 683
  clinical manifestations 564
  complications 564–80
    abdominal aortic aneurysm 566
    angina pectoris 565–6
    aortic obstruction 566
    cerebral 579–80
    cerebrovascular accident 566
    Charcot–Bouchard aneurysm 566
    decompensated benign nephrosclerosis 578–9
    hypertensive cardiomyopathy 579
    lacunar stroke/infarct 566
    malignant nephrosclerosis 578–9
    mesenteric vascular necrosis 580
    myocardial infarction **564**
    parenchymal changes 576–8
    renal disease 566–7, 576–9
    sudden death 565
    ventricular fibrillation 565
  complications of therapy 580–2
    antihypertensive agents 580, 581–2
  due to:
    cyclosporin A 553
    renal ischemia 76
  endothelial functional changes 558–60
  essential 571
  insulin role 553–4
  malignant 256–7, 571, 574–6
  pathophysiology 553–9
    endothelial control of vascular tone 537–9
    intracellular signal transmission mechanism 555
    kidney 559
    receptors 555
    renin–angiotensin system 556–7
    sympathetic nervous system 553–5
    vascular structural changes 555–6
  reactive changes in blood vessels 571–6
  secondary 571
  stroke related 439
  vascular causes 559–60
Hypertensive encephalopathy 482–3
Hypertrophic cardiomyopathy 162, 683
Hypoalphalipoproteinemias 144–5
Hypobetalipoproteinemia 146
Hypoprothrombinemia 481
Hypocomplementemic urticarial vasculitis 625

Imaging, diagnostic 699–720
Infection-related phlebitis 505
Infection-related vasculitis 625
Inflammatory cells 218, 329–31
  activation 330–1

intimal inflammation 329–30
Innominate (brachiocephalic) stenosis 444
Insulin 553–4
Intercellular adhesion molecule-1 333, 345–6
Interferon-γ 331, 332–3
Interleukins (cytokines) 331–3
  interleukin-1 121, 332
Internal auditory nerve 440
Internal carotid artery 440
  aneurysm 2
  injury 81
  kinking 453
  occlusion 452, 453
  rupture 541
  structures compressed by 440
  tortuosity 439–40
Internal-external carotid steal (external artery steal) 444
Intermediate density lipoprotein (IDL) 271
Interstitial collagenase *109*
Interventional angiography 720–3, 726–7
Intima 7
  thickening 17–18, 71
Intimal injury hypothesis 180, 204, 208, 242–3
Intracellular signal transduction mechanisms 555
Intracerebral haemorrhage 469–82
  primary 468–76
    aetiology 474–6
    associated lesions 472–3
    cerebellar 472
    cerebrum 470–1
    microscopy 473
    mortality 474
    pathology 470–6
  secondary 476–82
    adolescents 482
    blood dyscrasias 481–2
    cerebral amyloid angiopathy 477–80
    children 482
    eclampsia 482
    heat stroke 482
    inflammatory/infectious disorders 482
    neoplasms 480–1
    non-traumatic 476–80
    pontine 471–2
    post-endarterectomy 481
    ring haemorrhages 482
    traumatic 476
Intracranial-extracranial arteriovenous communications 541–2
Intrahepatic post-sinusoidal obstruction 582
Intraspinal haemorrhage 482
Intravascular papillary endothelial hyperplasia 503
Intraventricular haemorrhage 482
Isodesmosine 100, **101**

Jamaican bush tea 605
Jaundice, chronic obstructive 235

Kaposiform infantile hemangioendothelioma 763
Kaposi's sarcoma 512–13, 514, 740, 766–72
  clinical patterns 767
  differential diagnosis 770
  histogenesis 769
  lymphangioma-like variant 770
  nodular 771
  subtypes 766–7
  treatment 771

Kasabach–Merritt syndrome 752, 763
Kawasaki's disease (infantile polyarteritis) 239, 341, 361, 636
Keratan sulphate 106
Keshan disease 165
Keto-amines (oxo-amines) 93
Kidney, role in blood pressure 559
Kimura's disease 745–6
Klippel–Trenaunay syndrome 492–3, 525–6, 745
Klippel–Trenaunay–Weber syndrome 754
Krabbe's syndrome 489, 493
Kuf's disease 139–40

Lambl's excrescences 523–4
Laminin **102**, 104, 217
Laplace's law 202, 355
Larsen's syndrome 147, 150, 157
Lateral medullary syndrome (Wallenberg's syndrome) 449–50
Lathyrogens 118–19
Left atrium, both venae cavae terminating in 52
Left heart failure, acute 590
Left-to-right arterial shunt (systemic artery-pulmonary artery shunt) 524–5
Left ventricular hypertrophy 683
Leptomeningeal veins 10
Leucocyte-platelet thromboembolism 66, 70
Leukocytoclastic vasculitis (hypersensitivity vasculitis) 636–7, 649
Leukaemia 481
Levoatriocardiac vein 58
Ligament, stress deprivation of 18
Light-chain deposition disease 160–1
Lipid 211, 213–14, 438
  definition 313
  intralysosomal 213
  oxidized 335, 347
  smooth muscle cells containing 211
  source in intima/media 213
Lipid hypothesis 225–37
Lipid peroxidation 241
Lipid pneumonia 214
Lipid-rich particles 304–7
Lipoma, intracranial 398–9
Lipomucopolysaccharidosis (sialidosis; mucolipidosis I) 133
Lipoprotein 70, 71, 275, 438
  accumulation in human arteries 285–6
  chemical/physical characterization in human lesions 291–2
  cholesterol-containing 301
  deficiencies 144–7
Lipoproteinaemia type II 237–8
Livedo reticularis 417, 418
Lobular capillary hemangioma (pyogenic granuloma) 749–51
Löeffler's disease 502
Louis–Bar syndrome (ataxia telangiectasia) 489, 493, 544
Low density lipoprotein (LDL) 70, 234, 240, 241, 271–306, 334–5
  arterial proteoglycan complexes, enhanced macrophage uptake 302–3
  characterization in human arteries 286–8
  immune complex phagocytosis by macrophages 303–4
  localization in atherosclerotic lesions of animal models 273–4
  localization in human atherosclerotic arteries 271–2, **273**
  modification by macrophages 334–5

modification by mast cell secretory
        granules 304
modification by products of lipid
        peroxidation 302
oxidized 288–91, 293–301
    characteristics 288–90
    deficient processing in macrophages
        299–301
    extracted from human atherosclerotic
        lesions 290–1
    functional characteristics of aggregated
        particles 293–4, **295, 296**
    functional properties of monomeric
        particles 293
    lesion extracted, functional properties
        296–9
    role in atherogenesis 296
potential underlying mechanisms for
    specific localization 275–6
quantification in human arteries 276–80
quantification in lesions of experimental
    animals 280–2
spatial distribution/accumulation 282–4
ultrastructural, in human lesions 274
Lung carcinoma 252
Lung injury, acute 590
Lymphangiectasis 508
Lymphangitis 511
    filariasis-induced 511
Lymphangioendothelioma 512–13
Lymphangioleiomyomatosis 513
Lymphangioma 506–8
    cavernous 508
    simple 506–8
Lymphangiomatosis
    disseminated 508
    osseous 508
Lymphangiopericytoma 512–13
Lymphangiosarcoma 513–14
Lymphangiosclerosis 260
    primary 509–10
Lymphangiosis, inanimate irritant-induced
    511
Lymphedema 508–9
    congenital malformations associated 509
    primary 509
    secondary 509
Lymphocyte 218
Lymphomatoid granulomatosis 347, 652
Lymphotoxin 332
Lymph vessels
    congenital hypoplasia of superficial lymph
        collectors 489
    degeneration 509
    inflammatory diseases 511
    neoplasias 511–14
    thrombosis 510
    varices 510
Lysyl hydroxylase 91
Lysyl oxidase 92, 100, 116
Lysyl-pyridinoline (deoxypyridinoline) 93,
    94

Macromolecular haematologic syndrome of
    Hueper 73
Macrophage 121, 218, 333–4
    atherosclerotic plaques containing 331
    dead, harmful enzyme release 335
    growth promotion of production 332
    low density lipoprotein modification
        334–5
    response to injury hypothesis 335–6
    scavenger receptors on 335
Maffucci's syndrome 493, 753

Malignant angioendotheliomatosis 646
Mannosidosis 133–4
Marfan's syndrome 105, 112–13, 150–3,
    355
    aortic aneurysm 357, 360, 363
    berry aneurysm 398
    dissecting aneurysm of cervical arteries
        404
    neonatal 152
    progressive childhood form 152
    tortuosities 198
    vertebral artery aneurysm 369
Maroteaux–Lamy syndrome
    (mucopolysaccharidosis VI) 132
Martin–Bell syndrome (fragile X syndrome)
    157
Mastoiditis 457
Matrilysin 109
Matrix proteins (in blood vessel wall)
    215–18
    collagen 216–17
    elastin 215–16
    proteoglycans 217–18
Matrix vesicles 212–14
Mediastinal fibrosis 338
Medionecrosis (medial degeneration of aorta)
    252–3
Melanoma, haemorrhage into/about 468,
    481
Meningioma 398
    blood supply 547
    middle cranial fossa 547
Menkes' disease 119, 164–5, 223
Menstruation 220
Mesenteric vascular necrosis after surgical
    correction of aortic coarctation 580
Metalloproteinases **105**, 108–10
Methysergide maleate 347, 719
Mid-dermal elastolysis 115
Middle cerebral artery, ligation effect 451
Migraine 483
Mitral valve
    chronic rheumatic endocarditis 690, **691**
    infective endocarditis 690, **691**
    stenosis, erythrocyte life-span shortening
        212
Mixed essential cryoglobulinemia 625
Mönckeberg's sclerosis 206, 260–1, 573
Mondor's disease (phlebitis chronica
    obliterans filiformis) 505–6
Monoclonal hypothesis 243–4
Monocrotaline 605
Monocyte 218, 219, 331
Monocyte chemoattractant protein-1 333
Morquio's syndrome (mucopolysaccharidosis
    IV) 132
Moyamoya disease (multiple progressive
    intracranial arterial occlusion) 80,
    398, 456, 652
Mucolipidoses 133–4, 236–7
    I (lipomucopolysaccharidosis, sialidosis)
        133
    II (I-cell disease) 133
    III (pseudo-Hurler) 133
Mucopolysaccharidoses 129–33,
    236–7, 684
    induced 132–3
    I (α-L-iduronidase deficiency) 129–31
    II (Hurler syndrome) 129, 130, 131–2,
        236–7
    III (Sanfilippo syndrome) 132
    IV (Morquio syndrome) 132, 236
    VI (Maroteaux–Lamy syndrome) 132
    VII (Sly syndrome) 132

Mucosal associated lymphoid tissue (MALT)
    344
Mucosal ectasia 547
Multifocal fibrosclerosis 347
Multiple lipoprotein-type hyperlipidemia
    144
Multiple progressive intracranial arterial
    occlusion (moyamoya disease) 80,
    398, 456, 652
Murine macrophage elastase 110
Murmurs (bruits) 6–7
    aneurysm-induced 7
    arteriovenous anastomosis (fistula) 517,
        520
    cranial 6
    haemic 6
    orbital 6
    physiological 6
    spontaneous, in children 6
Myelomalacia 543
Myocardium 683
    hypertrophy 683
    infarction, right/left coronary artery
        dominance 12
    oxygen consumption 683
    oxygen-supply demand imbalance 683–4
Myxoedema 235–6
Myxoma, cardiac 403–4

Neck injury 81
Necrotizing angiitis 403
Necrotizing sarcoid granulomatosis 642,
    648
Nephrosclerosis 566–7
    decompensated benign 579
Nephrotic syndrome 236
Neurofibromatosis 563
    diagnostic angiography 720
Neuronal ceroid lipofuscinosis 139–40
Neuropeptide-Y 555, **556**
Neutral fat 214
Neutrophil collagenase 109
Nidogen (entactin) **102**, 104, 217
Nitric oxide 556, 557
Nitroglycerin (industrial) withdrawal 683
Nodal angiomatosis 771
Noonan's syndrome 508
Norepinephrine (noradrenaline) 554, 555,
    557

Obesity 438
Oblique vein of Marshall 50
Obliterated vein of Marshall 50
Occipital horn syndrome 114, 119
Ochronosis 147–9, 237
Oculomotor nerve, compression by aneurysm
    440
Oesophagus
    sharp foreign body effect 38, 80
    varices 13, 548
Oil, definition 313
Open lung biopsy 615–16
    congenital heart disease 616
    primary pulmonary hypertension 616
    unexplained chronic dyspnea 617
Optic chiasma compression 440
Optic nerve compression 440
Oral contraceptives 605, 686–7
    aseptic thromboembolism associated 70
    cerebral thrombosis associated 458
Oroya fever (Carrion's disease; verruga
    peruana) 740–2
Osler–Weber–Rendu disease (hereditary

haemorrhagic telangiectasia) 372, 545
Osteogenesis imperfecta 154–5, 409
Osteolathyrism 118
Oxalosis, see Hyperoxalurias
Otitic hydrocephalus 458
Oxo-imines (keto-amines) 93

Paget's disease of bone, murmur over 6
Pallidal siderosis (vascular siderosis; calcinosiderosis) 483–4
Papillary endothelial hyperplasia 742, **743**, 755
Paraplegia due to occlusion of large anterior artery of Adamkiewicz 363
Parkes–Weber syndrome 493, 753
Patent ductus arteriosus 21, **22**
D-penicillamine 115, 356–7
Peptides, pyrrolic crosslinks containing 94
Peri-aneurysmal retroperitoneal fibrosis 338, 340
Periaortitis, see Inflammatory aneurysm
Periarteritis nodosa 624
Peripheral vascular disease 195
Perivasculitis syndrome 419
Peroxidase-antiperoxidase 320
Persistent pulmonary hypertension of newborn 588–90
Persistent truncus arteriosus 23–5
  associated anomalies 24–5
Phantom bone (Gorham's disease; disappearing bone disease) 508, 756
Pheochromocytoma 399, 683
Phlebactasia 355, 491
Phlebitis 500
  granulomatous 506
  immune-mediated 506
  infection-related 505
  migrating (phlebitis migrans sive saltans) 505
Phlebitis chronica obliterans filiformis (Mondor's disease) 505–6
Phleboliths 80
Phlebosclerosis 79, 175, 258–9, 493–5
  secondary 495
  varicose veins associated 496
Phlebothrombosis 500
Phlegmasia alba dolens (white leg) 75
Phlegmasia coerulea dolens 502
Phosphoglycerides 427
Phospholipase C 555
Phospholipid 214
Physiological adaptation/remodelling 16–18
Pickwickian syndrome 602
Plaque cap 218
Plasma cell 218
Plasma cell dyscrasia (POEMS syndrome; Takatsuki syndrome; Crow–Fukase syndrome) 757
Plasma membranes, fragility 212
Plasminogen 73, 110
  activation 73
Plasminogen activator inhibitor-1 70, 120–1
Platelet 218–19
  aggregates, atheroembolism associated 417
  factor IV 417
  platelet-platelet adhesion 426
  reaction to atheroma contents 425–6
  thrombus 63, 64, 69
Platelet-derived growth factor 83, 211, 219, 332, 335, 417

release 574
Plexiform vascularization of lymph nodes 763
POEMS syndrome (Takatsuki syndrome; Crow–Fukase syndrome; plasma cell dyscrasia) 757
Polyarteritis
  infantile 636
  microscopic 635
Polyarteritis nodosa 341, 631–5, 649
  diagnostic angiography 709
Polycystic disease of kidney 396
Polycythaemia 451
Polycythaemia rubra vera 456, 481
Polygenic hypercholesterolemia 144
Polymyalgia rheumatica 529, 628
Polysplenic cardiac syndrome 55
Pontine haemorrhage, 471–3
Portal hypertension 582–3
  pulmonary hypertension associated 600
Portal venous obstruction 13
Post-endarterectomy haemorrhage 481
Posterior cerebral artery
  compression 440
  occlusion 449
  red infarction 451
Post-thrombotic syndrome 503–4, 511
Pregnancy
  aneurysmal rupture 375
  cerebral venous thrombosis 457
  puerperal hemiplegia/stroke 455
  puerperal venous thrombosis 457
  spiral arteries of placental bed 254
Presinusoidal obstruction 582
Primary (granulomatous) angiitis of central nervous system 645–8
Primary hyperlipoproteinemias of unknown origin 144
Prinzmetal's angina (variant angina pectoris) 682
Procollagen 91, 92
Pro-enzyme plasminogen 73
Progeria
  adult (Werner's syndrome) 147, 163
  carotid artery aneurysm 409
  childhood (Hutchinson–Gilford syndrome) 147, 162–3, 224–5
Prostacyclin **556**, 557
Prostaglandin H$_2$ 557, 558
Prostanoids 555
Prostatic cancer, oestrogen for 458
Proteoglycans 105–8, 217–18
  distribution in vascular wall 107–8
  function 107–8
  structure 105–7
  synthesis 105–7
Pseudo-Hurler polydystrophy (mucolipidosis III) 133
Pseudo-Kaposi sarcoma (acro-angiodermatitis) 770
Pseudotumour of orbit 347
Pseudovasculitic syndrome 625
Pseudoxanthoma elasticum 115–16, 153–4, 398, 684–5
Puerperal hemiplegia/stroke 455
Puerperium, venous thrombosis in 457
Pulmonary angiitis 637–45
Pulmonary arteries 47–50, 586
  absent 25
  aneurysm 21, 617
  banding 599
  branches 48–51
    anomalous origin 48–9
    atresia 50

pulmonary vascular sling 49
  stenosis 49–50
  dissections 618
  distal ductal origin 50
  idiopathic dilatation 47
  luminal obstruction 47–8
  neoplasms 617–18, 732–4
  origin from aorta 25–7
  rupture 617, **618**
  solitary aortic trunk 48
  surgical narrowing of trunk 599
Pulmonary arteritis, idiopathic non-granulomatous 612–13
Pulmonary arteriovenous communications 544–5
Pulmonary capillary hemangiomatosis 605, **606**
Pulmonary circulation 9–10
Pulmonary embolus 725
Pulmonary granulomatosis 637–9
Pulmonary hyalinizing granuloma 347
Pulmonary hypertension 10, 76, 582–3, 585–618
  acute/subacute 588–90
  chronic 590–4, **595**
    bronchial compression 592–3
    cardiac features 591–2
    co-existent forms 594
    laryngeal nerve compression 593
    liver changes 594
    pulmonary features 591
  chronic postcapillary 605–7
  classification 585
  dietary-related 605
  embolic 600–1
    chronic recurrent thromboembolism 601
    non-thrombotic embolic disease 601
  hypoxic 601–3
  pathophysiology 585
  plexogenic 596–600
    congenital left-to-right shunt 598–9
    Heath–Edwards classification 598, 599
    HIV-1 related 600
    irreversible 599
    microscopic features 596–8
    portal hypertension associated 600
    primary 600
    schistosomiasis related 600
    toxic oil syndrome related 600
  plus portal hypertension 600
  primary 608–15
    histopathology 611–13
    nomenclature 611
    open lung biopsy 616
    therapy 613–15
  pulmonary fibrosis associated **604**, 605
  thrombotic 602
  venae cavae dilatation 593–4
Pulmonary lymphatics 586–7
Pulmonary phlebitis 617
Pulmonary thromboembolism, acute 590
Pulmonary vascular sling 49
Pulmonary vasculature, normal 585–8
  age-related changes 587–8
  arteries, see Pulmonary arteries
  bronchial circulation 587
  microcirculation 586
  veins, see Pulmonary veins
Pulmonary vasculitis 617
Pulmonary veins
  atresia of individual veins 58
  partial anomalous connection 53–5
    anomalous right pulmonary veins/sinus

venosus atrial septal defect 53
  non-specific forms 53
  right pulmonary veins in polysplenic cardiac syndrome 55
  scimitar syndrome 53–5
  stenosis of individual veins 58
  total anomalous connection 55–8
    cardiac 56
    infracardiac 56–7
    supracardiac 55
    variations from usual types 57–8
Pulmonary veno-occlusive disease 58–9, 60
Pulmonary venous hypertension 607
Pulseless disease, see Takayasu arteritis
Purines 555
Pyogenic granuloma (lobular capillary haemangioma) 749–51
Pyridinium 118
Pyridinoline (hydroxylysyl pyridinolone) 93, 94
Pyrraline 95

Radiation fibrosis 712
Rat, sontaneously hypertensive 555, 572
Recklinghausen neurofibromatosis type I 369
Red cells, see Erythrocytes
Red (coagulation) thrombus 500
Refsum's disease 147
Reidel's thyroiditis 347
Reiter's syndrome 356
Relapsing polychondritis 341
Remodelling 17
Renal acute insufficiency 419
Renal artery
  accessory 3
  aneurysm 563
  atheroembolism 419–20
  injuries 81
  thrombosis 81
Renal biopsy 419
Renal failure, chronic 419
Rendu–Osler syndrome 489
Renin 557
Renin-angiotensin system 556–7
Renovascular vasculitis 563–7
Repetitive small stroke syndrome 419
Retroperitoneal fibrosis 343, 347
Reverse haemolytic plaque assay 345
Reynolds number 202
Rheumatic connective tissue disease 650
Rheumatic fever 341
Rheumatoid arthritis 341, 344, 356
Rheumatoid spondylitis 356

Sanfilippo syndrome (mucopolysaccharidosis III) 132
Sarcoidosis 341, 617
Scheie syndrome (MPS I-S) 129, 236
Schönlein–Henoch purpura 625, 645
Scimitar syndrome 53–5
Scleroderma 356, 605
Sclerosing cholangitis 347
Scurvy (vitamin C deficiency) 165
Selenium deficiency 165–6, 347
Senescence (aging) 224
Senility 484
Serotonin (5-hydroxytryptamine) 555, 556, 558
Serum sickness 221, 331, 649
Servelle–Martorell syndrome 493
Shock liver 594
Single umbilical artery 203, 206
Sinusoidal obstruction 582

Sly syndrome (mucopolysaccharidosis VI) 132
Small blood vessel diseases 253–7
Smoking 226, 438
Smooth muscle cell 210–12
  contraction 572
  extracellular matrix production 210
  lipid-containing 211
  lysosomes in 211
  proliferation stimulation 211
Sneddon syndrome 625
Spider naevi 220
Spinal cord
  arteriovenous communications 542–3
    glomus type 543
    juvenile type 543
    single-coiled vessel 543
  cavernous haemangioma 542
  extraspinal 542–3
  ischaemic lesions 458–60
    pathogenesis 459
    pathology of infarct 459–60
    venous infarction 460
  saccular aneurysms 543
  venous angioma 543
  telangiectases 542
Spinal haemangioblastoma 547
Spindle cell haemangioendothelioma 760–1
Spine, hyperextension effect on abdominal aorta 80
Splanchnic arteriovenous fistula 545–6
Sporadic hypertriglyceridemia 144
Steal syndromes 443–4
Sterol, purified 427
Sterol esters 427
Stewart–Treves angiosarcoma 512–13, 513
Streptavidin-biotin system 320
Straight sinus thrombosis 457
Stroke 437
Stromelysin 1 types 109, 110
Stromelysin 2 types 109, 110
Sturge–Weber syndrome 484, 489, 493, 526–8, 755
Subarachnoid haemorrhage 467–9, 579
  non-traumatic 467–9
    associated lesions 468–9
    pathology 467–9
    prognosis 469
  spinal 469
  traumatic 467
Subclavian artery 16
  right
    aberrant 38–9
    isolation 39
Subclavian lag 29, 42
Subclavian steal syndrome (brachial-basilar insufficiency) 443–4
Subdural hematoma 462–7, 473
  associated lesions 466
  pathology 464–6
  precipitating factors 463–4
  sequelae 466–7
  spinal 467
Subdural hygroma (hydroma) 465
Superficial arteriovenous tumor/hemangioma 753
Superficial siderosis of central nervous system 468
Superior longitudinal sinus thrombosis 457, 458
Superior mesenteric artery injury 81
Superior petrosal sinus thrombosis 457
Superior vena cava 50–1
  left superior vena cava to left atrium 51

occlusion 54
persistent left superior vena cava 50–1
Supratentorial pressure increase 455
Suramin 133
Sydecan 107
Sympathetic nervous system, systemic hypertension related 553–5
Syndrome X 675
Systemic angiodysplasias 492–3, 497
Systemic artery-pulmonary shunt (left-to-right arterial shunt) 524–5
Systemic fibrotic disorders 347
Systemic lupus erythematosus 341, 363, 399

Takatsuki syndrome (POEMS syndrome; Crow–Fukase syndrome; plasma cell dyscrasia) 757
Takayasu arteritis (aortic arch syndrome; pulseless disease) 341, 361, 444, 563–4, 624, 625–7
  diagnostic angiography 703–7
  synonyms 527–8
  types 626
Tangier disease 145–6
T cell 218, 329
  activated 332
  atherosclerotic plaques containing 331
  HAL-DR antigen expression 331
Telangiectasis 355, 528–9
Temporal arteritis, see Giant cell arteritis
Terminal vascular bed 9
Terminology misuse 16
Thoma's histomechanical laws 2, 14
Thoracic duct aneurysm 408
3-M syndrome 409
Thromboangiitis obliterans, see Buerger's disease
Thrombocytopenia 481
Thromboembolism 601
  chronic recurrent 601
  non-thrombotic 601
Thrombogenic hypothesis 83–5, 241–7
β-thromboglobulin 417
Thrombophlebitis 72, 500
Thrombophlebitis migrans 457, 661
Thrombosis 63–85, 499–504
  age estimation 501–2
  arterial 70–2
  atherosclerosis associated 68
  atypical 73
  basilar artery 450
  cardiac 72
  carotid sinus 71
  cerebral arteries 71
  cerebral veins 502
  coralline thrombus 64
  coronary artery 71
  deep leg veins 502
  dietary fat associated 70
  disturbed blood flow factor 69
  etiology 499–500
    coagulation disorders 499
    stasis 499
    vessel wall alterations 499–500
  fate 501
  haemostasis associated 64–5
  iatrogenic 503
  iliofemoral vein 75
  infection/inflammation associated 72
  inferior vena cava 502
  lower limb veins 63, 68
  marantic 68, 457
  mesenteric veins 502
  microthrombi 67

multiple 502
mural thrombi 63, 70–1
   aortic 68, 71
neoplastic disease associated 503
occlusive arterial 63
organization 501
pelvic veins 63
platelet thrombus 63, 64, 69
portal vein 502
post-mortem clots 63–4
postoperative 63
puerperal 63
red thrombus 61, 71
retinal veins 502
retrograde thrombus 65
secondary to inflammatory venous disease 503
sequelae 73–80, 502
   arterial thrombotic occlusion 73–4, 75
   collateral circulation 76–80
   pulmonary emboli 75–6
   venous thromboses 73
   white leg (phlegmasia alba dolens) 75
shear stress effect 69
splanchnic veins 502
spontaneous, lower animals 68
superior vena cava 502
thrombogenesis 65–7
   platelets 65–7
   Virchow's triad, see Virchow's triad
venous 72, 500–1
   course 500–1
   deep vein 72, 75
   elderly patients 68
   incidence 500
   localization 500
   morphology 500–1
upper extremity veins 502
venous valves 68
Thromboxane 374
   receptor 558
Thromboxane A_2 557
Thyrotoxicosis 683–4
   children 684
T lymphocytes, see T cells
Toxic oil syndrome 600, 605
trans fatty acids 240
Transforming growth factor-β 121, **556**
Transient ischaemic attacks 442–3
   endarterectomy for 443
   recurrent 443
Transplantation, chronic rejection 221–2
Transposition of great arteries 559
Transverse sinus thrombosis 457
Trauma 80–1
   extradural haematoma, see Extradural haematoma
   iatrogenic 82
   intimal proliferation 82–3
   repair 82–3
   subarachnoid haemorrhage 467
   subdural haematoma 463
Tropoelastin 99, 100, 118
Tuberculous aneurysms 357
Tuberous sclerosis 399

Tumour necrosis factor (cachetin) 121, 332, 345
Turner's syndrome 508
Type A personality 221

Unesterified cholesterol-rich particles 306–7
Unexplained renal failure-hypertension syndrome 419
Unifying hypothesis 244
Ureteric obstruction 347

Varicose veins 13, 495–8, 547–8
   epidemiology 495–6
   etiology 495–6, 548
   fatigue hypothesis 548
   morphology 497–8
   secondary 497
Vasa vasorum 184, 219
Vascular anomalies of central nervous system 528–30
Vascular calcification 260–1
Vascular cell adhesion molecule-1 333, 345–6
Vascular endothelial cells 319
Vascular malformation 489–93
Vascular patterns, peripheral anatomical variations 11–12
   in identical twins 12
Vascular siderosis (pallidal siderosis; calcinosiderosis) 483–4
Vascular steal 76
Vascular transformation of sinuses 771
Vasculitis 623–53
   cerebral 645
      drug use/drug abuse associated 651
   clinicopathological classification 623–5
   etiology 623
   definition 623
   diagnostic angiography 703–7, 710
   granulomatous 642, **648**
   necrotizing 623–5, 631–7
   pathogenesis 623
Vein of Galen aneurysm 533–4
Veins 9
   amyloidosis 498
   anastomoses 13
   anatomical variations 11–12
   aneurysms 491
   aplasia of deep veins 497
   arterialization 489
   chronic insufficiency 497
   circulatory venous disturbances 499–504
   cystic adventitial degeneration or disease 498
   degenerative diseases 493–5
   hemangiomas 491
   inflammatory diseases 504–5
   lipidosis 498
   malformations 490–3
      classification 490
      deep leg vein aplasia/hypoplasia 491
      etiology 489
      classification 490
      histopathology 489–90
      large veins 490–1
      pathogenesis 489

phlebectasia 355, 491
pressures 9
thrombosis, see Thrombosis
varicosities 79, 547–8
vertebral 13
Venae cavae terminating both in left atrium 52
Venization 16
Veno-occlusive disease of lung 502
Venous angioma 549
Venous bypass grafts 249–50
Venous gangrene 502
Venous malformation 489–93
Venous spur 495
Ventricular septal defect 32
   atresia of pulmonary trunk **48**
Versican 107
Vertebral arteriovenous fistula 542
Vertebral artery 2
   abducent nerve compression by 440
   dissecting aneurysm 453
   occlusion 449, 452, 452–3
Verruga peruana (Carrion's disease; Oroya fever) 740–2
Very low density lipoproteins (VLDLs) 271
   localization in human/animal models 274–5
Vibrating tool disease 81–2
Viral arteritis 222
Virchow's triad 67–70, 499
   blood flow 68–9
   changes in composition of blood 69–70
   vessel wall 67–8
Visceral ischaemia syndrome 419
Vitamin B_{12} metabolic defect with methylmalonic acidemia and homocystinuria (Cb1-C type) 150
Vitamin C 223
   deficiency (scurvy) 165
Vitamin D 260
Vitamin E deficiency 165–6, 347
Vasodilators 581–62
Voluntary muscle development 16

Wallenberg's syndrome (lateral medullary syndrome) 449–50
Watanabe rabbit 211, 234, 241
Wegener's granulomatosis 341, 639–40, **644, 645,** 649
Weibel–Palade bodies 496, 497, 498, 514
Werner's syndrome (adult progeria) 147, 163, 225
White blood cell trapping 498
White leg (phlegmasia alba dolens) 75
White thrombus (aggregation thrombus) 500
Willebrand factor 67, 69
Williams syndrome 28
Williams–Beuren syndrome (idiopathic infantile hypercalcemia) 163
Wilson's disease (hepatolenticular degeneration) 115, 164
Wolman's disease 139

Zahn's lines/striae 64, 65, 68
Zinc deficiency 223